PATHOLOGIC BASIS OF DISEASE

STANLEY L. ROBBINS, M.D.

Professor and Chairman, Department of Pathology,
Boston University School of Medicine

W. B. SAUNDERS COMPANY
Philadelphia • London • Toronto

W. B. Saunders Company: West Washington Square
Philadelphia, Pa.   19105

12 Dyott Street
London, WC1A   1DB

833 Oxford Street
Toronto, Ontario M8Z 5T9, Canada

Listed here is the latest translated edition of this book together with the language of the translation and the publisher.

Spanish (1st Edition) – NEISA, Mexico 4 D.F., Mexico

Pathologic Basis of Disease   ISBN   0-7216-7594-8

Print No.:   9   8   7   6   5

To
Sarah
to
Alexander
and to
Katharine
with love

PREFACE

On seeing the title of this volume, *The Pathologic Basis of Disease*, one might reasonably ask whether this is indeed a different book or merely a fourth edition of the author's earlier text, *Pathology*. This question can be answered confidently — it is a new book based, obviously, on the current body of pathologic knowledge. Despite a warm and satisfying acceptance of the earlier volumes, the need for a text more suited to present-day medical education and contemporary students of disease stimulated the preparation of this book.

Medical education, always in ferment, has undergone substantial change in the recent past, leading to many diverse forms and approaches. Common to all, I believe, is a deeper concern for the mechanisms of disease and for the applicability of basic sciences to the clinical processes of decision making. So, too, have contemporary medical and dental students changed. Increasingly, they are concerned with the question, "What does it mean to the patient and to society?" Students can no longer simply be assigned course programs and be expected unquestioningly to develop immediate enthusiasm for them. Rightfully, they wish to understand why the subject matter is important to learn. So this book attempts to present not only an adequate body of pathologic knowledge but also clear explications of the meaning of the subcellular, cellular and tissue changes to the patient and the physician. This emphasis in the writing is based on the premise that there is no sounder motivation to learn than an understanding of the goals of such learning.

The effort has been made to delve deeply into the "whys" and "wherefores" of disease. Much consideration has been given causes and mechanisms, since therein lie the origins of the pathophysiology of disease and the implications to the patient and the physician. For example, the chapter on heart disease begins with a discussion of the mechanisms and clinical presentations of cardiac failure, and the chapter on kidney disease with a consideration of the pathophysiology and clinical ramifications of renal failure. Considerable space has been accorded the biomolecular and ultrastructural origins of disease and the evolution of the cellular and tissue alterations from their incipiency to their full-blown stages of development. In this way, diseases are presented as dynamic processes changing with time, modified by therapy and by host and invader adaptive responses, all having effect on the ultimate clinical manifestations. Liberal citation of the literature not only duly acknowledges the origins of our present concepts, but also provides source material for deeper investigation of interesting subjects. Throughout, scrupulous effort is made to point out the gaps in our knowledge to make clear that much is still unknown and, possibly, to entice the student into joining the search for a greater understanding.

The text has been designed primarily for medical and dental students, clinicians and other students of disease. It is my hope that my peers will find it not adequately encyclopedic for their personal use or I shall have failed in my primary purpose of achieving a learning tool for those who are not professional pathologists. The organization into early chapters dealing with basic processes and later chapters devoted to a systematic presentation of the more important disease entities should provide general compatibility with most teaching programs in pathology. Many chapters open with pertinent comments on the normal, such as reviews of basic genetics, immunology and many features of the embryogenesis and structure of organ systems. To understand the abnormal, one must first know the normal. Diseases are accorded space consistent with their importance to society. Thus major entities such as atherosclerosis, myocardial infarction and diabetes mellitus are treated in some detail, while rare and exotic disorders are omitted. Value judgments, for which the author must assume full responsibility, are obviously involved. I cannot presume prescience; I can only hope that my judgments have been wise. Great effort has been expended to achieve clarity and lucidity in the writing and readily assimilable expositions in the hope that easy readability and the unfolding of a whole story will compensate, and indeed, offer rewards for length.

At the least, it can be said that every page has been prepared with the awareness that its worth stems ultimately from its usefulness to the reader. If any measure of success has been achieved, this book underscores the applicability of a sound knowledge of pathology to the care of patients while providing a not unpleasant means of obtaining such knowledge.

STANLEY L. ROBBINS, M.D.

ACKNOWLEDGMENTS

It is with pleasure and a deep sense of indebtedness that I acknowledge here the invaluable help of many colleagues, students and fellow workers who contributed so much to the completion of this text. It scarcely needs mention that, although a single name appears as author, the enormous task of data gathering, collating, writing, rewriting, editing and typing involves the labors, counsel and commitment of many. Indeed, were it not for their unstinting help, there would be no book. Although thanked below, no words can adequately express the depth of my gratitude and the significance to me of their graciously offered support and loyalty.

First and foremost among those to whom I am deeply indebted is Miss Kathy Pitcoff, my editorial assistant, typer of manuscripts, "eagle eye" for errors and organizer of the monumental stack of papers which represent a text in preparation. Far more lucid than the author and with uncompromising standards of excellence, she imparted to the writing much of any clarity and elegance it may possess.

To the contributors of special chapters, I express my many, many thanks for their willingness to lend their names and their expertise to the book. Drs. Violeta Arboleda and William Less skillfully and ably revised the chapter on The Oral Cavity prepared by the deceased and sorely missed Dr. Irving Glickman. Dr. Joseph Foley's The Nervous System is a masterwork, presenting an enormous body of information in succinct, lucid and delightfully readable style. The chapter on The Skin, by Drs. Herbert Mescon and Inta Grots, represents a superb contribution by two highly expert dermatopathologists. And Dr. Joseph Vitale's fine and comprehensive chapter on Nutritional Disease adds great strength in an area too long neglected. Although few in number, these chapters add great luster to this text. To all these contributors I can only express the hope and the wish that my contribution to this effort is worthy of theirs.

Many colleagues have offered wise counsel, editorial comment and choice illustrations. Dr. Marcia Angell, Dr. Henry Soto, Dr. Hugh Ryser, Dr. Michael Bennett, Dr. Vinay Kumar, Dr. Leonard Gottlieb, Dr. John Hayes, Dr. Richard Neiman, Dr. Ramzi Cotran, Nancy Chromey and Shirley Zajdel all are owed my heartfelt thanks. Dr. Henry Soto must be singled out for special gratitude. Without his generous help, keen eye and collection of excellent illustrative material, many more presentations in this text would remain unadorned. Similarly, I should express my gratitude to my photographer, Leo Goodman, for his skill and artistry which illume so many pages of this writing. To those inadvertently omitted, my sincere apologies.

Many heroes stand unsung in the shadows behind every large book—the medical students, secretaries and library assistants who help out in diverse and invaluable ways. All in small or large part put their shoulders to the wheel and, indeed, sometimes their "noses to the grindstone," to maintain the onward progress of the effort. Mary Kraft, Barbara Bjornson and Carol Winograd were invaluable student critics who freely gave of their time and "kept me honest" by mercilessly condemning loose statements and demanding clarity in exposition. Much as one becomes infatuated with one's own words, the keen analyses of these students, their devotion to me and to the text and their perceptive judgments as potential users of the book produced many changes in the writing, all good. They immeasurably enhanced such worth as this book may have. To Shari Paul and to Mary Leen, as well as other members of the library staff of Boston University School of Medicine, my grateful thanks for their valuable help and support in searching the literature for appropriate references.

In last analysis, a manuscript is completed by typist-secretaries. I have been most fortunate and blessed by a number of able and devoted helpers who more correctly might be called my associates-in-labor. Deserving of gratitude are Lori Feldman, Dorcas Weiler, Leslie Kaplan, Marcia Kipnes and especially Pamela Rook, who never failed to freely accept and graciously fulfill any extra burden imposed upon her.

Not to be forgotten is my personal family, and particularly my wife Elly, who patiently waited for the completion of this book and the return of the author to the land of the living. To them I can only offer my apologies and my deep appreciation for their willingness to put up with an obsessive writer.

These acknowledgments would be incomplete without citation of my continuing appreciation of my publishers, W. B. Saunders Company, and the many members of this organization, some of whom are unknown to me, who contributed wholeheartedly to the final format of this work. Particularly deserving of mention are Mrs. Daphne Moo-Young, manuscript editor, and Mr. John Dusseau, the Vice-President and Editor. To Mrs. Moo-Young goes all credit for shepherding the monstrous collection of manuscript pages, illustrations and tables through the intricate steps involved in publication. Only an expert could have so admirably succeeded while being so supportive and understanding of the author. And to Mr. John Dusseau, better known to me as long-time friend John, my many thanks for his generous enthusiasm for this text and his unflagging encouragement and support of its author.

It should be evident that such quality as this book may have is owed to many; any inadequacies must rest squarely on my shoulders.

STANLEY L. ROBBINS, M.D.

CONTENTS

1

THE NORMAL AND THE ADAPTED CELL

The emerging physician is told so often — be concerned with the *whole* patient — that he sometimes forgets that behind every organic illness there are malfunctioning cells. Indeed it is more correct to say that when a sufficient number of cells become sick, so does the patient. All illnesses, then, save those having emotional or functional causes, are expressions of cellular derangements; in turn, such cellular disorders result from biomolecular and ultrastructural dysfunctions. The day may not be far away when diseases will be grouped into categories according to their fundamental biomolecular derangement as, for example, those affecting oxidative phosphorylation or those resulting from impaired protein synthesis. It is appropriate, therefore, to begin the study of pathology with the consideration of derangements at the cellular and subcellular level before we turn to the diseases of whole organs and of the organism. The student of pathology is understandably impatient to get to the "people diseases." But, in this day of sophisticated medical technology, one cannot understand the etiology (cause), pathogenesis (development) and clinical implications of a disease without deep penetration into the cell.

Regrettably, much of our understanding of cells is derived from the fixed images offered by the light and electron microscopes.

The cell is no more static than is the ameba. Images of fixed tissues trapped at an instant in time, like still photographs, fail to provide a "living, breathing" conception of the cell's daily, perhaps hourly, adaptation to life's demands and stresses. Consider the mere act of running up stairs: the increased muscular activity requires increased cellular metabolic activity such as utilization of ATP reserves, mobilization of glycogen stores, increased cellular uptake of oxygen and perhaps adaptive alterations in organelles, to mention only a few of the many adjustments which occur in the daily life of the cell. Within limits, the cell is capable of adjusting to these varying demands. However, like the organism as a whole, its adaptive capability may be exceeded, and cellular injury or even death may follow. Even with our most sophisticated methods of study, the boundaries between the normal cell, the adapted cell, the injured cell capable of recovery and the irreversibly damaged cell are poorly defined. Our ability to discern varying morphologic states of cellular health and disease lags behind the deeper biochemical alterations leading to them. To the extent possible, these underlying biochemical lesions will be presented along with the morphologic changes they induce. We shall begin with a consideration of the normal cell and its limits of adaptation before turning

1

to the more marked deviations of reversible cell injury and the irreversible changes indicative of cell death.

THE NORMAL CELL

Although constantly adapting to changes in its environment, the normal cell is confined to a fairly narrow range of function and structure by its genetic programs of differentiation and specialization, the constraints of neighboring cells, the availability of metabolic substrates and the finite capacities of its primary and alternative metabolic pathways. Whole volumes in the field of cell biology are devoted to the full consideration of the normal cell (deRobertis et al., 1970). Here we can present only an overview to provide a point of departure for the consideration of the abnormal cell.

Despite widely varying specializations of cell types found in multicellular organisms, certain characteristics are common to all cells. They have a remarkably constant proportion of water, ranging from 75 to 85 per cent. The protein content is usually on the order of 10 to 20 per cent with lipids averaging 2 to 3 per cent, carbohydrates 1 per cent and inorganic solutes 1 per cent. Cell volumes, however, vary somewhat more widely, from about 500 to 15,000 cubic microns. It is quite remarkable that the individual liver cell is approximately the same size in all mammals. The differences in organ mass between the livers of the whale and the mouse derive from the number of cells. It may be of interest to know that these fundamental facts are used as an argument against a previously held theory of cancer causation. It was once postulated that some aberration in the mitosis of a single cell might give rise to a mutant which, having lost all controls, might grow into a cancer. If such were true and every mitotically dividing cell were at equal risk, consider the plight of the whale with its trillions of cells. In fact, cancers are less common in whales than in man.

The descriptions which follow will be confined to observations of fixed cells visualized under the light and electron microscopes. The particular instrument used for an observation will not be indicated since it should be obvious from the magnitude of the structure under consideration. Most cells appear as polyhedral solids of minimal surface. Only a sphere would provide a smaller surface for an equivalent volume. Close aggregation imposes this shape upon the cells just as the individual bubble in a soap foam assumes a polyhedral shape. But there are many deviations from the norm, such as the relatively free-living polymorphonuclear leukocyte which is as ameboid as its protozoal cousin, and the neuron in the spinal cord which may possess an axon process terminating in the toes. Much more subtle conformational specializations are found, such as microvilli, elaborately convoluted, interlocking cell margins, and the attenuated "fried egg" morphology of the endothelial and mesothelial cells lining the vessels and body cavities (Ma and Biempica, 1971) (Fig. 1–1).

PLASMA MEMBRANE

The plasma (cell) membrane which encloses all cells functions as a semipermeable barrier. The interior of the cell has an ionic composition quite different from that of the extracellular interstitial fluid. It is hardly necessary to emphasize the central role of the plasma membrane in the ecology of the cell. As the interface between the cell's interior and its environment, the plasma membrane is the barrier or gateway for all products entering and leaving the cell. Some substances, for example, water with its inorganic ions, pass through by simple diffusion, but traversal by macromolecules is more selective. Lipid soluble macromolecules pass more freely than water soluble ones, presumably by solution in the lipid constituents of the membrane. Other macromolecules, such as glucose, may require carriers which shuttle back and forth across the membrane picking up and delivering cargo to the interior. Normal membrane permeability is thus essential to the homeostasis of the cell.

With the light microscope, the plasma membrane appears as a single layered, marginal condensation but, with higher resolution, it appears much more complicated. The composition and molecular structure of this plasma membrane have become subjects of considerable controversy. The standard view has been that it is a trilaminar complex composed of two dark outer leaflets separated by an interposed paler layer. Each of these individual leaflets ranges from 20 to 40 microns in thickness so that the overall average thickness of the plasma membranes of most cells is about 100 Å. Danielli and Davson (1935) were the first to propose that the central pale zone was made up of an array of complex lipids, principally phospholipids, while the outer darker leaflets were protein in nature. The protein leaflets are held together by charges on amino acid side chains while the lipid molecules are presumed to be held together chiefly by ionic charged groups. Negative charges are present

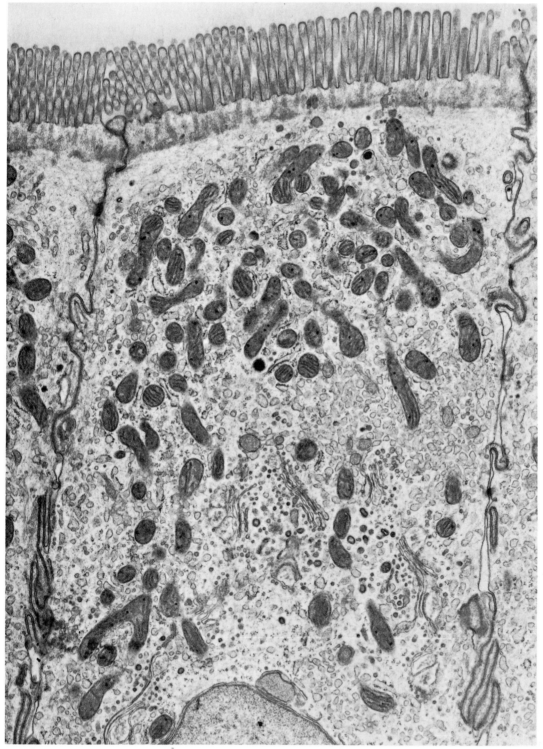

Figure 1–1. *Normal human jejunal cell with surface covered by microvilli. Also visible are the mitochondria, endoplasmic reticulum, Golgi complexes and the complicated interlocking lateral plasma membrane. × 17,000. (Through the courtesy of Dr. Leonard Gottlieb, Mallory Institute of Pathology.)*

on the exposed polar groups of the proteins, creating repellent forces on adjacent cells. A similar trilaminar construction was identified in all cells as well as in the membranes of mitochondria and endoplasmic reticulum (ER), giving rise to the view that all laminated membranes both within and around the cell were basically the same; hence, the term *unit membrane* was proposed by Robertson (1959).

Modifications in this conception were introduced as awareness of hydrophobic forces became apparent, and new models have now been proposed. In these proposals, it is held that clear separation of protein and lipid layers is no longer compatible with all of the evidence. Some protein molecules are thought to be present in the central pale lipid layer, presumably with their nonpolar portions oriented toward the center of the plasma membrane and their polar groups extending toward the hydrophilic interfaces of the plasma membrane. In this view, lipids are also thought to be present in the outer protein leaflets, with their charged polar groups contributing to the electrochemical forces of the outer cell membrane (Siekevitz, 1970). Thus Singer and Nicolson (1971) propose that the plasma membrane represents a lipid globular-protein *mosaic* made up largely of a discontinuous bimolecular array of phospholipids in which globular proteins are erratically embedded. The ionic and polar heads of the lipids are in contact with the aqueous phase as are the ionic residues of the proteins. The fatty acid chains of the lipids and the hydrophobic residues of the proteins are oriented toward the center of the membrane and provide an interior hydrophobic core. In this conception, the lipids do not compromise a continuous central layer but rather a mortar into which single protein molecules or aggregates of protein molecules are embedded as random stones. Such a conception emphasizes that membranes are, in reality, aggregations or concentrations of enzyme proteins involved in, for example, electron transport, oxidative phosphorylation, the tricarboxylic acid cycle and fatty acid oxidation (Korn, 1969). At the present time, then, attention is turning to the proteinous components of the membrane (Sjöstrand, 1967).

Much evidence supports this more flexible conception of membranes. The enzyme and protein content of membranes varies from one cell type to another and, indeed, varies among the organelles of the individual cell. For example, the composition of the cell membrane enclosing neurons is 75 per cent lipid and only 25 per cent protein while for the plasma membranes of epithelial cells in the intestinal villi,

the converse obtains. The varying enzyme content of membranes among the many cells of the body is well known. Perhaps the trilaminar pattern visualized by electron microscopy is, as it were, an artefact imposed by the fixatives employed. Artificial aggregations of osmium or other compounds along the inner and outer leaflets of the membrane might produce the apparent trilaminar structure. Indeed it has been shown that the three layers still persist even after the lipids have been removed by lipid solvents. These issues have not yet been resolved and, for the present, it is perhaps reasonable to conclude that membranes may have great variation in structure and function at different sites (Weinstein, 1969). The term *unit membrane* would then imply only the apparent uniformity of structure seen under the electron microscope.

Membranes are not static structures. Breaks can be repaired by the still viable cell. The phospholipids and fatty acid components of membranes are in a state of constant turnover. The life cycle of the rat liver cell is about six months, but the life cycle of some of the protein components of the membranes of mitochondria and the ER is about 9 days. Membranes, then, are in a state of continual synthesis and resynthesis and, although they appear well organized and static, their components are constantly being renewed.

INTERCELLULAR JUNCTIONS

Although cells appear to be directly apposed to each other, a closer look indicates a space of over 100 Å usually separating contiguous plasma membranes. This space is presumably maintained by electrostatic forces of repulsion. It is not a vacuum but probably contains a watery gel of uncertain composition. Although separated, the cells in such organized structures as epithelial surfaces are tightly held together by highly specialized cell organelles. For example, the columnar epithelial cells which line the small intestine have regions where the plasma membranes of adjacent cells appear to fuse, forming the so-called *tight junction* (zonula occludens). This tight junction is situated just below the luminal surface of the cell where it blocks the penetration of macromolecules between cells.

Other epithelial cells, such as those in the skin, produce specialized adhesion discs. These appear as darkly stained circular thickenings of the inner leaflet of the plasma membranes. The juxtaposition of these adhesion discs on contiguous cells produces the intercellular junction known as a *desmosome*. Within each cell, numerous fine tonofilaments, looking like guy wires, stretch out from the desmosome into the cell's interior, further securing cell-to-cell interadherence. Often the narrow gap between the discs on adjacent cells is filled with a substance more electron dense than the usual intercellular substance. The nature of this intercellular material is obscure but it apparently acts as a glue between the adhesion discs, thus locking cells into the special organization of the particular epithelial surface. Where a cell rests on a basement membrane, its basal surface may be anchored by a *hemidesmosome*. Other variations of the desmosomes exist, such as those without tonofilaments called terminal bars or intermediate junctions (zonulae adherentes).

These seemingly trivial structural details may have considerable importance. For instance, the individual tumor cells in cancers arising from epithelial surfaces often do not form desmosomes. Since these cells do not produce points of anchorage they are at greater liberty to invade contiguous tissues. As another example: physiologists have for years sought pores in cells such as those that line blood vessels to explain the permeability of blood vessels to plasma fluids and small molecules. Since few endothelial cells are fenestrated, perhaps the interendothelial cell junctions provide the very pores which physiologists have long sought. The theoretical calculations of permeability would require dimensions in the precise order of the interendothelial cell junctions found between these cells.

Many and perhaps all of the cells of man are coated by an amorphous fuzzy-looking polysaccharide substance which appears to be a product of the outer leaflet of the plasma membrane. This substance, termed the glycocalyx (Ito, 1969), is particularly well developed in the epithelial cells lining the small intestine where it has been shown to be rich in enzymes. It may well play an important role in further degradation of carbohydrates and proteins, aiding in their absorption by the microvilli. This glycocalyx about the cell may comprise the cement substance or gel which fills intercellular spaces.

CYTOPLASM AND ITS ORGANELLES

The deceptively bland-looking, finely granular appearance of the cytoplasm under the light microscope belies its busy heterogeneous content of organelles. The major types of organelles will be described in subsequent sections, but the reader might be delighted by the detailed but simply presented discussion found in *The Living Cell* (1965).

With stains such as hematoxylin and eosine (H & E stains), the cytoplasm assumes a pink (acidophilic) color. The cytoplasmic matrix in which all of the organelles are embedded can be best characterized as a polyphasic colloid. Within this gel, a variety of specialized filaments may be found. In epithelial cells, there are the tonofilaments attached to the desmosomes; in the cells lining the intestines, filaments just below the apical membrane form the so-called terminal web; in keratinizing epithelial cells, there are keratin fibrils. Muscle cells contain myofibrils within the cytoplasmic matrix. In addition, nonspecialized fine filaments can sometimes be found traversing the gel, presumably providing a structural framework for the organelles. The cytoplasmic matrix contains soluble enzymes of considerable importance to the functioning of the cell—e.g., those involved in anaerobic glycolysis and in the activation of amino acids prior to their linkage into polypeptides. Transfer RNA is also found in the cytoplasmic matrix.

The most important components of the cytoplasm are its numerous organelles (Fig. 1–2). The mitochondria are dispersed, independent units. Some of the organelles, the endoplasmic reticulum (granular and agranular) and the Golgi complex, comprise a continuous branching and anastomosing network of intracellular channels. These channels are continuous with the perinuclear space found between the double layered membrane which encloses the nucleus. Thus the perinuclear cistern is continuous with the channels of the endoplasmic reticulum and the latter, in turn, is continuous with the vesicles of the Golgi complex. It is tempting to speculate that this pathway serves as an intracellular circulatory system.

MITOCHONDRIA

With the exception of bacteria, all aerobically respiring cells possess mitochondria. Great variation exists in the size, shape and number of mitochondria among the many cell types in the body. In general the more metabolically active a cell, the more mitochondria it possesses. Whether round, oval or filamentous, all mitochondria are enclosed within an elaborately complex membrane having the complex structure characteristic of the plasma membrane. The outer leaflet is continuous around the periphery of the mitochondrion, but the inner leaflet is infolded to form cristae. These project into the interior of the mitochondrion creating ridges, but do not totally traverse the space and so do not wall off areas (Fig. 1–3). "Elementary particles" are attached to the inner membrane surfaces of the cristae at regularly spaced intervals. These particles

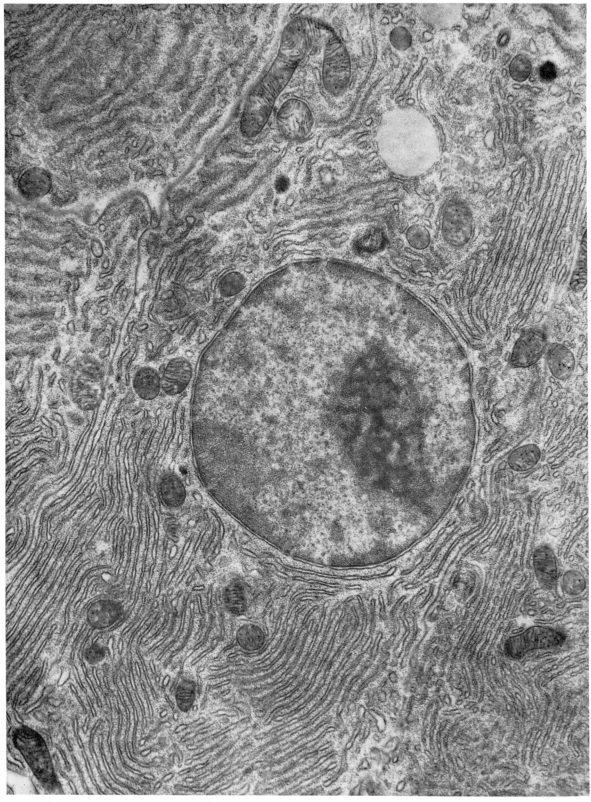

Figure 1–2. Bat pancreas. Clearly visible are the nucleus with its nucleolus; the double-layered nuclear membrane with its sharply defined pores; the numerous mitochondria in the cytoplasm with their laminated cristae mitochondriales; and the rich patterning of the cytoplasm with the membranes of the endoplasmic reticulum. A hand lens discloses the beading of ribonucleoprotein particles along the outer surfaces of the endoplasmic membranes. × 14,000. (Through the courtesy of Dr. D. W. Fawcett, Department of Anatomy, Harvard Medical School.)

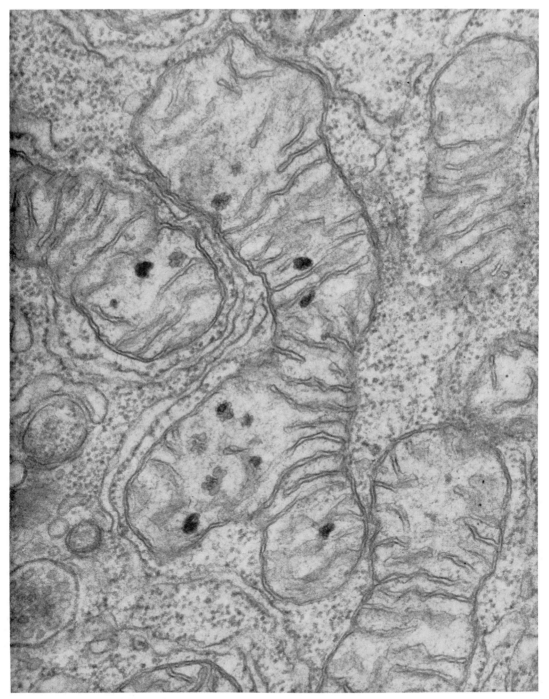

Figure 1–3. *Mitochondrion from crypt epithelium mouse duodenum with double limiting membrane and baffle-like cristae. Scattered nonspecific granules are enclosed. Approximately × 80,000. (Through the courtesy of Dr. Daniel Friend, Department of Pathology, University of California School of Medicine, San Francisco.)*

are thought to be the mushroom-like heads of a substructure whose stalks are buried within the cristae. The best evidence now suggests that these particles represent condensates of adenosinetriphosphatase (ATPase) or ATP synthetase involved in oxidative phosphorylation and electron transport (Kagawa and Racken, 1966). The interior of the mitochondrion is filled with a granular gel called mitochondrial matrix.

The function of mitochondria is well known to all students of biology. At the most elemental level, they can be considered as biochemical machines for the capture of the energy contained within food stuffs. Through the Krebs cycle and the electron transport respiratory chain, this energy is converted and stored into the high-energy phosphate bonds of ATP. It is beyond our scope to review the tricarboxylic acid cycle and the electron transport chains, but it will be remembered that through these pathways all three major foodstuffs enter as two carbon units bound to coenzyme A and leave as carbon dioxide and water, having yielded their energy reserves in the formation of ATP. Presently, about 70 enzymes and coenzymes are known to collaborate in a sequential and ordered fashion in this oxidative phosphorylation (Lehninger, 1964) (Hall and Palmer, 1969).

Although we are accustomed to visualizing mitochondria as apparently stable structures, they are in a continuous state of dynamic turnover. Mitochondria change their shape and volume; they may decrease or increase in number; some undoubtedly disintegrate, while others are formed. The actively metabolizing cell generates more mitochondria. The membranes of the mitochondrion are in a perpetual state of turnover. While the liver cell has a life span of many years, that of the protein component of the membranes of the mitochondria ranges between 5 and 12 days.

The mitochondrion has many of the characteristics of a completely independent unit, including its own chromosomal genetic apparatus. In fact, the mitochondrion can be considered as a subcell within a cell. There is good evidence that it is capable of dividing into two autonomous daughter mitochondria. Deoxyribonucleic acid (DNA) as well as DNA polymerase (required for DNA synthesis) have been identified within mitochondria (Nass, 1969). While there does not seem to be sufficient DNA to code for all of the numerous enzymes and coenzymes in mitochondria, this extranuclear DNA behaves as though it were a mitochondrial chromosome. It is not believed to originate in the nuclear DNA because it replicates at a different time in the life cycle of the cell, mainly during the late intermitotic G-2 phase in which there is no synthesis of nuclear DNA (Parsons and Simpsom, 1967) (Parsons and Rustad, 1968).

ENDOPLASMIC RETICULUM

The endoplasmic reticulum comprises a network of branching and anastomosing tubules 400 to 700 Å in diameter. The enclosing membranes are about 50 to 60 Å thick and have the same substructure as the plasma membrane. It has been calculated that 1 ml. of liver tissue contains about 11 square meters of endoplasmic membrane, indeed, more than enough to shroud the entire individual.

Two patterns are found in the cell: smooth or agranular (SER) and rough or granular (RER) endoplasmic reticulum (Weibel et al., 1969). As is well known, the rough ER is studded with an evenly spaced array of ribosomal granules, strategically located for the transfer of their synthetic products into the canals of the ER. From here, the proteins can pass freely into the Golgi complex where they are packaged for export (Bruni and Porter, 1965). The relative proportions of SER and RER vary among the many cell types in the body and are modified by the demands made upon the cells. Cells actively engaged in protein synthesis have a preponderance of RER. Thus one finds abundant granular ER in such cells as the hepatocyte, the primary site of the elaboration of plasma proteins, and in the plasma cell which synthesizes immunoglobulins.

The smooth ER, rich in a wide variety of enzymes, is most abundant in those cells involved in the synthesis of lipids, particularly triglycerides, lipoprotein complexes and steroids. Other functions of the agranular ER include conjugation of bile pigments, glycogenolysis and detoxification of many drugs and chemical agents (Rothschild, 1963). In striated muscle the ER, here called the sarcoplasmic reticulum, is thought to be involved in the conduction of contractile impulses from the surface membrane of the cell into the recesses of the muscle cell filled with myofilaments.

RIBOSOMES

These structural units on which proteins are synthesized are found studded along the membranes of the granular ER as well as in aggregates (polyribosomes) lying within the cytoplasmic matrix. The polyribosome, composed of ribosomes strung along a strand of messenger ribonucleic acid (RNA), is principally involved in the synthesis of proteins destined for use within the cells; intracellular enzymes and structural proteins for the maintenance of the cell as well as the buildup of proteins required for cell division. In contrast, enzymes packaged into lysosomes and proteins exported from the cell are probably synthesized on the ribosomes of the granular ER.

All ribosomes, whether attached to messenger RNA or to reticular membrane, have a remarkably complex substructure. The individual particle is composed of subunits. In bacteria, the whole ribosome particle has a sedimentation coefficient of 70S. It can be fractionated into 50S and 30S units. In the liver cells of man, the ribosomes are slightly larger (80S) and are composed of 60S and 40S subunits. The larger subunit is globoid and the smaller one sits on it as a cap. Indeed, these subunits may be further dissociated into ribosomal proteins and RNA particles (25S, 18S and 5S) made up of helical strands of RNA containing paired bases (Nomura, 1969) (Miller and Beatty, 1969). When a cell is rich in ribosomes, its cytoplasm stains darkly with the usual methods of tissue preparation, and so the plasma cell has basophilic cytoplasm. There has been some question as to whether ribosomes are fabricated in toto within the nucleus or RNA is synthesized intranuclearly and then finally assembled into ribosomes in the cytoplasm. Most evidence favors the latter view. But, in any event, it is clear that the nucleolus is the site of synthesis of the ribosomal RNA.

THE GOLGI COMPLEX

A well established substructure of the cell, the Golgi complex has several components: flattened vacuoles or cisternae, parallel membranes which may be the lateral boundaries of these cisternae, and many small vesicles (Fig. 1–4). It is usually situated in the periphery of the cell close to the plasma membrane. The vesicles are of variable size, from 400 to 800 Å in diameter. The flattened cisternae are often arranged in curved parallel stacks, giving convex and concave aspects to the entire complex. The concave margin, which is generally oriented toward the center of the cell, exhibits communications between the Golgi cisternae and the ER, while the vacuoles are disposed about the convex facade closer to the cell membrane.

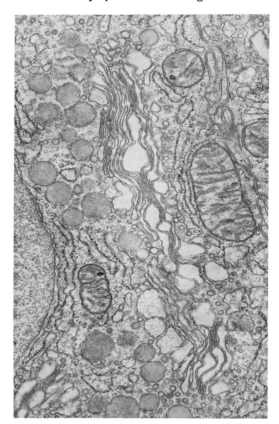

Figure 1–4. Golgi complex in center field from epithelial cell Brunner's gland mouse duodenum comprising parallel arrays of double membranes sometimes separated by vacuoles. Approximately × 20,000.

The organization of the Golgi complex is closely related to its presumed function. It is believed that the complex is largely involved in the segregation, aggregation and exportation of products formed within the cell. Thus, proteins synthesized in the RER pass down the anastomosing canals of the ER and accumulate within the parallel stacks of the cisternae. Here they are concentrated, and those scheduled for transfer across the plasma membrane may be transported to the cell surface within vesicles formed on the outer face of the Golgi. Lysosomes are created in this manner. Similarly, such substances as insulin and mucin pass through the Golgi complex. Thus, the connections between the Golgi complex and the ER at the so-called forming or concave face and the association of vesicles with the emitting convex face are ingeniously suited to serve the functions of this complex organelle (Ericsson and Glinsmann, 1966). In addition, it now appears likely that complex carbohydrate and polysaccharide synthesis occurs in the Golgi complex. Presumably, it is here that the complex carbohydrates are linked to protein to create glycoproteins (Neutra and Leblond, 1969).

LYSOSOMES

These organelles, first characterized by deDuve (1967), are best defined as membrane-bounded sacs containing hydrolytic enzymes. They range in size from 0.2 to 0.8 microns in diameter and contain more than a dozen acid hydrolases, principally acid phosphatase, glucuronidases, sulfatases, ribonucleases and deoxyribonucleases (deDuve and Wattiaux, 1966). The formation of these enzyme-filled sacs from vacuoles of the Golgi complex was described earlier.

The lysosome represents a means whereby destructive enzymes are sequestered and rendered harmless within the cell. Under normal conditions, the lysosomal membrane is impermeable to these enzymes but, if the pH of the cell falls sufficiently, the permeability of the membrane increases and permits diffusion of the enzymes into the cell substance. Such increased intracellular acidity, of necessity, is only encountered when there is serious cell injury or cell death. Thus the release of lysosomal enzymes facilitates autolytic removal of these obsolete cells. Release of lysosomal contents into the blood has been postulated as a possible cause of shock (Reich et al., 1965). Other fractions may be mediators of the inflammatory response (Janoff and Zweifach, 1964). Lysosomes also play an important role in the disintegration of foreign material, such as bacteria engulfed by cells, as well as in the removal of damaged organelles or cellular components. When bacteria are engulfed by a phagocytic cell, an ingenious sequence ensues in which the bacteria-containing vacuole fuses with a lysosome, forming an arena in which all of the lysosomal enzymes act directly on the offender without injury to the cell or its organelles.

When cells suffer a focal injury, the damaged organelles are enclosed within a membrane. The resultant structure is termed an *autophagic vacuole*. This sequestration of damaged organelles and its role in the adaptive response of cells to stress will be discussed in a later section (p. 13). It is enough to say here that the autophagic vacuole fuses with one or more lysosomes to accomplish the digestion of the damaged cellular structures.

Lysosomes are the wastebaskets in which cells sequester abnormal substances, particularly those of macromolecular nature. In some hereditary diseases known as inborn errors of metabolism, abnormal compounds may be synthesized which the cell cannot metabolize, and so they accumulate. The lysosomes of the cells of various tissues become filled with these abnormal products and, in this fashion, the cell sequesters these indigestible overloads. Other lysosomal disorders have been described, such as a familial metabolic disease in which there is a deficiency of lysosomal acid phosphatase (Nadler and Egan, 1970). Lysosomes have thus become organelles of considerable interest and clinical importance.

MICROBODIES

Microbodies or peroxisomes require only brief mention. These membrane-bounded particles are closely related to lysosomes. They are of the same approximate size, are found in man principally in kidney and liver cells and are rich in the enzymes peroxidase, catalase and, to a lesser extent, urate oxidase. They are distinguished from lysosomes by their dense, opaque, homogeneous cores called nucleoids.

OTHER CYTOPLASMIC COMPONENTS

Centrioles are found in the cytoplasm mostly in close relation to the nucleus. At low resolution, they appear as a pair of deeply stained rods sometimes referred to as the diplosome. Higher resolution indicates an immense complexity within each of these rods, comprising groups of microtubules arrayed about the periphery of the rod. Centrioles (diplosomes) come into play during mitotic division when the diplosome divides and both units migrate to opposite poles of the cells. Here they apparently provide anchorages for the mitotic spindle which will attach to the chromosomes or chromatids during mitotic or meiotic division. Microtubules, glycogen granules, pigment granules, secretory granules, lipid vacuoles and a host of cell products may also be identified in the cell cytoplasm.

NUCLEUS

The general features of the nucleus and its variable shape among the cells of the body are too well known to require repetition. Here we shall focus on some of the ultrastructural detail. The interphase nucleus has the following distinguishable features: (1) a distinct double nuclear membrane separated by a space of about 100 to 150 Å between the outer and inner leaflets, (2) a spheroidal body or nucleolus composed of RNA, (3) finely divided or filamentous chromatin (euchromatin), (4) clumps or flakes of chromatin (heterochromatin) usually most abundant about the nuclear membrane and the nucleolus, and (5) nuclear sap which fills up the space between these other nuclear components.

NUCLEAR MEMBRANE

The double nuclear membrane is principally of interest because of the suspected existence of pores. The two lamellae of the nuclear membrane fuse at the margins of the pores. An unsettled question is whether or not the pores are covered by a diaphragm. In protozoa, it has been shown that pores which have an apparent diameter of about 600 Å permit the passage, from the cytoplasm into the nucleus, of particles only up to about 85 Å in diameter. Apparently, in these primitive organisms the pores are largely closed, presumably by diaphragms which contain holes or perforations not larger than 100 Å. There is evidence of a similar type of partial covering for the pores of nuclei in animal cells as well (Afzelius, 1955).

The perinuclear space or cistern appears to communicate with channels of the ER. The existence of such communications should be no surprise, since there is considerable evidence that the nuclear membrane or envelope is made up of cisternae of the ER which collect around the chromosomes immediately at the completion of mitotic division. The outer leaflet of the nuclear membrane is studded with ribosomal granules, further supporting the view that RER forms the nuclear membrane. It is evident then that the nucleus has two channels of communication with the cytoplasm: the pores which presumably provide passageways directly into the cytoplasmic colloidal matrix, and the communications between the perinuclear cistern and the lumina of the ER. There is abundant evidence that the three main types of RNA—messenger, transfer and ribosomal—are all synthesized within the nucleus and pass to the cytoplasm of the cell where they participate in protein synthesis.

NUCLEOLUS

The nucleolus, with its complex substructure in which ribonucleoprotein granules, fibers and coiled bodies have been discerned, is directly involved in the synthesis of the ribosomal RNA. Nucleolar organizers control the synthesis of the RNA destined to form the ribosomes. It is no surprise then that cells engaged in active protein synthesis, particularly actively dividing cells, tend to have large nucleoli and may have more than a single nucleolus.

CHROMATIN

The finally divided euchromatin is genetically more active than the clumped heterochromatin. Its ultrastructural organization is still a matter of uncertainty, but observations in bacteria and animal cells suggest that the euchromatin exists as a fibrillar or filamentous strand of deoxyribonucleoprotein (DNP). These strands may obtain a length of several centimeters and presumably represent polymers of DNA complexed with protein in which the DNA-protein monomers are linked together end to end. The heterochromatin is presumed to represent tightly folded fibers or filaments. This conception of the heterochromatin is largely based on observations which suggest that the chromosome itself is a fiber of DNA, perhaps as long as 7 cm., in a tightly folded packed form. The chemical structure of DNA and the Watson-Crick model will be discussed in Chapter 6 (p. 172). In passing, we might note that in the female many of the cells contain a dense clump of heterochromatin known as the Barr body (sex chromatin) characteristically attached to the nuclear membrane (p. 180).

It is surprisingly difficult to determine with the light microscope when a cell has been irreversibly damaged. Changes in the nucleus are perhaps the most reliable indicators, although we must admit that such changes are probably late consequences of disrupted cytoplasmic and organellar function. The nuclear changes indicative of irreversible damage include pyknosis (irregular shrinkage, basophilic condensation and wrinkling of the nucleus), karyorrhexis (fragmentation of the nucleus) and karyolysis (fading of the nucleus as DNases and RNases catabolize the nucleoproteins). With this review of the normal cell, we can turn to the consideration of the adaptive responses of the healthy cell.

CELLULAR ADAPTATION

Cells adapt to alterations in their environment just as does the individual. Shivering is an adaptive response of the warm-blooded animal to low environmental temperatures. Unpleasant as the sensation may be, the increased muscular activity generates internal heat to compensate for that lost from the surface of the body. The cells do not shiver but it is their increased metabolic activity which is the ultimate source of the heat. Insofar as the body temperature is supported, no injury results to either the entire organism or its cells. In the same way, insofar as a cell can adapt to an alteration in its environment, it can escape injury.

The bulging muscles of the laborer engaged in heavy work are an excellent example of cellular adaptation. The increase in muscle mass reflects an increase in the size of individual muscle fibers, in turn, resulting from the synthesis of more mitochondria, sarcoplasmic reticulum and myofilaments (Richter and Kellner, 1963). The workload is thus shared by a greater mass of cellular components and each is spared excessive overwork so that the muscle cell escapes injury. The enlarged muscle cell achieves a new equilibrium permitting it to survive at a higher level of metabolic activity. Cellular adaptation, then, is a state which lies intermediate between the normal unstressed cell and the overstressed, injured cell. A few of the more important and well studied aspects of such cellular adaptation will be considered; these include: (1) the induction of increased amounts of endoplasmic reticulum, (2) sequestration of focal injuries in cells (autophagy), (3) increase in cell size — hypertrophy, (4) decrease in cell size — atrophy, (5) hyperplasia, and (6) metaplasia.

INDUCTION OF ENDOPLASMIC RETICULUM

The adaptive responses of cells involve both functional and structural changes. For example, when increased protein synthesis is required to replace destroyed cells or lost plasma proteins, more ribosomes are produced in the affected cell. In cells depending mainly on aerobic respiration, increased metabolic activity is associated with an increase in the number of mitochondria. Best studied, however, are the adaptive changes in the ER. Jones and Fawcett (1966), among others, have called attention to the hypertrophy of the agranular ER in hamster liver cells following the administration of phenobarbital to these animals. Protracted human use of this hypnotic drug has long been known to lead to a state of increasing tolerance to the medication. Repeated identical doses of phenobarbital lead to progressively shorter time spans of sleep. In effect, the patients have adapted to the medication. The basis of such adaptation has now been traced to the changes in the ER. In the hepatocyte where phenobarbital is detoxified via oxidative demethylation, there is extensive hypertrophy of the SER accompanied by a commensurate increase in the quantity of the hydroxylating enzymes found in the SER. Other drugs and agents are also detoxified or metabolized through pathways involving oxidative demethylation so that the cell adapted to phenobarbital exhibits an increased capacity for detoxifying other drugs such as steroids, carcinogenic hydrocarbons and carbon tetrachloride, as well as for metabolizing products such as bilirubin and bile acids (Popper and Schaffner, 1970).

The adaptive response is truly a protective one for the cell. Exposed to a foreign agent such as phenobarbital or, more dangerously, carbon tetrachloride, the cell protects itself by increasing its capability to metabolize the "intruder." Advantage is taken of this phenomenon in clinical practice. Among obstetricians, there is a great deal of interest in the administration of phenobarbital to pregnant mothers whose infant might have a hemolytic reaction after birth. Hemolytic disease in the newborn, called erythroblastosis fetalis, develops in infants having either an ABO or Rh incompatibility with the mother (p. 557). Maternal antibodies may develop to antigens "foreign" to the mother, which the infant inherited from the father. Some of these antibodies can pass the placental barrier and, once within the fetus, induce a reaction severe enough to cause neonatal death. Less severe hemolysis in the newborn is still dangerous because of the release of large amounts of hemoglobin and the formation of excessive quantities of bile pigments (jaundice). The administration of phenobarbital during the last stages of pregnancy, it is theorized, will induce adaptive changes not only in the ER of the liver cells of the mother but also in the fetus since the drug passes the placental barrier. The newborn should therefore have a greater capability for conjugating and excreting the bile pigments and thus be able to escape the deleterious effects of the severe jaundice. The therapy of hemolytic disease of the newborn (p. 557) demonstrates how a new and promising approach to medical management involves the adaptive response of subcellular organelles (Editorial, 1971) (Stiehl et al., 1972).

SEQUESTRATION OF FOCAL INJURY — AUTOPHAGY

Sequestration is a mechanism whereby a focal injury in the cell is isolated from the unharmed organelles. The membranes, mentioned earlier, which enclose such a focus of injury are derived from the ER (Ericsson, 1969).

The resultant membrane-bounded structure containing damaged organelles is known as an *autophagic vacuole* or *cytosegresome*. This autophagic vacuole then coalesces with a lysosome, causing the injured cellular structures to be digested by the lysosomal hydrolases. Some of the contained cellular debris within the autophagic vacuole may resist digestion or be incompletely digested and persist as membrane-bounded *residual bodies.*

Focal degradation of organelles or intracellular components is probably a common biologic process, and the sequestration of such injury represents an adaptive response by which the cells protect uninvolved areas (Swift and Hruban, 1964). Does the autophagic vacuole then persist in the cell? One of three pathways may be followed. In cell which border on a lumen or a duct, there is some evidence that the autophagic vacuoles or their residual bodies may be extruded by a process resembling reverse phagocytosis. Extrusion of residual bodies and autophagic vacuoles has been observed in liver cells and in epithelial cells lining kidney tubules. Alternatively, complete catalytic digestion may be achieved with disappearance of the autophagic vacuole. However, in some instances, the residual body persists within a sarcophagus in the cytoplasm.

Lipofuscin granules, seen as yellow-brown pigment with the light microscope, are residual bodies presumably derived from polymerized and partially degraded membranes of organelles. Lipofuscin has been called a *"wear and tear" pigment.* It is seen principally in the hepatocytes and the muscle fibers of the heart in aged individuals, and is often associated with atrophy of the cell and the affected organ. In sufficient amounts, it may impart a brown discoloration to the tissue—brown atrophy. The derivation of this pigment is discussed on p. 47. Here, however, we are principally interested in the phenomenon of sequestration as an expression of cellular adaptation. In later discussions, it will become evident that atrophy, along with its increased amount of pigment is also an adaptive response.

HYPERTROPHY

The adaptive response of a cell to a changed environment may involve the size of the cell. *Hypertrophy refers to an increase in the size of cells and, with such change, an increase in the size of the organ.* The hypertrophied organ has no new cells. The cellular enlargement is due to the synthesis of more ultrastructural components and is not due merely to an increased uptake of water. Hypertrophy as an adaptive response was cited earlier in the discussion of muscular enlargement (p. 12). The striated muscle cells, those in both the heart and skeletal muscles, are most capable of hypertrophy, perhaps because they do not adapt to increased metabolic demands by mitotic division and the formation of more cells to share the work. While the principal alteration in the striated muscle cell is an increased number of myofilaments, a greater number of mitochondria as well as a more abundant ER are produced. Nuclear enlargement is slight but not commensurate with the increased volume of the cell.

The environmental change which produces hypertrophy of striated muscle appears to be principally increased workload, implying an increased metabolic activity. The adaptation includes synthesis of more membranes, enzymes, ATP, higher levels of aerobic respiration and more myofilaments capable of achieving an equilibrium between the demand and the cell's functional capacity. The increased workload shared by a greater number of myofilaments achieves a level of metabolic activity per unit volume of cell not significantly different from that borne by the normal myofilament. The draft horse readily pulls a load that would "break the back" of a pony. Similarly, hypertrophy of the heart is an adaptive response encountered in a variety of cardiovascular diseases which place increased burdens on the heart. The best example is the cardiac enlargement encountered in patients with high blood pressure (hypertension) (p. 655). Because the heart must contract against increased pressures in the aorta and peripheral circulation, the heart may achieve a weight of 700 to 800 gm. as compared to the normal weight of 350 gm. (Braunwald et al., 1968).

Cardiac hypertrophy is also seen with valvular incompetence in which the heart becomes less efficient and adapts by greater work output (Fig. 1–5). When valves are damaged, there is incomplete emptying of the cardiac chambers referred to as increased end-diastolic volumes. Stretching of the myocardial chambers and cardiac muscle fibers results. The stretched fibers contract with greater vigor and so the strain of more work, more myofilaments and hypertrophy follows. This sequence is an expression of the Frank-Starling law of the heart which states that, as muscles become stretched, they contract with greater force. Unfortunately, the hypertrophied heart reaches a limit beyond which enlargement of muscle mass is no longer able to compensate for the increased burden, and cardiac failure ensues. The limiting factors are

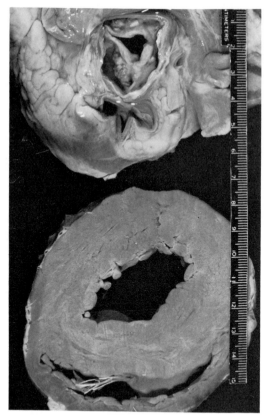

Figure 1–5. *Aortic stenosis with resultant myocardial hypertrophy. The narrowed valvular lumen is viewed from above, and the myocardial thickening is illustrated in the cross section of the ventricles (normal thickness of left ventricle is 1.2 to 1.4 cm.).*

muscle, the heart, secondary sex organs and brain. *The apparent causes of such atrophy are decreased workload, loss of innervation, diminished blood supply, inadequate nutrition or loss of endocrine stimulation* (Fig. 1–6). When a limb is immobilized in a plaster cast or muscles become paralyzed from loss of their innervation, as in poliomyelitis, atrophy of cells ensues (Fig. 1–7). In late adult life, the brain undergoes progressive atrophy, presumably as arteriosclerosis narrows its blood supply, and the gonads shrink with depletion of their endocrine stimulation (Figs. 1–8 and 1–9). In classic pathology, it was traditional to call such atrophy physiologic and to dignify the various circumstances in which pathologic atrophy might be encountered with such terms as disuse atrophy, neurogenic atrophy, vascular atrophy and endocrine atrophy. The fundamental cellular change is identical in all, representing a retreat by the cell to a smaller size at which survival is still possible within its constricted world. By bringing into balance cell volume and lower levels of blood supply, nutrition or trophic stimulation, a new equilibrium is achieved.

Atrophy represents a reduction in the

not well understood, but it has been proposed that enlargement in striated muscle cell size is not accompanied by a commensurate increase in the oxidative and phosphorylative capabilities of the mitochondria. The mitochondria of hypertrophied cells may be more numerous than in normal cells, but they appear to have inadequate cristae, the ultimate source of oxidative respiration. Presumably, then, at some point in cellular enlargement, the limiting factor becomes the energy-generating mechanisms within the cell and, when an imbalance occurs, cardiac failure ensues.

ATROPHY

Shrinkage in the size of a cell by loss of cell substance is known as atrophy. It is another form of adaptive response. When a sufficient number of cells are involved, the entire tissue or organ diminishes in size—becomes atrophic. Such diminution of cell and organ size may affect many organs but occurs principally in skeletal

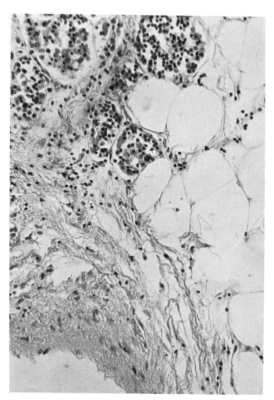

Figure 1–6. *Atrophic pancreas. The externally secreting acinar glands have atrophied, and only the islets remain in fat and fibrous tissue.*

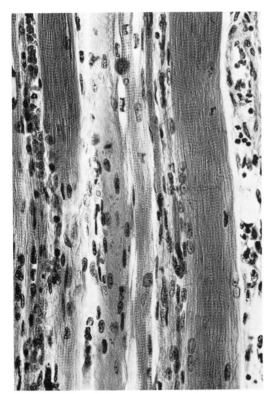

Figure 1-7. *Atrophic striated muscle cells in poliomyelitis. Contrast large normal cells with the intervening denervated shrunken cells which have indistinct cross striations.*

structural components of the cell. Fewer myofilaments, mitochondria and less endoplasmic reticulum are presumably present. But the most striking intracellular alteration is an increased number of autophagic vacuoles. As mentioned earlier, many of these autophagic vacuoles become converted to residual bodies containing lipofuscin pigment. The concurrence of atrophy and accumulation of lipofuscin is recognized by the term *brown atrophy*. The heart in the aged individual may weigh only 200 to 250 gm. and be dark brown in color—the so-called brown atrophy of the heart. The atrophic shrunken liver may likewise undergo brown atrophy. Obviously, atrophy may progress to the point where cells are injured and die. If the blood supply is inadequate even to maintain the life of shrunken cells, injury and cell death may supervene. The adaptive capability of the cell is limited and, when exceeded, is followed by more ominous consequences.

HYPERPLASIA

Just as enlargement of cells (hypertrophy) represents a response to increased functional demand, cells capable of mitotic division may divide when stressed or stimulated to increased activity. In this way, the load is shared among a greater number. *Hyperplasia comprises, then, an*

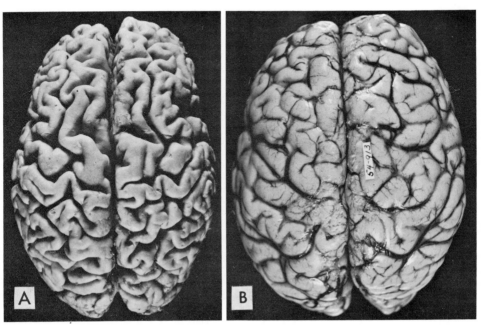

Figure 1-8. A, *Physiologic atrophy of the brain in an 82-year-old male. The meninges have been stripped.*
B. *Normal brain of 35-year-old male.*

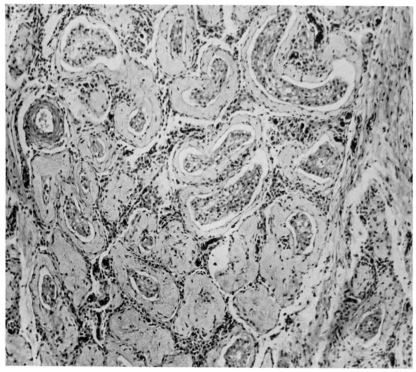

Figure 1–9. *Photomicrograph of atrophic testis. The tubules have walls thickened by fibrosis, and the atrophic germinal epithelium is pushed into small masses within the atrophied tubular lumina. The separation of the epithelium from its basement membrane is a fixation artefact.*

increase in the number of cells in an organ or tissue, which usually increases its volume. Hypertrophy and hyperplasia are very closely related and often develop concurrently. Both hypertrophy and hyperplasia will take place if the cellular population is capable of synthesizing DNA, thus permitting mitotic division. Hyperplasia in response to stress or endocrine stimulation may represent a physiologic process. It is best seen in the glandular epithelium of the breast of the female at puberty and pregnancy. Physiologic hyperplasia also occurs in the gravid uterus, and here it is accompanied by striking hypertrophy of preexisting smooth muscle cells. The enlargement of one kidney when the other is destroyed or removed is known as *compensatory hypertrophy* but, in reality, this phenomenon involves hypertrophy of individual nephrons produced by hyperplasia of tubular epithelial cells. The term compensatory hypertrophy is somewhat of a misnomer, alluding to the fact that new nephrons are not formed but that the increase in volume of the kidney is largely the consequence of enlargement and elongation of the nephric tubules, accompanied by stress-induced proliferation of tubular cells.

Little is known about the ultimate mechanisms which trigger physiologic hypertrophy.

In most instances, increased workload and hormonal stimulation underlie this response, but the mere knowledge of this does not provide insight into how these act (Malt, 1969). We know less about the circumstances that ultimately limit the extent of the hyperplasia. Once the cells of the breast or the kidney tubules begin to proliferate, what brings the process to a halt? It can be theorized that when a sufficient number of cells are available to bring the workload of the individual cell to a tolerable limit, some shut-off mechanism becomes operative or the stress stimulus, divided among the increased number of cells, falls at the individual cell level below some mystical threshold level.

In some circumstances, hyperplasia may assume pathologic proportions. Most forms of *pathologic hyperplasia* represent instances of excessive hormonal stimulation of target cells. The most common examples are cystic and adenomatous hyperplasia of the endometrium. Following every normal menstrual period, there is a rapid burst of proliferative activity which might be considered as reparative proliferation or physiologic hyperplasia of the endometrium. This proliferation is, as is well known, potentiated by pituitary FSH and ovarian estrogen. The rising levels of progesterone, usually about 10 to 14 days before the anticipated period, bring this proliferation to a halt. When the balance between estrogen and progesterone is disturbed, resulting in either an absolute or relative increase in the amount of estrogen, endometrial hyperplasia occurs. Sometimes the proliferative endometrial glands become cystically dilated and enlarged, inducing so-called *cystic hyperplasia.* At other times, because of more intense estrogen stimulation, there is proliferation of glandular epithelium, with outpouching of growing glands to form many more glands, thus producing *adenomatous hyperplasia.* Both forms of endometrial change are common causes of abnormal menstrual bleeding but, nonetheless, the hyperplastic process remains controlled within limits and so apparently responds to regulatory controls over the growth of cells. However, it should be stressed that such pathologic hyperplasia constitutes an important soil from which cancerous proliferation may arise. In various reported studies, it is estimated that 3 to 25 per cent of patients with adenomatous hyperplasia of the endometrium eventually develop endometrial cancer and, conversely, about half of all patients with endometrial cancer at one time suffered from adenomatous hyperplasia (Hertig and Sommers, 1949).

Pathologic hyperplasia is also seen in a variety of forms of thyroid disease known generically as goiter, and here the stimulus appears to be either an iodine deficiency in some forms of goiter (p. 1331) or a stimulatory factor known as "long-acting thyroid stimulator" (LATS) (p. 1334) in other forms of goiter. Other instances of pathologic hyperplasia might be cited, but it suffices here merely to indicate that although all hyperplastic processes, both physiologic and pathologic, are instances of controlled cellular proliferation, the mitotic and metabolic activities of the cell provide a soil for cancerogenic influences.

METAPLASIA

Metaplasia is a reversible change in which one adult cell type (epithelial or mesenchymal) is replaced by another adult cell type. It, too, may represent an adaptive substitution of cells more sensitive to stress by other cell types better able to withstand the adverse environment. Such adaptive metaplasia is best seen in the squamous metaplasia which occurs in the respiratory tract in response to chronic irritation or inflammation. In the habitual cigarette smoker, the normal columnar ciliated epithelial cells of the trachea and bronchi are often replaced focally or widely by stratified squamous epithelial cells. Similar changes may be encountered in chronic infections of the bronchi and bronchioles. Stones in the excretory ducts of the salivary glands, pancreas or bile ducts may cause replacement of the normal secretory columnar epithelium by nonfunctioning stratified squamous epithelium (Fig. 1–10). For less clear reasons, a deficiency of vitamin A induces squamous metaplasia in the respiratory epithelium. In all of these instances, the more rugged stratified squamous epithelium is able to survive under circumstances in which the more fragile specialized epithelium most likely would have succumbed.

In transformation of one adult cell to another adult cell type, presumably less differentiated reserve cells are conditioned by mysterious mechanisms to differentiate along divergent lines. Although the squamous metaplastic cells in the respiratory tract, for example, are capable of surviving, an important protective mechanism—mucus secretion—is lost. Thus, epithelial metaplasia is a two-edged sword and, in most circumstances, represents an undesirable change. Moreover, the influences which predispose to such metaplasia, if persistent, may induce cancerous transformation in the metaplastic epithelium. Thus, the common form of cancer in the respiratory tract is composed of squamous cells.

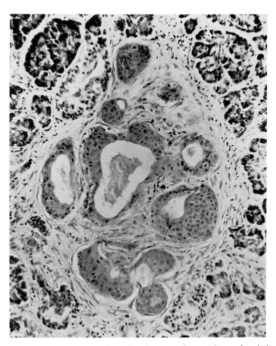

Figure 1–10. *Metaplastic transformation of adult columnar epithelial cells to adult stratified squamous cells in pancreatic ducts.*

Metaplasia may also occur in mesenchymal cells but less clearly as an adaptive response. Fibroblasts may become transformed to osteoblasts or chondroblasts to produce bone or cartilage where it is normally not encountered. For example, bone is occasionally formed in soft tissues, particularly in foci of injury. This process represents a form of "divergent differentiation." Similar abnormal differentiation is sometimes encountered in tumors in which genetic coding, apparently repressed in the normal cells from which the tumor derived, becomes expressed when the cells lose certain of their controls and become tumorigenic.

DYSPLASIA

Dysplasia is an alteration in adult cells characterized by variation in their size, shape and organization. It is a controversial term in pathology used both loosely and commonly. Strictly speaking, *dysplasia means deranged development; however, in common medical usage it is applied to either epithelial or mesenchymal cells, principally the former, that have undergone somewhat irregular, atypical proliferative changes in response to chronic irritation or inflammation.* It is not an adaptive process, but is considered here because it is closely related to metaplasia and, indeed, is sometimes called *atypical metaplasia.*

Epithelial dysplasia presents as a loss of normal orientation of one epithelial cell to the other, accompanied by alteration in cellular size and shape, nuclear size and shape, and staining characteristics. It is most commonly encountered in the uterine cervix following a long span of chronic cervicitis. The dysplastic stratified squamous epithelium is thickened by hyperplasia of basal cells, accompanied by disordered maturation of the cells as they proceed to the surface layers. Mitotic figures are found only in the basal layer in normal cervical mucosa but, in dysplastic cervical epithelium, they may be found in the mid levels or even toward the surface. The increased proliferative activity produces greater amounts of DNA and more intense basophilia of the nuclei (Figs. 1–11 and 1–12). Although mitoses are

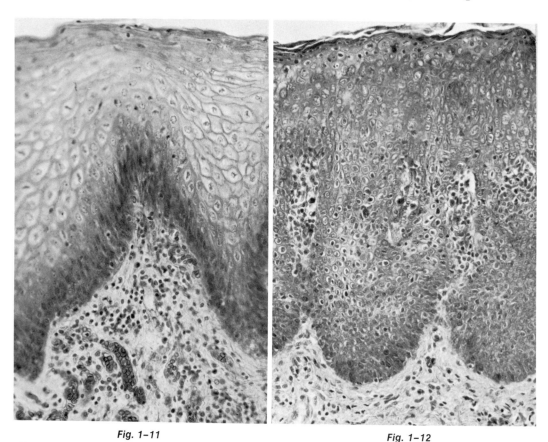

Fig. 1–11

Fig. 1–12

Figure 1–11. *Normal stratified squamous epithelium.*

Figure 1–12. *Dysplastic stratified squamous epithelium. The basal cells are hyperplastic and form a zone many cells thick. The dysplastic cells are deeply chromatic and disorganized.*

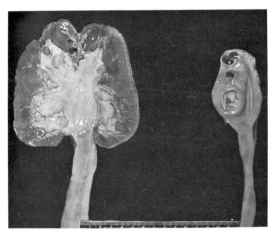

Figure 1–13. A normal and an aplastic kidney. Note that only the renal parenchyma is deficient. The pelvis and ureter, which develop from a separate anlage, are normal in size.

increased in number, they are not usually abnormal, such as are characteristic of cancer.

Dysplastic changes are also frequently encountered in the metaplastic squamous epithelium of the respiratory tract in habitual cigarette smokers. *In both the cervix and the respiratory tract, such dysplasia is strongly implicated in the causation of cancer.* Dysplastic changes are often found adjacent to foci of cancerous transformation and, in long-term studies of cigarette smokers, epithelial dysplasia almost invariably precedes in time the appearance of cancer (Auerbach et al., 1957, 1962). However, from many clinical studies it is known that dysplasia does not necessarily progress to cancer. *The changes are reversible and, with removal of the inciting causes, the epithelium may revert to normal.*

The term dysplasia is also used quite uncommonly, in its more rigorous syntax, to refer to the abnormal development of tissues or cells either from some embryologic rest sequestered in the body or from multipotential cells encountered most often in the deranged growth of a neoplasm.

HYPOPLASIA, APLASIA AND AGENESIS

All of these processes are mentioned here only for the sake of completeness. They are not adaptive in nature. They imply failure of an organ to develop, commonly encountered in one of the paired organs (kidney, ovary, testis). Hypoplasia represents a less severe developmental failure than aplasia and agenesis which imply total failure to develop. Thus, one kidney may be represented as a small 50 gm. organ in a case of hypoplasia, or as a mere nubbin of fibrous tissue in a case of complete agenesis or aplasia (Fig. 1–13). These phenomena are only of importance insofar as they imply reduction in the functional mass of the affected paired organs. The possibility of an aplastic kidney must always be borne in mind when unilateral nephrectomy is contemplated. More than one unfortunate patient has had a diseased kidney removed surgically by a physician who was not aware that the other kidney was aplastic. Obviously, aplasia of a vital single organ such as the heart or brain is not compatible with life, despite the fact that some politicians contend that their opponents suffer from such defects.

If the overall conception of this chapter can be captured in a few words, it is that the cell is by and of itself a unit of life. It is born, grows, respires, does its daily work and reproduces. Its adaptation to stress is in a sense a will to live. Confronted with adversity, it modifies its structure and function, and so adapts. When necessary, it may change its directions and become transformed from a fragile mucus-secreting factory to a less specialized, rugged scale-like squamous cell able to withstand the rigors of its microenvironment. Like its host, by daily adaptation it achieves a state of some harmony with its environment but, also like its host, it is limited in its adaptive capacity and may suffer injury and even die, as will be seen in the next chapter.

REFERENCES

Afzelius, B. A.: Ultrastructure of the nuclear membrane of the sea urchin oocyte as studied with the electron microscope. Exp. Cell Res., *8*:147, 1955.

Auerbach, O., et al.: Changes in the bronchial epithelium in relation to smoking and cancer of the lung. New Eng. J. Med., *256*:97, 1957.

Auerbach, O., et al.: Changes in bronchial epithelium in relation to sex, age, residence, smoking and pneumonia. New Eng. J. Med., *267*:111, 1962.

Braunwald, E., et al.: Mechanism of Contractility of the Normal and Failing Heart. Boston, Little, Brown and Co., 1968.

Bruni, C., and Porter, K. R.: The fine structure of the parenchymal cell of the normal rat liver. Amer. J. Path., *46*:691, 1965.

Danielli, J. F., and Davson, H. A.: A contribution to the theory of permeability of thin films. J. Cell. Comp. Physiol., *5*:495, 1935.

deDuve, C.: Lysosomes and phagosomes. Protoplasma, *63*:95, 1967.

deDuve, C., and Wattiaux, R.: Functions of lysosomes. Ann. Rev. Physiol., *28*:435, 1966.

deRobertis, E. D. P., et al.: Cell Biology. 5th ed. Philadelphia, W. B. Saunders Co., 1970.

Editorial: Jaundice of the newborn. Lancet, *1*:119, 1971.

Ericsson, J. L. E.: Studies on induced cellular autophagy, characterization of the membranes bordering autophagosomes in the parenchymal liver cells. Exp. Cell Res., *56*:393, 1969.

Ericsson, J. L. E., and Glinsmann, W. H.: Observations on the subcellular organization of hepatic parenchymal cells. I. Golgi apparatus, cytosomes, and cytosegresomes in normal cells. Lab. Invest., *15*:750, 1966.

Hall, D., and Palmer, J. M.: Mitochondrial research today. Nature, *221*:717, 1969.

Hertig, A. T., and Sommers, S. C.: Genesis of endometrial carcinoma. I. Study of prior biopsies. Cancer, *2*:946, 1949.

Ito, S.: Structure and function of the glycoclyax. Fed. Proc., *28*:12, 1969.

Janoff, A., and Zweifach, B. W.: Production of inflammatory changes in the microcirculation by cationic proteins extracted from lysosomes. J. Exp. Med., *120*:747, 1964.

Jones, A. L., and Fawcett, D. W.: Hypertrophy of the agranular endoplasmic reticulum in hamster liver induced by phenobarbital (with a review on the functions of this organelle in liver). J. Histochem. Cytochem., *14*:215, 1966.

Kagawa, K., and Racken, E.: Partial resolution of the enzymes catalyzing oxidative phosphorylation. J. Biol. Chem., *241*:2475, 1966.

Korn, E. D.: Current concepts of membrane structure and function. Fed. Proc., *28*:6, 1969.

Lehninger, A. L.: The Mitochondrion. New York, W. A. Benjamin Inc., 1964.

The Living Cell. Readings from Scientific American. San Francisco, W. H. Freeman and Company, 1965.

Ma, M. H., and Biempica, L.: The normal human liver cell. Amer. J. Path., *62*:353, 1971.

Malt, R. A.: Compensatory growth of the kidney. New Eng. J. Med., *280*:1446, 1969.

Miller, O. L., and Beatty, B. R.: Visualization of nucleolar genes. Science, *164*:955, 1969.

Nadler, H. L., and Egan, T. J.: Deficiency of lysosomal acid phosphatase, a new familial metabolic disorder. New Eng. J. Med., *282*:302, 1970.

Nass, M. M. K.: Mitochondrial DNA. Science, *165*:25, 1969.

Neutra, M., and Leblond, C.: The Golgi apparatus. Sci. Amer. (Feb.), *220*:100, 1969.

Nomura, M.: Ribosomes. Sci. Amer. (Oct.), *221*:28, 1969.

Parsons, J. A., and Rustad, R.: Distribution of DNA among dividing mitochondria of tetrahymena pyriformis. J. Cell Biol., *37*:683, 1968.

Parsons, P., and Simpson, M.: Biosynthesis of DNA by isolated mitochondria: incorporation of thymidine triphosphate-2-C[14]. Science, *155*:91, 1967.

Popper, H., and Schaffner, F.: Pathophysiology of cholestasis. Hum. Path., *1*:1, 1970.

Reich, T., et al.: Plasma cathepsin-like activity during hemorrhagic shock. J. Surg. Res., *5*:116, 1965.

Richter, G. W., and Kellner, A.: Hypertrophy of the human heart at the level of fine structure: an analysis and two postulates. J. Cell Biol., *18*:195, 1963.

Robertson, J. D.: Ultrastructure of cell membrane and their derivatives. Biochem. Soc. Sympos., *16*:3, 1959.

Rothschild, J.: The isolation of microsomal membranes. In Bell, D. J., and Grant, J. K. (eds.): The Structure and Function of the Membranes and Surfaces of Cells. Cambridge, Cambridge University Press, 1963, p. 4.

Siekevitz, P.: The organization of biologic membranes. New Eng. J. Med., *283*:1035, 1970.

Singer, S. J., and Nicolson, G. L.: The structure and chemistry of mammalian cell membranes. Amer. J. Path., *65*:427, 1971.

Sjöstrand, F. S.: The structure of cellular membranes. Protoplasma, *63*:248, 1967.

Stiehl, A., et al.: The effects of phenobarbital on bile salts and bilirubin in patients with intrahepatic and extrahepatic cholestasis. New Eng. J. Med., *286*:858, 1972.

Swift, H., and Hruban, Z.: Focal degradation as a biological process. Fed. Proc., *23*:1026, 1964.

Weibel, E. R., et al.: Correlated morphometric and biochemical studies on the liver cell. I. Morphometric model, stereologic methods, and normal morphometric data for rat liver. J. Cell Biol., *42*:68, 1969.

Weinstein, R. S.: The structure of cell membranes. New Eng. J. Med., *281*:86, 1969.

2

CELL INJURY AND CELL DEATH

Man's tolerance of adverse influences is limited by the ability of his cells and organelles to sustain injury. Whenever the cell's adaptive capability is overtaxed, damage results. Such damage may be sublethal and permit recovery, or more intense or prolonged, resulting in cell death. The adapted, the sublethally injured and the dying cell are merely three states along a continuum of progressive encroachment on the cell's homeostasis. It has been exceedingly difficult to define the boundaries which separate lethal from sublethal injury, and adaptive homeostasis from metabolic derangement. Should the parameter used as a criterion for cellular injury be the ability to visualize ultrastructural disorganization or, instead, the detection of some impaired biochemical function? For example, how much depletion of adenosine triphosphate (ATP) in an active muscle cell should be construed as normal, and what ATP level should be considered as reflecting too much activity, i.e., cellular derangement? All injuries, whether mild or lethal, ultimately occur at a biochemical level beyond our

present range of detection. For this reason, it has not been possible to determine the precise biochemical site of action of injurious agents or the extent of cellular injury compatible with reversibility or irreversibility. Four intracellular systems are thought to be particularly vulnerable: (1) aerobic respiration involving oxidative phosphorylation and production of ATP, (2) synthesis of enzymic and structural proteins, (3) maintenance of the integrity of cellular membranes on which the ionic and osmotic homeostasis of the cell and its organelles are dependent, and (4) preservation of the integrity of the cell's genetic apparatus.

Whatever the precise point of attack, injury at one locus leads to wide-ranging secondary effects. Because maintenance of the ionic and fluid balance of the cell is energy dependent, impairment of aerobic respiration and the synthesis of ATP soon leads to profound alterations in the intracellular content of ions and water. Loss of aerobic respiration is usually followed by reversion to anaerobic glycolysis with the production of excessive amounts of lactic acid. The falling pH has secondary effects on enzyme systems and biochemical reactions. Protein synthesis is impaired, preservation of membrane integrity hampered and progressive cellular dysfunction ensues. Important to our present consideration is the recognition that such a sequence of biochemical events does not occur instantaneously but is, rather, a dynamic process which evolves over a period of time—from minutes to hours. The precise time span involved depends on the particular characteristics of the injured cell, such as its metabolic activity and vulnerability to a specific lesion as well as the defensive mechanisms of the organism as a whole. *Morphologic changes become apparent only after some critical biochemical system within the cell has been deranged for some time.* As would be expected, the morphologic manifestations of lethal damage take more time to develop than those of reversible injury.

It is not difficult to distinguish morphologically a completely normal cell from a severely injured cell, but the transition zone is exceedingly subtle, even in hindsight. Equally obscure is the line between reversible cell injury and lethal cell damage. Some of these difficulties are exemplified in the following experimental model. The renal arteries of a series of animals were clamped for progressively lengthening time spans. When the clamps were removed and the animals permitted to live for an additional 24-hour period, the duration of loss of blood supply required to induce cell death was determined in retrospect. It could only be established on hindsight because the ensuing span of hours of enzymic activity was necessary to bring about unmistakable morphologic changes which marked the cell as dead.

Because experimental conditions do not exist in the clinical situation, the evaluation of cellular damage and the borderlines between normality, reversible injury and cell death are difficult if not impossible to delineate sharply. These complexities should come as no surprise. Well known in clinical practice is the problem of answering the question: when did the patient die? Brain function, as determined by the electroencephalogram, may cease hours to days before cardiac and respiratory functions stop. The heart may continue to beat for some time after respirations have ceased. Yet even after all vital signs such as pulse, respiration and body temperature indicate the death of the organism, most of the cells within the host continue to survive, as has been amply documented by the use of cadaver organs for transplantation. *The transition from life to death is as difficult to establish for the cell as it is for the whole organism.*

The extent of damage resulting from a given injury depends, on the one hand, on the severity and duration of the adverse influence and, on the other hand, on the capability of the cell to adapt. The adverse influence may be internal to the cell, such as genetic mutations leading to an inborn error of metabolism, or it may be some external alteration in the cell's milieu such as the clamping of a renal artery. Even more important are the cell's metabolic needs and the response to the injury. How vulnerable is the cell, for example, to loss of blood supply and hypoxia? The striated muscle cell in the leg can be placed entirely at rest when deprived of its blood supply; not so the striated muscle cell of the heart. On the whole, *with reversible cell damage, the cellular response is more critical than the precise nature and severity of the injury.* Exposure of two individuals to identical concentrations of carbon tetrachloride fumes may be without effect in one and may produce cell death in the other. Differences in the nutritional state or in potentiating factors such as alcohol consumption influence the ability of the two individuals (and their cells) to withstand the injury. We know that specialized cells have widely differing susceptibilities to the same injurious influences, yet we do not understand well those factors which determine how much impact a given injury will have on individual cells.

In the discussion which follows, first the causes or etiology of cell injury will be grouped into clinically applicable categories. Thereafter, the mechanisms or pathogenesis involved in the induction of injury to the cell will be considered. After this, the impact of cellular injury on structure and function will be discussed. The ultrastructural changes will precede the presentation of the alterations seen with the light microscope. Paradoxically, the morphologic differentiation between cell injury and cellular death can be better made with the light microscope than with the electron microscope. Perhaps the reason is that the significance of cell changes becomes more evident when viewed within the framework of the whole cell rather than in the minute detail of its substructures. The crude analogy might be drawn of the attempt to determine whether a tree is dead by viewing it in its entirety or by minutely examining a single leaf.

In classic pathology, reversible cell injuries are termed *degenerations*. When cells have suffered lethal injury, a series of irreversible biochemical reactions ensue, leading to changes unmistakably characteristic of cell death. The constellation of morphologic changes indicative of cell death is known as *necrosis.* When the necrosis results from the uninhibited action of intracellular catalytic enzymes, the process is referred to as *autolysis.* In some situations, extracellular enzymes of the lysosomes of polymorphonuclear leukocytes or blood enzymes contribute to the biochemical degradation of the cells, causing *heterolysis.* Ultimately, the autolytic or combined autolytic and heterolytic processes lead to the total destruction and digestion of the dead cell.

CAUSES OF REVERSIBLE AND IRREVERSIBLE CELL INJURY

Injury may be defined broadly as any adverse influence, external or internal, on the cell which deranges the cell's ability to maintain a steady normal or adapted homeostasis. It is understood that the steady state is in fact a fluid range within which the cell oscillates and is capable of optimal function. The causes of cell injury and death range from the gross physical violence of an automobile accident to the subtle genetic lack of a vital intracellular enzyme which impairs normal metabolic function. Most adverse influences can be grouped within the following broad categories: (1) hypoxia, (2) physical injuries, (3) chemical injuries, (4) injuries induced by biologic agents, (5) injuries induced by immune mechanisms, (6) genetic defects, (7) injuries induced by malnutrition, and (8) alterations associated with senescence.

HYPOXIA

Hypoxic injury to cells may be caused by loss of their blood supply, depletion of the oxygen-carrying capacity of the blood, or poisoning of the oxidative enzymes within the cells. Among these, loss of blood supply (*ischemia*) is most commonly encountered. It occurs whenever the arterial supply to or the venous drainage of a cell and its tissue is blocked. There are two common and important mechanisms by which vascular insufficiency causes cell injury and cell death. They involve the occlusion of arteries either by primary arterial disease (arteriosclerosis) or by intravascular clots (thrombi or emboli). Heart attacks (myocardial infarction) and strokes (cerebral infarction) from arterial occlusions are among the most frequent and lethal diseases of industrialized nations. Loss of oxygen-carrying capacity is exemplified by the many forms of anemia and by carbon monoxide poisoning in which a carbon monoxyhemoglobin is formed, blocking the normal oxygen transport of oxy-hemoglobin. Hypoxia may be produced at the intracellular level by agents which inhibit vital enzymes within the aerobic respiratory systems—e.g., inactivation of cytochrome oxidase by cyanide. All of these adverse influences ultimately affect cellular aerobic respiration, oxidative phosphorylation and synthesis of the high energy bonds of ATP.

PHYSICAL AGENTS

Physical injuries include mechanical trauma, extremes of temperature, changes in atmospheric pressure, radiation, and electrical shock. Mechanical trauma may be produced by such obvious means as the rupture of cells or by subtle intracellular dislocations resulting from the cell's absorption of kinetic energy. The well known concussion of the brain is a somewhat mysterious example of widespread neuronal reversible dysfunction induced by mechanical trauma.

Extremes of temperature are obvious causes of cell injury and, frequently, cell death. Low temperatures induce vasoconstriction and impairment of blood supply. If the drop in temperature is more profound, there is loss of vasomotor control of blood vessels, followed by marked vasodilation and increased permeability of the blood vessel wall with resultant extravasation of fluid and blood. The vascular injury may lead to intravascular clotting. If the temperature becomes sufficiently low, there may be actual crystallization of the intracellular water. However, less profound drops in temperature may induce more subtle injuries by slowing biochemical reactions with suboptimal temperatures for enzyme function. Abnormally high temperatures may, of course, combust cells but may also act by more insidious pathways—e.g., by inducing hypermetabolism beyond the capacity of the available blood supply and by coagulation of proteinous enzymes.

Sudden changes in atmospheric pressure mediate their effects through the gases dissolved in the blood. The deep-sea diver or tunnel digger works under increased atmospheric pressure. At these pressures, higher levels of atmospheric gases are dissolved in the blood. When the pressure is reduced too rapidly, these gases bubble out of solution and, while oxygen is rapidly resolubilized, bubbles of nitrogen may persist and block blood vessels. More is said about this phenomenon on p. 337. It is enough to mention that here the ultimate causes of cell injury are impairment of blood supply and cellular hypoxia.

In this atomic age, no one needs to be told of the injury-producing potential of radiant energy. This subject is discussed more fully on

p. 536. Here it is only necessary to point out that radiant energy in the form of sunlight, ultraviolet radiation, x-radiation, and that derived from radioisotopes and fission products is capable of causing severe cell injury and cell death. It may act on cells in one of two ways: by directly ionizing chemical compounds contained within the cell (the "target" action of radiation) or by indirectly ionizing cellular water, producing free hot radicals which then interact with the cellular constituents. The ionizing energy may break hydrogen and sulfhydryl bonds, oxidize compounds, break bonds within the helix of DNA, or cause dimerization of the purine and pyrimidine bases in DNA (Totter, 1968).

All cells are more or less vulnerable to radiation, but some are more radiosensitive than others. It is customary to divide the many cell types in the body into three categories: radiosensitive (e.g., lymphoid, hematopoietic cells and those of the germinal epithelium of the gonads), radioresponsive (e.g., those of the skin, blood vessels, epithelium, conjunctiva of the lens and cornea), and radioresistant (e.g., those of the kidneys, liver, endocrine glands, brain and striated muscle). The injurious effect of radiation is related to the amount absorbed. Hence, although the skin is radioresponsive and not radiosensitive, it most often suffers injury because, in the use of radiation for the treatment of deeply situated tumors, it lies in the pathway of the radiation.

Electrical injuries result from the heat generated in the passage of the current through the body and from the stimulation of tissues, principally nerves, which are responsive to electrical currents. The voltage, the amperage, the pathway traversed by the current, and the resistance of tissues to the flow of current determine the severity of the injury. There must obviously be a point of entrance and exit and, within limits, electrical energy follows the most direct route between these contact points (p. 536). High voltages tend to cause cardiac arrhythmias, low voltages tend to cause hyperexcitability and spasm of the muscles, and the amount of heat generated will depend on the interplay of voltage, amperage, and tissue resistance (Hyslop, 1946).

CHEMICALS

Chemical injury may be produced by virtually any chemical compound. Certain substances have a high level of toxicity and are known as poisons. Trace amounts of arsenic, cyanide and soluble salts of mercury may destroy sufficient numbers of cells within minutes to hours to cause death. But even innocuous substances such as glucose or saline in hypertonic concentrations may cause significant and even lethal damage by deranging the fluid and electrolyte homeostasis of cells. Not only do the many chemical poisons have different points of attack within cells, but the susceptibility to specific agents also varies widely among cell types in the body (p. 516). Mercuric salts, for example, affect principally the renal tubular epithelial cells and the mucosa of the stomach and colon.

BIOLOGIC AGENTS

Biologic agents have long been and continue to be important causes of cell injury and death. These agents range from the submicroscopic viruses to the gross, ugly tapeworms. How all these agents cause cell injury is still a mystery. Viruses and rickettsia can survive only within living cells which they parasitize. Here they subvert the metabolism of the host for their own survival and growth requirements. The host may be deprived of essential nutrients and so be injured. Alternatively, some of the viruses replicate rapidly within the cytoplasm of the cell, leaving only a destroyed carcass. The products of the dead cell then constitute a source of injury to contiguous healthy cells. Viral ribonucleic acid (RNA) or deoxyribonucleic acid (DNA) may become incorporated into the genome of the host cell. The cellular transformation may result either in stimulation of the growth activity of the host cell or in its death. In the former instance, the cellular proliferation may lead to tumor formation as in the viral causation of cancer in lower animals and in man (Chapter 4).

Extracellular parasites such as bacteria cause cell injury by a number of mechanisms. The most obvious pathway is the elaboration of an exotoxin by the microorganism. The diphtheria bacillus elaborates an exotoxin which inhibits oxidative processes and protein synthesis in cells. Bacteria, particularly those that are gram-negative, can cause cell injury by the elaboration of endotoxins. Endotoxins comprise complexes of phospholipids and polysaccharides which are released when the bacteria are killed. These damaging products are then absorbed by cells. Another pathway by which bacteria and other microbiologic agents cause cell injury is the induction of an allergic response to antigens contained within the microbiologic agent. The prime example is the *Mycobacterium tuberculosis.* Although the organism itself is relatively innocuous when first introduced into a susceptible host, in the course of a few weeks a hypersensitivity to the bacterial products develops in the sites of bacterial implantation. Allergic mechanisms are postulated for many of the higher forms of microbiologic agents such as protozoa, fungi and worms.

The invasive properties of the intruder will determine its ability to attack and invade the host, and its virulence will control the extent of injury produced. However, the extent and severity of cell injury are also related to the defenses of the host. The ability to mount an inflammatory or an immune reaction materially modifies the nature and extent of cell injury and cell death. But the inflammatory and the immune responses may themselves contribute to local cell injury while at the same time defending the rest of the body from generalization of the infection.

There is a remarkable organ specificity displayed by many microbiologic agents. Although the pneumococcus is a common inhabitant of the naso- and oropharynx, it rarely causes cell injury in this location but, instead, finds its most suitable environment for growth when it invades the lungs, producing serious respiratory infections. When typhoid organisms are swallowed in contaminated food or water, the *Salmonella typhosa* usually localizes in the small intestine. The basis for such organotropism is obscure.

DERANGEMENTS IN IMMUNE MECHANISMS

Immune responses may be life-saving or lethal. The role of the immune system in the defense against biologic agents is well known. But we must also consider the induction of cellular injury and cellular death by immune responses (Fig. 2–1). Immune reactions to both exogenous and endogenous antigens have come to be recognized as fairly common and important mechanisms of cellular injury. The anaphylactic reaction to a foreign protein or a drug is a prime example of the former. Reactions to endogenous ("self") antigens are now thought to be responsible for a number of so-called autoimmune diseases. Chapter 7 discusses more fully how cell injury is mediated in the immune response. Two mechanisms exist, one involving reactive lymphocytes belonging to the cell-mediated immune response, and the other involving circulating antibodies (p. 194) (Humphrey and Dourmashkin, 1969) (Cochrane, 1968) (Cochrane and Dixon, 1969).

GENETIC DERANGEMENTS

Genetic defects as causes of cellular injury and disease have become major interests of

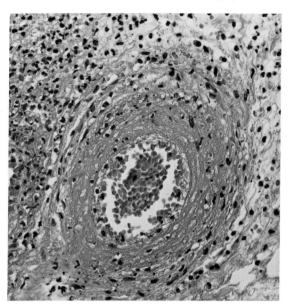

Figure 2–1. Acute hypersensitivity angiitis. The arterial wall is smudged by deposited fibrin, and there is an intramural as well as perivascular leukocytic infiltrate.

biologists today. The genetic injury may be as gross as the congenital malformations associated with Down's syndrome (Mongolian idiocy) or as subtle as the alteration in the coding of hemoglobin responsible for the production of hemoglobin S and sickle cell anemia. In general, the gross malformations are associated with chromosomal abnormalities and visible changes in the karyotype. The more subtle mutations occur at the level of the coding in DNA and are not associated with alterations in the karyotype. The host of inborn errors in metabolism arising from enzymic abnormalities, usually an enzyme lack, are excellent examples of cell damage due to exceedingly subtle mutations.

Some of these genetic abnormalities originate as mutations in the formation of the parental gametes, while others occur in utero during embryogenesis. There is a growing concern that environmental influences such as drugs, radiation and infections may underlie many of these so-called spontaneous mutations. Obviously, mutations so generated are not present in the parents, and hence the resulting disorders are not familial. However, if the affected patient survives into adult life and is capable of reproduction, he may be the forebear of affected generations. Other genetic abnormalities are transmitted from generation to generation as hereditary disorders. In general, these are the less serious defects which may, however, impair survival and fertility

(Carr, 1969) (Plotkin and Vaheri, 1967) (Smithells, 1966) (Chapter 6).

NUTRITIONAL IMBALANCES

Nutritional imbalances, even in the mid-twentieth century world, continue to be major causes of cell injury. Protein-calorie deficiencies still cause an appalling number of deaths, chiefly among underprivileged populations. Deficiencies in specific vitamins are found throughout the world. Avitaminoses are encountered even in the midst of abundance, but they abound in lower socioeconomic groups in all countries. While protein-calorie inadequacies affect virtually all cells of the body, the vitamin deficiencies have fairly specific cellular targets (Chapter 11).

Ironically, nutritional excesses have become important causes of cell injury and cell death among the "overprivileged." Excesses of calories, carbohydrates and lipids are thought to be important predispositions to the major form of arteriosclerosis known as atherosclerosis. Obesity is the external manifestation of the overloading of some cells in the body with lipids. But above and beyond such cellular change, obesity has been shown to have important associations with the production of pulmonary disease, hypertension and cardiac disease.

AGING OR SENESCENCE

Aging or senescence represents a somewhat controversial subject in the context of causes of cell injury and death. In the advanced years of life, widespread regressive alterations occur in such sites as the gonads, brain, skeletal muscles and heart. Some would interpret these either as manifestations of the normal physiologic processes of aging or as secondary attributes of the almost invariably present vascular disease of the aged. There is, however, evidence which suggests that aging may, in part, be the consequence of the progressive accumulation of metabolic deficits over the years. It must be remembered that individuals living under virtually identical environmental conditions age at widely varying rates. The nonagenarian who remains intellectually extremely acute contrasts sharply with the already senile septuagenarian. The influences involved in such a contrast are quite mysterious but are currently the subject of considerable interest. If we merely accept all of the changes of advanced years as inevitable modifications in cells, we shall never discover other mechanisms that may possibly exist.

PATHOGENESIS OF CELL INJURY AND CELL DEATH—MECHANISMS

The problem of unraveling the mechanisms and precise loci of attack of the many possible causes of cell injury has proved to be immensely complex. Cells may be injured by many influences, and the many specialized types of cells have their own particular vulnerabilities and responsive mechanisms. The many macromolecules, enzymes and biochemical systems within the cell are closely interdependent (Monod et al., 1963).

It was thought that a great insight had been gained when it was recognized that most injurious influences exert their effects ultimately by some impairment of enzyme activity. But did the injury directly inactivate the enzyme or, instead, did it modify its substrate or alter the optimal pH range of a specific biochemical reaction?

In certain forms of injury, the precise mechanisms and loci of attack have been fairly precisely elucidated. It is known, for example, that cyanide constitutes an intracellular asphyxiant by inactivating cytochrome oxidase. Actinomycin B inhibits RNA polymerase and hence blocks RNA and protein synthesis. Certain of the anaerobic bacteria such as *Clostridium perfringens* elaborate lecithinases which attack cell membranes and so cause injury or cell death. A number of other isolated observations could be cited but here we shall concentrate on the causes of cell injury which have been studied intensively: (1) the effect of hypoxia on cells and (2) the mechanism of action of carbon tetrachloride. These two model systems offer valuable insights into the mode of action of adverse influences on the cell. It is obvious that the same agent may cause reversible cell damage or may lead to a fatal outcome when applied for a longer period of time or in larger quantity. It is possible in the experimental animal model to titrate dosages which will produce only reversible injury or will pass the point of no return.

The primary point of attack of hypoxia is the cell's aerobic respiration and oxidative phosphorylation. We still do not know which of the many enzymes involved in such mitochondrial respiration is the primary target. Gallagher et al. (1956) propose that loss of respiratory cofactors involved in the Krebs cycle initiates the anoxic injury. Even though this problem is still unresolved, it is clear that as little as 2 minutes of hypoxia causes a 60 per cent loss of respiration in mitochondria derived from the brain (Ozawa et al., 1967). In contrast, mitochondria derived from the liver, kidney and heart were little affected after 10 minutes of hypoxia, an example of the varying vulnerability of specialized cells to one form of injury. Such observations help to explain the exquisite sensitivity of the brain to hypoxia. The loss of oxidative phosphorylation immediately slows or stops the generation of ATP. Some cells are then able to fall back on anaerobic glycolysis which, in part, sustains ATP levels. But anaerobic glycolysis cannot long suffice to maintain the levels of ATP. Loss of energy sources has widespread ramifications on many systems within the cell. The maintenance of cell membranes and the activity of their associated enzymes such as ATPase are impaired, resulting in increased permeability. The normal intracellular ionic and fluid balances are disturbed because they are so exquisitely dependent on a continuing supply of energy.

When the sources of energy are depleted, the "sodium pump" is slowed or stopped. Sodium continually leaks into the cell, facilitated by the hypoxia-induced cell membrane injury, but it can no longer be adequately "pumped out." The cell thus tends to become swollen, as fluid with dissolved solutes at concentrations equal to that in the extracellular phase seeps into the cell. ATP stores are further depleted by the increased demands for the extrusion of sodium. At the same time potassium leaks out of the cell. Membrane-bounded calcium also enters the cell through the damaged cell membranes (Trump et al., 1970). The calcium diffuses into the mitochondria and, in its ionic form, is a powerful inhibitor of oxidative phosphorylation, further depleting the energy resources of the cell.

These movements of fluid and ions cause swelling not only of the cell but also of its organelles. At the same time, the increased rate of anaerobic glycolysis depletes glycogen stores and leads to an intracellular lactic acidosis, further impairing enzyme function and the integrity of membranes. Concomitantly, the injury to cellular membranes causes separation of ribosomes from the granular endoplasmic reticulum and dissociation of polysomes. Protein synthesis thus becomes unhinged.

Ultimately, the falling pH or changing ionic composition of the intracellular environment leads to injury to the lysosomal membranes followed by leakage and activation of released acid hydrolases. Definite increases in the extra lysosomal levels of acid ribonuclease, acid phosphatase and beta glucuronidase have been found in cells which still possess intact lysosomes but which are already irreversibly injured. Undoubtedly, these enzymes participate in the digestion and

removal of the dead cell (*autolysis*). *It does not appear from present evidence that lysosomal rupture signals the point of no return; there is, in fact, evidence to the contrary.* At one time, lysosomes were referred to as "suicide bags," and it was postulated that their rupture represented the "coup de grace." Trump and Ginn (1969) have convincingly shown that the point of no return has already passed by the time these "suicide bags" rupture. However, this does not preclude the possibility that leakage of enzymes out of abnormally permeable lysosomes is important in the production of lethal cell injury. Consistent with this hypothesis, steroids and chloroquinone exert a protective action against many forms of cellular injury, and these agents act principally to stabilize lysosomal membranes (deDuve and Wattiaux, 1966).

At this point in the story, we should note that the leakage of intracellular enzymes across the abnormally permeable plasma membrane provides important clinical parameters of cell injury and cell death. These enzymes are absorbed into the blood and can be assayed by relatively simple techniques. The striated muscle cells of the heart, for example, contain glutamic-oxaloacetic transaminase (GOT), pyruvic transaminases, several isoenzymes of lactic dehydrogenase (LDH), and creatine phosphokinase (CPK). Normally, these enzymes are loosely bound to organellar membranes or are localized in the cell sap and are not diffusible across the plasma membrane. In any form of cellular damage with injury to membranes, these enzymes diffuse into the interstitial fluid and achieve detectable levels in the serum. Thus elevated levels of serum glutamic oxaloacetic transaminase (SGOT), LDH and CPK are valuable clinical criteria of myocardial infarction which is a hypoxic form of injury to the heart muscle. However, the lung, liver, pancreas and kidney, for example, also possess GOT and LDH. Elevated levels of these enzymes may therefore be produced by disease in a number of organs. In contrast, CPK is found only in the heart, skeletal muscle and brain; and since muscular and neurologic disorders rarely simulate myocardial infarction, elevations of CPK are far more definitive in the diagnosis of hypoxic injury to the heart.

The impact of hypoxic injury has been described from its initiation to the ultimate autolytic digestion of the lethally injured cell. But at what stage was the point of no return passed, and what represented the critical change? There have been many efforts to titrate the precise duration of hypoxia necessary to induce irreversible cell injury. As might be expected, it varies with the experimental animal used, the particular cells or tissue being studied and the parameters used to identify cell death. One study reports that at least one hour and, more certainly, two hours of ischemic anoxia (caused by clamping of the liver pedicle) are required to produce irreversible damage to liver cells (Bassi and Bernelli-Zazzara, 1964). In contrast, Vogt and Farber (1968) have reported that 25 minutes appears to be the critical time required for irreversible hypoxic injury to the renal tubular cells of the rat (induced by clamping of the renal pedicle). In this study, 20 minutes of ischemia failed to produce any evidence of renal cell death while 30 minutes produced widespread death among tubular epithelial cells in the distal portions of the proximal convoluted tubules, the cells most sensitive to hypoxia. Although the proximal convoluted tubules were severely injured, other portions of the kidney nephron showed no signs of irreversible cell damage, documenting once again the varying susceptibility of cells to specific forms of injury. In this particular study, the renal arterial clamp was removed at varying time intervals and the animals were sacrificed 2, 24 or 72 hours later. It was necessary to permit at least 24 hours to elapse following the injury in order for the degradative changes identifiable as cell death to develop.

These experiments are of interest since they not only determine the critical duration of hypoxia required to produce irreversible cell damage, but they also indicate that fatal injury could be recognized only in hindsight some hours after the fatal "biochemical lesion" had occurred. Myocardial cells have been shown to be lethally injured within 5 minutes of the institution of complete anoxia (Robbins, unpublished observations). Since the myocardial fiber is constantly at a high level of metabolic activity, it is understandably more vulnerable to hypoxia than other less active cells.

Although it would be reasonable to conclude that the critical parameter of such lethal hypoxic injury is progressive depletion of ATP levels, there are many suggestions that the availability of ATP is not the critical determinant. With the initiation of hypoxia, the concentration of ATP falls rapidly within a few minutes to a level approximately one-fifth that of the control. There is no progressive loss over the next 20- to 30-minute period when the vulnerable epithelial cells pass the point of no return. It remains at that low level for the next two hours without further change. The intracellular lactic acid levels continue to increase throughout the ischemic period. However, when anaerobic glycolysis was inhibited, the control of lactic acidosis did not protect the cell

from the damage induced by 20 to 30 minutes of ischemia. Intracellular acidosis therefore did not appear to be the crucial factor in the model of cellular death studied by Vogt and Farber. Attention has therefore been turned to other systems, and it has been proposed that hypoxia activates extramitochondrial lipolytic enzymes which cause irreversible damage to the inner membranes of mitochondria and so inflict a lethal blow to the respiratory apparatus (Ozawa et al., 1966). Here again, there are arguments against such a proposition. Isolated mitochondria can be shown to recover their phosphorylative abilities after 30 minutes of ischemia even though the cells from which they were obtained were destined to die. *At the present time, the precise molecular or biochemical event or events which signal irreversible cell damage are still unknown.* For now it must suffice that hypoxia affects oxidative phosphorylation and the synthesis of vital ATP supplies, and these changes in turn have widespread ramifications ending in possible fatal injury to cells.

For several reasons, carbon tetrachloride poisoning is a useful model of cellular injury to study. It provides an example in which the cellular damage is not caused directly by the absorbed agent but, many believe, by its metabolic derivatives. Toxic levels of carbon tetrachloride, whether absorbed through the lungs, the gastrointestinal tract or some parenteral injection site, principally affect the liver and kidneys. There is considerable controversy as to whether carbon tetrachloride (CCl_4) itself is capable of causing cell injury or whether it must first be metabolized. The toxicity of CCl_4 has been attributed to its direct action on the lipid components of the cell, particularly the cellular membranes. It has been pointed out that cell damage occurs within minutes of the intragastric administration of CCl_4, so rapidly that metabolic transformation could hardly have transpired. Moreover, CCl_4 is able to induce morphologic changes in isolated organelles when exposed to this agent in the test tube. Presumably, under such circumstances metabolic transformation could not have occurred. *While high dosage levels may exert such a direct effect, most of the evidence favors the view that the major toxicity of CCl_4 results from its metabolism in the liver, with the release of free radicals such as Cl and CCl_3.* There is good evidence that these products are toxic to cells (Recknagel, 1967). It has been shown that, among other actions, they induce peroxidation of lipids, shift double bonds in the polyunsaturated fatty acids throughout all cell membranes and are particularly damaging to organellar membranes and their attached enzymes.

In renal tubular epithelial cells, Striker et

al. (1968) report that the first demonstrable morphologic evidence of CCl$_4$ injury identifiable at two hours is swelling of the mitochondria. Subsequently, there is dissociation of polysomes and shedding of ribosomes from the rough endoplasmic reticulum, leading to impairment of protein synthesis (Smuckler and Benditt, 1965). Using the liver cell as a model, Reynolds and Ree (1971) suggest that the endoplasmic reticulum is the first organelle affected within minutes of the administration of the chlorocarbon. This is followed by the formation of small tubular aggregates, dilation of the cisternae of the endoplasmic reticulum and mitochondria, and increased plasmalemmal permeability, with influx of sodium, water and calcium. The sodium and water loads deplete the levels of ATP. Ribosomes dissociate from the membranes of the endoplasmic reticulum and polysomes are disrupted (Smuckler, 1968b) (Fig. 2–2). The disruption of the polysomes may be related to dissolution of messenger RNA. The loss of protein synthesis leads to the accumulation of lipids within the affected cells, presumably related to inability to synthesize lipoproteins. Thereafter, the sequence of events described in anoxic injury ensues.

Once again we should ask: what is the fundamental biochemical injury in CCl$_4$ that leads to cell death? Most of the evidence would point to a locus in cellular membranes. ATP reserves are depleted at an early stage, at a time when there is no observable mitochondrial change. Indeed, mitochondrial swelling does not appear in liver cells until two to six hours after ATP levels have been significantly reduced (Smuckler, 1968a). All this evidence is most compatible with the thesis of membrane injury affecting both endoplasmic reticulum (ER) and mitochondria, with irreversible injury to the cell's respiration, but other targets have not yet been excluded.

In concluding this discussion of the pathogenesis of cellular injury induced by hypoxia and CCl$_4$, several points should be made. Alterations in one intracellular locus have widespread ramifications on a host of additional systems. The tiny pebble cast into the pool causes only a minute splash, but the ripples propagate to ultimately affect the entire pool. The ultimate origins of life and the impact of adverse influences on these origins are being probed in the study of cell injury and, although penetrations have been achieved, they have often been only to deeper levels of ignorance. The fundamental lesion in most forms of in-

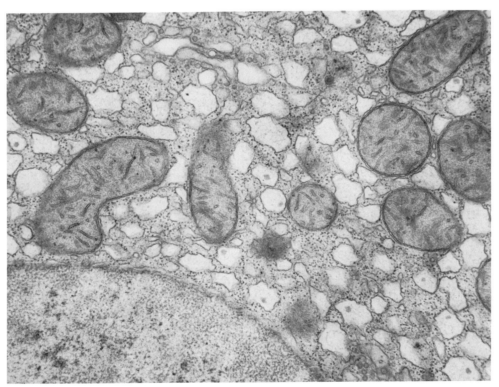

Figure 2–2. *Rat liver cell four hours after carbon tetrachloride intoxication with well developed swelling of endoplasmic reticulum and shedding of ribosomes. Mitochondria at this stage are unaltered. (Courtesy of Dr. Iseri.)*

jury is still unrecognized. It may well be that irreversible injury results not from damage to a single locus or system but, rather, may be the summation of many disruptions which eventually overcome the cell's capacity to adapt. Whatever the Achilles' heel or heels of the cell may be, they are undoubtedly biochemical processes which, when dislocated, lead in time to observable morphologic change. In summary, cells sustain biochemical injuries long before they undergo alteration in their structure.

ULTRASTRUCTURAL CHANGES IN CELL INJURY AND CELL DEATH

The ultrastructural changes of reversible and irreversible injury are presented here in time sequence as a continuum beginning with the initial mildest reaction to injury and progressing to those seen in the dead cell. Since only a broad overview is offered here, for more details, reference should be made to the writing of Trump and his collaborators (Trump and Ericsson, 1965) (Trump and Ginn, 1969) (Trump et al., 1965a) (Trump et al., 1965b) (Trump et al., 1962) (Smuckler and Trump, 1968) (Trump and Ginn, 1968) (Trump and Bulger, 1968a, 1968b). As stated earlier, it is not possible to determine the point of transition from the nonlethal to the lethal damage but, at some stage, the ultrastructural disorganization becomes so advanced as to unmistakably mark the cell as doomed.

Injury to the cell never affects only one type of organelle. The specific injurious agent, its toxicity or injury-producing potential, the type and degree of differentiation of the cell, its level of metabolic activity and its prior state of health and nutrition all to some extent modify the sequence. Despite these variations, the theme is basically the same in all forms of injury.

Mitochondrial and plasma membrane changes are usually the first observable evidence of cell damage. As soon as 15 minutes after many forms of injury, mitochondria swell and develop coarse matrical granules. These granules, probably representing structural components and calcium complexes, can be assumed to be the morphologic counterpart of the depressed oxidative phosphorylation which occurs early in most forms of cell injury. At about the same time, alterations appear in the plasma membrane which include thickening of the membrane, formation of blebs from the pinching off of endocytotic invaginations, creation of membranous whorls called myelin figures, blunting and distortion of microvilli and deterioration of desmosomes, resulting in loosening of intercellular attachments. The last mentioned alteration probably reflects the loss of membrane-bounded calcium which diffuses into the cell. The formation of myelin figures undoubtedly implies widespread damage to all cell membranes. They arise from dissociation of lipoproteins, with unmasking of hydrophilic phosphatide groups followed by their uptake of water to create strata similar to those in normal membranes. Similar changes occur in organellar membranes. Although increased cell membrane permeability occurs early in cell damage, enlargement of membrane pores prior to the development of permeability changes has not been detected. The one exception is found in erythrocytes undergoing complement mediated hemolysis, in which large pores up to 90 Å in diameter have been observed in the damaged red cell envelope. Beginning nuclear changes seen at this early stage of cell injury will be discussed after the cytoplasmic alterations.

More marked changes in the mitochondria as well as in the ER and polyribosomes begin at 30 minutes and are relatively fully developed in one hour. Mitochondria swell, appear to lose the matrix granularity aquired earlier in injury and then assume bizarre shapes and forms. The polysomes disaggregate, and the ribosomes are shed from the granular ER. These morphologic changes are associated with the previously described deterioration in the cell's capacity for oxidative phosphorylation and protein synthesis. The changes in the plasmalemma become more pronounced and, at this stage, membrane breaks can sometimes be seen in both the membranes enclosing the cell and those of the organelles. The smooth endoplasmic reticulum has by now become swollen and distorted. Many small vesicles and vacuoles appear within the cytoplasm, produced apparently by the pinching off of bits of smooth endoplasmic reticulum. These changes presumably accompany the influx of sodium and water into the cell. The smooth endoplasmic reticulum is often referred to as the "intracellular sponge" because it is the major site of uptake of water. It should be recalled from the earlier discussion that 30 to 60 minutes of anoxia represents the point of irreversible damage to most cells, and so the changes seen at this time are presumably lethal.

After the first hour, the intracellular disorganization progresses with ever-increasing rapidity. Swelling of the mitochondria and ER advances so that breaks and even rupture of their limiting membranes can be seen. The entire protein synthetic apparatus, including the polysomes and ribosomes, comes completely apart and such ribosomes as can be identified are found randomly scattered through the cytoplasmic gel. Myelin figures are now often abundant. But it is of interest to note that even after four hours of hypoxic injury, the lysosomes still appear to be intact.

By eight hours, the lysosomes have virtually disappeared as recognizable structures from the disfigured carcass of the long-dead cell. Most of these vanishing lysosomes must have ruptured but some may have fused with the numerous autophagic vacuoles (phagosomes) which now become apparent within the damaged cell. When death occurs abruptly, as with formalin fixation, the cell does not go through the adaptive protective response of sequestering focal cytoplasmic injury within phagosomes. So phagosomes only appear in significant numbers in cells which have passed through a long phase of sublethal injury and, indeed, are more characteristic of reversible injury.

Along with these basic changes seen in most injured cells, a variety of other alterations may appear in certain forms of injury. Some autophagic vacuoles may become filled with debris derived from the membranes of damaged organelles to create the residual bodies of *lipofuscin* pigment (p. 47). Lipofuscin is not seen in cells killed acutely but is more characteristic of cells which have undergone a long period of regressive change resulting from chronic injury or aging, hence the synonym "wear and tear" or aging pigment.

Minute droplets and later larger aggregates of fat appear in certain forms of cell injury. These accumulate first close to or within the endoplasmic reticulum. They are membrane-bounded and are called liposomes. In certain types of injury, the accumulation of lipids may be massive. In chronic alcoholism, clumps of fibrillar deposits occur within the cytoplasmic ground substance in a perinuclear location. With light microscopy and routine tissue stains, these aggregates have a glassy, pink, homogeneous appearance and so are referred to as *alcoholic hyalin*. Whether the hyalin represents aggregations of membranes derived from damaged organelles or is, instead, a fibrillar synthetic product of injured cells is still not clear, but most of the evidence suggests the latter (Iseri and Gottlieb, 1971). Many other changes are also encountered in injured cells but, since they are more visible by light microscopy, they will be described in the following sections.

Nuclear changes also occur in sublethally and lethally injured cells. However, there is abundant evidence that nuclear damage is not the critical determinant of cell death. Indeed it has been shown in unicellular animals that, following removal of the nucleus by microdissection, the organism continues to survive for several days. In the eukaryotic cells of man, nuclear changes appear in injured cells some time after cytoplasmic dislocations are well advanced. The earliest observable change is clumping of the euchromatin to create large aggregates attached to the nuclear membrane and the nucleolus. Such clumping can be produced by alteration in the pH of the cell and is reversible by restoration of the normal pH. Thus it is not a lethal alteration. Along with this clumping, the interchromatin nucleoplasm becomes cleared. As the degradative changes in the cell progress, the nuclear deterioration may follow one of two pathways. In some cells, the nucleus progressively shrinks and becomes transformed to a small, dense, wrinkled mass of tightly packed chromatin, an alteration called nuclear *pyknosis*. With time, this chromatin undergoes progressive dissolution (*karyolysis*) apparently as the result of the hydrolytic action of the DNases and catalases of lysosomal origin. In other cells, after undergoing pyknosis, the nucleus may rupture (*karyorrhexis*). In both pathways the nucleus disappears and, so far as we know, with the exception of the erythrocyte in man, no cell devoid of a nucleus is vital. However, by the time the nucleus has disintegrated, the cell is long dead.

LIGHT MICROSCOPIC PATTERNS OF REVERSIBLE INJURY

In classic pathology, the morphologic changes resulting from nonlethal injury to cells were termed *degeneration*, but today they are more simply designated reversible injuries. Several distinctive patterns can be recognized with the light microscope: cellular swelling, hydropic vacuolation and fatty change. The swelling is the primary expression of virtually all forms of nonlethal injury. It appears whenever cells are incapable of maintaining their ionic and fluid homeostasis. Hydropic change is merely an extension of cellular swelling, reflecting the intracellular accumulation of greater amounts of water. Fatty change may, under some circumstances, be another indicator of reversible cell injury. It is a less universal reaction, principally encountered in cells involved in and dependent on fat metabolism, such as the hepatocyte and myocardial cell.

CELLULAR SWELLING

The first manifestation of almost all forms of injury to cells is an increase in their size resulting from a shift of extracellular water into the cell. Aerobic respiration, synthesis of ATP and the proper function of the "sodium pump" are among the most vulnerable of all cellular metabolic functions (Ginn et al., 1968) (Saladino and Trump, 1968). As sodium accumulates within the cell and the osmotic pressure increases, water is passively imbibed and the cell swells. Increased permeability of plasma membranes contributes to the development of this form of cellular degeneration.

Cellular swelling is a difficult morphologic change to appreciate with the light microscope; it may be more discernible at the level of the whole organ. When it affects all cells in an organ, it causes some pallor, increased turgor and increase in weight of the organ. Microscopically, enlargement of cells is most often discernible by compression of the microvasculature of the organ as, for example, the hepatic sinusoids and the capillary network within the renal cortex. Likewise, the spaces of Disse in the liver may be narrowed.

Swelling of cells is a completely reversible alteration and, indeed, it may be without significant functional effect. It is, therefore, an indicator of mild injury and is of principal importance as a possible antecedent to more severe cell injury.

HYDROPIC CHANGE (VACUOLAR DEGENERATION)

If water continues to accumulate within cells, the further swelling is associated with the appearance of small cleared vacuoles within the cytoplasm. These vacuoles presumably represent distended and pinched off or sequestered segments of the endoplasmic reticulum. This pattern of nonlethal injury is encountered most often in the epithelial cells of the proximal convoluted tubules of the kidney, liver or heart, following chloroform or CCl_4 poisoning, as well as in certain infections, high fevers and hypokalemia.

Hydropic change in cells induces an increase in the size and consistency of the affected organ, accompanied by some pallor. Microscopically small cleared spaces are present within the cytoplasm but the nature of the vacuolar contents cannot be identified with certainty unless special histochemical procedures are employed to exclude fat and glycogen (other possible causes of clear vacuolation of cells) (Fig. 2-3). In minor injury, the small dispersed vacuoles do not displace the nucleus but, in more advanced stages, the vacuoles coalesce to create large solitary spaces which often push the nucleus to

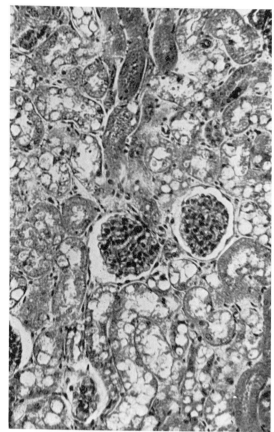

Figure 2–3. *Hydropic or vacuolar degeneration of the kidney. Many of the epithelial cells of the proximal convoluted tubules contain round vacuoles, which sometimes distend the cells and cause apparent narrowing of the tubular lumina. Note that all cells are not affected equally. Compare with glycogen nephrosis (Fig. 2–22) (p. 45).*

one side. Since hydropic change is an expression of a completely reversible injury, it is not accompanied by nuclear change.

Vacuolar degeneration or hydropic change denotes a moderately severe form of cell injury. When identified in the renal tubular epithelial cells, it should raise the suspicion of abnormally low levels of serum potassium. In extreme cases, it is associated with some renal functional impairment, but usually this alteration does not impair cellular or organ function. Liver or myocardial cells may also exhibit hydropic changes when injured, but again organ function is rarely impaired.

FATTY CHANGE

Fatty change refers to any abnormal accumulation of fat within parenchymal cells. *The term fatty change embraces the older terms fatty degeneration and fatty infiltration.* Fatty degeneration was used to refer to the accumulation of fat within the cells when prior injury rendered them incapable of metabolizing or mobilizing normal amounts of lipids. In contrast, the term infiltration was applied to the accumulation of fat within completely normal cells when excessive circulating levels of lipids flooded the cells. In starvation, for example, fat stores are mobilized and the blood lipid levels are elevated. As a consequence, fat appears within liver cells presumably because these cells are incapable of handling the overload. It was then assumed that such intracellular accumulation secondarily injured the cells. However, it is now appreciated that the appearance of even considerable amounts of fat within the cell may have little consequence and, judging by the function of the involved organ, the cells readily adapt. However, there are some instances in which excessive accumulation secondarily injures cells. The liver in the chronic alcoholic, for example, may become enormously enlarged by the accumulation of fat, and weights of 3 to 4 kilos (normal 1.5 kilos) are not unusual. Such extreme accumulation may indeed be associated with a hepatic functional deficit. So the term infiltration was interpreted to mean an intracellular accumulation of abnormal amounts of some substance in normal cells, while degeneration implied similar accumulations in previously injured cells. But both pathways may eventuate in cell damage. Because of these ambiguities, both terms have largely been dropped from the recent literature and have been supplanted by the more noncommital designation, fatty change. The interpretation of fatty change, then, requires an understanding of its pathogenesis.

Although quite different pathogenetic mechanisms may then underlie fatty change, several facts have emerged on which there is general agreement: (1) *The appearance of fat vacuoles within cells, whether small or large, represents an absolute increase in intracellular lipids.* It does not represent so-called unmasking of the normal fat content of cells. (2) The amount of contained fat is not dependent upon the pathogenetic mechanism but rather reflects some imbalance in production, utilization or mobilization of it. The injured cell is incapable of metabolizing or exporting even normal levels of lipids, while the normal cell may synthesize excessive quantities of fat when presented with excess substrate. (3) The derangements that lead to fatty change are varied, so this morphologic alteration is an expression of many types of cell injury or cell overload. (4) Fatty change is often preceded by cellular swelling. (5) While itself an indicator of nonlethal injury, fatty change is often the harbinger of cell death and, in many situations, it is encountered in cells adjacent to those which have died and undergone necrosis.

Fatty change is most often seen in the liver, heart, and kidneys.

Liver. In the liver, mild fatty change may not affect the gross appearance. With progressive accumulation, the organ enlarges and becomes increasingly yellow until, in extreme instances, the liver may weigh 5 to 6 kg. and be transformed into a bright yellow, soft, greasy organ. Such an extreme is most commonly encountered in chronic alcoholics and is often followed by the fibrous scarring of cirrhosis (cirrhosis of alcohol abuse). The pathogenetic relationship of the fat to the development of the cirrhosis is still controversial and is discussed in greater detail on p. 1025.

Fatty change begins with the development of minute membrane-bounded inclusions (liposomes) closely applied to the endoplasmic reticulum and probably derived from it (Lombardi, 1966). It is first manifested under the light microscope by the appearance of small fat vacuoles in the cytoplasm about the nucleus (Fig. 2-4). As the process progresses, the vacuoles coalesce to create sometimes solitary, large, cleared spaces which displace the nucleus to the periphery of the cell. However, until the advanced stages are reached, the nucleus itself is unaffected. The liver cell may thus come to resemble an adult adipose tissue cell (Fig. 2-5). Occasionally, contiguous cells rupture and the enclosed fat globules coalesce to produce so-called fatty cysts. Such ruptured cells are dead and have the nuclear changes of necrosis soon to be described.

Heart. In the heart, fatty change of myocardial cells occurs in two patterns. In one, prolonged moderate hypoxia, such as that produced by profound anemia, induces a "thrush breast" or "tigered" effect (Fig. 2-6). Here the intracellular deposits of fat create grossly apparent bands of yellowed myocardium, alternating with bands of darker, red-brown, uninvolved myocardium. This peculiar distribution is thought to be related to the vascularization of the myocardium. The uninvolved zones are presumed to be closer to blood vessels and are therefore less hypoxic than the yellowed bands. In the other pattern of fatty change such as that produced by more profound hypoxia or some forms of myocarditis (diphtheritic, for example), the myocardial cells are uniformly affected and the entire myocardium becomes yellowed and flabby. Histologically, the fat in the myocardial cell tends to be distributed in extremely minute cytoplasmic vacuoles which are readily missed on casual inspection of routine tissue stains. It is often necessary to perform special fat stains to unmask this change (Fig. 2-7).

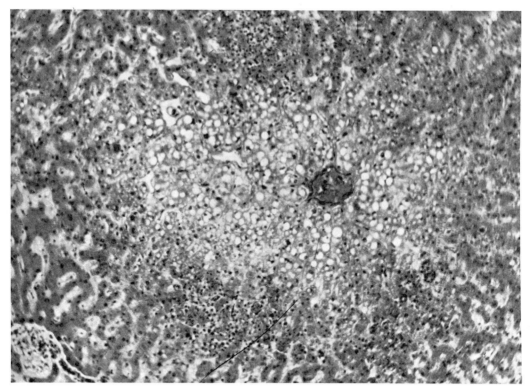

Figure 2–4. *Fatty change of the liver. The hepatic cells around the central vein are filled with small vacuoles of fat and appear paler than the surrounding hepatic parenchyma. Inflammatory cells surround the area of fatty deposition.*

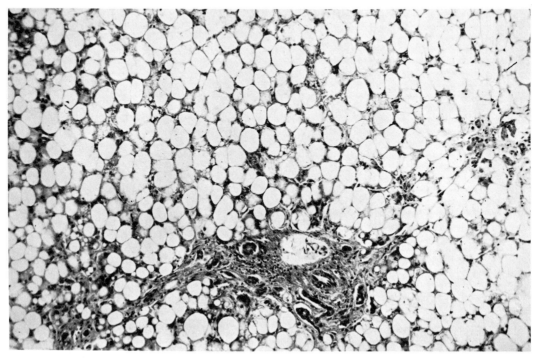

Figure 2–5. *Severe fatty change of the liver. The hepatic parenchymal cells are so loaded with fat that they appear totally cleared. Only the portal area below indicates the hepatic origin of the tissue section.*

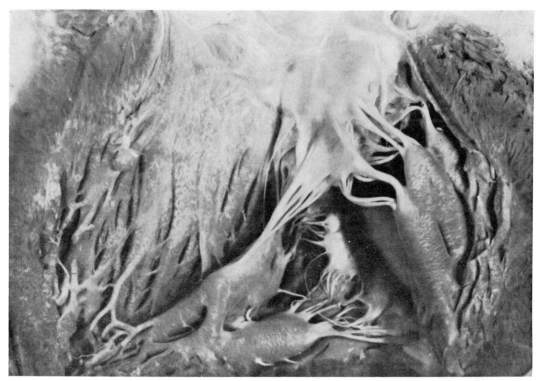

Figure 2–6. *"Thrush breast," fatty change (degeneration) of the myocardium, can be seen beneath the endocardium of the left ventricle.*

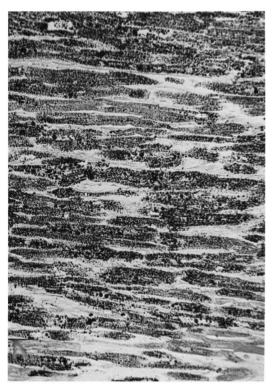

Figure 2–7. *Diffuse fatty change in diphtheritic myocarditis. The finely divided droplets of fat, appearing black, are dispersed throughout the cardiac muscle fibers (Sudan IV stain).*

Kidneys. Involved kidneys are often enlarged, pale and yellow. The cytoplasm of the proximal convoluted tubules is most often affected. When the injury is more severe, the distal convoluted and collecting tubules may also be affected. Chemical poisonings, profound anoxia and excessive reabsorption of lipoproteins in those renal diseases which have abnormal glomerular permeability are all productive of renal tubular fatty change. The fat usually manifests itself in the form of minute vacuoles within the cytoplasm surrounding the nucleus. Sometimes the fat-laden cells bulge into the lumina of the tubules and, occasionally, their rupture releases lipids into the urine, providing an important clinical indicator of tubular fatty change.

Parenchymal Cells. In all circumstances, fatty change appears as clear vacuoles within parenchymal cells. Intracellular accumulations of water or glycogen may also produce clear vacuoles, and it becomes necessary to resort to special techniques to distinguish these three types of clear vacuoles. The identification of lipids requires the avoidance of fat solvents commonly employed in paraffin embedding for routine hematoxylin and eosin stains. To identify the fat, it is necessary to prepare frozen tissue sections on either fresh or aqueous formalin-fixed tissues to preserve the lipid contents of the vacuoles. The sections may then be stained with Sudan IV or Oil Red-O, both of which impart an orange-red color to the contained lipids.

The periodic acid-Schiff (PAS) reaction is commonly employed to identify glycogen, although it is by no means specific. When neither fat nor glycogen can be demonstrated within a clear vacuole, it is presumed to contain water.

An understanding of the pathogenetic mechanisms involved in the accumulation of intracellular fat requires some familiarity with normal fat metabolism. The liver plays a central role in this metabolic activity. In skeletal detail, fat is brought to the liver cell predominantly in the form of free fatty acids released from depot storage fat by lipoprotein lipase or as chylomicrons from dietary sources which yield additional fatty acids. The synthesis of triglyceride from fatty acids occurs, as best we know, within the cisternae of the endoplasmic reticulum. Less certain is the site where these lipids are complexed with specific protein molecules to form lipoproteins, in which form they enter the circulation (Lombardi, 1966) (Isselbacher and Greenberger, 1964). *Fatty change may result from interference at any one of several points in the liver cell's metabolism of fat.* A host of agents, including chemicals (phosphorus, carbon tetrachloride, ethionine, puromycin, orotic acid and alcohol) as well as bacterial and viral infections, induce fatty change in liver cells. Each acts at a different point in the cell's metabolic process, but the various mechanisms can be grouped into the following categories: (1) excessive synthesis of triglyceride, (2) decreased utilization of triglyceride and (3) impaired exportation of lipoprotein. In some instances, a single agent may induce a combination of these disturbances.

Excessive synthesis of triglyceride usually results from the presentation of abnormal amounts of fatty acid or triglycerides to the liver cell. In starvation, for example, depot fats are mobilized and more fatty acids are brought to the liver where they are synthesized into triglycerides. Alcohol also induces elevation of the plasma triglycerides and, furthermore, appears to induce preferential esterification of fatty acids (Isselbacher and Greenberger, 1964). However, as will be noted, alcohol may act in other ways as well.

Impaired utilization of fats will result in intracellular accumulations, exemplified by the fatty change in the myocardium seen in patients suffering from diphtheria. *Corynebacterium diphtheriae* produces an exotoxin which interferes with the metabolism of carnitine, a cofactor in the oxidation of long-chain fatty acids.

Impaired exportation or decreased mobilization of fat may occur as a consequence of either diminished lipoprotein synthesis or impaired release of lipoprotein into the circulation. Some agents such as carbon tetrachloride, ethionine and phosphorus block the synthesis of the protein component of lipoprotein (Farber et al., 1964). In contrast, there may be an inability to synthesize lipoprotein because of impaired formation of the lipid moiety. Here the most striking example is a dietary deficiency of choline or its precursors (methionine). These substances, known as "lipotropes," are required for the formation of phospholipids. Diets low in protein are likely to be deficient in the lipotropes and so may impair lipoprotein synthesis, resulting in intracellular accumulation of fat within the liver cells. This pathway is held by some to be an additional cause of fatty liver in the chronic alcoholic (Porta et al., 1965). Even when there is adequate synthesis of both the lipid and protein moieties of the lipoprotein molecule, its assembly can be interfered with—the probable mechanism of action of orotic acid (Roheim et al., 1966). Alcohol may also act at this point in the normal metabolism of fat.

Although the previous discussion focuses on the hepatocyte, it is believed that fatty change in other cells, such as the epithelial cells of the renal tubule and muscle cells, involves similar pathogenetic mechanisms. It should be apparent that an individual etiologic agent may act at several loci within the complex process of fat metabolism. It is impossible from morphologic observation to discern the underlying metabolic derangement leading to the accumulation of fat. The normal cell may accumulate fat because of increased synthetic activity, but damage to one of the biochemical steps involved in the utilization or exportation of fat produces the same end result.

The significance and interpretation of fatty change depend on the pathogenetic mechanism (p. 33). It may have no effect on cellular function when mild. More severe fatty change may impair cellular function, but unless some vital intracellular process is irreversibly impaired, *fatty change per se is reversible.* In the chronic alcoholic who has not yet suffered the development of cirrhosis and is maintained on an alcohol-free balanced diet, it is quite remarkable to observe the return of an enlarged fatty liver to normal size, structure and function. However, as a severe form of injury, fatty change may be a harbinger of cell death. But it should be emphasized that cells may die without undergoing fatty change.

"NONDEGENERATIONS"

This somewhat facetious term refers to certain cellular and tissue alterations, loosely called degenerations, which do not represent morphologic expressions of cell injury.

HYALINE DEGENERATION

Hyaline degeneration has been applied to any cell or tissue change inducing a homogeneous, glassy, pink appearance in routine tissue stains. This tinctorial change is produced by a variety of alterations, none of which represents a specific pattern of degeneration. Collagenous fibrous tissue may appear hyaline, but it is clearly not a form of cellular degeneration. Amyloid, now known to be an abnormal synthetic product of cells, has a hyaline appearance. In longstanding hypertension, the walls of arterioles may become thickened and hyalinized. The change is not degenerative but results from reduplication of the basement membrane, collagenization and the precipitation within the vessel wall of plasma proteins, among them immunoglobulins.

In chronic alcoholism, droplets or tangled skeins of hyaline material which ultrastructural studies have shown to be composed of closely packed fibrils may appear within damaged liver cells. While a chronic ethanol intake may cause liver cell injury, it does not always induce the formation of alcoholic hyalin, and the severity of the liver cell injury is not always correlated with the amount of hyalin produced (p. 1026). (Fig. 2–8). Hyaline droplets may appear within the epithelial cells of the proximal convoluted tubules in mercury poisoning and in other forms of renal disease associated with severe proteinuria. The droplets represent reabsorption of excessive amounts of protein from the glomerular filtrate and are not a form of degeneration (Fig. 2–9). The involved cells are functionally unimpaired. Russell's bodies are spherical hyaline masses found within plasma cells in many forms of chronic inflammatory disease. These represent aggregates of

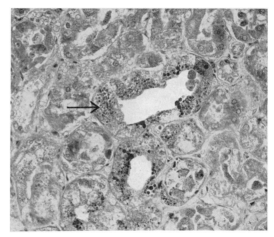

Figure 2–9. *Hyaline droplets in the renal tubular epithelium* (arrow).

immunoglobulins synthesized by the cell. Many viral infections are associated with the appearance of hyaline inclusions within cells. Thus, although one continues to hear the term hyaline degeneration, it is not a morphologic expression of cell injury.

MYXOMATOUS AND MUCOID DEGENERATION

Myxomatous and mucoid degeneration are equally inappropriate terms. The former is seen usually within connective tissue and represents accumulations or poolings of ground substance containing a variety of mucopolysaccharides synthesized by mesenchymal cells. Patently, it does not represent a cellular degeneration. Mucoid degeneration has been applied to the excessive elaboration of mucinous secretions by inflammatory or neoplastic cells, an example of which might be the production of large amounts of mucus by certain forms of cancer cells.

FIBRINOID DEGENERATION

Fibrinoid degeneration is another misnomer. Fibrinoid appears in tissue sections as a deeply eosinophilic clumped amorphous deposit usually within connective tissue or blood vessel walls. The term fibrinoid was drawn from the resemblance of this deposit to precipitated fibrin. Its composition is variable and depends on the circumstances in which it is deposited. But, in general, fibrinoid contains a variety of plasma proteins including fibrin, albumin, the globulins and, most importantly, the immunoglobulins and complement (Dixon, 1961).

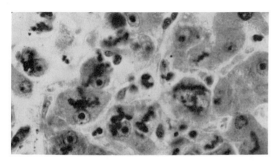

Figure 2–8. *The liver of alcohol abuse (chronic alcoholism). Hyaline inclusions in hepatic parenchymal cells appear as dark, irregular networks disposed about the nuclei.*

Fibrinoid most often appears in foci of immunologic injury, as in the Arthus reaction and other hypersensitivity states. The presence of complement and immunoglobulins within the deposits strongly supports the belief that it, in some way, represents an aggregate of antigen, antibody and complement. Fibrinoid may also be found in nonimmunologic injuries as in the base of chronic inflammatory peptic ulcers and, indeed, in some normal placental villi. In these nonimmunologic settings, the fibrinoid may be reasonably attributed to increased vascular permeability induced by either inflammation or hemodynamic influences. While fibrinoid is not an intracellular degeneration, the underlying causes for the precipitation of fibrinoid may also induce cellular injury, and so damaged or dead cells may be found in close association with it, explaining to some extent the basis for the inappropriate term fibrinoid degeneration.

STROMAL INFILTRATION OF FAT OR FATTY INGROWTH

Stromal infiltration of fat or fatty ingrowth should be discussed at this time merely to differentiate it from the condition already described as fatty change. Fatty ingrowth refers to the accumulation of lipids within stromal connective tissue cells. Parenchymal cells are *not* involved.

Fatty ingrowth is most commonly encountered in the heart and pancreas where adult adipose cells appear within the connective tissue stroma of these organs. In the heart, the right ventricle is usually more severely affected than the left. Usually, there is an increase of subepicardial fat which extends in continuity as finger-like projections between the muscle bundles (Fig. 2-10). These insinuations may extend throughout the thickness of the myocardium to appear beneath the endocardium as small yellow deposits. The adult fat cells separate but do not damage the adjacent myocardial cells (Fig. 2-11). In the pancreas, the fat is found in the connective tissue septa of the pancreatic lobules (Fig. 2-12). The glandular tissue may become so dispersed as to be almost invisible on gross inspection. However, if one were to extract the fat from such a pancreas, the normal size, shape and morphologic characteristics of the organ would be restored.

As far as is known, stromal infiltration of fat rarely affects cardiac or pancreatic func-

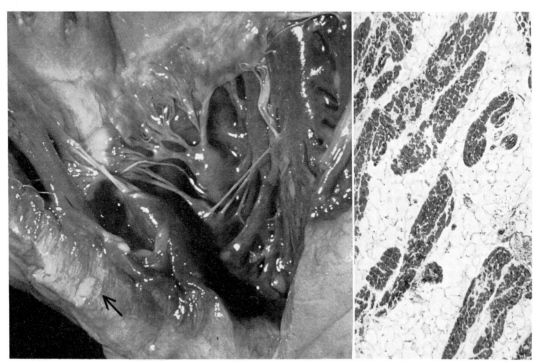

Fig. 2–10   *Fig. 2–11*

Figure 2–10. *Stromal fatty infiltration (fatty ingrowth) of the heart. Streaks of yellow fat extending through the myocardium are visible on cross section of the ventricular wall (arrow). Small, pale yellow deposits are also present subendocardially in the columnae carneae.*

Figure 2–11. *Stromal fatty infiltration (fatty ingrowth) of the heart. A microscopic detail to demonstrate normal myocardial fibers separated by adult fat tissue.*

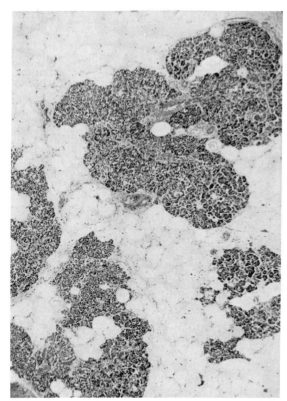

Figure 2–12. *Stromal fatty infiltration of pancreas (fatty ingrowth). Large fat cells separating normal acinar glands.*

tion. On extremely rare occasions, it has been said to be a cause of right ventricular failure but, even in these cases, there is still question about the relationship of the stromal infiltration to the impaired cardiac function. This lesion is a morphologic curiosity. It is more often encountered in obese individuals than in the lean. The origin of such an alteration is unclear but it should not be confused with fatty change in parenchymal cells.

MORPHOLOGIC PATTERNS OF NECROSIS (CELL DEATH)

Necrotic cells are dead cells, but dead cells are not necessarily necrotic. Recall for a moment the dead formalin-fixed "normal" cells studied in histology. *Necrosis is the sum of the morphologic changes caused by the progressive degradative action of enzymes on the lethally injured cell.* It already has been made clear that cells die some time before such lethal injury can be identified morphologically. Nor are there morphologic hallmarks at the level of the electron or light microscope which unmistakably indicate the point in time at which the cell has died. In the studies done by Majno and his

colleagues (1960), it was only possible to make light microscopic diagnoses of ischemic rat liver cell necrosis seven to eight hours after the cells had died. Ironically, the necrosis was apparent to the naked eye at three to four hours because the tissue became abnormally opaque and pale at this time. Yet, at this stage, the cells histologically appeared relatively well preserved and possibly viable.

It is paradoxical that the nucleus demonstrates the unequivocal morphologic hallmarks of cell death under the light microscope despite the extensive cytoplasmic disorganization which precedes these nuclear changes. The structural changes of necrosis result mainly from the activation and release of lysosomal enzymes, hence the process is called *autolysis*. However, the dead cells and their lysosomal enzymes evoke an inflammatory reaction which brings polymorphonuclear leukocytes to the area. These immigrant cells contribute their lysosomal enzymes to the cell's degradation and this action is referred to as *heterolysis*. The nuclear alterations have already been referred to as *karyolysis* (fading of nuclear basophilia), *pyknosis* (shrinkage and increased basophilia of nuclei) and *karyorrhexis* (nuclear fragmentation) (p. 31) (Fig. 2–13). The autolytic and heterolytic enzymes also affect the cytoplasm by inducing an increased cytoplasmic acidophilia as seen in the usual tissue stains employed in light microscopy. More correctly, the acidophilia represents a decreased basophilia as ribosomes in the cytoplasm are disorganized and lysed.

Death of cells is not always followed by immediate dissolution of the cellular carcass. Two pathways may be followed: in one, the cell undergoes progressive proteolysis and digestion called liquefaction necrosis. In the other, referred to as coagulative necrosis, the proteins are first denatured or coagulated and the cell is temporarily mummified, only later to undergo digestion.

LIQUEFACTION NECROSIS

Liquefaction necrosis results from the action of powerful enzymes which literally digest the cell and transform it into a proteinaceous fluid. It is particularly characteristic of anoxic destruction of brain tissue. Curiously, anoxic injury to other tissues usually produces coagulative necrosis. Why the brain should follow this somewhat unusual pathway is poorly understood. Liquefaction is commonly encountered in all focal bacterial lesions. Presumably, here, enzymes of bacterial and leukocytic origin contribute to the digestion of the dead cells.

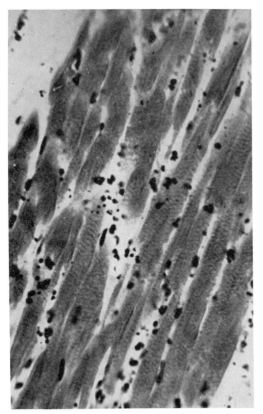

Figure 2–13. *Necrotic myocardial fibers. The nuclei have disappeared by karyolysis although the cellular shapes persist.*

Such liquefactive necrosis is particularly characteristic of pyogenic microorganisms (staphylococci, streptococci, *E. coli*, and others), and the leukocyte-containing proteinaceous fluid comprises a large part of what will be called pus (p. 57) (Fig. 2–14).

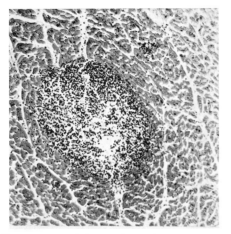

Figure 2–14. *A focus of liquefactive digestion in the myocardium. In the involved area, all muscle cells have been destroyed, and the focus is filled with inflammatory white cells.*

COAGULATIVE NECROSIS

Coagulative necrosis is characterized by conversion of the cell to an acidophilic opaque "tombstone," usually with loss of the nucleus but with preservation of the basic cellular shape permitting recognition of the cellular outline (Fig. 2–15). Presumably, this pattern results from denaturation of proteins soon after the cell has died. In time, further coagulation deforms the cellular outlines. The biochemistry of such denaturation is poorly understood but may be similar to the molecular transformations which occur when soluble proteins such as albumin are coagulated by heat, or when proteins are fixed by formalin. The proteins are rendered insoluble, thus blocking proteolysis and preserving, for a period of hours to days, the dense acidophilic coagulated cell. But, in the course of time, coagulated cells are either liquefied or removed by fragmentation and phagocytosis by scavenger white cells (Fig. 2–16). Coagulation is the usual pathway followed by all tissue cells killed by anoxia, save those of the brain.

CASEOUS NECROSIS

Caseous necrosis is a distinctive combination of coagulative and liquefactive necrosis encountered principally in the center of the soft granulomas seen (p. 412) in tuberculous infections (Fig. 2–17). The capsule of the tubercle bacillus (*Mycobacterium tuberculosis*) contains lipopolysaccharides which denature proteins, while others split lipids, transforming dead cells into clumped cheesy material, hence caseous necrosis. Because the cells are neither totally liquefied nor are their outlines preserved, they create a distinctive amorphous granular debris (Fig. 2–18). Characteristically, the caseous necrosis is enclosed within a granulomatous inflammatory wall. The recognition of this pattern of necrosis and its enclosing wall provides a histologic hallmark of tuberculosis although these findings may have other etiologies (p. 83).

ENZYMIC FAT NECROSIS

Enzymic fat necrosis is a highly specific morphologic pattern of cell death encountered in acute pancreatic necrosis. This disease represents one of the uncommon but calamitous causes of the so-called acute abdomen characterized by massive but patchy enzymic necrosis of the pancreas and lipid depots throughout the abdomen. Powerful lipases and proteases

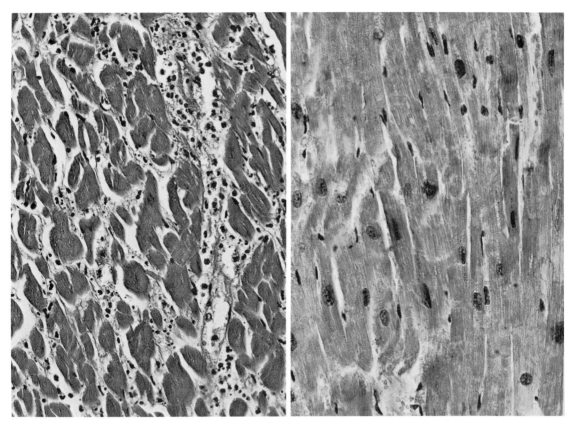

Figure 2–15. Left, necrotic cardiac muscle cells with well preserved outlines. The nuclei have disappeared and the cytoplasm is coagulated and granular. Right, preserved normal cardiac muscle for comparison.

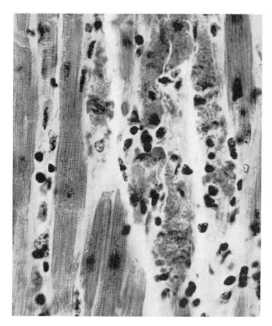

Figure 2–16. Individual cell coagulative necrosis of heart muscle. Many cells are normal. Others have undergone coagulation and are now transformed to fragmented debris being phagocytosed by leukocytes.

run amuck and enzymically destroy not only the pancreatic substance itself but also fat cells in and about the pancreas and throughout the peritoneal cavity. The enzymes may be absorbed into the blood and cause focal lesions of extra abdominal fat necrosis. In all sites, the fat necrosis takes the form of foci of shadowy necrotic outlines of fat cells, whose lipid content has been lipolyzed, surrounded by an inflammatory reaction (Fig. 2–19). The triglycerides are split by the action of lipases, with the release of fatty acids. These acids then complex with calcium to create soaps which appear in tissue sections as amorphous granular basophilic deposits. To the naked eye, the necrotic foci appear opaque and chalky white, and are rimmed by reddened inflammatory margins. Familiarity with the gross and microscopic features of this form of necrosis often enables the surgeon and the pathologist to identify the nature of the acute abdominal emergency.

"NON-NECROSES"

As in the case of the cellular degenerations, there are a number of commonly and

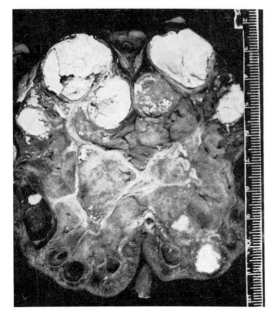

Figure 2–17. A tuberculous kidney with multiple discrete large foci of caseous necrosis. The caseous debris is yellow-white and cheesy.

loosely used terms which include the word necrosis but do not, in reality, represent distinctive patterns of cell death. Historically sanctified usage makes it necessary and desirable to be familiar with these terms.

GANGRENOUS NECROSIS

Gangrenous necrosis is a term still commonly used in surgical clinical practice. It is usually applied to a limb, generally the lower leg, which has lost its blood supply and has subsequently been attacked by bacterial agents (Fig. 2–20). The tissues have, in reality, undergone ischemic cell death and coagulative necrosis modified by the liquefactive action of the bacteria and the attracted leukocytes. When the coagulative pattern is dominant, the process may be termed *dry gangrene*. Alternatively, when the liquefactive action is more pronounced, it may be designated as *wet gangrene*. Gangrenous necrosis also may be applied to an appendix, gallbladder or other viscus suffering from the combined effects of coagulative and liquefactive necrosis. In these viscera, the usual course of events is a primary bacterial infection

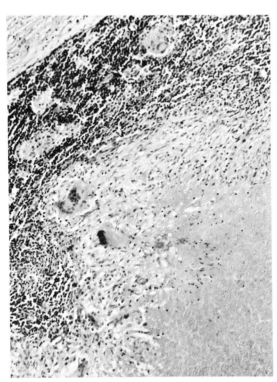

Figure 2–18. A tubercle. A large area of caseous tuberculosis is seen in lower right.

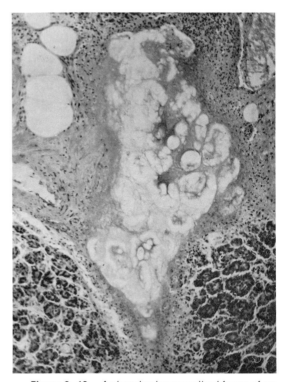

Figure 2–19. A sharply circumscribed focus of enzymic necrosis of fat. Shadowy outlines of fat cells persist, surrounded by a zone of inflammation. The focus is surrounded by normal pancreatic substance.

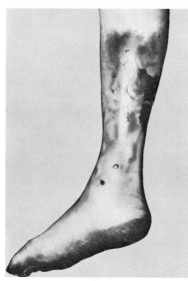

Figure 2–20. *Gangrene of the lower leg, sharply delineated from the proximal normal tissues. The affected areas are discolored and the superficial skin and tissues have begun to slough.*

skin retracts as the underlying lesion becomes more indurated and dense. Histologically, at the early stages there is a central focus of necrotic liquefied fat cells surrounded by an inflammatory rim containing large numbers of macrophages laden with granular lipid debris. Occasionally, foreign body giant cells may appear at this inflammatory rim and sometimes calcium is deposited apparently in response to released fatty acids. The reparative response to inflammation converts the lesion to a dense fibrous scar (Adair and Munzer, 1947).

Traumatic fat necrosis is not a distinctive pattern of cell death but is a distinctive clinical entity of significance since it produces an area of increased consistency within the breast which is easily mistaken for a tumor. Retraction of the overlying skin by the scarring heightens the similarity between this relatively innocuous lesion and certain forms of cancer of the female breast (see p. 1277), and thus it must be considered in the differential diagnosis of breast masses.

which causes sufficient swelling of the tissue to compromise the blood supply and thus induce some element of ischemia. Whatever the clinical setting, it is apparent that gangrenous necrosis does not refer to a specific pattern of cellular change.

TRAUMATIC FAT NECROSIS

Traumatic fat necrosis comprises an area of destroyed fat cells usually encountered in the subcutaneous fat depots of the body, most frequently in the female breast. This lesion comprises a focal area of necrotic liquefied fat cells surrounded by an acute inflammatory reaction which later is transformed to a depressed scar. At one time, this sequence of events was attributed to traumatic injury to the area. Its predilection for the breasts in the female was explained logically by their vulnerability to the relatively trivial trauma of daily life. However, *in perhaps half of the cases no history of trauma can be elicited, and the occurrence of this same lesion in the more protected areas of the body argues against the traumatic etiology of all such lesions.* Nonetheless, no better explanation has been offered for the causation of this form of fat necrosis.

The diameter of the lesion rarely exceeds a few centimeters and its morphologic appearance depends upon its age. The focus appears early as a tender subcutaneous nodule which may be hemorrhagic. With the passage of days, the nodule becomes increasingly firm and less tender. In time, the

INTRACELLULAR ACCUMULATIONS

Under a variety of circumstances, normal cells may accumulate abnormal amounts of various substances. The stockpiled substances fall into three categories: (1) normal metabolites such as lipids, protein and glycogen, (2) abnormal products of metabolism and (3) pigments. The intracellular accumulation is the consequence of either excessive synthesis or uptake of some substance by a cell on the one hand, or underutilization or undermobilization of the particular substance on the other.

Fatty change is an example of the accumulation of a normal product. Abnormal products of metabolism accumulate in many hereditary diseases generically referred to as *storage diseases.* In these inborn errors of metabolism, some enzyme lack usually blocks a specific metabolic pathway, creating an abnormal metabolite which cannot be used and so accumulates. The abnormal substance not only accumulates within the metabolically affected cells but also overflows and is transported via the blood to other cells, particularly to those of the reticuloendothelial system which also become overloaded. The resulting clinical entities are discussed more fully in a subsequent chapter (p. 295). Pigments accumulate within cells under a variety of clinical circumstances, some representing local derangements while others are systemic in nature.

Whatever the nature and origin of the intracellular accumulation, as this term is used, it implies the storage of some product by normal cells. If the overload is due to some systemic derangement and can be brought under control, the intracellular accumulation is usually reversible. For example, in diabetes mellitus control of the hyperglycemia may mobilize the abnormal accumulations of glycogen. In the genetic diseases, because the metabolic error is not correctable, the storage is progressive and the cells may become so overloaded as to cause secondary injury, leading to the ultimate death of the patient.

INTRACELLULAR ACCUMULATIONS OF LIPID

The overload of parenchymal liver cells by triglycerides has already been described (p. 33). In certain forms of glomerular disease, excessive leakage of proteins into the urine and reabsorption of lipoproteins by renal tubular cells lead to fat accumulations. By quite different mechanisms, phagocytic cells may become overloaded with triglycerides. Scavenger macrophages, whenever in contact with the lipid debris of necrotic cells, may become stuffed with neutral fats because of their phagocytic activities. Macrophages in the margin of an inflammatory focus may become so filled with minute vacuoles of lipids as to impart a foaminess to their cytoplasm (foam cells). Similar changes are encountered in areas of enzymic and so-called traumatic fat necrosis.

Intracellular accumulations of cholesterol and cholesterol esters are encountered in a variety of diseases associated with hypercholesterolemia. The most important disorder is atherosclerosis in which ballooned-out myointimal cells within the intimal layer of the aorta and large arteries develop as the result of the lipid accumulation. Such cells appear foamy, and aggregates of them in the intima produce the cholesterol-laden atheromas characteristic of this serious disorder. Like neutral fats, the cholesterol is dissolved out by the usual fat solvents and so requires special techniques for its demonstration, such as formalin-fixed frozen sections. The cholesterol takes up the usual fat stains but is differentiated from triglycerides by its birefringence in polarized light. Many of these overstuffed cells rupture, releasing the lipids into the ground substance of the intima. The extracellular cholesterol esters may crystallize in the shape of long needles, producing quite distinctive clefts in tissue sections. An inflammatory fibroblastic response ensues, creating the fibrofatty atherosclerotic lesion which causes permanent damage to the arterial wall.

Intracellular accumulations of cholesterol and cholesterol esters within histiocytic cells are also encountered in other hypercholesterolemic states. Usually, these lesions are found in the subepithelial connective tissue of the skin and in tendons, producing tumorous masses known as xanthomas. These curious lesions are also encountered in the hereditary disorders known as the hyperlipoproteinemias (p. 595) (Fredrickson et al., 1967).

INTRACELLULAR ACCUMULATIONS OF PROTEIN

Excesses of protein sufficient to cause morphologically visible alterations are encountered only in renal epithelial cells of the proximal convoluted tubules and in plasma cells. The former is seen in the group of renal diseases known as the nephrotic syndrome (p. 1102). All are characterized by heavy levels of proteinuria due to abnormal glomerular permeability. Reabsorption of the urinary proteins represents the basis of the intracellular excess. The protein deposits appear as pink hyaline droplets within the cytoplasm of the tubular cells. At the level of the EM, the protein is found within lysosomes. These aggregations do not impair cellular function. If the underlying cause for the proteinuria can be controlled, the protein excess is metabolized and the droplets disappear. Plasma cells engaged in active synthesis of immunoglobulins may become overloaded with their synthetic product to produce homogeneous, acidophilic, large inclusions (*Russell's bodies*). These develop whenever the endoplasmic reticulum becomes so overloaded and distended as to become visible under the light microscope (Gray and Doniach, 1970).

INTRACELLULAR ACCUMULATION OF GLYCOGEN

Excessive intracellular deposits of glycogen are seen in patients with a derangement of either glucose or glycogen metabolism. Whatever the clinical setting, the glucose first creates a fine foaminess in the cytoplasm of the affected cell. As the process advances, cleared vacuoles eventually appear. Occasionally, nuclear vacuolation is seen (Fig. 2–21). To differentiate glycogen vacuolation from other types of intracellular vacuolation (fat, water), aqueous fixatives and solutions should be avoided since glycogen is somewhat water soluble. Tissues are best fixed in absolute alcohol and stained with Best's carmine or the periodic acid-Schiff (PAS) reaction, which imparts a rose to violet color to the glycogen. Diastase digestion prior to staining will serve as a further control by hydrolyzing the glycogen.

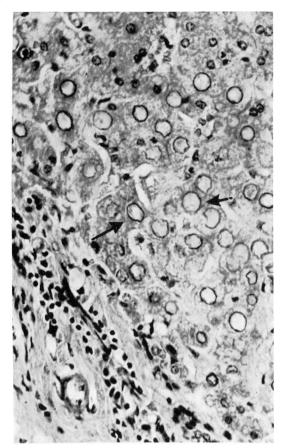

Figure 2–21. Glycogen accumulation in liver cell nuclei. The sharply defined circular nuclei are almost totally "cleared" by the glycogen (arrows).

Diabetes mellitus is the prime example of a disorder of glucose metabolism. In this disease, glycogen is found in the epithelial cells of the distal portions of the proximal convoluted tubules and, sometimes, of the descending loop of Henle, as well as within liver cells, beta cells of the islets of Langerhans and heart muscle cells. The mechanism involved in the renal change is: hyperglycemia resulting from impaired insulin function, glycosuria as the blood glucose levels rise above the renal threshold, and tubular reabsorption of the abnormal quantities of glucose in the glomerular filtrate. The glucose is stored in the form of glycogen. The intracellular glycogen produces marked vacuolation of the cytoplasm to the point where the cells appear to be entirely cleared (Fig. 2–22). The nuclei of such cells are often displaced basally. This morphologic change is also referred to as glycogen infiltration, glycogen nephrosis or Armanni-Ebstein cells. It does not impair renal tubular function and it is a reversible process which clears as

soon as the hyperglycemia and glycosuria are brought under control by the administration of insulin or some other hypoglycemic agent. For some obscure reason, glycogen deposition in hepatocytes appears principally within the nuclei which thus become swollen and cleared. Some reciprocal relationship appears to exist between the quantities of intranuclear and intracytoplasmic glycogen in these cells.

Glycogen may also accumulate within cells in a group of closely related disorders collectively referred to as glycogen storage diseases or glycogenoses. In these disorders, either some biochemical derangement impairs the ability of cells to mobilize normal glycogen, or some abnormal form of glycogen is synthesized which cannot be mobilized (Field, 1966) (Hsia, 1968). In the various syndromes (p. 296), the intracellular accumulations affect mainly myocardial, skeletal muscle, hepatic and renal cells. In all instances, the glycogen appears as clear intracytoplasmic vacuoles.

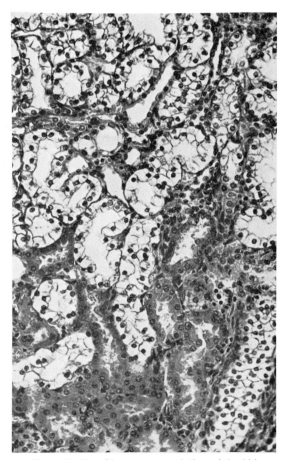

Figure 2–22. Glycogen vacuolation of the kidney. The epithelial cells of the affected tubules have distinct, well preserved nuclei and sharp cell membranes.

These glycogenoses provide instances in which massive stockpiling of substances within cells causes secondary cell injury and cell death and, indeed, some of the glycogenoses cause death of an affected infant or child.

INTRACELLULAR ACCUMULATIONS OF COMPLEX LIPIDS AND CARBOHYDRATES

In certain forms of storage diseases resulting from inborn errors of metabolism, abnormal complexes of carbohydrates and lipids which cannot be normally metabolized accumulate (p. 295). These substances collect within cells throughout the body, principally those in the reticuloendothelial system. In Gaucher's, Tay-Sachs and Neimann-Pick's diseases, the abnormal products are complex lipids while, in the mucopolysaccharidoses, they are complex carbohydrates. In the glycolipidoses and mucolipidoses, other more unusual products are accumulated. The abnormal metabolites in all of the storage diseases overflow into the blood and are phagocytized by reticuloendothelial cells which thus become enlarged and develop an apparent foaminess to their cytoplasm, often producing massive splenomegaly and hepatomegaly. The accumulations may also appear within parenchymal cells in the heart, liver and kidneys, and within ganglion cells of the brain and retina. The precise nature of the stored product rarely can be identified from morphologic examination and requires specific biochemical or enzymic analyses of affected tissues. These intracellular deposits may become extreme and cause death not only of the cell but also of the patient.

INTRACELLULAR ACCUMULATIONS OF PIGMENTS

Pigments are colored substances, some of which are normal constituents of cells (e.g., melanin and trace amounts of hemosiderin) while others are abnormal and collect in cells only under special circumstances (Wolman, 1969). Even the normal pigments, under certain circumstances, may accumulate in excess and possibly impair cellular function as discussed in the pathogenesis of hemochromatosis. But whether innocuous or not, pigments often provide valuable clues to the existence of an underlying disorder which leads to their accumulation. Exogenous pigments are derived from the environment while endogenous pigments are synthesized in the body.

Exogenous Pigments. Carbon or coal dust is the virtually ubiquitous air pollutant of urban life. When inhaled, it is picked up by macrophages within the alveoli and is then transported through lymphatic channels to the regional lymph nodes in the tracheobronchial region. Accumulations of this pigment blacken the tissues of the lungs (*anthracosis*) and the involved lymph nodes (Fig. 2–23). In general, anthracosis does not interfere with normal respiratory function nor does it predispose to infection. However, in coal miners and those living in heavily polluted environments, the aggregates of carbon dust in lymphatic and lymphoid tissue may induce a fibroblastic reaction or even emphysema (p. 792) and thus cause a serious lung disease known as "*coal miner's or black lung*" (p. 510). The blackness of the lungs of city dwellers is a grim reminder of man's devastation of his environment. While the anthracosis may be and usually is innocuous, more invidious air pollutants such as silica (p. 509) or hydrocarbon carcinogens (p. 833) usually accompany it.

Inhabitants living in iron-mining communities may develop a rust-like discoloration of the lungs (*siderosis*). This pigmentation itself is not associated with tissue damage but, in some areas, the iron dust is accompanied by silica dust (*siderosilicosis*). The silicotic component causes the serious lung disease, *silicosis* (p. 512).

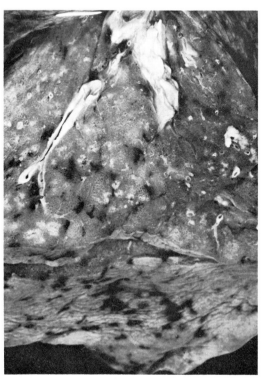

Figure 2–23. *Focal black deposits of anthracotic pigmentation in the lung.*

As is well known, *tattooing* is a form of localized pigmentation of the skin. The pigments inoculated are phagocytized by dermal macrophages in which they reside for the remainder of the life of the embellished. While the pigments do not evoke any inflammatory response, they have a distressing habit of persisting as a reminder of bygone follies.

Endogenous Pigments. Save for lipofuscin and melanin, all of the endogenous pigments are derived from hemoglobin.

Lipofuscin. Lipofuscin in tissue sections appears as a yellow-brown, granular, intracytoplasmic pigment. It is seen in cells undergoing slow regressive change such as that which occurs in the atrophy accompanying advanced age and in chronic injury. This form of pigmentation is particularly prominent in the liver and heart of aging patients and is usually accompanied by shrinkage in the size of the organ (*brown atrophy*) (Strehler et al., 1959). Lipofuscin may also accumulate within striated muscle cells in paralyzed or immobilized limbs as well as in hepatocytes in chronic forms of liver injury such as cirrhosis. In these circumstances, it may appear in younger patients. It is therefore better to consider lipofuscin as a form of metabolic or "wear and tear" pigment. However, certain cells of the body, such as the epithelial cells of the epididymis and the interstitial cells of the testis, as well as certain ganglion cells in the central nervous system, normally contain trace amounts of a granular yellow lipopigment which appears to be lipofuscin.

The genesis and composition of the pigment are still somewhat uncertain. When a cell suffers protracted stress, autophagic vacuoles are formed around degraded, cellular constituents (p. 13). These vacuoles fuse with lysosomes so that their contents are exposed to the degradative lysosomal enzymes. It is believed that lipofuscin derives from undigested membranous residues of the sequestered organelles. Presumably, the pigment results from the autooxidation of unsaturated lipids, yielding aldehydes and lipoperoxides which undergo further polymerization to create insoluble residues. It is worth noting, in passing, that deficiencies of antioxidants such as vitamin E are associated with the formation of increased amounts of lipofuscin. Chemical analyses of this pigment have not been very satisfactory. It appears to be composed of about 50 per cent lipid residues and 30 per cent protein residues, while the remainder is nonextractable and of unknown nature.

Lipofuscin itself is not injurious to the cell or to its function. It is principally an indicator of regressive change such as physiologic or pathologic atrophy, or chronic injury. Since it is membrane-bounded within residual bodies, it is isolated, as it were, from the remainder of the cell (Malkoff and Strehler, 1963). Sometimes, for obscure reasons, pigment which is both morphologically and biochemically indistinguishable from lipofuscin undergoes chemical or physical transformation and thus becomes acid-fast and autofluorescent. To this variant, the designation *ceroid* has been given but it is not believed to be different in any significant way from lipofuscin.

Melanin. Melanin is an endogenous, nonhemoglobin-derived, brown-black pigment synthesized from tyrosine in melanocytes. Tyrosinase catalyzes the oxidation of tyrosine to dihydroxyphenylalanine (dopa). Through a sequence of somewhat obscure steps, dopa is polymerized and then coupled with protein to produce melanin (Fitzpatrick et al., 1961). At the ultrastructural level, the dopa which is synthesized on the granular endoplasmic reticulum is aggregated or polymerized in the Golgi apparatus and incorporated there into a small membrane-bounded organelle known as a melanosome, comprising a pigment granule visible under the light microscope (Seiji and Iwashita, 1965).

This pigment is normally found in the basal malpighian layer of the epidermis and mucous membranes as well as in the uveal tract of the eye and the leptomeninges. The basal cells of the epidermis and mucous membranes acquire this pigment through a strange process. The melanocytes which synthesize the pigment are found in the dermis. They inject, as it were, the pigment into the epidermal cell through dendritic processes which form bridges between the epithelial cells and the melanocytes.

A similar phenomenon accounts for the pigmentation of the cells of the hair follicle. If this curious transfer of melanin from one cell to the other could be blocked in those persons who desire to be blond, imagine how much money would be saved on hair bleaches. Some of the normal pigmentation of the skin also results from the accumulation of melanin within melanophores. These are phagocytic cells which merely store the pigment they presumably acquire from nearby melanocytes. Aggregates of these dermal melanophores create freckles, and the accentuation of freckles after long exposure to sunlight results from the actinic stimulation of melanocytes and melanin synthesis. Occasionally, melanocytes are present in the ovary, adrenal medulla, bladder and substantia nigra of the brain.

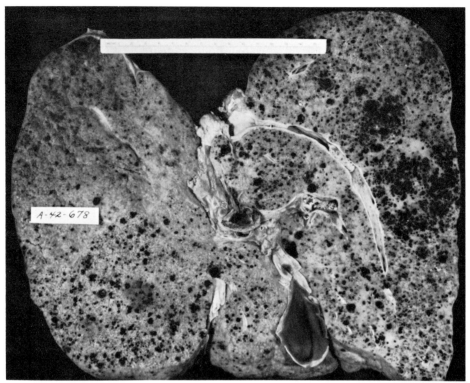

Figure 2–24. *Black nodules representing metastases of a melanocarcinoma in the liver; primary lesion was present in the skin.*

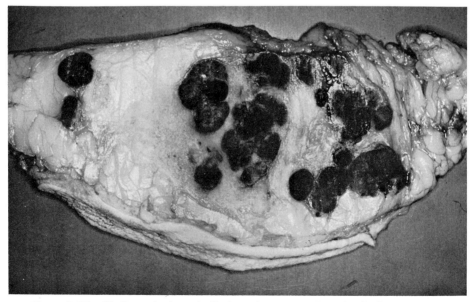

Figure 2–25. *Similar metastases to the breast seen on cut section in the same case.*

Melanin and melanocytes are of considerable importance for several reasons. Without melanin pigmentation of the skin, man could not tolerate exposure to the sun without fear of excessive sunburn or the development of skin cancers as a consequence of the actinic activity of the sun's rays. This pigment is sometimes referred to as a "light-absorbing mantle." Those with very fair skin are much more vulnerable to sunburn and actinic-induced skin cancers than those with more pigmentation. Indeed, the black race is virtually immune to these hazards. The *albino* born with a hereditary lack of tyrosinase is unable to convert tyrosine to 3,4-dihydroxyphenylalanine (dopa) necessary for the synthesis of melanin. He or she therefore has very blond hair, fair skin and blue eyes and is extremely vulnerable to actinic radiation, sunburn and skin cancers. The genetic defect is usually inherited as an autosomal recessive trait, but certain pedigrees suggest dominant transmission while others are sex-linked. Melanin also serves as a light shield in the iris of the eye. The albino is therefore extremely intolerant of bright light.

In addition to these functions of the pigment, melanocytes themselves are of considerable clinical importance. The very common "moles" (pigmented nevi) and their malignant counterpart, the melanocarcinoma (an often lethal form of cancer), arise from melanocytes or closely related cells. Since nevi and melanocarcinomas arise in melanocytes, they are usually pigmented and sometimes the massive accumulation of melanin imparts an intense black coloration to these lesions (Figs. 2–24 and 2–25). On occasion, perhaps because their cells of origin are less well differentiated and lack tyrosinase, these benign and malignant lesions may be nonpigmented.

Melanin synthesis in man is under adrenal and possible pituitary control. In animals, a melanocyte-stimulating hormone (MSH) has been identified in the pars intermedia of the pituitary. The existence of this hormone in man has been challenged and its role may be performed by adrenal corticotropic hormone (ACTH). Clearly, in man, increased levels of ACTH induce excessive melanin pigmentation. This occurs in Addison's disease, offering an excellent example of such pigmentation. In this condition, adrenal function is impaired or destroyed, and the unopposed pituitary elaborates increased amounts of ACTH, with subsequent darkening of the complexion. This endocrine-melanocyte interrelationship provides an important diagnostic feature in distinguishing the primary adrenal hypofunction of Addison's disease from the adrenal hypofunction associated with primary pituitary insufficiency. In the latter, there is decreased melanin pigmentation because of the lack of pituitary hormones, and so the skin appears unusually fair.

Hemosiderin. Hemosiderin, an iron storage substance, is a golden yellow to brown granular or crystalline pigment. Hemosiderin granules result from the aggregation of ferritin micelles. Ferritin is a normal constituent of most cells but, under normal conditions, it rarely accumulates in sufficient amounts to produce hemosiderin pigment except in the reticuloendothelial cells of the bone marrow, spleen and liver, all actively engaged in red cell breakdown. Iron metabolism and the synthesis of ferritin and hemosiderin are considered in detail on p. 273. Here it is enough to know that, in many pathologic states, excesses of iron cause hemosiderin to accumulate within cells, either as a localized process or as a systemic derangement. Under all circumstances, the hemosiderin contains trivalent iron which can be visualized by such histochemical procedures as the Prussian blue reaction (the application of colorless potassium ferrocyanide to gross or histologic sections of tissue, creating a blue-black insoluble iron salt wherever increased levels of hemosiderin are present). This reaction helps to differentiate, in tissue sections, the golden pigmentation of hemosiderin from that produced by lipofuscin.

Local excesses of iron and hemosiderin result from gross hemorrhages or the myriads of minute hemorrhages that accompany severe vascular congestion. The best example of localized hemosiderosis is the common bruise. Following the injury, the area is at first red-blue as a consequence of the hemorrhage. With localized lysis of the erythrocytes, the hemoglobin eventually undergoes transformation to hemosiderin. Macrophages take part in this process by phagocytizing the red cell debris, and then lysosomal enzymes eventually convert the hemoglobin, through a sequence of pigments, into hemosiderin. The play of colors which the bruise passes through reflects these transformations. The original red-blue color of hemoglobin is transformed to varying shades of green-blue, comprising the local formation of biliverdin (green bile), then bilirubin (red bile) which is in turn converted to the golden-yellow hemosiderin. The chronically congested lung and spleen in longstanding heart failure may become heavily pigmented. Capillaries may rupture or permit the escape of red cells. The erythrocytes are phagocytized by alveolar macrophages in the lung or by the reticuloendothelial (RE) cells of the spleen, and the hemoglobin is eventually converted to hemosiderin. The pigmented macrophages in the lung are often referred to as "heart failure cells."

Whenever there are causes for systemic overload of iron, hemosiderosis affects virtually all of the organs and tissues of the body. It is seen therefore with: (1) increased absorption of dietary iron, (2) impaired utilization of iron, (3) hemolytic anemias and (4) transfusions, since the transfused red cells have a short life span. Since the major consideration of iron metabolism is presented later (p. 273), only a few examples which illustrate the three pathways of excess iron accumulation are offered here.

The normal daily losses of iron are fairly rigidly limited in the range of 0.5 to 1.0 mg. per day. The normal daily requirement of iron is on the order of 1 mg. per day. Females, during active reproductive life, have a somewhat greater requirement resulting from the losses of iron in menstruation and pregnancy. The average daily diet contains quantities of iron far in excess of these requirements. Dietary overload is prevented by mechanisms, albeit somewhat obscure, which limit iron absorption. Failures in these mechanisms can lead to the accumulation of excessive quantities of iron, resulting in total body iron stores in the range of 60 to 80 gm. of elemental iron, as compared with the normal of 4.5 to 5 gm. Such dietary overload is considered by some to be the fundamental cause of hemochromatosis, the most extreme example of systemic overload (p. 277).

In certain hematologic disorders such as thalassemia, there is an inability to synthesize hemoglobin, and so the normal daily intake cannot be utilized and accumulates over the years. A wide variety of disorders—hemolytic anemias, multiple transfusions, red cell destruction by such toxic agents as heavy metals and phenylhydrazine, and a miscellaneous group of hereditary disorders with a deficiency of glucose-6-phosphate dehydrogenase (G6PD)—induce abnormal hemolysis, with the release of excessive amounts of iron.

The morphologic appearance of the pigment and its staining reactions are identical whatever the mechanism of its accumulation. It appears as a coarse, golden, granular pigment lying within the cell's cytoplasm. When the basic cause is the localized breakdown of red cells, the pigmentation is found at first in the RE cells in the area. In systemic hemosideroses, it is found at first in the RE cells of the liver, bone marrow, spleen and lymph nodes and in scattered macrophages throughout other organs such as the skin, pancreas and kidneys. With progressive accumulation, parenchymal cells throughout the body, principally those in the liver, pancreas, heart and endocrine organs, become pigmented.

In most instances of systemic hemosiderosis, the intracellular accumulations of pigment do not damage the parenchymal cells and so do not impair organ function. However, massive accumulations of hemosiderin may cause destruction of phagocytic cells in the spleen and lymph nodes, with release of the pigment into extracellular spaces. Fibrous proliferation may then occur about the pigment, particularly in the spleen, to create *siderofibrotic nodules.* The more extreme accumulations of iron in hemochromatosis are also associated with liver and pancreatic damage, but it is by no means certain that in this setting the hemosiderin itself is the injurious agent.

Hematin. Hematin is a hemoglobin-derived pigment of uncertain composition only encountered following a massive hemolytic crisis such as may occur with a severe transfusion reaction or in malaria, in which the parasite actively destroys red cells. It too is a golden-brown granular pigment which is virtually confined to RE cells. Because the iron is presumably bound into some organic complex, it fails to give a positive reaction with the Turnbull blue stain.

Bilirubin. Bilirubin is the normal yellow to green pigment of bile. While derived from hemoglobin, it contains no iron. Its normal formation and excretion are vital to health. Excesses of this pigment within cells and tissues cause jaundice as discussed on p. 989.

The normal metabolism of bilirubin, a tetrapyrrole, is a subject of some complexity and has been well reviewed by Robinson (1968). In skeletal outline, approximately 85 per cent is derived from the breakdown of red cells that have outlived their life span (100 to 120 days). These senescent erythrocytes are phagocytized by RE cells, principally in the spleen but to a smaller extent in the liver and bone marrow, where the envelopes are destroyed and the hemoglobin split into a heme pigment while the globin moiety is returned to the plasma. The heme pigment porphyrin ring is split; iron is released and, by a series of oxidation-reduction reactions in which heme-oxygenase participates, biliverdin (green) and then bilirubin (golden-yellow) is produced. A small amount of bilirubin (approximately 15 per cent), known as "shunt bilirubin," is directly synthesized in the bone marrow as a byproduct of hemoglobin synthesis, or in the liver as a result of the rapid turnover of cytochrome P-450 or the hemoproteins such as catalases and peroxidases.

Wherever formed, the bilirubin is transported in the blood to the liver, bound principally to albumin. It is then selectively taken up by the hepatocytes, but the exact details of this transport across the liver cell membrane are still obscure. Once within the hepatocyte, a molecule of bilirubin is conjugated to two molecules of glucuronide to produce bilirubin diglucuronide. Involved in such conjugation is the enzyme glucuronyl transferase. The bilirubin diglucuronide is then excreted into the biliary canaliculi. After its passage through the biliary tract, the bile flows into the duodenum and, within the gut, is converted by bacterial action to urobilinogen. This pigment is in some part reabsorbed into the portal circulation and thus returns to the liver, comprising the so-called enterohepatic circulation. Most of it, however, is excreted by the kidneys or is further transformed in the large intestine to urobilin (stercobilin). The normal brown coloration of stools is due to their content of stercobilin, accounting for the grey (putty-like) stools in diseases which obstruct the flow of bile into the intestines.

Normal plasma contains from 0.4 to 1 mg. of total bile pigments per 100 ml. This bilirubin is largely in the indirect unconjugated form in transport to the liver from its site of formation. Yellowing of the skin in jaundice becomes apparent when the bilirubin levels exceed 1.5 to 2 mg. per 100 ml. of plasma. Such hyperbilirubinemia is caused by a host of disorders which disrupt the normal metabolism of bile—e.g., increased breakdown of red cells (hemolytic jaundice), diseases affecting the liver cells, thus impairing the conjugation and excretion of bilirubin (intrahepatic cholestasis), and diseases which block the biliary outflow tract (extrahepatic or posthepatic cholestasis). The hemolytic and intrahepatic forms of jaundice result from elevated serum levels of unconjugated bilirubin. Posthepatic jaundice is due mainly to conjugated hyperbilirubinemia.

Bilirubin pigment within cells and tissues is only morphologically visible when the patient is rather severely jaundiced for some period of time. Even though this pigment is distributed throughout all tissues and fluids of the body, the accumulations are most evident in the liver and kidneys. In the liver, particularly with diseases caused by obstruction of the outflow of bile (such as cancers of the common bile duct or head of the pancreas), bilirubin is encountered within bile sinusoids, Kupffer cells and hepatocytes. In all of these sites, it appears as a mucoid green-brown to black, amorphous, globular deposit. In advanced cases of such obstructive jaundice, the aggregates of pigment may be quite large, creating so-called bile lakes. These may cause necrosis of hepatocytes in the focal area. Bilirubin pigment is encountered in the renal tubular epithelial cells in various forms of posthepatic jaundice.

CALCIFICATION

Both dead and dying tissues and sometimes normal tissues accumulate calcium salts together with smaller amounts of iron, magnesium and other mineral salts—a phenomenon referred to as calcification. When the deposition of calcium salts occurs in dead or dying tissues, it is known as *dystrophic calcification*; it may occur despite normal serum levels of calcium and in the absence of systemic derangements in calcium metabolism. In contrast, the deposition of calcium salts in vital tissues is known as *metastatic calcification*, and it almost always reflects some derangement in calcium metabolism, leading to hypercalcemia.

Dystrophic Calcification. This alteration is principally encountered in areas of coagulation, caseous and liquefactive necrosis and particularly in foci of enzymic necrosis of fat whenever the necrotic tissue persists for long periods of time. Thus, calcification is frequently encountered in chronic tuberculosis of the lungs or lymph nodes or in the centers of large infarcts. It also commonly develops in damaged heart valves, further hampering their function (Fig. 2–26). Calcification is almost inevitable in the aging atheromas of advanced atherosclerosis which, as will be seen, are focal intimal injuries in the aorta and larger arteries characterized by the accumula-

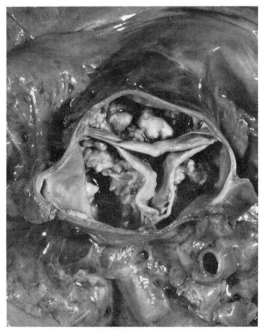

Figure 2–26. *Massive calcific nodules in the sinuses of the cusps of the aortic valve—dystrophic calcification of a previously injured tissue. (View is looking down on cusps from aortic side.)*

tion of lipids (p. 586). The coronary arteries may be converted virtually into pipe stems, and such damage is often the forerunner of coronary thrombosis and myocardial infarction. The anoxic, devitalized centers of tumors, particularly uterine leiomyomas, are prone to become calcified as well. Fetal tissues following fetal death are prone to undergo dystrophic calcification. Whatever the site of deposition, the calcium salts appear macroscopically as fine, white granules or clumps, often felt as gritty deposits. Sometimes, a tuberculous lymph node is virtually converted to stone.

Histologically, with the usual tissue stain, the calcium salts have a basophilic, amorphous granular, sometimes clumped appearance. In the course of time, heterotopic bone may be formed in the focus of calcification (Fig. 2–27). On occasion, single necrotic cells may constitute seed crystals that become encrusted by the mineral deposits. The progressive acquisition of outer layers may create lamellated configurations called psammoma bodies because of their resemblance to grains of sand. The extension of this phenomenon to necrotic cells shed into natural cavities may give rise to large stones or calculi, most frequently in the urinary bladder and calyceopelvic systems of the kidneys. Strange concretions emerge when calcium iron salts gather about long slender spicules of asbestos in the lung, creating exotic, beaded dumbbell forms.

The precise pathogenesis of dystrophic calcification is poorly understood and may involve different pathways in various settings and circumstances. One theory proposes that, in the progressive disintegration of dead cells, unfolding of the denatured proteins exposes groups capable of binding the phosphates contained within cells. In turn, the phosphate groups serve as nucleation sites for the precipitation of calcium (Glimcher and Krane, 1962). Most often, such depositions are amorphous and noncrystalline. These amorphous deposits may be in the form of phosphates, carbonates or oxalates, often admixed with iron salts. However, it has been shown that, occasionally, when the local circumstances are appropriate, crystalline formations of calcium phosphate are formed which are identical with the hydroxyapatite crystals of bone.

A different mechanism may be involved in the calcification of vessels. It has been speculated that alteration of the mucopolysaccharide of the ground substance predisposes to the binding of calcium ions. In the instance of enzymic necrosis of fat, it is postulated, as mentioned (p. 40), that the freed fatty acids combine with calcium to create insoluble soaps. Whatever the pathway, dystrophic calcification, although developing slowly, may be progressive with time, giving rise to ever larger "grave-stones" permanently marking the site of dead cells. Not infrequently, for reasons that are unclear, the calcification initiates bone formation and, indeed, sometimes the heterotopic bone accumulates islands of marrow.

Metastatic Calcification. This alteration may occur in normal tissues whenever there is hypercalcemia. Hypercalcemia will also accentuate dystrophic calcification. The causes of hypercalcemia include hyperparathyroidism, vitamin D intoxication, systemic sarcoidosis, milk-alkali syndrome, hyperthyroidism, idiopathic hypercalcemia of infancy, Addison's disease (adrenal cortical insufficiency), increased bone catabolism associated with disseminated bone tumors (such as multiple mye-

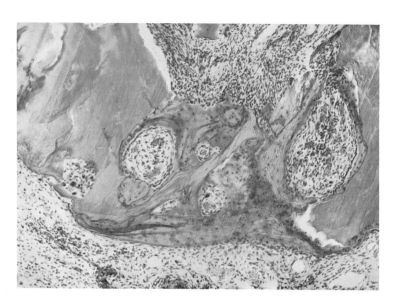

Figure 2–27. Heterotopic bone formation in an area of old fibrocalcific scarring of the lung.

loma and metastatic cancer) and leukemia and decreased bone formation as occurs in immobilization. Hypercalcemia also occurs in some instances of advanced renal failure with phosphate retention, leading to secondary hyperparathyroidism. Metastatic calcification may occur widely throughout the body but principally affects the interstitial tissues of the blood vessels, kidneys, lungs and gastric mucosa (Figs. 2–28 and 2–29). In all of these sites, the calcium salts morphologically resemble those described in dystrophic calcification. Thus they may occur as noncrystalline amorphous deposits or, at other times, as hydroxyapatite crystals. Metastatic calcifications tend to be more delicate than those encountered in dystrophic calcification, and rarely give rise to large concretions or calculi.

It has been customary to ascribe the precipitation of metastatic deposits in the lungs, kidneys and gastric mucosa to the excretion of acidic salts in these sites, thereby producing local alkalinity which favors the accumulation of the basic salts of calcium. Such an explanation, however, is probably simplistic since, under experimental conditions, metastatic calcium deposits often take the form of hydroxyapatite crystals and, in the kidney, for example, the calcium appears in the tubular basement membranes rather than in the epithelial cells, the site of renal secretory and excretory

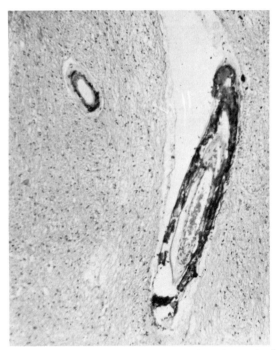

Figure 2–29. *Calcification of the wall of a cerebral blood vessel in a patient with hyperparathyroidism.*

activities. Nonetheless, we have no better explanation for the selective localization of metastatic calcific deposits. In general, the mineral salts cause no clinical dysfunction but, on occasion, massive involvement of the lungs produces remarkable x-ray films and respiratory deficits.

In closing this consideration of the various forms of cellular derangement, it is apparent that they cover a wide spectrum, ranging from the reversible and irreversible forms of cell injury to the less ominous forms of intracellular accumulations, including pigmentations. Reference will be made to all of these alterations throughout the entire book because all organ injury and, ultimately, all clinical disease arise from derangements in cell structure and function.

REFERENCES

Adair, F. E., and Munzer, J. T.: Fat necrosis of the female breast. A report of 110 cases. Amer. J. Surg., *74*:117, 1947.

Bassi, M., and Bernelli-Zazzara, A.: Ultrastructural cytoplasmic changes of liver cells after reversible and irreversible ischemia. Exp. Molec. Path., *3*:332, 1964.

Carr, D. H.: Chromosomal abnormalities in clinical medicine. Progr. Med. Genet., *6*:1, 1969.

Cochrane, C. G.: Immunologic tissue injury mediated by neutrophilic leukocytes. Advances Immun., *9*:97, 1968.

Cochrane, C. G., and Dixon, F. J.: Cell and tissue damage through antigen-antibody complexes. Calif. Med., *111*:99, 1969.

deDuve, C., and Wattiaux, R.: Functions of lysosomes. Amer. Rev. Physiol., *28*:435, 1966.

Dixon, F.: Discussion on composition of fibrinoid. Mechanism of

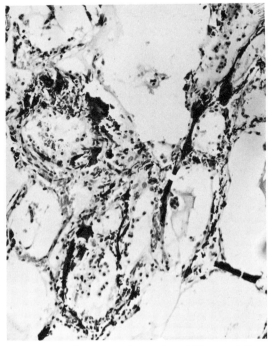

Figure 2–28. *Irregular dark calcific precipitates within the walls of the pulmonary alveolar septa in a patient with hyperparathyroidism.*

Cell and Tissue Damage Produced by Immune Reactions. IInd International Symposium Immunopathology. Basel, Benno, Schwabe and Co., 1961, p. 90.

Farber, E., et al.: Biochemical pathology of acute hepatic adenosine triphosphate deficiency. Nature (London), *203*:34, 1964.

Field, R. A.: Glycogen deposition disease. In Stanbury, J. B., Wyngaarden, J. B., and Fredrickson, D. S. (eds.): The Metabolic Bases of Inherited Disease. New York, Blakiston Division, McGraw-Hill Book Co., 1966, p. 71.

Fitzpatrick, T. B., et al.: Melanin pigmentation. New Eng. J. Med., *265*:328, 374, 430, 1961.

Fredrickson, D. S., et al.: Fat transport in lipoproteins. An integrated approach to mechanism and disorders. New Eng. J. Med., *276*:34, 94, 148, 215, 273, 1967.

Gallagher, C. H., et al.: Enzyme changes during liver autolysis. J. Path. Bact., *72*:247, 1956.

Ginn, F. L., et al.: Disorders of cell volume regulation. I. Effects of inhibition of plasma membrane adenosine triphosphatase with ouabain. Amer. J. Cell Biol., *53*:1041, 1968.

Glimcher, M. J., and Krane, S. M.: Studies on the interactions of collagen and phosphate. In McLean, F. C. (ed.): Radioisotopes and Bone, A Symposium. Philadelphia, F. A. Davis Co., 1962, p. 393.

Gray, A., and Doniach, I.: Ultrastructure of plasma cells containing Russell bodies in human stomach and thyroid. J. Clin. Path., *23*:608, 1970.

Hsia, D. Y.: The diagnosis and management of the glycogen storage diseases. Amer. J. Clin. Path., *59*:44, 1968.

Humphrey, J. H., and Dourmashkin, R. R.: The lesions in cell membranes caused by complement. Advances Immun., *11*:75, 1969.

Hyslop, G. H.: Effects of electrical injuries with particular reference to the nervous system. Occup. Med., *1*:199, 1946.

Iseri, O. A., and Gottlieb, L. S.: Alcoholic hyalin and megamitochondria as separate and distinct entities in liver disease associated with alcoholism. Gastroenterology, *60*:1027, 1971.

Isselbacher, K. L., and Greenberger, N. J.: Metabolic effects of alcohol on the liver. New Eng. J. Med., *270*:351, 402, 1964.

Lombardi, B.: Considerations on the pathogenesis of fatty liver. Lab. Invest., *15*:1, 1966.

Majno, G., et al.: Death and necrosis: chemical, physical, and morphologic changes in rat liver. Virchow Arch., *333*:421, 1960.

Malkoff, D. B., and Strehler, B. L.: The ultrastructure of isolated and in situ human cardiac age pigment. J. Cell Biol., *16*:611, 1963.

Monod, J., et al.: Allosteric proteins and cellular systems. J. Molec. Biol., *6*:306, 1963.

Ozawa, K., et al.: Biochemical studies on brain swelling. II. Influence of brain swelling and ischemia on the formation of endogenous inhibitor in mitochondria. Folia Psychiat. Neurol. Jap., *20*:73, 1966.

Ozawa, K., et al.: The effect of ischemia on mitochondrial metabolism. J. Biochem., *61*:512, 1967.

Plotkin, S. A., and Vaheri, A.: Human fibroblasts infected with rubella virus produce a growth inhibitor. Science, *156*:659, 1967.

Porta, E. A., et al.: Hepatic changes associated with chronic alcoholism in rats. Lab. Invest., *14*:1437, 1965.

Recknagel, R. O.: Carbon tetrachloride hepatotoxicity. Pharm. Rev., *19*:145, 1967.

Reynolds, E. S., and Ree, H. J.: Liver parenchymal cell injury. Membrane denaturation following carbon tetrachloride. Lab. Invest., *25*:269, 1971.

Robbins, S. L.: Unpublished observations.

Robinson, S. H.: The origins of bilirubin. New Eng. J. Med., *279*:146, 1968.

Roheim, P. S., et al.: Alterations of lipoprotein metabolism in orotic acid induced fatty liver. Lab. Invest., *15*:21, 1966.

Saladino, A. J., and Trump, B. F.: Ion movements in cell injury. Effects of inhibition of respiration and glycolysis on the ultrastructure and function of the epithelial cell of the toad bladder. Amer. J. Path., *52*:737, 1968.

Seiji, M., and Iwashita, S.: Intracellular localization of tyrosinase and site of melanin formation in melanocyte. J. Invest. Derm., *45*:305, 1965.

Smithells, R. W.: Drugs and human malformations. Advances Teratology, *1*:251, 1966.

Smuckler, E. A.: Cellular adenosine triphosphate levels in liver and kidneys during CCl$_4$ intoxication. Lab. Invest., *19*:218, 1968*a*.

Smuckler, E. A.: Structural and functional alteration of the endoplasmic reticulum during CCl$_4$ intoxication. In Campbell, P. N., and Campbell, F. C. (eds.): Structure and Function of the Endoplasmic Reticulum in Animal Cells. London and New York, Academic Press, 1968*b*, p. 11.

Smuckler, E. A., and Benditt, E. P.: Studies on carbon tetrachloride intoxication. III. A subcellular defect in protein synthesis. Biochemistry, *4*:671, 1965.

Smuckler, E. A., and Trump, B. F.: Alterations in the structure and function of the rough-surfaced endoplasmic reticulum during necrosis in vitro. Amer. J. Path., *53*:315, 1968.

Strehler, B. L., et al.: Rate and magnitude of age pigment accumulation in the human myocardium. J. Gerontol., *14*:430, 1959.

Striker, G. E., et al.: Structural and functional changes in rat kidney during CCl$_4$ intoxication. Amer. J. Path., *53*:769, 1968.

Totter, J. R.: Mechanism of radiation injury. Environ. Health Ser. (Radiol. Health), *33*:2, 1968.

Trump, B. F., and Bulger, R. E.: Studies of cellular injury in isolated flounder tubules. III. Light microscope and functional changes due to cyanide. Lab. Invest., *18*:721, 1968*a*.

Trump, B. F., and Bulger, R. E.: Studies of cellular injury in isolated flounder tubules. IV. Electron microscopic observations of changes during the phase of altered homeostasis in tubules treated with cyanide. Lab. Invest., *18*:731, 1968*b*.

Trump, B. F., and Ericsson, J. L. E.: Some ultrastructural and biochemical consequences of cell injury. In Zweifach, B. W., and Grant, L. (eds.): The Inflammatory Process. New York, Academic Press, 1965, p. 35.

Trump, B. F., and Ginn, F. L.: The pathogenesis of subcellular reaction to lethal injury. In Bajusz, E., and Jasmin, G. (eds.): Methods and Achievements in Experimental Pathology. Vol. IV. Chicago, Yearbook Medical Publishers, 1969, p. 1.

Trump, B. F., and Ginn, F. L.: Studies of cellular injury in isolated flounder tubules. II. Cellular swelling in high potassium media. Lab. Invest., *18*:341, 1968.

Trump, B. F., et al.: An electron microscope study of early cytoplasmic alterations in hepatic parenchymal cells of mouse liver during necrosis in vitro (autolysis). Lab. Invest., *11*:986, 1015, 1962.

Trump, B. F., et al.: Membrane structure: lipid-protein interactions in microsomal membranes. Proc. Nat. Acad. Sci., *66*:433, 1970.

Trump, B. F., et al.: Studies on necrosis in vitro of mouse hepatic parenchymal cells, ultrastructural and cytochemical alterations of cytosomes, cytosegresomes, multivesicular bodies, and microbodies and their relation to the lysosome concept. Lab. Invest., *14*:2000, 1956*b*.

Trump, B. F., et al.: Studies on necrosis of mouse liver in vitro, ultrastructural alterations in the mitochondria of hepatic parenchymal cells. Lab. Invest., *14*:343, 1965*a*.

Vogt, M. T., and Farber, E.: On the molecular pathology of the ischemic renal cell death. Reversible and irreversible cellular and mitochondrial metabolic alterations. Amer. J. Path., *53*:1, 1968.

Wolman, M.: Pigments in Pathology. New York, Academic Press, 1969.

3

INFLAMMATION AND REPAIR

Man owes to the inflammatory-reparative response his ability to contain injuries and reconstitute defects. This response has two themes, inflammation and repair, but they are so closely intertwined as to comprise a single story. *Inflammation may be defined as the response of the body to tissue injury involving neurologic, vascular, humoral and cellular reactions within the site of injury.* This response serves to destroy, dilute or wall off the injurious agent and the tissue cells it may have destroyed. The inflammatory response, in turn, sets into motion a complex series of events which, as far as possible, heal and reconstitute the damaged tissue.

Repair begins during the active phase of inflammation but reaches completion only after the injurious influence has been neutralized. Destroyed cells and tissues are replaced by vital cells, sometimes by regrowth of the native parenchymal cells, but more often by filling the defect with less specialized fibroblastic scar-forming cells. When the inflammatory reaction is prompt, effective and destroys or neutralizes the injurious agent before the latter causes much cell and tissue destruction, the need for repair is minimized and may lead to little or no scarring.

Both inflammation and repair generally

serve useful purposes. Without such protective mechanisms, bacterial infections would go unchecked, wounds would never heal and injured tissues and organs might retain permanently festering defects. Vital as these responses are to the maintenance of health, both are potentially harmful. Inflammatory reactions underlie the genesis of several forms of possibly fatal glomerular disease, crippling rheumatoid arthritis and life-threatening sensitivity reactions. Reparative efforts may lead to disfiguring scars, fibrous bonds which limit the mobility of joints, as well as masses of scar tissue that hamper the function of organs. Fortunately, such unwanted outcomes are the exceptions and not the rule. The following discussion will focus on the essential roles of inflammation and repair in the survival of the organism. Many excellent reviews, such as that of Schilling (1968) are available on this subject.

The inflammatory-reparative response involves a concatenation of events, some sequential, others virtually simultaneous but all overlapping and interdependent. An understanding of its complexity will be facilitated by first providing a hasty overview of the entire process which, in essence, comprises the order of consideration of the major features of the inflammatory-reparative response. (1) We begin our consideration with the initial changes—hemodynamic and permeability adjustments—which follow injury. Vessels thus changed readily exude fluids, plasma proteins and white cells. (2) The machinery activating such events comprises a constellation of chemi-cal mediators. (3) Once marshalled in a focus of injury, the various types of white cells contribute to the defensive reaction by virtue of their ability to migrate, release enzymes and phagocytose particulate matter. (4) In those inflammatory reactions evoking systemic responses, there is elevation of the white cell count in the circulating blood and the reticuloendothelial system throughout the body becomes involved. (5) Although all inflammatory responses tend to be alike in their early phases, many factors relating to both the inciting agent and the host modify the evolving reaction. (6) Other modifiers include the duration of the inflammatory response, the nature of the exudate, the specific cause of the inflammation and the location of the reaction. On the basis of these four variables, a classification of these reactions has developed. (7) At this point, repair, which has already begun during the inflammatory reaction, must be discussed to clarify the response of parenchymal cells and the connective tissue. (8) The factors that induce parenchymal cell and connective tissue proliferation, as well as the influences which bear on the rapidity of scarring and its strength, are considered. (9) Ultimately, attention is directed to systemic and local influences bearing on the quantity and quality of the inflammatory-reparative response. From this perspective, we first turn to a consideration of inflammation, followed by a discussion of repair, recognizing that such arbitrary separation is only justified in the interest of simplification.

INFLAMMATION

The basic character of the immediate inflammatory response is almost always the same, regardless of the location or nature of the injurious agent. It is common to think of bacteria or other living forms as the cause of inflammation, but many nonliving agents such as heat, cold, radiant energy, electrical or chemical injury and simple mechanical trauma may also act as destructive influences and evoke inflammatory reactions. Moreover, the necrotic products released serve as inflammatory stimuli.

While the basic pattern is stereotyped, the intensity of the reaction is determined by both the severity of the injurious stimulus and the reactive capability of the host. A single transient injury usually evokes a short-lived response. Repeated or persistent injuries usually result in a sustained reaction termed chronic inflammation. The intensity and duration of the inflammatory reaction may be viewed as a precarious balance between attacker and host. Even slight injury may produce a serious sustained response in a frail person. But even the robust may fall prey to a violent attack, as every victim of a severe burn well knows. Depending on the severity of the injury and the adequacy of the defense, the inflammation may remain localized to its site of origin and evoke no systemic reactions, or may call into play systemic responses. This point will become clearer in the following discussion of the clinical manifestations of acute inflammation.

CLINICAL MANIFESTATIONS OF ACUTE INFLAMMATION

Inflammatory involvement of an organ or tissue is designated by the suffix "itis"—e.g., tonsillitis, appendicitis, hepatitis. *Acute inflammation may evoke manifestations localized to the site of injury or may be accompanied by systemic changes.* The splinter in a finger causes only local signs whereas a severe tonsillitis may produce not only local signs but also a significant systemic reaction. We are far from understanding why a bacterial infection localized to the tonsils should produce such widespread symptoms as fever, listlessness, loss of appetite and some degree of debility. One would suspect the release of humoral agents and, indeed, a variety of substances of endogenous and exogenous origin have been identified. Endogenous pyrogens are released into the blood stream from neutrophils and monocytes when these cells contact injurious agents such as bacterial endotoxins, antigen-antibody complexes, particulate matter which stimulates phagocytic activity and products of necrotic cells (Atkins et al., 1967). Studies by Rafter et al. (1966) suggest that the pyrogen is a lipoprotein derived from cell membrane. It appears to act on the central nervous system, particularly on the thermal regulatory mechanisms in the hypothalamus which control the production and dissipation of body heat. During febrile reactions, the hypothalamic thermostat behaves "as though it were set at a higher level" (Atkins, 1960).

There are also exogenous pyrogens such as bacterial endotoxins, or whole bacteria which, when administered to rabbits, are capable of inducing fevers. These fevers develop after a longer latent period than those induced by endogenous factors. While these bacterial agents are termed exogenous pyrogens, there is a strong suspicion that their action is partially mediated by the release of endogenous pyrogens from the leukocytes of the host (Atkins and Wood, 1955). Although we have, therefore, some understanding of the genesis of the febrile reaction in inflammation, there is still no hint of the pathways involved in other commonly encountered systemic symptoms.

The local clinical signs of inflammation have classically been characterized as heat (calor), redness (rubor), swelling (edema), pain (dolor) and loss of function (functio laesa). To these might be added the potential appearance of pus in any injury. The local heat and redness result from dilation of the microcirculation in the environs of the injury. The swelling is largely produced by the escape of fluid, containing plasma proteins and other solutes, from the blood into the perivascular tissues, two processes known as transudation and exudation. The origin of the pain is somewhat more obscure but has been attributed to the pressure of extravascular fluid on nerve endings and/or to direct neural irritation by chemical mediators. Bradykinin, one of these mediators, is currently suspected as a major cause of pain.

We know very little about the causes of loss of function. At a simplistic level, the attempt to avoid pain evoked by movement of an inflamed finger may be adequate to explain cessation of motor function. But how does one explain impaired hepatic function in hepatitis? One may only postulate that fever produces a suboptimal temperature for biochemical reactions or that noxious metabolites are elaborated by injured or hypermetabolic liver cells.

Pus is an inflammatory exudate rich in proteins which contains viable white cells as well as cell debris derived from necrotic immigrant leukocytes and native parenchymal cells. A large variety of lysosomal enzymes are present in pus, and the extent of proteolysis which they induce determines the viscosity of such an exudate. But here we should define the terms exudate and transudate. An *exudate* is an inflammatory extravascular fluid with a specific gravity usually above 1.020, resulting from its high content of proteins and cellular debris. The white cells and cellular debris within it impart the yellow-white appearance of pus, more properly termed a purulent exudate. The escape of plasma proteins into the extravascular spaces implies significant alteration in the normal permeability of the microcirculation in the area of injury. In contrast, a *transudate* is a low-protein fluid with a specific gravity of less than 1.012. It is essentially an ultrafiltrate of the blood plasma and consists principally of water and dissolved electrolytes.

There is some correlation in man between the severity of the injury and the composition of the inflammatory exudate. Mild injuries produce a protein-poor watery transudate. With progressively more powerful stimuli, the exudate acquires higher and higher concentrations of plasma proteins (a process described as molecular sieving). Red cells appear only in the most severe forms of injury which cause necrosis of small vessels. The local manifestations of acute inflammation clearly highlight the three major components of the inflammatory response: (1) hemodynamic changes, (2) permeability changes and (3) events involving leukocytes. Each of these components will be discussed separately in following sections, but it should be emphasized that such separation is arbitrary (Spector, 1964). More accurately, the hemodynamic changes initiate the inflammatory response; very soon thereafter, alterations in the permeability of the affected vessels appear, followed in turn by reactions involving white cells. But there is much overlap, and all three major aspects of the reaction are well developed within two hours.

HEMODYNAMIC CHANGES

Most of the cardinal local signs of inflammation arise from changes in the microcirculatory bed in the area of the injury. Indeed, the acute inflammatory reaction requires an intact circulation capable of response. The hemodynamic alterations comprise an integrated chain of events activated by chemical mediators but perhaps transiently initiated by neurogenic mechanisms. These vascular events are manifested in the following order:

1. Arteriolar dilation sometimes preceded by transient vasoconstriction.
2. Increased rate of blood flow through the arterioles.
3. Opening of new capillary and venular beds in the area.
4. Congestion of the venous efflux.
5. Increased permeability of the microvasculature, with the outpouring of inflammatory fluid into the extravascular tissues.
6. Concentration or packing of red cells in the capillaries and venules.
7. Slowing or stasis of flow in these small vessels sometimes to complete stagnation.
8. Peripheral orientation of white cells in the capillaries (margination).
9. A sequence of subsequent white cell events to be discussed in a later section.

Many of these changes begin at the same time but develop at varying rates, depending on the severity of the injury. Following injury, there is a transient arteriolar constriction, probably neurogenic or adrenergic in origin, that usually lasts for seconds to a few minutes. Indeed, if the injury develops slowly, such as in the case of a sunburn, vasoconstriction may never occur. In any event, in all instances dilation of arterioles, associated with increased blood flow through the capillaries and venules, soon occurs.

The increased flow is largely associated with the release of precapillary sphincters and the opening of previously inactive capillaries and venules. But it may also result from some dilation of these small vessels. The overload of the venous efflux and the congestion of these drainage vessels undoubtedly contribute to this vasodilation. By this time, the permeability of the microcirculation is altered and fluid begins to leak out of the vessels. This leakage may comprise at first a watery transudate but, in significant inflammatory responses, the progressive increase in permeability permits the escape of ever larger macromolecules, forming a protein-rich exudate, a process referred to as molecular sieving. Loss of plasma fluid causes local hemoconcentration, and the small vessels become packed with erythrocytes which form rouleaux or agglutinated clumps of red cells. Such red-cell sludging also contributes to stagnation of flow which, when compounded by significant damage to the vessel wall, may lead to intravascular clotting (thrombosis).

Along with the slowing of blood flow, the clumped red cells collect in the central stream and the white cells assume a peripheral orientation along the endothelial surfaces of the affected vessels. The mechanisms which lead to this margination will be considered in the discussion of white cell changes. With mild stimuli, the stage of stagnation may not become apparent until 15 to 30 minutes have elapsed. With severe injury, there may be actual necrosis and rupture of small vessels, leading to hemorrhage or clotting of blood within a few minutes. However, even in such severe injury, more marginal venules and capillaries will reveal the characteristic chain of events just cited. It should be emphasized that, contrary to earlier beliefs, the venules are the principal actors in the early phases of the acute inflammatory drama. Capillaries play a larger role in the later phases of more severe injury.

PERMEABILITY CHANGES

Leakage of fluid as a consequence of changes in the permeability of the microvasculature, with resultant tissue swelling (edema), is a major characteristic of all significant acute inflammatory reactions (Fig. 3–1). The swelling results not only from the accumulation of fluid within the extravascular tissue spaces but also from cellular swelling. The fluid, as indicated earlier, is at first a transudate or ultrafiltrate of the plasma, but the permeability changes within the venules and capillaries soon permit the escape of plasma proteins, leukocytes and sometimes red cells. This protein-rich cell-containing exudate appears in all but the most trivial of inflammatory responses. It is worth pointing out here that transudates may also be encountered in noninflammatory congestion of vessels, but an exudate indicates inflammation. In congestive heart failure, a noninflammatory hemodynamic disorder, the transudate which may collect in the pleural cavity is designated pleural effusion. But, with infection within the pleural cavity, this fluid develops a much higher specific gravity. Therefore, the differentiation between these two forms of

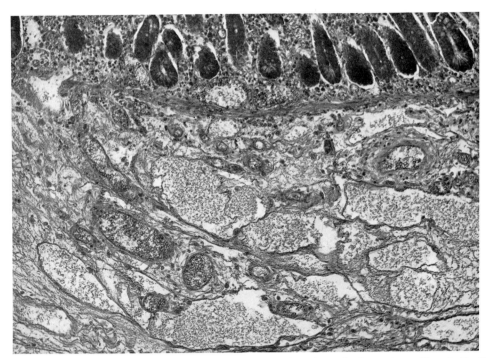

Figure 3–1. *Early acute inflammation in wall of small bowel. There is marked vascular and lymphatic dilatation. The submucosal connective tissue is spread apart by edema fluid. Many "polys" have migrated from the vessels into the interstitial tissue.*

fluid may be of considerable clinical diagnostic value.

The pathogenesis of inflammatory exudates involves an understanding of the normal permeability of the microcirculation. In biology, permeability refers to the ease with which a barrier can be penetrated by a substance. In the context of the inflammatory reaction, it refers to the ease with which plasma water, with its contained solutes and large molecules such as proteins and even blood cells, can pass through the walls of microvessels. Prior to electron microscopy, physiologists postulated the existence of pores in the endothelial cells (Pappenheimer, 1953). Two classes were proposed: (1) many pores of small diameter (in the range of 37 Å) which would permit the passage of an ultrafiltrate of plasma free of protein and (2) fewer pores of larger size (in the range of 120 to 350 Å) which would allow the passage of small amounts of larger molecules such as albumin with a molecular weight of approximately 70,000. Such a theoretical proposition would nicely explain the nature of the normal fluid exchange which is largely composed of plasma water and its contained electrolytes, with only a small amount of albumin.

Regrettably, the electron microscope has failed to reveal pores in the capillary structure of most tissues. As is well known, the endothe-lial lining of the microcirculation in most tissues is composed of an unbroken layer of endothelial cells. However, special endothelial patterns are encountered in the capillaries of a few organs. In the endocrine and exocrine glands, the cytoplasm of the endothelial cells is perforated by pores covered by thin diaphragms. Glomerular capillaries possess readily visible fenestrations, apparently devoid of diaphragms, through which small quantities of plasma proteins are filtered into the glomerular space and are then normally reabsorbed from the renal tubules. The bone marrow, spleen and liver are additional exceptions, a striking example of the "wisdom of the body." Here in the sinusoids, the endothelial lining is characterized by wide intercellular junctions and large fenestrations providing gaps for the easy passage of proteins and cells. Save for these special instances, the endothelial cells are tightly bound to each other by complicated interlocking cell junctions.

It was once thought that the plasma membranes of adjacent endothelial cells actually fused to produce a tight junction or zonula occludens. However, recent observations indicate that although the cell junctions are narrow, a space of about 40 to 60 Å separates contiguous cells (Karnovsky, 1967). Using particles of known molecular size (horseradish peroxidase, molecular weight, 40,000) visible in electron micrographs, Karnovsky was able to demonstrate their filtration through the normal intercellular junctions while larger molecules such as albumin were withheld. Perhaps it is incorrect to speak of an intercellular "space" since, in all probability, the crevice is filled with water-permeable, amorphous, acid mucopolysaccharides secreted by the endothelial cell. Similar material has been found covering the luminal surface of the endothelial cell (Luft, 1966). This glycoprotein appears to be analogous to the extraneous coat or glycocalyx found around many cells such as those lining the intestinal tract. The existence of these interendothelial slits may well represent the pores required to explain the previous theoretical calculations of capillary permeability.

Passage of fluid between the endothelial cells implies a passive role for the endothelium in the exchange of fluids. An active energy-dependent transport mechanism is also postulated. According to this proposal, endothelial cells have, on their luminal surfaces, small invaginations which become pinched off to create small endocytotic vesicles containing plasma. Transport of these vesicles across the endothelial cell, with discharge of the vesicular content on their basal aspects, would comprise an active transport mechanism. However, tracer studies using carbon and ferritin do not indicate significant transport via this pathway, certainly not sufficient to account for the volumes encountered in normal fluid exchange (Fawcett, 1963). It is possible that the vesicular transport contributes to the limited passage of the larger protein macromolecules characteristic of normal interstitial fluid.

Before leaving the fine structure of the microcirculation, a few words should be said about the still mysterious basement membrane on which the endothelial cells sit. As best we now know, it appears to be a mesh of fibers and filaments making up an unbroken layer varying from several hundred to over 1000 Å in thickness. No pores or defects have been visualized in it. Tracer particles, such as horseradish peroxidase introduced into the circulation, are sufficiently small to pass freely through the basement membrane. Larger particles such as carbon or ferritin, when they escape through abnormally widened endothelial cell junctions, are trapped against the basement membrane. Eventually, some penetrate this layer as well but the governing mechanism is still a mystery. Indeed, as we shall see later, much larger white cells are just as adept at this "escape act" by equally mysterious mechanisms or pathways known only to them.

Well known since the days of Starling is the normal fluid exchange which occurs across capillary walls. At the arteriolar end of the capillaries, the hydrostatic pressure of the blood (approximately 40 to 45 mm. Hg) is greater than the oncotic pressure of the plasma proteins (approximately 35 mm. Hg), and so water, with its contained electrolytes and trace amounts of albumin, is driven out of the vascular compartment into the perivascular spaces. At the venular end of the capillaries, the hydrostatic pressure falls to approximately 15 mm. Hg and so is lower than the plasma oncotic pressure. Fluid thus returns to the vascular compartment (Landis et al., 1932). However, the fluid balance is not perfect and there is a continuing loss into the extravascular spaces which are drained by lymphatic channels.

Against this background, it is now possible to consider the development of edema at sites of acute inflammation and the pathogenesis of inflammatory exudates. Two mechanisms are operative: the first is purely hydrostatic; the second involves alterations in permeability effected by the chemical mediators. Turning first to the hydrostatic mechanism, it will be recalled that arteriolar dilation leads to an increased blood flow in inflamed tissues. The pressure within skin capillaries at the arteriolar end has been shown by Landis to rise at sites of injection of histamine (a potent chemical mediator), from the normal of approximately 40 mm. Hg to levels above 50 mm. Hg. This increased intravascular pressure forces fluid, essentially an ultrafiltrate of plasma relatively free of protein, out of the vessels. Some albumin may escape but not enough to produce a characteristic exudate. However, exudation soon follows transudation as the permeability of the microcirculation increases.

Our understanding of the finer details of exudation was made possible by the development of techniques for demonstrating subtle alterations in the permeability of small vessels. The methods employ tracer particles of graded size. Commonly used are carbon and dyes such as trypan blue which bind to serum proteins, particularly albumin. The dye-protein complexes do not leak from normal vessels, but when there is an increase in permeability, albumin along with its marker dye escapes into the extravascular spaces and so stains the tissues. Using such a technique, Sevitt (1958, 1964) was able to demonstrate varying patterns in the rise and ebb of increased permeability when the skin of the guinea pig was exposed to graded severities of thermal injuries. He classified these responses into *immediate, delayed and sustained phases of vascular permeability*. Since that time, his observations have been confirmed by many others (Wilhelm, 1962). The time-response curves of the immediate, delayed and sustained responses vary somewhat, depending on the animal species studied and the nature of the injury. They are best demonstrated by fairly specific levels of thermal injury, and usually are not evoked by chemical or other forms of injury. Despite these variations, the three patterns are distinctive.

IMMEDIATE PERMEABILITY RESPONSE

Associated with mild thermal injury, this response usually begins 1 to 10 minutes after injury and phases out within 15 to 30 minutes. Rarely, it may persist for as long as 60 minutes. This immediate response is probably mediated by histamine or histamine-like substances and can be inhibited by antihistaminics (Wilhelm and Mason, 1960). Other mediators also participate (see p. 68). Ultrastructural studies have shown that *the principal vessels involved in this immediate reaction are the venules* while the capillaries are relatively unaffected (Cotran and Remensnyder, 1968). Majno and his coworkers have shown unmistakable widening of the endothelial cell junctions in these venules, resulting from contraction of the endothelial cells (Majno and Palade, 1961) (Fig. 3–2). These cells have been shown to contain myosin and myofibrils which provide a plausible explanation for the observed cellular contraction (Majno and Leventhal, 1967). Mild injuries elicit only this immediate response and proceed no further. Clinically, only redness and slight edema may be noted. However the width of the widened gaps does not appear to be related to the severity of the injury, and so this observation cannot explain the graded phenomenon of molecular sieving.

DELAYED RESPONSE

This response is best demonstrated in slightly more severe thermal injuries. In these circumstances, after the wave of immediate increased permeability, there is a period of low permeability which lasts for two to ten hours, followed in turn by the reappearance of increased permeability which may last for as long as 24 to 48 hours (Logan and Wilhelm, 1966). In this model, the permeability response is biphasic, having immediate and delayed peaks. Tracer techniques indicate that the sites of leakage in the delayed phase are in both venules and capillaries. *It is tempting to postulate, although it is as yet not well substantiated, that chemically mediated venular leakage on the less involved margins of the locus of injury is the origin of the immediate response, and that direct endothelial cell injury in capillaries and venules in the more severely* *damaged central focus underlies the delayed phase of increased permeability.* Presumably, more time would be required for the direct cell damage to develop to the stage of increased permeability. Electron micrographs tend to support such an explanation by revealing endothelial cell damage in the central focus of injury. If direct damage is not the basis for the delayed response, then we must confess that we do not understand its causation.

IMMEDIATE SUSTAINED REACTION

The third pattern of increased vascular permeability, referred to as a sustained response, is better characterized as an immediate sustained reaction. It is encountered in severe injuries usually associated with the immediate death of native cells. An immediate and persistent increase in permeability develops in the margins of such necrosis. The increased permeability does not follow a biphasic pattern but usually remains at sustained high levels for at least as long as the delayed phase encountered in milder injury. All levels of the microcirculation are affected, including venules, capillaries and arterioles. Endothelial cell necrosis of small vessels is often present. Frequently, intraluminal clots and extravascular hemorrhages are seen. Here the mechanism for increased permeability appears to be direct damage to vessel walls by severe injury. The inflammatory exudate is rich in white cells and proteins and may, in fact, have a protein content identical to that of plasma.

Although the *biphasic pattern* of permeability can be identified in experimental models and provides important insights into mechanisms, it should be stressed that in most human injuries no such sequence can be readily identified. *The significant injuries of man are generally so severe that they induce immediate sustained reactions.*

In closing this discussion of permeability, attention should be turned once again to the role of the basement membrane. No alterations in its structure can be identified during the height of inflammatory responses. However, when endothelial cells contract or are damaged, they sometimes separate from the underlying basement membrane. Since these cells are responsible for the formation and maintenance of the membrane, it is possible that subtle changes may be incurred which are undetectable by present-day methods of study.

WHITE CELL EVENTS

The massing of leukocytes, principally neutrophils and macrophages (derived from monocytes, as will be explained later), at sites

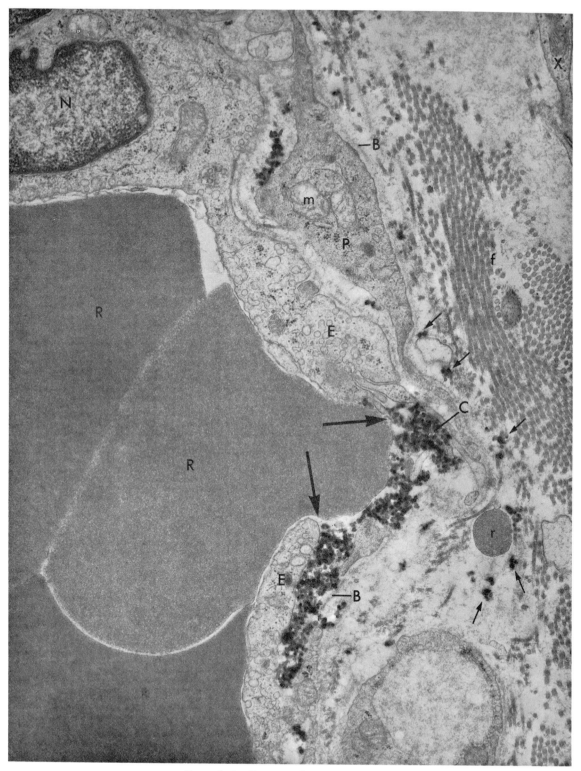

Figure 3–2. See opposite page for legend.

of inflammation may well constitute the prime defensive feature of the inflammatory response. Enzyme-rich phagocytic cells release powerful lytic juices and engulf foreign intruders, in most instances destroying or at least weakening the invaders. Lysosomes, particularly those of neutrophil origin, harbor a host of factors which play pivotal roles. Leukocytes thus constitute the third leg (along with the hemodynamic and permeability changes) of the tripod on which the inflammatory process stands. These white cell changes have been well reviewed by Hersh and Bodey (1970). How do these cells get to the precise focus of injury? The sequence of events can be divided into (1) margination and pavementing, (2) emigration, (3) chemotaxis, (4) aggregation and (5) phagocytosis.

MARGINATION AND PAVEMENTING

Margination or peripheral orientation of white cells in the moving blood stream has already been mentioned in the discussion of the hemodynamic changes. In the normally flowing blood, the red and white blood cells within microvessels are confined to the axial central column, leaving a relatively cell-free layer of plasma in contact with the vessel wall. As slowing and stagnation of the flow ensue, this laminar flow disappears. The white cells appear to fall out of the central column to assume positions in contact with the endothelium. Under phase microscopy, these cells appear to tumble slowly along the walls of the capillaries and venules to come finally to rest at some point. In time, the endothelium appears to be virtually lined by such cells, a phenomenon called pavementing. The mechanisms involved in such changes are still poorly understood.

The displacement of white cells to the periphery of the stream may be governed by the laws of physics. In the stagnated blood flow, the red cells tend to stick together and form small clumps or rouleaux, a process that has been referred to as *sludging*. These clumps thus become larger than the white cells and, in any moving column of fluid, the largest objects occupy the most rapidly moving central axis of the stream. Less clear is the reason the white cells stick to the endothelial surface.

There are three possible explanations for the adherence of white cells to the walls of blood vessels. Either the endothelium in some way becomes sticky, the white cell becomes abnormally adhesive or some substance extraneous to both serves as a glue. The numerous studies on this particular problem have led to observations in support of all possibilities and perhaps all are valid (Cliff, 1966). It has been repeatedly observed, since the early studies of Cohnheim (1889), that the white cell in a slow-moving stream intermittently adheres to the endothelial layer, then is swept off again and tumbles along for a distance, only to adhere once again outside the locus of injury. This stumbling course would suggest that whatever the nature of the change, it is intrinsic to the white cell. In support of this proposition, injury of individual leukocytes by micropuncture renders them more adhesive. Normally, the endothelium and the white cells are believed to repel each other by electrochemical negative charges. Perhaps in some way injury neutralizes such repellent charges. It has been observed that, following injury, white cells lose their essentially spherical shape and develop pseudopods. The pseudopods, carrying only relatively few charges, might be less repellent than the whole cell body and thus permit primary points of contact. Calcium may play some role in this adherence, serving as a bridge between the negative charges on the endothelium and the white cells. Treatment with EDTA (chelation of calcium) has been shown to block the gathering of white cells at sites of injury (Thompson et al., 1967). Endothelial changes may also participate. The layer of amorphous substance coating endothelial cells, known as a glycocalyx, could possibly be altered, rendering them more sticky (Luft, 1966). Allison et al. (1955) noted that white cells tend to adhere to the side of the vessel closest to the site of injury, suggesting changes in the endothelial cells. The third possibility which must be considered involves some constituent

---

Figure 3–2. *Wall of a leaking venule 6 minutes after local injection of histamine and intravenous injection of colloidal carbon black (rat, striated muscle). The lumen (left) is packed with red blood cells (stasis) as plasma is lost through leaks in the wall. One such leak is visible between the two large arrows. A red blood cell (R) is being squeezed into it. Shortly before this tissue was fixed, plasma loaded with carbon particles leaked between E, E; most of the carbon particles (C) were retained by the basement membrane (B), but a few managed to escape (arrows), possibly through a tear produced by an extravasating red blood cell, part of which is visible outside the vessel (r). E = endothelial cells. N = nucleus of endothelial cell. P = pericytes (cells contained within the vascular basement membrane). X = connective tissue cell, presumably histiocyte. (×26,000.) (Courtesy of Dr. Guido Majno, Department of Pathology, Harvard Medical School.)*

of plasma, so altered as to bind white cells to the endothelial layer. Cochrane and Aiken (1966) propose that the trimolecular complex of complement (C5, 6, 7) may play this role in certain immunologic reactions.

Perhaps the endothelium, the leukocyte and additional factors such as complement all participate in the production of leukocyte adherence. In any event, early in all acute inflammatory reactions, the white cells virtually pave first the endothelial surfaces of the venules and then the capillaries in the area of injury. It is worth noting at this point that pavementing of white cells can be largely blocked in vivo by the administration of large doses of adrenal steroids. Although the mechanism of such action is unclear, it may provide yet another means by which the inflammatory reaction is inhibited by these hormones. Moreover, this observation may also explain why bacterial infections are frequently worsened when patients are administered corticosteroids.

EMIGRATION

Emigration refers to the process by which motile white cells escape from blood vessels to reach the perivascular tissues. Neutrophils, eosinophils, basophils, monocytes and lymphocytes all use the same pathway. Little has been added to our knowledge of the morphodynamics of emigration since the brilliant descriptions of Cohnheim (1889). The motile cells insert large pseudopodia into the crevices between the endothelial cells and flow or crawl through the widened interendothelial junctions eventually to assume a position between endothelial cell and basement membrane. They then penetrate, via some mysterious byways, the seemingly impermeable barrier of the basement membrane to achieve an extravascular position. The elegant electron microscopic observations of Marchesi and Florey (1960) have shown the incredible plasticity of the relatively bulky white cells as they crawl through the narrow serpentine pathways opened by the contracted endothelial cells. The process is one of active motility rather than of passive extrusion by the hydrostatic pressure of the blood.

In the detailed study of emigration, it has become apparent that there are two separate waves of leukocytic activity. An immediate wave reaches massive proportions in the venules in 30 to 40 minutes; the delayed wave occurs in both capillaries and venules some hours later. *Neutrophils and monocytes both leave during the early wave but, in the delayed phase the continued recruitment of monocytes outpaces the neu-*

trophils. Moreover, the emigration of monocytes is dependent on neutrophils. A factor derived from these cells induces the emigration of monocytes. If animals are rendered neutropenic, monocyte emigration is inhibited. Although these two waves appear to coincide temporally with the biphasic permeability response of the microcirculation, it is quite clear that the two phenomena are independent. Many studies have shown that the early wave of emigration can be prevented in vessels which are nonetheless abnormally permeable, leaking a protein-rich exudate (Hurley, 1964a). It seems reasonable that the factors involved in leukocyte emigration are the same as, or at least very closely related to, the chemotactic factors detailed below.

For some time it was thought that lymphocytes did not leave vessels through interendothelial gaps. It was thought that, in some extraordinary fashion, they passed through endothelial cells, principally and perhaps solely in the postcapillary venules. It was proposed that endothelial pseudopodia extended out to embrace the adherent lymphocytes and eventually closed over them, thus incorporating them within the endothelial cell (Marchesi and Gowans, 1964). Recent studies by Schoefl (1972) spoil this picaresque notion. He has recently shown that lymphocytes use the same prosaic routes as do neutrophils.

Red cells may also leave blood vessels particularly in severe injuries. Unlike the white cell, the red cell seems to be passively and unwillingly shoved out of the leaky, injured vessels by intraluminal pressure in the wake of emigrating leukocytes—a process known as *diapedesis.* Such red cell diapedesis accounts for the development of hemorrhagic exudates in the more severe inflammatory reactions.

CHEMOTAXIS

Chemotaxis may be defined as the unidirectional migration of white cells toward an attractant. Granulocytes, including eosinophils and basophils, monocytes and, to a lesser extent, lymphocytes, respond to such stimuli. Once outside of their vascular imprisonment, they migrate at varying rates of speed to the inflammatory focus. Although there is still some question about the influences which control white cell migration, most investigators believe that cells are drawn to sites of injury by chemotactic influences (Hurley, 1964b). While the existence of such factors has been known for a long time, their clear delineation awaited the development of the micropore filter technique of Boyden

(1962). Leukocytes can be enclosed in one portion of a chamber, separated from the chemotactic substance by a millipore filter, and the migration of the leukocytes across the filter in response to the chemotactic influence can be readily identified and quantified. Furthermore, it can be shown that when different concentrations of the chemotactic factor are present on both sides of the filter the leukocytes will migrate in the direction of the greater concentration (Keller and Sorkin, 1968). The responsiveness of leukocytes to concentration gradients of chemotactic factors may readily explain why these cells continue to migrate until they reach the center of the inflammatory arena.

Some chemotactic factors operate on only polymorphonuclear leukocytes, others only on mononuclear cells, while a few affect both types of white cells. The term mononuclear cell is here used to refer to monocytes and macrophages. We shall soon discuss the origin of macrophages (p. 73). It will suffice at this point to indicate that, although a subject of some debate, it is generally believed that macrophages transform from blood monocytes which are, of course, marrow-derived. Known to be active on the polymorphonuclears are (1) the activated trimolecular complex of complement (C5, 6 and 7), (2) a plasmin-split fragment of C3, (3) fragments of C3 which are found after cleavage by tissue proteases and (4) soluble bacterial factors which can be isolated from filtrates of a variety of organisms including *Staphylococcus aureus*, *Diplococcus pneumoniae*, *E. coli*, *Proteus mirabilis*, *Pseudomonas aeruginosa* and alpha and beta hemolytic streptococci. Collectively, these bacterial agents represent the major pathogens of man. Ward (1970), in a recent study, suggested that a fragmentation product of the fifth component of complement, C5, may also be an attractant to polymorphonuclear leukocytes.

Specifically active for monocytes and macrophages but not neutrophils is a factor derived from serum treated with immune complexes. It is not the trimolecular complex of complement or a lysate of polymorphonuclears. An additional soluble factor that is chemotactic for monocytes and macrophages is derived from sensitized lymphocytes when activated by antigen release. This last factor could explain the aggregation of these mononuclears in hypersensitivity reactions. There are two factors to which both cell types respond: plasmin-split products of serum and the soluble bacterial factors already mentioned (Ward, 1968a and 1968b).

Several points are worthy of emphasis at this time. Complement plays a vital role in the massing of leukocytes at sites of inflammation. The chemotactic influences for mononuclears are critically dependent on polymorphonuclear leukocytes; indeed, in the clinical disorder, cyclic neutropenia, mononuclear aggregation at inflammatory sites does not develop during periods of neutropenia. An additional point of interest relates to the activated trimolecular complex of complement (C5, 6 and 7). This can be activated by immune complexes which evoke a sequential interaction of the first seven components of complement. But, in addition, this trimolecular complex may also be activated by esterases contained within polymorphonuclears. There are many suggestions that such enzymes are granule-bound and are found within the lysosomes of these white cells. It has been known for some time that steroids such as hydrocortisone and prednisolone have an anti-inflammatory effect, and it is highly likely that this is exerted by the stabilization of the membranes of lysosomes, thus blocking the release of those enzymes involved in the activation of complement (Ward, 1966).

Little is known about chemotactic influences for lymphocytes. Indeed, straight-line directed movement of lymphocytes to attractant substances has not been observed. Yet, if lymphocytes are sensitized to certain tissue cells, they cluster about these target cells when both are admixed in tissue culture flasks. The basis for this "togetherness" is obscure and, to date, no agents have been identified which will operate in the Boyden millipore chamber (Hersh and Bodey, 1970).

In concluding this discussion of chemotaxis, it is somewhat anticlimactic to interpose the cautionary note that, despite all of the evidence derived from in vitro systems, there is still some reason to be cautious about extrapolating these observations to the in vivo inflammatory response. There are still those who believe that, in the living animal, white cell migration is random, is not under the influence of chemotactic factors, and that the accumulation of white cells at sites of inflammation results from inhibition of migration once they have stumbled into the inflammatory focus (Harris, 1954).

AGGREGATION

Aggregation of white cells at the usual inflammatory focus follows a quite predictable pattern. Indeed, the accumulation of these immigrant leukocytes at a site of injury comprises a major morphologic hallmark of inflammation. Most agents such as staphylococci, streptococci, coliforms, and thermal and chemical injury evoke an initial neutrophil response in the acute phase of the inflammatory reaction; but in the later chronic stage of the response, monocytes, macrophages and lymphocytes come to predominate. This pattern is, however, not invariable and, in the inflammatory response to the tubercle bacillus and to immunologic injury, macrophages and lymphocytes predominate almost from the outset. Lymphocytes are particularly associated with immunology-induced injury and, in this context, receive major consideration in Chapter 7 dealing with disorders of immunity.

There are many reasons for the fairly predictable sequence of leukocytic aggregation at the site of an inflammation. While granulocytes and macrophages emigrate simultaneously, the granulocyte is more motile and so may arrive at the inflammatory site first. In addition, these cells are present in greater numbers in the circulating blood. They also emigrate over a shorter span of time than do the mononuclears. In the Boyden chamber, these cells require only 90 minutes to complete their chemotactic response. In contrast, mononuclear cells do not achieve maximal concentrations until five or more hours have elapsed. The rate of arrival of polymorphonuclears diminishes after the first few days, while the influx of mononuclear cells remains constant for weeks (Spector et al., 1967). Polymorphonuclear leukocytes are short-lived (3 to 4 days) and, unless their numbers are maintained by constant immigration, they progressively fall behind in the inflammatory white cell population. Moreover, the death of polymorphs releases enzymes which activate factors, chemotactic for mononuclear cells. In addition to all of these influences, it has been shown that mononuclear cells outnumber neutrophils in the later phases of the inflammatory reaction because some can persist in a functional state for months without dividing, and others that are more short-lived are capable of local proliferation (Spector, 1967) (Fig. 3–3).

PHAGOCYTOSIS

Phagocytosis and the release of powerful catalytic enzymes by both neutrophils and macrophages comprise two of the major benefits derived from the aggregation of leukocytes at the inflammatory focus (Zucker-Franklin, 1968). Turning first to the release of enzymes, it is well known that the lysosomal granules of neutrophils are rich in a wide variety of catalytic enzymes (see p. 72) as well as in less well characterized products such as phagocytin

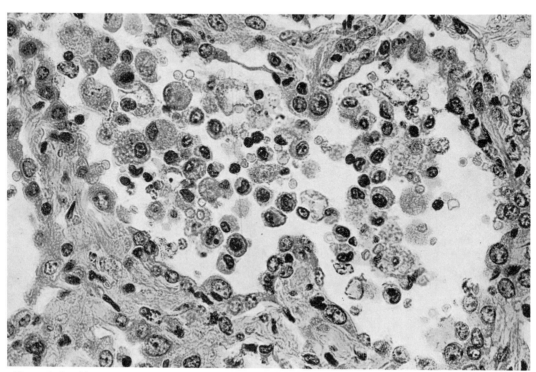

Figure 3–3. Monocytes and macrophages in an alveolus of the lung. The cells are slightly distended and the cytoplasm is granular and contains necrotic debris.

and bactericidal proteins (Weissmann, 1967) (Zeya and Spitznagel, 1968). These enzymes and antibacterial products are central to the bactericidal effectiveness of the phagocytic capacity of neutrophils. Monocytic granules, though less thoroughly characterized, also contain catalytic enzymes. These enzymes assume importance in two ways. Death of the leukocytes releases them into the site of inflammation where they may destroy susceptible invaders, but they also aid in the digestion of dead immigrant and native tissue cells.

Phagocytosis of particulate matter involves surface attachment of the leukocyte to the particle, engulfment, formation of a phagocytic vacuole and fusion of this vacuole with lysosomes, exposing the imprisoned object to the action of the lysosomal contents (Hirsch, 1962). This sequence of events is particularly important in the defense against bacterial invasion. In the course of this action, the neutrophil and the monocyte become progressively degranulated. The energy consumed in phagocytosis is derived from glycolytic pathways (Douglas, 1970). Inhibition of glycolysis significantly depresses phagocytosis, whereas inhibition of aerobic respiration is of much less consequence.

While both neutrophils and monocytes are active scavenger cells, the monocyte appears to be less fastidious in its dietary tastes (Cline and Lehrer, 1968). Certain matter such as polystyrene particles, red cells coated with antibody, certain bacteria and most fungi are readily engulfed by macrophages but not by neutrophils (Fig. 3–4). The macrophage then is the principal scavenger in clearing the inflammatory focus. These cells also have the major responsibility for the removal of the carcasses of their former allies, the neutrophils, which have made the supreme sacrifice in the defensive effort.

A number of influences modify the vulnerability of bacteria to engulfment. Perhaps the most important is the phenomenon of opsonization. *Opsonins* are naturally occurring and acquired substances which coat bacteria and render them more susceptible to phagocytosis. Included among these substances are IgG, IgM, complement components, noncomplement thermolabile factors and some polypeptides including lysozyme and basic polyamino acids (Rabinovitch, 1968). Indeed, certain opsonins are required for certain particles and bacterial species. As will be noted, some antibodies serve as opsonins, accounting in some part for the more effective defense of the body against organisms to which some immunity has been developed.

While phagocytosis may occur over a wide

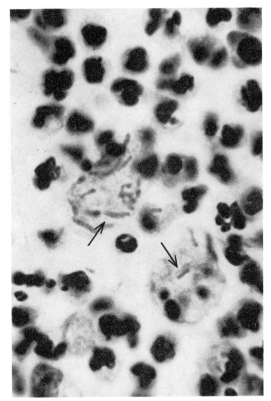

Figure 3–4. *Phagocytized bacteria within macrophages (arrows). The surrounding cells are neutrophils.*

pH range, it is favored by higher body temperatures. Febrile reactions in inflammations thus favor this phenomenon. Trapping of bacteria between some barrier and the scavenger cell facilitates phagocytosis by permitting a more firm attachment between the cell and its prey. For this reason, fibrin strands in an inflammatory exudate provide an effective support to the phagocytic process. This phenomenon becomes especially important in the lungs where the large alveolar spaces permit bacteria to escape the leukocytes until they become enmeshed in the fibrin coagulum (Wood et al., 1946). Bacteria vary in their susceptibility to phagocytosis. In general, the more virulent the organism, the more likely will it resist phagocytosis. Indeed, the virulence is often related to the presence of outer polysaccharide capsules which, in some way, hamper or even block phagocytosis.

Once a microorganism has been engulfed, what is its fate? Most are readily killed by the scavenger cells. Some, however, are sufficiently virulent to destroy their captor. Others, such as the tubercle bacillus, appear to survive happily within the phagocyte. Indeed, the persistence of organisms within phagocytes poses a problem in the eradication of such infections as tuberculosis. Thus enclosed, the microorganism is protected against the action of antibacterial drugs as well as other defense mechanisms. When these phagocytic cells migrate through lymphatic pathways, infections such as tuberculosis may be spread.

The significance of phagocytosis in the body's defense against bacterial infections is attested to by the vulnerability of patients who suffer from a deficiency of circulating white cells. Such clinical disorders as agranulocytosis, cyclic neutropenia, leukemia, and toxic depression of the bone marrow resulting either from radiotherapy or immunosuppressive chemotherapy are all associated with a markedly increased vulnerability to microbiologic infections. Such infections often cause the death of these predisposed individuals. In closing this discussion of phagocytosis, it should be remembered that the reticuloendothelial cells are also phagocytic, as is indicated in a later section.

CHEMICAL MEDIATORS OF THE INFLAMMATORY RESPONSE

Injury precipitates the inflammatory response but released chemicals mediate it. Their existence was long suspected for two reasons: (1) Whatever the nature of the injury, the ensuing inflammatory changes comprise a fairly uniform, almost stereotyped, reaction; and (2) the inflammatory process develops without apparent alteration in tissues deprived of their nervous connections. The search for mediators was given a major impetus in 1927 by Sir Thomas Lewis' description of his now classic "triple response." He pointed out that when the skin of a normal individual is firmly stroked by a dull instrument such as the tip of a lead pencil or the edge of a ruler, three separable changes can be observed. First, within seconds, a *dull red line* develops along the line of the stroke. It is followed by the second component, namely, the development of a bright red halo, often called the *flare*, about the stroke mark. Soon thereafter, the third feature appears—*swelling (edema)*—accompanied by blanching of the original stroke mark. This swelling is often described as a *wheal*. Lewis further observed that the flare, but neither the stroke mark nor the subsequent wheal, could be abolished by interruption of nervous pathways to the site. He postulated the release of a humoral histamine-like substance as the cause of the first and third components of the triple response and correctly attributed the flare to neurogenic reflex inhibition of vasoconstrictive impulses.

Some years later, it became apparent that histamine could not explain all the features of the inflammatory response. Indeed, histamine disappeared very early in the acute reaction and therefore could not explain its later phases. The active search for other mediators has uncovered a perplexing multitude of candidates. Now the questions must be asked: How many are significant in man, and what is the role of each? The best characterized of these mediators can be divided into four groups (Whilhelm, 1962).

1. Amines
    Histamine
    5-Hydroxytryptamine (serotonin)
    Inactivation of epinephrine and nor-epinephrine
2. Kinins
    Bradykinin (9 amino acids)
    Lysyl-bradykinin (10 amino acids)
3. Protein and Tissue Extracts
    Globulin permeability factor of Miles
    Cleavage fragments of complement
    Lymph node permeability factor
    Extracts of rabbit leukocytes (lysosomal cationic proteins, proteases)
4. Miscellaneous Group
    SRS (slow-reacting substance)
    Lysolecithin
    Esterases of complement

Histamine is generally conceded to be the principal mediator of the immediate inflammatory response to injury. It is stored and immediately available largely in the granules of mast cells and in platelets. More is said about this release in the later discussion of these cells (p. 73). Some may be synthesized at the inflammatory site by the decarboxylation of histidine. Local synthesis, however, would hardly explain its prompt appearance immediately following injury (Spector and Willoughby, 1964a). It causes dilation of arterioles and venules, constriction of veins and increased permeability principally in the venules. It has little effect on leukocyte function and does not participate in the escape of white cells from the micro-circulation. When antihistaminics are administered prior to the induction of injury, the immediate inflammatory response is delayed and, in fact, may be abolished (Wilhelm, 1962). This mediator has been isolated from the early phase of the acute inflammatory response, but it soon disappears and so is not believed to participate in the later, delayed phase of increased permeability (Kahlson and Rosengren, 1968).

Serotonin (5-hydroxytryptamine) causes vasodilation and increased permeability of the microcirculation only in the rat and mouse (Zweifach, 1964). In most species, including man, it is doubtful that mast cells contain significant amounts of 5-hydroxytryptamine, and so this agent probably plays little if any role in the inflammatory response in man.

Epinephrine and norepinephrine may play an indirect role in the inflammatory process. The catecholamines cause vasoconstriction and so, when administered prior to injury, inhibit the acute vascular phase of the inflammatory response. Conceivably, the destruction of epinephrine and norepinephrine by enzymes, such as monoamine oxidase released at the site of injury, might produce the vascular dilation and increased permeability encountered in the inflammatory response (Spector and Willoughby, 1964*b*).

The consensus is that *kinins* are major influences in the acute inflammatory response. They comprise a group of polypeptides (at least five have been identified in plasma) which dilate arterioles, increase vascular permeability, induce pain when injected subcutaneously or applied to the base of a blister, and cause margination of leukocytes within vessels (Lewis, 1964). In short, they reproduce many of the manifestations of the inflammatory response. The two most important are bradykinin, possessing nine amino acids and lysylbradykinin (kallidin), having ten amino acids. They occur naturally in the plasma in the form of inactive precursors called kininogens found in the alpha-2-globulin fraction. The vasoactive kinins are formed from their inactive precursors by kinin-forming proteases, principally plasma kallikrein. But this last mentioned kinin-forming enzyme also exists in inactive form in the blood plasma and so it too must be activated.

A number of pathways have been proposed for the activation of kallikrein. Plasmin activates it, as will simple dilution of plasma. Histamine might well provide such dilution by increasing vascular permeability, producing an inflammatory transudate in which the kallikrein precursors would undergo dilution. Hageman factor, one of the many clotting factors activated after escaping into the tissues, also releases kinins by activating the kinin-forming enzyme, kallikrein. It has also been suggested that histamine might directly activate the precursor of kallikrein. Alternatively, the inactive precursors of the kinins, kallikrein and Hageman factor may all enter the perivascular tissue spaces as the histamine-induced permeability of the microcirculation increases, thus sequentially activating Hageman factor, kallikrein and eventually the kinins (Zachariae et al., 1969). This sequence concurs with the observation that both histamine and the kinins are found together in major concentrations in the inflammatory fluids of the early response.

However, neither histamine nor the kinins persist very long in inflamed tissues and so could not mediate the delayed phase of the response.

The *globulin permeability factor* was described by Miles in 1961. Dilution of plasma by saline activates a factor in the globulin fraction which causes increased vascular permeability. Hence, this factor is often referred to as PF/dil. This globulin may also be activated through the participation of Hageman factor, suggesting the possibility that PF/dil and the kinins may be closely related or even identical and, indeed, PF/dil may participate in the activation of the kinins.

Several *cleavage fractions of the third and fifth components of complement constitute anaphylotoxins* (p. 219) which have the ability to increase vascular permeability indirectly by causing release of histamine from mast cells (Dias da Silva et al., 1967). Lysosomal cationic proteins (probably the pyrogenic factor) and proteases have been proposed as mediators of the early phase of the inflammatory process. These may be particularly important in immunologic injury in which neutrophils ingest immune complexes and then are destroyed or release their lysosomal contents. Patients suffering from a deficiency of circulating neutrophils often manifest a delayed and reduced inflammatory response. Extracts of the granules of neutrophils induce vasodilation and increased permeability of the microcirculation. Some of this action may result from the release of cationic proteins which have been shown to increase directly vascular permeability. Conceivably, the proteases could participate in two ways: by activation of kinin precursors or by direct injury to endothelial cells. Whether such agents are involved in the inflammatory process in man is not well established. However, we must still explain how these lysosomal enzymes are first released by injury; and here we come to a blank wall.

All the mediators mentioned up to this point are postulated as effectors of the early phase of the inflammatory reaction and thus are involved in the first wave of increased vascular (principally venular) permeability (Fig. 3–5). As mentioned earlier, in experimental models the increased vascular permeability and edema may be shown to follow a biphasic pattern. What can be said of mediators of the delayed phase of the reaction? Here we come to a controversial issue. Several mediators have been proposed but are far less well characterized than histamine and bradykinin and, indeed, none can be singled out clearly as a proven mediator of the delayed reaction. There is a strong suspicion that this delayed phase of vascular permeability results from

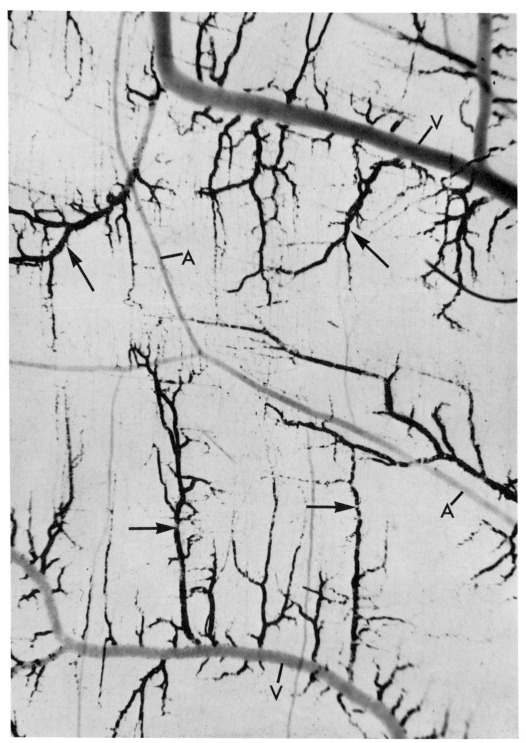

Figure 3–5. *Vascular leakage as induced by histamine, serotonin, bradykinin and PF/dil (Miles factor). This is a laminar muscle of the rat (cremaster), fixed, cleared in glycerin, and examined unstained, by transillumination. One hour prior to sacrifice, bradykinin was injected over this muscle, and colloidal carbon was given intravenously; bradykinin caused small gaps to appear between endothelial gaps in some vessels (see Fig. 3–2). Plasma, loaded with carbon, escaped; but most of the carbon particles were retained by the basement membrane of the leaking vessels, with the result that these became "labeled" in black. Note that not all the vessels leak—only the venules, and then only within a certain caliber range. The mechanism of this selectivity is not yet known. A = arteriole; V = small vein; arrows point to blackened, leaking venules. The capillary network is very faintly visible in the background. (Courtesy of Dr. Guido Majno, Department of Pathology, Harvard Medical School.)*

slowly developing, direct damage to endothelial cells caused by the injury itself. Despite this view, Willoughby and Spector (1964) described a factor, isolated from lymph nodes of animals exhibiting delayed hypersensitivity, which they termed *lymph node permeability factor*. They suggest that it plays a role in the delayed increased vascular permeability encountered in certain inflammatory processes of immunologic origin. An agent termed *slow reacting substance (SRS-A)*, which may be derived from neutrophils, when injected subcutaneously into appropriate experimental animals, increases vascular permeability after some delay. Another fraction, derived from the granules of rabbit neutrophils, which may be identical to the fever-inducing *endogenous pyrogen*, produces an increase of vascular permeability after a delay of about 45 minutes (Moses et al., 1964). *Lysolecithin* has also been suggested as a delayed mediator of the inflammatory response. Cotran and Majno (1964) demonstrated that injection of dilute solutions of lysolecithin induces increased permeability in venules and capillaries after some delay. Lysolecithin is of particular interest since it may be released by complement which is often present in inflammatory sites.

In summation, the multiplicity of proposed mediators is eloquent testimony to the fact that we still are unsure of the precise events involved in activation of the inflammatory response. No single unifying concept fits all of the collected observations. Best established is the fact that histamine plays a key role in the immediate response to injury. The kinins, particularly bradykinin, are also reasonably well established as mediators of this early acute reaction. It would be rational to propose that histamine-induced increased vascular permeability potentiates the escape of the kinin precursors into extravascular spaces where they are activated by simple dilution, by the Hageman-kallikrein system or by proteases derived from lysosomes. What then can be said of the other mediators? All is highly conjectural. Perhaps they are involved in special forms of inflammation, and agents such as the fractions of complement, SRS and lymph node permeability factor may be restricted in their roles as mediators to inflammatory responses of immunologic origin.

SUMMARY OF THE ACUTE INFLAMMATORY RESPONSE

The discussion of mediators culminates the basic description of the relatively stereotyped pattern of the inflammatory reaction encountered in most injuries. Recall that although hemodynamic, permeability and white cell changes have been described sequentially and may be initiated in this order, in the fully evolved reaction to injury, all of these phenomena are concurrent in a seemingly chaotic but remarkably organized multi-ring circus. As might be expected, many variables may modify this basic process. Particularly important are (1) nature and intensity of the injury, (2) site and tissue affected and (3) responsiveness of the host—nutrition, adequacy of the cardiovascular system, drug therapy, existence of predisposing disorders such as diabetes mellitus and cancer, and the possible presence of previously acquired immunity to the offender if it is indeed microbiologic in origin. These modifying influences will soon be considered. Table 3–1 highlights some of the principal characteristics of the inflammatory response in schematic form.

CELLS OF THE INFLAMMATORY EXUDATE

The basic types of white cells that take part in inflammatory reactions are (1) polymorphonuclear leukocytes or granulocytes (neutrophils, eosinophils, basophils), (2) monocytes, (3) lymphocytes and (4) plasma cells. All of these leukocytes, save the plasma cells, are normal inhabitants of the circulating blood. In the normal adult, the white cell count ranges from 4000 to 11,000 cells per mm.[3], having the following distribution (differential count): neutrophils, 50 to 65 per cent; eosinophils, 1 to 5 per cent; basophils, 0 to 1 per cent; lymphocytes, 30 to 40 per cent; and monocytes, 4 to 8 per cent. The total leukocyte count and the relative proportions of the various white cells may be materially modified in systemic responses to inflammation. Each cell type plays a fairly distinctive role and enters into the inflammatory response in a definite sequence as already indicated. The following discussion will concern itself principally with the morphologic and biochemical characteristics of these leukocytes.

NEUTROPHILS

These cells are usually the first to gather in the acute inflammatory response in which they play a key role. Unless otherwise designated, the terms poly and granulocyte are generally used as synonyms for neutrophilic polymorphonuclear leukocyte. Their morphologic features in usual preparations are too well known to require much detail. It is enough to say that they range from 10 to 12 microns in diameter

TABLE 3-1. SUMMARY OF THE ACUTE INFLAMMATORY RESPONSE

Temporal Sequence	Mediator	Site	Hemodynamic Changes	Permeability Changes	White Cell Changes	Visible Change
Immediate (transient:) 0 to 5 min.	Neurogenic	Arterioles	Vasoconstrictive ischemia	None	None	Blanching
Early Phase: 5 to 30 min.	Histamine ?Serotonin	Arterioles	Vasodilation	Increased	None	Rubor (redness) Calor (heat) Dolor (pain) Tumor (swelling)
	Kinins Proteases Miles factor Globulin permeability factor Complement esterases Other mediators	Venules and capillaries	New channels opened Engorgement— overall increase in blood flow	Increased— endothelial joints opened	Pavementing Adhesion Beginning emigration	
Delayed Phase: ½ to 2 hr.	?Lysolecithin ?Protein products Leukocyte emigrating factors	Venules Capillaries	Engorgement— overall increase in blood flow	Increased	Emigration Perivascular leukocyte aggregation	As above Formation of fluid and cellular exudate

and contain abundant granules which are neither eosinophilic nor basophilic—hence the designation neutrophil. In actual fact, three classes of granules have been identified, each of which has a distinctive profile of enzymes. All the enzymes are essentially catalytic, and so all the granules represent forms of lysosomes (Douglas, 1970).

Principal among the lysosomal enzymes are alkaline phosphatase, proteases, DNase, RNase and beta glucuronidase. In addition, these granules contain phagocytin and lysozyme which have specific antibacterial activity (Cohn and Hirsch, 1960). Extracts of the lysosomes of neutrophils derived from inflammatory responses have also been demonstrated to contain cationic basic proteins, which comprise a permeability factor, and pyrogens. But perhaps the major roles of neutrophils in the inflammatory response involve their participation in phagocytosis, the release of their lytic lysosomal enzymes and the formation of chemotactic factors. The trimolecular complex of complement (C5, 6 and 7) is activated by two neutrophilic esterases to yield an attractant for neutrophils. In addition, mononuclear cells respond to lysates of neutrophils, possibly to the liberated cationic peptides of lysosomal origin. The neutrophil with its lysosomes is therefore crucial to the entire inflammatory process (Page and Good, 1958).

EOSINOPHILS

Eosinophils are particularly abundant in sites of inflammation in diseases of immunologic origin. As is well known, the eosinophil is distinguished from the neutrophil by the affinity of its coarse cytoplasmic granules for the acid-dye eosin. It is an extremely short-lived cell with a total life span in the range of 8 to 12 days. Most of this brief interval is spent in the marrow, and virtually the entire remaining time is spent in the tissues, particularly the skin, lung and intestinal tract (Sweet, 1969). Its sojourn in the blood may be as short as one hour. The number of eosinophils in the circulating blood varies throughout the day, the highest levels being reached during the evening hours. Steroid hormones are known to induce eosinopenia, and the diurnal variation in the eosinophil count is attributed to the circadian rhythm of adrenal steroid secretion.

The capabilities and function of the eosinophil are still a matter of dispute. There is general agreement that the eosinophil is phagocytic; some would contend that it is as actively phagocytic as the neutrophil while others would say it is less so. The eosinophil responds to the same influences as the neutrophil, including soluble bacterial factors and activated components of complement (Ward, 1969). It is also responsive to antigen-antibody complexes, as was shown by Litt (1964). When antigen is injected into the footpad of guinea pigs, eosinophils appear at the injection site within minutes. This observation has been interpreted as indicating rapid local synthesis of antibody and the formation of chemotactic antigen-antibody complexes. However, the time interval for the response is extremely short, and it is possible that antigen alone may be chemotactic to eosinophils.

The lysosomal granules of the eosinophil contain a wide variety of catalytic enzymes very similar to those in the neutrophil, except that they lack lysozyme and phagocytin. Some investigators have contended that certain of these enzymes degrade histamine, and that the eosinophil represents some form of control mechanism for histamine release (Mann, 1969). Perhaps these antagonistic actions represent a delicate feedback regulation of histamine release. An additional feature of interest has been observed. Following phagocytosis, these cells release lysosomal enzymes as well as a protein substrate that crystallizes to produce Charcot-Leyden crystals which classically appear as two pyramids joined at their bases. These crystals are of interest since they are characteristically found in the sputum of patients with bronchial asthma, a respiratory disease often of allergic origin. Although the eosinophil is somewhat of a mystery cell, when present in inflammatory responses an allergic or immune causation should be suspected.

BASOPHILS AND MAST CELLS

These two cell forms are very closely related and have many similarities such as cytoplasm that is literally loaded with coarse granules which appear blue-black in usual blood stains. The granules are also metachromatic (they stain pink to blue with such stains as toluidine blue) because of their rich content of sulfated mucopolysaccharides, principally heparin. The basophil is of marrow origin and is a rare member of the white cell population of the blood. In the size and shape of their nuclei, they closely resemble neutrophils. In contrast, mast cells are granular connective tissue cells found throughout the connective tissues in virtually every organ in man. Mast cells are most numerous about small blood vessels and in serous membranes. They are slightly larger, and tend to have more polymorphous nuclei and somewhat more abundant cytoplasm than the basophil (Cruickshank et al., 1968). Both the basophil and the mast cell in man have been described as unicellular secretory glands. Their granules contain heparin,

histamine, as well as other proteolytic enzymes, some of which are chymotrypsin-like. After the release of these products, the cells become degranulated (Horsfield, 1965). In animals, they are also rich in serotonin, but human mast cells and basophils are devoid of this bioamine. These cells are intimately involved in the pathogenesis of some immunologic diseases since it is their release of histamine which triggers many of the manifestations arising from smooth muscle contraction and edema formation.

MONOCYTES AND MACROPHAGES

There is virtually unanimous agreement that the macrophages so prominent in the inflammatory reaction are derived from monocytes of marrow origin. This conclusion was first set on a solid foundation by Ebert and Florey (1939). Since that time, the use of isotopic labels such as tritiated thymidine has confirmed the identity of the blood monocyte and the tissue macrophage (Spector, 1969b).

All studies have invalidated the older concept that, under certain circumstances, small lymphocytes might become transformed to macrophages. Such a statement, however, does not preclude the possibility that, in immunologic reactions, lymphocytes may become enlarged and closely resemble macrophages. But with regard to our present concerns, in the inflammatory response, we may conclude that the macrophage is a transformed monocyte. Both of these cell types are slightly larger than neutrophils and, in routine tissue stains, possess a gray-blue cytoplasm filled with very fine granules. Their nuclei are large, usually centrally placed, and may be folded or bean shaped (Fig. 3–6). In the monocyte, the chromatin is scattered in a fine skein-like or lacy pattern, and nucleoli are not evident. Ultrastructurally, small cytoplasmic pseudopodia project from the margins of monocytes. The macrophage is virtually identical but contains more lysosomes, often has one or two small nucleoli and, at high resolution, has longer pseudopodia than the monocyte.

Ultrastructural changes in the course of transformation of monocytes to macrophages have been elegantly detailed by Sutton and Weiss (1966). Within inflamed tissues, the macrophages almost invariably contain phagocytic inclusions (phagosomes) that enclose bacteria and cell debris as well as lipid residues. In the course of such phagocytic orgies, these cells become swollen and ballooned. The major function of the macrophage has already been

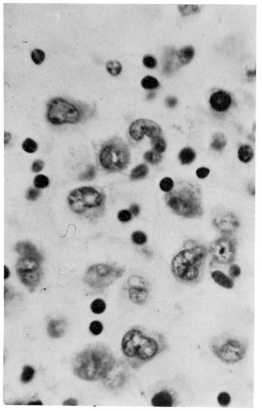

Figure 3-6. *High power detail of monocytes and macrophages in tissues. Note the bean-shaped and indented nuclei.*

tional mechanism of origin (Sutton and Weiss, 1966) (Spector, 1969*b*). These giant cells may achieve diameters of 40 to 50 microns and contain as many as 50 small nuclei. Two types are recognized. In the foreign body type, the nuclei are scattered erratically throughout the cytoplasm. In the Langhans' type, the nuclei are disposed about the periphery of the cell either in a complete circle or in a horseshoe-shaped pattern (Fig. 3-7). Classically, it has been taught that the Langhans' type giant cell is found in granulomatous inflammations, particularly those caused by the tubercle bacillus. The foreign body type with scattered nuclei is found whenever there is a large foreign structure such as a fragment of suture, wood, glass, steel or some crystalline material too large to be engulfed by a single macrophage (Fig. 3-8). Actually, there is no such sharp division between the settings in which these two forms are encountered, and little value in differentiating between the Langhans' and foreign body type giant cells. Both, however, should not be confused with tumor giant cells which have a very different morphology and clinical significance.

LYMPHOCYTES AND PLASMA CELLS

Both of these cell forms are principally involved in immune reactions and are the key mediators of both the immediate antibody response and the delayed hypersensitivity response. As such, they are discussed in detail in Chapter 7. Their roles in nonimmunologic injuries and inflammation remain very much a mystery. They appear late, usually in the chronic phase of most inflammations, and are particularly prominent in tuberculosis, syphilis, other granulomatous diseases and in viral and rickettsial infections (Fig. 3-9). Neither cell type is phagocytic, at least not for bacteria (Harris, 1953). Lymphocytes are less motile than are neutrophils and monocytes. The responsiveness of the lymphocyte to chemotactic agents is still uncertain as was cited on p. 65. It can only be speculated that the appearance of lymphocytes and plasma cells in chronic inflammations may reflect some local immunologic reaction which has evolved in the course of the long chronicity of the inflammatory response.

SYSTEMIC CHANGES IN WHITE CELLS

Inflammatory states, whatever their causation, if sufficiently intense or protracted to cause constitutional signs such as fever and malaise, almost invariably modify the white cell population of the blood. Most evoke an abso-

discussed on p. 67. These cells are sluggishly motile but are responsive to chemotactic influences. They are the major scavengers in the inflammatory site.

As was indicated earlier, monocytes and hence macrophages begin to accumulate very early in the inflammatory response. Both neutrophils and monocytes emigrate simultaneously, but the migration of the former occurs over a shorter time span and so macrophages dominate the inflammatory white cell population in the later phases of the reaction. They have a longer life span than do neutrophils and, indeed, macrophages may grow and divide at sites of protracted inflammation, accounting for their large numbers in longstanding reactions (Spector, 1968).

Whenever foreign bodies too large to be engulfed by a single macrophage are present in an inflammatory site, multinucleate giant cells are formed. Sutton and Weiss (1966) believe that a giant cell is formed by the coalescence of macrophages. Quite recently, DNA synthesis has been observed in the nuclei of these cells, suggesting that mitotic division without cytoplasmic cleavage may be an addi-

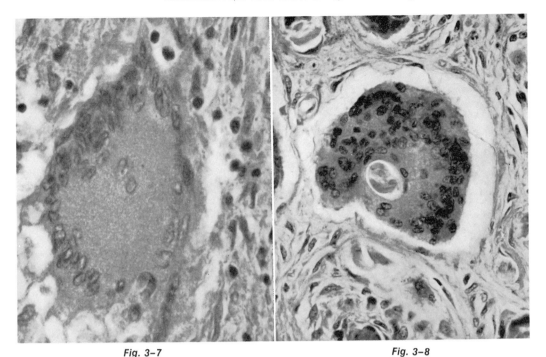

Fig. 3-7   Fig. 3-8

Figure 3-7. Detail of a Langhans' type giant cell in the margin of a tubercle.
Figure 3-8. Detail of a foreign body type giant cell containing a foreign body.

lute increase in the number of white cells (leukocytosis). The count may climb to 40,000 leukocytes per mm.³ of blood and, in rare instances, may achieve the extraordinary level of 100,000. The extreme elevations are referred to as leukemoid reactions since they simulate the white counts obtained in leukemia. The leukocytosis of acute inflammation is usually due to an absolute increase in the number of neutrophils, at the same time increasing their relative proportion in the differential count.

While most bacterial infections induce *neutrophilia*, infectious mononucleosis, whooping cough, mumps, German measles and undulant fever are exceptions and produce a leukocytosis by virtue of an absolute increase in the number of lymphocytes (*lymphocytosis*). On occasion, the absolute increase in the number of lymphocytes may be more than compensated for by a decrease in the neutrophils so that the total white count is not elevated. In an additional group of disorders such as bronchial asthma, hay fever, parasitic infestations and in many of the systemic necrotizing angiitides, there is an absolute increase in the number of circulating eosinophils, creating an *eosinophilia*. Generally, the magnitude of the eosinophilia is sufficient to raise the relative proportion of these cells in the differential count but it is not sufficient to induce a significant elevation of the total white count.

Certain systemic inflammatory states such as typhoid fever, paratyphoid fever, infections caused by viruses, rickettsiae and certain protozoal infestations decrease the number of circulating white cells (*leukopenia*). Leukopenia is also encountered in infections which over-

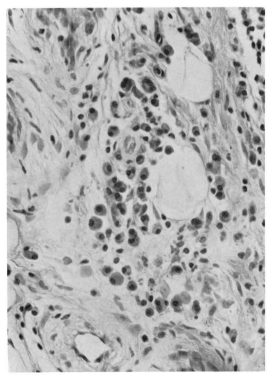

Figure 3-9. Plasma cells in tissue section.

whelm patients debilitated by disseminated cancer or rampant miliary tuberculosis. Under these circumstances, it is theorized that the massive assault upon the body depresses leukopoiesis.

The mediators and pathogenesis of the leukocytosis in inflammatory states are still poorly understood. The search for humoral stimulators has been in progress for almost a hundred years, but with little success. A number of factors have been proposed such as *leukocytosis promoting factor, neutropoietin, leukopoietin G,* as well as others, but none have been proven to be operative in the inflammatory state.

The only well documented humoral influences on the circulating white blood cells are the adrenal steroids. The administration of adrenal corticosteroids or ACTH in the animal with intact adrenals decreases the number of circulating lymphocytes and eosinophils. The mechanism of action of steroids on these white cells is poorly understood, but lymphocytes within lymph nodes as well as those in circulation exhibit pyknosis, karyorrhexis and inhibition of mitosis following the administration of steroids. The effect of these agents on eosinophilic leukocytes has been attributed to both prolongation of mitosis and lengthening of the intermitotic cycle, which slow their production. We are thus left with the fact that certain humoral agents can destroy white cells but none are known with certainty to stimulate white cell production. The origin of the leukocytosis associated with systemic inflammatory reactions is, then, unknown.

ROLE OF LYMPH NODES, LYMPHATICS AND THE RETICULOENDOTHELIAL SYSTEM

The lymphatic and reticuloendothelial systems comprise secondary lines of defense called into play whenever a local inflammatory reaction fails to contain and neutralize injury. The general system of lymphatics and lymph nodes essentially filters and "polices" the extravascular fluids. The reticuloendothelial system subserves this same role in the blood. Lymphoid tissues and lymphatic channels may be involved to some degree in virtually all injuries. In some, such as focal skin infections or minor burns, the involvement is minimal and not clinically manifest; but in more severe injuries, particularly those caused by invasive organisms, these secondary defense lines may be sufficiently implicated to give rise to clinically manifest signs and symptoms. Such involvement may, in fact, portend the spread of the

infection through the lymphatics to the blood. Before discussing these issues in greater detail, it might be well to point out some of their well known anatomic characteristics.

Lymphatics are extremely delicate channels, and are difficult to visualize in ordinary tissue sections because they readily collapse. Lined by fenestrated endothelial cells or continuous endothelium with loose cell junctions, they have a scant basement membrane and virtually no muscular support. Only the thoracic and right lymph ducts have a sufficient muscular and structural integrity to permit isolation by dissection. It has always been a mystery why the lymphatic channels, so dependent on perilymphatic tissues for their support, do not collapse under the pressure of the edema in the regions of inflammatory reactions. Recent studies may have clarified this enigma by demonstrating delicate fibrils attached at right angles to the walls of the lymphatic channels extending into the adjacent tissues (Leak and Burke, 1968). As an exudate is released into the extravascular tissues, fluid pressure mounts and exerts traction on these fibrils, maintaining the patency of the lymphatic channels. The traction may further widen the intercellular junctions and provide more ready access for macromolecules and cells. Commonly, then, in the vicinity of an inflammatory focus, these lymphatics fill with a protein-rich fluid as well as leukocytes and cell debris. Such drainage in the more minor involvements is relatively trivial, contains no organisms and evokes no reaction within either the lymphatic channels or the lymph nodes of drainage.

In more severe injuries, the drainage may contain the offending agent, be it chemical or bacterial. Indeed, certain virulent invasive organisms (e.g., the beta hemolytic streptococci) have a propensity for spreading beyond the confines of the local site of injury to gain access to these secondary structures. The lymphatics may become secondarily inflamed (*lymphangitis*) as may the regional lymph nodes of drainage (*lymphadenitis*). It is not uncommon, therefore, in focal streptococcal infections of the hand, for example, to observe red streaks up the entire arm to the axilla along the lymphatic channels, accompanied by painful enlargement of the axillary lymph nodes. Such nodal enlargement is usually caused by hypertrophy and hyperplasia of the lymphoblasts and reticulum cells in the cortical follicles. These germinal centers thus become enlarged and often their contained phagocytic cells engulf damaged leukocytes, cell debris and bacteria. The reticuloendothelial cells which line the sinuses of the lymph node similarly enlarge and become phagocytically active. This constellation of nodal histologic changes is termed reactive or inflammatory lymphadenitis. Hopefully, these secondary barriers will contain the spread of the infection but, in some instances, they too are overwhelmed and the organisms drain through progressively larger channels to gain access to the vascular circulation, thus inducing a *bacteremia*.

Potentially, bacteremia can seed any and all tissues of the body. The heart valves, meninges, kidneys and joint spaces are favored sites of implantation for blood-borne organisms. In such a fashion, bacterial endocarditis, meningitis, pyelonephritis and septic arthritis may develop, as may so-called metastatic abscesses in any other tissue. In the course of such dissemination, all of the lymphoid tissues of the body become involved, causing generalized lymphadenopathy, enlargement of the spleen (representing an acute splenitis) and enlargement of the liver (due to diffuse involvement of its Kupffer cells). It hardly needs to be pointed out that such spread of an infection represents a serious threat to life and, unless promptly and effectively treated with antibiotics, claims a high mortality.

The reticuloendothelial system (RES) plays a defensive role in bacteremia as well as in other septic assaults. It was characterized by Aschoff as a dispersed system of phagocytic cells capable of taking up dyes or particles from the blood. *These RE cells are found scattered in connective tissue throughout the body within the endothelial linings of blood vessels, but they are most abundant in the spleen, liver, bone marrow and lymph nodes.* Some investigators would include lymphocytes and plasma cells in the RES on the grounds that they are derived from mesenchymal precursors closely related to the fixed RE cells. But since the lymphocyte and plasma cells are not phagocytic, they are generally not considered reticuloendothelial elements.

The function of the reticuloendothelial system appears to be the removal by phagocytosis of "unwanted debris" floating about in the blood. Included are obsolescent or injured red cells, white cells and platelets, bacteria, coagulation products, antigen-antibody complexes and "foreign" macromolecules such as complex lipids and carbohydrates synthesized by the body in some of the inborn errors of metabolism (the basis for the so-called storage diseases). The phagocytosis of particulate matter purposefully introduced into the blood (such as carbon particles and vital dyes) is of course the means by which this system is identified. The Kupffer cells of the liver are the most active in the RES. It has been shown that when carbon particles of about 250 Å in diam-

eter are introduced into the experimental animal, about 80 per cent are removed in the liver.

The capacity of the RES to recognize "foreign" matter is remarkable. When red cells are coated with antibody, they are selectively filtered out by this surveillance system even though such cells do not appear morphologically abnormal. Thus, this system of phagocytic cells becomes extremely active in a wide variety of hemolytic diseases and anemias and in inflammatory reactions.

In some instances, the RES can become overloaded by its phagocytic activity, producing what is referred to as *reticuloendothelial blockade*. Such blockade can only occur if the phagocytic overload is continued and heavy, because these phagocytic cells can digest all biodegradable substances. But for as long as it lasts, it has the serious implication of removing the body's last line of defense, thus exposing all the other tissues of the body to the invader. In a real sense, then, the lymphatic and reticuloendothelial systems are the "ready reserves" called into play when the local inflammatory response is overwhelmed.

FACTORS THAT MODIFY THE INFLAMMATORY REACTION

Having discussed the fundamental events of the inflammatory response and its principal participants, we may now consider the various influences which often modify the course of events. Despite the virtually stereotyped nature of the acute inflammatory response, the extent of the tissue damage as well as its duration significantly modify the basic theme. These variables are dependent on both the invasive agent and the host.

THOSE RELATING TO THE INJURIOUS AGENT

Extent of the Injury. Obviously, small injuries evoke a lesser inflammatory response than large ones. Conditioning the amount of injury are a constellation of influences including the quantity, penetrance, resistance to neutralization and disease-producing potential of the intruder. This last variable involves, for example, the virulence of microbiologic agents, the toxicity of drugs and chemical agents and the cytotoxicity and penetrance of radiant energy. It is impossible to consider in detail all of these modifying influences since it would involve an individual consideration of the myriad of injurious agents lurking in man's environment. A few examples may suffice. A drop of dilute acid is obviously less dangerous than a similar quantity of concentrated acid, and the inflammatory response which follows depends, of course, on the amount of injury produced. On the other hand, repeated exposure to a large amount of dilute acid may be more serious than contact with a drop of concentrated solution. Bacteria vary enormously in their virulence. Many have no ability to produce disease, while others are of low pathogenicity and require great numbers or a predisposed host to evoke an inflammatory response. By contrast, it is said that one tubercle bacillus may produce disease even in the vigorous person. Carbon tetrachloride is more cytotoxic than chloroform. The considerations involved are virtually self-evident and need not be further belabored.

Duration or Persistence of the Injury. A pin prick evokes a trivial inflammatory reaction but an unremoved tiny splinter may cause a persistent, troublesome inflammatory reaction. The cellulose of the splinter resists digestion by the enzymes of the body and so can only be handled by sequestration within foreign body giant cells which, in effect, shield the surrounding cells and tissue from further injurious effects. But the persistence of such an intruder invites secondary bacterial invasion and so the duration of this injurious agent accounts for a far greater inflammatory response than the pin prick which initially may have injured as many cells.

Resistant microbiologic agents perpetuate and accentuate the inflammatory response. Some organisms such as the pneumococcus are resistant to phagocytosis perhaps because they form a capsule. Others, once phagocytosed, appear to live happily within their hapless host as has been described for the tubercle bacillus. Still others elaborate leukocidins which kill and, in some cases, lyse neutrophils. All of these attributes contribute to the persistence of the injury.

In this same context, we should mention susceptibility to therapy and drug resistance. The streptococci, for instance, are extremely vulnerable to penicillin and a number of other chemotherapeutic agents. Thus, infections by these organisms can be rapidly controlled, along with the resultant inflammatory reaction. In contrast, the chemotherapy for tuberculosis must be continued for months, and so one does not encounter a transient tuberculous infection. The development of microbial resistance to antibiotics materially influences the persistence of the agent and the severity of the inflammatory reaction. The staphylococci are the prime examples of organisms which have shown the ability to acquire resistance to commonly used antibiotics (discussed on p. 366),

and so resistant staphylococcal infections comprise serious forms of inflammatory disease. Duration of exposure to the offending agent significantly modifies the extent and nature of the inflammatory response. Some of these differences will be discussed in the later consideration of chronic inflammation.

THOSE RELATING TO THE HOST

The two sides of the inflammatory equation are the injurious agent and the host. A number of host factors significantly modify the inflammatory response. These same influences also come into play in the modification of the reparative response. Since they are discussed in detail on p. 99 it will suffice here merely to cite them: age of the host, nutritional status, hematologic derangements, immunity, underlying systemic disease (such as diabetes mellitus), therapy (particularly with steroids and antibiotics), and adequacy of blood supply.

MORPHOLOGIC PATTERNS OF INFLAMMATION

As the inflammatory response evolves, based on the many variables relating to both host and injurious agent, a variety of distinctive morphologic patterns develop. In every injury, there is variation in the: (1) duration of the inflammatory process, (2) nature of the exudate, a reflection of both the severity and etiology of the injury, (3) specific etiology (cause) of the reaction and (4) location of the injury. For example, we speak of an acute (duration) fibrinous (type of exudate) rheumatic (causation) pericarditis (location). In essence, such characterization specifies the individual inflammatory response. The modifications encountered within each of these four major subgroups are considered separately below.

TYPES OF INFLAMMATION BASED ON DURATION

Inflammations may be extremely short-lived with only an immediate transient response, or they may persist for months and years. They can be classified accordingly as *acute, subacute,* or *chronic.* There are no sharp lines between these divisions since acute inflammations may abate somewhat and become subacute or persist and become chronic. However, it must not be assumed that all subacute and chronic inflammations originate in preexistent acute reactions. Low-grade stimuli or microbiologic agents not possessing strong toxins may incite only subacute or chronic reactions without ever arousing a full-blown acute response. The following descriptions are therefore arbitrary in a sense, and represent the (full-blown) classic stages.

Acute Inflammation. In pathologic terms, *acute inflammation refers to an inflammatory reaction in which the dominant anatomic changes are vascular and exudative.* Therefore it may also be called an exudative inflammation. All non-immunologic acute reactions have in common vascular congestion and proteinous exudation containing variable numbers of neutrophils and macrophages but few, if any, lymphocytes (Fig. 3–10). Immunogenic reactions will demonstrate greater numbers of lymphocytes and macrophages. When nonspecific acute inflammations fail to subside, they accumulate large numbers of lymphocytes and must be considered to have entered a chronic phase. The acute inflammatory responses are manifested by the classic features of inflammation mentioned earlier—i.e., heat, redness, swelling, pain and loss of function. On rare occasion, acute inflammations begin insidiously and evoke few clinical signs or symptoms.

Chronic Inflammation. An injurious agent may persist for weeks to years, thus producing a chronic inflammatory response. From a morphologic viewpoint, *the chronic reac-*

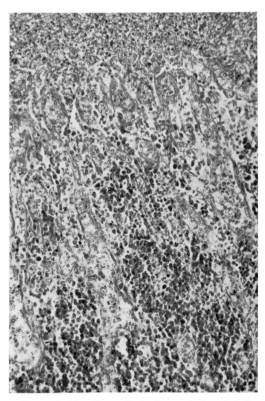

Figure 3–11. *The wall of a focus of chronic inflammation. The center of the focus of inflammation is oriented to the top of the photo and is occupied by necrotic polys and debris, enclosed by a zone of vascularized fibrosis, heavily infiltrated with lymphocytes and plasma cells.*

tion is characterized by a proliferative (fibroblastic) rather than an exudative response. The white cell population is predominantly mononuclear with a mixture of macrophages, lymphocytes and plasma cells. The latter two cell types often outnumber the macrophages. In addition, there is usually proliferation of fibroblasts in the involved stroma, leading to increased cellularity in the margins along with neovascularization (Fig. 3–11). It should be pointed out that, in some chronic inflammations, the persistence of a stronger or resistant irritant results in a continued neutrophilic reaction in the center of the injury, surrounded by a characteristic proliferative chronic inflammatory reaction.

Chronic inflammatory reactions are often followed by considerable scarring, with resultant deformities such as narrowing of the bowel, adhesions between serosal surfaces and permanent fibrous replacement of damaged parenchymal elements such as liver cells or kidney nephrons. Thus, chronic inflammatory reactions usually result in permanent damage to tissues and in persistent scars.

Clinically, chronic inflammation may ei-

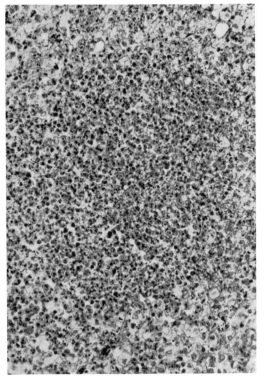

Figure 3–10. *A focus of acute inflammation. Massed polymorphonuclears fill the central region and are surrounded by a zone filled predominantly with macrophages.*

ther result from the perpetuation of an acute process or may begin insidiously as a low-grade, smoldering response which never has the classic features of the acute inflammation. Symptoms may persist for many months or even years as long as the chronic inflammation remains a site of persistent activity.

Subacute Inflammation. This term is uncommonly used in pathology because it is poorly defined. It is described after chronic inflammation because it represents an intergrade between acute and chronic inflammation. Subacute inflammatory foci have some elements of the exudative vascular response, modified by proliferation of fibroblasts and infiltration by eosinophils and the mononuclear inflammatory cells of the chronic reaction.

TYPES OF INFLAMMATION BASED ON CHARACTER OF EXUDATE

The exudates of inflammatory reactions vary in content of fluid, plasma proteins and cells. The precise nature of the exudate is largely dictated by the severity of the reaction and its specific causation. Despite the infinite number of variations that may be encountered, certain repetitive patterns can be segregated and differentiated morphologically.

Serous Exudation. Serous exudation is characterized by the extensive outpouring of a watery, low-protein fluid which, according to the site of injury, is derived from either the blood serum or the secretions of serous mesothelial cells—i.e., the cells lining the peritoneal, pleural and pericardial cavities, and the joint spaces. The skin blister which results from a burn is a simple example of a serous exudate in an inflammatory response (Fig. 3–12). In more specific morphologic terms, the blister represents a large accumulation of serous fluid, either within or immediately beneath the epidermis of the skin. This type of inflammatory exudate is seen early in the developmental phase of most acute inflammatory reactions. Thus it is classically encountered in the early stages of bacterial infections. It is the dominant pattern in mild injuries and is characteristic of certain causative agents such as tuberculous pleuritis, often referred to as pleurisy with effusion.

When the inflammatory reaction progresses and grows more severe, the serous exudate may become transformed to one of the other types to be described. The identification of serous exudation in tissue sections is somewhat difficult. The fluid itself is usually detected by the abnormal spaces it creates between cells in which is found a precipitate of fine, granular material, presumably protein, or

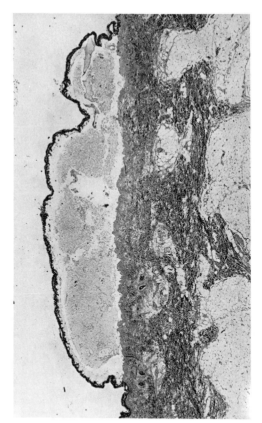

Figure 3--12. *A low power view of a cross section of a skin blister. The epidermis has been lifted off the dermis by the focal collection of fluid.*

by its spreading apart of the cells and fibers in connective tissue.

Fibrinous Exudation. The outpouring of large amounts of plasma proteins, including fibrinogen, and the precipitation of masses of fibrin are characteristic of certain inflammatory responses. This type of exudation tends to occur in the more severe acute inflammations associated with the marked increase of vascular permeability which permits the escape of the large fibrinogen molecule from the blood vessels. It is also characteristic of specific types of inflammation, such as rheumatic involvement of the pericardial cavity. Here the pericardial space may become virtually filled with large masses of fibrin. When the epicardium is stripped from the pericardium, the rubbery, adherent fibrin coats both surfaces, simulating the appearance of two slices of buttered bread when pulled apart (*bread and butter pericarditis*) (Figs. 3–13 and 3–14).

Fibrinous exudation is also quite characteristic of certain forms of bacterial infection in the lungs, such as pneumococcal pneumonia. In this disease, the pulmonary alveoli may be filled with masses of bacteria and white cells

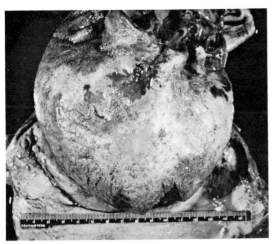

Figure 3–13. *A gross view of the heart with a massive, fibrinous, "bread and butter" pericarditis.*

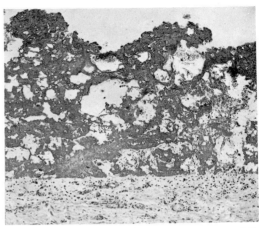

Figure 3–14. *The microscopic appearance of the shaggy amorphous fibrinous exudate.*

trapped within a coagulum of fibrin. Histologically, fibrin is readily identified by its tangled, thread-like eosinophilic meshwork, although it occasionally presents as large masses of solid amorphous eosinophilic coagulum. Cellular exudation usually accompanies this fibrinous exudation and, in almost all instances, the predominant leukocyte is the neutrophil. Fibrinous exudation may also be present in the more active zones of chronic inflammatory responses.

A fibrinous exudate carries implications not encountered with serous exudates. It invites ingrowth of fibroblasts and capillary buds which transform the proteinous precipitate into a vascularized connective tissue, a process referred to as *organization* of the exudate. Organization of a fibrinous pleuritis or pericarditis may obliterate these serosal cavities and hamper the function of the organs now tied down to surrounding structures. This sequence results in obliterative pericarditis or pleuritis. Happily, all fibrinous exudates do not follow such a path, and many are resorbed by fibrinolysis, referred to as *resolution* of the exudate.

Suppurative or Purulent Exudation. This form of inflammation is characterized by the production of large amounts of pus or purulent exudate. Certain organisms (the staphylococci, pneumococci, meningococci, gonococci, coliforms and certain nonhemolytic strains of streptococci) characteristically produce this localized suppuration, and are therefore referred to as pyogenic (pus-producing) bacteria. This type of exudate may be scattered diffusely within tissues, localized within a focus of infection, or spread over the surface of organs or structures. A common example of an acute suppurative inflammation is acute appendicitis. Here masses of polymorphonuclear leukocytes are found diffusely or in focal aggregates throughout the mucosa, submucosa, muscularis and subserosal regions, and coagulated pus may layer the surface as well as fill the lumen (Figs. 3–15 and 3–16). Abscesses (to be described more completely) are an example of a localized suppurative inflammation.

Hemorrhagic Exudation. A hemorrhagic exudate results whenever some form of severe injury causes rupture of vessels or diapedesis of red cells. This is not a distinctive form of exudation and is almost always a basic fibrinous or suppurative exudate, accompanied by the extravasation of large numbers of red cells.

Although the various types of exudative reactions have been described separately, mixed patterns develop in many inflammations and are termed serofibrinous or fibrinopurulent. Moreover, the exudation may begin as a serous response in any single inflammatory reaction and, with extension and increasing severity of the reaction, it may become predominantly fibrinous and ultimately change into a suppurative exudate. It is quite obvious that mixed patterns must be present during the transition stages.

Significant exudation usually denotes an acute response but the exudate may persist into the subacute or chronic stages of the reaction. The presence of fibrin or pus is not, therefore, an absolute indication of acuteness.

PATTERNS OF INFLAMMATORY REACTION BASED ON CAUSATIVE AGENT

Many of the injurious agents, particularly those of microbiologic nature, cause fairly dis-

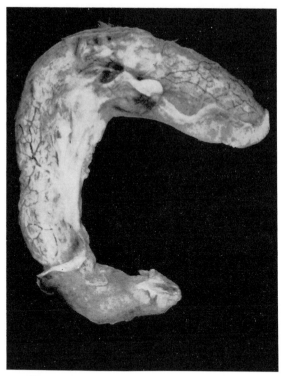

Figure 3–15. *A gross view of acute appendicitis. The covering serosa is heavily layered with a pale fibrinosuppurative exudate.*

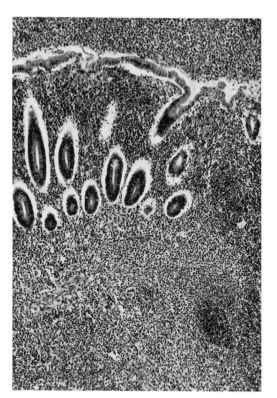

Figure 3–16. *A microscopic detail of the wall of an acute suppurative appendicitis. The lumen above the mucosal epithelium is filled with suppurative exudate and the wall is heavily infiltrated with neutrophils, most evident beneath the zone of mucosal glands.*

tinctive inflammatory reactions. These patterns are sufficiently constant, whatever the site of the reaction, to permit a shrewd guess as to the possible etiology. More accurately, groups of agents cause these distinctive patterns and so, for precise identification of the specific etiology, more exact methods such as bacteriologic or viral isolation must be used. But the morphology provides valuable guidance in such further studies.

Reactions to Pyogens. As has already been discussed, the pyogens (p. 81) classically cause elaboration of thick pus which tends to be confined within the site of implantation. These pyogens include the most common causes of bacterial disease in man. While they may infect any tissue in the body, certain of these organisms have a remarkable organotropism, usually localizing in predictable sites to produce quite characteristic disease. Thus, the Klebsiella enter through the upper respiratory tract, but classically cause widespread lung suppuration known as lobar pneumonia. The meningococci, as would be guessed, cause purulent meningitis although they, too, enter through the nasopharynx. The gonococci principally induce suppurative infections—gonorrhea—within the male and female genital tracts. However, as we shall see later, gonococci and meningococci rarely may infect other sites.

The staphylococci and gram-negative rods are less fastidious in their tastes and so are less predictable in their localization. Staphylococci are the common cause of skin infections, ranging from the trivial *folliculitis* of a skin hair follicle to the *furuncle* (known in layman's terms as a boil) to the more deeply seated larger *carbuncle* (a cluster of furuncles). The gram-negative rods (coliforms) are the common causes of infections within the bladder (cystitis), prostate (prostatitis) and kidneys (acute pyelonephritis). On rare occasion, the staphylococci and gram-negative rods may produce pneumonia or suppurative infections within the meninges, female genital tract, wounds (surgical or traumatic) or any other site where they gain a portal of entry. In addition, all of these pyogens may, as has already been mentioned, invade the blood to cause a bacteremia and seeding of sites that are distant from the primary infection, such as the heart valves, joint spaces or other tissues in the body.

Reactions to Spreading Infections.

Many *streptococci,* although they cause suppurative reactions, produce inflammatory patterns somewhat different from the other pyogens such as the staphylococci and *E. coli.* The highly virulent beta hemolytic Lancefield group A streptococci classically cause spreading infections so that the exudate treks between cells and dissects through the cleavage planes of the intersititial and tissue spaces. This pattern of reaction is referred to as a *cellulitis* or *phlegmon.* Other forms of streptococci, such as the enterococci and nonhemolytic strains, behave as typical pyogens.

The exudate in beta hemolytic infections, although replete with neutrophils, tends to be thin and watery. Here and there, small accumulations collect, but these are quite different from the thick focal aggregations of pus so characteristic of the abscesses caused by the other pyogens. An entire forearm or a large area of the lower extremity or abdominal wall characteristically become edematous, tense, red and painful. This spreading pattern of inflammation is attributed to the elaboration of fibrinolysins (streptokinase) and hyaluronidases by these bacteria which break down the ground substance of connective tissue and so permit the extension of the original nidus of infection. At the same time, these infections readily penetrate lymphatics to produce lymphangitis, lymphadenitis and, all too often, bacteremias. An even more important consequence of beta hemolytic streptococcal infections is their tendency to induce late-developing immunologic reactions, resulting in such extremely grave systemic diseases as diffuse glomerulonephritis (p. 1093) and rheumatic fever (p. 657). Certain of the clostridia, such as *C. botulinum,* cause spreading infections that are more severe than, but basically similar to, the spreading streptococcal infections.

Reactions to Salmonella Organisms.

Infections by the *Salmonella* organisms, the causative agents of typhoid and paratyphoid fevers, are characterized by early bacteremias. These diseases then comprise systemic inflammatory reactions in which the reticuloendothelial system is diffusely involved. This takes the form of swelling and hypertrophy of the RE cells in the spleen, liver and lymphoid tissues throughout the body, often accompanied by multiplication of these cells to produce focal aggregations or nodules of histiocytic cells, most evident throughout the liver. As might be guessed, these cellular changes result in enlargement of the liver, spleen and lymphoid tissues throughout the body.

Reactions to Viruses and Rickettsiae.

Viral and rickettsial infections produce inflammatory changes which are quite distinctive from those caused by bacteria. Classically, in involvements with these agents, the inflammatory infiltrate is almost entirely mononuclear (lymphocytes and macrophages) and is localized to interstitial sites, particularly about small blood vessels. The accumulation of these leukocytes about the blood vessels is descriptively referred to as "cuffing." Rarely, fulminating viral or rickettsial infections may cause neutrophilic exudates and, in these instances, the reaction may not only be interstitial but may also cause necrosis of parenchymal cells, resembling changes of bacterial origin.

Granulomatous Inflammatory Reactions.

A few agents evoke a distinctive pattern of reaction referred to as granulomatous inflammation. In a strict sense, *the term granuloma implies a tumor-like mass of granulation tissue (actively growing fibroblasts and capillary buds). However, the term should be restricted to a small 1 to 2 mm. collection of modified macrophages or histiocytes almost invariably surrounded by a rim of mononuclear cells, principally lymphocytes* (Fig. 3–17). Often Langhans' or foreign body type giant cells are present in the granuloma. The modified macrophages have been designated as *epithelioid cells* because of their abundant cytoplasm and their plumpness, creating a resemblance to epithelial cells. The basis for this transformation is still somewhat obscure. Spector (1969*a*) proposes that phagocytosis, with persistence of an irritant within the macrophage, produces this epithelioid transformation.

Tuberculosis is the prototype of granulomatous disease. In this entity, the granuloma is referred to as a tubercle. Other granulomatous disorders are syphilis, sarcoidosis, cat-scratch fever, lymphogranuloma inguinale, leprosy, brucellosis, berylliosis, some of the mycotic infections and reactions to irritant lipids. A few details on some of the major granulomatous diseases are given in Table 3–2.

In the experimental laboratory, a granulomatous reaction can be induced by the injection of such macromolecules as mineral oil, carrageenin, complex polysaccharides and polymers. The common denominator among these granulomatous disorders is the persistence of the irritant within macrophages. In tuberculosis, it is postulated that some of the lipids in the wall of the tubercle bacillus constitute macromolecular waxes which resist digestion by the enzymes of the macrophage. In support of such a proposition, lipid extracts of the tubercle bacillus have yielded mixtures of mycolic acid and polysaccharides which, when injected into the guinea pig, evoke characteristic granuloma formation (White, 1966).

Although, as indicated, a number of disorders are associated with granulomatous inflammation, each of these diseases produces a

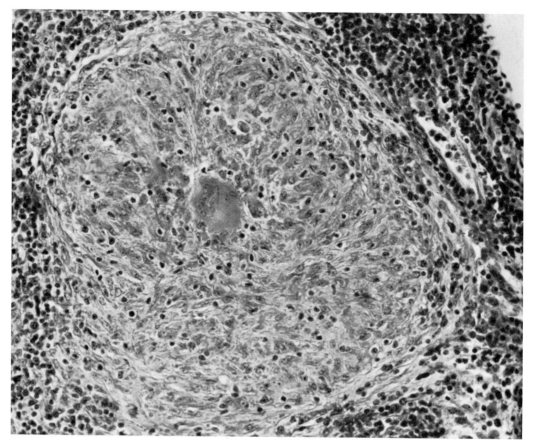

Figure 3–17. *A granuloma with a central Langhans' type giant cell surrounded by chronic inflammatory infiltrate.*

somewhat distinctive modification within the granuloma. Classically, tuberculosis is associated with caseous (cheesy) necrosis of the center of the granuloma to produce a caseating, soft tubercle, the hallmark of tuberculosis. In contrast, sarcoidosis almost never evokes central necrosis, and so the sarcoid granuloma is often called a "hard tubercle." The granulomatous reaction in syphilis is characterized by central gummatous necrosis. This term derives from the rubbery consistency of the central necrosis in large gummas. Histologically, there is persistence of shadowy outlines of the necrotic cells in the gumma. The other granulomatous diseases also evoke somewhat distinctive patterns as will become clear from their description in Chapter 10.

It must be apparent that the recognition of a granulomatous inflammation is of great help in separating this small group of chronic inflammatory disorders from the bulk of nonspecific chronic inflammations. The precise cytologic characteristics of the granuloma may permit a reasonably exact etiologic diagnosis, but there are a sufficient number of atypical presentations and overlaps to make such judgments precarious. As with most inflammatory conditions, it is necessary to identify the specific etiologic agent by more precise methods such as bacterial culture, serologic tests or chemical analysis.

Reactions to Immunologic Injury. *Immunologic injuries* evoke quite distinctive patterns of reaction, the principal hallmarks of which are the deposit of fibrinoid and the infiltration of lymphocytes and/or plasma cells in sites of tissue damage. Among the many disorders stemming from reactivity of the immune system to either endogenous or exogenous antigens, there is considerable variation in the tissues and organs affected as well as in both the humoral and cell mediated mechanisms involved.

In disorders involving the production of immunoglobulins, fibrinoid (described on p. 37) is deposited principally in blood vessel walls and in focal sites within the stroma of affected tissues or organs. The mechanism of accumulation of fibrinoid appears to be as follows: the localization of immune complexes in the walls of the blood vessels or in the interstitial tissue attracts neutrophils and comple-

TABLE 3–2. MAJOR GRANULOMATOUS INFLAMMATIONS

Disease	Cause	Tissue Reaction
Tuberculosis	*Mycobacterium tuberculosis*	Noncaseating tubercle (*Granuloma prototype*): A focus of epithelioid cells, rimmed by fibroblasts, lymphocytes, histiocytes, occasional Langhans' giant cell. Caseating tubercle: Central amorphous granular debris, loss of all cellular detail.
Sarcoidosis	Unknown	Noncaseating granuloma: Giant cells (Langhans' and foreign body types); asteroids in giant cells; occasional Schaumann's body (concentric calcific concretion).
Certain fungal infections		Granuloma usually larger than single tubercle with central granular debris; often contains causal organism and recognizable neutrophils.
	Cryptococcus neoformans	Organism is yeast-like, sometimes budding; 5 to 10 μ; large, clear capsule.
	Blastomyces dermatitidis	Organism is yeast-like, budding; 5 to 15 μ; thick, doubly refractile capsule.
	Coccidioides immitis	Organism appears as spherical (30–80 μ) cyst containing endospores of 3 to 5 μ each.
Syphilis	*Treponema pallidum*	Gumma: Microscopic to grossly visible lesion, enclosing wall of histiocytes, fibroblasts and lymphocytes; plasma cell infiltrate; center cells are necrotic without loss of cellular outline.
Cat-scratch fever	Virus ? Chlamydiae?	Rounded or stellate granuloma containing central granular debris and recognizable neutrophils; giant cells uncommon.
Actinomycosis	*Actinomyces bovis*	Granulomatous rim enclosing necrotic and viable polymorphonuclear leukocytes as well as "sulfur granules."

ment, and these cause increased vascular permeability (see p. 69). As a consequence, plasma proteins, including the immunoglobulins and fibrinogen, leak into the site of immunologic injury to create amorphous fibrin-like precipitates termed *fibrinoid*. The fibrinoid obscures the underlying histologic detail of the involved vessel wall and replaces it with an amorphous acellular pink deposit. The local injury also attracts leukocytes. Usually, some neutrophils in varying states of disintegration are trapped within the fibrinoid. As was cited earlier, these changes have erroneously been called fibrinoid necrosis; in reality, it is not a distinctive pattern of cell death but, rather, cell death caused by the cytopathic actions of complement and lysosomal enzymes, followed by the precipitation of fibrinoid in the areas of injury secondary to the increased vascular permeability.

The immunopathic mechanism of delayed hypersensitivity is the accumulation of sensitized lymphocytes which cause cell damage through pathways still imperfectly understood (p. 203). But in any event in grafting, for example, the transplant undergoing rejection is heavily infiltrated with these "killer" lymphocytes. Immunoglobulins may also participate in certain forms of immune disorders which are basically mediated by delayed hypersensitivity reactions such as graft rejection and, in these circumstances, the graft may exhibit not only aggregates of mononuclear cells but also acute vasculitis and deposits of fibrinoid.

In summing up the relationship of the pattern of the inflammatory reaction to its etiology, it is evident that the character of the reaction is significantly modified by its specific cause, a fortunate happenstance since it often provides useful clues to the etiology of obscure inflammatory states.

TYPES OF INFLAMMATORY REACTIONS BASED ON LOCATION

The morphology of an inflammatory reaction is significantly altered by the specific tissue and site involved. Five characteristic patterns are recognized.

Abscesses. *An abscess is a localized collection of pus* caused by suppuration buried in a tissue, organ or confined space. Abscesses are usually produced by the deep seeding of pyogenic bacteria into a tissue. In its early stages, an abscess is a focal accumulation of fairly well preserved neutrophils in an area created either by the separation of preexisting cellular elements or by the liquefactive necrosis of the native cells of the tissue or organ. As it develops, it may expand as a result of the progressive necrosis of surrounding cells. During this time some of the neutrophils, chiefly those in the older central regions, usually begin to deteriorate, becoming partially or completely necrotic. The central region at this time appears as a mass of granular, acidophilic, amorphous, semifluid debris composed of the necrotic white cells and tissue cells. There is usually a zone of preserved neutrophils about this necrotic focus and, outside this region, vascular dilation and parenchymal and fibroblastic proliferation occur, indicating the beginning of repair.

In time, the abscess may become walled off by highly vascularized connective tissue that serves as a limiting barrier to further spread. Containment of the abscess in this fashion is usually accompanied by a change in the cellular constituents of the exudate. Numerous macrophages appear within the fibroblastic zone in the margins of the active necrosis and, in the later healing stages, these cells may enter the central necrotic focus and eventually replace the neutrophils.

Healing of an abscess, to be described under repair, can occur only after the suppurative exudate and necrotic debris have been removed, since their presence still provokes inflammation. The removal may be accomplished through one of several pathways. The abscess may burrow to the surface of the organ or tissue and discharge its contents by rupture or "pointing." Since such spread or dissection of an abscess causes extensive tissue damage, surgical incision and drainage may be employed in abscesses which are readily accessible to operative intervention, such as those in the subcutaneous tissues. If evacuation of the abscess does not occur, healing may still take place after total proteolytic digestion of the accumulated tissue and cellular debris. This watery digestate may then be resorbed into the blood. Fluid sometimes remains loculated within its fibrous containment to create a cyst. Neglected abscesses frequently accumulate calcium salts to become converted into calcified masses.

Since abscesses are characterized by local destruction of parenchymal and stromal cells, they generally lead to scarring and permanent deformity of tissues.

Ulcers. *An ulcer is a local defect, or excavation, of the surface of an organ or tissue, which is produced by the sloughing (shedding) of inflammatory necrotic tissue.* Ulceration can occur only when an inflammatory necrotic area exists on or near a surface. It is most commonly encountered in three situations: (1) focal inflammatory necrosis of the mucosa of the mouth, stomach or intestines, (2) subcutaneous inflammations of the lower extremities in older individuals who have circulatory disturbances that predispose to extensive necrosis and (3) inflammation of the cervix or the uterus.

Such lesions are best exemplified by the peptic ulcer of the stomach or duodenum. The ulcer craters are usually circular to oval, 0.5 to 4.0 cm. in diameter, sharply punched out of the intestinal mucosa, with fairly perpendicular walls and a flat base (Fig. 3–18). The margins of the ulcer may be slightly elevated as a result of inflammatory edema, and the base may be flat or filled with shaggy necrotic debris. Microscopically, the pattern of the inflammatory reaction depends on the duration of the lesion. In the acute stage, serous and fibrinous exudation may be associated with an intense polymorphonuclear infiltration and vascular dilation in the margins of the defect (Fig. 3–19). With chronicity, the margins and base of the ulcer develop marked fibroblastic proliferation, scarring and the accumulation of lymphocytes, histiocytes and plasma cells. Eosinophils may also be very numerous, especially when foreign protein from the cavity of the stomach enters the ulcer and sensitizes the underlying tissues. In longstanding peptic ulcers, this mononuclear type of infiltrate extends into the deeper levels of the underlying tissue.

Even with long-term chronic ulceration, persistent acute activity may be present in the exposed base and margins of the crater so that an acute fibrinosuppurative exudate may line the ulcer base at the same time that a chronic reaction is present in the deeper levels. The healing of a chronic ulcer with fibrotic indurated margins requires first that the defect be filled, usually by scar tissue, and then that the epithelium of the stomach or duodenum be regenerated, reconstituting the continuity of the gastrointestinal mucosa.

Membranous (Pseudomembranous) Inflammation. As the name implies, this form of inflammatory reaction is characterized by the *formation of a membrane usually made up of precipitated fibrin, necrotic epithelium and inflam-*

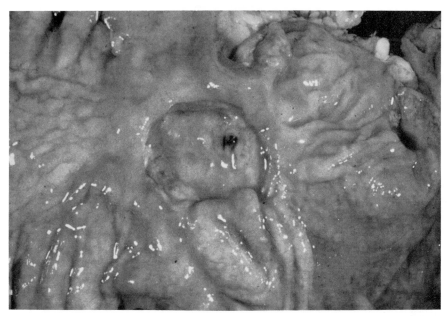

Figure 3–18. A gross view of an ulcer of the stomach.

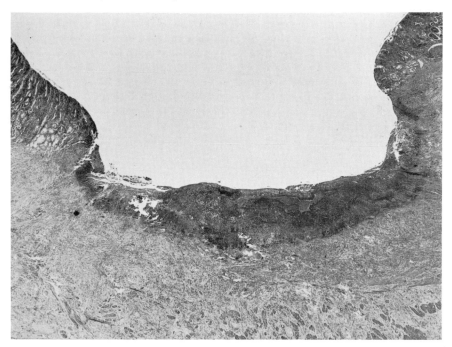

Figure 3–19. A low power cross section of an ulcer crater with a dark inflammatory exudate in the base.

matory white cells. Some prefer to call this reaction "pseudomembranous" since they reserve the term membrane for vital cells and structures. Whatever its designation, the reaction is encountered only on mucosal surfaces, most commonly in the pharynx, larynx, respiratory passages and intestinal tract (Fig. 3–20). The membrane formation results from an acute inflammatory response to a powerful necrotizing toxin—e.g., the diphtheria exotoxin which causes necrosis of surface epithelial cells and their desquamation. An exuberant outpouring of fibrinosuppurative exudate traps the necrotic and cellular debris, producing a dirty greywhite, rubbery membrane which layers the inflamed, eroded surface. A marked inflammatory response underlying the denuded surface will also be present. Membranous inflammation is quite characteristic of diphtheria, and frequently makes the clinical identification of this disease possible.

Catarrhal Inflammation. This pattern refers to excessive elaboration of mucin encountered in inflammatory states affecting any

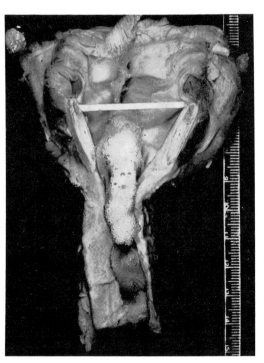

Figure 3–21. *A large plug of mucinous exudate lying within the larynx.*

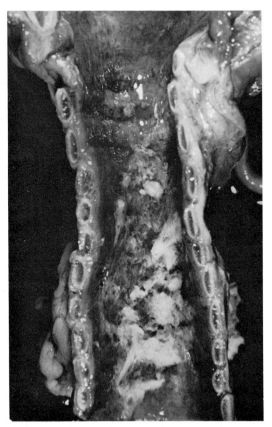

Figure 3–20. *Membranous inflammation in the trachea. The membrane appears as large patches of gray-white layered exudate.*

mucus-secreting mucosa (Fig. 3–21). It requires little further description since this pattern of reaction is all too well known to every person who has suffered from the common cold. The distinctiveness of this form of inflammation derives entirely from its location and its involvement of mucus-secreting cells. Presumably, the increased vascularization which occurs during the inflammatory reaction stimulates the formation and secretion of mucus.

In closing this discussion of inflammation, it is evident that, although the early reaction pattern of the inflammatory response is quite stereotyped, it is soon modified by a number of variables pertaining to both intruder and host which introduce striking departures from the basic theme. Perhaps the most important is the duration of the inflammatory process; but the causative agent, the location of the injury and the nature of the exudate all contribute heavily to the ultimate character of the reaction. Even these modifiers do not tell the whole story because an important component has, to this point, been omitted—the changes induced by the reparative response. The repair of injury begins almost as soon as the inflammatory changes have begun, and so constitutes a sequence of events as important as that of inflammation.

REPAIR

Repair comprises the replacement of dead or damaged cells by healthy cells. These new cells may be derived from either the parenchyma or the connective tissue stroma of the injured tissue. Parenchymal regeneration can completely reconstitute the defect, leaving no residual trace of the prior injury. However, in man such perfect reconstitution of the native architecture occurs only under very limited conditions (soon to be described).

The advantages that man may have gained in the evolutionary process have been accompanied by loss of the capacity to regenerate severely damaged organs. Because of these limitations, repair of tissue injury usually takes the form of connective tissue scarring. Such repair may fill defects and more or less restore morphologic continuity, but it usually replaces specialized functioning cells with nonfunctioning connective tissue. Such scarring depletes the functional reserve of an organ or tissue. The factors determining the pathways followed—parenchymal regeneration or connective tissue scarring—will emerge in the ensuing discussion. Parenchymal regeneration will be presented, followed by repair involving connective tissue scarring. Thereafter, consideration will be given to the mechanisms involved in both forms of repair.

PARENCHYMAL REGENERATION

The cells of the body have been divided into three groups based on their regenerative capacity; labile, stable and permanent cells. Labile cells continue to proliferate throughout life. Stable cells retain this capacity although they do not normally replicate. Permanent cells cannot reproduce themselves after birth. Many of the details which determine the regenerative capacity of various cells may be found in the authoritative review by McMinn (1967). It is obvious that perfect reconstitution of an injury can occur only in tissues composed of labile or stable parenchymal cells. When permanent cells are destroyed, repair can occur only by the proliferation of the simpler, less differentiated cells of the structure's connective tissue. It should be noted that, although labile and stable cells may replicate and reconstitute the cellular mass of the organ or structure affected, the original architecture is not always reproduced exactly.

LABILE CELLS

Under normal physiologic conditions, these cells continue to proliferate throughout life, replacing cells which are continually being destroyed.

Epithelial Cells. Epithelial surfaces throughout the body are made up of labile cells. These include the stratified squamous surfaces of the skin, oral cavity, vagina and cervix; the lining mucosa of all the excretory ducts of the glands of the body, e.g., salivary glands, pancreas and biliary tract; the columnar epithelium of the GI tract, uterus and tubes; and the transitional epithelium of the urinary tract. In all of these sites, the surface cells exfoliate continually throughout life, and the integrity of the epithelium is maintained by a continual proliferation of reserve cells, replacing lost elements. One has only to recall the regrowth of the endometrium following each menstrual period to appreciate the regenerative capacity of epithelial surfaces.

When epithelial cells are lost as a result of injury, almost perfect reconstitution may occur by replication of the marginal preserved cells. If the defect is small, the regenerative activity of the epithelial cells is prompt and remarkably rapid. Ordman and Gillman (1966) have shown that the epithelium in the skin of the pig completely closes over an incised wound within 24 hours. When injury produces a deep, excavated defect or ulcer, epithelial regeneration is completed only after the defect is filled. The regrowth of this supporting stroma is discussed more fully in the section on secondary union.

Splenic, Lymphoid and Hematopoietic Cells. The cells of splenic, lymphoid and hematopoietic tissues fall into the category of labile cells. Bone marrow cells are considered labile because marrow is in a state of active hematopoiesis throughout life. Destruction of hematopoietic cells is rapidly compensated for by proliferation of persisting elements. The embryonic precursors of splenic and lymphoid cells (primitive mesenchymal stem cells) survive postnatally, proliferating and differentiating to replace lost elements. Destruction of large areas of bone marrow, spleen or lymphoid tissues may radically reduce the population of stem cells, thus reducing the local potential for parenchymal reconstitution, giving rise to focal scarring. If an entire lymph node is destroyed, it will of necessity be replaced by scar tissue.

STABLE CELLS

It is postulated that injury to stable cells derepresses the genetic programs which repress mitotic processes in the quiescent cell. Two large categories of cells thus capable of functional reconstitution are: the parenchymal cells of virtually all the glandular organs of the body and the mesenchymal derivatives such as fibroblasts, osteoblasts, and chondroblasts.

Parenchymal Cells. Parenchymal cells of glands throughout the body, including the liver, pancreas, salivary and endocrine glands, kidney tubular cells and glands of the skin are stable cells. The regenerative capacity of stable cells is best exemplified by hepatocytes. Indeed, the liver possesses the most remarkable regenerative capacity of any parenchymal organ. When a two-thirds hepatectomy is performed on the mouse or the rat, an almost normal liver weight is restored in about a week (Bucher, 1967). It is remarkable that within an hour after hepatectomy, microscopic changes can be identified in parenchymal cells throughout the remaining liver. By 24 hours, cells, nuclei and nucleoli more than double in size. Thereafter, mitoses appear and the hepatic cell population enlarges at a rate parallel to the increase in tissue mass. In such a hepatectomy, it is obvious that whole liver lobules are destroyed and, indeed, an entire lobe may be removed.

Restoration of liver substance is accomplished largely by an increase in the size of the remaining liver lobules. There may be some disorderly proliferation of hepatocytes along the line of surgical incision, reproducing abortive liver lobules, but this marginal effort does not contribute heavily to the restoration of original liver weight. The enlarged regenerating liver lobules are capable of normal function. These observations have been extended to include man, and both McDermott et al. (1963) and Pack et al. (1962) have confirmed that normal liver function is restored three weeks postoperatively in patients who have had surgical hepatectomies for such diseases as cancer of the liver.

Hepatocytes are equally able to regenerate when liver cells have been destroyed by toxins or other diseases. Indeed, in carbon tetrachloride poisoning, for example, hepatocytes are selectively destroyed while the connective tissue framework of the liver is unaffected. As the following discussion indicates, such a situation is ideal for reconstitution of the original architecture.

Although labile and stable cells are capable of regeneration, it does not necessarily follow that injuries in organs or tissues composed of such cells will be repaired with restitution of the normal structure. *The underlying framework or supporting stroma of the parenchymal cells must be present to permit perfect replacement.* In the absence of this scaffold, cells may proliferate in a completely haphazard fashion and produce disorganized masses of cells which bear no resemblance to the original arrangement. Alternatively, scarring may ensue. To use the liver as an example, there are many types of hepatotoxins—e.g., viruses, which specifically destroy parenchymal cells without injuring the more resistant connective tissue cells of the stroma and framework of the liver lobule. Under these circumstances, regeneration of liver cells may reconstitute the liver lobule. By contrast, a liver abscess which destroys all the cells in the focus of injury is followed by scarring.

In most large injuries, the regeneration proceeds from the local margins where stable cells remain viable. Central regions where the framework is not preserved are usually replaced by scar tissue.

Complete destruction of a gland or organ obviously precludes the possibility of regeneration. This situation rarely pertains to the major glands of the body, such as the liver, pancreas and endocrine glands, since total ablation is usually incompatible with life. However, total destruction of the sweat and sebaceous glands and hair follicles is commonly encountered in full thickness skin injuries such as severe burns, large areas of infection or extensive physical trauma. Because of their small size, even slight injuries may destroy completely and permanently these anatomic units.

Connective Tissue Cells. *Connective tissue cells*, such as fibroblasts or their more primitive mesenchymal progenitors, are not only highly resistant to injury, but are also multipotential cells capable of proliferation throughout life. Connective tissue scars result from the proliferation of fibroblasts, with the subsequent deposition of intercellular collagen. Since most injuries destroy stromal as well as parenchymal cells, fibroblastic proliferation and scarring are consequences of almost all reparative processes. The multipotential fibroblast is further capable of differentiation into any other type of supporting tissue cell. By metaplastic transformation, it may be converted to an osteoblast or chondroblast and form bone or cartilage. By the accumulation of lipids, it or its progenitor becomes transformed into a lipid cell and so reconstitutes injured fatty tissue.

Muscle Cells. There is a growing body of evidence that *skeletal, cardiac, and visceral (smooth) muscle cells* are capable of regeneration (Reznik, 1969) (Hay, 1971). Most of the evidence is derived from studies of lower animals, but a number of reports dealing with human muscle cells confirm the applicability of these observations to man. The precise mode of regeneration of skeletal muscle is still somewhat uncertain. It appears that regeneration of skeletal muscle may occur: (1) from the budding of old fibers, (2) by the fusion of myoblasts or (3) by transformation of the mononucleated satellite cells found attached to the sheath of all multinucleated skeletal muscle cells (Shafiq et al., 1967).

The evidence in support of the regenerative capability of cardiac muscle and smooth muscle is less substantial and we must conclude that further study is necessary. Robledo (1956) claims that he has observed both sprouting and longitudinal splitting of cardiac muscle fibers at the edge of necrotic areas in the heart in rats. However, it must be pointed out that the heart also contains an abundant fibroblastic stroma and the precise identification of the regenerative cells may be difficult. It is probably fair to state that if cardiac muscle has regenerative capacity, it is limited, and most large injuries to the heart are followed by connective tissue scarring (Fig. 3–22).

Certainly, scarring follows the all-too-common myocardial infarction (ischemic necrosis of the myocardium) in man. This point is stressed because of its great clinical importance. Heart attacks are the most common cause of death in industrialized nations, and every heart attack implies some permanent loss of myocardial reserve. Regeneration of smooth

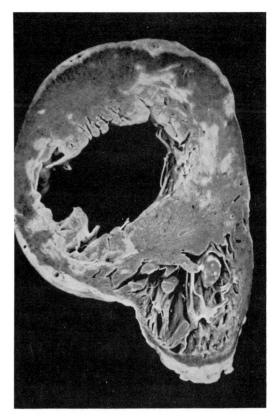

Figure 3–22. Myocardial fibrosis. The cross section of the ventricular myocardium is studded with pale scars of fibrous tissue that have been caused by ischemic necrosis of foci within the myocardium.

muscle has been observed in the wall of the gut, urinary bladder, uterus and blood vessel walls (McMinn, 1967). Here again, most injuries to smooth muscle inevitably induce some scarring. The regenerative capacity of the smooth muscle, therefore, must be considered to be limited.

PERMANENT CELLS

These highly specialized cells *cannot undergo mitotic division in postnatal life* presumably because the genetic programs involved in their division are irrevocably repressed. Severe injury in such tissue inevitably implies loss of specialized function.

Nerve Cells. Nerve cells, when destroyed in the CNS (central nervous system), are permanently lost. They are replaced by the proliferation of the CNS supportive elements, the glial cells. The situation is somewhat more complicated with respect to the neurons of the peripheral nerves (Lumsden, 1957). When the cell body is destroyed, the entire structure (i.e., the cell body and extended axon) totally degenerates. If the cell body is spared and only the peripheral axon is injured, regeneration of a new process may proceed from the cell body or from the remaining proximal axonal segment. In such injury, the distal segment degenerates entirely, and the proximal segment degenerates only to the nearest node of Ranvier. If the proximal segment, growing at a rate of 3 to 4 mm. per day, recontacts the channel of the original nerve fiber, the integrity of the neural innervation may be reestablished. In some injuries, however, the regenerating axonal process is isolated from the distal segment because tissues, coagulated blood (hematoma) or masses of fibrous scarring are interposed. The extending axonal process then gives rise to a tangled mass of fibers, sometimes termed an *amputation or traumatic neuroma.*

REPAIR BY CONNECTIVE TISSUE

Fibroblastic proliferation and scarring are the most ubiquitous features of repair, and are seen in all but the very few injuries in which only stable or labile cells are damaged and the connective tissue stroma remains intact. Since a connective tissue scar is a more primitive, simpler form of tissue than the specialized types that it replaces, scarring which is irreversible produces permanent loss of specialized function. Thus, fibrous replacement of kidney structure following an abscess or an infarct depletes renal function. Connective tissue repair is best presented in the context of wound healing. This will be divided into the events of primary union by which an incised wound such as a surgical incision closes, and those of secondary union by which an open tissue defect such as an ulcer of the skin heals.

PRIMARY UNION

The least complicated example of connective tissue repair is the healing of a clean surgical incision. The tissues are approximated by surgical sutures or tapes, and healing occurs without significant bacterial contamination and with a minimal loss of tissue. Such healing is referred to surgically as *"primary healing"* or *"union by first intention."* The incision causes the death of a limited number of epithelial cells as well as dermal adnexa and connective tissue cells; the incisional space is narrow and immediately fills with a scant amount of clotted blood. Dehydration of the surface clot forms the well known scab which covers the wound and seals it almost at once from the environment. The precise chronologic order of the subsequent events is still a subject of contention. Specifically at issue are the following questions: How soon does epithelial closure occur? How soon does subepithelial fibroblastic bridging take place? How rapidly does the incision achieve the full tensile strength of unwounded skin? What cells or extracellular products impart such strength? A reasonable consensus follows.

Within 24 hours, the characteristic changes of the acute inflammatory response appear in the subepithelial connective tissue in the margins of the incision. The gathering leukocytes are mainly neutrophils. The epidermis at its cut edges thickens as a result of mitotic activity of basal cells and, within 24 to 48 hours, spurs of epithelial cells from both edges grow both downward along the cut margins of the dermis as well as beneath the surface scab to fuse in the midline and thus produce a continuous but thin epithelial layer. This epithelial response is amazingly fast, and epidermal continuity is reestablished long before the subjacent connective tissue reaction has begun to evolve. The processes involved in such reepithelialization are discussed in detail on p. 96.

By *day 3*, the neutrophils have largely disappeared and are replaced by monocytes busily scavenging necrotic debris and removing red cells and fibrin. Hypertrophy of subepithelial fibroblasts becomes visible at this time, along with the initiation of fibroblastic replication and budding of capillary sprouts. This fibroblastic-vascular tissue progressively invades the incisional space. In time-lapse studies, Cliff (1965) has shown that this invasion advances at the remarkable rate of approximately 0.2 mm. per day into the blood clot which fills the incision. Such ingrowth is accomplished by mitotic division of both fibroblasts and endothelial cells. The major proliferative activity of the endothelium occurs just proximal to the growing tip of the capillary sprout, pushing the tip ahead. Demonstrable collagen fibers are now present in the margins of the incision but these are at first vertically oriented and do not bridge the incision (Ordman and Gillman, 1966). While this connective tissue response is taking place, epithelial cell proliferation and differentiation continue, thickening the epidermal covering layer.

By *day 5*, the incisional space is filled with a loose vascularized fibroblastic connective tissue rich in ground substance. The newly formed capillary sprouts from both sides have joined to create continuous channels and, at this stage of wound healing, the vascularization is maximal. Collagen fibrils become more abundant and begin to bridge the incision. During this 5-day interval, the epidermis usually recovers its normal thickness and differentiation of surface cells yields a mature epidermal architecture with surface keratinization.

During the *second week*, there is continued accumulation of collagen and proliferation of fibroblasts within the incisional connective tissue. Leukocytic infiltrate, edema and increased vascularity have largely disappeared, and the cellular connective tissue which fills the incision begins to compress the thin-walled, newly formed capillary channels. The surface scab is generally shed during this week.

At this time begins the long process of blanching, accomplished by the increased accumulation of collagen within the incisional scar, accompanied by shrinkage and disappearance of vascular channels. The tensile strength of the wound (see p. 97) is still well below that of normal skin and it will take months or even a year or more for the wound to attain its maximal mechanical strength.

By *the end of the first month*, the scar comprises a cellular, still excessively vascularized connective tissue devoid of inflammatory infiltrate, covered now by an intact epidermis. The slowed but continued proliferation of fibroblasts and the continued accretion of collagen build up the mechanical pressure on the vascular channels and, over the ensuing months, the vascularization is more and more reduced. It may require almost a year for the scar to be transformed to an acellular, avascular, pale, collagenous scar. The dermal appendages that have been totally destroyed in the line of the incision and the ensuing inflammatory response are permanently lost. Those that have only been injured or partially damaged along the lateral margins of the incision may regenerate.

In summary, *in the clean surgical wound, sealing occurs within hours by the formation of a blood clot, the surface of which becomes dehydrated to create the scab. Epithelial continuity is restored within 24 to 48 hours. Fibroblastic bridging does not become evident until 3 to 5 days following the incision, and demonstrable collagenization only begins to appear in the latter part of the first week.* Thereafter, the process is one of progressive proliferation of fibroblasts, the continued accumulation of collagen and the slow compression and devascularization of the newly formed connective tissue which fills the incisional space. Later, some of the details relating to the stimulation of proliferation, epithelialization and collagenization will be considered.

SECONDARY UNION

When there is more extensive loss of cells and tissue such as occurs in infarction, inflam-matory ulceration, abscess formation or surface wounds which create large defects, the reparative process is more complicated. The common denominator in all of these situations is a large tissue defect which must be filled. Regeneration of parenchymal cells may occur in the margins but, with loss of the stromal framework, it cannot completely reconstitute the original architecture. Vascularized connective tissue grows in from the margin to complete the repair. The inflammatory reaction is quite intense in such large wounds. The young vascularized connective tissue bearing a leukocytic infiltrate is known as *granulation tissue,* and so these defects are said to "granulate in." This form of healing is referred to as *"secondary healing"* or *"healing by second intention."*

The healing of a large tissue defect on the surface of the body, such as an excised wound, basically resembles the primary healing already described. Epithelialization can take place only from the margins. The subepithelial repair depends heavily on the "fibroblast-capillary system" (Grillo, 1964). Here of course, the ingrowth of granulation tissue and subsequent scarring are on a much grander scale than in the incised wound (Figs. 3–23, 3–24 and 3–25). As in the case of primary healing, epithelialization advances down along and over the edges of the wound while the granulation tissue grows upward from the floor and margins, filling the defect.

Secondary healing differs from the primary healing in several important respects. *Inevitably, large tissue defects have more necrotic debris and exudate which must be removed.* Consequently, the inflammatory reaction is more intense than in the incised wound. Healing cannot be completed until this inflammatory response has controlled the injurious agent and the necrotic debris and exudate have been removed at least sufficiently to permit ingrowth of the granulation tissue from the margins. The mechanisms of "cleanup" comprise proteolysis and resorption of the digestate, phagocytosis by scavenger cells, or drainage to the surface. The persistence of exudate in a tissue defect, as in an abscess in the liver, represents a serious obstacle to healing.

Other distinctive features of the secondary closure of surface wounds are: (1) ingrowth of granulation tissue and (2) wound contraction. When the large defect occurs in deeper tissues such as in a viscus, the fibroblastic-vascular system bears the full responsibility for its closure, since drainage to the surface cannot occur. Not only is the quantity of granulation tissue greater in secondary healing, it is also more heavily infiltrated with leukocytes as a result of the greater intensity of the inflammatory response.

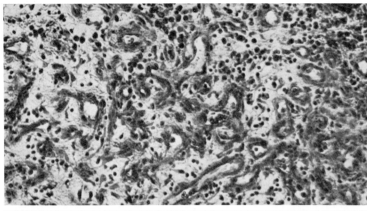

Figure 3–23. Active granulation tissue containing numerous dilated vascular channels and inflammatory white cell exudate in a loose fibrous tissue stroma.

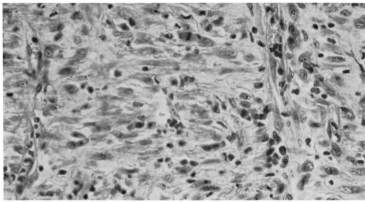

Figure 3–24. Cellular scar composed of packed fibroblasts with only scattered white cells and vascular channels.

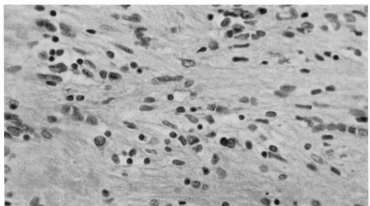

Figure 3–25. Dense collagenous scar. The widely scattered fibroblasts are separated by dense collagen. Only a few inflammatory white cells remain.

Perhaps the feature which most clearly differentiates primary from secondary healing is the phenomenon of *wound contraction* which occurs in large surface wounds. It can only occur in those sites where the skin is mobile. It has been shown by Billingham and Russell (1956) that a defect of about 40 cm.² in area in the skin of a rabbit is reduced in approximately six weeks to 5 to 10 per cent of its initial size largely by contraction. The margins of the wound are literally drawn together. It is estimated that all open skin wounds halve their surface area at the same rate and so all tend to approach the same size. Indeed, such contraction is largely responsible for the closure of skin wounds, and the granulation tissue sprouting from the base essentially provides a temporary covering which may, in fact, need to be resorbed in part to accomodate for the shrinkage in the size of the defect (Harkness, 1964).

The mechanism of wound contraction is still obscure and has excited great interest. Shortening of collagen fibers has been largely ruled out. The best evidence, provided by Majno and Leventhal (1967), indicates that fibroblasts within the granulation tissue develop characteristics of smooth muscle cells and shorten to provide the contractile forces (Gabbiani et al., 1972). These fibroblasts have considerable pull and it is of interest that efforts have been made to harness such forces as a source of energy (Higton and James, 1964). Whatever the mechanism, wound contraction contributes heavily to the repair of large surface defects, making it clear that whatever the dimensions of a scar the initial area of necrosis or tissue loss must have been much greater.

In summary, *second intention healing differs from first intention in the following respects:*

1. Loss of a greater amount of tissue.
2. Necessity for removal of greater amounts of inflammatory exudate and necrotic debris.
3. Formation of larger amounts of granulation tissue.
4. Contraction of surface wounds if there is mobility of the wound margins.
5. Production of larger amounts of scar.
6. Greater loss of skin appendages such as hair, sweat and sebaceous glands.
7. Slower completion of the entire reparative process.

As is the case with everything in life, sometimes things go wrong in the healing of wounds. Many of these aberrations (discussed on p. 99) relate to the management of the wound and the state of health of the wounded person. Two, however, may occur in the completely normal individual who received optimal care. The first comprises the formation of excessive amounts of granulation tissue. The excess, referred to as *"exuberant granulations"* or more grandiloquently as *"proud flesh,"* may protrude above the margins of the closing defect and block reepithelialization. Happily, the problem is readily managed by either surgical excision or chemical cauterization of the excess. The second abnormality, for mysterious reasons encountered most often in blacks, is *keloid* formation. Here, an abnormal amount of collagen is formed in the connective tissue, producing a large bulging tumorous scar (Fig. 3–26). The tendency to form keloids appears to be an individual genetic characteristic. It has only been recognized in skin wounds but the same excessive scarring may occur in deeper tissues as well, although we do not have substantial evidence that it does. Keloid formation can be a troublesome problem, particularly on exposed skin areas, since it is disfiguring and exceedingly difficult to manage medically; excision may be followed only by recurrence. It is encountered in both primary and secondary healing.

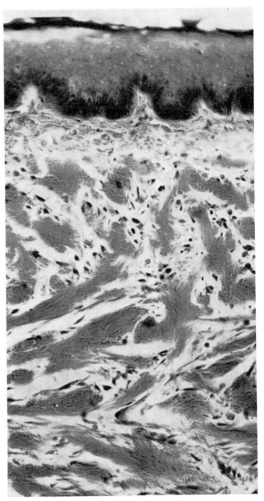

Figure 3–26. *Keloid. Deep to the overlying regenerated epithelium there are interlacing broad bands of dense collagen.*

INTEGRATION OF PARENCHYMAL REGENERATION WITH CONNECTIVE TISSUE SCARRING

Most bodily injuries are repaired by the regeneration of parenchymal cells, accompanied by more or less connective tissue scarring. Both of these processes have been considered separately, but it would be well to consider their respective contributions to the reparative process of most injuries. An abscess in the cortex of the kidney resulting from a bacterial infection might be used as an example. Reconstructive activities are initiated soon after the inflammatory phase has begun. Even during the acute stages of the response, there is proliferation of the marginal cells beyond the range of the toxic action of the microbial invader. At some point in the margin, there will be a zone where the epithelial cells lining the tubules are destroyed but the more resistant connective tissue framework is preserved. Here, regeneration of tubular cells may reconstitute the original architecture perfectly. At the same time, the focus of injury may have accumulated a considerable amount of suppurative exudate, filling the central space where all native architecture had undergone liquefactive necrosis.

Parenchymal regeneration cannot create new tubules where the framework has been destroyed. Here, the defect will be filled in by the process of removal of necrotic debris and exudate, followed by the ingrowth of granulation tissue. Glomeruli cannot be regenerated. The anatomic continuity of the tissue is thus restored by a combination of parenchymal regeneration and connective tissue scarring. Some of the lost functional capability may be partially compensated for by hypertrophy of residual preserved glomeruli as well as enlargement of surviving nephrons.

The quality and adequacy of the repair of any tissue loss is governed, then, by the regenerative capacity of the affected cells, by the extent of the injury, particularly since it may have destroyed the skeletal framework of the tissue, and by the proliferative activity of the connective tissue stroma which fills in the defects that remain after parenchymal regeneration has ceased. Although the example of an abscess in the kidney has been used, the essential details do not differ in any tissue composed of parenchymal cells capable of replication.

STIMULI TO CELL PROLIFERATION

Repeated references have been made in the previous discussion to the proliferation of parenchymal and connective tissue cells in the repair of an injury. What signal do these cells receive which initiates their proliferation? Is it a factor elaborated at the site of injury which stimulates cells to grow, and is this factor confined to the local area or is it a humoral, circulating principle? On the other hand, does the signal take the form of some loss of repression of cell division?

The vast literature on the subject of stimuli to cell proliferation can best be characterized as a welter of contradictions surrounded by confusion. *Most of the evidence supports the thesis that the trigger for cell proliferation consists of some local loss of inhibitory influences at the cell level, which thus permits affected cells to proliferate.* Nonetheless, certain findings suggest that stimulatory factors, so-called wound hormones, are produced following an injury and stimulate the mitotic division of cells. We must also concern ourselves with the question of whether the signal, be it in the form of stimulation or loss of inhibition, represents a generalized phenomenon applicable to all specialized cells, or is cell and tissue specific.

With regard to the existence of stimulatory wound hormones, most of the evidence derives from studies on the regeneration of the liver following hepatectomy. Many investigators have reported the existence of humoral circulating factors which stimulate the regeneration of liver parenchymal cells following hepatectomy. Among the experimental designs employed to support this thesis, perhaps the most critical is the use of hepatectomized animals, usually rats, linked in parabiotic union with normal animals, resulting in increased mitotic activity in the livers of the normal parabiont (Hurowitz and Studer, 1960). However, in a virtually identical experiment, the existence of such a humoral stimulatory factor has been denied by Heimann et al. (1963). The controversy continues.

The thesis of loss of mitotic inhibitory influences is not only attractive but is supported by a considerable body of evidence. Grisham et al. (1966) contend that, in the hepatectomized animal, a blood-borne influence which prevents proliferation of hepatocytes is lost. Their observations were derived from experiments in which total exchange blood transfusions were carried out between normal and hepatectomized rats, indicating the presence of a circulating inhibitor in the normal animal not found in the hepatectomized rat. These findings still require confirmation by others.

In contrast, there is a large body of evidence supporting the existence of intracellular controls which may be released at the site of injury. Most of this evidence derives from studies of the epidermal response to injury and of the behavior of cells cultured in vitro. The reepithelialization of wounds has provided the best model for studying these mechanisms of regenerative influences. As has been indicated in an earlier discussion, epidermal cells close over a surgically incised wound certainly within 48 hours and perhaps within the first day. Subsequently, there is progressive thickening of the epidermis and eventual differentiation into a keratinized surface. *Three distinctive processes are involved in such reepithelialization : (1) migration of cells, (2) proliferation and (3) differentiation.*

Migration is still a poorly understood phenomenon but appears to represent a mobilization of cells in the basal layers, followed by their sliding along the wound margins to advance toward the space created by the incision. As is well known, epidermal cells are attached to the basement membrane and to each other by desmosomes. Are these altered, detaching the cell from its anchorages, and are factors liberated which attract the cell? This question has not been resolved and, as Abercrombie and Ambrose (1962) put it: "It is likely to be difficult to decide whether when cells are mobilized, there is a primary change in their surfaces (or in the surfaces to which they are adhering) that is a decrease in the intensity of adhesion, or whether the primary change is the activation of the mechanism of movement." Within hours of the onset of migration, replication of cells commences. It is important to note that this proliferative reaction in the epidermis extends only about 1 mm. from the wound margin (Bullough, 1962). It is, therefore, a local phenomenon and not likely to be related to loss of circulating factors. Moreover, proliferative activity in the epidermis precedes, by several days, evidence of mitotic division in the subepithelial connective tissues, further suggesting some alteration in intracellular controls specific for cell types. *These observations have led to the general thesis that "control of mitotic activity, particularly in regeneration and repair, has swung away from the concept of stimulatory substance to one envisaging control by feedback mechanisms"* (Johnson, 1964).

The nature of the intracellular feedback control is still highly hypothetical and several postulations have been offered. Weiss (1955) proposes that cellular growth is dependent on cell-specific catalysts or *"templates"* which dictate the genetic programs for the reproduction of the living mass of new cells. Each cell also produces specific "antitemplates" which, unlike the templates, are free to diffuse into or out of the cell. The antitemplates block the action of the templates. With injury, loss of cells and the consequent inflammatory response, there is diffusion of the antitemplates out of the extracellular tissue spaces. The extracellular-intracellular concentration gradient then leads to diffusion of antitemplates from the cell, releasing the feedback controls on cell replication. As new cells are formed, antitemplates are synthesized by this progeny until the equilibrium is once again established.

Bullough (1962) refers to the intracellular control as a *chalone* (derived from a Greek maritime term implying "to reef the sails"). This thesis proposes that each tissue produces and contains its own specific inhibitor. With injury, chalones diffuse out of the cell, permitting regeneration. Iversen (1968) has extracted chalones from the skin of man and animals and has reported suppression of the mitotic rate of epidermal cells in tissue culture when this extract was added. The factor appears to be tissue specific since it has no effect on fibroblasts or liver cells, for example, but not species specific since an extract derived from human skin will act upon epidermal cells from lower animals.

Abercrombie (1966, 1967) has suggested another form of intracellular control of mitotic activity. He speaks of *contact inhibition* in which cells are inhibited from mitotic division by the interchange of signals or substances at their points of contact. It can be readily demonstrated in tissue culture. When cells grow out from two separate explants, they expand centrifugally until the two populations come into contact at some point. When contact is established, further migration and division ceases only at these points of contact. The nature of the message which passes from one cell to the other is still unclear. It could be the flow of electrochemical charges, soluble factors or modification of membrane receptors. More details on this interesting problem are available in the reports of Loewenstein (1969). Here this unsettled matter must rest for the present, but release of intracellular controls appears to be the initiator of cell replication in the reparative response.

Available evidence suggests that control mechanisms are tissue specific. What initiates the fibroblastic vascular response beneath the epidermis? Much less is known about this problem and, indeed, we cannot at the present time exclude the possibility that controls similar to those postulated for parenchymal cells also operate on stromal and vascular elements. Alternatively, it has been suggested that the blood vessels and fibroblasts may respond to local hypoxia. Conceivably, in the center of a wound, there is lower oxygen tension which stimulates proliferation in the marginal fibroblasts and blood vessels (Remensnyder and Majno, 1968). It must be apparent that the nature of the stimuli which initiate cell proliferation and regeneration in wounds is of utmost importance to the understanding of the nature of cancer. It is entirely conceivable that the mechanisms or stimuli which activate the controlled growth in repair may be further dislocated or permanently turned off or on to permit emergence of an uncontrolled cancerous growth.

DEVELOPMENT OF WOUND STRENGTH

It may come as a surprise to learn that, despite decades of study, there are still many gaps in our knowledge and numerous disagreements about several of the fundamental features of wound healing. There is still controversy over such basic issues as the following: What substances or structures within the wound impart to it its tensile strength in the first weeks of healing? What is the origin of the fibroblast, the backbone of all connective tissue repair? How is collagen synthesized? How rapidly does an incised wound regain the tensile strength of unwounded skin? These issues are examined in the following discussion.

Two viewpoints as to the origin of the fibroblast in the healing wound are still stoutly defended. The first proposes that some or many of the fibroblasts are derived from hematogenous cells, particularly monocytes and macrophages (Allgöwer, 1956) (Allgöwer and Hulliger, 1960). Alternatively, it is held that fibroblasts are derived from local fibroblasts or their immediate precursors. Underlying this problem is the well known fact that, in wound margins, the mature spindle-shaped fibroblast undergoes striking enlargement and becomes stellate or polymorphous, while the monocyte and macrophage develop larger pseudopods so that both cell types come to resemble each other to a considerable extent. Most of the evidence stems from in vitro cultures of mononuclear blood cells and the demonstration of collagen or collagen precursors in the culture flask. Opponents of this view contend that such cell cultures may well have been contaminated by connective tissue cells in the process of securing the blood cells (Grillo, 1963) (Ross, 1968). Most of the evidence supports the view that the fibroblast is derived from local fibroblasts (Grillo, 1964). Local irradiation of wounds suppresses collagen synthesis, which would not be anticipated if fibroblasts were derived from the circulating blood. Electron micrographic studies of the ultrastructural details of the cells in question reveal morphologic details of the cells consonant with the features of classic fibroblasts. Isotopic labeling experiments also indicate that newly formed cells are derived from local fibroblasts.

The amino acid composition of collagen is unique among the proteins of vertebrates. It is the only protein having significant amounts of hydroxyproline and hydroxylysine. Elastin may be a possible exception since it possesses small amounts of hydroxyproline. Three polypeptide chains possessing these hydroxylated amino acids are wound about each other in a helical fashion to form the tropocollagen macromolecule, the soluble precursor of collagen. The classic fibrillar structure of collagen results from the aggregation of these macromolecules to form fibrils which have periodic banding at approximately 600 to 700 Å intervals. Further details on the ultrastructure of collagen can be found in the review by Ramachandran (1963). The polypeptides, like all others, are synthesized on the ribosomes of the well developed, rough endoplasmic reticulum in the fibroblast.

There is general agreement that the fibroblast is responsible for the production of collagen, but the biomolecular pathways involved in its production are still debatable (Van Winkle, 1967). A major issue relates to where the collagen fiber is elaborated. One school of thought proposes that the tropocollagen macromolecules are aggregated into the collagen fibril in the peripheral cytoplasm of the fibroblast, and the fibrils are then extruded by some process that involves shedding of peripheral cytoplasm (Porter and Pappas, 1959). Another view proposes that the tropocollagen monomers are secreted outside of the cell, and aggregation into fibrils occurs in the extracellular ground substance (Ross, 1968).

It has been established that collagen fibrils can be created in the flask independent of cells from soluble precursors (Gross et al., 1955). It has been further shown that fibrils in extracellular locations enlarge in diameter with increasing age, strongly suggesting that the fibril develops outside of cells and is not born full grown within the fibroblast (Ross and Benditt, 1961). Most of the evidence therefore supports the notion that soluble collagen precursors are secreted by the fibroblast and that final aggregation or polymerization occurs extracellularly.

The ground substance of connective tissue is believed to play some important role in the production of collagen (Wagner and Siew, 1967). The substances found in connective tissue ground substance are derived from either the plasma or local cells, principally fibroblasts. They include a host of relatively water-soluble and water-insoluble components, the most important of which are mucopolysaccharides and glycoproteins (Spiro, 1966). The most important mucopolysaccharides are acidic and comprise two groups—those bound to sulfate and those which owe their acidity to carboxyl groups (hyaluronic acid and chondroitin). Because of their acidity, all have metachromasia when stained with toluidine blue. The mucopolysaccharides are largely synthesized locally in the wound area by connective tissue cells. The glycoproteins are elaborated principally in the liver and elsewhere. One might anticipate, therefore, that with the fibroblastic response of repair, increased amounts of acid mucopolysaccharides would, in the course of time, develop in the wound (White et al., 1961). It is postulated that this change in the composition of ground substance is important in the extracellular polymerization of collagen precursors into fibrils (Schilling, 1968).

We may now turn to the crucial clinical question: How long does it take a skin wound to achieve its maximal tensile strength? At the same time, consideration should be given to the factors or substances which contribute to this tensile strength. Both issues are highly controversial at the present time.

Observations in the literature vary widely on the rate and extent of recovery of wound strength. On the one hand, Adamsons et al. (1964), in studies of paramedian abdominal incisions in adult male guinea pigs, report that "the tensile strength of a wound reached the strength of the control side by the end of the fourth week." At the other end of the scale is the report of Douglas (1969) that, in both guinea pigs and man, skin wounds remain weak for many years and regain only about 30 per cent of their original strength at the end of one year. He further states that, in man, wounds have regained only about 50 per cent of their original strength at the end of three years; and even at the end of 14 years, a deficiency still exists. It is difficult to reconcile these startlingly different results, but perhaps the explanation may be found in a host of factors such as variations in the age of the animals, their diet, the depth of the skin incision, its length, methods of measurement and methods of suturing the original incision.

From the welter of opinions, a general impression emerges. Immediately after injury, there is a short lag phase perhaps lasting a few days and possibly lasting up to 10 to 14 days. Thereafter, there is a rapid increase in wound strength over the next four weeks. This rate of increase then slows and virtually plateaus at approximately the third month after the original incision. This plateau is reached at about 70 to 80 per cent of the tensile strength of unwounded skin and indeed, the plateau may persist for life.

Thus, Dunphy (1967) reports that "*most wounds involving skin, fascia or tendon never regain the initial strength of the tissue divided.*" The recovery of tensile strength comprises, therefore, a sigmoid curve terminating in a plateau below the original level of the unwounded skin (Levenson et al., 1965). The structural or biochemical explanation of this curve still eludes us. It is not merely a function of collagen synthesis since the curve of tensile strength does not parallel that of collagen increase in the wound. Immediately after injury, there is resorption of collagen. Thereafter, fibroplasia commences and the period of exponential rise in tensile strength is associated with a rapid increase in the number of fibroblasts as well as in the synthesis of collagen. But the later slower rise in tensile strength is not associated with a significant increase in the collagen content of the wound. Perhaps the collagen fibers are maturing or polymerizing at this time or there is remodeling of collagen to reorient the fibers across the wound, thereby increasing tensile strength. But collagen content alone cannot explain the curve.

In the light of these findings, one may properly ask: How can patients be discharged from the hospital within a week of surgery? An interesting study bears on this question. It has been shown that carefully sutured wounds have approximately 70 per cent of the strength of unwounded skin immediately following surgery (Lichtenstein et al., 1970). Indeed, eight weeks later there was no significant increase in tensile strength despite the presumed proliferation of fibroblasts and synthesis of collagen. The obvious conclusion is that, in the fresh wound, most of its tensile strength depends on surgical skill and the placement of sutures. When the latter are removed at the end of the first week, wound strength is only at approximately the 10 per cent level. But, in addition, it is reasonable to propose that reepithelialization which occurs within the first days of wounding provides some strength, and perhaps the early granulation tissue in some way serves as a binding agent or adhesive material. We must rest this discussion at this unsatisfactory point, recognizing that there is still much to be learned about this seemingly simple yet important surgical problem.

FACTORS MODIFYING THE QUALITY OF THE INFLAMMATORY-REPARATIVE RESPONSE

Many host factors influence the adequacy of the inflammatory-reparative response. Only a few of the more important will be discussed here under the headings of systemic and local influences.

SYSTEMIC INFLUENCES

Age. Age is probably not a major factor in the inflammatory-reparative response. It is mentioned here because there is a prevailing "general wisdom" that the elderly heal more slowly than the young; yet there is very little controlled data in the experimental animal to support this notion. Some years ago, it was reported that fibroplasia and collagenization occur more slowly in old rats than in young (Howes and Harvey, 1932). The validity of these observations when applied to man has not been established. It has been virtually impossible to rule out either the altered vascular supply due to the inevitable senile arteriosclerosis or the nutritional deficiencies due to eccentric dietary habits in the aged. In one of the few reports on aging as a factor in wound healing in man, no great differences were found among the various age ranges, nor were they linearly related to age (Abt and von Schuching, 1963).

Nutrition. Nutrition has a profound effect upon the inflammatory-reparative response, particularly in the healing of wounds. Many workers have confirmed the deleterious effects of prolonged protein starvation upon wound healing (Levenson et al., 1950). Fibroplasia and the synthesis of collagen both appear to be inhibited in protein-deficient animals. It has not been possible to isolate specific amino acids which are crucial to the healing process. It has been said by some and contradicted by others that methionine and cystine supplementations have a beneficial effect on the healing process in the protein-depleted animal (Rosenberg and Caldwell, 1965).

Of the many influences, the best documented is the necessity of adequate levels of vitamin C for the synthesis of normal collagen. Vitamin C in some manner enhances the conversion of proline to hydroxyproline and lysine to hydroxylysine. Deficiencies of this nutrient (scurvy) result in disorganizations in the ultrastructure of the fibroblast and impaired synthesis of normal collagen (Gould, 1966). Still unresolved is the precise point where vitamin C acts in the biosynthetic pathways of normal collagen formation. Many possibilities have been proposed. Vitamin C might be required for the formation of specific messenger or transfer RNA necessary for the delivery and incorporation of the hydroxylated amino acids into the polypeptides of the tropocollagen macromolecule. It might potentiate the activity of hydroxylating enzymes. Without hydroxyproline, the soluble collagen precursor (tropocollagen) may fail to undergo fibrillogenesis.

Yet another possibility is that vitamin C may be necessary for the maintenance of the normal ultrastructural integrity of the fibroblast (Ross and Benditt, 1964). Ross and Benditt (1965), after an intensive study of the problem, note that ribosomes are disorganized in the scorbutic animal and that normal cell integrity is restored within four hours after the administration of vitamin C. Their investigations suggest that the major role of vitamin C is in the maintenance of the normal protein synthetic apparatus within the fibroblast. Although the final word has not yet been said on this subject, it is clear that avitaminosis C profoundly inhibits normal wound healing.

A recent report, as yet unconfirmed, suggests that zinc may be important in the normal healing of wounds (Pories et al., 1967). It is proposed that marginal levels of zinc may be found in otherwise seemingly well nourished individuals and that this metal is crucial as a cofactor in the enzyme processes involved in wound healing.

Hematologic Derangements. Hematologic derangements may have a major effect on the inflammatory-reparative process. A deficiency of neutrophils in the circulating blood (granulocytopenia) is a well documented basis for increased susceptibility to bacterial infection. Deficiencies of neutrophils are encountered in a variety of hematologic disorders such as leukemia, pancytopenia and agranulocytosis; in all of these situations, the patients are rendered excessively vulnerable to bacterial infections and frequently succumb to these disorders because of an inability to bring them under control.

Currently, there is much interest in a number of genetic disorders in which there are lysosomal abnormalities, rendering the neutrophils inadequate in the inflammatory response. Bleeding disorders known as the hemorrhagic diatheses (p. 739) hinder the inflammatory-reparative process. Here there is a tendency toward excessive extravasation of blood during the inflammatory phase of the response, with the accumulation of large amounts of blood in the wounded areas. The blood serves as a substrate for bacterial growth and, as Ordman and Gillman (1966) have shown, significantly slows the reparative process. The red cells and fibrin must be removed before repair can be completed. The blood may also become enclosed within a fibroblastic wall to create an encysted collection of fluid which blocks healing until it is resorbed.

The impact of anemia has not been clearly established. Despite the prevailing clinical opinion that anemia impairs both the adequacy of the inflammatory response and the quality of the repair, it has not been possible to document this impression in rigorously controlled experiments. Almost invariably, there is a concomitant depletion of plasma proteins and possibly immune globulins which makes it difficult to isolate the effect of a single variable (Levenson et al., 1965).

Immunity. Immunity hardly needs to be mentioned as an important influence on the inflammatory phase of the response to injury. Natural or acquired antibodies may be paramount in the control of infectious diseases. This subject is of sufficient importance to be discussed in detail in Chapter 7 (p. 194).

Diabetes Mellitus. Diabetes mellitus comprises a serious handicap to the inflammatory-reparative process. Diabetics have a well known increased susceptibility to infections, but the biologic and biochemical mechanisms are still not understood. More accurately, it should be said that the diabetic is not more vulnerable to bacterial invasion but, once invaded, has greater probability of developing a clinically significant or even serious infection. They are particularly prone to tuberculosis, mycotic infections, skin infections and infections of the urinary tract. It is facile to say that the high levels of blood glucose favor bacterial growth, but the explanations are probably far more complicated. These patients are often dehydrated and have serious electrolyte disturbances. It has been shown that the skin in these patients has high levels of glucose and low levels of lactic acid, the latter removing one of the major inhibitory influences to bacterial growth. Neutrophils in the diabetic have decreased phagocytic capacity. All of these alterations would tend to render these patients more vulnerable to bacterial invasion; however, it is still not certain that they are the major or the ultimate causes of the increased susceptibility of these patients to infection and hence to more severe inflammatory reactions (Kandhari et al., 1969).

Hormones. Hormones, particularly the adrenal steroids (cortisone and hydrocortisone), have a well documented anti-inflammatory effect and also depress protein and polysaccharide synthesis (Kivirikko, 1963). However, where these steroids act is still somewhat uncertain. The anti-inflammatory action has been most clearly established. These steroids stabilize lysosomal membranes and so block the release of important proteolytic enzymes and permeability factors crucial to the evolving inflammatory response (Weissmann and Thomas, 1963). Another interesting suggestion has been offered that cortisone exerts its anti-inflammatory effect by hindering the action of histidine decarboxylase, thereby interfering with the local formation of histamine.

The action of steroids on the healing phase is more controversial. A number of conflicting reports may be found. Inhibition of the synthesis of connective tissues in vitro and in vivo, impairment of granulation tissue formation, decreased production of protein-bound hydroxyproline, as well as total collagen formation have all been reported (Nocenti et al., 1964). However, there is a strong suspicion that these inhibitory effects on the healing process result from suppression of the inflammatory response. If cortisone is administered to animals 2 days after injury, healing does not appear to be impaired, suggesting that it acts early in the response and probably does not primarily affect the healing phase (Sandberg, 1964). We may conclude by stating that steroids unquestionably block or retard the inflammatory-reparative response, but how they exert this effect is still uncertain.

LOCAL INFLUENCES

Adequacy of Blood Supply. The adequacy of the blood supply in an area of injury is an obvious important influence. From all that has been said before, it must be apparent that vascularization of the focus is a key factor in both inflammation and repair. Arterial disease which limits blood flow and venous abnormalities which retard drainage are well documented impairments to the healing of wounds. Indeed, in the aged individual, a trivial bruise on the lower extremity may give rise to an ugly, indolent, persistent leg ulcer. In these predisposed patients, arteriosclerosis narrows the inflow and varicose veins hamper the outflow of blood. While this generalization relative to blood supply holds true for virtually all tissues of the body, the cornea is a remarkable exception. It is virtually avascular and, nonetheless, exhibits great capacity for wound healing.

Foreign Bodies. Foreign bodies and, of course, sutures are included under this designation, and constitute impediments to healing. The surgeon is faced with the dilemma of an incision which has virtually no intrinsic strength during the immediate postoperative period save that conferred by sutures, while at the same time the sutures comprise an obstacle to healing. The puncture wounds in the epidermis invite bacterial contamination, and the suture material excites an inflammatory and foreign body reaction. One interesting study contends that a single suture enhances the invasiveness of staphylococci by a factor of 10,000 (Elek and Conen, 1957). Fragments of wood, steel, glass and even bone are equally undesirable. One must walk between Scylla and Charybdis by using sutures judiciously and by removing all extraneous foreign bodies.

Coaptation of Wound Margins. Careful coaptation of the wound margins greatly speeds the healing of an incision. Epidermal closure and sealing of the wound occurs within 1 to 2 days when the epidermal edges are properly coapted. On the other hand, deficiencies in such neat closure often permit depressed margins of the epidermis to grow downward into the wound and create buried nests of epithelium which may become transformed to small epidermis-lined cystic inclusions. Slowing of the reepithelialization keeps the door open for bacterial invasion.

Tissue in Which the Injury Has Occurred.

It is apparent that perfect repair can occur only in tissues made up of stable and labile cells, whereas all injuries to tissues composed of permanent cells must inevitably give rise to scarring and, at the most, very slight restoration of specialized elements. The location of the injury, or the character of the tissue in which the injury occurs, is also of considerable importance from yet another standpoint. There are many situations in the body in which inflammations may arise within tissue spaces or cavities and develop extensive exudates that fill these spaces. Despite these widespread extensive inflammatory responses, there may be no associated necrosis of fixed tissue cells. Under these circumstances, repair may occur by liquefactive digestion of the exudate, initiated by the proteolytic enzymes of leukocytes, and resorption of the dissolved exudate. This mechanism of dealing with an exudative inflammation is called *resolution.* Since no necrosis of fixed tissue cells has occurred, perfect restitution of the preexisting architecture is attained.

An example of resolution may make its meaning more clear. Bacterial infections in the lung cause inflammations which may solidly fill the alveolar spaces with exudate. In many instances, the alveolar septa are not damaged, although the lung becomes totally solidified by the inflammatory exudation. Proteolytic digestion of the exudate and resorption or coughing up of the watery digestate permit resolution of the pneumonia and restoration of normal lung structure and function. This same sequence of events is not inevitable in all pneumonias, since infections with more virulent pathogens may cause necrosis of alveoli and result in fibrous scarring and permanent pulmonary damage. Moreover, for completely obscure reasons, certain pneumonias with or without necrosis sometimes fail to resolve but, instead, granulation tissue grows from the septal walls into the exudate and converts it into masses of fibrous tissue, referred to as *organization* of the pneumonia (Fig. 3–27).

These processes of resolution or organization of inflammatory exudates are also observed in inflammations within other tissue spaces of the body—i.e., peritoneal, pericardial and pleural cavities and joint spaces. In the overall viewpoint, most injuries of the body do not resolve without tissue necrosis, and result in some connective tissue proliferation and therefore some degree of scarring. Finally, even when scarring is complete, there is another hazard consequent upon a lag in the return of tensile strength of the collagen fibers. A rise in tension may bring about undue stretching of

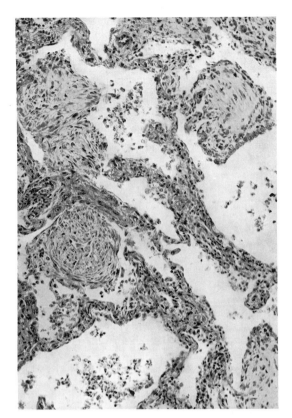

Figure 3–27. *Organized pneumonia. Large round masses of fibroblastic scar tissue are visible in the alveolar spaces.*

the scar, with hernia formation when the abdominal wall is affected. So, too, the thin-walled scar of syphilitic aortitis yields to blood pressure and fathers an aneurysm.

In concluding this discussion of host factors, it is hardly necessary to point out that many involve issues of considerable clinical importance. The correction of nutritional deficiencies, avoidance of steroid therapy, wise use of sutures, careful debridement and removal of foreign bodies and, in general, scrupulous attention to all of the influences which may hamper the inflammatory response are all responsibilities of the clinician.

PERSPECTIVE ON THE INFLAMMATORY-REPARATIVE RESPONSE

The full spectrum of events, from the initial reaction to injury to the ultimate tissue repair, has been presented. It must be obvious that an injury may have little consequence and

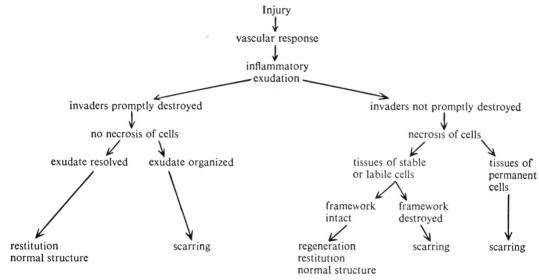

Figure 3–28. *Pathways of reparative response.*

may be dealt with readily or may culminate in severe destruction and damage. A perspective of the various pathways is offered in Figure 3–28. This overview makes clear that not all injuries result in permanent damage; some are resolved with perfect reconstitution of the native tissue. However, most often some residual scarring persists.

REFERENCES

Abercrombie, M.: Contact inhibition and its biological implications. Nat. Cancer Inst. Monog., 26:249, 1966.

Abercrombie, M.: Localized formation of new tissue in an adult mammal. Sympos. Soc. Exp. Biol., 11:235, 1967.

Abercrombie, M., and Ambrose, E. J.: The surface properties of cancer cells: a review. Cancer Res., 22:525, 1962.

Abt, A. F., and von Schuching, S.: Aging as a factor in wound healing. Arch. Surg., 86:627, 1963.

Adamsons, R. J., et al.: The relationship of collagen content to wound strength in normal and scorbutic animals. Surg. Gynec. Obstet., 119:323, 1964.

Allgöwer, M.: The Cellular Basis of Wound Repair. Springfield, Ill., Charles C Thomas, 1956.

Allgöwer, M., and Hulliger, L.: Origin of fibroblasts from mononuclear blood cells: a study on in vitro formation of the collagen precursor hydroxyproline in buffy coat cultures. Surgery, 47:603, 1960.

Allison, F., Jr., et al.: Studies of the pathogenesis of acute inflammation. I. The inflammatory reaction to thermal injury as observed in the rabbit ear chamber. J. Exp. Med., 102:655, 1955.

Atkins, E.: Pathogenesis of fever. Physiol. Rev., 40:580, 1960.

Atkins, E., and Wood, W. B., Jr.: Studies on the pathogenesis of fever. II. Identification of endogenous pyrogen in the bloodstream following injection of typhoid vaccine. J. Exp. Med., 102:449, 1955.

Atkins, E., et al.: Release of an endogenous pyrogen *in vitro* from rabbit mononuclear cells. J. Exp. Med., 126:357, 1967.

Billingham, R. E., and Russell, P. S.: Studies on wound healing, with special reference to the phenomenon of contracture in experimental wounds in rabbit skin. Ann. Surg., 144:961, 1956.

Boyden, S.: The chemotactic effect of mixtures of antibody and antigen on polymorphonuclear leukocytes. J. Exp. Med., 115:453, 1962.

Bucher, N. L. R.: Experimental aspects of hepatic regeneration. New Eng. J. Med., 277:686, 738, 1967.

Bullough, W. S.: The control of mitotic activity in adult mammalian tissues. Biol. Rev., 37:307, 1962.

Cliff, W. J.: Kinetics of wound healing in rabbit ear chambers. A time lapse cinemicroscopic study. Quart. J. Exp. Physiol., 50:79, 1965.

Cliff, W. J.: The acute inflammatory reaction in the rabbit ear chamber with particular reference to the phenomenon of leukocytic migration. J. Exp. Med., 124:543, 1966.

Cline, M. J., and Lehrer, R. I.: Phagocytosis by human monocytes. Blood, 32:423, 1968.

Cochrane, C. G., and Aiken, B. S.: Polymorphonuclear leukocytes in immunologic reactions. The destruction of vascular basement membrane in vivo and in vitro. J. Exp. Med., 124:733, 1966.

Cohn, Z. A., and Hirsch, J. G.: The isolation and properties of the specific cytoplasmic granules of polymorphonuclear leucocytes. J. Exp. Med., 112:983, 1960.

Cohnheim, J.: Lectures on General Pathology. Vol. I. McKee, A. D. (trans. from 2nd German ed.). London, New Sydenham Society, 1889.

Cotran, R. S., and Majno, G.: A light and electron microscopic analysis of vascular injury. Ann. N.Y. Acad. Sci., 116:750, 1964.

Cotran, R. S., and Remensnyder, J. P.: The structural basis of increased vascular permeability after graded thermal injury: light and electron microscopic studies. Ann. N.Y. Acad. Sci., 150:495, 1968.

Cruickshank, C. N. D., et al.: The responses of the basophil leucocyte. J. Invest. Derm., 51:324, 1968.

Dias da Silva, W., et al.: Complement as a mediator of inflammation. J. Exp. Med., 126:1027, 1967.

Douglas, D. M.: Wound healing. Proc. Roy. Soc. Med., 62:513, 1969.

Douglas, S. D.: Analytic review: disorders of phagocyte function. Blood, 35:851, 1970.

Dunphy, J. E.: The healing of wounds. Canad. J. Surg., 10:281, 1967.

Ebert, R. H., and Florey, H. W.: Extravascular development of monocyte observed in vivo. Brit. J. Exp. Path., 20:342, 1939.

Elek, S. D., and Conen, P. E.: The virulence of staphylococcus pyogenes for man: a study of the problems of wound infection. Brit. J. Exp. Path., 38:573, 1957.

Fawcett, D.: Comparative observations on the fine structure of blood capillaries. In Orbison, J. L., and Smith, D. E. (eds.): The Peripheral Blood Vessels. International Academy of Pathology. Monograph 4. Maryland, Williams and Wilkins Co., 1963, p. 17.

Gabbiani, G., et al.: Granulation tissue as a contractile organ: a study of structure and function. J. Exp. Med., 135:719, 1972.

Gould, B. S.: Collagen biosynthesis in wound healing. Proceedings of a workshop, National Academy of Sciences. U.S.A. National Research Council, 1966, p. 99.

Grillo, H. C.: Derivation of fibroblasts in the healing wound. Arch. Surg., 88:218, 1964.

Grillo, H. C.: Origin of fibroblasts in wound healing. An autoradiographic study of inhibition of cellular proliferation by local X-irradiation. Ann. Surg., 157:453, 1963.

Grisham, J. W., et al.: Effect of exchange transfusion on labeling of nuclei with thymidine-3H and on mitosis in hepatocytes of normal and regenerating rat liver. Cancer Res., 26:1476, 1966.

Gross, J., et al.: Extraction of collagen from connective tissue by neutral salt solution. Proc. Nat. Acad. Sci., 41:1, 1955.

Harkness, R. D.: The physiology of the connective tissue of the reproductive tract. Int. Rev. Connect. Tissue Res., 2:155, 1964.

Harris, H.: Chemotaxis. Physiol. Rev., 34:529, 1954.

Harris, H.: The movement of lymphocytes. Brit. J. Exp. Path., 34:599, 1953.

Hay, E. D.: Skeletal muscle regeneration. New Eng. J. Med., 284:1033, 1971.

Heimann, R., et al.: Liver cell proliferation due to biliary obstruction. Studies in parabiotic rats. Exp. Molec. Path., 2:442, 1963.

Hersh, E. M., and Bodey, G. P.: Leukocytic mechanisms in inflammations. Ann. Rev. Med., 21:105, 32, 1970.

Higton, D. I. R., and James, D. W.: The force of contraction of full-thickness wounds of rabbit skin. Brit. J. Surg., 51:462, 1964.

Hirsch, J. G.: Cinemicrophotographic observations on granule lysis in polymorphonuclear leucocytes during phagocytosis. J. Exp. Med., 116:827, 1962.

Horsfield, G. I.: The effect of compound 48/80 on the rat mast cell. J. Path. Bact., 90:599, 1965.

Howes, E. L., and Harvey, S. C.: The age factor in the velocity of the growth of fibroblasts in the healing wound. J. Exp. Med., 55:577, 1932.

Hurley, J. V.: Acute inflammation: the effect of concurrent leucocytic emigration and increased permeability on particle retention by the vascular wall. Brit. J. Exp. Path., 45:627, 1964a.

Hurley, J. V.: Substances promoting leukocyte emigration. Ann. N.Y. Acad. Sci., 116:918, 1964b.

Hurowitz, R. B., and Studer, A.: Effect of partial hepatectomy on mitosis rate in CCl4-induced liver damage of parabiotic rats. Arch. Path., 69:511, 1960.

Iverson, O. H.: Effect of epidermal chalone on human epidermal mitotic activity in vitro. Nature, 219:75, 1968.

Johnson, F. R.: The reaction of epithelium to injury. Sci. Basis Med. Ann. Rev.: 276, 1964.

Kahlson, G., and Rosengren, E.: New approaches to the physiology of histamine. Physiol. Rev., 48:155, 1968.

Kandhari, K. C., et al.: Investigations into the causation of increased susceptibility of diabetics to cutaneous infections. Indian J. Med. Res., 57:1295, 1969.

Karnovsky, M. J.: The ultrastructural basis of capillary permeability studied with peroxidase as a tracer. J. Cell. Biol., 35:213, 1967.

Keller, H. U., and Sorkin, E.: Chemotaxis of leukocytes. Experientia, 24:641, 1968.

Kivirikko, K. I.: Hydroxyproline containing fractions in normal and cortisone treated chick embryos. Acta Physiol. Scand., Suppl. 60:7, 1963.

Landis, E. M., et al.: Passage of fluid and protein through human capillary wall during venous congestion. J. Clin. Invest., 11:717, 1932.

Leak, L. V., and Burke, J. F.: Ultrastructural studies on the lymphatic anchoring filaments. J. Cell. Biol., 36:129, 1968.

Levenson, S. M., et al.: The healing of rat skin wounds. Ann. Surg., 161:293, 1965.

Levenson, S. M., et al.: The healing of soft tissue wounds, the effects of nutrition, anemia and age. Surgery, 28:905, 1950.

Lewis, G. P.: Plasma kinins and other vasoactive compounds in acute inflammation. Ann. N.Y. Acad. Sci., 116:846, 1964.

Lewis, T.: The Blood Vessels of the Human Skin and their Responses. London, Shaw, 1927.

Lichtenstein, I. L., et al.: The dynamics of wound healing. Surg. Gynec. Obstet., 130:685, 1970.

Litt, M.: Studies in experimental eosinophilia. VI. Uptake of immune complexes by eosinophils. J. Cell Biol., 23:355, 1964.

Loewenstein, W. R.: Transfer of information through cell junctions and growth control. Canad. Cancer Conf., 8:162, 1969.

Logan, G., and Wilhelm, D. L.: The inflammatory reaction in ultraviolet injury. Brit. J. Exp. Path., 47:286, 1966.

Luft, J. H.: Structure of capillary and endocapillary layer as revealed by Ruthenium red. Fed. Proc., 25:1776, 1966.

Lumsden, C. E.: Cell structure and cell physiology in relation to myelin. In Williams, D. (ed.): Modern Trends in Neurology. 2nd ed. London, Butterworth and Co., 1957, p. 148.

Majno, G., and Leventhal, M.: Pathogenesis of histamine type vascular leakage. Lancet, 2:99, 1967.

Majno, G., and Palade, G. E.: Studies on inflammation. I. The effect of histamine and serotonin on vascular permeability: an electron microscopic study. J. Biophys. Biochem. Cytol., 11:571, 1961.

Mann, P. R.: An electron-microscope study of the relations between mast cells and eosinophil leucocytes. J. Path., 98:183, 1969.

Marchesi, V. T., and Florey, H. W.: Electron microscopic observations on the emigration of leukocytes. Quart. J. Exp. Physiol., 45:343, 1960.

Marchesi, V. T., and Gowans, J. L.: The migration of lymphocytes through the endothelium of venules in lymph nodes: an electron microscopic study. Proc. Roy. Soc. Med. (Series B), 159:283, 1964.

McDermott, W. V., Jr., et al.: Major hepatic resection: diagnostic techniques and metabolic problems. Surgery, 54:56, 1963.

McMinn, R. M. H.: The cellular morphology of tissue repair. Int. Rev. Cytol., 22:63, 1967.

Miles, A. A.: Local and systemic factors of shock. Fed. Proc., Suppl. 9, 20:141, 1961.

Moses, J. M., et al.: Pathogenesis of inflammation. I. The production of an inflammatory substance from rabbit granulocytes in vitro and its relationship to leucocyte pyrogen. J. Exp. Med., 120:57, 1964.

Nocenti, M. R., et al.: Collagen synthesis and C-14 labeled protein uptake and conversion to hydroxyproline in steroid-treated granulomas. Proc. Soc. Exp. Biol. Med., 117:215, 1964.

Ordman, L. J., and Gillman, T.: Studies in the healing of cutaneous wounds. I. The healing of incisions through the skin of pigs. Arch. Surg. (London), 93:857, 1966.

Pack, G. T., et al.: Regeneration of human liver after major hepatectomy. Surgery, 52:617, 1962.

Page, A. R., and Good, R. A.: A clinical and experimental study of the function of neutrophils in the inflammatory response. Amer. J. Path., 43:645, 1958.

Pappenheimer, J. R.: Passage of molecules through capillary walls. Physiol. Rev., 33:387, 1953.

Pories, W. J., et al.: Acceleration of wound healing in man with zinc sulfate given by mouth. Lancet, 1:121, 1967.

Porter, K. R., and Pappas, G. D.: Collagen formation by fibroblasts of the chick embryo dermis. J. Biophys. Biochem. Cytol., 5:153, 1959.

Rabinovitch, M.: Phagocytosis: the engulfment stage. Seminars Hemat., 5:134, 1968.

Rafter, G. W., et al.: Studies on the pathogenesis of fever. XIV. Further observations on the chemistry of leukocytic pyrogen. J. Exp. Med., 123:433, 1966.

Ramachandran, G. N.: Molecular structure of collagen. Int. Rev. Connect. Tissue Res., 1:127, 1963.

Remensnyder, J. P., and Majno, G.: Oxygen gradients in healing wounds. Amer. J. Path., 52:301, 1968.

Reznick, M.: Origins of myoblasts during skeletal muscle regeneration. Lab. Invest., 20:353, 1969.

Robledo, M.: Myocardial regeneration in young rats. Amer. J. Path., 32:1215, 1956.

Rosenberg, B. F., and Caldwell, F. T., Jr.: Effect of single amino acid supplementation upon the rate of wound contraction and wound morphology in protein-depleted rats. Surg. Gynec. Obstet., 121:1021, 1965.

Ross, R.: The fibroblast and wound repair. Biol. Rev., 43:51, 1968.

Ross, R., and Benditt, E. P.: Wound healing and collagen formation. J. Cell Biol., 27:83, 1965.

Ross, R., and Benditt, E. P.: Wound healing and collagen formation. I. Sequential changes in components of guinea pig skin wounds observed in the electron microscope. J. Biophys. Biochem. Cytol., 11:677, 1961.

Ross, R., and Benditt, E. P.: Wound healing and collagen formation. IV. Distortion of ribosomal patterns of fibroblasts in scurvy. J. Cell Biol., 22:365, 1964.

Sandberg, N.: Time relationship between administration of cortisone and wound healing in rats. Acta Chir. Scand., *127*:446, 1964.

Schilling. J. A.: Wound healing. Physiol. Rev., *48*:374, 1968.

Schoefl, G. I.: Migration of lymphocytes across the vascular endothelium in lymphoid tissue. A reexamination. J. Exp. Med., *136*:568, 1972.

Sevitt, S.: Early and delayed edema: an increase in capillary permeability after burns of the skin. J. Path.Bact., *75*:27, 1958.

Sevitt, S.: Inflammatory changes in burned skin: reversible and irreversible effects and their pathogenesis. In Thomas, L., Uhr, J. W., and Grant, L. (eds.): Injury, Inflammation and Immunity. Baltimore, Williams and Wilkins Co., 1964, p. 183.

Shafiq, S. A., et al.: An electron microscopic study of regeneration and satellite cells in human muscle. Neurology, *17*:567, 1967.

Spector, W. G.: The acute inflammatory response. Ann. N.Y. Acad. Sci., *116*:749, 1964.

Spector, W. G.: The cytokinetics of chronic inflammation. Sci. Basis Med. Ann. Rev.: 163, 1967.

Spector, W. G.: The granulomatous inflammatory exudate. Int. Rev. Exp. Path., *8*:1, 1969*a*.

Spector, W. G.: The origin of mononuclear cells in inflammatory exudates. Res. Publ. Ass. Res. Nerv. Ment. Dis., *44*:1, 1968.

Spector, W. G.: Recent advances in the study of leucocyte emigration. Brit. J. Derm., Suppl. 3, *81*:19, 1969*b*.

Spector, W. G., and Willoughby, D. A.: Endogenous mechanisms of injury in relation to inflammation. In de Reuck, A. V. S., and Knight, J. (eds.): Cellular Injury. Boston, Little, Brown and Co., 1964*a*, p. 74.

Spector, W. G., and Willoughby, D. A.: Vasoactive amines in acute inflammation. Ann. N.Y. Acad. Sci., *116*:839, 1964*b*.

Spector, W. G., et al.: A quantitative study of leucocyte emigration in chronic inflammatory granulomata. J. Path. Bact., *93*:101, 1967.

Spiro, R. G.: Biochemistry of complex polysaccharides in ground substance. In Levenson, S. M., Stein, J. M., and Grossblatt, N. (eds.): Wound Healing Proceedings of a Workshop. Washington, D.C., National Academy of Science, National Research Council, 1966, p. 75.

Sutton, J. S., and Weiss, L.: Transformation of monocytes in tissue culture into macrophages, epithelioid cells and multinucleated giant cells. An electron microscope study. J. Cell Biol., *28*:303, 1966.

Sweet, L. C.: Eosinophils. Henry Ford Hosp. Med. J., *17*:209, 1969.

Thompson, P. L., et al.: Suppression of leucocytic sticking and emigration by chelation of calcium. J. Path. Bact., *94*:389, 1967.

Van Winkle, W., Jr.: The fibroblast in wound healing. Surg. Gynec. Obstet., *124*:369, 1967.

Wagner, B. M., and Siew, S.: Significance of extracellular hyaline substances. In Sommers, S. C. (ed.): Pathology Annual. Vol. 2. New York, Appleton-Century-Crofts, 1967, p. 299.

Ward, P. A.: The chemosuppression of chemotaxis. J. Exp. Med., *124*:209, 1966.

Ward, P. A.: Chemotaxis of human eosinophils. Amer. J. Path., *54*:121, 1969.

Ward, P. A.: Chemotaxis of polymorphonuclear leukocytes. Biochem. Pharmacol., Suppl. *17*(March):99, 1968*a*.

Ward, P. A.: Chemotaxis of mononuclear cells. J. Exp. Med., *128*:1201, 1968*b*.

Ward, P. A.: Neutrophil chemotactic factors and related clinical disorders. Arthritis Rheum., *13*:181, 1970.

Weiss, P.: Biological Specificity and Growth. Princeton, N.J., Princeton University Press, 1955.

Weissmann, G.: The role of lysosomes in inflammation and disease. Ann. Rev. Med., *18*:97, 1967.

Weissmann, G., and Thomas, L.: Studies of lysosomes. II. The effect of cortisone on the release of acid hydrolases from a large granule fraction of rat liver induced by an excess of vitamin A. J. Clin. Invest., *42*:661, 1963.

White, B. N., et al.: The glycoproteins and their relationship to the healing of wounds. Ann. N.Y. Acad. Sci., *94*:297, 1961.

White, R. G.: The effect of mycobacteria on macrophage mobilization and granuloma formation. In Illingworth, C. (ed.): Wound Healing. Boston, Little, Brown and Co., 1966, p. 27.

Wilhelm, D. L.: The mediation of increased vascular permeability in inflammation. Pharmacol. Rev., *14*:251, 1962.

Wilhelm, D. L., and Mason, B.: Vascular permeability change in inflammation: the role of endogenous permeability factors in mild thermal injury. Brit. J. Exp. Path., *41*:487, 1960.

Willoughby, D. A., and Spector, W. G.: The lymph node permeability factor: a possible mediator of the delayed hypersensitivity reaction. Ann. N.Y. Acad. Sci., *116*:874, 1964.

Wood, N. B., et al.: Studies on the mechanisms of recovery in pneumococcal pneumonia. J. Exp. Med., *84*:387, 1946.

Zachariae, H., et al.: Plasma kinins in inflammation: relation to other mediators and leukocytes. Scand. J. Clin. Lab. Invest., Suppl. *107*:85, 1969.

Zeya, H. I., and Spitznagel, J. K.: Arginine-rich proteins of polymorphonuclear leukocyte lysosomes: antimicrobial specificity and biochemical heterogeneity. J. Exp. Med., *127*:927, 1968.

Zucker-Franklin, D.: Electron microscopic studies of human granulocytes: structural variations related to function. Seminars Hemat., *5*:109, 1968.

Zweifach, B. W.: Microcirculatory aspects of tissue injury. Ann. N.Y. Acad. Sci., *116*:831, 1964.

4

NEOPLASIA

Cancer annually causes the death of over 300,000 persons in the United States. This number increases with each passing year. Only cardiovascular disease causes more deaths. The steady climb in cancer mortality may not only result from a real increase in attack rate, but may also reflect a decline in the death rates from such controllable diseases as tuberculosis, other infections, diabetes and malnutrition. By default, the stream of mortality has thus been diverted into the two channels of the still uncontrolled menaces of cardiovascular disease and cancer. Moreover, the increase in longevity in economically privileged societies exposes many more people to years of greater vulnerability to cancer. Whether the increased cancer mortality is real or spurious, the absolute number of cancer deaths increases yearly.

Although cancer is understandably of greater importance, both benign and malignant tumors are considered in the following discussion. Attention is focused principally on their basic characteristics, morphology and behavior as well as on a survey of where we currently stand in the search for their origins and causation(s). There follows in Chapter 5 the discussion of their clinical aspects and implications—in other words, the ultimate reasons for their great importance.

DEFINITIONS

Neoplasia literally means "new growth," and the mass of cells composing the new growth is a neoplasm. The term new growth does not adequately define a neoplasm. Much more meaningful is the definition of Willis (1952): "*A neoplasm is an abnormal mass of tissue, the growth of which exceeds and is uncoordinated with that of the normal tissues and persists in the same excessive manner after cessation of the stimuli which evoke the change.*" To this characterization we might add that the abnormal mass is purposeless, preys on the host and is virtually autonomous. It preys on the host insofar as the growth of the neoplastic tissue competes with normal cells and tissues for energy supplies and nutritional substrate. Inasmuch as these masses may flourish in a patient who is wasting away, they are to a degree autonomous. Later it will become evident that such autonomy is not complete. All neoplasms ultimately depend on the host for their nutrition, respiration and, indeed, their vascular supply; and many forms of neoplasia even require endocrine support.

The terms tumor and cancer should be clarified. Actually, *tumor* refers simply to swelling which is, in fact, one of the cardinal signs of inflammation. While a neoplasm near the surface of the body produces a tumorous swelling, all tumors, correctly speaking, are not neoplastic and may also be produced by hemorrhage or edema. Nonetheless, long historic precedent has equated the term tumor with neoplasm, and the other usages of tumor have now passed into limbo. Thus we have *oncology* (oncos = tumor) as the study of tumors or, more correctly, the study of neoplasms. *Cancer is the common term for all malignant tumors.* The term cancer has ancient origins, likening these obstinately clutching neoplastic masses to the crab: "Some say that it is so called because it adheres to any part that it seizes upon in an obstinate manner like the crab."

The terms benign and malignant, as applied to neoplasms, have clinical implications. The designation benign implies that the lesion is not life-threatening, is relatively slow-growing, will not disseminate through the body (metastasize) and is amenable to removal, with cure of the patient. Only rarely will a benign neoplasm kill, and then by virtue of its strategic location or function. For example, the benign neoplasm that obstructs the common bile duct or elaborates sufficient insulin to cause fatal hypoglycemia may not be so very benign. In contrast, nearly all malignant neoplasms have the ugly potentials of rapid growth, invasion and destruction of contiguous structures and dissemination throughout the body, leading to death.

NOMENCLATURE

The nomenclature of tumors unfortunately does not follow any single consistent scheme. *Most benign tumors are classified histogenetically by attaching the suffix "-oma" to the cell type constituting the neoplasm.* Thus, benign tumors composed of fibrocytes are termed fibromas and fatty tumors, lipomas. This system works well with mesenchymal benign tumors (those arising in muscle, bones, tendon, cartilage, fat, vessels, lymphoid and fibrous tissue) because the tumor cells usually closely resemble their normal counterparts, and the various adult mesenchymal cells are sufficiently distinctive to be readily differentiated from one another. However, benign tumors of epithelial origin defy such easy classification. For example, the cells that line the small intestine closely resemble those that line the ducts of the pancreas, the mucosal cells of the gallbladder and those of the fallopian tubes. Accordingly, benign epithelial neoplasms are variously classified, some on the basis of their cells of origin, others on microscopic architecture, and still others on their macroscopic patterns.

Adenoma is the term applied to the benign epithelial neoplasm which forms glandular patterns, as well as to the tumors derived from glands but not necessarily reproducing glandular patterns. On this basis a benign epithelial neoplasm that arises from intestinal lining cells growing in the form of numerous tightly clustered small glands would be termed an adenoma, as would a heterogeneous mass of adrenal cortical cells growing in no distinctive pattern but merely producing a small benign new growth. Benign epithelial neoplasms producing microscopically or macroscopically visible finger-like or warty projections from epithelial surfaces are referred to as *papillomas* or *polyps*. Those that form large cystic masses as in the ovary are referred to as *cystomas* or *cystadenomas*. Some tumors produce papillary patterns which protrude into cystic spaces and are called papillary cystadenomas (Fig. 4–1).

Malignant tumor nomenclature essentially follows the same schema used for benign neoplasms with certain additions. *Cancers arising in mesenchymal tissue are called sarcomas* (sarc = fleshy). A malignant neoplasm of fibrocytes is a fibrosarcoma, and one composed of lymphocytes is a lymphosarcoma. Sarcomas are then designated by their histogenesis. *Malignant neoplasms of epithelial cell origin, derived from any of the three germ layers, are called*

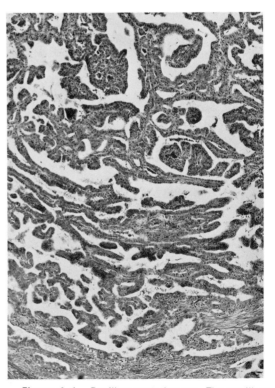

Figure 4–1. *Papillary cystadenoma. The papillary tumor fills a small cystic space.*

carcinomas. Thus, cancer arising in the epidermis of ectodermal origin is a carcinoma as is a cancer arising in the mesodermally derived cells of the renal tubules and the endodermally derived cells of the lining of the gastrointestinal tract. Carcinomas may be further qualified. One with a glandular growth pattern microscopically is termed an adenocarcinoma, and one producing recognizable squamous cells arising in any of the stratified squamous epithelia of the body would be termed a squamous cell carcinoma. It is further common practice to specify, when possible, the organ of origin—e.g., a renal cell adenocarcinoma or bronchogenic squamous cell carcinoma. Not infrequently, however, a cancer is composed of very primitive, undifferentiated cells and must be designated merely as a poorly differentiated or undifferentiated malignant tumor or, when possible, undifferentiated carcinoma or undifferentiated sarcoma.

Usually the proliferating cells of a tumor bear a close resemblance to each other as though all came from closely related forebears. Thus, all the cells of the adrenal adenoma resemble adrenal cortical cells, and the proliferating cells of the squamous cell carcinoma more or less resemble stratified squamous epithelial cells. Such neoplasms have been classified as *simple* merely to contrast them with *mixed* and *compound* neoplasms. In some tumors, divergent differentiation of the neoplastic cells gives rise to more than one cell type within the neoplasm. It should be emphasized that the divergent patterns all stem from common progenitors. Such neoplasms are categorized as *mixed,* the best example of which is the mixed tumor of salivary gland origin. Another designation of this lesion is a pleomorphic adenoma, indicating that it is basically a benign glandular tumor possessing divergent morphology—in some part, recognizable glandular epithelial formations, in other areas, apparent myxoid stroma, and in still other areas, perhaps islands of pseudocartilage (Fig. 4–2). Such mixed patterns should come as no surprise since ultimately all of the specialized cells of the body are derived from a single fertilized ovum and, understandably, under neoplastic influences repressed areas of the genotype may become expressed.

Another category which must be differentiated from the simple neoplasm is designated as *compound,* or *teratogenous,* to indicate a content of a variety of cell types representative of more than one germ layer. These neoplasms, called *teratomas,* arise from totipotential cells and so are principally encountered in the gonads. Rarely, teratomas arise from primitive cell rests sequestered in the midline of the body during embryogenesis. In the neoplastic proliferation of these totipotential cells, well differentiated tissues may be produced resembling skin, muscle, fat, gut epithelium, endocrine and exocrine glandular structures, tooth structures and, indeed, any structure of the body (Fig. 4–3). A particularly common pattern in the ovaries, the *cystic dermoid teratoma,* differentiates principally along ectodermal lines to yield a cystic tumor lined by skin replete with hair, sebaceous glands and tooth structures. Its true teratomatous origin is often disclosed by accompanying foci of muscle and cartilage. The cystic dermoid usually behaves as a benign neoplasm, but the solid (noncystic) more variegated teratoma is frequently malignant (p. 1248). The overwhelming preponderance of neoplasms, however, are composed of one cell type and so, unless otherwise specified, all neoplasms can be considered as simple. Yet the mixed tumors and the teratomas are of great conceptual interest since they indicate the depth of the fundamental change associated with oncogenesis. A classification of the more common forms of neoplasms is presented in the accompanying table:

TABLE 4–1. CLASSIFICATION OF TUMORS*

Tissue of Origin	Benign	Malignant
I. Simple (composed of one single neoplastic cell type)		
A. Tumors of Mesenchymal Origin		*sarcomas*
(1) Connective Tissue and Derivatives		
fibrous tissue	fibroma	fibrosarcoma
myxomatous tissue	myxoma	myxosarcoma
fatty tissue	lipoma	liposarcoma
cartilage	chondroma	chondrosarcoma
bone	osteoma	osteogenic sarcoma
notochordal tissue	chordoma	chordoma (or better, chordosarcoma)
(2) Endothelial and Related Tissues		
blood vessels	hemangioma: capillary cavernous sclerosing	angiosarcoma
	hemangioendothelioma	endotheliosarcoma (multiple sarcoma—Kaposi's sarcoma)

TABLE 4–1. CLASSIFICATION OF TUMORS* (*Continued*)

Tissue of Origin	Benign	Malignant
lymph vessels	lymphangioma	lymphangiosarcoma
	lymphangioendothelioma	lymphangioendotheliosarcoma
synovia		synovioma (synoviosarcoma)
mesothelium (lining cells of body cavities)		mesothelioma (mesotheliosarcoma)
brain coverings	meningioma	
glomus	glomus tumor	
? blood vessels of bone marrow		Ewing's tumor ? (endotheliosarcoma)
(3) Blood Cells and Related Cells		
hematopoietic cells		granulocytic leukemia
		monocytic leukemia
lymphoid tissue		malignant lymphomas
		lymphocytic leukemia
		plasmacytoma (multiple myeloma)
reticuloendothelial system		reticulum cell sarcoma (malignant lymphoma, histiocytic type)
		?Hodgkin's disease
(4) Muscle		
smooth muscle	leiomyoma	leiomyosarcoma
striated muscle	rhabdomyoma	rhabdomyosarcoma
B. Tumors of Epithelial Origin		*carcinomas*
stratified squamous	squamous cell papilloma	squamous cell or epidermoid carcinoma
skin adnexal glands:		
hair follicles		basal cell carcinoma
sweat glands	sweat gland adenoma	sweat gland carcinoma
sebaceous glands	sebaceous gland adenoma	sebaceous gland carcinoma
epithelium lining:		
glands or ducts—	adenoma	adenocarcinoma
well differentiated group	papilloma	papillary carcinoma
	papillary adenoma	papillary adenocarcinoma
	cystadenoma	cystadenocarcinoma
poorly differentiated group		medullary carcinoma
		undifferentiated carcinoma (simplex)
respiratory tract		bronchogenic carcinoma
		bronchial "adenoma"
neuroectoderm	nevus	melanoma (melanocarcinoma)
renal epithelium	renal tubular adenoma	renal cell carcinoma (hypernephroid)
liver cells	liver cell adenoma	liver cell carcinoma or hepatoma
bile duct	bile duct adenoma	bile duct carcinoma (cholangiocarcinoma)
urinary tract epithelium (transitional)	transitional cell papilloma	papillary carcinoma
		transitional cell carcinoma
		squamous cell carcinoma
placental epithelium	hydatid mole	choriocarcinoma
testicular epithelium		seminoma
		embryonal carcinoma
II. Mixed (more than one neoplastic cell type, usually derived from one germ layer)		
salivary glands	mixed tumor of salivary gland origin	malignant mixed tumor of salivary gland origin
renal anlage		Wilms' tumor
III. Compound (more than one neoplastic cell type derived from more than one germ layer)		
totipotential cells in gonads or in embryonic rests	teratoma, dermoid	One or more elements become malignant, e.g., squamous cell carcinoma arising in a teratoma (teratocarcinoma)

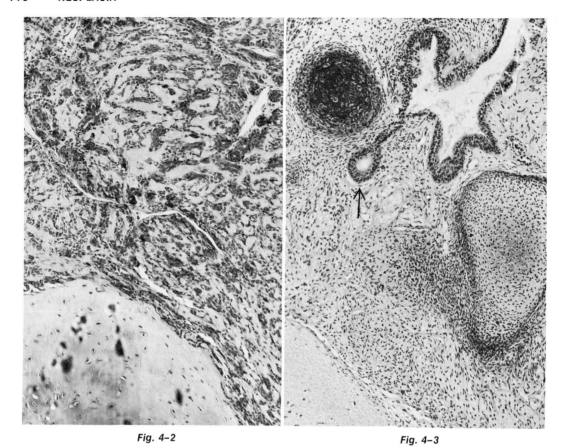

Fig. 4–2   *Fig. 4–3*

Figure 4–2. *A mixed tumor of salivary gland origin (pleomorphic adenoma). There is a large plate of pseudo-cartilage in the lower field. The remainder of the tumor is composed of small cords and nests of epithelial cells separated by pale areas of loose connective tissue.*

Figure 4–3. *A teratoma. Three distinct types of adult tissues are seen: a circular island of darkly stained cartilage (mesodermal) in the upper left, a large nest of stratified squamous epithelial cells (ectodermal) on the right, and in the center a gland space lined by columnar cells resembling intestinal tract mucosa (endodermal) (arrow).*

Since each tumor tends to have a specific behavior, its specific designation carries important clinical implications. Referring to the table, one finds that testicular seminiferous epithelium may give rise to either a seminoma or an embryonal carcinoma. Totipotential cells in the testes may also produce a choriocarcinoma if teratogenous development occurred along placental lines. Given a patient with a testicular tumor, the seminoma represents a form of carcinoma which tends to spread to lymph nodes along the iliac arteries and aorta. These cancers in their primary site tend to be resectable in almost all cases and the implants into the abdominal lymph nodes are remarkably radiosensitive and can be cured by irradiation. Very few of these patients die of their neoplasm. The embryonal carcinoma, by contrast, is not radiosensitive, and this tumor has a tendency to invade locally beyond the confines of the testis and to spread throughout the body. Despite all therapeutic efforts, over half of these patients are dead within two years of discovery of their neoplasm. The choriocarcinoma in the male is one of the most malignant neoplasms encountered. Specific terminology has specific clinical import.

It is necessary at this point to bring to attention certain inappropriate usages so deeply ingrained in medical parlance as to be virtually ineradicable. For example, malignant tumors arising in liver cells are usually called hepatomas although more properly they should be referred to as hepatocarcinomas. In the same way, the carcinoma arising in melanocytes is generally called melanoma rather than its proper designation, melanocarcinoma. Malignant tumors of lymphoid origin are generically designated lymphomas, but all possess varying levels of aggressiveness, and all are malignant in their clinical behavior. In these instances, innocent terms mask the malignant nature of the neoplasm. Perhaps it is irrational to expect man to be rational.

CHARACTERISTICS OF NEOPLASMS—CRITERIA FOR DIFFERENTIATING BENIGN FROM MALIGNANT

All neoplasms cause patients to be alarmed, but what comfort the diagnosis "benign tumor" brings. The differentiation of benign from malignant is the most important judgment the pathologist is called upon to make. Upon this decision are based the therapy of the lesion and the outlook for the patient. Many criteria are used to make such a distinction and the following discussion deals with the general characteristics of benign and malignant neoplasms and particularly those used as differential features. A chart at the conclusion of this discussion summarizes these differential points (p. 122).

Before entering this discussion of the differential characteristics of benign and malignant neoplasms, it should be emphasized that, although most tumors are clearly benign or unmistakably malignant, a few are borderline and cannot be categorized with certainty. As one wise pathologist once said, "All tumors need not of necessity be either benign or malignant." More accurately, such growths possess some feature which suggests a benign diagnosis while others point toward a malignant nature. These borderline lesions merely emphasize the ultimate subjectivity in the morphologic interpretation of the differential characteristics of benign and malignant tumors. It is also important to recognize that some deceptively benign-appearing neoplasms behave biologically like a cancer and vice versa. There is, therefore, not always perfect correspondence between morphologic predictions and biologic behavior. However, these tumors are the exceptions; in general, morphologic criteria can be established to distinguish the benign from the malignant, and the tumors behave correspondingly.

DIFFERENTIATION AND ANAPLASIA

All tumors, benign and malignant, have two basic components: (1) proliferating neoplastic cells which comprise their *parenchyma* and (2) supportive *stroma* made up of connective tissue, blood vessels and possibly lymphatics. The parenchymal cells are by far the most important since they not only make up the large bulk of most tumors, but also represent the proliferating "cutting edge" and so determine the nature of the neoplasm.

Parenchymal Cells. All parenchymal cells have certain characteristics in common since they have all undergone some funda-mental alteration (i.e., transformation) conferring upon them neoplastic capabilities. Nonetheless, they exhibit a wide range of altered morphology and function. This range extends from cells which are virtually indistinguishable from their normal forebears to wildly atypical cells bearing no resemblance to any normal cell. *The differentiation of parenchymal cells refers to the extent to which they resemble their normal cells of origin and includes the extent to which they achieve their fully mature morphologic and functional characteristics.* The closer the resemblance to their normal forebears, the better the differentiation; the greater the departure from the characteristics of the normal, the poorer the differentiation (Figs. 4–4 and 4–5). The poorly differentiated neoplasm may also be called undifferentiated. *In general, all benign neoplasms are well differentiated, but malignant neoplasms range from well differentiated to those consisting of primitive-appearing, anarchic, undifferentiated cells.*

Formerly, it was assumed that all neoplasms arose in fully specialized cells of the tissues and organs. Thus, it was assumed that when a totally undifferentiated carcinoma arose in the thyroid, the neoplastic transformation involved de-differentiation of the mature thyroid epithelial cells. At the present time, the concept of de-differentiation has been challenged and it is currently believed that undifferentiated tumor cells arise from undifferentiated reserve or stem cells found in virtually all organs. Similarly, the well differentiated cancer probably also arises from primitive reserve cells which undergo specialization as they proliferate to create the neoplasm. The conceptual issue is more than academic. While many specialized cells lose their capacity to replicate as they become fully mature (e.g., the upper layers of stratified squamous epithelium), in neoplasia specialization may occur without loss of replicative capability.

Anaplasia may be used as a synonym for undifferentiation of tumor cells. Literally, anaplasia means "to form backwards," a phenomenon that is now no longer believed to occur. Nonetheless, the term anaplasia has come to have specific connotations with regard to neoplasms. *Anaplastic tumors are invariably malignant and are composed of more or less undifferentiated cells that have lost some or all resemblance to their normal counterparts.* Both the cells and their nuclei characteristically display pleomorphism—variation in size and shape. Giant cells may be found that are many times larger than their neighbors, and other cells may be extremely small and primitive-appearing. Characteristically, the nuclei contain an abundance of DNA and are extremely dark staining (hy-

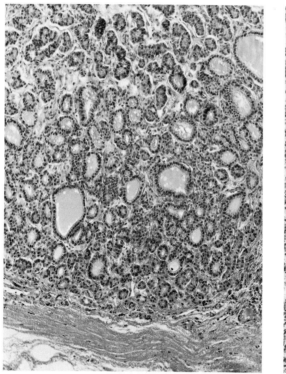

Fig. 4–4

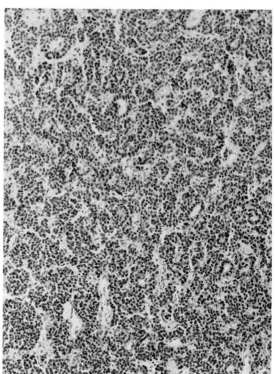

Fig. 4–5

Figure 4–4. *A well differentiated benign thyroid adenoma. The fibrous capsule is in the lower field. The tumor faithfully reproduces thyroid acini filled with colloid.*

Figure 4–5. *A moderately poorly differentiated thyroid carcinoma. The tumor cells form disorganized cords of cells and only occasional acinar spaces suggest a thyroid origin.*

perchromatic). The nuclei are disproportionately large for the cell and the nuclear-cytoplasmic ratio may approach 1:1 instead of the normal 1:4 or 1:6. The nuclear shape is usually extremely variable, and the chromatin is often coarsely clumped and is frequently distributed along the nuclear membrane. Large nucleoli are usually present in these nuclei, reflecting the synthetic activity of these cells. Anaplastic tumors usually possess large numbers of mitoses, reflecting the proliferative activity of the parenchymal cells. However, it must be stressed that the presence of mitoses does not necessarily indicate that the tumor is malignant.

More important as a diagnostic feature of malignant neoplasia are atypical and bizarre mitotic figures sometimes producing tripolar, quadripolar or multipolar spindles (Figs. 4–6 and 4–7). Often, the mitotic jumble possesses abnormally large spindles in one area and shrunken, puny spindles in other regions. Another important feature of anaplasia is the formation of tumor giant cells, some possessing only a single huge polymorphic nucleus, while others have two or more nuclei within the single cell. These giant cells are not to be confused with inflammatory Langhans' or foreign body giant cells which possess many small, normal-appearing nuclei. The cancer giant cell has hyperchromatism of the nucleus and too much nucleus for the cell (Figs. 4–8 and 4–9).

The orientation of anaplastic cells to each other varies among cancers. In some better differentiated lesions, the cells reproduce glandular patterns and a well defined architecture resembling, to some extent, the tissue of origin. Thus the acini in adenocarcinomas of the thyroid sometimes closely resemble the acini of the thyroid (Fig. 4–10). At the other end of the spectrum is the very anaplastic cancer, not only made up of very deviant cells but whose orientation to each other is helter-skelter. Sheets or large masses of tumor cells grow in an anarchic, disorganized fashion. While these growing cells obviously require a blood supply, often the connective tissue vascular stroma is scant and, indeed, in many anaplastic tumors, large areas undergo ischemic necrosis. *Anaplasia, when present, is an unmistakable hallmark of malignancy in a neoplasm.* In the

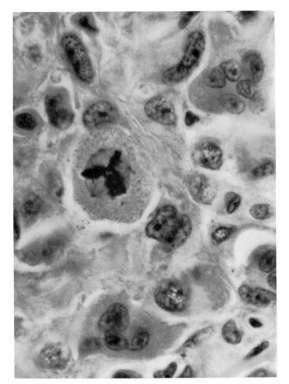

Fig. 4–6

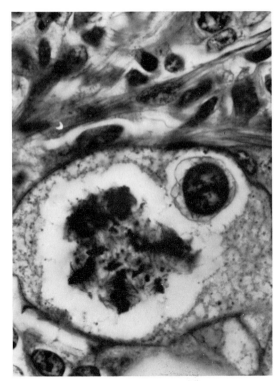

Fig. 4–7

Figure 4–6. *High power detail of anaplastic tumor cells to show cell and nuclear variation in size and shape. The prominent cell in the center field has an abnormal tripolar spindle.*

Figure 4–7. *High power detail of multinucleate tumor giant cell. One nucleus is in resting phase while the other nucleus is in abnormal mitotic division, with the formation of multiple poorly organized spindles.*

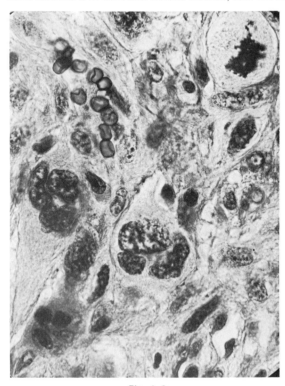

Fig. 4–8

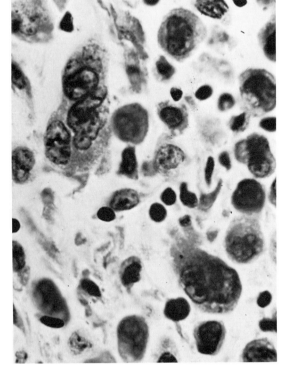

Fig. 4–9

Figure 4–8. *Anaplastic tumor cells with prominent multinuclear tumor giant cells and an abnormal mitotic figure in the upper right field.*

Figure 4–9. *Anaplastic tumor cells with prominent multinucleate tumor giant cells in which the nuclei virtually fill the cell.*

113

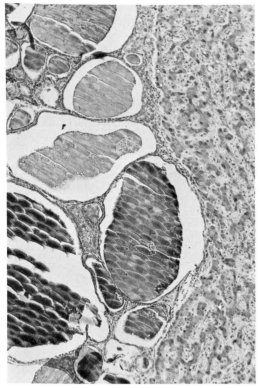

Figure 4–10. *Metastatic thyroid carcinoma in the liver. The tumor is formed of well developed acini filled with colloid and lined by flattened, innocent-appearing cells. Only its intrahepatic location discloses the true malignant character of the neoplasm.*

transformation to cancer, some level of anaplasia usually appears in tumor cells, although admittedly it is slight in some.

The electron microscope has added little to the characterization of neoplastic cells. Well differentiated tumor cells in benign neoplasms may have virtually all of the normal ultrastructural features of their normal forebears. Similarly, the well differentiated cancer cell deviates little from the normal. As these cells become progressively more undifferentiated, as would be anticipated, their ultrastructural organization departs from the normal. An entire spectrum of experimental carcinomas of the liver, misnamed hepatomas, have been induced in the rat (Hruban et al., 1972). Cells of well differentiated hepatomas called "minimum deviation hepatomas" are very similar to normal hepatocytes. They have few ultrastructural deviations from normal hepatocytes, principally simplification of the rough endoplasmic reticulum (RER) and variation in mitochondrial size and shape. In the more undifferentiated forms of hepatomas, there is an increase of free ribosomes, greater variation among the mitochondria and a further paucity

and simplification of the RER. All of these changes can be evoked by other forms of pathologic stress on normal hepatocytes. Changes paralleling the severity of anaplasia have also been described in the nuclei of tumor cells.

The tumor cell's functional sophistication correlates with its degree of differentiation. Deficiencies in enzymes such as esterases and phosphatases are encountered in cells showing disorganization of the endoplasmic reticulum, and deficiencies in respiratory enzymes are associated with mitochondrial alterations. In simple terms, the undifferentiated cell fails to mature along normal lines both morphologically and functionally.

Against this background, one can usually distinguish between benign and malignant neoplasms on the basis of their parenchymal differentiation. In general, all benign neoplasms are extremely well differentiated. The neoplastic cell in a smooth muscle tumor—a leiomyoma—so closely resembles the normal cell as to make it impossible, on high power examination of a leiomyoma, to recognize the smooth muscle cell as belonging to a tumor. Only the massing of these cells into a nodule discloses the tumorous nature of the lesion. One may get so close to the tree that one loses the forest. In such benign tumors, mitoses are extremely scant in number, and the few present are normal in appearance. Not infrequently, mitoses seem to be absent, raising the interesting question of how the tumor achieved its bulk. In contrast, cancers, although ranging from well differentiated to undifferentiated, generally have some degree of anaplasia. This histologic change, together with evidence of invasion of surrounding structures, constitute the two major criteria by which a diagnosis of cancer is made microscopically in the primary site of the neoplasm. Later, we shall see that cancers may disseminate (metastasize) and, when this has occurred, the nature of the primary lesion is no longer in doubt, since *benign tumors never metastasize.* Another correlate of anaplasia should be mentioned here although it will be discussed subsequently. In general, the rate of growth of a malignant tumor parallels its degree of anaplasia—i.e., the better the differentiation, the slower the growth.

A number of classifications of the degree of malignancy of a tumor have been proposed based on the level of differentiation of the parenchymal cells and the number of mitoses found in the neoplastic cells. One of the best known, that of Broders (1926), divides cancers into four grades. Grade I tumors are the best differentiated, have the highest proportion of relatively normal cells and the fewest mitoses, and should have the best prognosis. Grade IV are the most undifferentiated and have many mitoses and presumably the worst prognosis. While such a classification may have some use, too great dependence upon it is unwarranted since the behavior of tumors is, at best, unpredictable and every cancer has not read the classification and therefore does not know how it should behave. Some cancers that are well differentiated grow with surprising speed, while undifferentiated lesions may be unexpectedly sluggish. The classification offers little that is not provided by such qualifying terms as "very well differentiated apparently slowly growing adenocarcinoma" or "highly anaplastic apparently rapidly growing carcinoma." Moreover, far more important than the grade of malignancy is the extent of the carcinoma. For example, is it small and still confined to its epithelial site of origin or has it spread through the wall of the gut? Whatever the level of anaplasia, the cancer which has not invaded is usually resectable, resulting in cure of the patient, while the best differentiated lesion that has already invaded widely may be incurable.

The anaplasia of cancer cells has been usefully exploited in the cytologic diagnosis of cancer. The Papanicolaou smear test for cancer, described in some detail on p. 153, is based upon the facts that cancer cells are less cohesive than normal cells and so are readily shed, and anaplasia can be identified on careful microscopic examination of individual shed cells. Thus, in carcinoma of the cervix, anaplastic cells are desquamated into the vaginal secretions and examination of a smear of such secretions will, in almost all instances, disclose the presence of the primary lesion. The cytologic test is of great value in the diagnosis of cancer.

Stroma. The stroma, while critical to the survival and growth of a neoplasm, is not helpful in the differentiation of benign from malignant neoplasia. It is clear from experimental evidence that, in the inception of neoplasia, the development of a vascular supply and concomitant stromal support are vital to the evolution of the mass. Folkman (1971) has ingeniously shown that individual tumor cells will grow in tissue culture to minute masses, perhaps in the order of a few millimeters in diameter, and then cease growing. Adding fresh culture medium or oxygen to the flask permits no further growth. However, when grown in tissues, once they are able to develop a blood supply from the adjacent tissue, they rapidly enter a phase of logarithmic growth. Thus, the capacity of the parenchyma to proliferate is de-

pendent upon the adequacy of its blood supply and its stromal support. When parenchymal growth outpaces the blood supply, the central region of the neoplasm most remote from the peripheral blood supply undergoes ischemic necrosis and hemorrhage.

The richness of the connective tissue stroma determines the consistency of the tumor. Some cancers, particularly sarcomas (fleshy tumors), have very little fibrous stroma and have the consistency of raw fish flesh or brain substance. Carcinomas having such a soft consistency are designated as medullary. At the other end of the stromal spectrum are certain neoplasms which evoke a dense, collagenous stroma and thus achieve a gritty hardness. This stromal proliferative reaction is referred to as desmoplasia, and is particularly well exemplified in many cancers of the female breast designated as scirrhous carcinoma. Islands of metaplastic cartilage or bone are sometimes also found in the stroma and, in some cancers, a significant infiltrate of lymphocytes, plasma cells and histiocytes is seen. Later, it will be pointed out that such a mononuclear cell reaction is of great interest to the tumor immunologist, suggesting an immune response of the host against the intruder (Bell et al., 1969).

RATE OF GROWTH

In general, the rate of growth of a neoplasm correlates with its level of differentiation and with its clinical behavior. Most benign tumors which are well differentiated grow slowly over a period of years at a steady pace. Most cancers grow rapidly, sometimes at an erratic pace, eventually to spread and kill their hosts. Such generalizations must be extensively qualified. Benign neoplasms may enter periods of long dormancy when they apparently do not enlarge, and some achieve a certain dimension and apparently cease growing. Factors such as hormone dependence, compression of their blood supply with atrophy of the well differentiated neoplastic cells and, in all probability, other unknown influences may cause this halt in their growth. For example, uterine leiomyomas (benign smooth muscle tumors) are common. When of sufficient size, they are readily palpable on abdominopelvic examination. It is not infrequent to encounter women who have had leiomyomas which have not increased in size over the span of years or even decades. Not infrequently, such neoplasms are found to be largely replaced by collagenous fibrous tissue and, indeed, often are heavily calcified, both changes suggesting loss of growth vigor and, indeed, fibrocalcific atrophy of the lesion. On the other hand, the benign fibroadenoma (a tumor having an abundant fibrous stroma enclosing glands) of the female breast may undergo rapid increase in growth and size during pregnancy, presumably because of the increased levels of steroid hormones on which this neoplasm appears to have some dependency. Whether slowly increasing in size, dormant, or even appreciably enlarging over the span of time, mitoses are infrequent in benign neoplasms. Indeed, their mitotic activity is considerably less than that encountered in the striking regeneration of the proliferative menstrual endometrium and the constant growth and replacement of the lining epithelium of the gut.

In general, the growth rates of cancers parallel their levels of differentiation and the relative number of their cells in mitosis. Thus, mitoses are more abundant in the anaplastic variants. Although most malignant tumors grow rapidly, this growth rate varies widely. Radiographic studies of certain clinical cancers over a period of years have shown that some double their size in a week while others may require a year (Brenner et al., 1967). But it must be cautioned that such studies are only looking at the tip of the iceberg; they deal with clinically apparent masses.

When cancers arise, they are first identified as loci of anaplastic cells totally confined to their original location. Such early lesions do not produce masses nor can they be visualized radiographically. *Cancers that are confined to transformation of cells within their original location and have not spread across basement membranes into surrounding tissues are said to be in situ.* For example, an in situ gastric carcinoma would be confined to cancerous cells within the gastric glands, and an in situ skin cancer would still be confined to the epidermis. In terms of growth rate, the peak incidence of in situ cervical carcinoma occurs in women about 25 to 30 years of age. At this stage in their evolution, the lesions produce no grossly visible alteration in the cervical mucosa and can only be detected by histologic or cytologic examination. The average age of patients with clinically overt, visible cancer is 40 to 45 years. It must follow, therefore, that it requires 10 to 15 years for these neoplasms to evolve from the in situ stage to clinically apparent masses (Johnson et al., 1964). The same has been shown to hold true with other forms of clinical neoplasia. Thus, while we speak of rapid growth of cancers, we must appreciate that much of this growth becomes apparent only after long years of slow evolution.

The growth of cancer often pursues an erratic, unpredictable course. Although most progressively enlarge, some may suddenly shrink in size as they undergo ischemic necrosis resulting from outgrowth of their blood supply. Others may remain dormant for considerable periods of time and still others may enter phases of explosive enlargement. Cases abound in which the local cancer has remained extremely small and silent and is only discovered after it has disseminated widely throughout the body by a process soon to be described as metastasis. Small renal lesions have been observed by pyelographic study to remain dormant over years and decades and, indeed, have been thought to be benign but have been discovered, by virtue of their dissemination, to be cancers. Indeed, the renal cell carcinoma arising in tubular epithelial cells is a paradigm of erratic behavior. On occasion, removal of a kidney with a renal cell carcinoma in a patient who is otherwise apparently free of spread of tumor is followed 10 to 15 years later by the appearance of a renal cancer implant in the lungs. This may occur in the complete absence of local recurrence of the tumor at the operative site. Were the cancer cells lying dormant in the lungs all these years and, if so, what initiated their growth into demonstrable tumor?

Host factors undoubtedly influence the growth rate of cancers. There is much experimental evidence that the host may develop an immune reaction to tumors. Indeed, in the animal the immune response may destroy a tumor. Hints abound that immunity may comprise a controlling influence on tumor growth in man, a subject discussed more fully on p. 146. Reference has already been made to the necessity for developing an adequate blood supply if the cancer is to develop and expand. The cancer arising in the testis may so expand against the tunica albuginea as to compress its blood supply and so slow, or even contain, its growth for a period of time. Usually, however, such containment does not last long because of the invasive capacity of cancer. Many neoplasms arising in organs under hormonal control — e.g., the breast or prostate — retain a dependence upon a continued supply of hormones. If these hormone levels are augmented, the cancer may enter a phase of rapid growth. When the levels are lowered by ovariectomy or orchiectomy, the growth of these cancers is slowed. Thus cancer of the breast may widely proliferate if the woman becomes pregnant. Hormone dependence has been exploited clinically in the attempt to control tumor growth (p. 135).

Most cancer growth is achieved by an increased rate of proliferation — namely, shortening of the generation time of the neoplastic cells (Richart, 1963). However, increase in size of a tumor may also be accomplished by recruitment of normal cells immediately contiguous to the original focus. Conceivably, tumor cells elaborate factors that induce neoplastic transformation of cells in contact with the original focus. Notwithstanding, it is emphasized that most cancers are associated with an increased number of mitoses and growth rate of cells, and evidence will be presented later that such proliferative activity results from some apparent loss of normal controls. Nonetheless, few cancers can match the fetus in numbers of mitoses and rapidity of growth.

MODE OF GROWTH AND SPREAD

The mode of growth and capacity to spread most clearly differentiate cancers from benign neoplasms.

Encapsulation. *Nearly all benign tumors grow as localized expansile masses enclosed within a fibrous capsule.* They remain localized to their site of origin and cannot disseminate throughout the body. The capsule comprises an enclosing fibrous membrane in part derived from the fibrous stroma of the surrounding normal tissues and in part elaborated by the tumor. The slow, expansile pressure of the benign new growth causes atrophy of the surrounding normal parenchymal cells, leaving the more resistant fibrous stroma of the native tissue which thus envelops the tumor mass. In some part, however, the capsule is produced by the stroma of the tumor itself. Such encapsulation tends to contain the benign neoplasm as a discrete, readily palpable and easily movable mass that can be surgically enucleated (Figs. 4–11 and 4–12). However, the centrifugal growth does cause compression atrophy of contiguous structures. The benign adenoma of the anterior pituitary may destroy all residual normal pituitary parenchyma trapped between the expanding lesion and the sella turcica.

While encapsulation is a characteristic of benign neoplasms, lack of a capsule does not make a neoplasm malignant. Some benign tumors, such as the leiomyoma in the uterus, remain discrete but are not encapsulated; however, since it is surrounded by compressed myometrium, it can be enucleated. Similarly, benign hemangiomas (neoplasms composed of tangled blood vessels) are often unencapsu-

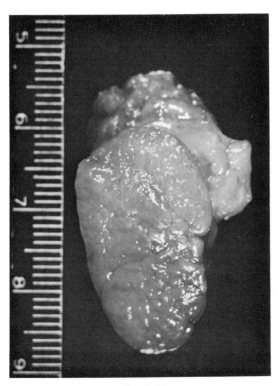

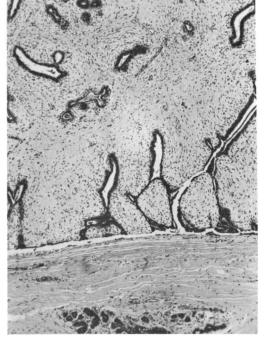

Fig. 4–11   *Fig. 4–12*

Figure 4–11. *A gross view of a fibroadenoma of the breast. The discrete tumor bulges above the level of the surrounding breast substance as it extrudes from its tight encapsulation.*

Figure 4–12. *A microscopic view of the fibroadenoma of the breast seen in Figure 4–11. The fibrous capsule separates the sharply delimited tumor mass from the surrounding breast substance.*

lated and may, indeed, appear to permeate the sites (commonly the dermis of the skin) in which they arise. Similarly, certain fibroblastic neoplasms of the dermis (dermatofibromas) are unencapsulated. Lymphangiomas commonly arising in the axillae, neck and mediastinum are classically unencapsulated and, indeed, have the disturbing characteristic of insinuating widely through normal cleavage planes. Despite their infiltrative growth and lack of capsule, these new growths never metastasize and so are considered benign.

Invasion. *Cancers are almost never encapsulated and are characterized by infiltrative, erosive growth* (Figs. 4–13 and 4–14). While on occasion the slowly expanding malignant tumor deceptively appears to develop an enclosing fibrous membrane, histologic examination will always disclose tiny crab-like feet penetrating such seeming encapsulation (Fig. 4–15). Most cancers, however, develop no semblance of a capsule and so, for example, may penetrate the wall of the colon or fungate through the surface of the skin as was once so common in the neglected cancer of the female breast. They recognize no normal anatomic boundaries and often permeate perineural spaces (Fig. 4–16). The advanced cancer of the cervix penetrates the vaginal walls, grows upward into the pelvis, into the urinary bladder, may occlude the lower ureters and continues to spread into surrounding structures. Such invasiveness makes their surgical removal, even in their local site of origin, exceedingly difficult. Excision of a cancer generally requires radical surgery involving the removal of a considerable margin of apparently normal tissues about the infiltrative neoplasm. Only in this way can the ramifying pseudopods beyond the range of visibility with the naked eye be encompassed.

Metastasis. Cancer cells, when carried to a site away from their origin, are able to implant—i.e., *metastasize*. The implant is called a *metastasis*. Metastases themselves may secondarily give rise to other metastases. The invasiveness of cancers carries them through not only tissues but also blood vessel and lymphatic walls. *Metastasis unequivocally marks a tumor as malignant because benign neoplasms cannot metastasize.* With few exceptions, all cancers may metastasize. The major exceptions are malignant neoplasms arising in glial cells in the central nervous system called gliomas and basal cell carcinomas of the skin. The latter were known in the older literature as rodent ulcers because of their invasive, destructive behavior, but they almost never metastasize.

In general, the more undifferentiated the cancer, the more rapid and infiltrative its growth and the more likely the possibility of metastasis. However, such a generalization has many exceptions, and mention has already been made of small primary cancers as well as of extremely well differentiated lesions, both with widespread metastases. From these exceptions has come the notion of "*biologic predeterminism.*" Based on the unpredictability of the behavior of cancers, some investigators believe that the malignant neoplasm acquires the ability to invade and to metastasize and its rate of growth as individual attributes. According to this concept, then, certain rapidly growing

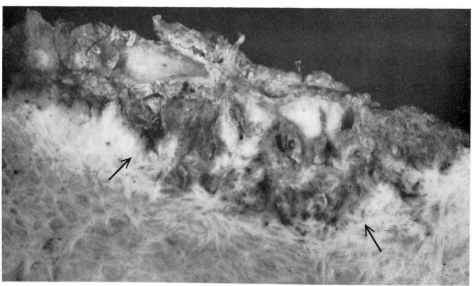

Figure 4–13. *Adenocarcinoma of the endometrium. A close-up. The malignant tumor (arrows) extends into the underlying muscular wall of the uterus. There is no sharp line of delimitation from the surrounding normal tissue.*

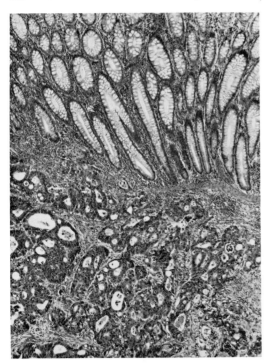

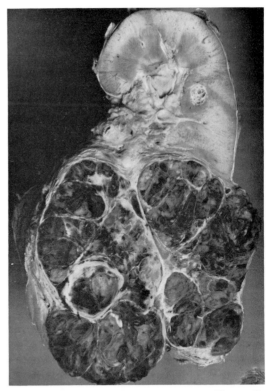

Figure 4–14. *Infiltrative invasive adenocarcinoma of the colon extending beneath the normal mucosa adjacent to the focus of origin of the cancer.*

Figure 4–15. *Renal cell carcinoma. The malignancy appears to be deceptively well encapsulated.*

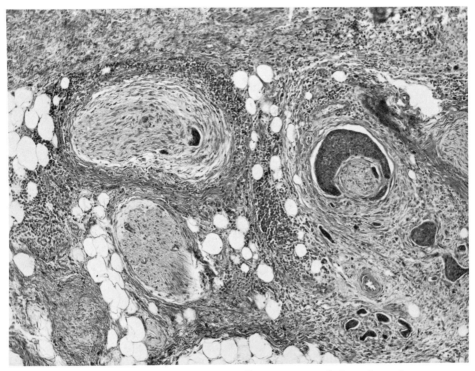

Figure 4–16. *Darkly staining nests of malignant tumor cells in perineural spaces.*

cancers might not have the ability to metastasize while other noninvasive lesions might have acquired metastatic capability. Hence, the biologic behavior would be predetermined, presumably by the genetic or epigenetic attributes of the cancer cell (MacDonald, 1951).

The dissemination of a cancer is obviously its most feared consequence. Once this has occurred, it is almost always beyond surgical extirpation—still the best hope for cure. Malignant neoplastic dissemination may occur through one of four pathways: (1) seeding throughout body cavities, (2) direct transplantation, (3) lymphatic permeation and (4) embolization through blood vessels. Each of these pathways will be described separately, followed by a discussion of the possible mechanisms which permit such tumor spread.

Seeding of Body Cavities. This may occur whenever a malignant neoplasm penetrates into a natural "open field." Most often involved is the peritoneal cavity, but any other cavity—pleural, pericardial, subarachnoid and joint spaces—may be affected. When, for example, a carcinoma arises in the mucosa of the stomach or colon, it may permeate the wall of the gut to appear on the serosal surface where small tumor seedlings may then reimplant anywhere in the peritoneal cavity. Such seeding is particularly characteristic of carcinomas arising in the ovaries where, not infrequently, all peritoneal surfaces may be coated with a heavy layer of cancerous glaze. Remarkably, in such seeding the tumor cells may all remain confined to the surface of the coated abdominal viscera without penetrating into their substance. Nonetheless, the widespread dissemination causes as much impact on the host as deeper seedings. Sometimes mucus-secreting ovarian and appendiceal carcinomas fill the peritoneal cavity with a gelatinous neoplastic mass referred to as "*pseudomyxoma peritonei.*" The reimplantation of cancer fragments from higher to lower levels of organ systems has always been a concern—e.g., the reimplantation of a renal cell carcinoma into the urinary bladder or the downstream dissemination of a gastric cancer into the colon. Such a theoretical possibility cannot be dismissed, but it is a practical rarity as judged by clinical experience.

Transplantation. This refers to the mechanical transport of tumor fragments by instruments or gloved hands. That this may occur is amply documented by the ease of tumor transplantation under appropriate conditions in animals. Transplantation of cancers has also occurred in the patient when, for example, a needle is inserted into a tumor to obtain an aspiration biopsy and the procedure is followed by implantation of tumor along the needle track. However, fortunately, mechanical transport is a rare pathway of tumor dissemination in man, a tribute either to judicious clinical care or the the inability of tumor fragments to survive when so artificially displaced. Conceivably, the immune response of the host to his neoplasm plays some role in suppressing the precariously situated fragments.

Lymphatic Spread. *Lymphatic spread is the pathway predominantly used by carcinomas, but sarcomas also use this route. More often sarcomas embolize through blood vessels.* However, the generalization applies that all forms of cancer may metastasize via lymphatics or blood vessels. The distribution of the lymphatic spread tends to follow natural channels of drainage. Carcinomas of the breast usually arise in the outer quadrants and, when they spread, it is almost always first to the axillary lymph nodes. Those of the inner quadrant may drain through lymphatics to the nodes within the chest along the internal mammary arteries. After these primary sites of spread, the supraclavicular and infraclavicular nodes may then be affected. Bronchogenic carcinomas arising in the major respiratory passages invariably spread first to the perihilar, tracheobronchial and mediastinal nodes. Growth of tumor within lymph nodes may block normal lymphatic channels of drainage and produce bizarre retrograde spread. In this fashion, the bronchogenic carcinoma, after it saturates the tracheobronchial nodes, may involve the chain of nodes along the aorta down into the abdomen. As mentioned earlier, any of these lymph node deposits may secondarily metastasize.

In some instances, nodal spread involves growth of the tumor in-continuity from its primary location through the lymphatic channels, eventually reaching the lymph node. In other instances, perhaps more commonly, tumor fragments drain through the lymphatics to arrest in the nodes as natural drainage depots (Fig. 4–17). Because regional lymph nodes are so commonly affected, it is fairly standard practice in surgery to excise them and the interposed lymphatic channels along with the primary growth. Thus, radical mastectomy for breast cancer has involved, since the time of Halsted, the removal of the entire breast, pectoral muscles because of their contained lymphatic channels and the axillary lymph nodes. Similarly, resection of a colonic carcinoma includes the adjacent pericolic fat and mesentery, where it is present, together with the regional nodes along the aorta.

Objection has been raised to the interpretation of dissemination to regional nodes as a form of metastasis. This concept would interpret regional nodal involvement as lymphatic

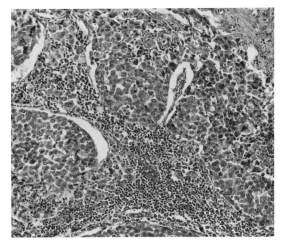

Figure 4–17. A portion of a lymph node with sinuses distended by metastatic tumor.

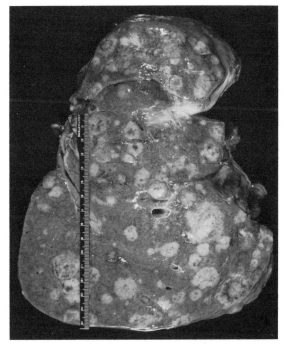

Figure 4–18. Metastatic carcinoma to the liver.

drainage no different from the inflammatory involvement of lymph nodes secondary to a nearby abscess. According to this view, then, nodal involvement does not necessarily imply metastatic capability. A rational argument could be made for not removing apparently uninvolved regional lymph nodes of drainage when a primary cancer is excised. They could serve as drainage traps for errant cancer cells freed at the time of surgery, and they might aid in the local immune response against any residual tumor cell nests left behind.

Blood Vessel Embolization. This is the typical pathway of spread of sarcomas but is also not uncharacteristic of carcinomas. Arteries, because of their thick, muscular walls, are less often penetrated than veins. The embolization follows the route of the venous flow draining the site. Understandably, the liver and lungs are most frequently secondarily involved in such hematogenous dissemination (Fig. 4–18). All of the portal area of drainage flows to the liver, and all of the caval blood leads to the lungs. Cancers arising in close proximity to the vertebral column—such as those of the thyroid and prostate—often embolize through the paravertebral plexus and thus frequently metastasize to the vertebral column.

Arterial spread may occur when pulmo-nary metastases themselves give rise to additional tumor emboli that flow through the left side of the heart. In such arterial spread, a number of factors, soon to be discussed, condition the patterns of distribution of the metastases, but perhaps most important is the quantity of blood flow through the organ. Understandably, then, the brain and kidney are favored sites of arterial dissemination. The spleen is less frequently involved by metastases than one would anticipate from the richness of its blood supply. Splenic metastases are less rare than was once thought, but they are much less frequent than adrenal and ovarian metastases for poorly understood reasons.

Certain cancers have a propensity for invasion of veins. The renal cell carcinoma often invades the branches of the renal vein and then the main renal vein to grow in a snake-like fashion up the inferior cava to sometimes reach the right side of the heart. Hepatocarcinomas display a similar behavior and often penetrate portal and hepatic radicles to grow within them into the main venous channels. Remarkably, such growth may not be accompanied by widespread dissemination, so unpredictable is the biology of cancer. On occasion, one witnesses a resected carcinoma of the kidney in which a cord of tumor lying within the

TABLE 4–2. COMPARISONS BETWEEN BENIGN AND MALIGNANT TUMORS

Characteristics	Benign Tumor	Malignant Tumor
Differentiation	Structure often typical of the tissue of origin	Structure often atypical, i.e., differentiation imperfect
Mode of growth	Growth usually purely expansive, and a capsule formed	Growth infiltrative as well as expansive so that strict encapsulation is absent
Rate of growth	Usually progressive, slow growth which may come to a standstill or retrogress; mitotic figures scanty, and those present are normal	Growth may be rapid with many abnormal mitotic figures
Metastasis	Absent	Frequently present

renal vein has been transected and the patient has subsequently suffered no recurrence nor developed metastases. Presumably, the intravascular mass of tumor left behind depended for its blood supply on the primary site of origin and so underwent ischemic necrosis following the removal of the primary growth. For these reasons, evidence of microscopic invasion of blood vessels or lymphatics in a primary neoplasm must be viewed guardedly. Understandably, such vascular invasion is not a happy portent, but neither does it indicate the inevitable development of widespread metastases.

The characteristics and differences between benign and malignant tumors have been discussed in considerable detail. It is now possible to summarize these briefly (Table 4–2).

MECHANISMS INVOLVED IN CANCER SPREAD

The factors that confer on cancers their erosive, destructive, metastasizing capabilities are still, to a large extent, mysterious. An enormous volume of literature dealing with these mysteries has developed, and a certain number of observations seem well founded. But we must admit that a complete understanding still eludes us. At one time, it was postulated that expansile pressure was the major force in the invasiveness and destructiveness of cancer, but ingenious experiments have made it clear that such a conception is an oversimplification. When a small cancer explant is placed into a tissue culture, close to but not in contact with an explant of normal tissue, the neoplastic cells preferentially grow toward and invade the normal explant and, indeed, expand very little in the opposite direction (Easty and Easty, 1963). The following observations have been made. *As compared with normal cells, cancer cells display: (1) decreased cohesiveness, (2) loss of contact inhibition, (3) increased motility and mobilization, (4) increased contact guidance, (5) the elaboration of enzymes or products injurious to normal cells and (6) the ability to survive translocation.*

DECREASED COHESIVENESS

Decreased cohesiveness helps to explain tumor embolization, the seeding of natural body cavities and the tendency of cancers to spread and penetrate normal tissues adjacent to their primary site of origin. Decreased cohesion also accounts for the shedding of cancer cells into natural channels, such as the desquamation of cervical carcinoma cells into vaginal secretions, bronchogenic carcinoma cells into bronchial secretions and renal carcinoma cells into the urine. A number of factors may be involved in such loss of cohesion (Coman, 1944). Cancerous tissue contains less calcium than normal tissues (DeLong et al., 1950). Calcium ions provide an anionic bond between exposed negative charges of adjacent cell membranes. The architectural integrity of many epithelial surfaces is maintained by the development of desmosomes which help provide cell-to-cell adherence. Cancer cells arising from such epithelial surfaces often fail to form normal intercellular junctions (nexus) (McNutt et al., 1971). An increase in the repulsive electrical charges between cells has been noted. This increased surface charge may be associated with the production of an abnormal amount of a sialo-mucopeptide possessing unopposed negative charges. All of these changes and others undoubtedly still unidentified result in decreased adhesiveness between cancer cells (Abercrombie and Ambrose, 1962) (Ambrose, 1966).

LOSS OF CONTACT INHIBITION

Loss of contact inhibition is an attribute of cancer cells that may well be important in explaining their behavior. The phenomenon of contact inhibition was discussed on p. 97. In cell culture, as normal cells grow out from a spare seeding, those cells which contact their neighbors stop proliferating. Once contact has been established, cell movement and cell growth ceases (Abercrombie and Heaysman, 1954). *Cancer cells exhibit no contact inhibition in vitro* and while this process is not easily recognized in vivo, there is no reason for doubting its applicability. With such a characteristic, cancer cells would continue to proliferate, whatever the pressure restraints, in their site of growth and progressively impinge on and undoubtedly destroy contiguous normal cells and tissue (Abercrombie et al., 1957).

MOTILITY

The motility in vitro of cancer cells exceeds that of most normal cells. They move away from the center of an explant more rapidly than do their normal forebears. In some part, such migration is due to increased rates of proliferation but it also involves cell motility. While such mobilization would be helpful in explaining extension of cancers into surrounding tissues and invasiveness, it must be remembered that cancer cells are no more motile than macrophages and neutrophils. Yet white cells do not destroy tissue cells and only permeate through preestablished interstitital tissue planes rendered accessible by inflammatory fluid exudation.

CONTACT GUIDANCE

Contact guidance deals with the property of growth of cells along a structural or architectural framework. In cell culture, normal fibroblasts grow out in radial orderly array from an explant. If lines are etched into the bottom of the culture flask, they will follow such grooves and will similarly grow along strands of fibrin. Cancer cells grow from explants in helter-skelter, tumbled masses. However, provided a framework such as grooves or other structural support, they rapidly advance along these guideposts. Such a phenomenon could explain the invasiveness of cancer between cells along fascial planes and other supporting framework of normal tissues (Weiss, 1958).

ELABORATION OF ENZYMES OR OTHER PRODUCTS

The elaboration of enzymes or other products that might open pathways or destroy normal cells is an enticing explanation of the invasive destructive nature of cancer. While widely spoken of, there is remarkably little "hard data" to validate this notion (Easty and Easty, 1963) (Easty, 1966). Hyaluronidase has been identified in a few cancers but not in all. The enzymes elaborated by cancer cells in general parallel those produced by their normal forebears. In explants, cancer cells invade normal cells but do not, on contact, destroy them. Perhaps competition for nutrients and the elaboration of waste products resulting from their increased metabolic activity might adequately explain such cytotoxic action as cancer cells have in tissue culture. In this context, it is worth noting that on occasion cancers do not destroy but rather stimulate the growth of adjacent normal cells. *The metastases to bone from a few cancers, particularly carcinoma of the breast and prostate, induce osteoblastic hyperactivity in the immediate locale of the tumor implant.* Such metastases are visualized radiologically as areas of increased bone density rather than the usual punched out, destructive lesions. Although osteoblastic metastases are the exception, they nonetheless indicate that all malignant tumors are not always destructive and, while most are, we do not know how and why.

TRANSPLANTABILITY

The ability of cancer cells to survive when translocated is obviously fundamental to their metastatic potential. Normal specialized cells from an adult are not readily grown in tissue culture, and some indeed cannot survive such translocation. Almost all cancers are readily explanted. By and large, cell suspensions derived from human cancers can be inoculated into appropriate laboratory animals where they will grow to produce tumors. It must be recognized that antigenic differences between donor and host found in all normal and cancerous cells provoke immune responses and sometimes render transplantation difficult or impossible. Nonetheless, it is abundantly clear that cancer cells have a survivability far greater than their normal counterparts. While such an attribute is, of course, critical to metastatic dissemination, the properties of the cancer cell that permit such independence are poorly understood. Reference has been made earlier to "biologic predeterminism" (p. 118), but such a concept merely expresses the problem and does not explain it.

FACTORS GOVERNING METASTATIC POTENTIAL

A number of factors influence the metastatic potential of a given cancer and condition the pattern of distribution and number of the metastases: (1) natural routes of spread accessible to the primary lesion, (2) size, rapidity of growth and anaplasia of the primary cancer, (3) number of tumor emboli, (4) richness of the blood supply of the various tissues and organs of the body, (5) mechanical trauma and movement of the primary lesion, (6) hormonal influences and (7) the immune response to the neoplasm.

It is obvious that the cancer arising in a tissue having a rich lymphatic and blood supply stands a far greater chance of disseminating than one arising in a less vascular location. However, surprisingly these factors do not appear to be of great importance, perhaps because ultimately all normal tissues have sufficient blood supply to sustain their vitality and to permit the neoplasm to gain access to vascular channels. Nonetheless, these natural channels of escape condition the pattern of distribution. Thus, carcinomas arising in the stomach almost invariably metastasize first to the perigastric lymph nodes and then to the liver, while the renal cell carcinoma usually first spreads to the lungs. But unpredictability is a characteristic of all cancers.

The size, growth rate and anaplasia of a malignant neoplasm in general correlate with the number of metastases encountered, but here again exceptions abound. Metastases have been found with in situ carcinoma of the cervix at a stage when the lesion was still microscopic, and many extremely well differentiated cancers have disseminated. Years ago, there was interest in normal lateral aberrant thyroid glands found adjacent to the carotid arteries and jugular veins. The aberrant thyroid appeared entirely normal in its architecture. Experience has taught that many of these lateral aberrant thyroids are metastases to lymph nodes of very well differentiated thyroid primaries. Despite these exceptions, large tumors, rapidly proliferating masses and undifferentiated growth patterns tend to have ugly attributes.

The number of tumor emboli would seem a priori to be an important influence on the number of metastases. While true, it is perhaps more important to note that *blood-borne dissemination of cancer cells cannot always be equated with the development of metastases*. The evolution of a metastasis involves: (1) liberation of cells from the primary, (2) transportation of liberated material, (3) deposition of transported fragments or cells, (4) establishment of deposits and (5) growth of deposits (Foulds, 1958). It can be shown in the experimental animal that the number of metastases generally correlates with the number of tumor cells injected (Fisher and Fisher, 1959). But even when several hundreds of thousands of cancer cells were introduced into the bloodstream, as many as one-fifth of the animals failed to develop metastases. Similarly, cancer cells have been identified in the bloodstream of patients who never developed metastases (Engell, 1959). Many of these emboli, although they may lodge, fail to survive because they are unable to attach to and invade the blood vessel wall. Following lodgement, the tumor cells are incorporated into secondary thrombi and are destroyed as the thrombus organizes or are killed along with the dissolution of the thrombus (Wood, 1958).

The number of metastases lodging in a given organ or tissue is largely related to the richness of its blood supply and its volume of blood flow. These are obviously determinants of the frequency with which the lungs, liver and kidneys are hit by metastatic implants. However, there are other still unknown influences which must be operative (Greene and Harvey, 1964). The spleen and striated muscles have rich blood flow and yet are relatively infrequently affected. Such tissues are spoken of as "barren soil" for metastatic growth. For the spleen, it is argued that tumor emboli are trapped in thick-walled penicilliary arterioles which resist penetration and so block the implantation and survival of cancer cells. But striated muscles have no such vascular supply and are rich in capillary beds. Here it is postulated that the constant mechanical movement of the emboli inhibits their implantation. But it should be noted that certain cancers, such as melanocarcinomas and lymphomas, frequently spread to the spleen and, on occasion, metastatic implants are found in striated muscles. Mechanical manipulation or movement of primary neoplasms may facilitate the breaking off of tumor fragments and favor metastatic dissemination. Yet if such influences are valid, they play at most a small role with most cancers. Long years of surgical experience have taught that incision into a carcinoma, as is done with a biopsy procedure, carries no significant threat of metastatic dissemination. Yet with highly vascularized sarcomas, manipulation is generally considered dangerous. Sometimes, however, such manipulation (e.g., a biopsy) is necessary in order to establish a definitive diagnosis before such radical surgery as amputation of a limb is instituted.

In the experimental animal, hormones can influence the number of metastases that will appear, and there are clinical reasons for believing the same to be true in man. The administration of cortisone or pituitary growth hormone increases the number of metastases in laboratory animals (Fisher and Fisher, 1964) (Fisher and Fisher, 1961). Conversely, the growth of certain forms of cancer and the frequency of metastasis are decreased in the experimental animal following hypophysectomy. Earlier it was noted that certain cancers arising in endocrine-dependent organs retain dependence, for their growth and spread, on these hormonal influences. So ovariectomy, adrenalectomy and even hypophysectomy are sometimes performed clinically in the attempt to slow the growth of metastatic breast carcinoma; similarly, orchiectomy may retard the growth of metastatic prostatic carcinoma. Lamentably, all that has been achieved to date is some alleviation of discomfort produced by the metastases and, in some instances, an increase in longevity, but the neoplasm, both in its primary and secondary sites, survives and almost invariably ultimately kills (Jessiman and Moore, 1956).

Finally, we come to the immune response and its influence on the growth and spread of cancer. Tumor immunology has become a vast and exciting subject. It is discussed in greater detail on p. 146. It suffices here to say that there is abundant experimental evidence that the host mounts an immune response against tumors, even those derived from the host's syngeneic cells. Cancers develop specific antigenic profiles known as tumor-specific antigens and these may induce an immune response. If the response is sufficiently strong, the tumor may be destroyed or metastatic spread may be inhibited.

There are hints that certain tumors, particularly carcinomas which arise in the testis and breast, evoke an immune response in the form of an intense lymphocytic infiltrate of the stroma of the tumor. Moreover, inflammatory nodes draining some neoplasms show striking hyperplastic responses interpreted as an immunologic reaction. Indeed, patients with these primary and secondary reactions have a somewhat better prognosis. While experimental models to document an immune reaction are readily produced, there are only a handful of clinical cases of spontaneous disappearance of cancer (Everson, 1964). However, these and other observations have raised the hope that the immune mechanism might be exploited in the control and cure of cancer. While this goal has not yet been achieved, it seems reasonable to speculate that immunity may play a role in conditioning the number of metastases.

But these speculations notwithstanding, the frequency and distribution of metastases are still unpredictable, quixotic phenomena. Why is it, for example, that bronchogenic carcinomas have a well defined propensity for specifically metastasizing to the adrenal glands along with their spread to the regional nodes? Isolated metastases from primary carcinoma in the prostate have been encountered in the brain without other organs being affected. The cervical carcinoma, which usually spreads locally to involve the pelvic nodes, on occasion implants in the eye. Thousands of bizarre instances could be cited and are well known to physicians, making it abundantly clear that there are no absolute rules governing metastatic dissemination.

FUNCTIONAL BEHAVIOR OF NEOPLASMS

Tumors retain the specialized functional characteristics of their cells of origin in proportion to their degree of differentiation. The well differentiated benign neoplasm may elaborate mucin, hormones and enzymes just as do the normal cells from which it arose. Adenomas of the colon usually secrete mucin, and adenomas of endocrine glands generally elaborate hormones. Indeed, because of certain loss of controls, they may be more productive than their normal counterparts. The minute parathyroid adenoma, less than a centimeter in diameter, may cause serious and even fatal hyperparathyroidism. The hyperinsulinism produced by a 1 cm. adenoma of the islets of Langerhans may cause hypoglycemic death. Indeed, such function is perhaps the greatest threat of benign neoplasms since they rarely cause much damage by their local growth.

The functional ability of malignant neoplasms is far more variable (Braunstein, 1966). In undifferentiated malignant tumors, all the metabolic activities appear to be turned to synthesis of cell substance and mitosis, and other specialized functions appear to be shut off. On the other hand, well differentiated thyroid carcinomas elaborate thyroid hormones, well differentiated adenocarcinomas of the colon elaborate mucin, and well differentiated cancers of the prostate elaborate acid phosphatase. The enzyme profiles of well differentiated tumors differ little from their normal counterparts. (Paul, 1966).

Cancers may elaborate products not produced by their normal cells of origin. *On occasion, tumors induce widespread effects on the host by the synthesis of hormones, suppression of immunity or the elaboration of poorly defined factors which alter central nervous system or bone marrow function.* Collectively, these systemic effects are referred to as *"paraneoplastic"* syndromes. The elaboration of hormones is of greatest interest. This aspect of neoplasia may provide some insight into the fundamental nature of neoplastic transformation since it suggests the activation or, more accurately, the expression of genetic information totally repressed in normal cell counterparts. Undifferentiated carcinomas of the lungs sometimes secrete ACTH while other lung tumors may elaborate antidiuretic hormone (ADH). Retroperitoneal fibrosarcomas have elaborated insulin (Lipsett et al., 1964). Some renal cell carcinomas elaborate erythropoietin and induce polycythemia in the host.

Of even greater interest is the elaboration of certain products normally produced only by primitive or fetal cells. About two-thirds of hepatocarcinomas elaborate alpha fetal globulin. Such globulins are normally produced by liver cells in fetal life, but this production ceases soon after birth. With the emergence of neoplasia, the functional characteristic, repressed at birth, also emerges (Abelev, 1968). Carcinomas of the colon sometimes elaborate an antigen identical to that produced by embryonic tissues, hence designated as the carcinoembryonic antigen (Zamchek et al., 1972).

One sometimes forgets that all cells of the body possess identical genes, since all cells are ultimately derived from the fertilized ovum. More surprising, then, is the fact that so few neoplasms elaborate exotic products. Indeed, these specialized functional attributes form the basis for a number of valuable clinical diagnostic procedures, as is discussed on p. 154.

CARCINOGENESIS

No one needs to be told that the cause of cancer is still unknown. Nonetheless, a vast amount of knowledge has been laboriously gathered in search of this elusive goal. All of the evidence points to the probability that there are many causes of cancer, perhaps acting through quite different mechanisms, and that cancer is not a single entity, but rather a constellation of neoplastic disorders arising out of these varied causes and pathways. In addition, many oncogenic factors may act in concert or in sequence over a long time span to result in the ultimate evocation of a single malignant neoplasm. The staggering variability noted among cancers may be due in part to the multiplicity of tissues from which tumors arise and to a plurality of etiologies.

The emergence of a cancer can be viewed from four vantage points: (1) In what cells do cancers usually arise? (2) What agents evoke cancer (the etiology) and how do they interact with living cells? (3) What are the events common to all cancerous transformation? (4) What critical events occur in the course of carcinogenesis (the pathogenesis)? Before entering this consideration, we should admit at the outset that much will be fact and some will be theory. However, more is known about malignant than benign neoplasia, whose origins remain virtually unknown.

ORIGINS OF CANCER AT THE CELL AND TISSUE LEVEL

Since benign tumors are composed of mature differentiated cells, it seems likely that they arise from adult cells. Cancers, however, are believed to arise from primitive precursor cells or from mature somatic cells whose homeostasis has already been disturbed by hyperplastic, metaplastic, dysplastic or regenerative changes. The common denominator among these settings is active cell replication or the potential for such. A great deal of clinical and experimental evidence suggests that the dividing cell is more susceptible to carcinogenic influences than the resting cell and that, indeed, cell division is a necessary requisite for carcinogenesis. For example, it is clear that hyperplastic processes in the endometrium and breast are common backgrounds for the emergence of cancer. Chronic cervicitis leading to mucosal dysplasia invokes a twenty-twofold increased incidence of subsequent cancer and it is of interest that, on the average, five years elapse between the appearance of dysplasia and the emergence of the cancer (Johnson et al., 1968). The bronchogenic carcinoma of the habitual cigarette smoker is usually a squamous cell carcinoma, and it almost invariably arises in a soil of dysplastic or metaplastic squamous epithelium in the respiratory passages. The contribution of cellular regeneration to oncogenesis is well exemplified also by the greatly increased incidence of carcinomas in patients having preexistent cirrhosis of the liver (p. 1019). This form of liver disease is associated with areas of liver cell necrosis and consequent active regeneration. Osteogenic sarcomas occur in children but only rarely in adults unless they have preexisting Paget's bone disease. Here again, the relationship between an active proliferative process—osteogenesis—and cancer is clear. All of these associations support the belief that *a restless soil is a fertile soil for oncogenesis.*

The high incidence of cancer in certain clinical conditions has given rise to the notion of predisposing or *"precancerous lesions."* Included under this designation are the atrophic gastritis of pernicious anemia, senile keratosis of the skin, hypertrophic leukoplakia of the oral cavity and vulva, xeroderma pigmentosum, familial polyposis of the colon and neurofibromatosis, the latter three being genetic disorders. Statistically, these designated conditions increase the risk of cancer developing in the affected organ or tissue. Thus, a patient with pernicious anemia and atrophic gastritis has a 10 per cent chance of developing a gastric carcinoma while, for others, the risk is much less than 1 per cent (Zamcheck et al., 1955). While the term precancerous is applied to these conditions, it must be appreciated that there can be no prediction that the individual patient will, of necessity, develop a cancer. For this reason, there is valid objection to the term precancerous as applied to a lesion in a given patient.

Does cancer arise in a single deviant cell *(the clone theory)* or, rather, in a field of simultaneously affected cells *(the field theory)*? This distinction, which was thought to be fundamental enough to give rise to different theories (clone vs. field theory), has now lost relevance since it is known from work in tissue culture that the two views are not mutually exclusive. When cancer is produced in vitro, it is possible on the one hand to identify clones of malignant cells. On the other hand (e.g., among a million cells exposed to the same carcinogenic conditions), several hundred may undergo similar changes within a defined time range and may give rise to a field of cancer cells.

Similarly, it is seen in the clinic that cancer may arise in separate foci within restless tissue presumably reacting to carcinogenic influences. The pernicious anemia patient with atrophic gastritis may develop multiple primary gastric carcinomas simultaneously just as multiple primary breast carcinomas have been observed. Multiple or sequential neoplasms are often encountered clinically in the urinary bladder. The medullary thyroid carcinoma (for which there is a genetic predisposition) (p. 1343) is frequently primary at more than one locus within the thyroid gland. Additional examples could be given, but it is important here only to emphasize that cancer may arise in a field of restless cells all simultaneously affected by carcinogenic influences whether they be genetic and/or environmental. Ultimately, however, carcinogenesis occurs at the individual cell level. The best clinical evidence of this is derived from the study of plasma cell neoplasias.

There is evidence that virtually all plasma cell neoplasms (multiple myeloma, plasmacytoma) synthesize abnormal globulins. Each tumor produces its own distinctive pattern of immunoglobulins with variable mixtures of light chains and heavy chains. This pattern remains constant throughout the life of the patient as though the dysproteinosis consisted of the synthetic product of a single cell. In reality, all the tumor plasma cells have identical protein synthetic programs, suggesting that all arose from a single common precursor. On these grounds, the plasma cell neoplasms have also been called *monoclonal gammopathies.* Other evidence for the clonal origin of neoplasms comes from cytogenetic studies. As will be seen later, most cancer cells exhibit karyotypic abnormalities. The changes may be structural (within the individual chromosome[s]) and/or numerical. The structural deviations may be so distinctive as to yield identical "markers" in almost all cells of a tumor, suggesting derivation from a single cell (Goh, 1968). It appears, then, that some cancers constitute clones derived from a single transformed cell; but others may arise in a field of cells simultaneously affected.

Of historic interest is a former conception that cancers originated in nests of embryonic cells sequestered during fetal development. On occasion, a tumor is found strongly suggesting such a sequence—e.g., the appearance of a teratoma in the mediastinum. Teratogenous tumors do arise, as best we know, from multipotential primitive cells barely more differentiated than gametes. Similar tumors are more often primary in the gonads. The ocurrence of such a lesion in the mediastinum can be explained only by the sequestration of embryonic totipotential cells. Despite this example, there is no evidence that the generality of tumors arise in sequestered embryonic cells. In fact, sequestration of embryonic cells must be a great rarity since they are almost never found in routine postmortem examinations.

A closely related issue proposes the possible origin of neoplasms in congenital malformations. Malformations take many forms. They may consist of an abnormal cluster of vessels dignified by the term *hemangioma.* These are not true neoplasms. They are usually present from birth, enlarge only along with the growth of the child and frequently spontaneously disappear. Rarely, if ever, does a congenital hemangioma give rise to a true neoplasm. Another form of congenital malformation is the *hamartoma*—a localized overgrowth of normal mature cells identical to the types constituting the organ in which the tumor is found. Thus, in the liver a discrete mass of disorganized hepatic cells, blood vessels, bile ducts and fibrous tissue discretely demarcated from the surrounding liver substance comprises a hamartoma of the liver. The cells within the hamartoma are mature, have no anaplasia, and only merit the designation of a congenital malformation by virtue of their lack of normal architectural organization.

A *heterotopic rest* of cells, also known as a *choristoma*, comprises another form of congenital malformation. Sometimes, this malformation is mistaken for a neoplasm. A small mass of pancreatic substance is not infrequently found in the submucosal connective tissue of the stomach, duodenum or small intestine. The pancreatic substance, on microscopic examination, is identical to that found in the normally situated organ and contains acinar glands and islets of Langerhans. Because it constitutes a small mass in an aberrant location, it is easily mistaken on radiographic study or surgical exploration for a true neoplasm. Hamartomas and heterotopic rests almost never give rise to cancers.

A more difficult question involves the nature of nevi and their role in neoplasia. The nevus—or common "mole"—is a small, brown pigmented lesion of the skin. From birth, virtually everyone has one or more nevi and, preponderantly, they are entirely innocuous, although some enlarge commensurate with the growth of the child. Some investigators consider nevi to be congenital malformations. The nevus contains melanocytes, and melanocytes may give rise to melanocarcinomas. About 25 per cent of these highly malignant cancers arise in one particular form of preexisting nevi (junctional nevi) as is discussed on p. 1400. Junctional nevi in certain locations of the body such as the external genitalia, hands and soles of the feet are much more likely to undergo malignant transformation than those situated elsewhere. If the nevus is a congenital malformation, as some believe, one can cite only this single exception to the generalization that malformations are not a fertile soil for oncogenesis.

It should also be pointed out here that, as far as we know, the origins of benign and malignant tumors are separate. In other words, only rarely does a cancer arise in a benign tumor (see p. 145).

CARCINOGENIC AGENTS AND THEIR CELLULAR INTERACTIONS

The numerous agents capable of inducing cancer in experimental animals can be grouped as follows: (1) oncogenic viruses, (2) carcinogenic chemicals, (3) radiation and (4) other agents. Under certain conditions, some may cause cancer in man (Berenblum, 1970) (Homburger, 1959).

Oncogenic Viruses. Approximately 150 viruses have been shown to be oncogenic in animals. About one-third of these are DNA viruses and the remainder, RNA viruses (Table 4–3). Among the DNA viruses, only polyoma (Py), simian vacuolating (SV 40), and the human adenoviruses have been studied in great detail. It should be pointed out that the *pa*pilloma, *po*lyoma and simian *va*cuolating viruses are often grouped together under the acronym of "papova" viruses. Both SV 40 and Py viruses are extremely small, the former having a molecular weight of 2.3 to 2.5×10^6, the latter 2.9 to 3.4×10^6. This amount of DNA constitutes about 5 to 10 genes. Most or the entire genome of SV 40 is required for

TABLE 4–3. ONCOGENIC VIRUSES

A. DNA Viruses (about 50)
  1. Papilloma Virus Group
      papilloma viruses of rabbit, man, dog, cows, and others
  2. Polyoma Virus Group
      polyoma virus (murine)
      (Py)
      (SV 40) simian virus
  3. Adenoviruses
      human adenoviruses (31 strains at least 12 of which induce tumors in newborn animals and/or transform cells in vitro)
      simian adenoviruses (6 viruses)
      avian adenoviruses (2 viruses)
      bovine adenoviruses
  4. Herpes Viruses (evidence not conclusive)
      Burkitt's lymphoma (human)
      Lucke's carcinoma (frog)
      Marek's disease (chicken)
B. RNA Viruses (about 100)
  1. Avian Leukemia-Sarcoma (Rous) Viruses (20 or more)
  2. Murine Leukemia-Sarcoma Viruses (number of types not established)
  3. Murine Mammary Tumor Virus (3 types)
  4. Leukemia-Sarcoma Viruses of Cat, Hamster, Rat and Guinea Pig

oncogenesis, but only some of the Py genes are similarly necessary (Greene, 1970).

The adenoviruses are still larger and, as with Py, only a small number of their genes are involved in oncogenesis. When cells are attacked by DNA viruses, one of two mutually exclusive pathways may be followed. Cells of the natural host (permissive cells) suffer a so-called *productive infection* in which virus is replicated, and the cell dies. Alternatively, cells belonging to a foreign host species block viral replication (nonpermissive cells) and, under appropriate conditions, up to 40 per cent of the cells may be transformed to cancer cells. *In this pathway, referred to as abortive infection, cells are not killed but are stimulated to replicate.* Presumably, nonpermissive cells lack some property or function essential for virus replication. Much evidence indicates that, in abortive infections, part of the genome of the DNA viruses is incorporated within the genome of the host cells.

The sequence of events in productive infections has been well documented with the Py and adenoviruses. (1) The virus attaches to the host cell membrane and is transported, partly uncoated, to the nucleus. (2) At the nuclear membrane or within the nucleus, the viral capsid is removed. (3) Transcription of specific regions of the viral DNA, probably by the cellular RNA polymerase, forms "early" messenger RNA. (4) The "early" mRNA is translated into proteins involved in viral DNA synthesis and in altering cell metabolism. (5) Viral DNA is replicated, utilizing cellular or possibly viral coded enzymes. (6) "Late" mRNA is transcribed from viral DNA molecules, possibly by a modified cellular or viral coded RNA polymerase. (7) "Late" mRNA is translated to viral structural proteins and other virus-specific proteins, some involved in regulatory functions. (8) Maturation of virus in the cell nucleus by "self assembly" from viral DNA and viral structural proteins is followed by lysis of the cell.

In abortive infections leading to tumor formation, only some of the first steps of productive infections occur. Viral DNA and capsular proteins are not assembled into virions. Instead, *the DNA of the infecting virus is inserted, at least in part, into the host cell genome and is replicated with it. Thus, the virus modifies the genotype of the host cell and leads to phenotypic expressions described later as neoplastic transformation.* Because viral DNA is incorporated into the host cell's genome, *infectious viral particles no longer exist in cells transformed by DNA viruses.* Thus, infectious virions cannot be recovered from cells so transformed. However, the virus can be "rescued" as in the case of SV 40 (where all of the viral DNA is incorporated) by fusion of transformed cells with permissive cells. With such cell fusion, the viral genome is replicated, the virus is assembled, the receptor permissive cell lyses and the mature infectious agent is released.

It is of interest that each transformed cell reproduces multiple copies of the viral genes, so amplifying the oncogenic influence of the virus. It is not known whether these copies are clustered, distributed singly or occur in a tandem sequence within the DNA of the host (Berg, 1971). Integration of viral DNA, it should be emphasized, is probably only the first of a sequence of changes involved in the ultimate emergence of a fully cancerous cell. Presumably, the first step produces sufficient derangement in the cell's regulatory controls so that it then enters a phase of active replication during which successive generations of cells acquire greater and greater cancerous potential (MacPherson, 1970). Later we shall consider the possible mode of action of these DNA viruses in their induction of neoplastic transformation (p. 139).

The oncogenic RNA viruses are of great interest because there is a growing suspicion that some of these agents may induce human cancer. In lower vertebrates as well as in mammals, the RNA viruses cause naturally occurring cancers such as chicken leukemia and sarcoma, mouse leukemia and mammary tumors in mice (the Bittner virus). Unlike the DNA viruses, *the RNA viruses may simultaneously replicate themselves and transform host cells without killing them.* It is thus usually possible to isolate the agent from most tumor lines and, with the electron microscope, to visualize C-type viral particles within the tumor cells. In some instances, the isolated virions are not infectious, but the virus can be complemented by the addition of a "helper" virus (Vigier, 1970). Usually in cell culture, the RNA virus must persist to maintain cell transformation (Marin and MacPherson, 1969). Oncogenic RNA viruses, then, live in a symbiotic relationship with their host cells.

Critical to the oncogenic action of RNA viruses is the requirement for continued DNA and RNA transcription within the host cell (Temin, 1964). If mitosis is blocked by such agents as actinomycin D, transformation of cells cannot be accomplished by RNA viruses. The key observation — that when DNA synthesis is blocked, cell transformation is irreversibly aborted — led to the realization that in oncogenesis *viral RNA modifies the host cell's DNA.* Temin proposed the genetic heresy that, in RNA viral oncogenesis, the RNA of viral origin modified the DNA code of the host cell. To make such a system work, it would be necessary to find an RNA-directed DNA polymerase, and such was documented by Temin and Baltimore virtually simultaneously (Temin and Mizutani, 1970) (Baltimore, 1970). Studies have now shown that *almost all oncogenic RNA viruses contain an RNA-directed DNA polymerase (known as a "reverse transcriptase").* Nononcogenic RNA viruses lack such a transcriptase. Later in the discussion of mechanisms of action, we shall pick up the story of how this reversed genetic sequence may induce neoplastic transformation.

The species specificity of viruses is singularly rigid. Indeed, sometimes the agent will act within cell culture but not within the living animal from which the cells were derived. SV 40, for example, is oncogenic in vivo in hamsters and multimammate mice. In vitro, it will transform cells from rats, mice, guinea pigs and rabbits, although it will not cause tumors directly in these animals. One would expect that, within susceptible animal strains, cross infection might occur with oncogenic RNA viruses, since transformed cells usually continue to elaborate infectious virions. Strangely, except for polyoma mice, cross infection (horizontal transmission) is rare in animal colonies. However, RNA viruses, particularly the Bittner agent, may be passed from one generation to the next (vertical transmission) perhaps through the ova and certainly through the milk of affected nursing females. Probably because of the species specificity and limited modes of transmission of the virus, there are no documented cases of cancer induction in laboratory workers.

Despite the irrefutable evidence of the oncogenicity of some viruses in animals, no cancer in man has been unequivocably linked to a viral causation. *The only documented viral tumor of man is the lowly wart (a skin papilloma).* Nonetheless, virtually every month some report adds suggestive evidence, and man after all is a member of the animal kingdom. Greatest excitement centers about the DNA herpes viruses. These agents are known to induce renal carcinoma in frogs, a lymphoma-like disorder of chickens (Marek's disease) and lymphatic leukemia and a form of lymphoma in owl monkeys and marmosets. Unlike other DNA viruses, the herpes virus may, after synthesis in the nucleus, be assembled at the nuclear membrane and pass into the cytoplasm as aggregates of mature virions enclosed within cytoplasmic vacuoles. In tumors of lower animals, therefore, the virions can be seen within the cytoplasm and the agent can be isolated from the tumor cells—a situation quite different from that of the other DNA viruses.

Perhaps the closest we have come to associating a herpes virus with a malignant human neoplasm is the evidence linking the herpes-like Epstein-Barr virus (EBV) and Burkitt's lymphoma. Virions characteristic of herpes virus have been identified in Burkitt's lymphoma cells grown in culture. The EBV has been isolated from the lymphomatous tissue in tissue culture. Antibodies against the virus are found in almost 90 per cent of affected patients as compared to 14 per cent of controls (Henle et al., 1969). The EBV can infect normal human lymphoid cells in vitro, change their morphology and induce a variety of behavioral and biochemical changes strongly suggestive of neoplastic transformation (Epstein, 1971). The EBV genome has been demonstrated as an integral portion of the host cell genome in Burkitt's tumor cells (Zur Hausan et al., 1970). Epidemiologic evidence adds further incriminating information. The lymphoma was first described in a limited geographic distribution in central Africa but, subsequently, cases have been identified throughout the world. The original locale was characterized by an abundant rainfall and a fairly high mean temperature, suggesting the possibility of insect vectors. The peak incidence of the lymphoma was found in children who might be expected to be less immune to microbiologic agents. It has been shown also that a high proportion of the population bear antibodies to the EBV, and it could be postulated that the agent is virtually endemic but is aroused to oncogenicity only by some other stimulus to proliferation in the reticuloendothelial system. A possible stimulus might be an infection such as malaria. In passing, it might be noted that the EBV has also been found in cases of infectious mononucleosis and nasopharyngeal carcinoma (Editorial, 1971). For ethical reasons, the ultimate experimental evidence is lacking—namely, viral inoculation to induce lymphoma in man.

A herpes virus has also been imputed to be the cause of cervical cancer (Aurelian, 1972). The epidemiology of this form of cancer resembles a venereal disease and is compatible with a transmissible agent. The prevalence of the cancer is related to the frequency of intercourse, number of consorts and age when sexual relations were begun. About 80 per cent of women having cancer of the cervix have antibodies against the type II herpes hominis strain as compared with 30 per cent of controls (Nahmias et al., 1970). However, this evidence must be interpreted with caution (Allen and Cole, 1972). It may well be that the cancer predisposes to secondary viral infection, as suggested by the facts that the prevalence of antibodies among cervical cancer patients has varied widely in published series and that patients with early lesions have antibodies less often than those with advanced disease (Rawls et al., 1970).

The possible association of herpes virus with Hodgkin's disease has been under intensive study. It will be remembered that this agent causes a lymphomatous condition in chickens, monkeys and marmosets. Although evidence in man is fragmentary, it includes identification of a herpes type virus from a patient with Hodgkin's disease, the finding of elevated titers of antibody in some patients, occasional instances of familial aggregations of Hodgkin's disease and one instance where 12 members of a school class developed the disease, suggesting horizontal transmission (Allen and Cole, 1972).

The RNA viruses have also been viewed as possible oncogenic agents in man. From their well documented connection with leukemia, breast cancer and sarcoma in animals, the most intense search has been made of the corresponding conditions in man. The evidence, with respect to human leukemia or lymphoma, has been summarized by Gross (1970) who states: "No experimental evidence is yet available to prove that human leukemia and malignant lymphomas are also of viral origin. However, the many different forms of leukemia and lymphomas developing in mice, rats or cats and those in man are so similar that it would be difficult to assume that leukemia in humans is a fundamentally different disease from that observed in other animal species. Furthermore in a few cases electron microscopic studies of human leukemia and lymphosarcoma revealed the presence of spherical virus particles similar in their morphology to those observed in mice, rats and cats."

In man, the link between RNA viruses and breast cancer is tenuous. Human milk in breast cancer populations has been searched for virus particles (Moore et al., 1971) (Schlom et al., 1971). Particles identical or similar to mouse mammary tumor virus have been found in breast milk in a larger proportion of women having a family history or ethnic predisposition to breast cancer than among control groups. Moreover, these particles have been shown to possess RNA-dependent DNA polymerase activity similar to that of other oncogenic RNA viruses. Milk lacking the particles also lacked the "reverse transcriptase." However, epidemiologic data have not shown an unequivocal relationship, suggesting vertical transmission of breast cancer among breast-fed offspring of afflicted mothers. The increased frequency of the disease among familial aggregations has been attributed to genetic influ-

ences. Despite the fact that it must be said that *no cancer in man has been proved to be of viral origin*, the bits of evidence keep adding up each year and there is a growing conviction that, in time, the sheer mass will be incontrovertible.

Chemical Carcinogens. Environmental agents causing cancer were first brought to light by Sir Percival Potts in 1775, when he astutely related the high incidence of scrotal cancer among chimney sweeps to their chronic exposure to soot. Indeed, few contemporary forms of prevention have been as successful in controlling a form of cancer as his simple but brilliant suggestion — cleanliness. More than a century passed before the full significance of Potts' observation became apparent. In 1915, Yamagiwa and Ichikawa developed the first chemical experimental model of cancer by repeatedly painting a rabbit's ear with coal tar, subsequently shown by British investigators to contain potent carcinogenic polycyclic aromatic hydrocarbons (Shimkin and Triolo, 1967). Since these pioneering observations, literally hundreds of chemicals have been proved to be carcinogenic in animals (Clayson, 1962) (Miller, 1970). Some of the major classes will be briefly discussed, followed by a consideration of the common properties which may be of significance in their carcinogenicity.

Polycyclic aromatic hydrocarbons were the first isolated and are some of the strongest known carcinogens. Best studied are: 7, 12-dimethyl benz(a)anthracene; dibenz(a,i) anthracene; benzo(a)pyrene; and 3-methylcholanthrene. All of these agents are capable of inducing in vitro neoplastic transformation of a variety of cell types derived from many species and of inducing cancer in vivo in most laboratory animals. When painted on the skin, the cancers appear locally; injected subcutaneously, they evoke sarcomas; introduced into a specific organ, they induce cancers at the locus of injection. Such constancy of action is a characteristic of strong carcinogens.

As will be seen, many chemical carcinogens must undergo metabolic conversion or activation before they exert their neoplastic influence. The active products are referred to as *proximate or ultimate carcinogens*. It is now established that the polycyclic hydrocarbons also undergo some form of activation at the local site to become "proximate" carcinogens (Grover and Sims, 1970). For dibenzanthracene, the activation may consist of oxidation of one of its double bonds to an epoxide. There is good evidence that such oxidations appear to be carried out by inducible microsomal enzymes present in the liver and several other tissues (Grover and Sims, 1970) (Gelboin, 1969). Whatever the conversion, *the hydrocarbons bind to cellular DNA, RNA and proteins.* In a comparison of several polycyclic hydrocarbons of different carcinogenicity, it has been shown that binding to DNA, but not to RNA and protein, correlates with carcinogenicity (Brookes and Lawley, 1964). While the exact position of the DNA-carcinogen bond is not yet established, it is known to be covalent. There are numerous examples of hydrocarbon-induced cancers in man, such as the scrotal cancer of chimney sweeps and, very likely, the lung cancers of cigarette smokers.

Certain *aromatic amines* are also powerful carcinogens. Best studied are: N-dimethyl-4-aminoazobenzene (DMAB), "butter yellow"; N-methyl-4-aminoazobenzene (MAB): 2-acetylaminofluorene (AAF); and 2-naphthylamine. These agents were the first to illustrate the requirement for metabolic conversion before they became carcinogenic (Miller and Miller, 1966a). For MAB and AAF, the proximate carcinogens are their N-OH esters or probably the sulfuric acid esters in the case of AAF (Miller, 1970). These conversions explain why the feeding of MAB to rats induces tumors in the liver but not in the gastrointestinal tract; MAB is metabolized in the liver. Most evidence now favors the view that the carcinogenicity of the "proximate" metabolites of MAB and AAF relates to their covalent binding to the 8-carbon of deoxyguanosine, although they also bind to RNA and proteins (Matsushima and Weisburger, 1969). Aromatic amines, then, like polycyclic hydrocarbons, can bind to DNA and alter its structure. It should be noted that DMAB was once used as a food additive to color margarine and that AAF was developed as a potential insecticide. While records do not prove their carcinogenicity in man, it is a fact that exposure to another aromatic amine, 2-naphthylamine, has been correlated with cancers of the bladder in man. Used in aniline dye and rubber industries, the compound is absorbed through the skin and lungs but induces its neoplasia in the bladder, suggesting that ultimately an excretory product in the urine is the proximate carcinogen.

Alkylating agents, such as betapropiolactone and epoxides, are both powerful carcinogens and mutagens. Unlike other carcinogens, the alkylating agents do not require metabolic conversion but bind directly to nucleophilic groups in DNA, RNA and proteins. The N-7 position of deoxyguanosine appears to be a preferred site of binding (Brookes and Lawley, 1961) (Colburn and Boutwell, 1966). Alkylated guanine is so modified as to pair with thymine rather than cytosine. Such mispairing constitutes, in essence, a point mutation. Other reactions between the alkylating agents and guanine and other bases of the nucleic acids have also been identified, further indicating that nucleic acids are likely to be a critical target of these agents (Loveless, 1969).

Other chemical carcinogens abound (Miller, 1970). Nitrosamines are transformed into agents that donate methyl and ethyl groups to RNA and DNA, again probably to guanine. Ethionine, carbon tetrachloride, urethane (ethylcarbamate) and a number of inorganic metals such as beryllium, cadmium, cobalt and nickel (their ionic forms are electrophilic) react with various compounds within the nucleus and induce tumors (Furst and Haro, 1969).

Some compounds found in the food of man are carcinogenic. Perhaps the most important is aflatoxin B_1, an alkaloid elaborated by a strain of Aspergillus mold which grows on improperly stored ground nuts and peanuts. Cycasin, another alkaloid found in cycad nuts of certain palm trees, also has oncogenicity. Safrol, an essential oil from the sassafras tree, used commonly as a flavoring agent, is no doubt the most delicious-tasting among the newly discovered carcinogens. The aflatoxin B_1 may be a major contributor to the high incidence of liver cell carcinoma in Africa. Ground nuts, many moldy, comprise a significant portion of the diet of many natives (Lin, 1970). Indirect evidence is at hand that aflatoxin B_1 may be activated by liver enzymes and may bind to DNA (see Miller, 1970). With respect to mold-derived carcinogens, it is of interest that actinomycin D is also carcinogenic and binds to DNA through hydrogen bonds (Svoboda et al., 1970). *The recognition that, when activated, almost all carcinogens react like arylating or alkylating agents and are thus capable of reacting with nucleophilic groups of critical macromolecules such as DNA represents a momentous step and a welcome simplification in understanding the mode of action of carcinogens* (Ryser, 1971). *On the one hand, it resolves the puzzle posed by the astounding chemical heterogeneity of carcinogens. On the other hand, it suggests how carcinogens may in some way act at the level of gene structure and gene expression.*

Before closing the citation of chemical carcinogens, it is appropriate to raise the subject of cigarette smoking and bronchogenic carcinoma. This is discussed in greater detail on p. 833, but it suffices here to say that condensate of cigarette smoke contains measurable amounts of several strongly carcinogenic polycyclic aromatic hydrocarbons. Habitual cigarette smokers have a fifty-fold higher incidence of lung cancer compared to nonsmokers. Extracts of cigarette smoke applied to the skin of mice, rats and rabbits induce skin cancers. Instillation of tobacco tar into the respiratory passages of rats has, in an occasional animal, induced a lesion purported to be a carcinoma. However, it should be pointed out that the numerous attempts to induce bronchogenic carcinoma in animals by having them "smoke" many thousands of cigarettes have not yielded unequivocal evidence of the induction of lung cancer. More details on this issue are available in the review by Shabad (1971). Condensates of car exhaust also contain carcinogenic hydrocarbons, which thus have become truly environmental carcinogens.

The study of chemical carcinogenesis has contributed more to our understanding of cancer than any other experimental approach. It may be useful, therefore, to discuss here the more salient biologic facts which have been brought to light by the experimental use of carcinogens. As has been outlined recently (Ryser, 1971), the following points are basic to the biology of carcinogenesis. *(1) The effects of carcinogens are dose-dependent, additive and irreversible. (2) Carcinogenesis does not occur immediately but emerges over a period of time. (3) Whatever the cellular changes involved in carcinogenesis, they are transmitted to daughter cells. (4) The ultimate creation of a cancer can be influenced by factors that are not themselves carcinogenic. (5) Chemical carcinogenesis requires cell proliferation.* These points will now be discussed.

Dose dependency has been established for chemical carcinogens. The number of tumors evoked in a series of animals increases with the size of the dose administered, and the number of cells transformed in vitro is proportional to increments of carcinogen. The sequential administration of small doses has been shown to have the same effect as a comparable total dose given in a *single administration*. The oncogenic effect of small doses, then, is additive; moreover, it indicates that the action of the carcinogen is fixed and apparently not subject to repair. *Whatever the change, it is proportional to the quantity of the carcinogen, is irreversible and can occur by the summation of numerous small impacts.*

All chemical carcinogens require time to exert their effect. They do not produce cancers immediately. The duration of the latent or lag period depends upon the potency of the carcinogen, the dose, the susceptibility of the cell or the host, and other factors. What is happening during this latent period is not clear, but it has prompted the concept that *cancer occurs by a sequence of changes imposed upon successive generations of cells.* In this context, it has been shown that all chemical carcinogens have an absolute minimal period of latency during which time the initiated cells are dividing. This latent period appears to be of comparable length in animal experiments and in tissue culture.

The first detectable morphologic changes in cells, following exposure of cultures to hydrocarbons, occur within hours or days, but such cells fail to produce tumors when inoculated into susceptible hosts. Tumor growth is attained only after 50 or more days of subculture in vitro, during which time successive generations of cells have appeared (Berwald and Sachs, 1963). Thus, neoplastic transformation occurs as a late event following a sequence of preneoplastic alterations. A few experimental systems, which use established nonmalignant lines as starting material, allow malignancies to develop faster and with higher yields than do primary tissue cultures. Such lines, however, are usually aneuploid and must be considered as partially transformed. The latent period in such cases appears to be shortened by a preexisting preneoplastic state.

It has been possible to grow clones starting from single cells exposed to carcinogens in vitro and to demonstrate that all subclones contain neoplastic cells (Mondal and Heidelberger, 1970). Such experiments clearly illustrate that *the initial event evoked by the carcinogen is transmitted from cell to cell. It is therefore a heritable characteristic.* With appropriate doses of carcinogen, it may take as long as a year for a skin cancer to be produced in the mouse following a single application of the agent, yet the generation cycle for skin cells in the mouse is approximately 6 days. Therefore, initiation must have occurred in the forebears of the ultimate cancer cells many, many generations ago, and these changes were transmitted to successive generations as irreversible, heritable alterations.

Berenblum (1941) has proposed a "two-stage" hypothesis of cancer. The first stage he called *initiation* and the second, *promotion*. The "two-stage" hypothesis must not be interpreted to mean that cancer evolution involves two well defined events. It is merely an expression of the probability that *sequential modifications occur in the conversion of the normal cell to a cancer cell.* Berenblum (1941) showed that substances not themselves carcinogenic may serve as promoters of carcinogenesis. Following initiation with the carcinogen, the application of croton oil (the active principle now identified as phorbol esters) increased the yield of tumors and significantly shortened the latent period (Berenblum, 1941). Identical doses of initiator and croton oil, given in reverse order, yielded no tumors. The action of croton oil is now believed to be transient stimulation of cell replication (Hennings and Boutwell, 1970).

That cell replication is a necessary requirement of carcinogenesis is self-evident, since the main pathologic feature of cancer is growth. It is important, nevertheless, to stress that *conditions enhancing cell replication also enhance cancer formation.* Cell proliferation is, then, a necessary requirement for the carcinogenic action of chemical agents. Hormones, tissue wounding, mechanical irritation, and possibly chronic infection also presumably contribute to carcinogenesis by acting as promoters of cell replication. The important role played by cell replication suggests either that in the course of cell division there is *clonal selection* for cells having the greatest growth vigor or, alternatively, that the changes of initiation require repeated mitotic divisions to become *amplified or fixed* within the cell.

The facts we have just discussed emphasize that the initial interaction of chemical carcinogens with tissue constituents is only the beginning of a long sequence of events. The deduction that these initial events must be inherited by daughter cells gives a firm guideline in the search for the critical events which initiate carcinogenesis. What are the critical targets of chemical carcinogens? To this point, we have emphasized the binding of the proximate carcinogen to DNA and the possibility that such binding might lead to point mutations. But carcinogens also bind to RNA and proteins, often even more strikingly than to DNA. Could such binding also lead to transmissible effects?

It has been suggested that some target proteins might be gene repressors (Pitot and Heidelberger, 1963). Carcinogens, by inactivating repressors, might lead to the expression of operator and structural genes involved in growth. While such a possibility cannot be ruled out, it is difficult to reconcile it with experimental facts, such as the transmission of initiation to daughter cells or the occurrence of long latent periods.

Several investigators have proposed tRNA as a critical target (Zamecnik, 1971) (Fujimura et al., 1972). The recent discovery and the wide occurrence of the enzyme "reverse transcriptase" offer a way to understand how messenger RNA, modified by a carcinogen, might lead to a permanent genetic effect. The enzyme would transcribe the modified RNA into a modified or "mutated" DNA (Ryser, 1971). The question of whether initiation is necessarily connected with a mutation is still debated, however, as will be discussed later on.

Radiation Carcinogenesis. Radiation is a potent carcinogen in both animals and man. Whether the radiation directly alters DNA or alters the phenotypic expression of the genome is still in contention. The weight of evidence favors the view that its oncogenicity is related to its mutagenic effect. Studies show that the tumor yield and number of mutations bear a linear relationship to each other, suggesting that oncogenicity involves mutation (Cole and Nowell, 1965). It is known that UV radiations may lead to changes in DNA structure in the form of thymine–thymine dimers. Such errors may, however, be excised and repaired by specific enzymes. Such repair may prevent carcinogenesis. Thus, when tissue cultures are subjected to x-rays, the carcinogenic effects of radiation are abolished unless cells divide soon after exposure (Borek and Sachs, 1966). Speculation persists that radiant energy merely: (1) accelerates aging, which inherently has a high incidence of spontaneous mutations and cancer, (2) activates oncogenic viruses, (3) alters the microenvironment of cells or (4) stimulates cells to proliferate, leading to mitotic errors and to growth of the most vigorous mutants into tumors (Warren, 1970).

The history of radiation-induced cancers in man goes back to the early radiologists, who often placed their hands in the x-ray beam to check the function of their crude instruments. Roentgen himself developed skin cancer. Radium painting of watch dials induced osteogenic sarcoma and antral cancer among the workers, who pointed their fine brushes by wetting them with their lips. The high incidence of bronchogenic carcinoma among the miners of radium in middle Europe, and of uranium in the United States indicates that radiation cancers may be induced by chronic inhalation of radon and its daughter products (United States Congress Joint Committee on Atomic Energy, 1968). Years ago, infants often received radiation to the thymic region on the then popular contention that thymic enlargement was responsible for sudden "crib" death. Unhappily, this therapy for a mythical disorder has led to a clear excess of thyroid cancer in the order of 100 times the anticipated attack rate (Hempelmann, 1968). Often these tumors appeared after a 20-year latent period. The effect of radiation on the bone marrow is discussed on p. 541. Radiologists once suffered a tenfold greater incidence of leukemia than other medical specialists but now better understanding of adequate protection has eliminated this hazard. The most critical evidence of the oncogenicity of radiation comes from a study of Hiroshima-Nagasaki survivors. Approximately five to 10 years following the atomic bombs, the incidence of leukemia (usually acute myelogenous) in exposed individuals rose to approximately 15 per 100,000, compared with the control rate of 1 or 2 per 100,000 (Bizzozero et al., 1966). All of this clinical evidence inescapably relates radiation to cancer production, but it does not indicate how radiation exerts its oncogenic effect.

Other Carcinogens. Other agents may induce cancer. However, there is a strong suspicion that they merely increase the yield of tumors by unleashing or facilitating some underlying oncogenic influence. There has long been a concern that an absolute or relative excess of estrogens might induce cancer in such target tissues as the breast and endometrium. The most critical study in this regard is that of Biskind and Biskind (1944), who demonstrated in rats that ovaries which had been grafted into the spleen developed neoplasms. Presumably, in this model, feedback inhibition of the pituitary is lost, since the ovarian hormones drain through the liver and are inactivated. Excessive levels of pituitary tropic hormones return to the spleen through the arterial system to induce proliferation of the transplanted target organ, followed by neoplastic transformation of the ovaries. In man, the presumed role of hyperestrinism in the induction of endometrial hyperplasia and endometrial carcinoma is further discussed on p. 1228. The increased incidence of breast cancer among Americans as compared to Japanese women has been attributed to the greater exposure of the former group to estrogens. Japanese women on the average have more children and nurse their children longer. Cyclic ovarian function is suppressed more frequently and longer, and so these women are less exposed over their lifetimes to estrogen stimulation.

Experimentally, tumors can be caused by other hormones. Cancer of the thyroid can result from excessive secretion of pituitary thyroid-stimulating hormone. Correspondingly, an excess of adrenocorticotropic hormone (ACTH) may lead to tumors of the adrenal gland. Cancer of the mammary gland can result from an excessive secretion either of gonadotropin or of mammotrope hormone. In all cases, the excessive secretion can be caused by an abolished or decreased negative feedback mechanism. As a rule, such endocrine tumors are at first hormone-dependent in that their growth can be stopped by withdrawing the tropic hormone. This observation forms the rationale for surgical procedures such as the ovariectomy and adrenalectomy in the treatment of cancer of the breast. These experimental and clinical observations suggest, but do not prove, a hormonal causation of cancer in man. It is conceivable that hormones simply maintain or stimulate cell replication and thus permit the emergence of neoplasia among cells already suffering from some preneoplastic changes due to a spontaneous mutation or a latent virus or other environmental carcinogen. In other words, *while it is not clear whether hormones may act as initiators, it is currently accepted that they may act as promoters* by stimulating the proliferation of their target organs.

In experimental systems, cancers have been induced by metal foils, methyl cellulose, synthetic polymer films fabricated of nylon, teflon and other plastics (Brand et al., 1967), macromolecules such as saturated iron oxide, asbestos fibers, and chronic irritation or injury. To date, there have been no reports of cancer in man following the use of such synthetic prostheses as heart valves or vascular grafts. Nonetheless, in the experimental animal, the subcutaneous implantation of plastic film induces cancer. It is speculated that the film blocks normal cell-to-cell communication and thus may lead to a selection of cells less reliant on such contacts, i.e., more autonomous. (Ryser, 1971). From well documented clinical observations, the chronic irritation or injury of poor dental hygiene, jagged tooth fragments and ill-fitting dentures seem to be important in the production of cancer of the oral cavity. In all likelihood, the chronic irritation or inflammation stimulates cell replication and may be considered a promoter of initiated cells. It might be well to comment, in this connection, that the contentious issue of whether a single physical blow is carcinogenic lacks all experimental confirmation. Repeatedly, the courts hear the claim that a blow to the body induced a cancer; far more likely, it called attention to the lesion.

At the end of this discussion of carcinogenic agents, the obvious conclusion is that there is no single etiology of cancer in man, but several possible etiologies. Even when the initial factor is defined, as in leukemia due to radiation or in bladder tumors due to naphthylamine, it appears certain that other parameters (promoters, host factors, etc.) play important roles. In addition, it is known that several agents may act synergistically to bring about initiation (Salaman and Roe, 1964) (Sachs, 1967). Radiation may potentiate the action of carcinogenic viruses or chemicals. Alternatively, chemical carcinogens may prepare the ground for viral oncogenesis (Casto et al., 1973) and act in concert with radiation (Salaman and Roe, 1964).

COMMON EVENTS IN CANCEROUS TRANSFORMATION OF CELLS

It is clear that the fully evolved cancer cell differs in many respects from the normal cell. These new characteristics permit it to escape control mechanisms and confer upon it enhanced growth potential. The sum of these changes is included under the term neoplastic transformation. *Transformation might be defined as an inheritable change in cells manifested by: escape from control mechanisms, increased growth potential, alterations in cellular membranes, appearance of new surface antigens, emergence of karyotypic abnormalities, development of morphologic and biochemical deviations from the norm, as well as other poorly characterized attributes conferring ability to invade, metastasize and kill.* Of all these characteristics, the ability to invade and to kill is, in the last analysis, the only one which is pathognomonic of malignancy. Frequently, cells transformed in culture look and grow like malignant cells in vitro but fail to show invasive and lethal potential when injected into isologous hosts. They may require additional subcultures in vitro to acquire true malignancy. It is important, therefore, to distinguish between "morphologic" transformation and "true malignant" transformation and to rely heavily on in vivo testing of malignancy.

Cancer cells derived from a malignant tumor of man or animals are thought to be irreversibly transformed, but recently it has become apparent that in some experimental systems, when the oncogenic influence is removed at the appropriate time, the cell transformation is reversible or aborted (Stoker, 1968). This observation is reminiscent of hormone-dependent tumors which stop growing in an unfavorable hormonal milieu. It has been known for a long time that skin papillomas arising where carcinogens are applied can either regress and disappear or develop into carcinoma. It has now been shown that tumors of established invasiveness, when subcultured in vitro, may also convert to levels of lesser malignancy. It would appear, then, that transformation is not always irrevocable.

The subsequent passages describe the evolution of cellular changes encountered after irrevocable transformation. It is to be *emphasized that the process of transformation involves the sequential acquisition of greater and greater deviations from the norm.* In the early stages, the alterations may be quite subtle. As the morphologic alterations encompassed under anaplasia have already been described, our attention now can be confined to: (1) loss of controls, (2) emergence of new antigenic profiles, (3) membrane changes, (4) biochemical changes and (5) karyotypic changes.

LOSS OF CONTROLS

The dominant functional attribute of the transformed and cancerous cell is its apparent escape from normal regulatory mechanisms. This is best demonstrated in cell culture. Many mature specialized types of cells cannot be grown in vitro. Those, such as fibroblasts, that can be cloned create small colonies characterized by radial linear cords of cells migrating out from the colony center. As mentioned earlier, when cells from neighboring colonies come into contact, their further growth and migration is inhibited — i.e., there is contact inhibition. Furthermore, normal cells tend to grow in monolayers and require an underlying framework to support their continued replication. In contrast, all transformed and cancerous cells can be cultured in vitro. When cloned, they form multilayered tangled masses, do not exhibit contact inhibition, will grow in suspension without contacting a supporting surface and are very much less restricted in their growth requirements. This behavior is attributed to loss of control mechanisms, but the precise nature of these controls is poorly understood.

Two types of cellular control might exist: long-range or extracellular mechanisms and short-range or intracellular mechanisms. A possible long-range control might be the chalones discussed on p. 97. These consist of tissue-specific inhibitors postulated to control the regenerative activity of cells following an injury. Some alteration in a cell, rendering it unresponsive to chalones, could lead to uncontrolled growth. Another form of long-range control might be immunologic in nature. It has long been hypothesized that the immune system maintains normal surveillance over cells and promptly destroys any aberrant forms not recognized as "self." New antigenic profiles composed of tumor-specific antigens appear in transformed cells, as is discussed below. Conceivably, then, the emergence of a tumor might imply breakdown of immunologic surveillance (Burnet, 1970). Despite such theoretical possibilities, the weight of evidence favors intracellular controls. New membrane characteristics, gene mutations, alterations in gene expression and increased activity or quantity of many enzymes involved in DNA synthesis are features of the transformed cell which provide a plausible background for the loss of intracellular regulatory circuits (Green, 1970) (Mazia, 1970).

CHANGES IN ANTIGENS

A new antigenic profile emerges in the transformed and cancerous cell which makes that cell immunologically distinctive from all of its normal forebears and from all of the normal cells in the host. This profile may result from either the production of new antigens or the deletion of some of the normal histocompatibility antigens (Haughton and Amos, 1968). Tumor-specific antigens (TSA) are found in most experimental neoplasms, however induced, and there is evidence that they occur in most human tumors as well. Tumors induced by oncogenic viruses have TSA that are common to all neoplasms induced by the same virus, regardless of the morphology of the tumor or the animal strain within which it is produced. Thus, all carcinomas, sarcomas and embryonal tumors induced by the polyoma virus share identical TSA. The morphologically identical sarcomas induced by the SV 40 virus have different antigens. Similarly, the RNA viruses produce tumor antigens unique for each virus; different tumors produced by one virus have cross reacting antigens. All these TSA are therefore virus-determined, although they are distinct from the antigens of the virion itself. The TSA persists in tumors induced by DNA virus even when the infecting virus is no longer detectable in the transformed cell line. These tumor-specific antigens are presumably coded for by the genome of the infecting virus integrated into the host's genome (Piessens, 1970). Chemical or radiation-induced tumors also possess TSA, but these antigens are different for each tumor and are not related to the carcinogen. Thus, several tumors induced in the same animal by methylcholanthrene would all be antigenically different and would not cross react (Klein, 1969).

Tumor-specific antigens are located at or in the plasma membrane and evoke an immune response in the host. They thus behave in the same fashion as histocompatibility antigens. Indeed, it is possible to immunize an animal against TSA so that it will reject a subsequent attempt to transplant the same tumor cells. Hence, these membrane-bounded tumor antigens are also referred to as *tumor-specific transplantation antigens (TSTA)*. In addition, the oncogenic DNA viruses induce virus-directed nuclear antigens referred to as T antigens (Greene, 1970). T antigens have not been identified in neoplasms induced by oncogenic RNA viruses, chemicals or radiation.

The existence of T antigens and TSA has opened new horizons in the study of carcinogenesis and tumor immunology in man. The question has been asked: "Is it the new antigenic profile which somehow renders the cell neoplastic, or is it merely a consequence of the change?" (Law, 1969). There is no firm answer, only the hint that cells, when first transformed by polyoma virus, may not always have detectable tumor-specific antigens. This evidence suggests that the antigenic change is not essential for transformation (Hare, 1967).

It might be asked why the host does not mount an immune response against the new antigens and destroy the tumor. It is clear that tumors evoke both circulating immunoglobulins as well as cell-mediated immune responses. While both mechanisms may operate against tumor cells, the delayed hypersensitivity, cell-based mechanism is probably more important, playing a role akin to its function in rejection of nonisogeneic transplants. Conceivably, the TSA are weak antigens and escape recognition, or the breakdown or inadequacy of immunologic surveillance might permit these neoplastic cells to survive. Alternatively, the tumor growth might be too vigorous to be overwhelmed. Hellstrom et al. (1971) have further helped to explain the paradox of a surveillance system that fails to eliminate "foreign antigens." They have demonstrated that at least some cancers elicit cell-mediated immunity and two types of circulating antibodies. One type of antibody can destroy neoplastic cells and another, in fact, protects tumor cells. The latter have been called "blocking antibodies" and their effect "immunologic enhancement." Blocking antibodies might complex with membrane-bounded tumor antigens and, while not destroying the cells, might mask their antigenic sites and thus protect them from recognition by sensitized lymphocytes. Such blocking antibodies have been identified in both animal and human patients with progressively growing tumors, but they are absent or low in titer when the tumors are regressing (Hellstrom et al., 1971).

As expected, the subject of tumor immunology has excited interest as a possible therapeutic tool. Whether all "spontaneous" tumors in man induce TSA and how these might be exploited for the benefit of the patient are discussed on p. 146. Here it suffices to emphasize that new antigens are characteristic of all fully evolved cancers and of all transformed cells in experimental systems, whether induced in vivo or in vitro. However, at the present time their significance in the production of cancer is questionable.

MEMBRANE CHANGES

Many observations point to the possibility that, *in the last analysis, cancer is a membrane disease* (Wallach, 1968). It will be recalled that characteristics of the cancer cell are decreased adhesiveness, usually increased repulsive negative surface charges, loss of contact inhibition, new membrane-bounded antigens and impaired intercellular junctional complexes (Abercrombie and Ambrose, 1962) (Curtis, 1967) (McNutt et al., 1971). Loewenstein (1969) has proposed that in cancerous transformation there is impaired transfer of information through cell junctions and between cells and that the loss of this signal underlies loss of growth control. The nature of the intercellular signal is not clear but might be electrochemical in nature and generated by membrane-bounded ions. The membrane alterations might not be confined merely to the cell surface but might affect all of the organelle membranes and account for many of the biochemical abnormalities observed in transformed and cancer cells (Wallach, 1969).

As is well known, membranes are lattices made up of lipids, proteins and hypoproteins. These are synthesized in accordance with the genetic code of the cell. It is tempting, therefore, to speculate that some genetic or epigenetic alteration in the cell alters membrane synthesis and so confers upon the cell the abnormal attributes so characteristic of neoplastic transformation. The profound nature of the membrane changes in cancer was recently underscored by the documentation that transformed cells have abnormal uptake or membrane transport of glucose and amino acids (Isselbacher, 1972). Their enhanced uptake of these nutrients might indicate a basis for the apparent priority possessed by malignant cells for the nutrients necessary for their growth and replication, even when the host himself is wasting.

BIOCHEMICAL CHANGES

A host of biochemical aberrations have been identified in cancer cells, but their significance is unclear (Potter, 1964). Without going into bewildering detail, certain generalizations can be made. (1) There are no biochemical changes which are hallmarks of cancer. (2) All cancer cells have biochemical deviations from their normal forebears. (3) All undifferentiated neoplastic cells undergo simplification of their metabolic capabilities and so converge toward a common profile. (4) Still unanswered is the question of whether the biochemical deviation contributes significantly to neoplastic transformation or is merely a secondary consequence.

At one time there was considerable interest in the tendency for neoplastic cells to utilize glycolytic mechanisms even in the presence of adequate supplies of oxygen, a phenomenon referred to as the "Warburg effect." While the glycolytic regulatory mechanism is defective in

tumors, it appears that the magnitude of the defect is proportional to the growth rate of the cell. The more rapidly dividing the cell, the more it relies on anaerobic glycolysis. Rapidly dividing normal cells, then, have respiratory patterns similar to those of well differentiated cancer cells. It now appears that the "Warburg effect" is due to mitochondrial malfunction, perhaps under the stress of high energy demands of the rapidly dividing cell population.

A variety of alterations in enzyme levels, specific enzyme deficiencies, increased activity of certain enzymes, and abnormalities in fatty acid and protein biosynthesis have all been found in one or another of the neoplasms intensively studied (Wallach, 1969). One alteration reported by Tallal et al. (1969) can be exploited therapeutically. These authors have reported remissions in patients with lymphatic leukemia when l-asparaginase is administered. Presumably, the leukemic cells suffer from low concentrations of asparagine or asparagine synthetase, and the administration of asparaginase exploits this enzyme deficiency (Whitecar, 1970). Other specific enzyme and biochemical defects have been reported, but none are universal for neoplasia. Nonetheless, the hope persists that, for tumors in general or for a specific form of tumor, a biochemical "Achilles' heel" may be found.

KARYOTYPIC CHANGES

The great majority of the primary cancers in man have either morphologic changes of one or more chromosomes and/or abnormal numbers of chromosomes. Three questions must be addressed: (1) What are the patterns of chromosomal abnormality? (2) Is there a specific "marker" for cancer? (3) What is the significance of the karyotypic change? Is it primary to the genesis of cancer or is it a secondary consequence?

The range of karyotypic abnormality is almost limitless, extending from hypodiploidy to hyperdiploidy, as well as all manner of aneuploidy (Sandberg and Hossfeld, 1970). Every conceivable form of abnormal chromosomal morphology has been identified, including deletions, translocations, fusions, breaks, satellites and multicentrics. Most clinically significant solid tissue cancers in man have such changes, but only some of the leukemias do (Porter et al., 1969). Chronic myelogenous leukemia is almost always associated with a karyotypic abnormality but, in all other forms of leukemia such as acute lymphatic and acute myelogenous leukemia, karyotypic abnormalities are found in only 50 per cent. In chronic myelogenous leukemia, the marker chromosome appears in all normoblastic, megakaryocytic and granulocytic cells. The abnormality is an abbreviated G-22 autosome known as the *Philadelphia (Ph) chromosome* (Nowell and Hungerford, 1960), with loss of part of one long arm (? translocation). It is germane to our later consideration to note that a substantial number of leukemic cells and rare malignant solid tissue tumor cells have normal karyotypes.

There is dispute in the literature about the issue of specific chromosomal markers indicative and diagnostic of cancer. It is generally held that, even among the cells of a single malignant neoplasm, there is great variation in the number of chromosomes. However, Porter and his colleagues (1969), among others, hold that "marker chromosomes are nearly always present in malignant cells." They further contend that all of the cells within a given neoplasm will have the same misshapen chromosome that thus constitutes a marker, despite any secondary mutations which may have altered the number of chromosomes. However, these "markers" not only vary in their morphology among the many forms of cancer but also vary among a group of similar types of cancer. *The only constant "marker" for cancer yet delineated is the Ph chromosome.* If identified in a single cell from the peripheral blood, the patient, with rare exception, has chronic myelogenous leukemia. It will later be pointed out that a few cases of chronic myelogenous leukemia do not have the Ph chromosome, and these may indeed be a genotypic and phenotypic variant of the usual form of myelogenous leukemia (p. 731).

Does karyotypic abnormality precede and initiate the cancerous transformation or is it a consequence? On balance, the evidence favors that it is a secondarily acquired phenomenon (Sandberg and Hossfeld, 1970) (Hsu, 1964). Occasional human cancers are diploid with completely normal chromosome morphology. About half of all acute forms of leukemia have no karyotypic abnormalities. In the experimental laboratory, "minimal deviation" hepatomas are euploid (Nowell and Morris, 1969). Early stages of chemically induced cancers are euploid. There is, therefore, considerable evidence that karyotypic abnormalities are not requisite for the cancerous state. This, however, in no way precludes the possibility that more subtle genetic alterations may underlie the initial changes of transformation. In the last analysis, demonstrable chromosomal deviations constitute gross mutations, but many subtle ones are beyond the range of cytogenetic detection.

Conceivably, mutations at the gene level initiate the process and permit further muta-tions to appear in the course of the subsequent cell divisions. In this context, it is of interest that patients and their families with preexisting chromosomal abnormalities have a strikingly high incidence of cancer. In patients with Down's syndrome (trisomy 21), the incidence of leukemia is almost twenty times that of the general population. Cells from patients with Down's syndrome are more readily transformed by SV 40 than cells from normal individuals (Todaro and Martin, 1967). Other genetic disorders, such as ataxia telangiectasia, also have an increased susceptibility to cancer. These genetic precancerous conditions imply that, once a mutation has occurred, the cell's genome is more vulnerable to further change.

Evidence supporting genetic aberrations as an early event in carcinogenesis is derived from the observations that, in premalignant lesions of the cervix, such as marked atypical dysplasia, and in the "precancerous" adenomas of the colon or rectum, occasional subtle chromosomal aberrations are identified. Indeed, these aberrations become more bizarre as the lesion advances to frank cancer (Atkin and Baker, 1969). Thus, while chromosomal abnormality cannot be considered as a critical initial event, there are many suggestions that at least one pathway for the development of cancer may be a process of clonal selection involving sequential chromosomal changes. *The initial event, whether imposed by viruses, chemicals or radiation, or spontaneous in origin, might merely be a base sequence disturbance which so alters the cell as to favor the superimposition of further mutational changes* (Zimmermann, 1971). Progression of the disease might involve, then, increasing complexity of genomic alterations.

PATHOGENESIS OF CANCER

The cellular origins of cancer, some of the etiologic agents known to induce cancer in animals and man, and some of the events involved in cancerous transformation have been discussed. Here we are concerned with how these agents act on cells to induce the described transformation. The fact that several theories have been competing for attention should come as no surprise and may simply reflect the complexity of the problem. We may be dealing with many lesions caused by a variety of agents acting through different, though possibly converging, pathways.

A sweeping simplification in the concept of carcinogenesis has been suggested by those virologists who suggest that x-rays and chemicals simply "unmask" or activate a latent oncogenic virus. This old concept has been revived recently by the discovery of C-type RNA viruses in an appreciable number of experimental tumors (Huebner and Todaro, 1969). Since it is known that nucleic acids of viruses can become integrated into host genomes, the viral theory has been refined by adding the suggestion that normal-appearing cells may possess within them, as an integral part of their DNA, a gene of an oncogenic virus, a so-called "oncogene" (Huebner et al., 1970). Chemicals and x-rays, it is suggested, would then merely activate this oncogene.

However welcome such a simplification would be in the confused field of cancer theories, it may not account for all the facts. It was pointed out earlier that virus-induced tumors possess surface antigens that are programmed by the viral agent so that all tumors caused by the same agent share the same antigen. In contrast, chemically induced tumors, even when caused by the same compound, have different antigenic profiles. Indeed, individual cells of the same tumor may have different antigenic profiles. Such antigenic heterogeneity is not consistent with the presence of a single "oncogene." If all cancers were due to viruses, one must postulate a phenomenal number of different viruses to account for the staggering number of antigenic profiles encountered in chemically induced tumors.

Now we come to the issue of whether oncogenesis always involves some mutation in the DNA code of neoplastic cells. The mutation may take the form of elimination of a gene, resulting in so-called gene simplification (Fahmy and Fahmy, 1970) or change in the information contained within existing genes. There is abundant evidence that viruses, chemicals and radiation are associated with somatic mutation. When viral genome, or a fraction thereof, is integrated into the host cell's DNA, the integration amounts to a genetic mutation, transmissible thereafter to daughter cells. Chemical carcinogens, by binding to DNA (or even to RNA later transcribed into DNA), alter the DNA code of the cell and cause errors in replication. Radiation is a well known mutagen.

Thus, all three main categories of etiologic agents affect the gene pool of animal cells, forming the basis for the "*mutational theory of cancer.*" The theory is consistent with the frequent occurrence of karyotypic changes in tumor cells. It easily accommodates observations such as "spontaneous tumors" observed in vitro, in animals and in man. For lack of known agents, it is postulated here that mutation occurs by chance in the course of normal cell division. Random mutations are more likely to occur during active cell replication.

This would explain, for instance, why certain clinical cancers, such as sarcomas, are most frequent in childhood, a period of active growth and cell replication. Proliferation, itself a promoter, may favor the occurrence of additional mutations. With advancing age, the random mutations which must occur among the millions of cell divisions in man occur against a background of ever longer exposure to environmental carcinogenic influences, heightening the chances of neoplastic initiation. The hereditary predisposition to certain forms of cancer discussed on p. 150 might merely be an expression of a genetic tendency to somatic mutation. In toto, there is much seduction in the mutation theory of carcinogenesis.

Despite its broad appeal, the mutation theory has not yet found complete acceptance. Arguments can be developed for an epigenetic causation of cancer. All the changes seen in cancer could be explained by modified gene expression which is not related to any changes in gene structure (Weinstein et al., 1971) (Gelboin, 1967). As Pitot and Heidelberger (1963) have stated, "By a suitable application of the Monod and Jacob theories, it is possible to explain how a cytoplasmic interaction of a carcinogen and a target protein could lead to a permanent and stable metabolic situation without the necessity of any direct interaction of the carcinogen and genetic material." It will be remembered that neoplastic transformations are not always stable and, under certain circumstances, the modified cells may revert to normal. Such instability is more compatible with a metabolic change than with some genetic alteration (Braun, 1970).

Interactions of carcinogens with messenger RNA might provide an explanation for alteration in phenotype, since normal cell differentiation is thought to entail the development of a particular set of stable mRNA templates (Pitot and Chou, 1965). The epigenetic hypothesis easily accounts for the expression by cancer cells of genes normally repressed. Thus, cancers of the liver and colon may express embryonic characteristics, such as the carcinoembryonic antigen or the alpha fetal globulin. Since the theory calls for changes in gene expression, it may explain the unexpected secretion of hormones by tumors of nonendocrine tissues (p. 126). The strongest appeal of the epigenetic theory resides in the hope that tumor cells could be made to redifferentiate to normal patterns and revert to normal cells.

As is often found with competing theories, they may not be mutually exclusive, and mutational events, as well as new functional states of gene expression, may both play important roles in carcinogenesis. It may be less important to pursue this argument than to ask the next critical question. How does an initial change, whether mutational or epigenetic, lead to cancer? *The accumulated evidence strongly suggests that cancerous transformation does not, and indeed cannot, occur during the lifetime of a single cell. It probably arises by the sequential acquisition of ever greater deviations from the norm by one generation after the other, ultimately leading to escape from normal growth controls.* These sequential changes continue even after tumors have become clinically detectable and then constitute tumor progression. In experimental systems, such progression might occur over a period of weeks or months, but in man, at least for some tumors such as cervical cancer, it might require years. We know very little about what is happening during this interval from initiation to frank cancerous expression. Some investigators believe that clonal selection for those cells which are most autonomous and have the greatest growth potential is occurring. In particular, Prehn (1964) postulates that chemical carcinogens exert greatest selective pressure against those cells having some postulated cell "control factor" but permit cells lacking this factor to grow without inhibition to become neoplastic front runners. Alternatively, Potter (1964) suggests that "the operationally defined initiated cell may be one in which two or more gene mutations have occurred but in which the number of gene mutations is not great enough to achieve autonomy." The first gene mutation might yield some escape from control and, successively, mitotic divisions might yield further mutations, leading eventually to the cancer cell. Promoters may play a role by stimulating cell replication, thus predisposing to further mutations. Selection in this case would favor mutants with growth advantages, and proliferation would further provide a fertile ground for clonal selection.

EPILOGUE

So we come to the end of our cancer story. Our cup is both half empty and half full. The etiology and pathogenesis of neoplasia are still clouded with many questions, and the prevention of this scourge is largely beyond our grasp. Nonetheless, many environmental hazards have been identified and some controlled. More is known about the biologic behavior of cancer, resulting in improved diagnosis and better understanding of approaches to treatment. Moreover, growing awareness of the many etiologic agents capable of inducing cancer in laboratory animals must one day bear fruit for man, because in the last analysis it is unreasonable to believe that the biologic laws relevant to lower animals are not applicable to men. Unhappily, today the outlook for most cancer patients is grim, but tomorrow, and with it answers, may arrive sooner than we know.

REFERENCES

Abelev, G. I.: Production of embryonal serum alphaglobulin by hepatomas: review of experimental and clinical data. Cancer Res., 28:1344, 1968.

Abercrombie, M., and Ambrose, E. J.: The surface properties of cancer. A review. Cancer Res., 22:525, 1962.

Abercrombie, M., and Heaysman, J. E. M.: Observations on the social behavior of cells in tissue culture. II. "Monolayering" of fibroblasts. Exp. Cell Res., 6:293, 1954.

Abercrombie, M., et al.: Social behavior of cells in tissue culture. III. Mutual influence of sarcoma cells and fibroblasts. Exp. Cell Res., 13:276, 1957.

Allen, D. W., and Cole, P.: Viruses in human cancer. New Eng. J. Med., 286:70, 1972.

Ambrose, E. J.: The surface properties of tumor cells. In Ambrose, E. J., and Roe, F. J. C. (eds.): The Biology of Cancer. London, D. Van Nostrand, 1966, p. 65.

Atkin, N. B., and Baker, M. C.: Possible differences between the karyotypes of preinvasive lesions and malignant tumors. Brit. J. Cancer, 23:329, 1969.

Aurelian, L.: Possible role of Herpesvirus hominis, type 2, in human cervical cancer. Fed. Proc., 31:1651, 1972.

Baltimore, D.: RNA dependent DNA polymerase in virions of RNA tumor viruses. Nature (London), 226:1209, 1970.

Bell, J. R., et al.: Prognostic significance of pathologic findings in human breast carcinoma. Surg. Gynec. Obstet., 129:258, 1969.

Berenblum, I.: The co-carcinogenic action of croton resin. Cancer Res., 1:44, 1941.

Berenblum, I.: The study of tumors in animals. In Florey, H. W. (ed.): General Pathology. Philadelphia, W. B. Saunders Co., 1970, pp. 645, 744.

Berg, P.: The viral genome in transformed cells. Proc. Roy. Soc. London [Biol.], 177:65, 1971.

Berwald, Y., and Sachs, L.: In vitro cell transformation with chemical carcinogens. Nature (London), 200:1182, 1963.

Biskind, M. S., and Biskind, G. R.: The development of tumors in the rat ovary after transplantation into the spleen. Proc. Soc. Exp. Biol. Med., 55:176, 1944.

Bizzozero, O. J., Jr., et al.: Radiation related leukemia in Hiroshima and Nagasaki 1946–1964. I. Distribution incidence and appearance time. New Eng. J. Med., 274:1095, 1966.

Borek, C., and Sachs, L.: In vitro cell transformation by X-irradiation. Nature (London), 210:276, 1966.

Brand, K. G., et al.: Carcinogenesis from polymer implants: new aspects from chromosomal and transplantation studies during premalignancy. J. Nat. Cancer Inst., 39:663, 1967.

Braun, A. C.: On the origin of cancer cells. Amer. Sci., 58:307, 1970.

Braunstein, H.: Histochemical study of the enzymatic activity of human neoplasms. III. Structural functional relationships in the hepatoma. Cancer, 19:939, 1966.

Brenner, M. W., et al.: The study by graphical analysis of the growth of human tumours and metastases of the lung. Brit. J. Cancer, 21:1, 1967.

Broders, A. C.: Carcinoma grading and practical application. Arch. Path., 2:376, 1926.

Brookes, P., and Lawley, P. D.: Evidence for the binding of polynuclear aromatic hydrocarbons to the nucleic acids of mouse skin: relation between carcinogenic power of hydrocarbons and their binding to deoxyribonucleic acid. Nature (London), 202:781, 1964.

Brookes, P., and Lawley, P. D.: The reaction of mono- and difunctional alkylating agents with nucleic acids. Biochem. J., 80:496, 1961.

Burnet, F. M.: The concept of immunological surveillance. Progr. Exp. Tumor Res., 13:1, 1970.

Casto, B. C., et al.: Enhancement of adenovirus transformation by treatment of hamster embryo cells with diverse chemical carcinogen. Cancer Res., *33*:819, 1973.

Clayson, D. B.: Chemical Carcinogenesis. London, J. A. Churchill, 1962.

Colburn, N. H., and Boutwell, R. K.: The binding of beta-propiolactone to mouse skin DNA *in vivo:* its correlation with tumor-initiating activity. Cancer Res., 26:1701, 1966.

Cole, L. J., and Nowell, T. C.: Radiation carcinogenesis, the sequence of events. Science, 150:1782, 1965.

Coman, D. R.: Decreased mutual adhesiveness. A property of cells from squamous cell carcinomas. Cancer Res., *4*:625, 1944.

Curtis, A. S. G.: In The Cell Surface. London, Academic Press, 1967, pp. 206, 211, 259, 266.

DeLong, R. P., et al.: The significance of low calcium and high potassium content in neoplastic tissue. Cancer, *3*:718, 1950.

Easty, G. C.: Invasion by cancer cells. In Ambrose, E. J., and Roe, F. J. C. (eds.): The Biology of Cancer. London, D. Van Nostrand, 1966, p. 78.

Easty, G. C., and Easty, D. M.: An organ culture system for the examination of tumor invasion. Nature (London), *199*:1104, 1963.

Editorial: E. B. Virus, Burkitt lymphoma and nasopharyngeal carcinoma. Lancet, *1*:218, 1971.

Engell, H. C.: Cancer cells of the blood: a five to nine year follow-up. Ann. Surg., *149*:457, 1959.

Epstein, M. A.: The possible role of viruses in human cancer. Lancet, *1*:1344, 1971.

Everson, T. C.: Spontaneous regression of cancer. Ann. N.Y. Acad. Sci., *114*:721, 1964.

Fahmy, O. G., and Fahmy, M. J.: Gene elimination in carcinogenesis: reinterpretation of the somatic mutation theory. Cancer Res., *30*:195, 1970.

Fisher, B., and Fisher, E. R.: Biologic aspects of cancer cell spread. Proc. Nat. Cancer Conf., 5:105, 1964.

Fisher, B., and Fisher, E. R.: Experimental studies of factors influencing hepatic metastases. I. The effect of number of tumor cells injected and time of growth. Cancer, *12*:926, 1959.

Fisher, B., and Fisher, E. R.: Experimental studies of factors influencing hepatic metastases. IX. The pituitary gland. Ann. Surg., *154*:347, 1961.

Folkman, J.: Tumor angiogenesis: therapeutic implications. New Eng. J. Med., *285*:1182, 1971.

Foulds, L.: The biological characteristics of neoplasia. In Raven, R. W. (ed.): Cancer. Vol. 1. London, Butterworth and Co., 1958, p. 37.

Fujimura, S., et al.: Modifications of ribonucleic acid by chemical carcinogens. Modification of *Escherichia coli* formylmethionine transfer ribonucleic acid with N-acetoxy-acetylaminofluorene. Biochemistry, *11*:3629, 1972.

Furst, A., and Haro, R. T.: Possible mechanism of metal ion carcinogenesis. In Bergmann, E. D., and Pullman, B. (eds.): The Jerusalem Symposia on Quantum Chemistry and Biochemistry, Physical Chemical Mechanisms of Carcinogenesis. Jerusalem, Israel Academy of Sciences and Humanities, Vol. 1. 1969, p. 310.

Gelboin, H. V.: Carcinogens, enzyme induction and gene action. Advances Cancer Res., *10*:1, 1967.

Gelboin, H. V.: A microsome-dependent binding of benzo(a)pyrene to DNA. Cancer Res., *29*:1272, 1969.

Goh, K.: Large abnormal acrocentric chromosome associated with human malignancies. Possible mechanism of establishing clone of cells. Arch. Intern. Med., *122*:241, 1968.

Green, M.: Effect of oncogenic DNA viruses on regulatory mechanisms of cells. Fed. Proc., *29*:1265, 1970.

Greene, H. S. N., and Harvey, E. K.: The relationship between the dissemination of tumor cells and the distribution of metastases. Cancer Res., *24*:799, 1964.

Gross, L.: Viral etiology of cancer, leukemia and allied diseases. Cancer, *20*:243, 1970.

Grover, P. L., and Sims, P.: Interactions of the K-region epoxides of phenanthrene and dibenz(a,h)anthracene with nucleic acids and histone. Biochem. Pharmacol., *19*:2251, 1970.

Hare, J. D.: Transplant immunity to polyoma virus-induced tumor cells. IV. A polyoma strain defective in transplant antigen induction. Virology, *31*:625, 1967.

Haughton, G., and Amos, D. B.: Immunology of carcinogenesis. Cancer Res., *28*:1839, 1968.

Hellstrom, I., et al.: Demonstration of cell-mediated immunity to human neoplasms of various histological types. Int. J. Cancer, 7:1, 1971.

Hempelmann, L. H.: Risk of thyroid neoplasms after irradiation in childhood. Science, *160*:159, 1968.

Henle, G., et al.: Antibodies to Epstein-Barr virus in Burkitt's lymphoma and control groups. J. Nat. Cancer Inst., *43*:1147, 1969.

Hennings, H., and Boutwell, R. K.: Studies on the mechanism of skin tumor promotion. Cancer Res., *30*:312, 1970.

Homburger, F. (ed.): Physiopathology of Cancer. 2nd ed. New York, Hoeber Division, Harper and Row, 1959.

Hruban, Z., et al.: Endoplasmic reticulum, lipid, and glycogen of Morris hepatomas. Comparison with alterations in hepatocytes. Lab. Invest., *26*:86, 1972.

Hsu, T. C.: Chromosome constitution in neoplasms. Proc. Nat. Cancer Conf., *5*:49, 1964.

Huebner, R. J., and Todaro, G. T.: Oncogenes of RNA tumor viruses as determinants of cancer. Proc. Nat. Acad. Sci. U.S.A., *64*:1087, 1969.

Huebner, R. J., et al.: Group specific antigen expression during embryogenesis of the genome of the C type RNA tumor virus: implications for ontogenesis and oncogenesis. Proc. Nat. Acad. Sci. U.S.A., *67*:366, 1970.

Isselbacher, K. J.: Sugar and amino acid transport by normal and malignant cells. New Eng. J. Med., *286*:929, 1972.

Jessiman, A. C., and Moore, F. D.: Carcinoma of the breast. New Eng. J. Med., *254*:846, 900, 947, 1956.

Johnson, L. D., et al.: Epidemiologic evidence for the spectrum of change from dysplasia through carcinoma in situ to invasive cancer. Cancer, *22*:901, 1968.

Johnson, L. D., et al.: The histogenesis of carcinoma in situ of the uterine cervix. Cancer, *17*:213, 1964.

Klein, G.: Experimental studies in tumor immunology. Fed. Proc., *28*:1739, 1969.

Law, L. W.: Studies of the significance of tumor antigens in induction and repression of neoplastic disease. Cancer Res., *29*:1, 1969.

Lin, T-Y.: Primary cancer of the liver. Scand. J. Gastroent., Suppl. *6*:223, 1970.

Lipsett, M. B., et al.: Humoral syndromes associated with nonendocrine tumors. Ann. Intern. Med., *61*:733, 1964.

Loewenstein, W. R.: Transfer of information through cell junctions and growth control. Canad. Cancer Conf., *8*:162, 1969.

Loveless, A.: Possible relevance of 0-6 alkylation of deoxyguanosine to the mutagenicity and carcinogenicity of nitrosamines and nitrosamides. Nature (London), *223*:206, 1969.

MacDonald, I.: Biological predeterminism in human cancer. Surg. Gynec. Obstet., *92*:443, 1951.

MacPherson, I.: Characteristics of animal cells transformed in vitro. Advances Cancer Res., *13*:169, 1970.

Marin, G., and MacPherson, I.: Reversion in polyoma-transformed cells: retransformation, induced antigens and tumorigenicity. J. Virol., *3*:146, 1969.

Matsushima, T., and Weisburger, J. H.: Inhibitors of chemical carcinogens as probes for molecular targets: DNA as decisive receptor for metabolite from N-hydroxy-N-2-fluorenylacetamide. Chem. Biol. Interactions, *1*:211, 1969.

Mazia, D.: Regulatory mechanisms of cell division. Fed. Proc., *29*:1245, 1970.

McNutt, N. S., et al.: Further observations on the occurrence of nexuses in benign and malignant human cervical epithelium. J. Cell Biol., *51*:805, 1971.

Miller, E. C., and Miller, J. A.: Mechanisms of chemical carcinogenesis, nature of proximate carcinogens and interactions with macromolecules. Pharmacol. Rev., *18*:805, 1966*a*.

Miller, J. A.: Carcinogenesis by chemicals: an overview. G. H. A. Clowes Memorial Lecture. Cancer Res., *30*:559, 1970.

Miller, J. A., and Miller, E. C.: A survey of molecular aspects of chemical carcinogenesis. Lab. Invest., *15*:217, 1966*b*.

Mondal, S., and Heidelberger, C.: *In vitro* malignant transformation by methylcholanthrene of the progeny of single cells derived from C_3H mouse prostate. Proc. Nat. Acad. Sci. U.S.A., *65*:219, 1970.

Moore, D. H., et al.: Search for human breast cancer virus. Nature (London), *229*:611, 1971.

Nahmias, A. J., et al.: Antibodies to herpes virus hominis types 1 and 2 in humans. II. Women with cervical cancer. Amer. J. Epidem., *91*:547, 1970.

Nowell, P. C., and Hungerford, D. A.: A minute chromosome in human chronic granulocytic leukemia. Science, *132*:1497, 1960.

Nowell, P. C., and Morris, H. P.: Chromosomes of "minimal deviation" hepatoma: a further report on diploid tumors. Cancer Res., *29*:969, 1969.

Paul, J.: Metabolic processes in normal and cancer cells. In Ambrose, E. V., and Roe, F. J. C. (eds.): The Biology of Cancer. London, D. Van Nostrand, 1966, p. 52.

Piessens, W. F.: Evidence for human cancer immunity. A review. Cancer, *26*:1212, 1970.

Pitot, H. C., and Chou, Y. S.: Control mechanisms in normal and neoplastic cells. Prog. Exp. Tumor Res., *70*:158, 1965.

Pitot, H. C., and Heidelberger, C.: Metabolic regulatory circuits and carcinogenesis. Cancer Res., *23*:1694, 1963.

Porter, I. H., et al.: Recent advances in molecular pathology: a review — some aspects of chromosome changes in cancer. Exp. Molec. Path., *11*:340, 1969.

Potter, V. R.: Biochemical perspectives in cancer research. Cancer Res., *24*:785, 1085, 1964.

Prehn, R. T.: A clonal selection theory of chemical carcinogenesis. J. Nat. Cancer Ins., *32*:1, 1964.

Rawls, W. E., et al.: Herpes virus type II antibodies and carcinoma of the cervix. Lancet, *2*:1142, 1970.

Richart, R. M.: A radioautographic analysis of cellular proliferation in dysplasia and carcinoma in situ of the uterine cervix. Amer. J. Obstet. Gynec., *86*:925, 1963.

Ryser, H. J.-P.: Chemical carcinogenesis. New Eng. J. Med., *285*:721, 1971.

Sachs, L.: An analysis of the mechanism of neoplastic cell transformation by polyoma virus, hydrocarbons and X-irradiation. Curr. Top. Develop. Biol., *2*:129, 1967.

Salaman, M. H., and Roe, F. J. C.: Cocarcinogenesis. Brit. Med. Bull., *20*:139, 1964.

Sandberg, A. A., and Hossfeld, D. K.: Chromosomal abnormalities in human neoplasia. Ann. Rev. Med., *21*:379, 1970.

Schlom, J., et al.: RNA-dependent DNA polymerase activity in virus-like particles isolated from human milk. Nature (London), *231*:97, 1971.

Shabad, L. M.: Review of attempts to induce lung cancer in experimental animals by tobacco smoke. Cancer, *27*:51, 1971.

Shimkin, M. B., and Triolo, V. A.: History of carcinogenesis: some prospective remarks. In Twentieth Annual Symposium on Fundamental Cancer Research. Baltimore, Williams and Wilkins Co., 1967, p. 1.

Stoker, M.: Abortive transformation by polyoma virus. Nature (London), *218*:234, 1968.

Svoboda, D., et al.: Invasive tumors induced in rats with Actinomycin D. Cancer Res., *30*:2271, 1970.

Tallal, L., et al.: L-asparaginase in ill children with leukemias and solid tumors. Proc. Amer. Assoc. Cancer Res., *10*:92, 1969.

Temin, H. M.: The participation of DNA in Rous sarcoma virus production. Virology, *23*:486, 1964.

Temin, H. M., and Mizutani, S.: RNA dependent DNA polymerase in virions of Rous sarcoma virus. Nature (London), *226*:1211, 1970.

Todaro, G. J., and Martin, G. M.: Increased susceptibility of Down's syndrome fibroblasts to transformation by SV-40. Proc. Soc. Exp. Biol. Med., *124*:1232, 1967.

United States Congress Joint Committee on Atomic Energy, Subcommittee on Research, Development and Radiation: Radiation exposure of uranium miners. Washington, D.C., Government Printing Office, 1968.

Vigier, P.: RNA oncogenic viruses: structure replication and oncogenicity. Progr. Med. Virol., *12*:240, 1970.

Wallach, D. F. H.: Cellular membranes and tumor behavior. Proc. Nat. Acad. Sci. U.S.A., *61*:868, 1968.

Wallach, D. F. H.: Generalized membrane defects in cancer. New Eng. J. Med., *280*:761, 1969.

Warren, S.: Radiation carcinogenesis. N.Y. Acad. Sci., *46*:133, 1970.

Weinstein, I. B., et al.: Chemical carcinogens and RNA. Cancer Res., *31*:651, 1971.

Weiss, P.: Cell contact. Int. Rev. Cytol., *7*:391, 1958.

Whitecar, J. P., Jr.: L-asparaginase. New Eng. J. Med., *282*:732, 1970.

Willis, R. A.: The Spread of Tumors in the Human Body. London, Butterworth and Co., 1952.

Wood, S., Jr.: Pathogenesis of metastasis formation observed in vivo in the rabbit ear chamber. Arch. Path., *66*:550, 1958.

Zamcheck, N., et al.: Immunologic diagnosis and prognosis of human digestive-tract cancer: carcinoembryonic antigens. New Eng. J. Med., *286*:83, 1972.

Zamcheck, N., et al.: Occurrence of gastric cancer among patients with pernicious anemia at the Boston City Hospital. New Eng. J. Med., *252*:1103, 1955.

Zamecnik, P. C.: Summary of symposium on transfer RNA and transfer RNA modification in differentiation and neoplasia. Cancer Res., *31*:716, 1971.

Zimmermann, F. K.: Genetic aspects of carcinogenesis. Biochem. Pharmacol., *20*:985, 1971.

Zur Hausan, H., et al.: EBV DNA in biopsies of Burkitt tumours and anaplastic carcinomas of the nasopharynx. Nature (London), *228*:1056, 1970.

5

CLINICAL ASPECTS OF NEOPLASIA

The ultimate importance of neoplasms is their effect on their hosts. The present chapter is concerned with certain general clinical aspects of neoplasia in man and some of the specific neoplasms arising in supporting tissues (e.g., connective tissue, fat and muscle) which are common to all organs. The three general areas of clinical importance are: (1) the interactions between tumor and host, (2) the factors involved in predisposition to neoplasia and (3) the diagnosis of neoplasia. The treatment of cancer is a subject beyond our scope since it falls within the provinces of the surgeon, radiotherapist and chemotherapist.

TUMOR-HOST INTERACTIONS

The neoplasm is essentially a parasite. Some cause only trivial mischief but others are catastrophic. Tumor-host interactions are, however, a two-way street, and the host impinges on the tumor as well. First we shall consider the effects of the tumor on the host, and then the converse.

EFFECTS OF TUMOR ON HOST

It is quite obvious that the impact of malignant tumors on their hosts is far greater than that of benign tumors. Nonetheless, benign tumors do not always constitute benign disease. Any mass must be investigated to rule out the possibility of malignancy. This issue comes into sharpest focus with benign tumors of the breast that often cannot be differentiated, on clinical grounds alone, from a carcinoma. In general, all "lumps" in the breast must be removed for pathologic examination to exclude the possibility of cancer.

While this general principle applies to benign neoplasms wherever they arise, clinical experience teaches that in certain locations some neoplasms are so characteristically benign as to permit a reasonably certain clinical diagnosis. Leiomyomas of the uterus are the commonest form of benign neoplasia in the woman. They typically present as spherical masses readily palpable on abdominopelvic examination. The leiomyosarcoma is so rare that most gynecologists do not consider the finding of spherical masses in the uterus an indication for immediate surgery. Nonetheless, the patient is not a statistic and any enlarging leiomyoma should be immediately removed because somebody has to be the "one in one thousand" patient. Soft, discrete subcutaneous lipomas and sebaceous gland cysts are commonplace and almost never transform to cancers; they do not signal immediate surgery. However, they do cause disfigurement and are better excised. Leisurely management is ultimately a gamble—in many instances, an educated gamble. The most benign lesion is the excised one.

144

Benign tumors may cause significant clinical disease. They may (1) exert pressure in a strategic location, (2) have functional activity such as hormone production, (3) superimpose complications such as hemorrhage or ulceration with secondary infection and (4) undergo malignant transformation. Regarding *location*, a very small benign tumor in the common bile duct, for example, may cause death due to obstructive jaundice. A leiomyoma can cause pain, a dragging sensation, abnormal vaginal bleeding and difficulties in delivery. A benign adenoma of the pituitary may or may not produce hormone, but its expansile growth can destroy the remaining pituitary and lead to serious endocrinopathy.

The elaboration of hormones and other products is, in fact, more characteristic of benign than malignant neoplasia. These functional attributes have been discussed in the endocrine chapter (p. 1297) and, while some are not life-threatening, many carry the potential of death. It is only necessary to emphasize that the underlying benign tumor may be minute and, indeed, many a parathyroid adenoma has required two or more surgical explorations before it was discovered.

Superimposed complications refers to such changes as hemorrhage due to a tumor, the ulceration of a benign tumor through a natural surface such as the skin or the mucosa of the gut, the development of secondary infection in such ulcerated surfaces, or the perforation of a hollow viscus. Intraductal papillomas of the female breast may cause bleeding from the nipple as papillomas of the urinary tract cause hematuria. A very common cause of bleeding into the stools is the benign adenoma (polyp) of the colon. In all these examples, the bleeding is trivial but always causes alarm as to its possible origin in a more ominous tumor. Ulceration caused by a benign neoplasm is exemplified by the leiomyoma arising in the wall of the stomach, which causes ischemic necrosis of the stretched-out overlying mucosas and thereby induces melena (blood in the stools). The large fibroadenoma of the female breast that erodes through the skin is inevitably followed by bacterial infection.

Another complication is twisting or torsion of a pedunculated tumor. Prime examples are cystic (dermoid) teratomas of the ovary which cause torsion of the broad ligament, thus cutting off the blood supply to the ovary and tumor and leading to ischemic necrosis. When the twist in the pedicle is not tight enough to occlude the thicker-walled arteries, the tumor and attached ovary suddenly enlarge, becoming extremely hemorrhagic with

venous infarction. Both complications give rise to acute abdominal symptoms that constitute clinical emergencies.

Malignant transformation of a benign tumor is more talked about than seen. While in the individual instance it is indeed a possibility, tumors that are benign at the outset rarely become malignant. Certain exceptions have been cited earlier (p. 127) which deserve careful note since they must be construed as "precancerous" lesions. Save for these, a tumor that is present for many years without increasing in size and later found to be malignant was more likely a dormant cancer from the outset rather than a benign tumor transformed to a malignant one. Nonetheless, there are exceptions, for example, where a focus of leiomyosarcoma is found within an otherwise benign-appearing leiomyoma and where a small nodule of carcinoma is encountered in a thyroid adenoma, so the possibility of malignant transformation of any benign neoplasm cannot be dismissed in the individual patient.

The clinical significance of a cancer is much greater than that of a benign neoplasm for reasons that must now be clear. Since most cancers are invasive, grow rapidly and are somewhat undifferentiated, they more often cause clinical symptoms because of location and superimposed complications than because of elaboration of hormones and other circulating products (Fig. 5–1). Nonetheless functioning carcinomas of the pituitary, adrenal cortex, thyroid, parathyroid, ovary and testis evoke wide-ranging endocrinopathies. Moreover, sometimes the undifferentiated carcinoma, arising within or metastatic to an endocrine gland, destroys it, provoking an endocrine insufficiency.

Systemic derangements associated with cancer may be mediated by ill-defined, non-hormonal circulating products of neoplasms. Acanthosis nigricans is a dermatologic condition characterized by increased pigmentation and hypertrophy of the skin. Its usual manifestation is darkening and roughening of the skin on the neck, axillae and groin. Almost always, these patients are found to have an abdominal cancer, usually in the stomach. Venous thromboses, known as migratory thrombophlebitis (p. 623), are encountered in cancer patients in whom the primary lesion most often occurs in the pancreas or lung. This curious association — Trousseau's sign — was first noted by the French physician who, ironically, diagnosed his own fatal disease as cancer of the pancreas when he developed migratory thrombophlebitis (Fusco and Rosen, 1966) (Dyck et al., 1958).

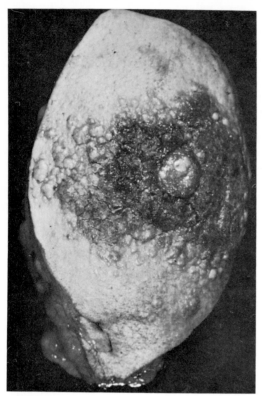

Figure 5–1. *Carcinoma of the breast. The tumor has eroded through the skin surface and produced a bleeding ulcerated, exposed mass.*

About 15 to 20 per cent of patients who develop dermatomyositis have an underlying visceral malignancy. These cancers may occur in virtually any organ, including the lungs, stomach, breast, kidney, uterus, ovary, lymph nodes and thymus. In some patients, the dermatomyositis becomes manifest before the tumor is discovered (Williams, 1959). Cancers of the lung sometimes cause disseminated peripheral neuropathy and myopathy. More often, they induce abnormal proliferative activity of the periosteum of the distal phalanges and of the subungual tissues of the nail beds, recognized clinically as *clubbing of the fingertips* (Brain and Henson, 1958). Thymic tumors may produce anemia, leukemia and a variety of other hematologic derangements. The substances or factors involved in these reactions have not been isolated and are poorly understood, but it is amply clear that once the primary lesion is removed, these systemic alterations disappear, only to reappear again if the tumor recurs. Tumors provide fascinating examples of deranged biology and divergent morphology and function.

The gravest implication of cancer is that it too often kills. It does so in a variety of ways,

some of which have already been mentioned with respect to its location, complications and possible function. While the final downfall of every patient with advanced cancer is in some way unique, all suffer *cachexia*, the constellation of progressive weakness, loss of appetite, anemia and wasting. Usually, but not always, there is a direct correlation between the size and extent of spread of the malignant tumor and the severity of the cachexia, and so the cachexia becomes more profound as the disease advances. Although small cancers are usually silent, it should be pointed out that, on occasion, remarkably small primary lesions have produced malignant cachexia.

Commonplace as cachexia is, it is still poorly understood. Cancers grow while the host is wasting, but it is not reasonable to ascribe the cachexia to the nutritional demands of the parasite. Cancers never grow as rapidly as the fetus, yet many a postpartal mother laments, on getting on the scale, that she did not suffer just a little bit of "cachexia." Grief, depression and anxiety, only too natural in the mortally ill patient, may be sufficient explanations for loss of appetite and weight. Anemia may, in part, be explained by bleeding from a fungating or ulcerated lesion such as is so typical of cancers of the colon. Bacterial infections, potentiated by the cancer, contribute to the cachexia. Bronchogenic carcinoma impairs drainage of the subtended respiratory passages and leads to chronic debilitating pulmonary infections. Cervical cancer which obtrudes on the ureters predisposes to bacterial pyelonephritis. The debilitated terminal patient often has an impaired immune response and so is prey to infections, particularly terminal bronchopneumonia. Vague and as yet unidentified toxic factors are postulated to be products of the necrotic malignant tumor, but they are hardly necessary to explain the cachexia of these unfortunate persons.

EFFECTS OF HOST ON TUMOR

Tumor-specific antigens (TSA) were described earlier (p. 136) (Richards, 1968) (Haughton and Amos, 1968). As best we know, the major defense of a host against his tumor takes the form of an immune response (Hellstrom et al., 1968). Clearly, animals mount immune responses against these TSA (Law, 1969). Evidence of tumor immunity in man is strong but not as incontrovertible as that in animals. Moral and ethical problems limit human investigation, and the constant presence of histocompatibility differences between individuals renders the study of tumor immunology in man difficult. Nonetheless, there is a growing body of evidence that (1) most, but perhaps not all, clinical cancers possess tumor-specific antigens, (2) tumor-specific circulating antibodies have been identified in cancer-bearing patients and (3) tumor-specific cell-mediated immunity occurs in man (Piessens, 1970). First, some of the clinical observations will be presented, followed by an overview of the immunologic data.

Spontaneous regression of cancers (p. 125), disappearance of metastases after surgical excision of the primary lesion, and failure to develop metastases despite the large numbers of tumor cells circulating in the blood all imply, but do not prove, host resistance to neoplasms (Jenkins, 1959) (Moore et al., 1957). One of the most exciting clinical findings, suggesting an immune response to cancer, relates to the once almost universally fatal choriocarcinoma. This neoplasm may arise in placental epithelium most commonly following an abnormal pregnancy (incomplete abortion, retained fragments of placenta following delivery, hydatidiform mole) (p. 1261). It may also arise in either sex from totipotential cells sequestered primarily within the gonads or in embryonic rests along the midline. The placental derivative can now be cured in almost all cases, with only moderate courses of tumor chemotherapy (Hertz et al., 1961). Those neoplasms arising as a result of parthenogenetic development of a totipotential cell do not respond to the chemotherapy and are usually fatal. It will be remembered that the placental epithelium is a product of the fertilized ovum. This zygote possesses normal histocompatibility antigens derived from both mother and father. Since the antigens of paternal origin are carried in these trophoblastic cancers, it has been speculated that the mother generates an immunologic response capable of destroying the cancer once its growth rate and vigor have been attenuated by chemotherapy. Indeed, patients have been cured by immunizing each with her husband's sperm, leukocytes and repeated skin grafts (Doniach et al., 1958).

Additional clinical evidence of an antitumor immune reaction comes from the increased frequency of malignant tumors in patients on long-term immunosuppressive therapy. Several reports attest to the higher than chance development of lymphomas and solid tissue tumors in patients following organ transplantation supplemented by immunosuppressive agents (McKann, 1969), and in those having a hereditary immune deficiency (Good, 1970). Here there is a strong suggestion that depression or an inborn deficiency of the immune mechanism potentiates the development

of neoplasms. Furthermore, autografting and homografting of cancers have been tried in man in the hope of documenting an immune response! (Nadler and Moore, 1965) (Southam et al., 1962). The grafting was performed on patients already having some form of cancer and even on normal volunteers (Southam et al., 1957). Fortunately, the autografts and homografts in most, but not all, instances failed to take. Extraordinary as these experiments are, they suggest that immunity may play some role in the rejections. The cancerous patients receiving tumor grafts rejected them more slowly than those suffering from some non-neoplastic yet debilitating disease; this is open to the interpretation that immunologic competence is reduced in the mortally ill cancer patient (Southam, 1968). A final line of clinical evidence suggesting host versus tumor reactions are the previously cited lymphocytic infiltrations found in the stroma of neuroblastomas, in some cancers of the breast, testis and digestive tract and in the histiocytic proliferative reactions in the lymph nodes about these neoplasms (Bill, 1969). A positive correlation has been shown between the intensity of the stromal lymphocytic infiltration and the length of survival of the patient. Accordingly, in Hodgkin's disease, lymphocyte depletion implies a poor prognosis (p. 760) (Lukes, 1964).

There is also abundant laboratory evidence for tumor immunity. Circulating tumor-specific antibodies have been demonstrated by immunofluorescence, cytotoxicity tests, complement fixation tests and other means in patients bearing Burkitt's lymphoma, melanocarcinomas, neuroblastomas and osteogenic sarcomas (Fairley et al., 1971). In many instances, there has been a positive correlation between the level of the immune response and the longevity and even cure of the patient.

In one series of patients having melanocarcinomas, about one-third who had autoantibodies to their neoplasms also had localized disease, suggesting better control of the new growth (Lewis et al., 1969). In three instances, antibodies disappeared when the disease suddenly began to generalize. The neuroblastoma of childhood provides further data of interest. Some children so afflicted have a rapidly progressive downhill course. In others, spontaneous regression occurs or the tumor transforms to a more benign neoplasm comprised of well differentiated ganglion cells (Bill, 1969). Perhaps here we are witnessing, in those children controlling their neoplasm, an effective antibody response referred to by Hellstrom as "repressor antibodies" while, in those whose tumor advances unabated, "persistor" or blocking antibodies might be present (Hellstrom and Hellstrom, 1971). Conceivably, in the unfortunate latter group, immunologic blockade mediated by IgG protects the tumor cells from the more lethal attack by sensitized lymphocytes as was discussed earlier (p. 137).

More crucial to the possible destruction of a cancer is cell-mediated immunity. Cytotoxic effects on tumor cells by sensitized lymphocytes have been demonstrated both in vivo and in vitro, and blast transformation of sensitized lymphocytes can be seen when these cells are exposed to their target tumor antigens (Andersen et al., 1969) (Hellstrom et al., 1971) (Jehn et al., 1970) (Hellstrom and Hellstrom, 1969). In terms of the possible causation of clinical cancers, it is of interest that lymphocytes from one patient bearing a melanocarcinoma will destroy cultivated melanocarcinoma cells from another source, but will not react against breast or colon carcinoma cells (Hellstrom et al., 1971). Analogous results have been found for Burkitt's lymphoma, neuroblastomas, colonic, breast and endometrial carcinomas, seminomas and certain sarcomas (Morton et al., 1969). The cross reactivity of the sensitized lymphocytes among patients bearing the same type of cancer raises the provocative possibility of a viral causation of these neoplasms. Recall that all tumors evoked by a single virus bear identical tumor-specific antigens.

It is important in interpreting this immunologic evidence to sound the caution that, in all instances, the cancer might be bearing passenger (nonetiologic) viral or bacterial antigens which evoke the immune response, and that attack of these "passenger" antigens by the humoral or cell-mediated mechanisms might secondarily injure the neoplastic cells. Clearly, in the Burkitt lymphoma, Epstein-Barr virus has been identified in the tumor cells and the immune response is directed to the viral antigens. It is important, therefore, to recognize that tumor immunology (1) does not prove viral causation of human cancers, (2) does not confirm that all clinical cancers have tumor-specific antigens as do experimental lesions and yet (3) does offer more than an enticing lead for the control and cure of cancers.

PREDISPOSITION TO NEOPLASIA

What considerations bear on the probability of an individual developing a neoplasm? Almost nothing is known in this regard about benign neoplasms. For cancers, it at least can be said that certain environmental and constitutional (genetic) factors have been identified which may be important in their causation. In one individual who develops a bladder tumor,

the influences might be largely constitutional in the form of a hereditary predisposition while, in another, the influence might be occupational exposure to beta naphthylamines. The World Health Organization (1965), after an extensive review of the problem, judged that there was strong evidence of environmental causation in about 50 per cent of all cancers.

The constitutional contribution to the genesis of cancer has been clearly shown in some highly inbred strains of lab animals (principally mice). Some strains with a high incidence of spontaneous cancers and others with a very low incidence have been bred, all maintained under identical environmental conditions. Certain strains have a high incidence of breast cancer; others, lung cancer; still others, gastric cancer; and the list of predisposition to forms of cancer does not end here. The constitutional factors for man can be segregated into age, sex, race and heredity. But before considering these influences, it may be well to review briefly some of the data on the epidemiology of cancer to provide a perspective of both the prevalence of cancer and the common forms encountered in the population at large.

EPIDEMIOLOGY

Cancers accounted for 16.8 per cent of all mortality, exceeded only by heart diseases which were responsible for 38.9 per cent (U.S. Dept. of H.E.W., 1967). The American Cancer Society (1968) expresses the problem on a more individual level by stating that one of every six deaths in this country is caused by cancer and one person in every four presently living may be expected to develop a neoplasm. This difference between mortality and morbidity is accounted for by the high incidence of nonfatal skin cancers representing 23 per cent of all cancers in the male and 13 per cent in the female. Only infrequently do skin cancers cause death since they are readily detected and usually cured by surgical excision.

The overall cancer death rates (age adjusted) per 100,000 population in the United States in the years 1964 to 1966 averaged 150.0 for males and 109.6 for females. In contrast, in 1949 to 1951, these rates were 129.8 and 120.2, respectively (U.S. Dept. of H.E.W., 1967). It is evident that the rate for males is mounting. These data express the magnitude of the individual's risk. Mortality rates alone do not express the complete scope of the cancer problem. In a study of a metropolitan population, it was shown that for every patient who dies of cancer in a given year, there are approximately two individuals newly diagnosed as having cancer (the incidence rate) and nearly three persons alive that year with cancer (the prevalence rate); so in the United States there are almost a million and a half cancer patients today. The mortality and morbidity caused by neoplasia, therefore, comprise a large part of medical practice.

ENVIRONMENTAL INFLUENCES

The term environment is here used broadly to include the vast array of external influences associated with the individual's habitat, life style, occupation, diet and social and cultural customs. Obviously, such a broad subject cannot be summarized and it will suffice merely to offer a few examples of the manner in which the environment contributes to the development of cancer.

The phrase "we swim in a sea of carcinogens" well describes the ecology of contemporary urban life, and its meaning should now be clear from the discussion of the many etiologic agents known to induce cancer in animals and in man. Chemicals recognized as carcinogens in man include certain soots, tars, oils, cigarette smoke, naphthylamines, benzidine, nickel, chromium compounds and asbestos (Miller, 1970) (Boyland, 1969). Some of these agents are essentially occupational hazards, but the soots, tars and oils resulting from auto exhausts, industrial fumes and cigarette smoke are virtually omnipresent. Radiation (even sunlight) and viral agents are everywhere. An example of dietary influence was discussed on p. 132, indicating the important role of mycotoxins in the production of liver cancer, particularly in regions of the world where moldy grains and cereals are consumed (Lin, 1970). The higher incidence of stomach cancer in Iceland and the Scandinavian countries poses the question of whether the heavy consumption of smoked meats and fish constitute chronic exposure to carcinogenic hydrocarbons. Liver flukes and bladder flukes are associated with a high incidence of cancer in their respective organs, and exposure to these parasites is a fact of daily life in many areas of Asia and Africa. Social and cultural customs have their input. Penile cancer is rare among Jews and those circumcised soon after birth and, similarly, cancer of the cervix is very infrequent among wives of circumcised husbands and among virgins. Indeed, the variable incidences of specific malignancies observed among economic and social classes are undoubtedly attributable to a host of environmental influences.

RACIAL AND GEOGRAPHIC FACTORS

The concept of racial and geographic pathology is a controversial one. Certainly the incidences of specific forms of cancer show striking differences in various regions and countries. For some time, these differences were attributed to racial predisposition, but with our expanding knowledge of the influence of the environment on the causation of cancer, as described above, it is much more likely that geographic variations are attributable to environmental rather than to individual and racial susceptibility.

Puzzling geographic problems remain. Breast cancer is far more common in the United States, Britain, the Netherlands and the Scandinavian countries than is cervical cancer, while in Japan the reverse obtains. Indeed, carcinoma of the breast is the commonest fatal malignancy in the female in the United States while it is far down the list in Japan. The question of vertical transmission of an oncogenic virus such as the Bittner agent is under intensive study but has not been established as a cause of the clinical disease. Perhaps these differences relate to the number of pregnancies and the corresponding lowered exposure to estrogens. Japanese women marry earlier and have larger families than American women (p. 1277). Why is gastric cancer more common among the Japanese living in Honolulu than among the general population of that area? These experiments of nature have meaning, but their message has not yet been deciphered. In any event, the environment makes a significant contribution to carcinogenesis and may, in fact, harbor the major influences of the causation of all human cancers.

AGE

With this consideration of the effect of the patient's age on the predisposition to cancer, we turn to influences inherent in the individual. Cancer is usually thought of as a disease of advancing age, but there is a small peak during the first four years of life, followed by a progressively increasing incidence which reaches a major peak in the age range of 55 to 74, with some drop off thereafter. The decline in the incidence of fatal cancer among the very aged is presumably due to their increased incidence of fatal heart disease and stroke. Despite these variable incidences, in terms of absolute numbers in the United States, over 80 per cent of all fatal cancers occur in individuals aged 55 and over.

The dominant forms of fatal cancer vary

with age. In men, in the third and fourth decades of life, bronchogenic carcinoma and lymphoid tumors dominate. In the fifth and sixth decades, the lymphoid tumors are displaced by those of the gastrointestinal tract. Later, prostatic carcinoma assumes increased importance, but never that of lung cancer. In women, breast and uterine cancers dominate the third and fourth decades but are soon joined by gastrointestinal tumors in the later decades (American Cancer Society, 1968).

It may come as a surprise to learn that with only two exceptional periods, cancer is the second leading cause of death from infancy to age 74. Homicide occupies second place in males aged 15 to 34 and, among females aged 35 to 54, cancer vaults to first place and supersedes heart disease. Among children aged 1 to 14, only accidents cause more deaths. These childhood cancers are discussed in more detail on p. 567.

SEX

As would be expected, there are distinct differences in the cancer death rates by site between males and females. These are plotted over the span of 38 years in the diagrams (p. 151) based on National Vital Statistics of the United States. Some of these differences are clearly due to cancers of the breast and the reproductive tracts. But, in addition, it is clear that lung carcinoma is almost ten times more common in males than it is in females, and this form of cancer alone accounts in large part for the progressive rise in the overall cancer death rate among males. Similarly, colorectal and stomach cancer are somewhat more frequent in males than in females. Indeed, excluding breast cancer, all forms of cancer occurring in both sexes tend to be more common among males. Interpretation of these results is uncertain. Men, in the course of their work, are exposed to many more occupational hazards. It has also been postulated that women have a more effective immunologic surveillance system which might be effective in destroying incipient neoplasms (Burnet, 1970). However, the striking rise in the importance of bronchogenic carcinoma among men overshadows all other differences. It remains to be seen whether changing mores will modify the sex difference or control this scourge.

HEREDITY

One frequently asked question is: "My mother died of cancer. Does that mean I'm likely to get it?" The answer is not simple, and a great deal more investigation is needed to accumulate sufficient data to provide an accurate response. The long generation cycle of man, the limited number of progeny, the lack of pathology-proven diagnoses on many death certificates, the difficulties in long-term follow-up of family groups and the many intercurrent deaths from other causes before the patient has reached the maximal cancer risk years make the study of inheritance difficult and often unrewarding. At the present time, certain understandings have been achieved. Mendelian inheritance patterns have been identified for a few cancers as well as for certain disorders predisposing to cancer. A list of these conditions, drawn from Lynch, is presented in Table 5-1 (Lynch, 1969). In the interpretation of this list, it is important to recognize that while any of the cited conditions may be inherited along mendelian lines, these same neoplasms occur in many patients who provide no background suggestive of hereditary transmission. Only about 3 per cent of all cases of melanocarcinoma have a familial setting. The great preponderance (97 per cent) occur sporadically (Lynch, 1967). Familial polyposis coli progresses to adenocarcinoma in about 40 per cent of the cases and affects about 50 per cent of the relatives of any patient (Lynch, 1971). Von Recklinghausen's disease, characterized by multiple neurofibromas, is associated with the development of sarcomas in some 8 to 20 per cent of the cases. So the genetic input in each of the above conditions varies.

Simple dominant or recessive mendelian

TABLE 5–1. CANCERS AND PRE-CANCEROUS DISEASES SHOWING MENDELIAN INHERITANCE PATTERNS

Autosomal Dominant Transmission
  Familial polyposis of colon
  Gardner's syndrome
  Hereditary exostosis
  Polyendocrine adenomatosis
  Medullary thyroid carcinoma with amyloid production and pheochromocytoma
  Peutz-Jeghers syndrome
  Neurofibromatosis of Von Recklinghausen
  Retinoblastoma
  Carotid body tumor
  Cutaneous melanocarcinoma
  Intraocular melanocarcinoma

Autosomal Recessive Transmission
  Xeroderma pigmentosum
  Ataxia telangiectasia
  Chediak-Higashi syndrome
  Albinism

From Lynch, H. T.: Genetic factors in carcinoma. Med. Clin. N. Amer., *53*:923, 1969.

Male Cancer Death Rates* by Site, United States, 1930–1968

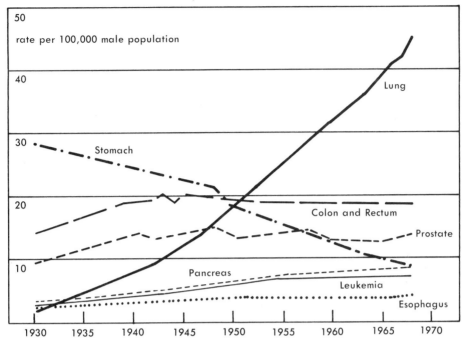

*Rate for the male population standardized for age on the 1940 U.S. population.
Sources of data: National Vital Statistics Division and Bureau of the Census,
United States.

Female Cancer Death Rates* by Site, United States, 1930–1968

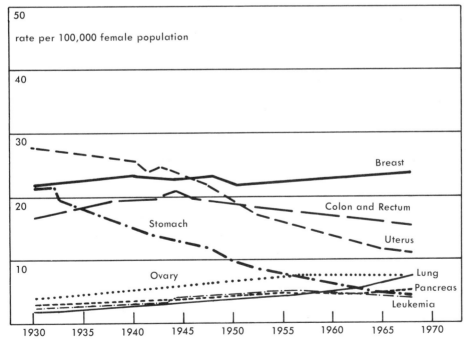

*Rate for the female population standardized for age on the 1940 U.S. population.
Sources of data: National Vital Statistics Division and Bureau of the Census,
United States.

patterns of transmission of cancer are the exception rather than the rule. For most forms of cancer, such inheritance as may exist involves the far more complex modes of polygenic transmission. Only six cancer families have been identified in which many members have suffered from a variety of forms of cancer (Lynch and Krush, 1967). All six groups have exhibited surprisingly similar patterns of cancer—i.e., increased frequency of adenocarcinoma, principally in the colon and endometrium, increased frequency of multiple primary cancers, early age of onset of the cancers and suggestions of an autosomal dominant mode of inheritance.

With the exception of these extraordinary families, *no familial predisposition to cancer in general has been identified. However, certain specific forms of cancer occur more frequently among families than can be accounted for by chance.* First-degree relatives of patients having a carcinoma in the breast, stomach, colon, prostate or endometrium have about a threefold increased risk of developing a similar tumor (Macklin, 1959). The most complete data now available relates to breast cancer. The following conclusions have been drawn: *the patient who has one breast cancer is at higher risk of developing a second primary breast cancer. Close relatives are at greater risk of developing a similar neoplasm.* However, the patient who has a carcinoma of the breast is not at higher risk of developing a carcinoma elsewhere, unless she happens to belong to one of the extraordinary cancer families.

There is other evidence that genetic factors influence the predisposition to cancer. The concurrence of leukemia in pairs of identical twins has been recorded sufficiently frequently to indicate a greater than chance probability of this phenomenon (Miller, 1968). Sibship aggregations of Wilms' tumor, hepatocellular carcinoma, adrenocortical carcinoma and neuroblastoma have been observed but not in sufficient numbers to permit genetic analysis. A number of diseases having a hereditary basis carry an increased predisposition to certain malignant neoplasms (Lynch, 1969). Hereditary disorders characterized by congenital malformations carry an increased risk, suggesting a possible common genetic factor leading to both the anomalies and the neoplasm. In closing this discussion, it is necessary to caution that all these genetic studies are plagued by the possibility that many instances of familial predisposition may merely reflect common exposure to environmental carcinogenic influences. But to attribute all of the above observations to the chance influence of the environment stretches the rules of probability.

DIAGNOSIS AND STAGING OF CANCER

A widely sought goal is the prevention of neoplasia. Since this "dream" seems unattainable in the immediate future, the early and certain diagnosis of cancer with reliable, nondisabling methods of cure would be highly acceptable in the interim. Man's technology has reached the moon and Mars but has not achieved completely objective methods for differentiating benign from malignant neoplasia or for identifying histologic patterns, sites of origin and anticipated biologic behavior of a new growth. The anatomic diagnosis of neoplasms is largely done by "eyeballing"—representing, in some part, a science and, in some considerable part, an art honed to fineness by long years of experience. Every surgeon has had, to his dismay and sometimes anger, the experience of removing a tumor which was judged to be borderline by the first pathologist, malignant by the second and benign by a third. It serves no purpose to attempt to answer in generalities for the patient and the surgeon what should be done in such a dilemma because there are no easy answers. Ultimately, every surgeon "must walk his own wilderness" guided by such considerations as the patient's age, the site and type of possible cancer, the risks and implications of undertreatment and overtreatment, the intelligence and reliability of the patient in returning for frequent follow-up visits and his level of confidence in the various opinions rendered. The example given merely emphasizes the fragility of the anatomic method of diagnosis. Fortunately, the preponderance of neoplasms do not straddle the fence and permit remarkably accurate anatomic diagnosis.

HISTOLOGIC DIAGNOSIS

Macroscopic and microscopic examination of a neoplasm by a competent pathologist may be expected to yield an accurate diagnosis in 95 to 98 per cent of neoplasms. To achieve such results, both surgeon and pathologist must be masters of their art and science. Obviously, the tissue submitted for anatomic diagnosis must contain the small neoplasm or a representative sample of a larger one. Ridiculous as this may sound, it may be exceedingly difficult to locate a small mass in the breast after its position becomes distorted by the operative procedure. Most biopsies, as contrasted with needle aspirations, are removed surgically. Such open biopsies involve anesthesia for the patient, medical expense, discomfort and the theoretical danger of spreading the neoplasm when the tumor is cut, as during subtotal excision. In all but the most malignant forms of sarcoma, as was indicated earlier, the dangers are more feared than real.

To avoid some of the undesirable aspects of open biopsy, needle aspiration biopsy is sometimes employed as, for example, with masses in the female breast, subcutaneous tumors, nodules in the liver, thyroid masses and, occasionally, lesions in the lung. Here the caveat becomes important—be sure to get a representative piece of the lesion. It is highly important that the biopsy contain representative non-necrotic tumor tissue. Most rapidly growing cancers undergo central necrosis; the practice of plunging into the center of a mass in order not to miss the tumor may merely secure only useless necrotic tissue that does not permit anatomic diagnosis. The margins of large tumors are the most viable regions since they contain the actively growing cutting edge of the expanding neoplasm. The other horn of the dilemma is that the "too marginal" biopsy may miss the lesion.

The surgeon further contributes to the accuracy of diagnosis by gentle and proper handling of the biopsy and by providing needed clinical information. All manner of cytologic distortions are produced by crushing, careless use of electric cautery, and improper fixation and preservation of specimens. The importance of adequate clinical data cannot be overly stressed. The unwary pathologist may easily misinterpret cellular abnormalities as indicative of cancer when he is not informed that the patient has had radiation therapy to the biopsy site in the past. Similarly, cervical biopsies in the pregnant female may show cytologic mucosal changes, easily mistaken for carcinoma in situ.

The pathologists' contributions to accurate anatomic diagnosis include meticulous care in dissecting and processing the specimen, in using the best methods of fixation, paraffin embedding, sectioning and staining. Techniques are now available for obtaining rapid paraffin sections within a few hours or, at most, 24 hours. In many instances, it is desirable to have an immediate anatomic diagnosis on a biopsy while the patient is still under anesthesia. Here, sections can be obtained by quick-freezing thin blocks of tissue (so called frozen sections) which are then rapidly stained and permit very satisfactory histologic diagnosis. But these frozen sections are inevitably thicker than paraffin sections; the cytologic detail is not as well preserved and the usual staining methods are less elegant than those employed in routine paraffin methods. Unfortunately, the technical problems result in greater diffi-

culty in establishing a diagnosis than with paraffin sections where better detail and greater clarity are available. Better to impose upon the patient the dangers and discomfort inherent in a second surgical procedure than to embark on surgery based on a wrong diagnosis. Consider the child who has a history of trauma to the leg and is then found to have a bone lesion that could be the result of injury or an osteogenic sarcoma. If the lesion is not clearly benign or certainly malignant on frozen section, it is inconceivable that amputation be performed on shaky evidence even though there are dangers of metastatic dissemination involved in the biopsy and delay of surgery with rapidly growing sarcomas in children.

CYTOLOGIC DIAGNOSIS

Next best to histologic diagnosis of cancer is the cytologic method first described by Papanicolaou in 1928 and confirmed in 1943 (Papanicolaou, 1928) (Papanicolaou and Traut, 1943). This method has been most widely applied in the detection of carcinoma of the cervix and carcinoma of the endometrium. The pooled secretions in the vaginal vault or those directly obtained from the cervical os are smeared onto a slide, quickly fixed and stained.

As was pointed out earlier, cancer cells have lowered cohesiveness and have a range of morphologic changes encompassed by the term anaplasia. Thus, shed cells can be evaluated for the features of anaplasia indicative of their origin in a cancer (Figs. 5–2 and 5–3). In contrast to the histologist's task, judgment here must be rendered on the basis of individual cell cytology or, at most perhaps, on that of a clump of a few cells without the supporting evidence of architectural disarray, loss of orientation of one cell to another and, perhaps most important, evidence of invasion. Despite the rigor involved in this diagnostic method, cells can usually be classified as falling into one of the following categories.

Class   I. Normal
Class   II. Probably normal (slight atypia)
Class III. Doubtful (more severe atypia representing possible dysplasia or possible cancer)
Class IV. Probably cancer (strongly suggestive of anaplasia)
Class V. Cancer (unmistakable anaplasia)

Under optimal conditions, with vaginal smears an 85 to 95 per cent correct positive diagnosis and a 95 to 98 per cent correct negative diagnosis can be achieved.

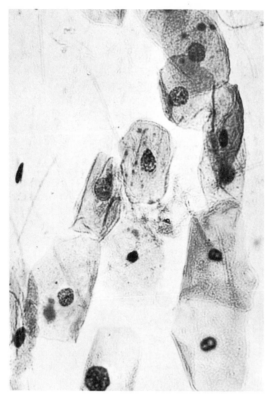

Figure 5–2. *Exfoliative cell smear showing normal cytologic flora of the genital tract. Cells are largely flattened surface squamous epithelial cells.*

The Papanicolaou method of diagnosis has also been applied to sputum, bronchial washings, abdominal, pleural, joint and subarachnoid fluids, discharges from the nipple, prostatic secretions, urinary sediment, gastric washings, and biliary and pancreatic duct aspirations. In all of these instances, cytology has proved its great worth, but the results are somewhat (not markedly) less reliable than those achieved for the female genital tract. The technique is particularly valuable since it permits the diagnosis of minute lesions which shed cells but are too small to be apparent even on direct visual inspection. A carcinoma high in the endometrial cavity might not produce abnormal vaginal bleeding, might be easily missed on curettage and yet be called to attention by the finding of abnormal cells on cytologic examination. Semi-yearly or yearly routine Papanicolaou smears have contributed greatly to the detection of early curable lesions and account in some part for the striking reduction in the mortality rates caused by carcinoma of the cervix and endometrium during the past five years in the United States.

OTHER DIAGNOSTIC TESTS

A variety of other diagnostic procedures are available that help in the diagnosis of

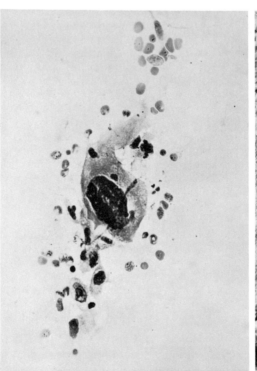

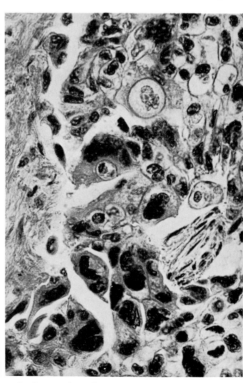

Figure 5–3. *On the left is an exfoliative cell smear of vaginal secretions from a patient with a cervical cancer. Contrast the large malignant anaplastic cell with the normal cells in Figure 5–2 (same magnification). On the right is a tissue section of the resected tumor showing the anaplastic cells in situ.*

cancer, but none have the specificity or accuracy of the histologic and cytologic methods. Identification of cancer cells in the circulating blood has been suggested as a diagnostic tool for cancer. This approach has proven of little value and is seldom used. Circulating cancer cells are found only when the primary cancer is large; even then the false-negative error is very high. Among patients with documented cancer, circulating cells are found in only one of five cases (Ericksson, 1962). Even when the test is positive, other means must be used to identify the location of the lesion. Other procedures for aiding in the diagnosis of cancer involve the detection of circulating hormones, enzymes or other products of the neoplasm. In many instances, these circulating substances are fairly specific for particular forms of neoplasia. Some of the more widely used diagnostic procedures involve the identification of elevated levels of the products listed in Table 5–2.

Every neoplasm among the various types listed does not, as has been indicated, elaborate its related product. A negative test, therefore, does not exclude the diagnosis. But in a patient having an enlarged prostate, for example, elevated levels of serum acid phosphatase would raise the suspicion of a prostatic carcinoma and would certainly suggest metastatic dissemination since the levels of enzyme correlate with the total mass of tumor in the patient. Similarly, abnormally high levels of chorionic gona-dotropin in the blood of a patient with some complication of pregnancy would strongly point toward a choriocarcinoma. On the other hand, about one-third of the hepatomas fail to produce alpha fetal globulin; carcinoembryonic antigen assay is positive in only 70 per cent of the patients with well advanced cancer of the colon and is negative in 50 per cent of the patients with small "early" lesions (Zamcheck et al., 1972). All of these tests, then, are not diagnostic of cancer but are merely aids. Moreover, despite their multiplicity, they relate to only a small fraction of the total spectrum of neoplasia. Yet to be achieved is the infallible method for the diagnosis of all forms of cancer or, indeed, any specific form of neoplasm.

STAGING OF CANCER

Over the years, there have been innumerable efforts to develop methods of expressing accurately the extent and gravity of cancer in a patient. Terms such as "operable" or "nonoperable," "localized" or "disseminated" are too subjective and diffuse to provide specific meaning. Some reasonably accurate method of staging the extent of cancer is crucial in evaluating the end results of therapy in different clinics. Many of the differences reported in the "cures" attained by one therapeutic modality or another stem from comparing different stages of the disease in various cancer populations. Obviously, if one deals with early localized disease, as against advanced cancers, the curability will be significantly modified. It is also necessary to develop methods of staging cancer for the selection of the most appropriate forms of treatment in cancer patients and to provide, as well, replicable prognostic criteria for the individual patient.

Several methods of classifying and staging cancer are now in current use. The Broders classification (p. 114) attempts to provide quantifiable grades of cancer aggressiveness based on the cytologic differentiation of tumor cells and the numbers of mitoses. Here the thrust is the prediction of biologic behavior based on morphologic features of the primary lesion. Regrettably, there is often considerable disparity between the morphology of cancers and their behavior in the individual patient. Many a highly anaplastic, undifferentiated cancer has advanced very slowly in the fortunate patient and, conversely, some apparently "tame" lesions have run wild. Prediction in the individual patient is chancy.

Of greater use are the methods which attempt to express in replicable terms the ex-

TABLE 5–2. ELEVATED LEVELS OF CIRCULATING PRODUCTS IN DIAGNOSIS OF NEOPLASM

Neoplasm	Circulating Product
	Enzymes
Prostatic carcinoma	Acid phosphatase
Cancer of digestive tract	Regan isoenzyme
Medullary thyroid carcinoma	Histaminase
	Hormones
Choriocarcinoma	Gonadotropins
Adrenal neoplasms	Steroids
Islet cell tumors	Insulin
Medullary thyroid carcinoma	Calcitonin
	Prostaglandins
	ACTH
Bronchogenic carcinoma	ACTH
	Insulin
	Growth hormone
	Calcitonin
	Gonadotropins
Fibrosarcoma	Insulin
	Other Products
Hepatoma	Alpha fetal globulin
Gastrointestinal carcinoma	Carcinoembryonic antigen
Plasmacytoma	Abnormal globulins

tent of the cancer (staging) in the patient. One method, that of Peters, is particularly applicable to Hodgkin's disease and the lymphomas and is presented on p. 759. Here the approach is to determine which lymph nodes and viscera are affected and whether the involvement is localized to one or several chains of nodes on one or both sides of the diaphragm. The most recent development in staging, applicable to all neoplasms, is known as the TNM system: T for primary; N for regional nodes; and M for metastases. These symbols are further quantified by defining the primary site as T_1, T_2, T_3 and T_4 for advancing disease, N_0, N_1, N_2 and N_3 for advancing nodal involvement and M_0 or M_1 for those without or with evidence of metastases. Obviously, the reliability of the TNM system depends on the accuracy of the observations relative to the extent of the disease in the individual patient. Imperfect as this method may be, it offers the possibility of a common language, which brings the promise of providing better data on the comparative results of treatment in different clinics. Hopefully, with such terminology, we shall not in the future be comparing "apples with oranges."

Other classifications for specific forms of cancer (an example is the Duke system for cancer of the colon) will be mentioned in the discussion of neoplasia in the individual organs in other chapters.

TUMORS COMMON TO ALL ORGANS

Connective tissue and some of its specialized derivatives, such as fat, are found throughout the body. Tumors of these tissues, therefore, belong to many organs and systems. They cannot be considered as falling into the category of any specific structure in the body, and for this reason are included here.

It is important to realize that connective tissue cells retain their capacity for proliferation throughout life. The fibroblast is a multipotential cell which can be transformed, under a variety of circumstances to other mesenchymal types, such as the chondroblast, osteoblast and lipoblast. As a consequence, mesenchymal tumors frequently display metaplastic tendencies with the formation of a variety of derivatives. The blood vessels and primitive blood cells are also of mesenchymal derivation and may form elements of these tumors. It is therefore not uncommon to find multiple elements of connective tissue, myxomatous tissue, bone, cartilage and sometimes blood vessels within a single neoplasm. Tumors with this variety of elements were for-

merly encumbered with such descriptive names as fibromyxochondrolipoma, in which the principal element was given the first position. More recently, such neoplasms have been designated as mixed mesenchymal tumors. In the following section, fibromas and fibrosarcomas, myxomas and myxosarcomas, lipomas and liposarcomas, mixed mesodermal tumors, leiomyomas and leiomyosarcomas are described in some detail, because they are common to all organs. The mesenchymal tumors composed of cartilage and bone are included in the chapter dealing with disease of the bone. Tumors of blood vessel origin are described in the chapter on blood vessels.

FIBROMA—FIBROSARCOMA

Grossly, fibromas are usually small (1 to 4 cm.), discrete, encapsulated, spherical to ovoid nodules of firm consistency, varying from soft, rubbery, pliable masses (fibroma molle) to extremely hard, unyielding nodules (fibroma durum). Occasionally, these benign neoplasms may grow to much greater size (15 to 20 cm.), particularly in certain organs such as the ovary. They may occur at any age and in any site in the body, although they show a definite predilection for the connective tissue sheaths of nerves, the sheaths and fascia of muscles, the periosteum of bones and the dermal connective tissue. On gross inspection, the discrete capsule is usually readily apparent, although the encapsulation may be poorly developed and the tumor may appear invasive when a fibroma arises in the dermal connective tissue. The cut section discloses a firm, white glistening surface, usually devoid of necrosis or hemorrhage.

Microscopically, typical spindle cell fibrocytes and fibroblasts are present. They have elongated nuclei with finely divided chromatin and long, tapering cytoplasmic processes on either end. The cells are characteristically laid down either in random patterns or in large, wavy ribbons made up of parallel bundles of cells. The cells are essentially normal and the nuclear-cytoplasmic ratio is not disturbed. Mitoses are rare and anaplasia is absent (Fig. 5-4). Between the fibroblasts, there may be scant to large amounts of collagen which give the tumor its characteristic firm consistency. Special silver impregnation techniques or phosphotungstic acid-hematoxylin stains will demonstrate fibrils called fibroglia. These are laid down by the fibroblasts and are seen between the cells. These fibrils are extremely helpful in distinguishing the three major types of spindle cells (fibroblasts, leiomyoblasts and endothelial cells), which may resemble one another on rou-

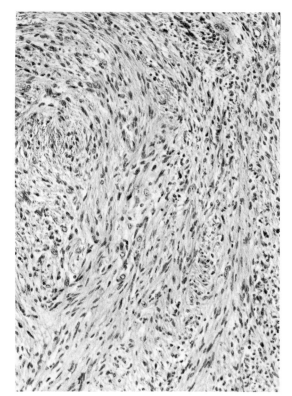

Figure 5–4. *Fibroma. The tumor is made up of regular, well formed fibrocytes and fibroblasts laid down in parallel bands.*

tine stains. Fibroblasts produce delicate wavy fibroglia; smooth muscle cells demonstrate thick, coarse, straight myoglia which may appear bent at one end; endothelial cells show no fibrils with these special stains. Fibromas having origin in nerve sheaths or perineurial connective tissue (perineurial fibromas) sometimes show distinctive arrangements of the nuclei which will be described in the section on tumors of nerves. In any principally fibromatous tumor, there may also be areas of other types of mesenchymal tissue.

Fibrosarcomas are the malignant analogues of the fibroma. These tumors tend to be bulky, poorly defined masses which may have origin in a benign fibroma, but more usually arise as a primary malignancy. They occur most frequently in the same sites as fibromas. On section, malignant fibromatous tumors show the characteristics of all sarcomas. They are soft, pearly gray-white tissue masses which, in appearance and consistency, resemble raw fish flesh. The tissue may assume a pulpy consistency in the frequent areas of necrosis. Hemorrhages commonly accompany the necrosis. Margins are poorly defined since no encapsulation exists, and extensions into sur-

rounding tissues may be evident. Histologic examination discloses all degrees of undifferentiation, from slowly growing tumors with cells which closely resemble benign fibromas to markedly anaplastic, rapidly growing tumors showing great variability in cell size and shape (Fig. 5–5). The more malignant fibrosarcomas display some of the greatest degrees of anaplasia encountered in oncology. Sometimes these tumors are so anaplastic that it is difficult to identify the cell of origin. Usually, however, examination of the better differentiated areas will establish the fibrous nature of the new growth. Large tumor giant cells with multiple nuclei and abundant cytoplasm may be present. Bizarre cell shapes are common, and the giant cells may show huge protoplasmic processes which extend across the high power microscopic field. In these anaplastic variants, mitoses may be quite numerous and atypical. These cancers are commonly extremely cellular with closely packed cells and little collagen. Just as in the benign fibromas, some fibrosarcomas may show varying admixtures of other types of mesenchymal tissue, such as myxomatous areas and cartilaginous areas.

One particular type of fibromatous tumor lies in the intermediate zone between benign

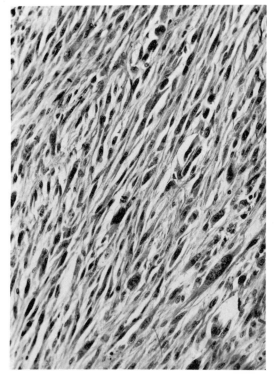

Figure 5–5. *Fibrosarcoma. There is considerable anaplasia of cells with marked variation in size and shape. Scattered giant cells are readily evident.*

fibromas and slowly growing well differentiated fibrosarcomas. It has received the special designation of *desmoid*. This tumor arises in the sheaths of muscles, usually of the anterior abdominal wall, but may arise in any other musculofascial area of the body. It may be described histologically either as a somewhat cellular fibroma or, more appropriately, as an extremely slow-growing, well differentiated fibrosarcoma. Encapsulation is not present. Invasion of the surrounding tissues may be evident, but dissemination and metastatic growth rarely occur.

Clinically, the benign fibroma usually presents no problem, save for the presence of a small tumor mass which may attract attention either because of its subcutaneous location or because of pressure on nerves or bone. Simple curative excision of these tumors is readily performed. The behavior of fibrosarcomas, however, is much more difficult to characterize. The wide variation in their significance depends upon their growth rate and degree of anaplasia. The more slowly growing, well differentiated lesions such as the desmoid are amenable to surgical excision, since they rarely produce metastatic spread or dissemination. Local recurrence may occur years later if the primary lesion has not been totally removed, but re-excision may produce cure even at this time. In the more rapidly growing variants, the malignancy may be of a high order with the possibility of successful extirpation precluded by blood and lymphatic spread. In general, fibrosarcomas which arise in superficial tissues, such as the subcutaneous connective tissue, have a better prognosis than tumors arising in the deeper structures. When these occur on extremities, radical excisions or amputations and local lymph node dissections are attempted, since tumors of fibroblastic origin are, in general, radioresistant. The duration of survival in the more anaplastic type may be limited to a few years or less.

MYXOMA – MYXOSARCOMA

True myxomatous tissue is present only in the developing fetus and does not appear in adults. There is much uncertainty about the interpretation of myxoid tissue in connective tissue tumors. These tumors are usually predominantly fibrous, but contain loose acellular areas with abundant ground substance. Formerly, such tumors were termed fibromyxomas. It is probable that the myxoid area merely represents a loose edematous region of the fibromatous lesion and not a separate neoplastic component of the tumor. Soft gelatinous polypoid tumors, sometimes termed myxomas, occur in the heart, but these lesions are thought to be derived from multipotential mesenchymal cells growing mainly along myxoid lines (p. 695). However, over and above these controversial lesions, there exist reasonably well documented true myxomatous tumors derived presumably from reversion of undifferentiated mesenchymal tissue. These occur predominantly subcutaneously and in contact with the muscular aponeuroses and fascia. Other locations include bones, the retroperitoneal area and the genitourinary tract.

Stout (1948), in his review of these tumors, points out that all true myxomas are locally infiltrative but do not metastasize. Because of this, he prefers the designation myxoma rather than myxosarcoma, with the understanding that these lesions are locally infiltrative, difficult to excise because of their gelatinous poorly defined consistency and have a strong tendency to recur each time, growing somewhat more actively.

In the subcutaneous areas, myxomas are generally small, but in retroperitoneal locations they may grow to masses over 30 cm. in diameter. All are pale gray, soft and jelly-like with poor delimitation. Histologically, there is much ground substance with scanty stellate or multipolar cells. Loose collagen is found between cells. Not infrequently, however, areas of more compact fibromatous cellularity are found, making it impossible to determine with certainty whether the lesion should be designated a myxoma or a fibroma. In most cases, the fibrous element is the more dangerous, justifying the latter designation.

The treatment for myxomas is wide surgical excision. This is often difficult to achieve when the tumors occur in regions other than the subcutaneous tissue.

LIPOMA – LIPOSARCOMA

These lesions are somewhat difficult to delineate pathologically, since many types of local overgrowths of fat or abnormal collections of fatty tissue exist that are frequently referred to as lipomas, but are not true new growths. Inasmuch as these are almost impossible to differentiate anatomically from true new growths, they are commonly referred to by pathologists as adipose tissue consistent with lipoma. Benign lipomas are common tumors particularly in adults. They may occur in any location of the body, but are perhaps most commonly found in the subcutaneous regions, particularly those which contain abundant amounts of fat, as well as in the retroperitoneal, mediastinal and omental fat. Grossly, a lipoma is characteristically a poorly delimited, thinly encapsulated, soft, multilobular mass of typical adult adipose tissue. Demarcation of the tumor may be very difficult because of its poor encapsulation and the tendency for the lobules to project into surrounding fatty tissue. These tumors are commonly composed of multiple discrete masses of fat separated only by thin septa of fibrous tissue. On cross section, the characteristic yellow translucence of adult fat is present. Hemorrhage and necrosis are uncommon.

On microscopic section, typical vacuolated adult fat cells are present, demonstrable only by the thin rim of cell membrane separating them from adjacent cells. Intercellular connective tissue stroma is usually quite scant and vascularization is not prominent. Because the usual techniques of paraffin embedding employ fat solvents, fat stains are of little aid in the diagnosis of routine specimens. Frozen section techniques with fat stains permit the identification of the vacuolar contents. Admixtures of fibrous tissue may be present in certain lipomas. However, since fat cells are probably derived from fibroblasts or their precursors, which accumulate lipid and assume the spherical appearance seen in adult fatty tissue, the fibrous tissue element is not included in the name of the tumor.

Liposarcomas are extremely uncommon tumors which tend to occur in older persons and to favor the retroperitoneal and mediastinal fat depots. On gross inspection, these tumors have a somewhat more opaque, gray-white to yellow appearance than lipomas, and are usually poorly delimited and not encapsulated. They may achieve massive size and invade surrounding structures, and they commonly grow about blood vessels and enclose neighboring organs. Microscopic detail in the liposarcoma shows the same variable qualities as in the fibrosarcoma. In the better differentiated liposarcomas, there may be normal-appearing fat cells interspersed among large anaplastic cells. The latter have abundant, commonly vacuolated cytoplasm and large, atypical nuclei. These cells tend to resemble anaplastic fibroblasts which can be identified as lipoblasts by their vacuolation. Other cells have many small vacuoles which impart a foaminess to their cytoplasm. As a general rule, cells tend to revert toward anaplastic fibroblasts in the more malignant types of liposarcomas. It is not uncommon to find areas in these malignant growths which may deserve the designation of fibroliposarcoma or to find other areas which include other types of mesenchymal derivatives.

Clinically, the benign lipoma is usually to-tally asymptomatic save for its presence as a tissue mass. Its soft, yielding quality frequently permits a correct clinical diagnosis. Deep-seated benign lipomas may cause concern by producing pressure distortion of surrounding structures, usually demonstrable by radiography or other techniques of visualization. The poorly differentiated liposarcoma has the same capacity to metastasize and invade as the fibrosarcomas. The well differentiated ones rarely metastasize. These malignancies are extremely rare lesions, however, and do not deserve primary consideration in the differential diagnosis of possible malignancy.

MESENCHYMOMA—MIXED MESODERMAL SARCOMA

These are rare malignant tumors apparently derived, as are the myxomas, from primitive mesenchyme which may differentiate into fibrous, adipose, angiomatous, osseous, cartilaginous or smooth and striated muscle elements. Such complete heterogeneity is rare, but often two or three of these lines of differentiation are present. In addition, there are often areas of undifferentiated mesenchymal tissue.

These lesions occur anywhere in the body but show a predilection for the vagina, uterus, bladder and striated muscle (p. 1213). They are all locally infiltrative and occasionally metastasize.

LEIOMYOMA—LEIOMYOSARCOMA

The benign tumor of smooth muscle origin, the leiomyoma, may arise anywhere in the body, in such tissues as the muscularis of the gut and the media of blood vessels, but by far its most common location is the uterus. Indeed, the leiomyoma of the uterus is the most frequent tumor in women. Here leiomyomas seldom occur singly, as they do in the other locations mentioned. They are firm, gray and circumscribed but not well encapsulated. In the gut and subcutaneous regions, they are generally small (2 to 5 cm. in diameter). In the intestinal tract, they appear as submucosal nodules or polypoid projections. In the uterus, however, they may achieve massive dimensions (over 30 cm. in diameter) (p. 1232). Enlargement to these proportions is often associated with pregnancy. It is generally believed that, when originating in the genital system, these tumors are stimulated to growth by high levels of estrogens. In the larger tumors, there may be areas of necrosis, cystic softening, hemorrhage and even calcification. When the tissue is vital, the cut surface reveals the wavy bundles of spindled smooth muscle cells by its whorled or "watered silk" appearance.

Microscopically, the leiomyoma presents broad intertwining bands of spindled smooth muscle cells exactly resembling their normal cells of origin (Fig. 5–6). Variations in cell or nuclear size are rare and mitoses are virtually absent. There is a scant fibrous stroma, sometimes overemphasized by the term fibromyoma which is, in turn, frequently shortened to the designation "fibroid."

The frequent statement that these tumors rarely become malignant (approximately 1 per cent) may even exaggerate the danger. Leiomyosarcomas are extremely rare relative to leiomyomas and it is conceivable that they arise de novo rather than in a preexisting leiomyoma.

Leiomyosarcomas are grossly virtually indistinguishable from leiomyomas, and show the same deceptively sharp delimitation from surrounding structure. However, they are often larger and tend to be softer. In addition, their more rapid increase in size may lead to larger areas of softening necrosis and hemorrhage as they outstrip their blood supply. Histologically, the cells show variable degrees of anaplasia ranging from those that still resemble smooth muscle cells to those demonstrating

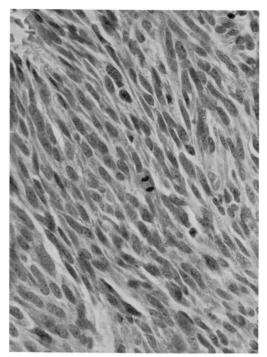

Figure 5–7. *A high power detail of the cytology of a well differentiated leiomyosarcoma for comparison with Figure 5–6. Note the slight variability in nuclear size and the mitotic figure in the center field.*

extreme cytoplasmic and nuclear pleomorphism and numerous mitoses (Fig. 5–7).

These sarcomas almost always occur in the uterus or retroperitoneal region and, from these locations, tend to metastasize via the blood to the lungs, liver and often the regional nodes of drainage.

THE LIFE HISTORY OF A MALIGNANT TUMOR

In the preceding chapters, the growth and differentiation of cells have been discussed, from normal growth to the most abnormal form of growth, neoplasia. While the clinical significance of these basic cellular concepts has been pointed out from time to time, the concepts are much more meaningful when they are examined as a part of a typical case history of a patient with a malignancy. An unfortunate case in which a patient neglected to follow advice provides an overview of the life history of a cancer and can serve as a prototype of malignancy in general. This patient, under observation for many years, presented an opportunity to follow the development of the cancer from its onset to the death of the patient. At the same time, the review of this case history

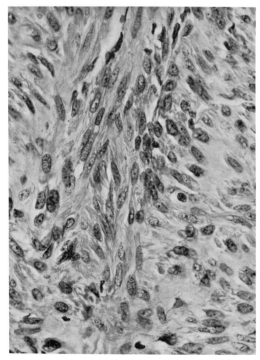

Figure 5–6. *A high power detail of the regular smooth muscle cells of a leiomyoma of the uterus for contrast with the leiomyosarcoma in Figure 5–7.*

provides an opportunity to observe the use of many of the diagnostic and therapeutic tools employed in the clinical management of a patient with a malignant tumor.

CASE HISTORY

First Clinic Visit. Mrs. L. W., a 38-year-old, white, married female, enters the clinic with the complaint of a vaginal discharge. Two months ago she noted the onset of a non-odorous, cloudy white vaginal discharge which has persisted to the present time. Although it was present throughout the menstrual cycle, it became more profuse prior to the onset of her periods. Her menstrual periods, which have always been regular, lasting four days, have not been affected by the appearance of the discharge. No intermenstrual bleeding has been noted nor has the secretion been blood-tinged. There have been no previous episodes of vaginal discharge.

Pertinent Past History. The patient has been married 16 years and has three children, all living and well, aged 12, eight and four years. Her menses began at age 14 and have always been regular. The pregnancies and postnatal periods have been entirely normal.

Physical Examination. The physical examination is entirely normal, except for the findings in the female genital tract. The external genitalia and vaginal inlet are normal and compatible with the three previous pregnancies. On palpation, the uterus is normal in size, shape and position, and there are no masses in either tubo-ovarian region. On digital examination, the cervix appears normal in size, shape and position. On direct visualization by speculum examination, the cervix is normal in shape and the external cervical os is normal in size and approximately 3 to 4 mm. in diameter. The covering exocervical mucosa is pale gray to red, intact and without deformity or scarring. The margins of the external os appear slightly reddened, granular and inflamed, and a scant amount of cloudy white secretion can be expressed by slight pressure from the external os. No focal areas of ulceration or apparent tumor formation are evident, and there is no suggestion of purulent or hemorrhagic exudate.

Treatment. Bacterial cultures and smears for the identification of *Trichomonas vaginalis* were taken from the cervix. Small, wedge-shaped biopsies of the cervix were taken at 12 and 6 o'clock for routine pathologic examination. A course of vaginal douches was outlined and the patient was instructed to return to the clinic one week later.

Bacteriologic Report. No significant pathogenic organisms were identified. No *Trichomonas vaginalis* organisms were present.

Pathology Report. Gross Examination. Specimens received consist of two wedge-shaped fragments of gray-red, firm tissue, each measuring approximately 1.5 cm. in length, 0.5 cm. in width and 0.5 cm. in depth. One surface is somewhat rounded and apparently covered by a reddened mucosa. The underlying tissue is gray-red, firm, homogeneous, and consistent with cervical fibromuscular stroma. There is no gross evidence of abscess formation, cysts or tumor masses.

Microscopic Examination. The two specimens are identified as uterine cervix. Both show essentially the same type of change and will be described together. On one surface, the tissue is covered by the junctional epithelium between the stratified squamous epithelium of the external cervical mucosa and the columnar mucin-secreting epithelium of the endocervical canal. The covering epithelium is intact throughout, without evidence of ulceration. There is, however, some evidence of thickening of exocervical epithelium, produced largely by the piling up of keratotic scales on the surface of the stratified squamous mucosa. The orderly organization of the stratified squamous epithelium is well preserved and there is no evidence of variability in cell size or orientation. Mitotic figures are scant, normal, and confined as usual to the stratum germinativum. The basement membrane of the mucosa is intact and there is no evidence of extension of epithelial cells into the underlying fibromuscular tissue. Underlying the endocervical columnar mucus-secreting epithelium, there is a fairly marked accumulation of lymphocytes, plasma cells and macrophages consistent with a chronic inflammatory reaction. These cells are found directly beneath the covering epithelium, about the endocervical glands and, occasionally, within the crypts of these glands. There is no evidence of ulceration, dysplasia or anaplasia of the cervical covering epithelium.

Diagnosis. Chronic, nonspecific inflammatory reaction of the endocervix, with moderate hyperkeratosis of the exocervical epithelium.

Follow-up. The patient failed to return for follow-up care.

Second Clinic Admission. Fourteen months after the first visit, the patient reentered the out-patient clinic because of the recurrence of vaginal discharge approximately five weeks ago. She states that the discharge cleared rapidly with the treatment outlined at the time of the first visit, and she therefore failed to return for further medical care. The present recurrence has more or less followed the pattern of the first attack, except that the discharge has been somewhat more copious.

Physical Examination. The uterus is normal in size, shape and position. The cervix is not enlarged and is without gross abnormality on palpation. Visual examination of the cervix confirms the presence of a thick, white, turbid secretion exuding from the external os. The external os is rimmed with granular red inflammation which extends onto the exocervical mucosa in a symmetrical, circular fashion for a distance of about 0.5 cm. There is no definite ulceration or evidence of tumor formation.

Treatment. Specimens for bacterial and protozoal studies were secured. A Schiller test was performed (the cervix is painted with Gram's iodine solution), and the uninvolved exocervical mucosa stained the characteristic normal red-brown color. The area of inflammation described failed to stain. Characteristically, inflammatory and neoplastic foci fail to stain with the Gram's iodine solution, since inflammation depletes the glycogen stores in the epithelial cells and tumor cells tend to be deficient in carbohydrate. Routine wedge-shaped biopsies of the exocervical os were again taken at 3, 6, 9, and 12 o'clock.

Bacteriologic Report. No significant pathogenic organisms or *Trichomonas* identified.

Pathology Report. GROSS EXAMINATION. Four apparently similar wedge-shaped pieces of red-gray tissue are received, 1.2 × 0.5 × 0.5 cm., covered on one surface by granular, slightly reddened, apparent mucosa. The underlying tissue is characteristic of uterine fibromuscular stroma and is not remarkable. No abscesses, cysts or tumors are evident.

MICROSCOPIC EXAMINATION. The tissue fragments represent exocervical os. All show essentially similar changes. While there is a marked chronic inflammation underlying the endocervical mucosa, the major changes involve the epithelial cells of the exocervical mucosa. The stratified squamous epithelium is moderately thickened, in part due to a keratotic layer on the surface and in part due to a thickening of the basal zone of the epithelium. There is an apparent proliferation of basal cells, composing a zone 3 to 4 cells deep. The basal layer of cells shows some disorganization of the normal parallel palisaded arrangement. In several foci in all four tissue specimens, the cells have lost their normal perpendicular orientation to the basement membrane of the epithelium, and lie in a slightly disorderly pattern at varying angles and, occasionally, even parallel to the basement membrane. These cells vary somewhat in size and shape, with ac-

companying variations in the nuclei. The nuclei stain darkly and show moderate numbers of normal mitotic figures. Mitotic figures are abnormally found above the basal layer of cells in the zone of apparent basal cell proliferation. The normal histologic pattern of the stratified squamous epithelium again becomes apparent above this layer, up to the flattened hyperkeratotic surface cells. No frank anaplasia, tumor giant cells or abnormal mitoses are present.

Diagnosis. Marked chronic cervicitis and endocervicitis with basal epithelial hyperplasia and dysplasia, consistent with marked chronic inflammation. There is no evidence of malignancy.

Treatment. The inflammatory condition cleared under appropriate treatment, and the discharge disappeared. Because of the cellular changes and their possible significance with respect to the development of frank neoplasia within the epithelium, the patient was instructed to return for a routine check-up visit four months later.

Follow-up. The patient returned as instructed for a routine follow-up four months after her last examination. There has been no recurrence of vaginal discharge, nor other symptoms or signs. The examination of the cervix reveals it to be normal in size, shape and position. There is no evidence of exudate, granularity or inflammation of the exocervical mucosa. Between 3 and 8 o'clock about the external os, the exocervical mucosa is gray-white, slightly wrinkled and opaque, extending out from the os for a distance of about 0.5 cm.

Treatment. Routine cytologic smears were made from the vaginal secretions as well as from the endocervical canal. A Schiller test revealed that the area of epithelial opacity remained uncolored, although the remainder of the cervix stained the normal red-brown. Biopsies were taken from the pale-staining area at 3 and 6 o'clock, as well as from 12 o'clock. The patient was instructed to return one week later for interpretation of the laboratory examinations.

Report of Cytologic Examination. The exfoliated cells show some variation in cell size and shape, with slightly enlarged nuclei showing some increased chromaticity. Interpretation: Class III (doubtful).

Pathology Report. GROSS EXAMINATION. The two wedge-shaped fragments from 12 and 3 o'clock have a pale pink, thin, flexible mucosal covering, with apparently normal underlying muscular tissue. The tissue from 6 o'clock presents a slight pallor, and apparent wrinkling and opacity of the mucosal surface. The mucosal epithelium, however, is not inflexible or unusually firm. The underlying fibromuscular tissue is not remarkable. There is no grossly visible evidence of inflammatory exudate or tumor formation.

MICROSCOPIC EXAMINATION. The biopsy taken from 12 o'clock shows an essentially normal exocervical os, with intact endocervical epithelium, stratified squamous exocervical mucosa and normal underlying fibromuscular stroma. The stratified squamous epithelial cells are entirely regular in architecture and cytologic detail. There is no evidence of hyperkeratosis in this fragment. The tissue taken from 3 and 6 o'clock discloses a fairly marked abnormality of the exocervical stratified squamous epithelial cells. The entire thickness of the epithelium is increased. The basal palisaded layer shows complete loss of the normal parallel arrangement of the cells, and many cells lie in haphazard groups and orientation. There is a fairly marked proliferation of these basal cells so that they extend approximately one-third of the way through the epithelium, but the basal cell proliferation does not extend up to the surface at any point. Within the basal cells, there is a moderate variation in cell and nuclear size and shape, with increased chromaticity of many of the nuclei. No frank tumor giant cells are present. Fairly numerous normal mitotic figures are scattered throughout. No abnormal mitoses are noted. There is moderate hyperkeratosis. The basement membrane is intact.

Diagnosis. Marked basal cell hyperplasia and dysplasia of exocervical epithelium. While the lesion is not clearly malignant, the cellular changes are sufficiently atypical to require close observation.

Follow-up. On return visit one week later, the results of the pathologic examination were discussed with the patient. It was emphasized that although no definite evidence of malignancy was present, the changes are similar to those which have been described in other individuals who have developed malignancy at a later date. It was made clear that no definite inevitable progression to tumor could be predicted and that such changes might be completely reversible so that the future course of the cervical lesion could not be prognosticated accurately. The need for close follow-up examinations was emphasized, and a return visit was scheduled for one month later.

First Hospital Admission. Seven years and eight months after the first visit, and approximately six years after the last observation, the patient entered the hospital with the chief complaints of generalized malaise, weakness, weight loss and irregular vaginal bleeding. A cloudy white vaginal discharge has been present for several years. Approximately five months ago, the patient noted the onset of occasional blood staining between menstrual periods. At first, this was minimal in amount and muddy brown but, within the past two months, the bleeding has become more excessive and bright red and has recurred every two or three days. Concomitant with this intermenstrual bleeding, her menstrual periods became more profuse, lasting 6 to 7 days. The patient thinks she has lost about 15 pounds. Her appetite has failed in the past two months and, in addition, she now complains of an increased frequency of urination, during the night as well as the day. About two weeks ago, she stopped her normal household activities because she felt too weak. The patient further stated that she failed to return for study after her last visit because she felt extremely well and was certain that "the doctors were alarmists."

Physical Examination. The patient is a pale, listless, middle-aged white woman, lying quietly in bed in no acute distress. Only the pertinent positive findings will be included. On palpation of the abdomen, the liver is enlarged, extending two fingerbreadths below the costal margin. There is a suggestion of irregularity of its anterior edge, but no definite nodules can be palpated. No other masses or abnormalities are palpable in the abdomen. On pelvic examination, the uterus is considerably enlarged to approximately twice its normal size, softer than normal, with apparent thickening of the tissues in the regions of the broad ligaments. The cervix is almost entirely replaced by a soft, friable, fungating, obvious tumor mass which bleeds readily on touch. On direct visualization, the external cervix is replaced by apparent tumor tissue which has a granular, gray-red, irregular, papillary appearance and extends onto the vaginal walls. Several small, 1 to 1.5 cm., firm lymph nodes are palpable in the left inguinal region.

Laboratory Examination. Hemoglobin, 9 gm.; white cell count, 14.3 thousand white cell per mm.^{3} of blood; catheterized urine; specific gravity, 1.015; sugar, 0; acetone, 0; albumin, 2+; and in spun sediment, 30 to 40 white cells and many red cells per high power field; blood urea nitrogen, 73 mg. per 100 cc.

Clinical Impression. The diagnosis of carcinoma of the cervix with extension into the vagina and broad ligaments was apparent at this time. The enlargement of the liver and lymph nodes strongly suggested metastasis to these organs. The urinary findings together with the elevated blood urea nitrogen were indicative of probable extension of the tumor into the ureters with possible urinary tract obstruction.

Course. Biopsy and pathologic examination confirmed the presence of a poorly differentiated, moderately rapidly growing squamous cell carcinoma. Both the probable widespread extension of the tumor into the surrounding pelvic tissues and the distant metastases precluded surgical excision of the tumor at this time. It was therefore elected to employ palliative radiation therapy.

Over the course of the next few days, it became apparent because of the patient's marked oliguria (low volume output of urine) that urinary tract obstruction existed. By the intravenous injection of radiopaque dye that is excreted through the kidneys into the urinary tract, marked narrowing of the ureters was demonstrated by x-ray and was attributed to malignant infiltration. Above these narrowings the ureters were dilated.

Despite the radiation therapy, the patient's condition continued to worsen over the next two weeks, with apparent progressive urinary tract obstruction, and rising blood urea nitrogen to a level of 145 mg. per 100 cc. Urologic consultation was requested to evaluate methods of alleviating the obstruction. At this time, however, the patient's condition began to deteriorate rapidly and she expired in apparent renal failure eight hours later. This was 21 days after entering the hospital.

Postmortem Examination. Only the relevant findings will be presented, in summary. At autopsy, a far advanced, fairly rapidly growing squamous cell carcinoma of the cervix was found. The tumor had almost entirely destroyed and replaced the cervix and lower uterine segment. It had extended into the fundus of the uterus, producing a large fungating growth totally filling the endometrial cavity and extending into the wall of the myometrium in many areas. Large gray-white plaques of tumor were found growing over the serosal covering of the dome of the uterus. Gray-white, firm tumor tissue had infiltrated into the broad ligaments and completely embedded the ureters at the level of the pelvic brim. The ureteral walls here were markedly thickened and firm, and the ureteral lumina were virtually occluded. The para-iliac and para-aortic nodes up to the level of the renal arteries were enlarged up to 2.5 to 3 cm. in diameter and totally replaced by gray-white obvious tumor tissue. The inguinal nodes were similarly replaced. Numerous 2 to 3 cm. gray-white metastases were found disseminated throughout the liver. There were no other sites of metastatic spread. The kidneys showed evidence of urinary tract obstruction, and the renal pelves, calyces and ureters were dilated above the points of obstruction.

COMMENT

Retrospectively, this case history provides an example of the total life history of a cancer. The initial inflammatory cellular changes progressed in atypicality until frank anaplasia eventually developed. Many years elapsed during this sequence of changes, and it was not until the malignancy was far advanced and produced marked hemorrhage from its eroded surface that the patient sought medical attention. Save for the complaints relative to the vaginal discharge and bleeding, the development of this cancer was relatively silent.

However, review of the case record reveals that there were some findings at an early date which suggested that the development of neoplasia was a real threat to this patient. When she was first observed, the cellular changes were confined to hyperplasia and dysplasia. These cellular changes, however, became progressively more marked over the course of the following years, until the pathologic interpretation indicated that the epithelial abnormalities were of sufficient severity to resemble closely the anaplasia of malignancy, but no frank anaplasia was present at the time of last observation prior to her final hospital admission. The later course of events strongly suggests that in this case these marked atypicalities in the cervical epithelium were indeed the forerunners of frank anaplasia and the development of a carcinoma. But it deserves reiteration that not all dysplasia progresses to malignancy, nor does all cancer arise in preexisting dysplastic changes. It is of interest that approximately six years elapsed between the time of the highly suspicious biopsy and her final hospital admission with an overt, markedly invasive, far advanced malignancy.

Two features of this case, however, must be stressed at this point. First, while chronic inflammation of the cervix has received considerable attention as a possible causal factor in the production of carcinoma in this site, there is no definite proof that the two processes are directly related. Second, there could have been no certain knowledge at the time of the third biopsy that the marked atypical hyperplasia and dysplasia signified the inevitable development of a later malignancy. With appropriate treatment, changes such as these have been observed to regress and cancer has not developed at the involved site.

REFERENCES

American Cancer Society: Statistics on cancer. Cancer, *18*:13, 1968.
Andersen, V., et al.: An in vitro demonstration of cellular immu-

nity against autologous mammary carcinoma in man. Acta Med. Scand., *186*:101, 1969.

Bill, A. H.: The implications of immune reactions to neuroblastoma. Surgery, *66*:415, 1969.

Boyland, E.: The correlation of experimental carcinogenesis and cancer in man. Progr. Exp. Tumor Res., *11*:222, 1969.

Brain, R., and Henson, R. A.: Neurological syndromes associated with carcinoma: the carcinomatous neuromyopathies. Lancet, *2*:971, 1958.

Burnet, F. M.: The concept of immunological surveillance. Progr. Exp. Tumor Res., *13*:1, 1970.

Doniach, I.: Attempted treatment of a patient with choriocarcinoma by immunization with her husband's cells. J. Obstet. Gynec., *65*:553, 1958.

Dyck, P. J., et al.: Carcinomatous neuromyopathy: a case of sensory neuropathy and myopathy with onset three and one-half years before clinical recognition of the bronchogenic carcinoma. Canad. Med. Ass. J., *79*:913, 1958.

Ericksson, O.: Method for cytological detection of cancer cells in blood. Cancer, *15*:171, 1962.

Fairley, G. H., et al.: Detection of tumor specific immune reactions in human melanoma. Ann. N.Y. Acad. Sci., *177*:286, 1971.

Fusco, F. D., and Rosen, S. W.: Gonadotropin-producing anaplastic large-cell carcinomas of the lung. New Eng. J. Med., *275*:507, 1966.

Good, R. A.: Immune Surveillance. Smith, R. T., and Landy, M. (eds.). New York, Academic Press, 1970, p. 439.

Haughton, G., and Amos, D. B.: Immunology of carcinogenesis. Cancer Res., *28*:1839, 1968.

Hellstrom, I., and Hellstrom, K. E.: Cellular immunity and blocking antibodies to tumors. J. Reticuloendothel. Soc., *10*:131, 1971.

Hellstrom, I., et al.: Blocking of cell-mediated tumor immunity by sera from patients with growing neoplasms. Int. J. Cancer, *7*:226, 1971.

Hellstrom, I., et al.: Demonstration of cell bound and humoral immunity against neuroblastoma cells. Proc. Nat. Acad. Sci. U.S.A., *60*:1231, 1968.

Hellstrom, K. E., and Hellstrom, I.: Cellular immunity against tumor antigens. Progr. Exp. Tumor Res., *9*:167, 1969.

Hertz, R., et al.: Five years experience with the chemotherapy of metastatic carcinoma: choriocarcinoma and related trophoblastic tumors in women. Amer. J. Obstet. Gynec., *83*:631, 1961.

Jehn, U. W., et al.: In vitro lymphocyte stimulation by a soluble antigen from malignant melanoma. New Eng. J. Med., *283*:329, 1970.

Jenkins, G. D.: Regression of pulmonary metastasis following nephrectomy for hypernephroma. Eight year follow-up. J. Urol., *82*:37, 1959.

Law, L. W.: Studies of the significance of tumor antigens in induction and repression of neoplastic disease. Presidential address. Cancer Res., *29*:1, 1969.

Lewis, M. G., et al.: Tumor specific antibodies in human malignant melanoma and their relationship to the extent of the disease. Brit. Med. J., *1*:547, 1969.

Lin, T-Y.: Primary cancer of the liver. Scand. J. Gastroent., Suppl. *6*:223, 1970.

Lukes, R. J.: Hodgkin's disease. Prognosis and relationship of histologic features to clinical stage. J.A.M.A., *190*:914, 1964.

Lynch, H. T.: Cancer genetics. Southern Med. J., Suppl. 1, *64*:26, 1971.

Lynch, H. T.: Genetic factors in carcinoma. Med. Clin. N. Amer., *53*:923, 1969.

Lynch, H. T.: Hereditary factors in carcinoma. Recent Results in Cancer Research. Vol. 12. New York, Springer Verlag, 1967, p. 186.

Lynch, H. T., and Krush, A. J.: Heredity and adenocarcinoma of the colon. Gastroenterology, *53*:517, 1967.

Macklin, M. T.: Comparison of the number of breast cancer deaths observed in relatives of breast cancer patients and the number expected on the basis of mortality rates. J. Nat. Cancer Inst., *22*:927, 1959.

McKann, C.: Primary malignancy in patients undergoing immunosuppression for renal transplantation. Transplantation, *8*:209, 1969.

Miller, J. A.: Carcinogenesis by chemicals: an overview. G.H.A. Clowes Memorial Lecture. Cancer Res., *30*:559, 1970.

Miller, R. W.: Deaths from childhood cancer in sibs. New Eng. J. Med., *279*:122, 1968.

Moore, G. E., et al.: Clinical and experimental observations of the occurrence and fate of tumor cells in the blood stream. Ann. Surg., *146*:580, 1957.

Morton, D., et al.: Immunologic and virus studies with human sarcomas. Surgery, *66*:152, 1969.

Nadler, S. H., and Moore, G. E.: Autotransplantation of human cancer. J.A.M.A., *191*:105, 1965.

Papanicolaou, G. N.: New cancer diagnosis. In Proceedings of the Race Betterment Conference. Battle Creek, Mich., Race Betterment Foundation, 1928, p. 528.

Papanicolaou, G. N., and Traut, H.: Diagnosis of Uterine Cancer by the Vaginal Smear. New York, The Commonwealth Fund, 1943.

Piessens, W. F.: Evidence for human cancer immunity. Cancer, *26*:1212, 1970.

Richards, V.: On the nature of cancer: an analysis from concepts in current research. Oncology, *22*:6, 1968.

Southam, C. M.: The immunologic status of patients with nonlymphomatous cancer. Cancer Res., *28*:1433, 1968.

Southam, C. M., et al.: Autologous and homologous transplantation of human cancer. In Biological Interactions in Normal and Neoplastic Growth (Henry Ford Hospital International Symposium). Boston, Little, Brown and Co., 1962, p. 723.

Southam, C. M., et al.: Homotransplantation of human cancer and normal cell lines into normal and cancer patient volunteers. Science, *125*:158, 1957.

Stout, A. P.: Myxoma, the tumor of primitive mesenchyme. Ann. Surg., *127*:706, 1948.

U.S. Department of Health, Education and Welfare: Vital Statistics of the United States. Vol. II, Mortality. Health Services and Mental Health Administration, National Center for Health Statistics, 1967.

Williams, R. C., Jr.: Dermatomyositis and malignancy. A review of the literature. Ann. Intern. Med., *50*:1174, 1959.

Zamcheck, N., et al.: Immunologic diagnosis and prognosis of human digestive-tract cancer: carcinoembryonic antigens. New Eng. J. Med., *286*:83, 1972.

6

GENETIC DISORDERS

All of the diseases of man might be grouped into three categories: (1) diseases almost entirely environmentally determined; (2) diseases almost entirely genetically determined; and (3) diseases in which both environmental factors and the genetic constitution play a role. The present chapter concerns itself principally with the diseases in category 2, but some of the interplay of nature and nurture will be considered briefly (Brock, 1972).

For all practical purposes, microbiologic infections and diseases caused by malnutrition represent instances in which the environment alone determines their development. Measles, for example, occurs no more often in both monozygotic twins (derived from a single fertilized ovum) than in both dizygotic twins (derived from separate fertilized ova). On the other hand, the problem is somewhat more complex in the case of tuberculosis. Blacks have a higher incidence of this disease than whites and, while this is in large part attributable to socioeconomic factors, the possibility of a racial predisposition has not been totally excluded. Malnutrition based on a lack of food is ironically an accident of birth, but only in the sense of the socioeconomics of one's parents. Into the group with mixed causation, where both nature and nurture play roles, go most of

the diseases of man. Peptic ulcer, diabetes mellitus, atherosclerosis, schizophrenia and probably most cancers are a few of the conditions in which genetic predisposition plays a significant role in potentiating the environmental influences.

Gregor (1967), in his life of Charles Darwin, expressed this nature-nurture interrelationship well:

> Between the environment and the genes that determine heredity there exists a highly complex relationship. It seems that genes cannot produce normal individuals unless the environmental factors are also normal. What is inherited is a packet of genes transmitted from the parents with the capacity to respond to environmental conditions in certain ways, some of which are called normal for the species in its normal environment.

We still have no complete appreciation of all the diseases which are almost entirely genetically determined. McKusick (1968) has catalogued over 1500 genetic traits. Some of these traits are trivial and confer no disadvantage on the individual; they might better be described as genetic aberrations in search of a disease. Others are as devastating as mongolian idiocy—Down's syndrome—resulting from a single extra chromosome. Heredity dictates the development of this syndrome since monozygotic twins always share this tragedy while both dizygotic twins are affected no more frequently than can be accounted for by the incidence of this disease in the population at large.

Genetic diseases may be divided roughly into three categories: (1) those having origin in chromosome mutations, (2) those having origin in gene mutations and (3) those showing marked deviations from the mean in polygenic systems (Carter, 1968). Chromosome mutations may affect either the autosomes or the sex chromosomes, as will be discussed in more detail presently. The chromosome mutations may take the form of aberrations in the number of chromosomes or abnormalities in the morphology of the chromosomes; both produce an abnormal karyotype. Gene mutations, unlike chromosomal mutations, are not visible even with the electron microscope. Such genotypic alterations are only detectable by the changes they induce in the phenotype. They account for modifications in the sequencing of a peptide or protein, resulting in diseases such as sickle cell anemia, or a specific enzyme deficiency provoking a host of inborn errors of metabolism such as galactosemia, phenylketonuria and the glycogenoses. Genic mutations also may affect the autosomes or the X (sex) chromosomes. It is intriguing that no disorders arising in mutations of the Y chromosome have yet been identified. Conditions arising in mutant genes may be divided into dominant, recessive and X-linked (McKusick and Milch, 1964). As is well known, dominant traits are those which are expressed in the heterozygote. When mutant genes have a large effect, the phenotypic expression is discontinuous—i.e, the expressed anomaly is either present or absent in the patient depending upon (1) whether the mutation is dominant or recessive, (2) whether the patient is heterozygous or homozygous, (3) the sex of the patient in X-linked recessive traits and (4) penetrance and expressivity of the mutation.

To this point, the discussion of gene mutation has mentioned some effects of single pairs of alleles of major genes having a large effect. A number of phenotypic characteristics such as hair color, height, weight, skin color and intelligence exhibit continuous variation in population groups, producing the standard bell-shaped curve of distribution. Such characteristics are controlled by the integration of individual small effects of many genes. Marked deviation from the mean in a polygenic system accounts for individuals 8 feet or 4 feet in height. Such deviations probably should not be regarded as disease. However, in the case of blood pressure, extreme deviation might represent hypertension and so could account for

significant malfunction and rightly deserve the label—disease. The polygenic mode of inheritance probably underlies the genetic predisposition to the common disorders of man previously mentioned, where both the genotype and the environment contribute. In all likelihood, the genetic predisposition depends upon the number of genes inherited which bear on the increased vulnerability to the specific malady.

Recently, it has become apparent that some polygenic variation may be discontinuous (Carter, 1969). At certain gene loci, allelic genes are present with frequencies that cannot be readily explained by chance mutation. To this phenomenon, the term "polymorphism" has been applied (Harris, 1966) (Lewontin, 1967). Despite the polygenic control of the characteristic, a threshold exists beyond which individuals are at risk. Consequently, genotype will be expressed or absent phenotypically in a discontinuous distribution. Undoubtedly, the environment plays some influential role in the emergence of the phenotypic change. Some of the lesions believed to be determined by polymorphic inheritance include cleft lip, pyloric stenosis, congenital hip dislocation, congenital heart defects and anencephaly.

It is important to clarify the commonly used and sometimes misused terms "hereditary," "familial" and "congenital." Genetic disorders may have their origins in some mutation passed from one generation to the next and, therefore, are hereditary and familial. Pedigrees of the proband's family will exhibit affected individuals dispersed throughout preceding generations. On the other hand, genetic disorders may not be familial and may arise from a mutation during gametogenesis or postzygotic development. Parents and previous generations, therefore, will be free of the trait. The mutation may be transmitted to the offspring of the proband if survival and fertility have not been reduced. On the other hand, many mutations disappear. Those affecting the karyotype and mutant genes of large effect may be lethal or may so reduce fertility that transmission is prevented. Polygenically induced disease may disappear as the many mutant genes are diluted by repeated matings with normal individuals. As is well known, the term congenital simply implies "born with." Obviously, all congenital diseases are not hereditary and may result from such prenatal influences as microbiologic infections in the mother or may be the consequence of drugs taken during pregnancy as is detailed on p. 175. Conversely, all genetic diseases are not congenital since patients with hereditary Huntington's chorea usually manifest none of their inheritance until the third or fourth decades of life.

CYTOPLASMIC OR EXTRACHROMOSOMAL INHERITANCE

Before pursuing the consideration of genetics, we should note that there has always been some suspicion (and evidence) that cytoplasmic factors may possibly act independently from the nucleus in controlling some heritable aspects of the cell. Examples have come mostly from fungi, protozoa and flowering plants. In higher animals, especially in vertebrates, it is more difficult to identify cytoplasmically inherited traits, and indisputable examples are hard to find. In order to prove that a trait is inherited on an extrachromosomal basis, one must demonstrate that the transmitting organelle has physical continuity (that it can reproduce or duplicate itself) and genetic continuity (that the trait is inherited, but not in a mendelian fashion). It should also be feasible to identify some "genetic unit" within a cytoplasmic organelle, or at least within the cytoplasm, which acts as a carrier of genetic information analogous to deoxyribonculeic acid (DNA) in the nucleus.

Three types of cellular organelles are thought to act more or less autonomously. These are the plastids, the mitochondria and the "fiber producers" (the latter includes the centrioles which are responsible for aster formation during mitosis as well as the basal granules which produce cilia, flagella and sperm tails). All three types of organelles are thought to divide by fission or to arise from preexisting membranes or granules in the cytoplasm near the "parent" organelle. All three organelles have shown altered characteristics which could only be explained by cytoplasmic inheritance. For example, in the plant *Mirabili jalopa* plastids may occasionally lose their capacity to produce chlorophyll, and involved sections of leaves will be white or albino. If a green *Mirabilis* plant is crossed with a variegated plant (one with leaves that have both green and white segments), then the type of offspring produced depends strictly on the female parent. If the female parent is green, the F_1 generation is likewise green; if variegated, the offspring is also variegated. When the F_2 generation is studied, the same holds true: the female parent still determines the color of the leaves and no mendelian ratios are produced.

Finally, it has been shown that these plastids, mitochondria and fiber producers do contain small amounts of DNA which, however, is not identical to nuclear DNA. The evidence is indirect, probably because of the minute amounts of DNA involved and the difficulties of chemical extraction and possible nuclear contamination. Whether this DNA acts as a genetic carrier has not been demonstrated. In some of these organelles, machinery for the synthesis of proteins and nucleic acids have been detected, but the extent to which the organelles use their own systems is not clear. In the mitochondrion, for example, development of the internal structure is apparently controlled by the mitochondrion itself while the outer membranes and soluble proteins seem to be controlled by nuclear genes. On the whole, evidence of cytoplasmic inheritance is fragmentary, but research indicates that some cellular organelles are directed in part by their own or other heritable factors in the cytoplasm. The interested reader is referred to the reviews of Gibor and Granick (1971), Kirk and Tilney-Bassett (1967) and Beale (1969).

THE NORMAL HUMAN KARYOTYPE

Although Mendel's work published in 1866 revealed the inheritance of discrete units, it was not until 40 years later that his work was rediscovered. Then it became apparent that these discrete units resided in special structures within the nucleus. Early in this century, cytogeneticists found that the number and types of chromosomes of plants and lower animals were species-specific. While the interphase chromosomes of these lower animals were technically easy to study, the interphase chromosomes of mammals, and especially of man, could not be visualized at all. Even if the cell were arrested in mitosis, the chromosomes were so crowded that a correct count could not be made. It is one of the ironies of medical history that, for over 30 years, students were taught that man had 48 chromosomes.

The correct count of man's 46 chromosomes by Tjio and Levan (1956) was achieved by improved techniques for spreading mitotic chromosomes. Over the ensuing years, several refinements have been added. The first involves the use of colchicine or one of its derivatives, which interferes with the development of the spindle and stops cell division during metaphase. Since the chromosomes cannot attach to the spindle, they remain distributed within the cell. The second step involves the use of a hypotonic solution, usually sodium citrate, which causes cells to swell and thus spreads the chromosomes. Then either a quick air-drying or a squashing technique is employed to spread the chromosomes still further and confine them within a single plane.

Theoretically, one can use any human tissue to analyze chromosomes, but many cells are difficult to grow in vitro and best results have been obtained from the culture of bone marrow, skin and the peripheral leukocytes. Bone marrow is an active mitotic tissue and, therefore, needs very little or no time in culture. In contrast, the outgrowth of cells from a fragment of skin takes approximately three weeks. Leukocytes and particularly small lymphocytes can be stimulated to undergo blast cell transformation and mitotic division within 3 days by the addition of phytohemagglutinin (PHA) to a cell culture. By any of these approaches, actively dividing cells can be obtained and a chromosome squash prepared. The squash is then microphotographed and with knowledge, diligence, care and a scissors, the karyotype can be arranged.

A metaphase chromosome consists of two strands of chromatids which are connected by a small pale-staining area known as the centromere or the kinetochore. *Chromosome types are differentiated by the position of the centromere: if it connects the chromatids in their center, the chromosome is said to be median or metacentric; if the centromere is eccentrically placed, the chromosome is said to be submedian or submetacentric. In some chromosomes, the centeromere is almost, but not quite, at the end of the chromatids. These are acrocentric chromosomes,* many of which bear small projections on their short arms. The projections are known as *satellites* and are involved in the formation of nucleoli. Probably because of this activity, acrocentric chromosomes are often seen in groups in the metaphase plate, a phenomenon described as satellite association.

The 46 chromosomes from a metaphase spread occur in homologous pairs. Twenty-two pairs are morphologically exactly alike in the two sexes and are known as the autosomes. The paired sex chromosomes in the female are alike (the two X chromosomes), but the sex chromosomes are different in the male, one being an X and the other a smaller Y chromosome. According to the international "Denver" classification, the pairs of chromosomes can be arranged according to size and centromere position. This is most easily done by numbering the pairs in descending order of size. Later, it was suggested that the pairs be segregated into seven groups (from A to G), depending more or less on type. This classification is now referred to as the cell karyotype. Table 6–1 describes the various chromosome groups which can be compared to the two normal karyotypes (Figs. 6–1 and 6–2).

Normal male and female karyotypes can be differentiated by the number of C group and G group chromosomes. The female has 16

TABLE 6–1. KARYOTYPE GROUPINGS OF HUMAN CHROMOSOMES

Group A (Nos. 1–3) Large metacentric chromosomes which differ sufficiently in size to be differentiated.
Group B (Nos. 4–5) Large submedian chromosomes which are hard to distinguish, but chromosome 4 is slightly longer.
Group C (Nos. 6–12+X) A large group of medium-sized, submedian chromosomes. Some are comparatively metacentric. The X chromosome belongs in this group.
Group D (Nos. 13–15) Three pairs of large acrocentric chromosomes; the first two pairs, Nos. 13 and and 14, are often satellited.
Group E (Nos. 16–18) Shorter chromosomes with submedian centromeres, except for No. 16 which is almost median.
Group F (Nos. 19–20) Short chromosomes which are median in type.
Group G (Nos. 21–22+Y) Very short acrocentric chromosomes, of which No. 21 is often satellited.

C group and 4 G group chromosomes, while the male has 15 chromosomes in the C group and 5 in the G group. The X chromosome cannot be identified from the metaphase spread or karyotype. However, the X is known to be a medium-sized, submetacentric chromosome which is similar to a C-6 or C-7 chromosome. The Y chromosome is usually a little larger than chromosome 21, is unsatellited and has long arms which are more or less parallel to each other. In 3 per cent of normal males, however, the Y chromosome is polymorphic. It is either very large (almost the size of a D group chromosome) or smaller than the G group chromosomes.

The use of radioactive precursors to DNA, particularly tritiated thymidine in the culture medium, has provided additional help in the identification of chromosomes. During the DNA synthetic period in interphase, many chromosomes become labeled at specific times and with characteristic patterns. For example, the D group chromosomes are large acrocentric chromosomes which are impossible to distinguish by routine karyotyping. After they have been exposed to radioactive thymidine, however, one pair (No. 15) completes synthesis very early, one pair (No. 14) completes synthesis late and labels primarily near the centromere, and the third pair (No. 13) also is synthesized late but labels more on its long arms. Other chromosomes may be identified in this

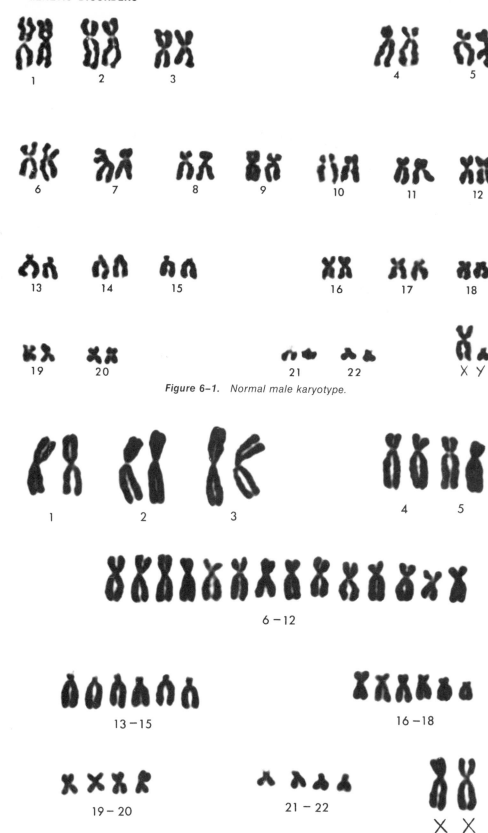

Figure 6-1. Normal male karyotype.

Figure 6-2. Normal female karyotype.

way (Nos. 1, 4, 5, 17 and 18, in particular), but autoradiography is most useful in the identification of X chromosomes. As a general rule, all X chromosomes in excess of one replicate later than the autosomes. This means that one X chromosome (the isocyclic X) in normal female cells replicates in time with the autosomes, and the other X chromosome (the allocyclic X) labels later than the autosomes. It is this allocyclic or late-replicating X chromosome which later forms the chromatin body. In the male cell there is, of course, only one isocyclic X chromosome, but the Y chromosome also replicates later, at least in comparison to the G group chromosomes. We can turn now to a closer look at the individual chromosome.

THE HUMAN CHROMOSOME

MORPHOLOGY

Many interphase nuclei studied with the light microscope show a few densely stained regions (heterochromatin), but most of the chromosomal material is lightly stained and is so diffuse as to appear amorphous (euchromatin). In many organisms, the heterochromatin is adjacent to centromeric regions, although large portions or entire chromosomes, such as the X and Y, may be heterochromatic. In man, the best example of heterochromatin is the Barr body (p. 180), but other chromocenters are often observed. The differential staining is attributed to differences in the coiling of the genetic strands, although the DNA is not altered chemically. Heterochromatin behaves differently from euchromatin in several respects. In some lower organisms, mendelian genes cannot be assigned to the heterochromatin. Also, its time of replication differs from euchromatin in that it occurs late in the DNA synthetic period. Nevertheless, heterochromatin does exert some genetic influence. In the absence of the Barr body in human female cells, abnormalities occur. Furthermore, the proximity of heterochromatin exerts a repressive effect on neighboring euchromatic genes. In cases where a heterochromatic segment can be translocated on a euchromatic chromosome, mendelian ratios for the euchromatic genes near that segment can no longer be obtained in the offspring. This is known as the variegated position effect. While little is known of the cellular effects of heterochromatin, it may be an important mechanism of inactivating or repressing whole areas of chromosome activity.

In general, the electron microscope has been a disappointment in the study of chromosome architecture. A great deal of effort has been expended on the attempt to resolve the DNA strand (unit fiber) of the interphase nucleus as well as in the isolated chromosome. Unfortunately, the results of these studies have not been consistent. Most investigators agree on a 100 Å (or 80 Å) interphase fiber, but the narrowest fibers of the isolated chromosome are reportedly in the range of 250 Å. This discrepancy in fiber size has not been resolved as yet, nor has the question of "strandedness" — i.e., whether many DNA fibers associate in parallel array or whether a single DNA fiber folds up on itself to form the typical chromatid.

CHEMICAL COMPOSITION

Chemically, chromosomes are known to consist of DNA, basic protein, RNA and other proteins variously referred to as acidic, neutral or residual protein. Other components include lipids and inorganic metals such as calcium and magnesium. Even the enzyme DNA polymerase thought to be necessary for DNA replication may be bound to the body of the chromosome. Recent analysis of metaphase chromosomes reveals 13 to 16 per cent DNA, 12 to 13 per cent RNA and 68 to 72 per cent protein. The protein fraction is surprisingly large and, in fact, may represent contamination. The RNA and residual protein are thought to have a transitory association with the chromosome. As will be seen later, some of the RNA plays a messenger role of transporting information from the chromosome to the cytoplasm. The role of the residual protein is not known, but it may play a part in the coiling or compacting of the chromosome. Only the basic proteins, notably histones (and in some sperm DNA protamines), have been shown to be an integral part of the structure of the chromosome. Histones exist in equimolar ratio to DNA, but the exact manner in which histones are bound to the DNA molecule is disputed. It may occupy the grooves of the DNA helix or surround the molecule like a coat. *Three possible functions have been ascribed to histones: (1) They may serve to stabilize DNA in rapidly dividing cells; (2) they may serve as a contractile element when the chromosome shortens; and (3) they may partially regulate genetic activity, repressing genes.*

The principal component of chromosomes, as is well known, is DNA (deoxyribose nucleic acid), the structure of which was brilliantly elucidated by Watson and Crick in 1953. Essentially, the backbone of the molecule, which is only 20 Å wide, is a double helix, each helix being composed of alternating deoxyribose and phosphate groups. The two helices wind themselves around a common axis in a parallel fashion but in opposite polar directions, making complete turns every 34 Å. The four nucleotide bases are bound to the deoxyribose in such a way that an adenine (A) and a thymine (T) are always linked together, as are a guanine (G) and a cytosine (C), forming, so to speak, the rungs of a ladder (Fig. 6–3).

The Watson and Crick model of DNA neatly satisfies the biochemical and physical data assiduously collected before and after 1953. It also explains how a large molecule such as DNA can be self-replicating. Radioactive experiments have confirmed the assumption that the two helices unwind, breaking the hydrogen bonds between the nucleotide pairs, and that each half forms a complementary strand, so that two new and identical molecules are formed. These are then passed on to the daughter cells or to the next generation.

PROTEIN SYNTHESIS AND THE GENETIC CODE

It is the sequence of nucleotide bases in the DNA molecule which provides the blue-

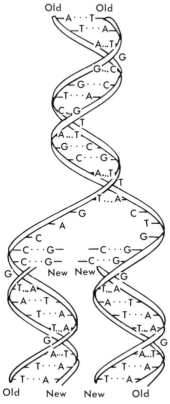

Figure 6–3. *The structure of DNA and its replication. (From Watson, J. D.: Molecular Biology of the Gene. New York, W. A. Benjamin, 1965.)*

print for the formation of the large number of enzymes and other proteins in the cell. The major steps from DNA structure to protein synthesis will be given here only in outline form.

The substance almost wholly involved in protein synthesis is RNA (ribonucleic acid) which is chemically and structurally similar to DNA, except for two alterations: the sugar component is ribose instead of deoxyribose and the base uracil (U) replaces thymine. Three classes of RNA can be identified in the cell. The first is *messenger RNA (mRNA)* which is present in small amounts and is remarkably unstable, having a half-life of hours to a few days. It is synthesized by an enzyme RNA polymerase which transcribes a complementary chain from one of the strands of the DNA molecule, the process being termed transcription. Control mechanisms, not yet identified, prevent the transcription of the second DNA strand in vivo and determine the length of DNA copied (that is, the final length of the mRNA molecule). Once formed, the mRNA leaves the nucleus via the nuclear pores and attaches to the ribosomes in the cytoplasm.

The amino acids destined to make up a specific protein or polypeptide chain have no inherent way of recognizing their place on the mRNA template. A second class of low-molecular weight RNA molecules, called *transfer or soluble RNA (tRNA and sRNA, respectively)*, have the specific task of identifying the necessary amino acids and transferring them to a site where the polypeptide is formed. Before this occurs, the amino acid must be linked to adenylic acid (AMP) requiring energy derived from adenosine triphosphate (ATP) and must bind to its tRNA in the presence of a specific enzyme (amino-acyl RNA synthetase), of which there are at least 20 different kinds. The specificity of each of these enzymes is incredible. They recognize both the appropriate amino acid and the specific transfer RNA and, in this linkage, account for the accuracy of protein or peptide synthesis.

The actual assembly of the polypeptide occurs on the surface of ribosomes. These specific cytoplasmic organelles are visible with the electron microscope either singly, in groups or lining the endoplasmic reticulum. *A single ribosome consists of two subunits. Each subunit contains its own kind of ribosomal RNA (rRNA) (23S or 16S) as well as approximately 20 kinds of proteins.* The mRNA attaches to the ribosome and, in the presence of several enzymes and GTP (guanosine triphosphate), forms peptide bonds between amino acids carried by the charged tRNA in the exact order prescribed by the mRNA. These processes by which protein is synthesized by the three types of RNA are called translation. A schematic view of these processes is given in Fig. 6–4.

Chemical analysis showed that there are four nucleotide bases (AUGC) in the mRNA which reflect the bases (TACG) in its complementary DNA. The problem then remained to determine how these four bases or letters code for 20 amino acids in the cell. Two major approaches have contributed to "breaking the code." One involved the induction of predictable mutations in bacteriophages in which the chemical sequence of the gene had been mapped out. The synthesized protein sequence could then be checked against the altered nucleotide sequence. The other approach involved the ,synthesis of proteins in vitro using specific mRNA or polynucleotides (especially trinucleotides) in the presence of all other necessary components (the 20 amino acids, tRNA's and their respective activating enzymes, ribosomes and an energy source such as ATP).

From these studies, it became apparent that three consecutive nucleotide bases (triplets) in the mRNA (and therefore in the DNA) make up the three letters (one codon) which code for *one* amino acid. The code is nonoverlapping, i.e., the nucleotides are read in sequence. Evidence also indicated that the code is very degenerate, that is, more than one codon and sometimes up to four or even six can code for a single amino acid. Furthermore, the code often does not distinguish between letters (or bases) in the third position; for example, UUU or UUC code for phenylalanine and CUU and CUC, for leucine. However, a study of the code (Table 6–2) will reveal that methionine and tryptophane each has a unique codon which will incorporate the respective amino acid into a protein. Combinations such as UAA, UAG and UGA (also referred to as ochre, amber and opal) do not code for any amino acid. Since there must be a way of indicating the start and finish of a polypeptide chain, it is thought that these combinations may code "begin" or "end" to the ribosome.

CONTROL OF GENETIC ACTIVITY

The multicellular organism, with all its differentiated cells, develops from a single diploid zygote. Every cell then in the body contains the same genetic information. A highly organized mechanism must be present to activate and repress genes at the proper time. At the cellular level, the intricate metabolism must accomodate new environmental stimuli. Sometimes these stimuli result in the activation or inhibition of an enzyme, but not at the gene

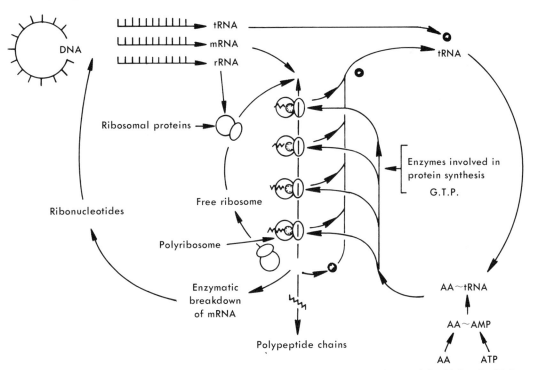

Figure 6–4.   *Schematic view of the role of RNA in protein synthesis. (From Watson, J. D.: Molecular Biology of the Gene. New York, W. A. Benjamin, 1965.)*

TABLE 6–2. THE GENETIC CODE

First Base	Second Base				Third Base
	U	C	A	G	
U	PHE	SER	TYR	CYS	U
	PHE	SER	TYR	CYS	C
	LEU	SER	*Ochre*	*Opal*	A
	LEU	SER	*Amber*	TRP	G
C	LEU	PRO	HIS	ARG	U
	LEU	PRO	HIS	ARG	C
	LEU	PRO	GLUN	ARG	A
	LEU	PRO	GLUN	ARG	G
A	ILEU	THR	ASPN	SER	U
	ILEU	THR	ASPN	SER	C
	ILEU	THR	LYS	ARG	A
	MET	THR	LYS	ARG	G
G	VAL	ALA	ASP	GLY	U
	VAL	ALA	ASP	GLY	C
	VAL	ALA	GLU	GLY	A
	VAL	ALA	GLU	GLY	G

level. In other instances, a substance may actually "turn on" a gene, with the result that an enzyme is produced in greater quantities, or a gene may be "turned off." These processes are known as induction and repression, respectively, and have been studied particularly in bacteria. The first such gene regulation model, analyzed by Monod and Jacob (1961), was based on the lactose system in *E. coli.* Known as the Operon Model, it is possibly applicable to man.

One result of mapping genes in bacteria was the discovery that, sometimes, genes involved in the formation of enzymes in one particular metabolic pathway (such as lactose utilization) were closely linked without intervening, unrelated genes. These and other genes concerned with the actual coding of the amino acid sequences of enzymes are known as *structural genes.* The Jacob-Monod Theory describes a second type of gene, the *operator gene* which is located at either end of the series of structural genes. The operator is thought to act as a switch, permitting or preventing transcription of the entire sequence of structural genes into perhaps one unit of mRNA. This linkage of related structural genes and their controlling operator gene is known as *"the operon."* At a distance from the operon, possibly on a different chromosome in higher animals, is a third type of gene, the *regulator gene* which manufactures a cytoplasmic repressor molecule (Ptashne and Gilbert, 1970). The repressor molecule can act in two ways. It can react with the end product of the biochemical

pathway, become activated and then combine with its specific operator gene to "switch off" the transcription of the mRNA controlled by the operon. Thus, the production of enzyme ceases. The repressor molecule can also react with an "inducer" molecule, if such be present, and become inactivated. Since it can no longer engage the operator gene, the operon will continue to transcribe and make more mRNA and more enzyme. In this way, the presence of "inducer" results in increased synthesis of enzyme. This theory of the Operon Model offers an explanation of the phenomena of induction and repression and appears as an efficient, economical system which makes enzymes when needed (Fig. 6–5).

With this overview of some of the fundamentals of the genetic apparatus, we can turn to the causes and consequences of genetic injury.

CAUSES OF MUTATION

Well known causes of genetic injury are ionizing radiation, drugs and viruses. Some of the mutagenic agents included in these categories are listed in Table 6–3. How much these agents contribute to the production of clinical disease remains uncertain. Unless alterations in the karyotype are induced, one must depend on expressed phenotypic change and, to confirm that such change is genetic in origin, successive generations within a pedigree must be followed. The long generation time of man, separation and migration of members of families, and the cost and complexity of the required clinical studies have all rendered difficult the study of genetic disease in man. Animal models have had only limited usefulness because of the remarkable variation in species susceptibility. For example, cortisone will induce congenital malformations in mice and rabbits, but not in rats (Hsia, 1968). Cortisone, as far as we know, has no effect on the genome of man.

The mutagenic potency of ionizing radiation has been clearly established and is discussed in some detail on p. 134. In animals, higher rates of abortion, increased frequency of congenital anomalies and a great variety of chromosomal aberrations can be produced by radiant energy (Green, 1968). In man, evidence of radiation injury comes from many sources. Leukocytes in 61 per cent of 77 heavily exposed survivors of the atomic bomb exhibited chromosomal aberrations as compared with 16 per cent of controls (Bloom et al., 1967). Translocations and pericentric inversions predominated. Infants born of mothers who had been pregnant when they received an

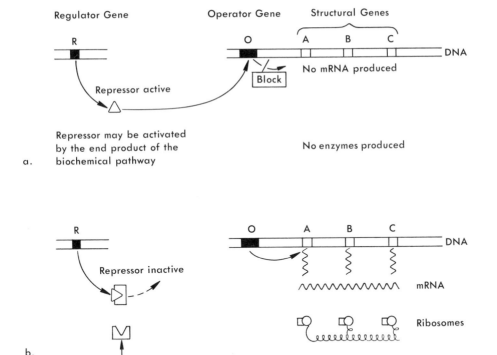

Figure 6–5. *The operon model in its simplest form. a, Repressor active, operator gene switched off. b, Repressor inactive, operator gene permits transcription of mRNA.*

TABLE 6–3. CHROMOSOMAL MUTAGENS

A. Radiation
   1. Human Cells in Vitro-Threshold 50 r
   2. Human Lymphocytes in Vivo-Threshold 12–35 r
B. Drugs
   1. Effect on Human Cells
      alkylating agents: triethylenemelamine, busulfan,
        N-mustards
      amethopterin
      azothiaprine
      methotrexate
      benzene
      ? lysergic acid (LSD)
      streptonigrin
      bromouracil
   2. Effects on Plant Cells
      caffeine and its analogues
      phenols, ethyl alcohol and other alcohols
      menadione, coumarin, etc.
C. Viruses
   1. In Vitro Effect on Mammalian Cells
      herpes simplex
      SV 40 virus
      adenovirus type 12
   2. In Vivo Effect in Humans
      poliomyelitis
      rubeola
      yellow fever vaccination
      ? mumps
      ? chickenpox

estimated 100 rads of total body irradiation from the atomic blast also suffered chromosomal mutations. In such infants, karyotypic abnormalities were encountered in approximately 0.52 per cent of their lymphocytes in contrast to a control rate of only 0.04 per cent (Bloom, 1968). An increased rate of abortion and stillbirths occurred among those exposed during pregnancy (Yamazaki et al., 1954). Mention has already been made of the increased incidence of leukemia and other forms of cancer in survivors (p. 134). Radiation injury, however, may follow even the relatively small exposures employed in radiotherapy as is detailed on p. 730 and, indeed, chromosomal abnormalities may persist for years after such exposure (Buckton et al., 1962).

The role of drugs and chemical agents in mutagenesis is a complex and controversial issue. Many compounds induce karyotypic aberrations in cell culture or, in animals, malform the fetus when sufficiently large doses are administered during pregnancy. In both settings, it has been impossible to segregate the metabolic and toxic effects of the drugs from their potential to induce direct genetic injury. In cell culture, karyotypic abnormalities can be produced by introducing into the nutrient medium a host of agents, even such seemingly innocent ones as aspirin. In almost all these instances, the evidence suggests that the genetic damage is a consequence of toxic cell injury and reflects irreversible damage to cells destined to die. Similarly, the tragic infants having "seal" deformities of their limbs (phocomelia), born of mothers who had taken thalidomide during pregnancy, have not had demonstrable karyotypic abnormalities in their leukocytes, suggesting again that the role of the drug was not that of a mutagen.

On the other hand, immunosuppressive compounds such as the nitrogen mustards, azothiaprine and amethopterin are clearly mutagenic both in vivo and in vitro (Jensen, 1967). As was discussed on p. 132, the alkylating agents are capable of binding directly to guanine in DNA, thereby altering the genetic code (Ryser, 1971). In this context, lysergic acid diethylamide (LSD) has been indicted by some as a mutagen (Cohen et al., 1967) (Irwin and Egozcue, 1967). Karyotypic abnormalities have been identified in the leukocytes of chronic users of this agent and in children born of mothers who had taken high doses of the drug during the early months of pregnancy. However, other investigators have questioned the meaning of these findings. Dishotsky et al. (1971), in a review of studies on LSD and genetic damage, suggested that the concentrations of the drug used in the in vitro experiments provided an exposure which could not be achieved with usual in vivo doses. Comparing studies of illicit drug users with those of subjects taking pharmacologically pure LSD, they recognized a significant difference in rates of chromosome breakage in the two groups, and so they suggested that impurities in illicit drugs, in addition to other stressful elements of the drug abuser's life style (poor nutrition, little sleep, etc.), might be responsible for the higher rate of chromosome damage noted in these individuals. The weight of evidence now available seems to indicate that LSD is unlikely to be a mutagenic agent in the concentrations used by human subjects.

Viruses have been clearly documented as mutagenic in animals and there is much suspicion of similar action in man (Nichols, 1966). It will be recalled that the DNA oncogenic viruses are incorporated within the genome of the transformed cell (p. 129). The cancerous transformation is attributed by some to the incorporation of this new viral genetic information into the affected cell. The RNA oncogenic viruses with their reverse "transcriptases" modify the genome of the host cell. Clearly, the virus induces a change in the genotype and phenotype of such cells. Nononcogenic viruses have also been shown to have mutagenic capacity both in vivo and in vitro (Stich and Yohn, 1967). An increased frequency of chromosome breaks has been reported in the leukocytes of patients suffering from measles, chicken pox, mumps and infectious mononucleosis (possibly of viral origin) (Gripenberg, 1965). However, the significance of such leukocytic changes is uncertain. Only rubella infections during pregnancy are clearly associated with congenital malformations in the infant. When mothers contract German measles in the first trimester of pregnancy, the infant may be born with cataracts, cardiac anomalies, deafness and even mental deficiency. However, it is not clear that these phenotypic abnormalities derive from genetic injuries. Ironically, no karyotypic alterations have been identified in the leukocytes of these malformed infants, and so it is suspected that direct viral infection of the developing fetus is the cause of the deranged embryogenesis.

So-called "spontaneous" mutations have been frequently identified in the cells of man both in vivo and in vitro. It would be surprising if mitotic errors did not occur among the many billions of cells which comprise the adult individual. These tend to be more common in the advanced years of life. Later we shall see that advancing maternal age is correlated with an increased frequency of chromosome mutations in the offspring. The term "spontaneous," however, must be viewed within the context of the many potentially mutagenic agents to which we are all exposed virtually daily; conceivably, the relationship of aging to mutation merely documents longer exposure to these hazards.

CHROMOSOMAL MUTATIONS

Mutations in chromosomes are seen as abnormalities in the karyotype either in the number or the morphology of chromosomes.

ABERRATIONS IN CHROMOSOME NUMBER – POLYPLOIDY AND ANEUPLOIDY

The survival of the species and its members is dependent on the orderly replication of the normal number of chromosomes in both somatic and sex cells. While mutations must provide for the variations involved in the evolution of the species, abnormalities in chromosome number constitute such gross genetic deviations as to confer on the organism a serious deficit and often death. The normal 46 chromosomal complement of a somatic or nonreproductive cell is diploid (2n). These chromosomes are actually the long chromatids of interphase. In preparation for *mitosis,* DNA is synthesized during the S phase, and the chromatids begin to replicate themselves, forming two long strands connected by the centromere. At the time of mitotic division, the long strands contract to produce the chromosomes having the familiar X or wishbone shapes. As is well known in the remaining stages of mitosis, the chromosomes line up at the equatorial plate during metaphase, the centromere divides longitudinally, and the chromatids so formed are either pulled or guided by the spindle fibers to opposite poles where they form the nuclei of two new daughter cells.

A variety of mishaps may occur in this orderly mitotic process. If all of the chromatids fail to separate and, instead, travel together to one pole, one of the daughter cells is then tetraploid (4n). If this same accident involves half of the chromosomes but the other half correctly divide, a cell having a triploid (3n) complement is formed. When the number of chromosomes is a whole multiple of n, the phenomenon is called *polyploidy.* Such gross aberrations in chromosome number are encountered in man virtually only in the anarchic divisions of cancer cells. Failure of a chromatid pair to separate normally at the proper time so that they travel together to one pole is known as *nondisjunction.*

Another process by which chromatids are incorporated into the wrong daugher cell constitutes *anaphase lag.* Here the chromosome attached to the spindle begins to move to the correct pole but lags behind and is incorporated into the wrong cell by the newly formed cell membrane. More often, nondisjunction or anaphase lag affects a single chromosome, yielding cells which contain one less or one more than the basic diploid complement. Such an aberration leads to a chromosomal complement which does not constitute a multiple of the basic chromosome number, termed *aneuploidy.* When nondisjunction affects a single chromosome (one daughter cell receives 47 and the other, 45 chromosomes), both cells are at a serious disadvantage and may die. Alternatively, the cell lacking one chromatid may die and the other may live and continue to multiply. The significance of mitotic accidents depends largely on the chromosome involved. In general, an extra sex chromosome or the absence of the usual second sex chromosome does not handicap a cell as much as one too few or too many autosomes. The larger the autosome, the more likely crucial genes are either lacking or are present in excess, and the more likely the affected cell will die.

Mitotic errors are common in cancer cells, but they are uncommon in somatic cells. While they undoubtedly must occur, the body probably selects against such cells' having an abnormal chromosome complement. As was cited previously, Court-Brown (1967) has shown that, in adults, the frequency of aneuploid cells increases with age. He found about 5 per cent aneuploid lymphocytes in women up to the sixth decade of life but, by age 75, such aneuploidy had reached a frequency of 13 per cent.

Germ or reproductive cells undergo a very specialized cell division—*meiosis*—reducing the diploid set (46) of chromosomes to the haploid (23). This is accomplished in the first division of meiosis—the reduction division—followed by a regular mitotic division which reproduces the haploid gametes.

In *meiosis I,* the chromosome behavior is different from that of mitosis in several respects. The chromosomes not only duplicate themselves but associate with their homologous partners side by side so that four chromatids with their two connecting centromeres lie closely together at the equatorial plate. At points where the two innermost chromatids overlap, they form bridges or chiasmata where an actual exchange of genetic material occurs. At metaphase, the two chromosomes separate, and an entire chromosome (rather than a chromatid) moves to the polar end of the cell. In this process, the number of chromosomes is halved. The new daughter cells then divide by mitosis in the male but, in the female, mitosis follows only if fertilization occurs. The details of meiosis I and mitosis are given in the following table:

TABLE 6–4. DIFFERENCES BETWEEN FIRST DIVISION MEIOSIS AND MITOSIS

Meiosis I	Mitosis
1. Homologous chromosomes align themselves and form chiasmata (synapsis).	1. Chromosomes align themselves at random (no synapsis).
2. Centromere does not divide. The entire chromosome moves to one pole.	2. Centromere divides. A chromatid moves to one pole.
3. Number of chromosomes is divided in half (n).	3. Number of chromosomes is the same as in parent cell (2n).
4. Nondisjunction results in aneuploidy of the zygote.	4. Nondisjunction results in mosaicism or, later in life, in clone formation.

Accidents in meiosis occur more often than previously suspected. The errant movement of a chromosome or a homologous chromosome pair results in gametes with unequal chromosome number (22 and 24). Although this may be caused by anaphase lag, nondisjunction is probably the more important pathway.

The cell division in which nondisjunction occurs is of great importance. After fertilization with a normal male gamete, a defective female gamete will give rise to an aneuploid individual with a complement of either 47 or 45 chromosomes if only one chromosome is affected. Nondisjunction after zygote formation yields a *mosaic individual* who has more than one chromosome count in his body cells. Some

nondisjunctional errors before and after zygote formation are presented in the accompanying diagram (Fig. 6–6).

The viability of aneuploid zygotes depends on the particular chromosome involved. With rare exception, the lack of a member of an autosome pair (monosomy) is virtually incompatible with survival. Similarly, the YO complement is lethal, but zygotes with a missing X chromosome may come to full term. Studies of abortuses indicate that many are aneuploid (World Health Organization, 1970).

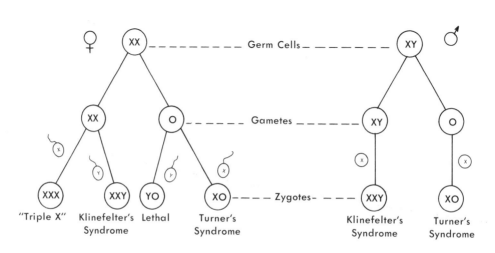

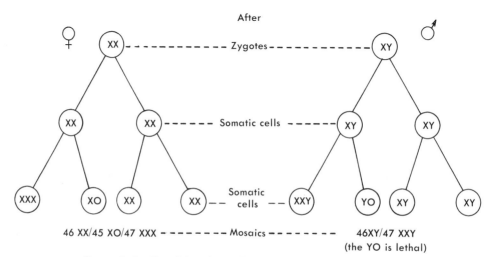

Figure 6–6. *Nondisjunction before and after zygote formation.*

An abnormal chromosome complement was demonstrated in approximately 20 per cent of spontaneous abortions and in only 2 per cent of induced abortions. Most of these aberrations (50 per cent) took the form of autosomal trisomy (an autosome is present in triplicate). Thirty per cent were related to monosomy and 12 per cent were related to triploidy. Mosaicism is seen only occasionally among human abortuses, perhaps because only one tissue is karyotyped in these early fetuses. Nevertheless, mosiacism has been found to be common in patients with sex chromosomal abnormalities.

ABERRATIONS IN CHROMOSOME MORPHOLOGY

The mutagenic agents already discussed, as well as possible unknown influences, may damage the structure of individual chromosomes. Most often, these adverse influences cause chromosomal fractures. Certain loci on the chromosomes, known as "hot spots," tend to be affected, but it is evident from the wide-ranging patterns of abnormal chromosome morphology that no rules are strictly followed. Five principal types of structural anomaly are recognized: deletion, duplication, inversion, translocation and isochromosome formation.

Deletion. A deletion involves loss of a portion of a chromosome. A single break may result in loss or deletion of the terminal segment of an arm. Intermediate segments may be deleted when there are two interstitial breaks. The proximal and distal segments rejoin but usually the isolated intermediate fragment, lacking a centromere, does not survive. As a consequence, many genes are lost. Indeed, the residual chromosome may be so deficient in genetic information as to preclude survival of the affected cell. If both terminal portions (telomeres) of a chromosome are lost, the sticky broken ends (but not their telomeric fragments) may reunite to form a *ring chromosome*. A ring chromosome breaks again when the spindle fibers at the succeeding mitotic division pull it apart.

Duplication. Duplication arises when a deleted portion of a chromosome either persists as a fragment or attaches to another chromosome of the normal complement. The genetic information contained in the fragment is duplicated since it is already present in the normal complement. In general, duplications are less harmful than deletions.

Inversions. Inversions may occur when there are two breaks in a chromosome. The intermediate fragment may not be lost but may reunite in its original site although in the reverse direction. Thus, if the genetic material on one arm of a chromosome could be designated as A, B, C. D, an inversion of the middle segment of this arm would yield A, C, B, D. When the segment does not include the centromere, the inversion is referred to as paracentric while those involving the centromere are pericentric. Paracentric inversions rarely produce visible change in the morphology of the chromosome, but pericentric inversions are usually recognizable under the microscope.

Translocation. Translocation designates the exchange of chromosomal parts between two nonhomologous chromosomes. The chromosome number remains unchanged, and the morphology may remain apparently normal. On the other hand, unequal breakage of the centromere region may block replication of one of the new chromosomes or may inhibit proper attachment to the spindle fiber, resulting in loss of the chromosome in the next cell division.

Isochromosomes. Isochromosomes, in which both arms are identical in length and gene composition, result when there is an error in centromere division, i.e., the plane of division is transverse rather than longitudinal. Obviously, isochromosomes are metacentric. Chromosomes may lack centromeres (*acentrics*), have two centromeres (*dicentrics*) or even three (*tricentrics*). These highly aberrant forms are usually encountered in cells suffering radiation injury, and most are lethal.

It is necessary to introduce, at this point, some cytogenetic shorthand to characterize the wide range of karyotypic anomalies involving changes in number or morphology. A normal female is 46 XX and a normal male, 46 XY. Such designations indicate the number of chromosomes in the karyotype, followed by the sex chromosome constitution. A Klinefelter's constitution would be represented as 47 XXY. As Figure 6–6 indicates, mosaicism is described as 46 XY/47 XXY or as 46 XX/45 XO/47 XXX. The trisomy 21 of Down's syndrome in a girl would be indicated as 47 XX 21+ or G+, implying an extra 21(G group) autosome. The short arm of the chromosome is designated p (petit) and the long arm, q. A plus or minus sign following such designation implies added or deleted material of the respective arm. Thus, 46 XY Bp– designates a male with a deletion of one of the short arms of one of the B chromosomes. Less commonly used nomenclature can be found in the report from the Chicago conference on standardization in human cytogenetics (Chicago Conference, 1966). In concluding this discussion of chromosome mutations, it is hardly necessary to point out that gross genetic alterations which can be recognized microscopically of necessity involve many genes and, if viability has not been precluded, result in significant clinical disorders.

CLINICAL DISORDERS ARISING IN SEX CHROMOSOME MUTATIONS

Sex-linked inheritance differs in some important aspects from autosomal inheritance. In the female, the two equal X chromosomes behave as a pair of autosomes, and recessive sex-linked traits are expressed only when the individual is homozygous for the trait. In the male, recessive traits on the unpaired X are always expressed since there is no homologous segment carrying a normal dominant gene on the Y chromosome. Specifically, the following pertains to sex-linked recessive traits:

1. A father can transmit an abnormal trait to his daughters only. If the mother is normal, all daughters will be carriers and phenotypically normal.

2. A carrier mother transmits the abnormal trait to 50 per cent of her daughters who will also be carriers if the father is normal. However, 50 per cent of her sons will manifest the disorder.

3. An affected male must have received the abnormal trait from his mother.

4. A female carrier may have received the abnormal trait from either her father or her mother.

More is known about the genetic information borne by the X than by any other chromosome. Estimates have been made that the X chromosome bears some 2000 genes and about 60 phenotypic characteristics are known to be controlled by it, including those related to gamma globulin formation, blood coagulation and color blindness. The X chromosome also has some bearing on intelligence, but in a fashion not warmly appreciated by female geneticists. The presence of extra X chromosomes in either females or males is associated with reduced intelligence and, indeed, as will be seen, there is a correlation between the severity of the mental retardation and the extent of the polysomy X. Unravelling the mysteries of the X chromosome has been simplified by the hemizygous state of the male, permitting expression of both dominant and recessive X-linked traits.

The only specific assignation to the Y chromosome is the control of the not altogether unpleasant "hairy ears." This holandric inheritance is transferred directly from father to son. Obviously, the Y chromosome dictates male differentiation and so must possess loci controlling male sex development. However many extra X chromosomes the individual may possess in his cells, the presence of a single Y results in male differentiation; conversely, the absence of the Y leads to female development. Turner's (XO) syndrome is an intriguing problem. Although these individuals are monosomic for the X chromosome, they are nonetheless phenotypic females, albeit bearing some stigmata from lack of the second X chromosome. The normal male has only a single X chromosome, and yet has none of the clinical features of Turner's syndrome. The Y chromosome, therefore, must bear some genes which block the development of an XO syndrome.

For some time, it puzzled geneticists that males and females had equal quantities of enzymes controlled by X-linked genes. It would be logical to assume that with their two X chromosomes, females should exhibit a dosage effect as a consequence of having twice as many genes as the male. Such, of course, is not the case, and we now believe we understand why. *One of the X chromosomes in the female is inactivated.*

The elucidation of the mystery concerning the equal quantities of X-linked enzymes in both males and females was begun by Bertram and Barr in 1949 when they described a distinctive clump of chromatin present in the nuclei of the neurons of female cats, which was not present in males. This chromatin clump (about 1 millimicron in width), lying within the nucleus immediately adjacent to the nuclear membrane in human female somatic cells, has since been called the "*Barr body*" or *sex chromatin* (Fig. 6–7). The simplest method for demonstrating sex chromatin is the buccal smear test. By gently scraping the inside of the cheek, a sufficient number of epithelial cells can be denuded to prepare a smear which, after appropriate fixation, can be stained by any one of the standard techniques. In normal females, 20 to 50 per cent of the cells will exhibit the sex chromatin. It should be cautioned that rare cells in the male will have chromatin clumps simulating a Barr body, and so a positive sex chromatin test requires that it be present in approximately a quarter to one half of all cells examined. Another normal female marker is the "drumstick," a nuclear appendage present in about 5 per cent of neutrophils in females. Subsequently, the Barr body was shown to represent a heterochromatic or heteropyknotic X chromosome which was genetically inactive.

Based on these observations, Mary Lyon (1961*a*, 1961*b*) presented her now famous

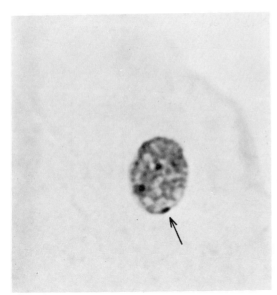

Figure 6-7. *Sex chromatin (Barr body) at 5 to 6 o'clock (arrow) in nucleus of squamous cell from buccal cavity. × 1200.*

"*Lyon hypothesis,*" proposing that such inactivation of one X chromosome occurs early in embryonic life (12th to 16th day) and is random among the many cells within the developing female embryo. By the law of averages, 50 per cent of the inactive X chromosomes would be derived from the father and 50 per cent, from the mother. The inactivation is irrevocable, and all progeny derived from this cell will maintain the same inactive X chromosome. In this way, all normal adults of both sexes have only a single dose of X-linked genes. Moreover, *all X chromosomes save one are inactivated and transformed into Barr bodies.* Thus, the XXX syndrome is characterized by two Barr bodies in somatic cells and the XXXX, by three. In this manner, compensation is achieved for extra X chromosomes. It follows that the XO karyotype of Turner's syndrome is characterized by a lack of sex chromatin in somatic cells.

The Lyon hypothesis carries some interesting implications. The female who is heterozygous for an X-linked trait has two different populations of cells. In some cells, the X chromosome carrying the mutant gene might be inactivated while, in other cells, the normal allele might be inactivated, permitting these cells to express their mutant gene. Consequently, if results of gene activity could be recognized only as normal or abnormal, female heterozygotes might show a mosaic comprising partial or occasional manifestation of the abnormality. The extent of phenotypic expression will depend on the proportion of cells with the abnormal genotype. A female heterozygote for X-linked traits may thus have a phenotype intermediate between that of the homozygous normal and the homozygous affected. Since the proportion of cells carrying the mutant gene varies from 0 to 100 per cent, a wide range of phenotypic expression is encountered (Francois, 1968) (Court-Brown, 1968).

If the Lyon hypothesis of the complete inactivation of one X chromosome in the normal female is correct, some mysteries remain. Why should individuals with an XO karyotype (Turner's syndrome) not be normal females? The parallel might be asked about the Klinefelter's syndrome (XXY): Why are they not normal males? The many efforts to explain these enigmas, although still somewhat unsatisfactory, propose that: (1) the second X chromosome exerts its effect prior to its inactivation early in embryonic life; (2) the process is not random and does not affect those cells involved in the phenotypic expression of Turner's syndrome and Klinefelter's syndrome; (3) inactivation is not total and segments of the involved X chromosome remain genetically active. The last possibility is the most appealing. Despite these problems, however, a large body of evidence supports the Lyon hypothesis.

The various disorders arising in aberrations of sex chromosomes are categorized in Table 6-5. Thereafter, each is described briefly.

KLINEFELTER'S SYNDROME

Also called testicular dysgenesis, Klinefelter's syndrome is one of the most common forms of genetic disease arising from aberrations in the sex chromosomes, as well as one of the most common forms of hypogonadism in the male. The incidence of this condition is estimated to be 1 in 500 live male births. Patients are usually eunuchoid with abnormally long legs, small atrophic testes, a small penis, gynecomastia (increase in breast size) and lack of such secondary male characteristics as deep voice, beard and pubic hair. Characteristic laboratory findings are (1) a positive sex chromatin test, (2) absence or striking reduction of sperm in the seminal fluid, (3) increased urinary excretion of the follicle-stimulating hormone and (4) lower than normal serum testosterone levels.

Klinefelter's syndrome has two important clinical significances: (1) It is an important cause of sterility in the male. and (2) it is associated with a slight decrease in intelligence. The reduced spermatogenesis is related to several patterns of

TABLE 6-5. DISORDERS ASSOCIATED WITH THE SEX CHROMOSOMES

Disorder	Karyotype	Chromatin Pattern	Approximate Incidence	Maternal Age	Clinical Signs
Klinefelter's syndrome with mosaicism	47,XXY 46,XY/47,XXY	+ +	1 in 500 male births	Slightly increased	1. Testicular atrophy and azoospermia 2. Increase in sole—os pubis length 3. Gynecomastia 4. Female distribution of hair 5. Mental retardation
Variants of Klinefelter's syndrome	48,XXXY 49,XXXXY 48,XXYY 49,XXXYY	++ +++ + ++	Rare	Increased	1. More severe mental retardation 2. Cryptorchidism 3. Hypospadias 4. Radio-ulnar synostosis
Gonadal dysgenesis (Turner's syndrome) defective second X chromosome	45,X 46,XXp— 46,XXq— 46,XXr 46,XXiq	Negative +(small) " +(large)	1 in 2000 female births	Normal Normal Normal Normal Normal	1. Short stature 2. Primary amenorrhea 3. Webbing of the neck 4. Cubitus valgus 5. Peripheral lymphedema 6. Broad chest and wide-spaced nipples 7. Low posterior hairline 8. Pigmented nevi 9. Coarctation of the aorta
Mosaicism	46,XX/45,X	Usually +		Normal	
Triple X females Variants	47,XXX 48,XXXX	++ +++	1 in 1000 female births Rare	Increased	1. Mental retardation 2. Menstrual irregularities 3. Many normal and fertile
Double Y males	47,XYY	Negative	Rare	Normal	1. Phenotypically normal 2. Most over 6 feet tall 3. "Increased aggressive behavior"
True hermaphrodites Most cases Some mosaics Rare case of double fertilization	46,XX 46,XX/47,XXY 46,XX/46XY	+ + +	Rare	Normal	1. Testicular and ovarian tissue 2. Varying genital abnormalities

morphologic change in the testis. In some patients, the testicular tubules are totally atrophied and are replaced by pink hyaline collagenous ghosts. In others, the dysgenesis is manifested by apparently normal tubules interspersed with atrophic tubules. In some patients, all tubules are primitive and embryonic-appearing, consisting of cords of cells which never developed a lumen or mature spermatogenesis. Hyperplasia of the Leydig cells is found in all of these variants.

The classic pattern of Klinefelter's syndrome has a 47 XXY karyotype, accounting for the positive sex chromatin test (Fig. 6–8). This complement has been explained by nondisjunction during the meiotic divisions in one of the parents and, in one recent study, it was shown that the extra X chromosome might be of either maternal or paternal origin (Race and Sanger, 1969). Advanced maternal age and irradiation of either parent have been suggested as relevant in the etiology of this condition (Ferguson-Smith, 1963). In addition to this classic karyotype, some cases of Klinefelter's syndrome have been found to have XXXY and XXXXY karyotypes as well as a variety of mosaic patterns including 46 XY/47 XXY, 47 XXY/48 XXXY and variations on this theme. With increasing numbers of X chromosomes,

patients exhibit a progressively greater reduction in intelligence. Concomitantly, such polysomic X individuals have further physical abnormalities including cryptorchidism, hypospadias, more severe hypoplasia of the testes and skeletal changes such as prognathism and radio-ulnar synostosis. Such severely affected individuals are likely to have had considerably older mothers.

TURNER'S SYNDROME OR GONADAL DYSGENESIS

Recently, this condition was more precisely defined as a disorder occurring in a female showing sexual infantilism, streak gonads, abnormally short stature and at least two of the following somatic anomalies: congenital webbed neck, cubitus valgus (an increase in carrying angle of the arm), shield-like chest with widely spaced nipples, coarctation of the aorta, webbing of the digits or of the axillae, senile facies, high-arched palate, low-set ears, peripheral lymphedema at birth, as well as other less frequent defects (Krmpotic et al., 1970). Turner's syndrome may be difficult to identify in young female children but, at puberty, they fail to develop normal secondary sex characteristics, the genitalia remain infantile, breast

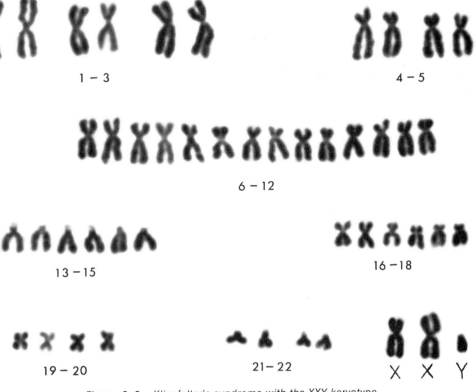

Figure 6–8. Klinefelter's syndrome with the XXY karyotype.

development is inadequate and little pubic hair develops. Primary amenorrhea characterizes many of these individuals. Morphologic examination of the ovaries shows that they are replaced by white "streaks" of fibrous stroma devoid of follicles. Many of the phenotypic characteristics are reflections of hypoestrinism. After puberty, the reduced levels of ovarian estrogens lead to elevated pituitary gonadotropin secretion. Mental retardation may be present in some patients, but it is usually not severe.

The classic karyotype of Turner's syndrome is 45 XO (Fig. 6–9). Approximately 60 per cent of patients have this typical karyotype and are, therefore, sex chromatin negative. Recent studies have confirmed that either the paternal or one of the maternal X chromosomes may be missing (De la Chapelle et al., 1964). It is the only recognized sex chromosome monosomy. To date, no YO syndrome has been found, presumably because it is incompatible with life.

Other cytogenetic variants of Turner's syndrome have been described, the most common of which is biclonal or triclonal mosaicism (e.g., 45 XO/46 XX, 45 XO/46 XX/47 XXX). Such patients are usually chromatin-positive

and range from those with a characteristic Turner's phenotype to those with an almost normal female phenotype. Some cases of phenotypic gonadal dysgenesis in females have been reported with a normal chromosome complement of 46 XX, or in males with a 46 XY karyotype. In these cases, it is presumed that one of the X chromosomes suffered a deletion. Turner's syndrome in males takes the form of abnormally short stature, webbed neck, congenital heart disease and mental retardation. The occasional cases with deletions of X chromosomes have provided important "experiments of nature" which have shed light on the location of genes in the X chromosome.

MULTI-X FEMALES

These facetiously dubbed "super females" may have trisomy X, tetrasomy X or pentasomy X karyotypes (Fig. 6–10). The most common variant is the triple X syndrome. The clinical features are quite variable. Some patients are fertile and have had normal children. Others have menstrual irregularity, amenorrhea or premature menopause (Johnston et al., 1961). Mental retardation is the common denominator among all of the karyo-

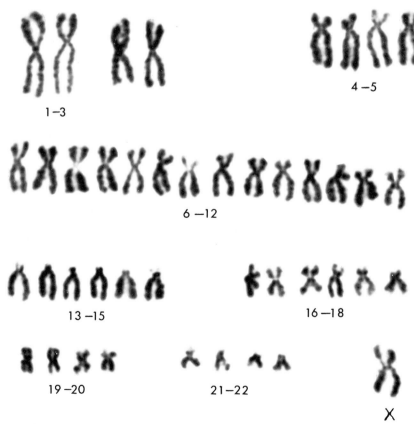

Figure 6–9. *Turner's syndrome with the XO karyotype.*

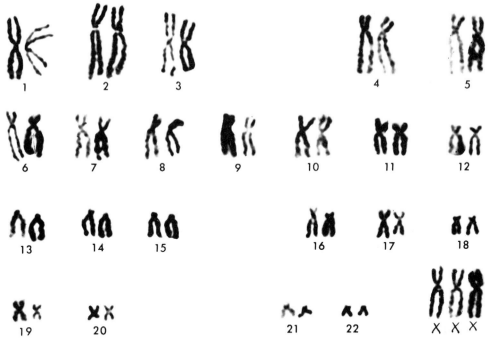

Figure 6–10. *So-called super female with XXX karyotype.*

types and, while this may be slight in the triple X individuals, it becomes progressively more marked the greater the number of X chromosomes. As would be anticipated in these polysomic X syndromes, somatic cells have multiple Barr bodies equal to one less than the number of X chromosomes.

XYY SYNDROME

Cytogenetic studies of males in maximum security prisons yielded the unexpected finding of an increased frequency of the XYY karyotype in 3 per cent of persons detained in the institution on account of their dangerously violent or criminal propensities (Jacobs et al., 1968). Furthermore, these males were found, on the average, to be about 6 inches taller than the XY males in the same institution. In men 6 feet or more in height, one in four had an XYY complement. It has been difficult to establish a baseline for the incidence of the XYY karyotype in the normal population. It is known that the XXY (Klinefelter's) syndrome has a frequency among live-born males of about 2 per 1000. It is argued that XYY males are not likely to be as common since an XXY zygote could be produced either at the first or second gametogenic division in the mother or at the first meiotic division in the father, while the error producing a YY sperm could occur only at the second mitotic division in the father. In a more direct study of random live-born male children, Court-Brown (1968) found only one instance of an XYY male in the examination of about 11,000 infants.

A question obviously arises: Is the extra Y chromosome related to the antisocial behavior of these imprisoned men? Possibly, these inmates represent a subgroup of a larger population with the XYY karyotype who may live normal lives undiscovered. Indeed, males with the XYY constitution have been identified who are neither overly aggressive nor antisocial. Fertility in XYY males appears unaffected and normal offspring result, seemingly because the second Y chromosome is selectively eliminated from spermatocytes in these patients. Variants of the XYY syndrome have been identified such as XXYY and XXXYY. These individuals have exhibited some of the features of Klinefelter's syndrome as well as aberrant behavior.

HERMAPHRODITISM

Disappointingly, karyotypic analyses have not shed much light on the difficult problems of intersex. The classification of these individuals into pseudohermaphrodites and true hermaphrodites is based on correlation of the male and female gonad with its respective karyotype. *Female pseudohermaphrodites* have immature ovaries, ambiguous external genitalia, are sex chromatin-positive and have a 46 XX karyotype. Masculinization in these patients has been attributed to adrenal hyperplasia with the elaboration of excessive quantities of androgens. *Male pseudohermaphrodites* have testes usually inguinal in location and their external genitalia and secondary sex characteristics are, to varying degrees, feminine. Most are sex chromatin-negative and have a normal male 46 XY karyotype. Recent evidence suggests that the disturbed male differentiation results from the excessive production of an antiandrogen, most probably 16-hydroxyprogesterone.

True hermaphrodites are rare and are cytogenic enigmas. The great majority of these patients are chromatin-positive and most have a 46 XX karyotype, yet these patients usually have both male and female gonads as well as mixed external genitalia. Some breast development is the rule and over half of these individuals menstruate and ovulate. The finding of testicular tissue in a hermaphrodite lacking a Y chromosome defies most genetic dogma. Some true hermaphrodites represent mosaics with a Y chromosome in one of the clonal lines, e.g., 46 XX/47 XXY. Even more intriguing are the rare cases of 46 XX/46 XY because here the mixed sexual development is matched by a female/male karyotype (Federman, 1967).

CLINICAL DISORDERS ARISING IN AUTOSOMAL MUTATIONS

Chromosomal mutations affecting the autosomes generally have devastating effects. It was previously pointed out that such aberrations are found in approximately 20 per cent of spontaneous abortuses. Those born alive represent the survival of the fittest, but even these, as will be seen, are severely handicapped. Autosomal mutations imply gross distortions of the genome, and phenotypic alterations accordingly affect many organs and systems. Only four syndromes are compatible with survival and these involve the G, E, D and B groups of chromosomes. Their major features are summarized in Table 6–6.

A vast array of autosomal mutations are also encountered in cancerous cells. Most of the evidence suggests that such mutations are late-occurring phenomena resulting from disturbances in intracellular growth controls which lead to shortened generation cycles and

TABLE 6–6. DISORDERS ASSOCIATED WITH THE AUTOSOMES

Disorder	Karyotype Examples	Approximate Incidence	Maternal Age	Clinical Signs in Newborns
Down's syndrome		1 in 600 births		1. Flat facial profile
Trisomy 21 type	47,XX,G+ or 47,XY,G+	Over 95% of cases	Increased	2. Muscle hypotonia 3. Hyperflexibility 4. Lack of Moro reflex 5. Abundant neck skin
Translocation type	46,XX,D-t(DqGq)+ 46,XY,G-t(GqGq)+	3–4% of cases	Normal	6. Dysplastic ears 7. Horizontal palmar crease 8. Dysplastic pelvis (by x-ray)
Mosaic type	46,XX/47,XX,G+	2–3% of cases	Normal	9. Dysplastic middle phalanx V (by x-ray) 10. Epicanthic folds
Edwards' syndrome Trisomy 18E	47,XX,E+ 47,XY,E+	1 in 5000 births	Increased	1. Mental retardation and failure to thrive 2. Prominent occiput 3. Micrognathia and low-set ears 4. Hypertonicity
Translocation type	46,XX,t(DqEq)+		Normal	5. Flexion of fingers (index over third) 6. Cardiac, renal and intestinal defects 7. Short sternum and small pelvis
Mosaic type	46,XX/47,XX,E+		Normal	8. Abduction deformity of hip
Patau's syndrome Trisomy 13D (arhinencephaly)	47,XX,D+ 47,XY,D+	1 in 6000 births Over 80% of cases	Increased	1. Microcephaly and mental retardation 2. Scalp defect 3. Microphthalmia 4. Harelip and cleft palate 5. Polydactyly
Translocation type	46,XX,D-t(DqDq)+	10% of cases	Normal	6. Rocker-bottom feet 7. Abnormal ears
Mosaic type	46,XX/47,XX,D+	5% of cases	Normal	8. Apneic spells and myoclonic seizures 9. Cardiac dextroposition and interventricular septal defect 10. Extensive visceral defects
"Le cri du chat" (Cat-cry) syndrome	46,XX,Bp– 46,XY,Bp–	Rare	Normal	1. Mental retardation 2. Microcephaly and round facies 3. Mewing cry 4. Epicanthic folds

frequent unregulated mitotic divisions. Most likely, the initiating events in the transformation of normal cells into cancer cells occur either at the gene level or are epigenetic, and so the karyotype is not intially affected. There is, in fact, a strong likelihood that the gross chromosomal mutations encountered in fully evolved cancer cells are lethal. For further details on this interesting problem, reference should be made to the earlier discussion (p. 139).

DOWN'S SYNDROME

This most common of all chromosomal disorders in man was known in years past as "mongolism" or "mongolian idiocy." It occurs in 1 in 600 live births and its incidence bears a strong relationship to maternal age. The incidence of Down's syndrome in offspring of women under 29 years of age is approximately 1 in 2000 and rises progressively to a 1 in 50 incidence for mothers over 45 years of age (Penrose, 1961).

The diagnosis of this unfortunate condition can usually be made on casual glance, based on the following anomalies: *short stature, flat occiput, flat facial profile, epicanthic folds, oblique palpebral fissures, protruding tongue, short broad hands with a single simian crease on the palm, short crooked fifth finger, hyperflexibility of joints and lack of Moro reflex. Mental retardation is severe* and approximately 80 per cent have an IQ of 25 to 50. Ironically, these severely disadvantaged children usually have a gentle, shy manner.

In a recent study, over 95 per cent of all cases of Down's syndrome had *trisomy 21 G* (Fig. 6–11). Although most of such identifications were not able to differentiate between 21 G and 22 G, the syndrome is accepted by convention as being a 21 G trisomy (Huang et al., 1967). With rare exception, the parents of such infants have normal karyotypes. However, a few women with Down's syndrome have reached adulthood and have had children, some with Down's syndrome and some completely normal (Finley et al., 1968). Approximately 2 per cent of "mongoloids" are mosaics (trisomy 21/normal). The phenotype of these mosaics depends upon how many cells are affected and may vary, therefore, from infants indistinguishable from the trisomy 21 to some that are virtually normal. Some of these pa-

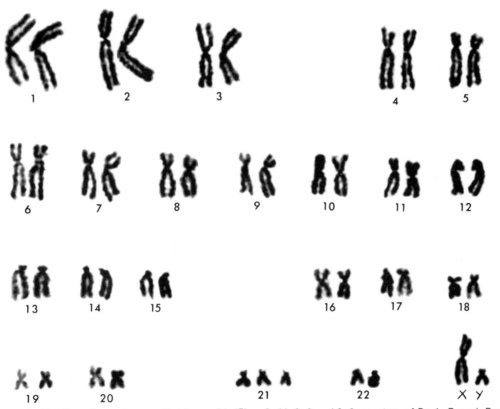

Figure 6–11. *Down's syndrome with trisomy 21. (Figs. 6–11, 6–8 and 6–9, courtesy of Dr. L. Razavi, Department of Bacteriology and Immunology, Harvard Medical School.)*

tients may have the Down's facies but normal intelligence (Carr, 1969). The third karyotypic variant consists of patients who have 46 chromosomes but who presumably have translocations of some material from 21 G or 22 G to another chromosome—almost always a member of group D or group G. This pattern is familial and is transmitted usually by the mother. The theoretical risk of a translocation carrier parent producing a child with Down's syndrome is one in three, but the actual risk calculated by Hamerton (1968) turns out about one in ten.

The outlook for these affected children is generally grim. About 40 per cent die in the first year of life and 60 per cent, within the first 10 years. However, with better care, increasing numbers are now reaching adult life and, as mentioned, some even have children. Their gentleness and unobtrusiveness, so often lacking in their normal siblings, make it possible to train many of these shy little people to perform quite admirably in life.

TRISOMY 18E — EDWARDS' SYNDROME

The congenital malformations in this condition are so numerous, severe, and wide-ranging that only 13 per cent of these infants live beyond the age of one year, and the mean age at death is little more than 10 weeks. The principal clinical features are severe mental retardation, cardiac defects (patent ductus arteriosus and interventricular septal defects), renal malformations, Meckel's diverticulum, micrognathia, low-set malformed ears, overlapping of the fingers (index with third finger) so that the middle finger is raised in a beckoning gesture, short sternum, small pelvis, abnormalities of the hips and feet and generalized muscular hypertonicity. Gross brain anomalies are common, especially absence of the corpus callosum and incomplete development of the cerebellum (Edwards et al., 1960).

The incidence of this anomaly is in the order of 1 in 5000 live births with a female/male ratio of 3 : 1. As in Down's syndrome, maternal age appears to be of etiologic significance, but most parents are normal and so presumably the chromosomal aberration arises in gametogenesis. Rare cases show mosaicism and translocations. In the latter instance, the disease may be familial.

TRISOMY 13D — PATAU'S SYNDROME

Infants born with Trisomy 13D are the most severely affected of all those with chromosomal abnormalities (Fig. 6–12). The peri-natal mortality is high and the mean survival is about 10 weeks. Slightly more than 10 per cent live longer than one year. Mental retardation is severe and many of these infants are thought by some to have arhinencephaly (congenital absence of those regions of the forebrain ontogenetically derived from the olfactory system). Other features include scalp defects, coloboma of the iris, microphthalmos, anophthalmos, cleft palate, hair lip, polydactyly and hemangiomas of the head, neck and lower back. Most of these patients have a regular trisomy D (47 XXD+), and again there is some relationship to the age of the mother at time of birth. Unlike trisomy 18, in trisomy 13 there is no female sex preponderance. Occasional patients have a normal 46 chromosome complement but represent translocations transmitted by carrier parents. Rare mosaics have been identified (Magenis et al., 1968).

"CRI du CHAT" (CAT-CRY) SYNDROME

The autosomal abnormality in this disorder consists of deletion of material from the short arm of a chromosome in group B. The syndrome derives its name from the characteristic mewing cry of these infants. In addition, these children have mental retardation which is severe, often accompanied by microcephaly, round facies, widely spaced eyes, low-set ears, epicanthic folds, hypertelorism, divergent strabismus and congenital heart anomalies (usually ventricular septal defect) in 25 per cent. Females are affected slightly more often than males. In general, these children thrive better than those with the trisomies, and some survive into adult life. As the infant grows older, the kitten cry and high vocal register improve, rendering the diagnosis more difficult.

Other deletion syndromes involving chromosomes 18, 13, 15 and 4 have been identified. A variety of congenital malformations are encountered in these deletion syndromes, including anomalies of the brain and mental retardation, microcephaly, hypertelorism, congenital heart disease and malformations of the face, hands and ears.

GENE MUTATIONS

The concept that a disease might be due to a hereditary deficiency of a specific enzyme dates back to the classic work of Garrod (1909). He astutely deduced that alkaptonuria, with its excessive excretion of homogentisic acid, was the consequence of some enzymic lack which blocked the further degradation of homogentisic acid, one of the metabolites of phenylala-

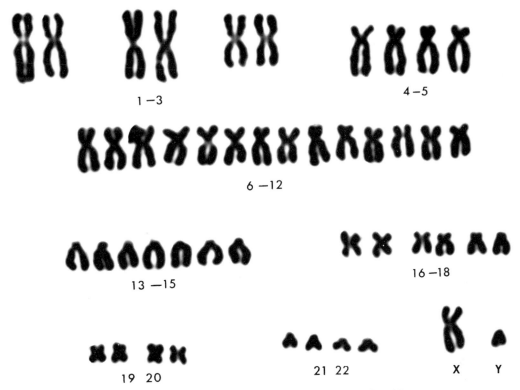

1–3

4–5

6–12

13–15

16–18

19 20

21 22

X Y

Figure 6–12. *Trisomy D with trisomy of group 13 to 15.*

nine and tyrosine. He further noted a characteristic familial distribution of these patients and, in consultation with a geneticist, Bateson, proposed that the defect was determined by a rare recessive "mendelian factor" which we now call a gene. So was born the important category of "inborn errors of metabolism" long before the science of cytogenetics had been developed.

The postulation that the hereditary deficiency of a specific enzyme might be caused by some abnormal "mendelian factor" set the stage for the "one gene one enzyme" theory of Beadle and Tatum (1941). In actual fact, while one gene may code for an entire enzyme, there is an increasing body of evidence that a single gene may control only a peptide chain comprising just a portion of a total protein (Hood, 1972). Soon thereafter, it was discovered that the gene mutation might be as subtle as the substitution of one base in the DNA code, leading to the synthesis of an abnormal protein or enzyme or, in some cases, to blocking of the normal synthesis of protein. As is now well known, the substitution of a single base in a triplet code for an amino acid may: (1) lead to no alteration in the structure of the protein since, as was pointed out on p. 172, several triplets may code for the same amino acid; (2)

result in the synthesis of an altered protein; or (3) code for polypeptide chain termination.

The range of gene mutations and phenotypic variations that have been identified boggles the mind (Harris, 1970). Over 100 variations of hemoglobin have been identified. The great majority differ from normal hemoglobin A by only a single amino acid, and each of these can be accounted for by a single substitution of a base within DNA. Some of these hemoglobin variants appear to be relatively harmless, but some may be as disastrous as hemoglobin S, causing sickle cell disease. Replacement of glutamic acid by valine in one of the peptides of the beta chain of hemoglobin results in hemoglobin S. This occurs when uracil is substituted for adenine in one triplet code of DNA in the gene controlling beta chain synthesis (Ingram, 1956). Here then is a common, frequently fatal disease arising from a single change in the base sequence of DNA.

The genetic heterogeneity underlying the "altered protein syndromes" and the inborn errors of metabolism is undoubtedly more extensive than the number of disorders identified. A particular metabolic disorder with a deficiency of an enzyme may be attributable to different abnormal genes, each causing the enzyme defect in its own characteristic manner.

At the most simplistic level of the operon, the structural or the operator or regulator gene might be affected, all impairing synthesis of a single product. Many enzymes are involved in a single metabolic pathway, and loss of any one of them could lead to the same apparent disorder of metabolism. The mutation might lead to a total enzyme lack by blocking synthesis. Alternatively, the mutation might lead to the synthesis of a structurally altered enzyme whose catalytic properties are not necessarily altered but whose inherent stability is reduced because its three-dimensional configuration is modified. Such an enzyme would have a curtailed half-life which constitutes an enzyme deficiency. Thus, many mutations can result in a deficiency of a specific enzyme, and many enzyme deficiencies may impinge on a single metabolic pathway to evoke a single disease. The number of genetic diseases recognized probably gives no real concept of the magnitude of the underlying genetic heterogeneity.

A few of the more common disorders will be briefly mentioned merely to indicate the nature and range of the conditions arising out of sex-linked and autosomal gene mutations. All are discussed in greater detail elsewhere.

CLINICAL DISORDERS ARISING IN SEX-LINKED GENE MUTATIONS

To date, no important disorders have been identified as being transmitted by sex-linked, dominant genes, but two—hemophilia and an anemia due to a deficiency of glucose-6-phosphate dehydrogenase in red cells—arise in recessive sex-linked inheritance. The hemizygous male always expresses such X-linked recessive genes but usually the female must be homozygous for the trait. On this account, these two disorders are encountered predominantly in males. On the basis of the Lyon hypothesis and because the normal dominant gene may be inactivated in the female, heterozygous recessive traits are sometimes expressed in the female, who is referred to as a "manifesting heterozygote."

HEMOPHILIA

Hemophilia (p. 743) is a hemorrhagic diathesis characterized by an abnormal tendency to bleed either spontaneously or following trauma, however slight. Queen Victoria propagated the most famous pedigree of hemophilia: she was heterozygous for this trait and expressed no bleeding tendency but transmitted it to nine titled male "bleeders." Hemophilia, in fact, is composed of two separate disorders, each transmitted as an X-linked recessive trait inducing a deficiency of a specific plasma-clotting factor. In one, there is a lack of antihemophilic globulin (factor VIII) while in the other, Christmas Factor (factor IX) is lacking. On rare occasion, either of these syndromes appears in a woman usually as a consequence of the mating of a heterozygous mother and a "bleeder" father. In the past, "bleeder" women were less frequently seen because most hemophilic males then died at an early age. Today, replacement of the missing clotting factor effectively controls the disease and permits these individuals to survive into adult life and have children.

Other plasma clotting factor deficiencies may occur as the consequence of a gene mutation. All of these, however, are inherited as autosomal recessive traits, with the exception of factor XII for which both X-linked and autosomal modes of transmission have been identified.

GLUCOSE-6-PHOSPHATE DEHYDROGENASE (G6PD) DEFICIENCY

Glucose-6-phosphate dehydrogenase (G6PD) deficiency is inherited as an X-linked recessive disorder. The lack of this enzyme in red cells predisposes them to hemolysis, often causing a severe anemia. Two major hereditary patterns of G6PD deficiency have been described. One occurs predominantly in whites in whom the anemia appears spontaneously. This disease is usually mild (p. 714). The other variant occurs predominantly in blacks but may be found in almost all ethnic groups. In this form of the disease, the hemolytic crises are usually triggered by the ingestion of drugs including aspirin, antibiotics and antimalarial agents. The resulting anemia may be quite severe, but removal of the offending drug stops the abnormal hemolysis. Other more rare variants of G6PD deficiency have also been described (World Health Organization Scientific Group, 1967).

CLINICAL DISORDERS ARISING IN AUTOSOME GENE MUTATIONS

No system in the body escapes the effects of mutation of autosomal genes. With rare exception, the mode of transmission is recessive. It would be fruitless to attempt to list all of these disorders, but a few large categories will be discussed briefly.

HEMOGLOBINOPATHIES

The hemoglobinopathies comprise a significant group of red cell diseases in which the

TABLE 6-7. GENETICALLY DETERMINED ENZYME DEFICIENCIES

Condition	Enzyme	Date of Discovery
Hypophosphatasia	Alkaline phosphatase	1948
Glycogen-storage disease I	Glucose-6-phosphatase	1952
Acatalasia	Catalase	1952
Phenylketonuria	Phenylalanine hydroxylase	1953
Galactosemia	Galactose-1-phosphate uridyl transferase	1956
Hemolytic anemia	Glucose-6-phosphate dehydrogenase	1956
Goitrous cretinism	Deiodinase	1956
Glycogen-storage disease III	Amylo-1,6-glucosidase (debrancher)	1957
Familial nonhemolytic jaundice	Glucuronyl transferase	1957
Adrenogenital syndrome	21 hydroxylase	1958
Alkaptonuria	Homogentisic acid oxidase	1958
Glycogen-storage disease VI	Phosphorylase (liver)	1959
Glycogen-storage disease V	Phosphorylase (muscle)	1959
Methemoglobinemia	NAD diaphorase	1959
Hemolytic anemia	Pyruvate kinase	1961
Orotic aciduria	Orotodine 5'-phosphate pyrophosphorylase Orotodine 5'-phosphate decarboxylase	1961
Fructose intolerance	Fructose-1-phosphate aldolase	1961
Histidinemia	Histidase	1962
Fructosuria	Fructokinase	1962
Hyperammonemia	Ornithine transcarbamylase	1962
Apnea	Pseudocholinesterase	1962
Hemolytic anemia	Glutathione reductase	1963
Glycogen-storage disease II	Alpha-1,4-glucosidase	1963
Maple-syrup-urine disease	Branched-chain ketoacid decarboxylase	1963
No disease	6-phosphate-gluconate dehydrogenase	1964
Xanthinuria	Xanthine oxidase	1964
Homocystinuria	Cystathionine synthetase	1964
Argininosuccinicaciduria	Argininosuccinase	1964
Citrullinuria	Argininosuccinic acid synthetase	1964
Hemolytic anemia	Triose-phosphate-isomerase	1965
Hemolytic anemia	2,3-diphosphoglycerate mutase	1965
Hemolytic anemia	Glutathione synthetase	1965
Glycogen-storage disease	6-phosphofructokinase	1965
Hydroxyprolinemia	Hydroxyproline oxidase	1965
Hyperprolinemia	Proline oxidase	1965
Metachromatic leukodystrophy	Aryl sulfatase	1965
Cystathioninuria	Cystathioninase	1965
Tyrosinemia	P-hydroxyphenylpyruvic acid oxidase	1965
Niemann-Pick disease	Sphingomyelin cleaving enzyme	1966
Isovaleric acidemia	Isovaleric acid CoA dehydrogenase	1966
Gaucher's disease	Glucocerebrosidase	1966
Glycogen-storage disease IV	Amylo 1, 4 ⟶ 1, 6 transglucosidase (brancher)	1966
Hypervalinemia	Valine transaminase	1967
Hemolytic anemia	Hexokinase	1967
Hyperuricemia	Hypoxanthine-guanine phosphoribosyl transferase	1967
Cataract	Galactokinase	1967
Hyperoxaluria	2-oxo-glutarate glyoxalate carboligase	1967
Fabry's disease	Ceramide trihexoseidase	1967
Central-nervous-system disease with cataracts	Sulfite oxidase	1967
No disease	NADP methemoglobin reductase	1967
Refsum's disease	Phytanic acid hydroxylating enzyme	1967
No disease	Erythrocyte NAD-ase	1968
Hemolytic anemia	Glutathione peroxidase	1968
L-glyceric aciduria	D-glyceric dehydrogenase	1968
Hemolytic anemia	Glucose phosphate isomerase	1968
No disease	Adenine phosphoribosyl transferase	1968
Generalized gangliosidosis	Beta-galactosidase	1968

From Childs, B., and Der Kaloustian, V. M.: Genetic heterogeneity. New Eng. J. Med., *279*:1205, 1267, 1968.

synthesis of an abnormal hemoglobin or impairment of hemoglobin production leads to significant and sometimes fatal anemias. The two most important prototypes are sickle cell disease and thalassemia. Both represent recessive traits in which the homozygote has the full-blown disease while the heterozygote expresses hematologic abnormalities usually without significant anemia.

DISORDERS OF THE IMMUNE SYSTEM

Disorders of the immune system may be inherited as recessive traits. They range from those affecting only immunoglobulin synthesis (sometimes only one class of immunoglobulin) to those principally affecting delayed hypersensitivity. Rarely, profound immune anomalies occur in which the patient appears to lack the capacity both to elaborate antibodies and to mount a cell-based immune response. More is said about these disorders on p. 215.

INBORN ERRORS OF METABOLISM

Inborn errors of metabolism, based usually on a deficiency of a specific enzyme, are perhaps the most important category of genetic diseases related to a mutant autosomal gene. Table 6–7, taken from the report of Childs and Der Kaloustian (1968) offers only a partial list of these "missing enzyme" diseases.

It is interesting to note in Table 6–7 the date of discovery of the various metabolic diseases. In the 1950's they were being uncovered at the rate of one or two a year. In the 1960's the number jumped to six to nine per year, and there is no end in sight. None of these disorders can be said to be common, but some are gravely important. Certain diseases such as the glycogenoses, lipidoses and mucopolysaccharidoses (p. 295) are almost always fatal. Galactosemia and phenylketonuria are also often fatal but, when recognized early, can be effectively controlled by diet, in most instances, preventing the development of progressive mental impairment and sparing the life of the child.

Genetic causation is found among the disorders of the skin (such as xeroderma pigmentosum), the skeletal system (such as multiple cartilaginous exostoses), the central nervous system (such as Huntington's chorea) and the vascular system (such as Ehlers-Danlos syndrome). The list could be extended for a great length. Certain neoplastic conditions such as hereditary multiple polyposis of the colon (p. 965) and retinoblastomas (p. 1319) comprise additional genetic disorders, in these instances, having autosomal dominant modes of inheritance.

Perhaps it is more accurate to conclude that, with a limited number of exceptions as was mentioned in the beginning of this chapter, all diseases have some genetic input. With all, the phenotype as expressed by the genome provides the soil on which the environment operates. The present consideration has cited only some of those in which nature plays a larger role than nurture.

REFERENCES

Beadle, G. W., and Tatum, E. L.: Genetic control of biochemical reactions in neurospora. Proc. Nat. Acad. Sci., 2:499, 1941.

Beale, G. H.: The role of the cytoplasm in heredity. In Bittar, E. E., and Bittar, N. (eds.): The Biological Basis of Medicine. Vol. 4. London and New York, Academic Press, 1969, p. 81.

Bertram, L. M., and Barr, E. G.: A morphologic distinction between the neurons of the male and female cat and the behavior of the nucleolar satellite during accelerated nuclear protein synthesis. Nature (London), 163:676, 1949.

Bloom, A. D.: Cytogenetics of the in utero exposed of Hiroshima and Nagasaki. Lancet, 2:10, 1968.

Bloom, A. D., et al.: Chromosome aberrations in leukocytes of older survivors of the atomic bombings of Hiroshima and Nagasaki, Lancet, 2:802, 1967.

Brock, J. F.: Nature, nurture and stress in health and disease. Lancet, 1:701, 1972.

Buckton, K. E., et al.: A study of the chromosome damage persisting after X-ray therapy for ankylosing spondylitis. Lancet, 2:676, 1962.

Carr, D. H.: Chromosomal errors and development. Amer. J. Obstet. Gynecol., 104:327, 1969.

Carter, C. O.: Genetics of common disorders. Brit. Med. Bull., 25:52, 1969.

Carter, C. O.: Genetics today. Public Health, 82:199, 1968.

Chicago Conference: Standardization in human cytogenetics. Birth Defects (Original Article Series II). New York, The National Foundation, 1966, p. 2.

Childs, B., and Der Kaloustian, V. M.: Genetic heterogeneity. New Eng. J. Med., 279:1205, 1267, 1968.

Cohen, M. M., et al.: In vivo and in vitro chromosomal damage induced by LSD-25. New Eng. J. Med., 227:1043, 1967.

Court-Brown, W. M.: Human population cytogenetics. In Newberger, A., and Tatum, E. L. (eds.): Frontiers of Biology. Vol. 5. Amsterdam, North Holland Publishing Co., 1967.

Court-Brown, W. M.: The study of human sex chromosome abnormalities with particular reference to intelligence and behaviour. Advance. Sci., 24:390, 1968.

De la Chapelle, A., et al.: Successive nondisjunction at first and second meiotic division of spermatogenesis: evidence of chromosomes and Xg. Cytogenetics, 3:334, 1964.

Dishotsky, N. I., et al.: LSD and genetic damage. Science, 172:431, 1971.

Edwards, J. H., et al.: A new trisomic syndrome. Lancet, 1:787, 1960.

Federman, D. D.: Abnormal Sexual Development. A Genetic and Endocrine Approach to Differential Diagnosis. Philadelphia, W. B. Saunders Co., 1967.

Ferguson-Smith, M. A.: Chromosome studies in Klinefelter's syndrome. Proc. Roy. Soc. Med., 56:577, 1963.

Finley, W. H., et al.: Down's syndrome in mother and child. Obstet. Gynec., 32:200, 1968.

Francois, J.: Basic principles of genetics. Int. Ophthal. Clin., 8:773, 1968.

Garrod, A. E.: Inborn Errors of Metabolism. London, Oxford University Press, 1909.

Gibor, A., and Granick, S.: Plastids and mitochondria: inheritable systems. In Levine, L. (ed.): Papers on Genetics. St. Louis, C. V. Mosby, 1971, p. 228.

Green, E. L.: Genetic effects of radiation on mammalian populations. Ann. Rev. Genet., 2:87, 1968.

Gregor, A. S.: Charles Darwin. London, Angus and Robertson, 1967.

Gripenberg, U.: Chromosome studies in some virus infections. Hereditas, 54:1, 1965.

Hamerton, J. L.: Robertsonian translocations in man: evidence for prezygotic selection. Cytogenetics, 7:260, 1968.

Harris, H.: Enzyme polymorphisms in man. Proc. Roy. Soc. Med., 164:298, 1966.

Harris, H.: Genetical theory and the "inborn errors of metabolism." Brit. Med. J., 1:321, 1970.

Hood, L. E.: Two genes, one polypeptide chain: fact or fiction? Fed. Proc., 31:177, 1972.

Hsia, D. Y.-Y.: Human Developmental Genetics. Chicago, Year Book Medical Publishers, 1968, p. 377.

Huang, S.-W., et al.: A cytogenetic study of 77 Chinese children with Down's syndrome. J. Ment. Defic. Res., 11:147, 1967.

Ingram, V. M.: A specific chemical difference between the globins of normal and sickle cell anemia hemoglobin. Nature, 178:792, 1956.

Irwin, S., and Egozcue, J.: Chromosomal abnormalities in leukocytes from LSD-25 users. Science, 157:313, 1967.

Jacobs, P. A., et al.: Chromosome studies on men in a maximum security hospital. Ann. Hum. Genet., 31:339, 1968.

Jensen, M. K.: Chromosome studies in patients treated with azothiaprine and amethopterin. Acta Med. Scand., 182:445, 1967.

Johnston, A. W., et al.: The triple X syndrome. Clinical, pathological and chromosomal studies in three mentally retarded cases. Brit. Med. J., 2:1046, 1961.

Kirk, J. T. O., and Tilney-Bassett, R. A. E.: The Plastids. London and San Francisco, Freeman, 1967.

Krmpotic, E., et al.: Sex chromosome abnormalities. Chicago Med. Sch. Quart., 29:99, 1970.

Lewontin, R. C.: An estimate of average heterozygosity in man. Amer. J. Hum. Genet., 19:681, 1967.

Lyon, M. F.: Gene action in the X chromosome of the mouse (Musculus L.). Nature, 190:372, 1961a.

Lyon, M. F.: Genetic factors on the X chromosome. Lancet, 2:434, 1961b.

Magenis, R. E., et al.: Trisomy 13 (D_1) syndrome: studies on parental age, sex ratio and survival. J. Pediat., 73:222, 1968.

McKusick, V. A.: Mendelian Inheritance in Man. 2nd ed. Baltimore, Johns Hopkins Press, 1968.

McKusick, V. A., and Milch, R. A.: The clinical behavior of genetic disease, selected aspects. Clin. Orthop., 33:22, 1964.

Monod, J., and Jacob, F.: General conclusions: teleonomic mechanisms in cellular metabolism, growth and differentiation. Sympos. Quant. Biol., 26:389, 1961.

Nichols, W. W.: Studies on the role of viruses in somatic mutation. Hereditas, 55:1, 1966.

Penrose, L. S.: Mongolism. Brit. Med. Bull., 17:184, 1961.

Ptashne, M., and Gilbert, W.: Genetic repressors. Sci. Amer., 222: June, 36, 1970.

Race, R. R., and Sanger, R.: Xg and sex chromosome abnormalities. Brit. Med. Bull., 25:99, 1969.

Ryser, H. J. P.: Chemical carcinogenesis. New Eng. J. Med., 285:721, 1971.

Stich, H. F., and Yohn, D. S.: Mutagenic capacity of adenoviruses for mamalian cells. Nature, 216:1292, 1967.

Tjio, J. H., and Levan, A.: The chromosome number of man. Hereditas, 42:1, 1956.

Watson, J. D.: Molecular Biology of the Gene. New York, W. A. Benjamin, 1965.

Watson, J. D., and Crick, F. H. C.: Molecular structure of nucleic acids. Nature, 171:737, 1953.

World Health Organization Scientific Group: Standardization of procedures for the study of glucose-6-phosphate dehydrogenase. W.H.O. Techn. Rep. Ser., 366:1, 1967.

World Health Organization: Five years of research on human genetics. W.H.O. Chron., 24:248, 1970.

Yamazaki, J. N., et al.: Outcome of pregnancy in women exposed to the atomic bomb in Nagasaki. Amer. J. Dis. Child., 87:448, 1954.

7

DISEASES OF IMMUNITY

Man's ability to mount an immune response is a two-edged sword. While immunologic competence is vital for survival in the sometimes hostile microbiologic environment, immune reactions may cause fatal disease as in the case of an overwhelming hypersensitivity reaction to the sting of a bee. Indeed, a host of disorders known collectively as the autoimmune diseases are thought to result from the abnormal emergence of immunity against one's own tissues and cells. The present chapter is devoted to a review of some of the fundamentals of the immune system followed by a consideration of its role in the production of disease.

IMMUNE SYSTEM

A recent W.H.O. report defines immunity: "The immune response comprises all the phenomena that result from the specific interaction of cells of the immune system with antigen. As a consequence of such interaction cells appear that mediate cellular immune responses (such as delayed sensitivity, or homograft immunity) as well as cells that synthesize and secrete one of several classes of immunoglobulins." (W.H.O. Scientific Group Report, 1970). Implicit in this statement is the now well established concept that the immune response of man involves two separate but interdependent mechanisms. One type, instigated by antigen-sensitive lymphocytes, is known as cell-mediated immunity or delayed-type hypersensitivity. This form of immunity is responsible for the rejection of foreign cells, and resistance to many viral and fungal infections. Circulating humoral antibody is not involved and the immune reaction is effected by mononuclear cells, some of which are immunologically competent lymphocytes. The other pattern is best

194

known as humoral immunity. It depends upon the synthesis of antibodies by plasma cells in response to some antigenic challenge. These antibodies are secreted into the circulation and extracellular fluids, and combine with the particular antigen wherever it is found. Because the humoral immunologic response usually manifests itself more promptly, following antigenic challenge of a sensitive animal, this reaction is also known as immediate-type immunity.

The major cellular component of both the immediate and the delayed types of immune response are lymphocytes. In the immediate-humoral reaction the lymphocytes, on antigenic challenge, become transformed, through a sequence to be detailed later, into plasma cells, the ultimate source of immunoglobulins. In the delayed response, the effector lymphocytes are transiently morphologically altered but revert to small lymphocytes. However, they are immunologically modified, as will be seen by the development of sensitivity to specific antigens. If antibodies are produced, they are closely bound to these lymphocytes and are thus termed cytophilic. Thus the lymphoid tissues of the body, including the circulating lymphocytes, spleen and bone marrow and especially the thymus, are the major structural components of the immune system. Two populations of lymphocytes are found within these anatomic sites as well as in the circulating blood. A third population, not involved in the immune response but involved in nonspecific inflammations, may also exist. This third family of lymphocytes is not well established and need not concern us further in this consideration. Of the two types of immunologically competent lymphocytes, those concerned with the cell-mediated reaction are dependent on the thymus for their function, while those involved in the plasma cell-humoral antibody system are thymus-independent. However, in certain immune reactions, cooperation must occur between the two populations and the two systems.

ONTOGENY OF THE IMMUNE SYSTEM

There is now general agreement that, in the individual, the entire immune system has its origin in primitive marrow stem cells of mesenchymal origin. These stem cells are multipotential and give rise to all the formed blood elements, i.e., erythrocytes, granulocytes, megakaryocytes as well as lymphoid cells. Their variable differentiation presumably reflects the action of local inducers in the sites colonized by the stem cells. Stem cells are first recognized in the blood islands of the yolk sac and then in the fetal liver and bone marrow. During the last half of embryogenesis, these cells colonize the rudimentary thymus. Here they divide and differentiate into lymphocytes, thus producing a well developed thymic cortex. In fowl, the bursa of Fabricius also appears during the last half of embryogenesis. Like the thymus, it is colonized originally by stem cells of marrow origin. In these animals, lymphocytes formed in the bursa migrate to the lymph nodes and spleen. *Thus, the thymus and bursa of Fabricius are known as primary or central lymphoid organs* (Craddock et al., 1971). Lymphocyte production, independent of antigens, occurs throughout life in these organs. Perhaps the bone marrow, although not prominent in lymphocyte production in man, should be considered also as a primary lymphoid organ since it is a continuing source of stem cells throughout life. At about the time of birth, there is seeding of cells from the thymus and the bursa of Fabricius to the secondary lymphoid organs (the lymph nodes and spleen).

The lymph nodes and spleen then comprise secondary or peripheral lymphoid organs. They develop later in fetal life and are colonized by two populations of lymphocytes, one thymus-dependent and a second thymus-independent. In fowl this second population is generated in the bursa of Fabricius. There is some evidence that in man the lymphoid tissues of the gut comprise the analogue of the bursa of Fabricius, and that cells generated in the gut lymphoid structures eventually colonize the spleen and lymph nodes. Although the evidence is still fragmentary, it is proposed that marrow stem cells migrate to bursa-equivalent tissue and then return to the marrow briefly before they eventually colonize. However, the evidence for such a sequence is still uncertain in man and it is generally proposed that stem cells migrate directly to the secondary lymphoid organs such as the lymph nodes and spleen (Nossal, 1969).

DUALITY OF THE IMMUNE SYSTEM

The lymph nodes and spleen are compound structures made up of cells under thymic control, known as T-lymphocytes, as well as cells from the marrow (bursa-equivalent), known as B-lymphocytes (Miller et al., 1967) (Balner and Dersjant, 1964). Within the secondary lymphoid organs, the two lymphocyte populations have fairly specific anatomic locations. The T-lymphocytes are found principally in the subcortical and paracortical areas of the lymph nodes and periarteriolar lympho-cytic sheaths of the spleen (Parrott et al., 1966). The bursa-equivalent system of B-lymphocytes is found principally in the cortex about the lymphoid follicles of the nodes and spleen but also diffusely throughout the marrow (Roitt et al., 1969). Thus, one can characterize the development of the immune system as a stream of cells which flow from the bone marrow; some either go through the thymus or are in some way modified by it before they go to peripheral lymph nodes and spleen, while others migrate from the marrow to bursa-equivalent tissue and then back to the marrow before they reach the peripheral lymphoid organs. This flow of cells probably continues throughout life (Moore and Owen, 1967).

Whether T-lymphocytes must physically pass through the thymus on their way to secondary lymphoid organs is a matter of some dispute. On the one hand, it has been reported that lymphocytes labeled locally in the thymus can later be identified in the "thymus dependent" areas of secondary lymphoid organs (Weissman, 1967). Metcalf (1966) on the other hand, has proposed that thymus-dependent lymphocytes do not of necessity require temporary residence in the thymus gland itself. He has isolated from calf thymus a humoral factor termed thymosin which is capable of reversing the immunologic deficit produced by thymectomy in newborn mice. Furthermore, implantation of thymic tissue within a millipore chamber in the peritoneal cavity of an animal corrects, to a large extent, the immunologic impairment produced by thymectomy in mice. Since cells can neither enter nor leave such a chamber, one must conclude that a circulating factor was elaborated which was capable, to a considerable extent, of substituting for normally situated thymic tissue. Thus the term "thymus-dependent" may not necessarily be synonymous with thymus-derived.

Much evidence in both animals and man supports the dual conception of the immune system. In animals, thymectomy at birth depresses the cell-mediated immune response but has no effect on immunoglobulin production. Thymectomy shortly after birth or in the adult animal has little effect at first, causing only a small drop in the peripheral lymphocyte count and some minimal temporary impairment of the cell-mediated immune mechanism. Presumably, by this time, the secondary lymphoid organs have been established and so there is less dependence on the thymus. However, in time, perhaps a year in the rat, these animals too become T-cell deprived. Removal of the bursa in chickens in ovo is followed by the depletion of the follicles of secondary lymphoid organs and complete inability to synthesize immunoglobulins. Recently, Percy et al. (1970) attempted the removal of all gut-associated lymphoid tissues such as the appendix and Peyer's patches from the rabbit. He found depression of the humoral antibody response and depletion of B-lymphocyte areas of the secondary lymphoid organs. The entire immunologic competence of an animal can be destroyed by total body radiation which is capable of ablating all lymphoid cells within the thymus, gut and secondary lymphoid organs. Such animals, if they survive the irradiation, develop a fatal wasting disease (runt disease) characterized by weight loss, weakness and diarrhea. It is thought to be due to their inability to resist infection since, when such animals are maintained in a germ-free environment, "runting" does not develop (McIntire et al., 1964). Immunologic competence can be restored by infusion of syngeneic stem cells from a normal donor.

A variety of immunologic deficiency syndromes in man have been identified that strongly support the duality of the immune system (Seligmann et al., 1968b). Infants may have severe deficiencies of both cell-mediated and humoral antibody responses. Presumably, the congenital derangement occurred early in embryogenesis, affecting the stem cell derivation of both arms of the immune system. DiGeorge's syndrome is characterized by the absence of the thymus and is associated with deficient cell-mediated immunity. These individuals are, however, capable of normal immunoglobulin synthesis and have no impairment of humoral antibody production. Transplantation of fetal thymic tissue restores their immunocompetence (Cleveland et al., 1968). Conversely, another disease is characterized by an absence of plasma cells throughout the lymphoid structures and an inability to synthesize humoral antibodies—the Bruton-type agammaglobulinemia (Bruton, 1952). Yet, in this syndrome, cell-mediated immunity is normal. Quite recently it was shown that grafting of marrow from histocompatible immunologically competent donors (presumably containing stem cells) restored, to a considerable extent, certain inborn immunologic deficiencies apparently arising in stem cell deficiencies (Gatti et al., 1968). These experiments of nature are discussed more fully on p. 215, but they provide unmistakable evidence of (1) the common origin, in stem cells, of both arms of the immune system, (2) the duality of the immune system and (3) the pivotal position of the thymus in cell-mediated immunity.

Here it is necessary to mention briefly

some new observations which raise the possibility of the existence of another population of immunocompetent lymphocytes relating to a system involved in the rejection of bone marrow cells. More is said about this system on p. 213, but it is entirely possible that, in the near future, we shall be talking about the "trinity" of the immune system. Since this new system is still in the exploratory stage, for the present we shall confine our consideration of the immune system to the T- and B-cells.

CELLS OF THE IMMUNE RESPONSE

Involved in the immune response are two categories of cells: (1) the immunologically competent cells of both the cell-mediated and humoral antibody systems and (2) those involved in the trapping, processing and recognition of antigen. The former comprise the effector or efferent limb of the immune response, the latter the afferent limb. We shall not concern ourselves here with the structural cells of the immune system such as the fibroblasts nor with the endothelial and reticuloendothelial cells which line the vessels and lymphatics.

IMMUNOLOGICALLY COMPETENT CELLS

These can be roughly divided into three morphologically distinguishable forms—lymphocytes, immunoblasts and plasma cells. All are interrelated and develop from one another, and so there are no sharp lines between them. Moreover, within each of these morphologically recognizable patterns, there are populations with significant differences in their function and role in the immune response which will become apparent in the following discussion.

The *lymphocytes* of the circulating blood and the fixed tissues of the immune system comprise two separate populations previously described. Most of the circulating lymphocytes belong to the T family and are long-lived. The B-lymphocytes are short-lived. These two populations are indistinguishable morphologically but can be identified immunologically and by isotopes. Using a DNA precursor, tritiated thymidine, it has been shown in rodents that one population of lymphocytes has a life span of less than 10 days and the other population, a life span of many months. In man, the long-lived lymphocytes may have a life span of many years, perhaps decades (Claman, et al., 1966). The two populations of lymphocytes are found not only in the circulating blood but in all of the lymphoid compartments of the body.

In order of increasing proportion of long-lived cells, the lymphoid structures can be arranged as follows: marrow and thymus, spleen, blood, lymph nodes and thoracic duct lymph. While the thymus contains very few long-lived cells, it is entirely possible that they are promptly exported after production. The thoracic duct lymph, however, contains largely long-lived lymphocytes which cycle through the lymphatic system, thymus and blood to constitute a recirculating lymphocyte pool.

The lymphocytes have the following functions: (1) They are antigen-sensitive cells; (2) some are capable of recognizing specific antigen and are referred to as "antigen recognition cells"; (3) some are carriers of the immunologic memory; (4) some are capable on specific antigenic challenge of "blast (immunoblast) transformation"; (5) some are capable of differentiation into plasma cells; and (6) some are the effector or "killer" cells of the delayed cell-mediated immune response. There continues to be some question as to whether the small lymphocyte may not also produce some antibody, particularly of the immunoglobulin M class (Sell and Asofsky, 1968). How they carry out these various functions will become clear in the following discussion.

Immunoblasts are large, weakly pyroninophilic cells (having affinity for pyronin—an indication of abundant RNA) resembling, to a considerable extent, other blast forms within the bone marrow. They contain large amounts of endoplasmic reticulum ribosomes and polyribosomes and, apparently, are capable of some protein (immunoglobulin) synthesis. They are formed by the blast transformation of small lymphocytes. The immunoblast itself is now believed to be committed to response to only one antigen and so its progeny of effector clones are similarly committed. An issue which has plagued immunologists involves the question of whether the immunoblast is derived from small lymphocytes which have already become committed to a specific antigen, thus specifying the immunologic reactivity of the immunoblast and its progeny, or whether the precursor lymphocyte is multipotential and the commitment occurs along with blastic transformation of the lymphocyte to the immunoblast. Involved here is the question of whether immunoblast transformation may be triggered by a variety of antigens or only occurs when an already committed lymphocyte receives its specific antigenic challenge.

It is of interest that several substances, particularly phytohemagglutinin (a kidney bean extract), possess the capability of nonspecifically inducing blast cell transformation. While blast cells have been demonstrated to contain small amounts of immunoglobulin, their primary role is that of proliferation and expansion of the clone. Those of the humoral system give rise, in turn, to plasmablasts or immature plasma cells which further divide or mature into antibody-forming plasma cells. Immunoblasts within the cell-mediated response produce large lymphocytes which, in turn, mature into the small sensitized lymphocytes of the cell-mediated response.

Plasma cells are the effector end organs of the humoral antibody system since they synthesize immunoglobulins. Their morphology has been described on p. 250. They are the principal source of antibody in the humoral response (Nossal, 1967). Electron microscopic studies have indicated a very highly developed endoplasmic reticulum with abundant ribosomes as well as numerous cytoplasmic polyribosomes and a well developed Golgi apparatus (Fig. 7–1). They are essentially specialized factories involved in the synthesis and export of antibodies. Plasma cells have a very short life span, less than one week, and thus a prolonged response to antigenic challenge implies proliferation of the clone with the production of successive generations of antibody-forming plasma cells, each generation contributing its share of the total response.

ANTIGEN-TRAPPING CELLS AND ANTIGEN PROCESSING

Macrophages within lymphoid tissues and dendritic or reticular phagocytic cells in the germinal centers play an important role in the immune response by trapping antigen. Their precise function is discussed in the next section, but it is clear that they are not directly involved with antibody production. Instead, they are crucial in the presentation of processed antigen to reactive lymphocytes.

Two separate sequences must occur in any immune reaction. The antigen must be presented to the immunologically competent cells in a form which they can recognize, and these cells must then respond. The response in the humoral system is the elaboration of circulating antibodies while, in the cell-mediated type of immunity, clones of specifically reactive (sometimes called "killer") lymphocytes must be generated. Our primary interest in this section concerns the first link in this chain, known as the afferent limb, involving antigen trapping, processing and transfer of appropriate information to the antigen-sensitive cells. Later we shall consider the effector response or the efferent limb.

There is great variation in the processing

of the many different antigens to which man is exposed. Some are soluble and of small size; others are large macromolecules. Some are naturally occurring; others may be synthetic. Proteins are the strongest antigens, but polysaccharides are also antigenic as may be some lipids. Despite this heterogeneity, all antigenic challenges result in one of three events. (1) The antigen, particularly if it is soluble, may fail to elicit an immune response because it remains extracellular (in the intra- and extravascular fluid compartment) where it is subjected to gradual catabolism and excretion. Indeed, as we shall see later, it may cause immunologic paralysis. (2) Aggregates, on the other hand, are phagocytized, perhaps by polymorphonuclear leukocytes, but also by macrophages as well as reticuloendothelial cells throughout the body. Within the granulocytes, the antigen is usually rapidly catabolized. Phagocytosis by macrophages or reticuloendothelial (RE) cells is particularly important because these cells in the lymph nodes and spleen are in immediate proximity to the cells of the efferent limb. Once engulfed, most of the antigen is incorporated within membrane-bounded sacs known as phagosomes where it is digested and destroyed. (3) A small fraction, possibly no more than 5 per cent, may persist for months, perhaps bound to the cell membrane where it retains its immunogenicity (Unanue and Askonas, 1968). Such antigen represents a continuing stimulus to the effector mechanism.

The material or information which passes from the macrophage with its trapped immunogens to the effector cells is still uncertain. One view proposes transfer only of a special type of RNA (Fishman et al., 1963). Whether it is messenger RNA which thus provides the code necessary for synthesis of a specific antibody has not been confirmed (Cohen, 1967). The weight of evidence suggests, rather, that the information or signal transmitted is a complex of RNA and fragments of antigen (Gottlieb and Doty, 1967). This latter view implies that the transmitted information is itself antigenic, perhaps an amplified antigen.

Preprocessing of antigen appears to be crucial to the induction of the efferent sequence in the immune response. (Frei et al., 1965). Lymphocytes respond poorly, if at all, to antigenic stimulation in macrophage free cultures (Cline and Swett, 1968). When such antigen is preprocessed in macrophages, it stimulates an effective immune response. Whether these reticuloendothelial cells are equally involved in the immune response to soluble antigens is not clear. But several observations suggest that perhaps even soluble antigen must first be

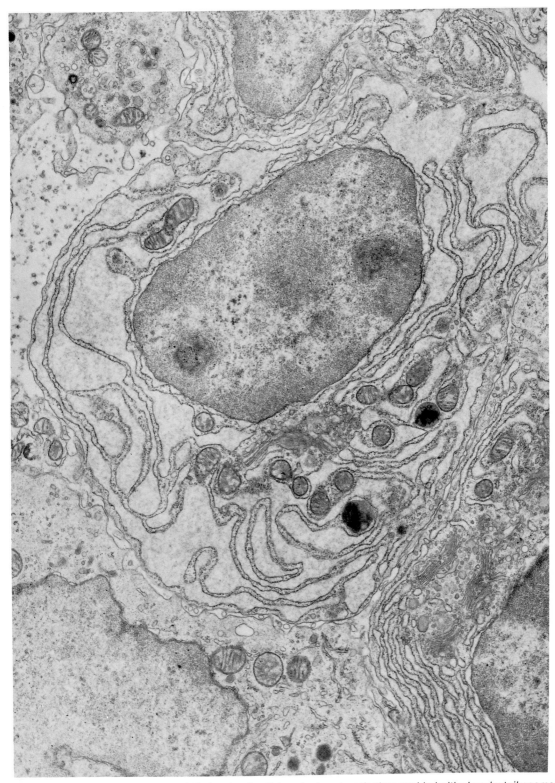

Figure 7–1.   *Plasma cell at × 13,000 showing the rich endoplasmic reticulum studded with abundant ribosomal granules. (Courtesy of Dr. Daniel Friend, Associate Professor of Pathology, University of California School of Medicine.)*

aggregated and processed after trapping (Dresser, 1962).

The dendritic reticular cells within lymphoid tissue function like macrophages and also trap antigen, presumably by binding it to their cell membranes. Here the antigen can be held for long periods. The glue that holds the antigens may be antibodies on the surfaces of these cells, because such localization of antigen is particularly prominent in so-called secondary responses in which the animal has had prior exposure to the same antigen. The accumulation of antigen on the dendritic cells provides a plausible means by which the lymphocytes, which move in and out of lymphoid tissues, come into intimate contact with it. Perhaps such exposure of lymphocytes is particularly important in secondary responses and accounts for the fact that secondary antibody responses are generally very much more powerful than primary responses.

Lymphocytes themselves bind or pinocytose antigen. The amount of antigen so held is relatively small and, sometimes, rather than inducing an immune response, this antigen may block the reactivity of the lymphocytes, a point discussed later. *The antigen receptor sites on the lymphocytes have been shown to be immunoglobulins.*

ANTIGEN RECOGNITION CELLS AND IMMUNOLOGIC MEMORY

Although the general nature of the antigen recognition mechanism seems reasonably well established, there is considerable uncertainty about which immunocompetent cells are the so-called "antigen recognition cells." There is good agreement that the primitive marrow stem cell does not respond to antigenic challenge and so possesses no antigen recognition system. But from this point, the trail is less clear as was mentioned earlier. It now appears that commitment occurs in the central lymphoid organs. Thus, in the T system, the commitment to a specific antigen occurs in the generation of thymic lymphocytes. When these lymphocytes colonize peripheral lymphoid organs, they are already committed. Similarly, commitment in the B system occurs in bursa-equivalent tissue. However, certain questions remain with this concept. Thymic lymphocytes in situ respond poorly to antigenic challenge. Whether the thymus is somehow sequestered from antigen or, instead, the lymphocytes are unresponsive remains uncertain. Since there is so much uncertainty, it is perhaps best merely to say that antigen recognition occurs in both forms of immune response, and immunologic specificity for a particular antigen develops somewhere along the line of sequential cellular transformations, leading to committed end organ cells, i.e., the plasma cell and sensitized lymphocyte (Sell, 1970).

Traditionally, the humoral system and the cell-mediated system are conceived of as possessing their own antigen recognition cells. First this view will be presented, but later we shall see that such total separation may not be entirely valid. *Most of the evidence supports the concept that the antigen-reactive or recognition cells are preprogrammed genetically for the synthesis of specific antibodies by having specific receptor sites.* Only those cells which possess the appropriate receptors respond to the antigen. Such antibody specificity implies genetic coding for the synthesis of the appropriate antibody. Thus, the antigen selects the preprogrammed cell. This, in essence, is the *clonal selection theory* of antibody formation proposed by Burnet (1959b). These responsive lymphocytes transform to immunoblasts. In the B system, some of the progeny of the immunoblasts are lymphocytes which do not develop into plasma cells, and these presumably comprise the memory of this "thymus-independent" system. In the T system, some of its lymphocytes comprise its memory cells.

The memory of the immune system is remarkable. It has been demonstrated to retain previous antigenic experience in man after 20 years (Gottlieb et al., 1964)! If B-cells are to have such a recall system, we must propose that some cells of the humoral response are long-lived; but most of the evidence suggests that the life span of B-cells is measured in terms of days. To resolve this problem, it has been suggested that the immunologic memory of immunoglobulin synthesis is perpetuated by continuous proliferation of successive generations of short-lived lymphocytes, all of which retain a record of initial exposure to an antigen. This concept has the particular advantage of maintaining, throughout the period of immunologic memory, the troops of cells ready to respond rapidly on second encounter with the antigen. The existence of such clones is also consonant with the well established fact that the secondary response to an antigen is more powerful than the primary response.

The cell-mediated reaction involves a parallel sequence of events. Here again, small "antigen recognition" lymphocytes presumably transform to immunoblasts which rapidly multiply and give rise to generations of small lymphocytes now specifically programmed for reaction with those antigens which activate the cell-mediated response. Some of these sensitized lymphocytes comprise the effector cells while others persist as memory cells. In the thymic system, these memory cells are proba-

Central Lymphoid Organ
Acquisition of antigenic specificity

Peripheral Lymphoid Organ
Acquisition of effector function

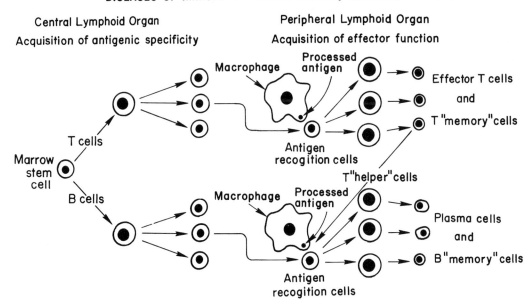

Figure 7–2. Development of immunocompetent cells.

bly the long-lived lymphocytes which constitute a large part of the recirculating pool of lymphocytes.

The clear-cut separation of the "thymus-dependent" and "thymus-independent" immune responses has been challenged recently (Nossal, 1969). B-cells cannot, by themselves, when infused into lethally irradiated animals, initiate humoral antibody production to some antigens. However, a mixed thymus-marrow infusion induces an immune response. When antigens, presumably evoking a humoral response, are introduced into animals, surprisingly, thymus-derived lymphocytes can be shown to undergo division (Davies et al., 1967) (Claman and Chaperon, 1969). These and other observations strongly indicate that, for some antigens, *the thymus system must help the thymus-independent system for the synthesis of immunoglobulins* (Nossal et al., 1968). Several explanations have been offered. One theory proposes that antigen recognition and immunologic memory for both forms of immune reactions reside in long-lived thymus-derived lymphocytes. These cells then serve as the storehouse of information for both the cell-mediated and humoral responses. In this view, the T memory cells would be required to help the B system. However, the clear demonstration of B memory cells suggests that the T "helper" cells are not involved in memory but, rather, in presenting certain kinds of antigens to the macrophages which collaborate with B recognition cells in the generation of immun-

oblasts and plasma cells. While these conceptions of immunologic memory and the role of T "helper" cells are still uncertain, all investigators agree that the thymic and marrow systems collaborate in some way in the induction of at least some humoral antibody responses (Miller and Mitchell, 1969). A summary of the concepts of T- and B-cell development, commitment and collaboration is offered in Figure 7–2.

HUMORAL ANTIBODY (IMMUNOGLOBULIN) SYNTHESIS

As is well known, immunoglobulins (Ig) are made up of polypeptide units of two sizes, light chains and heavy chains. These are linked by disulfide (SS) bonds. Each of these polypeptide chains, whether heavy or light, is composed of a portion with a constant sequence of amino acids characteristic of the particular class of immunoglobulin and a portion which is variable and which provides antigen specificity. For example, IgG has two heavy and two light chains linked by disulfide bonds. The molecule can be split by papain (protease) cleavage into three fragments as is diagrammed in Figure 7–3. The two Fab (antigen-binding) fragments constitute the two antigen-binding sites of IgG. The Fc (crystallizable) fragment binds complement.

The five major classes of Ig molecules are based upon the five major types of heavy-chain

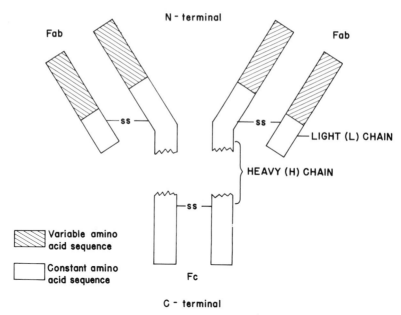

Figure 7–3. A single IgG molecule, schematically indicating cleavage into two Fab fragments and one Fc fragment.

polypeptides. In man, about 80 per cent of the gamma globulins are of the IgG class. The remaining 20 per cent of the gamma globulins of man are composed largely of IgM and IgA. IgM is of particular interest since it is the first and principal antibody produced phylogenetically and ontologically, and so is the first immunoglobulin to appear on primary antigen encounter. It is more effective at fixing complement and lysing cells than IgG whose main action is upon soluble antigens. IgA is found in two sites, principally in the external bodily secretions, i.e., salivary fluid, tears, respiratory and intestinal secretions and urine, but also in the blood. Secretory IgA differs from that of the blood by the presence of a secretory "piece," thus accounting for some variation in the molecular weight and sedimentation coefficient of this immunoglobulin. Much less is known about IgD and IgE. The latter is known as reaginic antibody and is principally involved in allergic reactions. It appears to attach itself to certain target cells such as mast cells, and so may bring about the release of histamine and other vasoactive compounds in the allergic response to antigens (Ishizaka and Ishizaka, 1968). A few details on these immunoglobulins are offered in Table 7–1. Further details on the structure of immunoglobulins can be found in several excellent reviews (Lennox and Cohn, 1967) (Franklin, 1968).

Immunoglobulin specificity is conferred by the precise amino acid sequence in the variable portions of the polypeptide subunits of the immunoglobulin molecule. The former view that specificity was achieved by secondary or tertiary folding of the molecule has been largely invalidated by sequential amino acid analysis of immunoglobulins and the growing evidence that all such specificity resides in the genetic programming of the synthesis of such proteins. The multiplicity of antibodies involved in the immunologic experience of man must imply, then, large numbers of antibody-forming clones, each having its own specificity (Makela, 1967) (Cosenza and Nordin, 1970). If this conception is valid as it now seems to be, then the role of antigen is to select and activate the specific clone bearing the appropriate receptors or antigen-binding sites known as the *clonal selection hypothesis of Burnet* (Burnet, 1959*b*). In this way, the antibody specific for the antigen is synthesized, and mitotic division within this specific clone provides adequate numbers of plasma cells for the immune response.

In the light of all of the antigens to which man may be exposed, how is all this genetic information incorporated within the antigen recognition cell, and how is the individual plasma cell programmed for the production of a specific antibody? Here we enter a gray uncertain area so well expressed by Sell (1970): "It is clear that there must be a multipotent stem cell with the potential to express all of the immunologic information in the genome of the individual. It is also clear that one end product of the immune response, the antibody-producing plasma cell, is severely restricted in its ability to express the immune information in the ge-

TABLE 7–1. IMMUNOGLOBULINS

Type	Where Formed	Where Found	Half-life	Sedimentation Coefficient	Complement Fixation	Chain Structure	Behavior
IgG	lymph nodes spleen	blood extracellular fluid	23 days	7 S	+		crosses placenta
IgM	lymph nodes spleen	blood	5 days	19 S	+++		does not cross placenta
IgD	lymph nodes spleen	blood extracellular fluid	3 days	7 S	0		does not cross placenta
IgA	mucus membranes of GI tract, Respiratory tract, Urogenital tract	a. secretions: tears mucus b. blood and extracellular fluid	6 days	7, 10, 14 S	0	a. _or_ b.	does not cross placenta secretory antibody
IgE	—	blood and extracellular fluid fixed to mast cells	1.5 days	7–8 S	0		does not cross placenta reaginic and cytotrophic antibody

nome. How this restriction occurs remains an enigma."

As best we now know, each polypeptide chain in the antibody molecule is genetically coded by two genes (Hood, 1972). The constant region of the polypeptide is under the control of one gene and the variable region, under the control of another. Where the joining of these separate functions occurs, at the DNA, RNA or protein level, is not known. If the plasma cell is so restricted, it must either possess only those genes necessary for such protein synthesis or repress all other genetic information relative to immunoglobulin synthesis.

Two model systems have been hypothesized for how this restriction of plasma cells is effected. One proposes that all stem cells and antigen recognition cells are totipotential and possess all of the possible genetic coding required for the elaboration of all possible antibodies required in life. In some way, the antigen-RNA complex which has been processed by a macrophage derepresses only those genes controlling the synthesis of the specific required immunoglobulin. This proposal is known as the _germ line concept_ since all cells are conceived of as multipotential. Obvious difficulties exist in this operational model. How does a single cell contain so much genetic information, and how does the preprocessed antigen complex derepress the genetic apparatus?

The other proposed model system invokes the concept of random somatic mutation among proliferating immunologically competent cells. Presumably, stem cells and antigen recognition cells are both multipotent.

The latter responds to a variety of antigenic challenges by proliferation and immunoblast transformation. In the course of this replicative activity, mutations occur, leading to some cells that are more responsive to the antigenic challenge than others. The antigen then selects for these more reactive cells and further stimulates their division again with the formation of mutants. Selective pressure by the antigen leads, ultimately, to the emergence of clones specifically reactive to the particular antigen. At the present, preference appears to lie in the somatic mutation rather than in the germ line model of immunologic specificity (Smithies, 1967) (Nordin et al., 1970) (Hood, 1972).

CELL-MEDIATED IMMUNITY

Thymus dependent cell-mediated immunity is involved principally in delayed hypersensitivity reactions such as tuberculosensitivity, allograft rejection and certain of the autoimmune diseases (McCluskey and Cohen, 1972). Less widely appreciated but no less important is the role of cell-mediated immunity in resisting many bacterial, fungal and viral agents (Editorial, 1969). This form of immunity differs from the humoral reaction in several respects. Although the immune response of the humoral and cell-mediated reaction is equally delayed on primary exposure to an antigen, the response on subsequent reencounter with the antigen evolves more slowly in the cell-mediated immunity and thus is referred to as _delayed hypersensitivity_. The reactions are effected by local infiltrations of sensitized lymphocytes and macrophages but do not involve plasma cells. Moreover, immunologic reactivity can be transferred from an immune to a nonimmune host by lymphoid cells and not by cell-free serum. Such transfer is called *adoptive immunity* rather than *passive immunity* which is effected by transfer of humoral antibody or serum containing such antibodies.

T-cells play many roles; they (1) cooperate with B-cells in the response to T-dependent antigens, (2) regulate the antibody response of B-cells, (3) participate in cell to cell destruction of target cells such as allogeneic grafted cells or tumor cells and (4) act as memory cells for the cell-mediated (T-cell) immune response. Because of these varied capabilities subsets have been proposed within the T-cell population called: (1) T-helper, (2) T-suppressor, (3) T-killer and (4) T-memory cells. Whether such a division of labor actually exists is unclear, but this terminology highlights the wideranging functions of T-cells.

How sensitized lymphocytes exert all these effects is still vague. It has been proposed that they produce circulating antibodies of very high affinity, but that the levels are below present methods of detection (Schlossman, 1967). However, such antibodies have never been clearly identified. Alternatively, a large number of nonimmunoglobulin factors known as *lymphokines* have been isolated from cell-free supernatants of sensitized T-lymphocytes. One is known as a macrophage *migration inhibitory factor (MIF)* because it agglutinates normal macrophages of animals and man in vivo and blocks their migration in cell cultures (David, 1968). A *lymphocyte mitogenic factor* is capable of causing normal lymphocytes to undergo blast transformation. A *cytotoxic factor* has been isolated that is capable of killing target cells to which the lymphocytes were previously sensitized (Granger and Williams, 1968). Also described recently is a *chemotactic factor* which attracts neutrophils and other factors which attract macrophages and eosinophils. *Interferon*, an antiviral substance (p. 430) is elaborated by T-cells (McCluskey and Cohen, 1972). All of these factors appear to be elaborated into the environment of the cells by the sensitized lymphocytes of cellular immunity.

Two additional nonimmunoglobulin factors have also recently been described. One is a so-called *inflammatory factor* capable of inducing increased vascular permeability and many of the classic features of inflammation (Panayi, 1970). The other is a so-called *transfer factor* capable of conferring on a nonsensitive human

recipient and his lymphocytes the pattern of delayed hypersensitivity possessed by the donor (Lawrence, 1970). These humoral factors may explain how cells of the thymus-dependent system exert their effect against antigenic targets (Perlmann et al., 1969).

Most cells in delayed hypersensitivity reactions are not sensitized T-lymphocytes (McCluskey et al., 1963). Some are non-sensitized lymphocytes, recruited perhaps by transfer factor. Macrophages contribute by virtue of a humoral substance known as "macrophage arming factor," elaborated by sensitized T-cells, which enables them to attach to such targets as tumor cells and "foreign" graft cells. In addition, recent evidence suggests that any cell with Fc receptors (macrophages, neutrophils and B-cells) may participate in cell to cell destruction. Antibody produced against target cells may coat them. Any Fc bearing cell may then attach to the Fc determinant in the antibody coating of target cells and thus destroy them. This phenomenon is called antibody dependent cellular cytotoxicity (ADCC). So a variety of cell types, in addition to T-cells, contribute to cell-mediated immune responses, including, paradoxically, B-lymphocytes.

FACTORS REGULATING THE QUALITY AND QUANTITY OF THE IMMUNE RESPONSE

The nature of the antigen, the prior experience of the immune system with the antigen and the genetic constitution of the host all modify the quality and quantity of the immune response.

The type, amount and physicochemical properties of an antigen such as its chemical nature (protein, polysaccharide, etc.), size, solubility and aggregation all condition the quality and quantity of the immune response. It has previously been pointed out, for example, that soluble protein antigens remain in the intra- and extravascular fluid compartments. Here they are rapidly catabolized or excreted. Since soluble antigen is not as effectively trapped by macrophages, it escapes preprocessing and may flood into effector lymphocytes where it binds to antigen receptors and, rather than inducing an immune response, may cause immune nonreactivity or tolerance. Larger aggregates are trapped by macrophages and so persist longer to induce a more effective response.

Certain agents, not themselves necessarily

antigenic, when administered either before or with an antigen, greatly enhance the magnitude of the immune response. Such agents, termed adjuvants, include oils, waxes and alum gels. Indeed, adjuvants are also effective in inducing an immune response to agents ordinarily nonimmunogenic. Adjuvants may not only increase the strength of an immune response to antigens but also affect the nature of the response. As an example, it was observed some time ago that the administration of killed mycobacteria, along with a soluble protein antigen, would evoke a delayed hypersensitivity reaction to the protein, whereas the protein alone induced a humoral circulating antibody response. This led to the discovery that a lipopolysaccharide component of the waxy capsule of tubercle bacilli *(Mycobacterium tuberculosis)* was responsible for the delayed hypersensitivity reaction to the protein even though the lipopolysaccharide was not itself antigenic. Thus came into existence *Freund's complete adjuvant*, essentially an oil detergent emulsion containing killed mycobacteria (Freund and McDermott, 1942). The incomplete Freund's adjuvant contains only the oil detergent emulsion. Although the mechanism of action of adjuvants is unclear, they may enhance antigenic potency by stimulating the activity of macrophages. The incorporation of antigens into oily waxy solutions so that the injection site comprises essentially a slowly resorbed depot of antigen also provokes a stronger immune response.

The most important consideration affecting the quantity and quality of the immune response is prior experience with the antigen. The first encounter in life with an antigen evokes a so-called *primary response*. The second or subsequent exposures result in a *secondary response*. The cellular changes which occur in both the primary and secondary responses differ somewhat, depending on whether the antigen causes a predominantly humoral immune reaction or a cell-mediated response. More is known about the former, and so most of the following remarks relate to the humoral system.

The primary response to an antigen evokes no histologic changes in the lymph nodes for at least 4 to 5 days (although the length of this lag phase is highly variable). Recently, Litt (1967) astounded everyone with his report of antibody production within 7½ minutes following the injection of red cells into the foot pad of guinea pigs. If his results are validated, then a great deal of previous work must be reevaluated. In any event, in most model systems, toward the end of the first week some antibody appears in the circulation, depending on many factors relating to the size, nature and quantity of the antigen. Thereafter, the rise in titer is exponential and, sometime toward the end of the second week, the antibody levels peak and begin to slowly decline over a period of months. The rate of climb of antibody level is a function of the number of active plasma cells and not the individual productivity of the cells. The decline in antibody level reflects waning of the antigen stimulus, death of the short-lived plasma cells and excretion, catabolism and complexing of antibody with antigen.

The first antibodies to appear in the serum after primary exposure to an antigen are of the IgM class. Later IgG appears to the same antigen while the level of IgM declines. Present evidence suggests that separate clones are involved in the synthesis of each of these immunoglobulins and that the precursors of the IgG antibodies in some way suppress the IgM clones.

There is a somewhat different cytologic change in nodes in the primary response when a cell-mediated immune reaction occurs. Here, as soon as 4 or 5 days after contact with the antigen, there is a rapid blast transformation and subsequent proliferation of lymphocytes in the thymus-dependent areas. These cells, at first large lymphocytes, mature into medium-sized and small lymphocytes of the cell-mediated reaction. The germinal centers of the lymph nodes and the plasma cells are not involved unless the response simultaneously evokes humoral antibodies.

The *secondary response* to a specific antigen, even months or years after the primary challenge, evokes a much more intense accelerated antibody production. This usually begins within 2 or 3 days, reaches a much higher level than the primary response, plateaus for a period of weeks and then, over the course of weeks and months, slowly declines. In Litt's (1967) sensational model system, this response is detected within 30 seconds. The antibody levels persist in the secondary response for some time and generally remain above those ever obtained in the primary response although, as before, the exact type and nature of the antigen modifies the secondary response. In general, smaller doses of antigen are required to produce a significant level of immunoglobulin synthesis than with the primary response. The antibodies are almost entirely of the IgG variety. Perhaps the most remarkable feature of the secondary response is the immunologic memory system which, as mentioned before, recalls a primary exposure to an antigen after 20 years have lapsed. For this reason, the secondary response is often referred to as a "memory response" or "anamnestic response."

What can be said of the secondary response in the cell-mediated reaction? Antigen, presumably after it has been processed, contacts small lymphocytes (antigen recognition cells) perhaps while they are in circulation. These cells settle in the thymus-dependent areas of peripheral lymph nodes and undergo blast transformation and division, giving rise to a population of sensitized lymphocytes. Further expansion of the number of responding cells may occur by recruitment of lymphocytes, not directly in contact with the antigen, mediated by humoral factors (such as transfer factor) elaborated by T-lymphocytes (p. 204). Some of these antigen-sensitive, recruited lymphocytes may be short-lived, but most are clearly long-lived. These differences in life span may merely reflect the rate of cell division and the rapidity of immunologic commitment and cell differentiation. Clearly, the long-lived cells constitute a significant proportion of the recirculating pool and provide the cytologic basis for immunologic memory. By their recirculation, they can mobilize for the secondary immune response all of the lymphoid tissues in the body.

Within the past few years, it has become evident that genetic controls of the immune response exist. These genetic controls appear to be closely linked to the genes controlling histocompatibility antigens (p. 226) (Benacerraf and McDevitt, 1972). Benacerraf and his colleagues have shown that C57 strain mice respond well to a specific branched multichain synthetic polypeptide, but C3H and CBA mice respond poorly (McDevitt and Benacerraf, 1969). Here we do not speak of general immunologic responsiveness but rather responsiveness to specific antigens controlled by *immune response genes*. There are many hints of this phenomenon in man which may provide important insights into individual vulnerability to certain diseases (McDevitt and Bodmer, 1972).

IMMUNOLOGIC TOLERANCE

Tolerance refers to a state of unresponsiveness of the immune system to an antigen. It can apply to foreign antigens such as bovine serum albumin or pneumococcal polysaccharide, or to the numerous antigens in cells and tissues. As will be seen, self-tolerance is as much an acquired characteristic as tolerance to foreign antigens.

Despite intensive study, the cellular and molecular mechanisms underlying immunologic tolerance are still poorly understood. Antigen-reactive cells are equipped with a restricted number of receptor sites. Tolerance might imply union between the receptor site and the antigen which failed to activate the cell, or alternatively led to its prolonged inactivation or even its destruction. There are reasons for believing that both mechanisms obtain.

Tolerance to foreign antigens can be induced both in vivo and in vitro by antigen given in two distinct quantitative zones (Mitchison, 1964). Extremely small doses given repeatedly will induce, in laboratory animals, a considerable amount of tolerance, perhaps not total, to a large variety of antigens. The dosage levels are critical. The same antigen can be given in much larger "paralyzing" doses to produce a much more profound and longer-lasting tolerance. Between these two zones, there is a wide zone in which the antigen will induce an active immune response without leading to tolerance. At the cellular level, a number of interpretations have been offered. It is proposed that, in the very low dosage range, the antigen is phagocytized by macrophages, but no signal or only a very weak signal reaches the effector cells. Repeated administrations may blockade the macrophage and thus prevent effective macrophage-lymphocyte interaction. Alternatively, trace amounts of antigen might, after processing, combine with only one of the receptor sites on the immune cell. Such a signal might be too weak to activate the cell. Repeated administration of minute amounts of antigen would eventually saturate all the receptor sites and block further immune responsiveness.

Large doses of antigen flood past the reticuloendothelial cells such as the macrophages and dendritic cells and come into direct contact with lymphocytes. Since such antigen has not been processed within macrophages, it evokes no immune reaction but instead binds all receptor sites on lymphocytes and thus has the effect of inducing immunologic paralysis of these cells. For this reason, small soluble antigens which remain in the fluid compartment of the body are particularly effective in inducing tolerance. Frei et al. (1965) demonstrated in the rabbit that biologic filtration of antigen, i.e., removal of aggregates by the reticuloendothelial system, leaves behind in the circulation small complexes which, on reinjection into other animals, produce tolerance. In terms of humoral immune responses, recent evidence suggests that *low zone tolerance* involves loss of T-helper cell function. In contrast, *high zone tolerance* appears to result from suppression or inhibition of function of both B-cells and T-helper cells. An additional highly speculative explanation of tolerance, particularly at the high zone level, raises the intriguing possibility that it may be the consequence of excessive T-suppressor cell function. Much is still uncertain.

Turning now to the subject of *self-tolerance, as mentioned earlier it is not merely an in-built genetic characteristic but rather an acquired phenomenon.* It has been shown in animals that removal of a piece of normal thyroid gland and injection of a macerate of this tissue into the same animal evokes an immune response. The animal failed to recognize the tissue as "self." In other words, there was no in-built recognition of self. The patient, too, may become sensitized to his own thyroid antigens. But we should point out that the thyroid is a special case, and most tissues when reintroduced to the host will not evoke an immune reaction. Nonetheless, no genetically programmed tolerance to thyroid tissue antigens exists.

In 1945, Owen made the epochal observation that, when bovine twins representing dizygotic embryos had an effective anastomosis of placental blood vessels permitting exchange of red cell populations, these animals freely accepted skin grafts from each other, despite marked differences in the antigenic composition of their tissues (Owen, 1945). It was concluded that cellular antigens to which the immune system was exposed during embryogenesis were recognized as "self." Such a conception proposes that *the presence of significant amounts of antigen during embryogenesis induces immune tolerance by one of the mechanisms discussed earlier.* Indeed, within limits, immunologic tolerance can be produced in animals by the administration of an antigen either before or immediately after birth (Smith, 1961). Presumably, the immune system is exposed to the totality of the tissue antigens of the fetus throughout embryogenesis. Blocking of T-helper cells might be involved or, as Burnet (1959*b*) proposes, unwanted clones may be destroyed. The mechanism by which such unwanted clones could be destroyed or repressed is speculative. It could be theorized that all antigen-sensitive cells programmed to react against "self" antigens might be stimulated into active proliferation. In the immature immune system, all of the precursors capable of giving rise to these clones would either be used up or exhausted and the entire line thereby eliminated. This phenomenon has been termed *terminal exhaustive differentiation.* Such exhaustion or elimination of specific clones would be difficult to accomplish in the adult animal with greater reserves.

Why then should introduction of thyroid tissue antigen into the host evoke an immune response? Here a controversial explanation is offered, namely, that during embryonic life the thyroid and its tissue antigens remain sequestered from the circulation and therefore never have contact with the immune system. Tolerance could never develop. Whether "sequestered antigens" truly exist, however, is not certain and there are reasons that will become clear in the discussion of autoimmune disease to suspect a more complicated process if, indeed, we have any satisfying explanation.

Before closing this discussion, tolerance breakdown should be mentioned. The perpetuation of tolerance to foreign antigens and, indeed, to "self" antigens may require the continued presence of low levels of antigen in the circulation. When the levels disappear or are reduced to nontolerogenic levels, new generations of antigen-reactive cells may once again appear capable of an immune response. In support of this hypothesis, it has been shown that sublethal irradiation of a tolerant animal or infusion of isogeneic immunocompetent cells from a nontolerant donor will be followed by the emergence of immune responsiveness. Presumably, the radiation caused destruction of many lymphoid cells, followed by a spurt of proliferation of new generations of cells, some mutants of which were capable of responding to the specific antigen to which tolerance had been induced. In addition, a cell rendered tolerant may itself revert to an antigen-sensitive state if new receptor immunolglobulins are synthesized during a time when antigen is not available to block the binding sites.

Breakdown of tolerance is commonly encountered in both animals and man. The line between the induction of tolerance and the initiation of an immune response is exceedingly fine. Clinical experience has taught how difficult it is to acheive. Effective immunologic tolerance in adult potential recipients of allografts has, to this time, been beyond our grasp, and it has been necessary to resort to immunosuppression (p. 209). Moreover, the risk of producing a secondary response is real, and constitutes a serious threat in any attempted induction of tolerance.

TISSUE-HISTOCOMPATIBILITY (H) ANTIGENS

The tissue cells of all species of animals including man possess histocompatibility (H) antigens which are either bound to or included in the plasma membrane of the cell. The antigenic systems are highly specific for each species and, moreover, the polymorphism within each species is so great that each individual has his own specific, virtually unique, antigenic profile which is genetically determined. At our present level of understanding, the histocompatibility system in man appears to be immensely complex. The transfer, therefore, of tissue or cell suspensions from one member of the species to another almost always induces an immune response. Thus, H antigens have also been referred to as "transplantation antigens." The cell-mediated system plays the principal role in such an immune reaction; however, the humoral system may also be activated, particularly when antigens are liberated from the cell membranes or when tissue extracts are introduced. Fortunately, from the clinical standpoint, H antigens are present on leukocytes. Thus, there is a readily available source of cells for the study of the histocompatibility profile of the individual. Obviously, it would be highly desirable to be able to type precisely the H antigens of donor and recipient, as is done with red cell antigens, and thus achieve a perfect or acceptable match for the transplantation of skin or kidneys.

Much has been learned about histocompatibility systems by the study of inbred populations of mice. Fifteen genetic histocompatibility systems have been identified which segregate as separate distinct loci. The major genetic locus in this species is referred to as H-2, controlling at least 30 or more antigenic determinants. This locus may in fact be comprised of five genetic subloci although it is entirely possible that many more exist. In addition to the H-2 system in mice there are other systems, but this one appears, at least, to be the major concern in determining transplantability of tissues from one animal to another.

At the present time, the major histocompatibility system of man is referred to as the human leukocyte antigen (HL-A) system and, on the basis of leukocyte typing, it appears to contain more than 30 distinctive transplantation antigens. This number is highly likely to be a gross oversimplification (Clarke et al., 1968). In man, this system is controlled by a single large chromosome region which consists of two subloci, each bearing a number of genes

and controlling a multiplicity of antigenic determinants (Dausett et al., 1969).

The HL-A antigens detected serologically behave as if they belong to two closely linked segregant series known as the LA or first and the 4 or second series. From serologic reactions, it is possible to deduce the inheritance of the HL-A alleles of "haplotypes." Each haplotype represents the LA and 4 alleles of the same chromosome. Because of the polymorphism of the HL-A region, the paternal haplotypes are designated A and B, the maternal haplotypes C and D, and the children AC, AD, BC, and BD. If two children inherit the same haplotypes, e.g., AC and AC, they are said to be HL-A identical. If they share only one haplotype, e.g., AC and AD, they are haploidentical; if they have neither haplotype, e.g., AC and BD, they are HL-A different. Kidney grafts from HL-A identical donors require less immunosuppressive drug treatment than grafts from HL-A different donors, and a bone marrow graft from an HL-A identical donor offers the best possibility for replacement therapy.

HL-A antigens are restricted to the cell surface of cells and are richest on lymphoid cells. Parenchymal cells, such as liver and kidney, are moderately rich in HL-A antigens. Fat and brain cells have very low levels of HL-A antigens. Since HL-A antigens are detected by serologic reactions, e.g., leukoagglutination or cell cytotoxicity, they must elicit a humoral antibody reaction. Another test for tissue compatibility is the mixed lymphocyte reaction, where one cultures blood leukocytes of the prospective donor and host together. The responding cell is a thymus-dependent T-cell which undergoes "blast transformation" with subsequent proliferation upon exposure to alloantigens. Recently, it was shown that the antigen which stimulates this response is coded for by a gene closely linked to but not identical with the genes determining the LA and 4 serotypable antigens of HL-A (Yunis and Amos, 1971). The gene is called MLR-S, mixed lymphocyte response-stimulation, and the antigen stimulates T-cell proliferation but does not initiate a humoral antibody response. Conversely, the LA and 4 antigens elicit a humoral antibody (B-cell) response but do not stimulate T-cells to proliferate in culture. Another distinctive gene in the HL-A region codes for antigen which sensitizes hosts for a hypersensitivity delayed reaction. Thus, as more distinct immunologic reactions are recognized and sorted out, more distinct antigens will probably be discovered. This may be a disturbing thought to classic immunologists who think only in terms of antibody reactions.

The genetics and immunology of this subject are complex enough, but the problem has been made even more confusing by the distressing practice of each major investigator giving his individual designations to the genetic loci and their antigenic determinants. So each locus and each antigenic determinant is known by many terms, and the literature has become an Augean stable. Here we shall adopt the terminology for the HL-A histocompatibility system used by Amos (1969).

The greater the antigenic difference between donor and recipient, often referred to as the "antigenic barrier," the more certain the immune response and the greater the likelihood of rejection of transplanted tissues or organs. However, certain considerations permit greater optimism. One can use the ABO red cell system as an analogy. It has been shown that there are more than 20 antigenic polymorphisms among the red cell antigens. Yet, despite this heterogeneity, clinical experience indicates that only the ABO and Rh antigens are sufficiently strong to be of major importance in blood transfusion. The remainder rarely cause significant immunologic reactions. Some of the red cell antigens such as the Kell and MNS antigens are either weak or rare, and so do not interfere. Hopefully, the majority of serologically demonstrable transplantation antigens will be shown similarly to be weak and so not to represent significant hazards in tissue transplantation.

Before closing, however, we should note that most of the usual methods employed for the typing of tissues utilize leukocytes. We do not know yet what fraction of the antigenic constituents of leukocytes represents histocompatibility antigens nor, conversely, that the antigenic profile of these circulating white cells is identical to that of solid tissue cells. Williams and his colleagues (1969a) have called attention to apparent antigenic differences between a donor's lymphocytes and his kidney cells. These antigenic differences could result from varying levels of expression of the genotype. Indeed, the various tissues within an individual have significant differences in the strength of their antigens. Leukocytes and the cells of the skin possess stronger antigens than, for example, the kidney and spleen. The antigenic barrier as determined by leukocyte typing may not, therefore, faithfully represent the magnitude of the antigenic differences between donor and recipient; but hopefully any discrepancy should be in the direction of exaggeration of immune differences since white cells possess strong H antigens. Obviously, ABO incompatibility must be reckoned with since these antigens are also present on tissue cells.

TRANSPLANTATION AND IMMUNOSUPPRESSION

In the mid-twentieth century, no subject in medicine has been more exciting or more frustrating than the transplantation of organs. Here appeared an avenue for prolongation of life by replacing a damaged organ with a healthy one. Indeed, enormous strides have been made in the surgical expertise necessary for the transplantation of virtually every viscus in man. The villain has been the immune mechanism with its implacable recognition of antigenic differences. The difficulties in obtaining a perfect or even acceptable "match" between donor and recipient have already been alluded to. It has therefore been necessary to retreat to methods of immunosuppression and to techniques which hopefully minimize the response of the immune system.

New discoveries will certainly outdate some of our present techniques but, currently, three approaches are commonly used to suppress the immune response: (1) irradiation, (2) drugs, (3) antilymphocyte and antithymocyte globulin, thoracic duct drainage and thymectomy. All lymphocytes are extremely radiosensitive and so irradiation is capable of destroying both the long-lived, sluggishly metabolic T-lymphocytes as well as the B-forms. The drugs may be divided into three classes: alkylating agents (e.g., nitrogen mustard, cyclophosphamide); antimetabolites (e.g., methotrexate, azothioprine also known as imuran, 6-mercaptopurine); and cortisone with its analogues. The alkylating agents block expansion of the clones by deranging mitotic division and inducing lethal mutations. The antimetabolites block DNA or RNA synthesis. Both drugs and irradiation then inhibit the proliferation or destroy immunocompetent cells and suppress the immune response. In addition to all of these actions, irradiation and the various cytotoxic drugs may impair phagocytosis in the macrophages of the immune system. It should be noted that all of these forms of treatment are completely unselective and so have effect on all rapidly proliferating cell systems in the body. They therefore have considerable toxicity for the bone marrow and gut epithelium and so they must be used cautiously in the attempt to achieve immunosuppression without serious secondary effects on other tissues. The corticosteroids are anti-inflammatory agents, as mentioned earlier in this book, presumably by virtue of their membrane-stabilizing action on lysosomes. But in addition, the steroids produce lymphopenia and deplete lymphoid tissue especially in the thymus and lymph nodes by lysis of lymphocytes.

Antilymphocyte (ALG) and antithymocyte

(ATG) globulins are two of the most interesting therapeutic agents employed for immunosuppression. They are prepared by immunizing an animal such as the rabbit with lymphocytes or thymocytes from man. Such sera appear to act preferentially on the lymphocytes in the recirculating pool. These are largely the long-lived T-lymphocytes. Thus the primary actions of ALG and ATG are on the cell-mediated immune response which plays the major role in homograft rejection. However, as was pointed out earlier, these same long-lived memory cells may also contribute in some way to the humoral antibody response, and so immunoglobulin synthesis may be impaired simultaneously (Berenbaum, 1965) (Berenbaum, 1967) (Levey and Medawar, 1966) (Makinodan et al., 1965). Both ALG and ATG may selectively destroy lymphocytes or alternatively act as antigens and so pre-empt the reactivity of immunocompetent cells from responding to other antigens. Possibly they coat the lymphocytes and block their receptor sites. Thoracic duct drainage and thymectomy have been particularly disappointing in clinical trials (Starzl, 1964).

The use of immunosuppression has had several undesirable side effects. The patient is rendered vulnerable to infections, even with organisms of very low virulence, usually incapable of inducing disease in normal hosts. Sometimes organisms usually considered to be nonpathogenic are productive of fatal disease in the patient deprived of immunologic capability. Under these circumstances, the disease is often referred to as an "opportunistic" infection. Thus, for example, uncommon agents such as fungi, *Pneumocystis carinii* and cytomegalovirus have been responsible for fatal infection in these severely predisposed patients (Hart et al., 1969) (Klainer and Beisel, 1969). Another unpleasant problem has emerged in patients receiving long-term immunosuppressive therapy, namely, an increased incidence of malignant tumors in organ transplant recipients. This subject is discussed on p. 754.

Regrettably, there is little evidence that even prolonged immunosuppression eventually induces tolerance to the transplanted tissue. However, it should be pointed out that the dosages of immunosuppressive agents can sometimes be reduced after some months, suggesting some level of adaptation between the allograft and its host (Brent, 1971). A number of ingenious methods have been employed to induce, in the adult recipient, immunologic tolerance to the antigens of the potential donor. To date, the results have been less than impressive. Calne et al. (1970) have recently reported that it has been possible to induce immunologic tolerance in pigs by the prior administration of "crude soluble extracts" of liver or spleen prior to transplantation of kidney allografts. This approach was completely unsuccessful in dogs and Rhesus monkeys. This striking difference among the species is as yet unexplainable. In man, few investigators have been intrepid enough to attempt this approach for fear of inducing the opposite and undesirable effect of enhanced reactivity. This area is, however, being actively explored and offers real hope.

It is clear that the magnitude of the antigenic differences between donor and recipient, i.e., the antigenic barrier, determines the likelihood of a successful "take" (Russell and Winn, 1970). Autologous grafting of skin from one site in the body to another presents no immunologic problem. Similarly, kidney transplantation between isogeneic monovular twins has proved to be highly successful with excellent long-term results. The same holds true for isogeneic highly inbred strains of animals. As one ascends the scale of antigenic differences, immunologic problems mount. Thus, it is apparent from the analysis of the thousands of kidney transplants that the results are better between related donors and recipients, i.e., between siblings and parents and children than between unrelated individuals. It is no surprise that xenografts across species barriers hold so little promise. Some of the results of organ transplantation reported to a national registry are given in Table 7–2.

It is evident that the success of kidney transplantation as measured by both survival of the patient and function of the transplant correlates with the probable "antigenic barrier" between donor and recipient. Sepsis (infection) is responsible for 30 to 40 per cent of the deaths of recipients, followed in importance by rejection (approximately 20 per cent). Cancer was the cause of death in about 1 per cent. The dominance of sepsis is an ironic tribute to the effectiveness of immunosuppression. The first human heart transplant was performed in December 1967, and the total number reported to the registry is about 170. As of the last half of 1971, still living were 22 recipients, ten of whom have survived for 24 to 28 months (Report, ACS/NIH Organ Transplant Registry, 1971). Approximately 150 liver transplants have been registered at the time of this writing. The longest survivor (29 months after surgery) is reported to be in excellent health. In addition lung, bone marrow, pancreas and, indeed, combined heart and lung transplantation have been performed, but the numbers are too small to provide useful data.

TABLE 7-2. RENAL TRANSPLANTS: TWO-YEAR PATIENT SURVIVAL AND
TRANSPLANT FUNCTION

Donor Type	Number of Transplants	Per Cent of Patients Surviving	Per Cent of Functioning Kidneys
Monozygotic twin	3	100	100
Sibling	171	76	68
Parent	163	76	66
Cadaver	644	61	47

Data taken from the ninth report of the Human Renal Transplant Registry of the American College of Surgeons/NIH Organ Transplant Registry, Chicago, Ill., 1971.

REJECTION REACTIONS

Rejection of nonisogeneic grafts involves principally cell-mediated mechanisms but also humoral antibodies (Najarian and Foker, 1969). Not only are sensitized lymphocytes involved, but there is evidence that granulocytes with their lysosomal enzymes and macrophages are involved in the cell-mediated reaction. Humoral antibodies appear in the more acute rejections where they induce an acute vasculitis closely resembling that found in serum sickness (p. 220). They have been eluted from rejected grafts and have been demonstrated by fluorescent techniques within grafted kidneys (Williams et al., 1969*b*) (Najarian and Perper, 1967). Humoral participation has been demonstrated also by the successful passive transfer of allograft immunity by sensitized allotypic plasma (Cochrum et al., 1969). But, in animals, it is easier to transfer allograft immunity with cells than with serum. This, however, might be attributed to the enormous quantities of antibodies absorbed by the tissue undergoing rejection. Very likely, humoral mechanisms play a major role in very acute rejections and only synergize the cell-mediated response in all others.

At one time, two morphologic patterns of rejection were recognized: "*first set rejection*," applied to primary grafts, and "*second set rejection*," applied to a subsequent graft from the same donor. It is apparent that "first set rejection" comprises a primary immune response while a "second set rejection" implies a secondary response. There are many objections to such terminology since recipients may become sensitized by pathways other than prior grafting. Mothers are sensitized to "foreign" antigens by the paternal antigens in the fetus. Transfusions are obvious sources of histocompatibility sensitization. Cross reactions between tissue antigens and bacterial antigens may presensitize recipients. For these reasons, current terminology favors the three terms "hyperacute," "acute" and delayed or "chronic" rejection.

Hyperacute rejection. This may be evident within minutes or hours of transplantation (Fig. 7-4). It results from acute vascular lesions induced by complexes of antibodies and histocompatibility antigens (released from cells injured or destroyed in the course of transplantation) which bind complement. *The principal anatomic hallmark of hyperacute rejection is acute necrotizing vascular lesions including vascular thromboses.* The rejection represents, therefore, failure of the graft to become vascularized. Immunofluorescent methods disclose gamma globulins belonging to the IgG, IgA and IgM classes, complement and fibrin in the vascular lesions. The mechanism of such acute vasculitis is described in detail on p. 219. In kidney transplants, glomerular capillaries and intertubular capillaries often contain fibrin thrombi characteristic of disseminated intravascular coagulation (DIC). A variety of ultrastructural glomerular alterations have been identified, including basement-membrane thickening with subendothelial focal and linear deposits of IgG, IgM, complement and fibrin, thickening of the mesangium, loss of foot processes, all suggestive of both ischemic and immunologic injury. Tubular cells undergo ischemic necrosis and the interstitial tissue is usually edematous and is often infiltrated with neutrophils and occasional lymphocytes, plasma cells and macrophages. An additional vascular lesion is often encountered in hyperacute rejections, comprising essentially a form of florid atherosclerosis in the larger arteries of the graft. It takes the form of massive accumulations of ballooned-out lipophages within the intima which cause marked thickening of the arterial wall and narrowing of the lumen. These changes are attributed to increased permeability of the endothelium with imbibition of lipoproteins or, alternatively, impaired lipid metabolism within the wall of the artery.

As a consequence of these vascular insults,

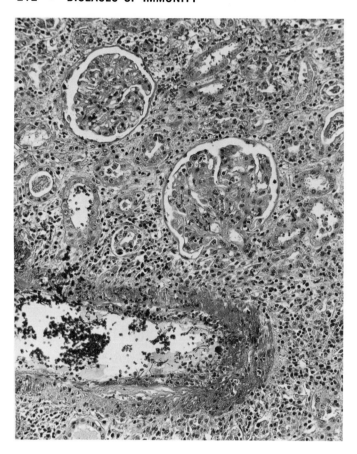

Figure 7–4. *Hyperacute rejection of the kidney 24 hours after transplantation. There is acute vasculitis in the artery below, and the glomerular capillary lumina are thrombosed. The leukocytic infiltrate is scant.*

the tissue never becomes vascularized and undergoes progressive ischemic destruction. Thus in skin grafts, the transplanted tissue remains pale white and progressively becomes ischemic and necrotic. In the case of kidneys, after the vascular connections have been established, the graft fails to develop the characteristic blush of the successful transplant and, moreover, it fails to produce urine. Under such circumstances, immune suppression may be intensified and, when these tissues are studied at a later date, fibro-obliterative arterial lesions comprise a major cause of the graft failure.

Acute Rejection. This generally implies loss of graft viability within several days to weeks, however it should be recognized that acute rejection may occur many months after the transplantation when immunosuppressive therapy is stopped. Acute rejection is mediated by both cellular and humoral mechanisms. In the words of Najarian and Foker (1969), "the result is histological confusion with lymphocytes, histiocytes, polys, plasma cells, and platelets all present. Antibody and complement are deposited within the graft. Interaction of all these factors produces perivascular edema, cellular infiltration, disruption of vessel en-

dothelium, and intravascular thrombosis." The more fulminant the acute rejection, the more it borders on the hyperacute vascular pattern just described.

At the other end of the spectrum, acute rejection resembles the cell-mediated pattern characteristic of chronic rejection. Vascular necroses are less florid and less abundant. In the kidney, glomerular thromboses may also be present but are not as widespread as in the hyperacute reaction. The interstitial edema tends to be more pronounced with a much heavier infiltrate of lymphocytes, plasma cells and macrophages. The renal tubular epithelium undergoes, as would be anticipated, regressive alterations characteristic of ischemic necrosis. The glomerular structural and ultrastructural changes are those already described in the more florid forms of rejection (Dammin, 1968). But in addition, endothelial and mesangial cell swelling and reduplication are more prone to occur, producing changes quite reminiscent of those encountered in proliferative glomerulonephritis. For this reason, it was at one time thought that these transplants were suffering from recurrence of the glomerulonephritic disease which had destroyed the recipients' own kidneys. However, it is now recognized that such glomerular lesions may occur in patients who never had glomerulonephritis, and so they are interpreted as *rejection glomerulopathy.*

In acute rejections, the graft at first becomes vascularized and assumes a characteristic pink blush only to develop progressive swelling and pallor and eventually undergo coagulative ischemic necrosis. If left in situ it undergoes, in time, atrophy and scarring (Andres at al., 1970).

Delayed or Chronic Rejection. This may occur years after transplantation. The dominant mechanism is cell-mediated but the anatomic changes are varied and undoubtedly reflect earlier episodes of acute rejection successfully suppressed by therapy and the progressive emergence of fibro-obliterative vascular lesions (Busch et al., 1971). In experimental systems, skin grafts first develop an adequate circulation, then over the course of weeks to months, become edematous and acquire a mononuclear infiltrate, principally of lymphocytes mixed with macrophages. Over the course of time, they undergo cell injury, cell death and fibrosis. It has not been possible to follow sequentially the changes in man as closely, but repeated biopsies have disclosed a similar sequence in the chronic rejection of kidneys (Busch et al., 1971) (Fig. 7–5). Most striking is the interstitial fibrosis and atrophy of parenchymal elements. All of the glomerular changes encountered in the acute rejection may be seen but are more advanced and often reach the stage of glomerular obliteration and fibrosis (Porter et al., 1967). Arterial walls are often markedly thickened and lumina may be obliterated. Often, the entire vascular architecture is replaced by fibrous cords barely recognizable as blood vessels. Even in kidneys undergoing delayed rejection, immunofluorescent studies have revealed fibrin and gamma globulin deposits indicative of the fact that humoral mechanisms are still operative at this late stage. Moreover, in renal grafts which have apparently functioned effectively for years, changes indicative of mild rejection are often found (Hamburger, 1967). The immune system never forgets and never seems willing to come to terms with the "foreign invader."

Rejection of Bone Marrow Allografts. Grafts of dispersed bone marrow cells are now given to patients with certain immunologic deficiency diseases, particularly Swiss agammaglobulinemia and marrow aplasia caused by drug reactions or therapy. There are two major problems associated with bone marrow transplantation: a graft-versus-host reaction or rejection of the transplanted cells. The graft-

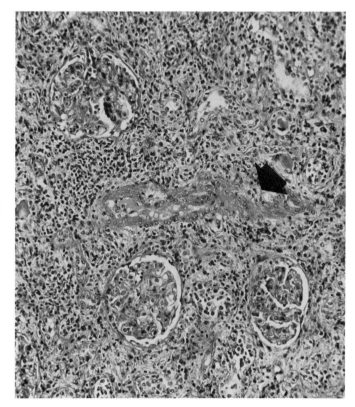

Figure 7–5. *Chronic rejection of the kidney. Tubular atrophy, increased interstitial fibrosis and a heavy mononuclear infiltrate are all evident. The transverse blood vessel (arrow) is sclerotic and markedly narrowed.*

versus-host reaction is a response by the grafted thymus-dependent T-cells to the alloantigens of the host. The mixed lymphocyte reaction mentioned earlier is its in vitro counterpart. An acute graft-versus-host reaction occurs especially when the marrow is admixed with peripheral blood as it is obtained from the donor. Acute reactions occur within 7 to 10 days after marrow grafting. Delayed graft-versus-host reactions occur during or after the third week following bone marrow transplantation; the delay is caused by the time required for the marrow stem cells to generate competent T-cells. In either case, there is a destructive lymphoid cell hyperplasia which drastically inhibits normal hemopoiesis and leads to marrow aplasia and death. Clinical signs of this reaction include hepatosplenomegaly and erythematous skin eruptions.

The marrow cells may also be rejected (Cudkowicz and Bennett, 1971). The exact process by which this occurs in man is not known. However, in the mouse it appears that *a separate class of immunocytes distinct from T- and B-lymphocytes are responsible for marrow allograft rejections*, particularly in situations where marrow grafts are performed. Marrow grafts are usually done in hosts who have been treated with ionizing radiation or cytotoxic drugs. Under these conditions, most of their immunocompetent lymphocytes are almost completely suppressed. Nonetheless, allogenic marrow grafts are often rejected. The antigens on marrow cells which elicit this reaction differ from all other transplantation antigens. The rejection may still occur in lethally irradiated recipients and is over within 1 to 3 days. In contrast, humoral antibody responses and rejection of solid tissue allografts take several days because cell proliferation is required. The cells responsible for this marrow rejection are thymus-independent even though this is a type of cell-mediated reaction. No humoral antibodies or other factors have been found to transfer this type of reaction. Treatment of mice with radioactive strontium, a long-lived bone-seeking isotope, prevents subsequent rejection of bone marrow allografts without disturbing T- and B-cell functions. Thus, it appears that bone marrow itself may be the central lymphoid organ for these particular immunocompetent cells.

SUMMARY OF THE IMMUNE RESPONSE

No better overview of the immune response can be given than to quote extensively from a recent report of the World Health Organization (Fudenberg et al., 1970):

Immunological responses are classically divided into those mediated by humoral antibodies and by cells. Both depend upon the activity of small lymphocytes which are themselves ultimately derived from stem cell precursors which in post natal life reside in the bone marrow. Neonatal thymectomy prevents the development of cell-mediated immunological reactions, such as homograft rejection and delayed hypersensitivity and also the humoral antibody response to certain antigens. In birds antibody production but not cell-mediated reactions, is dependent upon the bursa of Fabricius and it has been postulated that gut associated lymphoid tissue provides the mammalian analogue; however, no single or multifocal organ has yet been identified which can unequivocally be shown to exert a specific bursa-like function.

This suggests that stem cells originating in the bone marrow differentiate to form at least two distinct lymphocyte populations, one dependent on the presence of the thymus (T lymphocytes) and the other (B lymphocytes) independent of the thymus.

The T lymphocytes constitute the greater part of the recirculating pool of small lymphocytes, while the B cells appear to be more restricted to lymphoid tissue. Both populations contain antigen-sensitive cells, probably with specific antibody (or antibody-like molecules) on their surface.

The B lymphocytes can differentiate, proliferate and mature into plasma cells which synthesize humoral antibody. Any defect which limits the number and the differentiation of the B cell system will lead to deficiency in immunoglobulin synthesis.

The T cells can be nonspecifically stimulated in culture by mitogens such as phytohemagglutinin (PHA). T lymphocytes from a sensitized individual may also be stimulated by contact with specific antigen (which may have to be macrophage processed) in vivo and in vitro. These stimulated T cells which do not have intracellular immunoglobulins subserve many functions: (a) They divide further to form a standard population of primed antigen sensitive cells which make a major contribution to immunologic memory because of their long life spans. (b) They may be "killer" cells which are cytotoxic for graft target cells. (c) They release a number of soluble factors which are chemotactic for mononuclear cells, inhibit the migration of macrophages and possibly activate them, are mitogenic to other lymphocytes and increase vascular permeability. These characteristics taken from (b) form the basis for the phenomena of specific cell-mediated immunity. (d) They may cooperate during the immune response to certain antigens by stimulating the B lymphocytes to antibody production.

Failure to generate an effective T cell system will lead to defective cell-mediated immunity and also in the humoral antibody response in those circumstances where cooperation with T lymphocytes is important. In this case the B cell system may be intact yet the individual may show poor antibody responses.*

DISORDERS OF THE IMMUNE SYSTEM

The wide range of disorders of the immune system can be divided into four categories: (1) immunologic deficiency states; (2) hypersensitivity reactions; (3) autoimmune diseases; and (4) abnormal proliferations and neoplasia arising in the immune system.

---

*From Fudenberg, H. H., et al.: Classification of the primary immune deficiencies: W.H.O. recommendation. New Eng. J. Med., *283*:656, 1970.

IMMUNOLOGIC DEFICIENCY SYNDROMES

Many forms of immunologic deficiency have been identified in man. Most occur as primary hereditary disorders with fairly well defined genetic patterns of transmission. These presumably arise from some developmental defect in the formation of the immune system. The defect may be so fundamental as to affect both the thymic and marrow humoral immune responses, or less profound and involve only one of the two mechanisms. In addition to these genetic syndromes, there are a few usually much less severe immunologic deficiencies which occur as acquired disorders following some inflammatory or neoplastic disease which involves the lymphoid tissues of the body. Some concept of the scope of the primary immunologic deficiencies can be gained from Table 7–3 derived from a recent report of the World Health Organization (W.H.O. Scientific Group Report, 1968).

A survey of this classification indicates that some of the syndromes involve principally the immunoglobulins either in their quantity or distribution; others are characterized principally by cell-mediated immune deficits. In only a few are both forms of response totally impaired. All are quite uncommon, and it is only necessary to say a few words about several of the more significant syndromes.

ALYMPHOCYTIC AGAMMAGLOBULINEMIA (SWISS TYPE)

A severe form of hereditary immunologic deficiency, this syndrome is characterized by almost total lack of development of the thymus as well as the lymphoid follicles. The disease is transmitted as an autosomal recessive. There is virtually a total absence of lymphocytes throughout the body. Infants so affected can mount neither a humoral nor a cell-mediated immune response. They are predisposed to severe infections and most die within the first years of life.

GOOD'S SYNDROME

This syndrome is an equally severe immunologic deficiency state affecting both cell-mediated and humoral responses. It differs from the Swiss type by having a less clear genetic pattern of transmission and by the fact that the thymus is enlarged due to stromal or epithelial cell proliferation.

THYMIC APLASIA (THYMIC ALYMPHOPLASIA, DI GEORGE'S SYNDROME)

This syndrome is characterized by a constellation of clinical features all of which point to some failure in the development of the anlagen of the third and fourth bronchial pouches. The parathyroid glands are either hypoplastic or totally absent. The thymus is similarly hypoplastic or completely absent. The subcortical regions of the lymph nodes in the thymus-dependent areas are depleted. However, the follicles which are marrow-derived and thymus-independent are normal. Thus, these infants are characterized clinically by signs of parathyroid insufficiency (tetany) as well as by unusual vulnerability to those infections usually resisted by cell-mediated responses, particularly viral and fungal infections. Gamma globulins may be normal or somewhat deficient. The mode of genetic transmission is uncertain, but there is some suggestion that it is transmitted as an autosomal recessive. These children usually succumb to infection early in life. There have been several recent reports of transplantation of fetal thymus tissue into these patients, resulting in improvement in the immunologic deficit (Cleveland et al., 1968).

INFANTILE AGAMMAGLOBULINEMIA (BRUTON'S DISEASE)

Immunoglobulin deficiencies of hereditary origin may involve all classes of immunoglobulins or may be strikingly specific, affecting only a single class.

Bruton's disease is a sex-linked recessive disorder characterized by a deficiency in all classes of immunoglobulins, reflecting a failure of the entire humoral antibody-marrow system. The thymus is normal as is the cell-mediated response, but the lymph nodes and spleen lack the usual follicles. These lymphoid tissues, therefore, are somewhat hypoplastic, and there is a remarkable absence of plasma cells throughout the body. This disorder is not evident until the fourth to fifth month of infantile life when the transient normal hypogammaglobulinemia of infancy has abated. In some instances, slight improvement has been noted as these children have reached adolescence or young adult life, but most cases require a maintenance regimen of injections of gamma globulins to control their extreme vulnerability to bacterial infections. It is important that this condition be diagnosed early before these infections become so deep-seated and chronic as to resist antimicrobial therapy.

TABLE 7-3. IMMUNOLOGIC DEFICIENCY DISEASES

Syndrome	Pathologic Characteristics			Number of Circulating Lymphocytes	Immunoglobulin Deficiencies	Immunologic Defects		Genetics	Comments
	Thymus	Plasma Cells	Others			Humoral Antibody	Cell-mediated Responses		
Autosomal recessive alymphocytic agammaglobulinemia Swiss type agammaglobulinemia	Thymus hypoplastic, often undescended; lacks lymphoid cells and Hassall's corpuscles	Absent	Absence of lymphocytes in tissues	Very low	All extremely deficient	Absent or extremely deficient to all antigens (constant)	Deficient responses to all antigens (constant)	Autosomal recessive	Do not survive infancy
Autosomal recessive lymphopenia with normal plasma cells and immunoglobulins	Thymus hypoplastic, lacks lymphoid cells and Hassall's corpuscles	Present	Lymphocytes in tissues markedly deficient	Low	All normal	Antibodies present but responses not well studied	Decreased or absent responses to all antigens (constant)	Autosomal recessive	May be considered a disease entity but may be syndrome above + chimerism
Thymic aplasia Di George's syndrome	Failure of development of epithelium of 3rd and 4th pharyngeal pouch; no thymus	Present	Absence of parathyroid; lymphocytes lacking in thymus-dependent subcortical areas; germinal centers present	Low but variable; sometimes in normal range	All normal	Not yet well studied but many apparently deficient responses	Absent responses to all antigens (constant)	?Autosomal recessive	Usually recognized in neonatal period as tetany of the newborn
Infantile sex-linked recessive agammaglobulinemia Bruton's disease	Normal	Absent		Normal	All classes extremely deficient	Absent or extremely deficient to all antigens	Normal	X-linked	Recurrent infections with extracellular pyogenic pathogens
Selective deficiency IgA	Normal	IgA-producing plasma cells absent		Normal	Both secretory and serum IgA absent; other Ig levels usually normal	Normal except for IgA antibodies	Normal	Unknown; some may be autosomal recessive	Bronchitis, sinusitis, exudative enteropathy; some such subjects are still perfectly healthy
Transient hypogammaglobulinemia of infancy	?	Deficient		Normal	IgG primarily depressed	Antibody responses usually low or absent	Normal	Familial ? Genetic	May have low or low normal IgG later in life

Syndrome	Pathologic Characteristics			Number of Circulating Lymphocytes	Immunologic Defects			Genetics	Comments
	Thymus	Plasma Cells	Others		Immunoglobulin Deficiencies	Humoral Antibody	Cell-mediated Responses		
Non-sex-linked primary immunoglobulin deficiency of variable onset and expression (primary immunoglobulin aberrations)	?	Usually deficient but variable	Reticulum hyperplasia; tonsillar hyperplasia; infrequently giant follicular hyperplasia in nodes and spleen	Usually normal	Immunoglobulin deficit and abnormality invariably present but class involved, degree and direction of change variable	Deficient responses to most antigens but not others (constant)	Deficient responses to some antigens but not others (inconstant)	Possibly autosomal recessive in some, possibly multifactorial	This is possibly a large group from which specific forms may be removed as they are defined in etiologic or genetic terms
Thymic alymphoplasia with agammaglobulinemia Good's syndrome	Thymic enlargement of stromal epithelial spindle-cell type	Deficient or absent		Low and progressive decline often to extremely low level	All markedly reduced	Deficient responses to all antigens (constant)	Deficient responses to all antigens (constant)	May possibly be genetic factor	Eosinophils regularly absent or grossly deficient in blood and marrow; associated pure red cell aplasia in some cases
Immune deficiency with thrombopenia and eczema Wiskott-Aldrich syndrome	Normal	Normal	Lymphocytes depleted in thymus-dependent paracortical regions; progressive deficiency	Low and progressive decline	Immunoglobulin deficit invariably present but class, degree and direction of change variable (low IgM and high IgA frequent)	Deficient responses to some antigens but not others (isohemagglutins absent and failure to respond to carbohydrate membrane antigens)	Deficient responses to some but not all antigens (inconstant)	X-linked recessive	Associated disorders: eczema and central thrombocytopenia
Ataxia telangiectasia	Embryonic type lacking cortical and medullary organization; no Hassall's corpuscles	Variable	Lymphocytes deficient in thymus-dependent area	Slight decrease	Ig deficit usually present but classes involved and direction of changes variable; often involves IgA (inconstant)	Deficient responses to some antigens and not to others (inconstant)	Deficient responses to some antigens but not to others (constant)	Autosomal recessive	Associated disorders: progressive cerebellar ataxia, ovarian dysgenesis in females, telangiectasia in all tissues when present; may appear late
Hereditary lymphopenic immunologic deficiency	Thymus hypoplastic; gross deficiency of lymphoid cells and Hassall's corpuscles	Variable	Lymphocytes in tissues grossly deficient but foci of lymphocytes present in spleen and lymph nodes	Low but variable	Ig deficit and abnormality invariably present, but class and direction of change variable	Deficient responses to some antigens but not to others (constant)	Deficient responses to some antigens but not to others (constant)	X-linked recessive or autosomal recessive	Often die of fungal or viral infection in early childhood

Modified from W.H.O. Scientific Group Report. Genetics of the immune response. W.H.O. Technical Report Series No. 402, 1968, p. 28.

WISKOTT-ALDRICH SYNDROME

Immune deficiency with thrombocytopenia and eczema is known as the *Wiskott-Aldrich syndrome*. This curious entity is transmitted as a sex-linked recessive. It usually becomes apparent clinically because of the concurrence of an eczematous skin rash and a striking predisposition to infections. Occasionally, the hemorrhagic tendency resuting from the thrombocytopenia brings the patient to medical attention. Here the immunologic deficit appears to involve both the cell-mediated response as well as the ability to synthesize one or more of the immunoglobulin classes. Despite this immunologic deficit, the thymus appears relatively normal. The lymphoid tissues may be somewhat depleted but, in some cases, may appear normal. Often, there is a low peripheral lymphocyte count in the circulating blood which becomes more marked with progression of the disease. In the presence of seemingly normal-appearing lymphoid tissues, the primary mechanism of this disorder is obscure. It has been questioned whether the antigen recognition system or the macrophages which preprocess antigens or some protein synthetic defect in the plasma cell underlie the humoral deficit. The cell-mediated response which is also deficient has recently been shown to be improved by the administration of "transfer factor" to these patients. These experiments of nature based on genetic defects document in man the many observations made in animals of the existence of two quite distinct immune mechanisms.

ACQUIRED IMMUNE DEFICITS

Immunologic deficits are also encountered as acquired disorders. Most affect immunoglobulin synthesis. Only rarely is the cell-mediated system involved. Acquired hypogammaglobulinemia is seen in patients who have diffuse neoplastic involvement of the lymphoid system such as lymphatic leukemia or one of the lymphomas (p. 752). These neoplasms appear to be derived from B-cells. *Multiple myeloma* is a form of neoplasia of plasma cells. The neoplastic cells usually synthesize one class of immunoglobulin or only the light chains of the antibody molecule (proteoses). The abnormal proteins do not appear to have the antigen-binding sites of normal Ig and so are ineffective as antibodies. Thus, these patients may have a deficiency of antibodies despite the fact that they have high levels of gamma globulins.

In certain clinical disorders, there is extensive loss or catabolism of plasma proteins which results in an acquired hypogammaglobulinemia. This is encountered, for example, in certain renal diseases, the nephrotic syndrome (p. 1107), widespread desquamating lesions of the skin and in protein-losing enteropathies. In all of these circumstances, if the underlying disease can be controlled, the immunoglobulin synthesis which is unaffected will rapidly correct the deficit. An acquired deficit in the cell-mediated response is encountered principally in Hodgkin's disease and sarcoidosis. As a consequence, they have a reduced capacity for rejection of grafts as well as an increased vulnerability to viral and fungal infections. This deficit may be accompanied by some diminished effectiveness of the humoral mechanism, and so these patients are said to be anergic.

HYPERSENSITIVITY REACTIONS TO EXOGENOUS ANTIGENS

Man lives in an environment teeming with substances capable of producing immunologic responses. Antigens may be found in dust, pollens, foods, drugs, microbiologic agents, chemicals and in the many sera used in clinical practice. The immune reactions which may result from such exogenous antigens take a variety of forms, ranging from such annoying but trivial discomforts as itchiness of the skin to potentially fatal disease, such as bronchial asthma. Four prototype immune responses to exogenous antigens will be described in some detail: (1) the Arthus phenomenon, (2) serum sickness, (3) anaphylaxis and (4) the tuberculin reaction. The first three are models of cellular and tissue injury mediated by humoral antibodies. The tuberculin reaction is principally a model of cell-mediated tissue injury.

THE ARTHUS REACTION

This reaction may be defined as a localized area of tissue necrosis resulting from an immunologically induced acute necrotizing vasculitis. Essential to its pathogenesis is the local combination of antigen and antibody in vessel walls which then binds and activates complement at the site. Antibodies comprised of IgM and some IgG antibodies fix complement. IgA, IgD and IgE do not. Aggregation of the complement-fixing immunoglobulins by chemical means or heat also confers upon them the ability to fix and activate complement, and so formation of antibody aggregates is a key event. But ultimately it is the complement which mediates the tissue injury. For an understanding of the role of complement, we should review briefly some details about its substructure and function.

Complement (C), as is well known, is composed of nine components designated respectively, C1 to C9. The first component, C1, is made up of three subcomponents (r, s and q). All components have specific physical, chemical and immunochemical properties. When these components interact and thus become activated, they (1) promote phagocytosis of particles and organisms by opsonization or coating of these aggregates, (2) yield chemotactic factors which direct the migration of polymorphonuclear leukocytes, (3) yield so-called anaphylatoxins which effect the release of such vasoactive compounds as histamine and thus induce increased vascular permeability as well as contraction of smooth muscle and (4) cause cell membrane damage at least in red cells and even cytolysis.

The interactions of the complement fractions can be briefly presented as follows. The C1q subunit interacts with the immune complex aggregate. When bound to IgG or IgM, it activates C1s to C1 esterase. The C1 esterase then acts on C4 and C2 to form C4-2 complex which can cleave, enzymically, the C3 molecule. The activated C3, or certain cleavage fragments, constitute a chemotactic factor and other fragments, an anaphylatoxin. The cleavage products of C3 lead to the formation of a trimolecular complex of C5-6-7, another chemotactic factor. At the same time, fragments of C5 may be released as additional anaphylatoxins. In some manner, the trimolecular complex of C5-6-7 activates C8 and C9 or forms a complex of C8-9 which is capable of lysing red cell membranes and probably other cell membranes as well. A simplified view of this cascade is given in Figure 7–6.

Significant in this chain reaction are: (1) the release of chemotactic factors from C3 and C5, another being the C5, 6, 7 complex; (2) the formation of anaphylatoxins derived from C3 and C5; and (3) the cell membrane damaging (phospholipase) activity of either activated C8 or the C8, 9 complex (Humphrey and Dourmashkin, 1965) (Yachnin, 1966).

Returning to the Arthus reaction, we may now consider the role of complement in the induction of tissue injury. In the experimental animal, the Arthus reaction can be produced by the local subcutaneous injection of either antigen or antibody as long as the other is already present in the circulation. Thus, the Arthus reaction may be evoked by first inducing a systemic immune reaction to some antigen with the production of antibodies, followed at some interval by a challenge subcutaneous dose of the same antigen. Such a procedure, however, may also induce some delayed hypersensitivity or local anaphylaxis. Better models are the intravenous injection of antibody followed by a subcutaneous antigenic challenge or, conversely, intravascular administration of antigen followed by the subcutaneous injection of antibody derived from another animal. The latter combination is known as a reverse Arthus reaction. In both circumstances, *antigen-antibody complexes precipitate in the local subcutaneous vessel walls which bind and activate complement. The result is necrotizing angitis and tissue destruction at the site of the local injection* (Fig. 7–7). Polymorphonuclear leukocytes are attracted to the site by the chemotactic factors of complement. These white cells phagocytize the antigen-antibody complexes; some die and release their lysosomal enzymes.

Both the direct cytolytic action of complement and the lysosomal enzymes cause acute

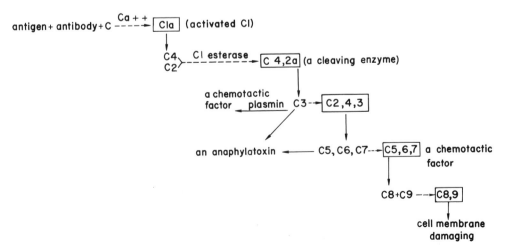

Figure 7–6. Interrelationship of components of complement (C).

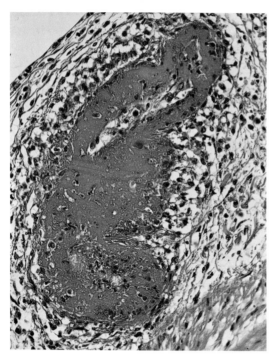

Figure 7–7. *Acute fibrinoid necrosis of walls of small vessels.*

necrosis of the vessel walls but, undoubtedly, the lysosomal enzymes are the more destructive influence since necrotizing reactions can be blocked by first rendering the animals neutropenic (Cochrane, 1967). Immunofluorescent stains disclose plasma proteins such as fibrinogen as well as the complement and immunoglobulins precipitated within the vessel wall, usually venules, producing a smudgy eosinophilic deposit which obscures the underlying cellular detail. *The combination of necrosis and precipitated plasma proteins induces so-called fibrinoid necrosis of the vessel.* Rupture of these vessels may produce local hemorrhages but, more often, the vascular lumina thrombose, adding an element of local ischemic tissue injury. The anaphylatoxins release vasoactive compounds which increase capillary permeability enhancing the inflammatory edema and neutrophilic exudation.

The sequence of events in the Arthus reaction is as follows. About 30 minutes to two hours following the challenge dose, local swelling appears. Within the next four to six hours, punctate hemorrhages appear and become confluent. Local ulceration may follow within the next 24 hours. Thus, the Arthus reaction is characterized by complement-mediated acute necrotizing angitis with consequent damage to cells and tissues in the local area. It is a model of the possible consequences of the union of antigen and antibodies in a local site.

SERUM SICKNESS (IMMUNE COMPLEX DISEASE)

Serum sickness is a systemic immune disorder caused by the formation of small soluble antigen-antibody aggregates within the circulation, hence its synonym, immune complex disease. Other disorders such as systemic lupus erythematosus and proliferative glomerulonephritis are also thought to result from the formation of soluble immune complexes in the circulation, and hence the consideration of serum sickness serves as a model of immune complex diseases. As in the Arthus reaction, humoral circulating antibodies are involved and complement plays an important role in the causation of the tissue injury.

Serum sickness may occur as an acute (one-shot), generally benign, self-limited disorder. In animals, it is best evoked by a large single I.V. injection of a foreign protein. In man, it may similarly follow the use of some therapeutic antiserum or, more commonly, may be initiated by a reaction to an administered drug. It is manifested by the appearance of urticaria, fever, edema and generalized lymphadenopathy after a latent period of about 8 to 12 days. In most cases, the illness is transient and is followed in the course of the next few days by complete recovery. Significant tissue or organ damage does not develop.

The chronic form of serum sickness usually results from repeated or prolonged exposure to an antigen. In this type of immunologic reaction, serious damage to the blood vessels, kidneys, joints and heart may occur, producing lesions reminiscent of those encountered in other immune complex diseases. The chronic form is initiated by fever, edema and lymphadenopathy, but the more serious sequelae become apparent in the next week or two. An understanding of the pathogenesis of these manifestations involves two considerations: (1) the circumstances which favor the formation of small, soluble, circulating immune complexes and (2) the mechanisms involved in their localization in specific sites in the body.

Most of our understanding of these problems concerning chronic serum sickness derives from the study of the model of this condition in rabbits (Dixon et al., 1958) (Dixon et al., 1961). When a foreign protein such as bovine serum albumin is administered to a rabbit, one of three responses may be evoked. The rabbit may be a poor antibody former or, for unknown reasons, may be relatively tolerant to the antigen; and so no antibody is formed, no immune complexes result and no disease appears. The second possibility is that the rabbit might have a vigorous antibody response to the antigen. Under these circumstances, large *insoluble*-antibody complexes are formed which are rapidly phagocytized and removed from the circulation by reticuloendothelial cells. However, while the antibody is developing, there is a critical period during which antibody is present in small amounts in the presence of antigen excess, and small soluble complexes are transiently produced. At this time, these small complexes may localize in blood vessel walls and the acute self-limited serum sickness may develop. The third possibility which may eventuate is seen in the rabbit which makes a poor antibody response that is too small to eliminate all antigen but sufficient to result in the formation of small soluble complexes which circulate in the presence of antigen excess. Repeated or large doses of antigen with an inadequate antibody response produce the same situation of antigen excess. These are the animals destined to develop immune complex disease.

There are no completely satisfactory explanations for the peculiar localization of immune complexes in certain tissues in the body while others are spared. First, how do the immune complexes leave the circulation and become trapped in tissues? Second, why are the kidneys, joints, heart and only focal segments of arteries affected? With respect to the trapping of the immune complexes, several possibilities must be considered: (1) phagocytosis of the complexes by endothelial cells lining the vessels, (2) alteration of endothelial cells which increases their stickiness and thus causes adherence of immune complexes or (3) filtration through endothelial cells and trapping of the aggregates against the basement membrane of the blood vessel wall. Studies have indeed shown that all three events may occur (Benacerraf et al., 1959).

When colloidal carbon is administered to an animal, it is first phagocytized by the RE cells throughout the body. When reticuloendothelial blockade develops, the carbon adheres and then begins to appear within endothelial cells. When large amounts of carbon are given, some is later found trapped between the endothelial cells and their underlying basement membranes. This sequence of events may transpire in the animal with large quantities of circulating small immune complexes. Vasoactive amines released by platelets may contribute to this intravascular localization by inducing increased vascular permeability as well as alterations in the endothelial cell itself (Humphrey and Jacques, 1955). Evidence has been offered that immune complexes cause clumping of platelets and subsequent release

of histamine and serotonin, increasing vascular permeability. Indeed, platelet depletion in animals prevents the vascular lesions of serum sickness (Knicker and Cochrane, 1968). Observations such as these provide a reasonable basis for the localization of the soluble complexes in blood vessels throughout the body, and acute necrotizing angitis might then ensue following the pattern already described in the Arthus phenomenon.

The localization of the small immune complexes in the kidney can be explained by their filtration through the capillaries of the glomeruli, following which they are first trapped between the endothelial cells and the glomerular basement membrane. Usually, however, they are small enough to squeeze through the basement membrane, only to accumulate along the outer aspect of the basement membrane, between it and the epithelial cells. Here they accumulate in "lumps or bumps." There is no clear understanding of this peculiar localization, but several explanations have been offered. As they pass through the basement membrane, the complexes may aggregate and become less soluble. On the endothelial side of the basement membrane, they may be more exposed to proteolytic enzymes in the plasma or to enzymes released from the endothelial cells themselves and thus may be catabolized. The polymorphonuclear leukocytes in the blood may aid in the degradation of the aggregates so situated. However, these postulations are quite theoretical because sometimes aggregates accumulate on both sides of the basement membrane.

The localization of immune complexes in segments of arteries of medium and small size as well as in the joints and heart is less easily explained. Perhaps local vascular damage predisposes to the curiously focal deposits of immune complexes which then initiate the chain of events described in the Arthus phenomenon. Conceivably, the formation of joint fluid by plasma filtration may provide a close parallel with the sequence described in the glomeruli. Similarly, there may be filtration of blood through the endocardium of the heart. We must admit that such explanations are tenuous and not totally satisfying. In any event, the lesions of chronic serum sickness cause serious and possibly progressive injury to arteries, kidneys, joints and heart.

The vascular lesions take the form of acute necrotizing vasculitis, with deposits of fibrinoid and intense neutrophilic exudation permeating the entire arterial wall, creating a great likeness to the changes in polyarteritis nodosa. Affected glomeruli are hypercellular because of swelling and proliferation of endothelial and mesangial cells, accompanied by a neutrophilic exudation. Electron microscopy and immunofluorescence disclose the immune complexes trapped along the glomerular basement membrane, usually on the epithelial side. The endocarditis takes the form of edema, and increased vascularity of the heart valves and the myocarditis have more than a passing resemblance to acute rheumatic lesions (p. 661).

Several points should be made in closing. The disease is always mediated by the accumulation of complement and polymorphonuclear leukocytes at sites of immune complex deposition as in the Arthus phenomenon. The tissues affected are essentially innocent bystanders in the immunologic reaction. There is usually no immunologic relationship between the offending antigen and the tissues damaged. The antigen may be of varied nature and only must exist in excess to evoke the tissue changes (Dixon, 1963). As will be seen in some of the immunologic diseases to be described, the antigen may be certain forms of streptococci, viruses or other microbiologic agents. And, finally, the antigenic trigger may rarely be the host's own tissues, producing what has been called autologous immune complex disease. Indeed, systemic lupus erythematosus may have such origins.

ANAPHYLAXIS

Anaphylaxis may be defined as a rapidly developing, severe immunologic reaction occurring within minutes of the combination of antigen and a special type of antibody in individuals or animals previously sensitized to the antigen. It may occur as a systemic disorder or as a local reaction. The systemic reaction usually follows an I.V. injection of an antigen to which the host has already become sensitized. Often within minutes, a state of shock is produced which sometimes is fatal. The local reactions, called passive cutaneous anaphylaxis (PCA), are usually mild and take the form of localized cutaneous swellings (urticaria, "the hives"). PCA is evoked by a subcutaneous administration of a challenge dose of antigen.

Other forms of severe immunologic reaction may induce shock and death. *The term systemic anaphylaxis should be restricted to those immune reactions in which the particular antibody, usually IgE, becomes adsorbed to specific membrane receptors on mast cells, triggering the release of powerful vasoactive compounds such as histamines, serotonin, the kinins and, possibly from neutrophils, SRS (slow reacting substance).* These vasoactive amines then exert powerful effects on smooth muscle throughout the body, particularly in blood vessel walls (Broder, 1971). For obscure reasons, the particular shock organs most severely affected by the vasoactive substances vary from one species to another. Thus, in man and the guinea pig, the musculature in the vessels and lungs are principally affected while, in the dog, it is the hepatic vasculature and, in the rat, the intestines and blood vessels. Several features of the systemic anaphylactic reaction deserve underscoring. The disorder erupts extremely rapidly and may lead to death within minutes or a few hours. The victim has had prior exposure to the antigenic trigger. Although man is usually first exposed by prior inoculation of the same agent, in some cases, sensitization to horse serum, for example, has been acquired by the inhalation of horse dander and sensitization to antibiotics has developed merely by the drinking of milk from antibiotic-treated cows.

It is beyond our scope to go into all the specificities of anaphylaxis in all animal species. These can be found in the excellent presentations of Becker and Austen (1968) and Broder (1971). The discussion here centers on anaphylaxis in man and only cites those animal observations which help in the understanding of the clinical problem. It is currently believed that certain particular classes of immunoglobulins are involved in the anaphylactic reaction of man (Ishizaka, 1967). One class has been identified as IgE; the other has not been clearly characterized. IgE appears to be responsible also for hayfever, food sensitivity, drug sensitivity and allergic asthma (Bloch, 1967). These immunoglobulins are also known as reagins and Prausnitz-Kustner (P-K) antibodies. They become fixed to tissue cells, principally mast cells, and are therefore known as cytophilic or cytotrophic antibodies. When the individual is exposed to the shock dose of antigen, it combines with the cell-bound antibodies. The question of whether complement participates in this immune reaction is unsettled. The contradictory observations tend to suggest that possibly only one of its components, such as C5, is involved. It will be remembered that this fraction may yield an anaphylatoxin. The mechanism of release of vasoactive compounds from particular target cells is still unclear. In animals, the major cell targets are the mast cells, and the same is thought to be true of man. However, platelets may also be involved. It is postulated that when the anaphylactic antibody unites with antigen, it undergoes some configurational change, unmasking some active site which, in some way, activates enzymes rendering the mast cell and possibly platelets permeable (Mongar and Schild, 1962) (Mota, 1963).

The clinical disorder in man varies, depending on the level of sensitization and the specific types and quantities of immunoglobulins present. However, in general it should be pointed out that the shock dose of antigen may be exceedingly small, as for example the tiny amounts used in ordinary skin testing for various forms of allergies. Usually within a few minutes, itching, hives and skin erythema appear, followed shortly thereafter by striking contraction of respiratory bronchioles and respiratory distress. Vomiting, abdominal cramps, diarrhea and laryngeal obstruction may follow, and the patient may go into shock and even die within the hour. At autopsy, some patients have pulmonary edema and hemorrhage while others have hyperdistention of the lungs, along with right-sided cardiac dilatation as a reflection of the constriction of the pulmonary vasculature (James and Austin, 1964).

It is obvious that the threat of anaphylaxis must always be borne in mind in the administration of therapeutic agents. While patients at risk can generally be identified by a previous history of some form of allergy, the absence of such a history does not preclude the possibility of an anaphylactic reaction. It is somewhat frightening to know that perhaps as many as one in five patients receiving penicillin develop some sensitivity to this drug and thus are potential candidates for an anaphylactic reaction. Remarkably, anaphylaxis is a rare clinical problem, but it is a model of immunologic disease in which the grave clinical consequences are ultimately effected by release of vasoactive compounds.

TUBERCULIN REACTION (DELAYED HYPERSENSITIVITY)

The tuberculin reaction is a prototype of the cell-mediated (delayed hypersensitivity) response. Delayed hypersensitivity is the principal pattern of immunologic response to a variety of microbiologic agents, particularly the organism causing tuberculosis (*M. tuberculosis*), as well as to most viruses, fungi, protozoa and parasites. So-called "contact sensitivity" to chemical agents and graft rejection are other instances of cell-mediated reactions.

The factors that determine which antigen will evoke a cell-mediated response are not entirely clear. Most foreign proteins such as bovine serum albumin evoke a humoral antibody response but, when administered with Freund's adjuvant, the same antigen evokes delayed hypersensitivity. Pure polysaccharides such as those derived from pneumococci usually do not evoke a delayed hypersensitivity

reaction. However, when complexed to protein or peptides, the polysaccharides elicit a delayed response. Similarly Benacerref and Levin (1962) have shown that when an antigenic hapten such as a chemical is coupled with a protein, the carrier protein evokes a delayed hypersensitivity reaction while humoral antibodies react with the hapten moiety. Much also depends upon the route of administration of the antigen. For example, streptococci, when administered intravenously, do not evoke delayed hypersensitivity but, when the same organisms are given intradermally, a cell-mediated response is evoked. The intradermal route is especially prone to induce delayed hypersensitivity. As mentioned earlier (p. 205), Freund's complete or incomplete adjuvant will generally cause a cell-mediated response to any antigen. The common denominator to all of these phenomena may be reduction of the potency of the antigen and prolongation of the period of absorption. Whole tissue cells, as in grafts, may therefore evoke cell-mediated reactions because the antigens are of low potency and are available over relatively long periods. The lipid moiety of cells may be a further contributing factor.

The classic tuberculin reaction is performed by intracutaneous injection of tuberculin (largely tuberculoprotein but containing a moiety of lipopolysaccharide). In a previously sensitized individual, reddening and induration of the site begins to appear in eight to 12 hours, reaches a peak in 2 to 7 days and, thereafter, slowly subsides. The extremely sensitive patient may indeed develop necrosis at the site of injection. This immunologic reaction is mediated by sensitized cells of the thymus-dependent system. Morphologically, it is characterized by the accumulation of mononuclear cells in the subcutaneous tissues at the site of the tuberculin injection. These cells accumulate principally about the blood vessels as well as the skin adnexa. Although a few polymorphonuclear leukocytes may be present, the principal components are lymphocytes and macrophages. Increased vascular permeability is a constant feature probably mediated by vasoactive substances and, in the more severe reactions, the vessels may themselves become necrotic with thrombosis of their lumina (Flax and Caulfield, 1963). Under such circumstances, tissue necrosis may ensue (Arnason and Waksman, 1964).

Despite intensive investigation, it has been surprisingly difficult to determine whether lymphocytes or macrophages predominate in the cellular infiltrate. Most investigators would favor a predominance of lymphocytes. Surprisingly, immunofluorescent techniques have demonstrated that in the early stages of the reaction only a minority of the cells can be shown to bear immunologic specificity to the specific antigen evoking the response (McCluskey et al., 1963). However, later in the reaction, a progressively larger number of sensitized cells are present, suggesting that only a few responsive cells are necessary to begin the reaction. But once initiated, other immunologically competent cells in the area become transformed. Such cellular transformation may involve the transfer factor described on p. 204. The other humoral factors elaborated by lymphocytes such as the lymphocyte-transforming factor, a cytotoxic factor and an inflammatory factor may also come into play in inducing the anatomic changes. It is hardly necessary to point out that, in the cell-mediated response, circulating humoral antibodies and complement are not involved. The tuberculin reaction is thus a prototype of cell-mediated immunity, and it should be emphasized that the same morphologic response is encountered in all allografts undergoing rejection.

AUTOIMMUNE DISEASE

The evidence is now quite compelling, although not absolute, that an immune reaction against "self" — autoimmunity — may cause disease in man. While this concept seems to be in direct contradiction to Ehrlich's (1906) "horror autotoxic," this pioneer astutely admonished at the turn of the century: "In the explanation of many disease phenomena it will, in the future, be necessary to consider the possible failure of the internal regulations." His prediction soon came to pass when Donath and Landsteiner (1904) described a complement-dependent autohemolytic serum antibody. Dameshek and Schwartz (1938) substantiated the existence of autoimmune diseases by describing a form of hemolytic anemia resulting from self-generated immune hemolysins. Subsequently, a form of thyroiditis was produced experimentally in rabbits by immunizing them against their own thyroid antigens, and spontaneous antithyroid antibodies were identified in the circulation of patients suffering from an essentially similar disease. Since then, a growing number of entities have been laid at the doorstep of autoimmunity. This list of probable and possible autoimmune diseases might include:

Probable Autoimmune Diseases
1. Autoimmune hemolytic anemia
2. Hashimoto's chronic thyroiditis
3. Systemic lupus erythematosus
4. Rheumatoid arthritis
5. Lupoid hepatitis
6. Myasthenia gravis
7. Glomerulonephritis (nephrotoxic)
8. Sjögren's disease
9. Autoimmune encephalomyelitis
10. Autoimmune thrombocytopenic purpura

Possible Autoimmune Diseases
1. Polyarteritis nodosa
2. Systemic sclerosis (scleroderma)
3. Polymyositis — dermatomyositis
4. Autoimmune adrenalitis
5. Autoimmune orchitis
6. Pernicious anemia
7. Rheumatoid arthritis

This listing is arbitrary and open to dispute. It has been difficult to establish criteria for classifying a disease as autoimmune. In almost all of the above entities, there is no clear understanding of the trigger which initiates the immune reaction against self, and the possibility continues to nag that the immune reaction may simply be the cart and not the horse. Conceivably, some underlying agent causes tissue damage, and the injured and dying cells then act as antigens to evoke an immune reaction. Antibodies to heart muscle can be found after myocardial infarction, but no one would suggest that myocardial infarction is an autoimmune disease. Moreover, when autoantibodies are present, do they play a pathogenetic role? They can be found in some individuals free of disease. In many animal models of autoimmune disease, transfer of antiserum will not evoke lesions in the recipient, and no correlation can be shown between serum levels of antibody and severity of the disease (Miescher et al., 1961). On these grounds, the issue has arisen as to whether cell-mediated mechanisms may be more important and, indeed, in certain animal models, immunologically generated lesions can be induced by cell transfer (Roitt and Torrigiani, 1967). Despite these complexities, there is considerable evidence that autoantibodies and sensitized lymphocytes do cause at least some of the changes seen in these diseases, whether they have a leading role or play only secondary parts.

INITIATING MECHANISMS OF AUTOIMMUNE DISEASE

Before seeking an explanation for the emergence of autoimmunity, we should consider the meaning of *"self-tolerance."* Earlier, it was pointed out that tolerance to one's own cells and tissues is an acquired characteristic achieved during prenatal life. An animal can be made tolerant to foreign proteins by prenatal exposure to the antigen and, indeed, dizygotic chimera sharing cross placental circulations will freely accept grafts from each other, exemplary of the embryogenetic development of cross tolerance (p. 207).

How man becomes tolerant of his own cells and tissues is still poorly understood. There are numerous theories. *Cellular antigens might be sequestered and therefore not be accessible to the immune system.* Such a concept may be valid for the proteins of the cornea or the lens, but it is highly unlikely that all cellular constituents in the body are "sequestered antigens." Alternatively, the *antigens might be present in the circulation or in contact with the immune system throughout life and induce immune paralysis.* Conceivably, certain antigens such as albumin may cause "high dose paralysis" and others such as insulin may induce "low dose paralysis." A third possibility relates to Burnet's concept of "forbidden clones." Here it is postulated that *any clone of immunocytes directed against self-antigens is destroyed during embryogenesis.* Presumably, self-reacting clones would be challenged by antigens from early embryogenesis, leading to exhaustive differentiation (Burnet, 1959a). In truth, the nature of self-tolerance is still mysterious.

Against this background, five possible pathways of autoimmunization can be postulated (MacKay, 1968) (Burnet, 1969). The first three involve normal immune responses to some alteration in the quantity or quality of self-antigens; the last two imply an abnormal immune response engendered by some change in the immune system.

1. Emergence of a Sequestered Antigen. Injury to one eye is sometimes followed several weeks later by an immunologically induced uveitis in the other eye. Surgery for cataracts of the lens is often followed by inflammatory reactions in the opposite eye. Trauma to the testes with the release of sperm into the tissues is followed by the appearance of antibodies to spermatozoa (Rumke, 1965). In all these instances, the immunologic response is quite appropriate to the sequestered antigen not recognized as "self." The sequestered antigen theory was also once applied to the causation of autoimmune thyroiditis, but has since been discarded with the demonstration that small amounts of thyroglobulin circulate freely in the blood. Seductive as this theory may be as an explanation of autoimmunity, it is probably not a major mechanism of autoimmune reactions in man, and is applicable only to a few special situations.

2. Change in the Level of Antigenic Challenge. The amount of autoantigen might fall below a "tolerogenic" level or, alternatively, may rise in level to initiate an immune response. It is clear from animal studies that tolerance requires the continued presence of the tolerated antigen. Even "low zone tolerance" can be abrogated by disappearance of circulating antigen. "Low zone tolerance" will also be broken by a rise in antigen level. Similarly, high zone tolerance can be terminated by a fall in antigen level. The amount of autoantigen might then be critical in breaking tolerance, but this hypothetical mechanism has not been clearly established as a cause of disease in man.

3. Modification of or Cross-Reactions with Self-Antigens. Loss of tolerance could result from some slight modification in self-antigens, resulting in antibodies reactive both to the altered antigen and to the native antigen (Weigle et al., 1967). Alternatively, exogenous antigens might induce cross reactions with self-antigens. Conjugation of cell proteins with a haptene, such as some drug, might yield antibodies against both haptene and carrier protein. Similarly, viral DNA or RNA may slightly alter the host genome and provide a rational basis for a new antigen that is cross-reactive with native self-antigens, one of the theories of causation of systemic lupus erythematosus (p. 231). Thus it is possible that inflammation, infections and trauma may subtly alter native antigens to evoke an immune response against both altered and native antigens. Exogenous antigens such as those of microbial origin might terminate self-tolerance because of their similarity to tissue antigens (Asherson, 1968). Rheumatic fever may result from a streptococcal infection which evokes antibodies reactive against cardiac muscle (Kaplan, 1965). A similar postulation is made for ulcerative colitis and *E. coli.*

4. Emergence of Forbidden Clones. Here we turn to theories relating to changes in the immune system. Autoimmune hemolytic anemia sometimes emerges in patients suffering from malignant diseases of lymphoid tissue such as chronic lymphatic leukemia and the lymphomas. This concurrence has been ascribed to somatic mutation in the proliferating neoplastic cells with the emergence of "forbidden" clones. In general, females develop autoimmune diseases more frequently than males. Burch (1965) suggests that this sex predisposition is linked with a stronger immunologic surveillance system in females, protecting them against cancer but rendering them more reactive immunologically and hence more prone to abnormal immune responses against "self." Viral infections would be another possible pathway for the emergence of mutations in immunocompetent cells. Such a conception has already been discussed with regard to the oncogenic viruses (p. 129). Incorporation of viral DNA into the genome of immunocytes or viral RNA with its viral reverse transcriptase could alter the genotype of cells, providing a basis for somatic mutation and the creation of forbidden clones. Enticing as this explanation of autoimmunity may be, it has neither been possible to prove nor disprove.

5. *Genetic Predisposition to Abnormal Immune Reactions.* Sound evidence now exists that immunologic responsiveness is genetically controlled not only for the broad range of all humoral and cell-mediated activities but also in highly selective immune responses against specific antigens. As mentioned earlier (p. 206), these immune response genes are closely linked to the histocompatibility genes (Benaceraff and McDevitt, 1972) (McDevitt and Bodmer, 1972). Individuals with specific histocompatibility antigenic profiles have an increased susceptibility to systemic lupus erythematosus, and the close link between the histocompatibility genes and the immune response genes suggests a possible parallel genetic predisposition to this form of autoimmune disease (Grumet et al., 1971). Conceivably, autoimmune diseases might result from genetically programmed heightened reactivity to specific self-antigens. Conversely, a genetic deficiency in synthesizing a specific immunoglobulin might in some way predispose to a disease—e.g., a deficiency of immunoglobulin A has been cited as predisposing to lupus erythematosus (Cassidy et al., 1969). How these genetic influences operate is unclear but, hopefully, will be clarified as further data are collected in this emergent area of immunology.

It must be clear that there is no dearth of speculation about the origins of autoimmunity, but it should also be clear that all theories are built on fragmentary observations held together by gossamer common threads.

The autoimmune diseases of man range from those in which the target is a single tissue or organ to those in which a host of self-antigens evoke a constellation of reactions against many organs and systems. The pathogenesis of two disorders—autoimmune hemolytic anemia and chronic thyroiditis—will be presented as prototypes of autoimmune reactions against a single tissue: in the former, red cells and in the latter, thyroid epithelium. Thereafter, some multisystemic disorders such as systemic lupus erythematosus and several others are discussed in some detail since they belong to no single organ or system. Nonetheless, they both evidence reactions principally targeted on con-

nective tissue and blood vessels. Many other diseases are suspected to be caused by autoantibodies, and so the present consideration should not be construed as exhausting the list.

AUTOIMMUNE HEMOLYTIC ANEMIA (AHA)

Autoimmune hemolytic anemia is characterized by antibody-mediated destruction of red cells. There are other causes for hemolysis of red cells including enzyme deficiencies, drug reactions and chemical hemolysins; but here our interest is in the immunologic pathways of red cell destruction. The general consideration of hemolytic anemias with all of their systemic consequences is presented on p. 704.

AHA may occur either as a primary disorder in the absence of underlying diseases or secondary to some underlying disease such as lymphatic leukemia, lymphoma, systemic lupus erythematosus, viral infections and sarcoidosis. Whether primary or secondary, the hemolysis is related to the appearance of circulating immunoglobulins. Three types of autoantibodies induce three distinctive patterns of autoimmune hemolytic anemia (Dacie and Worlledge, 1969):

1. A constellation of *warm antibodies* directed against Rh antigens, principally "e" antigens, which are most active at 37° C., belong to the IgG class, are usually incomplete and *do not agglutinate* or directly hemolyze red cells. Some fix complement while others do not.

2. *Cold antibodies* to the blood group antigen I, which are most active at 0 to 4° C., are progressively less active at higher temperatures and are complete IgM antibodies which cause hemolysis in the presence of complement at temperatures reached by the peripheral cooled parts of the body. It should be noted that the temperature of blood in the skin capillaries is of the order of 28 to 30° C. and is much lower when the body is chilled.

3. *Cold hemolysins* which are IgG antibodies against the blood group antigen P, which bind to red cells at low temperatures (close to 0° C.), fix complement and cause hemolysis when the temperature is raised to above 30° C.

The differentiation of AHA from other forms of hemolytic anemia depends upon the demonstration of the existence of autoantibodies. These are easily missed in the warm antibody syndrome since red cell agglutination does not occur here. *The major diagnostic criterion is the Coombs' or antiglobulin test* which depends on the use of an antihuman globulin serum prepared in rabbits. When red cells, previously sensitized by autoantibodies, are exposed to such serum they agglutinate. The temperature dependence of the autoantibodies will further help identify the specific type of autoantibody.

The mechanism of red cell destruction in the various forms of AHA is not simply red cell lysis. Autoantibodies, when present in high titer, may indeed cause hemolysis within the bloodstream, but often the red cell destruction takes more indirect paths. Phagocytosis is a major pathway of red cell destruction in the "warm" and "cold" antibody syndromes. Why the cells are rendered susceptible to such phagocytosis involves many considerations. Antibody may injure membranes and render the red cells spheroidal or rigid, leading to their fragmentation as they course through the microcirculation. Monocytes and macrophages have receptor sites for complement and IgG, facilitating attachment to and ingestion of coated red cells (Lo Buglio et al., 1967).

In the "warm" antibody form of the disease, the coated red cells are phagocytized in the RE system, particularly in the spleen, and so this form of anemia is characterized by moderate to marked splenomegaly (Mollison et al., 1965).

In the "cold" antibody disease, the antibody binds complement to the red cells when they are cooled in the distal parts of the body such as the extremities. This interaction with cold agglutinins is reversible and, as the temperature rises, the antibodies are dissociated; but the lytic complement firmly adfixed to the cell may complete the red cell lysis. In addition, red cells are agglutinated and rendered vulnerable to phagocytosis by the RE system, more so in the liver than in the spleen, for reasons that are not clear. Hence, splenomegaly is not a prominent part of this syndrome.

In the third variant caused by "cold" hemolysins, the destruction of red cells occurs within the intravascular compartment. The autoantibodies are said to be biphasic; they attach to red cells and bind complement at low temperatures and, when the temperature is elevated, cause lysis or increased permeability of the red cell envelope. This hemolytic action appears to be mediated by complement, probably by the activated lytic C8 and C9 components (Rosse et al., 1965). Cooling of the body permits the sensitization of red cells, followed by massive intravascular hemolytic crises and hemoglobinuria when the temperature is raised. Hence this syndrome is often referred to as *paroxysmal cold hemoglobinuria*.

What triggers the emergence of these autoantibodies? In some instances of warm-antibody hemolytic anemia, the patients give a history of having recently taken drugs such as penicillin, methyldopa, quinidine and Sedormid, suggesting that the antibodies are directed against the drug which presumably acts as a hapten with certain of the red cell antigens. However, in some of these drug-induced cases, the antibodies do not react with the drug but are directed against intrinsic red cell antigens, and so are true autoantibodies.

Hemolytic disease has occurred following syphilitic, viral and mycoplasmic infections, suggesting cross reactivity with microbial antigens (Feizi et al., 1969). Alternatively, it has been proposed that virus may be adsorbed onto the red cells and may evoke an immune reaction and that the binding of complement by the immune complex may cause lysis of red cells. The role of infections in inducing these anemias is further supported by the similarities between the clinical disease and a form of hemolytic anemia observed in experimental animals. In 1959 a strain of New Zealand black (NZB) mice were discovered to develop spontaneously, after the age of three months, a fatal hemolytic anemia associated with the appearance of warm autoantibodies against red cells (Howie and Helyer, 1965). Moreover, many of the animals developed a syndrome closely resembling systemic lupus erythematosus. Many of the tissues of these mice carried myxovirus. This murine disease could represent, then, an autoimmune disorder triggered by a viral infection in which the virus acted as a cross reacting antigen or induced somatic mutations in immunocytes with the emergence of forbidden clones.

Equally attractive is the possibility that this highly inbred strain of NZB mice might suffer from some genetic abnormality in their immune response genes, in some way predisposing to the autoimmune disease. Indeed, many patients with primary AHA have selective immune deficiencies, particularly diminished IgA levels, strongly suggesting a genetic background for the emergence of AHA. Thus, the autoimmune hemolytic anemia of man might be related to an infection which altered a red cell antigen, or it could be related to some genetic alteration of immunocompetent cells. The secondary forms of AHA associated with leukemia, lymphoma and the other lymphoproliferative disorders mentioned lend additional support to the concept of a primary abnormality in lymphoid cells. Despite the many mysteries still remaining in our understanding of the autoimmune hemolytic anemias, they comprise some of the purest examples of autoimmune disease evoked by humoral antibodies.

CHRONIC THYROIDITIS (HASHIMOTO'S DISEASE, STRUMA LYMPHOMATOSA)

Hashimoto's disease is a form of chronic thyroiditis characterized by thyroid enlargement, usually hypothyroidism, and several types of antithyroid antibodies in the circulation. The glandular enlargement is the result of massive aggregates of lymphocytes replete with active lymphoid follicles and a heavy infiltrate of plasma cells which virtually replace the native architecture to the point where the gland comes to resemble lymphoid tissue. This form of thyroid disease, like autoimmune hemolytic anemia, is an example of a disorder affecting a single organ or tissue probably caused by the appearance, albeit mysterious, of specifically directed autoantibodies. Other examples of single organ autoimmune disease are idiopathic adrenal atrophy and the atrophic gastritis of pernicious anemia, both also characterized by intense lymphocyte and plasma cell infiltrations of the specific target organ.

Morphologically, in Hashimoto's disease there is extensive destruction of the thyroid gland. Residual, often atrophic, acini remain as isolated nests within the mononuclear cell background. The thyroidal epithelial cells are usually transformed to large, acidophilic, granular so-called Hürthle or Askanazy cells. The striking female predisposition to this disease is evidenced by the 30:1 female to male ratio and, for obscure reasons, there is a strong peak incidence about the time of menopause. More will be said about the clinical syndrome of Hashimoto's disease on p. 1328, but here our attention is focused on its immunopathology.

Hashimoto's disease has long been a disorder of obscure etiology; light was thrown on its probable pathogenesis when Rose and Witebsky (1956) demonstrated that a very similar lesion could be produced in rabbits by immunizing them with homologous thyroid extract mixed with Freund's adjuvant. In the same year, patients with Hashimoto's disease were found to have serum precipitins to thyroid antigens (Roitt et al., 1956). Since then, *antibodies against three different thyroid antigens have been demonstrated: thyroglobulin, an antigen in the acinar colloid distinct from thyroglobulin, and a microsomal antigen apparently associated with the lipoproteins of the membranous component of microsomal vesicles* (Balfour et al., 1961) (Holborow et al., 1959). Despite all of these immunoglobulins, there are many reasons for doubting that they induce the thyroid damage. Only the microsomal antibody in the presence of complement is cytotoxic for thyroid cells, and then only in tissue culture. Passive transfer of serum

in experimental animals has failed to produce the disease in recipients. Although the microsomal antibody is in part IgG and might, theoretically, be expected to cross the placental barrier, it does not damage the thyroids of infants even when the mothers have active disease. Moreover, antithyroid antibodies, usually in low titer, have been demonstrated in a great many thyroid disorders such as focal thyroiditis, diffuse hyperplasia of the gland and thyroid cancer, in none of which are there the thyroid changes of Hashimoto's disease. Perhaps then the autoantibodies are secondary consequences of some primary thyroid damage.

The intense lymphocytic infiltration of the thyroid has strongly suggested a possible role for cell-mediated mechanisms. Chronic thyroiditis can be induced by transfer of lymphoid cells from animals suffering the disease to normal histocompatible hosts (McMaster and Lerner, 1967). However, lymphocytes from patients do not appear to damage thyroid cells in culture. Conceivably cooperation between humoral and cell-mediated mechanisms might be involved. Sharp and Irvin (1970) propose that some slight thyroid injury might first alter thyroglobulin and render it antigenic. Alternatively, you recall that low zone tolerance may result from tolerance induced in T-helper cells. If such T-helper cells become intolerant, antibodies to thyroglobulin might be produced through either pathway. The antibodies might then bind to thyroglobulin and thyroglobulin-secreting cells in the gland permitting Fc bearing cells to participate in antibody dependent cellular cytotoxicity, thereby causing the thyroid damage.

As with all autoimmune disease, the trigger mechanism initiating the immunologic reaction is obscure. It was once postulated that thyroglobulin was a sequestered antigen and that some trivial trauma, excessive metabolic activity or thyroid infection caused sufficient damage to permit the escape of thyroglobulin. Indeed, electron microscopy discloses apparent damage to the basement membranes of thyroid acini. However, thyroglobulin can be clearly identified in the venous effluent of the thyroid gland in normal individuals, and so the concept of sequestration must be discarded (Roitt and Torrigiani, 1967). Thyroglobulin might be rendered antigenic by some alteration induced by an infection or other form of thyroid injury. Genetic predisposition is also questioned. Hashimoto's disease and, indeed, the related conditions of autoimmune adrenal atrophy and gastritis occur together in one patient or in members of a family more often than can be accounted for by chance alone. Siblings and parents of patients with chronic thyroiditis often have elevated antithyroid globulins without manifest disease. Autoimmune thyroiditis has been reported in monozygotic twins (Hall, 1962). The 30:1 female preponderance might suggest some trait with greater penetrance in one sex. Thus, several observations point to some genetic derangement in the immune mechanism which, in some obscure fashion, predisposes to the emergence of reactivity to specific target antigens (DeGroot, 1970). But most of the evidence consists of plausibilities, and solid evidence for the etiology of the immune response and its mechanism of action is still lacking. Nonetheless, the immunologic data surrounding this form of thyroiditis are too abundant not to have some causative meaning.

SYSTEMIC LUPUS ERYTHEMATOSUS (SLE)

SLE is the classic prototype of a multisystem disease of presumed autoimmune origin. It can best be portrayed as a disorder in which the immune system appears to run wild, seemingly reacting to every antigen in the body with the production of a bewildering array of autoantibodies, particularly antinuclear antibodies. Acute or insidious in its onset, it is a chronic, remitting and relapsing febrile illness characterized principally by injury to the skin, kidneys, serosal membranes, joints and heart, although virtually every other organ in the body may also be affected. *Most of the lesions in these organs or tissues tend to occur in and about blood vessels and take the forms of focal pooling of ground substance, deposits of fibrinoid and acute vasculitis followed in time by collagenous fibrosis.* All of these changes are compatible with an immunologic causation although, as will be seen later, there is still much uncertainty about their precise etiology. At one time, it was felt that collagen was the primary target of the immunologic attack, when the deposits of fibrinoid within connective tissue were mistakenly interpreted as foci of "degeneration" of collagen. So SLE, along with polyarteritis nodosa, systemic sclerosis, rheumatic fever and polymyositis-dermatomyositis, all of which share features of SLE, were considered to be "collagen diseases" (Klemperer, 1950). However, ultrastructural and biochemical studies have proved that the collagen is not deranged in these disorders, save perhaps secondarily, and this group of entities are now referred to more noncommitally as *connective tissue diseases*

The development of sophisticated immunologic tests for identifying the many antibodies found in this disorder has disclosed a far greater prevalence of SLE than was formerly appreciated. It is estimated that perhaps its true incidence is in the range of one case per 10,000 population. The strong female preponderance is of the order of 6:1. The peak incidence occurs in the second and third decades of life, but no age is immune.

Etiology and Pathogenesis. Studies on the genesis of this disease have focused principally on immunologic mechanisms and on genetic predispositions. Because of the almost limitless number of antibodies in these patients against self-constituents, and because cell-mediated mechanisms may also be involved, one draws the conclusion that the *fundamental defect in SLE is an abnormal reactivity of the immune system expressed as total failure to recognize "self."* Antibodies have been identified against a host of nuclear and cytoplasmic components of cells which are neither organ- nor species-specific. The antinuclear antibodies (ANA) are directed against soluble and particulate nucleoprotein (NP), both double and single stranded deoxyribonucleic acid (DNA), histone, a saline extractable nuclear constituent (the Sm antigen), and RNA including double stranded RNA (could the double stranded RNA be of viral origin?). The following distinctive patterns of immunofluorescence are produced by some of these antibodies when tissue sections are stained with an SLE serum and counterstained with a fluorescent anti-immunoglobulin serum:

Anti-DNA (also soluble NP)	Rim or shaggy fluorescence; outlining the periphery of the nucleus
Anti-NP (particulate)	Homogeneous fluorescence; staining the entire nucleus
Anti-Sm	Speckled; numerous minute points of fluorescence throughout the nucleus
Anti-RNA	Nucleolar fluorescence

From these patterns of immunofluorescence, it is possible to judge which of the antibodies is present or predominant in an unknown SLE serum. ANA may be composed of the three major immunoglobulin classes — IgG, IgM, IgA. The cytoplasmic antigens evoking antibodies include mitochondria, ribosomes, lysosomes and a soluble cytoplasmic fraction (Wiedermann and Miescher, 1965). Antibodies have also been identified against red cells, white cells, platelets and blood-clotting factors which, as we shall see, may induce a variety of hematologic derangements. Every patient with SLE does not invariably have all of these antibodies. Anti-DNA is present in at least 99 per cent of patients (Schur, 1970). In contrast, anti-RNA globulins are found in only a small minority of patients.

Despite the impressive array of antinuclear autoantibodies, there is no evidence that any of them are directly cytotoxic and, indeed, their intracellular targets are probably inaccessible to the blood-borne immune globulins. Nonetheless, ANA are clearly responsible for two important features of SLE: (1) the production of LE bodies and LE cells and (2) the causation of the lupus nephritis. Although these immunoglobulins cannot penetrate healthy cells, they can attack the nuclei of damaged cells. The precise sequence of events transpiring in the formation of "LE bodies" and the LE cell has been subjected to intense scrutiny. Within 15 seconds of contact with ANA serum, nuclei in injured cells lose their chromatin pattern and become homogeneous. The nucleus concomitantly swells and is extruded to create an *LE body,* also known as a *hematoxylin body.* LE bodies are produced in vivo and when seen in tissue sections, are pathognomonic of this disease (Fig. 7–8). *This LE body is apparently extremely chemotactic for phagocytes. In the presence of complement, it is engulfed by a neutrophil or macrophage to create the LE cell* (Holman and Deicher, 1959). (Fig. 7–9). The LE cell is

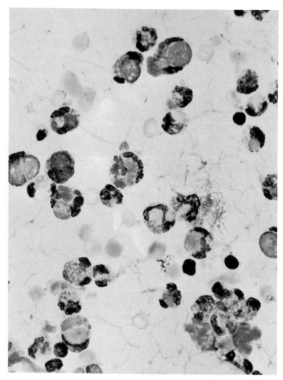

Figure 7–9. *A cluster of LE cells (in vitro reaction) demonstrating homogeneous inclusions that have distorted the enclosing polymorphonuclear leukocytes.*

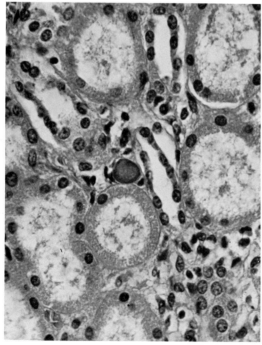

Figure 7–8. *A hematoxylin body within the interstitium of the kidney, presumably a residual of a former focus of inflammatory activity.*

rarely seen in blood smears, presumably because damaged nucleated cells are exceedingly rare in the circulating blood. Sometimes the LE body becomes surrounded by a cluster of neutrophils to produce a *"rosette."*

The LE cell test is performed in vitro because, in the act of withdrawing the blood, a sufficient number of leukocytes are injured to expose nuclei to the ANA. The LE cell test has been reported to be positive in 40 to 100 per cent of patients with this disease. Some of this variation is attributable to varying techniques and criteria. Undoubtedly, false-negative LE tests are encountered, but they are rare in the active stages of this disease unless the patient has been decomplemented by the development of widespread complement-binding tissue lesions. It should be noted that ANA (usually in low titers) are found in 60 to 80 per cent of patients with Sjögren's syndrome, 80 per cent with scleroderma, 15 to 25 per cent with adult rheumatoid arthritis; any of these conditions may also yield a positive LE cell test. Much more specific for SLE is the demonstration of antibodies to double stranded DNA which are not found in the other disorders (Levine and Stollar, 1968).

The nuclear autoantibodies are also clearly the

cause of renal lesions which take the form of an immune complex glomerulonephritis very similar to that encountered in serum sickness (p. 220). Free DNA has been identified in the serum in many patients with SLE. Patients with lupus nephritis have high titers of anti-DNA antibodies, and so circulating immune complexes are formed which bind complement. Immunoglobulins, complement and DNA can be demonstrated in the immune complex deposits distributed along the basement membrane of the glomeruli in lupus nephritis (Koffler et al., 1967). It should be noted that, in these renal lesions, the antibodies are not directed against glomerular basement membrane, and so the kidney is an innocent bystander, victimized by its trapping of circulating immune complexes (p. 1091).

The failure to document cytotoxicity for the circulating antibodies directed attention to possible cell-mediated mechanisms, and several observations implicate sensitized lymphocytes as contributing to the genesis of this disease (Roitt and Doniach, 1967). We can only query whether synergism between humoral antibodies and sensitized lymphocytes might be involved, but here the matter must rest.

Granted all the antibodies, what initiates their emergence, usually in the second and third decades of life? There is no clear understanding, but some evidence raises the possibility of alteration of native antigens perhaps by viruses, drugs or sunlight. The remarkable resemblance between SLE and the autoimmune disease of NZB mice (p. 227), possibly related to a virus infection, has raised the suspicion that viral agents may also act as the trigger of the autoimmune response in SLE. Particles thought to be viruses have been reported as intracellular inclusions in the vascular endothelium in muscle, skin, renal glomeruli and peritubular capillaries (Norton, 1969). These inclusions were only found in tissues having active lesions. While these intracellular particles somewhat resemble myxovirus, they are not identical. Immunofluorescent staining of the particles by antibodies prepared against myxovirus are generally negative, and serum antibody titers against the myxovirus are no more elevated in SLE patients than in control individuals. The antibodies against double stranded RNA provide some further fuel to the viral fire since such RNA could well be of viral origin. Nonetheless, myxovirus-like inclusions have been encountered in so many connective tissue diseases (SLE, systemic sclerosis, polymyositis-dermatomyositis) that there is a strong suspicion that the intracellular inclusions represent only an ultrastructural change in damaged cells (Whaley and Buchanan,

1970). The etiologic significance of these inclusions, then, remains questionable.

It is well established that many drugs either induce or activate lupus. Principally implicated are hydralazine, procainamide, anticonvulsants (such as dilantin), several antibiotics (including penicillin and tetracycline), reserpine, isoniazid and oral contraceptives (Alarcon-Segovia, 1969). In general, the drug-induced syndromes differ somewhat from the spontaneous disease. However, in some instances, relatives of patients developing drug-induced lupus have serologic abnormalities that suggest a familial "lupus diathesis," raising the possibility that the drugs triggered a genetic predisposition. Perhaps drugs act as haptenes which provoke antibodies reactive against the carrier protein as well; or, alternatively, they may alter nuclear antigens in such a way as to make them antigenic.

Frequently, patients date the onset of their disease to exposure to sunlight. Could ultraviolet light behave like drugs and so modify DNA as to make it antigenic? Radiation has been shown to alter DNA sufficiently to render it antigenic in its host. The amount of radiation required is perhaps not more than would be absorbed during a moderate sunburn (Tan et al., 1969). While such speculations offer a slender thread of explanation for the appearance of ANA, they cannot account for the wide array of antibodies and cell-mediated reactions encountered in these patients.

Favored today, in the genesis of this disease, is some in-built predisposition in the form of a genotypically directed abnormal immune response. SLE has been encountered in identical twins. Among 27 families, 60 cases of SLE have occurred. SLE and related disorders such as rheumatoid arthritis and polymyositis occur with greater than chance frequency among families. Patients with genetically determined agammaglobulinemia have an increased incidence of SLE (Wolf, 1962). In one study, 33 per cent of patients with SLE had the HL-A8 antigen as compared with 16 per cent of controls. Similarly, 40 per cent of SLE patients harbored an additional histocompatibility antigen (W15) as compared with 10 per cent of controls (McDevitt and Bodmer, 1972) (Grumet et al., 1971). The genetic linkage between the histocompatibility loci and those of the immune response genes has already been cited (p. 208). A selective deficiency of IgA has also been identified in some connective tissue diseases (Cassidy et al., 1969). *It is tempting to postulate, therefore, some genetic predisposition, presumably based on inherited patterns of immune response genes, as the fundamental immunologic defect in SLE.* Perhaps these patients are peculiarly vulnerable to some trigger such as haptenic drugs, viral infections or some other influence, slightly altering active antigens.

Morphology. The distinctive anatomic features of SLE are: (1) the apparent immunologic nature of the acute vascular lesions in all tissues and organs affected; (2) the multisystemic involvement of connective tissue and vessels; (3) the occasional development of a distinctive warty, vegetative endocarditis (Libman-Sacks endocarditis) and (4) the sometimes characteristic ultrastructural pattern of the lupus nephritis. No one of these features by itself is absolutely diagnostic, but collectively they establish an almost certain diagnosis. The acute vasculitis resembles that seen in serum sickness. Arterioles and small arteries (rarely large or medium) exhibit acute necrotizing destruction of their walls, accompanied by deposits of fibrinoid. At a later stage, the involved vessel undergoes fibrous thickening of its walls, narrowing of its lumen, and thus becomes a burned out, nondistinctive vascular sclerosis. Characteristically, a periarterial lymphocytic infiltration is present, sometimes accompanied by significant edema of the connective tissue and some apparent increase in ground substance. This infiltrate tends to persist for some long time in the collagenized connective tissue.

The distribution of organ involvement in several large series was as follows (Dubois, 1966) (Harvey et al., 1954):

	Approximate percentage of cases
Skin	80
Joints*	80–90
Kidneys*	60
Heart*	50
Serous membranes*	40
Lungs	10–20
Liver	25–30
Spleen	20
Lymph node enlargement	60
Gastrointestinal tract	30
Central nervous system	30
Peripheral nervous system	11
Eyes	20

*Lesions cause major clinical symptoms.

However, there are many deviations from the typical pattern and only one tissue or organ in the body may be affected, such as joints, lungs, gastrointestinal tract, central nervous system and lymph nodes throughout the body.

Pericarditis and Other Serosal Cavity Involvement. Inflammations of the serosal lining membranes may be acute, subacute or chronic. During the acute phases, the mesothelial surfaces are sometimes covered with fibrinous exudate. Later they become thickened, opaque and coated with a shaggy fibrous tissue that may lead to partial or total obliteration of the serosal cavity.

Even when the pericardial sac appears normal on gross inspection, microscopic evidences of edema, focal vasculitis with a perivascular, mononuclear, inflammatory infiltrate and fibrinoid necrosis, sometimes containing hematoxylin bodies, are evident in areas of acute involvement. These acute changes are replaced in time by fibroblastic proliferation, together with diffuse or focal lymphocytic and plasma cell infiltration.

Heart. In addition to the pericarditis, the cardiac valves or myocardium are affected in about half of these cases. The endocardial alterations (**nonbacterial verrucous endocarditis or Libman-Sacks endocarditis**), when present, constitute one of the most striking anatomic findings of lupus erythematosus. Vegetations occur on the mitral and tricuspid valves. These are small, warty excrescences or sometimes large, friable, berry-like masses of amorphous material that vary in size from less than 1 mm. to 3 or 4 mm. in diameter. They may occur singly, but more often multiply in random fashion anywhere on the valvular leaflets, usually on the surfaces exposed to the forward flow of blood. Uncommonly, these vegetations are located in the valvular intercommissures and extend behind the leaflets. Semilunar valves are less frequently affected. The involvement of the semilunar valves follows a similar pattern, with vegetations also occurring within the sinuses of the semilunar cusps. Infrequently, the vegetations extend onto the mural endocardium of the cardiac chambers or onto the chordae tendineae.

The vegetations of verrucous endocarditis must be differentiated principally from those formed in vegetative bacterial endocarditis and acute rheumatic endocarditis. In bacterial endocarditis, the vegetations tend to be considerably larger (0.5 to 2 cm.) than those in lupus, and only rarely are they as widely dispersed. More often, bacterial vegetations occur singly or in two or three discrete foci, and only very infrequently are they positioned behind the cusps. In rheumatic endocarditis, the vegetations are small and confined to the lines of closure of the leaflets on the surface exposed to the forward flow of blood and almost never extend behind the cusps.

Characteristic histologic alterations in Libman-Sacks endocarditis are found underlying the vegetations. Increased ground substance, "fibrinoid necrosis" and, in the later stages, increased vascularization, fibroblastic proliferation, and neutrophilic and mononuclear cell infiltration constitute the inflammatory changes. The vegetation itself may be composed in part of fibrin, but more characteristically is made up of necrotic debris, fibrinoid material and trapped, disintegrating, fibroblastic and inflammatory cells (Fig. 7–10). Within the fibrinoid material, darker, round to oval hematoxylin bodies

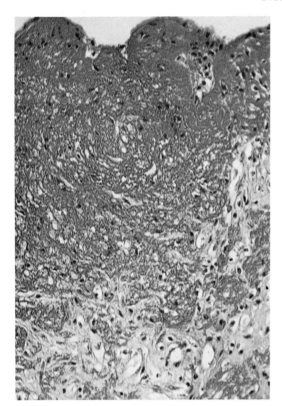

Figure 7-10. High power detail of a vegetation made up largely of fibrinoid with trapped fibroblastic and inflammatory cells.

are sometimes found. Organization may, in time, convert the vegetation into a nodule of organized connective tissue. The vegetations are sterile in the typical nonbacterial verrucous endocarditis, but occasionally they become infected by bacteria and are then converted in their gross and microscopic appearance to bacterial vegetative endocarditis. Focal areas of acute to chronic inflammation containing fibrinoid may be found throughout the heart in the connective tissue of the endocardium and myocardium, about blood vessels and in the interfascicular connective tissue planes. Surrounding these foci, there is usually a fibroblastic proliferation and infiltration of lymphocytes, macrophages and plasma cells. But giant cells, epithelioid cells and the striking fibroblastic proliferation characteristic of the Aschoff body are not present (p. 660). Myocardial arterioles and small arteries may suffer acute necrotizing injury with mural deposition of fibrinoid, but myocardial fibers are injured by resultant ischemia only in the florid, acute cases when the vascular damage is severe and causes thromboses of lumina.

Kidney. The kidneys are affected in approximately 60 per cent of these cases. When involved, the renal lesions are a major source of morbidity and mortality. Depending on the chronicity of the disease, the kidneys range from those slightly larger and heavier than normal, with a blotchy red-brown mottling, to the more chronically involved stages of overall contraction, with fine, granular, gray-brown external surfaces. Sometimes the kidneys are punctuated by small petechial hemorrhages. These gross alterations are the consequence of four possible histologic lesions: (1) proliferative (immune-complex) glomerulonephritis, (2) membranous glomerulonephritis, (3) focal glomerulitis with capillary thrombi and (4) acute "fibrinoid necrosis" of arterioles and small arteries within the kidney.

The **proliferative glomerulonephritis** is more or less identical with other forms of immune complex glomerulonephritis described in more detail on p. 1093. Here it will suffice to note that the glomeruli are the seat of an acute inflammatory lesion, resulting in swollen glomerular tufts, compressing the glomerular capillaries and filling the uriniferous space. The increased cellularity is due to swelling of endothelial and mesangial cells, proliferation of endothelial and mesangial cells and infiltration of the vascular tuft by neutrophils. Infrequently, proliferation of podocytic epithelial cells produces adhesions between the vascular tuft and the parietal layer of Bowman's membrane and/or masses of epithelial cells in the uriniferous space known as "crescents." The meaning of these histologic changes only becomes evident with electron microscopy and immunofluorescent staining. Deposits of immune complexes are usually found within mesangial cells and between the endothelial cells (lining the glomerular capillaries) and the glomerular basement membrane. This latter location is quite distinctive for lupus nephritis, and is not often seen in the other forms of immune complex glomerulonephritis. However, sometimes the antigen-antibody deposits are found within the glomerular basement membrane or trapped outside of it under the podocytes. The immune deposits in such involvements are usually focal and granular and are generally characterized as "humps" or "bumps" (Koffler et al., 1969). By immunofluorescence, it is possible to demonstrate immunoglobulins (principally IgG, but also IgM), complement and often fibrin in these deposits. Elution of this material has disclosed antinuclear antibodies as well as their antigenic trigger DNA. Such glomerular alterations tend to be widespread, involving virtually all glomeruli in both kidneys.

The **membranous glomerulonephritis** resembles that occurring as a primary renal disease (p. 1103). In lupus, it may occur as the sole glomerular lesion but, more often, it is accompanied by the other types of glomerular involvement mentioned. It usually takes the form of diffuse thickening of the glomerular basement membrane. Sometimes the involvement is patchy (both with respect to the number of glomeruli and the individual glomerulus) but, in general, all glomeruli in both kidneys are more or less uniformly involved. Such membranous thickening is best appreciated either with PAS or silver methenamine stains or with electron microscopy. It results from the uneven deposition of basement membrane matrix along the course of the basement membrane. In many cases, irregular deposits of immune complex are found along the outer surface of the basement membrane, between which "spikes" of basement membrane material accumulate. In the course of time, these immune deposits are either catabolized or mobilized and replaced by basement membrane matrix, causing more uniform and more striking thickening of the glomerular membrane. In such circumstances, the podocytes usually lose their foot processes and are transformed to an irregular cytoplasmic layer smeared along the outer aspect of the basement membrane. These membranes and cellular changes, as viewed with the light microscope, create an overall thickening of the walls of the capillary loops to produce the classic **wire loop** lesions (Fig. 7–11).

Focal glomerulitis, as the name implies, is an acute necrotizing focal change within the vascular tufts of glomeruli, accompanied often by the deposit of fibrin thrombi within the capillary lumina. The portion of the affected vascular tuft may have a heavy infiltrate of neutrophils, but often all architectural detail is obscured by the deposit of fibrin and other plasma proteins including immunoglobulins (Fig. 7–12). These focal lesions usually occur randomly among the glomeruli and within individual glomeruli. Frequently, this form of glomerulopathy is superimposed on the forms of glomerular involvement described above.

The acute vasculitis is that seen in all affected tissues or organs and is generally found within cortical arterioles as well as in small arteries. Accompanied by edema and a perivascular infiltrate, it is often responsible for ischemic necrosis of affected glomeruli or dependent tubules. Hematoxylin or LE bodies may be found in such areas of injury.

Spleen. Grossly, the spleen usually appears normal but, occasionally, it is slightly enlarged. In all other gross respects, it is not unusual. Histologically, a concentric, laminated, periarterial fibrosis involving the central and penicilliary arteries is one of the most distinctive findings in lupus erythematosus. This **"onion-skinning"** produces a wide collar of collagenous tissue about the vascular lumen many times the diameter of the patent lumen (Fig. 7–13).

Skin. In approximately 80 per cent of cases of SLE, a skin rash appears which may be quite distinctive or may be quite protean. In its classic form, it comprises a maculopapular, sometimes scaling erythema over the malar regions of the

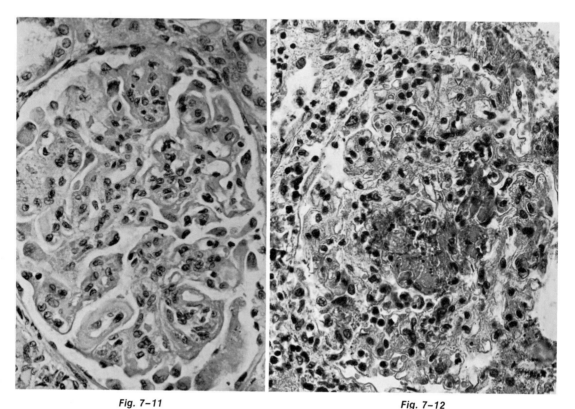

Fig. 7–11   *Fig. 7–12*

Figure 7–11. A glomerulus with diffuse "wire loop" thickening of the basement membranes. The capillary channels remain patent.

Figure 7–12. A glomerulus with focal necrosis and smudging of one of the lobules.

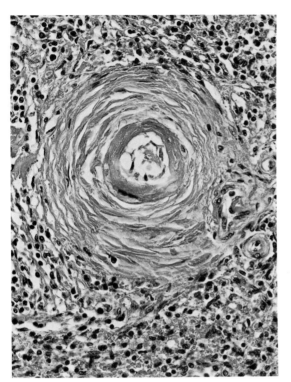

Figure 7--13. Lupus erythematosus—concentric periarterial fibrosis in the spleen.

cheeks and across the bridge of the nose to produce the so-called "butterfly" distribution. Generally, the area is slightly elevated and indurated and later may become somewhat depressed, atrophic and fibrotic. Histologically, the features are not diagnostic of SLE, but include liquefactive degeneration of the basal layer of the epidermis, edema at the dermal-epidermal junction with swelling and apparent fusion of collagen fibers, and acute necrotizing vasculitis with fibrinoid deposits in dermal vessels associated with the typical perivascular mononuclear inflammatory infiltrate. Occasional deposits of fibrinoid are found in the dermal connective tissue not associated with blood vessels. Immunofluorescence reveals gamma globulins in such fibrinoid, again suggesting the immunologic nature of the disease. Although the butterfly rash of the face is classic, skin lesions may occur in other locations such as the neck, chest, back or abdomen, and may be purpuric, bullous or vesicular. A subtle change which may be of help in establishing the diagnosis of SLE is the appearance of teiangiectasia on the upper eyelids.

Here it should be emphasized that the skin lesions of SLE must be differentiated from those of **discoid lupus erythematosus.** This similarity of name stems from the fact that both rashes assume the butterfly distribution just described. Discoid lupus generally appears as atrophic depressed hyperpigmented or depigmented lesions. There is much dispute over the relationship of discoid lupus to the systemic disease. Some authors favor the concept that discoid lupus is a purely dermatologic condition which rarely, if ever, leads to the systemic disease (Polak and Turk, 1969). However, most would take the position that discoid lupus is also an immunologic disorder (many patients have ANA) manifested by involvement of the skin only and that, in some fraction of such patients, the disease will progress to SLE.

Lymph Nodes. The lymph nodes may be enlarged and contain hyperactive follicles as well as plasma cells, changes that are of interest in view of the etiology of this disease. Focal fibrinoid necrosis in these organs may suggest the possibility of a collagen disorder.

Joints. Joint involvement usually takes the form of nonspecific swelling and mononuclear cell infiltration in the synovial membranes, occasionally accompanied by focal pooling of mucoid ground substance and areas of fibrinoid necrosis. Joint destruction such as occurs in rheumatoid arthritis is rare.

Other Organs and Tissues. Acute vasculitis may be seen in the portal tracts of the liver, accompanied by a lymphocytic infiltrate, creating a nonspecific portal triaditis. The bone marrow may be strongly indicative of lupus erythematosus if LE cells can be found. Although these cells are generally visualized in vitro, they have been unmistakably identified in tissue biopsies. Since the nuclear alterations characteristic of the homogeneous inclusions of the LE cell have been observed to occur within 5 seconds after cells have been incubated with the LE factor, it is possible that these in vivo LE cells develop in the interval between removal and fixation of the tissue. LE or hematoxylin bodies may be found at any site of immunologic injury. Vascular lesions may induce ischemic central nervous system lesions or peripheral neuropathies.

Clinical Course. The diagnosis of lupus may be readily evident when the disease presents in classic fashion but, in many cases, the diagnosis is extremely perplexing because of the many devious ways in which SLE begins. In some patients, the onset is acute while others first have an insidious febrile malaise without distinctive findings. Perhaps the most characteristic features are the triad of fever, "butterfly" skin rash and articular manifestations in a young woman. The skin rash frequently follows exposure to sunlight. Common additional findings are pericardial and pleural friction rubs, cardiac murmurs due to the Libman-Sacks endocarditis, splenomegaly, thrombocytopenia with bleeding tendency, anemia, leukopenia, generalized lymphadenopathy and usually urinary and biochemical findings, pointing toward some form of glomerular renal disease. The renal involvement may cause hematuria, proteinuria and, in some cases, the classic nephrotic syndrome (p. 1107). In some instances, the hematologic alterations are predominant, and patients may be discovered to have SLE in the investigation of thrombocytopenia which ushered in their disease. *It is, in fact, these multisystemic manifestations that are so typical of the disease.* In addition, these patients often have small retinal exudates (cytoid bodies), malaise, anorexia, vomiting and weakness sometimes so severe as to cause marked prostration.

However typical or atypical the clinical manifestations, the diagnosis of SLE rests heavily on laboratory evidence. The LE cell test is positive in the great preponderance of cases, but it must be remembered that an occasional false negative is encountered and, moreover, positive tests are encountered with rheumatoid arthritis, Sjögren's syndrome, other connective tissue disorders and certain forms of autoimmune hepatic disease (p. 1009). Moreover, drug-related lupus must always be considered as a possible cause of a positive LE test. Whether such drug-related cases represent activation of systemic lupus erythematosus or are iatrogenic syndromes related to drug sensitivity is still uncertain. Immunoglobulins are generally elevated in the serum and, more specifically, high titers of ANA are present in almost all cases. Here again, other conditions may also have elevated titers of ANA as mentioned on p. 230. Immunoglobulins to native or double stranded DNA have, to this date, only been reported in patients with SLE. The complement levels are often depressed and, while not diagnostic, are a highly valuable parameter of the severity of the lupus nephritis. Sudden lowering of complement may well be the first indication of the development of renal involvement.

The course of this disease is extremely variable and almost unpredictable. Rare acute cases go on to death within weeks to months. More often, with the correct diagnosis, therapy controls the acute flare-ups leading to long remissions which, in some instances, are followed by acute exacerbations, once again controlled by appropriate therapy. In general, with present methods of treatment and the early diagnosis of mild cases, the mortality has been reduced to less than 5 per cent. It is generally attributable to renal failure, cardiac failure, the development of bacterial endocarditis on the vegetative valvular lesions, and intercurrent infection probably related to immunosuppressive therapy (Bunim and Black, 1957).

POLYARTERITIS NODOSA (PERIARTERITIS NODOSA, PANARTERITIS NODOSA)

Polyarteritis nodosa (PN) is a subacute or chronic, remittent, disseminated vascular disease characterized by peculiarly focal, random and episodic necrotizing inflammation of the walls of medium and small-sized arteries. Vascular narrowing or obstruction results, leading to ischemic injury or infarction of dependent tissues. Larger arteries are involved in PN than in SLE. Although the name periarteritis nodosa is firmly entrenched in medical writing, the inflammatory process is not confined to the periarterial tissues but involves all of the vascular coats and, therefore, is more accurately called polyarteritis nodosa. The distribution and severity of the vascular lesions are completely haphazard, and so the resultant clinical manifestations are extremely varied and generally affect many systems.

Necrotizing arteritis is encountered in many clinical settings and diseases. Numerous attempts have been made to classify these acute angiitides (Zeek, 1952) (Alarcon-Segovia and Brown, 1964). The most recent is that of Wigley (1970):

Necrotizing Arteritis
    Acute polyarteritis (older term—hypersensitivity arteritis)
    Chronic polyarteritis (older term—periarteritis nodosa)
    Variants of Polyarteritis
        Wegener's granulomatosis
        Allergic granulomatosis
    Other Forms of Arteritis
        Temporal arteritis
        Takayasu's disease
    Arteritis in Other Diseases
        Rheumatic fever
        Rheumatoid arthritis
        Systemic lupus erythematosus
        Systemic sclerosis

Acute necrotizing arteritis is also a feature of the Arthus reaction, serum sickness, malignant hypertension, focal infections, as well as the other connective tissue disorders discussed in this chapter. Acute arteritis may occur locally in vessels adjacent to acute inflammatory processes such as an abscess. Regrettably, the acute vascular lesions in all of these settings are very much alike morphologically, and so the diagnosis of PN must be made cautiously with due regard for these differential problems. Indeed, PN may not be a true entity but rather a pattern of vascular reaction to a variety of insults.

Incidence. The exact clinical incidence of this disease is difficult to ascertain. The clinical diagnosis can be established only when lesions are fairly extensive and severe and the disease is full-blown. Undoubtedly, minimal involvements and bizarre patterns are missed and not included in incidence statistics. Moreover, from the anatomic standpoint, there is much disagreement over the precise morphologic criteria for the diagnosis, so that frequencies are reported in postmortem material, ranging from one to eight cases per 1000 autopsies. Probably the lower figure is more reasonable. In any event, the disorder is quite uncommon. While the disorder may occur at any age, the majority of patients are between 20 and 60 years old, and males are affected two or three times more commonly than females (reversal of the sex preponderance in SLE).

Etiology. Establishing the etiology of a poorly defined entity is, at best, precarious. It is only possible to present mechanisms which may lead to necrotizing inflammation of small- to medium-sized arteries. At one time, hypertension was thought to be a cause of PN, but necrotizing lesions in vessels of appropriate size are generally not found in most cases of hypertension, however severe the elevation of blood pressure. More often, hypertension develops subsequent to the acute vascular lesions, particularly when they affect the renal blood supply. A hypersensitivity reaction has been suspected, particularly since Rose (1957) drew attention to the frequency with which streptococcal infections of the upper respiratory tract preceded the onset of the acute vascular lesions in his cases. In many of his patients, the vascular lesions were virtually confined to the lungs, and there is some question as to whether such distributions should be designated as polyarteritis.

Relative to a possible sensitivity reaction triggered by a microbiologic agent, there are many similarities between the lesions of PN and those of the viral Aleutian mink disease. This animal disease is characterized not only by acute necrotizing vascular lesions, but also by renal changes which are virtually identical with those of lupus nephritis. Affected animals have elevated gamma globulins, and some have a positive Coombs' reaction and antinuclear antibodies (Barnett et al., 1968). One can only speculate that, in this disorder, the virus in some way evokes an immune reaction. Because of the likeness between Aleutian mink disease and PN, it has been argued that the latter may also have a viral etiology.

The notion that PN is an autoimmune disease is largely inferential. Its acute vascular changes are reminiscent of those encountered in other better established immunologic disorders. Prior sensitization of a rabbit to a foreign protein followed by a challenge dose evokes a necrotizing arteritis virtually identical to the florid lesions of PN (Rich and Gregory, 1943). Elevated levels of serum gamma globulins are found in some cases of PN. Immunofluorescent techniques have revealed a variety of plasma proteins including gamma globulins, complement and fibrinogen within the acute vascular lesions. Fibrinoid deposits of plasma proteins within affected arterial walls suggest an immunologic reaction, but it must be remembered that such changes may merely reflect some other basis for increased vascular permeability. In these patients, autoantibodies against vascular wall antigens have been identified by some investigators (Stephanini and Mednicoff, 1954) and denied by others (Asherson et al., 1968). Rare patients have antinuclear antibodies, but the titers are low and inconstant (Seligmann et al., 1965). Certain clinical cases follow apparent hypersensitivity reaction to drugs. However, such acute hypersensitivity vascular reactions are not good facsimiles of the chronic remitting disease of man, recognized by the earlier separation of acute from chronic polyarteritis. Nonetheless, at our present level of ignorance, the evidence favors an immunologic causation of PN in man. Whether the immune reaction is initiated by an exogenous agent or by an autoimmune response remains moot.

Morphology. The focal inflammatory lesions of polyarteritis nodosa may affect any artery of medium or small size or any arteriole in any organ or system of the body. The more usual sites of involvement are the kidneys (80 per cent), heart (70 per cent), liver (65 per cent) and gastrointestinal tract (50 per cent), followed by the pancreas, skeletal muscles, peripheral nerves and central nervous system. In the large series of cases reported by Rose (1957), approximately one-third of the cases had pulmonary involvement. Often, the lung lesions were present for years before systemic involvement occurred and, in some cases, systemic spread never occurred, raising the question of the identity of this disorder with systemic PN.

Grossly, the individual lesions are randomly distributed throughout the vascular tree, and involve curiously sharply localized segments of vessel separated by uninvolved zones. Even the focus of involvement may show a bizarre asymmetrical pattern so that only a part of the circumference of a vessel is affected. The lesions may be inapparent on macroscopic inspection but, in the classic cases, the affected vessels have nodular gray to red swellings. These may cause bead-like enlargements along the course of the artery. Rarely, small aneurysmal dilatations or perivascular hematomas may result from weakening or rupture of the wall. Intravascular thrombosis is a frequent sequel to the acute vasculitis. Ulcerations, infarctions, ischemic atrophy or hemorrhages in the parts supplied by these vessels may provide the first clue to the existence of the underlying disorder.

Microscopically, the inflammatory pattern can be divided into four stages that present the sequence of histologic events from the early to the final lesion. The **first stage** is characterized by acute necrosis and deposition of fibrinoid which begins in the media of an artery and extends to involve the intima, with consequent elevation and desquamation of the endothelial cells and narrowing of the vascular lumen. A few widely scattered neutrophils may be present in the inflammatory areas at this stage.

The **second stage** is chiefly characterized by an intense medial white cell infiltration, predominantly of neutrophils. These cells may aggregate to the point where they mask the underlying cytologic changes. The cellular exudation eventually extends to involve all three coats of the arterial wall and is particularly marked in the adventitia and perivascular tissues (Fig. 7–14). It is during this acute stage that the lumen becomes thrombosed and de-struction of the elastica, particularly the internal elastic membrane, can be demonstrated. In the last phases of the second stage, eosinophils become quite numerous and, in certain instances, may represent about one-half of all the white cells present.

The **third stage** is classically denoted by fibroblastic proliferation and the formation of granulation tissue. The acute cellular exudate subsides and is replaced by a mixed leukocytic population of eosinophils, lymphocytes and plasma cells. Fibroblastic proliferation replaces the areas of destroyed media and intima and extends out into the surrounding adventitia, producing the firm nodularity that is sometimes grossly apparent (Fig. 7–15). Thrombosis, if it is present, becomes organized and the entire vessel then becomes transformed into a fibrous cord.

The **fourth and end stage** is merely one of dense fibrous healing of the affected area with the disappearance of the inflammatory infiltrate. Scattered lymphocytes, plasma cells and occasional deposits of calcium may mark, for long periods, the site of the previous acute damage.

While these stages have been described separately, all four stages may coexist at one time in different loci, either within the same vessel or in different vessels. It is therefore evident that the focal

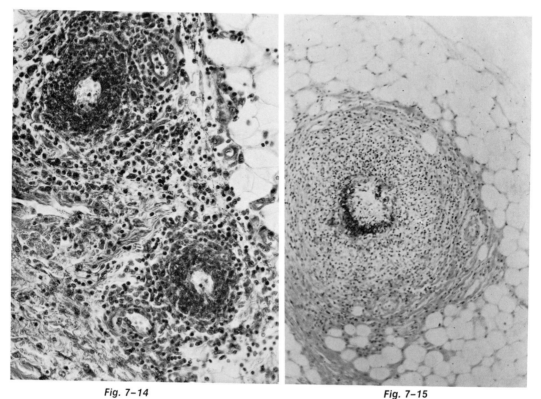

Fig. 7–14   Fig. 7–15

Figure 7–14. Intense leukocytic infiltration of walls of small vessels with permeation of infiltrate into perivascular tissues in stage 2.

Figure 7–15. Considerable fibroblastic organization of small vessel wall and surrounding fibro-fatty tissue in stage 3.

acute vascular reactions of polyarteritis nodosa do not all begin at one time. Only rarely are all lesions at one stage of inflammatory activity. When all signs of activity have regressed, it is impossible to establish the diagnosis of polyarteritis nodosa morphologically, since all that remains is fibrous scarring of nonspecific character.

Clinical Course. Since the vascular involvement is haphazard, widely scattered, occlusive and of differing ages and severity, it is obvious that the clinical signs and symptoms of this disorder must be extremely varied and puzzling. Indeed, the dominant clinical characteristics of polyarteritis nodosa are such nonspecific systemic reactions as low-grade fever, malaise, weakness, leukocytosis and a multiplicity of puzzling symptoms referable to many systems—hence the designation "multiple system disease." The course of the disease may be acute, subacute or chronic, and is frequently remittent with long intervals of freedom from symptoms. In accordance with the already cited frequency of organ involvement, disturbances in the kidney, liver and gastrointestinal tract are dominant (Griffith and Vural, 1951).

Involvement of the kidneys is manifested by hematuria and albuminuria and, if infarction occurs, the patient may suddenly complain of acute costovertebral angle pain. This is followed by showers of red cells into the urine. Vascular lesions in the alimentary tract produce abdominal pain, cramps, diarrhea and, many times, melena. These patients commonly complain of diffuse muscular aches and pains (Fig. 7–16). In somewhat over half the cases, peripheral neuritis or spinal cord involvement reflects vascular lesions in the nervous system. Lesions of the urinary tract, gastrointestinal tract and nervous system produce a characteristic variant symptom complex that, by virtue of the multiple system involvement, is suggestive of the diagnosis of polyarteritis nodosa. When present (12 to 50 per cent of cases), one of the helpful laboratory findings is eosinophilia in the peripheral blood. The clinical diagnosis can usually be definitely established only by the identification of the specific vascular lesions in biopsies of skin and muscle and by exclusion of other possible etiologies. Yet, because of the segmental, haphazard distribution of the lesions, it is apparent that a negative biopsy does not exclude the diagnosis. Since random biopsies may miss a lesion, a meticulous search should be made for some suggestion of nodularity along the course of a superficial vessel.

Death may occur during an acute fulminating attack, but more often follows a pro-

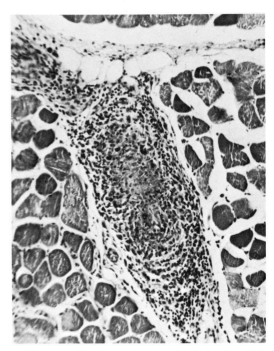

Figure 7–16. *An acute vascular lesion in striated muscle.*

tracted course, averaging five years. These fatal cases usually die of chronic wasting, terminated by cardiac or renal failure or, rarely, by massive internal or gastrointestinal hemorrhage from a ruptured vessel.

POLYMYOSITIS AND DERMATOMYOSITIS

Polymyositis and dermatomyositis describe the two major clinical presentations of a single nosologic entity. Muscular weakness is present in all cases but, in some, it is accompanied by a prominent skin rash. Because the diagnosis of all variants requires evidence of muscular involvement, they will all be included here under the term polymyositis.

The dominant feature which distinguishes this disorder from other myopathies is the nature of the pathologic lesions in the muscles, i.e., degeneration of individual or groups of muscle fibers, accompanied by a prominent interstitial infiltrate of chronic inflammatory cells (principally lymphocytes and histiocytes). The inclusion of this entity in a discussion of autoimmune diseases represents largely "guilt by association." As will become clear, there are a number of clinical and pathologic overlaps between polymyositis and the other connective tissue diseases, principally scleroderma and rheumatoid arthritis. It is of considerable clinical importance to note that some patients with polymyositis are found to have a visceral malignancy, raising speculation about possible immunologic cross reactions between tumor and muscle antigens.

The wide range of clinical presentations of polymyositis has been divided by Pearson (1971) into six syndromes.

1. Polymyositis in Adults. The onset is usually insidious, usually in females in the third to fifth decades, and is sometimes accompanied by: an atypical skin rash, Raynaud's phenomenon (paroxysmal vascular spasms in the digits, usually precipitated by cold, producing cyanosis and/or pallor), mild arthritis, as well as other manifestations common to the connective tissue diseases.

2. Typical Dermatomyositis. The onset is either acute or subacute, more common in women in the second to seventh decades, and is associated with a classic rash on the face as well as progressive muscular involvement.

3. Typical Dermatomyositis With Cancer. The clinical syndrome resembles that of Type 2, but occurs more commonly in males.

4. Childhood Dermatomyositis. The syndrome may occur as an acute intermittent or more often as a chronic disease leading, late in the course, to severe contractures, skin ulcerations and calcifications in affected muscles.

5. Acute Intermittent Myolysis. This syndrome is acute, catastrophic, often initiated by a viral infection and is characterized by rapidly progressive muscle destruction.

6. Polymyositis in Sjögren's Syndrome. Here the myopathy is essentially a part of the Sjögren's syndrome (p. 246).

Although the varying clinical presentations may become manifest at any age, overall, the peak incidence is in the fifth and sixth decades of life, females being affected twice as often as males (Pearson, 1962).

Morphology. An understanding of the morphologic lesions of polymyositis is necessary for the consideration of its etiology and pathogenesis.

Striated Muscle. Involvement of striated muscles is present in all cases of polymyositis and dermatomyositis. The first groups to be affected are almost always the proximal muscles of the lower and upper extremities. Thereafter, those of the pelvic and shoulder girdles, neck, posterior pharynx, intercostals and the diaphragm may be affected and, in severe cases, the involvement may be more generalized.

At the outset, the muscles are normal in gross appearance, possibly slightly enlarged due to diffuse edema. With advance of the disease, they become atrophic and yellow-gray as the muscle fibers are replaced by fibrous tissue and fat. Histologically, the early changes comprise a slight interfiber edema, perhaps accompanied by a scant interstitial infiltrate of lymphocytes and histiocytes. In the full-blown stage of the disease, focal or extensive muscle fiber death becomes apparent in the form of vacuolation and fragmentation of the sarcoplasm. Usually readily evident is invasion of necrotic fibers by scavenger phagocytic cells engulfing the cellular debris. At this stage, a prominent mononuclear interstitial inflammatory infiltrate is apparent, sometimes focal, sometimes widespread. Regeneration of injured but surviving muscle cells may become apparent in the later stages, producing large vesicular sarcolemmal nuclei accompanied by sarcoplasmic basophilia. The combination of muscle cell atrophy and regeneration leads to great variation in individual fiber size. In advanced cases, fatty ingrowth and dense fibrosis (containing irregular amorphous deposits of calcium) replace large areas of muscle substance (Fig. 7–17). Electron microscopy has only yielded the findings expected in cells undergoing severe injury and death. Focal degeneration of myofibrils, shredding of myofilaments, the formation of so-called "cytoplasmic" and "targetoid" bodies, increased numbers of autophagic vacuoles and residual bodies have all been noted (Mintz et al., 1968).

Skin. The typical skin rash of dermatomyositis occurs in about 40 per cent of all patients with polymyositis. It takes the form of a dusky erythematous eruption on the malar eminences and bridge of the nose in a butterfly distribution, quite similar to that seen in systemic lupus erythematosus. However, the facial rash is frequently accompanied by a similar eruption on the V of the neck, forehead, shoulders and front and back of the upper chest. Histologically, the early changes comprise slight edema in the dermis and a perivascular lymphocytic and histiocytic infiltrate, sometimes associated with overlying hyperkeratosis, parakeratosis and liquefaction degeneration at the epidermal-dermal junction. Increased dermal deposits of acid mucopolysaccharides have been demonstrated by the Alcian-blue reaction in both clinically involved areas of the skin and in uninvolved areas. In about 25 per cent of the cases, the rash is quite atypical and ranges from the sclerotic atrophy of scleroderma to scaly patches on the elbows, knees and knuckles. In some cases, a dusky lilac suffusion occurs on the upper eyelids, called the heliotrope rash (considered by some to be pathognomonic for dermatomyositis). In the late stages of skin involvement, dermal atrophy, fibrosis and calcification may ensue.

Other Systems. In common with the other connective tissue diseases, many organs and systems may be affected. Articular reactions are not usually prominent, but may closely resemble rheumatoid arthritis (p. 1466). Involvement of the gastrointestinal tract has been described in well documented cases of polymyositis, blurring the line between scleroderma and this entity (Kleckner,

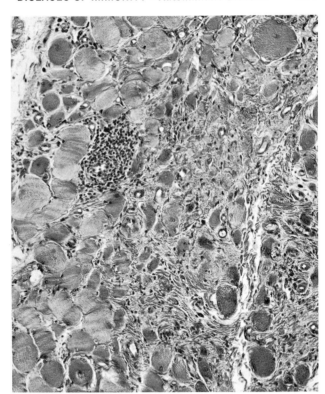

Figure 7-17. *A section of striated muscle with interstitial fibrosis, leukocytic infiltration, muscle cell atrophy and variability in muscle fiber size due to regenerative activity.*

1970). The visceral muscular involvement resembles that seen in striated muscles and basically comprises muscle injury and death accompanied by an interstitial inflammatory mononuclear infiltrate, followed by fibrous replacement. Such changes would be indistinguishable from those of systemic sclerosis. In childhood forms of the disease, an acute necrotizing vasculitis may be seen resembling polyarteritis nodosa.

It is apparent that there are many morphologic similarities among the so-called connective tissue diseases. Myopathy may be found in SLE, rheumatoid arthritis, systemic sclerosis and rheumatic fever as well as polymyositis. In all, an interstitial inflammatory reaction is present, but not the extensive muscle fiber injury and necrosis seen in dermatomyositis. Similarly, acute arteritis is common to many but, of course, is most characteristic of polyarteritis nodosa. While ischemic muscle damage may occur in polyarteritis, the myopathy is far more destructive in polymyositis and is disproportionate to the arterial involvement.

Etiology and Pathogenesis. The meaning of "guilt by association" must now be apparent with regard to the causation of polymyositis. The evidence that it has an immune basis derives largely from the many similarities between this disease and the other connective tissue disorders having more substantial evidence for an autoimmune origin. Antinuclear antibodies have been demonstrated in about a third of the cases but, generally, the titers have been low and of questionable significance (Seligmann et al., 1965).

The association of polymyositis, in about 15 to 20 per cent of the cases, with an underlying visceral malignant tumor has raised the possibility of some cross reaction between antigens in the tumor cells and the muscle fibers. However, these cancers may occur in virtually any organ, i.e., lung, stomach, breast, kidney, uterus and ovary, as well as lymphomas and thymomas; it would be quite remarkable if all such neoplasms bore antigens cross reactive with muscle antigens. Equally attractive are the notions that the tumors elaborate or release products having direct toxicity for muscle or that, indeed, the cancer and the myositis are unrelated. Nonetheless, rare cases of polymyositis have been reported where extracts of the tumor have elicited skin sensitivity reactions (Curtis et al., 1961). Despite all of this evidence, efforts to identify distinctive levels of antimyosin antibodies in these patients have led to negative or inconclusive results (Stern et al., 1967). Although some of these patients do, indeed, have such antibodies, they are not present in higher titers or more frequently than in other forms of muscular disease or among normal controls.

The etiology of this disease must be considered as uncertain.

The prominence of the inflammatory infiltrate in the muscles has understandably led to a search for possible microbiologic causations. A number of agents have been suspected, but of greatest interest today is the myxovirus. Inclusions closely resembling the myxovirus have been identified in affected muscle fibers (Sato et al., 1971). However, in these patients, only low to moderate levels of serum antibodies against the myxovirus were present and are also often present in normal controls. Efforts to isolate the virus have been unsuccessful to date. The intracellular inclusions may well be the consequence of muscle cell injury and not true virions. Thus, at the present time, the causation of polymyositis is unknown, and autoimmunity has certainly not been established.

Clinical Features. The major manifestations of polymyositis and dermatomyositis should be apparent from the preceding discussion. Muscle weakness, tenderness on palpation, muscular pain and eventually motor disability are the most important clinical findings. The proximal nature of the muscular involvement helps to differentiate this disease from some of the dystrophies (p. 1424). In chronic cases, the patient may be confined to a wheelchair or bed. The skin rash may be followed by sufficient dermal fibrosis and skin atrophy to cause stiffness of the fingers. Raynaud's phenomemon occurs in about one-third of the patients. The involvement of the joints is usually mild and rarely causes joint destruction. Dysphagia, due to involvement of the pharyngeal muscles, can be a very disabling and serious clinical problem. When visceral involvement occurs, colicky abdominal pain and constipation complicate the musculoskeletal disability. The diagnosis depends on: (1) demonstration of elevated serum enzymes derived from muscle (glutamic-oxaloacetic transaminase and aldolase); (2) detection of excessive creatinuria; (3) electromyographic evidence of muscle disease and (4) morphologic confirmation of the nature of the muscle involvement. With regard to the biopsy, it must be recalled that the disease may be focal, and careful search must be made for appropriate biopsy sites to avoid false-negative diagnoses.

SYSTEMIC SCLEROSIS, (PROGRESSIVE SYSTEMIC SCLEROSIS, SCLERODERMA)

Systemic sclerosis (SS) is a prime example of a connective tissue disease since it is characterized by inflammatory and fibrotic changes throughout the interstitium of many organs in the body, principally the skin. For a time, attention was focused on the sclerotic atrophy of the skin, hence the older name, scleroderma. Now it is appreciated that, in addition, the gastrointestinal tract, heart, lungs, kidneys and virtually every other internal organ may, in the progression of the disease, suffer similar sclerosis, justifying the designation, systemic sclerosis. Indeed, it is the visceral involvement which sometimes causes death from renal failure, myocardial failure or intestinal malabsorption and progressive inanition. Women are affected twice as often as men, usually in the third to fifth decades. However, no age is immune, and the disease has been identified in infants six months old and in the advanced years of life.

In systemic sclerosis, the skin usually becomes diffusely involved, beginning in the hands and extending proximally to eventually affect the neck, face, shoulders and possibly the entire body. Such diffuse scleroderma is, in the great majority of instances, followed in time by progressive systemic sclerosis. *A localized form of scleroderma, known as morphea, also exists.* Circumscribed scleroderma takes the form of yellow to white round or oval plaques demarcated on their periphery by red-blue hyperemia. Sometimes the plaques follow the distribution of a cutaneous nerve. This localized disease is only rarely associated with subsequent visceral involvement but, on occasion, disseminated visceral sclerosis develops in patients who first present with only a focal cutaneous lesion.

Etiology and Pathogenesis. SS is a disease of uncertain etiology. Three lines of investigation have long been pursued, one concerned with the metabolism of connective tissue and its ground substance, another with microvascular abnormalities and still another focused on some possible immunologic derangement.

Because of the widespread and striking overgrowth of connective tissue, it was natural to assume some derangement in the activity of fibroblasts or turnover of collagen. A host of studies have not, in the final analysis, disclosed any constant abnormality in fibrillogenesis, the chemical or physical structure of collagen or the composition of the ground substance (Winkelmann, 1971). An increase in the collagen content of affected skin, evidence of active fibrillogenesis and immaturity of collagen have all been demonstrated, but would be anticipated in any lesion undergoing active collagenization (Keiser and Sjoerdsma, 1969) (Uitto et al., 1969) (Hayes and Rodnan, 1968). Attention has been directed to the connective tissue ground substance. While there is some increase in hexosamines in the dermis, this finding is neither constant nor specific for this disease (Fleishmajer and Krol, 1967). Abnormalities in serotonin and tryptophane metabolism have been identified in rare patients, but are unsubstantiated as fundamental defects in all cases. As will be seen, vascular lesions are common in the sclerotic connective tissue of most organs, and so the issue arises as to whether the collagenization and atrophy might reflect ischemia. A number of studies have revealed narrowing of the microvasculature, but such changes might be secondary to the surrounding inflammatory sclerosis and might not be causal (Norton et al., 1968).

A great deal of evidence supports the view that SS is an immunologic disease. Many of its clinical and morphologic manifestations closely resemble and overlap other connective tissue diseases such as rheumatoid arthritis, SLE, serum sickness, Sjögren's syndrome, all having more reliable evidence of immunologic origins (Tuffanelli and Winkelmann, 1962). The inflammatory and vascular lesions which antedate the progressive sclerotic atrophy are entirely consistent with antibody-mediated lesions (Rodnan, 1963b). Immunofluorescent techniques reveal depositions of gamma globulin and complement in the acute vascular lesions (Toth and Alpert, 1971). A host of serologic abnormalities are seen in many but not all patients. Hypergammaglobulinemia, principally due to an increase in IgG, occurs in about one-half of patients. About a third of these cases have positive tests for rheumatoid factor, and some have positive LE cell tests (Rowell, 1962). Antinuclear antibodies may be found in the serum of up to 80 per cent of patients with SS, but the titers are relatively low as compared to those in SLE. However, there is little if any correlation between the levels of antinuclear antibodies and the clinical activity or severity of the disease (Rothfield and Rodnan, 1968). Antibodies to DNA are not found in SS, clearly differentiating this disorder from SLE.

Because of the lack of correlation between serum antibody titers and the activity of the disease, attention has been directed toward a possible cell-mediated mechanism. It has been reported that lymphocytes from two patients with SS destroyed human embryonic fibroblasts in tissue culture, but this observation has not yet been confirmed (Trayanova et al., 1966). Despite the wealth of immunologic data, no clear reason has been identified for activation of immune reaction. Recently, cytoplasmic inclusions resembling myxovirus particles have been identified in the endothelial cells in the kidneys of a few patients with systemic sclerosis (Becker, 1968). These inclusions are identical with those identified in the endothelial cells of patients with SLE and polymyositis, and in all of these situations, it has been impossible to confirm the true viral nature of the intracellular particles or to ascertain their pathogenetic significance (Haas and Yunis, 1970). Thus, with respect to the causation of this disease, we have an excess of theories and a dearth of facts.

Morphology. Virtually all organs may be involved in SS. The most prominent changes occur in the skin, musculoskeletal system and alimentary tract but, in addition, lesions are often present in the blood vessels, heart, lungs, kidneys and peripheral nerves.

Skin. The great majority of patients have diffuse sclerotic atrophy of the skin which usually begins in the fingers and distal regions of the upper extremities and extends proximally to involve the upper arms, shoulders, neck and face. In advanced cases, the entire back and abdomen, as well as the lower extremities, may be involved. In the early stages of the disease, affected skin areas are somewhat edematous and have a doughy consistency. Often, pigmentation resulting from increased melanin production in the basal layer of the epidermis darkens these areas. With progression, the edematous phase is replaced by progressive fibrosis of the dermis which becomes tightly bound to subcutaneous structures. In the long chronicity of the disease, the subcutaneous fat and soft tissues undergo sclerotic atrophy (Fig. 7–18). The fingers take on a tapered, claw-like appearance with limitation of motion in the joints, and the face becomes a drawn mask. Loss of blood supply may lead to cutaneous ulcerations. In some instances, dissolution of the bony substance of the finger tips results in autoamputations.

Microscopically, the edematous stage of SS is characterized by an increase in mucopolysaccharide ground substance, with separation and swelling of the collagen fibers of the dermis. This is usually accompanied by a scant lymphocytic and plasma infiltrate, principally about dermal vessels. With progression, there is a marked increase of compact collagen in the dermis, along with thinning of the epidermis, loss of rete pegs, atrophy of dermal appendages, and hyaline thickening of the walls of dermal arterioles and capillaries. Focal areas of calcification may produce calcinosis circumscripta or more widespread calcinosis universalis.

Musculoskeletal System. Inflammatory synovitis is common in SS. The changes comprise infiltrates of lymphocytes and plasma cells, sometimes gathered into focal aggregates, associated with hypertrophy and hyperplasia of the synovial soft tis-

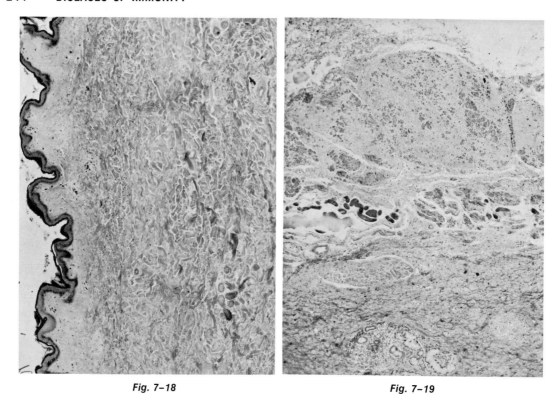

Fig. 7-18

Fig. 7-19

Figure 7-18. *Atrophy of skin with dense sclerosis of dermal tissue and atrophy of skin adnexae.*
Figure 7-19. *Extensive fibrous replacement of the musculature of the esophagus. Isolated striated muscle fibers of the pharyngeal constrictor muscles are present.*

sues. Later, fibrosis ensues. It is evident that these changes are closely reminiscent of rheumatoid arthritis, but joint destruction is not common in SS. As in polymyositis, the muscles may be affected, beginning usually with the proximal groups. Interfiber edema and perivascular infiltrates of lymphocytes and plasma cells comprise the early changes followed by progressive interstitial fibrosis and sometimes regressive alterations in the fibers themselves. However, in systemic sclerosis, the primary change involves the interstitium, while in polymyositis, fiber damage is a prominent early lesion. Thickening of the basement membrane of the microcirculation and microvascular sclerosis accompanies the interstitial fibrosis.

Alimentary Tract. The entire alimentary tract may be affected. Thickening of the skin of the face results in narrowing of the oral aperture. Progressive atrophy and collagenous fibrous replacement of the muscularis may develop at any level of the gut, but is most marked in the esophagus (Fig. 7-19). The lower two-thirds of the esophagus often develops a rubber hose inflexibility and usually has the most marked narrowing. The mucosa may be thinned and even ulcerated. Excessive amounts of collagen are present in the lamina propria and submucosa, and there is variable replacement of the muscularis by scar tissue. The walls of the small intestine and colon may likewise be-

come collagenized and atrophic. Loss of villi and microvilli in the small intestine provides the anatomic basis for the sometimes encountered malabsorption syndrome. Throughout the intestinal tract wherever there is fibrous atrophy, small vessels show perivascular infiltrates and hyaline collagenous thickening of their walls.

Blood Vessels. Along with the diffuse connective tissue changes in SS, there are prominent vascular lesions. These affect principally arterioles and small arteries. The vascular lesions take one of two forms. The most common pattern comprises intimal thickening caused by an increased deposition of acid mucopolysaccharides, accompanied by medial hypertrophy and proliferation. Perivascular lymphocytic and plasma cell infiltrations are seen about these involved vessels. The other pattern takes the form of acute necrotizing arteriolitis and arteritis characterized by fibrinoid deposits and neutrophilic and eosinophilic inflammatory infiltrates within the vessel wall. The first of these two patterns is quite typical of malignant hypertension and, in this context, many patients with SS have renal vascular lesions in the kidney which antedate the hypertension and, indeed, may cause it. However, cause and effect have not been clearly distinguished here. The more acute vascular lesions are very similar to those encountered in serum sickness and polyarteritis nodosa. Gamma globulins and complement can be identified in the fibrinoid deposits, along with fibrin. But here again, these proteinous precipitates may merely reflect increased vascular permeability. In the late chronic atrophic stages of the disease, both forms of vascular change eventuate in hyaline collagenous thickening of vessel walls.

Kidneys. The kidneys are a frequently damaged site, and renal failure accounted for nearly half of all deaths in one large series (Rodnan, 1963a). The changes take many forms. Localized or diffuse thickening of the glomerular basement membrane may be seen reproducing the wire loop lesions of lupus erythematosus. The diffuse basement membrane thickening is also identical with that seen in the primary disease membranous glomerular nephritis, and patients with such glomerular changes, whatever the etiology, almost always develop the nephrotic syndrome (p. 1107). The vascular lesions previously described are common in affected kidneys. When an afferent arteriole develops necrotizing arteriolitis, the glomerular vascular tuft frequently undergoes necrosis. Thrombosis of vessels may lead to microinfarcts. In still other patients, there is diffuse thickening of the axial framework of the glomerulus, producing changes reminiscent of diffuse intercapillary glomerulosclerosis (p. 268).

Lungs. The lungs are the site of diffuse interstitial and alveolar fibrosis, with varying degrees of small pulmonary vessel involvement. In some instances, the alveolar walls are thickened. In others, there is apparent distention of alveolar spaces and rupture of septa, leading to cyst-like cavities. Basement membrane thickening in the capillaries of the pulmonary alveolar walls has been identified, apparently antedating the appearance of interstitial fibrosis (Wilson et al., 1964).

Other Organs. Focal interstitial fibroses are encountered in the heart, accompanied usually by perivascular infiltrates of lymphocytes and plasma cells. Pericarditis and pericardial effusion may also occur, and there have been reports of valvular fibrosis and thickening, but it is not certain that such patients did not have coincidental rheumatic heart disease. The myocardial fibrosis may, with the progression of the disease, replace extensive areas of cardiac muscle and account for irregularities in rhythm and progressive cardiac failure. Rarely, a mono- or polyneuropathy appears due to loss of blood supply to the axis cylinders, resulting from the perineurial fibrosis and vascular sclerosis.

Clinical Course. Systemic sclerosis is obviously a multisystem disorder. In most cases, the disease presents with either symmetrical edema and thickening of the skin of the hands and fingers or with Raynaud's phenomenon. Occasionally, the disease presents with articular manifestations in the form of pain and stiffness of the finger and knee joints. Many patients are thus first diagnosed as having rheumatoid arthritis. Occasional cases attract attention because of visceral involvement with symptoms such as dysphagia, malabsorption, respiratory difficulties or elevated blood pressure. In the usual case, however, the skin manifestations progress to the sclerotic atrophy described and are associated with muscular weakness and atrophy, sometimes leading to marked motor disability and even total incapacitation (Fig. 7–20). Some fortunate patients have an indolent course or enjoy long remissions from progression of their disease (Tuffanelli and Winkelmann, 1961). In most patients, evidence of visceral sclerosis becomes apparent within a year. Malignant hypertension with renal involvement, progressive cardiac decompensation, progressive respiratory deficits, or marked malabsorption and inanition make their appearance. The patients with advanced pulmonary involvement may develop right-sided cardiac dysfunction. Generally, about 50 per cent of those with progressive disease are dead within two to three years.

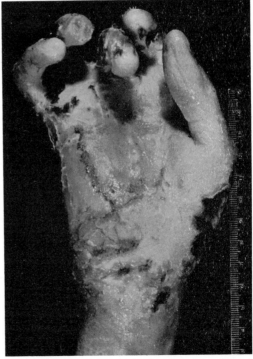

Figure 7–20. *Advanced scleroderma involving the hand. Flexion contractures, atrophy of substance and sloughing necrosis of skin are evident.*

Malignant hypertension, when it develops in patients with renal involvement, is ominous and usually is followed by death within weeks to months. For reasons that are not clear, this disease is most devastating in black females.

SJÖGREN'S SYNDROME

Sjögren's syndrome is a rare disorder usually characterized by (1) keratoconjunctivitis sicca (dryness of the eyes with lack of tears), (2) xerostomia (dryness of the mouth) with or without salivary gland enlargement and (3) rheumatoid arthritis. It occurs principally in menopausal and postmenopausal women, but may begin in childhood. Although it is a systemic, probably immunologic disease, some patients manifest only eye and mouth changes while, in others, these features occur together with rheumatoid arthritis, SLE, polymyositis, systemic sclerosis or polyarteritis nodosa. Of the 62 cases of Sjögren's syndrome studied by Bloch et al. (1965), 32 had rheumatoid arthritis, 3 had scleroderma, 4 had polymyositis and 23 had predominantly eye and mouth manifestations without evidence of systemic connective tissue disease.

The ocular and oral changes reflect a secretory failure of the lacrimal and salivary glands. But other secretory glands responsible for moistening the nose, pharynx, larynx, trachea, bronchi and vagina may also be affected. Because of the lack of tears, the corneal epithelium dries and becomes eroded, creating corneal ulcers. Secondary inflammatory changes follow. The dryness of the mouth is associated, in about half of the cases, with episodes of salivary gland enlargement. Whether enlarged or not, the glands undergo striking histologic changes reminiscent of the intense lymphocytic and plasma cell infiltration of Hashimoto's thyroiditis. This infiltrate may reach such proportions as to create germinal follicles and it is often accompanied by partial to complete atrophy of the secretory acini. Indeed, the total replacement of the native architecture is easily confused with a lymphoma. Inspissated secretions within the ducts and proliferation of ductal epithelium lead to the formation of myoepithelial islands within the mononuclear infiltrate.

The combination of lacrimal and salivary gland inflammatory involvement was once called Mikulicz's *disease* (Morgan and Castleman, 1953). More recently, the entity of Mikulicz's disease has been replaced by the more noncommittal Mikulicz's *syndrome* broadened to include lacrimal and salivary gland enlargement, whatever the cause (Sjögren's syndrome, sarcoidosis, leukemia, lymphoma, etc.).

Sjögren's syndrome is of interest because it represents a confluence of all of the presumed autoimmune, connective tissue diseases previously discussed. Perhaps it is more accurate to say that, in any of these connective tissue diseases, inflammatory involvement of the lacrimal, salivary and other secretory glands may occur to produce Mikulicz's syndrome. In any event, a host of immunologic changes are encountered in these patients. Nearly all have hypergammaglobulinemia due to a diffuse increase in the concentration of all three major classes of immunoglobulins—IgG, IgA and IgM. Nearly all patients have the rheumatoid factor; approximately 70 per cent have antinuclear antibodies; and about 25 per cent yield a positive LE cell test. In addition, a variety of other immunologic changes may be seen in these patients, such as complement fixing antibodies, and antithyroid antibodies. Interestingly, it has been noted that the circulating lymphocytes in a majority of patients fail to respond to phytohemagglutinin stimulation (Bloch et al., 1965) (Leventhal et al., 1967). Despite all the extraordinary immunologic abnormalities, the trigger evoking these reactions remains unknown.

Several other aspects of this syndrome are of considerable interest. Although glomerular lesions or renal failure such as occurs in many of the other connective tissue diseases is uncommon in Sjögren's syndrome, a number of more discrete renal abnormalities principally involving tubular function have been identified. A renal concentrating defect has been attributed to decreased permeability to water of the distal convoluted and collecting tubules (Kahn, 1962). Renal tubular acidosis, aminoaciduria and increased clearance of phosphate and urate, characteristic of the Fanconi syndrome, have also been described (Shearn and Tu, 1968). Late in the course of some patients with Sjögren's syndrome, disseminated lymphomas have appeared (Talal and Bunim, 1964). This increased incidence of lymphoma is considerably greater in Sjögren's syndrome than in other connective tissue diseases, suggesting that persistent immunologic and lymphoid hyperactivity may, in the course of time, be transformed to a malignant lymphoma. In support of such a notion, some patients have had disseminated lymphoid abnormalities designated as "pseudolymphoma." These may simply represent intergrades between the classic Sjögren's syndrome and the true malignant process (Talal et al., 1967).

WEGENER'S GRANULOMATOSIS

This rare disorder is characterized by: (1) acute necrotizing lesions of the respiratory tract, including the nose and upper airways; (2) disseminated, focal, necrotizing vasculitis principally in the lungs and upper airways but affecting other sites as well; and (3) renal disease in the form of focal glomerulitis or diffuse glomerulonephritis (Tuohy et al., 1958). It affects men and women of all ages, most frequently in middle life. In two-thirds of the cases, it begins as an apparent chronic sinusitis; in the remainder, as a persistent pneumonitis. However, in time the systemic nature of the disease becomes apparent, since most patients develop one or more of the following manifestations: skin rash, muscle pains, articular involvements, renal dysfunction and mono- or polyneuritis. Before present-day therapy, most cases went rapidly downhill to death within a year of the diagnosis. A limited form of this disease has been described by Carring-ton and Liebow (1966), restricted largely to pulmonary involvement (some with extrapulmonary involvement) but no extension to the kidneys.

Morphologically, the involvement of the respiratory tract takes the form of focal acute necroses in the nasal and oral cavities, paranasal sinuses, larynx or trachea, as well as focal lesions scattered throughout the lung parenchyma. These areas are generally surrounded by a zone of fibroblastic proliferation with Langhans' type or foreign body type giant cells and a leukocytic infiltrate. Sometimes the acute necrosis produces total granular disintegration of the background tissue, creating a more than superficial resemblance to a very acute tubercle (Fig. 7–21). These lesions undergo progressive fibrosis and organization and during this phase resemble the so-called hard tubercle. The lesions in the lungs are usually small but occasionally take the form of large (5 to 6 cm.) foci of consolidation.

The acute vasculitis affects arteries and

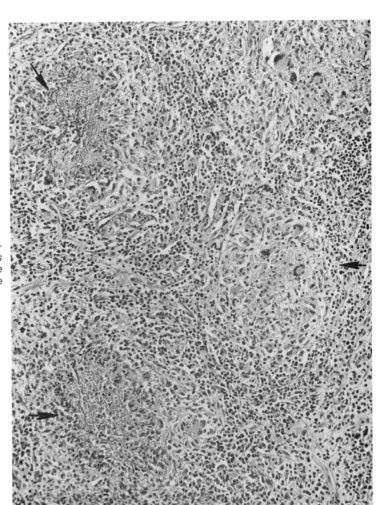

Figure 7–21. Multiple granulomas in the lungs in Wegener's granulomatosis (arrows). Note the central necrosis and multinucleate giant cells.

veins and has been described in virtually every vessel and organ of the body, favored sites being the respiratory tract, kidneys and spleen. These acute lesions are almost identical with those of the acute phase of polyarteritis nodosa with fibrinoid necrosis of the vessel wall and diffuse polymorphonuclear and eosinophilic infiltrations. The acute phase is followed by fibrous thickening of the arterial wall which may induce thrombosis and sometimes fibrosis of the vascular lumen (Budzilovich and Wilens, 1960) (Fig. 7–22).

The renal lesions consist of acute focal glomerular necroses with thromboses of isolated glomerular capillary loops. Sometimes the total glomerular tuft is affected, progressing to complete obliteration of the entire glomerulus. Proliferation of endothelial or epithelial cells may produce adhesions between the two layers of Bowman's capsule. These lesions are not at all dissimilar to those seen in bacterial endocarditis. When sufficiently diffuse, the changes resemble proliferative glomerulonephritis (p. 1093). Occasionally, the glomerulitis takes the form of a granulomatous lesion with granular disintegration of the entire glomerulus or of an individual capillary loop, accompanied by a neutrophilic infiltrate into the glomerular tuft as well as into the surrounding periglomerular tissue.

The nature and pathogenesis of this condition are still completely obscure. Because the acute vasculitis resembles, to a considerable extent, that seen in serum sickness, there is a prevalent belief that the etiology is some form of hypersensitivity, conceivably some form of autoimmune reaction. However, no autoantibodies have been identified. Recently, antigen-antibody complexes have been identified in the renal lesions (Castleman and McNeely, 1969). An abnormally high serum level of gamma globulin is frequent in these patients. Nonetheless, a specific microbiologic causation has not been ruled out. At one time, this disease was highly fatal with a mean survival on the order of half a year or less. Recently, highly gratifying prolongation of life has been achieved with the use of cytotoxic drugs (Novack and Pearson, 1971). Most patients have returned to work apparently in complete remission and some have even stopped therapy without recurrence (Editorial, 1972).

NEOPLASMS AND ABNORMAL PROLIFERATIONS OF THE IMMUNE SYSTEM

The cells of the immune system are no less vulnerable to neoplasia and abnormal proliferations than any of the other cells of the body. Many of the neoplasms of the lymphoreticular system are known as lymphomas and are discussed on p. 752. Our attention here is limited to those disorders in which the neoplastic cells are recognizable as plasma cells, their immediate precursors or the intermediate forms variously referred to as lymphocytoid plasma cells and plasmacytoid lymphocytes.

PLASMA CELL DYSCRASIAS

The generic term plasma cell dyscrasia embraces a group of disorders having in common an abnormal and frequently, but not invariably, neoplastic proliferation of plasma cells. All are characterized by the elaboration of excessive amounts of one of the immunoglobulins or their constituent units of light chains. Hence, these entities are also known as the *proteinopathies* or *dysproteinoses*. Because in the individual patient the abnormal proteins are always constant throughout the course of the disease, it would appear as though all of the neoplastic cells represented the clone of a single progenitor and, on this account, these disorders are sometimes referred to as *monoclonal gammopathies* (Cohen, 1968). The various patterns of these plasma cell diseases will first be presented briefly.

1. Multiple Myeloma (Plasma Cell Myeloma). This most common and, at the same

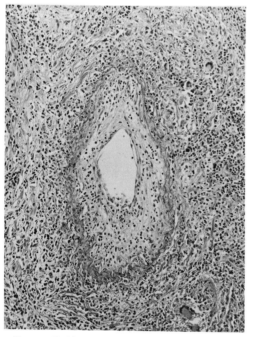

Figure 7–22. A small artery in the lung in Wegener's granulomatosis. The wall is markedly thickened, fibrotic and infiltrated with white cells.

time, most serious variant is basically a multifocal plasma cell cancer of the osseous system. The focal lesions may be disseminated throughout the skeleton, and progressively erode the bone in their growth, sometimes leading to pathologic fractures. Often, as the disease progresses, the cancerous plasma cells spread to extraosseous sites. Multiple myeloma probably comprises the disseminated end stage of all plasma cell dyscrasias.

2. Solitary Myeloma. In occasional cases, plasma cell myeloma presents as an apparently single skeletal lesion. Almost always, in the course of time, such solitary lesions disseminate more widely to other bones to become multiple myelomas.

3. Soft Tissue Plasmacytoma. Plasma cell neoplasms may occur in various extramedullary sites such as the gastrointestinal tract, spleen and lymph nodes, but most often in the oronasopharynx. By definition, skeletal lesions are not present, at least at the time the diagnosis of soft tissue plasmacytoma is made. However, in most instances, after a span of years, the localized primary tumor disseminates to other sites including the skeleton.

4. Plasma Cell Leukemia. This form of leukemia is exceedingly rare and probably represents, in almost all instances, spread into the circulating blood of neoplastic cells arising in lesions of bones or soft tissues.

5. Reactive Plasma Cell Proliferations. This pattern of plasma cell disease has also been called diffuse myelomatosis and asymptomatic plasma cell dyscrasia. It is a somewhat controversial entity, characterized by a diffuse plasma cell infiltration of the bone marrow, not associated with solitary discrete areas of bone destruction. The interpretation of this variant of the plasma cell dyscrasias is uncertain. Some patients have had an associated chronic inflammatory or infectious process, suggesting that the diffuse infiltrates of plasma cells were merely an immunologic reaction to systemic antigenic challenge. But, in other instances, the derangement has in time been transformed into a more overt neoplastic process (Kyle and Bayrd, 1965).

Collectively, plasma cell neoplasms account for about 11 percent of all deaths caused by malignant hematopoietic neoplasms. At least 95 per cent of such deaths result from disseminated multiple myelomas. Although myeloma may arise in young adults, it is principally a disease of those over 40 years of age, and its incidence increases with age.

One of the most intriguing and clinically important aspects of plasma cell neoplasms is their elaboration of a whole range of immunoglobulins. These are indistinguishable, biochemically and electrophoretically, from normal immunoglobulins and may belong to any one of the five major classes or the two types of light chains. Each patient usually produces one specific type of immunoglobulin and/or fragment which remains constant throughout the course of the disease, justifying the term monoclonal gammopathy. Rarely, patients produce more than one type, hence referred to as a polyclonal gammopathy. On electrophoretic analysis, the homogeneity of the elaborated serum immunoglobulin produces a single, narrow "spike" referred to as myeloma proteins, M-proteins or paraproteins, differentiating such globulin synthesis from the broad diffuse bands encountered in immune stimulation. M-proteins are present in approximately 90 per cent of patients with disseminated plasma cell neoplasms. As a consequence, total serum proteins are usually elevated in myelomatosis from 5 to 15 gm. per 100 ml. of serum (Hobbs, 1969a). The elevated serum globulins tend to cause rouleaux formations, induce sludging of the blood and tissue anoxia because of the hyperviscosity and, on occasion, lead to a bleeding diathesis. In the majority of patients, the globulins are of the IgG type, but in others they may be macroglobulins belonging to the IgM class. Occasionally, myeloma globulins exhibit cold precipitability (cryoglobulins).

About 50 to 60 per cent of patients with multiple myeloma also elaborate the light chain subunits of immunoglobulin. Because of their smaller molecular weight (in the range of 22,000), they are readily excreted through the glomeruli into the urine. These are known as Bence Jones proteins, and have the peculiar characteristic of coagulating when the urine is heated to 45 to 55° C. and redissolving at higher temperatures (Osserman and Takatsuki, 1963). In the individual case, immunoglobulins but no Bence Jones proteins may be synthesized; more rarely, only Bence Jones proteins are elaborated but most often the neoplastic clone both elaborates light chains and simultaneously incorporates these light chains into a complete immune globulin. Hence most patients have both M-proteins in the serum and Bence Jones proteins in the urine.

Either myeloma globulins or Bence Jones proteins or both were demonstrated in over 99 per cent of the patients in many large series of well studied cases of multiple myeloma (Hobbs, 1969b). The identification of these abnormal proteins is one of the most important means of diagnosing these diseases and, indeed, in many patients a dysproteinosis is discovered long before plasma cell lesions can be identified either clinically or radiographically. Although these myeloma proteins are indistinguishable from antibody immunoglobulins, they lack receptor sites and have no antibody activity. However, they have provided unique "experiments of nature" and made it possible to obtain and analyze immunoglobulins belonging to one pure class to thus unravel the precise amino acid sequencing of immunoglobulins and their molecular structure.

Systemic amyloidosis, generally conforming to the distribution called primary amyloidosis, is encountered in patients having plasma cell neoplasms, usually disseminated (p. 282). Osserman et al. (1964) long contended that the amyloid deposits comprise, at least in part, the interstitial deposition of abnormal gamma globulins or gamma globulin components. There is now strong evidence that the amyloid is produced in situ and is not a deposition of circulating proteins. However, the recent finding of a homology between amyloid proteins and immunoglobulins indicates that there is some definite association between amyloidosis and deranged immunoglobulin synthesis (p. 284).

Etiology and Pathogenesis. Although the genesis of plasma cell neoplasms is shrouded in the mystery of all cancer, many observations suggest that they may result from long-persisting stimulation of the reticuloendothelial system, operating either alone or in combination with genetic or viral influences. This evidence derives from both experimental and clinical studies. In C_3H strain mice, plasma cell tumors have been noted to arise in the iliocecal regions of the gut in animals having persistent cecal ulcerations (Pilgrim, 1965). Analogously, plasma cell tumors have been induced in mice by the intraperitoneal injection of a variety of irritant substances including Freund's adjuvant, mineral oil and plastic. At first, these substances evoke a chronic inflammatory reaction which progresses to granulomas and ultimately to lesions considered to be plasma cell tumors (Potter and MacCardle, 1964). The induced tumors are transplantable and produce myeloma proteins or Bence Jones proteins. These animal models are highly strain-specific, indicative of some genetic predisposition.

There are some parallels between these animal models and man. Plasma cell neoplasms have arisen with greater than chance frequency in patients suffering longstanding chronic infections such as osteomyelitis, tuberculosis, cholecystitis and nonspecific pneumonitis (Baitz and Kyle, 1964). Of interest, the tumor frequently develops in the site of the chronic inflammation. Perhaps relevant is the fact that about 15 per cent of plasma cell neoplasms arise in patients who have some form of soft tissue cancer (Weitzel, 1958). These associated malignant tumors have arisen in the biliary tract, breast, bowel and lung. The significance of this association is uncertain. Could it represent an immunologic response initiated by the tumor antigens of the visceral cancer which secondarily evoked a plasma cell tumor? Alternatively, could an oncogenic virus have been responsible for both? In this connection, virus-like particles have been identified in transplantable mouse plasma cell tumors (Howatson and McCulloch, 1958). However, it was not possible to transmit these tumors by cell-free extracts, raising the question about the interpretation and significance of these apparent cellular inclusions. Similarly, NZB mice and animals suffering from Aleutian mink disease have an increased incidence of plasma cell dyscrasias, providing yet another association between these tumors and viruses. In the last analysis, one can only speculate that persistent inflammatory reactive proliferation or possibly oncogenic viruses may induce a somatic mutation in those persons genetically predisposed leading to plasma cell neoplasia.

Morphology. Despite the abundance of abnormal biochemical findings, the ultimate diagnosis of plasma cell dyscrasias rests on the morphologic identification of the abnormal aggregates of plasma cells (Fig. 7–23). In many instances, the neoplastic cells are normal-appearing mature plasma cells, but all ranges of immaturity may be encountered to very undifferentiated cells resembling reticuloendothelial precursors as well as lymphocyte-plasma cell intermediates. It may be difficult to identify the neoplastic nature of the well differentiated plasma cell lesions from the cytology of the individual cells; more important is their abnormal aggregation or evidence of their destructive potential in the form of infiltration, invasion and erosion (Fig. 7–24). Sometimes bi- or even trinucleate cells are seen in these lesions, essentially reproducing cancerous giant cells. Electron microscopy has disclosed, in the myeloma cell, a highly developed endoplasmic reticulum, often stuffed with amorphous material compatible with protein aggregates (DePetris et al., 1963). Under the light microscope, the protein aggregates may appear as acidophilic inclusions known as Russell bodies. Intracytoplasmic crystals have also been found in these cells, apparently representing precipitated crystalline gamma globulin (Bessis, 1961). Virus-like particles have also been reported in one case but have not been confirmed by others.

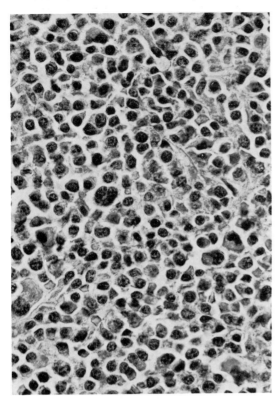

Figure 7–23. Multiple myeloma to show the masses of plasma cells, mostly mature but some with anaplasia and forming tumor giant cells.

Turning now to the various syndromes discussed at the outset, multiple myeloma presents as multifocal destructive bone lesions throughout the skeletal system. Although any bone may be affected, the following distribution obtains in large series of cases—vertebral column, 66 per cent; ribs, 44 per cent; skull, 41 per cent; pelvis, 28 per cent; femur, 24 per cent; clavicle, 10 per cent; and scapula, 10 per cent. These focal lesions generally begin in the medullary cavity, erode the cancellous bone and progressively destroy the cortical bone. On section, the bony defects are filled with red, soft, gelatinous tissue. Radiographically, the lesions appear as punched-out defects, usually ranging between 1 and 4 cm. in diameter (Fig. 7—25). In the late stages of multiple myeloma, plasma cell infiltrations of soft tissues may be encountered in spleen, liver, kidneys, lungs and lymph nodes, or more widely. Later, the development of myeloma kidneys will be discussed.

The solitary myeloma, as indicated earlier, appears as a unifocal lesion in any of the sites of involvement encountered in multiple myeloma. The solitary lesion is indistinguishable from one of the lesions of multiple myeloma.

The soft tissue plasmacytoma presents as a characteristic fleshy, red-brown neoplasm in the sites previously indicated. The cytologic detail con-

forms to that already described in the osseous lesions. Before such a diagnosis is entertained, it must be certain that latent osseous lesions are not already present. When these neoplasms occur in their favored locations, in the oronasopharynx or air sinuses, they are generally very insidious in their development and are highly erosive of adjacent bony structure.

The pattern previously referred to as abnormal reactive proliferation or diffuse myelomatosis presents as delicate, scattered focal infiltrates of plasma cells throughout the blood-forming bone marrow and the splenolymphoid tissues. The infiltrates do not create focal tumorous aggregates nor are they destructive of native architecture. Generally, the plasma cells are well differentiated and do not present evidence of anaplasia or giant cell formation. The interpretation of such infiltrates is exceedingly difficult, and they are readily mistaken for chronic inflammatory reactions. Rarely, such presentations evolve into symptomatic plasma cell

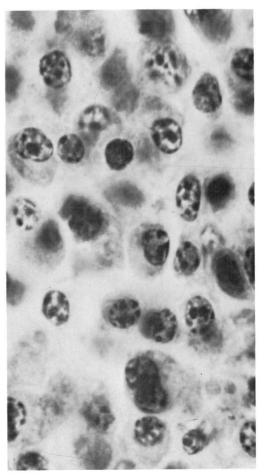

Figure 7–24. Plasmacytoma. A high power detail of the tumor composed of mature characteristic plasma cells.

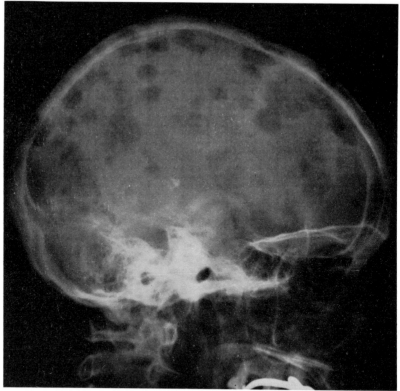

Figure 7–25. *Radiograph of the skull extensively involved by focal sharply punched-out lesions of plasma cell myeloma.*

tumors after a time lapse of 10 or more years (Osserman, 1958).

A clinical pattern consistent with the diagnosis of plasma cell leukemia is occasionally observed in patients having classic multiple myeloma or, more rarely, one of the other presentations of the plasma cell dyscrasias. The white cell counts are rarely in excess of 15,000 to 20,000 but may contain as many as 50 per cent plasma cells.

Renal involvement generally called myeloma nephrosis may occur in any of the plasma cell dyscrasias. Grossly, the kidneys may be normal in size or color, slightly enlarged and pale, or shrunken and pale because of interstitial scarring. The most distinctive features are microscopic. Interstitial infiltrates of abnormal plasma cells may be encountered. Even in the absence of these, proteinous casts are prominent in the tubules, principally the distal convoluted and collecting tubules. Most of these casts are made up of Bence Jones proteins, but some may be only albumen (MacKenzie et al., 1968). The epithelial cells within the tubules often become engorged with pale hyaline droplets (presumably of protein) or needle-like crystals. **Often, the cells lining tubules with casts become necrotic or atrophied while, in other instances, they apparently fuse to produce highly distinctive, multinucleate epithelial giant cells that encircle or engulf whole**

casts or fragments of casts (Fig. 7–26). About such tubules, there is often an inflammatory infiltrate of neoplastic cells and mature lymphocytes. Metastatic calcification may be encountered within the kidney as a reflection of the bone destruction and secondary hypercalcemia caused by the disseminated myelomatous lesions.

A myeloma neuropathy may develop due to tumorous infiltrations of nerve trunk roots. Fractures and compression of vertebral roots may add to these neurologic complications. Occasionally, a form of neuropathy occurs in the absence of obvious causes and may represent the nonspecific carcinomatous polyneuropathy discussed on p. 146. Pathologic fractures are sometimes produced by the plasma cell lesions; they are most common in the vertebral column, but may affect any of the numerous bones suffering erosion and destruction of their cortical substance.

Clinical Correlation. Enough has been said to make clear the protean manifestations of these derangements. Many times, these cases come to medical attention in the course of the investigation of an unexplained anemia, a proteinuria, or complaints of a nonspecific nature first considered to be psychoneurotic in origin. Bone pain, sometimes made more in-

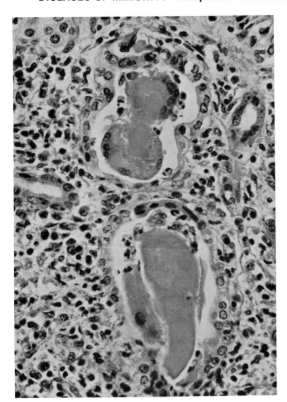

Figure 7–26. *Proteinous casts in the collecting tubules of the kidney in myeloma nephrosis. Note the epithelial cell reaction with formation of multinucleate giant cells about the casts.*

tense by complicating fractures, is perhaps the most common and characteristic feature. Usually, weakness and general debility mark the advanced stages of the disease. Although these patients have an excess of myeloma immunoglobulins, the latter do not function as antibodies, and enhanced susceptibility to bacterial infections characterizes these disorders. Anemia, rouleau formation, bleeding tendencies and clotting abnormalities are frequent accompaniments. The renal involvement may dominate the clinical problem in some cases, since it can produce progressive functional insufficiency. Uremia or azotemia, in the absence of hypertension or edema, is seldom found in primary renal disorders but is characteristically caused by myeloma nephrosis. Elevated nonspecific white counts may be encountered and are diagnostic in those cases of plasma cell leukemia. Hypercalcemia may lead to the diagnosis in some cases. The radiographic changes are quite distinctive and often permit a reasonably certain diagnosis. Classically, the individual lesions appear as sharply punched-out defects having a rounded, soap-bubble appearance on the x-ray. The finding, in a

biopsy, of an amyloid deposit in a patient with bone pain or vague manifestations of weakness and weight loss should dictate the need for further investigation. Abnormal gamma globulin peaks in the serum or Bence Jones protein in the urine comprise more important findings. However, *most reliable is the demonstration of abnormal masses of plasma cells on either bone marrow smears or sections.*

WALDENSTRÖM'S MACROGLOBULINEMIA

A form of plasma cell dyscrasia in which there is synthesis of only IgM macroglobulins is known as Waldenström's macroglobulinemia. Focal tumor formations do not appear but, instead, the clinical features comprise: anemia, bleeding tendencies and stagnant tissue anoxia, all related to the increased plasma viscosity caused by the serum macroglobulins (Fessel, 1962). Histologic studies of the bone marrow generally disclose a diffuse but scattered infiltrate of lymphocytic and plasmacytic forms, with many intermediate cell types (Imhof et al., 1959) (Fig. 7–27). Similar infil-

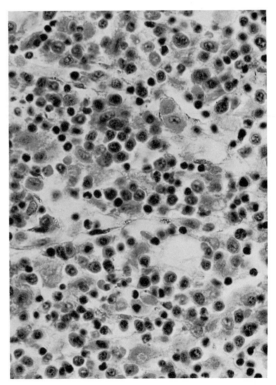

Figure 7–27. *Waldenström's macroglobulinemia. Detail of marrow with pleomorphic cellularity containing recognizable lymphocytes, histiocytes and plasma cells admixed with many hybrid forms. (From Cabot Case Record 26–1964. New Eng. J. Med., 270: 1190, 1964.)*

trates are found throughout the reticuloendothelial system and sometimes induce lymphadenopathy, splenomegaly and hepatomegaly. In none of the affected organs are tumorous aggregates encountered. Immunofluorescent stains confirm the synthesis of macroglobulins in these cells. Inclusions of PAS material (presumably glycoproteins) can sometimes be seen within these abnormal cells (Fig. 7–28). In rare instances, patients with such presentations have later developed more classic plasma cell tumors (Welton et al., 1968).

The differentiation of macroglobulinemia from reactive plasma cell proliferations or diffuse myelomatosis can only be made with certainty by electrophoretic demonstration of the nature of the serum globulins. In addition, the cellular composition of the infiltrate in macroglobulinemia tends to be more variable than that in myelomatosis. It is necessary in these cases to rule out chronic lymphatic leukemia and chronic inflammation as possible causes of the histologic changes. Once again, protein analyses may be required.

The circulating macroglobulins, as mentioned, account for most of the major clinical features of this disorder. Coating of red cells by IgM results in rouleau formation, autoagglutination, a positive Coombs' reaction, and further predisposes these cells to erythrophagocytosis throughout the RE system. The bleeding tendency is thought to be the result of interaction between IgM and coagulation factors (fibrinogen, prothrombin, factors V and VII). Platelet agglutination may contribute to bleeding manifestations. Bence Jones proteinuria is seen in a few cases, but renal functional impairment and myeloma nephrosis is much less common than in the other plasma cell disorders. Enhanced susceptibility to bacterial infections reflects the failure of the macroglobulins to serve as antibodies.

HEAVY CHAIN DISEASE

Two rare forms of plasma cell dyscrasia are characterized by the synthesis of heavy chain fragments of the immunoglobulins. One pattern known as Franklin's disease is associated with the heavy chain of IgG, the other with the heavy chain of IgA. The principal features of Franklin's disease are lymphadenopathy, hepatomegaly, splenomegaly and, indeed, manifestations strongly suggestive of a lymphoma. No skeletal involvement has been encountered in the few reported cases (Ellman and Block, 1968) (Osserman and Takatsuki, 1964). The infiltrates closely resemble those encountered in Waldenström's macroglobulinemia but, in addition, there is a prominent component of eosinophils and large reticulum cells. In essence, the infiltrate is very pleomorphic.

The IgA heavy chain disease closely resembles Franklin's disease, but the lymphomatous proliferations tend to be most severe in the small intestine and its mesentery (Seligmann et al., 1968a).

EPILOGUE

It is evident from the preceding chapter that disorders of the immune system range from "too little" (immunologic deficiencies) to "too much" (plasma cell dyscrasias), including every shade of hyper-reactivity and abnormal reactivity in between. Some of these disorders are as trivial as an allergy to strawberries, but obviously some are as ominous as the invariably fatal multiple myeloma. The immune system has for some years been the darling of medical investigators, but almost certainly all of its potential has not yet been recognized. It can be anticipated, therefore, that many more

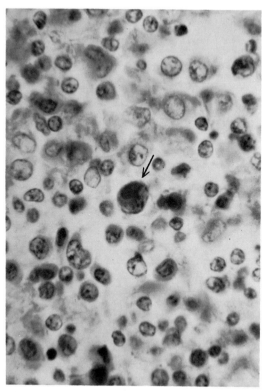

Figure 7–28. Waldenström's macroglobulinemia—high power detail of marrow infiltrate disclosing a PAS-positive inclusion (arrow) in a plasmacytoid cell in midfield. (Periodic acid-Schiff stain.) (Courtesy of Dr. Leonard Gottlieb, Mallory Institute of Pathology. From New Eng. J. Med., 270: 1190, 1964.)

disorders of this type will plague the medical student of the future.

REFERENCES

Alarcon-Segovia, D.: Drug induced lupus syndromes. Proc. Staff Meetings Mayo Clinic, *44*:664, 1969.

Alarcon-Segovia, D., and Brown, A. L.: Classification and etiologic aspects of necrotizing angiitides. An analytic approach to a confused subject with a critical review of the evidence for hypersensitivity in polyarteritis nodosa. Mayo Clin. Proc., *39*:205, 1964.

Amos, D. B.: Genetic and antigenetic aspects of human histocompatibility systems. Advances Immun., *10*:251, 1969.

Andres, G. A., et al.: Human renal transplants. III. Immunopathic studies. Lab. Invest., *22*:588, 1970.

Arnason, B. G., and Waksman, B. H.: Tuberculin sensitivity. Immunologic considerations. Advances Tuberc. Res., *13*:1, 1964.

Asherson, G. L.: The role of microorganisms in autoimmune responses. Progr. Allerg., *12*:192, 1968.

Asherson, R. A., et al.: Immunological studies in arteritis of the aorta and great vessels. Brit. Med. J., *3*:590, 1968.

Baitz, T., and Kyle, R. A.: Solitary myeloma in chronic osteomyelitis. Arch. Intern. Med., *113*:872, 1964.

Balfour, B. M., et al.: Fluorescent antibody studies in human thyroiditis: autoantibodies to antigen of the thyroid colloid distinct from thyroglobulin. Brit. J. Exp. Path., *42*:307, 1961.

Balner, H., and Dersjant, H.: Early lymphatic regeneration in thymectomized radiation chimeras. Nature, *204*:941, 1964.

Barnett, E. V., et al.: Nuclear antigens and antinuclear antibodies in mink sera. Arthritis Rheum., *11*:92, 1968.

Becker, E. L.: Structural Basis of Renal Disease. New York, Hoeber Medical Division, Harper and Row, 1968, p. 163.

Becker, E. L., and Austen, K. F.: Anaphylaxis. In Miescher, P. A., and Muller-Eberhard, H. J. (eds.): Textbook of Immunopathology. New York and London, Grune and Stratton, 1968, p. 76.

Benacerraf, B., and Levin, B. B.: Immunological specificity of delayed and immediate hypersensitivity reactions. J. Exp. Med., *115*:1023, 1962.

Benacerraf, B., and McDevitt, H. O.: Histocompatibility-linked immune response genes. Science, *175*:273, 1972.

Benacerraf, B., et al.: Localization of colloidal substances in vascular endothelium. A mechanism of tissue damage. I. Factor causing the pathologic deposition of colloidal carbon. Amer. J. Path., *35*:75, 1959.

Berenbaum, M. C.: Immunosuppressive agents. Brit. Med. Bull., *21*:140, 1965.

Berenbaum, M. C.: Immunosuppressive drugs. J. Clin. Path. Suppl. 20:471, 1967.

Bessis, M.: Ultrastructure of lymphoid and plasma cells in relation to globulin and antibody formation. Lab. Invest., *10*:1040, 1961.

Bloch, K. J.: The anaphylactic antibodies in mammals including man. Progr. Allerg., *10*:84, 1967.

Bloch, K. J., et al.: Sjögren's syndrome. A clinical, pathological and serological study of 62 cases. Medicine, *44*:187, 1965.

Brent, L.: Allograft and specific unresponsiveness. New Eng. J. Med., *284*:499, 1971.

Broder, I.: Anaphylaxis: In Movat, H. Z. (ed.): Inflammation, Immunity and Hypersensitivity. New York, Harper and Row, 1971, p. 333.

Bruton, O. C.: Agammaglobulinemia. Pediatrics, *9*:722, 1952.

Budzilovich, G. N., and Wilens, S. L.: Fulminating Wegener's granulomatosis. Arch. Path., *70*:653, 1960.

Bunim, J. J., and Black, R. L.: Connective tissue (collagen) diseases. Ann. Rev. Med., *7*:839, 1957.

Burch, P. R. J.: From mice to men. Lancet, *2*:589, 1965.

Burnet, F. M.: Autoimmune disease. I. Modern immunologic concepts. II. Pathology of the immune response. Brit. Med. J., *2*:645, 729, 1959*a*.

Burnet, F. M.: Cellular Immunology. London and New York, Cambridge University Press, 1969.

Burnet, F. M.: The Clonal Selection Theory of Acquired Immunity. Nashville, Tenn., Vanderbilt University Press, 1959*b*.

Busch, G. J., et al.: Human renal allografts. Analysis of lesions in long-term survivors. Hum. Path., *2*:253, 1971.

Calne, R. Y., et al.: Immunosuppressive effects of soluble cell membrane fractions, donor blood and serum on renal allograft survival. Nature, *227*:903, 1970.

Carrington, C. B., and Liebow, A. A.: Limited forms of angiitis and granulomatosis of Wegener's type. Amer. J. Med., *41*:497, 1966.

Cassidy, J. T., et al.: Selective IgA deficiency in connective tissue diseases. New Eng. J. Med., *280*:275, 1969.

Castleman, B., and McNeely, B. U.: Case records of the Massachusetts General Hospital weekly clinicopathological exercises. New Eng. J. Med., *280*:828, 1969.

Claman, H. N., and Chaperon, E. A.: Immunological complementation between thymus and marrow cells. A model for the two cell theory of immunocompetence. Transplant. Rev., *1*:92, 1969.

Claman, H. N., et al.: Human thymus cell cultures evidence for two functional populations. Proc. Soc. Exp. Biol. Med., *121*:236, 1966.

Clarke, C. A., et al.: The evolution of cellular immunity and the genetics of human organ transplantation. Quart. J. Med., *37*:242, 1968.

Cleveland, W. W., et al.: Foetal thymic transplant in a case of Di George's syndrome. Lancet, *2*:1211, 1968.

Cline, M. J., and Swett, V. C.: The interaction of human monocytes and lymphocytes. J. Exp. Med., *128*:1309, 1968.

Cochrane, C. G.: Mediators of the Arthus reaction and related conditions. Progr. Allerg., *11*:1, 1967.

Cochrum, K. C., et al.: Renal allograft rejection initiated by passive transfer of immune plasma. Proceedings of the Second International Congress of the Transplantation Society, *1*:301, 1969.

Cohen, E. P.: Conversion of non-immune cells into antibody forming cells by RNA. Nature, *213*:462, 1967.

Cohen, S.: The nature of myeloma proteins. Brit. J. Haemat., *15*:211, 1968.

Cosenza, H., and Nordin, A. A.: Immunoglobulin classes of antibody-forming cells in mice. III. Immunoglobulin antibody restriction of plaque-forming cells demonstrated by the double immunofluorescent technique. J. Immunol., *104*:976, 1970.

Craddock, C. G., et al.: Lymphocytes and the immune response. New Eng. J. Med., *285*:324, 378, 1971.

Cudkowicz, G., and Bennett, M.: Peculiar immunobiology of bone marrow allografts. J. Exp. Med., *134*:83, 1513, 1971.

Curtis, A. C., et al.: Study of the autoimmune reactions in dermatomyositis. J.A.M.A., *178*:571, 1961.

Dacie, J. V., and Worlledge, S. M.: Autoimmune hemolytic anemias. In Brown, E. B., and Moore, C. V. (eds.): Progress in Hematology. Vol. VI. New York, Grune and Stratton, 1969, p. 82.

Dameshek, W., and Schwartz, S. O.: The presence of hemolysins in acute hemolytic anemia. New Eng. J. Med., *218*:75, 1938.

Dammin, G. J.: The pathology of human renal transplantation. In Rapaport, F. T., and Dausset, J. (eds.): Human Transplantation. New York, Grune and Stratton, 1968.

Dausset, J., et al.: The HL-A system sub-loci and their importance in transplantation. Transplant. Proc., *1*:1, 1969.

David, J. R.: Macrophage migration. Fed. Proc., *27*:6, 1968.

Davies, A. J. S., et al.: The failure of thymus derived cells to produce antibody. Transplantation, *5*:222, 1967.

DeGroot, L. J.: Current concepts in management of thyroid disease. Med. Clin. N. Amer., *54*:1117, 1970.

DePetris, S., et al.: Localization of antibodies in plasma cells by electron microscopy. J. Exp. Med., *117*:849, 1963.

Dixon, F. J.: The role of antigen-antibody complexes in disease. Harvey Lect., *58*:21, 1963.

Dixon, F. J., et al.: Experimental glomerulonephritis: the pathogenesis of a laboratory model resembling the spectrum of human glomerulonephritis. J. Exp. Med., *113*:899, 1961.

Dixon, F. J., et al.: Pathogenesis of serum sickness. Arch. Path., *65*:18, 1958.

Donath, J., and Landsteiner, K.: Ueber paroxzsmale haemoglinurie. Munchen. Med. Wschr., *51*:1509, 1904.

Dresser, D. W.: Specific inhibition of antibody production. Paralysis induced in adult mice by small quantities of protein antigen. Immunology, *5*:378, 1962.

Dubois, E. L.: Lupus Erythematosus: A Review of the Current

Status of Discoid and Systemic Lupus Erythematosus. New York, Blackiston Division, McGraw-Hill Book Co., 1966.

Editorial: Cellular immunity in infectious diseases. Lancet, 2:253, 1969.

Editorial: Wegener's granulomatosis. Lancet, 2:519, 1972.

Ehrlich, P.: Collected Studies on Immunity. Translated by C. Bolduan. New York, Wiley, 1906.

Ellman, L. L., and Block, K. J.: Heavy chain disease: report of a seventh case. New Eng. J. Med., 278:1195, 1968.

Feizi, T., et al.: Cold agglutinin production in rabbits immunized with mycoplasma pneumoniae-treated human erythrocytes. Clin. Res., 17:366, 1969.

Fessel, W. J.: Clinical analysis of 142 cases with high molecular weight serum proteins. Acta. Med. Scand., Suppl. 391, 173:1, 1962.

Fishman, M., et al.: In vitro transfer of macrophage RNA to lymph node cells. Nature, 198:549, 1963.

Flax, M. H., and Caulfield, J. B.: Cellular and vascular components of allergic contact dermatitis. Amer. J. Path., 43:1031, 1963.

Fleischmajer, R., and Krol, S.: Chemical synthesis of the dermis in scleroderma. Proc. Soc. Exp. Biol. Med., 126:252, 1967.

Franklin, E. C.: Structure and function of immunoglobulins. Relation to allergy. New York J. Med., 68:411, 1968.

Frei, P. C., et al.: Phagocytosis of the antigen, a crucial step in the induction of the primary response. Proc. Nat. Acad. Sci. U.S.A., 53:20, 1965.

Freund, J., and McDermott, K.: Sensitization to horse serum by means of adjuvant. Proc. Soc. Exp. Biol. Med., 49:548, 1942.

Fudenberg, H. H., et al.: Classification of the primary immune deficiencies: W.H.O. recommendation. New Eng. J. Med., 283:656, 1970.

Gatti, R. A., et al.: Immunological reconstitution of sex-linked lymphopenic immunological deficiency. Lancet, 2:1366, 1968.

Gottlieb, A. A., and Doty, P.: Studies on macrophage RNA involved in antibody production. Proc. Nat. Acad. Sci. U.S.A., 57:1849, 1967.

Gottlieb, S., et al.: Long term immunity to tetanus. A statistical evaluation and its clinical implications. Amer. J. Public Health, 54:961, 1964.

Granger, G. A., and Williams, T. W.: Lymphocyte cytotoxicity in vitro: activation and release of a cytotoxic factor. Nature, 218:1253, 1968.

Griffith, G. C., and Vural, I. L.: Polyarteritis nodosa: a correlation of clinical and post mortem findings in seventeen cases. Circulation, 3:481, 1951.

Grumet, F. C., et al.: Histocompatibility (HL-A) antigens associated with systemic lupus erythematosus. A possible genetic predisposition to disease. New Eng. J. Med., 285:193, 1971.

Haas, J. E., and Yunis, E. G.: Tubular inclusions of systemic lupus erythematosus: ultrastructural observations regarding their possible viral nature. Exp. Molec. Path., 12:257, 1970.

Hall, R.: Immunologic aspects of thyroid function. New Eng. J. Med., 266:1204, 1962.

Hamburger, J. A.: Reappraisal of the concept of "organ rejection" based on the study of homotransplanted kidneys. Transplantation, 5:870, 1967.

Hart, P. D., et al.: The compromised host and infection. J. Infect. Dis., 120:169, 1969.

Harvey, A. M., et al.: Systemic lupus erythematosus. Review of the literature and clinical analysis of 138 cases. Medicine, 33:291, 1954.

Hayes, R. L., and Rodnan, G. P.: Ultrastructural study of skin collagen fibrillogenesis in progressive systemic sclerosis. Arthritis Rheum., 11:487, 1968.

Hobbs, J. R.: Immunochemical classes of myelomatosis. Brit. J. Haemat., 16:599, 1969a.

Hobbs, J. R.: Paraproteinaemia. Proc. Roy. Soc. Med., 62:773, 1969b.

Holborow, E. J., et al.: Cytoplasmic localization of "complement fixing" autoantigen in human thyroid epithelium. Brit. J. Exp. Path., 40:583, 1959.

Holman, H., and Deicher, H. R.: The reaction of the lupus erythematosus (LE) cell factor with deoxyribonucleoprotein of the cell nucleus. J. Clin. Invest., 38:2059, 1959.

Hood, L. E.: Two genes, one polypeptide chain: fact or fiction? Fed. Proc., 31:177, 1972.

Howatson, A. F., and McCulloch, E. A.: Virus-like bodies in transplantable mouse plasma cell tumour. Nature, 181:1213, 1958.

Howie, J. B., and Helyer, B. J.: Autoimmune disease in mice. Ann. N.Y. Acad. Sci., 124:167, 1965.

Humphrey, J. H., and Dourmashkin, R. R.: Electron microscope studies of immune cell lysis. In Wolstenholme, G. E. W., and Knight, J. (eds.): Ciba Foundation Symposium on Complement. London, J. and A. Churchill Ltd., 1965.

Humphrey, J. H., and Jacques, R.: The release of histamines and 5-HT (serotonin) from platelets by antigen-antibody reaction (in vitro). J. Physiol., 128:9, 1955.

Imhof, J. W., et al.: Clinical and hematological aspects of macroglobulinaemia of Waldenström. Acta Med. Scand., 163:349, 1959.

Ishizaka, K.: Induction of passive cutaneous anaphylaxis in monkeys by human gamma E antibody. J. Allerg., 39:254, 1967.

Ishizaka, K., and Ishizaka, T.: Human reaginic antibodies and immunoglobulin E. J. Allerg., 42:330, 1968.

James, L. P., Jr., and Austin, K. F.: Fatal systemic anaphylaxis in man. New Eng. J. Med., 270:597, 1964.

Kahn, M.: Renal concentrating defect in Sjögren's syndrome. Ann. Intern. Med., 56:883, 1962.

Kaplan, M. H.: Autoantibodies to heart and rheumatic fever: the induction of autoimmunity to heart by streptococcal antigen cross-reactive with heart. Ann. N.Y. Acad. Sci., 124:904, 1965.

Keiser, H. R., and Sjoerdsma, A.: Direct measurement of the rate of collagen synthesis in skin. Clin. Chim. Acta, 23:341, 1969.

Klainer, A. S., and Beisel, W. R.: Opportunistic infection: a review. Amer. J. Med. Sci., 258:431, 1969.

Kleckner, S. S.: Dermatomyositis and its manifestations in the gastrointestinal tract. Amer. J. Gastroent., 53:141, 1970.

Klemperer, P.: The concept of collagen diseases. Amer. J. Path., 26:505, 1950.

Knicker, W. T., and Cochrane, L. G.: The localization of circulating immune complexes in experimental serum sickness. The role of vasoactive amines and hydrodynamic forces. J. Exp. Med., 127:109, 1968.

Koffler, D., et al.: Immunological studies concerning the nephritis of systemic lupus erythematosus. J. Exp. Med., 126:607, 1967.

Koffler, D., et al.: Variable patterns of immunoglobulin and complement deposition in the kidneys of patients with systemic lupus erythematosus. Amer. J. Path., 56:305, 1969.

Kyle, R. A., and Bayrd, E. D.: Benign monoclonal gammopathy: a potentially malignant condition? Amer. J. Med., 40:426, 1965.

Lawrence, H. S.: Transfer factors and cellular immune deficiency disease. New Eng. J. Med., 283:411, 1970.

Lennox, E. S., and Cohn, M.: Immunoglobulins. Ann. Rev. Biochem., 36:365, 1967.

Leventhal, B. G., et al.: Impaired lymphocyte transformation and delayed hypersensitivity in Sjögren's syndrome. J. Clin. Invest., 46:1338, 1967.

Levey, R. H., and Medawar, P. B.: Nature and mode of action of antilymphocytic antiserum. Proc. Nat. Acad. Sci. U.S.A., 56:1130, 1966.

Levine, L., and Stollar, B. D.: Nucleic acid immune systems. Progr. Allerg., 12:161, 1968.

Litt, M.: Studies of the latent period. I. Primary antibody in guinea pig lymph nodes 7½ minutes after introduction of chicken erythrocytes. Cold Spring Harbor Sympos. Quant. Biol., 32:477, 1967.

LoBuglio, A. F., et al.: Red cells coated with immunoglobulin G: binding and sphering by mononuclear cells in man. Science, 158:1582, 1967.

MacKay, I. R.: Autoimmune disease in humans. Proceedings of the 11th Congress of the International Society of Blood Transfusion, Sydney, 1966. Bull. Haemat., 29: Part 2, 463, 1968.

MacKenzie, M. R., et al.: Rapid renal failure in a case of multiple myeloma: the role of Bence-Jones proteins. Clin. Exp. Immun., 3:593, 1968.

Makela, O.: Specificity of antibodies produced by single cells. Cold Spring Harbor Sympos. Quant. Biol., 32:423, 1967.

Makinodan, T., et al.: Suppression of immunological responses. Med. Clin. N. Amer., 49:1569, 1965.

McCluskey, R. T., and Cohen, S.: Mechanisms of delayed hypersensitivity. In Ioachim, H. L. (ed.): Pathology Annual 1972. New York, Appleton-Century-Crofts, 1972, p. 111.

McCluskey, R. T., et al.: Studies on the specificity of the cellular infiltrate in delayed hypersensitivity reactions. J. Immun., 90:466, 1963.

McDevitt, H. O., and Benacerraf, B.: Genetic control of specific immune responses. Advances Immun., 11:31, 1969.

McDevitt, H. O., and Bodmer, W. F.: Histocompatibility antigens, immune responsiveness and susceptibility to disease. Amer. J. Med., 52:1, 1972.

McIntire, K. R., et al.: Pathogenesis of the post natal thymectomy wasting syndrome. Nature, 204:151, 1964.

McMaster, P. R. B., and Lerner, E. M.: II. The transfer of allergic thyroiditis in histocompatible guinea pigs by lymph node cells. J. Immun., 99:208, 1967.

Metcalf, D.: The thymus: its role in the immune responses, leukaemia development and carcinogenesis. Recent Results in Cancer Research. Vol. V. Berlin, Springer, 1966.

Miescher, P., et al.: Studies on the pathogenesis of experimental immune thyroiditis. Proc. Soc. Exp. Biol., 107:12, 1961.

Miller, J. F., and Mitchell, G. F.: Thymus and antigen-reactive cells. Transplant. Rev., 1:3, 1969.

Miller, J. F., et al.: Cellular basis of the immunological defects in thymectomized mice. Nature, 214:992, 1967.

Mintz, G., et al.: Ultrastructure of muscle in polymyositis. Amer. J. Med., 44:216, 1968.

Mitchison, N. A.: Induction of immunological paralysis in two zones of dosage. Proc. Roy. Soc. Med., Series B,161:275, 1964.

Mollison, P. L., et al.: Rate of removal from the circulation of red cells sensitized with different amounts of antibodies. Brit. J. Haemat., 11:461, 1965.

Mongar, J. L., and Schild, H. O.: Cellular mechanisms in anaphylaxis. Physiol. Rev., 42:228, 1962.

Moore, M. A. S., and Owen, J. J. T.: Stem cell migration in developing myeloid and lymphoid systems. Lancet, 2:658, 1967.

Morgan, W. S., and Castleman, B.: A clinicopathologic study of Mikulicz's disease. Amer. J. Path., 29:471, 1953.

Mota, I.: The behavior of mast cells in anaphylaxis. Int. Rev. Cytol., 15:363, 1963.

Najarian, J. S., and Foker, J. E.: Mechanisms of kidney allograft rejection. Transplant. Proc., 1:184, 1969.

Najarian, J. S., and Perper, R. J.: Participation of humoral antibodies in allogeneic organ transplantation rejection. Surgery. 62:213, 1967.

Nordin, A. A., et al.: Immunoglobulin classes of antibody-forming cells in mice. IV. The incorporation of tritiated thymidine into IgM and gamma 1 plaque-forming cells during the primary immune response. J. Immun., 105:154, 1970.

Norton, W. L.: Endothelial inclusions in active lesions of systemic lupus erythematosus. J. Lab. Clin. Med., 74:369, 1969.

Norton, W. L., et al.: Evidence of microvascular injury in scleroderma and systemic lupus erythematosus: quantitative study of the microvascular bed. J. Lab. Clin. Med., 71:919, 1968.

Nossal, G. J. V.: The cellular basis of immunity. Harvey Lect., 63:179, 1969.

Nossal, G. J. V.: Mechanisms of antibody production. Ann. Rev. Med., 18:81, 1967.

Nossal, G. J. V., et al.: Cell to cell interaction in the immune response. III. Chromosomal marker analysis of single antibody-forming cells in reconstituted, irradiated or thymectomized mice. J. Exp. Med., 128:839, 1968.

Novack, S. N., and Pearson, C. M.: Cyclophosphamide therapy in Wegener's granulomatosis. New Eng. J. Med., 284:938, 1971.

Osserman, E. F.: Natural history of multiple myeloma before radiological evidence of disease. Radiology, 71:157, 1958.

Osserman, E. F., and Takatsuki, K.: Clinical and immunochemical studies of four cases of heavy (H-gamma₂) chain disease. Amer. J. Med., 37:351, 1964.

Osserman, E. F., and Takatsuki, K.: Plasma cell myeloma: gamma globulin synthesis and structure. Medicine, 42:357, 1963.

Osserman, E. F., et al.: The pathogenesis of "amyloidosis." Studies on the role of abnormal gamma globulin and gamma globulin fragments of the Bence-Jones (1-polypeptide) type in the pathogenesis of "primary" and "secondary amyloidosis" and the "amyloidosis" associated with plasma cell myeloma. Seminars Hemat., 1:3, 1964.

Owen, R. D.: Immunogenetic consequences of vascular anastomoses between bovine twins. Science, 102:400, 1945.

Panayi, G. S.: Unified concept of cell-mediated immune reactions. Brit. Med. J., 2:656, 1970.

Parrott, D. M. V., et al.: Thymus dependent areas in the lymphoid organs of neonatally thymectomized mice. J. Exp. Med., 123:191, 1966.

Pearson, C. M.: Polymyositis and dermatomyositis. In Samter, M. (ed.): Immunological Diseases. Boston, Little, Brown and Co., 1971, p. 1039.

Pearson, C. M.: Polymyositis: clinical forms, diagnosis and therapy. Postgrad. Med., 31:450, 1962.

Percy, D. V. E., et al.: The mammalian homologue of the avian bursa of Fabricius. Lab. Invest., 22:212, 1970.

Perlmann, P., et al.: Cytotoxic effects of leucocytes triggered by complement bound to target cells. Science, 163:937, 1969.

Pilgrim, H. I.: The relationship of chronic ulceration of the ileocecal junction to the development of reticuloendothelial tumors in C₃H mice. Cancer Res., 25:53, 1965.

Polák, L., and Turk, J. L.: Genetic background of certain immunological phenomena with particular reference to the skin. J. Invest. Dermat., 52:219, 1969.

Porter, K. A., et al.: Human renal transplants. I. Glomerular changes. Lab. Invest., 16:153, 1967.

Potter, M., and MacCardle, R. C.: Histology of developing plasma cell neoplasia induced by mineral oil in BALB/C mice. J. Nat. Cancer Inst., 33:497, 1964.

Report, ACS/NIH Organ Transplant Registry. J.A.M.A., 217:1520, 1971.

Rich, A. R., and Gregory, J. E.: The experimental demonstration that periarteritis nodosa is a manifestation of hypersensitivity. Bull. John Hopkins Hosp., 72:65, 1943.

Rodnan, G. P.: The natural history of progressive systemic sclerosis (diffuse scleroderma). Bull. Rheum. Dis., 13:301, 1963a.

Rodnan, G. P.: A review of recent observations and current theories on the etiology and pathogenesis of progressive systemic sclerosis (diffuse scleroderma). J. Chronic Dis., 16:929, 1963b.

Roitt, I. M., and Doniach, D.: Delayed hypersensitivity in autoimmune disease. Brit. Med. Bull., 23:66, 1967.

Riott, I. M., and Torrigiani, G.: Identification and estimation of undegraded thyroglobulin in human serum. Endocrinology, 81:421, 1967.

Roitt, I. M., et al.: Autoantibodies in Hashimoto's disease. Lancet, 2:820, 1956.

Roitt, I. M., et al.: The cellular basis of immunological responses. A synthesis of some current views. Lancet, 2:367, 1969.

Rose, G. A.: The natural history of polyarteritis. Brit. Med. J., 2:1148, 1957.

Rose, M. R., and Witebsky, E.: Studies on organ specificity. V. Changes in the thyroid glands of rabbits following active immunization with rabbit thyroid extract. J. Immun., 76:417, 1956.

Rosse, W. F., et al.: Membrane defects in lysis of normal paroxysmal hemoglobinuria (PNH) red cells by complement. Clin. Res., 13:282, 1965.

Rothfield, N. F., and Rodnan, G. P.: Serum antinuclear antibodies in systemic sclerosis (scleroderma). Arthritis Rheum., 11:607, 1968.

Rowell, N. R.: Lupus erythematosus cells in systemic sclerosis. Ann. Rheum. Dis., 21:70, 1962.

Rumke, P.: Autospermagglutinins: a cause of infertility in men. Ann. N.Y. Acad. Sci., 124:696, 1965.

Russell, P. S., and Winn, H. J.: Transplantation. New Eng. J. Med., 282:786, 1970.

Sato, T., et al.: Chronic polymyositis and myxovirus-like inclusions: electron microscopic and viral studies. Arch. Neurol., 24:409, 1971.

Schlossman, S. F.: The immune response. New Eng. J. Med., 277:1355, 1967.

Schur, P. H.: ANA. New Eng. J. Med., 282:1205, 1970.

Seligmann, M., et al.: A new immunoglobulin abnormality. Science, 162:1396, 1968a.

Seligmann, M., et al.: A proposed classification of primary immunological deficiencies. Amer. J. Med., 45:817, 1968b.

Seligmann, M., et al.: Studies on antinuclear antibodies. Ann. N.Y. Acad. Sci., 124:816, 1965.

Sell, S.: Development of restrictions in the expression of immunoglobulin specificities by lymphoid cells. Transplant. Rev., 5:19, 1970.

Sell, S., and Asofsky, R.: Lymphocytes and immunoglobulins. Progr. Allerg., 12:86, 1968.

Sharp, G. C., and Irvin, W. S.: Autoantibodies. Friend or foe? Amer. J. Med. Sci., 259:365, 1970.

Shearn, M. A., and Tu, W. H.: Latent renal tubular acidosis in Sjögren's syndrome. Ann. Rheum. Dis., 27:27, 1968.

Smith, R. T.: Immunological tolerance of nonliving antigens. Advances Immun., 1:67, 1961.

Smithies, O.: Antibody variability. Somatic recombination between the elements of "antibody gene pairs" may explain antibody variability. Science, *157*:267, 1967.

Starzl, T. E.: Experience in Renal Transplantation. Philadelphia and London, W. B. Saunders, 1964, p. 211.

Stephanini, M., and Mednicoff, I. B.: Demonstration of antivessel agents in serum of patients with anaphylactoid purpura and periarteritis nodosa. J. Clin. Invest., *33*:967, 1954.

Stern, G. M., et al.: Circulating antibodies in polymyositis. J. Neurol. Sci., *5*:181, 1967.

Talal, N., and Bunim, J. J.: The development of malignant lymphoma in the course of Sjögren's syndrome. Amer. J. Med., *36*:529, 1964.

Talal, N., et al.: Extrasalivary lymphoid abnormalities in Sjögren's syndrome (reticulum cell sarcoma, "pseudolymphoma," and macroglobulinemia). Amer. J. Med., *43*:50, 1967.

Tan, E. M., et al.: Ultraviolet light and antibodies to DNA. J. Clin. Invest., *48*:83A, 1969.

Toth, A., and Alpert, L. I.: Progressive systemic sclerosis terminating as periarteritis nodosa. Arch. Path., *92*:31, 1971.

Trayanova, T. G., et al.: Destruction of human cells in tissue culture by lymphocytes from patients with systemic lupus erythematosus. Lancet, *1*:452, 1966.

Tuffanelli, D. L., and Winkelmann, R. K.: Scleroderma and its relationship to the "collagenoses": dermatomyositis, lupus erythematosus, rheumatoid arthritis and Sjögren's syndrome. Amer. J. Med. Sci., *243*:133, 1962.

Tuffanelli, D. L., and Winkelmann, R. K.: Systemic scleroderma: a clinical study of 727 cases. Arch. Dermat., *84*:359, 1961.

Tuohy, J. E., et al.: Wegener's granulomatosis. Amer. J. Med., *25*:638, 1958.

Uitto, J., et al.: Protocollagen proline hydroxylase activity in the skin of normal human subjects and of patients with scleroderma. Scand. J. Lab. Invest., *23*:241, 1969.

Unanue, E. R., and Askonas, B. A.: Persistence of immunogenicity of antigen after uptake by macrophages. J. Exp. Med., *127*:915, 1968.

Weigle, W. O., et al.: Autoimmunity and termination of immunological unresponsiveness. Arch. Path., *84*:647, 1967.

Weissman, I. L.: Thymus cell migration. J. Exp. Med., *126*:291, 1967.

Weitzel, R. A.: Carcinoma coexistent with malignant disorders of plasma cells. Cancer, *11*:546, 1958.

Welton, J., et al.: Macroglobulinemia with bone destruction. Amer. J. Med., *44*:280, 1968.

Whaley, K., and Buchanan, W. W.: Immunologic mechanisms in the pathogenesis of systemic lupus erythematosus. Scot. Med. J., *15*:261, 1970.

W.H.O. Scientific Group: Report. Factors regulating the immune response. W.H.O. Technical Report Series No. 448, 1970, p. 7.

W.H.O. Scientific Group: Report. Genetics of the immune response. W.H.O. Technical Report Series No. 402, 1968, p. 28.

Wiedermann, G., and Miescher, P. A.: Cytoplasmic antibodies in patients with systemic lupus erythematosus. Ann. N.Y. Acad. Sci., *124*:807, 1965.

Wigley, R. D.: The aetiology of polyarteritis nodosa: a review. New Zeal. Med. J., *71*:151, 1970.

Williams, G. M., et al.: Antibodies and human transplant rejection. Ann. Surg., *170*:603, 1969a.

Williams, G. M., et al.: Participation of antibodies in acute cardiac-allograft rejection in man. New Eng. J. Med., *281*:1145, 1969b.

Wilson, R. J., et al.: An early pulmonary physiologic abnormality in progressive systemic sclerosis (diffuse scleroderma). Amer. J. Med., *36*:361, 1964.

Winkelmann, R. K.: Classification and pathogenesis of scleroderma. Mayo Clin. Proc., *46*:83, 1971.

Wolf, J. K.: Primary acquired agammaglobulinemia with a family history of collagen disease and hematologic disorders. New Eng. J. Med., *266*:473, 1962.

Yachnin, S.: Functions and mechanisms of action of complement. New Eng. J. Med., *274*:140, 1966.

Yunis, E. J., and Amos, D. B.: Three closely linked genetic systems relevant to transplantation. Proc. Nat. Acad. Sci. U.S.A., *68*:3031, 1971.

Zeek, P. M.: Periarteritis nodosa. A clinical review. Amer. J. Clin. Path., *22*:777, 1952.

8

SYSTEMIC DISEASES

This chapter concerns itself with an important group of diseases that have two principal characteristics: (1) They result from some derangement in metabolism principally of one of the three major foodstuffs of the body—carbohydrates, proteins or fats. (2) The body as a whole is affected, resulting in changes in many organs and structures. Since each disease tends to evoke its own pattern of involvement, it is usually possible to identify the disease on morphologic and biochemical grounds.

DIABETES MELLITUS

Diabetes mellitus is a genetic metabolic disorder characterized by a lack (absolute or relative) of insulin which results in impaired utilization of carbohydrates and altered lipid and protein metabolism. This hereditary disease must be differentiated from acquired pancreatic diabetes which appears whenever some significant portion of the pancreas and its islets is surgically removed or destroyed by disease. Another form of nonhereditary diabetes is seen in certain forms of hyperadrenalism, acromegaly and with pheochromocytomas. While these endocrinopathies affect carbohydrate metabolism and induce hyperglycemia and diabetes, control of the basic endocrine dysfunction corrects the metabolic derangement. These nongenetic forms of diabetes mellitus are not associated with the striking predisposition to generalized vascular disease characteristic of the genetic disease. The hereditary form of diabetes mellitus is by far the most common, and is the focus of the subsequent discussion.

Glucose and free fatty acids are the primary and the immediate sources of energy for the body. In diabetes mellitus, not only is carbohydrate metabolism seriously deranged, but simultaneously fatty acid synthesis is impaired. The diabetic relies, therefore, for his energy needs on the metabolism of lipids, stored or dietary, and so produces excessive amounts of acetyl-CoA and ketone bodies (acetoacetic acid, beta-hydroxybutyric acid and acetone). Ketosis and acidosis result and, in the neutralization and excretion of the organic acids, potassium and sodium are lost. Some of the accumulated acetyl-CoA is diverted to excess synthesis of cholesterol. Thus, hypercholesterolemia is a prominent feature of diabetes mellitus and, as will be seen later, is associated with the grave consequence of accelerated atherosclerosis. Anabolic processes such as synthesis of glycogen, proteins and triglycerides are slowed while proteins and glycogen are catabolized for gluconeogenesis and sources of energy. The impaired carbohydrate, fat and protein metabolism eventually involves all of the endocrine glands but principally the anterior pituitary and the adrenals. Growth hormone is necessary for mobilization of stored triglycerides but, unfortunately, the liberated fatty acids act as insulin inhibitors. Adrenal steroids are involved in gluconeogenesis. *Thus, diabetes is a complex metabolic pluriglandular systemic disorder manifested principally by glycosuria, hypercholesterolemia and, often, ketoacidosis.*

Significant as the metabolic derangements are to the survival of the diabetic, they are generally controllable with the use of insulin or oral hypoglycemic agents. A greater threat to life is the increased susceptibility of the diabetic to generalized vascular disease, principally atherosclerosis and small vessel disease (microangiopathy). The atherosclerosis pursues an accelerated course even in the very young so that, in the course of 10 to 15 years, it often becomes sufficiently advanced to cause ischemic lesions in many organs, principally the heart, brain and kidneys. Nearly 80 per cent of diabetics die of some form of cardiovascular disease (including renal vascular disease) — roughly twice the number of nondiabetics (Entmacher et al., 1964) (Kessler, 1971). Most of these deaths result from myocardial infarction caused by coronary atherosclerosis, but cerebral strokes, renal failure, mesenteric occlusions with intestinal infarctions and gangrene of the lower extremities also exact their toll.

For years, there has been a dispute as to whether control of the metabolic derangements and, more specifically, the blood glucose levels will simultaneously control the predisposition to atherosclerosis. The Joslin Clinic points with pride to "gold medal" (carefully regulated) diabetic patients who have had their disease for up to 45 years without having developed vascular complications (Chazan et al., 1970). Many others, however, disagree and deny the value of rigid metabolic control in protecting against the onward march of the cardiovascular lesions (Conn, 1964) (Ellenberg, 1963). Central to this controversy is the question: Is the predisposition to atherosclerosis the consequence of the deranged carbohydrate and lipid metabolism or is the genetic insulin-carbohydrate disorder somehow associated with, but separate from, a hereditary predisposition to vascular disease? We shall return to this controversy but, in any event, diabetes mellitus is more than a disorder of carbohydrate metabolism; it is simultaneously associated with a striking predisposition to atherosclerosis and small vessel disease.

Classification. The diabetic state varies over a wide range of clinical expressions in terms of age of onset, severity of biochemical defect, clinical manifestations, rate of progression and response to therapy. Indeed, the basic genotype may not be the same in all patients and there may be a multiplicity of hereditary factors. Within this spectrum of phenotypes clearly established is the existence of two forms of hereditary disease: juvenile (growth onset) and adult (maturity onset) diabetes. No arbitrary age divides these forms but they are clearly separable by a difference in islet cell function. The juvenile diabetic has an absolute deficiency of insulin secretion, the adult has a less clear basis for the relative lack of insulin function. Pragmatically, most patients with manifest diabetes before the age of 25 are probably juvenile diabetics.

The variable expression of the carbohydrate metabolic derangement in both the growth onset and maturity onset forms of hereditary diabetes makes it possible to establish stages of the disease. One widely used classification recognizes four stages: (1) prediabetes, (2) latent or subclinical diabetes, (3) chemical diabetes and (4) overt or manifest diabetes (Lister, 1966) (Danowski, 1964).

Prediabetes is a theoretical state through which all individuals who eventually develop overt diabetes pass. It implies the existence of a hereditary predisposition to the disease and is applicable only to offspring of two diabetic parents or to monovular twins, one of whom is diabetic. Some investigators would add to this category the mother of many unusually large babies, a characteristic of the diabetic state.

Latent or subclinical diabetes refers to the stage wherein the glucose tolerance test is normal under usual conditions, but becomes abnormal under such stresses as pregnancy, emotional disturbances, infections and physical trauma. The administration of cortisone will provoke an abnormal glucose tolerance test (Fajans and Conn, 1959).

Chemical diabetes refers to the stage where the patient is asymptomatic, usually has normal fasting blood glucose levels but has a postprandial hyperglycemia and a clearly abnormal glucose tolerance test. Chemical diabetes may be transformed to overt disease during periods of stress and by excessive weight gain. This stage may exist unchanged for many years and it is estimated that perhaps 50 to 60 per cent of such patients never develop the overt disease (Fajans et al., 1969). However, the patient with chemical diabetes is at high risk, and the existence of this stage should be suspected whenever parents, siblings or close relatives are diabetic.

Overt or manifest diabetes represents the full-blown clinical symptom complex. Fasting and postprandial hyperglycemia are regularly present and the patient has all the metabolic and vascular problems already mentioned. Many patients with a mild form of overt diabetes shift back and forth between the chemical and overt stages.

There is no certainty that patients with one stage of the disease will inevitably develop the next more serious stage; however, the hereditary trait undoubtedly underlies all stages and so implies the possibility of such progression. Environmental factors — obesity, pregnancy and some endocrine dysfunctions are diabetogenic and unmask the hereditary trait or worsen the diabetic state. Similarly, stress, particularly infections, physical trauma and emotional disturbances are diabetogenic in those with the trait.

The relationship between increasing body weight and the development of clinical diabetes is well documented by the fact that approximately 80 per cent of maturity onset diabetics are obese and, conversely, about 60 per cent of grossly obese adults have carbohydrate intolerance, usually in the form of slightly abnormal glucose tolerance tests. The carbohydrate intolerance tends to return to normal following weight loss (Yalow et al., 1965) (Solomon et al., 1968). Reduction of body weight in the diabetic is usually followed by reduced insulin requirements and may, indeed, convert diabetes to the chemical stage. The nature of this association is not clearly established, but it has been attributed to increased rates of mobilization of fatty acids with their antagonism of insulin. An increased resistance to insulin in the fatty peripheral tissues has also been postulated as contributing to the diabetogenic action of obesity.

An increased insulin resistance is found in the later stages of pregnancy, but its precise nature is still uncertain. Increased estrogen and progesterone levels may contribute, but recent evidence suggests that it is largely due to the release of placental lactogen which, like growth hormone, accelerates lipolysis (Turtle and Kipnis, 1967) (Josimovich and MacLaren, 1962). Women who develop overt diabetes during pregnancy and who are presumably genetically predisposed often return to the stage of chemical diabetes or subclinical diabetes following delivery, only years later to become overt diabetics. The diabetogenic effect is enhanced with increasing parity.

The association between hyperglycemia and certain endocrine disorders is well established. These patients have diabetes mellitus, but not the hereditary form, and so can be cured of their deranged carbohydrate metabolism if the primary endocrinopathy can be controlled. The increased secretion of growth hormone in acromegaly is diabetogenic. Indeed, it has been shown by Young (1937) that administration of anterior pituitary extract may produce permanent diabetes in dogs by causing prolonged hyperglycemia and exhaustion atrophy of the beta cells. The mechanism of action of growth hormone is not established but may be the induction of excessive lipolysis and insulin antagonism by the released fatty acids, or the hormone may directly inhibit insulin release (Mayhew et al., 1969). It should be stressed that there is no evidence that the anterior pituitary plays a primary role in the production of genetic diabetes. It may, however, precipitate the disease in those having a hereditary predisposition (Luft et al., 1967).

Excess glucocorticoids, such as occur in Cushing's syndrome and in those persons receiving steroid therapy, increase the need for insulin by accelerating gluconeogenesis. The resulting hyperglycemia is steroid-dependent and the adrenal hyperfunction only leads to permanent diabetes in those with the trait (McKiddie et al., 1968). Hyperaldosteronism is also thought to be a possible cause of abnormal carbohydrate metabolism, presumably by impairing insulin release. Thyroxin appears to modify the responsiveness of the islets to glucose. Because pheochromocytomas elaborate catecholamines, hyperglycemia and glycosuria are encountered in about 10 per cent, but here again this deranged glucose metabolism returns to normal when the tumor is excised (Freedman et al., 1958). These endocrinopathies could, over the course of years, lead to classic diabetes by prolonged stress on the pancreatic islets, particularly in those persons with the genetic trait.

All forms of physical stress, including trauma, infections, hypoxia and hyperthermia are diabetogenic in those harboring the hereditary trait. All probably act by stimulating the release of catecholamines which, in turn, induce hepatic glycogenolysis and lipolysis, thus uncovering the existence of prediabetes or subclinical diabetes. It is no surprise, then, that the insulin requirements of the overt disease almost always mount during periods of stress.

Incidence and Inheritance. While the exact prevalence of diabetes is not known, no one would challenge the statement that it is a very common disease. As a reasonable estimate, approximately 2 per cent of Americans have diabetes, but only about half of them have been diagnosed. It is further estimated from projections of known diabetics and their family trees that perhaps 5 per cent of the American population are potentially diabetic because they harbor the genetic trait (Sharkey, 1971). Because the disease may appear at any age, the prevalence in each decade rises progressively throughout life and is greater than 10 per cent in the eighth decade (O'Sullivan et al., 1967).

The genetic study of diabetes has been called a "geneticist's nightmare" (Neel, 1969). The problem is made complex by lack of uniform diagnostic criteria, the variable clinical expression of the disease and the likelihood that the basic genetic mutation may be polygenic. Most recent views reject the older hypothesis of transmission by a single recessive autosomal gene with reduced penetrance. Favored today is polygenic inheritance involving the small additive effects of at least several alleles at different chromosomal loci. Such a mode of transmission would be most compatible with the wide variation in clinical expression. But, in addition to the hereditary trait, many environmental influences, particularly obesity and pregnancy, condition the expression of the metabolic defect (Simpson, 1964). Whether there is a basic genetic difference between the childhood and adult forms of the disease has not yet been established.

Pathogenesis. Frustration has dogged the search for the fundamental defect in diabetes. The following is well established. Administration of insulin to diabetics promptly corrects the hyperglycemia and controls the carbohydrate defect with its attendant metabolic ramifications. The precise biochemical structure of insulin is known and has been synthesized in the test tube (Katsoyannis, 1964). The intracellular morphologic and biosynthetic pathways of its formation have been elegantly delineated (Lacy and Hartroft, 1959) (Renold and Burr, 1970). Precise immunoassay methods are now available for its quantitation in plasma and the pancreas (Yalow and Berson, 1960). Notwithstanding these gains, the basis for the insulin lack in maturity onset diabetes is still unkown as is the precise role of insulin in carbohydrate metabolism. Some understanding of insulin biosynthesis and release is necessary even to consider working hypotheses of the pathogenesis of diabetes mellitus.

Insulin, with a molecular weight of 5700, is derived from proinsulin, a large single chain protein having a molecular weight of about 9000 (Sanger, 1959) (Steiner et al., 1967). Conversion of the precursor into insulin is effected by peptidases in both beta cells of the islets and plasma, which "chop out" of the long chain a 30-amino acid connecting segment. The two terminal segments, together containing 51 amino acid residues, are then linked together by disulfide bonds to form insulin. Proinsulin is secreted into the plasma by the pancreas and, although it has a high degree of cross reactivity in the insulin immunoassay tests, it has low biologic activity in terms of its effect on glucose metabolism. It probably represents less than 15 per cent of the plasma insulin as measured by immunologic assays. It should be noted that there is no evidence that the fundamental defect in hereditary diabetes represents excessive secretion of proinsulin (Goldsmith et al., 1969).

As with all polypeptides, proinsulin synthesis takes place on the ribosomes of the endoplasmic reticulum. Passing along the endoplasmic reticulum to the Golgi apparatus, it is packaged into membrane-bounded sacs which comprise the granules of the beta cells of the pancreatic islets (Lacy, 1968). Crystalline structures have been resolved within these granules, but whether they represent proinsulin or insulin is not yet clear, and the precise site of the conversion of proinsulin to insulin has not been established. In any event, in response to insulin demands, these granules migrate to the plasma membrane of the beta cell and, by a process of emiocytosis, their contents are solubilized and discharged into the plasma, representing insulin release. The beta cell is freely permeable to its prime physiologic stimulus — glucose. After phosphorylation, glucose initiates both insulin release and synthesis. In contrast, the sulfonylureas (oral hypoglycemic agents) such as tolbutamide only effect release, but do not stimulate synthesis of more insulin. When insulin is released into the circulation, it must traverse the basement membrane on which the beta cells rest, then the vascular basement membrane and finally the endothelial cells themselves. In maturity onset diabetics, the vascular basement membrane becomes thickened, but there is no evidence that this basement membrane alteration exerts a blocking effect on the secretory process. Once in the circulation, insulin is degraded by cleavage of the disulfide bonds, yielding A and B chains having low biologic activity. There is no evidence that the hereditary diabetic trait represents a block in the conversion of proinsulin to insulin or excessive cleavage of insulin (Levine, 1967).

Insulin is secreted in a biphasic process. There is an initial rapid and transient secretory response, probably representing release of stored insulin, followed by a more sustained secretion thought to represent active beta cell synthesis and release of more insulin. Although many stimuli trigger insulin release from the beta cell, glucose more specifically glucose-6-phosphate is the most potent stimulus. Orally administered glucose is more effective than a similar load given intravenously even though the latter produces an immediate higher blood glucose level. This observation led to the recognition that several intestinal hormones—gastrin, secretin, pancreozymin and enteroglucagon—all have insulin-releasing activity (Creutzfeldt et al., 1970). These hormones stimulate insulin release following ingestion of food, thereby anticipating the rise in blood glucose levels resulting from the digestion of food. Several amino acids, particularly arginine, lysine, phenylalanine and leucine, stimulate insulin release (Floyd et al., 1966). How these act is unclear, but they may possibly release intestinal hormones. They also appear to enhance glucose stimulation of the beta cell (Jarrett et al., 1969). Inorganic cations, particularly calcium, are necessary for the insulin release secondary to glucose-6-phosphate stimulation. Other cations, including potassium, sodium and possibly magnesium, also modify the release of insulin, possibly because of their roles in the maintenance of the normal permeability of the plasma membrane of the beta cell (Renold, 1970).

Pancreatic glucagon plays a complex role in carbohydrate metabolism. It stimulates hepatic glycogenolysis, thereby raising blood glucose levels but, at the same time, it is a potent stimulator of insulin release. Pancreatic glucagon is itself elaborated in response to the secretion of the intestinal hormone pancreozymin and it could well be important in maintaining normoglycemia following a largely protein meal. The protein meal is not immediately converted to glucose and yet it would stimulate intestinal mechanisms which release insulin. Thus, the glucagon would support the blood glucose levels by glycogenolysis and the later-occurring postprandial hyperglycemia would be compensated for by the direct glucagon-insulin release mechanism (Lawrence, 1969). It now seems likely that many of the hormones, including glucagon and gastrin, act by stimulation of adenyl cyclase and the formation of intracellular cyclic adenosine monophosphate (AMP) from adenosine triphosphate (ATP). *Cyclic AMP probably represents the ultimate intracellular signal of insulin release and it is probable that all mediators converge on this pathway* (Sussman and Vaughan, 1967).

Turning to the role of insulin in carbohydrate metabolism, it is surprising that it is still a matter of some controversy. That it facilitates transport or entry of glucose into some cells, particularly fibroblasts, muscle and fat cells, is well established. It is postulated that insulin acts as a carrier shuttling back and forth across the membrane, delivering glucose to the interior of the cell (Levine, 1967). Insulin also suppresses glycogenolysis and gluconeogenesis (Madison, 1969). It inhibits lipolysis and favors synthesis of fatty acids and lipogenesis from excess dietary carbohydrates. More controversial is the question of whether insulin is necessary for the intracellular metabolism of glucose. At one time, it was proposed that insulin was necessary to permit the conversion of glucose to glucose-6-phosphate, catalyzed by glucokinase. This activity has been fairly well ruled out, but whether insulin might facilitate other reactions in the glucose metabolic pathway has not yet been excluded.

Against this background, we can turn to some of the current hypotheses of the pathogenesis of the hereditary form of diabetes mellitus. Least controversial is the evidence that *juvenile diabetics have an absolute or at least severe insulin deficiency* (Kipnis, 1970). They have pathologic evidence of beta cell destruction (Ogilvie, 1964), decreased quantities of insulin extractable from the pancreas (Wrenshall et al., 1952) and severely deficient or totally absent insulin secretory response to oral glucose as measured by the immunoreactive assay methods (Parker et al., 1968). They also fail to show a secretory response to glucagon. Thus, a juvenile diabetic derives no benefit from the administration of oral hypoglycemic drugs since his pancreas lacks insulin (Chiumello et al., 1968). A variety of inflammatory changes may be found in and about the islets in juvenile diabetics, suggesting destruction of beta cells. Destruction of beta cells by an autoimmune reaction or overwork has been proposed as the trigger of the inflammatory response, but without proof. Animal models of "insulitis" and diabetes mellitus have been developed by immunizing rabbits against insulin (Grodsky et al., 1966). The suggestion has been made that insulin is a sequestered antigen in the fetus and immunization occurs postnatally in the juvenile diabetic. How such a notion fits the hereditary nature of the disease is unclear. Synthesis of an "abnormal" insulin has been offered as an alternative pathogenetic mechanism (Elliot et al., 1965). Whatever the cause of the initial insulin deficiency, the strain on the residual functioning cells undoubtedly is injurious and the insulin deficit of juvenile diabetics worsens over the course of years, reflecting progressive loss of islet cell mass and ability to elaborate insulin. It might be noted that occasional adults have this juvenile pattern of the disease.

The pathogenesis of the maturity onset form of the disease is much more uncertain. The following proposals have been made: (1) There is an absolute or relative deficiency of insulin, perhaps because the insulin release mechanism is deranged or delayed; (2) insulin circulates in the blood in a biologically ineffective form; (3) an abnormal nonfunctional insulin is elaborated or there is antagonism to the action of insulin, either in the circulation or in the peripheral tissues. Other theories exist but are not given wide credence (Renold and Burr, 1970) (Clarke, 1970). With respect to an absolute deficiency of insulin, maturity onset diabetics, paradoxically, respond to glucose challenge with abnormally high levels of insulin. To explain this apparent paradox, the term "relative lack" has been introduced.

There is a growing conviction that, *in the maturity onset form of the disease the insulin response is either delayed, inappropriate or is relatively deficient in terms of the duration-level of the hyperglycemia* (Luft, 1968). With regard to the delayed insulin response, in normal persons following glucose loading there is a prompt release of insulin which reaches its peak in 30 to 60 minutes and returns to normal in about two hours. In the maturity onset diabetic, the insulin secretion does not peak before 60 minutes and fails to return to basal levels for three to four hours. Thus in the normal, the blood glucose and insulin curves remain in phase, but in the diabetic the insulin delay leads first to hyperglycemia and then to hypoglycemia (Perley and Kipnis, 1966). Relative to the level and duration of the hyperglycemia, the total insulin output is deficient, and these patients are said to have a "low insulinogenic index" (Seltzer et al., 1967). Further evidence that the secretory capacity or responsiveness of the beta cell in maturity onset diabetes is diminished has been derived from determining the plasma insulin response to intravenous tolbutamide. This shows a marked impairment in the early phase of insulin secretion in the maturity onset diabetic (Perley and Kipnis, 1966). Thus, most experts favor the view that *the essential feature of maturity onset genetic diabetes is a delayed and inappropriate secretory response to hyperglycemia and so, in both the juvenile and adult forms of the disease, there is a deficiency of insulin production perhaps resulting from genetically determined defects in the beta cells* (Seltzer, 1969).

The proposition that a maturity onset diabetic suffers from a biologically ineffective insulin has not yet been excluded. It is believed that in the normal individual, when insulin is released into the circulation, it is in part loosely bound to albumin, the so-called free insulin, and in part bound more tightly or complexed in some form which impairs its activity (Antoniades et al., 1961). In diabetics, it has been suggested that most of the insulin is in the tightly bound form, impairing its participation in carbohydrate metabolsim (Antoniades et al.,

1962). These claims have not been substantiated. For a time, it was suspected that the problem lay in the secretion of proinsulin due to some beta cell inability to form the biologically effective insulin. This view has now been excluded because studies of the relative biologic effectiveness of endogenous insulin in diabetics and nondiabetics fail to disclose any differences (Kipnis, 1970).

Although most of the evidence supports the view that the major defect in hereditary diabetes represents an abnormal secretory response of beta cells, insulin antagonists have not been completely excluded as contributing to the diabetic state. Vallance-Owen et al. (1955) have for years contended that a pituitary-adrenal dependent and genetically determined antagonist, normally present in plasma, is increased in amount in diabetes. The antagonist is called synalbumin and it has been proposed that genetic coding determines the amount produced. This hypothesis has been challenged by many but cannot be totally discounted (Davidson and Goodner, 1967). As well known, the diabetic mobilizes excessive amounts of lipids and releases increased amounts of fatty acids which are, indeed, insulin antagonists (Hales and Randle, 1963). It is unclear which is cause and which is effect.

The notion that diabetics elaborate an abnormal insulin (to be distinguished from a normal but complexed insulin) cannot, at the present time, be discounted. Some diabetics, untreated with insulin, habor insulin antibodies, suggesting a response to a "foreign" protein (Mancini et al., 1964). Moreover, immunofluorescent studies indicate the existence of apparent insulin antibodies in some of the vascular lesions found in adult diabetic patients (Blumenthal, 1968). Such immunologic reactions support the possibility of the secretion of an abnormal insulin evoking an immune response, and so autoimmunity once again rears its head as a possible pathogenetic mechanism (Sharkey, 1968).

In conclusion, the pathogenesis of the maturity onset form of the disease is still not settled. On balance, it would seem most reasonable to believe that the juvenile and adult forms of the disease have similar origins conditioned by hereditary traits. If such be the case and if the juvenile suffers from an absolute lack of insulin, it would be rational to believe that the adult has inherited a less severe expression of the defect and thus has a relative lack of insulin, perhaps residing in an inappropriate response to demand. It should be recognized, however, that all of the above provides no insights into the translation of the genotypic alteration into the phenotypically modified beta cell.

Morphology. The diagnosis of diabetes mellitus on morphologic grounds alone can be made only in some patients; most have lesions that are only suggestive, and some have no distinctive lesions. While many organs may be affected, the major changes are found in the pancreas, blood vessels, kidneys and eyes. With a few exceptions, the juvenile onset and maturity onset forms of the disease cannot be distinguished on morphologic grounds. The growth onset form of the disease is more likely to have diagnostic changes in the islets. The maturity onset form of the disease is often associated with islet lesions, but these are not usually distinctive and, indeed, may be absent. After 10 to 15 years of both forms of the disease, large and small vessel lesions are almost inevitably present in the kidney and eye grounds as well as in other tissue and, while these vascular lesions are not qualitatively different from those in nondiabetics, their exaggerated severity should arouse suspicion of the existence of genetic diabetes. Moreover, their stage of advancement will correlate with the duration of the disease although, as has been pointed out, some believe that rigid therapeutic metabolic control blocks the advance of these vascular changes (Ricketts, 1960). This view, however, is not widely held.

Pancreas. In their study of diabetics, including juveniles and adults, Warren and LeCompte (1952), using routine methods of light microscopy, found at post mortem the following islet changes: hyaline (amyloid) degeneration (41 per cent), fibrosis (23 per cent), hydropic degeneration, as well as glycogen accumulation (4 per cent), lymphocytic infiltration (1 per cent), hemochromatosis (2 per cent), hypertrophy (8 per cent), adenoma (7 per cent) and normal islets (33 per cent). More will be said about the so-called normal islets which, indeed, often disclose beta cell degranulation when more intensive methods of study are used.

Hyaline deposits are the most common alteration in the islets of maturity onset diabetics. Pink amorphous material is found in intercellular locations and in and about the capillaries compressing and distorting the islet cells (Fig. 8—1). Under the electron microscope, this hyaline material shows masses of interlacing small fibrils characteristic of amyloid. However, in other tissues apparently similar hyaline deposits are observed that do not appear to be fibrillar, so that at the present time the nature of this substance remains uncertain. Because of the known association of amyloid with immunologic derangements (p. 283), the composition of the pancreatic hyalin may point to a possible autoimmune pathogenesis of this disease. Progressive ac-

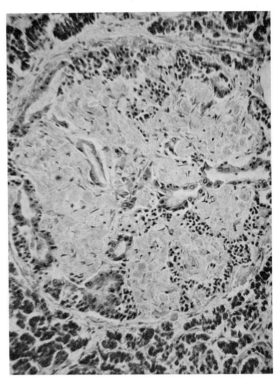

Figure 8–1. Hyalinization of an islet in the pancreas.

cumulations of this hyaline material may reduce the beta cell mass, but there is no clear correlation between the severity of the metabolic derangement and the extent of the hyalinization. The severity of these deposits is better correlated with the duration of the disease and, in the late stages, the islets may be virtually totally replaced (Lacy, 1964). Such hyaline (amyloid) deposits have been reported in nondiabetics by some investigators, but others insist that these changes are pathognomonic of diabetes and their presence in patients without hyperglycemia merely indicates the prediabetic stage. This controversy remains unresolved.

Fibrosis implies thickening of the capsule and stroma of the islets by fibrous connective tissue, ultimately leading to collagenization and replacement of the islet cells. The severity of the fibrosis is correlated with the duration of the diabetes. Fibrosis, however, is without question also encountered in nondiabetics with severe atherosclerosis, so that the change is not diagnostic of diabetes.

Glycogen accumulation and hydropic degeneration are both manifested in the diabetic pancreas by distended foamy vacuolated beta cells. The alpha cells are not affected. The glycogen accumulation is related to the level and duration of the hyperglycemia in the last days of life. Sometimes, the clear vacuoles are devoid of glycogen. These water-containing vacuoles can be produced in the experimental animal by inducing hyperglycemia and presumably overworking the beta cells.

"Ballooning" degeneration, as this hydropic vacuolation is called, may be a portent of cell death to come.

Leukocytic infiltrations into and immediately about the islets are found in some juvenile diabetics. The term "insulitis" has been applied to this lesion, seen usually in growth onset diabetics who come to autopsy within days to weeks of the onset of their disease. The well known involvement of lymphocytes in immunologic reactions and the rapidly progressive nature of the juvenile form of the disease both raise the suspicion that, whatever the nature of the fundamental genetic weakness of the beta cell, cell death from overwork or an immune reaction contributes to the relatively rapid downhill course of this form of diabetes. Very similar changes have been found in the islets of cows and rabbits immunized with heterologous insulin. A second type of leukocytic infiltrate comprises a mixture of lymphocytes and eosinophils usually found in infants born of diabetic mothers. Here it is postulated that beta cell death occurs in the infant as a consequence of the overwork imposed by the hyperglycemia of the mother. Lending support to this interpretation is the marked hypertrophy and hyperplasia of the islets associated with this leukocytic reaction, a further indication of a compensatory reaction to hyperglycemia.

Adenomas of the pancreas were found in a few cases in the series of diabetics studied by Warren and LeCompte (1952). Their occurrence bore no relationship to the duration of the diabetes or the age of the patient. Presumably, the adenomas were noninsulin secreting.

Islets appearing **normal** with routine light microscopy were present in 33 per cent of the patients reported by Warren and LeCompte (1952). However, when some of these so-called "normals" are submitted to quantitation of either the beta cell mass or extractable insulin, abnormalities are usually found. Moreover, degranulation of the beta cells can also be seen. It is possible, then, that in the course of diabetes the pancreas undergoes first beta cell degranulation, then loss of beta cells themselves and ultimately loss of islet cell mass. It is only when rigorous quantitation and electron microscopy are performed that the extent of the loss becomes apparent. Using such techniques, it is highly likely that the great preponderance of diabetics have abnormalities in their islets (Ogilvie, 1964).

Vascular System. The diabetic is particularly prone to the development of vascular lesions in vessels of all sizes. The large vessel disease, namely atherosclerosis, accounts for the heavy toll exacted by myocardial infarction, cerebral strokes and gangrene of the lower extremities in these patients. **Significant coronary atherosclerosis and myocardial infarction is up to five times more prevalent in diabetics than in the normal popula-** tion (Goldenberg et al., 1958) (Thomas et al., 1956). In one postmortem survey, the incidence of coronary thrombosis in diabetic subjects ranged from 20 to 64 per cent, depending on the age at death of the patient, and in nondiabetic subjects from 2 to 23 per cent (Liebow and Hellerstein, 1949). Whereas myocardial infarction is uncommon in nondiabetic females during reproductive life, it is almost as common in diabetic females as in diabetic males. Gangrene of the lower extremities is a hundred-fold more common in diabetics than in nondiabetics. The other common form of vascular disease in diabetics is microangiopathy—thickening of the walls of arterioles, capillaries and venules. It contributes to the increased mortality rate of diabetes principally by damaging the kidneys, but it also induces significant morbidity by involvement of retinal, neural and skin vessels as well as those in other tissues.

Arteries. Atherosclerosis begins to appear in diabetics, whatever their age, within a few years of the onset of the disease. Only 2 to 5 per cent of nondiabetics but approximately 75 per cent of diabetics below the age of 40 have moderate to severe atherosclerosis (Robertson and Strong, 1968). The vascular lesions do not differ qualitatively from those found in nondiabetics. This form of arterial disease is discussed in detail on p. 586, but to understand its clinical significance, it is necessary only to point out that it comprises the development of raised intimal lipid-laden plaques called atheromas (Fig. 8—2). These at first may be widely scattered in the aorta, coronary arteries or any artery but, with progression of the disease, they become larger and more numerous, encroach on the un-

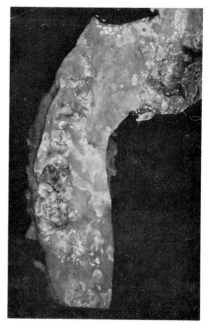

Figure 8–2. Atherosclerosis of the aorta.

derlying media and undergo a constellation of superimposed alterations, e.g., the endothelial surface of the atheroma may ulcerate and so provide a prime site for thrombosis. They may become fibrotic or calcify and thus render the vessel inelastic and rigid or, by causing medial damage, they may predispose to aneurysmal dilatation (Fig. 8–3). Thus, atherosclerosis may lead to arterial narrowing or occlusion and attendant ischemic injury to organs or, alternatively, it may induce aneurysmal dilatation seen most often in the aorta with its grave potential of rupture (p. 615).

The susceptibility of the diabetic to atherosclerosis remains an enigma. It does not correlate with severity of the disease, but rather with its duration. Pragmatically, all diabetics who have had their disease for at least 10 years are likely to have moderate to severe atherosclerosis. Elevated blood lipid levels—be it in diabetes, the nephrotic syndrome, hypothyroidism or some genetic lipid derangement—are always associated with an increased predisposition to atherosclerosis.

Nonetheless, the doubt still persists that in genetic diabetes the predisposition to vascular disease stems from a hereditary trait separate from the trait involved in carbohydrate metabolism. There are numerous reports of diabetics having premature atherosclerosis long before deranged carbohydrate or lipid metabolism became evident (Herman and Gorlin, 1965) (Ellenberg, 1963). However, before dismissing the causal relationship between the vascular disease and the metabolic derangements, it should be noted that the cause of atherosclerosis is unknown. There may be hidden causal metabolic derangements in diabetes, and the elevated levels of blood glucose and lipids may be only the top of the iceberg of the biochemical disruption in the diabetic state (New et al., 1963) (Kagan et al., 1963). In this context, abnormal levels of circulating insulin (Mahler, 1966) and deranged mucopolysaccharide metabolism have also been suspected as playing some role in the development of the arterial disease (Yudkin and Roddy, 1964).

Arterioles. Thickening of the walls of arterioles—arteriolosclerosis—is not only more common among diabetics than normals, but it also tends to be more severe (Siperstein et al., 1964). The mural thickening is a consequence of many changes: an amorphous hyalinization of the arteriole wall, basement membrane thickening, endothelial proliferation, pericytic proliferation and deposits of PAS-positive mucopolysaccharides (Blumenthal, 1968). Indistinguishable arteriolosclerosis can also be found in nondiabetic hypertensive patients (p. 602). In the diabetic it may be found in the absence of hypertension (Bell, 1953). The arteriolosclerosis affects all vascular beds, particularly those in the kidneys. There is a vigorous controversy as to whether this arteriolar lesion is a manifestation of an immune disorder.

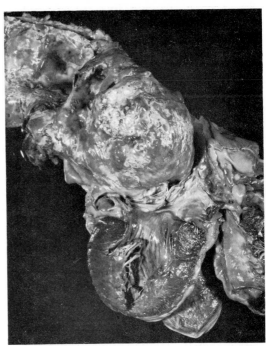

Figure 8–3. Atherosclerosis of the aorta with irregular, pale calcific deposits in the aortic intima.

Plasma proteins, among them immunoglobulins, have been identified in the thickened arteriole walls (Bloodworth, 1963). However, others interpret these changes as merely reflecting increased permeability of damaged vessels and point out the presence of similar plasma proteins in the arteriolosclerosis of nondiabetics (Larsson, 1967).

Capillaries. Thickening of the walls of precapillaries, capillaries and venules—microangiopathy—is a characteristic finding in most diabetics. These changes are particularly evident in the vessels of the skin, muscle, peripheral nerves and eye. Save for the lesions in muscles, similar microangiopathy may be encountered in nondiabetics, and so it is not pathognomonic of the disease. The microangiopathy of muscle capillaries is rarely observed in the nondiabetic. The severity of involvement of all capillary beds, save those in muscle, is related to the duration of the disease. Microangiopathy has been observed in patients with chemical diabetes and biochemically normal close relatives of diabetic persons, raising once again the spectre of a separate but parallel hereditary trait for vascular disease (Siperstein et al., 1968). The thickening is largely the consequence of uneven thickening and splitting of the basement membrane of the small vessels, accompanied by the deposit of a PAS-positive material rich in mucopolysaccharides. In addition, immunoglobulins and complement have been identified in these thickened capillaries, and Blumenthal (1968) raises the possibility that the immunoglobulins are bound to insulin and so represent some form of immune causation of the microangiopathy. However, others, principally Larsson (1967), challenge this concept. The renal microangiopathy, as will be seen, is responsible for significant glomerular damage.

Kidneys. The kidneys are usually the most severely damaged organs in the diabetic. Renal failure, usually due to renal microvascular disease, accounts for many of the diabetic deaths in both juveniles and adults. Any one or any combination of the following lesions may be found: (1) glomerular involvement with three distinctive patterns—diffuse glomerulosclerosis, nodular glomerulosclerosis and exudative lesions, (2) arteriolosclerosis inducing so-called benign nephrosclerosis, (3) pyelonephritis, sometimes with necrotizing papillitis, (4) glycogen accumulation in tubular cells and (5) fatty change of tubular cells.

Glomerular Lesions. **Diffuse glomerulosclerosis** is the most common form of nephropathy in the diabetic and is present in at least 90 per cent of patients who have had their disease for more than 10 years. It is not limited to diabetes mellitus since it is encountered in nondiabetic aged patients, particularly those with hypertension, advanced atherosclerosis and arteriolosclerosis. However, it occurs to a more extreme degree in diabetic patients. Diffuse glomerulosclerosis comprises an overall thickening of the basement membranes of the capillaries throughout their entire length, associated with the proliferation of mesangial cells and the deposition of excess amounts of mesangial matrix which may engulf and, in fact, obliterate the mesangial cells (Kimmelstiel et al., 1966). Both the matrix depositions and membrane thickenings are PAS-positive. The membranes may be widened up to tenfold. All capillaries are more or less affected, although not entirely uniformly. These changes almost always begin in the vascular stalk and sometimes seem continuous with the almost invariably present hyaline thickening of arterioles. In more marked glomerular involvements, the foot processes of the epithelial cells are lost and the lumina of the glomerular capillaries are narrowed. Eventually, the entire glomerular tuft may undergo sclerosis.

Nodular glomerulosclerosis is also known as intercapillary glomerulosclerosis or Kimmelstiel-Wilson disease. Whereas diffuse glomerulosclerosis is commonly found in nondiabetics, the nodular pattern is widely held to be pathognomonic of diabetes mellitus, although a few dissenting opinions may be found (Brown et al., 1968). **The glomerular lesions take the form of ovoid or spherical, often laminated, hyaline masses situated in the periphery of the glomerular tuft.** They lie within the mesangial core of the glomerular lobules and often are surrounded by peripheral patent capillary loops (Fig. 8–4). One, several or all of the lobules in the individual glomerulus may be involved as may any num-

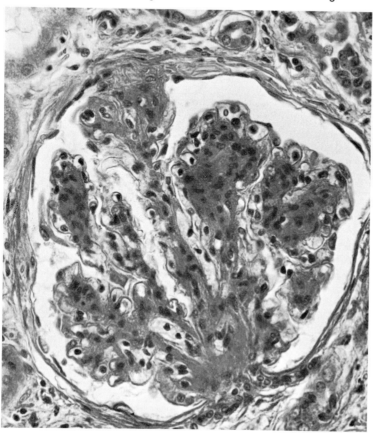

Figure 8–4. Nodular intercapillary glomerulosclerosis (Kimmelstiel-Wilson disease). The large deposits of homogeneous hyaline material are apparent in the central regions of each glomerular tuft. The capillary loops about these deposits are patent.

ber of glomeruli up to total involvement of the entire kidney. The nodules are PAS-positive, contain mucopolysaccharides, lipids and fibrils, and have the same composition as the matrix deposits of diffuse glomerulosclerosis. Often they contain trapped mesangial cells. Diffuse glomerulosclerosis and arteriolosclerosis usually accompany the nodular lesions. As Kimmelstiel-Wilson disease advances, the individual nodules enlarge and eventually compress and engulf capillaries and so obliterate the glomerular tuft. The glomerular space may become filled with laminated crescents of hyalinized fibrous tissue so that eventually the entire glomerular structure assumes a hyaline, sclerotic appearance.

As a consequence of the glomerular involvement, whether it be diffuse or nodular, the kidney suffers from ischemia and so develops tubular atrophy and increased interstitial fibrosis and undergoes overall contraction in size. Accompanying this contraction, pallor and a fine granularity appear on the cortical surface. For totally mysterious reasons those with nodular glomerulosclerosis undergo less contraction than those with only the diffuse form of the glomerular involvement.

The relationship of the nodular lesions to the diffuse basement membrane thickening continues to be a subject of dispute (Bloodworth, 1968) (Kimmelstiel et al., 1966). One view proposes that the nodules merely represent an extreme stage of diffuse glomerular basement membrane disease. Alternatively, it is held that the nodular lesion is a product of mesangial or deep endothelial cells and is distinctive from but may fuse with the capillary basement membrane lesion. In any event, nodular glomerulosclerosis is almost always associated with diffuse glomerulosclerosis. The nodular lesion is limited or virtually limited to the diabetic, yet diffuse glomerulosclerosis is encountered by itself in aged nondiabetics. Approximately 15 to 30 per cent of long-term diabetics develop nodular glomerulosclerosis and, in most instances, it causes renal failure. It is rarely encountered in those who have had diabetes for less than 10 years, save perhaps juvenile diabetics with rapidly advancing disease (Gellman et al., 1959).

"Exudative lesions" (fibrin caps and capsular drops) comprise the third form of glomerular involvement seen in the diabetic. The "fibrin cap" appears as a homogeneous brightly eosinophilic crescentic deposit overlying a peripheral capillary of a lobule. With high resolution, the deposit is found to lie either trapped between the endothelial cells and the basement membrane of the capillary or, alternatively, outside of the basement membrane under the visceral epithelial cells. It appears to represent a condensate of plasma proteins and may be merely a reflection of the heavy proteinuria sometimes encountered in the diabetic as a consequence of the widespread glomerular membrane alterations. Fibrin caps are also encountered in the nondiabetic. The capsular drop appears as an eosinophilic, focal thickening of the parietal layer of Bowman's capsule, which apparently hangs into the uriniferous space. The capsular drop is PAS-positive and may be merely an exaggeration of the widespread basement membrane alterations so characteristic of this disease. However, it also contains plasma proteins and so its precise genesis awaits further clarification. Neither the fibrin cap nor the capsular drop has significance in terms of causing renal functional impairment, but the capsular drop, when identified in tissue sections, is virtually diagnostic of diabetes.

Atherosclerosis and arteriolosclerosis, while generalized in the diabetic, often involve the kidneys more severely than other organs. The development of atheromas within the renal arteries and its major branches may, at times, cause either generalized renal ischemia and contraction or, at other times, focal infarcts. More regularly, however, the kidney is the seat of advanced arteriolosclerosis which affects not only the afferent **but also the efferent arterioles.** Such arteriolosclerosis is almost inevitably accompanied by diffuse glomerulosclerosis and the combination of impediments to blood flow induces mild diffuse scarring of the kidney known as benign nephrosclerosis. It should be emphasized that arteriolosclerosis and benign nephrosclerosis are also encountered in nondiabetics, particularly aged hypertensives but, in the nondiabetic, efferent arterioles are rarely if ever affected.

Pyelonephritis is an acute or chronic inflammation of the kidneys encountered in both diabetics and nondiabetics. However, it tends to take a more severe course in diabetics and may be somewhat more common in these predisposed individuals than in the general population. Acute pyelonephritis is clearly a bacterial infection of the kidney by organisms which either ascend via the ureters from the bladder or seed the kidneys from a bacteremia. Chronic pyelonephritis is usually a persistent bacterial infection but may also have other etiologies (p. 1122). Excretion of organisms in the urine (bacteriuria) occurs in both the acute and chronic forms of bacterial pyelonephritis. Studying the outpatient population of a large municipal hospital, Kass (1960) noted bacteriuria to be three times more common in diabetics than in nondiabetics, suggesting a significantly higher incidence of pyelonephritis in the diabetic population. These kidney infections are merely one manifestation of the vulnerability of the diabetic to all forms of bacterial infection.

Pyelonephritis, described in detail on p. 1117, is a nonspecific suppurative inflammation which generally begins in the interstitial tissue and rapidly extends into tubules and sometimes glomeruli. It essentially causes cortical and medullary abscesses or focal suppurations (Fig. 8–5). Chronic pyelonephritis, like all chronic inflammations, is manifested by interstitial scarring, a heavy infiltrate of lymphocytes, histiocytes, plasma cells and some neutrophils and tubular atrophy.

One special pattern of acute pyelonephritis, known as **necrotizing papillitis or renal medullary necrosis,** is particularly prone to develop in diabetic patients. It is only encountered in the nondiabetic when there is obstructive uropathy or in association with chronic analgesic abuse (p. 1125). In necrotizing papillitis, the acute bacterial infection within the renal pyramids in some way embarrasses the blood supply of the tips of the renal papillae and induces an infarct-like necrosis of the distal segment. One or more papillae may be involved, unilaterally or bilaterally (Fig. 8–6). When both kidneys are totally involved, the selective destruction of the collecting tubules almost always leads to acute renal insufficiency. Occasionally, when there is subtotal involvement, the necrotic papillae may slough off and be found within the urinary sediment, permitting a clinical diagnosis of this condition. Cortical suppuration and abscesses, characteristic of nonspecific acute pyelonephritis, usually accompany renal medullary necrosis.

Glycogen accumulation in tubular epithelial cells is seen in the diabetic who has had marked

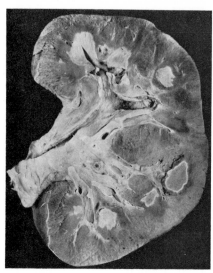

Figure 8–6. *Necrotizing papillitis in the kidney of a diabetic. Discrete, pale areas of ischemic necrosis, rimmed by sharp margins of inflammatory exudation, are present in almost every renal pyramid.*

hyperglycemia and glycosuria in the last days of life. It is believed to be caused by reabsorption of the urinary glucose, with the accumulation of glycogen within the epithelial cells of the distal portions of the proximal convoluted tubules and the descending limb of the loop of Henle. This alteration has been called **glycogen infiltration, glycogen nephrosis or the Armanni-Ebstein lesion.** The cells have cleared cytoplasm, distinct cell membranes and basally displaced nuclei. The glycogen content of the vacuoles yields a positive PAS reaction. In the experimental animal rendered diabetic by the administration of alloxan, glycogen accumulation appears following several days of heavy glycosuria. Control of the hyperglycemia and glycosuria by insulin brings about prompt mobilization of the glycogen and disappearance of the epithelial cell vacuolization. Thus, these tubular alterations are thought to be reversible and so are only encountered in the diabetic who has been out of control for at least some time prior to death. It is now encountered only rarely at postmortem examination. The Armanni-Ebstein lesion does not appear to cause tubular malfunction. When present, the lesion is virtually diagnostic of diabetes. It must be differentiated only from the glycogen accumulations in the renal tubular epithelial cells found in the glycogenoses or glycogen storage diseases (p. 296).

Fatty change in the epithelial cells of the proximal convoluted tubules is sometimes encountered in diabetes mellitus. It is a trivial lesion causing no tubular malfunction and probably represents tubular reabsorption of lipoproteins in patients suffering from diabetic glomerulosclerosis and heavy proteinuria and lipoproteinuria.

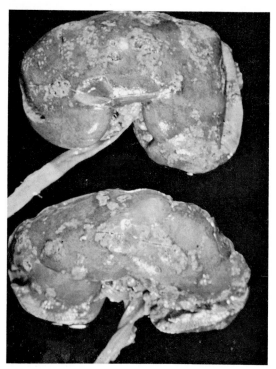

Figure 8–5. *Acute pyelonephritis in the kidneys of a diabetic. The kidney substance is seeded with numerous widely scattered small pale abscesses.*

Eyes. One of the most threatening aspects of diabetes mellitus is the development of blindness as a consequence of retinopathy, cataract formation or glaucoma. The retinopathy is the most common of this triad and, in a large study of more than 2500 diabetics who developed their disease in the first decades of life, more than half had developed retinopathy after 15 years of their disease (Colwell, 1966). Diabetes alone is responsible for at least 10 per cent of the blindness in the United States and, as the other causes are brought under control, it is growing in importance every year. Diabetic retinopathy is characterized by microangiopathy, exudates, proliferative changes and vitreous hemorrhages. The microangiopathy consists of **microaneurysms**, intraretinal or preretinal hemorrhages, retinal edema and venous dilatations. Among these, the microaneurysms are of particular interest. They comprise discrete, saccular dilatations of retinal-choroidal capillaries which appear as small red dots through the ophthalmoscope. Their nature and genesis are still in dispute. Cogan et al. (1961) proposed that they resulted from specific destruction of mural pericytes in diabetics, thus causing focal weaknesses and aneurysmal dilatations. Others disagree and suggest that the systemic angiopathy leads to focal collapse of the capillary bed in the retina, followed by the development of dilated, circuitous capillary shunts. The tortuous capillaries kinked upon themselves may create the microaneurysm. The latter thesis does not truly explain aneurysm formation and, on balance, the evidence favors Cogan s explanation.

Microaneurysms are generally thought to be virtually diagnostic of diabetes mellitus. It is of interest that about half of the patients with retinal microaneurysms have nodular glomerulosclerosis. Conversely, if a patient has nodular glomerulosclerosis he is almost certain to have retinal microaneurysms. For obscure reasons, the capillaries of the glomerulus and the retina are particularly predisposed to such microangiopathy. The retinal and preretinal hemorrhages are attributed to dilatation and rupture of venules, as these thin-walled structures are compressed and partially blocked by the thick-walled, rigid arterioles suffering from diabetic arteriolosclerosis. Retinal exudates are of both "soft" (microinfarcts) and "hard" (deposits of plasma proteins, lipids) varieties. Fibrovasoproliferative lesions may appear in the diabetic retina and extend into the vitreous body. These are presumably reactions to focal hemorrhages (Friedenwald, 1950) (Cogan, 1964).

Nervous System. The peripheral nerves, brain and spinal cord may all be damaged in long-standing diabetes (Colby, 1965). The most commonly encountered change consists of a symmetrical peripheral neuropathy affecting both motor and sensory nerves of the lower extremities. It is characterized by myelin degeneration which, in time, may injure the axon processes as well. The peripheral neuropathy is infrequently accompanied by disturbances in the neural innervation of the pelvic organs, leading to sexual impotence and bowel and bladder dysfunction. The neuropathy is generally associated with poorly controlled diabetes and may be caused by microangiopathy of the vascular supply of the nerves. Neuronal degeneration in the brain and spinal cord may appear as a consequence of the widespread angiopathy. In addition, the diabetic has some predisposition to cerebral infarctions and brain hemorrhages, the latter related to the hypertension seen so often in these patients. It is worth noting that neurons are vulnerable to hypoglycemia encountered in insulin reactions and to the ketoacidosis of the uncontrolled diabetic state.

Other Organs. A variety of lesions are encountered in the skin in long-term diabetics. Perhaps most common are skin infections, reflecting the diabetic's predisposition to infections. Localized collections of lipid-laden macrophages (foam cells or xanthoma cells) in the dermis and subcutaneous fat create so-called **diabetic xanthomas.** These appear as firm, yellow nodules directly beneath the epidermis, usually on the extensor surfaces of the elbows and knees and on the back and buttocks. Other distributions may also occur. Xanthomas are thought to result from the hyperlipemia of diabetes and are seen in other disorders associated with high blood lipid levels.

Necrobiosis lipoidica diabeticorum comprises another form of skin lesion. It constitutes a focal area of necrosis occurring within the subcutaneous fat depots anywhere on the body. On clinical examination, these lesions take the form of slightly tender, irregular plaques or focal depressions having somewhat pale to yellow centers surrounded by a red-violet margin. Histologically, the lesion is characterized by a central region of necrosis of fat cells and fragmentation of collagen, surrounded by a nonspecific inflammatory reaction. Prominent in the inflammatory infiltrate are lipid-laden macrophages stuffed with the debris of necrotic fat cells. The margin may have a granulomatous appearance and contain foreign body type giant cells. The origin of this necrobiosis is obscure but has been attributed to microangiopathy in the subcutaneous small vessels. Its name notwithstanding, necrobiosis lipoidica diabeticorum is not limited to the diabetic.

The liver is often fatty in long-term diabetics and is indistinguishable from the fatty change induced by many other causes. **Glycogen vacuolation is occasionally found in the nuclei of hepatic cells.** It causes clearing of the nucleus but no other retrogressive alteration. **Diabetic myopathy** with injury or death of muscle cells is sometimes seen in longstanding diabetes, particularly when it has been poorly controlled. It may be related to the generalized disease of the microvasculature or to motor neuron damage.

In conclusion, it is evident that, although diabetes is a disorder of insulin function, paradoxically the pancreas does not exhibit the most impressive morphologic changes and, indeed, in many maturity onset diabetics, it may be virtually normal. Much more impressive is the accelerated atherosclerosis and the nephropathy, retinopathy and neuropathy, sometimes designated as the triopathy of diabetes. The common denominator among these "opathies" may be microangiopathy. It must also be evident that, among all of the potential morphologic changes to be encountered in this disease, only a few can be considered as pathognomonic. Leukocytic infiltrations of the islets in the infant or juvenile diabetic are virtually diagnostic of the growth onset form of the disease. Nodular glomerulosclerosis, glycogen accumulation in renal tubular epithelial cells, efferent arteriolosclerosis in the kidney and the full-blown retinopathy are, individually, highly suggestive and, collectively, virtually diagnostic of diabetes mellitus.

Clinical Course.
The clinical manifestations of "early diabetes" stem from the metabolic derangements. Those of the "chronic diabetic syndrome" relate to the development of vascular changes as well as to the deranged carbohydrate metabolism. Hyperglycemia, glycosuria and abnormal glucose tolerance tests comprise the only diagnostic features of the early stages of diabetes. Since the patient cannot be aware of his biochemical abnormalities, his first presenting symptoms are often polyuria, polydipsia and polyphagia. The polyuria represents an obligate osmotic diuresis related to the glycosuria. The polydipsia probably arises as a consequence of increased urinary output and, more importantly, the effect of the hyperosmolarity of the blood (hyperglycemia) on the osmoreceptors in the thirst centers. The polyphagia is less easy to understand but may be related to inability to utilize glucose as a source of energy. Weakness is an additional prominent manifestation, perhaps related to the catabolism of muscle proteins for glyconeogenesis. Obviously, metabolic acidosis when it supervenes, introduces its own set of signs and symptoms. The onset of these symptoms may be exceedingly subtle and delayed until middle to later life in the maturity onset form of the disease. In the juvenile diabetic, they may appear quite abruptly.

In both the growth onset and maturity onset diabetes over the span of 10 to 15 years, the complications of the "chronic diabetic syndrome" make their appearance in most patients. At this point, the signs and symptoms of the metabolic derangement are complicated by the generalized vascular disease, particularly coronary artery disease, and the likely emergence of nephropathy, retinopathy and neuropathy. There is little merit to further discussing the issue of whether rigid control of the carbohydrate defect will prevent the onward march of the "chronic diabetic syndrome" since insufficient data are available to resolve this most important but complex problem (Hardin et al., 1956) (Keiding et al., 1952). Nonetheless, it should be emphasized that since answers are not available, the more optimistic attitude should be maintained in the treatment of the patient (Lukens, 1967). There is also a significantly increased incidence of hypertension in diabetics and, among adult diabetics, elevated blood pressure levels are found in up to 80 per cent. The hypertension is often accompanied by obesity but is probably also related to the generalized vascular disease and possibly to secondary pituitary hyperactivity and overproduction of adrenal corticoids (Editorial, 1967).

Diabetic nephropathy as a cause of morbidity and mortality is superceded only by coronary artery disease (myocardial infarction and/or arteriosclerotic heart disease). Diffuse and nodular glomerulosclerosis, along with the almost ever-present arteriolosclerosis, cause progressive impairment of renal function. Long before renal insufficiency becomes evident, these patients usually manifest proteinuria and hypertension. The proteinuria is generally mild but, in some cases, it may exceed 4 gm per 24 hours and induce the nephrotic syndrome (p. 1107).

Kimmelstiel and Wilson (1936) called attention to the occurrence in diabetes of hypertension, albuminuria and edema, often designated as the Kimmelstiel-Wilson syndrome. At one time, it was thought that this syndrome was peculiarly associated with nodular glomerulosclerosis, but it has become evident that it is more likely attributable to the diffuse form of glomerulosclerosis with its widespread basement membrane alterations (Gellman et al., 1959). It should be pointed out, however, that sometimes diabetics as well as nondiabetics free of glomerulosclerosis have proteinuria, edema and hypertension due to the combination of elevated blood pressure levels and cardiac decompensation. The syndrome then is neither specific for glomerulosclerosis nor limited to the diabetic. The ocular and neurologic problems such as visual impairment, total blindness and a variety of sensory and motor nerve deficits do not contribute to the mortality, but they are probably the most distressing burdens imposed upon the long-term diabetic.

An increased vulnerability to microbiologic infections is one of the serious problems of chronic diabetes. It is not clear whether diabetics have a higher incidence of infections or whether, once contracted, infections tend to be more difficult to control even with therapy. Tuberculosis, bacterial pneumonia, pyelonephritis and skin infections together cause the death of about 5 per cent of diabetics. This vulnerability to microbiologic agents is not simply related to the hyperglycemia but is much more complex. The combination of microangiopathy, metabolic acidosis and ineffective phagocytosis by macrophages are all believed to contribute to the vulnerability to infections (Kandhari et al., 1969).

Before closing this discussion, it is worthwhile to point out that there is a considerable amount of experimental evidence that prolonged hyperglycemia throws a burden on beta cells. Indeed, in the experimental animal, permanent diabetes can be produced by prolonged administration of growth hormone which, in effect, causes sustained hyperglycemia (Young, 1937). Similarly, in man it has been observed that the mild overt diabetic may revert to a latent form of the disease with weight reduction, dietary restriction and supportive insulin therapy when needed. A strong case can therefore be made for the therapeutic control of the hyperglycemia to relieve the beta cells of excess work. In this connection, *the sulfonylureas (tolbutamide and orinase) have little effectiveness in the juvenile form of the disease since these patients have an absolute deficiency of insulin.* With respect to the adult form of the disease, the American Diabetes Association and the University Group Diabetes Program issued the following statement: "Although tolbutamide and other oral preparations will continue to be useful for treatment of patients who are unable to take insulin... when dietary treatment fails to control the disease in usual adult onset diabetes of mild to moderate severity, insulin should be used in preference to oral agents. Insulin is essential in severe diabetes regardless of age of onset."

The outlook for the patient with diabetes depends on the age of onset of the disease. A recent analysis of over 20,000 diabetics, followed for a 26-year period, indicated a significant excess mortality in both sexes and at all ages (Kessler, 1971). The overall picture, including diabetics of all ages at the time of onset of their disease, showed an approximate 40 per cent excess mortality for diabetic males and about 60 per cent for females. The greatest excess was encountered in patients in the age range of 20 to 39 years, most of whom can be considered to have had growth onset disease. In those who manifest overt diabetes prior to 20 years of age, life expectancy is shortened by as much as 20 to 25 years (Knowles et al., 1965) (Larsson et al., 1962). However, about two-thirds of the cases of diabetes become manifest after 40 years of age and, in these adult onset patients, longevity may only be slightly shortened, but unfortunately it is not free of restrictions, discomfort and disability. It is discouraging to report that the diabetic's life expectancy has not improved over the past three decades.

IRON STORAGE DISORDERS

The total body content of iron in the normal adult ranges between 2 and 5 gm., depending chiefly on body size and hemoglobin level. For the individual, his total body iron constitutes one of the closely guarded homeostatic constants maintained by balancing absorption and excretion. In two conditions, large amounts of iron (10 to 80 gm.) accumulate in the body. In both, the iron is stored in the form of hemosiderin pigment in many organs. One condition, *systemic hemosiderosis, is characterized by widespread accumulations of hemosiderin in tissues or organs, but it produces little or no tissue or organ damage.* In *hemochromatosis, on the other hand, the accumulation of iron is generally larger than in systemic hemosiderosis and, furthermore, it is associated with damage to many organs, principally the liver.* Thus, hemosiderosis is essentially a morphologic expression of iron overload but does not produce clinical signs or symptoms. Hemochromatosis, in contrast, is a well defined syndrome having wide-ranging manifestations arising in injury to organs, particularly the liver. The consideration of these two iron storage disorders is facilitated by a review of ferrokinetics.

NORMAL AND ABNORMAL IRON METABOLISM

Iron is distributed in the body in two general types of compounds. In the first, the iron is present in the porphyrin ring of the heme complex. In the second, it is directly bonded to protein, and no heme is present. The former compounds (hemoglobin, myoglobin, cytochrome) are concerned with the handling of oxygen, i.e., its transport, storage and activation. The latter are involved in the transport and storage of iron (iron-binding protein, ferritin, hemosiderin). Ferritin is a macromolecular complex of protein and colloidal ferric hydroxide-phosphate enclosed within a protein shell arranged in micelles. These contain about 17 to 23 per cent by weight of iron. The complexes vary somewhat in size and configuration and are readily mobilizable when iron is needed (Crichton, 1971). Small amounts of ferritin are stored in the liver, spleen, bone marrow and muscle but, since it is somewhat water-soluble, it is dissolved out in the usual processes of tissue fixation. Hemosiderin is generally believed to represent aggregates of ferritin. These aggregates are water-insoluble and less mobilizable than ferritin. Ultrastructural studies indicate that hemosiderin granules vary somewhat in size and shape, presumably because of variation in the number of ferritin micelles incorporated into the individual hemosiderin granule as well as the physical state of the aggregation (Woehler, 1960). With normal iron stores, only trace amounts of hemosiderin are found along with the stored ferritin.

The maintenance of iron balance depends largely on mechanisms controlling excess absorption since the pathways for excretion are very limited and inflexible. The daily requirement of iron in the adult male, about 1 mg., is needed to balance a similar loss arising in gastrointestinal seepage of blood, desquamation of cells from the skin, gastrointestinal tract and other body surfaces, and the iron losses in sweat and bile. To the best of our knowledge, all of the losses in the male are limited to these pathways. The daily average requirement for females, taking into consideration all ages, is slightly higher — on the order of 1 to 2 mg. per day — because of the additional drains occasioned by menstruation, pregnancy and lactation. It is estimated that as much as 20 to 23 mg. of iron are lost in a single normal menstrual period. Average American diets contain in the range of 10 to 15 mg. of iron daily. Only about 10 per cent of the daily iron in the diet can be absorbed if a balance is to be achieved.

While mechanisms must exist to control absorption of dietary iron, their nature still eludes us. A number of theories have been propounded, but none are entirely satisfactory. Granick (1949) proposed a "mucosal block" residing in the epithelial cells lining the small intestine, principally the duodenum and jejunum where the major portion of iron is absorbed. It was postulated that these cells synthesize a specific iron-binding protein — apoferritin. The amount of apoferritin harbored by these cells would be sufficient, once saturated with dietary iron, to provide for the daily

losses of iron. Apoferritin saturated with iron becomes ferritin. Iron for the body's daily needs would be made available by its transfer from the saturated apoferritin (ferritin) to specific transport plasma proteins known as transferrin (siderophilin). In the normal individual, there is sufficient transferrin (a beta-1-globulin) to carry about 250 to 350 microgm. of iron per 100 ml. of plasma, but normally the transferrin is only about 33 per cent saturated and so carries about 100 microgm. of iron. By transferring the iron to the carrier transferrin, the ferritin in the mucosal cells becomes unsaturated and so permits further absorption of iron from the gut.

While this version of a "mucosal block" was of great value in calling attention to the role of the intestinal mucosal cells in maintaining iron balance, it requires revision for many reasons. Newer information indicates a more complex pathway of iron absorption and, moreover, the Granick theory failed to provide a ready explanation for adjustments in iron absorption in response to abnormal losses. More recent observations suggest that iron absorption involves two separate pools within the intestinal mucosal cells (Manis and Schachter, 1962) (Boender and Verloop, 1969). One pool involves an energy-dependent active transport system capable of rapid transfer of iron from the lumen of the gut across the cell to transferrin in the blood (Jacobs et al., 1966). The other pool, having a considerably slower turnover, is associated with some storage form of iron in the mucosal cell, presumably saturated apoferritin. The active transport pathway is capable of delivering iron to the plasma within two to four hours of the onset of absorption. The precise nature of the compounds or complexes involved in such transfer is still unknown (Pearson and Reich, 1969). The other storage pool, perhaps complexed with apoferritin, represents a ready reserve which can be delivered to the plasma if needed. When not needed, this iron would be retained in the intestinal mucosal cells and be shed as these cells are desquamated. (Their average life span is 3 days.)

Iron absorption must be responsive to the body's needs. To explain flexible control, a circulating "messenger iron" has been proposed. The "messenger iron" may be the transferrin-iron complex found in the plasma. It is postulated that as mucosal epithelial cells are being formed in the intestinal mucosa, "messenger iron" is delivered to the cell and complexes with its apoferritin. When iron is lost from the body, as in a hemorrhage, the need for iron in the erythropoietic tissues drains the iron from the plasma, and so the level of saturation of transferrin falls. Thus, less is delivered in the form of "messenger iron' to the mucosal cell which then has reduced iron stores and can absorb more from the intestinal lumen. Conversely, when body iron stores are normal, the amounts of "messenger iron' delivered to the developing mucosal cells are such that iron absorption is limited to the daily losses (Wheby and Jones, 1963) (Wheby et al., 1964). It is postulated that once having received its content of "messenger iron' at the time it was formed, the absorptive capacity of the mucosal cell is fixed for its lifetime of 3 days. The flexibility of this system resides, then, in the rapid turnover of intestinal mucosal cells.

Intriguing as these conceptions of the control of iron absorption are, there is considerable evidence that the blocking mechanisms are less than perfect and are vulnerable to a host of influences. When either iron salts or hemoglobin iron are ingested in increasing amounts, there is a progressive rise in the *amount* retained although the *percentage* absorbed decreases with increasing dose (Bothwell and Finch, 1957). If the mucosal block were impeccable, one would not expect the amounts absorbed to be dependent on the amount ingested. Moreover, absorption of excessive amounts of iron can persist with high dietary levels of iron, despite the level of saturation of transferrin (Taylor and Gatenby, 1966) (Schade et al., 1969).

A number of dietary factors influence iron absorption. Man absorbs ionic iron chiefly or entirely in the divalent state. For absorption to occur, iron must be split from its complex and chemically reduced. Despite the controversy in the past, it now seems well established that acid gastric juice has a potentiating effect on the absorption of ferrous and ferric iron in man since it also aids in reducing iron to the divalent state (Jacobs et al., 1968). Patients with achlorhydria absorb iron less effectively than those with normal gastric secretion and, moreover, cannot increase their levels of absorption as flexibly as normals. Alcohol augments absorption, presumably by increasing flow of acid gastric juice. Ascorbic acid, citrates and fructose in the diet favor absorption. Increased levels of absorption are seen in patients with underlying liver disease. Conversely, absorption is impeded by phosphates, phytates, calcium and fat in the diet. The iron in eggs and green vegetables is less readily absorbed than that from bread and meat. The mucosal controls of iron absorption are thus subject to a welter of conflicting influences but, nonetheless, although we do not understand these controls perfectly, they must function more or less well in most normal individuals or else iron overload would be universal in the presence of so much dietary excess.

It must be appreciated that, in addition to exogenous sources of iron, there is a daily breakdown of red cells with the release of approximately 25 to 30 mg. of iron. As best we know, serum transport iron is called upon first for the body's need, followed in turn by the release of iron from the recycled heme pigment; only when these sources are inadequate is the iron stored in the body in the forms of ferritin and trace amounts of hemosiderin called upon.

We may now turn to a consideration of the pathways by which excessive amounts of iron accumulate in the body. Excesses of iron may result from: (1) increased absorption, (2) abnormal breakdown of erythrocytes and (3) impaired utilization. We know very little about the possibility of decreased excretion of iron which, theoretically, might lead to a positive balance. The mechanisms of shedding iron are rigidly limited in the male and almost as limited in the female, save for the additional losses occasioned by menstruation, pregnancy and lactation.

Increased absorption of iron has already been discussed, and among the many dietary influences best established is a high dietary intake of iron. Large stores of iron and the consequent accumulation of iron in the form of hemosiderin pigment is common among Bantu natives in South Africa who prepare their food and beer in crude iron cooking pots (Walker and Arvidsson, 1950). Excessive stores have been noted in patients following the ingestion of large amounts of iron medications over the span of years (Wallerstein and Robbins, 1953). A habitually high dietary intake of iron and alcohol, such as is encountered in wine, may lead to excessive iron stores in the body. The alcohol not only augments iron absorption but also carries the threat of liver injury and the possible development of cirrhosis associated with alcohol abuse. The cirrhosis, in turn, appears to augment iron absorption (MacDonald, 1961) (Sabesin and Thomas, 1964). These individuals, therefore, are in double jeopardy. Genetic defects in iron absorption have been postulated as will be discussed in the consideration of hemochromatosis.

Excess breakdown of red cells with release of iron from heme pigment may lead to an iron excess. The iron is usually stored in the form of ferritin or hemosiderin and could be mobilized for the metabolic pool. However, the latter is relatively inert and so the erythropoietic response called forth to replace the lost red cells depends largely on the more immediately available sources of iron in the plasma and, in turn, on increased dietary intake. Thus, systemic hemosiderosis is encountered in all forms of hemolytic anemia (p. 704). Similarly, patients receiving large numbers of transfusions accumulate excesses of iron because the transfused red cells have a short life span. Each transfusion represents an infusion of about 200 to 250 mg. of iron per 500 ml. of blood.

Impaired utilization of iron will lead to an iron excess since, as was pointed out earlier, absorption of iron from the gut continues despite adequate body stores. When marrow aplasia is produced in animals by the destruction of the bone marrow by radiant energy, they continue to absorb iron (Mendel, 1961). In certain anemias of man, such as thalassemia (p. 711) and the anemia of marrow failure (p. 721), there is impaired production of hemoglobin and red cells and consequent accumulation of iron in the body.

HEMOSIDEROSIS

Whatever the underlying basis, excess iron is stored in the form of ferritin and hemosiderin. The deposits may be body-wide or localized in distribution depending on the genesis of the iron excess. Localized hemorrhages, hemorrhagic infarcts or longstanding congestion or stagnation of the blood in an organ will lead to localized hemosiderosis. In contrast, the systemic pathways of iron accumulation discussed above induce widespread hemosiderosis. *Whether localized or body-wide, hemosiderosis causes little, if any, tissue injury and hence no functional impairment of affected organs.*

Morphology. Hemosiderin has been described as variable aggregates of ferritin micelles which produce a golden brown, granular, cytoplasmic pigment. Its content of iron is demonstrable by such histochemical procedures as the Prussian blue reaction (p. 49). Under the electron microscope, the granules are membrane-bounded within phagosomes (Sturgeon and Shoden, 1969). Localized he-

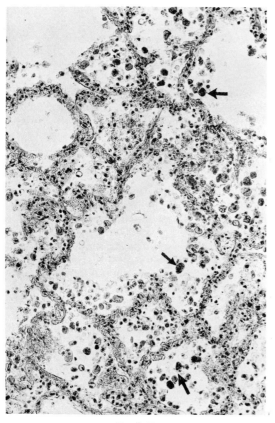

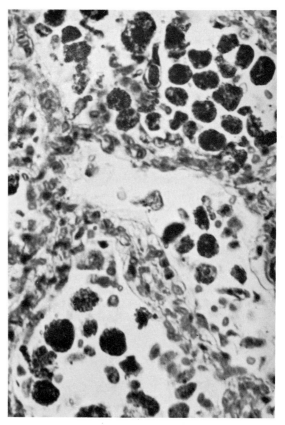

Fig. 8–7　　　　　　　　　　　　　　　　*Fig. 8–8*

Figure 8–7. *Low power view of lung containing granular edema precipitate and scattered dark hemosiderin-laden macrophages in the alveolar spaces (arrows).*
Figure 8–8. *High power detail of similar hemosiderin-laden macrophages.*

mosiderosis is well exemplified in chronic passive congestion of the lung where hemosiderin may be found lying within macrophages in the alveolar spaces as well as within lymphatic channels draining the lungs (Figs. 8—7 and 8—8). Such a sequence of events gives rise to the "heart failure" cells in the lungs of patients with longstanding cardiac decompensation and pulmonary congestion. The production of hemosiderin pigment in areas of hemorrhage accounts for the yellowish discoloration which develops late in the course of the resorption of the extravasated blood in bruises and hematomas (p. 49). Similarly, in old hemorrhagic infarcts, the resulting scar is often pigmented by the accumulation of hemosiderin.

Systemic hemosiderosis is most often caused by hemolytic disorders. In these, the hemosiderin localizes first in the reticuloendothelial (RE) system where red cell breakdown is accomplished. Thus, the Kupffer cells of the liver and the RE cells of the bone marrow, spleen, lymph nodes and scattered macrophages throughout other organs such as the skin, pancreas and kidneys accumulate deposits of hemosiderin. Massive accumulations of pigment may cause destruction of these cells with the release of the pigment into the intercellular spaces in the area. In the pulp tissues of the spleen and lymph nodes, deposits tend to localize about the endothelial sinuses. Fibrous proliferation then ensues about the pigment to produce focal areas of pigmented scarring known as **siderotic nodules.**

With progressive accumulation of iron, whatever the pathway, parenchymal cells of many organs are eventually affected. It is sometimes said that dietary excesses go directly into parenchymal cells, but it is not possible in most instances to identify the pathway of accumulation of iron from the distribution of the hemosiderin within the tissues. It is found within the cytoplasm of hepatic parenchymal cells, the islet and acinar cells of the pancreas, the epithelium of the salivary glands, the lining epithelial cells of thyroid acini, the adrenocortical cells and the epithelial cells of the renal tubules. Rarely, it may also collect in the muscle fibers of the myocardium and about the skin adnexal glands in the fibroblasts of the dermis. When the accumulations are sufficiently advanced, they impart a brown color to the affected organ. It should be noted that **parenchymal cell injury, interstitial fibrosis and scarring are not usually associated with the pigmentation of systemic hemosiderosis.**

Hemosiderin, of course, implies abnormal accumulations of iron, either due to local breakdown of red cells or systemic causes of excess iron accumulation. In the great majority of instances, it is purely a morphologic finding, not associated with clinical manifestations of organ dysfunction. However, whether hemosiderin in massive amounts may cause functional or morphologic damage is a vexing issue, as is discussed in the following presentation of hemochromatosis.

HEMOCHROMATOSIS

The most important iron storage disorder, hemochromatosis, is a well defined clinical syndrome characterized by (1) a heavily hemosiderotic "portal" cirrhosis known as pigment cirrhosis, (2) siderosis of other organs, (3) pancreatic fibrosis and siderosis and (4) pigmentation of the skin. The combination of the last two features has given rise to the clinical designation *bronze diabetes* (Marble and Bailey, 1951). Additional characteristics of the usual case are greatly increased body stores of iron (up to 80 gm.), elevated levels of plasma iron in the range of 200 to 250 microgm. per 100 ml. of plasma and excessive saturation of transferrin on the order of 60 to 70 per cent. *Most constant among these various features are the iron overload, systemic siderosis and pigment cirrhosis.* Diabetes may be absent in one-third, and the pigmentation is so subtle (a summer tan) as to be readily missed or absent in about one-half. The classic form of hemochromatosis is preponderantly a male disease in the ratio of 9 to 1, rarely becoming manifest under the age of 40. The sex distribution is attributed to the protection against iron overload afforded to females by menstruation and pregnancy, while the age range is compatible with the many years required to accumulate the ten to twentyfold increases of total body iron. In patients receiving multiple transfusions or having other exogenous sources for their iron overload, there is no sex predilection.

Pathogenesis. Despite the enormous amounts of iron accumulated by these patients, it has been impossible, to date, to establish the nature of the fundamental defect leading to the iron storage. This mystery has led to two widely held but opposing conceptions: (1) that the disease is a hereditary inborn error of iron metabolism, or (2) that no genetic defect need be invoked since there are adequate grounds for accepting hemochromatosis as an acquired or environmental disorder.

Support for the genetic, metabolic theory is provided by the occasional familial distributions of this disease (Sheldon, 1935) (Crosby, 1966). Elevated levels of plasma iron and excessive saturation of transferrin have been identified in immediate relatives of patients with hemochromatosis (Morgan, 1961) (Walsh et al., 1964). However, no unequivocal pattern of mendelian inheritance has been established. Some investigators suggest transmission by an autosomal dominant gene with incomplete penetrance while others favor an autosomal recessive mode of inheritance with manifesting heterozygotes. Perhaps both modes of transmission are valid and families having this disease vary in their inheritance patterns. Some increased mucosal uptake and retention of iron has been reported in certain patients with this disorder (Boender et al., 1967). This increased transfer of iron across the mucosal cells is attributed to some enzyme abnormality in intestinal mucosal cells, but the evidence for such is at best meager (Mazur and Sackler, 1967). Other studies have suggested an increased tissue avidity for iron in the form of excessive synthesis of tissue iron-binding proteins (Goldberg and Smith, 1960). However, this conception is also not well established. A deficiency of a specific gastric inhibitor of iron absorption is offered as another possible genetic defect, but here again the evidence is contradictory (Davis et al., 1966) (Smith et al., 1969). If there is a genetic defect, its existence and nature have, to this date, not been clearly elucidated (Powell, 1970) (Boender and Verloop, 1969), and so this presentation of the disease is called "idiopathic" or "primary" hemochromatosis.

The opposing view of the nature of hemochromatosis contends that the evidence for a genetic defect in iron metabolism is at best fragmentary. It proposes instead that hemochromatosis is an acquired or environmental disease developing on the basis of (1) the known imperfections in mucosal controlling mechanisms (p. 274) or (2) excesses of dietary iron or (3) prolonged parenteral administration of iron (drugs, transfusions). It is pointed out that only about 2 per cent of reported cases of hemochromatosis have a definite familial background (MacDonald, 1970). Emphasis is placed on variation, among individuals, in the amount of iron absorbed following even relatively normal levels of dietary intake. It has been pointed out, with increasing loads of dietary iron, the absolute amount of iron absorbed increases. Presumably, South African Bantus develop systemic hemosiderosis on this basis and others, a disorder quite similar to if not identical with hemochromatosis (Walker and Arvidsson, 1950). A higher than anticipated incidence of hemochromatosis has been observed among wine-drinking populations (MacDonald, 1963). Here it is argued that the alcohol first induces cirrhosis of the liver (p. 1025) which, in turn, leads to the absorption of the relatively large amounts of iron contained in the wine. Patients receiving transfusions or iron-containing drugs throughout their life, such as those having some form of chronic anemia, have sometimes developed hemochromatosis. Thus it is held that a mysterious genetic defect need not be invoked since the "mucosal block" is not impeccable and, in some circumstances, the iron is delivered directly to the body (as in transfusions) bypassing any theoretical block.

These somewhat conflicting theories have been reconciled by postulating two forms of the disease: a primary and a secondary or "exogenous" syndrome. Indeed, it is contended that "exogenous" hemochromatosis and the primary disease have many dissimilarities (Charlton and Bothwell, 1966). In general, the idiopathic disease is characterized by larger stores of body iron which are more mobilizable and chelatable than the deposits in the "exogenous" forms (Powell, 1970). Moreover, in the exogenous form of the disease, the liver may have only little fibrous scarring in contrast to the clear-cut cirrhosis of the primary disease. Perhaps we are dealing with two separate diseases or the same (or virtually the same) end point of two pathways. One pathway might involve a genetic defect in mechanisms controlling iron absorption while the other might be nongenetic and simply involve dietary excesses or bypassing normal controlling mechanisms.

Still another issue remains in the pathogenesis of this controversial disease: Is the iron overload in the tissues responsible for the organ injury? In particular, what is the cause of the pigment cirrhosis of the liver? According to the "geneticists," the "iron gradually accumulates *causing siderosis and injury* of the organs in which the iron is stored" (Crosby, 1966). However, it has been virtually impossible to induce pigment cirrhosis in rats by prolonged heavy administration of iron. While some investigators would argue that these experiments have only been continued for two years, insufficient time for the changes found in man to develop, this criticism seems vitiated in the context of the average life span of man and the rat. The "environmentalists" suggest instead that cirrhosis is possibly the fundamental defect and it, in turn, leads to the increased iron absorption and hemosiderosis. In support of this contention is the high incidence of alcoholism with all of its attendant nutritional deficiencies (plausible grounds for the development of cirrhosis) in patients with hemochromatosis (p. 1025) (Saint, 1963). Alternatively, the hemosiderosis, whatever its cause, may overload and blockade the RE system with pigment, thus exposing the liver to endotoxins or bacteremias as the cause of the cirrhosis (MacDonald et al., 1968). Where there is so much speculation, it must be apparent that the

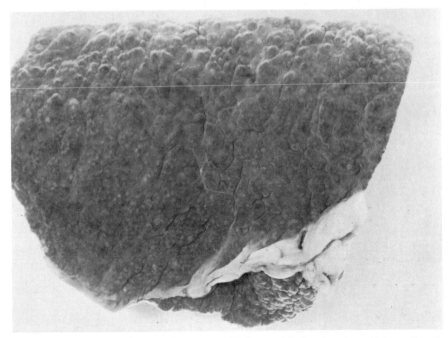

Figure 8–9. *Pigment cirrhosis. Intermediate stage with fine nodularity of surface. Note scattered pale nodules of regeneration.*

relationship of the iron overload and pigment to the cellular and organ damage is still obscure. But recent therapeutic measures such as repeated venesections shed some light on this problem as will be seen later.

Morphology. The major morphologic features of hemochromatosis are the pigment cirrhosis of the liver and the systemic hemosiderosis. Pigment deposits and fibrotic reactions are also found in the pancreas, spleen, lymph nodes, endocrine glands, myocardium, skin and, indeed, in virtually all tissues in the body.

The **liver** is finely nodular, chocolate brown and slightly enlarged. The weight usually ranges between 1500 and 3000 gm. and is increased out of proportion to the volume of the liver owing to the increased density imparted by the iron deposits. The individual nodules vary in diameter from several millimeters to 1 cm. and are of the same order of magnitude as those encountered in the cirrhosis associated with alcohol abuse (Fig. 8–9). The nodules are created by fine interlacing strands of connective tissue which tend to interconnect portal triads but which also penetrate the individual lobules to segregate small islands of liver substance (Fig. 8–10). Large accumulations of golden brown granular hemosiderin are found within hepatocytes, Kupffer cells, bile duct epithelium and in the interlacing fibrous scars (Fig. 8–11). The pigment is often extracellular within the scars as well as within the fibroblasts. Lipofuscin may also be present in

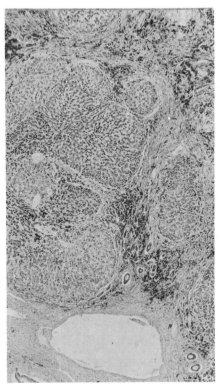

Figure 8–10. *Pigment cirrhosis. Low power magnification. Liver tissue is divided up into many nodules of varying size by fibrous tissue. Large amounts of pigment appear in fibrous tissue and liver cells.*

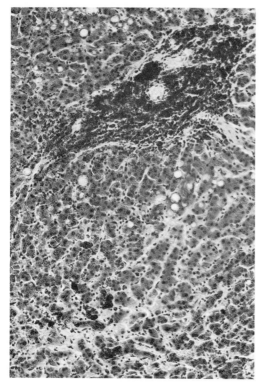

Figure 8–11. Pigment cirrhosis in hemochromatosis—a low power view of a liver containing pigment in the periportal fibrous tissue and in scattered hepatic cells near the center of the lobule (at bottom of illustration).

the liver as it is in all forms of cirrhosis. The hemosiderin is readily differentiated from the lipofuscin by special stains for iron.

The **pancreas** is extensively pigmented and brown but rarely as severely as the liver (Fig. 8–12). Hemosiderin is found in the stroma, in the acinar cells of the exocrine glands, in the columnar lining epithelium of the ducts and in the islet cells. The severity of the pigmentation bears no correlation to the severity of the diabetic state nor is there any evidence that the pigment deposits in the beta cells of the islets constitute the basis for the diabetes. A diffuse interstitial fibrosis is also often present throughout the exocrine and endocrine glands of the pancreas.

The **spleen, lymph nodes and reticuloendothelial cells** throughout the body are heavily pigmented. The hemosiderin may accumulate to a sufficient degree to cause a brown coloration of the spleen and lymph nodes. As a consequence of the cirrhosis, the spleen may be enlarged and somewhat fibrotic, representing the congestive splenomegaly of longstanding portal hypertension (p. 771).

The **heart** often has brown coloration as a consequence of the deposition of hemosiderin within the myocardial fibers. In passing, it should be noted that occasional patients with hemochroma-

tosis develop signs and symptoms of heart disease attributed by some authors to the myocardial hemosiderosis. However, interstitial myocardial fibrosis and evidence of myocardial cell necrosis is notably absent in uncomplicated hemochromatosis. But since many of these patients are of advanced age and have coronary arteriosclerosis, it is understandable that myocardial changes may be present on the basis of vascular insufficiency.

Many of the **glands** in the body develop hemosiderosis, particularly the cortical cells of the adrenal, the thyroid acini, the germinal epithelium in the testis and the parenchymal cells of the salivary glands. Usually, there is no evidence of cellular destruction or interstitial fibrosis.

Hemosiderin may be found in fibroblasts in the corium of the skin, chiefly about the dermal gland appendages. However, the bronze coloration which comprises one of the diagnostic features of this disease is, in large part, attributable to an increased production of melanin within the basal layer of the epidermis.

Hemosiderosis may be found in virtually any other cell and tissue in the body, particularly the epithelial cells of the renal tubules, the fibroblasts in the lamina propria of the intestinal tract and, occasionally, in skeletal muscle fibers.

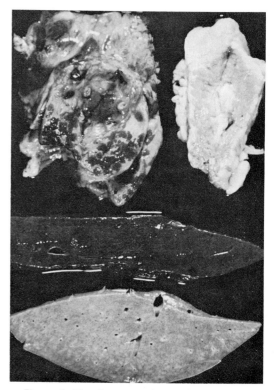

Figure 8–12. Cross sections of the pigmented liver and pancreas from a case of hemochromatosis alongside paler cross sections of liver and pancreas from a normal control.

Clinical Correlation. Patients with hemochromatosis come to clinical attention with one of four symptom complexes: (1) They may be discovered to be diabetic and investigation discloses the underlying iron storage disease; (2) hepatomegaly or portal hypertension calls attention to the existence of the liver involvement; (3) a variety of endocrine dysfunctions may become apparent, such as sterility, impotence or adrenal dysfunction; and (4) manifestations of cardiac disease or cardiac failure arise which respond poorly to conventional therapy. The skin pigmentation is sometimes helpful but often subtle. It may take the form of the classic bronzing due to the combination of increased melanin and hemosiderin but, in many cases, the pigmentation has a blue-gray cast when the iron deposits are predominant. The pigmentation is usually most evident over the face, arms, genitals and in the skin folds. The combination of skin pigmentation and manifestations of cirrhosis of the liver points strongly to the diagnosis, particularly when diabetes mellitus is also present. However, usually it is necessary to document the presence of increased levels of serum iron and excessive saturation of the serum iron-binding capacity. Sometimes liver needle biopsy or skin biopsy is necessary to document the presence of excessive hemosiderin deposits.

Prior to the advent of venesection (withdrawal of blood) therapy, the mean survival after diagnosis averaged approximately five years. A study at that time indicated that almost 50 per cent of these patients died of infections, 17 per cent of heart failure, 10 per cent of liver cell carcinoma, 7 per cent of gastrointestinal bleeding, 5 per cent of liver failure and the remainder of miscellaneous causes (MacDonald and Mallory, 1960). *Special note should be made of the development of primary hepatocarcinoma in pigment cirrhosis,* variously cited as occurring in 8 to 42 per cent of these cases. Venesection therapy for these patients has significantly altered their prognosis. Currently, clinical, biochemical and histologic improvement has been achieved in patients with this form of treatment (Williams et al., 1969). Five hundred milliliters of blood contain about 200 to 250 mg. of iron. The mean survival with such management averages 8.2 years. Lessening of the skin pigmentation, reduction in the hepatosplenomegaly, improvement in liver function tests, improved carbohydrate tolerance (in about one-third of the patients with diabetes) and, more remarkably, apparent regression of the scarring in the liver occur. Indeed, in two patients who had documented cirrhosis, "an almost normal lobu-

lar pattern" was demonstrated after four and 15 years of such therapy (Williams et al., 1969).

Such reversal of liver damage following drainage of the iron is of great interest pathogenetically. It certainly suggests a causative role for the iron overload and hemosiderin in the production of the cirrhosis. Similar remarkable results have been reported by others (Powell and Kerr, 1970). However, it should be pointed out that if these patients continue to imbibe excessive amounts of alcohol no reversal of the cirrhosis or improvement in survival is afforded by the venesections, implying that alcohol abuse and its attendant nutritional imbalances may also play some role in the origins of the liver disease. Further studies on the effectiveness of venesection in the treatment of hemochromatosis may well shed significant light on the pathogenesis of this disorder.

AMYLOIDOSIS

Amyloid is a pathologic homogeneous translucent hyaline deposit laid down between cells in various tissues and organs of the body in a wide variety of clinical settings. When first observed by Virchow, it was erroneously considered to be starch-like and hence the designation amyloid. It is distinguished in tissue sections from other hyaline materials by the following properties: it is acidophilic in usual tissue stains but yields a positive PAS reaction and assumes a rose-violet color with metachromatic dyes such as methyl violet or toluidine blue. It has an affinity for congo red dye. When examined with the polarizing microscope, it is weakly birefringent, but congo red staining intensifies its green birefringence. The gross deposits in whole organs develop a mahogany brown color when stained with iodine and dilute sulfuric acid. Under the electron microscope, it has a quite characteristic fibrillar substructure. It is of interest and clinical importance not only because its precise composition and pathogenesis are still unknown but also because accumulations of amyloid, when sufficiently advanced, engulf and obliterate parenchymal cells and so injure affected organs.

Most often, amyloidosis is encountered in patients suffering from some protracted underlying disease, causing extensive tissue breakdown. It also appears as a primary disorder. In other instances, it seems to have hereditary origins and so may be familial. In most of these settings, it is systemic in distribution. However, occasionally it occurs mysteriously in a single site, such as in the heart in aged patients and in the pancreatic islets in diabetes mellitus. Many attempts have been made to categorize these presentations on the basis of its distribution among organs and the clinical setting in which it occurred. But all classifications have proven to be artificial and plagued by numerous cases which failed to fit into one category or another. Despite these difficulties, it is helpful in understanding the spectrum of amyloidosis to provide the following classification:

A. Systemic amyloidosis with recognized predisposing disease *(secondary amyloidosis)*
  1. Associated with chronic infections—principally tuberculosis, osteomyelitis, bronchiectasis and syphilis
  2. Associated with chronic inflammatory diseases of uncertain etiology—principally rheumatoid arthritis, ulcerative colitis, regional enteritis, lupus erythematosus and other connective tissue diseases
  3. Associated with neoplasms—principally plasma cell myeloma, Hodgkin's disease and renal cell carcinoma
B. Systemic amyloidosis not associated with known predisposing disorders *(primary amyloidosis)*
C. Heredofamilial amyloidosis
  1. Familial Mediterranean fever with systemic amyloidosis
  2. Familial amyloid polyneuropathy
  3. Familial amyloid nephropathy
  4. Familial cardiac amyloidosis
  5. Familial amyloidotic medullary thyroid carcinoma
D. Isolated organ amyloidosis
  1. Senile amyloidosis—heart, brain, seminal vesicles
  2. Tumor amyloid of the tongue
  3. Amyloidosis of the islets of Langerhans in diabetes mellitus

In *secondary amyloidosis*, the deposits tend to affect abdominal viscera such as the spleen, kidneys, adrenals, liver, lymph nodes and pancreas, but the gastrointestinal tract, heart, blood vessels and gingiva are sometimes also affected. This pattern of amyloidosis tends to have the most massive deposits which often cause considerable organ dysfunction. Secondary amyloidosis appears only after the predisposing disease has been present for many years. In *primary amyloidosis*, the sites of deposition are principally small blood vessel walls, heart, lung, tongue and gingiva, but abdominal visceral involvement also sometimes develops. The overlap is apparent. In the *heredofamilial syndromes*, one particular organ or system is usually most severely attacked, save in familial Mediterranean fever where the distribution is systemic. However, in all of these familial syndromes, amyloid can be found in many organs and tissues when assiduously sought. *Isolated organ amyloidosis* is a mysterious condition. Tumor-like masses of amyloid have been described in the tongue, respiratory tree, pharynx, thyroid and other sites. Not understood yet is whether the solitary organ involvement would have been followed by a more widespread systemic distribution had the patient lived longer. However, at the time of autopsy, no other deposits may be found in patients having such localized patterns of involvement.

Whatever the anatomic site or clinical setting, amyloid deposits have a uniform appearance under the light and electron microscope. In general, in secondary amyloidosis, the characteristic staining reactions mentioned are strong, and so this form of amyloid has been called "typical." In some cases of primary amyloidosis, certain of the histochemical reactions may be weak and the amyloid has been called "atypical." However, as more is learned about the biochemistry and ultrastructure of amyloid, the conviction grows that amyloid is amyloid and such subtle variations as have been found may be attributable to adsorbed products or to the matrix in which it is deposited (Bonar et al., 1969).

Nature and Origin of Amyloid. Although it has a remarkably bland, uninteresting amorphous appearance under the light microscope, high resolution has disclosed a remarkable complexity to the substructure of amyloid (Fig. 8–13). All amyloid contains, or indeed may be entirely made up of fibrils or fibers of two types. Most of the fibers are fine, nonbranching fibrils about 75 Å in diameter. These, in turn, are composed of smaller filaments which are themselves made up of protofilaments. Twisting of these component filaments imparts a periodicity to the parent fiber (Shirahama and Cohen, 1965) (Cohen and Calkins, 1959). The nonbranching, filamentous fibril has been characterized as possessing cross-beta proteins having amino acid sequences that suggest a strong homology with immunoglobulin light chains (Glenner, 1971). This homology with light chains is of considerable interest in terms of the possible origin of amyloid.

The second type of major fiber presents as a rod composed of numerous stacked ringed units, much in the fashion of a stack of donuts. The external diameter of the rings are on the order of 100 Å and the stacks may measure up to 1500 Å in length (Hirschl, 1969). The stacked rods appear to have a totally different

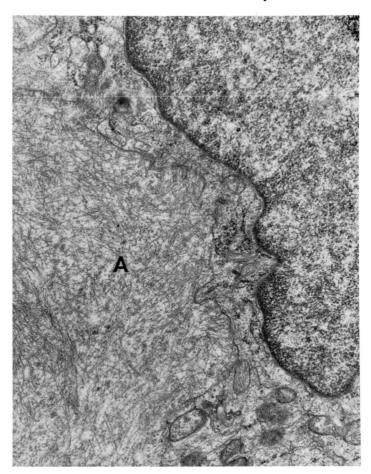

Figure 8-13. *Amyloidosis of the spleen under the electron microscope. The amyloid deposit (A) adjacent to a reticular cell contains a feltwork of delicate fibrils. × 22,500. (Courtesy of Cohen, A. S.: The constitution and genesis of amyloid. In International Review of Experimental Pathology, Vol. 4. New York, Academic Press, 1965.)*

origin from the nonbranching fibrils, and most of the evidence suggests that they are composed of an alpha globulin derived from plasma proteins (Bladen et al., 1966). The nonbranching fibrils and the rods have also been shown to have totally distinct antigenic profiles (Cathcart et al., 1971). A small content of carbohydrate is found on biochemical analysis of crude amyloid deposits, but it is uncertain as to whether this represents ground substance in which the fibrils and rods are embedded or a native component of the amyloid itself. Gamma globulins, complement and mucopolysaccharides are not found within amyloid except as they may be adsorbed to the depositions.

The origin of amyloid is truly an enigma wrapped in mystery. Years ago, it was thought to be a deposition of circulating gamma globulins. There seemed to be a great deal of evidence to support such a postulation. Secondary amyloidosis followed chronic infections and inflammatory diseases with elevated levels of circulating gamma globulins. Horses used for the production of diphtheria antisera often

died of advanced amyloidosis. The association of amyloid deposits with plasma cell myelomas lent further support to the concept of an association with gamma globulins. Animal models of amyloidosis can be produced by the injection of a variety of antigens such as casein, bacteria and other foreign proteins. Such a postulation, however, could not explain the appearance of amyloid deposits in isolated organs or primary amyloidosis not associated with known predisposing disease. The notion of deposition of circulating globulins was further weakened by the demonstration that immune tolerance to casein could be induced in mice soon after birth but, nonetheless, the tolerant animals were found to develop as much amyloidosis as a control group of nontolerant mice (Clerici et al., 1965). Furthermore, by the use of splenic explants from amyloid-bearing rabbits, Cohen et al., (1965a) demonstrated the in vitro deposition of amyloid in the absence of a blood supply and circulating gamma globulins.

Currently, and tentatively, it is proposed that *amyloid is a direct product of immunocompetent cells suffering from some abnormality in their normal immune response* (Muckle, 1968). Perhaps a genetic enzymic defect, the protracted antigenic challenge associated with chronic inflammatory disease, or the neoplastic transformation of immumocompetent cells as in plasma cell tumors all derail the normal synthetic pathways of one or many of the cellular components of the immune system (reticuloendothelial cells, macrophages, lymphocytes, plasma cells). If the normal pathways of immunoglobulin synthesis are blocked, perhaps fibrillar proteins so closely resembling immunoglobulin light chains are synthesized instead. Direct evidence that amyloid is induced by immunologically compentent cells has been provided by the induction of amyloid in normal syngeneic recipient mice following transfer of splenic cells from amyloidotic donors (Hardt, 1971). Here it would appear clear that the production of amyloid occurs locally and by cells of the immune system. Consonant with this proposition, Cathcart et al. (1970) propose that amyloid may be deposited when immunologic responsiveness is suppressed, and thus amyloidosis might be an expression of immunologic tolerance. They suggest "that experimental amyloidosis in the guinea pig is the end product (or one of the end products) of a specific clone of inactivated lymphocytes." We can come no closer at the present time to the precise origin of this still mysterious substance.

Morphology. Since there are no consistent systemic distributions of amyloid in the clinical syndromes mentioned, each of the major organ involvements will be described separately. Certain common features characterize amyloidosis wherever it is deposited. When present in only small amounts, it produces no apparent gross abnormalities. Often the presence of small amounts of amyloid is not suspected macroscopically until after the surface of the cut organ is painted with iodine and sulfuric acid. With larger amounts, the involved organ often assumes a rubbery, firm consistency and a waxy gray appearance.

Histologically, the depositions always begin between cells, often closely adjacent to basement membranes. Congo red staining followed by polarizing microscopy will often disclose trace amounts of amyloid not readily evident under the light microscope with usual tissue stains. With these techniques, the deposits become birefringent (Fig. 8–14). With progression, and as the amount of amyloid accumulates, nodular masses fuse and encroach on neighboring cells. In the advanced stages of this process, large masses of amyloid completely entrap and, in time, destroy the cellular constituents of the involved organ. All depositions of amyloid are identical at the ultrastructural level and are composed of the nonbranching fibrils and rods described.

Amyloidosis of the kidney is the commonest and potentially the most serious form of organ involvement. In most reported series of patients with

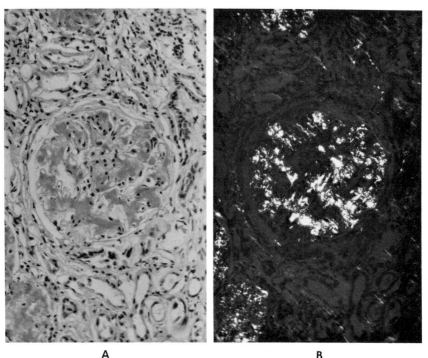

A **B**

Figure 8–14. A and B, *Amyloidosis of the glomerulus. Illustrating birefringence of the deposits after Congo red staining. (Courtesy of Cohen, A. S.: The constitution genesis of amyloid. In International Review of Experimental Pathology. Vol. 4. New York, Academic Press, 1965.)*

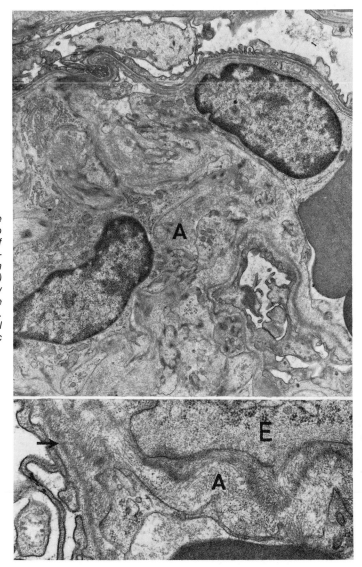

Figure 8-15. Amyloidosis in the kidney under the electron microscope to illustrate the subendothelial location of the amyloid deposit (A). In the lower figure (at 23,000 magnification), the location between the basement membrane (arrow) and the endothelial cell (E) is clearly shown. (Courtesy of Cohen, A. S.: The constitution and genesis of amyloid. In International Review of Experimental Pathology. Vol. 4. New York, Academic Press, 1965.)

amyloidosis, renal amyloidosis is the major cause of death (Lindeman, et al. 1961). On gross inspection, the kidney may appear normal in size and color or it may be enlarged, pale gray and firm. Often the cortical surface shows a slight undulation owing to subcapsular masses of amyloid. It is not unusual, however, for the kidney to be shrunken and contracted even in the absence of other intercurrent nephropathies. This contraction is attributable to vascular narrowing induced by the deposition of amyloid within arterial and arteriolar walls.

Histologically, the selective sites of amyloid involvement are primarily the glomeruli, but the interstitial peritubular tissue, arteries and arterioles are also affected. The glomerular deposits first appear as subtle thickenings of the mesangial matrix, accompanied usually by barely discernible uneven widening of the basement membranes of the glomerular capillaries. In time, the mesangial depositions and the depositions along the basement membranes cause capillary narrowing and distort the glomerular vascular tuft. With the electron microscope, the fibrillar accumulations begin on the endothelial side of the basement membrane and then appear to flood over the basement membrane to abut on the contiguous podocytes (Fig. 8–15). In many instances, the epithelial cells lose their foot processes and are fused to the membranous deposits. With progression of the glomerular amyloidosis, the endothelial cells are enveloped, the capillary lumina are obliterated and the obsolescent glomerulus is flooded by confluent masses or interlacing broad ribbons of amyloid (Fig. 8–16). Often the enlarged damaged vascular tufts obliterate the

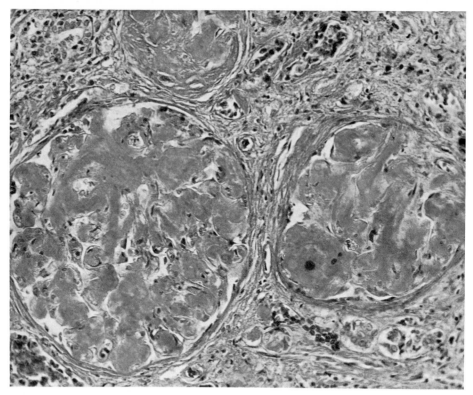

Figure 8-16. *Amyloidosis of the kidney. The glomerular architecture is almost totally obliterated by the massive accumulation of amyloid.*

urinary space and, with time, all normal architecture is wiped out.

While amyloidosis is widespread throughout the kidneys, for obscure reasons some glomeruli are more severely affected than others, but in end stage disease virtually all become involved. The peritubular deposits also begin in apposition to the tubular basement membranes and progressively extend into the tubular connective tissue as well as encroach on the tubular lumina. The overlying tubular epithelium may be unaffected or may undergo regressive changes. Often, proteinous casts fill these tubular lumina. The vascular involvement takes the form of pink hyaline thickening of arterial and arteriolar walls, often with narrowing of the lumina. With such ischemia, widespread tubular atrophy and interstitial fibrosis superimposes itself upon the basic deformity produced by the amyloidosis.

Amyloidosis of the spleen may be inapparent grossly or may cause moderate to marked splenomegaly (up to 800 gm.). For completely mysterious reasons, the deposits tend to follow one of two patterns. In one, the deposit is largely limited to the splenic follicles producing tapioca-like granules on gross inspection, designated "sago" spleen. Under the light microscope, the amyloid is laid down in a lacy pattern surrounding individual or nests of follicular cells. With progression, the amy-

loid encroaches on the follicular cells and eventually fuses into conglomerate masses which replace the follicles, giving rise to the small discrete granules visible to the naked eye on the cut surface. In the other pattern, the amyloid is laid down first in the walls of the splenic sinuses and connective tissue framework. The pulp is therefore affected, rather than the follicles (Fig. 8–17). Here again, the early deposits fuse eventually to cause large map-like areas of increased consistency, giving rise to the designation "lardaceous" spleen (Fig. 8–18). Ultrastructural studies indicate that the earliest deposits always occur in immediate apposition to the basement membranes of the reticuloendothelial cells of the splenic sinuses and within the walls of small blood vessels (Cohen et al., 1965b).

Amyloidosis of the liver was found in 52 of 53 patients with secondary, and in 17 of 20 patients with primary disease in one large series (Briggs, 1961). Here again, the deposits may be grossly inapparent or may cause moderate to marked hepatomegaly. Enlargements of up to 9000 gm. have been recorded (Rukavina et al., 1956). With enlargement, the liver assumes a pale, waxy-gray firm appearance. The amyloid appears first in the space of Disse and then progressively encroaches on adjacent hepatic parenchymal cells and sinusoids. In time, deformity, pressure atrophy and eventual dis-

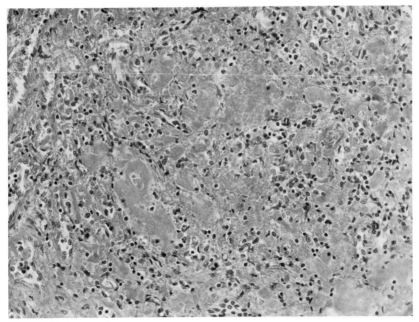

Figure 8-17. Amyloidosis of the spleen. The coalescent masses of amyloid surround the spleen cells.

appearance of hepatocytes occur, causing total replacment of large areas of liver parenchyma (Fig. 8—19 and Fig. 8—20). Vascular involvement and Kupffer cell depositions are frequent. It is difficult to believe that normal liver function is usually preserved despite sometimes quite severe involvement of the liver.

Amyloidosis of the heart is a major feature of primary amyloidosis but is also encountered in the secondary patterns and in association with multiple myeloma (Lindsay, 1946). In some patients, it represents an isolated organ involvement and, almost invariably, the patient is older than 80 years of age **(senile cardiac amyloidosis).** The heart may be enlarged and firm but more often shows no significant changes on cross section of the myocardium. Somewhat distinctive findings, when present, are pink to gray pinpoint or nodular elevations of the endocardium having a dew-drop appearance. Histologically, the deposits begin in focal subendocardial accumulations and within the myocardium between the muscle fibers. Expansion of these myocardial deposits eventually causes pressure atrophy of myocardial fibers (Fig. 8-21). Vascular and subepicardial accumulations may also occur. In most cases, the deposits are separated and widely distributed but, when subendocardial, the conduction system may be damaged and account for the electrocardiographic abnormalities encountered in some patients (Eliot et al., 1961). It should be emphasized that, in many cases of so-called isolated cardiac amyloidosis, special stains and polarizing microscopy have disclosed involvement of

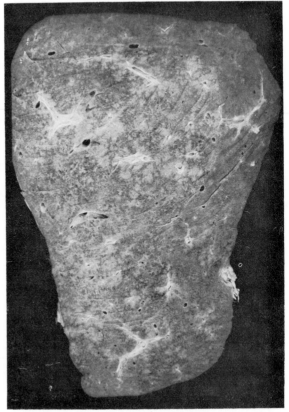

Figure 8-18. Amyloidosis of spleen. The focal deposits appear paler than the surrounding substance and in areas are confluent. The pattern is that known as "lardaceous."

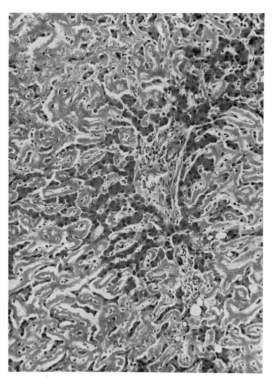

Figure 8–19. *Amyloidosis of the liver. A high power detail of the massive accumulation of amyloid and consequent pressure atrophy of liver cells.*

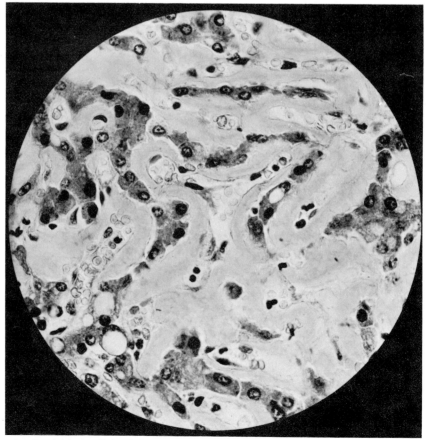

Figure 8–20. *Amyloidosis of the liver. Pressure atrophy of hepatic cords by amyloid. Some cells are compressed and distorted, while others have been replaced by the amyloid deposit.*

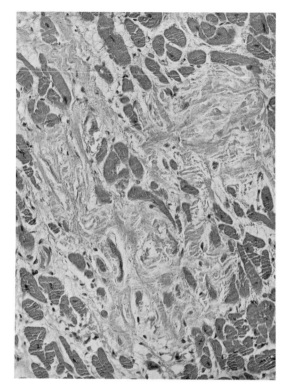

Figure 8–21. Primary amyloidosis of the heart. The amyloid surrounds isolated myocardial fibers and has caused atrophy of others.

other organs, raising the issue of whether isolated organ amyloidosis is not merely an early stage of a systemic disease. It is of interest that senile cardiac amyloidosis is rarely the cause of clinical manifestations while cardiac involvement in systemic amyloidosis may, indeed, produce serious cardiac irregularities and even fatal decompensation.

Amyloidosis of other organs is generally encountered in systemic distributions. The adrenals, thyroid and pituitary are common sites of involvement. In the adrenals, the intercellular deposits begin adjacent to the basement membranes of the cortical cells, usually first in the zona glomerulosa. With progression, the deposits encroach on cortical cells and advance into the deeper layers of the cortex. Large sheets of amyloid may replace considerable amounts of the cortical parenchyma. Similar patterns are seen in the thyroid and pituitary. The gastrointestinal tract may be involved at any level, from the oral cavity (gingiva, tongue) to the anus. The early lesions are largely perivascular in origin but eventually extend to involve the adjacent areas of the submucosa, muscularis and subserosa. Coalescence of these small deposits may produce plaques or bands of firm gray substance. Depositions in the tongue may cause macroglossia, giving rise to the designation **"tumor-forming amyloid of the tongue."** The respiratory tract may be involved focally or diffusely from the larynx down to the smallest bronchioles. Once again, the deposits are often perivascular in location, located in the submucosa, but enlargement may yield plaques, nodules or polyps that protrude directly beneath the covering epithelium. Amyloidosis of the central nervous system has been reported within the so-called plaques in the brain in patients having senile dementia and, occasionally, has been found in peripheral neuropathies. The peripheral nerve involvement is quite characteristic of one of the familial syndromes. In conclusion, no tissue in the body is immune (Cohen, 1967).

Clinical Correlation. Amyloidosis may be found as an unsuspected anatomic change having produced no clinical manifestations, or it may cause death. The symptomatology depends, of course, on the particular sites or organs affected. In the overall spectrum of cases with manifestations, renal disease, hepatomegaly, splenomegaly, cardiac abnormalities and alterations in immunoglobulins are the most consistent and suggestive findings (Cathcart et al., 1972). The renal involvement is usually manifested by proteinuria, protein and cellular casts and rarely red cell casts. Some patients develop massive proteinuria and the nephrotic syndrome (p. 1107). Azotemia and fatal uremia may develop in advanced cases, and it is worth noting that, unlike most forms of renal failure, amyloidosis is usually not associated with hypertension. The hepatosplenomegaly rarely induces organ dysfunction, but its occurrence along with nephropathy should suggest the diagnosis of amyloidosis in the appropriate clinical setting. Cardiac amyloidosis manifests in a variety of ways including conduction disturbances, coronary artery insufficiency due to arterial narrowing, myocardiopathy and cardiac failure, not responsive to the usual therapeutic measures. Not infrequently, cardiac amyloidosis masquerades as chronic constrictive pericarditis (p. 684). A few words are in order about the more common clinical syndromes.

Amyloidosis associated with other diseases (secondary amyloidosis) most commonly follows (1) chronic tuberculosis, (2) rheumatoid arthritis and (3) chronic osteomyelitis, although other associations have already been noted. Since the advent of the chemotherapy of tuberculosis, amyloidosis is seen less often in these patients, and rheumatoid arthritis is becoming the commonest predisposing condition. The reported prevalence of amyloidosis in those with rheumatoid arthritis is as high as 60 per cent but a more reasonable estimate might be 30 per cent (Calkins and Cohen, 1960).

There is recent experimental evidence that amyloid may be resorbed in virtually all sites of deposition save the kidneys. DeLellis et al. (1970) demonstrated that the generalized amyloidosis induced in mice by a single intraperitoneal injection of mycobacteria mixed with Fruend's adjuvant would regress from the spleen, liver, intestines, lymph nodes, heart and tongue but not from the kidneys. Whether similar mobilization might occur in man if the predisposing disease could be controlled has not yet been established.

Primary amyloidosis is more difficult to diagnose clinically because there are no predisposing conditions to arouse suspicion. The diagnosis of primary disease should be made only when all possible associations, such as a hidden plasma cell myeloma or latent infection, have been ruled out. In the primary category are found most of the exotic sites of localization such as the eyes, skin and genitourinary tract, usually accompanied by the systemic distribution described.

Amyloidosis associated with neoplasms, particularly plasma cell myeloma, is one of the best established of the "amyloid syndromes." It has been reported in 6 to 15 per cent of patients having multiple myeloma (Kimball, 1961). Less frequently, amyloidosis occurs with other forms of neoplasms and lymphomas such as renal cell carcinoma and Hodgkin's disease.

Senile amyloidosis is most often clinically significant when it affects the brain. Schwartz (1965) reported an unusually high prevalence of amyloid in the brain, pancreas or heart (89.5 per cent) of patients who died with senile dementia over the age of 60. Only rarely is senile cardiac amyloidosis as an isolated organ involvement responsible for clinical manifestations.

Among the heredofamilial syndromes, that associated with familial Mediterranean fever is most common. The predisposition is apparently transmitted as an autosomal recessive. In a series of 400 patients with this febrile disorder, 40 per cent developed amyloidosis affecting the kidneys, blood vessels, spleen, respiratory tract and rarely the liver (Heller et al., 1961). The other familial patterns are far less common, but of particular interest are the now well defined families having a hereditary predisposition to medullary thyroid carcinoma and pheochromocytomas, bearing amyloid deposits within the stroma of the tumors (Schimke and Hartmann, 1965). More details on these familial syndromes are available in the report of Cohen (1967).

The diagnosis of amyloidosis may be suspected by the signs and symptoms mentioned or by the clinical setting, but more specific tests must be employed for definitive diagnosis. Since amyloid has an affinity for congo red, it is possible to detect the presence of significant amounts of amyloid in the patient by the intravascular injection of known amounts of dye and by determining the amount removed from the circulation. The so-called congo red test, however, is only of value in instances where there is 80 per cent or more extraction of the circulating dye and, even at this level, false-positive results are sometimes encountered. Most experts would agree that retention of less than 80 per cent is of uncertain diagnostic value. Gingival biopsy was positive in 11 of 19 patients known to have amyloid (Calkins and Cohen, 1960). Rectal biopsies are positive in 60 to 75 per cent of patients with systemic amyloidosis (Blum and Sohar, 1962). With biopsy procedures, only a positive result is of value since a negative biopsy may merely indicate sparing of that particular site in an otherwise widespread disorder.

In the overall spectrum of patients diagnosed as having amyloidosis, the mean survival after diagnosis was reported to be approximately 11 months (Brandt et al., 1968). Obviously, for the diagnosis to have been made ante mortem, the disease must have been more than incipient. No effective therapy has yet been discovered, and still to be determined is whether control of a predisposing disease will be followed by regression of the deposits.

GOUT

Gout is a disorder of uric acid metabolism characterized by hyperuricemia and recurrent attacks of acute arthritis which may progress to chronic deforming arthritis. The acute arthritis is manifested by redness, pain and swelling of affected joints which typically completely subside only to flare again weeks, months or even years later. Over the span of years, urates may be deposited in and about the joints producing chronic arthritis, sometimes with total destruction of the articular surfaces and permanent disability. *The focal urate deposits in tissues with their attendant inflammatory reaction are known as tophi.* In some cases, tophi also occur in heart valves and the kidneys. Rarely, gout is manifested by hyperuricemia and renal involvement without significant accompanying arthritis. Hypertension and accelerated atherosclerosis are frequent concomitants.

It has become clear that serum uric acid levels in the population at large fall along a characteristic bell-shaped curve of distribution, and it is impossible to establish a specific level above which hyperuricemia may be said to exist. In clinical practice, 7.0 mg. per 100 ml. for males and 6.0 mg. per 100 ml. for females (enzymic spectrophotometric method) have proven to have pragmatic usefulness (Seegmiller et al., 1963). About 5 to 10 per cent of nongouty individuals will have serum uric acids above these limits and, conversely, about 5 to 10 per cent of gouty patients will have lower levels (Wyngaarden, 1970). Nonetheless, at some specific level for the individual the solubility of monosodium urate in biologic fluids is exceeded, and urate deposition in the tissues follows. A host of influences, both inborn and acquired, affect the serum uric acid levels and induce hyperuricemia. These can be divided into two large categories and, therefore, two forms of the disease are recognized: primary gout associated with genetic metabolic defects leading to hyperuricemia and secondary gout resulting from some acquired cause for hyperuricemia.

Primary gout represents an inborn error of metabolism. In some instances, it is clearly familial; in others, it may represent a genetic mutation in the individual. The study of gouty families indicates polygenic control of uric acid metabolism. Familial transmission patterns suggest that some of the genes may be autosomal dominant, others recessive, and still others sex-linked, dominant or recessive (Haughe and Harvald, 1955) (O'Brien et al., 1964). The hereditary disease has a strong male preponderance attributed to greater penetration in this sex; less than 5 per cent of the cases occur in females.

Secondary gout develops whenever some underlying disease causes increased production or inhibits excretion of uric acid, leading to hyperuricemia. Among the disorders causing increased production of uric acid are polycythemia, leukemia, hemolytic anemias, psoriasis and rapidly growing tumors. All of these diseases are associated with an increased breakdown of cells and turnover of nucleoprotein. Cytolytic agents used in the treatment of cancer and leukemia may augment the hyperuricemia. Decreased excretion of uric acid may be encountered in any form of renal insufficiency, but is also induced by drugs (thiazides, mercurials, aspirin) which inhibit renal uric acid excretory mechanisms. Secondary gout has also been observed somewhat mysteriously in association with a wide range of clinical conditions including obesity, sarcoidosis, glycogen-storage disease, alcoholism, thyroid dysfunction and many others (Kelley, 1969) (Sorensen, 1969).

Pathogenesis. The basis for the hyperuricemia of secondary gout has been mentioned already. The pathogenesis of primary gout is still somewhat unclear although much has been learned about its pathophysiology. Wyngaarden (1970) states: "No definite conclusion regarding the biochemical lesion or lesions responsible for overproduction in gout is possible at the present time." Nonetheless, certain understandings have been achieved. Uric acid is liberated from nucleotides by the enzymic degradation of tissue and dietary purines. The immediate precursors of uric acid are hypoxanthine and xanthine. The oxidation of hypoxanthine to xanthine and that of xanthine to uric acid are both catalyzed by the enzyme xanthine oxidase. The nucleotides adenylic acid (AMP) and guanylic acid (GMP), essential components of nucleic acids, are synthesized through two pathways: (1) de novo from basic precursors through a common intermediate, inosinic acid (IMP), or (2) from their respective preformed purines in the presence of phosphoribosylpyrophosphate (PRPP) and PRPP amidotransferase. AMP and GMP control these two synthetic pathways by feedback inhibition of certain essential enzymes. They inhibit both PRPP amidotransferase, the rate-limiting enzyme of purine biosynthesis de novo, as well as the phosphoribosyl transferase enzymes which catalyze the "salvage" or "reutilization" of free bases, reconverting them to their nucleotides. These interactions are set out in Figure 8–22.

Once formed, uric acid is excreted through the kidneys by a complex process involving glomerular filtration, reabsorption in the proximal convoluted tubule and then secretion back into the distal tubule.

Primary gout may be caused by a number of genetic metabolic defects which lead to increased production of uric acid and hyperuricemia. Several pathways may be involved: (1) increased production of one of the substrates, PRPP or glutamine necessary for the de novo synthesis of nucleotides; (2) decreased production of either of the purine nucleotides, AMP or GMP with release of feedback controls; or (3) an inappropriate increase in the amount or activity of PRPP amidotransferase relative to the concentration of the inhibitory end products. *Thus, primary gout actually represents a heterogeneous group of genetic disorders.*

The most clear-cut example of a hereditary defect leading to hyperuricemia is found in the Lesch-Nyhan syndrome in which there is a total deficiency of hypoxanthine-guanine phosphoribosyltransferase. This enzyme, it will be remembered, is involved in the salvage

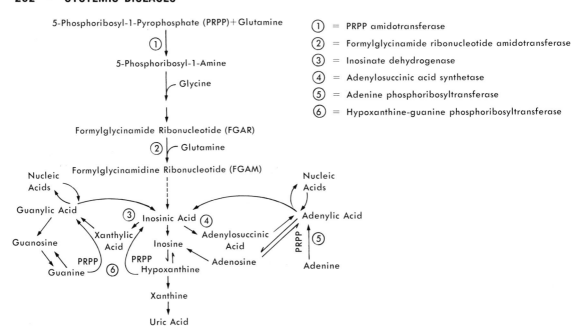

Figure 8–22. *Schematic outline of purine metabolism in man. (Adapted from Kelly, W. N.: Recent progress in the pathogenesis and treatment of gout. Med. Times, 97:230, 1969.)*

pathway of reconverting free purine bases to their respective nucleotides and, when it is congenitally lacking, there is impaired synthesis of AMP and GMP and this, in turn, leads to an accelerated purine biosynthesis through the de novo pathway (Seegmiller et al., 1967). The Lesch-Nyhan syndrome is characterized by neurologic derangements and clinical manifestations of gout including acute arthritis, tophi, and gouty nephropathy, all becoming manifest in infancy. Most patients die from uremia or wasting before they reach adolescence. To date, all patients have been males and the inheritance of the defect conforms to an X-linked recessive mode of transmission (Lesch and Nyhan, 1964) (Shapiro et al., 1966). The Lesch-Nyhan syndrome is relatively rare and does not account for the preponderance of cases of primary gout but, soon after its delineation, it was found that other patients with gout had a partial deficiency of this enzyme (Kelley et al., 1967).

An additional metabolic defect leading to hyperuricemia involves the rate-limiting enzyme PRPP amidotransferase. In some patients, it is postulated that this enzyme retains its function but is no longer susceptible to feedback inhibition. Conceivably, some mutation in the gene controlling the synthesis of this enzyme underlies this aberration (Henderson et al., 1968). However, many patients with primary gout with excessive levels of purine synthesis have no identified enzyme defect, and the basis for the increased purine synthesis is

unclear. Sorenson (1969) alludes to such a mystery in his statement: "Thus primary gout, characterized by overproduction of uric acid, is merely the phenotypic expression of a heterogeneous group of genetic abnormalities."

Primary gout may also be caused by impaired renal handling of uric acid. It has been proposed, although not documented, that the renal mechanisms of uric acid processing are under genetic control, and so primary gout with underexcretion may also represent an inborn error of metabolism. In support of this hereditary notion is the well known fact that the Dalmation coach hound possesses a hereditary recessive trait in the form of failure of tubular secretion of urate (Bunim et al., 1962). Thus, primary gout may result from overproduction or underexcretion of uric acid or, of course, both.

Granting the existence of hyperuricemia, what accounts for the acute attacks of arthritis and the selective sites of deposition of tophi? The mechanism for the acute gouty attack has been fairly well established by Seegmiller et al. (1962). It is clear that hyperuricemia is the manifestation in the blood of an increased uric acid pool throughout the body. All biologic fluids share in the elevated levels of uric acid. When the level of urates rises in the body fluids and its solubility coefficient is exceeded, needle-like crystals of monosodium urate monohydrate precipitate out in the joint fluids. Factors other than simple chemicophysical considerations may underlie this precipitation.

Alvsaker (1966) noted that urates may be maintained in solution by reversible interactions with certain plasma proteins. He has further suggested that synthesis of these proteins is under genetic control and may be impaired in gouty patients, thus predisposing them to precipitation of urates into tissues (Alvsaker, 1968). Another factor contributing to the precipitation of crystals may be the local pH in the joint fluid which is lower than that in the blood because of the high rates of glycolysis in the relatively avascular joint tissues. In any event, in the acutely involved joint, minute crystals have been identified within the synovial membranes and these excite an acute inflammatory reaction characterized by the infiltration of neutrophils. The leukocytes phagocytize the crystals, and their increased glycolytic metabolic activity and increased lactate production further lower the pH and so augment the crystallization of urates. Death of some of the neutrophils releases lysosomal enzymes, and the combination of intra-articular acidosis, accumulation of lysosomal enzymes and release of inflammatory kinins all evoke the acute inflammatory response so characteristic of the rapidly developing arthritis of acute gout (McCarty, 1964).

When the hyperuricemia has been present for long periods of time, urates may deposit in tissues. The basis for the localization of tophi in and about joints, in the kidneys and in heart valves is not clearly understood. One theory proposes that relatively avascular tissues having ground substance rich in acid mucopolysaccharides predispose to tophus formation (Sokoloff, 1957). Tophi are also prone to form in acral parts of the body such as the earlobes or toes, and here lower body temperature may decrease the solubility of urates in the body fluids and predispose to precipitation (Seegmiller et al., 1963).

Morphology. The acute arthritis of gout is nondistinctive morphologically. It comprises a nonspecific acute inflammation within the synovial tissues made distinctive only by the microcrystals of urate. These however, would be lost in the usual aqueous solutions employed in the fixation and staining of tissues. For their demonstration, special methods must be employed. Chronic gout is characterized morphologically by masses of urates on articular surfaces and by tophi in the capsular and tendinous connective tissues about the joints and in the connective tissues of the kidney pyramids, heart valves and ear lobes (Fig. 8—23). The urates are usually laid down in parallel bundles of needle-like crystals, but occasionally occur as completely amorphous granular masses. **The tophus comprises a mass of urate crystals surrounded by an inflammatory response composed of young fibroblasts intermingled with lymphocytes, plasma cells, macrophages and foreign body giant cells** (Fig. 8—24). The giant cells are one of the most distinctive features since, in the process of surrounding large masses of urates, these cells are distorted and stretched out and so may extend across half a high power microscopic field. **The tophus constitutes a virtual hallmark of gout.** The deposition of urates on joint surfaces first appear as minute, irregular, chalky white granular foci. With progression, these foci become larger and coalesce eventually to form large, irregular plaque-like encrustations. The plaques frequently become polished and smooth from joint motion and so resemble encrusted white enamel (Fig. 8-25). Expansion of these precipitates

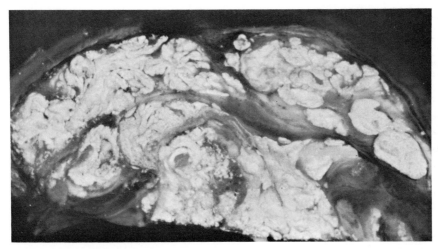

Figure 8–23. *A cross section of the periarticular tissues of the metatarsophalangeal joint with massive white amorphous urate deposition in all layers up to the skin.*

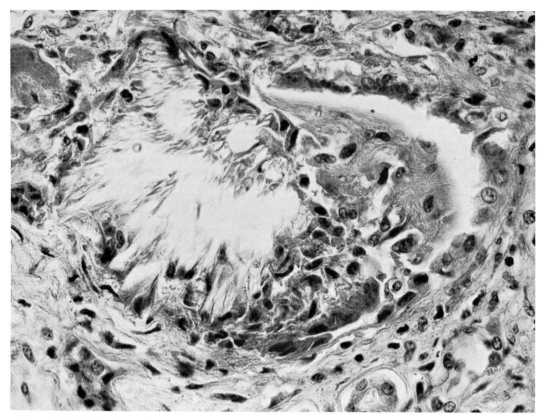

Figure 8–24. *A tophus of gout. The group of slender urate crystals is surrounded by a reaction of fibroblasts, occasional lymphocytes and giant cells.*

may erode the articular surface and the underlying bone eventually to destroy the entire joint surface. Thus, chronic tophaceous gout leads to crippling deformities. Secondary osteoarthritis often supervenes (p. 1470).

Generalized atherosclerosis and arteriolo-sclerosis is found in 30 to 40 per cent of gouty patients to a far more advanced level than would be anticipated in age-matched controls. The basis for such predisposition has been attributed to some concomitant abnormality in lipid metabolism (Barlow, 1966). Hypertension is a frequent concomi-

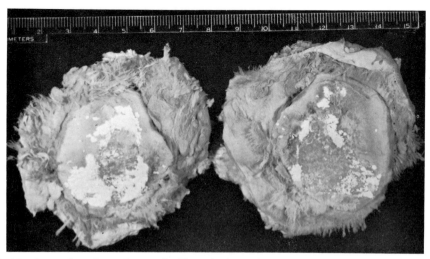

Figure 8–25. *Gouty deposits on the patella. The articular surfaces of the patellas are encrusted with white deposits of urates.*

tant, but it is still not clear whether the blood pressure levels are the cause or the effect of the arteriolosclerosis (p. 1128).

The kidneys are damaged in almost all cases of gout. In a review of 191 cases, Talbott and Terplan (1960) found only four patients free of renal disease. The most distinctive renal change was the formation of tophi within the pyramids but, in addition, tubular precipitates of uric acid, nephrosclerosis and pyelonephritis were commonly present. Recent studies have indicated that the earliest structural abnormality in the kidney is tubular damage followed by an interstitial reaction. Thus, the morphologic lesion that has been interpreted as pyelonephritis may not be of infectious origin (Gonick et al., 1965). A variety of other renal lesions may also be found, including acute tubular necrosis, several forms of glomerular disease and amyloidosis. About 10 per cent of gouty patients develop uric acid renal stones. It should be emphasized that the renal changes may not necessarily parallel in severity the arthritis, and it has been repeatedly observed that, in some patients, the only consequence of the hyperuricemia has been the development of renal disease.

Tophi are occasionally encountered in more exotic locations such as the central nervous system, eyes, tongue, larynx, penis and testes (Chung, 1962).

Clinical Correlation. Clinical gout may appear in any hyperuricemic patient. Primary gout is familial in approximately 75 per cent of cases. It is far more common than secondary gout in the ratio of approximately 20 to 1 (Yu and Gutman, 1959). The mean age of onset of the primary disease is approximately 40 years while the secondary has a later onset, approximately 50 years. Whatever the basis, three stages have been delineated. *Stage one* is designated as hyperuricemic asymptomatic gout. Silent hyperuricemia has been identified in about 25 to 33 per cent of relatives of gouty patients and only about one-third of these individuals will ever develop disabling disease. Most will have only persistently elevated serum uric acid levels throughout life without resulting tissue damage. *Stage two* comprises acute gouty arthritis. It is characterized by the sudden onset of joint pain, redness and swelling affecting the following sites in order of frequency: great toe, ankle, foot, knee, finger, elbow, wrist and other joints (Grahame and Scott, 1970). The arthritis may be monoarticular but, as the disease advances, more often several joints are affected concomitantly. Characteristic of this stage are asymptomatic intercritical periods ranging from months to years, punctuated by the sudden onset of another attack of arthritis. *Stage three* is chronic tophaceous gout, the likely consequence of recurrent acute arthritis. Disabling joint disease may develop within a few years or only after many decades of acute gout. In the chronic disease, the development of renal changes is manifested by proteinuria, pyuria, renal stones, renal colic and hypertension. Indeed, renal failure usually associated with hypertension was the second most common related cause of death in the series of patients studied by Grahame and Scott (1970). The most common related cause was myocardial infarction, presumably associated with the augmented atherosclerosis which accompanies this disorder.

The diagnosis of gout should not be missed by the clinician because it affords him the splendid opportunity of doing good. A wide armamentarium of drugs is available to (1) abort or prevent acute attacks of arthritis by such agents as colchicine, (2) mobilize tophaceous deposits by such uricosuric agents as probenecid and (3) inhibit uric acid synthesis with allopurinol, for example. In general, gout does not materially shorten life expectancy, but it certainly may impair the quality of life (Talbott and Lilienfeld, 1959).

URATE DEPOSITS IN THE KIDNEYS

Yellow-white streaks are occasionally observed in the tips of the kidney pyramids in newborn infants and rarely in leukemic or polycythemic adults. The lesions have erroneously been called uric acid infarcts. Since there is no evidence of tissue necrosis or infarction, there appears to be no justification for the perpetuation of the term infarct. The lesions consist of deposits of amorphous or crystalline urates in the collecting tubules of the kidney (Fig. 8–26). With progressive deposition, the lining epithelial cells and the peritubular connective tissue may be affected. The urates are derived from the excessive breakdown of nucleoprotein, presumably from the destruction of red cells in infants, and from the destruction of white and red cells in affected adults.

There is no associated clinical evidence of renal damage. These lesions are anatomic changes which have importance only insofar as they must be differentiated grossly from deposits of calcium in the interstitial tissue of the pyramids of the kidneys.

STORAGE DISEASES

The growing sophistication of biochemical and ultrastructural studies has yielded an ever

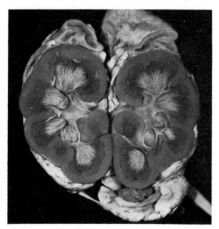

Figure 8-26. *Urate deposits in the kidney. The crystalline deposits in the tubules and peritubular connective tissue form linear white streaks in the renal pyramids.*

enlarging list of inborn errors of metabolism characterized by the excessive formation and storage of a variety of macromolecular substances in the tissues of the body. Almost all of these genetic disorders represent a lack of a specific enzyme which thus blocks a normal metabolic pathway and consequently either leads to the pileup of a normal metabolite or forces the synthesis of an abnormal product through some biosynthetic shunt. The metabolic error is presumably the expression of a gene mutation and thus these storage diseases are examples of the "one gene-one enzyme" concept of Beadle and Tatum (1941). Most storage diseases are familial and breed true insofar as affected members of a family suffer the same enzyme defect and accumulate the same storage product. Transmission is almost always as a recessive, although a few patterns have been found to be dominant and some sex-linked. The recessive traits only become manifest in homozygotes.

Undoubtedly, a block in every known metabolic pathway must have been described at one time or another in the world's literature, but fortunately only a few result in morphologically demonstrable storage diseases. Moreover, individually and even collectively, these disorders are uncommon, and so only a few will be described: the glycogenoses (sometimes called glycogen-storage diseases), three lipidoses—Gaucher's disease, Niemann-Pick disease and Tay-Sachs disease, and the two mucopolysaccharidoses—Hunter's syndrome and Hurler's syndrome.

In all of these storage diseases, the stored product is macromolecular, and so its accumulation becomes apparent by distention and vacuolation of affected cells. The specific sites

of storage depend upon the metabolic pathway involved and the dependence of the various tissues of the body upon this particular biochemical pathway. So some storage diseases are quite distinctive because mainly local sites of production or utilization of the abnormal product are affected as, for example, the CNS in Tay-Sachs disease. In others, however, the abnormal product overflows into the circulation and so is picked up by the RE scavenger cells, leading to splenomegaly, hepatomegaly, lymphadenopathy and marrow involvement. In these "reticuloses," the patterns of tissue and organ involvement tend to merge, and it is impossible from morphologic examination alone to identify the nature of the stored macromolecule. In all, biochemical analysis of affected tissues, serum and urine is necessary to identify with certainty the specific nature of the metabolic error. Histochemical procedures may be helpful in differentiating lipidoses from mucopolysaccharidoses, for example, but they cannot always identify the individual entities within a group of closely related disorders. In some, circulating white cells and epidermal cells are affected, providing readily accessible sources of biochemical assay materials. Amniotic fluid with its shed fetal epidermal cells thus provides a source for the prenatal diagnosis of storage diseases, permitting therapeutic abortion in those instances with a tragic, hopeless prognosis.

GLYCOGENOSES (GLYCOGEN-STORAGE DISEASES)

Six well defined syndromes have been identified resulting from a genetic defect in the catabolism or synthesis of glycogen. Each is associated with an inborn deficiency of one of the enzymes involved in the complex buildup or breakdown of glycogen, and hence this product accumulates in cells suffering the enzyme lack. A seventh syndrome, although included with the glycogen-storage diseases, actually represents a metabolic block in the synthesis of glycogen, and so the cells of the body lack this product. All are designated by roman numerals. Table 8–1 provides a brief characterization of the seven most common syndromes, although other more rare forms have been described.

It is apparent that among the seven syndromes, four are characterized by the accumulation of normal glycogen, two by the accumulation of abnormal glycogen, and one indeed by a lack of glycogen. All are transmitted as autosomal recessive traits only expressed in the homozygote, but type VI may be sex-linked and therefore more often expressed in the

TABLE 8–1. GLYCOGENOSES

Type	Synonym	Enzyme Deficiency	Glycogen	Organ Involvement
I	Von Gierke's disease	glucose-6-phosphatase	normal	liver, kidney, intestine
II	Pompe's disease	alpha-glucosidase	normal	heart, striated muscles
III	Limit dextrinosis	amylo-1, 6-glucosidase (debrancher)	abnormal	liver, kidneys, heart, muscles, leukocytes
IV		amylo-1, 4-1, 6-trans-glucosidase (brancher)	abnormal	liver, spleen, lymph nodes
V	McArdle's syndrome	muscle phosphorylase	normal	striated muscle
VI		liver phosphorylase	normal	liver, spleen
VII		glycogen synthetase	deficient synthesis	principally liver with hypoglycemia

male (Hsia, 1968). All become manifest soon after birth and generally cause progressive illness leading to death during childhood. The gravity of the disease and the rapidity of its course depend on the specific enzyme involved, the severity of the enzyme lack, and the specific tissues and organs principally affected. With respect to the enzyme lack, in some patients it is total, and in others, partial. For this reason there is a belief that the critical gene mutation may involve either the structural gene, in which case no enzyme can be synthesized, or the regulator genes, which control quantity.

The significance of a specific enzyme deficiency is best understood from the perspective of the normal metabolism of glycogen. As is well known, glycogen is a storage form of glucose. Glycogen synthesis begins with the conversion of glucose to glucose-6-phosphate by the action of a hexokinase. A phosphoglucomutase then transforms the glucose-6-phosphate to glucose-1-phosphate which, in turn, is converted to uridine diphosphoglucose. A highly branched, very large polymer is then built up (molecular weight up to 100,000,000) containing up to 10,000 glucose molecules linked together by alpha-1,4-glucoside bonds. The central spine gives off many branches joined by alpha-1,6-glucoside linkages requiring brancher enzymes. The glycogen chain and branches continue to be elongated by the addition of glucose molecules mediated by glycogen synthetases. Mobilization of glycogen involves a number of steps requiring glucosidases, phosphorylases and debrancher enzymes. Eventually, the fundamental building block of glucose-1-phosphate is recovered which is interconverted to glucose-6-phosphate from which glucose is liberated. Some of these details are presented in Figure 8–27.

Type I (Von Gierke's disease) is principally characterized by an excess storage of glycogen in the liver and kidneys and hence is often known as the *hepatorenal form of glycogenosis*. It results from a deficiency of the microsomal enzyme glucose-6-phosphatase, and so glucose cannot be mobilized from glycogen. The disorder usually becomes manifest during the first year of life by the appearance of convulsions related to hypoglycemia. Because of the deranged glucose metabolism, hyperlipemia may develop often leading to xanthomatous deposits. The hepatomegaly is the consequence of excess storage of glycogen and fat within liver cells. Striking deposits of glycogen cause renal tubular cell vacuolization throughout the cortex and renomegaly. These infants fail to thrive, develop progressive enlargement of their abdomens, have retarded growth, and many die of infections. Rare cases having, presumably, less profound enzyme deficiencies survive into adult life (Brown and Brown, 1968).

Type II (Pompe's disease) is manifested by glycogen storage within striated muscles principally in the heart, hence this syndrome is best remembered as *cardiac glycogenosis*. It results from a hereditary deficiency of the lysosomal enzyme alpha-glucosidase transmitted as an autosomal recessive trait. Alpha-glucosidase is involved in hydrolyzing the outer branches of glycogen to free glucose, as well as in hydrolyzing maltose. Because of the enzyme lack, glycogen accumulates within skeletal and cardiac muscle cells, principally within ballooned-out lysosomes which appear as cleared vacuoles under the light microscope. Other organs are affected—e.g., the tongue, diaphragm, kidneys and RE cells. Pompe's disease is one of the more virulent variants of the glycogenoses and usually causes death during the first year of life. The major clinical manifestations comprise muscular weakness, cardiac enlargement and progressive heart failure. To diagnose definitively this form of glycogen-storage disease, it is necessary to confirm biochemically the deficiency of glucosidase in affected tissues (Hers, 1965). Heterozygotes not manifesting

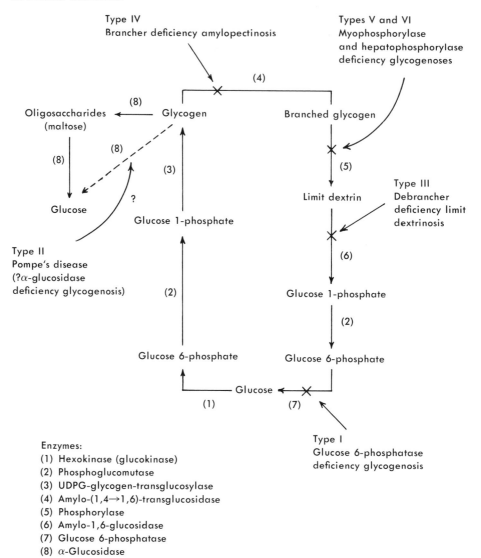

Figure 8–27. *The glycogen cycle (schematic) and sites (marked with an x) of genetically determined enzyme "lesions" causing excessive glycogen deposition. (Adapted from Field, R. A.: Glycogen deposition diseases. In Stanbury, J. B., Wyngaarden, J. B., and Fredrickson, D. S. (eds.): The Metabolic Basis of Inherited Disease. New York, The Blakiston Division, McGraw-Hill Book Co., 1966, p. 171.)*

the disease can be detected by assay of phyto-hemagglutinin-stimulated lymphocytes for alpha-glucosidase (Hirschhorn et al., 1969).

Type III (Limit dextrinosis) resembles Von Gierke's disease clinically but, in general, is milder. The metabolic abnormality sometimes clears with age. It too is transmitted as an autosomal recessive and is characterized by a deficiency of amylo-1, 6-glucosidase, the debrancher enzyme. This deficiency blocks the degradation of glycogen beyond the branching points, and so the stored glycogen is abnormal in configuration. Like Von Gierke's disease, accumulated glycogen is found in the liver and kidneys but is also present in this syndrome

within the heart, skeletal muscles and white cells. For obscure reasons, the hepatic involvement is sometimes accompanied by a mild periportal fibrosis.

Type IV is one of the most lethal patterns and almost invariably causes death in infancy. It is characterized by a deficiency of the brancher enzyme amylo-1, 4-1, 6 transglucosidase necessary for the creation of the branch points in glycogen. As a consequence, elongated configurations are produced, resembling plant amylopectins. The abnormal glycogen accumulates within the liver, spleen, lymph nodes and intestinal mucosa. These severely affected infants fail to thrive from early life, almost invariably develop a diffuse portal cirrhosis and die of liver failure (Pearson, 1968).

Type V (McArdle's syndrome) is made distinctive by striking muscular weakness which becomes manifest early in life. The fundamental defect is a deficiency of muscle phosphorylase which catalyzes the cleavage of the alpha-1, 4-glucoside linkages. Glycogen therefore accumulates within striated muscle and, at the same time, the inability to liberate glucose induces profound motor weakness after brief intervals of physical activity. Cases are on record where the motor deficit is less profound and patients have survived into adult life (Pearson, 1968).

Type VI is caused by a deficiency of liver phosphorylase also involved in the catalysis of glycogen and, as would be expected, it causes marked hepatic enlargement and hypoglycemia. Unlike the other glycogenoses, it may be sex-linked (Hsia, 1968). Studies of these infants have yielded some insight into the possible mechanisms responsible for mild deficiencies of an enzyme rather than its total lack. Infants with type VI glycogenosis have been shown to lack activation or regulation of pathways involved in hepatic synthesis of phosphorylase.

Other variants of these hereditary disorders of glycogen metabolism have been described but are even more rare than the uncommon forms cited above (Hug et al., 1966). Only one need be briefly recalled, namely, type VII which differs from those just described by having a lack of glycogen synthetase and hence an inability to fabricate glycogen.

GAUCHER'S DISEASE

This inborn error of metabolism is characterized by the storage of glucocerebrosides in massively distended reticuloendothelial cells throughout the body, principally in the liver, spleen and bone marrow. *A deficiency of glucocerebroside-cleaving enzyme, capable of splitting glucose from the ceramide residue, has been demonstrated in the spleen and liver of these patients* (Brady et al., 1966). As a consequence, the complex lipid accumulates in phagocytic histiocytes or reticuloendothelial cells. Three genetic and clinical patterns have been identified: (1) transmission as a mendelian recessive with clinical expression in adult life; (2) transmission as a mendelian dominant; (3) transmission as a mendelian recessive with neurologic manifestations (Hsia et al., 1959) (Groen, 1964).

The most common pattern of Gaucher's disease is the autosomal recessive becoming manifest in adult life, not associated with neurologic complications. The glucocerebrosides in this disorder may be derived from globosides contained within senescent red cells. In the usual adult, the liver and spleen progressively enlarge, sometimes to enormous size (the liver up to 5000 gm. and the spleen up to 10,000 gm.). The splenic substance appears pale gray and is literally replaced by masses of Gaucher's cells measuring up to 100 microns in diameter, often containing three or more small, eccentrically placed nuclei. The cytoplasm may appear cleared or vacuolated but often has a quite characteristic irregular streaking, resembling crumpled tissue paper (Fig. 8–28). Ultrastructural studies indicate that the irregular linear configurations are produced by large cytoplasmic elongated bodies containing tubular elements. The cytoplasmic bodies are presumably massively distended lysosomes, and the tubular elements are thought to be complexes of glucocerebrosides (Hibbs et al., 1970). Phagocytized erythrocytes are often found in the cytoplasm of the large Gaucher's cells and may represent the source of the glucocerebrosides since these lipids are abundant in their envelopes. For reasons that are not clear, Gaucher cells are rich in acid phosphatase. The liver may have a mottled or uniform, pale gray, cut surface due to focal or massive infiltration of Gaucher's cells. Involvement of the bone marrow may produce small focal areas of softening or large soft gray tumorous masses composed of Gaucher's cells. These may erode the normal bony architecture and cause skeletal deformity. Occasionally, aggregates of distended histiocytes are found in the lungs and in other organs, particularly the endocrine glands.

The clinical course of Gaucher's disease depends upon the age when symptoms first become apparent. It generally first comes to attention by manifestations related to the splenomegaly or hepatomegaly. Bone marrow involvement may produce skeletal pain or disability in motor function. Anemia, leukopenia and thrombocytopenia, often with a hemorrhagic diathesis, either reflect the marrow involvement or are the consequence of a hypersplenic syndrome. Although the disease is progressive in the adult, it is compatible with long life. The diagnosis can be suspected by the characteristic clinical setting, particularly the association of bone lesions with the massive splenic and hepatic involvement but, for definitive diagnosis, biopsy and biochemical analysis of affected tissues may be required. Recently, it has been shown that the adult type of Gaucher's disease and its carrier state can be

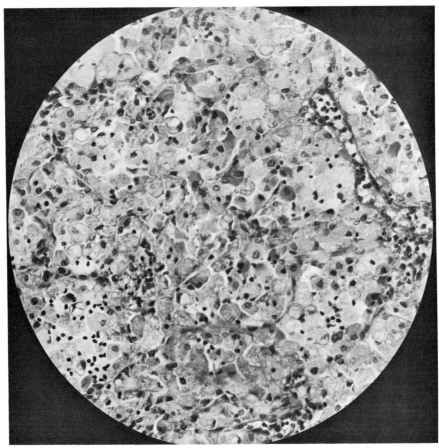

Figure 8-28. *Gaucher's disease involving the spleen. The entire field is made up of lipid-laden cells of varying size with sharp cell boundaries, abundant granular cytoplasm and small eccentric nuclei. A few cells are vacuolated, an unusual feature of this disease.*

diagnosed by the demonstration of a deficiency of beta-glucosidase in peripheral blood leukocytes (Beutler and Kuhl, 1970).

The infantile form with neurologic involvement is associated with the accumulation of cerebrosides in neurons possibly derived from cerebrogangliosides. It may represent a metabolic block quite different from that in the usual adult form of the disorder. In any event, the diseased children usually die in infancy or childhood.

NIEMANN-PICK (NP) DISEASE

Niemann-Pick disease is characterized by the accumulation of sphingomyelin in the reticuloendothelial cells of the liver, spleen, bone marrow and lymph nodes. In most cases, central nervous system involvement becomes manifest in infancy but, in some patients, there is no involvement of the brain. Because of this variation in presentation, many believe that NP disease is not a single clinical and biochemical entity but a constellation of four metabolic defects having in common tissue storage of sphingomyelin (Frederickson, 1966). About 85 per cent of the patients have the classic disease characterized by hepatosplenomegaly and intellectual deterioration which become manifest during the first year of life, leading to death within a year or two. The other variants essentially comprise more benign disorders appearing later in life, some free of neurologic symptoms (Philippart et al., 1969).

In classic cases, a deficiency of the sphingomyelin-cleaving enzyme, sphingomyelinase, has been identified in the kidneys, liver and spleen (Schneider and Kennedy, 1967). The metabolic error is transmitted as an autosomal recessive. In the classic disease, the metabolic block results in the storage, within histiocytes throughout the body, of lipids—predominantly sphingomyelin but also cholesterol and other phosphatides. Indeed, the lipid-laden cells may contain more cholesterol than sphingomyelin. The stored lipid causes some enlargement of the cells but not as great as that in Gaucher's disease, and creates a fine, reticulated foaminess to the cytoplasm caused by numerous minute vacuoles (Fig. 8–29). The storage cells are usually uninuclear and are not significantly different from macrophages filled with fatty debris in areas of necrosis or inflammation. Histochemical stains performed on these cells disclose a positive periodic acid-Schiff reaction and strong uptake of fat soluble dyes such as Sudan IV. At higher resolution, the minute vacuoles can be resolved as lamellar configurations closely resembling myelin figures (Lynn and Terry, 1964).

In the usual infantile form of NP disease, the liver and spleen are moderately enlarged by infiltrations and aggregations of these storage cells. Less severe involvement is found in the bone marrow, lungs, skin and other organs. The hepatic and splenic enlargement is less marked than that encountered in Gaucher's disease and usually causes only slight pale gray mottling of the cut surface of these organs. The bone marrow involvement is usually diffuse and does not produce the tumorous masses or distortion of the bone structure so characteristic of advanced stages of Gaucher's disease. Most crucially, however, ballooned ganglion cells are seen in various areas of the brain, primarily in the cerebellum, brain stem and spinal cord (Ivemark et al., 1963). Ganglion cells throughout the body are also affected, such as those in Auerbach's plexus and Meissner's plexus. It should be noted that, in some cases, macular degeneration results in the retinal cherry red spot often considered to be diagnostic of Tay-Sachs disease.

When NP disease becomes manifest in infancy, it usually follows a rapid downhill course over the span of one to two years. Wasting and mental deterioration become evident very early, leading to progressive inanition usually brought to an end by an intercurrent infection. Although the diagnosis is usually evident from the clinical findings, it can be confirmed by demonstration of vacuolation and degeneration of ganglion cells in biopsies of the rectal wall. Biochemical analysis of affected tissues is a more certain way of confirming the diagnosis.

Other less fulminating forms of NP disease have been segregated from the classic form just described. In one of these sub groups, there is massive visceral involvement similar to the classic disease, but the patients remain free of neurologic symptoms. Another variant differs from the classic pattern only in having no demonstrable deficiency of sphingomyelinase. The nature of this variant is poorly understood, and one might question whether it should be characterized as a form of NP disease. Still another clinical pattern is sometimes encountered in which the neurologic abnormalities do not become evident until middle childhood and, in these patients, the lipid accumulations are largely nonesterified cholesterol with only small amounts of sphingomyelin. There is much yet to be learned about the altered metabolic pathways underlying such variable presentations of this group of closely related but possibly dissimilar disorders.

GANGLIOSIDE-STORAGE DISEASES (TAY-SACHS DISEASE)

Five ganglioside-storage diseases have been delineated, all characterized by progressive mental and motor deterioration beginning in infancy and resulting from the accumulation, in neurons, of a specific ganglioside and/or structurally related glycolipids, polysaccharides or glycoproteins. In each of these variants, there is an absence or severe deficiency of specific lysosomal hydrolytic enzymes involved in the catabolism of the stored product. All five variants are transmitted as autosomal recessive traits. A survey of these syndromes is provided in Table 8–2 (O'Brien,

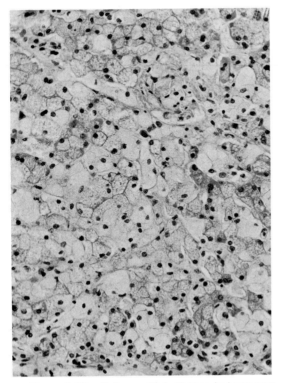

Figure 8–29. *Neimann-Pick disease in bone marrow. The marrow space is virtually filled with fairly regular lipophages.*

TABLE 8–2. GANGLIOSIDE-STORAGE DISEASES *

Common Name	Year Discovered	Chemical Classification	Ganglioside Stored in Brain	Age at Onset	Age at Death (Year)	Enzyme Defect	Carrier Detection	Prenatal Diagnosis	Organ Involvement
Tay-Sachs disease	1881	GM_2-gangliosidosis, type 1	ganglioside GM_2 (100–300 times normal value)	3–6 mo	2–4	nearly absent hexosaminidase A	reliably established (serum)	reliably established	Central and autonomic nervous systems
Sandhoff's disease	1968	GM_2-gangliosidosis, type 2	ganglioside GM_2 (100–300 times normal value)	3–6 mo	2–4	nearly absent hexosaminidase A & B	possible (leukocytes)	possible	Central and autonomic nervous systems; occasionally viscera
Juvenile GM_2-gangliosidosis	1968	GM_2-gangliosidosis, type 3	ganglioside GM_2 (40–90 times normal value)	2–6 yr	5–15	partial deficiency of hexosaminidase A	reliably established (serum or skin)	possible	Central and autonomic nervous systems
Generalized gangliosidosis	1965	GM_1-gangliosidosis, type 1	ganglioside GM_1 (10 times normal value)	At birth	½–2	nearly absent β-galactosidase A, B & C	reliably established (skin or leukocytes)	possible	Systemic; including brain, liver, spleen and bone marrow
Juvenile GM_1-gangliosidosis	1968	GM_1-gangliosidosis, type 2	ganglioside GM_1 (10 times normal value)	½–2 yr	3–10	nearly absent β-galactosidase B & C	reliably established (skin or leukocytes)	possible	Central and autonomic nervous systems; reticuloendothelial cells

*All five disorders are transmitted as autosomal recessive traits with a 25 per cent risk for recurrence in families who have had one or more affected children.

Adapted from O'Brien, J. S.: Ganglioside storage disease. New Eng. J. Med., 284:893, 1971.

1971). It is evident from Table 8–2 that each of the variants involves a specific ganglioside and a specific enzyme defect. It is also evident that the brain is prominently involved in all, leading to death usually during early childhood.

Tay-Sachs (TS) disease is the most common form of these quite rare disorders. It is more prevalent among those of Eastern European Jewish stock in contrast to the other variants which do not appear to have an ethnic predilection (Schneck et al., 1969). These tragically affected infants give evidence of mental and motor deterioration by six to nine months of life in the form of progressive loss of muscle strength and exaggerated "startle reaction," motor incoordination and general mental obtundation. Deafness and blindness soon follow, accounting for the descriptive clinical designation of *amaurotic (having blindness) familial idiocy.* The best known clinical feature of TS disease is the appearance of a cherry red spot in the macula resulting from swelling and degeneration of the retinal ganglion cells with masking of the underlying vascular choroid.

The clinical manifestations of this disorder stem from the progressive destruction of neurons throughout the body secondary to their ever-increasing burden of gangliosides. Small cytoplasmic vacuoles become evident within the cytoplasm of the ganglion cells, leading to complete cytoplasmic clearing in massively distended cells (Fig. 8–30). Histochemical stains disclose that the accumulated storage products yield a positive periodic acid-Schiff reaction but are only weakly positive with routine fat stains such as Sudan III or IV. The nuclei of the ganglion cells are often displaced to the periphery and undergo all levels of regressive alteration to complete pyknosis and disappearance. Most striking, however is the development of whorled membranous cytoplasmic inclusions made up of onion skin layers of membranes (Terry and Weiss, 1963). Similar aggregates of concentric membranes are found sometimes in the axis cylinders and the ballooned-out dendrites of affected neurons. It should be cautioned that such inclusions have been encountered in rare cases of other forms of lipid-storage disease. As a consequence of the diffuse neuronal lipidosis, these infants develop marked enlargement of the brain (up to 50 per cent greater than normal) and expansion of the skull producing striking macrocephaly. Other organs are not affected in TS disease.

The other forms of ganglioside-storage disease are too rare to merit description, but it should be pointed out that the generalized variants bear more than a passing resemblance to NP disease and, for definitive diagnosis, biochemical characterization of the stored lipid and enzyme defect may be necessary. Because

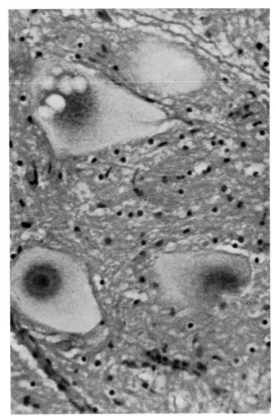

Figure 8–30. *Ganglion cells in amaurotic familial idiocy. The large neuron at the top has obvious lipid vacuolation with karyolysis and granularity of the nucleus.*

all of the ganglioside-storage diseases are invariably fatal, great efforts have been made to detect affected heterozygous parents. Assay of serum, leukocytes or skin biopsies has revealed a partial deficiency of hexosaminidase A in carriers of the Tay-Sachs trait. Prenatal diagnosis has been successfully established in many instances by amniocentesis permitting therapeutic abortion. But more importantly, carrier parents have been reassured that their unborn child was unaffected. Women who have previously borne a child with the disease have a 25 per cent risk of bearing another affected infant. But conversely, 75 per cent of pregnancies are free of this tragic metabolic genetic error (O'Brien, 1971).

WOLMAN'S DISEASE

This rare inborn error of lipid metabolism is also known as "primary familial xanthomatosis with calcified adrenals." It appears to result from a deficiency of a lysosomal lipase leading to the accumulation of cholesterol esters and triglycerides in many organs, particularly the liver. (Patrick and Lake, 1969). The hepatocytes become enlarged and vacuolated as do the Kupffer cells, and often in the portal areas, there are collections of macrophages and cholesterol-like crystals. Further details are available in the report of Crocker et al. (1965).

FABRY'S DISEASE

Fabry's disease is also known by the imposing appellation—angiokeratoma corporis diffusum universale. The angiokeratoma comprises a dermal cavernous hemangioma (p. 629) with overlying hyperkeratotic thickening of the epidermis. They present clinically as red blue, slightly elevated nodules rarely over 1 cm. in diameter. Underlying this disorder is a genetic error in the metabolism of the glycolipid ceramide trihexoside, resulting in its systemic accumulation in endothelial, perithelial and smooth muscle cells of blood vessels; in ganglion cells; in perineurial cells of the autonomic nervous system; in reticuloendothelial, myocardial and connective tissue cells; in epithelial cells of the cornea; and most dramatically in the kidney glomeruli and tubules. This rare disease is transmitted on the X chromosome and may be incompletely recessive. The storage product creates a foaminess to the affected cells which, on higher resolution, can be resolved as lamellated whorls reminiscent of myelin figures (Bagdade et al., 1968). In adolescence and young adult life, skin lesions

(angiokeratomas) and central nervous system symptoms dominate the presentation of this disease, but most patients die in middle life of progressive renal failure due to the kidney involvement. The recent evidence suggests that the metabolic block is due to an absence of a catabolic enzyme ceramide trihexosidase (Krivit, 1970).

MUCOPOLYSACCHARIDOSES (MPS)

There are several phenotypically distinct syndromes characterized by defects in the catabolism of mucopolysaccharides resulting in their accumulation in storage cells throughout the body. All are genetic disorders, and all presumably have a specific catabolic enzyme deficiency although the precise enzyme lack has not been identified in most. The two major (albeit rare) forms of the MPS are Hurler's syndrome (autosomal recessive) and Hunter's syndrome (X-linked). These and some closely related variants are briefly characterized in Table 8–3.

Hurler's syndrome is more descriptively known as "gargoylism" for reasons that will soon become clear. A deficiency of a lysosomal alpha-L-iduronidase has been identified in these patients, which presumably blocks the catabolism of mucopolysaccharides, leading to their accumulation in cells throughout the

TABLE 8–3. THE GENETIC MUCOPOLYSACCHARIDOSES*

Designation		Clinical Features	Genetics	Excessive Urinary MPS	Substance Deficient
MPS I H	Hurler syndrome	Early clouding of cornea, grave manifestations, death usually before age 10	Homozygous for MPS I H gene	Dermatan sulfate Heparan sulfate	α-L-iduronidase (formerly called Hurler corrective factor)
MPS I S	Scheie syndrome	Stiff joints, cloudy cornea, aortic regurgitation, normal intelligence, ?normal life-span	Homozygosity for MPS I S gene	Dermatan sulfate Heparan sulfate	α-L-iduronidase
MPS I H/S	Hurler-Scheie compound	Phenotype intermediate between Hurler and Scheie	Genetic compound of MPS I H and I S genes	Dermatan sulfate Heparan sulfate	α-L-iduronidase
MPS II A	Hunter syndrome, severe	No clouding of cornea, milder course than in MPS I H but death usually before age 15 years	Hemizygous for X-linked gene	Dermatan sulfate Heparan sulfate	Hunter corrective factor
MPS II B	Hunter syndrome, mild	Survival to 30's to 50's, fair intelligence	Hemizygous for X-linked allele for mild form	Dermatan sulfate Heparan sulfate	Hunter corrective factor
MPS III A	Sanfilippo syndrome A	Identical phenotype: Mild somatic, severe central nervous system effects	Homozygous for Sanfilippo A gene	Heparan sulfate	Heparan sulfate sulfatase
MPS III B	Sanfilippo syndrome B		Homozygous for Sanfilippo B (at different locus)	Heparan sulfate	N-acetyl-α-D-glucosaminidase
MPS IV	Morquio syndrome (probably more than one allelic form)	Severe bone changes of distinctive type, cloudy cornea, aortic regurgitation	Homozygous for Morquio gene	Keratan sulfate	Unknown

*Adapted from McKusick, V. A.: Heritable Disorders of Connective Tissue. 4th ed. St. Louis, C. V. Mosby Co., 1972, p. 525.

body, principally those of the RE system (Mac-Brinn et al., 1969). The spleen, liver, lymph nodes and bone marrow are principally affected but, in addition, endothelial cells and fibroblasts throughout the body are also involved. Excessive cerebral storage of gangliosides is also encountered in some patients, accounting for the progressive mental deterioration. The stored mucopolysaccharides apparently spill out of the intracellular compartment to appear in the blood and are excreted in excessive amounts in the urine. During blood transport, these macromolecules are picked up by subintimal histiocytes in blood vessels to produce subendothelial plaques which may, when the coronary arteries are affected, lead to myocardial ischemia and myocardial infarction or heart failure. The cardiac valves may be similarly affected and deformed. Massive distention of phagocytic cells with mucopolysaccharides in the liver and spleen cause enlargement of both organs. The accumulations of these storage cells in the bone marrow lead to a variety of skeletal deformities, particularly enlargement of the skull, widening and lengthening of the bones of the limbs, distortion of the small bones of the hands and feet, and deformities of the first or second lumbar vertebrae. In all sites affected, the storage cells are monstrously distended and vacuolated by PAS-positive mucopolysaccharides. Higher resolution discloses the vacuoles to be massively distended lysosomes (Lagunoff and Gritzka, 1966).

Coarsening of the facial features, enlargement of the head and an ape-like body habitus transform these unfortunates into likenesses of the storied gargoyles. Deafness, corneal clouding and mental deterioration (resulting from the accumulation of gangliosides within neurons) further plague their lives. These clinical manifestations usually become evident within the first years of life and are followed by death, as a rule within the first decade, due to cardiorespiratory complications.

Hunter's syndrome is essentially a milder variant of Hurler's syndrome. Although it is inherited as a sex-linked recessive, the same mucopolysaccharides appear to be stored. Involvement of the eyes does not occur, nor do these patients develop the gibbus habitus and mental deterioration so characteristic of Hurler's syndrome (Gerich, 1969).

Here, as in the other storage diseases, biochemical analyses must be used to identify the precise storage product. The clinical diagnosis is often supported by the observation of metachromatic granules (Reilly bodies) in white cells of the blood or bone marrow.

Nowhere in the field of medicine is the fragility of health and its exquisite dependence on a normal genetic inheritance more graphically displayed than in these storage diseases, where a single gene mutation, not visible in the karyotype, leads to lack of a single enzyme and tragic fatal disease. Recently a ray of hope has been raised. Reasoning that the storage product in the mucopolysaccharidoses is normal and only accumulates because of blocks in its utilization, several attempts have been made to supply the needed enzyme(s). The administration of purified enzymes, normal plasma and leukocytes possessing a normal enzyme complement has been tried. Some benefit has been obtained, but the problem becomes one of long-term provision of adequate amounts of enzyme. However, the goal should be attainable and, hopefully, one day these storage diseases will become as controllable as diabetes mellitus (Knudson et al., 1971) (Di Ferrante et al., 1971).

HAND-SCHÜLLER-CHRISTIAN DISEASE (HISTIOCYTOSIS X)

Three overlapping yet somewhat distinctive syndromes are included under the designation of HSC *disease*: Letterer-Siwe (LS) *syndrome,* Hand-Schüller-Christian (HSC) *syndrome* and eosinophilic *granuloma.* All are of unknown etiology, and all are characterized by abnormal proliferation, sometimes tumorous, of histiocytes which contain varying amounts of lipids, principally cholesterol. Thus the generic designation *histiocytosis X.*

LS is a highly fatal, rapidly progressive disease usually affecting infants, characterized by widespread lymphoma-like proliferation of histiocytes throughout the body which usually contain little lipid, hence its other designation *nonlipid reticuloendotheliosis.* Rarely, it occurs in adults. It principally affects the skin and the reticuloendothelial organs (including bones). The HSC syndrome also affects infants and occasionally adults. It is systemic in distribution, involving mainly the skull bones but in addition the skin, liver, lungs and spleen. Somewhat more chronic in its course, it allows more than half of the patients to survive for 10 to 15 years; and they are often cured with appropriate therapy. Eosinophilic granuloma generally presents as a benign unifocal destructive lesion in bone (favored sites: skull and facial bones, ribs and femurs) but sometimes it presents as a multifocal involvement of bone. Patients with unifocal lesions have an invariable excellent prognosis. While the outlook for those with multiple lesions is somewhat more guarded, few deaths occur in this group.

Whether all three syndromes of HSC disease comprise a spectrum of clinical presentations of a single nosologic entity is a moot issue. The clinical and morphologic overlaps among the three and the occasional cases which appear to begin as one pattern and then become transformed into another provide the major justifications of the unitarian view (Green and Farber, 1942). On the other hand, many, including Siwe himself, contend that the abnormal proliferation of histiocytes represents only an inflammatory response to an infectious agent or possibly a neoplastic disorder akin to a leukemia or lymphoma. They point out that some cases are quite benign while others pursue a fulminant, fatal course, raising the strong possibility that many discrete entities have been lumped together unjustifiably because of attenuated clinical and morphologic similarities (Siwe, 1949) (Lieberman, 1969). Recognizing the controversy, these three syndromes will be presented as variations of a single theme since they have many similarities (Dennis and Rosahn, 1951) (Nyholm, 1971).

Although the cause of these entities is unknown, there are many features pointing to an infectious etiology. The histiocytic proliferation could represent an inflammatory response to some exogenous agent. Age of the patient has some influence on the severity and distribution of the lesions. The LS variant tends to occur in the youngest group and, in fact, may be present almost from birth. The lesions are usually widespread throughout the osseous and visceral systems. Presumably in this age range, there would be little immunity yet acquired to exogenous agents. With advancing years, more benign variants are encountered until the unifocal, rarely fatal eosinophilic granuloma is reached, usually occurring in young adults. As its name implies, the granuloma has many histologic resemblances to an infectious lesion and is replete with inflammatory cells, particularly eosinophils and lipid-laden histiocytes. The significance of this lipid in these entities is obscure. It is generally believed to result from the imbibition of lipid-rich debris derived from neighboring necrotic cells; but increased intracellular synthesis has not been ruled out. These patients are normocholesterolemic, and so clearly accumulation of lipids does not represent a storage disease. With this overview, we can turn to the individual syndromes.

Letterer-Siwe Syndrome (Nonlipid Reticuloendotheliosis). This is the *skin, visceral and widespread osseous variant most often encountered in infants one year of age or under. It is infrequently encountered in older children, and only rare cases have been reported in adults.* Both sexes are affected equally. The clinical course is usually rapidly fatal, particularly in infancy, but survivals of up to 15 years have been recorded in older children.

Anatomically these patients present a rather typical syndrome. The infants usually develop a single or a few firm red to brown skin nodules often thought to be insect bites. Very soon there follows a rather severe generalized cutaneous involvement in the form of a maculopapular rash or multiple discrete nodules often with ulceration, scaling and hemorrhages. Generalized lymphadenopathy is almost invariably present at this time. Usually at the time when the disease is first recognized bone lesions are absent, but in most cases these appear in the course of months. Splenomegaly, hepatomegaly and low-grade fever are frequent. Anemia, leukopenia and thrombocytopenia almost always are present, the last-mentioned derangement accounting for a hemorrhagic diathesis. The dominant histologic change is that of a pure histiocytic proliferation throughout the reticuloendothelial sites of the body, i.e., the skin, spleen, liver, lymph nodes and, later, bones. The lungs, kidneys and virtually any other organ are sometimes affected. Usually these histiocytes contain no lipid, and usually there is little eosinophilic or lymphocytic infiltration. However, all these features may be present in the individual case—not often in the infant, more often in older patients with the disease of longer duration.

Hand-Schüller-Christian Syndrome. This is a *more chronic disorder than that just presented, with multiple system, soft tissue and bone involvements. It may arise in infancy but also affects adults.* It generally runs a more prolonged course. In the 40 cases reported by Oberman (1961) about half the patients were living, some well, some with persistent disease, for 10 to 15 years after the diagnosis was first made.

Said to be characteristic of this variant is the occurrence of bony lesions in the skull and orbit, providing **the triad of diabetes insipidus, exophthalmos and radiolucent bone defects principally in the skull.** In actual fact the classic triad is rarely present. The diabetes insipidus and exophthalmos occur in only about half the cases, and even the bone lesions are absent from 20 per cent of the cases. The bony defects are produced by local accumulations of lipid-laden histiocytes, while the exophthalmos and diabetes insipidus are caused by aggregations of the same tissue in the base of the skull and orbit expanding beyond the bone and causing pressure on the brain and retro-orbital tissues (Fig. 8–31). In addition to these sites, the skin, liver, spleen, lymph nodes and lungs are also involved, recalling the changes of Letterer-Siwe disease. New foci may appear from time to time in the progressive case, creating changing symptomatology.

The clinical course of Hand-Schüller-Christian syndrome is difficult to predict. In general, the younger the age of onset the more rapid the progression, the more widespread the lesions and the poorer the prognosis. However, these generalizations may be

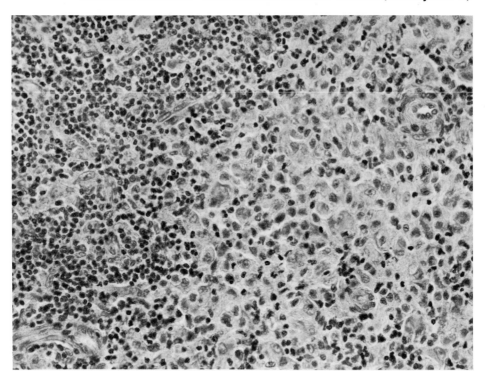

Figure 8–31. Hand-Schüller-Christian syndrome. The typical round and oval macrophages (at right) are most numerous and are interspersed with scattered lymphocytes, plasma cells and eosinophils.

wrong in the individual case, and there are reports of patients having all the clinical and anatomic manifestations of Hand-Schüller-Christian syndrome with onset at age 1 who are alive and well 20 years later.

One point is clear: it is not possible to predict the course of the disease from the histology of a lesion. It was once believed that much lipid and many eosinophils augured well, but reviews prove the fallacy of such a concept.

Eosinophilic Granuloma. This represents the most benign variant of the Hand-Schüller-Christian complex, in which the involvement at the onset is usually confined to one or several bones with no evidence of diffuse visceral involvement. The disease is encountered predominantly in older children and adults, the age ranging from the first year of life to the seventh decade, with a strong male preponderance.

The bones of the skull are often first affected, but virtually all the other bones of the skeletal system have, at one time or another, been affected. The classic radiographic appearance is of a sharply circumscribed focal area of bone destruction simulating a tumor. Soft tissues, particularly the skin, have also presented monofocal histiocytic proliferations that have been designated eosinophilic granuloma. Lymph node enlargement is sometimes reported but is not a prominent feature, and splenohepatomegaly and diffuse skin involvement are usually absent.

The prognosis in this condition is generally good and most of these patients have a long survival. Complete remission of the disease either spontaneously or with appropriate therapy is not infrequent. Occasionally, a solitary lesion characteristic of eosinophilic granuloma is found in cases of otherwise classic Hand-Schüller-Christian syndrome, supporting the proposition that the eosinophilic granuloma is merely one pattern of these histiocytic proliferations. This is well illustrated by the following case:

A 14-year-old child was brought to medical attention because of fairly severe, persistent pain in the right upper arm. On complete clinical study, an area of bone destruction 2 to 3 cm. in diameter was found in the right midshaft of the humerus, interpreted by the radiologist as either a bone cyst or an eosinophilic granuloma. The remainder of the clinical findings were negative. On surgical exposure, the soft gray-red tissue that filled the focus was removed and a diagnosis of eosinophilic granuloma was established morphologically. Following operation, the bony defect apparently filled. On follow-up roentgenograms the child appeared perfectly well. However, six years later, headaches, progressive weakness and debilitation occasioned further study, and multiple bony defects in the skull, enlargement of the liver and spleen, and anemia were found, all characteristic of Hand-Schüller-Christian disease.

Morphology. The histologic changes in each of these three entities are somewhat distinctive, but basically they are more alike than different. The common denominator is a focal or diffuse proliferation of large mononuclear histiocytes in the organs already mentioned. These cells may appear as slender spindle cells resembling fibroblasts or as large rounded mononuclear cells. The nuclei in these cells tend to be vesicular and lobulated with clearly demarcated nucleoli. These cells appear in masses and sheets in the bony lesions described, in aggregates within the skin and diffusely throughout such solid organs as the spleen, liver and lymph nodes. Multinucleated giant cells are sometimes present, presumably representing fused histiocytes. Vacuolated histiocytes containing lipid can be found in all three variants. These occur in the more protracted cases of Letterer-Siwe disease but are particularly abundant in Hand-Schüller-Christian syndrome and eosinophilic granuloma. As mentioned, acute cases of Letterer-Siwe disease may have no lipid. Eosinophils are present in all three variants. They are most prominent in the eosinophilic granuloma but are abundantly present in the Hand-Schüller-Christian variant. They are a less frequent finding in Letterer-Siwe disease. Lymphocytes and plasma cells are also characteristic of eosinophilic granuloma and Hand-Schüller-Christian syndrome and sometimes are found in scanty numbers in Let-

terer-Siwe disease (Fig. 8-32). Thus we may summarize the anatomic changes in the following manner. In Letterer-Siwe syndrome, the changes are basically a pure proliferation of histiocytes throughout many if not most of the organs of the body, usually unrelieved by other histologic features. In a few instances, however, scattered eosinophils, plasma cells, lymphocytes, multinucleate giant cells and lipid-laden foam cells are present. In the Hand-Schüller-Christian variant, the histiocytosis takes the form of masses or sheets of lipid-laden foam cells abundantly interspersed with eosinophils, lymphocytes and plasma cells. Fibrosis may occur in the periphery of these lesions, creating the appearance of a chronic inflammatory granuloma. Central necrosis may heighten this resemblance. The eosinophilic granuloma does not differ from the granuloma just described in the Hand-Schüller-Christian variant, but sheets and masses of eosinophils produce the somewhat distinctive pattern characteristic of the longstanding chronic involvement. When these lesions occur in bones, there is resorption of the underlying bone and sometimes reactive bone formation in the margins.

WEBER-CHRISTIAN DISEASE

This entity, also known as *relapsing nonsuppurative panniculitis*, is characterized principally

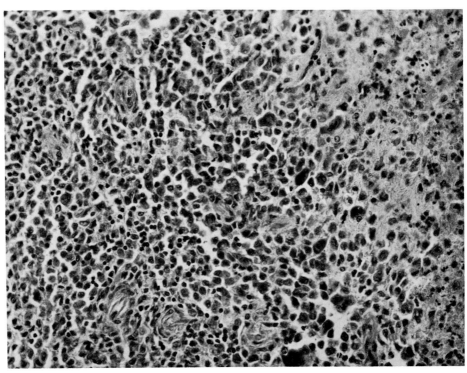

Figure 8–32. *Eosinophilic granuloma. The granulomatous pattern is made up of round to oval macrophages and long, slender fibroblasts, intermingled with occasional plasma cells, lymphocytes, giant cells and large numbers of eosinophils (at left).*

by the spontaneous occurrence of foci of non-suppurative necrosis of fat, principally in the subcutaneous fat depots. Although these lesions had been described earlier, it was Weber in 1925 who called attention to the distinctive characteristics of this disorder. In his case the focal areas of fat necrosis were limited to the subcutaneous depots of the abdomen, and for some time it was believed that the lesions were limited to this region; hence the designation nodular panniculitis. Subsequently it became evident that *deeper fat depots such as the omentum, mesentery of gut and the fat deposits about the heart, pancreas, adrenal glands and kidneys might also be affected.* In these systemic distributions the condition might indeed be fatal. Cases are also on record in which only the mesentery has been involved, and to these the designation of *"mesenteric panniculitis"* has been given. In other instances, the reticuloendothelial cells throughout the body have been loaded with fat, with resultant enlargement of the liver, spleen and peripheral nodes, sometimes followed by focal lesions in the bone.

For these reasons the condition is better considered as some curious abnormality in the homeostasis or metabolism of fat cells. Possibly the fat depots are target organs of some allergic or hypersensitivity reaction, leading to focal excessive mobilization of fat, injury to cells and widespread phagocytosis of fat in the reticuloendothelial cells of the body. If hypersensitivity were involved, then this entity would be related to the rheumatic, polyarteritis and lupus erythematosus disorders (Spagnuolo and Taranta, 1961). But to date no concurrence between these hypersensitivity disorders and Weber-Christian disease has been identified.

Histologically the focal necroses of fat pass through three stages. In the first phase there is a nonspecific acute inflammatory reaction within fat characterized by extensive infiltration of polymorphonuclear leukocytes, lymphocytes and macrophages (Fig. 8-33). Occasional lipid-laden macrophages are present at this time. At this stage of the lesion, the focal subcutaneous area is red, slightly swollen and more firm and tender. In the second, more well developed phase, there is collapse of the cell membranes of the fat cells with extensive phagocytosis of fat droplets by macrophages (Steinberg 1953). The inflammatory infiltrate is still fairly acute with numbers of leukocytes as well as accompanying lymphocytes and plasma cells. Foreign body giant cells and needle-like cholesterol spicules are sometimes present. In addition, one occasionally sees acute vasculitis with intimal proliferation in local affected vessels. At this stage, the individual lesion continues to be firm, red and painful. From this

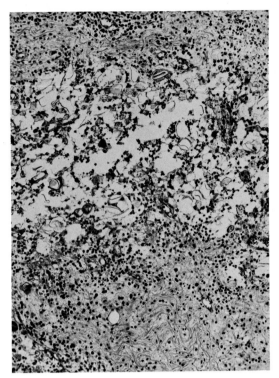

Figure 8–33. Nodular panniculitis (Weber-Christian disease). The focus of necrosis is marked by a collection of fat-laden macrophages, mononuclear leukocytes and fibroblasts. Ruptured cell membranes of necrotic fat cells are evident.

point, the third phase of the disease follows in which the inflammatory focus becomes progressively fibrotic. The acute leukocytic infiltrate subsides and is replaced by fibroblasts, mononuclears and prominent foreign body giant cells. Progressive organization leads to an area of increased induration. Fibrous scarring causes retraction of the overlying skin. In the course of time, the depressed area of skin may again become filled out as new fat cells are formed.

Clinically the acute focal involvements tend to appear in crops in the subcutaneous fat, characteristically over the abdomen and lower extremities, over an interval in time as long as several years. Even as older lesions undergo progressive fibrosis, new lesions may appear; hence the name "relapsing." When the process is fairly widespread, fever and leukocytosis may be present. The cause of death in patients having a systemic distribution is still obscure.

REFERENCES

Alvsaker, J. O.: Genetic studies in primary gout. Investigations on the plasma levels of the urate binding alpha 1-alpha 2 globulin in individuals from gouty kindreds. J. Clin. Invest., 47:1254, 1968.

Alvsaker, J. O.: Uric acid in human plasma. Isolation and identification of plasma proteins interacting with urate. Scand. J. Clin. Lab. Invest., 18:227, 1966.

Antoniades, H. N., et al.: Studies on the state of insulin in blood, "free" insulin and insulin complexes in human sera and their in vitro biologic properties. Endocrinology, 69:46, 1961.

Antoniades, H. N., et al.: Studies on the state, transport and regulation of insulin in human blood. Diabetes, 11:261, 1962.

Bagdade, J. D., et al.: Fabry's disease: a correlative clinical, morphologic and biochemical study. Lab. Invest., 18:681, 1968.

Barlow, K. A.: Lipid metabolism in gout. Proc. Roy. Soc. Med., 59:325, 1966.

Beadle, G. W., and Tatum, E. L.: Genetic control of biochemical reactions in neurospora. Proc. Nat. Acad. Sci., 2:499, 1941.

Bell, E. T.: Renal vascular disease in diabetes mellitus. Diabetes, 2:376, 1953.

Beutler, E., and Kuhl, W.: The diagnosis of the adult type of Gaucher's disease and its carrier state by demonstration of deficiency of beta-glucosidase activity in peripheral blood leukocytes. J. Lab. Clin. Med., 76:747, 1970.

Bladen, H. A., et al.: The ultrastructure of human amyloid as revealed by the negative staining technique. J. Ultrastruct. Res., 14:226, 1966.

Bloodworth, J. M. B., Jr.: Diabetes mellitus, extrapancreatic pathology. In Bloodworth, J. M. B., Jr. (ed.): Endocrine Pathology. Baltimore, Williams and Wilkins Co., 1968, p. 330.

Bloodworth, J. M. B., Jr.: Diabetic microangiopathy. Diabetes, 12:99, 1963.

Blum, A., and Sohar, E.: Diagnosis of amyloidosis: ancillary procedures. Lancet, 1:721, 1962.

Blumenthal, H. T.: The relation of microangiopathies to arteriosclerosis, with special reference to diabetes. Ann. N.Y. Acad. Sci., 149:834, 1968.

Boender, C. A., and Verloop, M. C.: Iron absorption, iron loss and iron retention in man. Studies after oral administration of a tracer dose of $^{59}FeSO_4$ and $^{131}BaSO_4$. Brit. J. Haemat., 17:45, 1969.

Boender, C. A., et al.: Iron absorption and retention in man. Nature (London), 213:1237, 1967.

Bonar, L., et al.: Characterization of the amyloid fibril as a cross-B protein. Proc. Soc. Exp. Biol. Med., 131:1373, 1969.

Bothwell, T. H., and Finch, C. A.: The intestine in iron metabolism. Amer. J. Dig. Dis., 2:145, 1957.

Brady, R. O., et al.: Demonstration of a deficiency of glucocerebroside-cleaving enzyme in Gaucher's disease. J. Clin. Invest., 45:1, 112, 1966.

Brandt, K., et al.: A clinical analysis of the course and prognosis of forty-two patients with amyloidosis. Amer. J. Med., 44:955, 1968.

Briggs, G. W.: Amyloidosis. Ann. Intern. Med., 55:943, 1961.

Brown, D. I., and Brown, D. H.: Glycogen storage diseases: type I, III, IV, V, VII and unclassified glycogenoses. In Dickens, F., Randle, P. J., and Whelan, W. J. (eds.): Carbohydrate Metabolism and Its Disorders, II. New York, Academic Press, 1968, p. 123.

Brown, J., et al.: Diabetes mellitus: current concepts and vascular lesions (renal and retinal). Ann. Intern. Med., 68:634, 1968.

Bunim, J. J., et al.: Biochemical abnormalities in hereditary diseases. Ann. Intern. Med., 57:472, 1962.

Calkins, E., and Cohen, A. S.: Diagnosis of amyloidosis. Bull. Rheum. Dis., 10:215, 1960.

Cathcart, E. S., et al.: Amyloidosis: an expression of immunological tolerance? Lancet, 2:639, 1970.

Cathcart, E. S., et al.: Immunogenicity of amyloid. Immunology, 20:945, 1971.

Cathcart, E. S., et al.: Immunoglobulins and amyloidosis. An immunologic study of 62 patients with biopsy proved disease. Amer. J. Med., 52:93, 1972.

Charlton, R. W., and Bothwell, T. H.: Hemochromatosis: dietary and genetic aspects. In Brown, E. B., and Moore, C. V. (eds.): Progress in Hematology. New York, Grune and Stratton, 1966, p. 298.

Chazan, B. I., et al.: 25 to 45 years of diabetes with and without vascular complications. Diabetologia, 6:565, 1970.

Chiumello, G., et al.: Effects of glucagon and tolbutamide on plasma insulin levels in children with ketoacidosis. Diabetes, 17:133, 1968.

Chung, E. B.: Histologic changes in gout. Georgetown Med. Bull., 15:269, 1962.

Clarke, B. F.: The pathogenesis of diabetes mellitus. Scot. Med. J., 15:339, 1970.

Clerici, E., et al.: Experimental amyloidosis in immunity. Path. Microbiol., 28:806, 1965.

Cogan, D. G.: Current concepts in diabetic retinopathy. New Eng. J. Med., 270:787, 1964.

Cogan, D. G., et al.: Retinal vascular patterns. IV. Diabetic retinopathy. Arch. Ophthal., 66:366, 1961.

Cohen, A. S.: Amyloidosis. New Eng. J. Med., 277:522, 574, 628, 1967.

Cohen, A. S., and Calkins, E.: Electron microscopic observations on a fibrous component in amyloid of diverse origins. Nature (London), 183:1202, 1959.

Cohen, A. S., et al.: The constitution and genesis of amyloid. Int. Rev. Exp. Path., 4:159, 1965a.

Cohen, A. S., et al.: Light and electron microscopic autoradiographic demonstration of local amyloid formation in spleen explants. Amer. J. Path., 47:1079, 1965b.

Colby, A. O.: Neurologic disorders of diabetes mellitus. Diabetes, 14:424, 1965.

Colwell, J. A.: Effective diabetic control of retinopathy. Diabetes, 15:497, 1966.

Conn, J. W.: Expanding concepts of diabetes mellitus. Mod. Med., 32:130, 1964.

Creutzfeldt, W., et al.: Effect of gastrointestinal hormones on insulin and glucagon secretion. New Eng. J. Med., 282:1139, 1970.

Crichton, R. R.: Ferritin: structure, synthesis and function. New Eng. J. Med., 284:1413, 1971.

Crocker, A. C., et al.: Wolman's disease: three new patients with a recently described lipidosis. Pediatrics, 35:627, 1965.

Crosby, W. H.: Heredity of hemochromatosis. In Ingelfinger, F. J., Relman, A., and Finland, M. (eds.): Controversy in Internal Medicine. Philadelphia, W. B. Saunders Co., 1966, p. 261.

Danowski, T. S.: Diabetes Mellitus: Diagnosis and Treatment. New York, American Diabetes Association, 1964.

Davidson, M. B., and Goodner, C. J.: Failure of synalbumin to exhibit insulin antagonism in vivo. Diabetes, 16:386, 1967.

Davis, P. S., et al.: Reduction of gastric iron-binding protein in haemochromatosis. Lancet, 2:1431, 1966.

DeLellis, R. A., et al.: Amyloid IX. Further kinetic studies on experimental murine amyloidosis. Int. Arch. Allerg., 37:175, 1970.

Dennis, J. W., and Rosahn, P. D.: Primary reticulo-endothelial granulomas with report of a typical case of Letterer-Siwe disease. Amer. J. Path., 27:627, 1951.

Di Ferrante, N., et al.: Induced degradation of glycosaminoglycans in Hurler's and Hunter's syndromes by plasma infusion. Proc. Nat. Acad. Sci., 68:303, 1971.

Editorial: Diabetes and hypertension. J.A.M.A., 202:358, 1967.

Eliot, R. S., et al.: Cardiac amyloidosis. Circulation, 23:613, 1961.

Ellenberg, M.: Diabetic complications without manifest diabetes. J.A.M.A., 183:926, 1963.

Elliot, R. B., et al.: An abnormal insulin in juvenile diabetes mellitus. Diabetes, 14:780, 1965.

Entmacher, P. S., et al.: Longevity of diabetic patients in recent years. Diabetes, 13:373, 1964.

Fajans, S. S., and Conn, J. W.: Early recognition of diabetes mellitus. Ann. N.Y. Acad. Sci., 82:208, 1959.

Fajans, S. S., et al.: The course of asymptomatic diabetes in young people as determined by levels of blood glucose and plasma insulin. Trans. Ass. Amer. Physicians, 82:211, 1969.

Floyd, J. C., et al.: Stimulation of insulin secretion by amino acids. J. Clin. Invest., 45:1487, 1966.

Frederickson, D. S.: Sphingomyelin lipidosis: Niemann-Pick disease. In Stanbury, J., Wyngaarden, J., and Frederickson, D. S. (eds.): The Metabolic Basis of Inherited Disease. New York, McGraw-Hill Book Co., 1966, p. 586.

Freedman, P., et al.: Phaeochromocytoma, diabetes and glycosuria. Quart. J. Med., 27:307, 1958.

Friedenwald, J. S.: Diabetic retinopathy. Amer. J. Ophthal., 33:1187, 1950.

Gellman, D. D., et al.: Diabetic nephropathy: a clinical and pathologic study based on renal biopsies. Medicine, 38:321, 1959.

Gerich, J. E.: Hunter's syndrome. Beta galactosidase deficiency in skin. New Eng. J. Med., 280:799, 1969.

Glenner, G. G.: Amyloid fibril proteins: proof of homology with immunoglobulin-like chains by sequence analyses. Science, *172*:1150, 1971.

Goldberg, L., and Smith, J. P.: Iron overloading and hepatic vulnerability. Amer. J. Path., *36*:125, 1960.

Goldenberg, S., et al.: Sequelae of arteriosclerosis of the aorta and coronary arteries. A statistical study in diabetes mellitus. Diabetes, *7*:98, 1958.

Goldsmith, S. J., et al.: Significance of human plasma insulin sephadex fractions. Diabetes, *18*:834, 1969.

Gonick, H. C., et al.: The renal lesion in gout. Ann. Intern. Med., *62*:667, 1965.

Grahame, R., and Scott, J. T.: Clinical survey of 354 patients with gout. Ann. Rheum. Dis., *29*:461, 1970.

Granick, S.: Iron metabolism and hemochromatosis. Bull. N.Y. Acad. Med., *25*:403, 1949.

Green, W. T., and Farber, S.: Eosinophilic or solitary granuloma of bone. J. Bone Joint Surg., *24*:499, 1942.

Grodsky, G. M., et al.: Diabetes mellitus in rabbits immunized with insulin. Diabetes, *15*:579, 1966.

Groen, J. J.: Gaucher's disease: hereditary transmission and racial distribution. Arch. Intern. Med., *113*:543, 1964.

Hales, C. N., and Randle, P. J.: Effects of low carbohydrate diet and diabetes mellitus on plasma concentrations of glucose, non-esterified fatty acid and insulin during oral glucose-tolerance tests. Lancet, *1*:790, 1963.

Hardin, R. C., et al.: Development of diabetic retinopathy: effects of duration and control of diabetes. Diabetes, *5*:397, 1956.

Hardt, F.: Transfer amyloidosis: I. Studies on the transfer of various lymphoid cells from amyloidotic mice to syngeneic nonamyloidotic recipients. II. Induction of amyloidosis in mice with spleen, thymus and lymph node tissue from casein-sensitized syngeneic donors. Amer. J. Path., *65*:411, 1971.

Haughe, M., and Harvald, B.: Heredity in gout and hyperuricemia. Acta Med. Scand., *152*:247, 1955.

Heller, H., et al.: Amyloidosis in familial Mediterranean fever: Independent genetically determined character. Arch. Intern. Med., *107*:539, 1961.

Henderson, J. F., et al.: Variations in purine metabolism of cultured skin fibroblasts from patients with gout. J. Clin. Invest., *47*:1511, 1968.

Herman, M. V., and Gorlin, R.: Premature coronary artery disease and preclinical diabetic state. Amer. J. Med., *38*:481, 1965.

Hers, H. G.: Inborn lysosomal diseases. Gastroenterology, *48*:625, 1965.

Hibbs, R. G., et al.: Biochemical and electronmicroscopic study of Gaucher's cells. Arch. Path., *89*:137, 1970.

Hirschhorn, K., et al.: Pompe's disease: detection of heterozygotes by lymphocyte stimulation. Science, *166*:1632, 1969.

Hirschl, S.: Electron microscopic analysis of human amyloid. J. Ultrastruct. Res., *29*:281, 1969.

Hsia, D. Y.: The diagnosis and management of the glycogen storage diseases. Amer. J. Clin. Path., *50*:44, 1968.

Hsia, D. Y., et al.: Gaucher's disease: report of 2 cases in father and son and review of the literature. New Eng. J. Med., *261*:164, 1959.

Hug, G., et al.: Glycogen storage disease: types II, III, VIII and IX. Amer. J. Dis. Child., *111*:457, 1966.

Ivemark, B. I., et al.: Niemann-Pick disease in infancy: report of two siblings with clinical, histologic and chemical studies. Acta Pediat., *52*:391, 1963.

Jacobs, P., et al.: The influence of gastric factors on the absorption of iron salts. S. Afr. J. Med. Sci., *33*:53, 1968.

Jacobs, P., et al.: Intestinal iron transport: studies using a loop of gut with an artificial circulation. Amer. J. Physiol., *210*:694, 1966.

Jarrett, R. J., et al.: Proteins and insulin release: a dual role of amino acids and intestinal hormones. Brit. Med. J., *4*:598, 1969.

Josimovich, J. B., and MacLaren, J. A.: Presence in the human placenta and term serum of a highly lactogenic substance immunologically related to pituitary growth hormone. Endocrinology, *71*:209, 1962.

Kagan, A., et al.: The coronary profile: heart disease epidemiology study. Framingham, Mass. Ann. N.Y. Acad. Sci., *97*:883, 1963.

Kandhari, K. C., et al.: Investigations into the causation of increased susceptibility of diabetics to cutaneous infections. Indian J. Med. Res., *57*:1295, 1969.

Kass, E. H.: Bacteriuria and the pathogenesis of pyelonephritis. Lab. Invest., *9*:110, 1960.

Katsoyannis, P. G.: The synthesis of the insulin chains and their combination to biologically active material. Diabetes, *13*:339, 1964.

Keiding, N. R., et al.: Importance of control of diabetes in prevention of vascular complications. J.A.M.A., *150*:964, 1952.

Kelley, W. N.: Recent progress in the pathogenesis and treatment of gout. Med. Times, *97*:230, 1969.

Kelley, W. N., et al.: A specific enzyme defect in gout associated with overproduction of uric acid. Proc. Nat. Acad. Sci., *57*:1735, 1967.

Kessler, I. I.: Mortality experience of diabetic patients. A 26 year follow up study. Amer. J. Med., *51*:715, 1971.

Kimball, K. G.: Amyloidosis in association with neoplastic disease: report of unusual case and clinico-pathologic experience at Memorial Center for Cancer and Allied Diseases during 11 years (1948–1958). Ann. Intern. Med., *55*:958, 1961.

Kimmelstiel, P., and Wilson, C.: Intercapillary lesions in the glomeruli of the kidney. Amer. J. Path., *12*:83, 1936.

Kimmelstiel, P., et al.: Glomerular basement membrane in diabetics. Amer. J. Clin. Path., *45*:21, 1966.

Kipnis, D. M.: Insulin secretion in normal and diabetic individuals. Advances Intern. Med., *16*:103, 1970.

Knowles, H. C., Jr., et al.: The course of juvenile diabetes treated with unmeasured diet. Diabetes, *14*:239, 1965.

Knudson, A. G., Jr., et al.: Effect of leucocyte transfusion in a child with type II mucopolysaccharidosis. Proc. Nat. Acad. Sci., *68*:1738, 1971.

Krivit, W.: Recent advances in Fabry's disease. Trans. Ass. Amer. Physicians, *83*:121, 1970.

Lacy, P. E.: The islets of Langerhans. In Bloodworth, J. M. B., Jr. (ed.): Endocrine Pathology. Baltimore, Williams & Wilkins Co., 1968, p. 316.

Lacy, P. E.: Pancreatic beta cell. In Ciba Foundation Colloquia on Endocrinology, Volume 15. Aetiology of Diabetes Mellitus and Its Complications. Boston, Little, Brown and Co., 1964.

Lacy, P. E., and Hartroft, W. S.: Electron microscopy of the islets of Langerhans. Ann. N.Y. Acad. Sci., *82*:287, 1959.

Lagunoff, D., and Gritzka, T. L.: The site of mucopolysaccharide accumulation in Hurler's syndrome. An electron microscopic and histochemical study. Lab. Invest., *15*:1578, 1966.

Larsson, O.: Studies of small vessels in patients with diabetes. Acta Med. Scand., Suppl. *480*:5, 1967.

Larsson, Y., et al.: Longterm prognosis in juvenile diabetes mellitus. Acta Paediat., Suppl. 130, *51*:1, 1962.

Lawrence, A. M.: Glucagon. Ann. Rev. Med., *20*:207, 1969.

Lesch, M., and Nyhan, W. L.: A familial disorder of uric acid metabolism and central nervous system function. Amer. J. Med., *36*:561, 1964.

Levine, R.: Insulin: the biography of a small protein. New Eng. J. Med., *277*:1059, 1967.

Lieberman, P. H.: A reappraisal of eosinophilic granuloma of bone. Hand-Schüller-Christian syndrome and Letterer-Siwe syndrome. Medicine, *48*:375, 1969.

Liebow, I. M., and Hellerstein, H. K.: Cardiac complications of diabetes mellitus. Amer. J. Med., *7*:660, 1949.

Lindeman, R. D., et al.: Renal amyloidosis. Ann. Intern. Med., *54*:883, 1961.

Lindsay, S.: Heart in primary systemic amyloidosis. Amer. Heart J., *32*:419, 1946.

Lister, J.: The clinical spectrum of juvenile diabetes. Lancet, *1*:386, 1966.

Luft, R.: Some considerations on the pathogenesis of diabetes mellitus. New Eng. J. Med., *279*:1086, 1968.

Luft, R., et al.: Studies in the pathogenesis of diabetes in acromegaly. Acta Endocrin., *56*:593, 1967.

Lukens, F. D. W.: Diabetes mellitus: 1967. Perspect. Biol. Med., *11*:136, 1967.

Lynn, R., and Terry, R. D.: Lipid histochemistry and electron microscopy in adults: Niemann-Pick disease. Amer. J. Med., *37*:987, 1964.

MacBrinn, M., et al.: Beta galactosidase deficiency in the Hurler's syndrome. New Eng. J. Med., *281*:338, 1969.

MacDonald, R. A.: Hemochromatosis: a perlustration. Amer. J. Clin. Nut., *23*:592, 1970.

MacDonald, R. A.: Idiopathic hemochromatosis: a variant of portal cirrhosis and idiopathic hemosiderosis. Arch. Intern. Med., *107*:606, 1961.

MacDonald, R. A.: Idiopathic hemochromatosis: genetic or acquired? Arch. Intern. Med., *112*:184, 1963.

MacDonald, R. A., and Mallory, G. K.: Hemochromatosis and hemosiderosis: autopsy study of 211 cases. Arch Intern. Med., *105*:686, 1960.

MacDonald, R. A., et al.: Studies of experimental hemochromatosis. Disorder of the reticuloendothelial system and excess iron. Arch. Path., *85*:366, 1968.

Madison, L.: Role of insulin in the hepatic handling of glucose. Arch. Intern. Med., *123*:284, 1969.

Mahler, R. F.: Insulin action on arterial tissue in relation to diabetes and atheroma. In Duncan, L. J. P. (ed.): Diabetes Mellitus. Edinborough, Edinborough Press, 1966, p. 41.

Mancini, A. M., et al.: Human insulin antibodies detected by immunofluorescent technique. Lancet, *1*:726, 1964.

Manis, J. G., and Schachter, D.: Active transport of iron by intestine: features of the two step mechanism. Amer. J. Physiol., *203*:73, 1962.

Marble, A., and Bailey, C. C.: Hemochromatosis. Amer. J. Med., *11*:590, 1951.

Mayhew, D. A., et al.: Regulation of insulin secretion. Pharm. Rev., *21*:183, 1969.

Mazur, A., and Sackler, M.: Haemochromatosis and hepatic xanthine oxidase. Lancet, *1*:254, 1967.

McCarty, D. J., Jr.: The pendulum of progress in gout: from crystals to hyperuricemia and back. Arthritis Rheum., *7*:534, 1964.

McKiddie, M. T., et al.: The relationship between glucose tolerance, plasma insulin and corticosteroid therapy in patients with rheumatoid arthritis. Metabolism, *17*:730, 1968.

Mendel, G. A.: Studies on iron absorption. I. The relationship between the rate of erythropoiesis, hypoxia and iron absorption. Blood, *18*:727, 1961.

Morgan, E. H.: Idiopathic hemochromatosis: a family study. Aust. Ann. Med., *10*:114, 1961.

Muckle, T. J.: Impaired immunity in the etiology of amyloidosis: a speculative review. Israel J. Med. Sci., *4*:1020, 1968.

Neel, J. V.: Current concepts of the genetic basis of diabetes mellitus and the biological significance of the diabetic predisposition. In Östman, J., and Milner, R. D. G. (eds.): Proceedings of the Sixth Congress of the International Diabetes Federation, Stockholm, 1967. Diabetes, Supplement. Amsterdam, Excerpta Medica Foundation, 1969, p. 68.

New, M. I., et al.: The significance of blood lipid alterations in diabetes mellitus. Diabetes, *12*:208, 1963.

Nyholm, K.: Eosinophilic xanthomatous granulomatosis. Acta Pathol. Microbiol. Scand., Suppl. *216*:21, 1971.

Oberman, H. A.: Idiopathic histiocytosis: a clinico-pathologic study of forty cases and review of the literature on eosinophilic granuloma of bone, Hand-Schüller-Christian disease and Letterer-Siwe disease. Pediatrics, *28*:307, 1961.

O'Brien, J. S.: Ganglioside storage disease. New Eng. J. Med., *284*:893, 1971.

O'Brien, W. M., et al.: The genetics of hyperuricemia in Blackfeet and Pima Indians. Arthritis Rheum., *7*:335, 1964.

Ogilvie, R. F.: The endocrine pancreas in human and experimental diabetes. In Ciba Foundation Colloquia on Endocrinology, Volume 15. Aetiology of Diabetes Mellitus and Its Complications. Boston, Little, Brown and Co., 1964, p. 49.

O'Sullivan, J. B., et al.: The prevalence of diabetes mellitus and related variables: a population study in Sudbury, Mass. J. Chronic Dis., *20*:535, 1967.

Parker, M., et al.: Juvenile diabetes mellitus, a deficiency in insulin. Diabetes, *17*:27, 1968.

Patrick, A. D., and Lake, B. D.: Deficiency of an acid lipase in Wolman's disease. Nature (London), *222*:1067, 1969.

Pearson, C. M.: Glycogen metabolism and storage diseases of types III, IV and V. Amer. J. Clin. Path., *50*:29, 1968.

Pearson, W. N., and Reich, M. B.: Studies of ferritin, a new iron-binding protein found in the intestinal mucosa of the rat. J. Nutr., *99*:137, 1969.

Perley, M., and Kipnis, D. M.: Plasma insulin responses to glucose and tolbutamide of normal weight and obese diabetic and nondiabetic subjects. Diabetes, *15*:867, 1966.

Philippart, M., et al.: Niemann-Pick disease: morphologic and biochemical studies in the visceral form with late central nervous system involvement (Crocker's group C). Arch. Neurol., *20*:227, 1969.

Powell, L. W.: Changing concepts in haemochromatosis. Postgrad. Med. J., *46*:200, 1970.

Powell, L. W., and Kerr, J. F.: Reversal of "cirrhosis" in idiopathic haemochromatosis following long-term intensive venesection therapy. Aust. Ann. Med., *19*:54, 1970.

Renold, A. E.: Insulin biosynthesis and secretion: a still unsettled topic. New Eng. J. Med., *282*:173, 1970.

Renold, A. E., and Burr, I.: The pathogenesis of diabetes mellitus. Possible usefulness of spontaneous hyperglycemic syndromes in animals. Calif. Med., *112*:23, 1970.

Ricketts, H. T.: Cardiovascular disease. In Williams, R. H. (ed.): Diabetes. New York, Paul B. Hoeber Medical Division, Harper and Row, 1960, p. 549.

Robertson, W. B., and Strong, J. P.: Atherosclerosis in persons with hypertension and diabetes mellitus. Lab. Invest., *18*:538, 1968.

Rukavina, J. G., et al.: Primary systemic amyloidosis: review and experimental and genetic clinical study of 29 cases with particular emphasis on familial form. Medicine, *35*:239, 1956.

Sabesin, S. M., and Thomas, L. B.: Parenchymal siderosis in patients with pre-existing portal cirrhosis. A pathologic entity simulating idiopathic and transfusional hemochromatosis. Gastroenterology, *46*:477, 1964.

Saint, E. G.: Haemochromatosis. Med. J. Aust., *1*:137, 1963.

Sanger, F.: Chemistry of insulin. Science, *129*:1340, 1959.

Schade, S. G., et al.: Normal iron absorption in hypertransferrinanaemic rats. Brit. J. Haemat., *17*:187, 1969.

Schimke, R. N., and Hartmann, W. H.: Familial amyloid-producing medullary thyroid carcinoma and pheochromocytoma: a distinct genetic entity. Ann. Intern. Med., *63*:1027, 1965.

Schneck, L., et al.: The gangliosidoses. Amer. J. Med., *46*:245, 1969.

Schneider, P. T., and Kennedy, E. P.: Sphingomyelinase in normal human spleens and in spleens from subjects with Niemann-Pick disease. J. Lipid Res., *8*:202, 1967.

Schwartz, P.: Senile cerebral pancreatic insular and cardiac amyloidosis. Trans. N.Y. Acad. Sci., *27*:393, 1965.

Seegmiller, J. E., et al.: Biochemistry of uric acid and its relation to gout. New Eng. J. Med., *268*:712, 1963.

Seegmiller, J. E., et al.: Enzyme defect associated with a sex-linked human neurological disorder and excessive purine synthesis. Science, *155*:1682, 1967.

Seegmiller, J. E., et al.: Inflammatory reactions to sodium urate: its possible relationship to genesis of acute gouty arthritis. J.A.M.A., *180*:469, 1962.

Seltzer, H. S.: Insights about diabetes and hyperinsulinism gained from the insulin immunoassay. Postgrad. Med., *46*:72, 1969.

Seltzer, H. S., et al.: Insulin secretion in response to glycemic stimulus: relation of delayed initial release to carbohydrate intolerance in mild diabetes mellitus. J. Clin. Invest., *46*:323, 1967.

Shapiro, S. L., et al.: X-linked recessive inheritance of a syndrome of mental retardation with hyperuricemia. Proc. Soc. Exp. Biol. Med., *122*:609, 1966.

Sharkey, T. P.: Diabetes mellitus: present problems and new research. I. Prevalence in the United States. J. Amer. Diet. Ass., *58*:201, 1971.

Sharkey, T. P.: Recent research developments in diabetes mellitus: Part IV. J. Amer. Diet. Ass., *52*:108, 1968.

Sheldon, J. H.: Haemochromatosis. London, Oxford University Press, 1935.

Shirahama, T., and Cohen, A. S.: Structure of amyloid fibrils after negative staining and high resolution electron microscopy. Nature (London), *206*:737, 1965.

Simpson, N. E.: Multifactorial inheritance. A possible hypothesis on diabetes. Diabetes, *13*:462, 1964.

Siperstein, M. D., et al.: Small Blood Vessel Involvement in Diabetes. Washington, American Institute of Biological Sciences, 1964.

Siperstein, M. D., et al.: Studies of muscle capillary basement membranes in normal subjects, diabetic and prediabetic patients. J. Clin. Invest., *47*:1973, 1968.

Siwe, S.: The reticuloendothelioses in children. Advances Pediat., *4*:117, 1949.

Smith, P. M., et al.: Postulated gastric factor enhancing iron absorption in haemochromatosis. Brit. J. Haemat., *16*:443, 1969.

Sokoloff, L.: The pathology of gout. Metab. Clin. Exp., *6*:230, 1957.

Solomon, S. S., et al.: Effect of starvation on plasma immunoreactive insulin and non-suppressable insulin-like activity in normal and obese humans. Metabolism, *17*:528, 1968.

Sorensen, L. B.: Hyperuricemia and gout. Advances Intern. Med., *15*:177, 1969.

Spagnuolo, M., and Taranta, A.: Post-steroid panniculitis. Ann. Intern. Med., *54*:1181, 1961.

Steinberg, B.: Systemic nodular panniculitis. Amer. J. Path., *29*:1059, 1953.

Steiner, D. F., et al.: Insulin biosynthesis: evidence for a precursor. Science, *157*:697, 1967.

Sturgeon, P., and Shoden, A.: Haemosiderin and ferritin. In Wolman, M. (ed.): Pigments in Pathology. New York, Academic Press, 1969, p. 93.

Sussman, K. E., and Vaughan, G. P.: Insulin release after ACTH, glucagon and 3-5 cyclic AMP in the perfused isolated rat pancreas. Diabetes, *16*:449, 1967.

Talbott, J. H., and Lilienfeld, A.: Longevity in gout. Geriatrics, *14*:409, 1959.

Talbott, J. H., and Terplan, K. L.: The kidney in gout. Medicine, *39*:405, 1960.

Taylor, M. R. H., and Gatenby, P. B. B.: Iron absorption in relation to transferrin saturation and other factors. Brit. J. Haemat., *12*:747, 1966.

Terry, R. D., and Weiss, M.: Studies on Tay-Sachs disease. II. Ultrastructure of the cerebrum. J. Neuropath. Exp. Neurol., *22*:18, 1963.

Thomas, W. A., et al.: Fatal acute myocardial infarction in diabetic patients: a comparative study of 94 autopsied diabetics with acute myocardial infarction and 406 autopsied non-diabetics with acute myocardial infarction with special reference to age and sex distribution. Arch. Intern. Med., *98*:489, 1956.

Turtle, J. R., and Kipnis, D. M.: The lipolytic action of human placental lactogen. Biochim. Biophys. Acta, *144*:583, 1967.

Vallance-Owen, J., et al.: Plasma insulin activity in diabetes mellitus; measured by the rat diaphragm technique. Lancet, *2*:583, 1955.

Walker, A. R. P., and Arvidsson, U. B.: Iron intake and haemochromatosis in the Bantu. Nature (London), *166*:438, 1950.

Wallerstein, R. O., and Robbins, S. L.: Hemochromatosis after prolonged oral iron therapy in a patient with chronic hemolytic anemia. Amer. J. Med., *14*:256, 1953.

Walsh, R. J., et al.: A genetic study of hemochromatosis. Abstracts of the Tenth Congress of International Society of Hematology, F-16, 1964.

Warren, S., and LeCompte, P. M.: The Pathology of Diabetes Mellitus. 3rd ed. Philadelphia, Lea and Febiger, 1952.

Weber, F. P.: A case of non-suppurative nodular panniculitis, showing phagocytosis of subcutaneous fat cells by macrophages. Brit. J. Dermat. Syph., *37*:30, 1925.

Wheby, M. S., and Jones, L. G.: Role of transferrin in iron absorption. J. Clin. Invest., *42*:1007, 1963.

Wheby, M. S., et al.: Studies on iron absorption. Intestinal regulatory mechanisms. J. Clin. Invest., *43*:1433, 1964.

Williams, R., et al.: Venesection therapy in idiopathic haemochromatosis. Quart. J. Med., *38*:1, 1969.

Woehler, F.: On the nature of hemosiderin. Acta Haemat.,*23*:342, 1960.

Wrenshall, G. A., et al.: Extractable insulin of pancreas. Diabetes, *1*:87, 1952.

Wyngaarden, J. B.: Gout. Advances Metab. Dis., *46*:1, 1970.

Yalow, R. S., and Berson, S. A.: Immunoassay of endogenous plasma insulin in man. J. Clin. Invest., *39*:1157, 1960.

Yalow, R. S., et al.: Plasma insulin and growth hormone levels in obesity in diabetes. Ann. N.Y. Acad. Sci., *131*:357, 1965.

Young, F. G.: Permanent experimental diabetes produced by pituitary (anterior lobe) injections. Lancet, *2*:372, 1937.

Yu, T. F., and Gutman, A. B.: Secondary gout: observations in 20 cases. Proceedings of the Second Pan American Congress of Rheumatic Disease, Washington, D.C., 1959, p. 44.

Yudkin, J., and Roddy, J.: Levels of dietary sucrose in patients with occlusive atherosclerotic disease. Lancet, *2*:6, 1964.

9

FLUID AND HEMODYNAMIC DERANGEMENTS

A normal fluid environment and an adequate blood supply are critical to the homeostasis of cells and tissues. Either or both supporting systems may be deranged in a wide variety of clinical settings, and so fluid imbalances (edema or dehydration) and vascular disturbances such as thrombosis, embolism and infarction are everyday clinical problems. Regrettably, they are not only commonplace; they are also life threatening. Vascular insufficiency of the heart is the dominating cause of death in industrialized nations (p. 643). Edema of the brain or lungs is not an infrequent cause of death. Hemorrhage causing shock is encountered virtually daily in all large hospitals. Before considering these important derangements, it may be well to review briefly the maintenance of fluid balance and the maintenance of the fluidity of the blood.

FLUID BALANCE

The cell lives in an aqueous milieu and is itself largely composed of water. Its entire ecology depends on this watery environment through which all products entering and leav-

314

ing the cell must pass. The body, then, is largely composed of water, about 70 per cent of the lean body mass. Total body water is distributed between intracellular and extracellular compartments, the latter subdivided into plasma water and interstitial fluid. The relative sizes of the compartments is given in the following table:

TABLE 9–1. DISTRIBUTION OF TOTAL BODY WATER

Compartments	Volume (liter)	Percentage of Lean Body Weight
Total body water	49	70
Extracellular water	14	20
Plasma	3	4–5
Interstitial	11	16
Intracellular water	35	50

The amounts and distribution of these body fluids are closely guarded homeostatic constants maintained by balanced intake and losses. When total body water is depleted either because of water deprivation or increased losses resulting from excessive sweating, hyperventilation, vomiting or diarrhea, the intracellular compartment is most rigidly conserved. The compensatory depletion of interstitial fluid and, principally, the plasma results in hemoconcentration. With hyperosmolarity of the blood, two renal compensatory mechanisms are called into play. The first mechanism is mediated by the antidiuretic hormone (ADH). Hyperosmolarity of the blood causes ganglionic osmoreceptors in the supraoptic hypophyseal axis to shrink, thereby activating impulses which stimulate pituitary secretion of ADH. This hormone increases reabsorption of water in the distal and collecting tubules of the kidney and so conserves water. The thirst centers are also found in the hypothalamus closely related anatomically to the supraoptic osmoreceptors. Stimuli activating the ADH mechanism simultaneously initiate thirst impulses, increasing water intake. Aldosterone secretion regulating renal tubular reabsorption of sodium and water is the second important mechanism for conserving water. This steroid increases reabsorption of sodium in the distal collecting and Henle's tubules. When water is lost, increased levels of aldosterone are elaborated and sodium, followed by water, is retained. The precise events involved in such secretion of aldosterone are beyond our scope but involve direct action on the adrenal by the sodium levels of the blood and action mediated by the angiotensin-renin system related to the juxtaglomerular apparatus in the kidney (p. 1082).

Maintenance of the intracellular and interstitial compartments is largely accomplished indirectly through mechanisms dependent on the blood volume and its osmolarity. The adult of average size has a blood volume of approximately 5 liters made up of plasma (3 liters) and blood cells (2 liters). An absolute reduction in the normal blood volume may be produced by loss of whole blood (hemorrhage), deficiency of red cells (anemia) or loss of plasma (anhydremia). A relative reduction in the circulating blood volume can result from increasing the volume capacity of the vascular system. Dilatation of the arterioles, venules and capillaries may trap blood in the periphery of the vascular system and diminish the effective circulatory blood volume without actual loss of blood. Increases of blood volume are usually less marked than losses but are, nonetheless, of great clinical significance. Cardiac congestive failure and renal failure are undoubtedly the most important clinical states in which increased blood volume (hypervolemia) occurs.

In both conditions, there is retention of salt and water and the resultant hypervolemia leads to a secondary increase in interstitial fluid. Decreased renal blood flow results in increased levels of ADH and aldosterone which contribute in both of these syndromes to the retention of salt and water (Merrill, 1946). High temperatures, muscular exercise and emotional excitement also produce hypervolemia through mechanisms that at this time are poorly understood.

Maintenance of the balance between the various fluid compartments is as important to health as the maintenance of their absolute volumes. There is constant ebb and flow of fluids between the cells and the interstitial fluid. The rates of such water exchange are different for the various cells of the body. The red cells, brain and liver have rapid exchanges, while the supporting tissues (muscle and bone) are much more static. Some concept of the forces involved in the transfer of water across the cell membrane can be gained by the estimate that if a cell were placed in distilled water, the osmotic force drawing water into the cell would be in the range of 5500 mm. Hg, and the equilibration of osmotic gradients would occur within seconds to, at most, a minute. To prevent intracellular hypertonicity (p. 27), a constant expenditure of energy is necessary to maintain a "sodium pump." Decreases in intracellular water are immediately compensated for by the reservoir of interstitial fluid. This balance between cells and their watery milieu is greatly influenced by the osmotic tension of the interstitial fluid which, in turn, is largely a function of its sodium ion concentration.

Fluid also passes freely between the interstitial and plasma compartments, and each buffers losses or excesses in the other. This exchange is mainly dependent on the hydrostatic pressure within the microcirculation and the osmotic tensions of the blood and interstitial fluid as was discussed on p. 60. In the ebb and flow of water from the plasma, there is always a small net loss which remains within the interstitial fluid. This is drained off through the lymphatics and is ultimately returned to the vascular compartment.

In closing this discussion of normal fluid balance, the role of the endothelium should be understood. It behaves as a semipermeable membrane permitting the free passage of water and crystalloids while opposing the passage of colloids. Increases in its permeability lead to loss of plasma colloids, principally albumin, which both decreases the osmotic pressure within the vascular compartment and simultaneously increases the osmotic pressure of the interstitial fluid. As is clear from the discussion of the inflammatory response, a host of injuries may increase endothelial permeability, but perhaps most important in terms of clinical disease is hypoxia.

FLUIDITY OF THE BLOOD – THE CLOTTING MECHANISM

Nowhere in the body is there a more graphic example of the delicate balances involved in homeostasis than the preservation of the fluid state of the blood. *Many factors such as the elegant streamlined architecture of the blood vessels, the normal laminar flow of the blood and the flexibly controlled cellular and colloidal composition of the blood contribute to this fluidity. But most important is the control of blood clotting.* Two views of this control mechanism are equally strongly held. One proposes a continuous physiologic intravascular coagulation in which minute amounts of clot are constantly being formed and removed at the same rate (Stormorken and Owren, 1971). The other view maintains that clotting does not occur unless triggered by some appropriate stimulus (Deykin, 1970*b*). Both views imply a state of dynamic equilibrium between opposite forces. This delicate balance between normal fluidity and clotting is a two-edged sword. On the one hand, it is life-saving when it prevents exsanguinating hemorrhage from a severed vessel but, on the other hand, intravascular clots are capable of cutting off the blood supply within a coronary artery to cause fatal myocardial infarction. To understand the derangements which may cause such unwanted intravascular coagulation, it is desirable to review our current understanding of hemostasis (control of hemorrhage).

Three processes are involved in hemostasis: (1) vasoconstriction, (2) the formation of a temporary hemostatic plug and (3) the formation of a permanent hemostatic plug or clot (Deykin, 1967) (Deykin, 1970*b*) (Sherry et al., 1969). The first response of a muscular artery or arteriole to injury is vasoconstriction which may suffice to close off incised wounds in large arteries and may even totally obliterate the lumen of small arteries and arterioles. This response is so prompt that it is believed to be mediated by a reflex axon pathway. Vasoconstriction cannot occur in capillaries which lack a well developed musculature, nor is it entirely effective in thin-walled veins. In any event, even in the muscular arteries the wave of vasoconstriction soon passes, and hemorrhage would resume were it not for the concurrent development of a hemostatic plug.

During the period of temporary vasoconstriction, an aggregate of platelets builds up at the site of injury to form the temporary hemostatic plug. The stimulus to such aggregation is endothelial injury or disruption, exposing collagen (Zucker and Borelli, 1962). Further details on the specific stereochemical characteristics of collagen crucial to its aggregating function are available in the studies of Spaet and Zucker (1964) and Wilner et al. (1968). Ultrastructural studies indicate that at first the platelets are relatively little changed but nonetheless firmly bound to each other and so are effective in sealing small vessels or closing all but the large defects in larger arteries and veins (Hovig, 1962). Such platelet aggregation is reversible and may be dissociated by the continuing flow of blood past the aggregate except when a second mechanism intervenes. The platelets adherent to the collagen release adenosine diphosphate (ADP) inducing further platelet aggregation and the buildup of the temporary hemostatic plug (Hovig, 1963). An autocatalytic chain reaction develops in which further platelet aggregation releases more ADP and consequently aggregation of platelets continues. In contrast to the collagen-initiated reaction, ADP-induced aggregation requires the presence of divalent cations, fibrinogen in trace amounts and a heat-stable plasma protein (Marcus, 1969). Webber and Johnson further suggest that thrombin in trace amounts must be formed to effect this ADP release (Webber and Johnson, 1970). It should be noted that while the platelets are firmly interadherent and now have undergone ultrastructural changes, they are nonetheless intact and the ADP aggregation would be capable of dissociation were it not for intercurrent events which stabilize the platelet plug (as will be discussed below) and convert it into a permanent clot (Ashford and Freiman, 1967) (Hovig et al., 1967).

The buildup of the permanent hemostatic plug or definitive blood clot begins virtually contemporaneously with the temporary aggregation of platelets. The permanent hemostatic plug is essentially a firm mass of precipitated polymerized fibrin in which platelets and blood cells are enmeshed. This coagulum is insoluble and irreversible. The complex sequence of interactions in such clot formation involves principally the platelets and clotting factors (Table 9–2), and the critical events are the conversion of prothrombin to thrombin and the subsequent conversion of soluble fibrinogen to the fibrin polymer.

The interaction of the coagulation factors in clot formation has been likened to a "waterfall" or cascade in which a trigger initiates the

TABLE 9–2.   CLOTTING FACTORS

International Classification Number	Commonly Used Terms
I	fibrinogen
II	prothrombin
III	tissue thromboplastin
IV	calcium
V	accelerator globulin, labile factor
VI	(none identified at present)
VII	serum prothrombin conversion accelerator (SPCA), stable factor, convertin
VIII	antihemophilic globulin (AHG)
IX	plasma thromboplastin component (PTC), Christmas factor
X	Stuart factor
XI	plasma thromboplastin antecedent
XII	Hageman factor
XIII	fibrin stabilizing factor

factor (XII) with exposed collagen or some other wettable or electrically charged surface such as glass. Once factor XII is converted from an inactive precursor to an activated enzyme, factor XI and factor X are activated in a chain reaction terminating in the conversion of fibrinogen to fibrin. Alternatively, thrombin and hence the remaining factors can be activated through the "extrinsic" pathway. Here a microsomal lipid-protein complex termed tissue thromboplastin (factor III) is released from injured tissues (blood vessel walls, lung, brain) which, in the presence of a cofactor, factor VII, directly activates factor X, and the subsequent steps to fibrin formation are the same as in the intrinsic system. These sequences are presented in Figure 9–1.

Several features of these cascades are noteworthy. The first two steps in the intrinsic system develop slowly. Vigorous blood flow may block the buildup of sufficient concentration of activated factor XI to convert factor IX, and so progressive clotting may be inhibited. However, once factor IX undergoes conversion, the sequence is autocatalytic and virtually explosive. Some concept of this geometric pro-

first step and, thereafter, sequential conversion of other factors ensues. Thrombin may be formed by two major sequences—an "intrinsic" and an "extrinsic" pathway. The intrinsic pathway is initiated by the contact of Hageman

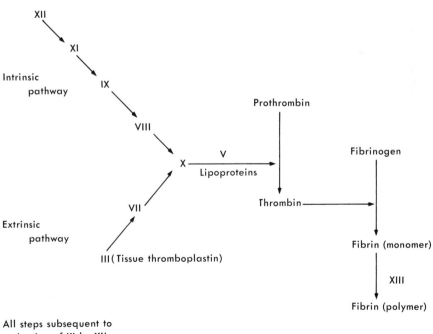

All steps subsequent to
activation of XI by XII
require the presence of
ionized calcium.

Figure 9–1.   The clotting mechanism. Intrinsic and extrinsic pathways in the formation of thrombin and fibrin.

gression is gained from the estimate that 15 ml. of blood contains sufficient prothrombin, if totally activated, to completely precipitate the fibrinogen in 2500 ml. of blood within 15 seconds. Indeed, later we must ask, what checks this chain reaction? Calcium ions are critical at every step in the pathway once factor XI has been activated and are still necessary in the last step, i.e., the conversion of fibrin monomer by the enzymatic action of thrombin in the presence of activated factor XIII into the insoluble precipitated fibrin polymer. Thus, calcium precipitants are effective anticoagulants in the test tube. Further to be noted are the roles of factor V and platelet lipoproteins in catalyzing the conversion of prothrombin to thrombin by activated factor X. Platelets contribute in other ways to the formation of the permanent hemostatic plug as will now be discussed.

Platelets not only form the temporary hemostatic plug, but they also contribute heavily to the permanent blood clot. It was noted that during the phase of the temporary hemostatic plug, the platelets remained essentially unchanged and might have undergone reversible disaggregation. Soon thereafter, however, they undergo second-phase aggregation or viscous metamorphosis. ADP alone will not cause this second phase, and viscous metamorphosis involves contact with collagen or thrombin (Berger, 1970). In such permanent aggregation, the platelets are degranulated and then rupture, creating amorphous masses (Spaet, 1964; 1966). In this manner, they release (so-called "release action") more ADP and vasoactive amines, principally 5-hydroxytryptamine (5-HT). This bioamine undoubtedly contributes to the neurogenic vasoconstriction described earlier. Lipoprotein components of the platelet plasma membrane are, as has been pointed out, necessary cofactors in the conversion of prothrombin to thrombin. This lipid component has been called platelet factor III (Marcus, 1969). In addition, platelets also possess a protein which has many of the properties of actomyosin and so serves as a contractile force in the developing fibrin meshwork. This contractile protein known as *thrombasthenin* causes clot retraction, increasing its density while at the same time squeezing out serum and other activated clotting factors from the interstices of the fibrin meshwork, thereby extending the coagulation process into the immediately adjacent, still fluid blood (Luscher, 1967). Once a definitive hemostatic plug has been produced, more platelets become adherent, the concentration of activated coagulation factors increases in the local area, and a vicious circle is set up which requires control mechanisms lest the entire vascular tree be eventually involved. These control measures will be considered in the subsequent discussion of abnormal intravascular clotting (thrombosis). With these considerations of some of the normal physiology of the body fluids and blood, we may now turn to their derangements.

EDEMA

Edema is the abnormal accumulation of fluid in the intercellular tissue spaces or body cavities. It may occur as a localized process as, for example, when the venous outflow to the leg is obstructed, or it may be systemic in distribution as in chronic congestive heart failure or renal failure. When the edema is severe and generalized, it produces diffuse marked swelling of the subcutaneous tissues and is called *anasarca.* Collection of edema fluid in the peritoneal cavity is known as *ascites,* in the pleural cavities as *hydrothorax,* and in the pericardial sac as *pericardial effusion* or *hydropericardium.* Noninflammatory edema fluid, such as is encountered in heart failure and renal disease, is a *transudate*; it has a specific gravity usually below 1.012 and contains less protein and other colloids than inflammatory exudates which generally have specific gravities above 1.020 (p. 57). This difference in specific gravity is at times a very useful clinical aid. For example, in a patient with cardiac failure, it may be important to exclude the possible coexistence of bacterial pneumonia as a cause of pleural exudation. The specific gravity of the fluid obtained by pleural tap may help in making the appropriate diagnosis.

Pathogenesis of Edema. Edema results from an imbalance between the forces (discussed on p. 60) that tend to retain fluid in the intravascular compartment and those that tend to move and retain fluid within the interstitial tissue spaces or body cavities, e.g., hydrostatic pressure and osmolarity of the interstitial fluid opposed by the colloid osmotic pressure of the blood and the interstitial pressure (Chinard, 1962) (Gauer et al., 1970). Guyton (1963) has recently presented evidence that the interstitial tissue spaces are actually under negative pressure and so, as fluid collects, it at first produces no visible increase in the volume of the tissue, but merely obliterates the negative pressure. Only when the interstitial pressure rises to atmospheric levels do volume changes become apparent. Up to a point, increased lymphatic drainage may compensate for the accumulation of interstitial fluid. Although this compensatory mechanism is limited, its role in the prevention of edema must not be overlooked.

Systemic Derangements Causing Edema.
Important associations between certain systemic disorders and edema are pointed out here.

INCREASED HYDROSTATIC PRESSURE OF THE BLOOD. Cardiac failure is the most important cause for increased venous pressure. As the heart fails, the venous pressure at the level of the right atrium may rise from a norm of 0 to 3 mm. Hg up to levels between 10 and 20 mm. Hg. This elevation is inevitably reflected in elevation of the blood pressure in the venular end of the capillary, leading to excessive transudation of fluid. It is by no means certain, however, that this is the only or, in fact, the principal mechanism by which cardiac failure causes edema. Edema develops in heart failure before there is a significant increase in venous pressures. Cardiac decompensation leads to reduced glomerular filtration with retention of salt and water. There is also an augmented production of aldosterone leading to increased sodium retention. There may also be an increased elaboration of ADH when circulatory failure causes decreased arterial pressures in the various baroreceptors of the body which then transmit signals to the supraoptic nuclei. As a consequence, there is expansion of the blood volume (hypervolemia) as well as of the interstitial fluid compartment. All of these mechanisms contribute to the accumulation of systemic edema in well advanced heart failure.

DECREASES IN OSMOTIC PRESSURE OF THE BLOOD. Renal disease with excretion of plasma proteins is the most common clinical cause of a marked decrease in the osmotic tension of the blood. In many forms of glomerular disease, the glomerular basement membrane becomes abnormally permeable, permitting the escape of large amounts of albumin into the urine. Systemic edema usually develops when the serum level of proteins falls below 4 gm. per 100 cc.

Decreases in plasma osmotic tension may also be caused by inadequate formation of serum proteins. This situation is sometimes encountered in patients with cirrhosis of the liver, in whom disturbed albumin synthesis results in hypoproteinemia. At the same time, the cirrhosis may lead to increased secretion of ADH, worsening the water retention. Starvation or malnutrition may at times also result in inadequate formation of plasma proteins. In these cases, other somewhat more obscure mechanisms, such as nutritional disease affecting the heart and electrolytic imbalances, may underlie the development of the edema. Alternatively, it has been suggested that extreme atrophy of the muscles, as in war hunger cases, may cause loss of normal tissue turgor and the appearance of edema without actual increase in the interstitial water volume.

INCREASED OSMOTIC TENSION OF THE INTERSTITIAL FLUID—SODIUM RETENTION. Sodium is the principal regulator of extracellular fluid volume. Although cardiac failure causes sodium retention, the most extreme instances are found in renal insufficiency whatever its basis. Several forms of adrenal disease, particularly those in which there is increased elaboration of aldosterone (hyperaldosteronism), likewise induce retention of sodium. Indirectly, the salt content of the diet is a further influence, but only in the patient who has impaired renal function, since normal kidneys are perfectly capable of excreting such dietary excesses. Recently, a "volume regulating system" has been described which modifies proximal tubular sodium reabsorption independent of the glomerular filtration or adrenal steroid hormone levels (Rector et al., 1968).

As mentioned earlier, a variety of agents or conditions may increase vascular permeability and thus permit the escape of plasma colloids to increase the osmotic pressure of the interstitial fluid. Systemic causes for endothelial and basement membrane damage are bacterial toxins, various chemicals and, most important, hypoxia.

Local Derangements Causing Edema.
Localized edema may be caused by a local increase in the hydrostatic pressure of the blood or capillary permeability as well as by local obstruction to lymphatic drainage.

INCREASED HYDROSTATIC PRESSURE OF THE BLOOD. Obstruction of a vein by an intravascular clot, tumor or external pressure (enlarged organs, encircling tight garments, surgical dressings, casts) may produce localized edema. Clinical situations in which edema occurs are: (1) pregnancy in which the gravid uterus produces sufficient pressure upon the iliac vessels to cause increased venous pressures and consequent edema in the lower extremities, (2) venous thromboses in the lower extremities (p. 332) and (3) varicose veins in which incompetence of the venous valves induces an increased hydrostatic pressure in the veins of the lower legs.

INCREASED VASCULAR PERMEABILITY. Localized edema is a manifestation of many forms of immunologic disease. Reference is made here to such conditions as hives, urticaria and angioneurotic edema, all of which have their origin in increased vascular permeability mediated by immune mechanisms, discussed in greater detail in Chapter 7. Mast cells, histamine, immunoglobulins and complement comprise the mediators of the increased vascular permeability in these reactions. The edematous manifestations tend to follow repetitive patterns in the individual with each exposure to the same antigen or allergen. Presumably, certain circulatory beds are target organs for the antigen and hence react following each challenge.

LYMPHATIC OBSTRUCTION. Under normal conditions, the lymphatics constantly drain small amounts of interstitial tissue fluid with its low protein content. Obstruction to the lymphatics by traumatic, surgical, inflammatory, radioactive or neoplastic injury may produce edema. Edema is a common sequel to cancer surgery when regional lymph nodes are excised to control the spread of tumor. For example, the axillary dissection of lymph nodes performed in the excision of cancer of the breast quite often results in edema of the arm.

The most striking cause of inflammatory obstruction to the lymphatics is encountered in the parasitic infestation known as *filariasis*. These parasites penetrate the skin, usually in the feet, and migrate to the inguinal nodes where they cause inflammatory fibrosis and lymphatic obstruction. Massive subcutaneous edema develops in the legs and genitals with accompanying epidermal thickening (p. 459). The deformed legs come to resemble those of the elephant, hence the clinical designation of this condition as *elephantiasis*.

Congenital malformation or absence of the lymphatics such as is encountered in Milroy's disease (p. 626) produces a form of localized lymphedema of the extremities.

Morphology of Edema. The anatomic changes produced by edema depend upon its severity, the rapidity with which it occurs and the underlying cause. The two most common systemic causes, namely cardiac failure and renal disease, tend to produce slightly differing patterns of edema. In **cardiac edema**, the accumulation of fluid is basically due to increased pressures (along with the generalized tendency to retain salt and water resulting in hypervolemia) and is most severe in the dependent portions of the body. Hence this form of edema is referred to clinically as **dependent edema.** When the patient is ambulatory, the edema collects first in the lower extremities, particularly over the dorsal aspects of the feet and lower legs. If the patient is confined to bed, the edema may accumulate over the sacral region. Changes in the position of the patient may cause the edema to shift in its distribution and most severely affect the lowermost regions of the body.

Edema of renal origin is generally of greater severity than cardiac edema. Here the edema is due to many factors: sodium retention, expansion of the extracellular fluid volume and loss of plasma col-loids through proteinuria. This last factor is most important and accounts for the most severe forms of renal edema known as the **nephrotic syndrome.** This syndrome is seen in those diseases that particularly affect the glomerular membranes, i.e., glomerulonephritis (p. 1107), amyloidosis (p. 284) and diabetic glomerulosclerosis (p. 268). All regions of the body are affected equally in the renal mechanisms of fluid retention and so the edema tends to be generalized throughout the body. It may, however, be most manifest in those tissues which have a loose connective tissue matrix. Renal edema, therefore, is classically identified by edema of the face, particularly of the eyelids. However, even in this form of edema, posture modifies the distribution and, with the erect position, the facial edema may slowly subside, only to accumulate again on confinement to bed.

In those cases in which the edema is due to localized disturbances, the distribution, of course, depends upon the location of the underlying disorder. Whatever the mechanism of its origin, finger pressure over edematous subcutaneous tissue will displace the interstitial fluid from the dermal and subcutaneous connective tissues to leave pitted depressions, often referred to clinically as "pitting edema" (Fig. 9-2). When the subcutaneous tissue is incised, a free ooze of tissue fluid and a gelatinous slippery consistency may be apparent.

While considerable emphasis has been placed upon subcutaneous edema, the visceral tissues like-

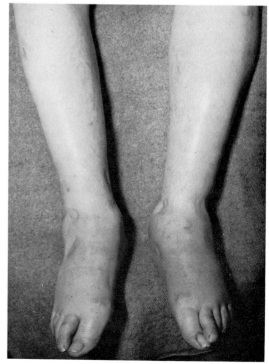

Figure 9-2. *Dependent edema of the lower legs, illustrating "pitting" about the ankles.*

wise participate in generalized edema. Edematous viscera are slightly enlarged, pale, heavier than normal, show somewhat tense capsules and, on section, have a glistening wet appearance.

When well defined, edema is apparent microscopically as a granular acidophilic interstitial precipitate which separates the cellular and fibrillar elements of the tissue. This pink, amorphous deposit represents the protein and solutes of the edema fluid. As the parenchymal cells swell, gland lumina and small vessels are compressed. The edema may infiltrate between parenchymal cells to separate them slightly or may accumulate between cells and their basement membrane, lifting the cells off their basal attachments. Parenchymal cells may also become edematous, but this change is referred to as cellular swelling (p. 31).

Edema of the brain and lungs are the most life-threatening forms of abnormal fluid retention.

Edema of the brain is encountered with brain trauma, infections within the cranial vault (meningitis, brain abscesses, encephalitis), hypertensive crises and obstruction to the venous outflow of the brain. The edematous brain is heavier than normal; the sulci are narrowed, and the swollen gyri are flattened where they press against the skull. On section, the white matter may appear unusually soft and gelatinous and the peripheral layer of gray matter is widened. The ventricles are usually compressed. Histologically, there is considerable widening of the interfibrillar spaces of the brain substance; this gives a loose appearance to the white and gray matter. Swelling of the neuronal and glial cells may also be present. The perivascular (Virchow-Robin) spaces become unusually widened and form clear halos about the small vessels.

Pulmonary edema is a principal manifestation of left ventricular failure, but it is also encountered in renal disease, shock, infections within the lung and in hypersensitivity states where the lungs are target organs. The lungs are particularly susceptible to edema because they are composed of large alveolar spaces lined by thin flattened cells which exert no tissue resistance against the collection of edema fluid. The large volume of exposed capillary wall also predisposes to the formation of edema. The edema is usually confined to, or is most marked in, the lower lobes. In far advanced edema, however, all lobes may be involved and take on a rubbery, gelatinous consistency. Sectioning of the lobes permits the free escape of frothy, sanguineous fluid representing a mixture of air, blood and edema. On histologic examination, there is the precipitation of a granular pink protein coagulate within the alveolar spaces (Fig. 9–3). More important in causing respiratory dysfunction is the accumulation of fluid within the alveolar walls interposing a blanket of fluid between the alveolar air and the septal capillaries. These changes are accompanied by congestion and widening of the alveolar capillaries. When present for any period of

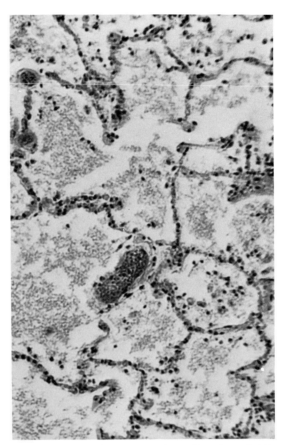

Figure 9–3. *Pulmonary edema. The edema fluid in tissue section appears as a granular pink precipitate within the alveoli.*

time, edema fluid is prone to become secondarily infected to produce pneumonia, in this setting called **hypostatic pneumonia.**

Clinical Significance of Edema. In the brain and the lungs, the edema may be fatal, but subcutaneous edema and edema of other viscera are usually of little functional significance. Swelling of the brain leads to increased intracranial pressure with resultant headaches, projectile vomiting and convulsive seizures. Herniation of the brain stem or cerebellar tonsils into the foramen magnum may precipitate death. Cerebral edema may develop within hours of brain injury, requiring immediate corrective steps if the patient's life is to be saved. Pulmonary edema is important because the alveolar fluid and, more importantly, the fluid blanket which surrounds the alveolar capillaries impedes the normal ventilatory function of the lungs. In functional terms, this alveolar septal edema produces an alveolocapillary block. Characteristically, as the respired air bubbles through the proteinous fluid within the alveolar spaces, a variety of abnormal breath sounds called rales are produced. In severe pulmonary edema, the collection of fluid in the respiratory passages gives rise to extremely loud rales popularly but appropriately termed the "death rattle." Edema of the lungs (with the attendant hazard of *hypostatic pneumonia*) is one of the most serious complications of cardiac and renal insufficiency and frequently triggers the demise of these vulnerable patients.

HYPEREMIA OR CONGESTION

Hyperemia may be defined as increased redness of a tissue caused by dilatation of its microvessels. The volume of contained blood in the affected part is obviously increased.

Types and Pathogenesis. *Active hyperemia* occurs in muscular exercise, in inflammatory or toxic conditions which produce vascular dilatation, and in neurogenic blushing. *Systemic passive congestion* is virtually always the consequence of cardiac failure. Depending on its cause, only the right ventricle or only the left ventricle may decompensate for a period of time. Right ventricular decompensation, so-called backward failure, causes progressive venous stasis throughout the systemic circuit manifested principally by peripheral edema, ascites and congestion of the abdominal viscera. Left ventricular failure or insufficient cardiac output, so-called forward failure, causes venous congestion within the pulmonary circuit. However, in all well established cases of cardiac decompensation, both sides of the heart are affected and give rise to generalized congestion.

Passive hyperemia may also be produced locally when there is obstruction to the venous return of the blood, as by tumors, clots and external pressures. Varicosities of the extremities are common causes of venous congestion of the lower extremities. Cirrhosis of the liver may produce a form of localized vascular obstruction of the abdominal viscera. *Congestion of capillary beds is closely related to the development of edema, and congestion and edema commonly occur together.*

Morphology of Hyperemia or Congestion. Cut sections of hyperemic organs are excessively bloody. In longstanding passive congestion, the stasis of blood causes chronic hypoxia which may lead to degeneration or even death of parenchymal cells. Minute hemorrhages from capillary rupture may be converted in time to hemosiderin-laden scars. The lungs, liver and spleen develop the most obvious manifestations of congestion.

Chronic passive congestion of the lungs and consequent pulmonary edema are encountered in all forms of cardiac decompensation or whenever there is reduced left ventricular output. The most extreme form is associated with rheumatic mitral stenosis. Microscopically, the alveolar capillaries become engorged with blood, and often they develop tortuosity with small aneurysmal dilatations (Fig. 9–4). Rupture of distended capillaries may cause minute intra-alveolar hemorrhages and the breakdown and phagocytosis of the red cell debris eventually leads to the appearance of hemosiderin-laden macrophages ("heart failure" cells) in the alveolar spaces. In severe forms of chronic passive congestion, the alveolar septa are widened both by the dilatation of alveolar capillaries and by edema fluid which collects around the capillaries within the alveolar septa (congestion and edema). In time, the edematous septa become fibrotic which, together with the hemosiderin pigmentation, comprise the basis for the designation "brown induration." The longstanding congestion and consequent pulmonary hypertension may cause progressive thickening of the walls of the pulmonary arteries and arterioles (p. 789).

Chronic passive congestion of the liver results from right-sided heart failure or, more rarely, from obstruction to the inferior vena cava or hepatic veins. The first changes are a dusky red cyanosis and an increase in liver size and weight. On cut section, there is an excessive ooze of blood and the central veins may appear prominent. With longstanding chronic congestion, the central regions of the lobule become red-blue, surrounded by a yellow-brown zone of uncongested liver substance, descriptively referred to as the "**nutmeg liver**" (Fig. 9–5). Microscopically, the central vein and the vascular sinusoids of the centrilobular regions are distended with blood. Chronic distention of these vessels may cause atrophy of the central hepatocytes. If the chronic passive congestion is sufficiently severe or suddenly worsens, rupture of the capillary sinusoids may cause hemorrhage into the hepatic cords and acute necrosis of the central parenchymal cells, i.e., **central hemorrhagic necrosis** (Fig. 9–6). In time, fibrous thickening of the walls of the central veins appears. Extension of this fibrous tissue into the surrounding lobule creates the distinctive anatomic pattern called cardiac sclerosis or sometimes "cardiac cirrhosis" (p. 1036).

Chronic passive congestion of the spleen produces a slightly enlarged, tense, cyanotic organ which, on section, freely exudes blood and collapses slightly so that the capsule becomes wrinkled. The pulp is red, soft and semifluid, and almost flows out of the cut section. In the early stages, the spleen usually does not exceed 250 to 300 gm. in weight (normal, 150 gm.). Microscopically, marked sinusoidal dilatation is present, accompanied by foci of recent hemorrhage and possible hemosiderin

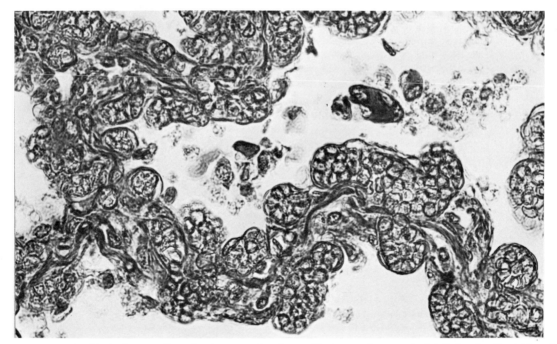

Figure 9–4. *Marked congestion of pulmonary alveolar capillaries, a microscopic detail showing the widened and tortuous capillaries. Their lumina now permit the passage of two to three red cells abreast of each other.*

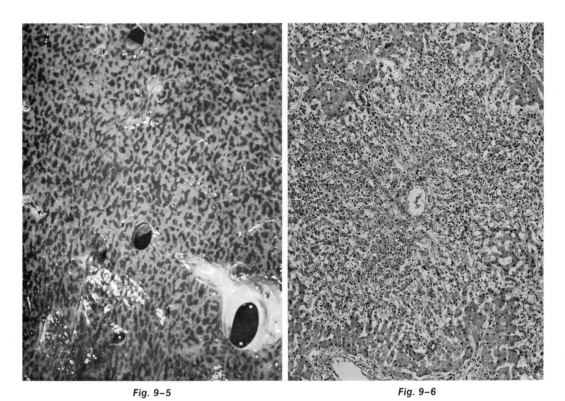

Fig. 9–5   Fig. 9–6

Figure 9–5. *Chronic passive congestion of the liver. On the cut surface, the central congested areas appear darker than the pale peripheral portions of the lobules, and thus compose the so-called "nutmeg" pattern.*

Figure 9–6. *Central hemorrhagic necrosis of the liver. The extravasation of blood into the hepatic parenchyma is accompanied by destruction and disappearance of the centrilobular liver cells.*

deposits. In longstanding chronic congestion, the organ progressively enlarges and may weigh up to 500 to 700 gm. Fibrous thickening and hemosiderin depositions within the edematous, congested sinusoidal walls produce the characteristic anatomic pattern of **congestive splenomegaly** (p. 771). Sometimes focal hemorrhages followed by repair yield **siderofibrotic** nodules of scar tissue laden with hemosiderin.

DEHYDRATION

Abnormal losses of body water may take place through one of three pathways: (1) decreased intake, such as may occur with coma, psychosis or lack of available drinking water; (2) increased losses via the skin, lungs, gut and kidneys; and (3) excessive excretion of urinary solutes with obligate polyuria (as with uncontrolled diabetes and in Addison's disease). Excessive losses commonly result from persistent vomiting, chronic diarrhea and the marked polyuria (5 to 25 liters per day) found in diabetes insipidus with its insufficient elaboration of ADH.

Depletion of total body fluids is first reflected in diminution of the blood volume. If the reduction in blood volume is sufficiently sudden, shock (p. 345) may supervene and cause death. Withdrawal of water from the interstitial fluid compartment then occurs and, eventually, water is withdrawn from the cells. This cellular dehydration, most threatening in the infant, may be of sufficient magnitude to impair normal metabolic function and cause death.

Anatomic changes consequent to fluid depletion are usually quite minimal. The normal small quantities of free fluid in the pleural, pericardial and peritoneal cavities may be absent. Excessive dryness of the serosal membranes may cause loss of their glistening character. The body tissues as a whole show slight contraction, and the blood becomes thicker and more viscous.

HEMORRHAGE

Rupture of a blood vessel is the obvious cause of hemorrhage. If the released blood accumulates within a tissue, it may produce a massive clot, referred to as a *hematoma* (Fig. 9–7). For example, with rupture of the aorta, usually due to some underlying aortic disease, large mediastinal or retroperitoneal hematomas may be produced. If the blood escapes into a serous cavity, it is referred to as *hemothorax, hemopericardium* or *hemoperitoneum.* Smaller hemorrhages, usually encountered in

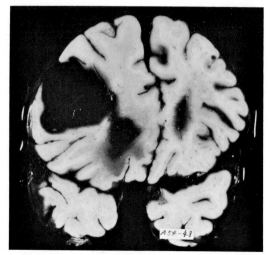

Figure 9–7. *Intracerebral hemorrhage. In the transection of the cerebral hemispheres, the large hematoma extends to the cortical surface as well as into the ventricular system, and blood is visible in the lateral ventricle on the opposite side.*

the skin, mucous membranes and serosal surfaces, are known as *petechiae* (minute), *purpura* (up to approximately 1 cm.) or *ecchymoses* (when large and blotchy).

The causes of hemorrhage are as numerous as the diseases which primarily (such as atherosclerosis) or secondarily (such as an extending erosive cancer) attack vessel walls. These are discussed in Chapter 15. Worthy of special mention in this context are hypertension and the hemorrhagic diatheses. Retinal and, more ominously, cerebral hemorrhages are encountered in hypertensive patients. The latter is a frequent cause of death in patients having marked (malignant) hypertension. The hemorrhagic diatheses comprise a group of clinical disorders having in common an increased bleeding tendency. Platelet deficiencies and a lack of any one of the clotting factors discussed earlier provide examples of the causes of the hemorrhagic diatheses (p. 739).

Clinical Significance of Hemorrhage. The significance of hemorrhage depends upon the amount of blood loss, its rate of escape and the site of the hemorrhage. Acute losses of up to 10 to 20 per cent of the blood volume and slow losses of even greater amounts may have no clinical significance. Larger or more rapid losses may cause hemorrhagic (hypovolemic) shock. But even relatively small amounts of hemorrhage in the brain or pericardial sac may produce sufficient increases of pressure to cause death. It is obvious that external bleeding or hemorrhage into the gastrointestinal tract represents a permanent loss of vital iron. However, if the bleeding occurs into a body tissue or cavity (peritoneal, pleural), progressive breakdown of the hemoglobin permits the resorption of the iron and its reutilization. In the course of this resorption of the hemoglobin, increased amounts of bilirubin are formed which may cause transient jaundice. This sequence is associated particularly with massive gastrointestinal bleeding because even though much of the red cell mass is excreted, some is rapidly digested with rapid resorption of large amounts of the hemoglobin precursor of bilirubin.

THROMBOSIS

The process of formation of a solid clot in blood vessels or in the heart from the various constituents of the blood is known as *thrombosis*, and the coagulated mass is termed a *thrombus*. There is no better way to introduce this subject than to quote from a recent editorial (Stengle, 1970):

To place thrombosis in proper perspective, it is interesting to compare it with other biological enigmas which also represent major health problems. The problems of neoplasia are in many ways comparable. Biologically both thrombosis and neoplasia are aberrations of important normal survival mechanisms; both are failures of homeostatic mechanisms whose functional details are not clearly understood. Clinically the two processes are alike in having as targets all the major organs and systems of the body. And, in the public health sense, the two problems are of similar magnitude, although if one admits a major role for thrombosis in myocardial infarction, stroke and a variety of peripheral diseases, it appears a more important health problem than cancer by one or two magnitudes.

The entire clinical and pathologic significance of a thrombus lies in its capacity to (1) produce ischemic injury and (2) become dislodged or fragmented and generate emboli. An embolus is an intravascular body or mass carried in the bloodstream to some site of lodgment removed from its origin or entrance into the cardiovascular system. The overwhelming preponderance of emboli arise in thrombi. Thrombosis and embolism are therefore so closely interrelated as to justify the designation *thromboembolism*. Thrombi may partially obstruct vessels and cause only ischemic atrophy or focal necroses, but total occlusion of a vessel often causes necrosis (*infarction*) of the tissues served by the vessel. Although these consequences are particularly true of arterial thrombi, venous thrombosis may have the same effect. Since emboli are carried by the bloodstream to a vessel too small to permit their further transport, they generally cause total vascular occlusion and infarction of the dependent tissues. Together, thrombosis and embolism constitute

the usual decisive fatal occlusive event in most patients with advanced atherosclerosis, and such an unhappy sequence constitutes "the leading health hazard facing the aging population of the western world" (Sherry, 1969*b*). In the following discussion, the morphology of thrombi will be presented first since it provides a basis for understanding their pathogenesis.

Morphology of Thrombi. Thrombi may occur anywhere in the cardiovascular system: within the cardiac chambers, arteries, veins or capillaries. **A thrombus is a layered or conglutinated mass containing varying amounts of red cells, granular leukocytes and masses of platelets bound together by fibrin** (Hume et al., 1970). They may have any size and shape dictated by their site of origin and the circumstances leading to their development. Because somewhat dissimilar pathogenetic mechanisms are involved, arterial thrombi differ in appearance from those arising in sluggishly flowing veins. Arterial thrombi usually appear as dry, friable gray masses composed of tangled pale layers of fibrin and platelets irregularly mixed with scant amounts of darker red coagulated blood. Sometimes they are brownish due to hemosiderin staining. It is usually possible to delineate on their exposed surfaces and more certainly on their cross sections paler gray lines interspersed with layers of darker red coagulated blood. These laminations, known as the **lines of Zahn**, result from the irregular deposition, in rapidly moving arterial streams, of layers of platelet masses and fibrin alternating with layers of red cells which become enmeshed in the precipitated fibrin. Because they are largely composed of platelets and fibrin, arterial thrombi are referred to as **white or conglutination thrombi**.

In slower moving streams such as are found in the veins, the thrombus appears to form as an intravascular clot, closely resembling the clotting of blood in a test tube. Such thrombi have a more gelatinous moist appearance and are called **stasis or red coagulation thrombi.** Coagulation thrombi closely resemble postmortem clots, but they differ in having some tangled fibrin layers and usually the primary origin of the thrombus is firmly attached to the underlying endothelium or endocardium.

Arterial white thrombi differ in other respects from stasis venous thrombi. In the rapidly moving stream of blood encountered in arteries or the heart, the thrombus usually begins at some site of alteration of the endothelial or endocardial lining. At the outset, it comprises a mass attached to the wall which does not occlude the lumen, hence their designation as **mural thrombi** (Fig. 9–8). The flow of blood past the evolving intravascular mass creates a buildup of more clot. The surface exposed to the flowing stream tends to accumulate platelets

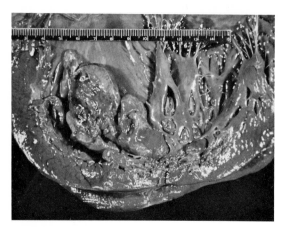

Figure 9–8. *Numerous fresh dark mural thrombi attached to the ventricular endocardium.*

Occlusive arterial thrombi are encountered, in order of frequency, in the coronary, cerebral, iliac and femoral arteries. Almost always, the soil on which the arterial thrombus develops is atherosclerotic involvement of the artery. Uncommonly, other forms of vascular disease such as that produced by syphilis, the many forms of necrotizing arteritis (p. 612) and traumatic injury of vessels underlie arterial thrombus formation.

Mural thrombi tend to arise in the more capacious lumina of the heart chambers and aorta. A myocardial infarct or cardiac arrhythmia are the common soils on which thrombi form in the heart, while atherosclerosis is the almost invariable precursor to aortic thrombus formation. In these sites, mural thrombi are generally formed which do not fill the entire lumen since total occlusion would be incompatible with survival except in extraordinarily rare instances.

Venous thrombi (phlebothromboses) rarely constitute mural masses. Rather, the process comprises total coagulation of blood in some predisposed segment of vein, much like clotting in the test tube. Because of the manner of their formation, venous thrombi are almost invariably occlusive and, in fact, often form quite accurate casts of the vessel in which they arise. Such phlebothrombosis is encountered preponderantly in the veins of the lower extremity (90 per cent occur in leg veins) in approximately the following order of frequency: deep calf, femoral, popliteal and iliac veins (Fig. 9–9). Less

and fibrin, creating a white head while the downstream surface accumulates a dark red stasis tail because of the slowing of the blood flow and turbulence in the lee of the obstructing mass. In this fashion, a large propagating tail may build up to eventually fill the lumen and thus produce an **occlusive thrombus.** The developing head and long snake-like tail may not be firmly attached to the underlying endothelium and, since they literally wave in the bloodstream, they sometimes unfortunately fragment and embolize.

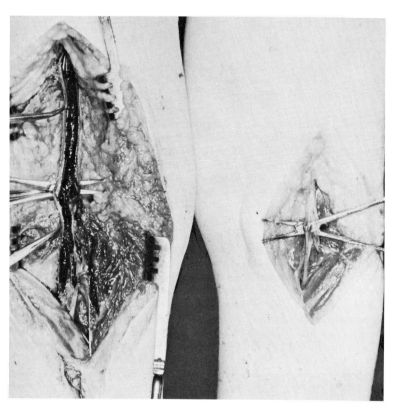

Figure 9–9. *The popliteal veins exposed to demonstrate a large thrombus on the left and the normal vein for comparison on the right.*

commonly, venous thrombi may develop in the periprostatic plexus and the ovarian and periuterine veins. This order of frequency varies considerably among the many series of patients reported (Hume et al., 1970).

In addition to arising within the cardiac chambers, under special circumstances, thrombotic masses may build up on the heart valves, particularly the mitral and aortic valves. In this setting, the thrombi are referred to as **vegetations**. The most common antecedent is a blood-borne bacterial infection which seeds the heart valves and thus provides a site of injury on which a thrombotic mass of fibrin and platelets builds up to produce so-called **bacterial vegetative endocarditis** (p. 673). Less commonly, **nonbacterial bland thrombotic vegetations** (verrucous endocarditis) appear, particularly in patients having systemic lupus erythematosus (p. 232) and in those gravely debilitated by some fatal illness such as disseminated cancer, advanced tuberculosis or some lymphomatous-leukemic disorder. In these settings, hypercoagulability of the blood appears to initiate the formation of the bland vegetations (Wooley, 1970).

Thrombi must be differentiated from postmortem clots. This may be particularly difficult with venous thrombi formed in a sluggish circulation and, therefore, having a large component of red cells. The thrombus is generally somewhat friable and firm while the postmortem clot is usually a rubbery, gelatinous coagulum. Thrombi, even stasis thrombi, usually yield evidence of their origin within flowing blood in the form of a layering or lines of tangled fibrin. Thrombi may or may not nicely fit their vascular enclosure but, in all instances, they will have some attachment to the underlying wall. In contrast, postmortem clots almost always form a perfect cast of the vessel in which they arise, and they can usually be gently lifted out because they have no attachment to their site of origin. The postmortem clot may be a cyanotic dark red "currant jelly" or it may have a supernatant portion of coagulated clear plasma "chicken fat" overlying a portion of darker hue where the red cells have settled. It is not necessary to emphasize the significance of differentiating such postmortem clotting in, for example, the coronary artery from a valid thrombus which may, indeed, have been the cause of death. The development of postmortem clots is a highly variable phenomenon since, in many patients, activation of the fibrinolytic system prior to or immediately after death prevents postmortem clotting while, in others, such does not occur and postmortem clots are abundant.

Pathogenesis of the Thrombus.

The formation of a thrombus involves the interplay of two opposing sets of influences; those predisposing to and those preventing or limiting intravascular clot formation. Virchow in 1856 was the first to clearly delineate the major predisposing influences (Virchow, 1860). Remarkably little has been added to his observations save perhaps for some refinements made possible by the electron microscope. These predisposing influences comprise a triad of (1) changes in vessel walls, particularly endothelial alterations; (2) disturbances in blood flow such as turbulence and stasis; and (3) alterations in the blood inducing a thrombotic diathesis or hypercoagulability. One or more of these influences may be critical in the particular vascular site and patient involved.

Changes in the underlying wall generally underlie most thrombi arising in arteries and in the heart, amply substantiated by the fact that thrombi on the arterial side of the circulation generally overlie lesions in the walls of the vessels or heart. In these settings, its seems reasonable to postulate that the vascular disease or cardiac lesion damages the overlying endothelium or endocardium and exposes collagen which then initiates platelet aggregation (Ashford and Freiman, 1967) (Spaet and Gaynor, 1970). Thereafter, the platelet nidus sets into motion the train of events described in the formation of a permanent hemostatic plug. Such an explanation, however, may not suffice for the understanding of thrombosis in an artery merely adjacent to an abscess. Perhaps here the biochemical mediators of the inflammatory response induce sufficient increase of the endothelial permeability to expose collagen in the widened interendothelial cell junctions. Alternatively, it is suggested that with injury there is breakdown of ATP within cells to produce ADP sufficient to initiate platelet aggregation at the site. It has been shown experimentally that inhibition of ADP production by pretreatment of animals with enzyme poisons inhibits platelet aggregation even in severely injured vessels (Honour and Mitchell, 1964).

The contribution of changes in the underlying vessel wall to the formation of venous thrombi is far more mysterious. As will become clear, venous thrombi usually begin in the sinuses behind the cusps of venous valves. Why should they select these particular sites of origin? As we shall see, stasis and alterations in the blood itself undoubtedly are the major contributors to the coagulation process in these settings. But presumably some local influence dictates their initiation or else stasis thrombosis would occur throughout the length of the affected vein. A number of theories have been offered regarding the possible nature of the local triggering influences but clearly no primary readily evident vascular disease is usually found at sites of venous thrombosis. It has been proposed that the endothelial lining is nonwettable and therefore provides no site of attachment for platelets which initiate intravascular clot formation. Some alteration in this attribute would then predispose to thrombosis. In vitro it can be shown that nonwettable surfaces such as silicones prevent or at least remarkably slow clotting. But the problem of wettability versus nonwettability of the endothelium is probably of little consequence in the induction of thrombosis. Another theory proposes that changes in the electronegative charges of the endothelium are induced by some subtle injury permitting the negatively charged platelets to adhere (Sawyer et al., 1965). Alternatively, alterations in some coating of the endothelium might be induced by stasis and local hypoxia. A heparin-like anticoagulant (coating the endothelial cells) has been proposed but has never been firmly established (McGovern, 1955). Quite recently, however, Cotran (1965) identified an electron dense, extraneous coat covering endothelial cells and observed adherent platelets in sites of mild thermal injury. Interesting as these observations are, perhaps we are seeking nonexisting mechanisms; certainly within veins stasis and hypercoagulability may provide adequate mechanisms for venous thrombosis.

Changes in the normal flow of the blood such as stasis or turbulence are probably instrumental in the development of arterial thrombi of significant size and are requisite for venous thrombosis (Wessler and Yin, 1969). Stasis and turbulence (causing countercurrents and local pockets of stasis) provide three important dimensions: (1) They prevent the dilution and clearance (by the liver and reticuloendothelial system) of the activated coagulation factors by the fresh flow of blood. (2) They disrupt laminar blood flow and bring platelets into contact with the endothelium. (3) The turbulence could lead to injury to the endothelium and the formed elements of the blood.

In the heart and arteries, the normal rapidly moving laminar flow sharply limits the buildup of the elements necessary to produce an intravascular mass. This fact is readily demonstrated in the experimental animal where a thrombus may be initiated by some injury to a vessel wall but, unless the blood flow is altered, the small thrombus is swept off and does not evolve. Indeed, if such were not the case, imagine the consequences of the innumerable minor injuries of everyday life. In normal blood flow, the largest formed elements occupy the central axial stream. A clear plasmatic sleeve is juxtaposed between the endothelial lining and the formed elements. Platelets gen-

erally lie within the interface between the cleared plasma and the larger formed elements in the central column. With turbulence and stasis, the laminar flow is disrupted and the formed elements contact the endothelium where the platelets may adhere (Deykin, 1967). Furthermore, turbulence might damage the endothelial lining, as well as the formed elements such as red cells and platelets. Release of ADP would lead to aggregation of platelets and would set into motion the chain of events leading to thrombosis (Jorgensen, 1971).

The roles of turbulence and stasis are clearly documented in many clinical situations. Thrombi often form in the aorta and arteries with aneurysmal dilatations and overlying atheromatous ulcerations. In the heart, myocardial infarctions not only provide sites of endocardial injury but the necrotic muscle does not contract, and so some element of stasis is added. In disorders causing mitral stenosis, the left atrium balloons and fails to empty and, when arrhythmias such as auricular fibrillation (common in rheumatic heart disease) supervene, the stage is set for atrial and auricular thrombosis. In the same way, abnormal venous dilatations (varicose veins), which render the valves incompetent, induce stasis, sometimes to the point of minimal flow. The dependent position of the lower legs adds to the hydrostatic pressure. Cardiac decompensation, immobilization of an extremity in a cast, bed rest with the loss of the milking action of the leg muscles, as well as local pressures on veins such as the pregnant uterus pressing on the iliac veins all constitute situations where venous stasis may predispose to thrombosis.

The origin of venous thrombi in the sinuses behind valve cusps has been elegantly documented (Hume et al., 1970). These small thrombi act as temporary hemostatic plugs which then trigger the coagulation mechanism. Presumably, the earliest step is aggregation of platelets which then release ADP. But this temporary aggregation would not survive unless thrombin were generated and fibrin were precipitated. There is much evidence that the intrinsic system is activated in this situation, but how it is done remains unclear (Deykin and Wessler, 1964). The local stasis and turbulence prevent the generated thrombin from being washed away and so clotting progresses. Clot retraction thereafter squeezes out more activated factors, and a vicious cycle is established.

Thrombi are also prone to form at arterial branchings and venous junctions. Here again, turbulence probably plays a major role. In plastic models of the vascular system, suspended particulate matter within the circulating fluid silts out at branch points and junctions (Murphy et al., 1962). The deposits which simulate a thrombus are obviously not the result of changes in the vessel wall but rather the consequence of eddy currents and local stasis permitting the settling of the particles.

It is important to point out that stasis alone will probably not induce thrombosis. In the experimental animal, when a segment of vein is carefully and gently sequestered by ligatures causing total stasis of the trapped blood, clotting does not follow (Wessler, 1968). When aged serum from the same animal was injected into the isolated segment of vein, thrombosis followed, suggesting the necessity for some simultaneous alteration in the blood toward a hypercoagulable state. Wessler (1962) has proposed the appearance, during periods of stasis, of a thrombogenic factor which he calls serum-thrombotic accelerator that serves as the trigger of the coagulation sequence.

Changes in the blood in the form of hypercoagulability or some *thrombotic diathesis* have been suspected since the time of Virchow as contributing to the predisposition to thrombosis. The literature on this subject is as contradictory as it is plentiful. Most studies report changes in the blood found in patients who have already had a thrombosis. Here the changes might well result from the thrombus, since the first event would reasonably be expected to activate procoagulant factors. The most critical studies are those done in prospect, attempting to identify in high-risk clinical disorders hematologic changes which might lead to thrombosis, with extended followup of these patients to necropsy, to determine the actual development of thrombi. In such studies, a number of thrombopotentiating changes in the blood have been noted which collectively might induce a hypercoagulable state. The changes are extremely wide-ranging and include, among others, a rise in the platelet count, increased adhesiveness of the platelets, hyperfibrinogenemia, hyperprothrombinemia, elevations of factors VII and VIII and a decrease in fibrinolytic activity (Ham and Slack, 1967) (Sandrock and Mahoney, 1948) (Innes and Sevitt, 1964) (Izak et al., 1967). Despite all of these findings supporting the validity of a hypercoagulable state, the subject is kept in perspective by the quotation from Hume et al. (1970): "Whether or not there is a prethrombotic state in the blood before venous thrombosis has not been settled."

In the individual patient, one or more of the three major predisposing influences to thrombosis, i.e., vascular changes, stasis, and alterations in the blood, may be operative. An aneurysmal dilatation with endothelial damage, eddy current formation and stasis might not require the presence of hypercoagulable changes. Severe ulcerative atherosclerosis in the coronary arteries might induce thrombosis by exposure of collagen perhaps coupled with some element of turbulence. In the veins of the lower legs, stasis and perhaps hypercoagulability might constitute the driving forces. It might be said then that the risk of thrombosis is commensurate with the number of collaborating thrombotic influences.

An understanding of the pathogenesis of thrombosis involves more than a consideration of the predisposing influences. It is reasonable to ask why it does not occur more frequently in the light of the precarious balance involved in the maintenance of the fluidity of the blood. Moreover, once a thrombus begins, why does the process not continue to solidify the entire vascular system? Trivial injuries, long periods with the legs in a resting dependent position, broken bones requiring immobilization and surgical procedures happily are not always followed by thrombosis. The mechanisms involved in maintaining the fluidity of the blood and in limiting the extension of thrombi are (1) the normal blood flow, (2) mechanisms inhibiting the clotting cascade and (3) the fibrinolytic system.

The cardiovascular system of man is ingeniously contrived to present an uninterrupted smooth endothelial surface. Vessels subtly diminish in caliber on the arterial side and equally subtly enlarge on the venous side, thus providing streamlined laminar flow. The rate of flow confines the formed elements to the central column of the blood and, at the same time, tends to sweep off any wandering platelets which enter the clear plasmatic layer. The valves in the veins of the lower portions of the body break the long hydrostatic columns of blood and thus prevent excessive stasis and venous dilatation. Muscular movements and the one-way venous valves milk the veins of the lower extremities and force the fluid column in the direction of the heart. The flow of blood also dilutes and permits clearance of activated coagulant factors to prevent their buildup to critical threshold levels. At the same time, the flow brings in fresh supplies of inhibitors. Normal flow, the obverse of stasis, is a significant factor in preventing and limiting thrombosis.

Dilution, removal and inhibition of activated procoagulants are important protective mechanisms against thrombogenesis and enlargement of a nidus. There are many naturally occurring circulating inhibitors capable of inactivating or neutralizing each of the precursors of thrombin as well as thrombin itself (Soulier, 1962). As many as six antithrombic activities have been identified. The coagulation mechanism itself has built-in rate-limiting reactions. Fibrin, once precipitated, absorbs large amounts of thrombin which serve to brake the continued precipitation of fibrin. The liver and the RE system clear activated factors IX and X from perfused serum (Deykin et al., 1968). Moreover, dilution by the blood flow further prevents the local buildup of activated factors.

The fibrinolytic system is perhaps the most important mechanism involved in the protection against thrombosis. Virtually all tissues including endothelium possess activators of plasminogen. Furthermore, activated factor XII and thrombin itself convert plasminogen to plasmin. The activated form, plasmin, is a potent proteolytic capable of digesting factors V, VIII and fibrinogen, as well as fibrin. Proteolysis of fibrin produces degradation products known as fibrin split products (FSP). FSP also exert an anticoagulant effect by: (1) the inhibition of polymerization of fibrin monomer to fibrin, (2) the formation of unclottable complexes with fibrin monomer, (3) a direct antithrombin effect and (4) the inhibition of platelet aggregation (Deykin, 1970b). There are, however, circulating antiplasmins which, to some extent, neutralize the fibrinolytic system. On balance, there is much evidence that fibrinolysin is an important inhibitor of thrombosis and is particularly active in limiting the extension of the thrombotic nidus (Sherry, 1969a). In perspective, the mechanisms operating to induce and prevent thrombosis are so finely balanced that a relative dominance, at any given point in time, of the inductive or the protective influences spells the difference between thrombosis and its absence.

Evolution of the Thrombus. If a patient survives the immediate ischemic effects of a newly developed thrombus, what happens thereafter? One of a number of pathways may be followed. *The thrombus may (1) propagate and, by its enlargement, eventually cause obstruction of some critical vessel, (2) give rise to an embolus (discussed in the next section), (3) be removed by fibrinolytic action or (4) become organized.* The last two potentials deserve further consideration. As already indicated, a thrombus provokes a prompt activation of the plasminogen-plasmin system. Indeed, in animals it is difficult to create a persistent thrombus because of the prompt and effective fibrinolytic response. Such a happy outcome may also occur in man, and pulmonary thromboemboli have been observed by angiography to shrink rapidly and, indeed, to disappear

within days of the appearance of the intravascular obstruction (Fred et al., 1966) (Sabiston, 1968). Resolution occurs mostly within the first few days of the development of the coagulum, probably because freshly formed fibrin is more susceptible to lysis than older fibrin. The efficacy of this response depends, of course, on the size of the thrombus, the adequacy of the blood flow in its environs and the level of the fibrinolytic activity. Blood flow is crucial since the occlusive thrombus may induce sufficient stasis to block the delivery of the necessary activated enzymes. Fortunately, as is well known, fresh clots retract under the action of thrombasthenin of platelet origin. In this manner, even an occlusive thrombus generally leaves a slit-like channel through which some flow continues. However, if the early fibrinolytic response does not totally resolve the coagulum, the continued buildup may outpace the fibrinolysis. Despite these uncertainties, fibrinolysis may suffice to reopen an occluded channel and, optimally, may digest the entire mass.

When a thrombus is formed, it acts as a foreign body and, almost from the outset, excites an inflammatory reaction in the underlying wall of the heart or blood vessel. This reaction takes the form of a neutrophilic infiltration of the vessel wall with subsequent migration of the inflammatory cells into the thrombic mass. These changes have considerable significance. The neutrophilic invasion may be sufficiently intense to induce enzymic digestion of the center of the coagulum where the concentrations of lysosomal enzymes achieve their highest levels. Such a sequence is referred to as *puriform softening* and is particularly likely to occur in large thrombi within the cardiac chambers or aneurysmal sacs. Bacteremic seeding of such a digestate may convert the softened thrombus to a mass of pus. Fortunately, puriform softening and bacterial seeding are uncommon sequelae. Far more commonly, the inflammatory reaction is followed by the inevitable reparative response and fibroblasts and capillary buds invade the thrombus. In this way, the thrombus becomes more firmly attached to its site of origin. In the course of time, the entire intravascular mass is populated by fibroblasts and capillary channels, and the thrombus becomes converted essentially into a vascularized connective tissue. This process is referred to as *organization of the thrombus.* The capillary channels may anastomose to produce thoroughfares which traverse the thrombus and, indeed, provide new channels through which blood flow may at least in part be reestablished, a process known as *canalization of the thrombus* (Fig. 9–10). Concomitantly, the endothelial cells grow over the

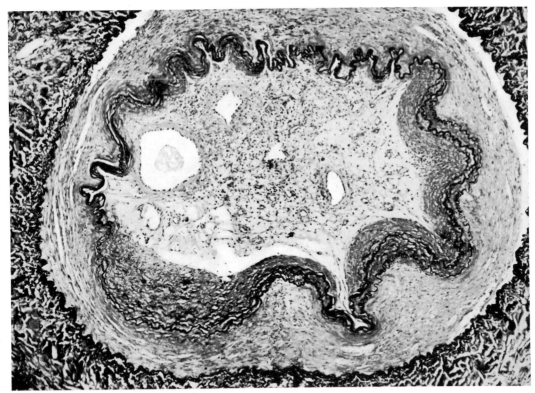

Figure 9–10. *A low power view of a thrombosed artery stained for elastic tissue. The lumen is delineated by the partially degenerated internal elastic membrane and is totally filled with organized clot, now traversed by many newly formed recanalized channels.*

external surfaces of the thrombus to reendo-thelialize it and thereby exclude it from the flow of blood. Since fibrous tissue contracts in the course of weeks to months, the thrombus is virtually incorporated within the vessel wall or cardiac chamber as a fibrous lump or thickening (Fig. 9–11).

We should return for a moment to the stage of the early inflammatory reaction. In the past, much attention was directed to the differentiation of bland venous thrombosis *(phlebothrombosis)* from *thrombophlebitis* (p. 622). The latter was considered to be some obscure primary inflammatory disease of veins which subsequently excited thrombogenesis. Thrombophlebitis was considered to be a not uncommon complication of pregnancy and visceral cancer, and the subsequent formation of an intravascular clot was held to be less threatening than bland phlebothrombosis since the thrombotic mass would presumedly be firmly attached to the inflamed vessel wall and thus would be unlikely to embolize. The existence of the entity thrombophlebitis has now been seriously questioned, and it seems more likely that it represents a standard form of thrombosis followed by the invariable inflammatory

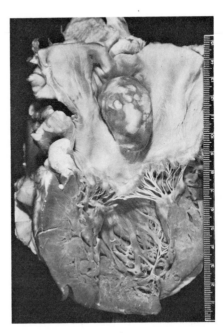

Figure 9–11. *An endothelialized mural thrombus within the left atrium of the heart. The surface is smooth and the clot has been converted into a firmly attached globular mass.*

response in the underlying wall. The hazard of embolization in all such situations is real and will be discussed later. These remarks should not be construed to deny that inflammation in a vessel wall will not excite a thrombus. Indeed, an abscess contiguous to a vein or artery or primary inflammatory arterial disease frequently induces thrombosis and, in such circumstances, the site of origin of the intravascular coagulum is usually firmly attached but the subsequent buildup may still provide a loosely attached head or tail capable of embolization.

Clinical Implications of Thrombosis. The major concerns of the clinician with respect to thrombotic disease are: (1) What are its possible consequences? (2) Where is it most likely to occur in the cardiovascular system? (3) In what clinical settings is it most apt to develop? The first issue is by now apparent. Thrombotic disease has grave significance since it causes vascular occlusion and is a ripe source of emboli. Depending on the extent of vascular occlusion, it may cause only atrophy or only focal necrosis of the dependent tissues or organ. More often, it induces massive ischemic necrosis (infarction) which is more characteristic of arterial than venous lesions. Venous thrombosis, although occlusive, may not cause severe ischemia since opening of collateral channels of venous drainage may sustain some level of blood flow. Under these circumstances, edema may be the only manifestation of the phlebothrombosis. This sequence is particularly common when the major venous outflow channels of the lower extremity are involved, such as the femoral and iliac veins, since widened‛ bypass venous channels permit some venous drainage. However, the veno-occlusive disease produces not only edema but also painful swelling and tenderness on palpation of the affected vein. Thus, thrombosis of deeply situated veins within the calf muscles, one of the most frequent sites of origin of this disease, can often be detected by forced dorsiflection of the foot. This maneuver, which compresses the affected veins, elicits pain known as *Homan's sign.* Simple squeezing of the calf muscles will also be painful. Often, however, *deep vein thromboses are entirely silent,* causing neither pain nor edema, and their presence first becomes known when they give rise to a pulmonary embolus.

The sites of origin of thrombi depend largely on the predisposing influences but ultimately are not totally predictable. Nonetheless, certain locations are favored and were presented on p. 326. In addition to these sites, venous thrombosis is sometimes seen in the radicles of the portal vein when there is an infection within the peritoneal cavity and following pelvic or upper abdominal surgery (splenectomy, gastrectomy, pancreatectomy). Thrombosis is also prone to appear in the superficial veins of the leg when they develop varicosities. These thrombi are painful, disabling and may cause edema, but only rarely do they embolize. However, the edema and impaired venous drainage predispose the skin of the lower leg to infections following trivial trauma and to the development of indolent *varicose ulcers* that are most difficult to control.

Turning to the question of the clinical settings in which thrombosis is apt to occur, patients with certain disorders are at high risk of developing thrombi. Some concept of the magnitude of the risk can be derived from the numerous studies indicating deep vein thrombosis of the lower limbs at necropsy in 60 to 80 per cent of hospitalized patients suffering from burns, trauma, fractures and other medical and surgical diseases. Moreover, pulmonary embolism arising in venous thrombi has been reported to be responsible for or significantly contributory to death in 3 to 10 per cent of seriously ill patients (Coon and Coller, 1959) (Kucera, 1968) (Roberts, 1963). Whatever the underlying disease, age and bed rest are two important predisposing factors. The effect of age may be related to the virtually inevitable development of atherosclerosis, the greater tendency for some cardiac insufficiency and the general loss of muscle tone, vigor and physical activity. Bed rest adds the dimension of sluggish venous return.

Heart disease, particularly congestive heart failure, myocardial infarction and rheumatic heart disease are associated with a high incidence of thrombosis. Heart failure has the obvious implications of advanced age, bed rest, atherosclerosis, sluggish venous return and generalized hypoxia, rendering the tissues more vulnerable to further vascular embarrassment. Myocardial infarction produces not only a prime site of injury for the development of a thrombus, but also involves impaired circulation, bed rest and the possible development of hypercoagulable changes in the blood. Indeed, thrombotic occlusion of an atherosclerotic coronary artery may be the cause of the infarct. Because patients with myocardial infarction often develop arrhythmias of the heart and diskinetic contractions of the left ventricle, the risk of embolization of the mural thrombus is heightened. Rheumatic heart disease is frequently characterized by a myocarditis and the development of a tight stenosis of the mitral valve. Several factors become operative; the left atrium enlarges, fails to empty during diastole, and the myocardial lesions predispose to auricular fibrillation, a concatenation of events providing an ideal setting for auricular thrombi and subsequent embolization. We should also mention here the various forms of vegetative endocarditis since, by definition, they are characterized by thrombotic lesions on the cardiac valves.

Rampant atherosclerosis, particularly common in diabetes mellitus, and aneurysmal dilatations of the aorta or any other vessel are ripe settings for mural thrombosis. Sometimes the thrombus which fills a saccular aneurysm has the beneficial effect of acting as a blowout patch. Indeed, the entire sac may thrombose up to the original level of the arterial wall. Regrettably, as the clot retracts, it often separates from the underlying wall of the aneurysm, providing a slit-like space for fresh thrombus formation. Cross section of such a thrombosed aneurysm may reveal distinct laminations with the oldest layers farthest removed from the wall of the sac.

A high risk of venous thrombosis is associated with congestive heart failure, varicosities of the lower legs, severe burns or other forms of trauma, postoperative and postpartum states, disseminated cancer and, in fact, all serious illnesses and prolonged bed rest. Most of the influences predisposing to thrombosis in these clinical settings are fairly obvious but a few deserve further consideration. Many factors act in concert to predispose to thrombosis in the postoperative, puerperal and postpartum states. Surgery invokes trauma to vessels and hypercoagulable changes in the blood. In several large surveys, thrombosis and embolism were found to be unmistakably more frequent following surgical procedures in the upper abdomen and female pelvis than in other forms of surgery and in nonsurgical patients (Barker et al., 1940) (Belding, 1965). It must be remembered that, in these patients, other important concurrences such as age, bed rest, the possibility of coincidental atherosclerotic and heart disease all must be weighed. During delivery, there is similar trauma to vessels, and the amniotic fluid contains thromboplastic substances providing an obvious basis for the hypercoagulability. But, in addition, there is an increased tendency for thrombosis in the third trimester of pregnancy. Iliofemoral thrombosis is so commonly encountered in the puerperium and post-delivery as to have received the specific designation *"milk leg"* or *"phlegmasia alba dolens" (painful white leg)* (p. 623). Here an increase in both the number and adhesiveness of platelets, accompanied by an increase of fibrinogen, factors VIII, VII and other clotting factors, have been

indicted as the causative mechanisms of the thrombosis (Todd et al., 1965). In addition, some obscure basis for inhibition of fibrinolysis contributes to the hazards imposed on the pregnant woman (Shaper et al., 1968). Venous thrombosis following extensive burns, fractures (particularly of long bones) and, in fact, all forms of significant trauma is now a well established association (Hamilton and Angevine, 1946) (Sevitt, 1968) (Sevitt and Gallagher, 1961). Bed rest, immobilization of extremities and hypercoagulability appear to be the dominant influences in these settings.

The association of phlebothrombosis with cancer was first noted over a hundred years ago by Trousseau. Since his time, many have confirmed the appearance of venous thrombi, often multiple, sometimes disappearing at one site only to reappear elsewhere, in patients with various forms of cancer, justifiably now designated as *Trousseau's sign or migratory thrombophlebitis* (Coon and Coller, 1959) (p. 623). The pathogenesis probably involves a number of influences including confinement to bed, surgical interventions, age and coincidental heart disease but, in addition, it has been suggested that the necrotic products of the tumor may have thromboplastic properties. Other hypercoagulable alterations have been described as well (Sise et al., 1962).

Very few subjects are more timely, more vexing and have aroused more impassioned writings than the relationship of *oral contraceptive medications to thrombosis.* A number of reports contend that users of contraceptive pills have from a four- to ninefold increased risk of thromboembolic disease as compared with nonusers (Vessey and Doll, 1969) (Inman and Vessey, 1968) (Inman, 1970) (Sartwell et al., 1969). An equally impressive array of reports can be found that refute this contention just as vehemently (Food and Drug Administration, 1963; 1966) (World Health Organization, 1966) (Goldzieher, 1970) (Drill and Calhoun, 1968). Each of these writings and the subsequent correspondence which they aroused painstakingly points out the flaws in the previous reports: inadequate number of cases, inadequate controls, unreliability of clinical diagnosis of thrombosis, etc. It is equally impossible to detail succinctly the contradictory evidence as it is to reconcile the conflicting conclusions. Two of the most recent reports published within months of each other, having the benefit of all of the earlier writings, are still in complete disagreement; one states a fourfold increased incidence of thromboembolic disease in users of contraceptive pills and the other stoutly denies the justification for indictment of this form of contraception as having any thrombogenic potential (Goldzieher, 1970) (Sartwell et al., 1969).

Before commenting on this perplexing and important controversy concerning the thrombogenic potential of contraceptive pills, several points need to be made. The hormonal content of contraceptive pills has been undergoing constant change. In most reported studies to date, the "users" have taken "combined products" (mixtures of estrogenic and progestational agents) or sequential products in which tablets containing only an estrogenic compound are taken for 14 to 16 days of the cycle followed by 5 to 7 days of tablets containing mixtures of estrogens and progestogens. Estrogen has long been known to induce hypercoagulable changes in the blood when given in sufficiently high dosages (Poller, 1969). Recent contraceptive preparations have lowered or omitted the estrogen content but they have not been in use long enough for evaluation. Progesterone has not been implicated in changes in the blood. Against this background, it seems reasonable to conclude that, at least for sequential products, there is some increased risk of thromboembolism. The magnitude of the risk may be on the order of three- to fourfold (Sartwell et al., 1969). The issue with respect to combined medications is less clear but appears to involve some increased risk, and the newer low-estrogen products must still be surveyed. However, it should be pointed out as Goldzieher reports that the death rate in pill users, if one assumes the highest level of increased risk, is still considerably below the death rate from the complications of pregnancy, delivery and the puerperium. Indeed, it is said that the death rate encountered in unwanted pregnancies representing failures in the use of contraceptive methods still exceeds the thromboembolic fatality rate in users of the pill.

In closing this discussion of thrombosis, it is important to point out that although many "high-risk" disorders are known, thrombogenesis is a quixotic phenomenon. It may occur at any time, in any setting and, indeed, has developed in young vigorous individuals without apparent provocation or predisposition.

MICROCIRCULATORY THROMBOSIS—DISSEMINATED INTRAVASCULAR COAGULATION (DIC)

In a variety of clinical settings, widespread thromboses form in the microcirculation, principally within the capillaries. The thrombi are largely composed of aggregated platelets and fibrin and the disorder is known as *disseminated intravascular coagulation* (DIC). DIC may follow obstetric complications (premature separation of the placenta, retained dead fetus and amniotic fluid infusion), mismatched blood transfusions, acute hemolytic crises from any cause, extensive burns and trauma, extracorporeal circulation, advanced cancer, infections (bacterial, viral, mycotic, parasitic), postinfectious immunologic reactions and acidosis. To this list might be added the obscure entity of thrombotic thrombocytopenic purpura (TTP) (p. 742) which is considered by some to be based on immunologic injury to the microcirculation. Others, however, do not believe that TTP is a distinct entity and consider it a form of DIC having one of the many trigger mechanisms found in the variety of disorders just mentioned. The pathophysiology of DIC is discussed in more detail on p. 744.

It suffices now to say that the weight of evidence favors hypercoagulability of the blood as the chief mechanism of DIC, although primary endothelial damage in the capillaries may also be a factor. Whatever the basis, a complicated sequence of events follows. The widespread occlusion of the microcirculation may induce shock, signs of acute respiratory distress, central nervous system depression, heart failure or renal failure. Affected tissues may show, besides the small white thrombi, focal necroses. On the other hand, the intravascular coagulation may give rise to the seeming paradox of a hemorrhagic diathesis. The pathophysiology of the bleeding tendency is complicated but lies principally in the rapid consumption of fibrinogen, platelets, prothrombin and factors II, V, VII and X, hence the synonym *consumption coagulopathy*. Activation of the fibrinolytic system by the widespread thrombosis and inhibition of the clotting mechanism by the release of fibrin split products further contributes to the bleeding tendencies (Deykin, 1970a) (Bachmann, 1969). We may thus have the apparent contradiction of widespread coagulation causing a hemorrhagic diathesis. To carry the paradox further, DIC may not have a significant number of thromboses because, in some patients, fibrinolysis removes the thrombi as they are formed. More is said about this complex and challenging syndrome on p. 744. It is of significance in our present context since it represents the diffuse formation of myriads of white thrombi.

EMBOLISM

An embolus has been defined as a detached intravascular mass (solid or gaseous) that is carried by the blood to a site distant from its point of origin. Inevitably, these lodge in vessels too small to permit their further passage, resulting in partial or complete occlusion of the vessel. Ninety-nine per cent of all emboli arise in thrombi (thromboembolism). Rare forms of emboli include fragments of bone or bone marrow, bits of tumor, foreign bodies such as bullets and bubbles of air or nitrogen. Unless otherwise qualified, the term embolus implies thromboembolism. Depending on their site of origin, they may come to rest anywhere within the cardiovascular system and are best discussed from the standpoint of whether they lodge in the pulmonary or systemic circuits, thus producing differing clinical effects.

PULMONARY EMBOLISM

Embolic occlusion of the large or small arteries of the pulmonary arterial tree is not only the most common form of embolism in man, it is also one of the most lethal. Postmortem studies of the general population of hospitals reveal that 6 to 8 per cent have grossly recognizable emboli within the pulmonary tree (Hume et al., 1970). In patients suffering from severe burns, trauma or fractures, these numbers rise to 25 to 30 per cent. Fatal pulmonary embolism is said to occur in 3 to 5 per cent of hospitalized patients found in the general wards of large hospitals, rising to 5 to 10 per cent in selected older groups who have suffered trauma (Sevitt and Gallagher, 1968) (Hume et al., 1970).

Approximately 95 per cent of all pulmonary emboli arise in thrombi within the veins of the legs (Fig. 9–12). As mentioned earlier, the deep veins of the calf muscles are the most common sites of origin, followed by the larger veins of the lower legs (p. 326). Uncommonly, involvement of the veins in the pelvis — i.e., the periprostatic, broad ligament, periovarian and uterine veins — gives rise to emboli. Dislodgement of such thrombi, in part or whole, produces an embolus, which flows with the venous drainage through progressively larger vessels to the right heart. Unless the blood clot is very large, it passes through the capacious chambers and the valves of the right side of the heart, and enters the pulmonary arterial circulation. Infrequently, long masses impact astride the bifurcation of the main pulmonary artery to create a *saddle embolus* (Fig. 9–13). More often, they occlude a major pulmonary vessel or pass further out into the periphery of the pulmonary vasculature to occlude smaller vessels. Occasionally, showers of small emboli may have the same effect as a large embolus.

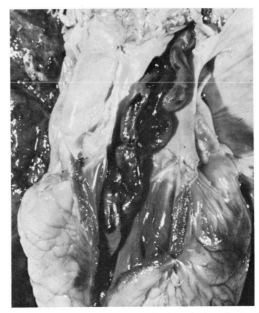

Figure 9–12. *A large coiled embolus from the veins of the lower legs lies in the right ventricle and pulmonary artery, and almost completely covers the pulmonary valve.*

Rarely, emboli may enter the right side of the heart and pass through interatrial or interventricular septal defects to gain access to the arterial side of the circulation (*paradoxical embolism*).

The clinical significance of pulmonary embolism depends upon the size of the occluded vessel and the general status of the cardiovascular system. Large emboli are commonly

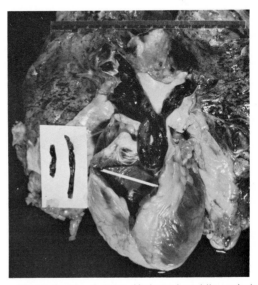

Figure 9–13. *A large Y-shaped saddle embolus from the femoral veins fills the pulmonary artery and its two major divisions.*

fatal. They cause sudden death due to systemic anoxia or massive strain on the right side of the heart with resultant sudden right-sided cardiac failure. Young patients with sufficient cardiac reserve may survive this insult, but death usually follows in elderly people with underlying cardiopulmonary disease. The suddenness of death may be extremely dramatic. A patient may stand up after a period of confinement to bed and suddenly topple over silently with a massive embolus. One well remembered patient appeared to be eating her meal cheerfully when she suddenly gasped in the middle of a spoonful of food and died within minutes. A massive pulmonary embolus had arisen silently from the femoral vein of the right lower leg and occluded the main pulmonary artery. Such massive pulmonary emboli rarely cause infarction. Either the patient suddenly dies or, if there is sufficient blood flow to sustain life, it is generally adequate to sustain the vitality of the lung tissue.

Many emboli, although large, permit some flow about their margins. If the patient survives the initial impact, the embolus may contract as do all blood clots. Fibrinolytic activity may then further reduce its size and, in this fashion, an adequate blood flow is reestablished (Soloff and Rodman, 1967). Serial angiograms have shown, in some patients, remarkable resolution of such pulmonary emboli with total lysis in the course of a few days of the vascular obstruction, particularly in the relatively young patient capable of surviving the initial blow (Sabiston, 1968).

When pulmonary emboli are smaller, they are less likely to cause sudden death. Smaller emboli travel out into the more peripheral areas of the lung where they become impacted and cause either pulmonary hemorrhage or infarcts. At the same time, the increased resistance to flow which they induce may be responsible for hypertension within the pulmonary circuit (p. 789). In the relatively young patient without cardiac or circulatory insufficiency, the bronchial circulation suffices to sustain the vitality of the tissue which has lost its pulmonary arterial flow. Such emboli cause intra-alveolar hemorrhage, as well as signs of respiratory difficulty, but there is no ischemic necrosis of tissues. *Pulmonary embolism, therefore, is not synonymous with infarction.* In the older patient with an impaired cardiovascular circulation, the bronchial arteries cannot adequately compensate for the loss of the pulmonary supply, and infarction ensues. In two series of cases, the frequency of infarction in the presence of embolism ranged from 60 to 30 per cent (Parker and Smith, 1958) (Freiman et al., 1965). It should not be forgotten that the pa-

tient who has had one pulmonary embolus risks having a second or multiple events resulting from fragmentation of the primary thrombus or from multiple primary sites. It is generally held that a previous episode of embolism carries a greater than 50 per cent chance of recurrence.

SYSTEMIC EMBOLISM

This term refers to emboli which travel through the arterial circulation. Such emboli arise almost always in thrombi within the left ventricle (myocardial infarction or other forms of myocardiopathy) or within the left atrium (rheumatic heart disease, postsurgical cardiotomy). Emboli less often arise in thrombi overlying severe atherosclerotic disease of the aorta and major arteries. Such thrombi are usually firmly attached to the severely eroded and damaged arterial wall. Fortunately, the various forms of vegetative endocarditis (bacterial and nonbacterial) are uncommon diseases. However, when present, the vegetations are extremely prone to fragment and embolize. Since the valves of the left side of the heart are much more frequently involved than those on the right, the emboli affect the systemic arterial circulation. Rarely, smaller arteries may give rise to emboli, but usually intravascular thrombosis of these secondary vessels produces a firm, occlusive thrombus which blocks the flow of blood and therefore minimizes the likelihood of embolization.

By contrast with venous emboli, arterial emboli follow a much shorter and more varied pathway since they travel through vessels of progressively diminishing caliber. *The brain, lower extremities, spleen and kidneys are most often the victims of arterial embolism.* The blood supply to the brain arises from major arterial trunks which receive a large portion of the total left ventricular output. Embolic masses entering these large vessels assume a central position in the laminar stream of flow, fail to enter lateral vessels and ultimately are halted in the vessels of the brain, the fairly direct terminus of the flow of the innominate and carotid arteries. Infarction of the brain may or may not occur, depending upon the level at which the vascular occlusion occurs. Within the circle of Willis, collateral supply may prevent infarction. However, impaction within the cerebral and cerebellar arteries causes ischemic necrosis within the dependent brain substance.

The legs also represent a major terminus of the arterial flow in the descending aorta. Emboli frequently affect the spleen and kidneys, owing mainly to the large volume of blood flow through these organs. Approximately one-fourth of the left ventricular output passes through the kidneys, and a large fraction passes through the spleen. *Unlike emboli in the lungs, those that impact in the systemic arterial circulation almost always cause infarction of the affected parts.* Bacteria-laden emboli from bacterial vegetative endocarditis cause septic infarcts which may be rapidly converted to large abscesses.

AIR OR GAS EMBOLISM (CAISSON DISEASE)

Bubbles of air may gain access to the circulation during delivery or abortion when it is forced into ruptured uterine venous sinuses by the powerful contractions of the uterus. Air embolization may also occur during the performance of a pneumothorax when a large artery or vein is ruptured or entered accidentally. It may also be observed when injury to the lung or the chest wall opens a large vein and permits the entrance of air during the negative pressure phase of inspiration. These bubbles of air act as physical masses. Many small bubbles may coalesce to produce frothy, gaseous masses, sufficiently large to occlude a major vessel, usually in the lungs or brain. The resulting symptoms are as would be expected —signs of acute respiratory distress or sudden neurologic disturbances such as convulsions or deep coma. Aggregates of larger size may become trapped in the chambers of the right heart and block the orifice of the pulmonary artery. Sudden death may result in any of these circumstances (Barley, 1956). From animal experiments, it appears that large quantities of air, probably somewhere in the neighborhood of 100 cc., are required to produce significant disease in man, and the small amounts which are commonly introduced during intravenous therapy are of no significance, since they rapidly dissolve in the plasma.

When air or gas embolism is suspected, it is necessary at autopsy to open the heart and major pulmonary trunks under water to detect the escaping gas. At times the frothy appearance of the blood calls attention to the presence of the air.

A specialized form of gas embolism, known as *caisson disease* or *decompression sickness,* occurs in divers, underwater construction workers and in those otherwise exposed to increased atmospheric pressures. The high pressure causes increased amounts of the atmospheric gases to dissolve in the blood and tissue fluids. If the patient then passes too rapidly from high to low pressures (decompresses too rapidly), the dissolved oxygen, carbon dioxide and nitrogen will come out of solution as minute bubbles. The oxygen and carbon dioxide will be rapidly reabsorbed, but the nitrogen, which is of low solubility, may remain as minute bubbles or may coalesce to form large masses of gas within the blood vessels and tissues. The same sequence may occur in air flight in unpressurized cabins with rapid ascent from ordinary barometric pressures to extremely high altitudes.

Clinical symptoms are produced either by the numerous minute emboli of nitrogen gas within vessels or by the formation of bubbles within the interstitial tissues of the body. The muscles, tendons and ligaments are particularly affected, attributed by Catchpole and Gersh (1947) to the sudden and constantly changing local tissue tensions characteristic of these supporting tissues. The embolic occlusions and interstitial gas in and around the joints and skeletal muscles cause the patient to double up in pain, a phenomenon known as "the bends." The bubbles of gas may affect the brain and cause mental disturbances and even coma. A similar process in the lungs produces sudden respiratory distress, "the chokes." Embolization and infarction of the highly vascularized bones cause destruction of articular surfaces and joints. The heart may also be affected. These symptoms are promptly relieved by placing the individual in a compression chamber where the solution of the bubbles of nitrogen is accomplished by raising the barometric pressure.

FAT EMBOLISM (CIRCULATING FAT MICROGLOBULES)

An uncommon form of embolism is caused by the occlusion of small vessels of the microcirculation by fat globules. This curious phenomenon is encountered most often in patients suffering from severe traumatic injuries to fat-laden tissues such as fractures of bones containing fatty marrow or extensive damage to the subcutaneous fat depots. In a study by Scully (1956) of battle casualties dying within the first four weeks of wounding, fat embolism could be identified at necropsy in approximately 90 per cent. However, in only 1 per cent of these individuals could clinical manifestations be attributed to the microembolism.

The pathogenesis of this condition is considered to be injury to fat-bearing tissues, rupture of small venules and entrance of fat globules into the circulation (Peltier, 1957). Model systems have been developed which support such a possible sequence of events. Moreover, in traumatic cases, the not infrequent finding of bits of bone marrow bearing hematopoietic cells along with the fat globules supports this mechanical conception of fat embolism.

Fat embolism may also be encountered in nontraumatic cases. Usually it is an incidental autopsy finding and has not caused serious clinical dysfunction. In such cases, the appearance of fat microglobules in the blood is thought simply to represent emulsion instability of the chylomicrons of fat conceivably following a large or fatty meal. Alterations in the blood induced by stress or trauma might favor such coalescence (Tedeschi et al., 1968). Grossly demonstrable globules of fat have been visualized in the circulation in the absence of trauma in a variety of medical disorders including fatty liver, acute alcoholism, the hyperlipemia of diabetes and, indeed, in up to 20 per cent of randomly tested healthy individuals. In most instances, these minute globules, identified at necropsy, were completely without clinical significance since the patients had had no manifestations of microembolism during life (Tedeschi et al., 1971).

The significance of fat embolism depends largely on the size and quantity of the microglobules as well as the extent of the systemic involvement. At one end of the spectrum, the emboli are small and few in number, cause no symptoms and are discovered only by a careful search at autopsy As will be recalled, the demonstration of fat requires special techniques (p. 35). At the other end are the fatal cases in which the globules are larger, ranging from 10 to 20 microns in diameter Depending on their precise dimensions, they may obstruct the pulmonary vascular bed or pass through the lungs to enter the systemic arterial circulation and produce microcirculatory disturbances in the central nervous system Between these two extremes are occasional cases in which embolization causes respiratory or neurologic symptoms but permits survival.

The two potential pathways for the appearance of fat globules in the circulation are not mutually exclusive (Ellis and Watson, 1968). Traumatic fat embolism is probably the more sinister form clinically However, microglobules derived from chylomicrons have been held responsible for death in nine cases of human pulmonary fat embolism (LeQuire et al., 1959). While fat embolization is an uncommon clinical problem it has theoretical significance since it demonstrates the capability of showers of microemboli to induce serious clinical symptoms and even death from widespread microcirculatory arrest.

AMNIOTIC EMBOLISM—AMNIOTIC FLUID INFUSION

Amniotic fluid embolism, a potentially fatal maternal obstetric complication, has been described within the past 30 years. In the first cases of sudden death, attention was focused on the solid contents of the amniotic fluid (keratotic squames and lanugo hairs mixed with mucous and amorphous debris) which were found in the pulmonary vessels and alveolar capillaries (Fig. 9–14). Sufficient trauma occurs in labor to rupture venous sinuses and presumably the uterine contractions force the amniotic fluid into the opened venous sinusoids. It was presumed that death was due to widespread embolic obstruction of the pulmonary capillary bed. It is now appreciated that the clinical features do not derive from simple embolic phenomena, and it has been suggested that a better name for this disease might be *amniotic fluid infusion*. The solid and formed contents of the infusion may, indeed, contribute to circulatory blockade but amniotic fluid is rich in a thromboplastin-like substance, and the manifestations of vascular occlusion are now believed to be due mainly to disseminated intravascular coagulation (DIC). Amniotic fluid infusion is, then, one of the many causes of DIC discussed on p. 744. Some of the patients die in respiratory distress or shock (usually during the first stage of labor) as a consequence of the widespread vascular occlusion. Others may have an episode of respiratory distress, then improve only to develop profuse bleeding, sometimes fatal, principally from the placental site because of the consumption coagulopathy (Bachmann, 1969).

INFARCTION

An infarct is a localized area of ischemic necrosis in an organ or tissue resulting from occlusion of either its arterial supply or venous drainage. The vascular occlusion is usually caused by thrombosis and/or embolism. However, vascular occlusion does not necessarily produce ischemic necrosis, as will soon be seen. It may cause only atrophy or focal cell death.

The great majority of infarcts result from embolic occlusion of the vital arterial supply to some tissue or organ. Systemic emboli arising in the heart or major arteries always impact in arteries, and venous thromboemboli likewise lodge in the pulmonary arterial system. In contrast, infarction due to venous occlusion is usually the consequence of an in situ thrombosis of a vein. *Interruption of the arterial blood*

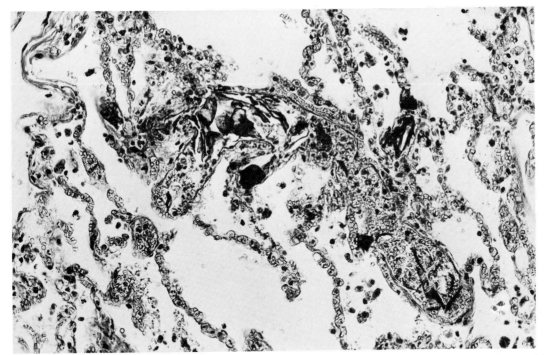

Figure 9–14. *Amniotic embolism. Masses of dark mucous debris and desquamated squames are present in the pulmonary vessels and alveolar capillaries.*

supply to a tissue produces ischemic necrosis more certainly than does venous obstruction. Thrombosis of veins may lead to pulmonary arterial embolism but, if the thrombus remains in situ, it may cause only stasis for a brief period of time until the increased venous pressure distal to the obstruction leads to dilatation of bypasses which at least partially restore the vascular flow in the affected tissue. However, in organs having a single venous outflow channel devoid of bypass channels, occlusion of this outflow may induce infarction. Examples of this are seen when the venous drainage of the testis or ovary is blocked. Arterial flow must soon come to a standstill since it has no escape through venous bypasses and infarction often develops.

Much more rarely, occlusion of a vessel and infarction may be caused by other forms of vascular disease, such as a large atherosclerotic plaque in the wall of a medium or small-sized artery, compression of vessels by expansile tumors, or inflammatory fibrous adhesions. Vascular occlusion may also result from the twisting of the pedicle of a mobile viscus, such as a loop of bowel or the ovary. The venous drainage or arterial supply of loops of bowel which become trapped in narrow-mouthed hernial sacs may also become severely narrowed or totally compromised. External pressures and torsions usually lead to embarrassment of venous flow, since the veins

are more readily compressed than the arteries. In all of these instances, the final occlusive episode is thrombotic closure of the narrowed vessel.

Types of Infarcts. Infarcts are classified on the basis of their color and the presence or absence of bacterial contamination. Infarcts are either *anemic (white) or hemorrhagic (red). Venous infarcts (such as occur in the testes and ovaries) are almost invariably intensely hemorrhagic. When a solid tissue is deprived of its arterial circulation, the infarct may be transiently hemorrhagic, but most become pale in a very short time* (Sheehan and Davis, 1958). The reasons for the development of pallor in most organs are as follows. In the area of ischemia, vessels, particularly the capillaries, as well as parenchymal cells are destroyed. At the moment of vascular occlusion, blood from anastomotic peripheral vessels flows into the focus of injury, producing the initial hemorrhagic appearance. If the tissue affected is solid, the seepage of blood is minimal. Soon after the initial extravasation, the red cells are lysed and the released hemoglobin pigment either diffuses out or is converted to hemosiderin. In solid organs, therefore, the arterial infarct will soon (24 to 48 hours) become pale. The heart, spleen and kidneys are representative of solid, compact organs which tend to have pale infarcts (Fig. 9–15).

In contrast, arterial infarcts in loose tissue

are usually so hemorrhagic that they remain red. The loose honeycombed tissue of the lung provides an example of hemorrhagic infarction secondary to arterial obstruction. At the moment of infarction, large amounts of hemorrhage collect in the spongy pulmonary parenchyma, and so the arterial infarction remains red (Fig. 9–16). However, this pattern is not invariable and, occasionally, pale infarcts may be encountered in the lung or hemorrhagic infarcts in the compact organs. The small intestine is another exception to the general rule. Here arterial occlusions may cause hemorrhagic infarction of long segments of the

Fig. 9–15

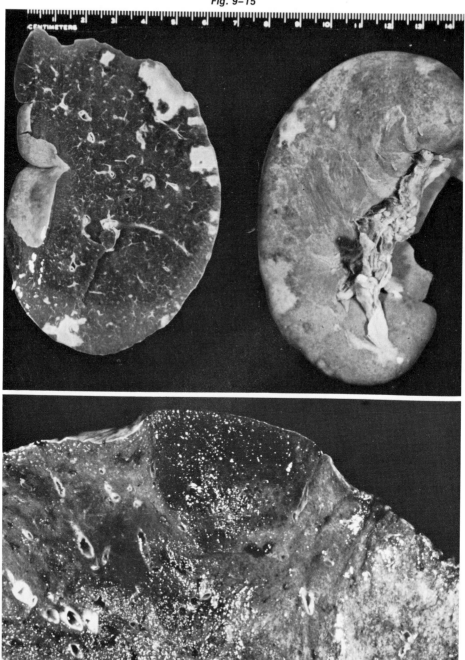

Fig. 9–16

Figure 9–15. Multiple small, peripheral, pale infarcts in a spleen viewed from the capsular surface and cross section.

Figure 9–16. A sharply circumscribed hemorrhagic infarct in the lung.

intestine. The explanation lies in the rich arterial anastomoses between the many branches of the superior mesenteric artery which permit arterial flow to the injured segment through anastomosing arcades. Indeed, this type of vascular supply may well protect against ischemic damage (p. 343). Hemorrhagic arterial infarction is sometimes encountered in the brain as well. An embolus to a large artery such as the middle cerebral may produce a nonhemorrhagic area of cerebral infarction. Soon thereafter, the embolus may shatter and the fragments may move into smaller more peripheral branches. Reflow through the major trunk may yield extensive hemorrhage into the primary area of ischemic necrosis.

Infarcts are also classified as either *septic* or *bland*, depending upon the presence or absence of bacterial infection in the area of necrosis. Bacterial contaminations may be due to organisms present in the tissue prior to the development of the ischemic necrosis, as in infarction of a lung already affected by bacterial pneumonia, or may be brought to the area by an infected blood clot, as occurs with embolization of a fragment of bacterial vegetation from a heart valve; or they may result from bacteremic seeding of the margins of the area of ischemic necrosis.

Morphology of Infarcts. Whether hemorrhagic or pale, all infarcts tend to be wedge-shaped, with the apex of the wedge pointing toward the focus of vascular occlusion. The external aspect of the organ forms the base of the wedge. The exact outline of the infarct may be quite variable, and sometimes map-like patterns result from the preservation of small marginal areas of tissue which have different and unaffected sources of blood supply.

A few hours after onset, all infarcts are somewhat poorly defined, are only slightly darker in color than normal and have a firmer consistency than surrounding normal tissue. During the next 24 hours, the demarcation between normal and infarcted tissue becomes better defined, and the color change is more intense. In the solid organs, the infarct may then appear paler than normal, as the small amounts of hemorrhage are lysed, whereas in the spongy tissues the massive hemorrhage makes the lesion red-blue. The increased consistency of the infarct is due to the suffusion of blood and inflammatory exudation (Karsner and Austin, 1911).

In the course of several days, pale infarcts become yellow-white and sharply demarcated from the surrounding tissue while the appearance of the pulmonary hemorrhagic infarcts remains relatively unchanged. The margins of both types of infarcts tend to become better defined by a narrow rim of hyperemia due to the marginal inflammatory response (Fig. 9-17). The involved surface of the organ is usually covered by an inflammatory exudation which is commonly fibrinous. In venous thrombosis and infarction, the areas of hemorrhagic necrosis may be somewhat poorly delimited because the intense, edematous, hemorrhagic response tends to blend gradually into the adjacent normal tissue. In venous occlusions of the small intestine, for example, it is sometimes quite difficult to clearly delimit the border between viable and nonviable gut.

The characteristic cytologic change of all infarcts save those in the brain is ischemic coagulative necrosis of the affected cells (p. 40) (Fig. 9-18). The tissue cells undergo the progressive changes of coagulative necrosis, and resorption discussed in Chapter 2. These basic changes may be considerably masked or modified by the extensive hemorrhage in hemorrhagic infarcts and by the bacterial suppuration in septic infarcts. In the infarct that has occurred only a few hours prior to the death of the patient, there may be no demonstrable cellular change since there may have been insufficient time for enzymic transformation of the dead cells. If the patient lives for less than 12 to 18 hours, only hemorrhagic suffusion may be present.

Inflammatory exudation begins after the first few hours and becomes better defined over the next few days (Fig. 9-19) (Sheehan and Davis, 1958). The inflammatory reaction is followed by a fibroblastic, reparative response beginning in the preserved margins. Some parenchymal regeneration

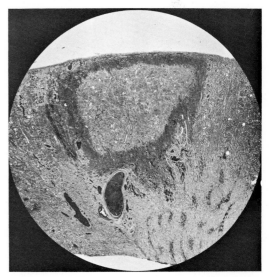

Figure 9–17. *A low power view of a small renal infarct enclosed within a zone of dark hyperemia and hemorrhage.*

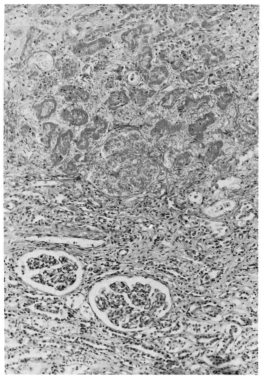

Figure 9–18. *The margin of a renal infarct in detail. Outlines of coagulated tubules remain (above) and are separated from the normal renal substance by a wide band of fibrosis.*

may occur at the periphery where the underlying framework of the organ has been spared. However, in most cases the necrotic focus is replaced by scar tissue. In very large infarcts, the replacement of the central necrotic tissue may be long delayed, probably because the blood supply to the advancing margin of granulation tissue becomes constricted by the previously formed peripheral dense scar. On this basis, in some infarcts, months-old, dense fibrous scar may be found enclosing areas of persistent ischemic necrosis. Ultimately, however, these infarctions end up as fibrous scars, just as do all areas of extensive tissue destruction (Fig. 9-20).

Septic infarction complicates the sequence by adding a more marked element of acute suppurative inflammatory necrosis. The infarct is then converted to an abscess and, if seen at a very late stage, may be unrecognizable as an infarct. The inflammatory reaction is correspondingly greater, but the eventual sequence of organization follows the pattern already described.

The brain is an exception to these generalizations. When it suffers ischemic necrosis, the affected area promptly and rapidly undergoes liquefaction (p. 39). The microglia constitute the scavenger cells of the brain, and these phagocytize the cellular debris while the other glial cells in the margins proliferate and invade the area (gliosis) to comprise the reparative scar.

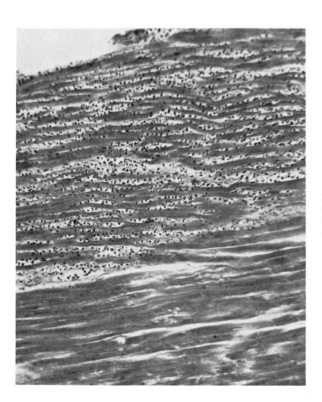

Figure 9–19. *A high power microscopic detail of infarcted myocardium. All the fibers are coagulated and their nuclei have disappeared. Inflammatory exudation has infiltrated only part way into the necrotic focus.*

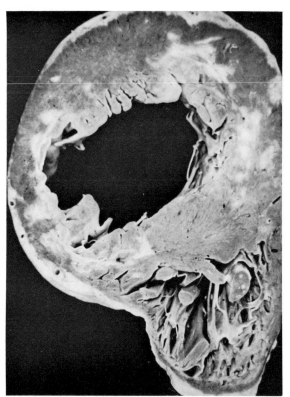

Figure 9–20. Numerous old myocardial infarcts have resulted in scattered pale fibrous scars through the myocardium.

Factors Conditioning the Severity of Injury Resulting from Vascular Occlusion.

Most often, loss of the arterial supply of a tissue or organ results in infarction. Obstruction to the venous outflow less predictably causes ischemic necrosis. But both arterial and venous vascular obstructions may be without effect or may cause only atrophy or single cell necroses. The extent to which a tissue is disturbed by occlusion of its venous or arterial connections depends upon a number of factors: (1) the general status of the blood and the cardiovascular system, (2) the anatomic pattern of the vascular supply, (3) the rate of development of the occlusion and (4) the vulnerability of the tissue to ischemia.

General Status of the Blood and the Cardiovascular System. Any systemic alteration which reduces the oxygen-carrying capacity of the blood or the velocity and volume of blood flow through the tissues predisposes to infarction. Severe anemia or reduced oxygenation of the blood (as in chronic cardiac or lung disease) predisposes to tissue anoxia. Anemia may exert its effect not only by reduction in the hemoglobin mass, but in other ways as well. Sickle

cell anemia is characterized by logjamming of the misshapen erythrocytes, and the stasis creates tissue hypoxia. Infarctions are common in these patients. In the very aged patient with marked coronary atherosclerosis, myocardial infarction may occur subsequent to the development of severe anemia or sudden drops in blood pressure, even in the absence of total occlusion of a vessel. Blood loss and shock impair the oxygenation of all tissues and thereby render tissues vulnerable to further diminution of their vascular supply.

Anatomic Patterns of Arterial Supply. The various tissues and organs of the body receive their arterial supply through one of four patterns: (1) a double blood supply, (2) parallel arterial systems, (3) "single" arterial supply with rich interarterial anastomoses and (4) "single" arterial supply with few anastomoses, insufficient to provide adequate bypass channels, so-called "end arteries." Obviously there are many gradations between the last two patterns. The lungs and the liver are examples of organs fortunately provided with dual blood supplies. In individuals having a normal hematologic and cardiovascular status, the bronchial circulation is capable of preventing ischemic necrosis when a radicle of the pulmonary artery is obstructed. Similarly, infarction is extremely uncommon in the liver because the portal supply of blood may be adequate even when the hepatic arterial flow is compromised. However, in the presence of cardiac failure, severe anemia or reduced oxygenation of the blood, occlusion of one system may precipitate ischemic necrosis.

Parallel arterial systems are encountered in the forearm and brain. Either the radial or the ulnar artery is sufficient to sustain the vitality of the tissues of the forearm when the other is occluded. The brain with its circle of Willis is protected from ischemic injury resulting from an occlusion at any point *in* the circle of Willis or in one of the major arteries *supplying* the circle. Such a proposition, of course, implies the absence of preexisting vascular disease within the circle of Willis. These comments should not be construed to apply to the arterial supply to the brain *derived from* the circle of Willis. Occlusion of one of the cerebral or cerebellar arteries will, of course, cause infarction of the dependent region of the brain. Indeed, cerebral infarction (encephalomalacia), more popularly known as a "stroke," is a major cause of disability and death.

The small intestine is the prototype of a tissue enjoying an arterial supply with rich interarterial anastomoses. The branches of the superior mesenteric artery are interconnected by looping arcades enabling blood to bypass focal occlusion. If, however, one of the primary divisions of the superior mesenteric artery or the main artery itself is obstructed, the arcades cannot provide compensation.

The kidney is the unfortunate victim of an arterial supply composed of "end arteries." The major branches of the renal artery supply well defined segments of the kidneys, and occlusion of one of these major branches or, of course, the main renal artery is almost invariably followed by ischemic necrosis. Obviously, if the occlusion occurs at the terminal ramifications, there may be sufficient blood flow from contiguous capillary beds to prevent tissue injury, but such a happenstance applies only to extremely small vessels on the order of arterioles.

The heart is an example of an organ having an intermediate pattern of fairly rich interarterial anastomoses which are not adequate to compensate for occlusion of one of the three main trunks of the coronary arterial system. Perfusion techniques have confirmed the presence of fine interarterial anastomoses joining each of the major coronary trunks to the others (Robbins et al., 1966). In the normal heart, these are usually less than 40 microns in diameter. While anatomically present, they are inadequate to prevent ischemic necrosis in most hearts when a major trunk is suddenly obstructed, as is attested to all too graphically by the frequent occurrence of myocardial infarction with occlusion of only one of the coronary arteries. However, when slow narrowing of one coronary artery occurs, these small anastomoses may enlarge to augment the blood supply to the myocardium dependent on the partially obstructed artery. Under these circumstances, if the stenosis eventually reaches total occlusion, the enlarged bypass channels may prevent ischemic necrosis.

It is apparent that the anatomic pattern of the vascular supply of a tissue materially modifies the consequence of a vascular occlusion.

Rate of Development of Occlusion. Slowly developing occlusions are far better tolerated than those occurring suddenly. Reference to this situation has just been made above in regard to the coronary arterial system. Although best studied in the heart, this same phenomenon must occur elsewhere since it is not uncommon to find at necropsy small arterial obstructions without infarction of the dependent tissues.

Vulnerability of Tissue to Ischemia. Tissues of the body vary widely in their susceptibility to ischemic hypoxia. The ganglion cells of the central nervous system are undoubtedly the most sensitive, and complete anoxia for a period of only a few minutes may produce irreversible changes. Indeed, a hierarchy of vulnerability to ischemia has been described for the varying cell types within the brain (Krainer, 1958). Cerebral cortical neurons are most sensitive to hypoxia followed in order by those in the cerebellum and by those in the basal ganglia. The glial cells are more resistant than ganglion cells, but also have differing sensitivities. The epithelial cells of the proximal convoluted renal tubules (more so than the other tubular segments) and the myocardial cells are likewise exquisitely sensitive to hypoxia. By contrast, the mesenchymal tissues of the body are in general quite resistant. The robustness of the fibroblast permits the axial framework and stroma of a tissue to remain vital despite ischemic necrosis of its more sensitive parenchymal cells.

Clinical Significance of Infarction. The clinical importance of infarctions cannot be overstated. In the U.S. in 1967, over half of all deaths were caused by cardiovascular disease. Most of these cardiovascular deaths resulted from myocardial and cerebral infarctions. Coronary heart disease alone accounts for about 30 per cent of all the mortality, and myocardial infarction is by far the predominant cause of fatal coronary heart disease (Fig. 9–21). Cerebral infarction (encephalomalacia) is also the most frequent type of central nervous system disease. Pulmonary infarction is an extremely common complication in a variety of clinical settings, as has been indicated, and is a major cause of death in hospitalized patients. Renal infarction does not have the paramount importance of these other forms mentioned. It is, nonetheless, an occasional cause of renal failure and death, and is a not uncommon cause of clinical signs and symptoms. Ischemic necrosis (gangrene) of the lower extremities is a relatively unusual clinical problem in the population at large, but is a major concern in diabetics. Infarction of tissues, therefore, is a commonplace cause of clinical illness.

The clinical course of a patient suffering from a myocardial infarction provides an excellent insight into the potential seriousness of thromboembolic complications. The usual myocardial infarction is due to atherosclerotic narrowing of the coronary arteries, and in most instances the final occlusion is produced by thrombosis superimposed on an area of narrowing (Friedman, 1970). In such atherosclerotic vessels, all the appropriate conditions exist for retrograde extension of the thrombus, enlarging the area of myocardial necrosis as more and more branches are

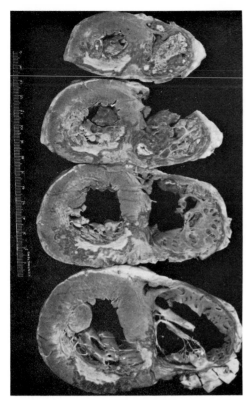

Figure 9–21. *The heart is cut in cross sections to disclose the large area of relatively fresh, pale infarction that resulted from coronary occlusion.*

blocked. Prevention of such extension is of ultimate importance. Moreover, in this disease the area of myocardial necrosis may extend to the endocardium and initiate mural thrombosis within the cardiac chambers. This is an obvious source of emboli that may scatter throughout the arterial tree, possibly lodging in such vital areas as the brain or kidneys. The attendant circulatory stasis, arrhythmias, confinement to bed and numerous other factors already cited in this chapter make thromboses within the veins of the lower extremities and possibly pulmonary embolization additional considerations of grave significance in these patients. Thrombosis, embolism and infarction comprise a lethal triad that stalks every ill, bedridden and aged patient, regrettably those least able to cope with them.

SHOCK

Shock is a complex syndrome appropriately discussed here because it is basically a form of low perfusion circulatory insufficiency. In reality, shock is not a single clinical syndrome as the name would imply, but a con-

stellation of syndromes encountered in a variety of clinical settings such as severe hemorrhage, trauma, burns, myocardial infarction, cardiac tamponade, massive pulmonary embolism and uncontrolled bacterial sepsis, to mention only the most important precursors. It is apparent that these disorders are quite varied, but all produce massive insult to the body and severe stress. The signs and symptoms of shock encountered in these diverse settings are inconstant. The most familiar syndrome consists of hypotension, weak thready pulses, cool clammy skin, tachycardia, alterations of respiration and sensorium, peripheral cyanosis and oliguria. But all shock patients do not have these findings. Some are flushed with a warm dry skin; others have no sensory alterations and are alert and indeed anxious; and all patients have changing signs and symptoms with the progression of this syndrome. One must delve down to the metabolic and cellular level to find commonalities among the many forms of shock.

Most fundamentally, *shock can be defined as a state of hemodynamic circulatory failure leading to impaired perfusion of tissues with resultant inadequate cellular oxygenation or oxygen utilization.* The anticipated chain of metabolic changes then ensues. Deprived of aerobic respiration, the cells revert, to the extent possible, to anaerobic glycolysis, but such energy sources are not adequate to indefinitely maintain normal levels of NAD, ATP and protein synthesis (Schumer and Sperling, 1968). In the absence of oxygen, pyruvate cannot be decarboxylated to acetic acid and so is reduced to lactate by lactate dehydrogenase. The pyruvic and lactic acids accumulate in the blood causing an acidosis, and the intracellular acidosis releases powerful lysosomal enzymes contributing to the cellular injury. While the brain and the heart are most dependent on aerobic respiration and, therefore, are most vulnerable to such disturbed homeostasis, reflex compensatory mechanisms partially protect these vital centers. But the impact of severe shock soon reaches them and so accelerates the downward spiral. How does this hemodynamic collapse and cellular oxygen deficit come about in the varied clinical settings cited? Several pathophysiologic pathways may be involved, but to understand them it is necessary to first consider in some detail the clinical circumstances in which the shock syndromes are encountered.

Classification. The frequent association of shock with certain disorders has given rise to a subdivision of shock into several clinical patterns.

Hemorrhagic shock follows acute loss of

some critical volume of blood. Massive hemorrhage is the most obvious and predictable cause of shock. The extent of blood loss necessary to induce shock varies with the rate of loss, the cardiopulmonary status of the patient prior to shock, the preshock oxygen-carrying capacity of the blood and the amount of tissue trauma associated with the hemorrhage. Slow loss of even 40 per cent of the blood volume is better tolerated than a sudden loss of 10 to 20 per cent. Such patients may go into shock within minutes or hours of the hemorrhage and are readily recognized with the familiar face of shock already described. Here the loss of blood volume underlies the inadequate perfusion of cells and presumably accounts for the cellular oxygen deficit.

Extensive body burns and severe trauma may both induce shock. *Burn shock* is largely the result of massive loss of fluids and electrolytes into the injured tissues. While the depth of the burn is important, of greater import is the amount of surface area involved. If a single lower extremity of man is denuded, up to six liters of fluid escape in a relatively short time. The resultant depletion of blood volume may be as extreme as in massive hemorrhage. *Traumatic* or *wound* shock may follow extensive physical trauma to tissues even in the absence of significant amounts of hemorrhage. Clearly, if there is massive bleeding, then the shock is attributable to the loss of blood volume. In the absence of such bleeding, the explanation of the hemodynamic collapse is less clear. It may be related to pain and neurogenic mechanisms postulated to cause alterations in the vasomotor control of the peripheral circulation with peripheral pooling of blood. Blood so sequestered in the periphery is removed from the effective circulating blood volume. *Surgical shock* is merely professionally precipitated wound shock.

Cardiogenic shock, sometimes called central failure, represents circulatory collapse resulting from suddenly developing insufficiency of the cardiac pump. Myocardial infarction is by far the most common cause of such pump failure, but it is also encountered in cardiac tamponade, serious cardiac arrhythmias, massive pulmonary embolism and rupture of papillary muscles or cardiac valves.

Septic shock is encountered in patients having overwhelming bacterial infections. The most common causative agents are the gram-negative rods with their elaboration of endotoxins, hence the designation *gram-negative endotoxic shock.* Uncontrolled gram-positive coccal infections may also cause septic shock. The pathophysiology of the circulatory collapse here is most unclear as will become evident in the following presentation.

Pathophysiology. The pathophysiology of the hemodynamic and metabolic alterations of the shock state encountered in the varied clinical disorders is still incompletely understood. It is best to admit at the outset that each patient is a problem unto himself. While certain common denominators may be found in the majority of instances, each patient develops his own constantly changing sequence of events. At the risk of oversimplification, three basic patterns of deranged physiology can be identified: (1) hypovolemia, (2) central or cardiogenic failure and (3) microcirculatory derangements.

Hypovolemia is the major operative factor in the pathophysiology of the shock state encountered with hemorrhage and burns. With the fall in blood volume, there is diminished venous return to the right heart, low central venous pressure, tachycardia, reduced stroke volume, low cardiac output and a drop in peripheral blood pressure (Hopkins et al., 1965). Mechanisms come into play to support the falling blood volume and blood pressure. Reflex sympathetic vasoconstriction triggered by baroreceptors initiates peripheral and splanchnic vasoconstriction and increased peripheral resistance. The skin thus assumes its ashen gray pallor and coldness, often admixed with an element of cyanosis. But the sympathetic mediated vasoconstriction does not cause significant constriction of either the cerebral or coronary arteries. In fact, it may cause slight vasodilatation of the latter. In this manner, blood is shunted from noncrucial areas to the heart and brain. The sympathetic peripheral vasoconstriction is supported by mechanisms involving the medullary vasomotor centers, adrenal catecholamines, aldosterone, ADH and the renin-angiotensin system. All of these compensations act both to conserve fluid and support the falling blood volume and blood pressure (Shoemaker, 1971) (Watts, 1965). In this manner, while the heart and brain are temporarily protected, the widespread vasoconstriction further worsens the perfusion of the peripheral tissues and the anaerobiosis, reflected in the progressive buildup of lactacidemia. Accompanying the elevated arterial blood lactate is a decreased cellular oxygen consumption as well as a decreased arterial venous oxygen difference indicating either some impaired utilization of oxygen by the cells or the opening of arteriovenous shunts.

A major consequence of the fall in blood pressure and peripheral vasoconstriction is impairment of renal function. Oliguria or even anuria can be important clinical problems demanding careful management and, indeed, the renal output is one of the reliable parameters of the depth of the circulatory collapse. The volume of urine produced varies almost in direct proportion to the effectiveness of the compensatory mechanisms and the therapy. When the urinary flood appears, the patient is on the road to recovery. If the compensatory mechanisms and appropriate therapy (particularly replacement of blood volume) do not, within the first day or two, bring the hemodynamic decline to a halt, the patient will go into a progressively rapidly deteriorating state erroneously called "irreversible shock" and will probably die. The basis of this turn for the worse is discussed on p. 349.

Central or cardiogenic shock might more descriptively be called pump failure. It may follow any disease producing acute cardiac failure, but the predominant cause is myocardial infarction. The importance of cardiogenic shock can be appreciated from the report of Friedberg (1969). Of 100 patients suffering an acute myocardial infarction, approximately 20 die before they reach the hospital, usually within four hours of the onset of their catastrophe. Of the remaining 80, approximately 10 to 15 die in the hospital even under optimal management. Most of these early hospital deaths are due to pump failure or cardiogenic shock. Primary arrhythmias, at one time almost as important a cause of death as pump failure, have largely been controlled by better monitoring and treatment. But once the pump begins to fail, there are no effective means of supporting the circulation and pump-assist devices have unfortunately proved to be of limited value.

Cardiogenic shock carries about a 75 to 80 per cent mortality rate. These patients present with a clinical symptom complex very much like that encountered in hypovolemic shock. Most are characterized by hypotension, pallor, cold skin, rapid thready pulse, oliguria or anuria, depressed sensorium and many go into coma and die. The hemodynamics of this syndrome are very similar to those encountered in hypovolemic shock, but certain differences should be noted, and there are many variations among patients. The basic hemodynamic defect is a great decrease in myocardial strength, reduction in stroke volume and cardiac output and consequent fall in blood pressure. In contradistinction to hypovolemic shock, the central venous pressure is usually elevated because of the reduced cardiac output. Compensatory mechanisms are now activated, such as were described in hypovolemic shock. Sympathetic vasoconstriction, increased peripheral resistance, tissue underperfusion, low urine output, reversion from aerobic to anaerobic metabolism, elevated blood lactate levels and fall in blood pH all follow (Haddy, 1970). It is confusing to report, however, that some patients present a somewhat different hemodynamic pattern. While most have a low cardiac output and elevated peripheral resistance, some have a normal or even high cardiac output and a normal or low peripheral resistance (Weil and Shubin, 1968). Much of this variability reflects the size of the infarct, the duration of the shock and the vigor and durability of reflex compensatory mechanisms. For example, a low peripheral resistance might be found late in the course when vasomotor control of arterioles had finally collapsed. Here, as in hypovolemic shock, unless the hemodynamic crisis can be brought under control, the patient will go into ever-deepening shock and die.

The term *microcirculatory derangements* refers to a variety of pathophysiologic alterations in the peripheral circulation which secondarily cause profound disturbances in the overall hemodynamic homeostasis of the patient. Some of the operative mechanisms are pooling of blood volume in the periphery (peripheral pooling), disseminated intravascular coagulation and abnormal permeability of capillaries with loss of plasma water and blood volume. These mechanisms are thought to underlie the shock encountered in patients with sepsis, endotoxinemia and trauma unassociated with hemorrhage; they may also contribute to cardiogenic shock. Peripheral pooling refers to the trapping of large volumes of blood in the capillary and venular beds. Lillehei and his colleagues (1964) have called attention to this mechanism in a variety of forms of shock. They postulate that, as the shock continues, the initial sympathetic vasoconstriction is followed by a phase of relaxation of the precapillaries as a consequence of the appearance of refractoriness of the arteriolar receptors to continued catecholamine stimulation. However, the postcapillary venous beds do not develop such refractoriness since they are capable of functioning normally in a lower pH range. Constriction at this locus continues after the arteriolar spasm has abated. As a result, the capillary beds become congested with blood, producing "stagnant anoxia." In this manner, a large volume of blood is sequestered in the periphery with reduction in the effective circulating blood volume, reduced venous return to the heart, low cardiac output, low blood pressure and reduced cellular perfusion. The stagnant anoxia in the periphery further contributes to the oxygen deficit in the cells with the consequent metabolic abnormalities already detailed (Rhoads and Dudrick, 1966).

Disseminated intravascular coagulation (p. 744) of the microcirculation is sometimes encountered in shock. Hardaway et al. (1967) contend that it is a major factor in the evolution of most forms of shock. It probably is not an initiating mechanism, but may play an important role in the hemodynamic deterioration of all forms of shock and undoubtedly contributes to the high mortality rate of persistent shock. Similarly, increased permeability of the microcirculation and vascular atony may be a mechanism of induction of shock, but it is more likely to be a late phenomenon that worsens the situation. Here it is proposed that the hypoxic injury to autonomic control centers and release of vasoactive substances including histamine, bradykinin and acetylcholine underlie the loss of peripheral resistance and expansion of the microcirculation (Weil and Shubin, 1967). In effect, paralysis of the peripheral vascular bed is postulated, along with an increased permeability leading to transudation of large volumes of fluid. Release of lysosomal enzymes may contribute directly to such microcirculatory injury as well as to the release of vasoactive agents such as bradykinin with its well known effects on capillary and venular permeability (Janoff et al., 1962).

We are far from understanding how sepsis or endotoxinemia induces microcirculatory derangements. Gram-negative endotoxins are lipoprotein carbohydrate complexes found in the O somatic antigens of the bacterial cell wall. It is clear from animal experimentation that endotoxin induces, in the dog for example, profound shock characterized by hypotension, decreased cardiac output, impaired peripheral perfusion and all of the metabolic alterations already described. While many patients with gram-negative sepsis present similar hemodynamic derangements, some, especially those with marked hyperthermia, have a low peripheral resistance, dilatation of the capillary beds in the skin and a flushed hot skin. It is true that later these patients may lapse into the more familiar syndrome with the cold, clammy skin and increased peripheral resistance. This variation in the presentation of septic shock illustrates the many faces by which this syndrome may be manifested. That endotoxin is a powerful shock agent is unchallenged, but how it acts is still obscure. One theory proposes that it triggers the release of vasoactive substances and thus causes peripheral pooling (Spink, 1962). Others propose that it reproduces a Shwartzman-like reaction characterized by

DIC (Corrigan et al., 1968). Still others suggest that endotoxin may damage the myocardium and thus cause hemodynamic collapse due to central failure (Kwaan and Weil, 1969). But even those who attribute endotoxic shock to central failure agree that gram-positive organisms, while causing shock, cause no reduction in the cardiac output. At this time, then, the understanding of the hemodynamic basis is far from clear (Christy, 1971) (Hardaway, 1965) (McKay, 1967).

The genesis of shock in nonhemorrhagic trauma is also thought to lie in microcirculatory derangements. However, undoubtedly other mechanisms such as some loss of blood and transudation of fluid in the wound also contribute. How the peripheral pooling is effected remains unclear. Pain and neurogenic mechanisms might lead to increased elaboration of catecholamines. While these at first might cause vasoconstriction, in time vascular atony might develop and lead to peripheral pooling. Neurogenic mechanisms, although poorly delineated, are undoubtedly capable of affecting the circulation as is well documented by individuals who experience a transient drop in blood pressure and faint at the mere anticipation of an injection. In the experimental animal, tourniquets applied to crushed extremities to prevent fluid loss do not prevent circulatory collapse if the nerves of the extremity remain intact. Whatever the pathways, neurogenic reflexes may mediate hemodynamic collapse, and such may be the explanation of traumatic shock.

It should be stressed that, in the individual patient, several mechanisms may act conjointly to bring about the hemodynamic deterioration. The patient with a serious infection not only has the microcirculatory changes described, but may also have some element of cardiac failure as well as losses of fluid into the site of infection. In cardiogenic shock, the perfusion deficit in the periphery may ultimately invoke peripheral pooling. We should conclude this discussion of pathogenesis of shock by emphasizing the complexity of the tangled changes encountered when the body is subjected to a massive assault. The lactic acidosis, for example, may lead to reduced arterial pCO_2 which, in turn, slows the respiration and precipitates a respiratory alkalosis. Changes in the gut, to be described later, may produce mucosal hemorrhages and loss of blood and fluids in all forms of shock. Intracellular changes in electrolytes are compounded by renal failure with its effect on fluid and electrolytic imbalances. In the shocked patient, homeostasis virtually comes apart.

"Irreversible" Shock. Whatever the form and cause of the shock state, it has long been known that unless the hemodynamic and metabolic deterioration can be promptly halted, there comes a point in time at which the patient's condition precipitously worsens and, despite all efforts, death is very likely to ensue (Lillihei et al., 1964). Regrettably, this phase of rapid decline has been called "irreversible" shock. The term derives from an experimental model of shock devised by Wiggers (1950). He showed that when a dog is bled to shock levels and the blood is not replaced for approximately four hours, total return of the original blood volume will be to no avail in 90 to 95 per cent of the animals. After an initial brief period of improvement following restoration of the original blood volume, most animals suddenly go into progressively deepening shock and die. Earlier replacement of the withdrawn blood brings about complete recovery of all but a few animals. At a crucial point in time, some irreversible change occurs in the shocked dog. Although some patients indeed pursue a similar clinical course and die despite all measures, there is no evidence to justify the extrapolation of the animal model to man. *No known clinical, biochemical or metabolic parameters have been found by which it can be determined unequivocably that the point of no return has passed for the patient.*

The pathophysiology of this phase of rapid hemodynamic and metabolic decline is, in part, explicable and, in part, obscure. Often it lies in the inability to control the primary cause of shock. As mentioned earlier, there is no adequate method of supporting or substituting for a massively damaged heart. Septic shock cannot be managed unless the bacterial infection is controlled. But, in addition to these obstacles, there is evidence that after a period of oxygen deficit the once constricted microvasculature and its vasomotor control become paralyzed, presumably as a result of serious hypoxic injury. Fine and his colleagues (1959) contend that absorption of bacterial products from the hypoxic injured gut plays an important role in this microcirculatory collapse. Whatever the precise mechanism, it is clear that in this agonal phase of shock, peripheral resistance falls and the capillaries become massive pools of stagnant blood. At the same time, the hypoxic injury increases capillary and venular permeability, and fluid is lost into the tissues. The fall in circulating blood volume becomes profound. All aerobic metabolism ceases and lactic acidosis rapidly mounts. Administration of more fluid or blood is followed by greater sequestration in the periphery, and

the clinician is faced with the dilemma of trying to fill a bucket with an ever-enlarging hole in its bottom. The metabolic deficits ultimately affect the heart even in those cases where there was no primary myocardial injury. Arteriovenous shunts further add to the therapeutic nightmare (Shoemaker, 1967). Perhaps release of lysosomal enzymes contributes to the deterioration. Despite the murkiness of the pathways involved, it is crystal clear that the patient in shock must be promptly and effectively treated if this phase of progressive decline is to be averted. But it is to be emphasized that the term "irreversibility" should never be put on the patient's chart until death writes it.

Morphology of Shock. The description of the anatomic changes is limited to those resulting from the shock state and does not include the lesions which induced the shock. Most of the changes encountered in shock are thought to result from the impaired perfusion of tissues and oxygen deficits, to which the intracellular metabolic derangements perhaps contribute. Although all tissues are adversely affected, the principal organs involved are the lungs, kidneys, heart, liver, gastrointestinal tract and brain.

The **lungs** manifest a variety of morphologic changes which collectively are referred to as "the shock lung." On gross inspection, they are wet, heavy, boggy and somewhat airless, changes indistinguishable from marked congestion and edema. Histologic examination confirms that, indeed, most of the gross appearance is the result of congestion and edema. The edema is not only intra-alveolar in location but is often interstitial as well. The accumulation of pericapillary and interstitial fluid produces widening of the alveolar septa and lifting of the alveolar lining cells from the underlying capillary wall. When the hypoxic injury is severe, increased capillary permeability permits plasma proteins to escape and form hyaline membranes lining the septa. Ultrastructural studies indicate that the escape of fluid occurs principally through venules. It also reveals considerable ultrastructural disorganization of the endothelial cells similar to that encountered in all hypoxic cells (Teplitz, 1968). In those forms of shock that develop disseminated intravascular coagulation, microthrombi may be found within the alveolar circulation.

The **kidneys** are perhaps the most severely injured organs in shock although, as shall be discussed later, the reasons for this are not entirely clear. At one time it was thought that the principal site of injury was the distal tubule within the nephron; hence the kidney lesions were called **lower nephron nephrosis** (Lucke, 1946). Later it was recognized that similar morphologic changes might be produced by mismatched transfusions or acute hemolytic crises, giving rise to the term **hemoglo-binuric nephrosis.** Still later, similar alterations were encountered in all forms of shock, adding such designations as **hypoxic nephrosis, shock kidneys and crush kidneys.** Today the preferred designation is **acute tubular necrosis (ATN).** It should, however, be made clear that acute necrotizing lesions of the tubules (nephrotoxic ATN) may be caused by toxic agents such as chloroform, mercury and sulfonamide overdosage. In our usage, the term ATN will be restricted to the renal lesions of shock and massive hemolytic disorders. The renal changes begin within 24 hours and become progressively more marked over the next 7 to 10 days, but then may undergo reversible regeneration in the surviving patient.

Grossly, acutely affected kidneys are usually somewhat enlarged and have somewhat pale, slightly widened cortices and deep red congested, cyanotic pyramids (Fig. 9–22). Sometimes the kidneys appear remarkably bland despite obvious clinical evidence of impaired renal function. The distal convoluted tubules are affected first. Early the cells appear swollen then undergo fatty change but, with progression, some are desquamated into tubular lumina and many die and disintegrate. Ultrastructurally, nonspecific organelle changes are inevitably present. These include swelling, distortion and rupture of mitochondria, vesiculation and disruption of endoplasmic reticulum, plasma membrane and tubular basement membrane breaks.

Soon thereafter, the damage extends more widely. Oliver and his colleagues (1951) in a scholarly study documented focal patchy destruction of segments of **all levels of the nephron** in the full-blown involvement. These focal injuries comprise tubular cell death and rupture of the tubular basement membranes designated by these re-

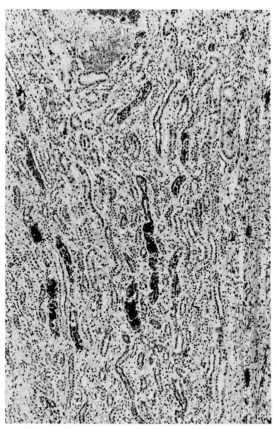

Figure 9–23. A low power detail of the medulla of a shock kidney with deeply pigmented casts in the collecting tubules.

searchers as **tubulorrhexis.** Accompanying these focal lesions are proliferation of marginal vital cells to create multinucleate tubular giant cells and edema with mononuclear infiltration of the circumambient interstitium. Additional common and prominent findings are dilatation of the proximal convoluted tubules and numerous scattered pigment casts, composed of hemoglobin or myoglobin, in the collecting tubules (Fig. 9-23). The epithelial cells about these casts often become necrotic (Fig. 9-24). Less distinctive but also present are proteinaceous casts. All of the changes described to this point become manifest within the first 3 to 4 days. On the assumption that the patient survives, implying control of the shock, the renal lesions progressively evolve. Beginning about day 5 or 6, mitotic activity can be found in the vital tubular epithelial cells adjacent to the focal areas of epithelial necrosis. These newly formed cells stretch out to cover long reaches of the denuded basement membrane. Over the course of the next week or two, depending upon the severity of the initial injury, the tubules are remarkably reconstituted. As will be seen, this regenerative activity is accompanied by return of renal function. Notably absent in ATN are glomerular and vascular lesions save in those forms of shock

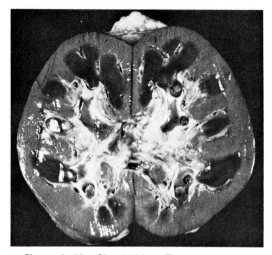

Figure 9–22. Shock kidney. The cortex is pale and the pyramids darkly pigmented by congestion and by the deposition of hemoglobin casts in the tubules.

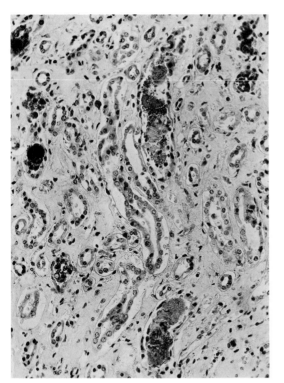

Figure 9–24. Shock kidney. Granular pigment casts are seen in the collecting tubules. Some of the tubular epithelial cells in the affected tubules are necrotic, while others are flattened, stretched-out and regenerating.

which develop DIC. In the latter circumstance, the microcirculatory thromboses are particularly prominent in the glomerular capillaries (Dalgaard, 1960).

The **adrenal** lesions encountered in shock constitute the reaction of this gland to all forms of stress and hence might be designated as the "stress response." Histologic changes occur at about 24 hours and by the third to fourth day are well established. These consist of focal depletion of lipids within the cortical cells, transforming them from their usual clear vacuolated state to nonvacuolated, so-called compact cells (p. 1298). The transformation to compact cells begins within the zona reticularis and then spreads toward the capsule into the adjacent zona fasciculata. It is uncommon for the entire zona fasciculata to be converted, presumably because of the acute short-term duration of the stress, if the patient is to survive. Scattered necrosis of isolated cortical cells may create apparent lumina or "pseudotubules." The loss of corticolipids has erroneously been interpreted as adrenal exhaustion. Ultrastructural studies indicate increased numbers of organelles in these compact cells indicative of increased functional activity with mobilization of the steroids in response to the stress. Confirming this interpretation is the finding of normal,

sometimes slightly lowered or even elevated levels of circulating adrenal steroids in the blood in these individuals. All of the adrenal alterations are completely reversible if the patient survives.

The **heart** demonstrates the anticipated changes of hypoxic and toxic injury. Myocardial cell swelling, fatty change and the organelle alterations described on p. 30 are often present. More severe alterations would probably be incompatible with survival. If the patient survives the acute episode, the myocardial alterations are completely reversible.

The **liver** similarly suffers hypoxic injury and sometimes accumulates fat within the hepatocytes in shock patients. Fatty change appears within the first day or two but is rarely of sufficient magnitude to alter either the gross appearance of the liver or its function. With survival the fat disappears.

The **gastrointestinal tract** in shock suffers patchy mucosal hemorrhages and necrosis designated as **"hemorrhagic gastroenteropathy"** (Bachrach and Thorner, 1963). The lesions are most common in the small intestine but may occur anywhere within the entire tract. Microscopically, the changes range from focal dilatation of submucosal capillaries and venules, accompanied by submucosal edema, to hemorrhagic extravasation of red cells and, in some cases, massive hemorrhage and necrosis of the mucosal lining cells of the intestine so that the entire surface of the gut appears to be a mass of disintegrating agglutinated red cells. Local superficial ulcerations may develop accompanied by an acute inflammatory infiltrate. It should be noted that the muscularis and serosa of the affected areas of the bowel are entirely normal, differentiating hemorrhagic gastroenteropathy from infarction due to either arterial or venous occlusions (Ming, 1965).

These intestinal lesions are reasonably ascribed to hypoxic injury to the mucosa reflecting the hemodynamic and metabolic deteriorations so characteristic of shock. Presumably, the reflex sympathetic splanchnic vasoconstriction first induces hypoxia but, with the continuation of the shock state, vascular atony leads to peripheral pooling and the reflow of blood into the injured areas of the intestine. Alternatively, it has been suggested that the lesions of the mucosa result from hypoxia-induced death of cells complicated by the lytic action of the intestinal enzymes.

The **brain**, as is well known, is extremely vulnerable to oxygen deficit and suffers widespread neuronal damage referred to as **anoxic** or **hypoxic encephalopathy** (p. 1505). Such neuronal damage accounts for the profound changes in the sensorium encountered in most patients in shock.

Clinical Course. The patient in shock walks a veritable tightrope. Early in the course, the major problems stem from the circulatory insufficiency and consequent cerebral ischemia. Cardiac failure may also become manifest at this stage due to the hypoxic injury to the myocardium. Soon thereafter, the progressive acidosis leads to serious electrolyte disturbances, and with the metabolic acidosis comes an increased respiratory rate which introduces new hazards. Even if all of these problems are surmounted, the renal functional deficit remains and, indeed, comprises one of the major threats to life after the crisis of the first few days has passed. While the urine output is diminished during the first 24 to 48 hours, in many patients it begins to fall dramatically anywhere from the second to sixth day to levels of perhaps a few milliliters per day. The BUN and creatinine which had been slowly rising now begin to increase rapidly concomitant with the appearance of life-threatening disturbances in fluid and electrolyte balance.

The dilemma is presented of a circulation which is volume depleted, requiring the administration of fluids to sustain the blood volume while, at the same time, there is virtually no urine output. The widespread cellular injury results in massive loss of intracellular potassium and ever-mounting levels of serum potassium with all of its potential sequelae (p. 690). Happily, judicious management of the fluid and electrolyte imbalances and dialysis, when necessary, can tide patients over this period; if the patient survives, some return of urine output may be anticipated toward the end of the second week. But the return of renal function does not begin slowly; it commences with a flood and, soon after the oliguric phase, the urinary output may reach levels of 3 or more liters per day. Because tubular epithelial cell function has not yet been completely restored, quantities of electrolytes, principally sodium and chloride, are washed out with the massive diuresis, causing a new set of electrolyte imbalances. The gastrointestinal lesions, melena and diarrhea add to the fluid and electrolyte losses. Indeed, about 25 per cent of deaths from ATN occur during this diuretic phase. In addition to these problems, for reasons that are not clear but perhaps are related to the widespread cellular hypoxia, these patients are extremely vulnerable to bacterial infections, particularly in the lungs, and these constitute yet another threat to life. Traversing the tightrope may require as long as three or four weeks but, if the underlying cause of the shock can be brought under control, the patient who survives this period may be expected to leave the hospital.

The mechanisms which underlie the oliguria are poorly understood. It is simplistic to ascribe it entirely to hypotension and reduced glomerular filtration. If this were the explanation, one would anticipate production of small amounts of concentrated urine, but such is not the case. The pathetically small volumes of urine have a low specific gravity. Moreover, many patients have a very transient or relatively minimal hypotensive episode and yet become oliguric, and the same clinical and anatomic changes are seen in ATN caused by massive hemolysis, in which there may be no hemodynamic deficit. A host of explanations for the oliguria have been offered, their very number indicating our lack of understanding. Juxtamedullary arteriovenous shunts have been invoked by Trueta and his associates (1947). They suggest shunting of the blood through juxtamedullary glomeruli and away from the renal cortex caused by neurovascular reflexes activated during the initial period of hemodynamic collapse or hemolysis. Persistence of such shunts in the corticomedullary junction would explain the marked hypoxic and tubulorrhectic injury to the cortical tubules and would likewise account for the reduced glomerular filtration.

Other explanations for the oliguria have been offered. Neurogenic impulses are postulated which increase renal vascular resistance, further decrease perfusion of the cortex and increase the flow in the medulla (Pomeranz et al., 1968). Such redistribution of renal blood flow might play a role in initiating the tubular injuries and reducing glomerular filtration, leading in turn to oliguria and anuria. Leakage of glomerular filtrate from tubules with ruptured basement membranes could account for both the reduced volume output and the increase in interstitial edema in ATN. On this same level of reasoning, the severe interstitial edema might cause blockage of tubules. Recently, yet another attractive hypothesis has been offered invoking increased renin secretion, afferent arteriolar constriction and hence reduced glomerular filtration (Wilson et al., 1969). With so many theories, it is evident that the mechanism of the renal failure is still not clear.

None of these mechanisms explains the characteristic low specific gravity of the urine or the appearance of pigment, usually hemoglobin casts, in the collecting tubules. Very recently, it has been proposed that the failure in the concentration mechanism in the shocked kidney results from impairment of the counter-current mechanisms within the renal medulla and papillae (Selkurt, 1969). Under normal circumstances, urinary concentration is largely achieved by osmotic equilibration of the urine with the hypertonic electrolyte levels of the peritubular interstitial tissue in the papillae. Such hypertonicity is normally achieved by the counter-current mechanism deep in the papillae. The buildup of the hyperosmolarity of the interstitium in the papillae is dependent upon a slow but stable flow of blood through the papillae and a normal volume of urine flow through the tubules. In shock, reduction in the glomerular filtration rate accompanied by reduced vascular perfusion of the papillae blocks this buildup of interstitial electrolytes and so the counter-current mechanism breaks down and we have both low urine volume and low specific gravity.

The origin of the pigment casts in ATN is unknown. Myoglobinuria and hemoglobinuria are not characteristic features of most forms of shock. Hemolysis of red cells in the stagnant anoxia of the peripheral pools has been invoked as well as lysis of red cells due to marked acidosis, but the evidence remains fragmentary, and it is better to admit the mystery of the origin of the pigment casts. It is apparent that much is still unknown about ATN but, whatever its origins, it is a reversible clinical and anatomic change, and complete restoration of function and structure are achieved in most surviving patients. It should be emphasized that this is a reversible form of renal failure.

It is evident that shock and its attendant lesions create a therapeutic nightmare. Underperfusion of the peripheral tissues invites the use of vasodilator agents (a stormy controversy at the time of this writing), but such agents expand the capacity of the circulatory bed and worsen the relative hypovolemia. Vasopressor agents which might support the blood pressure decrease the peripheral circulation. Blood transfusions and fluids are needed to sustain the effective circulating blood volume in patients critically vulnerable to fluid overload because of the renal shutdown. The metabolic acidosis often induces tachypnea with the production of respiratory alkalosis. But irreversibility of shock does not exist and, with modern methods of treatment, particularly careful management of fluids, electrolytes and the use of dialysis if necessary, 90 to 95 per cent of the patients with all forms of shock recover if its initiating cause can be managed.

REFERENCES

Ashford, T. P., and Freiman, D. G.: The role of the endothelium in the initial phases of thrombosis. Amer. J. Path., 50:257, 1967.

Bachmann, F.: Disseminated intravascular coagulation. D. M.,; 3, December, 1969.

Bachrach, W. H., and Thorner, M. C.: Hemorrhagic enteropathy complicating myocardial infarction. Amer. J. Cardiol., 11:89, 1963.

Barker, N. W., et al.: A statistical study of post operative venous thrombosis and pulmonary embolism. Proc. Mayo Clin., 15:769, 1940.

Barley, H.: Air embolism. J. Int. Coll. Surg., 25:675, 1956.

Belding, H. H.: Use of anticoagulants in prevention of venous thromboembolic disease in post operative patients. Arch. Surg., 90:566, 1965.

Berger, S.: Platelet function: a review. I. Normal function. Canad. Med. Ass. J., 102:1271, 1970.

Catchpole, H. R., and Gersh, I.: Pathogenetic factors and pathological consequences of decompression sickness. Physiol. Rev., 27:360, 1947.

Chinard, F. P.: Starling's hypothesis in the formation of edema. Bull. N.Y. Acad. Med., 38:375, 1962.

Christy, J. H.: Pathophysiology of gram-negative shock. Amer. Heart. J., 81:694, 1971.

Coon, W. W., and Coller, F. A.: Some epidemiological considerations of thromboembolism. Surg., Gynec., Obstet., 109:487, 1959.

Corrigan, J. J., et al.: Changes in the blood coagulation system associated with septicemia. New Eng. J. Med., 279:851, 1968.

Cotran, R. S.: The delayed and prolonged vascular leakage in inflammation. II. An electron microscopic study of the vascular response after thermal injury. Amer. J. Path., 46:589, 1965.

Dalgaard, O. Z.: An electron microscopic study on glomeruli in renal biopsies taken from human shock kidney. Lab. Invest., 9:364, 1960.

Deykin, D.: The clinical challenge of disseminated intravascular coagulation. New Eng. J. Med., 283:636, 1970a.

Deykin, D.: Local and systemic factors in the pathogenesis of thrombosis. Calif. Med., 112:31, 1970b.

Deykin, D.: Thrombogenesis. New Eng. J. Med., 276:622, 1967.

Deykin, D., and Wessler, S.: Activation product, factor IX, serum thrombotic accelerator activity and serum induced thrombosis. J. Clin. Invest., 43:160, 1964.

Deykin, D., et al.: Hepatic removal of activated factor X by the perfused rabbit liver. Amer. J. Physiol., 214:414, 1968.

Drill, V. A., and Calhoun, D. W.: Oral contraceptives and thromboembolic disease. J.A.M.A., 206:77, 1968.

Ellis, H. A., and Watson, A. J.: Studies on the genesis of traumatic fat embolsim in man. Amer. J. Path., 53:245, 1968.

Fine, J., et al.: The bacterial factor in traumatic shock. New Eng. J. Med., 260:214, 1959.

Food and Drug Administration: Final report on Enovid by the ad hoc committee for the evaluation of a possible etiologic relationship with thromboembolic conditions. Department of Health, Education and Welfare, Washington, D.C., 1963.

Food and Drug Administration: Report on oral contraceptives. Advisory Committee on Obstetrics and Gynecology, Washington, D.C., 1966.

Fred, H. L., et al.: Rapid resolution of pulmonary thromboemboli in man: an angiographic study. J.A.M.A., 196:1137, 1966.

Freiman, D. G., et al.: Pathologic observations on experimental and human thromboembolism. In Sasahara, A. A., and Stern, M. (eds.): Pulmonary Embolic Disease. New York, Grune & Stratton Inc., 1965, p. 81.

Friedberg, C. K.: General treatment of acute myocardial infarction. Circulation, Suppl. 4, 40:252, 1969.

Friedman, M.: Pathogenesis of coronary thrombosis intramural and intraluminal hemorrhage. Advances Cardiol., 4:20, 1970.

Gauer, O. H., et al.: The regulation of extracellular fluid volume. Ann. Rev. Physiol.,32:547, 1970.

Goldzieher, J. W.: Oral contraceptives: a review of certain metabolic effects and an examination of the question of safety. Fed. Proc.,29:1220, 1970.

Guyton, A. C.: Concept of negative interstitial pressure based on pressures in implanted perforated capsules. Cir. Res., 12:399, 1963.

Haddy, F. J.: Pathophysiology and therapy of the shock of myocardial infarction. Ann. Intern. Med., 73:809, 1970.

Ham, J. M., and Slack, W. W.: Platelet adhesiveness after operation. Brit. J. Surg., 54:385, 1967.

Hamilton, T. R., and Angevine, D. M.: Fatal pulmonary embolism in 1,000 battle casualties. Milit. Surg., 99:450, 1946.

Hardaway, R. M.: Microcoagulation in shock. Amer. J. Surg., 110:298, 1965.

Hardaway, R. M., et al.: Intensive study and treatment of shock in man. J.A.M.A., 199:779, 1967.

Honour, A. J., and Mitchell, J. R. A.: Platelet clumping in injured vessels. Brit. J. Exp. Path., 45:75, 1964.

Hopkins, R. W., et al.: Hemodynamic aspects of hemorrhagic and septic shock. J.A.M.A., 191:731, 1965.

Hovig, T.: Release of a platelet aggregating substance (adenosine diphosphate) from rabbit blood platelets induced by saline "extract" of tendons. Thromb. Diath. Haemorrh., 9:264, 1963.

Hovig, T.: The ultrastructure of rabbit blood platelet aggregates. Thromb. Diath. Haemorrh., 8:455, 1962.

Hovig, T., et al.: Experimental hemostasis in normal dogs and dogs with congenital disorders of blood coagulation. Blood, 30:636, 1967.

Hume, M., et al.: Venous Thrombosis and Pulmonary Embolism. Cambridge, Mass., Harvard University Press, 1970, p. 25.

Inman, W. H. W.: Role of drug-reaction monitoring in the investigation of thrombosis and "the pill." Brit. Med. Bull., 26:248, 1970.

Inman, W. H. W., and Vessey, M. P.: Investigation of death from pulmonary, coronary and cerebral thrombosis and embolism in women of child bearing age. Brit. Med. J., 2:193, 1968.

Innes, D., and Sevitt, S.: Coagulation and fibrinolysis in injured patients. J. Clin. Path., 17:1, 1964.

Izak, G., et al.: Studies on hypercoagulable state. II. The application of ^{131}I-labelled fibrinogen for the estimation of intravascular coagulation in human subjects. Thromb. Diath. Haemorrh., 18:544, 1967.

Janoff, A., et al.: Pathogenesis of experimental shock. IV. Studies on lysosomes in normal and tolerant animals subjected to lethal trauma and endotoxinemia. J. Exp. Med., 116:451, 1962.

Jorgensen, L.: Mechanism of thrombosis. In Ioachin, H. L. (ed.): Pathology Annual for 1971. New York, Appleton-Century-Crofts, 1971, p. 139.

Karsner, H. T., and Austin, J. H.: Studies in infarction. Experimental bland infarction of the kidney and spleen. J.A.M.A., 57:951, 1911.

Krainer, L.: Pathological effects of cerebral anoxia. Amer. J. Med., 25:258, 1958.

Kucera, M.: Some problems of venous thromboembolism in patients with heart disease. Rev. Czech. Med., 14:1, 1968.

Kwaan, H. M., and Weil, M. H.: Differences in the mechanism of shock caused by bacterial infections. Surg., Gynec., Obstet., 128:37, 1969.

LeQuire, V. S., et al.: A study on the pathogenesis of fat embolism based on human necropsy material and animal experiments. Amer. J. Path., 35:999, 1959.

Lillehei, R. C., et al.: The nature of irreversible shock: experimental and clinical observations. Ann. Surg., 160:682, 1964.

Lucke, B.: Lower nephron nephrosis. The renal lesions of the crush syndrome of burns, transfusion and other conditions affecting the lower segments of the nephrons. Milit. Surg., 99:371, 1946.

Luscher, E. F.: Platelets in hemostasis and thrombosis. Brit. J. Haemat., 13:1, 1967.

Marcus, A. J.: Platelet function. New Eng. J. Med., 28:1213, 1278, 1330, 1969.

McGovern, V. J.: Reactions to injury of vascular endothelium with special reference to the problem of thrombosis. J. Path. Bact., 69:283, 1955.

McKay, D. G.: Endotoxin shock. Trans. Coll. Physicians Phila., 34:137, 1967.

Merrill, A. J.: Edema and decreased blood flow in patients with chronic congestive heart failure: evidence of forward failure as primary cause of edema. J. Clin. Invest., 25:389, 1946.

Ming, S. C.: Hemorrhagic necrosis of the gastrointestinal tract and its relation to cardiovascular status. Circulation, 32:332, 1965.

Murphy, E. A., et al.: Encrustations and atherosclerosis: the analogy between early lesions and deposits in extracorporeal circulations. Canad. Med. Ass. J., 87:259, 1962.

Oliver, J., et al.: The pathogenesis of acute renal failure associated with traumatic and toxic injury: renal ischemia, nephrotoxic damage and the ischemuric episode. J. Clin. Invest., 30:1307, 1951.

Parker, B. M., and Smith, J. R.: Pulmonary embolism and infarction: a review of the physiologic consequences of pulmonary arterial obstruction. Amer. J. Med., 24:402, 1958.

Peltier, L. S.: An appraisal of the problem of fat embolism. Int. Abstr. Surg., 104:313, 1957.

Poller, L.: Progesterone oral contraception and blood coagulation. Brit. Med. J., 1:554, 1969.

Pomeranz, B. H., et al.: Neural control of intrarenal blood flow. J. Physiol., 215:1067, 1968.

Rector, F. C., Jr., et al.: Demonstration of a hormonal inhibitor of proximal tubular reabsorption during expansion of extracellular volume with isotonic saline. J. Clin. Invest., 47:761, 1968.

Rhoads, J. E., and Dudrick, S. J.:Hypovolemic shock. Postgrad. Med., 39:3, 1966.

Robbins, S. L., et al.: Demonstration of intercoronary anastomoses in human hearts with a low viscosity perfusion mass. Circulation, 33:733, 1966.

Roberts, G. H.: Venous thrombosis in hospital patients: a post mortem study. Scot. Med. J., 8:11, 1963.

Sabiston, D. C.: Pulmonary embolism. Surg., Gynec., Obstet., 126:1075, 1968.

Sandrock, R. S., and Mahoney, E. B.: Prothrombin activity: a diagnostic test for early post-operative venous thrombosis. Ann. Surg., 128:521, 1948.

Sartwell, P. E., et al.: Thromboembolism and oral contaceptives: an epidemiologic case-control study. Amer. J. Epidem., 90:365, 1969.

Sawyer, P. N., et al.: Irreversible electrochemical precipitation of mammalian platelets and intravascular thrombosis. Proc. Nat. Acad. Sci., 53:200, 1965.

Schumer, W., and Sperling, R.: Shock and its effect on the cell. J.A.M.A., 205:215, 1968.

Scully, R. E.: Fat embolism in Korean battle casualties: its incidence, clinical significance and pathologic aspects. Amer. J. Path., 32:379, 1956.

Selkurt, E. E.: Primate kidney function in hemorrhagic shock. Amer. J. Physiol., 217:955, 1969.

Sevitt, S.: Fatal road accidents: injuries, complications and causes of death in 250 subjects. Brit. J. Surg., 55:481, 1968.

Sevitt, S., and Gallagher, N. G.: Venous thrombosis and pulmonary embolism. A clinopathological study in injured and burned patients. Brit. J. Surg., 48:475, 1961.

Sevitt, S., and Gallagher, N. G.: Venous thrombosis and pulmonary embolism: a clinico-pathological study in injured and burned patints. Brit. J. Surg., 55:481, 1968.

Shaper, A. G., et al.: The platelet count, platelet adhesiveness and aggregation and the mechanism of fibrinolytic inhibition in pregnancy and the puerperium. J. Obstet. Gynaec. Brit. Comm., 75:433, 1968.

Sheehan, H. L., and Davis, J. C.: Complete permanent renal ischemia. J. Path. Bact., 76:569, 1958.

Sherry, S.: Fibrinolysis and thrombosis. In Sherry, S., Brinkhous, K. M., Genton, E., and Stengle, J. M. (eds.): Thrombosis. Washington D.C., National Academy of Sciences, 1969a, p. 585.

Sherry, S.: Thrombosis. Circulation, 40:755, 1969b.

Sherry, S., et al.: Thrombosis. Washington D.C., National Academy of Sciences, 1969.

Shoemaker, W. C.: Sequential hemodynamic patterns in various causes of shock. Surg., Gynec., Obstet., 132:411, 1971.

Shoemaker, W. C.: Shock. Chemistry, Physiology and Therapy. Springfield, Ill., Charles C Thomas, 1967.

Sise, H. S., et al.: On the nature of hypercoagulability. Amer. J. Med., 33:667, 1962.

Soloff, L. A., and Rodman, T.: Acute pulmonary embolism. Amer. Heart J., 74:710, 1967.

Soulier, J. P.: Inhibition of blood coagulation. IV. Natural inhibitors. Thromb. Diath. Haemorrh., Suppl. 1, 7:38, 1962.

Spaet, T. H.: Hemostatic homeostasis. Blood, 28:112, 1966.

Spaet, T. H.: The platelet in hemostasis. Ann. N.Y. Acad. Sci., 115:31, 1964.

Spaet, T. H., and Gaynor, E.: Vascular endothelial damage and thrombosis. Advances Cardiol., 4:47, 1970.

Spaet, T. H., and Zucker, M. B.: Mechanism of platelet plug formation and role of adenosine diphosphate. Amer. J. Physiol., 206:1267, 1964.

Spink, W. W.: Endotoxin shock. Ann. Intern. Med., 57:538, 1962.

Stengle, J. M.: Thrombosis. Blood, 35:867, 1970.

Stormorken, H., and Owren, P. A.: Physiopathology of hemostasis. Seminars Hemat., 8:29, 1971.

Tedeschi, C. G., et al.: Fat macroglobulinemia and fat embolism. Surg., Gynec., Obstet., 126:83, 1968.

Tedeschi, L. G., et al.: Fat particles in plasma. The macroglobule:

its relevance to the concept of fat embolism. Hum. Path., 2:165, 1971.

Teplitz, C.: The ultrastructural basis for pulmonary pathophysiology following trauma. J. Trauma, 8:700, 1968.

Todd, M. E., et al.: Changes in blood coagulation during pregnancy. Proc. Mayo Clin., 40:370, 1965.

Trueta, J., Barclay, E., Daniel, P. M., Franklin, K. J., and Prichard, M. M. L. (eds.): Studies of the Renal Circulation. Springfield, Ill., Charles C Thomas, 1947.

Vessey, M. P., and Doll, R.: Investigation between use of oral contraceptives and thromboembolic disease. A further report. Brit. Med. J., 2:651, 1969.

Virchow, R.: Cellular Pathology as Based upon Physiological and Pathological Histology. London, Churchill, 1860, pp. 197, 203.

Watts, T. D.: Adrenergic mechanisms in hypovolemic shock. In Mills, L. C., and Moyer, J. H. (eds.): Shock and Hypotension. Pathogenesis and Treatment. New York, Grune and Stratton, 1965.

Webber, A. J., and Johnson, S. A.: Platelet participation in blood coagulation aspects of hemostasis. Amer. J. Path., 60:19, 1970.

Weil, M. H., and Shubin, H. S.: Diagnosis and treatment of shock. Baltimore, Williams and Wilkins Co., 1967.

Weil, M. H., and Shubin, H. S.: Shock following acute myocardial infarction. Current understanding of the hemodynamic mechanism. Prog. Cardiovasc. Dis., 11:1, 1968.

Wessler, S.: Experimental thrombosis. Clin. Obstet. Gynec., 11:197, 1968.

Wessler, S.: Thrombosis in the presence of vascular stasis. Amer. J. Med., 33:648, 1962.

Wessler, S., and Yin, E. T.: On the mechanism of thrombosis. In Brown, E. B., and Moore, C. V. (eds.): Progress Haematology. New York, Grune and Stratton, 6:201, 1969.

Wiggers, C. J.: Physiology of Shock. New York, Commonwealth Fund, 1950.

Williams, W. J.: Recent concepts of the clotting mechanism. Seminars Hemat., 5:32, 1968.

Wilner, J. D., et al.: Aggregation of platelets by collagen. J. Clin. Invest., 47:2616, 1968.

Wilson, D. R., et al.: The role of the concentration mechanism in the development of acute renal failure: micropuncture studies using diabetes insipidus rats. Nephron, 6:128, 1969.

Wooley, C. F.: Nonbacterial thrombotic endocarditis, clinical recognition. Arch. Intern. Med., 125:126, 1970.

World Health Organization. Technical report series No. 326, 1966.

Zucker, M. B., and Borelli, J.: Platelet clumping produced by tissue suspensions and by collagen. Proc. Soc. Exp. Biol. Med., 109:779, 1962.

10

INFECTIOUS DISEASES

GENERAL FEATURES

Although in economically developed countries microbiologic diseases are no longer major causes of death, they are still rampant in many parts of the world. They are of particular importance to the physician because they represent a form of illness in which correct diagnosis and appropriate treatment can effect "miracles." With the discovery of the potent antibacterial drugs, the erroneous impression at first prevailed that these diseases were a thing of the past. It was said jocularly: "When a patient has a fever you give him penicillin and if he hasn't recovered in two days you examine him." As every physician knows, nothing is further from the truth. Every chemotherapeutic drug has limits to its usefulness and is more effective with some agents than with others. It is more important than ever to establish the precise etiology of microbiologic diseases if merely to select the most effective antibacterial treatment.

Before considering microbiologic diseases in detail, certain fundamentals are worthy of consideration: (1) the general characteristics of microbiologic agents responsible for causing disease in man, (2) the reaction of the host to these invading agents and (3) the features which distinguish diseases caused by living agents from those produced by other forms of injury.

CHARACTERISTICS OF MICROBIOLOGIC AGENTS

Evolution has taught that all forms of life on this planet struggle for a suitable environment for their survival. Microbiologic organisms cause disease only incidentally in the competitive biology of life. Man is surrounded by these biologic forms; happily, only relatively few cause disease. Among the microorganisms parasitizing man, some are commensals which coexist happily with their host, causing no evidence of injury. In some instances, the coexistence is of mutual benefit; for example, the *E. coli* flora of the gut is requisite for the production of vitamin K. Such a relationship is known as symbiosis. Only relatively few are predators and cause disease, i.e., are pathogenic in man. But a microorganism cannot be categorized as a commensal or a predator without recognizing the importance of the parasite-host relationship. *E. coli* may well cause disease in the abnormally vulnerable host or when it spreads outside of its normal habitat in the gut. The relationship then between the microorganism and man is a delicate balance established by the adaptation of the parasite to its environment and the resistance of the host to further incursion. Some biologic agents such as the plague bacillus have not adapted at all and destroy their host and ultimately themselves. Death of the host deprives them of their required environment for survival. At the other end of the spectrum are the many commensals living in the mouth, nose and vagina, seeking only moisture and nourishment for their harmless existence. *Clinical disease results, then, only when the microorganism evokes anatomic and functional damage in the course of obtaining the necessary requirements for its survival.*

Some determinants involved in the disease-producing potential of organisms are: (1) the agent's need to find a portal of entry; (2) its ability to survive in the host—i.e., to resist the immediate defensive reaction of the host and to invade; and (3) the virulence of the agent.

PORTALS OF ENTRY

Portals of entry of microbiologic agents are the lungs, skin and the membranes which line the various orifices and tracts of the body. The skin, mouth and nose comprise the important exposed areas. The last two are the gateways through which countless microorganisms pass daily, in air and food. While the surface of the skin and mucous membranes are heavily contaminated, the immediately subjacent tissue is normally sterile. Even when these barriers are breached, as they so commonly are, defensive mechanisms of the host such as the inflammatory reaction with its leukocytes and secretory IgA provide defenses against most trivial invasions. We probably have little awareness or appreciation of the innumerable transient invasions which are efficiently controlled by the host. Indeed, autopsy studies indicate that trivial incursions are very common since microorganisms can be isolated from apparently normal tissues having no evidence of microbiologic disease (DeJongh et al., 1968). Involved in disease production following an invasion are the size of the inoculum and the ability of the invaders to achieve an environment suitable for their survival. The critical mass of inoculum, i.e., the number of microorganisms required to induce disease, varies with each agent and with the susceptibility of the host. For most, relatively large numbers are probably required, but we have few precise data on this problem. With some, for example the organisms causing tuberculosis, only a very few may initiate disease.

SURVIVAL OF ORGANISMS

Having achieved a portal of entry, biologic agents must be capable of surviving within the host. The most important immediate hazard to the invader is phagocytosis by leukocytes. If a local tissue reaction is evoked, the inflammatory response brings more white cells, immunoglobulins and fibrin meshes to ensnare and destroy the invader. Surviving these defenses, most agents invade to find the optimal environment for their survival and replication. Some, such as the staphylococci, find any tissue acceptable as a home. Other more fastidious agents, for example, the neurotropic viruses, are only capable of survival and replication in nervous tissue. In this section then we shall consider (1) the attributes of organisms that protect them against phagocytosis and enhance their invasiveness and (2) their preferential localization.

Most pathogenic microorganisms must invade tissues to produce disease. There are a few rare exceptions such as the tapeworm which may live happily within the lumen of the intestinal tract and produce intestinal obstruction without actual invasion of tissue. Similarly, certain flukes such as *Fasciola hepatica* may cause fatal obstructive jaundice by growing within the lumen of bile ducts and producing mechanical blockage. Agents which invade are immediately exposed to phagocytic neutrophils and macrophages.

A common bacterial defense against phagocytosis is the formation of a capsule. Most capsules contain complex polysaccharides. The fungus *Cryptococcus neoformans* is one of the most heavily encapsulated microorganisms. Pneumococci possess capsules composed of a high molecular weight polymer of glucose and glucuronic acids. Similarly, the *Klebsiella pneumoniae* is richly endowed with a capsule. The manner in which such capsules inhibit phagocytosis is poorly understood. It has been suggested that the hydrophobic lipid plasma membrane of neutrophils is inhibited from making intimate contact (necessary for phagocytosis) with the hydrophilic polysaccharide capsule. Whatever the mechanism, it is clear that for these specific organisms, their ability to elaborate a capsule is related to their pathogenicity. So-called rough strains of pneumococci are incapable of forming capsules and these organisms have a very low virulence as compared with the fully encapsulated

strains. However, capsular antigens evoke powerful antibody responses and so their presence represents for the organism a two-edged sword. Other surface products possess antiphagocytic activity. Certain streptococci elaborate M-proteins which are both pathogenic and, at the same time, antiphagocytic. The M-proteins of group A streptococci are probably primary determinants of virulence.

Invasion is a poorly understood attribute of most pathogenic agents, but certain observations have been made. Some bacteria elaborate extracellular enzymes which facilitate their spread in host tissues. Hyaluronidases are produced by some gram-positive bacteria. By depolymerizing hyaluronic acid in the ground substance, these enzymes enhance the spread of the organism. Certain streptococci elaborate coagulases which convert fibrinogen to fibrin. Such clotting might produce a film about the staphylococci, protecting them from phagocytosis. At the same time, coagulase-induced thromboses in the blood supply to the area would inhibit the defensive reactions of the host and produce a sequestered focus in which the organisms might proliferate. Thus these coagulases would enhance the tendency for infections by these organisms to remain localized and produce abscesses. Counterbalancing the coagulases, staphylococci and streptococci both elaborate kinases that activate plasminogen, converting it to plasmin. We might speculate that by the time plasmin has digested the fibrin clots, the staphylococci have had an opportunity to proliferate and gain a foothold and, thereafter, fibrinolysis favors their spread. The causative agent of gas gangrene, *Clostridium perfringens*, synthesizes collagenase which contributes significantly to the spread of this agent and its pathogenicity. With the exception of these few examples, we little understand the biomolecular mechanisms of bacteria invasion.

A microbiologic agent's requirements for growth and replication determine to a considerable degree the nature of the disease it can produce. Some can survive (i.e., grow and replicate) extracellularly, but others are intracellular parasites and, indeed, cannot replicate in extracellular locations. Most pathogenic bacteria are extracellular parasites and these in general evoke humoral immune responses (Table 10–1).

Some microbiologic agents have the capacity to thrive within living cells and some, in fact, require intracellular localization for growth and replication. The former are referred to as facultative and the latter as obligate intracellular parasites. Intracellular par-

TABLE 10–1. EXTRACELLULAR PATHOGENS OF MAN

Gram-Positive Bacteria	Gram-Negative Bacteria
Staphylococcus	Meningococcus*
Streptococcus	Gonococcus*
Pneumococcus	Coliforms
Diphtheria	Hemophilus
Clostridia	Shigella
Anthrax	Cholera

*These are also facultative intracellular parasites.

TABLE 10–2. INTRACELLULAR PATHOGENS OF MAN

Facultative		
Bacteria	*Fungi*	*Protozoa*
Mycobacteria	Blastomyces	Toxoplasma
Salmonella	Coccidiomyces	Leishmania
Brucella	Histoplasma	Trypanosomes
	Candida	Pneumocystis
	Cryptococcus	
	Nocardia	

Obligate		
Rickettsiae	*Viruses*	*Protozoa*
All	All	Malarial plasmodia

asites, partially listed in Table 10–2, evoke cell-mediated immune responses.

Intracellular existence is a fascinating biologic phenomenon which has important clinical implications. The *Mycobacterium tuberculosis*, for example, may survive within the macrophage after phagocytosis and thus be spread along with the migration of the leukocyte. In this intracellular location it is protected, as it were, from antibacterial drugs and so intracellular parasitism often implies disease resistant to antibiotic therapy. While extracellular parasites generally cause tissue reactions characterized by outpourings of neutrophils, intracellular parasites evoke largely mononuclear reactions and some produce granulomatous inflammation, i.e., tuberculosis.

Much has been learned about the determinants of obligate intracellular parasitism. Rickettsiae, for example, do not possess the well developed, stable cell membranes found generally in extracellular bacteria. Vital intracellular constituents of the microorganisms such as ADP readily diffuse out. Moreover, they lack enzymes necessary for certain metabolic pathways. They are deficient in glycolytic enzymes and cannot metabolize glucose or glucose-phosphates. Thus, rickettsiae are fragile biologic forms which depend on the metabolism of the host cell for their sources of energy and are only able to replicate in highly specialized settings.

Viruses are even more dependent on the host cell than are rickettsiae. As is well known, they are essentially composed of genetic material (DNA or RNA) surrounded by a protective protein capsid. They lack virtually all metabolic machinery. Viral replication is carried out by the host cell although it is directed by the genetic information derived from the virus. The viral DNA- or RNA-directed ("reverse") transcriptase inserts instructions into the genome of the host cell for replication of the viral DNA or RNA and the protein units which are assembled into the viral capsid. If infectious mature virions are released from their intracellular prison (usually by rupture and destruction of the host cell), it is designated a *productive infection*. When infectious virions are not assembled and the virus cannot be recovered from the host cell, it is an *abortive infection*. Most oncogenic DNA viruses cause abortive infections in which the virus cannot be recovered from the tumor without special "rescue" procedures while, by contrast, oncogenic RNA viruses can be recovered from tumors since complete virions are produced.

Preferential localization of organisms extends beyond the cellular level to specific organotropism and specific animal species. The leprosy bacillus is only pathogenic for man and it has been impossible, to date, to establish an animal model of the disease because the organism cannot survive in other hosts. Organ or tissue preference is best exemplified by *Bordetella pertussis*, the cause of whooping cough. These bacteria preferentially and selectively localize on the ciliated epithelium of the trachea and bronchi. Indeed, when introduced into chick embryos, they invade to localize eventually on the ciliated epithelium of the bronchial mucosa. If inoculated in the early embryo before ciliated cells have appeared, the bronchial epithelium does not become infected. Numerous examples of tissue and organ selectivity might be offered. Meningococci use the nasopharynx as a portal of entry but selectively localize in the meninges. The poliomyelitis virus, although it enters through either the oropharyngeal or intestinal gateway, preferentially localizes within the central nervous system although sometimes the cardiac muscle is also affected. On the other hand, as mentioned before, many agents (staphylococci, streptococci and the enteric bacteria) are more catholic in their tastes and happily implant and replicate in any tissue or organ they reach.

VIRULENCE

The virulence of a microbiologic agent, or its pathogenicity (i.e., its disease-producing potential), is the summation of a number of factors relating to the predator and the host. Highly virulent organisms such as those causing plague are able to destroy virtually any host unfortunate enough to be attacked. On the other hand, extremely vulnerable, perhaps debilitated or immunodeficient patients may suffer rampant infections from organisms that would be nonpathogenic to those more robust. The considerations involved in the virulence of an agent are complex and are often poorly understood but include resistance to destruction (e.g., encapsulation), ability to invade (e.g., enzymes), the elaboration of toxic products and induction of hypersensitivity. The first two attributes have already been discussed. The elaboration of toxic products might apply to a host of substances synthesized by bacteria but, classically, has been limited to those substances which are liberated from living bacteria (exotoxins) capable of causing disease at a distance from the site of implantation and endotoxins only released on disintegration of the organisms.

Exotoxin production is principally an attribute of gram-positive organisms such as those causing diphtheria, tetanus, botulism and staphylococcal food poisoning. Shigella dysenteriae is, however, a gram-negative bacillus which produces a very potent neurotoxin. All of these exotoxins are heat-labile proteins which are highly antigenic. Their potency is almost beyond belief, and it has been estimated that 1 ounce of diphtheria toxin could kill 10 million people. How it acts is uncertain; it is thought to be an inhibitor of protein synthesis, and thus should affect all growing cell systems in the body. However, as will be seen, the effects of diphtheria exotoxin are exerted principally on myocardium and nerves. The basis for such preferential damage is at the present time obscure. On the other hand, the causative agent of gas gangrene, Clostridium perfringens, elaborates a virulent alpha toxin in the form of a lecithinase which splits lecithin and thereby destroys cell membranes, rapidly destroying all cells. Here there is good correlation between the bacterial exotoxin and its resultant disease, i.e., lytic destruction of all tissues exposed to high concentrations of the exotoxin. Other exotoxins will be encountered in the consideration of the specific diseases.

Endotoxins are usually lipopolysaccharides contained within the cell walls of most gram-negative bacteria. They are released only after bacterial lysis, are less potent than exotoxins, have less specific target organs than exotoxins and are, at best, weak antigens. It is indeed uncertain that they play any role in the local induction of tissue injury at sites of bacterial invasion. Rather, it is suspected that they may have systemic effects when released and absorbed into the blood, such as the induction of fever and endotoxic shock discussed on p. 346. Endotoxemia may also trigger disseminated intravascular coagulation (DIC) (p. 744).

How microbiologic agents which do not elaborate either exotoxins or endotoxins cause disease is even more mysterious. In some instances, the emergence of hypersensitivity to organismal antigens is suspected. Tuberculosis is an instance where the organism itself is of relatively low toxicity, but it induces hypersensitization which is responsible for much of its destructive effects. In others, for example rickettsiae, with their obligate intracellular existence, competition for substrate may injure the host cell. Elaborated enzymes or other products may also have injury-producing potential.

The virulence of viruses is another area of mystery. An agent such as the herpes virus can be found in the nasopharynx of many individuals without inducing injury. Why should excessive exposure to sunlight or an intercurrent respiratory infection trigger the formation of herpetic blisters on the lips (cold sores), and how did these stresses activate the virus or predispose the host? Other viral infections only emerge months to years after initial exposure to the agent. These are referred to as slow virus infections. Are the slow viruses replicating at a leisure pace until the cell is destroyed, and is it the cellular debris which initiates the inflammatory reaction recognized as the infection? Much is yet to be learned about the disease-producing potential of microbiologic agents.

As stated at the outset, bacterial virulence and disease-producing potential are relative to the resistance of the host. Man lives in a relatively delicate state of balance with his microbial environment. He is in constant contact with a wide range of bacteria, viruses, fungi and, indeed, all manner of microbiologic agents with whom he lives in a state of commensalism. This endogenous flora is present on every body surface and in every orifice in contact with the environment. Under normal conditions, this endogenous flora is harmless. But any disturbance of the delicate balance, i.e., modification of the endogenous flora or impairment of normal defenses, may lead to disease. Previously innocuous agents may produce serious and, indeed, often fatal disease called *opportunistic infections.*

Most *opportunistic infections* result from artificially induced modifications in the usual endogenous flora of the individual. Antibacterial drugs are the chief culprit in this respect. They have two effects: (1) suppression of drug-sensitive organisms, permitting others that are more resistant to proliferate free of competition for nutrients and (2) induction of drug-resistant mutants. Staphylococcal enterocolitis provides a good example of a disease caused by an endogenous commensal which runs riot after its more drug-sensitive neighbors have been suppressed by antibacterial therapy. The fecal stream always contains scant numbers of staphylococci. Broad-spectrum antibiotics may wipe out the coliform flora of the gut and thus permit staphylococci to multiply wildly, inducing an enterocolitis which can lead to a staphylococcal bacteremia and death. Indeed, when the enterocolitis begins to make its appearance, cessation of drug therapy and regrowth of coliforms will control the disease if it is not too advanced.

Sponsoring drug-resistant mutants is another untoward effect of antibacterial therapy (Finland et al., 1959). How this comes about is not clear. Chance mutation with the survival of the most drug-resistant is one possibility. There are, however, observations which suggest that drug resistance may be mediated by extrachromosomal genetic elements known as R or resistance factors (Watanabe, 1963). These factors appear to be composed of DNA, are transferable between bacteria by conjugation and apparently are not related to bacterial growth and mutation. Drug-resistance can be transferred without cell replication. Other pathways for the development of resistance have been described, such as the acquired ability to synthesize penicillinase, the agent responsible for penicillin resistance (Novick, 1967). The message is clear: the use of antibacterial drugs, especially in less than bacteriocidal or bacteriostatic dosages, permits organisms to adapt to their unfavorable environment and so predisposes to the emergence of drug-resistant strains. Drug-resistant bacterial strains have now emerged as major causes of disease. Cross infections within hospitals have become serious problems, as the patient with an infection caused by a drug-resistant organism contaminates his environment and, all too often, his neighbor.

In the parasite-host equation, lowering of the defenses of the host may lead to opportunistic infections. The unusually vulnerable patient is prey to all forms of microbiologic disease, including infections by organisms having little pathogenicity in normal individuals. Depression of host defense mechanisms can be related to old age, underlying debilitating disease (particularly diabetes), alcoholism, heart failure, the presence of foreign bodies such as artificial heart valves and prosthetic grafts, but the two dominant causes are the hereditary or acquired immunodeficiency states and the use of immunosuppressive drugs such as corticosteroids, antimetabolites and alkylating agents. This problem is particularly important in patients receiving organ transplants who are maintained on immunosuppressive drugs for long periods of time. In these individuals, opportunistic infections with such uncommon low-virulence agents as fungi, cytomegalovirus and *Pneumocystis carinii* have induced fatal disease (Hart et al., 1969) (Klainer and Beisal, 1969). In the instance of renal transplantation, infection is a more important cause of death than transplant rejection. It is apparent, then, that the terms virulence and pathogenicity, when used with regard to the microbiologic organism alone, have little meaning in this day of opportunistic infections.

REACTIONS OF THE HOST TO BIOLOGIC AGENTS

The host factors involved in resistance to infections have already been discussed in the earlier consideration of inflammation (p. 99). Here those particularly pertinent to microbiologic disease will be briefly detailed.

The importance of the intact integument and mucosal linings of the body as barriers needs no further comment in the light of the earlier discussion of portals of entry (p. 357).

A host of physiologic mechanisms protect the body. Only a few examples will be cited. The vibrissae in the external nares filter out particulate matter from the inspired air. Organisms passing through this barrier may then be trapped in the mucous secretions of the respiratory tract, where ciliary action and the cough reflex come into play. The normal pH and secretions of the skin are unfavorable environments for the growth of many microorganisms. The gastric acidity destroys most swallowed organisms. Secretory IgA in mucosal surfaces undoubtedly contributes to the defense of the host. The mucosal lining of the urinary bladder in some way protects itself against bacterial invasion (p. 1118). The reticuloendothelial system is one of the most important protective mechanisms (p. 76). A much longer list might be cited.

The inflammatory reaction is, of course, a major bulwark against predators, bringing to bear many protective influences, principal among which are the phagocytic neutrophils and macrophages, opsonins which facilitate phagocytosis of bacteria, immunoglobulins and sensitized lymphocytes. The immune system and immune responses are, of course, crucial in overcoming infections once established. Immunity, or the lack of it, dictates to a considerable extent the age distribution of infectious diseases. Chickenpox, mumps, measles and whooping cough are classically referred to as the "childhood diseases," because of the lack of immunity in this age group to these common biologic agents. Such diseases are uncommon in adults merely because of the prior experience of the individual with the causative agents and acquired immunity. The epidemics that ravaged the world in years past, such as smallpox, diphtheria and poliomyelitis, have been controlled by effective immunization programs.

The importance of these host reactions to microbiologic agents has already been made clear but, to provide some perspective on the problem, a few examples might be cited. In patients with hereditary immunodeficiency states, the major causes of death are microbiologic diseases. The unfortunate use of steroids in a patient with a localized infection, such as pulmonary tuberculosis, often permits the bacteria to proliferate wildly and spread throughout the body to produce so-called miliary tuberculosis. Rampant infections are classic hallmarks of hematologic disorders characterized by deficiency of normally functioning neutrophils (such as granulocytopenia). So it is that the reactions of the host determine, to a considerable extent, the disease-producing potential of microbiologic organisms.

DISTINCTIVE FEATURES OF INFECTIOUS DISEASE

Clinical Features. Diseases induced by biologic agents are characterized by a time lag between the invasion and the development of clinical manifestations, i.e., the incubation period. It may vary from minutes to hours in botulism to months and years in leprosy and slow virus infections.

Infections tend to be manifested by distinctive local and systemic signs and symptoms. These have been detailed in Chapter 3. It will suffice merely to recall the term "cardinal signs" and the systemic reactions of fever and leukocytosis or leukopenia. As will become apparent, all infections do not evoke a neutrophilic leukocytosis; some are characterized by lymphocytosis or even leukopenia. In addition, serious infections are generally manifested by malaise, increased fatigability, muscular aches and pains, sweating and, in those with bacteremia or viremia, shaking chills. Many hemodynamic and metabolic adjustments also occur. Associated with the fever, there is a marked reduction in blood volume with a shift in intravascular fluid into the interstitial spaces and tissues, accompanied by sodium retention. These changes are mediated by increased synthesis of adrenal steroid hormones, particularly aldosterone. The low blood volume leads to oliguria. With the return of the temperature to normal, the retained chlorides and water are excreted through the skin and kidneys in the form of increased sweating and polyuria. The elevated body temperature leads to generalized catabolism of all tissues with resultant increased urinary excretion of nitrogen, negative nitrogen balance and sometimes weight loss. An increased pulse (tachycardia), respiratory rate (tachypnea) and caloric requirement are all associated with the hypermetabolism of the elevated temperature levels. While the pulse rate increases in most febrile diseases, in a few, such as typhoid fever, tularemia and psittacosis, the rate may slow (bradycardia), comprising an important clinical finding suggesting such infections. Also encountered in most febrile infections is an increase in gluconeogenesis and hypercoagulability of the blood. The latter is seen particularly in gramnegative infections. In blood-borne infections, particularly with gram-negative endotoxic organisms, abnormalities in the electrocardiogram may appear, suggesting direct injury to the myocardium. Indeed, cardiac failure may develop, or even cardiogenic shock (p. 346).

Microbiologic infections have profound effects on certain preexisting disease states, particularly diabetes mellitus, hyperthyroidism and adrenocortical insufficiency. Latent diabetes may be converted to clinically overt disease, and insulin requirements are greatly increased. Similarly, subclinical adrenocortical insufficiency may flare into overt manifestations requiring the administration of adrenal steroids to prevent fatal electrolyte and water imbalances (p. 1311). In febrile reactions, there is an increase in thyroid activity aggravating preexisting hyperthyroidism.

It is evident that diseases caused by microbiologic agents have wide-ranging ramifications, not the least of which is their ability to disseminate from their local site of implantation to distant sites. In this sense, infections resemble cancers. Not only is the primary site a problem, but its potential for spread is an ever-present danger. Thus, the lung abscess caused by staphylococci may lead to blood-borne metastatic abscesses throughout the body. Implantation on the heart valves may give rise to a vegetative endocarditis, or seeding of the meninges may induce meningitis. Similarly, the parasitic infection of the gut may spread to produce a hepatic abscess, as occurs in amebiasis. The immune response may lead to systemic hypersensitivity reactions, exemplified by poststreptococcal glomerulonephritis and rheumatic fever. Indeed, the potential immunologic sequellae of streptococcal disease are more threatening than the bacterial infection itself. Prompt diagnosis and immediate control, if possible, are requisite then for all microbiologic diseases.

Morphologic Features. Diseases caused by groups of biologic agents tend to fall into certain morphologic tissue patterns of reaction, dependent upon the specific causative agent. Bacteria usually evoke either *focal, suppurative, necrotizing infections,* characterized by the abscess, or *diffuse, spreading inflammations (cellulitis)* also possessing leukocytic infiltrations but not necessarily marked by focal necroses. The pathogenic staphylococci, alpha hemolytic streptococci, coliforms, Hemophilus group, *B. proteus, P. aeruginosa,* pneumococci, meningococci and gonococci all characteristically produce frank suppurative, purulent exudate and, when embedded within solid tissues, create abscesses.

In contrast, the exotoxic organisms tend to evoke spreading, nonlocalized infections, manifested by interstitial inflammation associated with an infiltration of mixed neutrophils, plasma cells, lymphocytes, and histiocytes or monocytes. From the standpoint of morphologic response, the spirochetes tend to behave as do the exotoxic organisms, and thus cause chiefly a diffuse inflammatory reaction with mononuclear infiltration, which is limited for the most part to the interstitial tissue. These morphologic patterns are by no means invariable. It is also to be understood that *many bacteria evoke fairly specific tissue responses, such as the granulomatous reaction of the tubercle bacillus,* not included in the categories just cited.

The rickettsiae are obligate intracellular parasites and classically evoke a diffuse interstitial reaction, which is more prominent in and about blood vessels. Most of the rickettsial infections are also characterized by striking vascular lesions, which include parasitization of the endothelial cells and varying degrees of damage to the vascular walls, sometimes to the point of complete necrosis, accompanied by striking perivascular infiltrations of mononuclear leukocytes. Viral infections likewise cause predominantly interstitial reactions that are usually fairly specific in distribution and pattern of involvement, depending upon the precise agent. The diseases caused by yeasts, molds and various types of worms do not permit any characterization, since the tissue responses are very variable.

It should be emphasized that, throughout the entire range of biologic disease, it is virtually impossible to be completely certain of the precise etiology of a disease from the observed histologic response. Granted an abscess may be suspected as staphylococcal in origin, it can also be caused by gonococci, meningococci, coliforms, *H. influenzae* and a host of other organisms. Striking reticuloendothelial hyperplasia is characteristic of typhoid fever, but is also found in brucellosis. The classic tubercle comes close to a pathognomonic tissue lesion, but it too may be confused with sarcoidosis, syphilis, tularemia and other infections. The incidence of certain infections, and associated clinical findings, may permit a reasoned guess as to the etiology of many clinical problems. But ultimately the microscope is of limited differential value, and cultural, biochemical and serologic techniques must be used for complete certainty.

In the following consideration of the various diseases caused by bacteria, viruses and other forms of parasites, primary attention is focused on: the causative agent, the method of spread, the pathogenesis of the lesions and the resultant clinical infections. Morphologic descriptions of tissue changes are confined to those which are reasonably specific for the particular agent under discussion. When the tissue damage is of a nonspecific nature, e.g., the formation of an abscess, no repetitious description is given. The following presentation of diseases of biologic origin does not pretend to be an exhaustive treatment. The biologic agents and their diseases are accorded space in proportion to their incidence and clinicoanatomic significance. Many of the "medical curiosities" encountered only in localized endemic areas of the world are considered as disorders better relegated to reference sources.

BACTERIAL DISEASE

PYOGENIC COCCI

Staphylococci, streptococci, pneumococci, meningococci and gonococci are designated *pyogenic cocci because they classically evoke suppurative exudations and cause abscesses.* All have in common the capacity to localize in many sites in the body and to destroy cells locally. Except for the identification of the organism bacteriologically, it is impossible to distinguish the purulent exudation of staphylococci from that produced by streptococci, meningococci, or any of the others. While other bacteria and biologic agents may also evoke suppurative reactions, at least 80 per cent of clinical infections characterized by the formation of pus are produced by the pyogenic cocci. However, the various members of this group have predilections for different tissues or organs in the body as well as other differences. These differences evoke sufficiently distinctive clinical diseases to require separate consideration.

STAPHYLOCOCCAL INFECTIONS

Staphylococci characteristically cause localized suppurative infections in the skin and less frequently in the lungs, kidneys, bones and brain. However, no organ or tissue of the body is immune so that suppurative infection in any site must be suspected as staphylococcal in origin until proved otherwise.

Causative Agent. The staphylococci are gram-positive organisms. Of the various staphylococci, *the S. aureus is the most significant pathogen for man.* The usual clinical criteria applied to determine the pathogenicity of staphylococci are: *their capacity to produce hemolysis on blood agar plates and their capacity to coagulate blood (coagulase reaction).* Almost all staphylococci isolated from tissue lesions are hemolytic and coagulase-positive. The coagulase has the capacity to clot plasma in vitro and presumably may cause thrombosis of vessels in the region of an infection, thereby tending to produce the *localized infections so characteristic of the staphylococci.*

Staphylococcus aureus elaborates many powerful toxins and enzymes. A soluble *necrotizing exotoxin* is probably responsible for the local cytolytic action of the organism in tissues. Three or four *hemolysins* account for its hemolytic action on blood agar plates and may be responsible for some of its systemic toxic manifestations. A substance toxic to leukocytes, *leukocidin,* appears to be distinct from the ne-

crotizing exotoxin and undoubtedly contributes to the virulence of *Staphylococcus aureus* by the destruction of defensive white cells. A few strains of staphylococci elaborate an *enterotoxin* responsible for symptoms of acute food poisoning. The acute gastroenteritis that it causes is at times as severe as the food poisoning caused by *Clostridium botulinum.* Some virulent staphylococci also elaborate *fibrinolysins and mucolytic enzymes—hyaluronidases.* A *staphylokinase* can activate plasminogen. However, these enzymes either are produced only in small amounts or do not have the potency of similar enzymes elaborated by the streptococci. Whereas the fibrinolysins of streptococcal origin are capable of dissolving clots within minutes, staphylococcal fibrinolysin does not exert material effect for many hours to days.

Method of Spread. Staphylococci are widely distributed in the environment in virtually all media with which man comes into daily contact, e.g., air, water, food and articles of everyday life. Most such staphylococci are of the nonpathogenic variety. However, pathogenic strains are unquestionably contacted daily. In fact, *Staphylococcus aureus* of disease-producing virulence can be isolated from the skin of about 20 per cent of the population and from the upper respiratory tract of 50 per cent. These carriers provide a large reservoir for the dissemination of infections. The skin is the common portal of entry for staphylococcal infections, but some trauma must provide the pathway of ingress, since the organism cannot penetrate the intact epidermis.

Pathogenesis. In the usual skin infection, the organisms penetrate into a sebaceous gland or hair shaft and there find adequate nutrition to incite a minute infection and necrosis, which provides a pathway for further invasion. Less common portals of entry are the oropharynx, respiratory tract, urogenital tract and gastrointestinal tract. In all instances, some form of injury prepares the pathway. The defensive or resistive factors of the host and the size and virulence of the infecting inoculum clearly condition the likelihood of the development of a staphylococcal infection, even in the presence of a portal of entry. It is on this basis that staphyloccal infections tend to occur in the two extremes of life and are particularly common in diabetics, alcoholics and the malnourished.

Infections. Having gained access to the body, the staphylococcus may be responsible for a variety of infections, such as a furuncle, carbuncle, osteomyelitis, bacterial pneumonia, endocarditis, meningitis, tonsillitis, sinusitis, otitis media, bacterial enteritis, colitis and localized abscesses in any tissue or organ of the body. Since there is an essentially similar reaction in all these sites, only a few prototypes will be described.

Furuncle and Carbuncle. Most suppurative infections of the skin are due to *Staphylococcus aureus. The furuncle, more generally known as a boil, is a focal suppurative inflammation of the skin and subcutaneous tissues.* It may occur singly or multiply, and frequently recurs in successive crops of new infections. *The carbuncle is a more deeply situated infection that spreads laterally beneath the deep subcutaneous fascia and then burrows superficially to create multiple adjacent draining skin sinuses.* While other bacteria occasionally give rise to these lesions, they are usually due to *S. aureus.* Furuncles may be found in any location, but are most common in hair-bearing, moist areas of the body, as on the face, neck, axillae, groin, legs and breasts. In contrast, carbuncles are essentially confined to the back and to the posterior aspect of the neck, where appropriate fascial planes permit the lateral spread described.

Furuncles and carbuncles generally begin in hair follicles and at this stage are recognized as *folliculitis.* From this origin, the infection penetrates more deeply to create a subcutaneous abscess, the furuncle, or, on the nape of the neck or back, the larger but nonetheless localized carbuncle. Both these infections have the characteristic macroscopic and microscopic features of an abscess with local tissue destruction and accompanying vascular and exudative reactions (p. 86). In the characteristic progression of the abscess, the central focus undergoes liquefaction. The inflammatory necrosis often burrows toward the surface ("points") and frequently produces one or several draining sinuses that aid the healing response by evacuation of the necrotic debris. The only distinction between the furuncle and the carbuncle, therefore, is in the depth of the tissue lesion and the resultant development of one or more sinuses (Fig. 10–1). When spontaneous rupture fails to occur, these infections are often best handled by incision and drainage.

The furuncle and carbuncle are responsible for considerable pain and discomfort. Invasion of the circulating blood with the production of metastatic abscesses (pyemia) and infections elsewhere in the body is an invariable threat of all staphylococcal spread. This course is uncommon in the young, healthy adult, and these complications are more apt to occur in diabetics and debilitated patients. Favored sites for such secondary localization are the lungs, meninges, kidneys and heart valves.

Bacterial Pneumonia. The staphylococcus is a fairly common *primary cause of bacterial*

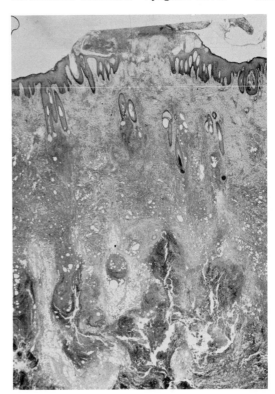

Figure 10–1. *Staphylococcal carbuncle at low power showing deep-seated suppuration and a sinus tract through the overlying epidermis.*

pneumonia and is an even more frequent secondary invader of other forms of lung disease. Staphylococcal secondary infection is particularly common in viral pneumonias, longstanding congestion and edema of the lungs, bronchiectasis, bronchial asthma, cystic fibrosis, and in the pneumonias that develop in the course of childhood communicable diseases, such as whooping cough and measles (Wolleman and Finland, 1943). The hazard of superinfection and antibiotic-resistant strains is always a grave threat. Irrespective of whether *S. aureus* is a primary or secondary invader, the resultant bacterial pneumonia is of serious significance, because of the tendency for these organisms to evoke abscess formation in the lung with destruction of pulmonary parenchyma.

The bacterial pneumonia may be patchy and focal in the pattern known as bronchopneumonia (p. 809) or, less commonly, it may consolidate large confluent areas of the lung to produce lobar pneumonia (p. 811).

Pharyngitis, Tonsillitis and Sinusitis. These infections of the oropharynx and upper respiratory tract are less commonly caused by *Staphylococcus aureus* than by the streptococci. The staphylococcal lesions are characterized by intense inflammatory responses accompanied by edema, hyperemia and usually copious suppurative exudation. The mucosal epithelium is frequently destroyed with resultant superficial or penetrating crypt abscesses. The necrotizing inflammation in the confines of a paranasal sinus may cause virtually total destruction of the respiratory mucosa (p. 848).

Acute Enteritis. The normal *E. coli* flora of the colon may be virtually destroyed by therapeutic levels of broad-spectrum antibiotics as discussed on p. 361. Concomitantly, the occasional resistant staphylococcus found normally in the feces overgrows and totally replaces the coliforms. No untoward reactions are encountered in most of these patients. However, tissue lesions develop in a small but unknown percentage. In certain of these cases, abscesses and ulcers develop in the gut. (For further details on the anatomic changes, reference should be made to p. 961. The patients develop the characteristic manifestations of acute colitis, consisting of abdominal cramps, diarrhea sometimes leading to febrile reactions, dehydration and electrolyte imbalance. In addition, extremely grave systemic reactions may be encountered, such as pyemia with metastatic foci of infection on the heart valves, in the lungs, brain, kidneys and elsewhere. This iatrogenic enterocolitis is a serious disorder that should be guarded against by repeated fecal cultures in patients receiving antibacterial drugs.

Osteomyelitis. Osteomyelitis is a suppurative infection of bone most often caused by *Staphylococcus aureus*. This condition is discussed in Chapter 31, since it is a primary disorder of bones.

Staphylococcal Food Poisoning. Staphylococcal food poisoning does not represent a true staphylococcal infection, but rather is an intoxication due to the ingestion of preformed enterotoxins. Symptoms of acute poisoning develop within one to several hours after the ingestion of contaminated food. Nausea, vomiting, abdominal cramps, diarrhea and prostration are the usual clinical manifestations. These symptoms are usually transient and the patient recovers with or without therapy in about 24 hours. Only rarely have fatalities been recorded. Morphologic lesions are ordinarily not demonstrable, and in fact viable staphylococci cannot be demonstrated in most cases.

Staphylococcal Bacteremia. Invasion of the blood by *Staphylococcus aureus* is the most serious complication of any localized infection (Lyons, 1942). About half of these blood infections arise from primary foci in the skin. The primary focus in the remaining half is found in the intestinal tract, kidneys, lungs or bones. The bacteremia may follow one of two courses. It may consist principally of an extremely severe blood infection without the development of focal lesions, presumably because the patient does not live long enough. This overwhelming invasion is therefore as fulminating and as serious as streptococcal or meningococcal bacteremias. These patients die within days unless the infection is controlled.

In the other pattern, the bacteremia pursues a less fulminating course, but is accompanied by metastatic foci of infection in many tissues and organs. The most frequent sites of these metastatic abscesses are the skin, subcutaneous tissues, lungs, kidneys, heart and skeletal muscles. The brain and its coverings may be seeded to produce meningitis or a brain abscess; the pleural, pericardial and peritoneal cavities may become contaminated; and no structure is immune. Both these clinical bacteremic syndromes are extremely grave and the mortality is variously reported as between 50 and 90 per cent.

Infections Due to Antibiotic-Resistant Staphylococci. As has been mentioned, staphylococci perhaps more than any other organism have demonstrated a remarkable and alarming capacity to acquire resistance to virtually every form of antibiotic yet discovered. Thus, infections that begin as perhaps streptococcal in origin may be successfully controlled by appropriate therapy only to have a "resistant" staphylococcus become superimposed and cause a more serious infection than the original organism. The staphylococcus has therefore become an important and major cause of fulminant forms of bacterial endocarditis. Enterocolitis in postoperative patients being treated with broad-spectrum antibiotics, which wipe out the *E. coli* flora of the bowel and permit the recalcitrant staphylococcus to flourish, is an additional major clinical problem. Frequently in these vulnerable patients, spread from the bowel to other sites may occur to cause a fatal disseminated disease. The management of these antibiotic-resistant staphylococci is a major problem today.

STREPTOCOCCAL INFECTIONS

The large group of streptococci includes many organisms capable of causing pyogenic infections. However, these infections differ in many respects from those caused by staphylococci. Within the group of streptococci, many organisms are nonpathogenic for man and others are pathogenic chiefly for animals. Only a few are chiefly pathogenic for man, but these are responsible for some serious infections. The diversity of the infections and their totally dissimilar clinical and anatomic features make it difficult to believe that all are caused by essentially similar organisms. Important as streptococcal infections may be, even more grave are rheumatic fever (p. 657) and acute glomerulonephritis (p. 1093), representing diseases resulting from the immune response to the original bacterial infection—hence their designation as poststreptococcal disorders. These hyperergic states are presented later in the consideration of the heart and kidneys. The present discussion is confined to those diseases directly attributable to streptococcal invasion.

Causative Agent. There are at least 30 different types of streptococci which have in common only their gram-positive, chain-like morphology. This large number has been subdivided by many techniques. The oldest classification is based upon their capacity to hemolyze blood. Those organisms that cause total destruction of erythrocytes when grown on blood agar plates with clearing around the colony are the *beta hemolytic streptococci;* those that produce green pigment about the colony, *alpha hemolytic;* while the remainder that cause no alteration in the erythrocytes are the *gamma streptococci.* This old classification retains some clinical usefulness, since the highly virulent streptococci tend, on the whole, to fall in the beta hemolytic group. The alpha hemolytic group comprises the less virulent but nonetheless somewhat pathogenic members, and the gamma streptococci are in general of low virulence, if not entirely nonpathogenic for man.

More recently, Lancefield, on the basis of specific carbohydrates, divided the streptococci into 12 groups, designated by the letters A, B, C, D, E, F, G, H, K, L, M and N. The organisms in group A are almost entirely beta hemolytic and are the most important as far as human infections are concerned. While most of the other Lancefield groups are also beta hemolytic, these are generally of less clinical importance. The Lancefield group D includes the streptococci commonly known as enterococci. These are frequently the causative agents of genitourinary tract infections, and occasionally they initiate intestinal, respiratory and endocardial disease. The viridans division of streptococci is not included in the Lancefield groups. In general, the viridans organisms cause alpha hemolysis and are chiefly of importance in the causation of low-grade bacterial infections of the heart valves, known as subacute bacterial endocarditis.

Many enzymes are produced by the streptococci. Streptolysins are hemolysins. Two types have been identified: streptolysin O and streptolysin S. The former is antigenic and evokes antibodies that can be titered in the serum. Elevated levels of antistreptolysin are important indicators of an active streptococcal infection. *Streptokinase* may be a distinct enzyme or may be identical with streptolysin. It is elaborated by the group A organisms and activates *plasminogen* to its active proteolytic *plasmin* form. Deoxyribonucleases, also known as *streptodornases,* are capable of depolymerization of deoxyribonucleoproteins. This latter complex of enzymes is probably important in the causation of rheumatic fever, known to occur as a poststreptococcal sequel. Streptokinase and streptodornase have also been found to be of therapeutic value. The administration of these enzymes to patients with thick, viscid, inflammatory effusions, such as suppurative infections of the pleural cavity, aids in the liquefaction of the exudate and renders its resorption more rapid. Certain streptococci, *when phage infected,* are also capable of producing an *erythrogenic toxin* that is responsible for the erythematous eruption characteristic of scarlet fever. In addition to these fractions, streptococci also elaborate *hyaluronidases,* which are quite specific for the organism of origin. The capacity of these hyaluronidases to degrade the mucopolysaccharides of ground substances adds to the invasiveness and spread of streptococcal infections.

No one specific streptococcal disease is induced by one variety of streptococcus. At one time it was believed that scarlet fever was caused by a specific organism designated as *Streptococcus scarlatinae.* It was also postulated that erysipelas was due to *Streptococcus erysipelatis.* It has become clear with our increased knowledge of the serologic and biochemical typing of streptococci that many of the group A and occasional members of groups C and G are capable of causing identical clinical diseases. This lack of correlation between the clinicoanatomic response and specific strains of streptococci may be related to the fact that many strains elaborate essentially similar antigenic patterns and thus cause similar clinical and morphologic reactions.

Method of Spread. Most streptococcal infections are contracted directly from patients with clinical disease or asymptomatic carriers. Of these two sources, the carrier is probably more important. About 5 to 20 per cent of the general population harbor group A hemolytic streptococci in the oropharynx. The viridans streptococci are almost universally present. The carriers may themselves fall prey to these symbionts when their resistance is lowered by intercurrent illnesses, malnourishment or exposure. Hemolytic streptococcal infections may also be transmitted indirectly through contaminated dust, water, foods and articles of daily life. Such contamination of the environment must have its origin in human or animal disease.

Pathogenesis. Bacterial infections induced by the streptococci may assume any of the following characteristics: (1) *a local infection* that usually remains fairly well localized to the primary portal of entry, e.g., acute tonsillitis and acute nasopharyngitis; (2) a *spreading infection* that extends rapidly from a primary portal of entry to cause lymphangitis or cellulitis; (3) *hematogenous dissemination* from some local or spreading infection (the primary portal may be very insignificant and the major clinical disease may take the form of bacteremia or endocarditis); (4) *exanthematous disease*, such as scarlet fever due to the elaboration by phage-infected streptococci of an erythrogenic toxin, or (5) *poststreptococcal hypersensitization* responsible for such serious systemic disorders as rheumatic fever, glomerulonephritis and skin lesions known as erythema nodosum and erythema multiforme.

The Infections. *Upper Respiratory Tract Infections.* The usual portal of entry for streptococci is the nasopharynx, and infections in and about the nasopharynx comprise one of the more common forms of streptococcal disease. While most of these infections are caused by the group A hemolytic streptococci, occasional, usually mild, attacks have been attributed to the other groups. Some of these strains may elaborate erythrogenic toxins and thus compound the clinical syndrome and produce scarlet fever.

The streptococcal infections in the upper respiratory tract may be subdivided on the basis of the anatomic distribution of the inflammation. The inflammation may be confined to the nasopharyngeal mucosa (*nasopharyngitis*). Almost invariably, the infection drains through the lymphatics to involve the tonsillar tissue in and about the nasopharynx (*acute tonsillitis*). Spread to the peripharyngeal and peritonsillar tissue may cause a *peritonsillar abscess*, also known as *quinsy sore throat*. Spread to the base of the tongue, floor of the mouth, neck and laryngopharynx may produce a very serious infection known as *Ludwig's angina*. The organisms commonly disseminate through the eustachian tube to involve the middle ear (*otitis media*). Spread may then occur to the *mastoid, adjacent dural venous sinuses, and even to the meninges or brain.* In the same way, streptococcal sinusitis may develop. Acute lymphadenitis in the regional nodes of drainage is characteristic of many streptococcal infections.

All these infections are characterized by an intense, acute neutrophilic exudation, accompanied by prominent edema and vascular dilatation. The infection tends to infiltrate through the tissue planes and intercellular spaces, spreading them apart, and in many instances does not produce localized pockets of pus. The inflammatory exudation is not purely neutrophilic and frequently is admixed with macrophages. This spreading infection is presumably attributable to the active hyaluronidases and fibrinolysins elaborated by most of the group A streptococci.

On the basis of these histologic reactions, streptococcal infections are characterized clinically by intense erythema and edema. Focal gross collections of pus may or may not be evident. In the characteristic acute tonsillitis of children over the age of 2 or 3, pus accumulates within the crypts of the tonsils to produce *crypt abscesses (cryptitis).* When the infection penetrates into the deeper tissues to produce a peritonsillar abscess and sinusitis, the pus is often thin and watery and resembles a cloudy serous fluid.

Streptococcal infections are of grave importance because of their local and systemic effects. In the infections described in the pharyngeal region, the involved tissues may be exquisitely tender and produce agonizing pain on swallowing. When the edema occurs in the base of the tongue, as in Ludwig's angina, or laryngopharynx, as in a retropharyngeal abscess, there may be sufficient narrowing of the airway to produce serious respiratory difficulty, and before the advent of antibiotics many of these patients died. In the same way, peritonsillar abscesses may cause serious encroachment upon the airway. Even when these infections remain localized to the upper respiratory tract, the elaboration of powerful antigens is responsible for severe systemic reactions such as fever, chills, malaise and even prostration. Moreover, dissemination of these organisms via the lymphohematogenous routes carries the potential of metastatic focal infections such as meningitis, endocarditis, arthritis, pyelonephritis or pneumonia. Above and beyond these complications, streptococcal infections are particularly ominous because of the possibility of the nonsuppurative sequelae of rheumatic fever, nephritis, erythema nodosum and erythema multiforme.

Infections of the Skin. Streptococcal diseases of the skin run the gamut from such relatively innocuous but highly contagious lesions as impetigo contagiosa through skin abscesses, rapidly spreading erysipelas, skin lesions caused by erythrogenic toxins, to the other lesions that are essentially allergic reactions to streptococcal products. Despite the wide variety of clinical and anatomic reactions, most of these skin lesions are caused by the group A streptococci.

Impetigo contagiosa is frequently considered a staphylococcal disease, but there is considerable evidence to implicate the streptococci as the primary invaders and the staphylococci as secondary contaminants. It is a highly contagious, autoinoculable disease of the superficial skin, encountered almost entirely in children. It will be presented in detail in Chapter 30 (p. 1392).

Erysipelas is caused chiefly by the beta hemolytic streptococci of group A and occasionally by organisms in group C. It is *a rapidly spreading, erythematous, edematous, cutaneous infection,* which usually begins on the face and less frequently on the body or other areas. The disease is uncommon before the age of 20 and occurs chiefly in middle adult life; occasional cases have been described in the two extremes of life. Certain individuals appear to be predisposed and have repeated exacerbations. It is of interest that spread of this streptococcal strain to other individuals may not produce erysipelas, but rather acute upper respiratory tract streptococcal infections or even scarlet fever.

Anatomically, the disease is characterized by an irregular, spreading, map-like area of brawny erythema which has a sharp, well demarcated, serpiginous border. The skin of the affected part is thickened and has a consistency described as tallow-like. Gross areas of suppuration are uncommon. Red streaks of lymphangitis will occasionally extend from the margins to the local nodes of drainage, and these nodes are often enlarged by acute inflammation (p. 750). Histologically, there is an acute edematous, neutrophilic, interstitial reaction in the dermis and epidermis with some reaction deeper in the subcutaneous tissues (Fig. 10–2). This infiltration is often more intense about vessels and the skin adnexa. Microabscesses are often formed, but the tissue necrosis is usually small in amount. The intervening areas often have a mononuclear infiltrate. Occasionally there are large abscesses with tissue destruction. Since the inflammation rarely causes significant tissue destruction, resolution permits apparent complete restitution of normal architecture. In addition to the local symptoms, regional adenopathy and constitutional reaction, toxigenic skin rash, bacteremia, and metastatic foci of infection may all follow.

Wound and Hair Follicle Infections. Streptococci, as well as staphylococci, are common wound contaminants and frequently cause hair follicle infections. At one time, postoperative streptococcal infections were considered ex-

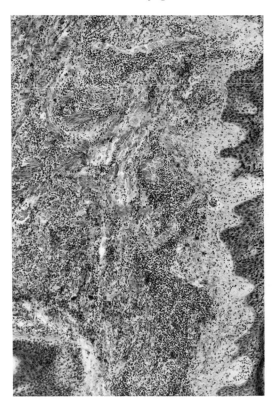

Figure 10–2. *Streptococcal erysipelas. The section is oriented with the epidermis to the right and the dermal inflammatory infiltrate to the left.*

tremely serious. With the present effectiveness of antibiotics, streptococcal contamination is now of less concern than staphylococcal. Wound infections in both traumatic and surgical cases are usually caused by a variety of bacteria. Such mixed infections are characterized by suppurative exudation, hyperemia and edema and, unless the streptococcal organisms are controlled, erysipeloid patterns, lymphangitis and severe regional lymphadenitis may develop. When the streptococcal component leads to a spreading extension, a diffuse inflammatory reaction may ensue within the deep subcutaneous tissues and muscles, characterized as usual by striking edema, diffuse suppurative infiltrate, and occasionally by small loculated pockets of pus. This pattern of deep-seated, diffuse inflammation is known as a *cellulitis* or a *phlegmon*. Streptococcal hair follicle infections when improperly treated are of considerably graver potential than staphylococcal, since the organisms are more capable of spread into the lymphatics, regional nodes and blood. The morphologic and clinical aspects of lymphangitis are presented on page 625.

Scarlet Fever. Scarlet fever is a group A hemolytic streptococcal infection characterized by acute nasopharyngitis and tonsillitis, accompanied by a diffuse erythematous exanthem and enanthem. No longer is the causation attributed to a single strain, *Streptococcus scarlatinae*, but rather to the production of erythrogenic exotoxins by phage-infected streptococci. Scarlet fever is rare before the age of 3 and after 15. This upper age limit reflects prior exposure and development of immunity against the *erythrogenic toxin*. Protection is thus conferred against the rash, but not necessarily totally against other patterns of streptococcal infection. Scarlet fever is contracted from active cases, carriers and, in many instances, indirectly from the environment. The pathogenesis of the rash is still somewhat uncertain. It may be produced by the direct toxic action of the erythrogenic antigen but, alternately, there is reason to indict an allergic phenomenon potentiated by previous contact with this toxin.

Morphologically, the disease begins essentially as a streptococcal nasopharyngitis and tonsillitis. The diffuse rash appears approximately 1 to 3 days later. The nasopharyngitis and tonsillitis evoke a fiery red color in the pharyngeal mucosa and frequently small crypt abscesses with punctate exudate in the enlarged tonsils. The tongue is bright red, and the papillae are edematous to produce the "raspberry tongue" or, when the mucosa is coated and the papillae protrude, the "strawberry tongue." The rash is a diffuse, bright, violaceous red with punctate erythema, most abundant over the trunk and inner aspects of the arms and legs. The face is also involved, but usually a small area about the mouth remains relatively unaffected, to produce the so-called circumoral pallor. In the early stages, the rash blanches on slight pressure but, in later stages, small petechiae and ecchymoses occur from rupture of vessels and then the lesions do not blanch. Toward the end of the first week, the nasopharyngitis and rash begin to subside and the skin begins to scale and desquamate.

Accompanying these macroscopic alterations, there is a characteristic acute, edematous inflammatory reaction within the affected tissues, i.e., oropharynx, skin and lymph nodes. The inflammatory involvement of the epidermis is usually accompanied by increased cellular proliferation of the skin with consequent hyperkeratosis. It is this accelerated epidermal growth that accounts for the scaling and desquamation during the defervescence of the disease.

Clinically, the disease has an incubation period of 2 to 5 days. It is usually ushered in by headache, nausea, vomiting, fever, and chills or chilly sensations. The sore throat soon makes evident the probable streptococcal nature of the infection. There is usually little further doubt as to the diagnosis when the characteristic exanthem and enanthem appear. The fever usually spontaneously subsides in the course of one week. Control of the infection can be effected by adequate antibiotic therapy. During the height of the skin rash, application of a tourniquet to the arm for 5 minutes will produce multiple petechiae distal to the obstruction, the so-called *Rumpel-Leede* test. This test is not diagnostic of scarlet fever and here indicates increased fragility of capillaries due to a vasculotoxin. The Rumpel-Leede test is therefore also positive in many other diseases such as scurvy and thrombocytopenic purpura. A further diagnostic test to establish the nature of the rash is the *Schultz-Charlton* reaction, which is of diagnostic value only if positive. Injection of convalescent human serum or scarlet fever antitoxin into an area where the rash is full-blown will be followed by blanching in approximately 12 hours. This test consists merely of the local neutralization of the erythrogenic toxin.

In the usual case, progressive improvement follows without further complication. However, local spread of the nasopharyngitis may cause suppurative complications in the middle ear and sinuses, and occasionally in the dural venous sinuses and central nervous system. Alternately, peritonsillar abscesses, Ludwig's angina and suppurative cervical adenitis may follow. A streptococcal bacteremia may cause seeding of other organs in the body. The most important, but fortunately infrequent, complications that may follow scarlet fever are rheumatic fever and glomerulonephritis. Usually, recovery induces a permanent immunity against recurrent attacks of full-blown scarlet fever. This immunity is measured by the *Dick* test, the intradermal inoculation of a measured amount of streptococcal erythrogenic toxin. If protective levels of antibodies are present, the toxin is neutralized. If the patient is not immune, an erythematous reaction follows.

Other Streptococcal Infections. The hemolytic group A streptococci may also cause puerperal sepsis, acute endocarditis, bacterial pneumonia and meningitis, and may be secondary invaders in any other type of bacterial disease. The viridans streptococci are capable of evoking less severe clinical disease such as infections of the urinary and upper and lower respiratory tracts, and also cause focal abscesses in any site. Many cases of subacute bacterial endocarditis are caused by the viridans streptococcus.

There is a small group of streptococci that do not fall into any of the categories already mentioned. These are distinctive in that they require strict or almost complete anaerobic conditions for their growth. These microaerophilic streptococci are of principal importance clinically as secondary invaders of wounds and as causes of puerperal sepsis. In wounds they cause deep, undermining, spreading infections (*Meleney's ulcers*) that are resistant to usual forms of therapy.

PNEUMOCOCCAL INFECTIONS

The pneumococci are gram-positive diplococci which characteristically evoke suppurative exudations and are responsible for the majority of cases of bacterial lobar pneumonia. The pneumococcus may also cause pyogenic infections in the middle ear, paranasal sinuses, mastoids and joint spaces. It is a not uncommon cause of meningitis and brain abscess. Endocarditis and peritonitis are uncommon patterns of pneumococcal infection.

Causative Agent. At least 75 separable strains of pneumococci have been identified. These can be distinguished by type-specific capsular polysaccharides, which are not solely responsible for the virulence of the organism, although antigenic and capable of evoking antibody reactions. These specific soluble substances (SSS) are found only in the virulent pneumococci that possess a thick mucoid capsule. The mucoid hydrophilic capsules apparently protect the organism against phagocytosis and thus permit its rapid growth in any situation in which it becomes implanted.

Of the great number of types identified, types I, II and III account for at least 50 per cent of bacterial pneumonias caused by pneumococci, and the first eight types account for 80 per cent. Antibodies to these organisms are highly specific for the SSS in the capsule, and therefore immunity to one type does not confer protection against any of the other types.

Method of Spread. The common portal of entry for the pneumococcus is the respiratory tract. The infection may be contracted either from patients with active disease or from carriers. As many as 70 per cent of normal individuals harbor pneumococci in their throats but, for the most part, these are nonpathogenic.

Pathogenesis. Although pneumococci are classically said to cause primary bacterial pneumonias, some evidence suggests that often some underlying injury or adverse influence, such as a viral infection, predisposes to the bacterial implantation. Other contributing factors are chilling, fatigue, chemical or physical irritation to the respiratory mucosa due to the inhalation of noxious fumes or dust, al-

coholism and debilitating illnesses. These predisposing forces presumably lower the resistance of the lung and thus permit the cocci to gain a foothold.

The Infections. *Pneumonia.* Pneumococci are responsible for about 95 per cent of lobar pneumonias and also account for a considerable number of the patchy bronchopneumonias. As lung diseases, these processes are considered in detail in Chapter 19. However, it should be emphasized at this point that (1) other organisms may also cause both these forms of bacterial pneumonia, and (2) the pneumonias are characterized by total solidification of large tracts of alveolar spaces. A variety of complications may stem from the bacteremias that accompany the bacterial pneumonias. Many of these have already been listed, including focalized suppurative infections in the meninges, paranasal sinuses, middle ears, mastoids, dural venous sinuses, heart valves and joints. Empyema (infection of the pleural cavity) occurs in about 10 per cent of the cases of pneumococcal pneumonia.

MENINGOCOCCAL INFECTIONS

Meningococci are gram-negative diplococci which characteristically evoke suppurative reactions in their selective sites of localization. For obscure reasons, the meningococcus appears to find the meninges of the brain or, more properly, the cerebrospinal fluid, the most favorable environment in the body for its growth. Hence, meningitis is the most common clinical disease caused by this organism. However, endocarditis, suppurative arthritis, otitis media, pericarditis and other suppurative infections have been caused by these organisms. Since the usual portal of entry is the nasopharynx, meningococcal nasopharyngitis usually precedes these more serious infections, but often the nasopharyngitis is of such transient or trivial character as to escape clinical detection.

Causative Agent. These diplococci have a fairly distinctive morphology in smears. While the individual coccus is ovoid, the paired forms are frequently compressed at their points of apposition to create paired kidney shapes. The organism closely resembles *Micrococcus catarrhalis, Neisseria flava* and the gonococcus, and since the first two forms are common inhabitants of the nasopharynx and skin, care must be exercised in making a diagnosis of meningococcal infection merely on the basis of a gram-stained smear. One of the most important attributes of the meningococcus is its tendency to *invade the walls of small blood ves-*

sels, causing their rupture and thus leading to hemorrhages.

Method of Spread. The oral cavity is almost invariably the portal of entry for the meningococcus. Organisms are either inspired directly from active clinical cases and carriers or, far less often, are derived indirectly from contaminated dust and articles of daily use.

Pathogenesis. Meningococcal infections follow a fairly standard pattern in their development. *The initial stage is a localized naso-pharyngitis*, which may be extremely insignificant and evoke little anatomic change or clinical signs, or at times may produce manifest tissue reaction and symptomatology. From this primary focus, the organisms directly invade the blood to produce a *bacteremia*. This systemic dissemination may pass unnoticed, may appear as an acute fulminating disease *(acute meningococcemia)* or may be a very insidious, chronic disorder that persists for months and even years *(chronic meningococcemia)*. During the course of the bacteremia, widespread skin petechiae and ecchymoses are common and, occasionally, massive hemorrhage occurs into the adrenals (the Waterhouse-Friderichsen syndrome) (Chapter 29). The third phase that may or may not develop is that of a meningeal infection *(meningitis)*, presumably as a metastatic focus of seeding. The prominence of each of these phases, their duration and their temporal relationship to each other are extremely varied.

The Infections. *Nasopharyngitis.* When a clinically manifest nasopharyngitis is caused by the meningococci, it is entirely banal in character and is characterized by hyperemia, edema and mucopurulent exudation in the mucous membranes of the nasopharynx. The bacteremia that follows the nasopharyngitis sometimes produces no clinical reaction but at other times leads to an obvious meningococcemia. In chronic meningococcemia, there may only be mild bouts of recurrent fever *without* striking prostration, chills, elevation of the white count or other systemic signs of infection. This chronic form may at times produce scattered, isolated petechial or ecchymotic lesions on the skin that resemble in miniature the lesions found in the more acute fulminating forms of the disease.

Meningococcemia. In its more dramatic and usual form, the *acute meningococcemia* is evidenced as a sudden febrile illness of sharp onset with fever, chills, malaise, muscle aches and pains, nausea and vomiting, arthralgia, and sometimes severe prostration. The most striking clinical finding is the rash, which becomes evident within the first day or two of the illness.

The rash takes a variety of forms; the most common patterns are petechial, purpuric or ecchymotic hemorrhages scattered over the entire body surface. The individual lesions vary from a few millimeters to sometimes large, coalescent, irregular, map-like, violaceous discolorations. The centers of these hemorrhagic areas occasionally develop small, pinpoint, yellow-white necroses (Fig. 10–3). In other cases, the skin manifestations may appear as vesicles, bullae, allergic wheals, or even deep-seated firm nodules resembling erythema nodosum.

Histologically, these skin lesions are the result of *acute vasculitis* in the minute vessels, followed by suppurative necrosis and hemorrhage into the dermal connective tissue. There is marked perivascular cuffing of leukocytes, particularly neutrophils and macrophages, with occasional lymphocytes about the affected vessels. Many of these vessels are thrombosed. In some cases, organisms can be identified within the walls of the vessels, in the contained

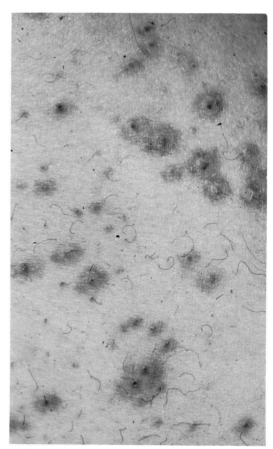

Figure 10–3. *The characteristic petechial rash of meningococcemia with small central foci of necrosis.*

blood clot and in surrounding leukocytes, but such identification is frequently difficult. It has been postulated that the acute vasculitis is due not to direct bacterial virulence, but rather to hypersensitivity reactions to bacterial seeding. The small white foci of necrosis occasionally found represent small abscesses that provide an ideal site for the possible isolation of bacteria. In the more acute, fulminating bacteremias, it is sometimes possible to visualize meningococci in the plasma and in white cells, and in most cases the organisms are readily cultured from the blood.

Not infrequently, adrenal involvement occurs in the acute meningococcemias. This combination of meningococcemia, and adrenal medullary hemorrhage is known as the *Waterhouse-Friderichsen syndrome* (Martland, 1944) (p. 1312). However, identical clinical syndromes are caused less often by other organisms, and there is some question whether this term should be confined only to meningococcal infections.

Meningitis may or may not be present in these cases. These patients classically have a very fulminating disease that may cause vascular collapse and death within 24 hours. It is still not clear whether this collapse is due largely to acute adrenal insufficiency or to the overwhelming toxemia. Most authors favor the latter concept. The mortality rate of this form of meningococcal infection is in the range of 90 per cent.

Meningitis. *The third and most characteristic stage of infection with the meningococcus is the development of meningitis.* In most patients, meningitis occurs without obvious meningococcemia. In others, the meningitis becomes manifest first and is followed by acute or chronic meningococcemia while, in still others, meningococcemias are punctuated by the onset of meningitis. However, it is well to recognize that all meningococcal infections do not eventuate in meningitis, and meningococcemias and the Waterhouse-Friderichsen syndrome are not invariably accompanied by infections within the central nervous system. The meningitis is classically an acute suppurative type, described in Chapter 32.

In addition to the lesions in the adrenals and in the central nervous system, meningococci may seed the heart valves, the pericardium, the joints, lungs or any other tissue of the body in the course of the bacteremia. Such additional sites of localization are rarely encountered in the absence of the meningitis and are not of grave clinical import save for the endocarditis.

GONOCOCCAL INFECTIONS

In common with other pyogenic cocci, the gonococcus evokes inflammatory reactions characterized by copious purulent exudation. In its growth requirements, the gonococcus evidently finds the mucous membranes of the male and female genital tracts the most appropriate environment. Clinical infections with this organism almost invariably begin in the anterior urethra in males and in the urethra, vulvovaginal glands and cervix in the female. These acute conditions are distressing, but not often of long-term significance. However, the infection may extend in the genital tract to cause serious sequelae, and metastatic infections through the circulating blood may spread to the joint spaces, heart valves, meninges and, far less commonly, to other organs and tissues.

Causative Agent. The gonococcus is a gram-negative diplococcus that very closely resembles the meningococcus. On gram-stained smears, it would be impossible to differentiate these organisms without knowing more about their cultural and biochemical characteristics. The gonococcus is capable of fermenting glucose but not maltose while the meningococcus ferments both maltose and glucose. Gram-negative intracellular diplococci found in the exudate of a genital tract infection must be interpreted as the *N. gonorrhoeae* until proved otherwise. One of the major factors contributing to the frequency of gonococcal infections is the failure of the development of immunity following an infection. Chronicity is thus a common characteristic of gonococcal disease, and reinfection may occur virtually as frequently as the individual is exposed.

Method of Spread. Gonorrhea is a universal infection that affects all races. There is considerable individual variation in resistance to the infection. Certain individuals are remarkably resistant, while others are extremely susceptible. Transmission is almost entirely by venereal exposure to active clinical cases. Nonvenereal transmission is responsible for two special forms of gonococcal infection: *gonococcal ophthalmia neonatorum* and *epidemic vulvovaginitis* in female children. In the days before the prophylactic use of penicillin or silver compounds in the eyes of newborn infants, gonococcal ophthalmitis was a prevalent condition in infants born of mothers having active infections. It was one of the principal causes of blindness, but present standard prophylaxis has virtually wiped it out. Epidemic vulvovaginitis is attributed to indirect, nonsexual contamination of the genital tract of female infants, usually over the age of six months and before puberty. Between these ages, the vagina has lost the keratinized maturity induced by the maternal hormones and has not yet developed the full-scale mucosal growth of puberty. The immature stratified squamous epithelium is susceptible to gonococcal invasion.

Pathogenesis. The stratified squamous epithelium of the external genitalia and the vagina *in the adult* is highly resistant to gonococcal infection. The organism finds its most favorable environment in the epithelium of the anterior urethra, prostate, seminal vesicles, epididymides and accessory urethral glands in the male and in the Bartholin's and Skene's glands, cervix and fallopian tubes in the female. For obscure reasons, the endometrium is apparently quite resistant to these infections.

The Infection. Gonorrhea. The initial infection becomes manifest approximately 2 to 7 days after an exposure by the appearance of suppurative exudation in any of the sites just mentioned. In the male, gonorrhea is manifested by the appearance of a mucopurulent exudate from the anterior urethra and meatus. This infection appears to be limited largely to the superficial mucous membranes and accessory glands. The meatus becomes hyperemic, edematous and obviously inflamed, and the reaction is characterized histologically by a superficial inflammatory neutrophilic reaction. The infection is of little consequence if the disease is effectively treated or does not spread upward in the genital tract. However, in the usual course of the untreated disease, it extends into the posterior urethra and major glands of the male genital tract. Although gonococcal epididymitis is characteristic of the neglected case, the testis is remarkably resistant to this organism and orchitis rarely develops, save for a superficial reaction to the adjacent epididymal lesion. The secondary infections in the prostate, seminal vesicles and epididymides give rise to chronic, persistent, deep-seated suppuration, abscess formation and destruction of the local structures, which may eventuate in urethral strictures and permanent sterility.

In the female, the disease is ushered in by reddening and edema of the urethral meatus. Similar acute suppuration and abscess formations may occur in the Bartholin's and Skene's glands. The cervix is initially or soon involved and, when improperly treated, gonococcal salpingitis eventuates in the usual course of events. A localized pelvic peritonitis commonly ensues. In the course of time, the fimbriated ends of the tube seal or become adherent to the ovaries to create a *pyosalpinx (pus tube)*. The infection may thus become sealed off and chronic, and eventuate in hugely distended tubes, *tubo-ovarian abscesses* and pelvic adhesions. This pattern of advanced inflammatory disease is often designated as pelvic inflammatory disease (P.I.D.). Purulent exudation and extensive adhesions characterize the neglected case and may also lead to permanent sterility in the female, detailed on p. 1206.

From the clinical standpoint, the early case of gonorrhea with involvement of only the lower genitourinary tract is of importance largely because of the pain and discomfort that it produces and because of its transmissibility. However, when upper level infections develop, persistent discharge, painful urination, impotence in the male and chronic leukorrhea in the female may eventuate. Salpingitis causes severe lower abdominal pain, menstrual cramps, pain on defecation, intestinal disturbances and signs and symptoms of pelvic peritonitis. In addition to these problems relating to the local infection, transient bacteremias may occur either with or without clinical symptoms. Very infrequently, the gonococcemia may produce a fulminating disease that is extremely difficult to differentiate from acute meningococcemia. More often, the transient bacteremia passes unnoted and only becomes known by the appearance of metastatic infections such as suppurative arthritis, vegetative bacterial endocarditis and meningitis. These complications have become extremely uncommon since the advent of effective chemotherapeutic measures.

HEMOPHILUS BACILLI

The Hemophilus bacilli are gram-negative, nonmotile, aerobic coccobacilli of which only *H. influenzae, H. pertussis* and *H. ducreyi* are important pathogens for man. The clinical infections caused by the first two are chiefly limited to children. The inflammatory reaction to the Hemophilus organisms tends to be suppurative in nature irrespective of the tissue involved. Because this form of reaction is entirely nonspecific and resembles those caused by pyogens, the Hemophilus causation cannot be confirmed in tissue sections unless appropriate organisms can be visualized. Preferably, cultural and serologic methods are necessary to identify the precise bacterial agent.

H. INFLUENZAE INFECTIONS

Hemophilus influenzae is an important primary and secondary invader in children and is responsible for a variety of suppurative infections such as meningitis, laryngotracheobronchitis, nasopharyngitis, otitis media, sinusitis, pneumonia and, less commonly, foci of suppuration in other organs or tissues.

Causative Agent. Six strains of *H. influenzae* bacilli have been identified by specific serologic and biochemical characteristics. Only type B is an important pathogen. This organism has both encapsulated and unencapsulated variants. While the organisms without capsules are believed to cause clinical disease occasionally, significant infections are almost invariably due to the more virulent encapsulated forms. The capsule presumably blocks the phagocytosis of the *H. influenzae*, thus enhancing its pathogenicity and invasiveness.

Method of Spread. The route of infection in man is not well understood. It is probable that it occurs by fairly direct airborne contamination of the upper respiratory tract by organisms derived from clinically active cases, convalescent patients, or possibly from carriers. *H. influenzae* can be isolated from the nasopharynx of about 30 to 50 per cent of children. Most of these organisms are unencapsulated and probably not of great clinical importance, but some of the carriers harbor virulent, encapsulated type B bacilli. It is not known whether these individuals are long-term carriers of this virulent pathogen or whether they have recently recovered from an unrecognized or possibly subclinical infection.

Pathogenesis. It is believed that the organisms are directly implanted on the nasopharyngeal mucosa where clinical or subclinical local infections may develop. Although organisms are not readily identified in the blood, it is assumed that transient bacteremias must occur in some cases, because visceral organs are sometimes involved, for instance, the brain, joints, heart valves and other sites. In respiratory infections, the organisms probably spread by continuity from the upper to the lower respiratory tract.

H. influenzae infections are virtually limited to children between the ages of two to three months and eight years, the period when passive immunity from the mother is lost and an acquired immunity has not yet been gained. However, adults may become predisposed by debilitating influences, and therefore *H. influenzae* is an occasional secondary invader in the wake of viral infections of the lung, chronic debilitating disease and chronic alcoholism. Once implanted within the tissues, the organisms characteristically evoke a nonspecific, acute, neutrophilic exudation. These exudates tend to be quite rich in fibrin and therefore have a plastic quality, which may be important in protecting the organisms and may be of further significance insofar as the exudates are less easily resolved and thus tend to become organized.

The Infections. *Infections of the Upper Respiratory Tract.* *H. influenzae* may cause trivial or extremely serious infections in or about the pharynx, including mild or severe pharyngitis, otitis media, sinusitis and occasionally tonsillitis. While these infections are accompanied by variable levels of fever and are sometimes resistant to simple therapeutic measures, they are not extremely serious save as sites for the seeding of the blood. However, one form of upper respiratory infection (*laryngotracheobronchitis* and *epiglottitis*) is important in young children and infants. It can be extremely fulminating, with sudden onset of fever and subsequent hyperemic edema of the epiglottis and larynx leading to respiratory obstruction. These manifestations may become full-blown within 24 hours, creating an acute pediatric emergency that often requires prophylactic tracheotomy to prevent total respiratory obstruction. Without appropriate treatment, death may follow within 1 to 4 days. The anatomic changes consist of an inflammatory response that differs in no way from the acute responses to the pyogens.

Meningitis. *H. influenzae* is one of the two most common causes of meningitis in infancy and childhood, the other being the meningococcus (Neal et al., 1934). Influenzal meningitis begins with a prodromal period of an upper respiratory tract infection, which becomes complicated within the first week by the development of meningitis. The meningitis is of a nonspecific, suppurative form. It is somewhat distinctive by the heavy plastic nature of the exudate, which is rich in fibrin. This exudate is limited for the most part to the subarachnoid space; but invasion of the superficial brain substance, particularly about the perivascular spaces, is sometimes encountered. The exudate collects most heavily about the base of the brain and brain stem. In this location, it may obstruct the foramina and aqueducts of the ventricular systems and produce progressive dilatation of the ventricles of the brain (internal hydrocephalus). Hydrocephalus is a grave hazard in persistent infections because the exudate tends to organize rather than resolve. Precise identification of the cause of the pyogenic meningitis requires bacteriologic and serologic procedures. In unrecognized cases, there is an 80 to 90 per cent mortality rate, similar to the rate in the preantibiotic era.

Pneumonia. *H. influenzae* pneumonia may result from the direct spread of an infection from the upper respiratory tract or may occur as a blood-borne localization. These pulmonary infections may develop as primary diseases in both infants and adults. However, in adults there is more often some preceding, usually viral, respiratory infection. While at one time it was believed that *H. influenzae* was responsible for the extremely lethal pandemics of influenza that scourged the world in 1890 and again in 1918, it is now known that these pandemics were caused by the influenza virus, although the clinical disease was aggravated and made more lethal by *H. influenzae*, streptococcal and staphylococcal superinfections. *H. influenzae* pneumonia may appear in the pattern of patchy focal consolidations or confluent total lobar consolidation. The histologic reaction is indistinguishable from that produced by the pneumococcus or other pyogens, and therefore specific identification requires adjunct laboratory procedures.

Other Infections. Pyogenic infections due to *H. influenzae* may occur in many other sites of the body, presumably due to the bacteremic spread of bacilli. These diverse localizations include bacterial endocarditis, pyelonephritis, suppurative arthritis, cholecystitis, and a form of acute purulent conjunctivitis known as "pink-eye" in children. This ocular infection has long been attributed to the Koch-Weeks bacillus. According to present opinion, however, the Koch-Weeks bacillus is indistinguishable from *H. influenzae*.

H. PERTUSSIS INFECTIONS—WHOOPING COUGH

Hemophilus pertussis causes an acute, infectious, communicable disease, virtually limited to children, known as *whooping cough or pertussis*. This disease is characterized by violent, asphyxiative paroxysms of coughing. But it must be appreciated that the characteristic "whoop" may be absent in the less severe forms, and often such cases go unrecognized.

Causative Agent. *H. pertussis* is a gram-negative coccobacillus having the pleomorphism of the influenzal organisms. Of the four variants that have been identified, the so-called "phase one" organisms are the most virulent. However, all variants may induce disease, and these subgroups are chiefly of importance in epidemiologic and public health studies. These organisms produce a variety of antigenic fractions, the most important of which is *a heat-labile toxin which is capable of strong necrotizing action* when injected intradermally into a rabbit. This toxin presumably accounts for the cellular destruction found in whooping cough. Good antibody response follows infections with this organism, and recurrent infection following a full-blown clinical case of pertussis is uncommon.

Method of Spread. *H. pertussis* is extremely sensitive to drying, and on this basis the disease is most often contracted by direct exposure to active clinical cases. Whooping cough is extremely communicable, and transfer of infection occurs in about 80 to 90 per cent of the nonimmune members of a family and in up to 25 per cent of the exposed susceptible students in a classroom. The disease is apparently transmissible during the incubation period of two weeks, and the catarrhal stage of two weeks, when patients do not yet have characteristic clinical features of whooping cough. This disease also occurs in epidemic form. It is probable that carriers maintain a reservoir of pathogenic strains that potentiate widespread transmission of organisms and epidemic outbreaks.

Pathogenesis. Aspiration of contaminated droplets is followed by localization of the organisms in their favored site—the ciliated epithelium of the upper respiratory tract (p. 359). The usual case follows a fairly standard clinical pattern of a *two-week incubation period, two weeks of catarrhal developmental disease, and two weeks of full-blown paroxysmal coughing, followed by a final convalescent period of two weeks' duration*.

The Infection. Following the incubation period, the catarrhal period of coughing, sneezing and signs of an upper respiratory tract infection develops. These symptoms are caused by a superficial mucosal infection in the upper respiratory tract, evidenced by a neutrophilic exudation limited largely to the lining epithelium and the superficial submucosal connective tissues. Large numbers of organisms are now demonstrable, lying on the surface of the epithelium and entangled within the cilia of the columnar lining cells (Fig. 10–4). As the disease enters the stage of paroxysmal coughing, necrosis of the midzonal and basal portions of the pseudostratified columnar mucosa is evident, accompanied by an outpouring of a mucopurulent exudate and a mild leukocytic infiltrate in the submucosal tissues. As the disease progresses, the inflammatory reaction permeates the walls of the trachea and bronchi, and peribronchiolitis and interstitial pneumonitis ensue. A more copious exudate accumulates within the air passages at this time.

In the more severe cases, the necrotic epithelium of the air passages may desquamate, but deeper ulcerations are not common. Exudative consolidation of the alveoli occurs infrequently and is usually due to secondary bacterial invaders. Other pulmonary parenchymal changes may occur, secondary to the violent paroxysms of coughing and consequent asphyxia. Hemorrhage and edema may be found in the alveoli, and patchy atelectasis occurs distal to totally obstructed bronchi and

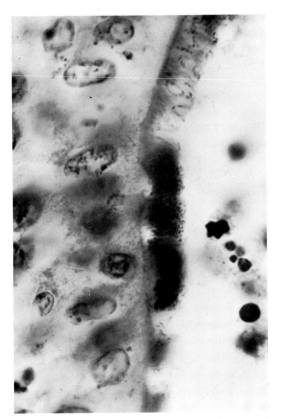

Figure 10-4. *Whooping cough—a high power detail of the columnar epithelium of a bronchus with bacilli entangled within the cilia.*

bronchioles. In rare cases, the violent coughing may rupture alveolar walls and may permit air to escape into the stromal framework of the lung with the development of interstitial and subcutaneous emphysema (p. 800).

Nosebleeds, rupture of superficial vessels in the mucosa of the alimentary tract, hemorrhages into the sclera or conjunctiva, petechial hemorrhages into the serosal linings of the body cavities, petechiae in the skin of the face and neck, and punctate hemorrhages in the brain sometimes appear as a consequence of the explosive coughing and hypoxia. Convulsions appear in about 10 per cent of the full-blown cases, probably related to the hypoxia and intracerebral hemorrhages. Post-tussis encephalitis is an infrequent complication of obscure nature, probably not directly attributable to either the organism or its toxins. Characteristically, there is a striking lymphocytosis with total white cell count sometimes up to 100,000 cells per mm.³ of blood. This hematologic change may well be due to endotoxin released by the death of organisms trapped in the respiratory tract epithelium.

Convalescence usually follows the paroxysmal stage and is accompanied by the progressive development of permanent immunity. Whooping cough is a serious disease in the very young. About 5 per cent of hospitalized cases terminate in death. The majority occur in patients below one year of age. Fatalities after 10 years of age are distinctly uncommon. The usual cause of death is a bacterial pneumonia due to a secondary invader, i.e., staphylococci, streptococci, *A. aerogenes* and sometimes the Proteus bacillus. Less commonly, an influenzal interstitial pneumonitis or otitis media develops.

H. DUCREYI INFECTIONS—CHANCROID (SOFT CHANCRE)

Chancroid is an acute venereal disease caused by *Hemophilus ducreyi* and characterized by the development of a necrotic ulcer, *the soft chancre*, at the site of inoculation on the genitals. The causative organism is a very short, plump, gram-negative coccobacillus about 1 to 2 microns in length. The disease is transmitted by sexual intercourse, and inoculation of the organism occurs through abrasions or injuries of the skin and mucous membranes. The organism may be a normal saprophyte of the vaginal tract, and carriers may be responsible for a considerable part of the incidence of this condition. Chancroid is somewhat uncommon in the United States and is particularly localized to the Orient, West Indies and North Africa. Poor personal hygiene and promiscuity favor its spread. It is highly infectious, and autoinoculation frequently leads to multiple chancres.

The soft chancre usually occurs on the penis and about the labia minora and majora. A small macule or vesicle that becomes papular and then forms an intradermal abscess or pustule develops at the site of invasion. The overlying skin sloughs to produce a draining ulcer. This ulcer is at first shallow and less than 1 cm. in diameter, but may enlarge up to 2 to 3 cm. in diameter. The well developed ulcer is covered with a necrotic, purulent slough and bears a superficial resemblance to the chancre of syphilis, but does not have the characteristic induration of the syphilitic hard chancre. In the course of one to two weeks, the regional nodes undergo painful inflammatory hyperplasia in about half the cases. Suppuration may occur in these sites to produce fluctuant masses that drain to the skin surface, producing lesions (sometimes designated as *buboes*) resembling those found in bubonic plague.

Histologically, the soft chancre presents

three distinctive zones. The surface of the ulcer is composed of coagulated proteinous exudate, necrotic debris, and disintegrating leukocytes and red cells. Deep to this level, there is a zone of granulation tissue which is somewhat distinctive in the marked involvement of the small capillaries. There is considerable hypertrophy and hyperplasia of the endothelial cells, as well as a marked inflammatory reaction both within and about the vessel wall. This vasculitis often leads to intravascular thrombosis or frank necrosis of the vessel wall. Deep to the granulation tissue, there is a third zone of more chronic inflammatory reaction with fibroblastic proliferation infiltrated with mononuclear leukocytes. The changes in the regional nodes of drainage are essentially similar and present the same characteristic alterations of the involved vessels. Abscesses may form in the centers of these inflammatory nodes and, by coalescence, form large areas of suppurative necrosis. The walls of the abscess reproduce the histologic changes of the skin lesion. The disease usually remains localized to the genital tract and its nodes of drainage, and widespread dissemination has not yet been reported.

Clinically, the local macule or papule usually appears within the first two weeks following the exposure, and from this stage the characteristic ulcer develops in the course of the succeeding 3 to 5 days. The ulcer is not particularly painful; however, the regional nodes of drainage are extremely tender, presumably due to tension on the capsule of the nodes produced by the inflammatory response. The constitutional symptoms that accompany this disease are extremely mild and of little significance.

The diagnosis of chancroid can be established by the isolation of *Hemophilus ducreyi* or by tissue biopsy with the demonstration of the more or less characteristic histologic changes just mentioned (Sheldon and Heyman, 1946). A skin test for chancroid is available, but remains positive for as long as several years after an acute infection and therefore does not have critical value in identifying the nature of an acute lesion. This condition runs a relatively short course and subsides spontaneously or with therapy, to leave behind only fibrous induration of the affected nodes and a local scar at the site of the skin lesion.

SPIROCHETES

Three genera in the order of Spirochaetales cause clinical disease. The most important genus is the Treponema, of which *T. pallidum* causes syphilis; *T. pertenue*, yaws; and *T. cara-* *teum*, pinta. In the genus Borrelia, several species cause relapsing fever. The third genus, the Leptospira, is responsible for Weil's disease and related disorders. It is useful to group spirochetoses together, because *the spirochetes tend to cause widespread interstitial inflammations associated with proliferative vascular changes and prominent perivascular lymphocytic and plasma cell infiltrations.* While they sometimes cause focal necrosis of tissues, as in a gumma, in general these organisms do not cause suppurative exudations or lesions that resemble those produced by the pyogens. *Infections caused by the spirochetes also differ from many bacterial diseases in the apparent paucity of microorganisms in tissue lesions and in the extreme difficulty in identifying the causative agents by bacterial cultural methods.* Moreover, the organisms are not revealed by usual bacterial stains. Identification of spirochetes in bacterial smears or tissue sections requires darkfield examinations, contrast stains in which the organisms are visualized against the black background of India ink, or silver impregnation techniques which coat the organisms. Organisms are so sparse even in active lesions as to make it difficult to understand the manner in which they injure tissue. *The histologic identification of spirochetal diseases therefore requires a knowledge of the relatively nonspecific changes that these organisms induce, the pattern of lesions associated with each organism, and the appropriate special studies to detect the possible existence of a spirochetosis.*

SYPHILIS

Despite the great improvements in the control and treatment of syphilis, this infection remains one of the most important communicable diseases in man. Syphilis is of particular clinical importance because the initial lesion and subsequent widespread systemic dissemination are often not accompanied by disturbing signs or symptoms. The disease may then enter a period of latency, to be followed much later by serious crippling or fatal lesions. It is estimated that about 80 per cent of these patients come to medical attention for the first time when these late visceral lesions have already developed. While most of these late manifestations are localized to a relatively few systems, principally the cardiovascular and central nervous systems, infrequently other organs or structures are affected. This random unpredictable localization leads to a multiplicity of clinical symptom complexes. Many clinicians, Osler among them, have therefore dubbed this disease "the great mimic."

For many years, the incidence of syphilis has progressively declined, but in the past few years it has begun to show a sharp and significant climb. Syphilis is a serious disorder, since it causes the death of approximately 5 to 10 per cent of those infected.

Causative Agent. *Treponema pallidum* is a slender, spiral, motile organism up to 20 microns in length and about one-fifth micron in thickness. Little is known of the toxicity and antigenicity of this organism. Most of its virulence is probably attributable to its invasiveness. It must be assumed that tissue lesions are caused by a weak, but nonetheless existent, endotoxin, since no other antigens have been identified.

Immunity is conferred by a syphilitic infection. However, complete immunity can be blocked by subcurative treatment in the early stages of the disease. *Immunity begins to develop shortly after infection, since two distinct antibodies appear in the serum at this time.* One of these is *syphilitic reagin.* It is closely associated with the plasma gamma globulins and provides the basis for the complement fixation and flocculation tests for syphilis.

The serologic tests for syphilis usually become positive about one month after the contraction of the disease, but sometimes not until three to four months later. Once detectable levels of reagin have developed, they usually persist in the untreated cases for the remainder of the patient's life. Appropriate therapy may convert the test to negative. In a small but significant number of cases, *spontaneous reversal* occurs in untreated cases, usually only 10 to 15 years after the development of the infection, so that a negative serologic test does not exclude the possible existence of an untreated latent case of syphilis. Reagin, however, is *not* responsible for the immunity to reinfection and does not, as far as we know, contribute to the destruction of treponemas.

The other antibody identified in syphilitic infections is known as the *treponemal immobilizing antibody* (T.P.I.). This antibody can be demonstrated by an *in vitro test.* In the presence of complement, syphilitic serum causes the progressive immobilization and eventual death of pathogenic *T. pallidum.* This and other similar tests are quite specific although cross reactions occur with the other treponematoses. It becomes progressively stronger with the age of the infection. *The T.P.I. test is considerably more reliable than the usual reagin serologic test.* False-positive reactions to the reagin serologic tests occur in a number of unrelated clinical states, such as infectious mononucleosis, the other spirochetal infections, measles, chickenpox and, in fact, during or soon after any febrile disease. In most of these false positives, the T.P.I. test would be negative. It is tempting to speculate that the T.P.I. antibody is indeed responsible for the destruction of spirochetes in the host as well as for the development of the active immunity to this disease.

Method of Spread. Syphilis occurs in both acquired and congenital forms. The acquired infection is almost invariably transmitted by sexual contact. *T. pallidum* is extremely vulnerable to drying and it is highly unlikely that indirect transmission ever occurs. The usual primary site of infection occurs on the penis in the male and on the vulva or cervix in the female. In approximately 10 per cent of the cases, the infection may be extragenital, transferred to the lips, fingers, oropharynx or some other site from a chancre or from some secondary infectious lesion. When the chancre occurs on the cervix, the initial lesion may pass unnoticed. In about 50 per cent of females and 30 per cent of males, primary lesions either never develop or are not recognized by the patient. The organism presumably enters through a break, possibly microscopic in size, in the continuity of the skin or mucous membranes, since the organism cannot penetrate the intact epidermis, and it is highly doubtful that it can penetrate even the thinner mucosa.

Pathogenesis. Once the organism gains access to the tissues of the host in acquired syphilis, local multiplication and sharply localized regional invasion occur almost immediately. The treponemes penetrate the lymphatics and are drained to the regional nodes. A total systemic spirochetemia follows within the first 24 hours by drainage through lymphatics or by direct invasion of veins. In the course of this bacteremia, organisms undoubtedly penetrate small vessels to become implanted throughout the body. This spirochetemia may persist for weeks or months, possibly even years, and is terminated only by the development of immobilizing antibodies. Thus, new localizations and superficial infectious lesions appear during the prolonged spirochetemia long after the initial contact.

On the basis of this pathogenesis, *three classic stages of the acquired disease are recognized* (Martland, 1932). The *primary stage* consists of the local development of the chancre between the end of the first week and the subsequent three months following the contact. From two to 12 weeks thereafter, the *secondary stage* becomes manifest in the form of a generalized skin rash, sometimes accompanied by involvement of the mucous membranes. An asymptomatic period follows the secondary stage which lasts up to several decades. The subsequent fate of these patients is quite unpredictable. About one-third achieve apparent spontaneous cure and most develop negative serologic tests, even without treatment. One-third remain seropositive, but never develop structural lesions or definite anatomic stigmata of syphilis. The remaining third or less develop late lesions characteristic of tertiary syphilis, but not all these patients develop symptoms from their tissue involvements. *About 80 to 90 per cent of these tertiary lesions involve the cardiovascular system and the central nervous system.* The other tertiary lesions consist principally of gummas in the skin, liver, bones, spleen and, less commonly, in other sites. Later, ocular manifestations may also develop. The cardiovascular involvement is the principal cause of death today. Occasionally, several tertiary localizations occur concurrently in the same patient.

Syphilis may also be transmitted to the fetus in utero by an infected mother. The disease can be transmitted for a variable period of months to even years, presumably until the spirochetemia has abated. Congenital syphilis may result in intrauterine fetal death any time after the fifth month of gestation. When the child survives, a widespread, fulminating type of infection may result, which usually does not have the classic stages of acquired syphilis and is further manifested by anatomic changes dissimilar to those of the adult disease. Occasionally, prenatally acquired syphilis may first become manifest in youth or adult life and, in this instance, may be mild or severe, paralleling the acquired form of the disease.

The Infections. *Acquired Syphilis.* *Primary Stage.* The primary chancre usually begins as a solitary, slightly elevated, firm papule, which varies in size up to several centimeters in diameter, on the penis or on the vulva or cervix. Multiple chancres are rarely found. When the chancre occurs at some extragenital site, it may not be recognized. It then superficially erodes to create a clean-based, shallow ulceration on the surface of the slightly elevated papule. *The contiguous induration characteristically creates a button-like mass directly subjacent to the eroded skin or mucosa.* Superimposed secondary bacterial infection may impart a suppurative exudation.

Histologically, the chancre is characterized by an intense mononuclear leukocytic infiltration, chiefly of plasma cells with scattered macrophages and lymphocytes (Fig. 10–5). This inflammatory infiltrate is found within a proliferative vasofibroblastic response that comprises the margins of the ulcer. There is concentric endothelial and fibroblastic proliferative thickening of the small vessels in the area, to produce a lesion known as *obliterative endarteritis, a characteristic but not pathogno-*

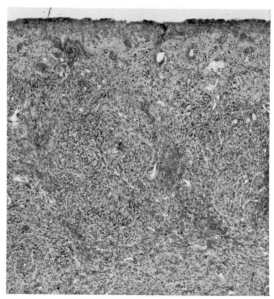

Figure 10–5. *The base of a syphilitic chancre with loss of epithelium and a deep-seated inflammatory reaction.*

monic change in syphilis. In the deeper regions, the inflammatory reaction is less intense, and the mononuclear infiltrate is more sharply limited to *perivascular cuffing,* accompanied by the vascular thickening described. The immediate surface of the chancre may have a neutrophilic infiltration. In usual tissue sections, treponemes are not evident, but with silver impregnations, characteristic spiral microorganisms are found in large numbers in the areas of active inflammation. In the course of approximately two months, the chancre completely heals with reepithelialization of the surface defect. The regional nodes are usually enlarged and somewhat tender, and have evidence of nonspecific acute or chronic lymphadenitis (p. 750). Not infrequently, even at this early stage of the disease, there is a generalized lymphadenopathy.

The primary stage of syphilis and its accompanying early spirochetemia are remarkable for the absence of systemic signs and symptoms. The patient is entirely well, is usually free of fever, and may have only some slight local pain in the region of the superficial erosion. These lesions are readily recognized as chancres by the classic anatomic features, when they occur in the usual genital sites. Recognition becomes particularly difficult in extragenital sites and when secondary bacterial invasion transforms the clean granulation tissue base into a suppurative ulcer. The final diagnosis can often be made by identification of treponemes in the exudate of the chancre or in the fluid aspirated from the enlarged regional nodes. At this stage of the disease, both the reagin serologic tests and the Treponema immobilization test are usually negative.

Secondary Stage. The generalized spirochetemia is usually manifested by the appearance of widespread mucocutaneous lesions about one to three months after the primary stage. These cutaneous lesions are extremely protean, and can be characterized as having *any form other than vesicular.* In the usual case, the rash is maculopapular and varies from scattered lesions, perhaps involving a single region of the skin surface, to diffuse involvement of the entire skin, including the mucous membranes of the oral cavity and involvement of the palms of the hands and soles of the feet. The individual macule has a red-brown appearance and rarely exceeds 5 mm. in diameter. In other cases, follicular, pustular, annular and scaling lesions may predominate. Histologically the inflammatory reaction in the foci of mucocutaneous involvement resembles that found in the chancre. However, there is less intensity to the mononuclear leukocytic infiltrate and it is ordinarily confined to perivascular cuffing. When the rash is distinctly papular, it is usually accompanied by thickening of the epithelium and elongation of the rete pegs. Ulceration modifies the macroscopic and microscopic appearance by the development of suppurative exudation.

One type of secondary lesion merits special mention. Papular lesions in the region of the penis and vulva may become large, elevated, broad plaques. These flat, red-brown elevations (up to 2 to 3 cm. in diameter) are designated as *condylomata lata (venereal warts)* and are distinct from the nonvenereal papillary condylomata acuminata. They sometimes occur on the lips and perianal region. The overlying epithelium is intact unless secondarily traumatized or infected. Histologically, there is a striking hyperplasia of the epithelium, with superficial hyperkeratosis and deep prolongation of the rete pegs into the underlying dermis. There is an accompanying characteristic plasma cell and mononuclear infiltrate, as well as the characteristic, but not full-blown, vascular obliterative endarteritis. Spirochetes may be found in these mucocutaneous lesions and condylomata. The generalized adenopathy of secondary syphilis is of a nonspecific character.

The lesions of secondary syphilis are not of themselves pathognomonic since there is such variability in their form. However, the diagnosis of syphilis must at least be suspected when such a disseminated rash develops in a patient who appears to be entirely well, save possibly for generalized adenopathy. In the other bacteremic states associated with rashes, such as meningococcemia, typhoid fever and the rickettsial diseases, systemic constitutional signs of fever, chills, malaise and even prostration almost invariably accompany the skin lesions. Uncommonly, three types of ocular disease are found during the stage of generalization: iritis, neuritis or retinitis. The mucocutaneous lesions abound with spirochetes, and when ulcerated, these lesions and their secretions are infective. In this stage of the disease, the serologic and Treponema immobilzation tests are usually positive.

Tertiary Stage. Tertiary lesions develop in about 30 per cent of patients, but clinical disease results in only half these cases. The cardiovascular system bears the brunt of these tertiary lesions (80 to 85 per cent). The central nervous system accounts for about 5 to 10 per cent. Gummas in the liver and other sites make up the remainder of the tertiary syphilitic lesions. These localizations are not mutually exclusive, as was mentioned.

Cardiovascular Syphilis. Luetic involvement of the aorta may become manifest years to several decades after the initial infection. Presumably, the organisms have localized in these tissues during the primary and secondary stages of the spirochetemia and have remained latent. Alternatively, it is possible that these lesions develop extremely slowly over the course of many years. *Cardiovascular syphilis is an extremely serious disorder that causes considerable inflammatory scarring and weakening of the media of the aorta (mesaortitis) with weakening and dilatation of the aorta (aneurysm formation), widening of the aortic valve ring, and narrowing of the mouths of the coronary ostia* (p. 616).

Central Nervous System Syphilis. Central nervous system syphilis, neurosyphilis, is another late manifestation, apparently also initiated by invasion of the central nervous system and its meningeal covering during the early stages of spirochetemia. Neurosyphilis differs somewhat from the other tertiary lesions in that even though spirochetes can be demonstrated in the spinal fluid of many patients, only about one-third eventually develop demonstrable tissue damage. *Neurosyphilis takes one of several forms designated as meningovascular syphilis, tabes and paresis.* Focal gummas occur very infrequently. All these variants present as central nervous system disorders and are considered in Chapter 32.

The Gumma. The gumma is a late-appearing *focal area of nonsuppurative inflammatory destruction caused presumably by the localization of spirochetes in a tissue, characterized by a peculiar rubbery, gray-white total necrosis known as gumma-*

tous necrosis. While they may occur anywhere, they are most commonly found in the mucocutaneous tissues, liver, bones and testes. They may occur singly or multiply. They vary in size from microscopic defects to large tumorous masses of necrotic material. Characteristically, the gumma is enclosed within a wall of fibroblastic scarring. Erosion of a superficial cutaneous or submucosal gumma may yield a ragged, shaggy ulcer that is extremely persistent and resistant to usual local therapeutic measures.

In the liver, gummas may cause nodular enlargement during the stages of acute necrosis, but later yield depressed scars that cause a type of cirrhosis known as *hepar lobatum* (p. 1036). Gummas in bones cause focal areas of destruction. They may erode the cortical surfaces and lead to fractures, and sometimes they extend into joints to destroy the articular surfaces and the joint function. A testicular gumma may cause enlargement early and simulate tumor but later produce fibrous replacement of the testis or focal area.

Histologically, the active gumma consists of a center of coagulated, necrotic material which differs from frank caseation necrosis in the faint persistence of shadowy outlines of underlying tissue cells (Fig. 10–6). There are no

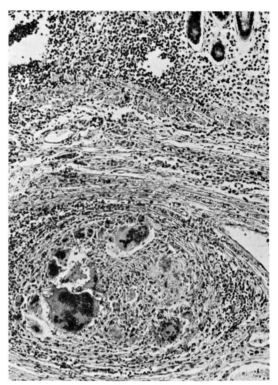

Figure 10–7. *A microscopic detail of a minute gumma in the submucosa of the bowel illustrating the characteristic granuloma with foreign body type giant cells.*

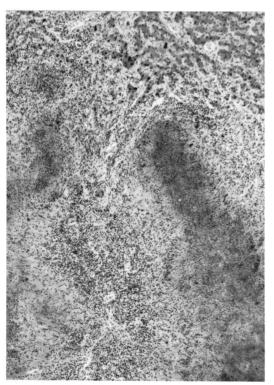

Figure 10–6. *Gumma of the liver with central necrosis.*

vital native or leukocytic cells in these necrotic centers. The center is avascular and appears to have undergone ischemic necrosis. The margins of the gumma are composed of plump fibroblasts that resemble the epithelioid cells in tuberculosis, infiltrated with the characteristic mononuclear leukocytes, chiefly plasma cells and lymphocytes. The small vessels in the wall are narrowed by the obliterative endarteritis found in other syphilitic lesions. Typical perivascular cuffing may be evident. Treponemes are scant in these gummas and are extremely difficult to demonstrate. When present, they are most abundant in the enclosing inflammatory wall.

The gumma at times may be microscopic in size, producing a lesion which is virtually indistinguishable from the granulomas of tuberculosis and Boeck's sarcoid without additional evidence of the causative agent (Fig. 10–7). Although in the majority of cases the reagin serologic test and the T.P.I. test are positive in these late stages of syphilis, such serologic evidence does not preclude the possibility of intercurrent tuberculosis or sarcoidosis.

Gummas are of clinical importance either as causes of local destruction or as enlargements that are often confused with neoplasms. In many areas such as the liver or spleen, they are of little clinical significance save for their differentiation from a tumor. However, in bones the gumma may cause severe clinical disease.

Except for tissue biopsy, the most valuable diagnostic test of a gumma is its response to antisyphilitic treatment. With adequate therapy, the gumma progressively shrinks in size and becomes a fibrotic scar.

Congenital Syphilis. Congenital syphilis may be contracted by the fetus as long as the spirochetemia persists in the mother. The treponemes do not invade the placental tissue or the fetus until the fifth month of gestation, and therefore syphilis is an uncommon cause of early abortion. Instead, it causes late abortion, stillbirth or death soon after delivery, or it may remain as a latent infection to become apparent only in childhood or adult life. This variable outlook depends entirely upon the severity of the infection in the infant. It is worthy of note that treatment of the syphilitic mother before the fourth month of pregnancy will result in a nonsyphilitic child in over 90 per cent of the instances.

In the perinatal and infantile form of congenital syphilis, the characteristic lesions follow a fairly well defined pattern. The most striking lesions affect the *mucocutaneous tissues* and the bones. A diffuse, maculopapular, desquamative rash develops, which differs from that of the acquired secondary stage in that there is extensive sloughing of the epithelium. This desquamation affects the entire body surface, but is particularly prominent on the palms and soles and about the mouth and anus. These lesions teem with spirochetes and have the characteristic mononuclear leukocytic infiltrate and obliterative endarteritis found in all syphilitic lesions. There is a generalized luetic *osteochondritis* and *perichondritis* that affects all bones of the skeletal system, most prominently the nose and lower legs. Destruction of the vomer causes collapse of the bridge of the nose and the characteristic *saddle deformity.* Periostitis of the tibia leads to excessive new bone growth on the anterior surfaces and produces *anterior bowing, or "sabre shin."* In addition to these findings, there is widespread disturbance in the endochondral bone formation. The normal orderly replacement of cartilage by osteoid tissue is disrupted. The epiphyses become widened as the cartilage overgrows. Cartilage is found as displaced islands within the metaphysis. Throughout this disorderly area, there is an overall increase in fibrous tissue accompanied by the characteristic mononuclear leukocytic and vascular changes of syphilitic infec-

tions. This deranged epiphyseal growth results in separation of the epiphyses and sometimes marked deformity of bone growth.

The *liver* is usually severely affected in the case of congenital syphilis. The diffuse spirochetemia causes an overall inflammatory reaction, which is at first interstitial and diffuse and eventuates in extensive scarring and disruption of the normal architecture. As a consequence of the inflammatory fibrosis, the liver is enlarged, somewhat more pale than normal, and has a typical fibrotic consistency. The diffuse fibrosis is at first limited to the interstitium of the liver substance, but in the course of its progression and extensive fibrous overgrowth, it permeates lobules to isolate hepatic cells and nests of cells. A very diffuse form of hepatic fibrosis (cirrhosis) results, accompanied by the characteristic white cell infiltrate and vascular changes. Gummas are occasionally found in the liver even in these very early cases.

The *lungs* may be affected by a diffuse interstitial fibrosis that produces a marked increase in their consistency. When severely affected, they appear as pale, virtually airless organs *(pneumonia alba)*. The alveolar spaces are decreased in size and the septa widened. There is hypertrophy of the cuboidal lining epithelium and a permeation throughout the lungs of mononuclear leukocytes accompanied by obliterative endarteritis. Secondary infections by other bacteria may modify the histologic pattern.

The generalized spirochetemia may lead to diffuse interstitial inflammatory reactions in virtually any other organ of the body, for example, the pancreas, kidneys, heart, spleen and the endocrine organs. Central nervous system *meningovascular syphilis* may develop. Changes in the eye consist of an *interstitial keratitis* or a *choroiditis* with focal or diffuse inflammatory scarring of the choroid. Abnormal pigment production in focal areas may produce the *spotted retina of congenital syphilis.*

The late-occurring form of congenital syphilis usually resembles the tertiary stage of acquired syphilis. However, it is distinctive in that interstitial keratitis is found in the congenital form and is often accompanied by the periostitis, sabre shins and saddle deformity of the nose. In addition, there are characteristic alterations in the formation of the teeth due to spirochetal infection during the stages of tooth development. The incisor teeth are somewhat smaller than normal, and have a "screwdriver" shape or are sometimes even more pointed, to produce a peg-shaped deformity. The defective formation of enamel results in notching of the biting margins of the incisors. Other tertiary lesions may develop, such as gummas in any tissue or organ of the body or neuro-syphilis, but, for unknown reasons, cardiovascular syphilis is quite uncommon. On the basis of the meningovascular involvement, eighth nerve deafness and optic nerve atrophy may develop as these cranial nerves are damaged by the surrounding inflammatory reaction.

YAWS

Yaws, caused by *Treponema pertenue*, is a tropical and semitropical disease that bears many strong resemblances to syphilis. The disease is characterized principally by cutaneous and mucous lesions that form large warty granulomas (frambesiomas) and by late, gumma-like, destructive lesions in the skin and bones. However, it is not venereal in origin, is not transmitted to the fetus through the placenta and rarely, if ever, involves visceral structures such as the cardiovascular and central nervous system.

Causative Agent. *T. pertenue* is morphologically indistinguishable from *T. pallidum*, and has many biochemical and immunologic similarities. There is therefore some question whether it is not actually a variant of *T. pallidum* that has been modified by its long survival in a different environment.

Method of Spread. Yaws is endemic in the tropics. It is most often found in the South Pacific islands, the Netherlands, East Indies, the Philipines, India, Ceylon and Africa, but also occurs in areas of Central and South America and in the West Indies. Sporadic cases have been reported in the northern hemisphere. The endemic foci are particularly sharply localized.

The disease frequently becomes manifest in children under the age of 5 and, in the majority of instances, is well established before adulthood. Transmission is apparently by direct contact, with active clinical cases having open skin lesions. Some break in the continuity of the epidermis prepares the portal of entry since the organism is incapable of penetrating the intact epithelium. Transmission is not sexual as with syphilis. Congenital yaws has not yet been observed. Several reports implicate an intermediate insect vector, but this observation is not yet established. No animal reservoir has been identified.

Pathogenesis. As with syphilis, a lesion, the "mother yaw," appears at the site of the initial invasion three to four weeks following the introduction of the organism. A secondary stage develops some weeks to months later, characterized by mucocutaneous secondary lesions (frambesiomas) distributed over the entire body surface and mucous membranes.

Some time later, tertiary manifestations may develop, generally restricted to the skin and bone. Spirochetemias may persist for two to four years following the onset of the disease and, during this stage, secondary skin lesions appear and reappear at any time. Eventually, after approximately 10 years, most infected persons become immune and the bacteremia and fresh lesions subside.

The Infection. The lesion that represents the analogue of the chancre in syphilis is known as the "mother yaw." This red-brown papule increases up to 2 to 3 cm. in diameter and eventually creates an elevated, strawberry-like, red mass, from which the term frambesia (strawberry) is derived. The surface sloughs to form a dirty, granular, eroded ulcer which crusts over. Often the crust is scratched off or desquamates, and the lesion further erodes and frequently becomes extensively secondarily infected. This primary stage may undergo spontaneous healing or may persist until the stage of generalized secondary lesions develops. Histologically, the yaw is a papillary, inflammatory granuloma composed of marked hypertrophy and thickening of the epidermis with extensive underlying chronic granulation tissue in the dermal and subcutaneous connective tissues. There is hyperkeratosis of the surface of the epithelium and widening and prolongation of the epidermal rete pegs. In the nonulcerated phase, the inflammatory infiltrate is largely mononuclear, and is accompanied by endothelial cell hypertrophy and proliferation to produce a vascular lesion very similar to that of syphilis. Spirochetes abound in the inflammatory focus.

About two to three months later, generalized skin lesions usher in the secondary stage. In this disseminated phase of the disease, the lesions vary from scaly macules to papules, and eventually most lesions become large granulomas (4 to 5 cm. in diameter) that more or less resemble the mother yaw. Crops of these lesions may develop recurrently over a period of years until relative immunity is developed. Histologically, these secondaries are entirely similar to the mother lesion described. Less commonly, these secondaries involve the mucous membranes of the body in the form of papillomatous condylomas resembling, to a considerable extent, the condyloma latum of syphilis. The secondary lesions of yaws regress after a period of months, and are eventually reduced to fibrous scars. During the active stages, serum from these lesions usually yields large numbers of viable treponemes.

The tertiary lesions appear after an interval of months to years and primarily involve the skin and bones. These late lesions may resemble the frambesiform masses of the secondary or may take the form of cutaneous gummas that produce large subcutaneous masses. Such lesions are likely to occur on the soles of the feet but, instead of producing the protruding, strawberry-like masses, the papules are eroded by trauma to create small to large painful ulcerations. Long, fissured, deep clefts result with dirty necrotic bases and extensive secondary infection. The lesions of bone consist of osteoperiostitis and gummatous foci of necrosis. The sabre shin deformity may develop in the tibia. Gummatous nodules may erode or protrude from the surfaces of bone into the subcutaneous tissues and sometimes ulcerate through the epithelium. These bone lesions account for several of the characteristic mutilating deformities produced by yaws. *Gangosa* is the term applied to destruction of the cartilage and bone of the nose. Large egg-shaped gummatous masses may protrude from the supramaxillary bone. Visceral gummas have been described, but are extremely rare. Infections of the central nervous system and cardiovascular system are extremely uncommon. When they occur, they are thought by many to be due to intercurrent syphilis.

The cutaneous manifestations of yaws are sufficiently dramatic to permit the ready identification of this disease and its differentiation from syphilis. Because of the plantar lesions, the patients develop a peculiar waddling, crab-like gait. Frequently, this stage of the disease is referred to as "crab yaws." Accompanying these skin lesions, there is regional and frequently generalized adenopathy. The age of the patient, the endemic foci of prevalence, positive serologic tests and treponemal immobilization tests for either syphilis or yaws, and the mutilating destructions of the face in the later stages make the diagnosis readily apparent.

PINTA

Pinta is a nonvenereal, chronic disease chiefly of the skin, caused by the *Treponema carateum*. While the disease has three stages and resembles syphilis to a considerable extent, it is nonvenereal in its transmission, tends to affect the young, rarely causes death, and is principally responsible for the development of variegated hyper- and hypopigmentations of the skin. The causative organism, *T. carateum*, is morphologically indistinguishable from *T. pallidum* and apparently has many antigenic similarities. Patients with pinta develop positive serologic and treponemal immobilization tests to syphilis. The disorder is endemic in certain areas of Central and South America, but has also been reported in Africa, the South Pacific and other tropical climates. Transmission is from person to person from open skin lesions. The infection usually begins in children and young adults, but the disease persists into the advanced years of life. Transplacental transmission is not believed to occur. Flies and insects have been suggested as intermediate vectors, but this hypothesis has not been established.

The disease begins approximately two to three weeks after the inoculation, with the appearance of a primary papular lesion at the site of inoculation. This primary papule progressively enlarges and assumes an irregular shape with a serpiginous, hyperpigmented border. Sometimes the lesion is violaceous or red. Scaling or superficial ulceration with weeping and crusting of the surface may further modify its appearance. In the course of time, this initial lesion may assume giant proportions up to 15 to 20 cm. in greatest diameter. Small daughter or satellite papules may appear about the margins, and these may coalesce to expand the primary lesion.

This initial lesion is characterized by epidermal thickening, hyperkeratosis of the surface and some prolongation of the rete pegs. There is a diffuse, scattered, dermal mononuclear infiltrate, chiefly localized about the blood vessels and adnexal structures. This infiltrate often extends into the epidermis and is accompanied by some intraepidermal edema. One of the more prominent histologic features of the early lesion of pinta is the increased numbers of melanophores in the dermal connective tissue and an increase in the pigmentation of the basal cells of the stratum germinativum. These account for the hyperpigmentation of the early skin lesions known as *pintids*. Treponemes can be identified in these lesions. As the lesion becomes more chronic and fibrotic, its vascularity diminishes, the inflammatory reaction is replaced by fibrous scarring, and eventually a depigmented splotch remains, composed of thin, atrophic skin. The regional nodes are usually enlarged as in syphilis and yaws.

The secondary stage follows within the subsequent year and is characterized by a variable maculopapular rash that is distributed over the body with a particular predilection for the exposed areas. The secondary lesions vary greatly in color. Some are rose-pink because of increased vascularity; others become brown to black with the accumulation of melanin pigment; and as the lesions get older, they progressively blanch. Histologically, the changes are essentially similar to those described in the primary stage.

When the lesions have assumed the variegated piebald pigmentation described, the disease is said to have entered the tertiary stage. There is no sharp clinical, anatomic or temporal division between the secondary and tertiary stages of this disease. In the long chronicity of pintids, lasting over many years, the acute and chronic inflammatory components subside, and the lesions eventuate in bizarre, mottled areas of vitiliginous depigmentation with sometimes immediately adjacent areas of deep brown-black hyperpigmentation. Palmar and plantar hyperkeratosis also develops, and, in rare cases, mesaortitis and cardiovascular lesions have been described, furthering the close similarity of this disease to syphilis.

BEJEL

Bejel is a nonvenereal treponemal disorder of the Arabian and Middle Eastern populations, caused by an organism that is indistinguishable from *T. pallidum.* The disease may in fact represent a modified form of syphilis that is acquired, usually in childhood, by direct contact with active cases or indirect transmission by articles of daily life. In the endemic areas, as many as 90 per cent of the inhabitants of certain communities are infected. The initial lesion, analogous to the chancre, is particularly common about the lips and within the oral cavity, presumably because of the transmission of the treponemes on drinking utensils. A subsequent generalized secondary mucocutaneous dissemination appears, and in later stages there is involvement of the skin, mucous membranes and bones in a fashion closely resembling that described in syphilis and yaws. Many times the skin lesions have the blotchy, irregular pigmentation found in pinta. Gummatous ulcerations of the skin and mucous membranes and periostitis further the similarity to syphilis. However, visceral lesions have not yet been described.

RELAPSING FEVER

Relapsing fever is an acute, febrile, infectious, world-wide disease, caused by the Borrelia. The disease is transmitted chiefly by ticks and lice, but may also be spread by the bites of fleas and bedbugs. The genus Borrelia includes ten strains, all of which are believed to produce an essentially similar disease. The most important strains are *B. recurrentis, B. duttonii* and *B. novyi.* These organisms are irregularly wavy spirochetes, approximately 20 mi-

crons in length and one-half micron in diameter. Unlike the treponemes, the Borrelia can be stained with ordinary aniline dyes and therefore can be detected in tissue and bacterial stains.

While the Borrelia have been identified in many rodents, including rats, mice and squirrels, it is not known whether these animals represent the natural reservoir for these organisms or whether man himself is the natural host. Most clinical cases have followed the bite of an infected tick or contamination from an infected louse. These insects presumably become infected by biting a diseased animal or human, although ticks may transmit organisms to their offspring. Crushing of an infected tick may contaminate the skin and permit the organism to penetrate either the intact or injured epidermis. The louse-borne disease is also spread by crushing the louse against the intact or abraded skin. The disease is widespread in its distribution. The tick-borne form occurs mainly in the western regions of the United States and in Central America and South Africa. The louse-borne disease is more worldwide. It frequently occurs in epidemic form, particularly when a population has been predisposed by war and famine.

Following their introduction, the organisms rapidly gain access to the blood and apparently are able to proliferate there since large numbers are readily found in the blood in the acute, febrile stages of the disease.

While the tick-borne and louse-borne fevers are sometimes distinguished clinically, the two variants are basically similar. The incubation period is believed to vary from 5 to 11 days, and is followed by an abrupt onset of fever, chills, headaches, diffuse muscle aching and pains, nausea and vomiting. The fever usually rises to 103° to 105° and remains elevated for a period of 2 to 7 days. During the fever, flushed facies, conjunctival injection and reddening of the pharyngeal mucous membranes, dizziness, confusion and even delirium become prominent. In the classic case, there is pronounced tenderness of the calf muscles and the appearance of an erythematous rash around the neck, upper abdomen and inner aspects of the thighs and arms. The rash is maculopetechial in type and bears many resemblances to the skin manifestations of typhoid and typhus fever. Jaundice may appear during this acute febrile episode and almost invariably does in all fatal cases.

Characteristically, the fever drops sharply by crisis at the end of the initial bout, and the patient rapidly regains his well-being until a relapse occurs, usually several days to one week later. This subsequent relapse follows more or less the pattern of the initial attack, but is more often accompanied by jaundice and hemorrhagic skin manifestations, as well as by bleeding from the nose and gastrointestinal tract. The fever recurs four to five times in the usual case but, in some variants, may reappear over a period of several months. During each of these febrile attacks, large numbers of organisms can be found in the blood by Wright's or Giemsa's stains. If the organisms cannot be found in the blood, intraperitoneal inoculation of mice provides an in vivo culture. False-positive serologic tests to syphilis develop in about 10 per cent of these cases, and many of these patients develop agglutination antibodies for *Proteus* OX-K.

The fatality rate is quite variable. About one in 20 patients may be expected to succumb, but intercurrent pneumonia and other predisposing conditions, such as famine and debilitating disease, elevate this rate.

The cadavers are usually jaundiced. The most prominent anatomic alterations are found in the spleen, liver, gastrointestinal mucosa and serosal linings of the body cavities. The spleen characteristically weighs in the range of 300 to 400 gm., and may contain small infarcts or small abscesses. Histologically, these abscesses consist of agglomerated histiocytes, plasma cells and scattered neutrophils, surrounded by a zone of basophilic amorphous debris. Numerous Borrelia may be found in these lesions, principally in the outer margins. There is in addition an overall splenic congestion, accompanied by hypertrophy of the sinusoidal reticuloendothelial cells. These phagocytic cells are frequently stuffed with hemosiderin granules and intact and disintegrating red cells.

The liver is enlarged due to marked congestion, which produces increased vascular markings on gross inspection. Histologically, the congestion occurs throughout the lobule with marked widening of the vascular sinusoids and compression and apparent atrophy of the intervening hepatic cords. Miliary abscesses may likewise be found in this organ.

Petechial hemorrhages are found in the gastrointestinal mucosa, pericardium, pleura and peritoneum. At autopsy, the lungs commonly have bacterial pneumonic infections that are probably due to secondary invaders. Glomerular congestion, petechial hemorrhages in the oral cavity, meningeal and cerebral congestion, and acute meningitis have all been described in occasional cases. Interstitial nephritis sometimes accounts for renal disturbances.

The diagnosis of this condition is usually apparent from the characteristic relapsing nature of the fever, but the differential diagnosis must include malaria, Weil's disease, typhoid and typhus fever, and other acute, febrile illnesses. Recovery from an attack confers only a transient immunity and reinfections have been reported.

RAT-BITE FEVER

Rat-bite fever is an acute, febrile, infectious disease caused by *Spirillum minus*. There is a totally distinct form of rat-bite fever caused by one of the Bacteroideae that must not be confused with this spirochetal disorder (p. 422). The spirochetal disease causes relapsing fever, skin eruption and involvement of the joints. *Spirillum minus* is a short, loosely coiled organism, 2 to 5 microns in length. The disease is most often contracted by the bite of wild rats, but it has been transmitted by apparently healthy laboratory animals, such as the guinea pig, rat and mouse. In the usual case, the initial rat bite heals promptly, but about two to three weeks later there is an abrupt onset of fever with reactivation of inflammation at the site of the bite. This site becomes reddened, edematous and indurated, and may even ulcerate. The regional nodes become enlarged and painful. Febrile episodes which last several days are spaced by afebrile periods of similar length. These recur over a period of weeks. In about half the cases, reddening and swelling of one of the large weight-bearing joints occurs and, in a similar proportion of cases, a maculopapular rash appears. Usually the relapsing fever spontaneously subsides in a few months, but occasionally it may persist for as long as a year.

Histologically, the initial location of the rat bite presents evidence of a chronic inflammatory reaction, consisting largely of vascular congestion, edema and mononuclear leukocytic infiltration. Similar changes may be found in the skin lesions, and a variety of regressive alterations have been described in the kidneys, liver, heart, spleen and brain. These consist principally of interstitial edema, interstitial mononuclear leukocytic infiltration, cloudy swelling and fatty degeneration of parenchymal cells in the liver, kidneys, heart and adrenals. Organisms can often be demonstrated in these involved organs.

The disease is nonfatal in the absence of intercurrent or complicating infections so that the data on anatomic changes are extremely limited and not entirely conclusive.

WEIL'S DISEASE (LEPTOSPIROSES)

Of the more than 20 strains of Leptospira identified, three are of major importance to man: *L. icterohaemorrhagiae* (reservoir — rats and mice), *L. canicola* (reservoir — dogs) and *L. pomona* (reservoir — pigs). The last two strains generally cause in man mild subclinical febrile reactions. Similarly, *L. icterohaemorrhagiae* infections may be mild, but more often are severe in the form known as Weil's disease.

Weil's disease is characterized by fever, widespread petechial skin hemorrhages and generalized muscular aches and pains. Later signs of renal insufficiency and jaundice develop. These clinical manifestations are based upon widespread lesions in the skin and muscles and acute diffuse parenchymal damage to the kidneys and liver (Ashe et al., 1941).

Causative Organism. *Leptospira icterohaemorrhagiae* is a tightly wound spirochete that is from 4 to 20 microns in length. These organisms are widely found in wild rats and mice. In these animals, the organisms may cause little or no disease or acute or chronic, fatal or nonfatal disease. Organisms can be transmitted from one animal to others, creating a large potential reservoir. They are difficult to stain and are best visualized by silver impregnations or in living preparations by darkfield microscopy.

Method of Spread. The principal source of clinical infection is the rat. These animals excrete large numbers of microorganisms in their urine. Contact with this excreta provides the pathways of spread. Fishermen, fish cleaners, slaughterhouse employees, dock workers, farmers and miners are particularly vulnerable. Cases have been reported from bathing in contaminated water. A bite, skin injury or abrasion provides the portal of entry. Reports persist that leptospira can penetrate the unbroken skin or mucosa. The organisms may also enter through the digestive and respiratory tracts. Once within the body, the organisms rapidly permeate the blood vessels, leading to a leptospiremia in the earlier stages of the clinical disease. Organisms thus invade many organs and tissues.

The Infection. The disease usually begins about one to two weeks after exposure, and is *classically divided into three stages: septicemia, toxic or icteric stage and convalescent stage.* The onset is acute and is ushered in by fever and chills. During the septicemic stage, the patient suffers greatly from generalized muscular aches and pains, with exquisite tenderness of the muscles, particularly the gastrocnemius muscles. Headache, nausea and vomiting, and stiffness of the neck reflect meningeal irritation. One of the characteristic clinical findings is intense conjunctival congestion and hemorrhage. Petechial and ecchymotic hemorrhages occasionally occur on the skin, but these are not frequent and may not appear until later. Between the third and seventh days, the toxic or icteric stage usually begins. Jaundice appears in about two-thirds of the cases. The liver may be enlarged and tender at this time. The jaundice lasts for a few days and then subsides gradually over the course of the next several weeks. Toward the end of the first week, oliguria may appear and progress to total anuria and lead to a uremic death. In the convalescent stage, in those who recover, the fever slowly falls, the urine output gradually returns to normal during the second week and the jaundice progressively fades.

The anatomic changes of Weil's disease are fairly striking and virtually pathognomonic (Jeghers et al., 1935). Jaundice is almost invariably present in fatal cases. There are widespread petechial and ecchymotic hemorrhages in the skin, gastrointestinal mucosa, serosal membranes, and possibly in visceral organs. However, the major specific alterations are found in the liver, kidneys and striated muscles of both skeletal and cardiac origin. The *liver* is usually slightly enlarged with a tense capsule and frequently subcapsular and parenchymal hemorrhages. Histologically, there is widespread hepatocytic intracellular and intercellular edema. The cellular swelling leads to apparent disorganization of the lobular architecture. Rare, isolated, liver cell necrosis is present, along with infrequent mitoses. Accompanying this destruction of liver parenchyma, there is a mononuclear leukocytic infiltrate, most marked about the periportal areas. No bile duct proliferation or bile stasis can be seen. Kupffer cells are usually enlarged. With silver impregnation techniques, numerous leptospira can be demonstrated in the interstitial tissue, hepatic cells and throughout the liver substance.

The *kidneys* are grossly enlarged, tense, and bulge above the levels of the cut capsule. Subcapsular and intraparenchymal hemorrhages may be present. Histologically, there is widespread, interstitial edema and inflammatory infiltration of mononuclear white cells in the interstitium. The glomeruli are frequently markedly congested with blood and may have well preserved or disintegrating red cells within the capsular spaces. In the later, convalescent stage, most of these acute changes disappear. *Striated muscle* of both skeletal and cardiac origin contains focal hemorrhages and vacuolization and swelling of individual muscle fibers. In these affected fibers, cross striations are lost and the sarcoplasm takes on a pink, hyaline, coagulated appearance (Zenker's hyaline degeneration). Many of these cells may disappear and are replaced by a proliferation of the sarcolemmal cells. There is surprisingly little inflammatory reaction to these focal muscle injuries, and most of the leukocytes present are of the mononuclear variety. In the more chronic stages, fibroblastic scarring occurs, and frequently trapped muscle cells become transformed into atypical masses of pink cytoplasm containing multiple nuclei or muscle giant cells. A mononuclear meningitis has been described, as well as vegetative endocarditis and fibrinous pericarditis. Focal interstitial inflammatory foci may be found in other organs or tissues of the body. The lymph nodes are characteristically enlarged and have fairly nonspecific, acute or chronic lymphadenitis. Leptospira can be demonstrated by silver stains in any of the involved tissues or organs.

While these features characterize the full-blown classic case, it is now appreciated that many less severe involvements may also occur with slight or even no hepatic or renal involvement. Some of these milder forms are influenza-like with fever, diffuse aches and pains but no evidence of jaundice or renal disease. The diagnosis may well be suspected by the clinical combination of fever, muscle pain, petechial hemmorhages, conjunctival hemorrhages, and signs of liver and renal disease, but absolute confirmation may necessitate identification of microorganisms or specific antibodies. Anemia is frequently present. The jaundice is held by Thomson (1964) to be due to hemolysis rather than hepatic failure. Leptospira can be found in the blood during the first week of the disease, and these organisms can be cultured by intraperitoneal inoculation of immature guinea pigs, mice or hamsters. Organisms can also be isolated from the urine of the patient during the second to fourth weeks of the disease. Specific antibodies for these leptospira begin to develop during the second week and subsequently reach extremely high titers. It is worthy of note that organisms can rarely be cultured at postmortem 24 hours after death of the patient.

In the usual case, progressive improvement occurs after about two to three weeks of illness, but relapses have been reported in as many as 20 per cent. The fatality rate of severe cases may be as high as 20 per cent. However, this level of mortality is based upon only the more severe cases since many mild or abortive infections undoubtedly go unrecognized. Death is usually due to uncontrolled systemic infection and the generalized febrile toxemia.

DONOVANIA GRANULOMATIS—GRANULOMA INGUINALE

Granuloma inguinale is a chronic granulomatous disease, usually of the genital region, caused by *Donovania granulomatis.* In lesions these agents appear as encapsulated coccobacilli or rod-like forms within phagocytic mononuclear cells, referred to as *Donovan bodies.* The disease is uncommon but is worldwide in distribution. It is only occasionally encountered in Europe and the United States. Because granuloma inguinale is often found associated with other venereal infections and because the usual site of involvement is the genital region, it is considered a venereal disease. However, this classification is challenged since transfer of the infection does not necessarily occur to the coital partner. This observation may, however, merely reflect low infectivity and invasiveness. The incubation period varies from 3 days to several months.

The initial lesion is an inflammatory papule at the site of inoculation, on the perineum, perianal region, anus, vagina, cervix or penis. Extragenital lesions are encountered, however, in many sites such as the lips, oral cavity, esophagus and larynx. The pathways followed in these extragenital localizations are not well understood, and it is possible that they represent either autoinoculation or hematogenous dissemination. Wherever it develops, the original papule of granuloma inguinale enlarges, ulcerates and becomes a chronic spreading lesion having a necrotic center and a raised, inflammatory border. Characteristically, this border has a rounded, red succulence, due to the piling up of granulation tissue. In other instances, the granulation tissue may pile up to produce a broad, irregular, elevated plateau. Satellite papules and their ulcers may appear along the course of the lymphatic drainage. In the long chronicity of this infection, the ensuing fibrosis may cause large, irregular, nodular scars and lesions that resemble keloids (Fig. 10–8).

Histologically, the dominant feature is that of a fairly nonspecific, acute and chronic inflammation accompanied by an exuberant granulation tissue. There is an intense infiltrate of plasma cells and macrophages throughout the granulation tissue and, near the surface, an admixture of polymorphonuclear neutrophils. Microabscesses form in the advancing margins of the lesion. The most distinctive characteristics are the large vacuolated macrophages loaded with the gram-negative Donovan bodies described. This inflammatory ulcerative and cicatricial pattern is followed in any of the sites of localization. Drainage occurs

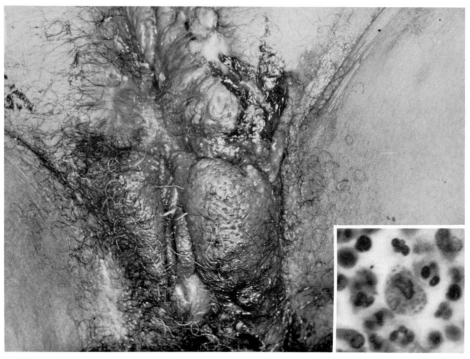

Figure 10--8. *Granuloma inguinale of the vulva. The inset shows a macrophage in high power detail filled with faintly visible Donovan bodies.*

along the lymphatics to the regional nodes and leads to suppurative necrosis and fluctuant enlargements resembling buboes. Rarely, metastatic hematogenous dissemination may give rise to similar foci of granulomatous inflammation in the skin, subcutaneous tissues, bones, joints and other organs.

The clinical diagnosis is usually readily evident from the nature of the skin lesion. The ulcer itself is relatively painless except in the presence of an acute superinfection by other bacterial agents. The long chronicity and regional node enlargement further substantiate the diagnosis. The extensive inflammatory scarring may cause many late sequelae, such as lymphatic obstruction and various types of elephantiasis of the external genitalia resembling those described in lymphogranuloma venereum (p. 440). The diagnosis is principally based upon the characteristic pattern of the ulcer, but is supported by the demonstration of Donovan bodies either in smears or tissue biopsies. Further confirmatory evidence is available in the form of complement fixation tests and skin tests. The disease is more disabling than fatal, but death has been produced by the systemic dissemination of the primary infection.

CORYNEBACTERIUM DIPHTHERIAE — DIPHTHERIA

Diphtheria is an acute, communicable disease caused by the strongly exotoxic *Corynebacterium diphtheriae*. The disorder is characterized by local pseudomembranous inflammation, usually in the upper respiratory tract, and systemic dissemination of toxin that evokes lesions in many organs of the body. The control of diphtheria by extensive immunization campaigns has been one of the triumphs of preventative medicine. In the U.S., in 1880, the death rate from this disease was approximately 100 per 100,000 population; in 1960, this rate was only 0.4 per 100,000.

Causative Agent. The causative organism is a gram-positive, club-shaped bacillus that commonly manifests barred metachromatic granules or terminal masses at the poles. While many *strains* have been identified serologically, these variants have little clinical importance as compared with the separation of diphtheria bacilli into gravis, intermedius and mitis *groups*, based on their exotoxin production. Recent studies indicate that exotoxin production is dependent on phage infection of the bacilli. Despite the implication that the gravis organisms are more dangerous, there is no absolute relationship between these forms and the severity of the resultant clinical disease. The great preponderance of clinical disease is caused by the intermedius and mitis groups. The mitis organisms assume significant pathogenicity in the chronically debilitated, weakened individual.

Method of Spread. These pathogens are usually transmitted by sneezing or coughing. Virulent strains are derived from either carriers or active clinical cases. Approximately 1 per cent of the population are said to carry virulent bacilli. No age is completely immune, but the disease most commonly affects children before the age of 5. The usual portal of entry is the oral cavity, although the organism may find a suitable substrate for growth on any mucosal surface, such as the mucous membranes of the eye or genital tract, and rarely may implant on open wounds in any part of the body surface creating chronic ulcers. The significance of these ulcers is often not appreciated until the systemic spread of the exotoxin evokes manifestations reminiscent of the more usual forms of diphtheria.

Pathogenesis. The organism usually establishes itself superficially on the surface of the mucous membrane of the nasopharynx, oropharynx or laryngopharynx, but occasionally it first affects the larynx or trachea. Reimplantation may occur at several sites that usually coalesce in the course of the disease. Satellite infections occur rarely in the esophagus or lower airways. The growth of organisms remains localized, but the exotoxin is absorbed into the blood and evokes a severe systemic reaction. There is some suggestive evidence that

the exotoxin exerts its injurious effect by interference with the cytochrome system of cells.

The Clinical Infection. The incubation period varies from 1 to 7 days, during which the organism proliferates at the site of implantation. Edema and hyperemia of the affected epithelial surface appear first. In the next few days, the elaboration of exotoxin causes necrosis of the epithelium, accompanied by an outpouring of large amounts of a fibrinosuppurative exudate. The coagulation of this exudate on the ulcerated necrotic surface creates the almost diagnostic, tough, dirty gray to gray-white, superficial pseudomembrane (Fig. 10–9). The pseudomembrane also harbors necrotic sloughed epithelial cells as well as the *Corynebacterium diphtheriae*. Caution should be exercised in the histologic establishment of a positive diagnosis, because nonvirulent diphtheroids are normal inhabitants of the oral cavity and may also become enmeshed within a pseudomembrane caused by other organisms. Mild neutrophilic infiltration in the underlying tissues becomes progressively more severe with the continuance of the bacterial invasion, and is accompanied by marked vascular congestion, interstitial edema, fibrin exudation and *intense* neutrophilic infiltration. When the pseudomembrane is torn off this highly vascularized bed, fairly active oozing of blood occurs. By centrifugal spread the pseudomembrane may reach the larynx, trachea and even the lower respiratory passages to sometimes cause laryngeal or nasal obstruction. Occasionally intense suppurative inflammation and necrosis of the subjacent tissues permit spontaneous dislodgement and aspiration of the membrane. Similar pseudomembrane forma-

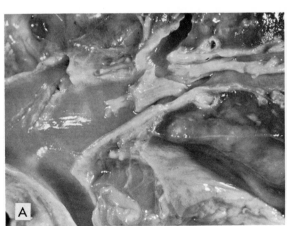
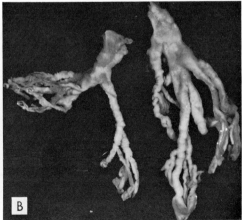

Figure 10–9. *The pseudomembrane of diphtheria: in A, lying within the transverse bronchus: in B, forming a perfect cast (removed from the lung) of the branching respiratory tree.*

tion and inflammatory reactions are produced in any other site of localization of the organisms. With control of the infection, the membrane may slough or may be removed by enzymic digestion. The inflammatory reaction subsides and the local mucosal defect is closed by regeneration.

The regional nodes of drainage respond with a nonspecific acute lymphadenitis. Although the bacterial invasion remains localized, generalized systemic effects, i.e., nonspecific generalized reticuloendothelial hyperplasia of the spleen and lymph nodes, are caused by the absorption of the soluble exotoxin into the blood. The exotoxin may cause fatty myocardial change (p. 33), inflammatory polyneuritis with degeneration of the myelin sheaths and, less commonly, fatty degenerative changes or even focal necroses of parenchymal cells in the liver, kidneys and adrenals. Occasionally, Zenker's hyaline degeneration or necrosis occurs in the striated voluntary and cardiac muscle fibers in the more severe cases. The systemic alterations are reversible and are rarely followed by permanent scarring. Permanent degeneration of nerve fibers, which fail to regenerate adequately, and minimal interstitial myocardial fibrosis may persist as residuals of the diphtheritic infection.

The clinical manifestations of diphtheria result from both the local bacterial invasion and the systemic absorption of exotoxin. The local lesions usually evoke an insidiously developing sore throat accompanied by fever, malaise, chills and weakness. During the full-blown pathognomonic stage of pseudomembrane formation, laryngeal and tracheal involvement may cause severe respiratory distress, crowing respiration, cyanosis, and even sudden death from the dislodgement and aspiration of the necrotic membrane. Involvement of the heart usually does not become manifest until 5 to 7 days after the local changes have developed, and electrocardiographic changes can be demonstrated in up to three-quarters of clinically overt cases of diphtheria. When sufficiently severe, the cardiac involvement may cause signs of cardiac decompensation and may cause death from myocardial insufficiency. The neurologic manifestations usually develop considerably later, and frequently are not demonstrable clinically until the acute infection has subsided (referred to as postdiphtheritic neuritis). Weakness and paralyses of the soft palate, extraocular muscles of the eye, and even of the peripheral nerves of the extremities occur in less than one-quarter of the cases. Many of these neurologic disturbances slowly subside, but some

may persist. While the myocardial, neural and other visceral affections are frequently listed as complications of diphtheria, these are more properly considered as integral aspects of the infection that result from the blood dissemination of the highly potent soluble exotoxin.

The clinical diagnosis is usually fairly apparent from the characteristic pseudomembrane. However, direct bacteriologic smear and, more specifically, identification of pathogenic organisms by culture on Loeffler's and tellurite mediums may be required to confirm the clinical impression. It is to be remembered in the interpretation of a throat smear that diphtheroids are normal inhabitants of the oral cavity and are indistinguishable morphologically from C. diphtheriae.

The mortality rate of present-day treated cases is extremely low. Death is usually due to respiratory obstruction, myocardial failure, or overwhelming toxemia and shock. Both the local morphologic changes and systemic injuries may be effectively curtailed or even prevented by adequate and prompt therapy.

CLOSTRIDIA

TETANUS

Tetanus is a highly fatal disease characterized by convulsive contractions of *voluntary* muscles, caused by the absorption into motor nerves and the central nervous system of the powerful exotoxin elaborated by the *Clostridium tetani*. Tetanus resembles diphtheria insofar as there is a local site of bacterial invasion and systemic absorption of the locally produced exotoxin. The neural tissues are chiefly affected and produce the major clinical features of this infection.

Causative Organism. *Clostridium tetani* is a gram-positive, fairly slender, motile rod up to 5 microns in length. Large terminal endospores are often formed and lend a tennis racket shape to the organism. Low oxygen tensions are required for the germination of spores and the growth and multiplication of the vegetative forms. The exotoxin is one of the most violent poisons known to man. However, *Cl. tetani* has little invasiveness; it is virtually saprophytic in its growth requirements. Spores may remain dormant in wounds, unless other organisms or trauma produce the necessary anaerobiosis and soluble nutrients.

Method of Spread. The spores of the organism have unlimited capacity for survival outside man. They are widely distributed in all material contaminated by the excreta of horses, man and many other animals. The spores are often ingested with plants and vegetables, but are incapable of germinating in the gut and hence elaborate no exotoxin. The disease is usually contracted by the contamination of wounds with the spores. Owing to the requirement of low oxygen tensions, the hazardous wounds are those that are penetrating and permit the development of deep-seated infections, which become sealed off at the surface. Soluble nutrients are also necessary for the germination of spores, and it has been repeatedly demonstrated *that the spores are entirely harmless in clean, debrided wounds, devoid of tissue necrosis.* These facts provide the basis for careful surgical debridement of all tissue injuries, and for the "laying open" of deep wounds suspected of harboring spores.

Pathogenesis. The development of vegetative organisms and exotoxins requires from a few days to as long as two to three weeks, and hence clinical manifestations may be delayed. However, this time sequence is not invariably followed. Spores may totally fail to germinate because of an unfavorable environment. At other times, the spores may remain dormant for weeks and even months, and then begin to develop. Thus, tetanus may begin in a person who has no active local infection and who may even have failed to take note of the original lesion because of its triviality.

The Infection. The usual incubation period is one to two weeks. The disease is ushered in by *stiffness of voluntary muscles,* usually first in the muscles of the jaw, followed by spasm of the facial muscles and then of the muscles of the trunk. As a consequence, there may be difficulty in opening the jaw (trismus), giving rise to the lay term of "lockjaw." Facial involvement sometimes causes a sardonic smile (risus sardonicus) and contractions of the back muscles produce opisthotonos. Minimal stimuli, such as a noise or even gently moving the patient, may set these affected muscles into violent, painful convulsions. The patient remains mentally clear throughout this course and suffers greatly from the spastic contractions. Respiratory difficulty develops with the progression of the disease and frequently is the immediate cause of death. It is still not certain whether the respiratory difficulty is due only to spastic contraction of the respiratory muscles or muscles of the larynx or to central involvement of the respiratory center.

The morphologic changes found in such patients are usually quite minimal and nonspecific. Examination of the local injury discloses only a nonspecific inflammatory reaction and tissue necrosis, due usually to a mixed bacterial flora which may contain bacilli suggestive of *Clostridium tetani.* The neurologic changes are equally nonspecific and inconstant, and consist of swelling of the motor ganglion cells of the spinal cord and medulla associated with nuclear swelling and chromatolysis. The manner in which the exotoxin reaches these selected sites is still somewhat controversial. The water-soluble exotoxin may diffuse from the initial focus of infection through contiguous skeletal muscles to reach the myoneural end plates, or alternatively the exotoxin may be absorbed into the lymphatics and blood and be selectively taken up by the motor ganglion cells in the spinal cord and medulla, possibly in the same manner affecting the respiratory center. It is still not known whether the toxin acts at the myoneural plate or at the cell of origin of the motor fibers, but there is evidence that the toxin stimulates the elaboration of acetylcholine.

Active immunization with tetanus toxoid protects against this disease, and prompt administration of antitoxin may block the development of clinical disease by effective neutralization of circulating exotoxin. If treatment is delayed, the antitoxin is ineffective in neutralizing toxin already fixed in tissue and hence is of no value in blocking the development of neurologic disease. The toxin is strongly bound to the myoneural junction and once the patient begins to convulse, antitoxin is not effective in controlling these seizures.

BOTULISM

Botulism is an extremely grave *food poisoning* caused by the ingestion of the preformed exotoxin of the *Clostridium botulinum. Cl. botulinum* is a gram-positive anaerobic bacillus, a normal inhabitant of the soil, which is capable of elaborating a powerful exotoxin when provided with adequate anaerobiosis. Appropriate conditions for germination and toxin production are provided in canned fruits and vegetables or preserved meats such as sausages and hams, which are kept for long periods of time without refrigeration. The contaminated food may not appear to be spoiled since pure cultures of this organism fail to produce gas bubbles or apparent alterations in the character of the food. However, in many instances the food is obviously altered, possibly by accompanying bacterial infection. The organism or its spores are found in soils and on fruits and on vegetables. Spores are commonly ingested, but are of no concern since they cannot germinate without anaerobiosis.

Five immunologic varieties (A, B, C, D and E) of *Cl. botulinum* have been identified. Each produces an immunologically specific exo-toxin, but all toxins evoke identical clinical manifestations. The spores are extremely resistant to drying and boiling, and can withstand boiling for many hours. The preformed toxin is more heat-labile and is destroyed by boiling for 10 minutes. When absorbed, it affects the central nervous system and peripheral nerves and causes motor paralysis, chiefly of the muscles of the orbit, pharynx, and larynx and muscles of respiration, probably because the toxin has an anticholinergic action blocking the elaboration of acetylcholine. These symptoms may develop rapidly, since the disease is purely a toxemia and manifestations may appear within two hours. Sometimes they are delayed as long as two weeks. Nonspecific complaints may accompany these paralyses, such as headache, dizziness, nausea and vomiting and diarrhea.

The anatomic findings are poorly defined and nonspecific. They consist of visceral and central nervous system hyperemia, accompanied by minute thromboses of small vessels, chiefly in the brain and brain stem. Similar thrombi may be found in other organs. When the thrombosis is sufficiently extensive, regressive changes in the motor ganglion cells may be present. Variable degrees of hypoxic damage may be found in the kidneys and heart muscle. Even effective prompt administration of antitoxin has failed to lower the mortality below 50 per cent in clinically overt cases.

GAS GANGRENE

Gas gangrene is a rapidly spreading, necrotizing inflammation that begins in a local area of tissue injury and rapidly disseminates to affect contiguous connective tissue and muscle (Eliason et al., 1937). This local damage is accompanied by a systemic reaction to the absorption of exotoxins. The disease is caused by a large group of gram-positive anaerobic clostridia, most commonly *Clostridium perfringens (welchii)*, *Clostridium novyi (oedematiens)*, and *Clostridium septicum (vibrion septique)*. One or several forms may be present in the individual case. The disease is usually contracted by soil contamination of a tissue injury. The most dangerous wounds are those involving large areas associated with sufficient cell destruction to produce an inflammatory reaction with the release of nutrients and anaerobic conditions. In most instances other aerobes, such as staphylococci and the Proteus bacillus, are present to add to the local injury and anaerobiosis by causing suppuration. Under these conditions, the implanted spores may germinate. Gas gangrene is partic-

ularly prone to occur in compound fractures, where the splinters of bone provide foreign bodies which enhance the infection, as well as permit the solution of small amounts of calcium that lower the oxidation-reduction potential. In the same way, embedded debris or dirt provides both the required foreign particulate matter and small amounts of calcium. Gas gangrene infections have occasionally begun in the uterus following criminal abortion. The mere presence of spores in a wound is of no great concern since germination is impossible with sufficient oxygenation. Adequate debridement of tissues and the resultant ample supply of oxygen in the depths of wounds thus prevent the growth of these organisms. In this sense gas gangrene resembles tetanus. However, the organisms of gas gangrene are highly "invasive."

The spreading tissue injury results from the elaboration of a variety of *enzymes and toxins,* the most important of which are fibrinolysins, hyaluronidases, collagenases, hemolysins, cytolysins, and variable amounts of lecithinase. The collagenases aid in the spread of the infections by destruction of the connective tissue framework of tissues. The lecithinases attack membranes, known to be rich in lecithin. The lecithinase also reduces the succinoxidase activity of mitochondria, forcing a shift in the intracellular metabolism to glycolysis. It is possible that in this way the intracellular accumulation of organic acids further injures the cell. The destroyed tissue provides additional substrate for further microbial growth with consequent augmentation of the infection in a geometric progression.

Infection, if it is to occur, usually becomes manifest within 1 to 3 days of the injury. The morphologic reaction is characterized by marked edema and enzymic necrosis of involved muscle cells (Fig. 10–10). A nonspecific, mild leukocytic exudation follows. The extensive exudation and edema cause spreading and swelling of the affected region, and the overlying skin becomes tense and pale from pressure. Necrosis or rupture of the skin may follow the formation of large bullous vesicles as the contained exudation bursts out through all points of weakness. The wound at this time contains large amounts of a serosanguineous exudate, but because the tissue destruction is largely enzymic in character, there is surprisingly little suppurative reaction.

Gas bubbles caused by fermentative reactions appear early in the gangrenous tissues, accompanied usually by local lysis of red cells with the release of hemoglobin pigment into the exudate and affected tissues. The endothelial linings of the local blood vessels are stained

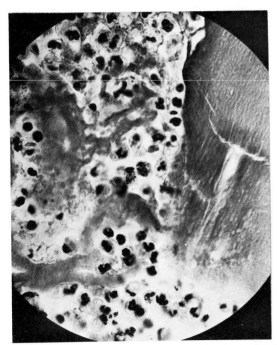

Figure 10–10. Gas gangrene—a histologic detail of enzymic lysis of muscle cells with accompanying leukocytic exudation.

by this hemolytic reaction. Injury to vascular walls may cause local thromboses. At this time, numerous vegetative bacilli are present within the exudate and within the affected tissue cells. As the infection progresses, the inflamed muscles become soft, blue-black, friable, and sometimes almost semifluid as the result of the massive proteolytic action of the released bacterial ferments. The infection spreads rapidly to contiguous structures, manifested by the spread of edema formation and gas bubbles. Absorption of the elaborated enzymes and invasion of the blood by the bacteria terminally give rise to the striking disseminated anatomic changes found in most postmortem cases, i.e., hemolytic discoloration of the endothelial lining of the entire cardiovascular system and the formation of gas bubbles throughout the body, principally in the liver (p. 1017).

The initial symptom of the clinical infection is almost invariably pain, presumably caused by the rapid exudation and distention of tissues. Profuse, serosanguineous, slightly foul-smelling fluid exudes from the area of tissue injury, and very soon gas bubbles cause *crepitus* in the region of bacterial growth. The absorbed toxins cause systemic manifestations, chiefly in the form of a rise in the pulse rate, sometimes markedly out of proportion to the rise in the temperature. Active hemolysis may cause rapid drops in the red cell count and

hematocrit. The pulse rate and fever progressively rise with continuance of the disease, and death is usually preceded by a short period of prostration and shock. Prompt, adequate administration of antitoxin, effective debridement of devitalized tissues, surgical incision of involved areas to increase aerobiosis, and the administration of antibiotics, such as bacitracin and penicillin, are the most effective methods of treatment. Far better than therapy, however, is the prevention of this highly fatal infection by adequate debridement and cleansing of extensive tissue injuries, particularly those associated with fractures and soil contamination.

ENTERIC GRAM-NEGATIVE BACILLI

The enteric organisms comprise a large variety of gram-negative bacilli that resemble each other to some extent morphologically, but are readily separated by biochemical and serologic tests. The group spans a wide range of pathogenicity for man, varying from such relatively avirulent organisms as *Aerobacter aerogenes* to the powerful pathogen, *Salmonella typhosa*. Certain members of this group, *E. coli* and *A. aerogenes*, are normal inhabitants of the intestinal tract in man, while the others are strictly invaders that use the gastrointestinal tract as their portal of entry. Thus, these organisms are known as the enteric group.

E. COLI AND A. AEROGENES INFECTIONS (COLIFORM BACILLI)

Escherichia coli and *Aerobacter aerogenes* are normal inhabitants of the intestinal tract in man. *A. aerogenes* is presumably a transient derived from air and its ubiquitous habitation on vegetables and grains. *E. coli* sets up its symbiotic residence in the gut almost at birth. It is an important cause of urinary tract infections, but rarely induces disease elsewhere in man, save possibly on the basis of opportunism. All of the gram-negative rods have certain resistance to common antibiotics such as penicillin and so may give rise to serious infections in those patients receiving such therapy. Similarly, in infancy and senescence, periods of increased vulnerability, the coliforms may assume pathogenicity. Several serologic strains of *E. coli* (particularly O 111 and O 55) may induce severe diarrhea in infants and occasionally cause death.

E. coli may become implanted in tissues via the lymphohematogenous routes or may be introduced into injuries by contamination of the body surface. This organism is an important cause of focal pyogenic skin infections, urinary tract infections such as acute pyelonephritis and cystitis, and peritonitis, acute appendicitis, cholecystitis, cholangitis and infectious biliary cirrhosis. In all its sites of localization, it evokes an entirely nonspecific suppurative reaction with abscess formation that is indistinguishable from that caused by staphylococci. In addition, specific strains of *E. coli* may be responsible for a severe form of epidemic diarrhea, usually encountered in hospitalized children. Pneumonic and bacteremic complications may follow these localized infections, particularly in children and in very aged individuals. While most of the generalizations presented for *E. coli* organisms also obtain for *A. aerogenes*, the latter organism is of lower virulence and usually confines its pathogenicity to the production of infections of the urinary tract. However, as a close relative and neighbor to *E. coli*, it is frequently present as one of the components of a mixed infection in the sites commonly invaded by *E. coli.*

Mention should also be made here of the similar role that the Proteus and Pseudomonas organisms play. In the present antibiotic era, these bacteria along with *A. aerogenes* and *E. coli* have come into a new prominence since they are all frequently antibiotic resistant. They are therefore important secondary invaders and are capable of producing the same kinds of infection as have already been detailed with respect to *E. coli*. The pseudomonas organisms are particularly common invaders of burn wounds and, because of their propensity for invading blood vessel walls, such infections often lead to bacteremia and endotoxic shock. In today's medicine, the "gram-negatives" have become important causes of serious resistant forms of urinary tract infections, pyelonephritis and peritonitis, and have also become important causes of postoperative wound infections. In those patients in whom broad-spectrum antibiotics are used postoperatively, all the sensitive strains are destroyed, leaving the field open for the unrestricted proliferation of these "gram-negatives."

SALMONELLA INFECTIONS

The salmonellae are gram-negative, nonsporing, motile bacilli closely related to but much more pathogenic than the coliform organisms. As a group, they cause fairly characteristic anatomic changes and equally characteristic clinical infections. When these organisms gain access to the body, *the inflammatory response consists principally of a striking systemic reticuloendothelial hyperplasia* with hypertrophy of lymph nodes and lymph follicles throughout the body and enlargement of the spleen and liver (Stuart and Pullen, 1946). *Histologically, active phagocytosis of organisms and red cells by these reticuloendothelial cells is a further characteristic of Salmonella infections.* Clinically, this group of organisms tends to cause one of three types of disease: enteric fevers (the prototype being typhoid fever), gastroenteritis, and focal infections of the body secondary to septicemic dissemination of the organisms.

Causative Organisms. The many species of Salmonella have been divided into *three groups*. The *first* contains those that are principally pathogenic to man alone, including *S. typhosa, S. paratyphi* A and B, *S. schottmülleri* and *S. hirschfeldii. S. typhosa* is the most important and virulent pathogen in this group. The *second group* is composed of a large number of bacilli, such as *S. typhimurium, S. choleraesuis* and *S. enteritidis*, that are primarily pathogens for animals, but occasionally produce clinical disease. The third group is pathogenic only for animals and is of no clinical concern.

All these organisms possess O somatic antigens and H flagellar antigens. The somatic antigens are powerful endotoxins that are released on the dissolution and death of the bacteria.

Method of Spread. The Salmonella organisms enter the body through the gastrointestinal tract. *S. typhosa* is entirely confined to man and infections are transmitted by human contamination of water, milk, food or other articles of daily life. Although active clinical cases may provide this contamination, the far more important reservoirs of the disease are "carriers" who have recovered from clinical infections but who continue to harbor bacteria, principally in the biliary tract. These apparently healthy individuals are particularly hazardous when employed as cooks and food handlers. The other Salmonella organisms may be derived from active infections in both man and animals by the contamination of foods, water and other objects. Flies may be a vector in the transmission of the Salmonella.

Pathogenesis. It is believed that many ingested organisms are destroyed in the stomach, but when the infective dose is large enough, some enter the small intestine where they are phagocytized by the mucosal lymphoid tissue, particularly in the ileum. The lymphoid tissues of the oropharynx and nasopharynx are additional potential sites of localization of these organisms. Rapid microbial multiplication in these localized sites occurs during the incubation period. The organisms then flood into the circulating blood and, in the more serious forms of these diseases, produce a bacteremia that may persist for a week or longer. These bacteremias subside with the progressive development of immunity.

With certain of the less virulent forms, e.g., *S. paratyphi* and *S. choleraesuis*, both the onset of clinical disease soon after the ingestion of contaminated food and the short duration of the illness point to the possibility that the clinical manifestations may be due merely to absorption of bacterial products from the lumen of the gut. It is doubtful that sufficient time elapses between the exposure and the onset of symptoms to permit the development of lesions. The organisms at most gain only a superficial foothold in the gut.

The Infections. *Typhoid Fever.* Typhoid fever is the most serious of the salmonelloses. The incubation period of this infection varies considerably, but averages about one and a half to two weeks. Organisms are usually focalized during this time to the Peyer's patches of the ileum, where they cause the lymphoid follicles to swell. As the proliferation of organisms and phagocytic cells continues, plateau-like elevations up to 6 to 8 cm. in diameter result which clearly delineate the Peyer's patches (Fig. 10–11). These changes may affect not only the ileum but also the lymphoid foci in the more proximal levels of the small intestine, as well as in the colon. As these lesions in the bowel mature during the second week of the disease, the mucosal coverings of the greatly hypertrophied lymphoid masses slough, presumably due to pressure ischemia (Fig. 10–12). Ulcerations are thus produced in the small intestine and possibly in the colon. *These are usually oval in shape with their long diameters in the long axis of the bowel,* conforming to the distribution of the Peyer's patches. In a small percentage of cases, these ulcers perforate and produce peritonitis. When the disease subsides, these ulcers heal and the mucosa regenerates.

Histologically, at first, there is marked proliferation of the reticuloendothelial cells of the lymphoid follicles locally and systemically (Mallory, 1898). *The reticulum cells, reticuloendothelial cells and immigrant macrophages in the resultant aggregations are plump, round to oval, and have abundant cytoplasm* (Fig. 10–13). They often contain bacteria, cellular debris and red cells in their cytoplasm. The *erythrophagocytosis* is a prominent microscopic detail that virtually marks the lesion as being due to a Salmonella infection, probably typhoid fever. There is in addition a scattered infiltrate of lymphocytes and plasma cells in and about these foci, but to be particularly noted is the conspicuous absence of polymorphonuclear leukocytes. As these lesions progress, the central areas of the accumulations of phagocytic cells may undergo necrosis, particularly when there has been ulceration of lesions in the bowel. At this time, some polymorphonuclear infiltration may occur.

These changes just described in the primary site of infection, namely the intestinal tract, also occur in nodes of drainage as well as in all the lymphoid tissues of the body, i.e., the spleen, liver and more distant lymph nodes. The *spleen* is markedly enlarged, not uncommonly up to 1000 gm. The capsule is tense, and the organ has a soft mushiness which on cut section is due to a soft, red, pulpy, splenic substance. The parenchyma of the spleen may literally flow out after the organ is sectioned. Histologically, the dominant features are those of hyperemia and striking proliferation of the reticuloendothelial cells of the lymphoid sinuses, accompanied by hypertrophy of the reticulum cells in the splenic follicles. *The agglomeration of these cells forms small "typhoid nodules" of active phagocytic cells replete with erythrophagocytosis* exactly resembling that already described. The rapid enlargement and engorgement of the spleen may lead to its rupture and serious, if not fatal, hemorrhage.

The *liver* reflects these same changes, and

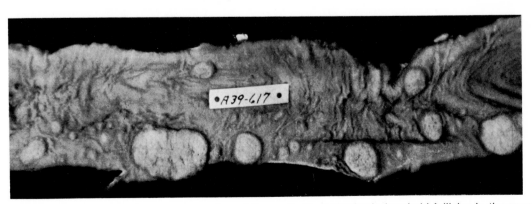

Figure 10–11. *Typhoid fever—a gross view of the markedly hyperplastic lymphoid follicles in the opened ileum.*

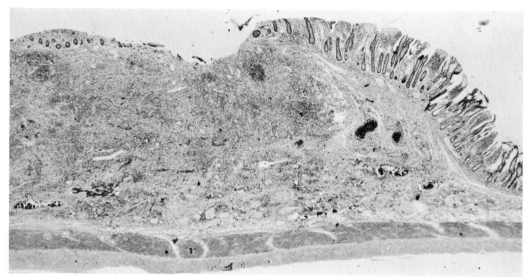

Figure 10–12. *Typhoid fever—a low power view of the cross section of a markedly enlarged lymphoid follicle in the ileum with necrosis of the overlying mucosa.*

may also become enlarged. Marked hypertrophy and proliferation of the Kupffer cells, producing typhoid nodules, causes necrosis of isolated or focal nests of hepatic cells. These foci do not bear a constant relationship to the architecture of the hepatic lobule. Such necrosis may indeed be due to the striking proliferation of the Kupffer cells with the occlusion of minute vascular sinusoids and consequent infarction of dependent cells. Similar focal lesions develop in the marrow.

Swelling of the epithelial cells of the proximal convoluted tubules has been described in the kidneys. Swelling and fatty change may be found in the cardiac muscle cells. The striated muscle fibers may undergo hyaline change or coagulation necrosis both in the heart and in the voluntary muscles. Such changes are particularly prone to occur in the most active voluntary muscles, i.e., the diaphragm, intercostal muscles, prevertebral muscles and muscles of the anterior abdominal wall. Sometimes these cellular necroses lead to hemorrhage and produce localized pain in the site affected.

The clinical manifestations that stem from these anatomic changes vary considerably from one case to another and depend entirely upon the severity of the invasion, the virulence of the organism and the resistance of the host (Stuart and Pullen, 1946). Certain cases are extremely mild and apparently have only minimal lymphoidal involvement without such omi-

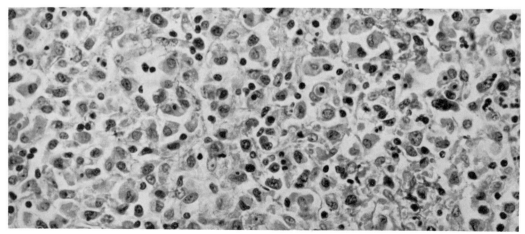

Figure 10–13. *Typhoid fever—a high power detail of the massed phagocytic cells in the center of a reactive lymphoid follicle. Scattered cells contain phagocytized red and white cells.*

nous features as ulceration of the bowel wall and enlargement of the spleen. These patients usually have a brief febrile illness that spontaneously subsides with or without treatment. In other instances, the disease may be overwhelming, with massive tissue changes that rapidly lead to ulceration, severe hemorrhages, perforation of the bowel or overwhelming toxemia. Such patients pursue a fulminating course terminated by death in a few days. In the usual case, the disease is ushered in by malaise, headache and fever that is characteristically of a spiking variety with peaks up to 103° to 105°. This fever usually persists for as long as a week, during which time the patient may have recurrent chills, reflecting the bacteremia and a variety of symptoms (i.e., distention, colicky pain and constipation followed usually by severe diarrhea) pointing to intestinal disease. Because of the high fever and diarrhea, the patient is markedly prostrated.

During the second week, a characteristic skin rash may appear that is described as "rose spots." These lesions are found most often on the lower anterior chest and upper abdomen as 1 to 5 mm. red macules that blanch upon pressure. This eruption is widely distributed in the more severe illnesses, but in many cases the few spots are readily missed. Splenohepatomegaly reflects the inflammatory involvement of these visceral organs. Characteristically, the patients have bradycardia and leukopenia. It will be recalled that the polymorphonuclear leukocytes in this disease participate but little in the defensive response. The brunt of the attack is borne by reticuloendothelial cells and macrophages.

This combination of bradycardia and leukopenia in a patient who has an apparently severe septic, febrile illness is sufficiently unusual to suggest the possibility of typhoid fever.

The diagnosis can be confirmed by *isolation of the organism from the blood* during the first and possibly the second weeks. *Bacilli do not appear in the stools until the second or third week of the disease.* They reside within macrophages up to this time and ulceration of the bowel has not yet occurred. However, stool cultures become positive in about three-quarters of the cases by the end of the third to fourth weeks as open ulcerative lesions develop. Antibodies, as demonstrated by the Widal reaction, become demonstrable during the second week of the illness with progressively rising titers during the illness. Cross reactions may occur with other Salmonella organisms so that the Widal test is not completely specific.

Many complications may modify this clinical picture. The most common serious complication is *intestinal hemorrhage.* It may be suffi-

ciently profuse to produce obvious gross bleeding in as many as one-fifth of the cases. Occult blood can be found in the third and fourth weeks of the disease in almost all cases. *Perforation of the bowel wall with generalized peritonitis* is an uncommon complication, particularly since the advent of therapy. *Rupture of the spleen* may occur. *Pneumonia* may complicate typhoid fever, due either to an extension of the typhoidal bronchitis often found in the early stages of this disease or to intercurrent bacterial infection.

S. typhosa may localize in many other sites in the body and be responsible for conjunctivitis, sinusitis, meningitis, suppurative arthritis, cholecystitis and pyelonephritis. Save for the cholecystitis, these complications are distinctly uncommon. The invasion of the biliary system bears special mention, since it commonly gives rise to a low-grade chronic infection that provides a mechanism for the continuing dissemination of organisms into the intestine during and long after the active stages of the disease. About 2 per cent of patients with active clinical cases become carriers.

Other Salmonella Infections. The diseases produced by the other pathogenic Salmonella organisms fall into one of several clinical patterns. One pattern can be designated as *enteric fevers*, usually caused by *S. paratyphi* A, *S. paratyphi* B or *S. choleraesuis*, which may resemble typhoid fever but tends to be less severe. The clinical and anatomic changes are virtually indistinguishable from those of typhoid fever, save for their lesser severity. These less virulent salmonelloses are uncommon causes of death.

Gastroenteritis—food poisoning—is a second pattern of clinical disease caused by any of these less virulent organisms. As mentioned earlier, these infections may well be caused by extremely superficial invasion of the gastrointestinal tract or mere absorption of endotoxins. The anatomic changes and clinical manifestations then are largely limited to the intestinal tract and regional nodes of drainage. There is usually an abrupt onset of mild to severe nausea, vomiting, colicky pain and diarrhea, sometimes within hours to days following the ingestion of the contaminated food. In the more severe instances, generalized involvement of the reticuloendothelial system may produce a disease that begins to resemble typhoid fever. There is no sharp line of distinction between the gastroenteritis variant and the enteric fever pattern. These disorders are rarely fatal and few anatomic data are available. Reticuloendothelial cell hyperplasia gives rise to the lymphoid hypertrophy in the bowel along with the splenohepatomegaly and lymphadenopathy.

Ulcerative lesions are uncommon, and the anatomic changes promptly revert with subsidence of the infection.

The third pattern of these infections comprises *a febrile septicemia*. Organisms apparently invade the bowel wall and directly permeate blood vessels without causing local manifestations in the intestinal tract. In children, the bowel wall may be involved in passing, but in adults, the portal of entry may be surprisingly unaffected and most of the clinical signs and symptoms relate to the hematogenous dissemination of the organisms. In addition to a severe constitutional febrile reaction, the organisms localize in a variety of sites in the body and give rise to pyelonephritis, cholecystitis, meningitis, pericarditis, endocarditis, salpingitis and other local lesions. This pattern of disseminated disease is most characteristic of *S. choleraesuis*. The histologic reaction in all these sites is the accumulation of macrophages and striking cyto- and erythrophagocytosis, the characteristic hallmark of Salmonella infections. These focalized lesions undoubtedly provide reservoirs for the continued dissemination of organisms into the blood and thus perpetuate the bacteremic state.

BACILLARY DYSENTERY

The shigellae are a large group of gram-negative enteric bacilli that produce acute enteritis and are closely related to the salmonellae and coliform organisms. *These infections differ from those caused by the salmonellae in at least one important respect. There is little tendency for bacteremic spread of the organisms and few, if any, reactions in tissues outside the gut.* Lesions remain fairly well localized to the intestinal tract, principally the colon, and produce a clinical syndrome known as *bacillary dysentery*. These forms of bacterial diarrhea vary in severity depending upon the resistance of the host, the size of the infecting dose and the virulence of the particular strain of Shigella involved. Thus, the diseases may be so insignificant as to escape clinical detection or may be severe, prostrating and even fatal. These infections generally cause localized ulcerations of the mucosa of the colon, which as a rule do not penetrate deeply into the wall and rarely perforate. The Shigella dysenteries are therefore not accompanied by the ominous complications characteristic of typhoid fever and, while the clinical disease may at times be equally severe, the prognosis on the whole is better.

Causative Organism. The shigellae morphologically resemble the other enteric pathogens described, but they can be differentiated from the salmonellae and coliforms by a variety of cultural and serologic techniques. A great many species have been identified. The most important pathogens for man are *Shigella dysenteriae* type I (Shiga bacillus) and type II (Schmitz bacillus), *Shigella flexneri* (Flexner group of paradysentery bacilli), *Shigella boydii* (Boyd subgroup of paradysentery bacilli), and *Shigella sonnei* (Sonne bacillus).

All these organisms produce endotoxins. Only the Shiga bacillus (*S. dysenteriae* I) produces a powerful neurotropic exotoxin. In animals the Shiga toxin produces intestinal and central nervous system disease, but similar lesions have not yet been identified in man. It is probable that the exotoxin does not play a dominant role in the clinical dysentery caused by the Shiga bacillus. A variety of additional antigens have been identified within these bacilli, some of which are found in only one strain and others with considerable overlap. These antigens may have importance in epidemiologic and public health studies, but are probably not germane to the consideration of clinical diseases. There is even considerable question as to the role of the clearly identified endotoxins in the causation of disease.

Method of Spread. The dysentery bacilli are confined to the gut of man and animals. Man is probably the natural reservoir of the organisms and animals are only incidentally involved by their contact with man. The organisms are transmitted by the same indirect routes as the salmonellae, presumably in contaminated food, milk, water and articles of daily life. Flies and other insects undoubtedly aid in the dissemination. The gastrointestinal tract is virtually the only portal of entry. In the temperate climates, bacillary dysentery is usually sporadic in occurrence and is contracted from active cases of the disease. Epidemics are more often initiated by unsuspected carriers who disseminate the organisms to a number of susceptible hosts. However, other factors, such as poor sanitation, a susceptible crowded population and a virulent organism, contribute to this epidemic spread. Bacillary dysentery has been one of the major serious forms of epidemic disease in military groups, and in the past has been responsible for a mortality rate of about 50 per cent in these predisposed populations.

Pathogenesis. The Shigella organisms limit their tissue damage almost entirely to the mucosa of the colon, although the ileum is sometimes involved. While the inflammatory changes may be severe and extensive, they are relatively superficial and not usually accompanied by bacteremia. Localized infections occur infrequently in other sites in the body, presumably due to transient invasion of the blood. The sequence of events that leads to the tissue changes and clinical manifestations is still poorly understood. According to one view, most of the systemic changes are due to absorbed endotoxin that is liberated as the organisms proliferate and die within the lumen of the gut. However, as mentioned, some coliforms produce an analogous endotoxin without evoking a reaction that is at all comparable to bacillary dysentery.

The Infection. While the Shiga strain of Shigella tends to produce the most severe forms of dysentery, there is no close correspondence between clinical patterns of disease and specific agents. Ultimately all the shigelloses resemble each other a great deal more than they differ. The incubation period of most infections is as little as 1 day. They begin with the acute onset of cramps, distention and diarrhea. The first signs of inflammation are usually found in the cecum and ascending colon. Later the entire colon and ileum may become involved. The organisms presumably invade the crypts of glands and lymphoid tissue in the colon. The mucosa becomes hyperemic and edematous, and enlargement of the lymphoid follicles creates small, projecting nodules. *Within the course of 24 hours, a fibrinosuppurative exudate covers the mucosa and sometimes produces a dirty gray to yellow pseudomembrane.* This does not have the internal strength of the classic fibrinous pseudomembrane of diphtheria, but more nearly resembles coagulated pus. The inflammatory reaction within the intestinal mucosa builds up, the mucosa becomes soft and friable, and superficial irregular ulcerations appear. If the infection is severe, large mucosal tracts may be denuded, leaving only islands of preserved mucosa. Usually these ulcerations are very superficial and rarely extend below the mucosa; occasionally they become deeper. These mucosal defects are not totally distinctive from the lesions of nonspecific ulcerative colitis or typhoid fever. Rarely the ulcers extend into the underlying muscularis, particularly when the infection becomes chronic. Perforation is an uncommon complication, contributed to by secondary infection (Felsen, 1936).

Histologically, the reaction is dominantly that of a mononuclear leukocytic infiltrate within the intestinal mucosa, but the surfaces of the ulcer are covered with an acute suppurative, neutrophilic reaction accompanied by congestion, marked edema and thromboses of small vessels, chiefly confined to the mucosa. At a later stage, when the ulcerations are more fully developed, the cellular exudation, infiltration and edema become more intense and the inflammatory infiltrate extends more deeply into the submucosa. In these deeper levels, the immigrant white cell population is principally made up of mononuclear leukocytes. However, polymorphonuclears are still found rimming the ulcer defects. As the disease progresses, the ulcers deepen and their margins are transformed into active granulation tissue. As the disease remits, this granulation tissue fills the defect, and the ulcers heal by regeneration of the mucosal epithelium. Often there is considerable distortion of the regenerated mucosal glands as well as of the marginal preserved glands involved by the inflammatory reaction, manifested by cystic dilatation, loss of orderly parallel arrangement and mucinous hypersecretory activity.

Degenerative, loosely termed toxemic, changes have been described in other organs, such as the central nervous system, epithelial cells of the proximal convoluted tubules of the kidney and hepatic cells, but these changes are inconstant, equivocal, and are almost certainly not related to direct invasion by bacteria. Occasionally, hematogenous spread does result in local pyogenic infections, such as acute suppurative arthritis, acute pyelonephritis, and rarely vegetative endocarditis. Very infrequently, acute pylephlebitis or liver abscesses develop.

The nonspecific character of the macroscopic and microscopic alterations described requires bacteriologic and serologic studies to identify the precise etiology.

The clinical course of bacillary dysentery is very variable, as has been mentioned. Disease due to the Shiga organisms may be extremely fulminating and result in a mortality rate as high as 20 to 50 per cent. Such severity is unusual, however. The classic case is initiated by the abrupt appearance of diarrhea that usually precedes the appearance of a fever of 102° to 103°. Usually nausea and vomiting accompany the diarrhea, and headache appears with the onset of fever. Crampy abdominal pain soon becomes evident, associated temporally with diarrheal movements. The excreta at first consist of a watery fecal material. Soon, as the bowel is emptied of feces, the diarrheal movements are composed only of scant mucoid slime stained with blood or pus. As many as 50 or more bowel movements may occur each day, to the point of prostrating the patient and rapidly producing a state of fluid and electrolyte imbalance. Signs of meningeal irritation develop in certain cases, presumably reflecting the systemic toxemia of obscure nature.

While the diagnosis can be suspected from these clinical findings, certain identification of this condition can only be accomplished by bacteriologic and serologic studies. Organisms can be isolated in the stool during the early stages of the disease. During the second week, specific agglutinins can be demonstrated in the patient's blood, but there is considerable variability in antibody response in individual cases and only low titers may be produced in certain cases. Moreover, cross reactions occur with other Shigella organisms. Blood cultures are usually of little avail in this disease, since the organism does not consistently pass through a bacteremic phase. It is important to stress that staphylococci, botulinus organisms and many of the "gram-negative rods" all induce bacterial diarrheas, and the differential diagnosis requires precise cultural and serologic studies (Grady and Keusch, 1971).

As with typhoidal infections, relapses occur in about 10 per cent of the cases, and these cases may become chronic. With the exception of the high mortality rate in the Shiga infections, the other shigelloses do not result in more than a 5 per cent mortality, and even this figure is subject to revision with the current use of chemotherapeutics.

CHOLERA

Cholera is an acute diarrheal disease of man caused by either *Vibrio comma* or *Vibrio El Tor.* The disease is largely confined to Southeast Asia and the Western Pacific where approximately 60,000 cases are seen each year. The overall mortality rate from this disease is currently 33 per cent but during the nineteenth century there were five pandemics of cholera in which millions of people died of the disease. The causative agent is a comma-shaped, gram-negative motile bacillus with a single polar flagellum. The organisms contain both an H flagellar and an O somatic antigen in common with the Salmonella organisms.

This disease affects the poor, the undernourished and those living under poor sanitary conditions, and classically is characterized by severe vomiting, abdominal cramps and massive diarrhea of slightly yellowish fluid, containing flecks of mucus (the rice water stool), with resultant dehydration, anuria, metabolic acidosis and hypovolemic shock. The patients when seen initially demonstrate severe dehydration with soft, shrunken eyeballs and with skin that has lost its elasticity and is severely wrinkled.

Until recently, it was thought that the vibrio caused the diarrhea by two mechanisms, i.e., elaboration of a potent endotoxin released upon lysis of the bacterial cell, and denudation of the small bowel epithelium with the diarrheal fluid simply pouring forth from this "sloughed surface." Recently, it has been shown that the cholera vibrio remains in the lumen of the bowel and that enterotoxin elaborated by the organisms penetrates the intact mucosal epithelial layer and acts on the vasculature of the bowel, with resultant outpouring of tremendous amounts of fluid causing the diarrhea and dehydration.

Using intestinal biopsy, it has been shown that while the epithelium is intact, there is an inflammatory response in the lamina propria of the bowel characterized by engorgement of the capillaries, dilatation of the central lacteals and a sparse infiltrate composed predominantly of mononuclear cells, plasma cells, lymphocytes and histiocytes. Neutrophils are usually absent. No ulceration occurs, and therefore it is unusual to find blood or pus in the intestinal contents. Increased vascular leakage and epithelial cell hypersecretion are the major features. During the disease and subsequent recovery, there is a marked increase in the rate of mitotic activity in the intestinal lining epithelium, particularly in the crypts. Because the organism does not invade the body, bacteremia is not seen. With early and intensive care centered primarily around the infusion of massive amounts of intravenous physiologic saline (5 to 20 liters per day), the disease will be self-limited in approximately 5 to 7 days with a mortality rate of 0.1 per cent. Almost all fatalities attributable to the disease stem from the metabolic and fluid imbalance, rather than from a specific anatomic lesion or systemic toxemia. In the state of peripheral vascular collapse, renal glomerular filtration practically ceases, and azotemia and acidosis complicate the clinical management.

FRIEDLÄNDER'S BACILLUS

The Friedländer bacillus (*Klebsiella pneumoniae*) is a gram-negative, nonmotile rod that is morphologically very similar to the coliform bacilli, but differs principally in that it has an extremely large, mucoid capsule. However, since occasional coliforms are encapsulated, the morphologic distinction is not always easy. *Klebsiella pneumoniae (B. mucosus capsulatus)* is an uncommon cause of bacterial pneumonia. This organism may also localize in other organs to produce pyelonephritis, cholecystitis, cholangitis, sinusitis, mastoiditis, meningitis and endocarditis. However, considering all the various etiologies for such infections, a

Friedländer's causation is most unusual. In all sites of localization, the organism evokes a suppurative inflammatory reaction with abscess formation that is morphologically not distinctive from those due to other pyogenic organisms (Hyde and Hyde, 1943). One possible distinguishing feature is the *mucoid character of the exudate* that is produced by the heavy gelatinous capsules of *Klebsiella pneumoniae*. While many type-specific, capsular polysaccharides have been identified in various strains, these antigenic differences do not result in distinctive clinical and morphologic infections. Most clinical disease is produced by variants that have been classified in the group A. The organisms are normal inhabitants of the respiratory passages in up to 25 per cent of the population. Whether these organisms are of high virulence and have been degraded by their symbiotic existence has not been clearly established.

Infections are probably transmitted directly from active cases to the new host by droplet contamination. Presumably the organism is inhaled and implants either in the upper respiratory passages or within the lung itself. From here, it may evoke a bacterial pneumonia that greatly resembles pneumococcal lobar pneumonia. At other times, the organism may enter the blood directly to produce a bacteremia with localized infections in the organs and tracts mentioned. A respiratory infection usually precedes the hematogenous dissemination.

Klebsiella pneumoniae is responsible for about 1 to 2 per cent of bacterial pneumonias. The disease tends to occur in the fifth to seventh decades of life and is particularly apt to develop in debilitated individuals, i.e., the malnourished, chronic alcoholics and those suffering from some chronic illness.

The organism apparently evokes an acute inflammatory exudation in the lung that is responsible for an extremely sudden onset of respiratory symptoms. A characteristic widespread pneumonic consolidation develops within the lung which may be limited to a portion of a lobe, but more often affects a whole lobe or multiple lobes. The affected regions are solidly filled with exudate, and the lung has the solidified "plaster cast" appearance described in pneumococcal pneumonia (p. 811). Each lung may weigh up to 1500 to 2000 gm. The pleural surfaces are consistently covered by a fibrinosuppurative exudate. On transection, the lung parenchyma is usually uniformly gray to gray-red punctuated by small foci of apparent abscess formation. Copious, mucoid, slimy pus exudes from the cut surface and clings to the sectioning knife and hands.

Histologically, the pneumonic consolidation is characterized by filling of the alveoli with a mucoid suppurative exudate heavily laden with large numbers of encapsulated bacilli. Neutrophils and macrophages comprise the dominant leukocytic response. One of the characteristic features of *Klebsiella pneumoniae* is the production of *numerous small focal abscesses*. Fibrin is generally not so copious in amount in the Friedländer's pneumonia as in the pneumococcal pneumonias. (For further details, reference may be made to Chapter 19.)

The pulmonary disease usually begins suddenly with the onset of chills, fever, pleuritic pain, cough and the expectoration of a copious amount of at first sanguineous, then frankly sanguinopurulent, mucoid sputum. When the consolidation is widespread, shortness of breath, dyspnea and cyanosis may become evident within the first 48 hours of the disease. Patients classically have difficulty in raising the thick, tenacious sputum. When such material is examined, it is usually loaded with the encapsulated bacilli of the morphologic form described. If the patient survives, particularly when the infection is aborted by therapy, considerable resolution may follow. But in almost all full-blown infections, residual scarring occurs in the areas of abscess formation, and many times widespread organization of the exudate leaves dense, fibrous pleural adhesions and permanently solidified parenchyma as sequelae.

Prior to the advent of the chemotherapeutic agents, the mortality rate was over 50 per cent. Considerable improvement has been accomplished since that time in the prognosis, but the disease remains a highly fatal illness, particularly in the predisposed. Occasionally an acute pneumonia is followed by a chronic persistent pulmonary infection so that these organisms are sometimes identified in chronic bronchitis, bronchiectasis and lung abscesses. A widespread septicemia occurs many times in the course of the pneumonia and in other instances without the development of full-blown pneumonia, evidenced by chills, fever, malaise and prostration. These septicemic cases are extremely fulminating, and the patients usually succumb without the development of localized tissue lesions. However, in other cases the bacteremia may be less fulminating and the various organs mentioned are seeded.

BRUCELLA — UNDULANT FEVER

Brucellosis is usually a chronic, insidious, infectious disease caused by a small, gram-negative, pleomorphic coccobacillus, the Brucella. The organisms are found in many domestic farm animals. Although it is usually thought that the organism is transmitted to humans by the ingestion of contaminated milk, and such indirect transfer does occur, most cases now seem to be contracted by direct contact with infected animals or their excreta (Spink, 1954). *Bacterial infections by Brucella are characterized principally by invasion of the reticuloendothelial system, with resultant widespread generalized reticuloendothelial hyperactivity and hyperplasia and the formation of small miliary granulomas that resemble those found in sarcoid and tuberculosis* and, to a lesser extent, the lesions of tularemia. The clinical manifestations are extremely protean, but in all instances the histologic changes are believed to be fairly uniform.

Each species of animal harbors chiefly one strain of organism, i.e., cattle, *Brucella abortus;* hogs, *Brucella suis;* and goats, *Brucella melitensis.* However, infection of any species of animal may occur by any strain of organism. While there is some correspondence between the clinical pattern of the disease and the specific strain of Brucella responsible, there is no absolute correlation.

Little is known about the pathogenesis of these infections. However, it is clear that *once the organism gains a foothold within the body, it rapidly invades the reticuloendothelial cells.* This intracytoplasmic localization may account for the great chronicity of this disease, since many patients remain ill for months and even years. Clinical manifestations usually appear within three to four weeks, but occasional cases have been recorded in which symptoms have been delayed for as long as a year.

By the time the tissues were available for study in the few cases that ended in death, parasitization of the reticuloendothelial cells was found in the liver, spleen, lymph nodes and bone marrow (Sharp, 1934). Usually there is no macroscopic alteration, but sometimes small gray-white foci indicate the sites of reaction. These foci consist principally of *accumulations of macrophages and reticuloendothelial cells surrounded by a collar of mononuclear leukocytes and proliferating plump fibroblasts.* Often there are giant cells within this inflammatory collar. The similarity between the Brucella nodule and the focal granulomas of sarcoid and tuberculosis is thus evident. Central caseation of these granulomas heightens the similarity to tuberculosis.

As a consequence of these inflammatory alterations, the lymph nodes are enlarged throughout the body, along with splenohepatomegaly. Similar lesions may occur in any tissue of the body. Of the less common sites, the testes, brain, joints, heart valves, intestines, kidneys, spinal cord and vertebral column merit special mention.

The clinical manifestations are so protean as to defy brief description. Occasionally, the disease begins abruptly with chills, fever, sweats, generalized muscle aches and pains, and marked prostration. Alternatively, the disease may be extremely insidious in onset, and the patients may suffer from vague malaise, weakness and general debilitation for many months. These cases have often been diagnosed as neurasthenia. These vague infections are often characterized by night sweats and transient pains in the abdomen, extremities and joints. Severe neuritis and radiculitis may develop. The symptoms may persist for weeks to many months, and recovery may not occur for a year or more unless the disease is recognized and treated. The fever in this condition follows many patterns. Usually it is intermittent, with diurnal temperature spikes up to 100° to 104°, giving to this condition the designation of *undulant fever.*

The diagnosis almost always depends on the demonstration of specific antibodies by complement fixation tests and upon skin tests. Blood cultures may disclose the organisms during the height of the febrile reaction, particularly if the patient is having chills. While these organisms are unquestionably excreted in the feces and urine intermittently in patients having lesions within the intestinal tract and urinary tract, these localizations are too inconstant to render bacterial cultures of much value. The mortality rate is low even in the untreated case, on the order of 2 to 5 per cent.

PASTEURELLA

Two strains of Pasteurella are responsible for highly destructive clinical disease. *Pasteurella pestis* is the causative agent of bubonic plague and *Pasteurella tularensis* produces tularemia. Both these infections are characterized by animal reservoirs in which the microorganisms abound in nature, permitting transfer to man either directly or indirectly through insect vectors. These infections are distinctive in several regards. *Both P. pestis and P. tularensis produce powerful necrotizing toxins that lead to extensive tissue destruction in the sites of bacterial localization, and both microbial agents are extremely invasive and are thought to be capable of penetrating the intact skin.*

Quite recently a third strain of Pasteurella has been identified as a pathogen for man. *Pasteurella multicida* has been identified as the causal agent of localized infections in the skin, bones and sinuses and has even been responsible for pleuritis and meningitis.

TULAREMIA

Tularemia is an extremely acute infectious systemic disorder characterized by focal suppurative and granulomatous inflammatory reactions in many sites in the body (Goodpasture and House, 1928). Depending upon the dissemination or localization of the infection, several clinical patterns are distinguished, known as *ulceroglandular, glandular, oculoglandular, typhoidal and pleuropulmonic.* These variants are not mutually exclusive and combinations are often encountered.

Causative Agent. *P. tularensis* is a tiny, gram-negative, extremely pleomorphic coccobacillus. At times its morphology is virtually indistinguishable from that of the pyogenic cocci, while, at other times the organisms appear as distinct rods that resemble the gram-negative enteric bacilli. Various antigenic components have been identified, but the specific toxic fraction that accounts for their extreme pathogenicity and invasiveness is still unknown. The organism is readily destroyed by heating, and thorough cooking of food renders infected meat and water safe. When dried in vacuo and held at room temperature, the organisms are viable for as long as four years and, in infected carcasses, bacteria remain viable for months.

Method of Spread. The organism is widely distributed in rabbits, rats, squirrels and other fur-bearers and, in these animals, is responsible for an endemic transmissible disease. Transfer to man occurs as an incidental offshoot from this animal-to-animal chain of infection. The clinical disease may be contracted through several portals of entry. Ninety per cent of human cases are the result of direct contact with infected animals, and the disease is particularly common among butchers, hunters, farmers, cooks and housewives. The organisms may be abraded into the skin, rubbed into the eye, inhaled or ingested. Rare cases have occurred from the bite of diseased animals or the ingestion of contaminated water or meat. To *P. tularensis* is attributed the capacity to penetrate the unbroken skin, and therefore skin injuries are not necessary to provide a portal of entry. Insects, such as ticks, deerflies and horseflies, may transmit this organism. It is quite remarkable that despite the apparent invasiveness and infectiveness of the organism, man-to-man transmission has not been recorded, even in the presence of fulminating pneumonic forms of this disease with undoubted contamination of the air and surrounding articles.

Pathogenesis. The disease usually becomes manifest about 2 to 5 days following the introduction of the organism. However, the incubation period may vary from 1 to 21 days. In about 10 per cent of the cases, a local lesion develops at the site of the original portal of entry. A bacteremia is usually present during the first week of the disease. With the appearance of antibodies the bacteremia disappears, but subsequent spread of the disease may occur via the lymphatics or by local contiguity.

The Infections. *Ulceroglandular Form.* This designation refers to the most common clinical pattern in which a local ulceration develops at the site of the original invasion and is followed by regional or generalized lymphadenopathy. It begins abruptly with fever, chills, sweats, headache, nausea and vomiting, and generalized muscular aches and pains. About 1 or 2 days later, a painful, red, papular lesion develops at the site of entry, and the lymph nodes draining the site become painfully enlarged. The primary lesion usually is located on the hands, arms or face, but may also be situated in the conjunctivae or in the oropharynx. The papule rapidly enlarges to 1 to 2 cm. in diameter, becomes pustular, and eventually ruptures to cause an extremely painful ulcer.

Grossly, the local ulceration is a nonspecific, acute inflammatory lesion, while the lymph nodes are usually extremely soft and matted together. At other times the nodes of drainage are tense and of increased firmness, apparently due to considerable edema. Transection of these nodes will disclose small to large, confluent, yellow-white foci of necrosis in most instances.

Histologically, the tularemic reaction is characterized by *focal, intense suppurative necrosis, reproducing to a considerable extent the granulomatous pattern found in tuberculous infections.* The central area of necrosis consists largely of polymorphonuclear leukocytes and macrophages in varying stages of preservation. In the larger or older lesions, the central white cells may have undergone total coagulative granular necrosis, resembling caseation. Surrounding the intense reaction, there is a wall of plump fibroblasts that in many places assume the appearance of epithelioid cells as well as occasional Langhans' or foreign body type giant cells. Smaller, non-necrotic lesions may be present, resembling the so-called hard tubercles. The lesion may be extremely difficult to differentiate from a classic tubercle. Bacteria can be visualized in these lesions only with great difficulty if at all. However, they are readily isolated by cultural methods.

Glandular Form. In many cases, no localized skin lesions can be found, and the disease takes the form of a regional or generalized adenopathy alone. This pattern of the disease is sometimes referred to as the glandular variant. When the adenopathy is distributed throughout the body, it is almost invariably accompanied by marked enlargement of the spleen and liver. The lesions in this diffuse form of the disease are similar to those described in the regional nodes. However, the spleen often does not contain discrete tularemic nodules and presents only a generalized hyperplasia of the reticuloendothelial cells accompanied by increased numbers of polymorphonuclears and macrophages within the splenic sinuses with central necrosis of the follicles rimmed by a polymorphonuclear and histiocytic infiltration.

In about one-half of the ulceroglandular and glandular cases, the nodes subsequently slowly decrease in size and the lesions undergo total fibrous scarring. In the remainder of the cases, individual nodes may become progressively large, soft and fluctuant, and may eventually ulcerate through the skin to produce draining sinuses. The skin lesion follows a similar pattern of slow regression with ultimate scarring of the deeper tissues and superficial reepithelialization.

Oculoglandular Form. The oculoglandular form of the disease differs only in the initial portal of entry which involves the conjunctival surfaces with the production of tiny papules that eventually become pustular and ulcerate. When these pustules occur on the bulbar conjunctiva, they may perforate the eyeball to produce extensive infections in the anterior and sometimes posterior chambers of the eye. Occasionally, the entire eye is destroyed and the optic nerve becomes involved by the contiguous spread of infection. In almost all these cases, the regional nodes of drainage, particularly the preauricular, submaxillary and anterior cervical nodes, undergo the characteristic gross and microscopic changes described. The oculoglandular variant of the disease may also be accompanied by generalized adenopathy and splenomegaly.

Gastrointestinal Form. When the disease is contracted by the ingestion of contaminated food or water, the local ulceration may appear anywhere in the oropharynx, or the portal of entry may occur out of sight in the lining of the alimentary canal. In addition to the nonspecific features of fever, chills, sweats and headaches, these patients suffer predominantly from acute abdominal symptoms, such as vomiting, diarrhea, and abdominal pain and cramps. Melena may become an important manifestation, presumably owing to the occurrence of ulcerative lesions in the intestinal mucosa. Regional and generalized adenopathy, accompanied by splenomegaly, is also present in this clinical symptom complex.

Typhoidal Form. This designation is given to cases of tularemia that are manifested chiefly by acute septicemia without a localizing skin lesion and frequently without striking peripheral adenopathy. In this pattern of the disease, the patients are acutely ill with extremely high fever, drenching sweats, headache, prostration and sometimes shock, all reflecting the overwhelming bacteremia and toxemia. In this form, the disease may be extremely difficult to identify without a careful history of contact or exposure, and the diagnosis rests almost completely upon the identification of organisms by blood cultures. Focal tissue lesions may or may not develop, depending upon how long the patient lives.

Pleuropulmonic Form. Pleuropulmonic tularemia is manifested chiefly by the development of patchy, bacterial pneumonia or sometimes confluent pneumonia. Pleuropulmonic tularemia may occur as a primary infection, but more often it develops in the course of one of the other variants already mentioned. Pulmonary involvement is encountered in about 50 per cent of the cases of the typhoidal form. It occurs less often in the ulceroglandular form. The pneumonic involvement is most often localized about the hilus of the lung and appears grossly as small to large areas of yellow-white consolidation in which central foci of necrosis can sometimes be seen. When the disease is more florid, large portions of a lobe or entire lobes may become solidified.

Histologically, these lesions differ from the usual bacterial pneumonia by the presence of characteristic tularemic nodules that sometimes strikingly simulate tuberculosis. In contrast to many of the other bacterial pneumonias, the pulmonic involvement in this disease is almost invariably accompanied by necrosis of alveolar walls and lung substance so that complete resolution is not possible and scarring and fibrosis are virtually inevitable residuals. A serous or seropurulent pleuritis is present in about half the cases of pulmonary infection. Sometimes the effusion is modified by hemorrhages, and in occasional cases characteristic tularemic nodules develop on the pleural surfaces. The hilar nodes of the lung are almost inevitably enlarged owing to inflammation.

Although various clinical patterns have been singled out for special description, tularemia is quite protean in its behavior and occasionally localizations are found in the meninges, peritoneal cavity, pericardium and bone. It cannot be assumed, therefore, that the variants described exhaust the possible clinical expressions of this disorder. The course of this disease is one of fairly striking chronicity, and patients are frequently sick for as long as one to two months. Occasionally, relapses occur along with reexacerbation of lymphadenopathy, which may progress to the stage of forming new draining sinuses. In the usual case, the acute phase begins to subside about two to three weeks after the onset of fever, or sooner if appropriately treated, and the convalescence, although prolonged, is uneventful. The diagnosis frequently can only be suspected by the clinical manifestations and anatomic changes described. Agglutinating antibodies can be demonstrated in the blood, usually following the second or third week of illness. There is some cross reaction between tularemia and brucellosis, but the levels of antibody against the specific disease are usually sufficiently high to indicate the true nature of infection. Although organisms can usually be cultured from the areas of necrosis and sometimes from the blood, this diagnostic study is fraught with danger because of the great communicability of these organisms and so is best carried out under a hood. A diagnostic skin test that is of fairly high specificity is available.

This disease is of considerable gravity and approximately 4 per cent of the cases succumb. This mortality rate is greatly enhanced when pulmonary involvement develops.

PLAGUE

Plague is an extremely severe, acute infection caused by *Pasteurella pestis*. Fortunately, this disease is uncommon today, but its possible reappearance and its overwhelming impact on the world in years past make requisite a brief consideration. Plague is basically an infection of a great variety of wild animals, principally rats, which serve as the reservoir of infective material. In the western part of the U.S., ground squirrels and chipmunks constitute an additional reservoir of infection. The disease is usually transmitted to man indirectly by the bite of fleas (rodent or human), but sometimes it is transferred by direct contact with infected animals or active clinical cases. The disease may express itself in man in one of three clinical patterns: *bubonic, pneumonic* and *septicemic*.

Causative Agent. *P. pestis* is an encapsulated, gram-negative, nonmotile, markedly pleomorphic bacillus, which may assume bacillary to coccal shapes. Although the organism produces no exotoxin, a very strong endotoxin has been identified within the somatic proteins. *P. pestis* is readily killed by sunlight in three to

four hours and is inactivated by heating at 55° C. in only 15 minutes. Nonetheless, it may remain viable at room temperature in animal feces, sputum and tissues for as long as five weeks. Colder temperatures permit an even longer survival, recorded as lasting up to 25 years.

Method of Spread. Plague should be considered principally as an animal infection that only occasionally is diverted to man. Approximately 38 species of wild rodents and other fur-bearers are known to be susceptible, but the most important reservoir for man is the wild rat. The disease may be transmitted from rat to rat, either directly or through the rat flea. It may also be transmitted from the wild rat to laboratory rats and other laboratory animals, usually through the intermediate vector of the rat flea.

Most human infections are acquired by the bite of infected fleas. The hazard of human contamination depends upon: (1) the size of the infected rat population, (2) the availability of uninfected rats to provide a continuing appropriate environment for the survival of the rat flea and (3) the intimacy of the coexistence of man, rats and their fleas. Other insects may serve as vectors, namely, the human flea, lice, ticks and even bedbugs. Infected flea feces may be abraded into the skin even in the absence of a bite, or the organism may penetrate the intact epidermis. Infection may also be contracted by handling infected animals or by the ingestion of infected material. Direct man-to-man, air-borne contamination may occur, particularly during epidemics. Animals other than the rat do not constitute such an important reservoir of infection merely because man does not ordinarily come into such close contact with these other species.

Pathogenesis. *P. pestis* infection in man is characterized by: (1) severe fibrinous and leukocytic (neutrophilic) exudation, (2) invasion of blood vessels and lymphatics and (3) necrosis and thrombosis of vessels, leading to hemorrhages and infarction of tissues. While the term "plague" usually conjures up the concept of an overwhelming, invariably fatal infection, the disease may vary from a mild disorder to an overwhelming invasion, depending upon the size and virulence of the infecting inoculum and the resistance of the host. In the mild case, the plague bacilli may be largely localized to the initial site of inoculation and produce only a local vesicle or pustule. Inflammation of the regional nodes of drainage usually follows. However, the organism may overwhelm the nodes of drainage and enter the lymphatics and blood vessels to be spread throughout the body. Generalized reticuloendothelial hyperplasia follows with enlargement of nodes, liver and spleen and localization of the organism in any organ or tissue. If the organism is highly virulent and the patient particularly vulnerable, the organism may multiply rapidly in the body to cause an overwhelming septicemia, followed by death so quickly that local tissue lesions may not become fully developed.

The Infections. *Bubonic Form.* The bubonic pattern of plague is the most common variant. It usually begins abruptly with high temperature, chills, tachycardia and headache, soon followed by mental confusion, delirium and prostration. The site of entry of the organisms may be unaffected, but at times is marked by a vesicle, pustule or small necrotizing ulceration. The regional nodes of drainage are usually involved and characteristically become enlarged, sometimes to the extreme diameter of 5 cm. In the course of a few days, the individual nodes become matted together to form the characteristic "*bubo*." Macroscopically, the nodes are soft, pulpy and frequently hemorrhagic and plum-colored. A plastic, fibrinous, hemorrhagic exudate surrounds the nodes. At later stages, the suppurative necrosis floods over into the perinodal tissue and the nodes themselves may undergo total infarction and suppurative necrosis. As the suppurative reaction involves the subcutaneous tissues, the infection may rupture through the skin and produce draining sinuses.

Histologically, the inflammation is characterized by extensive hemorrhagic exudation, marked dilatation of blood vessels, intravascular thromboses, necrosis of vessel walls and total necrosis of the tissues (Fig. 10–14). This inflammatory necrosis is a mixture of suppuration and infarction and apparently reflects the extreme necrotizing action of the bacteria, as well as the vascular injury induced by these organisms. Large numbers of bacteria can be identified with appropriate stains within the necrotic material. The spreading inflammation may create a diffuse, spreading cellulitis. Other reticuloendothelial sites undergo nonspecific inflammatory hyperplasia and swelling, and in many cases the nodes throughout the body develop localized areas of necrosis similar to those in the regional nodes.

In the more fulminating cases, the bacteremia induces widespread, disseminated hemorrhage and necrosis in the skin, spleen, liver, mucous membranes of the body, and linings of the alimentary, respiratory and urinary tracts. Often these hemorrhagic necroses create ecchymotic or large map-like areas. Sometimes small secondary foci of ulcerative

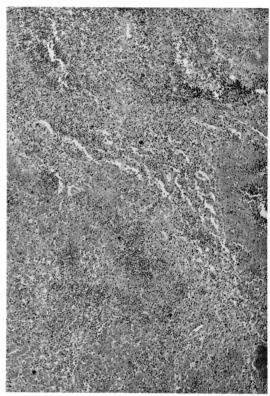

Figure 10–14. *Plague—a low power view of the total hemorrhagic necrosis of an area in a lymph node.*

necrosis develop within these lesions. It is this overwhelming hemorrhagic discoloration of the skin that provides the basis for the descriptive term, "*black death*." Hemorrhages and necrotic lesions may also be found in the serous cavities and the endocardium and epicardium.

Pneumonic Form. About 5 per cent of the cases of the bubonic variant develop a secondary pneumonia, while in other instances the pneumonia may occur as a primary pattern, usually in epidemics with man-to-man, airborne contamination. The lungs are heavy, red and edematous and have patchy to confluent areas of hemorrhagic, gray consolidation. Fibrinous pleuritis is present in most cases. The characteristic necrotizing, hemorrhagic, exudative inflammation of plague is evident in these sites. The alveolar spaces are filled with bloody serous fluid, containing but little fibrin. The white cell response is chiefly neutrophilic. Organisms abound in the lesions, causing an almost unrestricted destruction and necrosis of underlying architecture. These patients have the same systemic febrile reactions as the bubonic pattern and, in addition, have prominent signs related to the respiratory infection. The sputum is abundant and blood-stained, and teems with *P. pestis.*

Septicemic Form. The septicemic form essentially results from an overwhelming infection with a highly virulent organism that proliferates wildly in the blood and leads to death so quickly that tissue localizations do not have a chance to develop. Early pneumonic involvement, generalized reticuloendothelial hyperactivity and acute lymphadenitis may be present, along with vascular engorgement, congestion throughout the body and widespread hemorrhages into the various sites described.

Prior to the advent of antibiotics, the mortality rate of the bubonic form varied between 50 and 90 per cent, and the pneumonic and septicemic forms were almost invariably fatal.

PASTEURELLA MULTOCIDA INFECTIONS

Quite recently, it has become apparent that this third strain of Pasteurella may also be pathogenic for man as well as the highly pathogenic tularensis and pestis. The multocida strain is a nonmotile, gram-negative coccobacillus having a large reservoir in both domesticated and wild animals. The organism is transmitted to man either by an animal bite or without any obvious pathway. A local nonspecific and suppurative inflammation with abscess formation occurs at the site of the bite. When the organism is transmitted by less obvious mechanisms, sinusitis, pleuritis and meningitis have been described. These are all entirely nonspecific, acute suppurative infections. Twenty-five such cases have been collected and reported from the Mayo Clinic (Schipper, 1947).

B. ANTHRACIS — ANTHRAX

Anthrax is an acute infectious disease caused by *B. anthracis*, a highly pathogenic organism found in many species of animals, particularly the herbivora. The disease is extremely uncommon, but is of great severity when encountered. The organism characteristically evokes a striking hemorrhagic, edematous, inflammatory response accompanied by ischemic necrosis of tissues. In its usual clinical pattern (approximately 95 per cent of the cases), anthrax is contracted as a skin infection by contact with infected animals. The local lesion is graphically described as a *malignant pustule*. However, the organism or its spores may be air-borne, resulting in a diffuse pneumonic consolidation. This clinical variant is designated as *"woolsorters' disease."* In both forms, bacteremia may ensue if the body defenses are overwhelmed with the development of meningitis or localized infections in other sites.

Causative Agent. *B. anthracis* is a large, gram-positive, nonmotile, encapsulated bacillus that characteristically grows in long chains. The organism forms spores that are extremely resistant to adverse influences, persist in soil and in other sites for years, resist ordinary boiling for at least 10 minutes, and withstand many of the common chemical disinfectants. Much of the virulence of the anthrax bacillus is due to its capsular polypeptides, which in some way block or overcome the protective mechanisms of the host.

Method of Spread. The chief reservoirs of these bacilli are sheep, cattle, horses and pigs, but occasionally other animals are affected. The disease is transmitted to man by direct or indirect contact either with infected animals or their products. In the usual cutaneous form of the disease, the organism apparently gains entry through a skin injury.

Pulmonary anthrax (woolsorters' disease) is particularly apt to occur in industries dealing with the raw wool products. Man-to-man transmission or contamination by the ingestion of infected meat occurs extremely infrequently, if at all.

The Infection. Following an incubation period of several days, a small, red, macular lesion appears, resembling a flea bite. The macule enlarges and becomes edematous to create a papule. Further progression rapidly produces a vesicle that is filled first with hemorrhagic fluid and then with thin, bloody, purulent exudate, imparting a dark purple-black color to the skin blister. A frank pustule develops and the surrounding tissues become edematous. *The combination of the relatively small hemorrhagic pustule and extensive brawny edema creates the malignant pustule that should arouse suspicion as to the nature of the infection.* In the course of the first week of the disease, these vesicles rupture and ooze a serosanguineous fluid. A tough black eschar forms over the ruptured vesicle, but the circumferential edema continues to expand. Satellite vesicles commonly appear about the primary lesion. The regional nodes become moderately enlarged due to a nonspecific lymphadenitis. Reddened lymphatics can often be found along the course of this drainage.

Histologically, the inflammatory reaction in the skin lesion consists principally of intense edema, vascular congestion with hemorrhages, and necrosis of tissues resembling infarction necrosis, presumably due to the compression and embarrassment of the local blood supply. The leukocytic response is relatively deficient in contrast to the amount of tissue necrosis and consists of a mixture of neutrophils and mononuclear white cells. The involved lymph nodes have similar changes. In the usual case, the inflammatory process slowly subsides following this stage, and the disease remains localized to the initial site of entry and the regional nodes of drainage. However, if the invasion is more extensive, bacteremia may follow and give rise to meningitis or localizations in the lungs or other tissues.

A diffuse pneumonia develops in the disease contracted by the inhalation of spores, characterized by an extensive serofibrinous exudation throughout large areas of the lung fields that may produce total lobar consolidations. The striking characteristics of this pneumonia are the relative paucity of neutrophils, the tendency to develop hemorrhagic necrosis of alveolar septa and the overwhelming abundance of bacteria within the inflammatory exudate. Occasionally an overwhelming septicemia develops and causes death within such a short space of time that frank recognizable anatomic lesions do not develop.

The systemic manifestations may be relatively mild in the cutaneous form, but in the pneumonic form the reaction is intense and is accompanied by high fever, signs of respiratory distress and often severe prostration. As might be anticipated from the paucity of leukocytic reaction, there is only a slight elevation of the white cell count and sometimes leukopenia develops. In all variants, the diagnosis rests upon the identification or cultivation of bacteria in the tissue lesions or from the blood. Since the organisms are large and distinctive in their morphology, they are readily identified. The fatality rate in this disease is quite high and may reach levels of about 20 per cent even in the milder forms. Fatalities are even more common in the pneumonic and septicemic involvements.

MALLEOMYCES MALLEI—GLANDERS

Glanders is an extremely acute, severe, infectious disease caused by *Malleomyces mallei*, an organism that finds its natural reservoir among horses and donkeys and is transmitted to man by contact with these animals. *The disease consists essentially of a rapidly developing, overwhelming pyemia in its acute form, but in some instances it takes a more insidious course that may resemble such chronic infections as tuberculosis.* The organism is a small, gram-negative, nonmotile, nonsporing bacillus. As this is an infectious disease of equines, man is only involved incidentally by contact with these animals. However, Malleomyces is extremely pathogenic for man. Transmission occurs by contamination of the intact or abraded skin, by implantation on the conjunctiva, by eating contaminated food or by inhalation. Most clinical disease results from a cutaneous portal of entry, since this organism is credited with the capacity to penetrate the intact epidermis.

Acute glanders is characterized by an incubation period of only a few hours to a few days, followed by the rather sudden onset of severe, prostrating infection with constitutional signs, i.e., fever, malaise, chills, nausea, vomiting, and generalized aches and pains. A local papular abscess develops at the site of inoculation, and the organism spreads from this site along the lymphatics to the regional nodes. Multiple satellite abscesses may occur along the pathways of drainage. The organism rapidly invades the blood to cause generalized pyemic abscesses in many organs and tissues, particularly in the liver, spleen, lungs and muscles. Meningitis, osteomyelitis and polyarthritis may all develop in the course of a few days. Subcutaneous and superficial abscesses may develop anywhere on the body.

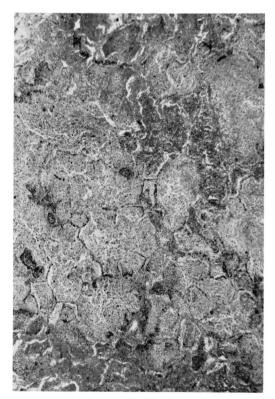

Figure 10–15. Glanders pneumonia with extensive exudation and necrosis in the pulmonary parenchyma.

The anatomic characteristics are those of non-specific suppuration, reflecting an overwhelming pyemia (Fig. 10–15). Bacteria can be identified in many of these lesions, and the diagnosis is frequently made by the demonstration of the small gram-negative bacilli in the skin lesions.

Chronic glanders is seen less frequently and takes the form of a low-grade, febrile, infectious disease characterized by chronic draining abscesses of the skin, lymphadenopathy, splenomegaly and hepatomegaly with the formation of chronic granulomatous abscesses in any of these sites or elsewhere. These granulomas often simulate tubercles. The lesions are not pathognomonic, and the diagnosis rests upon the cultural and serologic identification of the organism.

In the acute form of the disease, 80 to 90 per cent of the patients die within the first or second week of illness. In the more chronic variant, a remitting, relapsing or persistent infection may continue for months to even a year. Over half of these patients eventually die of their infection.

MYCOBACTERIA

TUBERCULOSIS

Tuberculosis is an acute or chronic communicable disease caused by Mycobacterium tuberculosis *which usually involves the lung but may affect any organ or tissue in the body.* Five strains of *M. tuberculosis* have been identified: human, bovine, avian, murine and piscine, but only the human and bovine strains are pathogenic to man. Thus the disease is perpetuated throughout the world by man-to-man transmission and the drinking of infected milk. Improved living standards, public health measures and more effective therapy have brought about a remarkable decline in the prevalence of this disease in economically developed nations. In the United States in 1900, tuberculosis was the leading cause of death accounting for approximately 200 deaths per 100,000 population. In 1965, this death rate had fallen to the vastly improved level of 4.1 per 100,000, representing the 18th most frequent cause of death (National Health Education Committee, 1966). However, in many of the underdeveloped nations, the death rate still exceeds 200 to 300 per 100,000 population. It is estimated that as many as 5 million people around the world die annually of this disease.

Although the control of tuberculosis has been satisfactory in many parts of the world, it persists as a major clinical problem. Even in economically developed countries, the crowded slums of virtually every urban center as well as the economically deprived rural areas continue as high-incidence pockets of disease. Occupational hazards account for a markedly increased prevalence of tuberculosis among physicians, hospital personnel and laboratory workers. Silicosis, diabetes mellitus, congenital heart disease and, in fact, any chronic debilitating illness greatly predispose to tuberculosis. In many regions of the world where pasteurization of milk is not routine, bovine tuberculosis is still rampant.

Fortunately, man has a relatively high natural resistance to *M. tuberculosis*. As a consequence, on the first exposure the organism may gain a portal of entry, cause relatively trivial lesions but never produce significant disease. Probably no more than 5 per cent of Americans now infected with *M. tuberculosis* will ever develop clinical disease. Thus with tuberculosis we must distinguish between infection and disease. In older individuals, the disease usually represents activation of latent infections acquired during childhood. It is estimated that about 75 per cent of symptomatic cases in the United States represent activation of such latent childhood infections (Trauger, 1963). The past 50 years have witnessed significant changes in the distribution of tuberculous disease in low-incidence nations. Tuberculosis has been transformed from a disease of children and young adults to a disease primarily of those in the later years of life. The number of young adults and children now infected has declined remarkably from past years. Whereas at one time the majority of the young had been exposed and infected, now those who have never had contact with *M. tuberculosis* outnumber those who have (Mitchel, 1967).

Causative Agent. *M. tuberculosis* is only one of a fairly large group of gram-positive acid-fast bacilli which includes both pathogenic and saprophytic organisms. Almost all human disease is caused by the human and bovine strain as mentioned. Rare cases have been attributed to *M. kansasii*. All mycobacteria are characterized by the slow uptake of ordinary bacterial dyes at room temperature. Staining is hastened by heating or by introducing wetting agents into the bacterial dyes. Once stained, the mycobacteria resist decolorization with acid alcohol and hence the designation of this group as *acid-fast* organisms. This acid-fastness is probably attributable to the high lipid content of the bacilli, in the range of 50 per cent of the organism. This lipid fraction includes long-chain waxes, neutral fats and phosphatides. *M. tuberculosis* is a slender curved rod averaging 4 microns in length and less than 1 micron in diameter. It is more acid-fast than the saprophytic forms and the degree of acid-fastness appears to correlate with the virulence of the pathogen. As a consequence of its high lipid content, the organism is poorly penetrated by aqueous bactericidal agents and, moreover, it is resistant to drying and can survive and remain infective for long periods of time in dried sputum, feces or other bodily secretions.

M. tuberculosis has certain biologic characteristics that contribute materially to an understanding of the disease in man. Tubercle bacilli are aerobic organisms which multiply at a significant rate only between 35° C. and 41° C. While the organism grows best in fairly high oxygen tensions, it is nonetheless capable of retarded growth at low oxygen tensions. However, *progressive anaerobiosis eventually reaches a limiting level at which further growth is inhibited.* This characteristic may be important in limiting the proliferation of these bacilli in the somewhat anaerobic centers of tuberculous foci of caseation. At the same time, the oxygen requirements help to explain the sudden multiplication of bacilli in infective foci when the caseous lesions erode into a natural passage or surface, and thus expose the deeply situated organisms to increased supplies of oxygen. Conceivably, the same concept might be offered to explain the favored localization of tuberculous infections in the well aerated lung. By cultural methods, it has been well substantiated that these organisms are susceptible to many organic and inorganic materials, such as soaps, heavy metals and phenol. Most important, from the standpoint of the clinical disease, *aliphatic fatty acids from the lowest to the highest members of the series inhibit the growth of tubercle bacilli in synthetic media.* It has been shown in vitro that acetic, butyric and lactic acids have inhibitory effects upon multiplication of the tubercle bacilli, particularly at a pH of 6.5. These laboratory observations may have considerable importance in the pathogenesis of tuberculous infection. The pH of 6.5 is frequently reached in inflammatory foci, and in caseous areas it is believed that lipases may release short- and long-chain aliphatic acids that are instrumental in slowing the reproduction, or even injuring or destroying exposed bacilli. *These fatty acids, the progressive local acidosis, and the increasing anaerobiosis in a focus of tuberculous inflammation together may account for the progressive disappearance of tubercle bacilli within the central regions of caseous lesions.*

Method of Spread. In industrialized nations, tuberculosis is usually spread from man to man by inhalation of airborne organisms coughed or sneezed into the environment by so-called "open cases." Organisms may also be transmitted through the stools in patients with gastrointestinal lesions and through the urine in cases having infections within the urinary tract. Transmission may be direct or indirect. The bacilli are so resistant to drying that they may remain viable for months in dust and on articles of daily use. With widespread pasteurization of milk, tuberculosis due to the bovine strain has become very infrequent in the United States and probably accounts for less than 5 per cent of tuberculous disease. However, in other areas of the world, nonpasteurized milk from infected cows accounts for the preponderance of cases. Thus, for the tubercle bacilli there are four possible portals of entry into the body: (1) the respiratory tract, (2) the lymphoid tissue of the oropharynx, (3) the gut and (4) the skin (in the rare case of contamination of a wound). Among these, inhalation into the lung is responsible for the great preponderance of tuberculous clinical infection in the low-incidence countries while the alimentary tract pathway makes a substantial contribution in the high-incidence countries.

Pathogenesis. Tuberculosis is the prototype and the most important granulomatous infection of man. *Wherever the tubercle bacilli become implanted in the body, they evoke a characteristic granuloma known as a tubercle.* Other granulomatous infections include sarcoidosis, brucellosis, tularemia, syphilis, leprosy, glanders, lymphogranuloma inguinale, cat scratch fever, berylliosis and some of the mycoses. Collectively, these other granulomatous diseases are still far less common than tuberculosis. The basic characteristics of granulomatous inflammation were discussed on p. 83. Here it suffices to recall that *the tubercle comprises a microscopic aggregation of plump rounded histiocytes that vaguely resemble epithelial cells and are therefore called epithelioid cells.* These cells in usual tissue stains have an abundant, pink, faintly granular cytoplasm and sometimes they contain ingested, intact or fragmented bacilli (Fig. 10–16). In the margins of this cluster of epithelioid cells and sometimes within the center, there may be characteristic multinucleate giant cells usually of the Langhans variety (p. 74). About the granuloma, a peripheral collar of plump fibroblasts interspersed with lymphocytes is found. The description just given comprises the so-called "*hard*" tubercle so designated because of the absence of central necrosis and softening. In the course of days, the central region of epithelioid cells undergoes a characteristic form of granular caseous necrosis (p. 40). It is, in fact, the central caseation and the production of a "*soft*" tubercle that create the most characteristic hallmark of tuberculosis

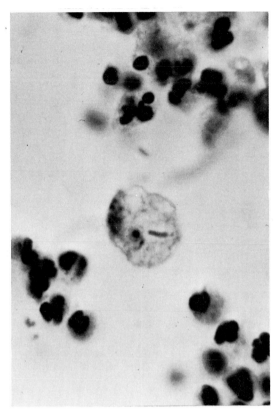

Figure 10–16. *A phagocyte with an engulfed tubercle bacillus thus creating an epithelioid cell.*

(Fig. 10–17). When caseation is absent, most of the diagnostic distinctiveness of the tubercle is lost.

Here we should ask—why does *M. tuberculosis* evoke a granulomatous inflammation? *The pathogenicity of the tubercle bacillus does not derive from any inherent toxicity but rather from its capacity to induce hypersensitivity in its host.* The bacilli elaborate no known endotoxins or exotoxins and, when introduced into a laboratory animal, evoke at first only a non-specific neutrophilic response. A carbohydrate fraction has been extracted from these organisms that induces a neutrophilic outpouring in the experimental animal and is presumably chemotactic in man. Soon thereafter, histiocytes follow the neutrophils and become enlarged to assume the characteristic epithelioid appearance. It is currently believed that it is the persistence of viable or fragmented tubercle bacilli within the phagocytes which induces the epithelioid transformation of the macrophages (Spector, 1969). Models of granulomatous reactions can be induced in experimental animals by the injection of such macromolecules as carrageenin and complex polysaccharides. Presumably, macromolecular substances such as the bacillary waxes are the immediate source of the epithelioid transformation. Thus, hard tubercles are created in the early response to implanted bacilli. After

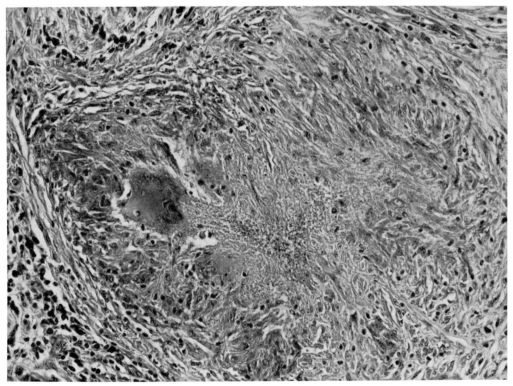

Figure 10–17. *A typical tubercle with giant cell and central caseous necrosis.*

several weeks, *the character of the host reaction abruptly changes as cell-mediated delayed hypersensitivity to the tubercle bacillus develops.* The precise antigen which induces such hypersensitivity is not completely understood, but appears to be tuberculoproteins derived from the bacillus. When tuberculoprotein is injected into the skin of the patient who has been sensitized by prior contact with the bacillus, it evokes a typical hypersensitivity reaction at the injection site. However, tuberculoproteins themselves are not capable of the initial induction of sensitivity. Only live bacilli or the injection of tuberculoprotein and some adjuvant (such as Freund's adjuvant) will induce tuberculin sensitivity. Concomitant with the appearance of such tuberculosensitivity, the centers of hard tubercles undergo caseation necrosis to create the typical "soft" tubercle.

Tuberculosensitivity provides the basis for the widely used Mantoux's test to determine whether an individual has ever acquired a tuberculous infection. A positive tuberculin test comprises an area of induration and redness 48 to 72 hours following the intracutaneous inoculation of a measured amount of tuberculoprotein, either O.T. (old tuberculin) or P.P.D. (purified protein derivative). In general, the larger the area of induration, the more recent the infection and the greater the likelihood of active tuberculosis. Tuberculosensitivity, which first appears several weeks after the organism becomes implanted in the host, usually persists for the life of the patient. Whether such a positive tuberculin reaction implies the persistence of live bacilli possibly sequestered in some tiny focus, or merely indicates past experience with the organisms (possibly completely destroyed) remains a controversial issue. Preponderant opinion now favors the view that once the patient is infected, viable bacilli probably persist. However, it should be emphasized that tuberculous infection and tuberculopositivity do not imply active disease. *The tuberculin test does not distinguish between infection and active disease.* In most asymptomatic cases, the bacilli are deeply sealed off in some fibrotic or calcified focus and are not communicable, but these lesions may provide the source for endogenous activation of the disease. *A negative tuberculin test does not always imply the absence of infection.* Anergy is seen with overwhelming illnesses, *including rampant tuberculosis*, acute illnesses such as measles, extreme old age or debility, corticosteroid and other immunosuppressive therapy, sarcoidosis, Hodgkin's disease and lymphomas.

Concomitant with the development of delayed hypersensitivity, the host acquires a heightened resistance or partial immunity to the disease. This resistance appears to reside in the acquired capacity of histiocytes to destroy phagocytized bacilli. The resistance or partial immunity is obviously not complete since active disease may flare up years after acquiring an initial infection.

In the belief that previous exposure and the acquisition of some resistance protects against tuberculous disease, one school of thought favors inoculation of tuberculonegative individuals with a vaccine of living but avirulent tubercle bacilli, known as BCG (bacille Calmette Guérin). The vaccine converts the patient to a positive skin reactor. Although BCG is widely used in Europe, prophylactic inoculation has not been popular in the United States.

The Infections. *Two forms of tuberculosis are recognized, primary tuberculosis representing the initial infection by the bacillus and secondary or reactivation tuberculosis resulting either from reinfection from an exogenous source or more likely from reactivation of a primary infection.* Obviously, the patient with secondary tuberculosis has already acquired tuberculosensitivity as well as some resistance. The tuberculosensitivity leads to more florid caseation necrosis in tissues; the resistance favors localization of the process. Which of these two influences predominates in the individual is variable, unpredictable and impossible to estimate.

What are the factors that determine the likelihood of active disease and the influences which condition its severity? The two extremes of life, childhood and senility, are periods of increased vulnerability. There is both clinical and experimental evidence of some genetic predisposition to this disease. Blacks appear to be more susceptible than whites. To some degree, this is related to socioeconomic conditions but, apart from this, there still remains a racial predisposition (Lurie, 1950). Tuberculosis in identical twins tends to follow exactly parallel courses and distributions whereas, in fraternal twins, there is a lower incidence of parallel disease. Animal experiments confirm that there may be a genetic susceptibility. Malnutrition, fatigue, debilitation and intercurrent diseases, particularly diabetes mellitus, silicosis and Hodgkin's disease, all materially influence the likelihood of developing active disease. Particularly important are steroid and immunosuppressive therapy which permit quiescent infections to flare into rampant disease. In such individuals, focal pulmonary lesions may disseminate throughout the body to produce miliary tuberculosis (p. 416). The magnitude of the infecting dose, virulence of organisms and extent of the primary lesion with its contained organisms may all contribute to the likelihood of developing active disease, but how large a role these factors play is poorly understood.

Primary Tuberculosis. *Primary tuberculosis is the phase of the tuberculous infection that directly follows the first seeding of the tissues of the body by the tubercle bacilli.* During the first 10 to 14 days of this process, the patient is tuberculin-negative but, following this period, sensitization develops and modifies the nature of the primary tuberculosis. The development of this sensitization does *not* mark the end of the primary tuberculosis. This type of infection generally is found in infancy or childhood, but it may also occur in adults when they have not been exposed to tubercle bacilli during their early life.

In primary infections, the source of the organism must always be exogenous, i.e., outside the body, and the usual portal of entry is the respiratory system. Rarely in the United States, and more often in other countries, the primary infection begins in the oropharynx or intestinal tract from the ingestion of milk contaminated with the bovine strain of *M. tuberculosis.*

Inhaled tubercle bacilli become implanted upon the alveolar surfaces of the lung parenchyma in a fairly standard pattern. The primary focus of parenchymal infection is usually found immediately *subjacent to the pleura in the lower part of the upper lobes or upper part of the lower lobes of one lung.* Bilateral lesions are very infrequent. This primary lesion is called the *Ghon focus* or lesion. Less commonly it is situated in other regions of the lung. Generally it is a 1 to 1.5 cm. area of gray-white inflammatory consolidation, which is sharply circumscribed from the surrounding lung parenchyma. As sensitivity develops in the course of the second week, the consolidated focus becomes caseous and develops a soft, cheesy, necrotic center. Usually the initial infection is handled well by the patient and progressive fibrosis walls off the focus. In the course of time, this lesion is totally replaced by fibrous tissue and may also become calcified and even ossified. Inevitably, however, with the first infection there is immediate lymphatic drainage of the tubercle bacilli, either as free agents or within phagocytes, along the regional peribronchial lymphatic channels. In this way, tubercles are usually found in the peribronchial lymph nodes and particularly in the tracheobronchial nodes draining the affected region. The combination of the primary lesion and lymph node involvement is classically recognized as the *Ghon complex.* In the majority of patients, the primary tuberculosis undergoes progressive fibrosis with arrest of the progression of the disease.

In the course of healing, these subpleural Ghon lesions frequently cause subpleural fibrous scars with puckering of the pleural surface. Occasionally the pleural reaction may become calcified. At the same time, fibrocalcific scarring replaces most of the tuberculous foci in the regional tracheobronchial nodes. The nodal involvement is often unilateral with fairly sharp limitation of lymphatic drainage to the affected side only.

However, in many of these cases, the infection is not totally eradicated and viable bacilli persist for months and years. In a few patients, probably less than 10 per cent, the initial complex progresses and spreads by contiguity or by erosion into bronchi and thus disseminates through these natural channels. Multiple patchy areas of tuberculosis, or large consolidations known as *tuberculous pneumonia, may develop* (Fig. 10–18). These areas that erode into bronchi may cavitate. In still fewer instances, the initial lymphatic invasion reaches the venous blood and is thus disseminated to other sites in the body, or a tuberculous focus may erode into a blood vessel to produce hematogenous dissemination. In this fashion,

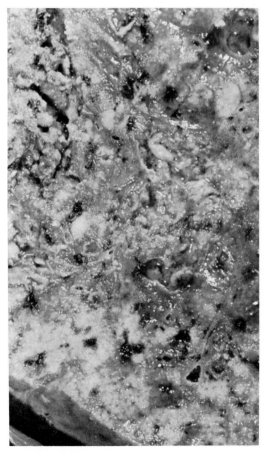

Figure 10–18. *Caseous pneumonic spread of a primary tuberculosis with small foci of cavitation in a 4-year-old child.*

other regions of the lung, or distant organs, may develop *miliary tuberculosis* and also *isolated organ tuberculosis*, to be described. These progressive primary infections are in general the exceptional cases.

The histology of the early stages of primary tuberculosis has been described in the pathogenesis of tuberculous infections and includes the development of classic caseous tubercles followed by fibrosis, calcification and ossification of the healed foci. It should be emphasized at this time that the entrance of tubercle bacilli into the blood is not necessarily followed by the development of tuberculous lesions in the sites of localization. It is, in fact, believed that in most instances of primary infection, organisms frequently drain via the lymphatics into the venous system and are widely disseminated but rarely give rise to anatomic lesions. Presumably, these organisms are promptly destroyed at their sites of localization. In the experimental animal, tubercle bacilli may be obtained from the blood within 24 hours after subcutaneous inoculation of virulent organisms, and it might be assumed that a similar process also occurs in man. However, in the susceptible individual, such organisms are capable of producing disseminated lesions, and it is therefore not uncommon to find, even in infants, isolated, focal, fibrous scars in the liver, spleen or in scattered nodes that are consistent with healed tuberculous foci.

When the primary tuberculous infection occurs at the less common portals of entry cited, the gross and microscopic sequence of events parallels those already described.

Reinfection, "Adult" or Secondary Tuberculosis. Reinfection tuberculosis is *that phase of the tuberculous infection that follows reactivation of a primary tuberculosis or reinfection of a previously exposed individual.* Accordingly, the tubercle bacilli may be derived either from *endogenous* or *exogenous* sources. Reinfection tuberculosis is most common now in middle to later life. It is well known that viable organisms may persist in caseous, partially fibrotic, and even calcified primary lesions for many years, and perhaps even for life. Recall may be made, in fact, of the statement that the persistence of a tuberculin-positive reaction is believed by some to be an indication of the sequestration in the body of living bacilli. Endogenous reinfection is believed to be responsible for most cases of adult-type tuberculosis (Trauger, 1963).

Reinfection pulmonary tuberculosis is almost invariably localized to one or both apices of the lungs. Far less commonly, particularly in debilitated and diabetic susceptibles, the adult type of tuberculosis begins in other areas, such as about the hilar regions. The cause of this usual apical localization is completely obscure. Innumerable explanatory theories have been proposed, based upon circulatory, ventilatory, mechanical and drainage mechanisms but, to date, the basis for the apical localization continues to elude discovery. It is, however, of interest that when rabbits are experimentally exposed to contaminated air, they fail to develop apical localization when they live in their normal four-footed posture. However, when these animals are forced to maintain an erect position upon their hind legs and are similarly exposed, apical localization parallels the clinical disease. In man, the minimal pulmonary lesion in the apex consists of a 1 to 3 cm. focal area of caseous consolidation, usually within 1 to 2 cm. of the pleural surface. Because of the altered character of the inflammatory response in the sensitized individual, drainage to the regional nodes is distinctly less common than in the primary complex.

Histologically, the reaction consists classically of tubercle formation with emphasis on the formation of epithelioid cells, Langhans' giant cells, caseation, fibrosis and lymphocytic infiltration. Further details on pulmonary tuberculosis may be found on p. 818. The *potential course* of this apical infection is extremely varied. (1) The pathologic process may undergo healing, scarring and calcification to yield apical, fibrocalcific, healed or perhaps more appropriately termed "*arrested*" *tuberculosis*. (2) The initial parenchymal infection may spread to the other areas of the lung through one of many pathways to create many forms of pulmonary tuberculosis (progressive pulmonary tuberculosis), to be described under the lungs (p. 821). (3) It may extend to the pleura to produce pleural fibrosis, focal pleural adhesions, inflammatory *pleural effusions* or, by direct extension of the bacilli into the pleural cavity, lead to a *tuberculous empyema*. (4) When the pulmonary lesions erode into bronchi, the material may be coughed up and seed the mucosal lining of the bronchioles, bronchi and trachea (*endotracheobronchial tuberculosis*), or organisms may become implanted in the larynx to produce laryngeal tuberculosis. (5) Swallowed bacilli can become trapped by the lymphoid patches of the small and large bowel to cause *intestinal tuberculosis* (Fig. 10–19) (p. 939).

(6) *Miliary tuberculosis* may result when the organisms gain access to the lymphatics and blood to seed distant organs. The term miliary is descriptive of the character of the minute lesions. These small, yellow-white, barely visible foci resemble canary bird seeds, or millet seeds, in the sites of localization. The *spleen and liver* are most commonly affected in such miliary dissemination. Occasionally, when the or-

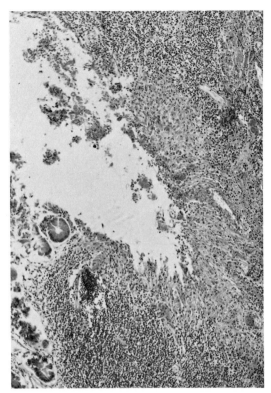

Figure 10–19. *A low power view of a tuberculous ulcer in the ileum rimmed by granulomatous reaction.*

ganisms erode into a *pulmonary artery,* the miliary dissemination may be limited to the lungs as the organisms are trapped in the alveolar capillary circulation. When the seeding of the pulmonary arteries is heavy and organisms get through the alveolar capillaries, or when a caseous focus erodes into a *pulmonary vein,* systemic dissemination follows and miliary lesions may develop in virtually any organ of the body. It is, however, well known that certain tissues are remarkably resistant to tuberculous infection, and therefore it is rare to find tubercles in the heart, striated muscle, thyroid and pancreas. Favored sites of miliary localization are the lymph nodes, liver, spleen, kidneys, adrenals, prostate, seminal vesicles, fallopian tubes, endometrium and the meninges. It is worthwhile to point out at this time that miliary dissemination often involves the bone marrow, liver and retina. These sites offer valuable clinical opportunities to diagnose miliary tuberculosis. The tubercles can be visualized in many instances in the eye grounds by simple funduscopic examination, and bone marrow and liver aspiration biopsy provide the opportunity of identifying, by both cultural and histologic techniques, the miliary dissemination.

(7) *Isolated-organ tuberculosis* may occur.

This term implies the development of a progressive tuberculous infection in any of the organs or tissues commonly affected by miliary dissemination. The explanation of isolated-organ tuberculosis rests on the assumption that in the course of the lymphatic or hematogenous dissemination of bacilli, organisms are rapidly destroyed in all other sites save for the particular tissue involved in the isolated tuberculous process. The *most common sites* of such isolated-organ tuberculosis are the meninges (tuberculous meningitis), kidneys (renal tuberculosis), adrenals, bones (tuberculous osteomyelitis) and the fallopian tubes and epididymides (genital tuberculosis). From such organ tuberculosis, subsequent dissemination or seeding may occur, and thus, in renal tuberculosis, it is common for infective material to drain through the urine and cause tuberculous cystitis. In the same way, tuberculous salpingitis is frequently followed by tuberculous endometritis and tuberculous pelvic peritonitis. Tuberculous epididymitis may be followed by extension of the tuberculous infection into the testes, and spread from the prostate and seminal vesicles may affect other organs in the genitourinary tract.

Before concluding the discussion of the pathology of tuberculosis, attention should be drawn to the *need for positive identification of acid-fast tubercle bacilli in these anatomic lesions.* While the characteristic tubercle with caseation necrosis is virtually pathognomonic of tuberculosis, granulomatous reactions are not confined to tuberculosis, and caseation necrosis may be mimicked in other infections. The most difficult granulomas to distinguish from the tubercle are those of Boeck's sarcoid, syphilis and the nonspecific granulomatous responses to foreign bodies, lipids and certain of the fungi. If caseation does not develop in the tuberculous lesion, the hard tubercle may be completely indistinguishable from other granulomatous lesions. Because of the gravity of a diagnosis of tuberculosis, this final diagnosis should never be made unless tubercle bacilli have been unmistakably identified in histologic sections or have been cultured either from infected sputum, gastric washings or tuberculous lesions.

The clinical signs and symptoms manifested by patients with pulmonary tuberculosis are as *varied* as the nature, site, distribution and extent of tuberculous anatomic lesions. It is apparent that a minute focus of tuberculosis may be totally occult, while extensive tuberculosis is almost invariably accompanied by systemic reactions to the inflammatory destructive process. In general, primary tuberculosis is usually an entirely silent process. Occasionally the child may have a low-grade fever and lack of appetite, accompanied by failure to gain weight and grow at the normal rate. Occasionally extension to the pleura may produce pleuritic pain, especially on deep breathing or coughing. When the primary lesion is in the lung, spread to a bronchus may be heralded by the onset of a persistent dry cough, which eventually becomes productive of a scanty, mucopurulent sputum. In most instances, however, the primary tuberculous infection goes unnoted, and its existence, past or present, is detected only by tuberculin testing of the individual or by routine roentgenography with visualization of a focus of scarring or calcification in the lung parenchyma or tracheobronchial nodes.

Reinfection tuberculosis may also be asymptomatic when the condition is confined to minimal lesions within the lung apices. However, when the disease progresses beyond this early localization, the more extensive tissue destruction and inflammatory reaction give rise to many systemic changes. Characteristically, these patients have the *insidious* onset of temperature elevations, usually most marked in the mid-afternoon, night sweats, weakness, fatigability, and loss of appetite and weight, manifestations that are presumed to reflect a systemic toxemia. The exact basis for such toxemic symptoms is still not clear. These constitutional reactions are attributed to the absorption of nitrogenous breakdown products from areas of caseation necrosis. Superimposed upon these nonspecific signs and symptoms are the many manifestations occasioned by the destructive tuberculous lesions in the particular site of reinfection. When, as is usual, the lungs are the site of attack, cough, production of a mucopurulent sputum, hemoptysis and, in farther advanced lesions, dyspnea and orthopnea may be present. When the process affects other organs, the clinical manifestations are accordingly altered, and therefore reinfection tuberculosis may present as a form of meningitis or as a form of renal disease. When the disease is miliary in its dissemination and does not produce focalizing signs or clear-cut macroscopic lesions, the symptom complex may be that of a fever of unknown origin.

The diagnosis of all forms of tuberculosis depends on historic data (a possible source of infection), appropriate clinical evidence, x-rays, and eventually identification and/or isolation of the causative organism. X-ray examination may disclose the consolidation, cavitation, scarring calcification or destructive nature of the lesion. Tuberculin testing of the individual can establish the existence of tuberculosensitization. Most children are tuberculonegative. A positive tuberculin test in a child is therefore highly suggestive. In the adult the skin reaction is of little diagnostic value for reasons given earlier. A negative reaction is evidence against the existence of a tuberculous disease, but the problem of anergy cannot be overlooked. Ultimately, in all cases it is required that tubercle bacilli be identified on direct smear, by cultivation on artificial media, or by inoculation of the infective material into guinea pigs. It should once again be cautioned that all acid-fast organisms are not necessarily *Mycobacterium tuberculosis*, and that nonpathogenic strains are sometimes found in the oral and vaginal cavities, as well as in the intestinal contents. The failure to demonstrate tubercle bacilli in sputum, gastric washings or other secreta does not rule out the diagnosis of tuberculosis since, in many instances, the lesions may not be in contact with natural channels of drainage, and the case may fall into the so-called "closed" type of infection.

It is impossible, in such a consideration, to outline a satisfactory differential diagnosis of tuberculous infections. It will be apparent later that tuberculosis must be considered in the differential diagnosis of any type of meningitis, must always be considered in any form of pulmonary disease, is a plausible cause for renal disease and at times may simulate a bone tumor. Inasmuch as tuberculosis is one of the leading causes of death, its presence must be suspected in any FUO (fever of unknown origin). In general, the prognosis for tuberculosis is now quite favorable. Primary tuberculous disease is usually benign. Secondary or adult type tuberculosis is far more ominous but, in all but advanced cases, it is readily managed with appropriate chemotherapy in those free of predisposing influences such as intercurrent disease or immunosuppressive therapy. Indeed, most patients with localized apical lesions are managed on an ambulatory basis usually after an initial short period of hospitalization. In the more advanced cases requiring long-term hospitalization, death results in 16 to 20 per cent. Secondary systemic amyloidosis may supervene in those with longstanding disease.

LEPROSY

Leprosy is a low-grade, indolent infection which is unusual in many regards. Although it is attributed to *Mycobacterium leprae*, Koch's postulates have never been fulfilled since the disease has not been transmitted to man or animals experimentally. The manner of spread, the genesis of the lesions, and the precise pathways of dissemination of the organisms in the host have never been clearly established. Clinically, *the disease is characterized by an extremely prolonged incubation period, a long course lasting over many years, and eventual involvement of the skin, mucous membranes or peripheral nerves. The anatomic lesions, while not pathognomonic, are distinctive in the production of either lepromatous nodules that contain large, lipid-laden, phagocytic macrophages and giant cells, often filled with bacilli (lepra cells) or microscopic granulomas that resemble hard tubercles.* Mycobacterium leprae is a pleomorphic, acid-fast bacillus that is found in tissues in matchstick bundles, packets or globular masses (globi). In lesions, the organisms are present both intra- and extracellularly. They decolorize in the acid-fast stain much more readily than does *M. tuberculosis* and, moreover, stain more readily with the usual aniline dye techniques.

It is believed that the organism is of low invasiveness and low virulence, and that many years of fairly intimate exposure are required for its transmission from man to man. In the usual clinical disease, a history can be obtained of contact with a lepromatous individual from childhood. Leprosy is not transmitted in utero and children removed from their infected parents do not contract the condition. The disease is twice as common in males. The incubation period may be as long as five to 10 years. The bacilli produce lesions on the skin and mucous membranes, and therefore exudate from these lesions harbors the bacilli. Similarly, secretions from the oral cavity and nose in cases with lesions in the oropharynx are infective. Presumably, the organisms enter through abrasions in the skin or mucous membranes, and it is probable that spread from the initial site via the lymphatics and the blood vessels evokes the systemic manifestations so often encountered. The basis for the principal localization in the skin and nerves is still not understood, but it must be recognized that other organs, such as the liver, spleen and viscera, are sometimes involved.

Two variants of the disease are recognized: *lepromatous and tuberculoid.* These variants probably reflect differences in susceptibility of the host (Fete, 1943). *Tuberculoid leprosy occurs in more resistant hosts and is principally characterized by symmetrical maculopapular lesions of the skin and peripheral nerves.* This variant is frequently designated by such descriptive terms as *neural, anesthetic* or, more properly, *maculoanesthetic leprosy.* The individual skin macule is a nonelevated, red-brown focus surrounded by an indurated, elevated, more deeply hyperemic border. These lesions vary from 1 cm. up to large coalescent areas that may involve large parts of the face, trunk and limbs. Histologically, the nonelevated central areas contain a nonspecific mononuclear inflammatory infiltrate chiefly about blood vessels and the skin adnexa. *The papular indurated borders harbor characteristic hard tubercles composed of epithelioid cells surrounded by a collar of lymphocytes and plasma cells, often accompanied by scattered giant cells. Central caseation is usually not present.* Leprosy bacilli are extremely scant if they are present at all in these lesions. The peripheral nerve filaments in the area are involved in a similar process. The neural involvement extends centripetally to affect progressively larger nerve tracts. Tuberculoid granulomas form in and about the nerves and, in the long chronicity of the disease, become fibrotic and indurated. As a consequence, the nerves are sometimes palpable as thick, ropy cords. At times, these focal lesions in the nerves may undergo central necrosis to produce lesions virtually indistinguishable from tuberculosis. The lymph nodes draining these skin lesions are sometimes involved by similar granulomas.

Lepromatous leprosy apparently develops in more susceptible individuals. The disease begins with a macular skin rash which is symmetrical and resembles that present in the tuberculoid type. However, the rash rapidly changes into nodular lesions in the dermis (lepromas) that vary from less than 1 cm. in diameter to large masses that may cause considerable disfigurement. These lepromas may occur anywhere on the body, but have a particular predilection for the face and extensor surfaces of the extremities. Lepromas on the forehead, malar prominences, nose and lips produce the characteristic wrinkled, leonine expression. These nodules are yellow-gray-white and situated in the dermis directly underneath the epidermis. The overlying skin often sloughs to cause chronic draining, disfiguring ulcerations. *They are composed of large aggregations of macrophages and giant cells that contain lipid and, in addition, numerous bacteria* (lepra cells). These bacteria are disposed in the bundles and globi described. Sometimes these globi reach a diameter of 50 microns or more and also are found within tissue spaces, lymphatics or even huge giant cells (Figs. 10–20 and 10–21). Interspersed between the lepra cells are scattered mononuclear leukocytes, principally lymphocytes and plasma cells.

The lymph nodes are almost invariably af-

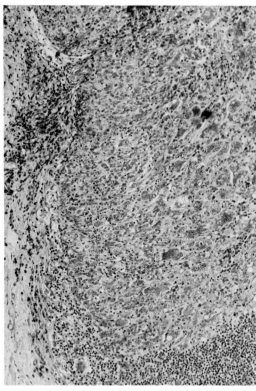

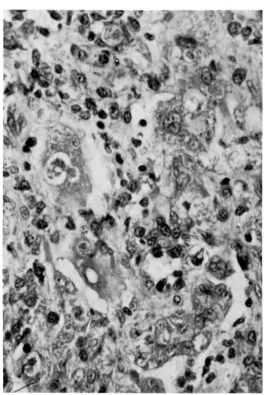

Fig. 10–20   **Fig. 10–21**

Figure 10–20. Leprosy—a portion of a lepromatous mass composed of typical lepra cells.
Figure 10–21. Leprosy—high power detail of lepra giant cells, one with a phagocytized mass of organisms.

fected in lepromatous leprosy, and contain foci of lepra cells similar to those just described. Lepra cells appear among the nerve bundles in the regions affected and progressive inflammatory permeation of these fibers develops and leads eventually to diffuse scarring in and about the nerves, producing the same end result as in the tuberculoid variant. Lepromas may also occur in the nasal and oropharyngeal mucous membrane and, in some cases, extend into the epiglottis, larynx and upper respiratory air passages. Lepromatous infiltrations have also been identified in the liver, spleen, bone marrow, lungs and gonads. The orbit may be invaded by lesions arising in the adjacent skin.

In both forms of leprosy, involvement of the peripheral nerves gives rise to a variety of secondary changes. Incident to the loss of the sensory innervation, anesthesia occurs and is frequently followed by ulcerations and skin infections that reflect both trophic atrophy and excessive trauma to the insensitive parts. The denervated skeletal musculature undergoes atrophy and the bones may show considerable mobilization of calcium.

The additional clinical manifestations of leprosy depend upon the clinical variant and

the localization of lesions. With the tuberculoid type, the disease is of insidious onset with a diffuse maculopapular rash that is sometimes accompanied by fever and can be mistaken for one of the contagious exanthemas of childhood. Usually, however, the persistence of the rash, followed by the development of neurologic manifestations, such as tingling, hyperesthesia and eventual numbness, distinguishes this disease from less serious skin conditions. Over the course of weeks, the anesthesia progresses and is followed by trophic changes in the skin, muscles and nails. Contractures in the hand muscles may result in the so-called claw hand or "main en griffe." Facial paralyses, atrophy of extremities, resorption of bone, and even autoamputations of totally denervated fingers and toes may develop.

The lepromatous variety has a similar onset, accompanied sometimes by fever. However, it is distinguished from the previous variant by the progression of the maculopapular lesions to subcutaneous nodules and masses. The leonine facies and similar nodules over the body make this condition quite distinctive. Involvement of the nasal mucosa and oropharynx may give rise to a hemorrhagic serous discharge and, when the larynx is involved, hoarseness and cough become evident. Neurologic involvement in the lepromatous variant may give rise to the sequence of changes just described in the maculoanesthetic form of leprosy.

The diagnosis of leprosy is usually readily made from the clinical findings. When in doubt, tissue biopsy or scrapings of lesions should disclose either the fairly characteristic histologic tuberculoid nodule or acid-fast bacilli. It is to be remembered that, in the tuberculoid variant of the disease, few organisms are present. A lepromin skin test, using an extract of the lepra bacilli, produces an inflammatory reaction in normal individuals and those with tuberculoid leprosy, but is negative in lepromatous cases.

Both forms of the disease are characterized by great chronicity with long periods of remission, by apparently spontaneous, sometimes permanent arrests, and by repeated reexacerbations in most instances. The mortality rate is not high. The tuberculoid form has the better prognosis, and in most cases does not materially shorten the longevity. Lepromatous leprosy may lead to death from intercurrent diseases, such as tuberculosis, pneumonia or other infections due to the debilitating effects of the chronic underlying disease.

BACTEROIDES AND RELATED ORGANISMS

The Bacteroides are a group of gram-negative, nonsporing, anaerobic coccobacilli. These organisms in man are normal inhabitants of the mouth, intestinal tract and vagina. However, they may invade tissues to evoke completely nondistinctive, suppurative infections. The most common sites of localization include the lung, middle ear and abdominal cavity. However, in occasional cases the Bacteroides may also be responsible for tonsillitis, suppurative arthritis and endometritis. They are rarely present in these infections in pure culture and are often accompanied by other pyogenic bacteria, such as the coliforms and the pyogenic cocci. Although the organisms are of apparent low antigenicity and are responsible for persistent, chronic, suppurative infections, they may at times invade the blood to produce metastatic abscesses in the lungs, liver and other sites. Bacteroides infections are frequently unrecognized clinically because of the great difficulty in the isolation of these obligate anaerobes. Consequently, they often pass unrecognized and so sometimes account for the failure of focal infections to respond adequately to the usual antibiotics. Even when they cannot be isolated in culture, the diagnosis can often be made clinically by the demonstration of rising levels of agglutinins in the patient's serum.

MYCOPLASMA—PLEUROPNEUMONIA-LIKE ORGANISMS (PPLOs)

Only relatively recently have the mycoplasma been conclusively proved to cause disease in man. These comprise a group of extremely small coccobacillary organisms ranging in size from 125 to 150 millimicrons. They are the smallest free-living organisms known, having a size almost identical with that of the myxoviruses. They do not have a rigid cell wall as do other bacteria and therefore tend to be pleomorphic. They are bounded instead by a so-called triple layered unit membrane. Of clinical significance is the fact that they are completely resistant to penicillin but appear to be readily inhibited by the tetracyclines.

From the clinical standpoint, these organisms are extremely interesting because it is now apparent that they are capable of causing suppurative infections in a number of sites but are extremely difficult to isolate and to identify in these sites. Hence they are possible causes of infections of apparently obscure origin. *Pneumonia* is one of the more important types of clinical disease these organisms may cause. The specific member of the group most often involved is the *M. pneumoniae,* and this organism is in fact the only one of the mycoplasma definitely established to be pathogenic for man in any of the sites of infection. The pneumonia does not resemble the usual bacterial pneumonia and is similar or even identical to the viral pulmonary infections known as *primary atypical pneumonia* (p. 815). *Genito-urinary tract disease* of a nonspecific suppurative nature may be produced by the mycoplasma. This may take the form of urethritis, Bartholin's abscess, salpingitis, cervicitis or vaginitis. In some instances, the infection is closely similar to that of gonorrhea, and therefore careful studies must be made to establish the correct etiology. *Rheumatoid arthritis* was at one time reported to be due possibly to the PPLOs. Much excitement attended these early reports in which the mycoplasma were identified in the synovial fluid of patients with rheumatoid arthritis. However, isolation of these organisms indicated that they were a type consistent with *M. hominis,* an organism not thought to be pathogenic for man and a common tissue culture contaminant. At present, therefore, the role of the PPLOs in rheumatoid arthritis must be considered as unestablished (Chanock, 1965).

Best for the identification of the myco-plasma are serologic studies, immunofluores-cent techniques and complement fixing anti-body tests.

RAT-BITE FEVER AND HAVERHILL FEVER

There is one form of clinical disease caused by organisms closely related to the Bacteroides that merits a few words. *Streptobacillus moniliformis* is also known as the *Haverhillia multiformis*. These very pleomorphic organisms may be transmitted to man either by the bite of an infected rat or by the ingestion of contaminated milk. When spread by the rat vector, the disease is known as *rat-bite fever*. When spread by infected milk, it is known as *Haverhill fever*. (This form of infection was first recognized in Haverhill, Massachusetts.) The rat-bite pattern is usually evidenced by a slight inflammatory reaction at the site of the puncture wounds, followed by regional adenopathy, followed in turn by a systemic, febrile illness characterized by malaise, headache, arthritis and a cutaneous, maculopapular, erythematous rash. The disease usually lasts from several days to several weeks, and is followed by spontaneous recovery. The pattern spread by contaminated milk resembles that just described save for the absence of the bite. There is also a greater tendency to generalized adenopathy rather than regional adenopathy in relation to the bite. The diagnosis can usually be made by specific agglutinins and also by identification of the organism in exudate derived from mice injected with the patient's blood. There are few recorded histologic observations in these entities, but mild inflammatory changes in the myocardium, liver and kidneys have been described, as well as microinfarcts of the spleen.

LISTERIOSIS

Within the relatively recent past, human infections have been described due to *Listeria monocytogenes*. These organisms are known to have a reservoir in both domestic and wild animals. The organism itself is a gram-positive, small rod that has been cultivated from throat washings, the urethra, and from the placenta and vagina of both humans and animals. The method of transmission is still not understood, although it is believed that animals may contract the disease by drinking infected water. There is some possibility that it may be transmitted by contaminated milk. In man, the infections have usually taken the form of non-specific encephalitis or meningoencephalitis.

In addition, in the few autopsy cases, focal necroses of the liver, pneumonia and acute splenitis have been identified (Wright and MacGregor, 1939).

RICKETTSIAL DISORDERS

Rickettsial infections are caused by microorganisms intermediate between the bacteria and the viruses. We should pause for a moment to pay homage to one of the early pioneers, Dr. H. T. Ricketts, who contracted an infection and died while studying Rocky Mountain spotted fever and typhus fever, accounting for the generic designation of these agents. All are obligate intracellular parasites capable of multiplication only within certain cells of susceptible hosts. All are transmitted to man by insect vectors, with the possible exception of the respiratory disease, Q fever, which is spread directly from man to man in the same fashion as the common cold. Virtually all cause acute febrile self-limited illnesses and, again, with the exception of Q fever, all are characterized either by a skin rash (spotted fever group) or central nervous system involvement (typhus group). All evoke strong immunologic reactions conferring long-lasting immunity against reinfections. These antibodies also provide highly specific complement fixation or rickettsial agglutination tests. By chance, most rickettsial infections evoke antibodies cross reactive with certain strains of the bacillus, *Proteus vulgaris*. Such cross reactivity comprises the basis of the Weil-Felix test. While this test denotes some form of rickettsial infection, it does not differentiate among the specific causative agents.

Rickettsial infections are relatively uncommon. They usually occur sporadically but one, typhus fever, tends to occur in epidemics. Indeed, typhus fever has probably influenced world history more than any man. In all probability, Napoleon's army was more devastated by this disease than by the British. Travel by air and the wanderlust of contemporary man have brought rickettsial infections from endemic areas to all parts of the world. Despite its name, there are more cases of Rocky Mountain spotted fever on the eastern seaboard of the United States than in the Rocky Mountains purely on the basis of population distribution. An overview of the rickettsial diseases of man is provided in Table 10–3.

The pathology produced by the rickettsiae is characteristic. All cause systemic febrile reactions

TABLE 10-3. RICKETTSIAL DISEASES OF MAN

Group	Principal Diseases	Synonyms	Etiologic Agent	Reservoir	Usual Mode of Transmission to Man	Known Occurrence
Typhus	Epidemic typhus	Classic, historic, European, louse-borne typhus	*Rickettsia prowazeki*	Man	Human body louse	Winter and spring in cold climates over most of world
	Brill-Zinsser	Brill's disease, recrudescent typhus	*Rickettsia prowazeki*	Man	See text for explanation	Can be world-wide
	Murine typhus	Endemic typhus, flea-borne typhus	*Rickettsia mooseri*	Rats	Rat flea	World-wide
Spotted Fever	Rocky Mountain spotted fever	Spotted fever, tick fever, tick typhus, etc.	*Rickettsia rickettsi*	Rabbits and other mammals (possibly dogs) and ticks	Ticks	North and South America
	North-Asian tick-borne rickettsiosis	Siberian tick typhus	*Rickettsia siberica*	Wild rodents and ticks	Ticks	Asiatic USSR and Mongolia
	African tick typhus	Boutonneuse fever; S. African, Kenya and Indian tick typhus	*Rickettsia conori*	Dogs, wild rodents and ticks	Ticks	Africa, India and the basins of the Black Sea, Caspian Sea and Mediterranean
	Queensland tick typhus		*Rickettsia australis*	Marsupials, wild rodents, (? ticks)	Ticks	Queensland, Australia
	Rickettsialpox	Kew Gardens fever	*Rickettsia akari*	Mice	Mites	USA, USSR and Korea
Tsutsu-gamushi Disease	Scrub typhus	Mite-borne typhus, Japanese river fever, tropical typhus, Sumatran mite fever; etc.	*Rickettsia tsutsugamushi (orientalis)*	Rats, other rodents and mites	Mites	South Asia and Western Pacific
Q Fever	Q fever	Nine mile fever, Balkan grippe	*Coxiella burnetii*	Cattle, sheep, goats, marsupials, other mammals and ticks	Principally air-borne; occasionally ticks; possibly milk	World-wide
Trench Fever	Trench fever	Wolhynian or 5-day fever	*Rickettsia quintana*	Man	Human body louse	Europe, USSR and Mexico

From Snyder, J. C.: Introduction to rickettsial diseases. In Beeson, P. B., and McDermott, W. (eds.): Cecil-Loeb Textbook of Medicine. 12th ed. Philadelphia. W. B. Saunders Co., 1967, p. 126.

which are self-limited and are almost always accompanied by a prominent skin rash. With the exception of Brill-Zinsser disease and sometimes Q fever, the diseases are contracted by the bite of an insect which inoculates the microorganism into the new host. In some, as will be indicated , a local skin lesion referred to as an eschar develops at the site of the insect bite. In others, there is only a transient local lesion, but in all instances the rickettsial organisms disseminate from this portal of entry through the blood to invade the endothelial cells of the finer vessels, principally the capillary beds throughout the body. Sometimes parasitization of the underlying smooth muscle cells in these vessels also occurs. The microorganisms can be visualized in infected cells by Giemsa or Macchiavello stains. Once within the endothelial cells, a characteristic acute vasculitis is produced, manifested by swelling and proliferation of these cells, often followed by thrombosis of the vascular lumen. Almost invariably, a perivascular leukocytic inflammatory infiltration ensues. While these lesions may occur in virtually any organ or tissue of the body, the brain, heart, testes, skin, serosal membranes, skeletal muscles, lungs and kidneys are favored locations. The vascular lesions may lead to focal necroses and proliferative responses in the surrounding tissue and organs, creating, for example, the "typhus nodule." Thus, all the rickettsial infections are characterized by basically similar microscopic changes in the same organs and tissues. Moreover, all are characterized by a paucity of gross anatomic changes save for the foci of necroses and hemorrhages attendant on the vascular changes described. In the following presentation, attention will be focused on the prototype diseases in each of the first four groups presented in Table 10–3.

EPIDEMIC TYPHUS FEVER

Epidemic typhus fever is an acute rickettsial infection that occurs sporadically throughout the world and may, under appropriate conditions, become epidemic. Prevention of epidemics depends not only on prompt recognition of active infections but, more importantly, on control of the insect vector responsible for transmission of the organism. The causative agent, *Rickettsia prowazeki*, has a diameter of approximately 0.3 micron and a life cycle limited to man and his lice. The disease is transmitted by the human head louse (*Pediculus humanus capitis*) and the human body louse (*Pediculus humanus corporis*). These insects are themselves infected by biting a typhus patient, particularly during the early febrile period of the disease. The organisms multiply within the cells lining the gut of the louse and then escape into the intestinal lumen to pass out with the feces. When the louse feeds on the next human host, it makes a small puncture in the skin, which is irritated by the secretions of the insect. The human host scratches the irritated site, thereby introducing the infective feces into the skin puncture. A local area of hemorrhage may mark the site of the bite, but an ulcerated or crusted eschar is not common. It is important to note that it is possible to contract the disease without being infested by lice. The rickettsiae are deposited on the garments of patients, and transfer has occurred merely by contact of a skin abrasion or defect with contaminated clothing. Alternatively, inhalation of fomites blown into the air has caused respiratory infection. Apparently, the organisms are able to penetrate the intact respiratory epithelium, or perhaps phagocytic macrophages aid in this transfer.

After a 7- to 14-day incubation period, headache, weakness, chills and fever appear, followed in a few days by a generalized skin rash. Presumably, throughout the incubation period, the microorganisms are proliferating at the local site of the bite. During the period of chills and fever, blood-borne dissemination is taking place. The onset of the rash (which occurs in 90 per cent of patients) implies the invasion of the endothelial cells of the capillaries and small vessels. At first the rash is maculopapular and pink to bright red, the individual lesions varying in size up to 0.5 cm. in diameter. At this time, pressure will blanch these lesions, but during the second week of the rash, lesions become darker, more hemorrhagic and no longer will blanch on pressure. Characteristically, the rash begins on the trunk and extends centrifugally. In very severe cases, the individual macules and papules coalesce to produce irregular mottling and map-like hemorrhagic blotches. During the second week, there is usually central nervous system involvement in the form of apathy, progressing to dullness, stupor and even coma in severe cases. Frequently, this progression is punctuated by episodes of wild delirium. If the patient recovers, the rash begins to fade and the temperature begins to subside toward the end of the third week. Most fatalities occur during the second and third weeks of the illness. During some epidemics, the mortality from typhus has risen to as high as 50 per cent, but today, with effective antibiotics, the death rate is probably below 10 per cent.

In the milder cases, the macroscopic changes are limited to the skin rash and small internal ecchymoses or hemorrhages incident to the vascular lesions. In the more severe cases, there are often large areas of necrosis of the skin with gangrene of the tips of the fingers, nose, ear lobes, scrotum, penis and vulva. In such cases, irregular ecchymotic hemorrhages may be found internally, principally in the brain, heart muscle, testes, serosal membrane, lungs and kidneys.

The microscopic findings in all cases tend to be far more widespread than the gross alterations would suggest. Most prominent are the small vessel lesions that underlie the rash and the focal areas of hemorrhage and necrosis in the various organs and tissues affected. Endothelial proliferation and swelling in the capillaries, arterioles and venules may severely narrow the lumina of these vessels. Rickettsia can usually be demonstrated in these intimal cells, using the special staining techniques mentioned. The vascular lumina are often thrombosed but, generally, necrosis of the vessel wall is less prominent in typhus than in the spotted fevers. It is these vascular thromboses that lead to the gangrenous necroses of the skin and other structures. Surrounding these acutely involved vessels, a cuff of lymphocytes, plasma cells and histiocytes with an admixture of polymorphonuclear leukocytes is usually present (Fig. 10–22).

In the brain, the small vessel lesions tend

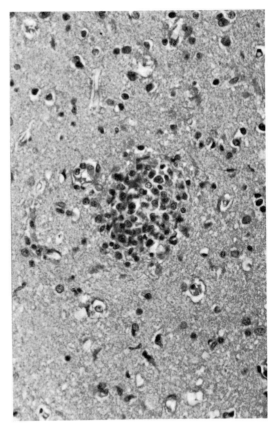

Figure 10–23. A typhus nodule in the brain.

to be limited to the gray matter and are often associated with focal glial proliferations mixed with mononuclear leukocytes to produce the characteristic "*typhus nodule*" (Fig. 10–23). There are sometimes a mononuclear cell meningitis, ring hemorrhages about the small vessels and, occasionally, degenerative changes in ganglion cells, presumably on an ischemic basis. Typhus nodules may occur in other tissues, approximate to the microvascular lesions already mentioned. In addition, an interstitial pneumonitis sometimes accompanied by exudative consolidation of alveoli may be present. Although this pneumonitis may be rickettsial in origin, it is more likely due to secondary bacterial invaders. A generalized, nonspecific lymphadenitis and splenitis are usually present (Wolbach, 1948).

Because all the rickettsial infections resemble one another, the diagnosis of typhus fever is extremely difficult to make on either clinical or anatomic grounds. Moreover, such bacterial diseases as typhoid fever, meningococcemia and measles, to mention but a few, produce quite similar febrile reactions with a rash. Specific serologic tests (complement fixa-

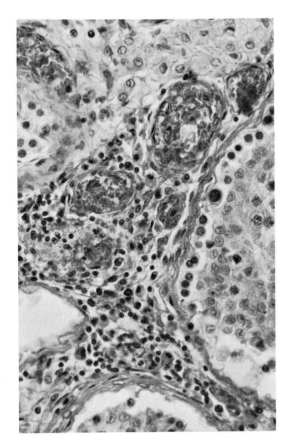

Figure 10–22. Testis in typhus fever with a focus of interstitial leukocytic infiltrate and acute vascular lesions.

tion and agglutination) are therefore very important in establishing the precise diagnosis.

OTHER DISORDERS IN THE TYPHUS GROUP

Brill-Zinsser disease is a recrudescent form of epidemic typhus, appearing as a relatively mild febrile illness years after the initial attack of typhus. The factors that precipitate such recrudescence are unknown. The causative agent is, of course, that of epidemic typhus. Because the disease is milder and does not often cause death, there is a paucity of data on the histopathologic changes. Such lesions as have been observed do not differ in any significant way from the milder lesions of the primary epidemic pattern, but only rarely are focal necroses and gangrene encountered in these cases.

Murine typhus is an endemic form of rickettsial infection, milder than epidemic typhus. It is transmitted to man by rat fleas, and has a natural animal reservoir in rats and mice. The causative agent, *R. mooseri*, closely resembles the rickettsia of epidemic typhus. Although the anatomic changes are probably similar to those of epidemic typhus, here again few recorded observations are available since most of the cases are not fatal. Specific serologic tests are required to differentiate this disease from epidemic typhus.

ROCKY MOUNTAIN SPOTTED FEVER

Rocky Mountain spotted fever is an acute febrile rickettsial infection transmitted to man by ticks and characterized by a prominent hemorrhagic rash. The causative agent, *R. rickettsi*, is somewhat larger than *R. prowazeki* and, in culture, is usually seen in pairs apparently surrounded by a clear zone forming a halo. A broad range of small mammals including squirrels, chipmunks, rats, mice and particularly cottontail rabbits serve as reservoirs for the infectious agent. Ticks provide the usual vector between this "wild world" and man. Although cases have been described in all parts of the world, the principal endemic areas are North and South America.

The disease is contracted by the bite of an infected tick. A primary lesion which becomes hemorrhagic, necrotic, and may lead to an eschar is sometimes observed at the site of the bite. This sequence, however, is infrequent in Rocky Mountain spotted fever, as compared with rickettsialpox, in which an eschar is quite characteristic. After multiplying at the local

site for some 7 to 14 days, the organisms are blood-borne throughout the vascular system, in the same fashion as with typhus fever, and invade the endothelial cells of the small blood vessels. A full-blown rash ensues. This is at first maculopapular, pink and predominantly peripheral in distribution, in contrast to the centrally distributed rash of typhus fever. The patients at this time are markedly febrile with chills, mental apathy and sometimes stupor. In the course of the next few days, the rash extends centripetally and becomes hemorrhagic. In the more severe cases, coalescence of lesions produces large, mottled ecchymoses or geographic map-like patterns. Because the vascular lesions which underlie the rash often lead to acute necrosis and thromboses of the small blood vessels, the rash may contain central foci of necrotic skin. Such vascular necrosis and thrombosis are far more frequent with Rocky Mountain spotted fever than with typhus. The disseminated vascular lesions evoke a perivascular inflammatory response similar to that of typhus, particularly in the brain, skeletal muscle, lungs, kidneys, testes and heart muscle. A pneumonitis is present in severely affected patients which may be of primary rickettsial origin but is more often due to a secondary bacterial infection. Despite the widespread microscopic changes, the only grossly demonstrable anatomic alterations are hemorrhages and microinfarcts in affected organs and tissues. The overall mortality from Rocky Mountain spotted fever was once about 20 per cent, but antibiotic and supportive therapy has markedly improved this result. Deaths are due to shock, central nervous depression and renal failure.

It is apparent from the previous description that the anatomic changes of Rocky Mountain spotted fever resemble, to a considerable extent, those of typhus, and for clear differentiation of the diseases, serologic studies are necessary. Recognition of the vector of transmission is helpful, but much more definite are identification of the organisms by culture, complement fixation reactions and other serologic tests capable of demonstrating the specific antibodies.

SCRUB TYPHUS (TSUTSUGAMUSHI FEVER)

Scrub typhus (Tsutsugamushi fever) closely resembles the infections already described. It is characterized clinically by fever, chills, the development of an eschar right at the site of the bite of a mite, and by a transient rash which is much less prominent than that found in typhus fever and spotted fever. This disease occurs in a rather well defined geographic area encompassing Japan, China, India, Korea, Formosa, the Philippines and Australia. It probably does not occur outside this region of the world. The causative agent, *R. tsutsugamushi*, is morphologically similar to those of spotted fever and typhus fever. The disease is transmitted by several species of chigger-like mites which have a wide animal reservoir in rodents, particularly rats and mice. At the site of inoculation, an indurated lesion about 1 cm. in diameter appears. It vesiculates centrally, then ulcerates and is followed by a black scab. This eschar formation is a hallmark of tsutsugamushi fever and is seen similarly only in rickettsialpox. The organisms multiply at the portal of entry, then disseminate through the blood system as with the other rickettsioses described. Once again, the brain, lung, kidney and heart are among the organs principally affected. Vascular lesions develop similar to those of typhus fever and spotted fever, but only rarely is there necrosis of the blood vessel walls as with the spotted fevers. Also, the perivascular inflammatory response is far less prominent. In the brain, the lesions usually consist of a few minor vascular and perivascular reactions with the occasional formation of glial nodules such as occurs with typhus fever. In a few instances, a scant meningitis is present, characterized principally by an accumulation of mononuclear cells in the subarachnoid space. Hemorrhagic pneumonia of rickettsial origin, sometimes with a superimposed bacterial pneumonia, is encountered in the more severe cases. The mortality rate in this infection has been variously reported as 1 to 60 per cent but, on the whole, the disease is milder than either epidemic typhus or Rocky Mountain spotted fever, and fatalities are rare.

The diagnosis rests with identification of the causative agent and with specific serologic tests.

Q FEVER

Q fever is caused by the *Coxiella burnetii (R. burnetii)*, and presents clinically as an acute pneumonia. Unlike the other rickettsial diseases, it is not accompanied by a rash and it does not produce agglutinins against any of the various strains of *Proteus vulgaris.* The organisms have a wide reservoir in a variety of animals, including rats, rabbits, mice, hedgehogs, tortoises, cattle, sheep, goats, horses and dogs, as well as in a host of arthropods, including ticks, lice, mites and parasitic flies. There is, however, strong suspicion that it may also be transmitted to man without an animal or arthropod vector via contaminated milk or placental material. In some dairies, cows are maintained on the open range where they contract the infection, and so man is contaminated in handling their tissues.

The disease begins with fever, chills, headache and generalized malaise, but very promptly shows respiratory symptoms of variable severity. Some patients demonstrate few pulmonary findings, while others have fever and difficulty in breathing, characteristic of a full-blown pneumonia. The disease is rarely fatal but, in a few autopsy cases, lobar consolidation of the lungs quite similar to that seen in pneumococcal pneumonia has been found. Macroscopically a gray to red hepatization (p. 811) may be present, produced by an alveolar exudate consisting principally of mononuclear cells. This pattern is in striking contrast to the pneumonias of bacterial origin, in which the reaction is primarily neutrophilic. Superimposed bacterial infection, however, may obliterate this differential feature. In other cases, the pneumonia resembles that of psittacosal or viral origin. In the viral pattern, there is a prominent interstitial inflammatory reaction within the walls of the alveoli, manifested by an infiltration of macrophages, lymphocytes and plasma cells, with occasional neutrophils. Occasionally, areas of septal necrosis are present (Whittick, 1950). The bronchioles contain a leukocytic exudate that is more often neutrophilic. Vascular lesions have been reported in Q fever but are not as prominent as those in patients suffering from typhus fever or Rocky Mountain spotted fever. When they occur, they affect the same group of organs involved by the other rickettsioses. Fatalities are rare with a death rate of less than 1 per cent.

Two uncommon manifestations of Q fever have been reported within the recent past. One takes the form of vegetative endocarditis, involving the mitral and aortic valves, producing vegetations, ulcerations and gross deformity of the affected leaflets (Marmion et al., 1960). The other atypical pattern involves miliary granulomas in the liver. Rarely, the hepatitis is the sole manifestation of the rickettsial infection (Picchi et al., 1960).

As with the other rickettsioses, serologic tests are required to confirm the diagnosis of Q fever. No agglutinins against any of the Proteus organisms are produced.

VIRUS DISEASES

At one time considered only biologic curiosities, viruses have recently become the darlings of oncologists and of those interested in communicable diseases. Their role in neoplasia was discussed in Chapter 4. Here we are concerned with their causation of communicable disease. Understandably, only the more important disorders can be considered here. For more complete data, reference should be made to such standard texts as (1) Davis et al. (1968) (2) Horsfall and Tamm (1965) and (3) Jawetz et al. (1970).

As pointed out earlier (p. 128), all viruses are microscopic aggregates of either DNA or RNA enclosed within a protein-bearing capsid. All are obligate intracellular parasites. They are only capable of replication within a host cell which provides them with their required energy and the necessary machinery for replication. Thus, for their survival and multiplication, the following steps are requisite (Tamm and Eggers, 1965):

1. Attachment to the appropriate host cell involving specific plasma membrane receptors.
2. Penetration of the cell and shedding of the capsid envelope.
3. Transport of the viral genetic material to the appropriate site within the host cell.
4. Synthesis of required viral components by the host cell.
5. Assembly of these components.
6. Release of the mature virions in productive infections.

While the host cell provides the means, viral DNA or RNA directs the synthesis of the viral components. In the course of their intracellular existence, viruses have a variety of effects on the host cell, as will be apparent in the subsequent discussion.

Classification of Viruses. More than 300 immunologically distinct viruses have been identified as having significance in the causation of human disease. These have been classified in a number of ways and, regrettably, no single classification is suitable for all purposes. Here we shall follow the classification suggested by the International Sub-Committee of Virus Nomenclature (1963). The RNA viruses and DNA viruses have each been divided into four major groups as follows.

DNA Viruses. *Poxvirus group* are relatively large agents responsible for smallpox in man and for cowpox.

Herpes virus group is responsible for chickenpox, shingles, keratoconjunctivitis and herpetic vesicles (coldsores, fever blisters). As will be recalled, this group has lately come under suspicion in the induction of cervical cancer in the female.

Adenovirus group comprises a large assortment of immunologically distinct entities often isolated from upper respiratory infections and pharyngitis.

Papovavirus group is chiefly known for the ability to induce neoplasms in lower animals but, in man, has only been established as the cause of warts.

RNA Viruses. *Myxovirus group* includes the agents responsible for mumps, measles, rubella, rabies and influenza, and undoubtedly contributes to the causation of some common colds.

Arbovirus group is associated with the induction of a variety of forms of encephalitis, dengue and yellow fever.

Reovirus group is thought to be involved in the causation of upper respiratory infections and possibly the common cold. However, such causation has not been clearly established.

Picornavirus group embraces two major subgroups, enteroviruses and rhinoviruses. The enteroviruses include the Coxsackie agents, the ECHO viruses (Enteric Cytopathogenic Human Orphan viruses) and polio viruses. The rhinoviruses have also been isolated from upper respiratory infections and may contribute to the common cold.

A large number of additional viruses have not yet been clearly classified, for example, the cytomegalovirus and the Epstein-Barr virus. The latter closely resembles a herpes virus and so is often referred to as herpes-like. Some agents of disease now known as Chlamydiae (Bedsoniae) lie in the border zone between bacteria and viruses. Diseases caused by such agents are discussed in a separate section (p. 438).

Pathogenicity. The impact of viral invasion on a host cell and the mechanisms by which viruses cause cell injury are extremely variable. At one end of the spectrum is the apparent symbiotic relationship in which viral replication may continue within a cell without inducing any apparent morphologic change or ill effect. Infections caused by the cytomegalovirus, for example, may be very subtle or, indeed, may be entirely silent. At the other end of the spectrum are the viral invasions that rapidly destroy the cell (cytocidal). Smallpox is a destructive disease associated with extensive cellular necrosis. In between are the slow virus infections which require months or years to come to full maturation, and the slow proliferative effects of the oncogenic viruses. Some viruses exert both necrotizing and proliferative effects.

As with bacteria, viruses must be transmitted from an external source to a susceptible host. Viral infections are transmitted in the same fashion as bacterial infections, by direct man-to-man spread or indirectly. Some agents are spread by insect vectors, for example, yellow fever. They must then achieve a portal of entry, usually the same as those involved in bacterial infections (e.g., skin, respiratory system and gastrointestinal system). Very rarely, as in the case of rabies, the nervous system constitutes a portal of entry. The inhaled virus may ascend the olfactory nerve and, following nerve trunks, reach the central nervous system. As was made clear at the outset, however, viruses differ from bacteria in requiring intracellular localization for their replication, and have greatest cytopathic effects in specific types of cells. To reach such cells, they must spread from the portal of entry, whatever it may be. From the studies of animal models of disease, much has been learned about such localization (Frenkel, 1969).

In the instance of poliomyelitis, we now know that the usual events in infection relate to direct spread of the polio virus from person to person. The portal of entry is the oral cavity, leading to alimentary tract infection. Usually the virus is transmitted by fecal, oral or droplet pharyngeal contamination. Within the gut, the virus multiplies but produces no visible lesions. Only in a very few patients does it enter the bloodstream and even more rarely is the brain seeded by such blood-borne spread. Thus the viremia reaches out to all cells in the body. Since neurons cannot regenerate, replication of the poliovirus eventually causes its principal effects here, giving rise to the neurologic lesions of poliomyelitis (Bodian and Horstmann, 1965). Thus, the polio virus might be more accurately said to be *neuropathic* rather than neurotropic. It appears that cytopathogenicity is a function not only of the invader, but also of the ability of the host cell to survive the physiologic interference resulting from the "uninvited guest." However, we still do not understand why the virus of smallpox causes largely a cytopathic effect on epidermal cells, while the Shope papilloma virus evokes a tumor in these same cells. The mysteries reside within the viral-genetic information and the mode of its expression within the cell.

The visible morphologic lesions of viral infections can be categorized as: (1) regressive changes within parasitized cells, (2) proliferation of cells and (3) secondary inflammatory reactions. The cytopathic changes characteristic of acute viral infections consist primarily of cytoplasmic vacuolization (ballooning degeneration), nuclear chromatolysis and cellular lysis. Obviously, cell lysis is the most serious effect of cytocidal viruses. Proliferation may be produced by cytocidal viruses, but usually it is more characteristic of oncogenic viruses. Proliferation within viral lesions may also be a secondary response of contiguous cells to the necrotic products of destroyed cells. Secondary inflammatory reactions in viral infections consist essentially of the infiltration of mononuclear cells (lymphocytes and histiocytes). Very acute infections with extensive cell death may evoke a neutrophilic response.

One of the most characteristic morphologic changes seen in some viral infections is the production of *inclusion bodies* in cells. Inclusions represent either viral aggregations (basophilic inclusions) or focal regions in which viral replication has been completed (acidophilic inclusions). These may be located either within the nucleus or the cytoplasm and, in some infections, are present in both sites. Viral inclusions may be very large, approximating the size of an erythrocyte and, when located in the cytoplasm, are often surrounded by a cleared halo. When present, they are of considerable diagnostic aid. For example, the Negri body in neurons (cytoplasmic) is virtually pathognomonic of rabies. Inclusions are of considerable help in differentiating smallpox from chickenpox because, in the former, there are multiple inclusions within the cytoplasm while in chickenpox the inclusions are found within the nucleus. Interestingly, one cannot judge from the DNA or RNA content of the virus whether the inclusion will be nuclear or cytoplasmic, since DNA viruses may assume cytoplasmic localizations and RNA viruses, nuclear locations.

Host Resistance. The outcome of a viral invasion depends, as with all microbiologic infections, not only on the invader, but also on the response of the host. Some of the defense mechanisms include an intact skin or mucous membrane, phagocytosis by leukocytes and reticuloendothelial cells, and the protective roles of mucous secretions and ciliary action in the respiratory tract. Likewise, the immune system, particularly cell-mediated immunity, is important in controlling and eradicating viral infections. Macrophages and sensitized lymphocytes and their elaborated factors ("lymphokines") play the major roles here. Thus, viral lesions tend to be characterized by mononuclear inflammatory infiltrates. Humoral antibodies may also participate by coating viral antigen, rendering it susceptible to phagocytosis and destruction. The antibody coating may also block the attachment sites of the virion and block its adsorption and penetration of susceptible cells.

Interferon is probably the most distinctive form of protective host response against viral infections. Interferon is a generic name for certain cell proteins that inhibit viral replication. These proteins are synthesized by host cells (including lymphocytes) in response to intracellular virus, but other substances such as polysaccharides and certain bacterial and fungal products may also induce the elaboration of interferon. These interfering proteins are species but not virus specific. Thus, interferon induced by one agent may protect against others. The precise nature of the protection is uncertain. As is best known now, interferon exerts cellular resistance by evoking the synthesis of a cellular mRNA which, in turn, directs the synthesis of new proteins. Whether the induced proteins are inhibitory or whether instead, the role of interferon is to pre-empt the synthetic machinery of the host cell and thus block viral synthesis remains unknown. These antiviral proteins appear to be synthesized by cells early in infection, even before immune mechanisms are mounted. Recent studies suggest that interferon may be transferred from one cell to another, rendering them resistant to viral infection. Presumably, the transfer of the messenger RNA is involved. In any event, interferon apparently acts by interfering with the translation of viral messenger RNA and thus viral replication is inhibited (Joklik and Merigan, 1966) (Marcus and Salb, 1966) (Merigan, 1967). It may well be that interferon comprises the first host response to viral invasion, serving to control the replication and spread of the infection, thus providing the immune mechanism with sufficient time to achieve effective response levels.

Clinical Categories of Viral Diseases. In contrast to the microbiologist, the clinician and pathologist are primarily concerned with a grouping of the viral agents that permits a differential diagnosis of diseases as they appear in man. For example, it is necessary to have an understanding of those agents capable of causing nonbacterial meningitis or to know the possible etiology of a diffuse skin rash that may be measles, chickenpox, smallpox or any of the other microbiologic agents that affect the skin. On this basis, the following presentation will divide the viral diseases into groups based upon the principal organ affected. For example, the dermatopathic viruses such as smallpox, chickenpox and measles will be grouped under viral diseases that affect principally the skin, although it must be understood that, in many instances, other organs may also be affected in these systemic diseases. Poliomyelitis, as another example, primarily affects the central nervous system and will be listed under such a heading. The virus is also responsible in some cases for a myocarditis. In the same way, while the cytomegalovirus is listed under salivary glands, where it causes its principal anatomic alterations, there is an accompanying systemic dissemination of the virus that produces changes in many other organs. Recognizing these difficulties, the major viral diseases can be divided as follows:

1. Viral diseases affecting principally the skin and mucous membranes (dermatopathic viruses)—measles, rubella, chickenpox, smallpox, vaccinia, herpes simplex, herpes zoster, molluscum contagiosum and warts.

2. Viral diseases of the respiratory tract—influenza, primary viral atypical pneumonia, the common cold and a host of ill-defined upper respiratory diseases caused by the adenoviruses, rhinoviruses and occasionally Coxsackie viruses.

3. Principal viral diseases of the nervous system—poliomyelitis, viral meningitis, encephalitis, meningoencephalitis, rabies and lymphocytic choriomeningitis.

4. Viral diseases of the liver—infectious hepatitis and serum hepatitis.

5. Viral diseases of the salivary glands—mumps and salivary gland virus disease (cytomegaloviruses).

6. Miscellaneous viral diseases—yellow fever.

The more important viral diseases will now be presented in accordance with the classification just given, indicating where necessary any additional discussion of these entities that may be found under specific organs.

DERMATOPATHIC VIRAL INFECTIONS

SMALLPOX (VARIOLA)

Smallpox is an acute, highly communicable, febrile viral disease, principally characterized by a widely disseminated vesicular, then pustular skin eruption. Since the epochal introduction of vaccination by Jenner, this disease has become virtually extinct, particularly in those countries where vaccination is compulsory. In the United States, where vaccination is not compulsory, there are still occasional minor outbreaks and epidemics still occur sporadically in Asia and Africa.

The variola virus belongs to the group of poxviruses. Its portal of entry is the mucous membranes of the upper respiratory tract; the agent probably multiplies in the lymphoid tissue here and then is disseminated through the blood by a transient viremia. About 12 days following exposure, the patient develops fever, sometimes chills and, in the course of the next 1 to 5 days, the characteristic rash. In general, the rash tends to occur as a single crop of lesions, but at times one area of the body may be affected before another, producing successive waves of new lesions. However, *characteristic of smallpox is the tendency for all lesions in the area to be of the same age.* The rash begins as small red macules and rapidly becomes papular and vesicular. Over the course of 5 to 10 days, these vesicles become pustular and rupture or else begin to subside and dry, forming a surface crust.

The mucous membranes of the body have accompanying changes consisting principally of marked focal areas of erythema that become vesicular briefly, and then rupture to form shallow, superficial ulcers. Full-blown vesicles and pustules are rarely encountered in these moist surfaces, presumably because of the wet maceration of the mucosal surfaces and the greater tendency to early rupture.

The *severity of the infection* is roughly correlated with the severity of the skin and mucosal eruption. In the milder cases, the individual pocks remain discrete; in the more severe cases, they may become confluent; and in the very fulminating cases that are often fatal, the lesions become hemorrhagic. It is these atypical hemorrhagic lesions that are often not recognized as smallpox which provide the greatest danger in the dissemination of this disease.

An intraepidermal vesicle develops in the skin and mucous membranes (Councilman et al., 1904) presumably by the vacuolar or ballooning degeneration of the prickle cell layer of the epidermis. Individual cells enlarge because of intracytoplasmic edema, producing "clearing" of the cytoplasm. In this focus, intercellular fluid accumulates and separates the cells, thus creating a network of these cells. As the vesicle enlarges, the strands of cells rupture and a clear, fluid-filled space, completely enclosed within the epidermis, is formed. Occasionally the accumulation of fluid causes degeneration of the basal layer of epidermis so that the vesicle comes in direct contact with the corium. At a later stage, leukocytes infiltrate the vesicles, principally macrophages (Fig. 10–24). In the frank pustule stage, a thick, purulent exudate fills the vesicles. There is an accompanying infiltrate of macrophages, lymphocytes and plasma cells in the dermis underlying these vesicles and pustules. If the lesion ruptures and becomes secondarily in-

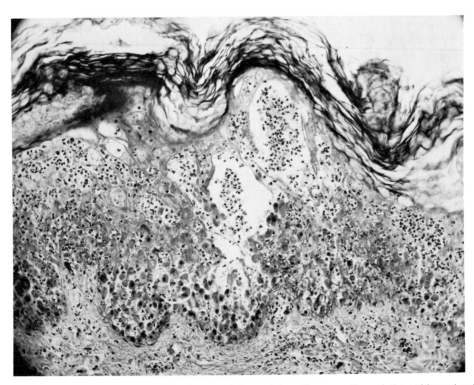

Figure 10–24. *Smallpox—a view of a characteristic vesicle with separation of the epidermal cells and a leukocytic exudate within the vesicle.*

fected, the inflammatory reaction in the dermis is heightened. If the pustule does not rupture, the fluid within the pustule is resorbed, and the inspissated residue and necrotic epithelial cells are sequestered and then eventually exfoliated along with the outer layer of cornified cells. In the mucous membranes, the full-blown stage of vesiculation and pustulation is replaced by the development of a superficial ulcer with accompanying neutrophilic and mononuclear inflammatory reaction.

The *cytoplasm* of epithelial cells within and about the vesicle and pustule usually contains *acidophilic Guarnieri inclusion bodies.* These are large acidophilic structures up to 10 microns in diameter, surrounded usually by a pale halo. As these cells degenerate, the inclusions may shift to or develop within the nuclei. There is some question whether the intranulcear inclusion should be designated as a Guarnieri body and, equally, some doubt that it represents viral substance in the same way as the cytoplasmic body.

Accompanying these more or less specific alterations in the epithelium, there is usually a generalized nonspecific hyperplasia of the reticuloendothelial system, manifested principally by nonspecific splenitis and lymphadenitis. Scattered focal fatty changes, petechial hemorrhages and interstitial mononuclear leukocytic infiltrates have been described in the liver, kidney, adrenal gland and testis. Distinctive within the inflammatory infiltrate are abnormally large lymphoid cells. These inflammatory changes are said to cause sufficient pressure upon vessels to produce localized ischemic necroses. Focal hemorrhages are found in the bone marrow, mucosa of the intestinal tract, mucosa of the urinary tract and sometimes in serosal membranes. Granulocyte formation may be depressed in the bone marrow, thus providing the apparent anatomic basis for the leukopenia so commonly identified in this condition. Secondary bacterial infections lead to bronchopneumonia in the lung, although some propose that the bronchitis and pneumonia are directly due to the viral invasion. Encephalitis, frequently fatal, is an additional complication.

The diagnosis can often be made from the rather characteristic skin lesions. However, when there is doubt, electron microscopic examination of the cells from vesicles should easily disclose the typical virus particles. The viruses are found in the vesicular fluid and may also be present in the blood and can be isolated from these sources. A simple test that is positive in a high percentage of cases is the examination of smears of cells from the vesicle

lesions, disclosing the cytoplasmic Guarnieri bodies that are readily evident in the active stages of the vesiculation.

Death is usually attributable to pulmonary complications. The mortality rate in epidemics may be as high as 80 per cent.

CHICKENPOX (VARICELLA)

Chickenpox is an acute but mild communicable "childhood" disease. It is characterized by minimal to moderate constitutional symptoms and a maculopapular vesicular eruption. The exanthem resembles to a considerable degree that of smallpox, but is usually less marked in severity. The individual vesicles tend to remain discrete and frequently do not develop into pustules.

The varicella virus, one of the DNA-herpes virus group, is apparently identical with the agent causing herpes zoster and is therefore often referred to as the varicella-zoster virus. It is composed of a DNA core, polyhedral in shape, surrounded by an icosahedral capsid constituting an envelope having an outer diameter of about 180 millimicrons.

The route of infection is not definitely established, but is assumed to be through the upper respiratory tract. The incubation period is usually 12 to 16 days. The virus then gains access to the blood and a viremia ensues, followed by vague malaise and fever, in turn followed by the appearance of a rash. Lesions appear first on the trunk and then involve the face and extremities. In the course of the succeeding days, some of these lesions assume a definite vesicular character. The individual vesicle is slightly elevated and surrounded by a narrow rim of erythema, the areola. *These vesicles appear in successive crops over the same area of skin involvement, so that lesions of different ages are found in any given locus.* Unlike smallpox, the rash of chickenpox tends to be centripetal with a greater distribution of lesions over the trunk than over the face and extremities. Lesions also appear in the mucous membrane of the mouth. In the course of the succeeding week, the thin-walled vesicles rupture or begin to resorb, and the vesiculation is replaced by dry-crusted scaling of the skin. Secondary infection may convert the vesicles into pustules.

Anatomically, these skin lesions consist of intraepithelial vesicles. However, their development differs slightly from that in smallpox. One of the earliest changes found is the development of *acidophilic intranuclear inclusions.* These precede the stage of frank vesiculation. In the affected focus, the epidermal cells then undergo ballooning degeneration and as they disintegrate, small fluid-filled spaces appear. In most of the lesions there is an intact underlying layer of basal epithelial cells. However, occasionally the vesicle is in direct contact with the underlying corium. Accompanying the development of the vesicle, there is a tendency for amitotic division of the epithelial cells with the formation of bizarre-shaped, multinucleate forms. At this stage, the nuclei may degenerate and the inclusions thus shift to the cytoplasm. The dermis underlying the vesicle is infiltrated with mononuclear leukocytes, chiefly about the vessels. As the vesicle reaches its full maturity, the fluid is progressively resorbed or escapes, and the epithelial cells at the margins regenerate the damaged epithelium.

Since most of the cases are benign, little is known of the visceral lesions in this disease (Cheatham et al., 1956). According to one report, focal necroses are found in the pancreas, liver, lungs, spleen, gastrointestinal tract and adrenals, suggesting that, like smallpox, varicella may in its more florid manifestations cause injury to internal viscera as well as the epithelium. In these areas of necrosis, inclusions may be seen in the various involved cells. Occasionally an encephalitis of indefinite character follows chickenpox, but it is not believed to be due to direct invasion of the central nervous system by the varicella virus. Generalized lymphadenopathy usually accompanies the disease.

In the usual case, the infection runs a relatively short course and, following the crusting stage, progressive recovery is the rule. Secondary infection of the vesicles and the development of vesicles in the larynx and on the conjunctival surfaces produce some of the more difficult problems in the management of these cases. Deaths are extremely rare, even when complicating intercurrent pneumonia, otitis media and encephalitis develop.

HERPES ZOSTER

Herpes zoster is an acute infectious disease which, as has been indicated, bears many close resemblances to chickenpox. There is a strong suspicion that, in many instances, it arises by reactivation of a latent herpes virus, or by exogenous reinfection of a host having antibodies from a previous bout of chickenpox. Herpes zoster is characterized by localization of the virus within dorsal root ganglia or cranial nerve ganglia, resulting in extremely painful neuritic complaints and simultaneous viral invasion of the epidermis with the development of vesicles usually along the course of the nerve. The skin vesicles are almost identical grossly and microscopically with those of chickenpox. Occasionally, the vesicles may be widely scattered over the skin to heighten the similarity to chickenpox. Similar vesiculation may occur in viscera supplied by the affected nerve, helping to explain some of the bizarre symptom complexes seen in this condition. The lesions in the ganglia consist of a severe infiltration with mononuclear leukocytes and regressive alterations in the ganglion cells to the point of their total destruction. The loss of the nerve cell body leads to degeneration of the myelin of the sensory nerve fibers and of the posterior nerve root. Occasionally, intranuclear and later intracytoplasmic inclusions are found in the vesicle of herpes zoster, indistinguishable from those in chickenpox.

HERPES SIMPLEX

The virus of herpes simplex is the prototype of the herpes virus group and has the same morphology as the agent described in chickenpox.

The herpes virus may cause a variety of clinical entities depending upon whether it is a primary infection or a recurrent infection, implying in the latter instance some partial immunity. Primary infections may be systemic in distribution and may be quite serious; recurrent infections are rarely of great consequence. The various clinical patterns that may all be present in the primary systemic disease include herpes labialis, herpetic gingivostomatitis, meningoencephalitis and parakeratoconjunctivitis.

Because the virus is virtually ubiquitous in the general population, most individuals have some prior exposure and some partial immunity. Many of these individuals continue to harbor the virus in a latent form. Active disease takes the form of the well known *fever blister* or *coldsore* with the production of a small vesicle on a mucous membrane. Histologically, this vesicle almost exactly resembles those found in chickenpox and herpes zoster and is replete with ballooning degeneration of epidermal cells, giant cell formations and intranuclear inclusions. In the gingivostomatitis pattern occurring most often in infants and children, there is a vesicular eruption throughout the oropharyngeal cavity. The meningoencephalitis takes the form of other viral invasions of the central nervous system and produces a mononuclear benign meningitis but, when involvement of the brain substance itself is present, there may be extensive involvement of ganglion cells to produce meningoencephalitis.

MEASLES (RUBEOLA)

Measles is an acute, infectious, highly communicable "childhood" disease, characterized by coryza, conjunctivitis, the appearance of characteristic focal lesions in the mouth known as Koplik's spots, and a generalized exanthem. The disease, however, may also affect nonimmune adults, and in this age range it may be much more severe.

The causative agent is an RNA-containing myxovirus. It is transmitted by droplet infection through the respiratory tract and becomes implanted here. During the incubation period (about 10 days), the virus is present in the blood and upper respiratory tract. It has been isolated from nasal, pharyngeal, tracheal and bronchial secretions. It is worth noting that the virus may be transmitted through the placenta to produce congenital measles.

Early in the disease there is photophobia, burning pain in the eyes and considerable lacrimation. Several days later, characteristic small red macules appear in the buccal mucous membrane, usually close to the points of opening of the excretory ducts of the parotid gland. These later develop central vesicles or white foci of necrosis to create the virtually pathognomonic *Koplik's spots*. At this stage of the disease, generalized lymphadenopathy and sometimes splenomegaly appear. As the Koplik's spots recede, a generalized, blotchy erythematous rash appears. It begins on the face or behind the ears and then spreads downward to cover the trunk and finally the extremities. The individual lesion is a red-brown maculopapule that is only slightly elevated and is for the most part discrete. In the course of the subsequent day or two, these lesions may coalesce to produce irregular map-like areas of discoloration. This typical rash blanches on pressure, but occasionally hemorrhages create a nonblanching exanthem ("black measles"). The rash usually fades within the subsequent week and is followed by scaling desquamation of the epithelium. Throughout the course, there is characteristically a cough which is at first dry but is later productive of a mucoid or purulent sputum.

Anatomically, the principal lesions of measles are found in the skin and in mucous membranes, the lymphoid tissues of the body and in the lungs. The skin lesions consist principally of vascular dilatation, edema and perivascular infiltrates of mononuclear leukocytes. In the more severe hemorrhagic rashes, there is extravasation of blood in the interstitial tissue. Occasionally, abortive small vesicles may form within or immediately beneath the epidermis. There may be endothelial proliferation of the capillaries in the affected foci. The Koplik's spots have a similar histologic pattern, but are more often accompanied by pronounced endothelial proliferation and frank necrosis creating the small, white foci described previously. These necrotic lesions may ulcerate and are then accompanied by a neutrophilic infiltration. No characteristic inclusion bodies are found in measles. The lymphoid tissues of the body are uniformly enlarged and contain cellular alterations which are virtually pathognomonic of the disease. The diagnosis of measles is sometimes made by examination of the lymphoid follicles in the appendix or other lymphoid tissue. There are hypertrophy and hyperplasia of the germinal follicles and the formation of large, multinucleate measles giant cells. These measure up to 100 microns in diameter and contain multilobate or more usually myriads of small nuclei, sometimes up to the number of 50 to 100 (Fig. 10–25). These giant cells often contain nonspecific nuclear and cytoplasmic inclusion bodies. In the uncomplicated pulmonary involvement, the lesions consist principally of peribronchiolitis and interstitial pneumonia that strongly resemble those found in other viral infections of the lung. Sometimes hypertrophy of septal

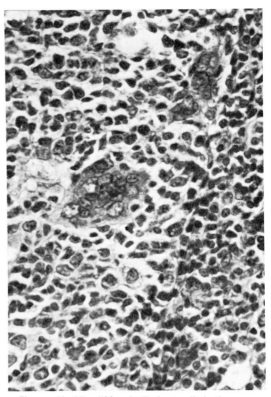

Figure 10–25. *"Measles" giant cells in the appendix.*

lining cells creates a likeness to cytomegalic inclusion disease (p. 563). However, in the majority of fatal cases, there is superimposed bacterial infection that leads to patchy focal bronchopneumonic consolidations characterized by exudation into the alveoli. Inflammatory changes in the laryngeal, tracheal and bronchial mucosa are also found, but it is difficult to determine whether these are the result of the uncomplicated viral infection or are due to the almost invariable secondary bacterial contamination. Often, the epithelial lining cells of the respiratory tract undergo apparent mitotic division without separating, creating epithelial giant cells. Such cells can occasionally be identified in the sputum.

Measles encephalomyelitis is an uncommon complication that develops in less than one in 200 cases. In these instances, there is perivascular mononuclear infiltration within the brain substance, accompanied by perivascular hemorrhage. Demyelinating lesions may appear in the brain and cord. These central nervous system changes closely resemble those encountered in some of the chronic demyelinating disorders such as subacute sclerosing panencephalitis. Furthermore, the antigenic similarities between the measles virus and inclusions found in subacute sclerosing panencephalitis strongly suggest that the measles virus may be the cause of some of these "idiopathic" central nervous system disorders. In the usual case of measles, the course is one of progressive improvement following the blanching of the skin rash. However, in the very young and the very old, fatalities may occur, usually due to an intercurrent bacterial pneumonia. Otitis media is a not uncommon complication in children.

GERMAN MEASLES (RUBELLA)

German measles is an extremely mild constitutional disease characterized by fever and a transient eruption that closely resembles the exanthem of measles. Like measles it is caused by a myxovirus. The disease is almost invariably benign, and there are virtually no data available on the characteristics of the lesions. The important role of maternal rubella infection during the first trimester of pregnancy in causing malformations in the fetus is discussed on p. 552.

MOLLUSCUM CONTAGIOSUM

Molluscum contagiosum is a skin lesion caused by a virus. Since the anatomic changes are totally confined to the epithelium, this lesion is described in Chapter 30.

VIRAL INFECTIONS OF THE RESPIRATORY TRACT

Viral infections of the respiratory tract cover a broad range of anatomic and clinical patterns. The clinical diseases vary from the extremely mild, transient common cold to the fulminating, severe forms of pneumonitis caused by the influenza viruses.

Between these two extremes, there is a continuum of increasing severity that encompasses a large number of overlapping and poorly defined clinical syndromes. In 1953, a virus was isolated from surgically removed adenoids that could be grown in tissue culture of adenoidal origin. Because this virus caused degeneration of the tissue culture cells, it was designated as the adenoid degeneration (AD) agent. Subsequent to this observation, virus was isolated from a number of cases of acute respiratory disease, and hence was called the ARD virus. Another group has been designated as RI for respiratory illness. Agents extracted from adenopharyngeal-conjunctival infections are called the APC viruses. Together all these agents are generally referred to as the adenoviruses. But, in addition, these agents have likewise been isolated from cases of conjunctivitis and keratoconjunctivitis.

Upper respiratory infections including the common cold and other ill-defined upper respiratory illnesses are included here. The etiology of these banal infections, despite their frequent and commonplace occurrence, ironically remains unknown. These diseases may be responsible for more time lost from productive work than all the other viral diseases together and, although intensive efforts have been directed toward establishment of their nature and prevention, we are still in as much doubt about the genesis of these harassing disorders as ever. A great many viruses have been isolated from the nasal and oral pharyngeal secretions of patients suffering from these illnesses, including adenoviruses, rhinoviruses and other picornaviruses such as the Coxsackie viruses and ECHO viruses, to mention a few of the most common ones.

At the opposite end of the spectrum, the more serious primary atypical pneumonias and viral influenzas are found. In the case of influenza, the problem is a little less complicated, since four fairly clearly defined subgroups have been identified, classified as types A, B, C and D. From the anatomic standpoint, all these infections principally involve the upper respiratory tract or lungs, and so are considered in Chapter 19.

VIRAL DISEASES AFFECTING PRINCIPALLY THE CENTRAL NERVOUS SYSTEM (NEUROPATHIC VIRUSES)

A number of viral diseases manifest themselves principally by involvement of the central nervous system. Most important among these are poliomyelitis and rabies. As such these disorders are taken up in Chapter 32. It is important, however, to remember that poliomyelitis, before localizing in the central nervous system, enters the body presumably through the oropharynx and then becomes disseminated through the blood. In the course of this viremia the agent may cause rather widespread, lymphoidal involvement of the tonsils, Peyer's patches of the small intestine and other lymph nodes, particularly in the neck. Rarely the virus may localize in the heart to produce a *myocarditis* (p. 686). Rabies, in contrast, appears to confine its damage to the central nervous system in the form of nerve cell destruction in the cerebral and cerebellar cortices as well as in the midbrain, basal ganglia, pons and medulla. For further details, reference should be made to p. 1500. In addition to these two specific disorders, there are a host of viral forms of meningitis, lymphocytic choriomeningitis and meningoencephalitis produced by a great variety of agents. Perhaps most important are the arborviruses that produce various patterns of encephalitis (p. 1497). In addition, encephalitis and meningoencephalitis may be encountered following mumps, measles, herpes infection, chickenpox, Coxsackie illnesses and quite rarely after ECHO virus infections. In all these cases, the anatomic changes are quite similar and have given rise to the speculation that the viral agent itself may be less important in causing the central nervous system damage than an accompanying immunologic reaction to the damaged brain substance itself.

VIRAL DISEASES AFFECTING THE LIVER

It has been well known that transmissible agents, presumably viruses, are capable of causing diffuse hepatocellular damage. Two clinical patterns are encountered called infectious hepatitis or hepatitis A and serum hepatitis or hepatitis B. Whether these two patterns are caused by two distinctive viral agents is not certain, but present evidence tends to support such a view. It is possible that the same agent might be responsible for the two clinical patterns based on variable host responses. Since these disorders are limited to the liver, they are discussed in Chapter 22 (p. 1004). While the transmissible agent (or agents) is known to be a virus, it has not been isolated in crystalline form and its precise nature is still not known.

VIRAL DISEASES AFFECTING PRINCIPALLY THE SALIVARY GLANDS

The two principal diseases included here are mumps and cytomegalic inclusion disease caused by the cytomegalovirus. Since this last entity is principally confined to infants, it is discussed in Chapter 13 (p. 563).

MUMPS

Mumps is an acute, contagious viral "childhood" disease characterized principally by involvement of the parotid glands and, less often, other organs, i.e., the submandibulars, sublinguals, pancreas, ovaries and testes. Sometimes the central nervous system is involved as well. In addition to these more characteristic sites of localization, the breast, prostate and heart may be affected.

The etiologic agent is an RNA myxovirus. The disease is contracted by droplet infection. Whether the virus travels from the mouth directly through Stensen's duct to the parotid gland as the primary site of multiplication or, instead, replicates in the respiratory tract and is then blood-borne to the specific organs mentioned is unclear. The latter mechanism is more likely since, in occasional cases, gonadal localization is seen without involvement of the salivary glands. Most patients are in the 5 to 15-year-old age range, because beyond this time it is believed that the greater part of the population has already been exposed and developed an immunity. However, rarely the disease is encountered in adults, usually in a more severe form.

The incubation period is generally three weeks, but occasionally it may appear as soon as two weeks after exposure or may be delayed as long as four weeks. The enlargement of the parotid glands is usually preceded by headache, malaise and fever. Bilateral parotitis occurs in about 70 per cent of the cases and is combined with involvement of the submandibular and sublingual glands in about 10 per cent of these instances. Unilateral parotitis occurs in about 20 per cent of the cases. It should be particularly noted that mumps may exist without parotid involvement, and the secondary structures that are attacked may be involved either before, synchronously with, or after the parotid swelling becomes evident. Moreover, as mentioned, sometimes mumps pancreatitis or orchitis is encountered in patients who never have parotitis, producing a bizarre clinical pattern (Warren, 1955). The most common secondary complication is orchitis, which occurs in about 20 per cent of patients with mumps. Most often this testicular involvement is unilateral. In passing, it should be noted that mumps pancreatitis may induce elevated levels of serum amylase and lipase as do the other forms of acute pancreatitis. The parotitis causes considerable tenderness, swelling of the affected gland and pain on mastication. The skin overlying the gland is tense but usually not reddened. The involved gland has a doughy, rubbery consistency and on transection is moist, glistening and red-brown.

Histologically, there is a diffuse, serofibrinous, interstitial exudation, accompanied by a heavy infiltration principally of mononuclear leukocytes, plasma cells and macrophages. The inflammatory reaction is largely confined to the interglandular stroma, but occasionally degenerative changes are found in the compressed acini and in the ductal epithelium. Similar interstitial lesions are present in the affected pancreas. In the testis there are diffuse interstitial edema and mononuclear as well as scattered polymorphonuclear leukocytic infiltration. In addition, there may be considerable regressive alterations or necrosis of the epithelium of the testicular tubules. The affected tubules fill up with a neutrophilic exudate in these more severely damaged loci. Hemorrhages into the interstitium accompany these changes. In other instances apparent microinfarctions develop, presumably because of edematous compression of the blood supply within the tight enclosing tunica albuginea. The central nervous system encephalitis or encephalomyelitis is of nonspecific character and cannot be distinguished from other forms of viral infection. Splenomegaly and lymphadenopathy, when they develop, are not severe and are due to the systemic toxemia. Characteristic inclusions have not been found in the lesions of mumps.

In the usual clinical case occurring in a child, the parotid swelling persists for one to two weeks, during which time there is a variable temperature that tends to fall after about one week of illness, followed by progressive improvement. The involvement of the testis and of the pancreas is perhaps more common in adults and may have much greater clinical significance than the parotitis. Some residual fibrosis and atrophy of the testis occur in about 50 per cent of the cases, but in the majority of these instances the disease is unilateral or only patchy and focal so that permanent sterility is a rare residual. The pancreatitis may give rise to acute abdominal symptoms that may be difficult to distinguish from acute pancreatic necrosis or other causes of an acute abdomen. However, the attack is usually transient and subsides fairly promptly. Neither the encephalitis nor the encephalomyelitis is of lethal significance. The mortality rate is very low in both children and adults.

MISCELLANEOUS VIRAL INFECTIONS

Included here are those viral diseases that produce changes in many organs and systems of the body. Cat-scratch fever, although possibly of viral etiology, will be discussed under the chlamydial infections (p. 441).

YELLOW FEVER

Yellow fever is an acute, infectious viral disease, virtually limited now to Africa and South America, which is transmitted by the bite of an infected mosquito. It is characterized clinically by high fever, a hemorrhagic diathesis, and signs of renal and liver damage. There is a wide range in the severity of this infection, varying from cases which are extremely mild and may be unsuspected to those cases that run a fulminating course to death within a week. The virus of yellow fever belongs to the arbovirus group. Through the epochal investigations of Reed, Carroll, Agramonte and Lazear, it was proved that the disease was transmitted from man to man by the *Aedes aegypti* mosquito. Since that time, however, other types of mosquitoes have also been implicated. After the bite of the insect, the virus presumably spreads to the local nodes and multiplies and shortly thereafter permeates the blood to cause a viremia.

The classic case has a short incubation period, in the range of 3 to 6 days, followed by a sudden onset of chills and fever. This febrile reaction is accompanied by a stage of so-called active congestion, manifested by flushing of the face and injection of the conjunctivae and sclerae. During this stage the fever is quite high, but the pulse is notably slow. Jaundice usually appears at this time and, synchronously, the hemorrhagic diathesis becomes evident in the form of ecchymoses in the skin and gingival bleeding. Bleeding into the stomach gives rise to the "black vomit." Sometime during the height of the illness, there is evidence of renal damage in the form of a progressive fall in urine output along with marked proteinuria and some pyuria. The renal involvement may become sufficiently marked to produce total anuria and death in renal failure. Although there are few adequate anatomic data on marrow changes, there is a striking leukopenia, due usually to a depression of granulopoiesis.

As can be anticipated from these clinical features, the major damage is found in the liver and kidneys, but in addition the heart, spleen and lymph nodes are involved. The liver is slightly enlarged or is of normal size and has a pale, soft, flabby consistency. Subcapsular and parenchymal focal hemorrhages are found in the classic case. The lobular pattern is usually preserved, but is sometimes blurred and indistinct.

On microscopic examination, there is an acute coagulation necrosis, midzonal in mild cases, but involving almost the entire lobule in the severe cases. Usually a small rim of peripheral cells is spared. The necrosis is coagulative in type, but the less severely affected cells have only increased granularity of their cytoplasm and sometimes fatty degenerative changes as well. The nuclear alterations vary from increased chromaticity to frank pyknosis, karyorrhexis and karyolysis. Total hyalinization of the cytoplasm of necrotic cells gives rise to the so-called *Councilman's bodies*. These rounded hyaline bodies are sometimes present within the faintly discernible outlines of the necrotic liver cells but, in many places, they are extruded into the adjacent sinusoids. The Kupffer cells are hypertrophic and the sinusoids are dilated. There may be considerable interstitial exudation of fluid and some hemorrhage, but there is a remarkable absence of inflammatory cell infiltration. In the very severe fulminating case, the hepatic necrosis may resemble that produced by chemical hepatotoxins with destruction of entire regions of the liver.

The involvement of the kidney is principally localized to the proximal tubules, which have cell swelling and fatty change and, in more marked involvements, frank coagulative necrosis. There is an accompanying interstitial edema and scant leukocytic infiltrate. Hemorrhages may also be present in this organ. On the basis of these changes, the kidneys are usually enlarged and tense and have a pale yellow fatty cortex.

Focal Zenker's hyaline degeneration and necrosis of cardiac muscle are described as well as a marked hyperplasia of the germinal follicles of the spleen. Follicular hyperplasia occurs in the lymph nodes. In almost all postmortem studies, the patient is jaundiced, and there are petechiae and hemorrhages into the skin, gingiva and the mucosa of the gastrointestinal tract, principally the stomach. Intranuclear inclusions are reported in the damaged liver cells in monkeys, but these are not a frequent finding in man.

The fulminating forms of this disease are highly fatal, but many milder expressions are encountered so that the overall mortality is perhaps not over 5 per cent. Death, when it occurs, is usually due to renal failure, overwhelming toxemia, liver failure, or sometimes intercurrent infection potentiated by the striking leukopenia.

DISEASES CAUSED BY CHLAMYDIAE

The Chlamydiae (Bedsoniae) comprise a small group of microorganisms lying intermediate between bacteria and viruses. The effective particles—"elementary bodies"—are smaller than most cocci and larger than most viruses. They subdivide by fission and contain both RNA and DNA. Like viruses, they are obligate intracellular parasites. Human diseases of chlamydial origin are: lymphogranuloma venereum, psittacosis (ornithosis), trachoma, inclusion conjunctivitis and possibly cat-scratch disease. Only the more important and frequently encountered entities follow (Moulder, 1964).

PSITTACOSIS (ORNITHOSIS)

Psittacosis is a chlamydial infection of birds that occasionally is transmitted to man to produce an acute interstitial pneumonitis. However, since lesions are produced in other viscera and sites in the body, this disorder is more appropriately considered as a systemic disease. The infective agent can be visualized within cells as spherical elementary bodies about 300 to 400 millimicrons in diameter which are readily stained by the Macchiavello or Castaneda technique.

The agent infects many birds, including canaries, parrots, parakeets, sparrows and pigeons, but it can be transmitted to mice, guinea pigs, rabbits and monkeys. When the disease is transmitted by parrots, it is referred to as psittacosis. When transmitted by other birds, it is designated as ornithosis. The usual pathway of transmission is the handling of diseased birds. It is important to realize that apparently healthy birds may harbor the virus and thus induce clinical disease. Less often, the infection is contracted by the bite of a bird or by the inhalation of infective material, such as dried feces, from the contaminated environment of animals. Spread may also occur from person to person during the height of active clinical disease.

The incubation period varies from one to two weeks and is followed by the relatively sudden onset of fever and chills, malaise, headache, sore throat and cough. The cough persists throughout the height of the disease and is relatively nonproductive. The active stage of the disease usually lasts for about one to two weeks, and during this time there may be central nervous system disturbances, such as drowsiness, delirium or stupor.

The respiratory involvement is remarkable in several respects. The cough, as has been mentioned, does not produce significant sputum. At times, despite apparent hyperpnea and dyspnea, there may be little cough. Physical examination may be remarkably negative, and roentgenograms of the chest, while positive, may fail to disclose the extent of the pneumonic involvement. These apparent paradoxes are readily explained by the anatomic characteristics of the lesions in psittacosis. The pulmonic lesions are similar in certain respects to those found in viral pneumonias. The inflammatory reaction is principally confined to the interstitial tissue and alveolar septa.

Grossly, the lung has focal areas of increased consistency and hyperemia. These focal areas are slightly elevated on cross section and are darker than the intervening normal pulmonary parenchyma. The pleural surfaces are usually not affected. When the involvement is extensive there may be some increase in the weight of the lung. The bronchi and bronchioles are little affected in certain cases, but in others there is considerable hyperemia, edema and mucopurulent exudation. However, in most of these involvements, secondary bacterial contamination complicates the interpretation of the changes.

Histologically, the alterations consist principally of edema and mononuclear leukocytic infiltration of the alveolar septa in foci of involvement. As the disease advances, seroproteinous fluid accumulates in the alveolar spaces, accompanied by scattered numbers of mononuclear leukocytes (Fig. 10–26). In the affected foci, the alveolar septal cells are often hypertrophic and cuboidal. Occasionally, intracytoplasmic elementary bodies can be identified in these alveolar cells in sections stained by the Giemsa technique. If the process is ex-

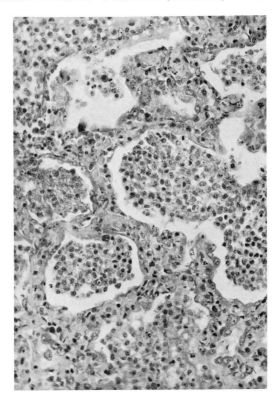

Figure 10–26. *Psittacosis of the lung with thickening of the alveolar septa and accumulations of mononuclear cells in the alveoli.*

tremely severe, there may be frank necrosis of alveolar septa with the formation of apparent abscesses accompanied by neutrophilic infiltration. In these severe instances, hemorrhages and fibrin masses may fill the air spaces. There is a considerable variability in the severity of the involvement of different foci. In some areas, the reaction may consist principally of an interstitial septal involvement, while in others there is considerable outpouring of fluid within the alveolar spaces, and in still others, the frank necrotizing lesions already described. Frank purulent exudation has been described in the alveoli in some cases, but it is always possible that these alterations may be due to intercurrent bacterial invasion. The nodes of drainage are usually enlarged and edematous and show reticuloendothelial hyperplasia and acute lymphadenitis.

The blood-borne infection is reflected in focal necroses in the liver and spleen and diffuse mononuclear infiltrative changes in the kidneys and heart and sometimes in the brain. The reticuloendothelial cells of the liver may contain the intracytoplasmic elementary bodies that were described in the lung. Similar foci are present in the spleen and are accompanied by diffuse reticuloendothelial hyperactivity with desquamation of large numbers of mononuclear phagocytes into the splenic sinuses. Swelling of cardiac muscle fibers, interstitial edema and mononuclear leukocytic infiltrates are described in the heart. The changes in the central nervous system consist of nonspecific edema, congestion and occasional foci of hemorrhage, both in the brain substance and in the meningeal coverings. It is not known whether these central nervous system alterations are due to direct viral invasion or are merely a reflection of the tissue destruction in other sites and the generalized toxemia.

In spite of the widespread anatomic lesions, the principal clinical manifestations stem from the involvement of the lungs. In the usual case, after a period of two to three weeks of illness, the condition spontaneously improves and most patients recover. The prognosis is dependent on the magnitude of the exposure and the virulence of the infective agent. Patients infected by parrots have a higher mortality (20 per cent) than those who contract their disease from other species of birds.

LYMPHOGRANULOMA INGUINALE (LYMPHOGRANULOMA VENEREUM, LYMPHOPATHIA VENEREUM)

Lymphogranuloma inguinale is a disease of uncertain etiology usually transmitted by sexual intercourse. The agent is related to that of psittacosis, and has been variously classified as being bacterial, viral or more likely chlamydial in nature. The disease spans a wide range of clinical patterns and tissue changes. Basically, it may be considered as a genital infection that involves the skin in and about the external genitalia and then rapidly spreads to the regional nodes. Despite this usual localization, constitutional symptoms may result. In a few cases, the infection extends beyond this local drainage to become a systemic disorder with more distant lesions in the brain, meninges, lungs, kidneys, bones and joints.

The clinical disease is best considered by dividing it into various stages. First, there is invasion which is usually not accompanied by symptoms. This stage may only last a few days. The second stage is heralded by the appearance of a genital or anorectal lesion at the site of introduction of the agent. Such lesions, however, are not invariably present and, in fact, in more than one-half of the reported cases, they are either inapparent or never develop. About one to two weeks later, the third stage is initiated by the progressive swelling and enlargement of the regional nodes of drainage, either unilaterally or bilaterally. This stage may last from days to many weeks. Much later, a fourth stage is encountered in a small percentage of the patients, consisting of either elephantiasis of the genitals due to lymphatic obstructions or fibrous strictures in the rectum due to inflammatory scarring.

The genital or anorectal lesion comprises a small intraepidermal or subepidermal vesicle that soon ruptures to create a shallow inflammatory ulcer. This occurs most often on the glans penis and prepuce of the penis, the labia, vaginal walls or cervix, but is also found sometimes within the urethra or the anus. Nonsexual accidental contamination of laboratory workers and physicians has resulted in initial lesions in other locations.

Histologically, the surface of the ulcer is often bathed in a neutrophilic exudate. The ulcer is characterized by a fairly nondescript mononuclear leukocytic infiltration accompanied by edema, fibroblastic proliferation, some vascular engorgement and endothelial cell hyperplasia. Occasionally some granulomas occur in the base of these ulcerations similar to those that occur in the lymph nodes. Cellular inclusions have been recorded in the phagocytes within these lesions.

The regional adenitis is characterized by the progressive swelling of the node to create large, painful, tense masses. These at first are discrete, but as the inflammatory reaction extends into the perinodal tissue, the nodes become matted together in the characteristic "bubo." Early in the disease, the nodes have a pink, hyperemic, succulent appearance, but as the inflammatory reaction matures, suppurative necrosis transforms them into fluctuant sacs in the severe involvements. These nodes may rupture through the skin to produce draining sinuses. In the male, the adenopathy is almost invariably localized to the inguinal regions and is usually bilateral. However, in the female, the adenopathy may or may not affect the inguinal nodes, depending on the location of the primary lesion. If the inoculation occurs on the external genitalia, the inguinal nodes are apt to be affected. If the vagina or the posterior perineum is the site of the origin, the pelvis and perirectal nodes are involved.

Histologically, the nodes in the developmental stages of the disease have a fairly nonspecific, diffuse reticuloendothelial hyperplasia and permeation by mononuclear leukocytes. However, aggregates of macrophages and reticuloendothelial hyperplasia may soon develop into small granulomas. The centers may then become necrotic to create minute abscesses. As these small lesions coalesce, they form irregular linear or branching stellate abscesses consisting of focal areas of suppuration enclosed within a granulomatous wall distinctive but not pathognomonic of this condition. The centers of the abscess contain polymorphonuclear leukocytes in varying stages of preservation, about which there is a radially arranged palisade of fibroblasts, reticuloendothelial cells and altered macrophages that closely resemble epithelioid cells. Occasional Langhans' or foreign body giant cells are found in this zone. About the enclosing wall there is an intense infiltrate of plasma cells and lymphocytes. Blood vessels in this inflammatory wall are dilated and often have endothelial proliferation. The small focus of lymphogranulomatous inflammation may closely resemble the granuloma of syphilis and tuberculosis. The radial palisade and the central accumulation of polymorphonuclears, when well developed, provide points of differentiation. In the long chronicity of this infection, which may last for many weeks or months, considerable fibroblastic proliferation eventuates in marked scarring of the nodes.

The late sequelae of lymphogranuloma venereum stem from the inevitable lymphangitis and severe lymphadenitis just described. As a consequence of lymphatic blockage, there is marked edema and elephantiasis of the female external genitalia known as esthiomene. Elephantiasis of the penis may develop for the same reason. Because of the drainage of the infection to the perirectal nodes and deeper pelvic nodes in the female, chronic fibrosis about the rectum produces strictures that are sometimes difficult to differentiate from rectal carcinoma (Cole, 1933). It is to be emphasized therefore that, in the female, rectal obstruction may be attributable to this inflammatory disorder.

The diagnosis of this condition can usually be established by the clinical finding of the large, fluctuant "bubos" or draining sinuses. The tissue lesions may be sufficiently well developed to be virtually diagnostic. In addition, the Frei skin test is of value. A positive Frei test, however, is of limited significance, since it merely demonstrates the presence or previous existence of an infection, and in certain regions of the United States between 10 to 40 per cent of the adult population have been exposed to this microorganism. A complement fixation test is more specific, particularly when progressively rising titers can be demonstrated during the active disease. Fatalities are extremely rare, and most of the importance of this disease centers about the serious late sequelae.

CAT-SCRATCH DISEASE

Cat-scratch disease is a benign infectious process of uncertain etiology characterized by a striking regional lymphadenitis following, usually, the scratch of a cat. The causative agent may be either viral or chlamydial (one of the Bedsoniae). This entity is of significance because the nodal enlargement may be enough to arouse suspicion of some more serious form of lymphadenopathy. Almost invariably a history can be obtained of contact with a cat as the presumed vector of transmission, but in a few instances inoculation has been associated with splinters or thorns. In the usual case, the local skin injury is relatively trivial, but sometimes it is followed by the development of an erythematous papule at the site of trauma, often surmounted by a pustule or crust. One or two weeks later, but occasionally delayed for several months, the regional nodes of drainage become painfully enlarged. The most common regions affected are, in order of frequency, axillary, head and neck, and inguinal or femoral nodes. Occasionally other nodes may be involved, such as those under the pectoral muscles, in the scalp or even the mesenterics. The lymph nodes may sometimes reach a size of 8 to 10 cm. in diameter. In approximately half the cases, they suppurate and become soft and fluctuant. Constitutional symptoms are common but not invariable. Quite rarely, the systemic manifestations may be quite severe, and temperatures as high as 105° F. have been recorded. A very few cases of encephalitis have developed in the course of this condition, but in most instances the disease constitutes a mild febrile illness that subsides spontaneously in weeks to months.

Morphologically, the nodes are tense, red and soft and, when suppuration ensues, small microabscesses or sometimes large confluent collections of pus appear. The histologic reaction is fairly distinctive and can be characterized as *"granulomatous abscess formation."* The reaction at first consists of focal reticuloendothelial hyperplasia. Soon these foci accumulate large numbers of macrophages, and the centers collect increasing numbers of polymorphonuclear leukocytes. Central necrosis then ensues so that the lesion in its full-blown stage represents an irregular, round or ovoid abscess containing central debris with fragmented nuclei of polymorphonuclear leukocytes. This focus is enclosed within a rim of reticuloendothelial cells and fibroblasts including giant cells of the foreign body or Langhans' type creating the epithelioid pattern. Plasma cells and lymphocytes often surround these granulomas.

From this anatomic description, it is apparent that the tissue reaction closely resembles those of lymphogranuloma venereum, tularemia, and even tuberculosis or sarcoidosis. When suppuration does not ensue, the reticuloendothelial hyperplasia may create a likeness to Hodgkin's disease.

The diagnosis of this condition requires the exclusion of tuberculosis and other bacterial agents by cultural methods as well as the confirmation of the nature of the process by a skin test. The skin test antigen is essentially a heat-treated dilution of the suppurative exudate from a known case. When injected into the skin of suspected patients, a positive test comprises redness and induration 48 hours after the intradermal injection. Histologic examination of excised nodes permits only confirmation of the clinical diagnosis since the tissue changes described are not pathognomonic and may be simulated by some of the other entities already mentioned (Spaulding and Hennessy, 1960; Winship, 1953).

DISEASES CAUSED BY FUNGI AND PROTOZOA

Infections produced by fungi and protozoa still loom large as clinical problems in many regions of the world. In the United States, fungal and protozoal diseases must still be considered as uncommon. However, it is of interest that recent reports indicate some increase in their number. The movements of troops to and from arenas of war and air travel have brought pockets of endemic disease to all parts of the world. Diagnoses of malaria, amebiases or leishmaniasis can no longer be disregarded in economically advanced countries. But in addition to this consideration, a striking fivefold increase has been shown in the frequency of fungal diseases in the United States in the recent past (1948 to 1955) as compared with the preceding six years (Key and Magee, 1956). The increased frequency is attributable to opportunistic infections in patients who have been rendered particularly vulnerable because of debilitating influences such as preexisting malignancy, lymphoma, leukemia, total body irradiation, treatment with cytotoxic or immunosuppressive drugs or prolonged treatment with some broad-spectrum antibiotic that destroys bacteria and leaves the field open for the growth of fungi. Only the salient features of these diseases are presented here. For further details, reference may be made to the monographs by Ash and Spitz (1945) and Marcial-Rojas (1971).

Fungi are closely related to bacteria; in fact, bacteria are themselves fungi (Kurung, 1942). However, most fungal diseases differ from those caused by bacteria in their chronicity and resistance to usual chemotherapy. The fungi produce neither exo- nor endotoxin and are weak antigens. Most of the tissue damage evoked by these organisms is due to the *progressive development of sensitization to the parasitic proteins* with resultant allergic necroses in the local areas of implantation (Baker, 1947). While all pathogenic fungi are capable of causing lesions in the skin, some virtually limit their involvement to the skin. The more significant of these skin infections, i.e., epidermophytosis, microsporosis, maduromycosis and sporotrichosis, will be considered in Chapter 30. Only the more important of the fungi that also produce lesions in deeper structures which fall into the category of generalized disease are presented here.

ACTINOMYCOSIS AND NOCARDIOSIS

Actinomycosis and nocardiosis are two closely related disorders caused by somewhat similar organisms. The causative agents of actinomycosis are usually *A. israeli* or *A. bovis* (anaerobic fungi), while that of nocardiosis is *Nocardia (Actinomyces) asteroides*, an aerobic fungus. Both agents grow in tangled, branching, filamentous threads and are gram-positive. The *Actinomyces* are weakly and inconstantly acid-fast and tend to grow in colony formation within tissue lesions. They thus create a dense central mass of tangled threads, surrounded by radiating, sometimes terminally clubbed, filaments that create a fuzzy border to the colonial formation. This colony is sometimes grossly visible, *thus giving rise to the characteristic "sulfur granules" found in infections.* In contrast, the Nocardia are usually acid-fast, rarely grow in colony formation, and do not form well defined terminal clubs. Little is known about the pathogenesis of the Nocardia infections, but *A. israeli* is believed to be a *normal inhabitant of the oral cavity of man.* Presumably, infections arise when these organisms gain a portal of entry through an injury either in the oral cavity or in the respiratory or intestinal tract. As a consequence of this route of invasion, three clinical forms of actinomycosis are encountered: cervicofacial, abdominal and thoracic. These three forms are not mutually exclusive.

Cervicofacial actinomycosis is the most frequent pattern (approximately 50 per cent of cases). It usually originates in some injury within the mouth, such as the extraction of a tooth. At first the gingiva and adjacent soft tissues become swollen and tensely indurated, but the lesion is not extremely painful because it develops insidiously. In the course of time, *a large, woody swelling develops, characteristically over the angle of the jaw.* This hard induration eventually becomes soft and fluctuant as the lesion matures and suppurates centrally. These infections are characterized by great chronicity and by burrowing, invasive spread; thus, in the cervicofacial disease the inflammation often extends to the skin to perforate and produce chronic draining sinuses. Periostitis and osteomyelitis with extensive destruction of bone are common accompaniments. The burrowing sinus tracts may penetrate the vertebral column, cranium, air sinuses and facial bones. The lesion consists at first of a diffuse edema and leukocytic infiltration that is principally mononuclear, surrounded by considerable fibrovascular proliferation that creates a granulomatous pattern. In the course of time, a central focus of suppurative necrosis develops. Usually at this stage, some secondary bacterial invasion is present. The suppuration often contains "sulfur granules" (Fig. 10–27). The character of the suppuration is entirely nonspecific and the diagnosis must be made by the identification of the causative agent. Often the

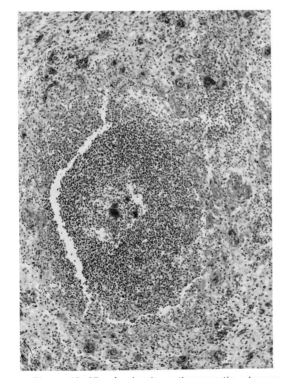

Figure 10–27. *A classic actinomycotic abscess containing colonies of fungi (sulfur granules) appearing as black masses within the center of the abscess.*

appropriate diagnosis can be made clinically. The gross impression can be confirmed by merely crushing the sulfur granules between glass slides to visualize the branching filamentous mycelial growth. For more certain identification, culture techniques may be required.

Abdominal actinomycosis arises from invasion of the intestinal mucosa, most commonly of the *appendix* or *colon.* There ensues a characteristic acute and chronic inflammatory reaction that invariably penetrates the wall of the bowel to produce a localized peritoneal abscess which then may extend into adjacent loops of bowel, the retroperitoneal tissues and anterior abdominal wall and may sometimes dissect to the skin surface with the formation of draining external sinuses. In many instances, organisms reach the liver either via the lymphohematogenous routes or by direct continuity, and cause extensive liver abscesses. Further spread may then lead to subdiaphragmatic infections and eventual penetration of the diaphragm and intrathoracic infections.

Thoracic actinomycosis results either from aspiration of the fungus or from direct penetration of a subdiaphragmatic infection. Lung abscesses, pulmonopleural fistulas and suppurative empyema result, and further spread erodes the ribs and anterior chest wall or extends into the vertebral column and the pericardial cavity. Thus, from any primary lesion, spread in virtually any direction may occur.

Nocardiosis may evoke the same pattern of tissue lesions, but more commonly gives rise to infections of the lungs and lower extremities. In the lungs, focal areas of suppuration occur that sometimes progress to total caseous necrosis. Cavitation and surrounding fibroblastic proliferation heighten the similarity to tuberculosis. This pulmonic pattern may cause death within weeks to months. Both causative agents have been reported to permeate blood vessels and give rise to widespread metastatic areas of suppurative necrosis.

Neither actinomycosis nor nocardiosis is attended by significant local or systemic reactions. However, as the tissue destruction increases in extent, pain and tenderness and systemic febrile symptoms appear. Further secondary signs may be the development of intra-abdominal masses, intestinal dysfunction or, in thoracic lesions, cough, the raising of copious amounts of sputum when the infection extends into a bronchus, and varying degrees of respiratory difficulty. Signs of bony destruction are common in almost all localizations because of the unrelenting invasiveness of the infection. Because the organisms are resistant to most chemotherapeutic drugs, the infections are characteristically persistent and difficult to heal, leading to extensive tissue destruction and secondary scarring.

CRYPTOCOCCOSIS (TORULOSIS)

Cryptococcosis is a communicable disorder caused by *Cryptococcus neoformans (Torula histolytica)*. Although the organism can cause skin lesions and infections in the subcutaneous tissue, joints and lungs, it most commonly localizes in the *meninges*. The causative agent is a round to oval yeast about 5 to 10 microns in diameter that reproduces by budding. It has *a distinctive, very prominent, heavy, gelatinous capsule* that creates a clear halo or space about the agent in tissue sections or exudate. A useful laboratory aid in the identification of this organism is the introduction of *India ink* into exudate suspected of harboring these fungi. The ink provides a contrast medium which clearly outlines the heavy, translucent, gelatinous coat.

It is not clear whether cryptococcosis begins as an endogenous or an exogenous infection. Fungi have been found on the surfaces of fruits and in animals but, equally significant, the organisms have been found on the skin and in the feces of healthy individuals. One of the most frequent patterns is the development of cryptococcosis in patients already suffering and debilitated from some leukemia or lymphoma. In the report by Zimmerman and Rappaport (1954), one-third of their cases were of such an opportunistic nature.

The organisms evoke an insidious chronic disease. Lesions may appear first in the skin and spread through the blood to the lungs or vice versa. Systemic dissemination from either of these sites may seed any other organ in the body. When the organisms are aspirated or spread through the blood, focal or more usually disseminated miliary consolidations may develop that resemble tuberculous granulomas. Fungi are scattered through this chronic inflammatory and granulomatous reaction (Fig. 10–28). Large giant cells appear in the margins of these areas, thus furthering the similarity to tuberculosis. Occasionally the pulmonary lesions consist only of gelatinous masses of fungi with little or no inflammatory response. There is strong evidence that these infections may resolve spontaneously and leave only quiescent foci of pulmonary fibrosis.

Meningitis may also be associated with very little inflammatory reaction. In these cases, large, gelatinous, fungal masses are present in the subarachnoid space accompanied by only a scattered mononuclear, chiefly macrophagic, exudation. In other instances

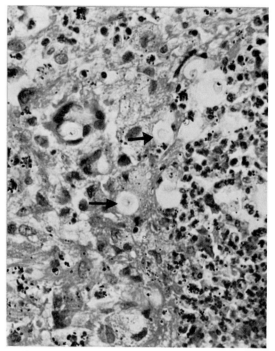

Figure 10–28. *Cryptococcosis—several fungi are visible as pale organisms surrounded by a clear zone created by the mucinous capsule* (arrows).

there is a more pronounced mononuclear and scattered neutrophilic exudation along with the formation of chronic granulation tissue that sometimes reproduces the focal granulomas described in the lung. The infection may extend into the brain substance about the perivascular spaces and sometimes enters the gray matter to produce small microcysts filled with organisms and their mucinous secretions. Metastatic foci of involvement have been described in the skeletal muscles, male urogenital tract and adrenals.

A major point of differentiation of cryptococcosis from blastomycosis, to be described, is *the relatively scant inflammatory response* evoked by the cryptococci, whereas the Blastomyces cause intense tissue destruction, cellular exudation and inflammatory fibrosis.

Cutaneous cryptococcosis takes the form of multiple or single isolated abscesses or subcutaneous infections that cannot be differentiated from bacterial infections except by isolation and identification of the fungus. Occasionally the diagnosis can be made by tissue biopsy. *Pulmonary* cryptococcosis usually masquerades as either primary carcinoma of the lung or tuberculosis. The correct clinical diagnosis can sometimes be established by identification of the cryptococci in the coughed-up sputum and exudate. *Central nervous system* cryptococcosis appears as a meningitis of insidious onset, characterized by headache, dizziness and stiffness of the neck. Usually the patient has little febrile reaction, and most often the meningeal involvement is mistakenly interpreted as tuberculous meningitis. The intracranial infection is usually resistant to treatment and leads to a variety of cranial nerve palsies, and in the majority of cases terminates in the death of the patient.

NORTH AMERICAN BLASTOMYCOSIS

North American blastomycosis is an infection by *Blastomyces dermatitidis*, an organism that assumes a yeast-like form in tissue lesions, but has also been identified as mold bearing conidia in the soil (Denton and DiSalvo, 1964). The yeast form is round to oval, varying between 5 and 15 microns in diameter, having a thick, double-contoured wall. The organism reproduces by budding (Fig. 10–29).

North American blastomycosis is an infection of exogenous origin. The organism enters the body either by inhalation or by its introduction into the skin through a wound. The clinical patterns of disease divide themselves fairly

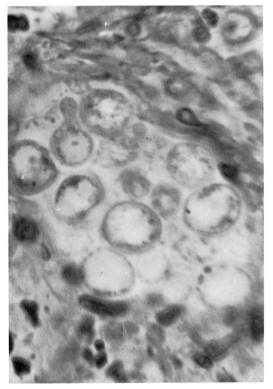

Figure 10-29. *North American blastomycosis with a cluster of organisms, one in the process of reproduction by budding.*

sharply into *cutaneous blastomycosis* and *pulmonary blastomycosis*, often complicated by systemic dissemination. The term cutaneous blastomycosis implies that the organism invades through a skin injury. However, a primary pulmonary infection may be disseminated through the blood to secondarily involve the skin.

In primary *cutaneous blastomycosis*, lesions are found on the exposed parts, such as the hands, face, feet, wrists and ankles. The lesion begins as a small papule and, over the course of weeks, months or even years, becomes a larger, irregular, flat papule, having red to violet raised margins studded with microabscesses and a central depressed area of older scarring. This lesion may spread slowly over the course of months or years and sometimes causes large geographic lesions with sharply defined serpiginous borders. Satellite lesions may begin in remote areas, presumably due to autoinoculation.

Histologically, there are microabscesses within the dermis, many of which extend up to the epidermis. In the surrounding tissues, there is a marked inflammatory reaction which is both acute and chronic. One of the most striking features is a pseudoepitheliomatous hyperplasia of the epidermis. The epithelium is extensively thickened. The rete pegs are broadened and extend down into the underlying subepidermal connective tissue. Often the rete pegs appear to anastomose deeply to enclose microabscesses. There is some variability in the size and shape of the epithelial cells. However, there is no true anaplasia and no disorderly growth, differentiating this form of inflammatory proliferation from true neoplasia. The surface of the epithelium is usually covered by a dry crust of blood, exudate and serum. Occasionally these areas of suppuration harbor small granulomatous foci containing large giant cells which produce lesions that are quite similar to those of tuberculosis. Blastomyces may be found in these giant cells as well as in macrophages in the inflammatory foci.

Pulmonary blastomycosis usually develops from the inhalation of fungi, and is manifested by miliary abscesses throughout the lung. Granulomatous reactions may also occur here. Occasionally the involvement is localized to a single region to produce a solid consolidation resembling tumor infiltration. Histologically, these lesions take the form of either minute abscesses or tubercle-like granulomas. Characteristic double-contoured fungi can usually be demonstrated in these lesions. Systemic dissemination may lead to metastatic sites of infection, particularly in the skin and bones, or in any other tissue of the body.

The clinical manifestations stemming from these lesions are fairly apparent from the anatomic description. The spreading skin infection can usually be correctly recognized clinically, but may require isolation or cultivation of the fungus for confirmation of the diagnosis. *Pulmonary blastomycosis is usually confused with either carcinoma of the lung or pulmonary tuberculosis.* The patients have fairly marked systemic reactions in the form of fever, night sweats, malaise, weakness, weight loss, and frequently a bloody, purulent sputum. The final diagnosis requires the identification of the causative agent.

SOUTH AMERICAN BLASTOMYCOSIS

South American blastomycosis is a chronic infection caused by *Blastomyces (Paracoccidioides) brasiliensis.* This disease has been reported only in South America. The causative organism is much larger than the North American variant. The anatomic lesions produced by this infection closely resemble those of North American blastomycosis. The usual manifestations of this disease are a *mucocutaneous* lesion, usually in the mouth, a spreading *lymphangitic* infection, pulmonary lesions and sometimes systemic dissemination. Infection of the mucous membrane of the mouth takes the form of an inflammatory papilloma that resembles the early stages of North American blastomycosis. Drainage from this lesion may give rise to a striking involvement of the regional nodes. This lymphadenopathy is sometimes encountered in patients who do not have a well defined mucocutaneous primary lesion. In disseminated blastomycosis, these lesions are present in the skin, gastrointestinal tract, lungs, liver and other organs. In all these sites of localization, microabscesses or a chronic granulomatous inflammatory reaction develops which resembles that of North American blastomycosis. The chief differential point is the demonstration of the much larger, double-contoured organisms that produce buds.

COCCIDIOIDOMYCOSIS

Coccidioidomycosis is a highly communicable disease caused by *Coccidioides immitis.* This disease is most prevalent in the Southwest and Far West of the United States and is particularly common in the San Joaquin Valley of California. In this locale, this disorder is sometimes known as "valley fever" or "San Joaquin fever." The causative organism is a fungus whose arthrospores, when inhaled, grow into a large, thick-walled sporangium 10 to 80 microns in diameter. This fungus reproduces by endosporulation, and as many as 100 to 200 small endospores between 2 to 5 microns in diameter may be seen within one parent sporangium (Fig. 10–30). However, in tissue lesions, there may be few spores within a spherule, creating a likeness to the causative organism of blastomycosis. Infection is transmitted by inhalation of spores but also, uncommonly, by the inoculation of spores into a cutaneous injury.

The clinical disease is quite variable in severity and has a *cutaneous or pulmonary localization* (Schwarz and Muth, 1951). In many patients, the infection is confined to the development of focal skin lesions. More often, the disease is acquired by inhalation and presents as a pulmonary disease. In some patients, it evokes only a minimal febrile reaction, a cough, and later small calcified lesions in the lung parenchyma or hilar nodes. These can be identified only as coccidioidomycosis because the patients develop a positive skin coccidioidin test. In its more severe expressions, an acute and chronic respiratory disease is produced. It usually remains localized to the lungs

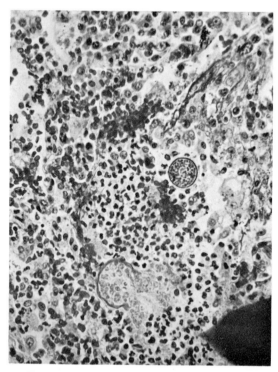

Figure 10–30. *Coccidioidomycosis with several microorganisms filled with endospores. One has been caught at the moment of rupture with release of daughter spores.*

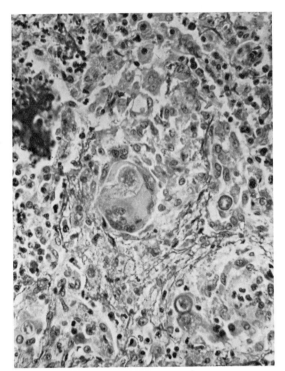

Figure 10–31. *Coccidioidomycosis — a rather typical tubercle-like granuloma.*

but, in about one in 500 cases, the infection is disseminated to other tissues and organs. This systemic or progressive coccidioidomycosis is a highly fatal disorder. The pulmonary form of the disease may be confined to involvement of only the hilar nodes, it may affect fan-shaped areas of lung parenchyma about the hilar nodes, or it may be more diffusely scattered through the lung substance.

Anatomically, the lesions consist of either focal suppurative abscesses that are entirely nonspecific in character save for the presence of the causative agent, or the development of rather characteristic, tubercle-like granulomas (Fig. 10–31). As these lesions progress or coalesce, large areas of cavitation and caseation evolve. Histologically, the tissue lesions appear as leukocytic infiltrates about areas of frank suppurative necrosis or as characteristic epithelioid granulomas replete with giant cells and central caseation. The Coccidioides may be found within the liquid exudate. The anatomic changes caused by this disorder, therefore, are similar to those found in North American blastomycosis and in tuberculosis. The recognition of such an infection depends upon the isolation or demonstration of *Coccidioides immitis*. When the disease enters a progressive form with hematogenous dissemination, similar foci of necrosis are found throughout the body in the spleen, liver, lymph nodes, bone, skin and occasionally the meninges. In the course of their healing, these lesions became calcified so that in many subclinical cases mysteriously developing calcifications appear in the lung parenchyma or elsewhere.

Positive coccidioidin skin tests have been found in as many as three-quarters of the population of some areas of the Southwest and California. Most of these individuals have not had a recognized clinical infection. When symptoms appear, they closely simulate those of tuberculosis, i.e., chills, fever, night sweats, weakness and weight loss, accompanied by a cough productive of mucopurulent sputum. This sputum may harbor the pathognomonic microorganisms and thus permit the appropriate diagnosis. When the fungi cannot be identified, the skin test may be of value, but obviously is of limited value in the endemic areas. In some patients, the infection is limited to skin lesions and is descriptively referred to as "the bumps." The prognosis in coccidioidomycosis is in general very good, but becomes increasingly grave with the systemic dissemination of the organism and the development of focal infections in the bones or central nervous system.

HISTOPLASMOSIS

Histoplasmosis, caused by *Histoplasma capsulatum*, is a highly communicable disease encountered in many parts of the world. All ages and all races are affected. The causative organism in tissues is a round to oval, budding, yeast-like fungus that varies between 2 and 4 microns in diameter. The disease is contracted by the inhalation of fungal spores that are usually phagocytized by intra-alveolar macrophages. Within these phagocytes, the spores germinate into yeast forms and rapidly multiply. A primary nonspecific pneumonitis develops, but is soon transformed into a granulomatous reaction, exactly resembling tuberculosis. Drainage to the hilar nodes further heightens the resemblance to the Ghon complex of tuberculosis. Usually, such primary pulmonary lesions spontaneously fibrose and calcify, and the nature of the lesion can only be suspected by a positive skin test to histoplasmin (a filtrate of the yeast culture). Occasionally systemic dissemination of such solitary pulmonary lesions occurs without significant clinical manifestations, yielding calcified lesions in the liver, spleen, nodes, brain and other viscera. In predisposed patients, particularly in infants, the pulmonary process is progressive and followed by massive dissemination of the yeast forms. In others, the primary lesion heals, only to become reactivated into clinically overt disease some years later (endogenous reinfection).

Hepatomegaly, splenomegaly and *generalized lymphadenopathy* may be seen in the acutely disseminated cases. Small, gray-white infiltrations can sometimes be distinguished on the cut surface of these organs. Adrenal, bone marrow, meningeal, kidney and gastrointestinal involvement are also present in such disseminated disease. Histologically, the infiltrates in all sites are composed of collections of macrophages and prominent hypertrophy of the reticuloendothelial cells. If the nodule is large, there may be central necrosis and, with the development of multinucleate giant cells, a striking similarity to tuberculosis results. The macrophages and reticuloendothelial cells usually contain large numbers of the round to oval, yeast-like forms (Fig. 10–32). The central necrosis in the histoplasma lesion is a bland, infarct-like necrosis that closely resembles caseation. Careful search for the fungal forms may be necessary to avoid misinterpretation of these lesions as tuberculous. Lymphoid hyperplasia characterizes the intestinal tract involvement, and usually the overlying mucosa ulcerates. These ulcers apparently develop from the progressive inflammatory enlargement of the lymphoid tissue of the mucosa with eventual ischemic necrosis of the overlying surface epithelium. As a consequence, the walls and bases of the ulcer are composed of masses of macrophages and reticuloendothelial cells, many of which are hugely distended with the fungi. Vegetative endocarditis has been recorded.

In the usual adult pulmonary form of the disease, the clinical manifestations closely resemble those of tuberculosis. Dissemination may masquerade as miliary tuberculosis. In immunodeficient adults or infants, acute dissemination is reflected in lymphadenopathy, splenohepatomegaly, anemia and leukopenia (simulating leukemia). In endemic regions, such as the Mississippi Valley, the finding of a single cavitary pulmonary lesion, or a calcified focus, must be strongly suspected as representing this disease.

Special mention should be made of the diagnostic use of bone marrow smears. In the widespread dissemination of the fungus, it is usually possible to identify fungi within phagocytic cells in the bone marrow on ordinary Giemsa or Wright's smears.

MONILIASIS (CANDIDIASIS)

Moniliasis is principally a superficial infection of the moist cutaneous areas of the body caused by *Candida (Monilia) albicans.* The most common sites of involvement are the mouth, urinary tract and the folds beneath the breast, axillae and perineum. Occasionally infections are also encountered between the toes and fingers, about the bases of the nails and around poor fitting dentures. Vulvovaginal candidiasis is an occasional complication of pregnancy and is sometimes encountered in young girls in apparent good health. Only rarely are the esophagus and respiratory tract affected.

The fungus is an extremely common inhabitant of the oral cavity and the skin of normal individuals. The basis for its initiation of clinical disease is obscure. Probably the affected individual is predisposed in some fashion to the low virulence of this fungus. Visceral infections are therefore classically encountered in *diabetes, lymphoma, leukemia, severe malnourishment, avitaminosis and in individuals who have received antibiotic, steroid or immunosuppressive therapy.* By the destruction of antibiotic-sensitive bacteria, uncontrolled growth of the Monilia is permitted. Of recent date, this disease is encountered frequently in drug addicts.

Moniliasis is called "thrush" when it occurs in the oral cavity. However, in all its mucocutaneous localizations, an apparently consistent pattern of reaction is followed. The lesions

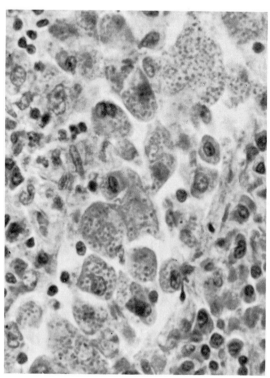

Figure 10–32. *Histoplasmosis in a lymph node. The central phagocytes are stuffed with histoplasma.*

consist of superficial, *confluent, white patches based upon a red, moist, inflammatory surface.* The white membrane is a diffuse mycelial growth of fungus which often penetrates deeply into the subjacent tissues. The resultant inflammatory reaction is slight and nonspecific. Secondary infection may modify this anatomic reaction.

In the particularly predisposed, systemic lesions may occur in the esophagus and respiratory tract. In the esophagus, long, slender, filamentous fungi penetrate deeply into the wall (Fig. 10–33). Thus, long, filamentous, basophilic, mycelial strands are found permeating the submucosa and muscularis, as though they were growing in a culture medium, with little accompanying inflammatory reaction. In the lung, focal, consolidative, granulomatous lesions that closely resemble those of tuberculosis result. Rarely, systemic dissemination of the Monilia produces lesions in other organs, and even vegetative endocarditis has been caused by these fungi. The diagnosis is usually readily evident from the characteristic white patches on the inflammatory surface. Identification of the filamentous mycelia or budding yeast-like forms in the absence of a capsule differentiates them from cryptococci

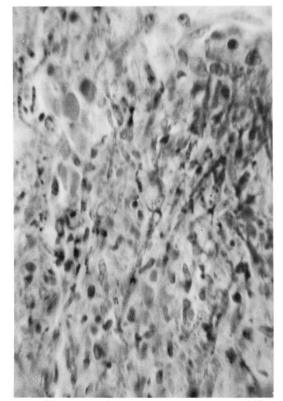

Figure 10–33. *Moniliasis of the esophagus with slender fungal filaments permeating the esophageal wall.*

and confirms the diagnosis. It should be remembered that the Monilia organisms are often secondary invaders in other infections and in these circumstances are presumably entirely saprophytic and play no role in the underlying disease. The mere presence then of *Candida albicans* in oral or pulmonary lesions does not necessarily indicate a primary monilial infection.

MUCORMYCOSIS

Mucormycosis infections are uncommon clinical problems caused by the Phycomycetes, ubiquitous fungi of low virulence. These infections have recently shown an increased incidence, because they tend to occur in chronically, frequently fatally, debilitated patients who are kept alive now by intensive therapy. In patients with severe diabetes, in terminal malignancy, in leukemic, lymphomatous and transplantation cases receiving chemotherapy, and in patients receiving broad-spectrum antibiotic therapy that suppresses competitive bacterial growth, these fungi are apparently able to invade and cause disease. The lungs, brain, paranasal sinuses and middle ear are favored sites of involvement. Presumably the fungus spreads from the last mentioned sites into the cranial vault.

The tissue lesions consist of foci of suppurative necrosis in which large, wide branching, *nonseptate* hyphae are readily demonstrated particularly with the periodic acid-Schiff staining technique. The fungi permeate the tissues and often invade vessels as though they were of high pathogenicity and invasiveness, but it must be remembered that these lesions only occur in the predisposed, debilitated patient. Occasionally, the fungi can be seen growing in tissues as in a culture medium without evoking an inflammatory reaction. The basis for this inconstant tissue reaction is obscure, but may only reflect the totally depressed responsiveness of a fatally ill patient.

ASPERGILLOSIS

Diseases caused by this fungus take one of two forms: trivial but persistent infections about the fingernails and toenails, or severe pulmonary and sometimes systemic infections. These more serious infections are almost always of an opportunistic nature. Curiously, aspergilli, mucormyetes and candida cause secondary infections superimposed on preexisting pulmonary disease or opportunistic infections more commonly than other far more virulent pathogens. Frequently, this fungal infection is encountered in sites of preexisting lung disease, such as nonspecific pulmonary abscesses, infarcts or bronchiectasis. The aspergillus grows with *septate* filaments branching at more acute angles than mucormycetes. Tangled masses of mycelia may produce so-called "fungus balls." Involvement of the lung may cause focal areas of consolidation or abscess cavities whose walls are diffusely permeated by the mycelia. Its presence should be suspected in any severely debilitated patient who suddenly takes a turn for the worse, and particularly in those on long-term, broad-spectrum antibiotic, steroid or immunosuppressive therapy.

PNEUMOCYSTOSIS

In premature infants and in particularly vulnerable adults, the *Pneumocystis carinii* may induce a curious interstitial pneumonitis accompanied by protoplasmic masses of the causative organism lying within the alveolar spaces. These masses are so amorphous they often resemble coagulated proteinous edema fluid. However, the septal wall mononuclear leukocytic infiltrate and the abundant macrophages surrounding these masses should suggest an inflammatory process. On careful examination under reduced light, the amorphous masses have a honeycombed appearance, which may require silver methenamine stains to more clearly highlight the organisms. With such special techniques, the parasitic masses, sometimes 50 microns in diameter, can be seen as aggregates of organisms quite similar to histoplasma. Although this agent is of extremely low virulence, it may lead to a fatal outcome because it attacks only when host resistance is severely depressed.

AMEBIASIS

Amebiasis is an infection by *Entamoeba histolytica*, primarily of the colon, followed in some cases by secondary spread to the liver, lungs and brain (Clark, 1925). The primary localization manifests itself principally by a chronic, remittent diarrhea, accompanied by variable constitutional symptoms. There is an age-old controversy about the prevalence of amebiasis and the meaning of amebic organisms in the stools of otherwise healthy individuals—carriers. In the United States, particularly in the southern regions, it is estimated that about 3 to 5 per cent of the population harbor amebas in their stools. Some would place the frequency at 10 per cent. The great preponderance of these individuals have no clinical manifestations. Careful studies of the stools in these cases have revealed that the amebas are unusually small and may, indeed, not represent *E. histolytica*. Some would classify such small forms as *E. hartmanni*. Large- and intermediate-sized amebas are probably found very infrequently in asymptomatic individuals. In most instances they are associated with intestinal lesions and clinical manifestations. In general, there is a linear relationship between the size of the motile form and its pathogenicity.

Man contracts the disease by ingesting cysts in contaminated food and water. These cysts may persist and be viable for prolonged periods, as long as adequate conditions of humidity prevail. Once ingested, the cysts pass the unfavorable environment of the stomach, and the cystic wall is dissolved in the alkaline contents of the small intestine, where the vegetative trophozoites emerge to parasitize the colon.

The cecum and ascending colon are affected most often, followed in order by the sigmoid and rectum. However, in severe, full-blown cases, the entire colon is involved along with the terminal segment of small intestine. The amebas invade the crypts of the colonic glands by virtue of their motility and elaborate *strong proteolytic enzymes* and *hyaluronidases* that lyse the surface epithelium. They then burrow through the tunica propria, but are usually halted in their forward progress by the muscularis mucosae. At this level, they fan out laterally to create an undermined minute ulceration having a *flask shape*, i.e., a narrow neck and broad base. As the undermining progresses, the overlying surface mucosa is deprived of its blood supply and sloughs. In this fashion, progressively larger ulcerations are produced that classically have undermined margins and fairly clean bases.

Histologically, a remarkable feature of the amebic ulcer is the *relative absence of inflammatory infiltration*. Since the destruction is caused by the cytolytic effects of the parasitic enzymes, the necrosis is essentially one of *chemical digestion* and is not accompanied by intense suppuration. However, usually some secondary bacterial infection modifies this histologic appearance. Characteristically, these ulcers do not penetrate the bowel wall and only rarely do they coalesce. Occasionally, however, such perforation does occur and an amebic peritonitis ensues. (For further details on the bowel lesion, reference may be made to Chapter 21.)

In about 40 per cent of autopsied cases of amebic colitis, trophozoites penetrate vessels and are drained to the liver to produce solitary or multiple discrete *abscesses*. These again result from local proteolysis of tissues with scant inflammatory reaction. The walls are composed of a shaggy fibrin lining surrounded by a scant fibrovascular response that is infiltrated with a few mononuclear leukocytes. Because of hemorrhage into the partially digested debris, the abscess cavities are filled with a chocolate, pasty material that is graphically represented as "anchovy paste." Secondary bacterial infection may convert these areas into frank suppurative abscesses. The lung may become involved, following the development of hepatic lesions, either by drainage of parasites through the blood vessels or by direct penetration through the liver capsule and diaphragm into the pleural cavities and then the lung parenchyma. Extension into the pericardial sac or the formation of bronchopleural or pulmonopleural fistulas occurs in this fashion. In other cases, the hepatic abscesses may spread into the kidney, stomach, duodenum or reenter the colon. From the lung, the brain may become secondarily involved and occasionally the meninges. In all its sites of localization, the reaction is that of local lysis of tissues accompanied by a scant inflammatory infiltrate principally of mononuclear cells.

The appropriate histologic diagnosis cannot be established by the character of the tissue changes alone. It is necessary to identify the trophozoites. These appear as large, round to oval, sometimes ameboid forms averaging 20 to 25 microns in diameter. It is to be remembered that the vegetative form contains a single nucleus that is small in comparison to the abundant, finely granular cytoplasm. One of the distinctive features of the pathogenic *E. histolytica* is its classic *tendency to engulf whole red cells* (Fig. 10–34). Since nonpathogenic amebas inhabit the colon, one cannot equate the finding of trophozoites with disease. Characteristically, nonpathogens do not phagocytize red cells.

Clinical manifestations may or may not appear in amebiasis dependent on the extent and severity of tissue lesions. In acute cases, symptoms may begin almost explosively a few days after infection. In others, the amebas may be of smaller size and produce only trivial lesions and few manifestations. As mentioned above, amebas of small size may be nonpathogenic and, indeed, represent a different species of protozoan.

Amebic colitis is reflected in a completely nonspecific form of dysentery with abdominal cramps, diarrhea and melena in certain cases. Constitutional symptoms may be minimal or absent. Localization in the liver may cause considerable enlargement of this organ and signs

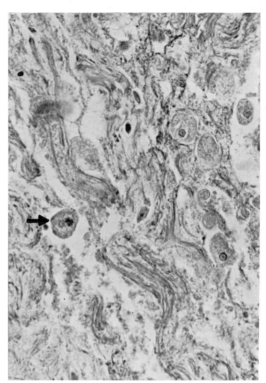

Figure 10–34. *Amebiasis of the colon—a histologic detail of the vegetative parasites is shown. The arrow points to an ameba with a phagocytized red cell.*

of hepatic insufficiency. Upper abdominal symptoms may indicate penetration of liver abscesses into the peritoneal cavity or subdiaphragmatic space. Respiratory symptoms, such as cough, chest pain and fever, develop in cases that involve the lung. Since secondary bacterial infection is almost inevitable in this organ, constitutional febrile reactions usually make their appearance in these cases. Occasionally patients with pulmonary abscesses cough up large amounts of characteristic pasty, brown material that may suggest the diagnosis, and parasites may be identified in such sputum. From the description of the anatomic lesions, it is evident that the leapfrog spread of this parasite may give rise to a varied and puzzling clinical disease.

MALARIA

Because of its world-wide distribution, malaria is one of the most important communicable diseases of man. It is estimated that between 15 and 20 million persons are affected around the world. At one time uncommon in Europe, Great Britain, Australia, New Zealand and the United States, this disease has been spread from endemic areas into regions where it was formerly little encountered, as a result of air travel and mass migration of military personnel. Four species of plasmodia commonly infect man. P. falciparum *is the most virulent and causes malignant tertian malaria or falciparum malaria.* P. vivax *and* P. ovale *cause benign tertian malaria, and* P. malariae *produces quartan malaria.* Recently *P. knowlesi,* a simian parasite, was identified as the cause of some cases of malaria. Man contracts the disease from the bite of an infected mosquito. Over 65 species of anopheline mosquitos may transmit the plasmodia. These insects acquire the plasmodia by biting an infected person and ingesting blood containing the sexual forms called gametocytes.

Details of the life cycle of the malarial parasite are beyond our scope and may be found in Marcial-Rojas (1971). Briefly, it has two phases: (1) asexual reproduction, or schizogony, which occurs in man and (2) sexual reproduction, or sporogony, which occurs in a female mosquito. Within the midgut of the mosquito, the gametocytes mature and form a zygote. The zygote releases sporozoites which penetrate into the body cavity of the mosquito eventually to reach the salivary glands. Thus the salivary secretion of the mosquito laden with sporozoites is injected with the bite of the insect.

Introduced into the blood of the new host, the sporozoites of the malarial parasite circulate briefly and then invade liver cells in the so-called preerythrocytic cycle. This comprises the incubation period of malaria before the parasites enter the blood and evoke the classic manifestations of fever and chills. The incubation periods for the four types of malaria are: *P. falciparum,* 8 to 20 days; *P. vivax,* 12 to 15 days; *P. malariae,* approximately 24 days; and *P. ovale,* 16 to 18 days. Within the liver, the sporozoites evolve through a sequence yielding a schizont, which ruptures the liver cell and frees cryptozoites to enter red cells. Within the erythrocyte, the parasite ingests hemoglobin and converts the heme portion to malarial pigment called hemozoin. During the erythrocytic cycle, further development can be seen yielding trophozoites, somewhat distinctive for each of the four forms of malaria. In this way, the specific form of malaria can be recognized in appropriately stained thick smears of the peripheral blood. For details on such parasitology, reference should be made to specialized texts. It suffices for our consideration to know that when the trophozoite is fully grown within the red cell, it divides into merozoites which rupture the erythrocyte and may then reenter other red cells to develop into gametocytes ready for the bite of the next mosquito. When, erythrocytes rupture, not only mero-

zoites are released but also malarial pigment, unused hemoglobin and, of course, the metabolites of the parasite. Liberation of these products initiates the chills and fever. More red cells are destroyed, however, than can be explained by parasitization alone, and it has been hypothesized that immune hemolytic processes may also be involved. Conceivably, antibodies developed against parasitized red cells destroy not only these red cells but also nonparasitized cells.

The distinctive clinical and anatomic features of malaria are related to the following. (1) The completion of the asexual life cycle in the erythrocyte releases showers of merozoites. This cycle is repeated approximately every 48 hours for *P. vivax,* 72 hours for *P. malariae,* and 36 hours for *P. falciparum.* The recurrent clinical spikes of fever and chills encountered in malaria may be timed with these cycles and thus occur daily or every 2, 3 or 4 days. (2) The red cell destruction causes anemia. (3) The malarial pigment released from the parasitized red cells is picked up by the reticuloendothelial system and gives rise to the marked pigmentation seen classically in the spleen, lymph nodes, liver and bone marrow. (4) The phagocytic defense mechanisms of the host lead to marked reticuloendothelial hyperplasia, reflected in splenomegaly, hepatomegaly and lymphadenopathy. (5) The parasitized red cells, particularly in *P. falciparum* malaria, plug the peripheral microcirculation and induce severe tissue hypoxemia or ischemic necrosis. This is particularly destructive in the small vessels of the brain. The malignant nature of falciparum malaria may be related to the production, during the preerythrocytic cycle, of vastly greater numbers of sporozoites than is encountered in the other forms of malarial disease; and so there is greater parasitization of red cells, more severe anemia and more severe microcirculatory blockade.

There are few data available on the anatomic changes in the benign forms of malaria, since these types are rarely fatal. It will be remembered that *P. vivax, P. malariae* and *P. ovale* all produce this pattern of disease. *P. falciparum* is a highly fatal type of malaria in which there are well described anatomic changes (Greaves, 1946). The *spleen* is the principal organ affected. Depending upon the duration of the infection and the patient's resistance, the spleen may undergo varying degrees of enlargement up to 1000 gm. or more. During the acute stage of the infection, the splenic enlargement is moderate and the substance hemorrhagic. The capsule is thin, predisposing to rupture. As the disease becomes more chronic, there is increased fibrosis and cellularity, creating a solid enlargement. The capsule is thickened, and on cross section the splenic substance is brown to gray-black and often has the consistency of dried cake—"ague cake."

Histologically, in the acute stages there are few specific changes other than marked congestion, along with hypertrophy and moderate phagocytic activity of the reticuloendothelial and reticulum cells. Parasites may be found within the erythrocytes in the splenic sinuses. In the chronic stages there is extreme congestion of the sinuses, particularly in falciparum malaria. Parasites are found within the red cells. There is considerable pigmentation of the hypertrophied reticuloendothelial cells, the phagocytes within the splenic sinuses and the reticulum cells within the splenic pulp. These enlarged phagocytic cells accumulate in great numbers to produce solid masses of heavily pigmented cells. The finely divided pigment is yellow-brown. When it accumulates, it assumes a brown-black, dense, granular appearance. Accompanying the phagocytosis of pigment, there is engulfment of parasites, leukocytic debris and red cell debris so that the entire spleen becomes transformed in time to a mass of phagocytic cells with markedly thickened fibrous trabeculae and capsule, and considerable compression and narrowing of the vascular sinusoids.

The *liver* is likewise enlarged in malaria. In acute malaria, this enlargement is only slight and is accompanied by considerable hyperemia. As the infection becomes more chronic or reinfections occur, the increase in size progresses and the organ becomes more firm and pigmented. The principal changes are found in the *Kupffer cells*, which are enlarged and hyperplastic. These become heavily laden with malarial pigment, parasites and cellular debris (Fig. 10–35). Pigment is rarely found in the parenchymal cells. The changes in the bone marrow and lymph nodes are of the same general nature. Phagocytic cells may be found dispersed throughout the body in the subcutaneous tissues, in the lung and in other sites, particularly when infection has overwhelmed the principal reitculoendothelial organs.

In malignant falciparum malaria, there are many changes in the *brain*. One of the most prominent features is *extreme congestion of the vessels* so that they become plugged with parasitized red cells. Such stasis is augmented by an increased stickiness of the erythrocytes. About these vessels, there are ring hemorrhages that are probably related to the weakening of the vessel walls and supporting contiguous tissue by local hypoxia incident to the vascular stasis.

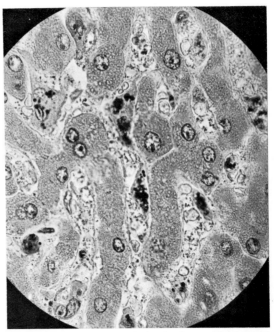

Figure 10–35. *Malaria in the liver with pigment-laden Kupffer cells.*

Small focal inflammatory reactions (called malarial or Dürck's granulomas) may occur about these vessels. These granulomas consist principally of a small focus of ischemic necrosis surrounded by a glial reaction. With more severe hypoxia, there is degeneration of ganglion cells, focal ischemic softenings and infarcts and occasionally a scant inflammatory infiltrate in the meninges. Nonspecific hypoxic focal lesions in the heart and kidneys may be induced by the progressive anemia and circulatory obstructions in chronically infected patients. The kidneys are often enlarged and congested and sometimes discolored by the hemozoin pigment. A dusting of pigment is often present in the glomeruli and the tubules frequently contain hemoglobin casts, particularly in falciparum malaria, hence the term "blackwater fever."

As has been mentioned, malaria may be relatively benign, particularly in those living in endemic areas with acquired immunity; or it may be a viciously fatal disease and kill within days (the malignant falciparum form). The patient experiences chills, fevers, sweats, muscular aches and pains, and classically severe headache. The fever is recurrent and takes the form of high spikes followed by severe, prostrating, shaking chills and drenching sweats. The spleen undergoes progressive enlargement along with the liver. Occasionally jaundice appears. For an indefinite period of time, the patient pursues this febrile course and then, in the usual course of events, undergoes spontaneous recovery, or is dramatically benefited by antimalarial drugs. These apparently benign courses are sometimes punctuated by sudden rupture of the spleen. Few patients, however, die of benign malaria. The acute malignant form of malaria may begin suddenly or slowly, but is rapidly progressive with the development of high fever, chills, convulsions, shock and vascular collapse with death. Death may occur within a few days or weeks, and is usually accompanied by extreme hyperpyrexia. Malaria may take one of several other clinical forms known as chronic malaria, the pattern usually encountered in native populations who have developed some resistance to this infection. In this pattern, the disease occurs as repeated attacks of benign malaria accompanied by progressive enlargement of the liver and spleen. It is in such patients as these that the most massive types of splenomegaly and hepatomegaly are encountered.

Blackwater fever is the dramatic complication which may occur during the course of malaria, usually of the falciparum type. It is found most often in the white man living in an endemic area. The syndrome may appear within weeks or not until a year after the onset of the disease. Characteristically, this complication is ushered in by the sudden onset of severe chills, fever, jaundice, vomiting, and the passage of dark red to black urine. Although the mechanism is poorly understood, there appears to be *sudden hemolysis of red cells with the liberation of great amounts of hemoglobin* into the serum. The excretion of this hemoglobin gives rise to the discoloration of urine. The massive production of bilirubin cannot be excreted by the liver, and jaundice therefore develops. The best treatment of all forms of malaria is prevention by the use of the now widely available antimalarial drugs.

LEISHMANIASIS

Three clinical patterns of disease are caused by three distinctive species of Leishmania. *Leishmania tropica* is responsible for *cutaneous leishmaniasis*, also known as *"oriental sore"*; *Leishmania braziliensis* causes *mucocutaneous leishmaniasis*; and *Leishmania donovani* is responsible for *visceral or systemic leishmaniasis*, better known as *kala-azar*. Only visceral leishmaniasis will be described.

Visceral leishmaniasis *(kala-azar)* may be categorized as a diffuse parasitization of the reticuloendothelial system of man by *L. donovani.* These parasites are readily visualized (with Giemsa stain) within RE cells and macrophages as round to oval bodies approximately 4 to 5 microns in diameter containing nuclei about 1 to 2 microns in diameter. The parasites literally stuff the phagocytic cells. The disease is encountered principally in Asia, the Middle East, about the Mediterranean, Africa and South America. The method of spread is thought to be through the bite of certain species of blood-sucking sandflies. The reservoir of infection is infected humans and dogs. Other mammals, such as squirrels and foxes, may also harbor the organisms.

The disease is principally characterized by profound splenomegaly, hepatomegaly, lymphadenopathy and parasitization of all phagocytic cells throughout the body. In addition, the lungs, gastrointestinal tract, kidneys, pancreas, testes, skin and other organs are also involved in florid cases. In all these organs, the phagocytic cells are markedly swollen and stuffed with parasites (Fig. 10–36). With the distention of the phagocytic cells and their proliferation, marked enlargement of affected organs may be anticipated. The spleen is most severely af-

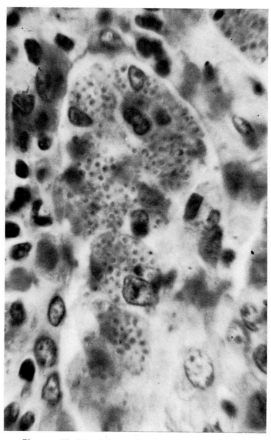

Figure 10–36. *Visceral leishmaniasis (kala-azar). Phagocytes within a lymph node are laden with the Leishmania.*

fected and may increase in weight up to 3 kilos or more. The capsule is thickened and the organ is hyperemic, dark red and firm. There is total loss of architectural detail, both macroscopically and microscopically. The dominant histologic pattern is that of total suffusion of the splenic substance by the distended phagocytic cells described. The liver is enlarged but relatively less severely than the spleen. The Kupffer cells in the liver show the principal pathognomonic alterations. The lymph nodes, bone marrow, and other sites mentioned may all present the characteristic stimulated growth of phagocytic cells.

The clinical course is one of constitutional reaction to the parasitic invasion in the form of fever, weakness and weight loss. The striking *visceromegaly* becomes apparent in the long chronicity of this infection. Presumably because of the bone marrow involvement, anemia and leukopenia become progressively more severe in these cases and 80 to 90 per cent of untreated patients die of intercurrent infections incident to the granulocytopenia. The diagnosis depends upon the identification of the causative agent either by its cultivation or in histologic sections.

TRYPANOSOMIASIS

Trypanosomiasis, also known as *"sleeping sickness,"* is a parasitic disease caused by a variety of trypanosomes that is endemic in Central Africa. *Chagas disease* (p. 687) of South America is a closely related trypanosomal infection. These parasites appear in man as slender, spindle-shaped organisms, approximately 15 microns in length and 1 to 3 microns in width, having a central nucleus and a flagellum with an undulating membrane. The parasites are inoculated into man by the bite of the *tsetse fly*, which is required for the extramammalian completion of the life cycle of the parasite. The inoculated parasites circulate and, in African cases, localize principally in the *lymph nodes and brain.* The lymph nodes are heavily parasitized and become enlarged, soft and hyperemic.

Histologically, the nodes have the striking reticuloendothelial hypertrophy and hyperplasia that are found in kala-azar, and these cells are filled with the parasites. In the brain, there is thickening of the meninges and diffuse cerebral edema with multiple scattered petechiae and hemorrhages throughout the brain substance. The meninges and perivascular spaces contain both mono- and polymorphonuclear leukocytes; the vessels often have marked endothelial thickening, sometimes to the point that the lumina are virtually occluded. These vascular occlusions presumably give rise to the ring hemorrhages and microinfarcts described. In the foci of brain damage, there is a glial reaction and the appearance of so-called "morular cells." These are altered mononuclear cells which have ingested large amounts of fatty debris, to produce peripheral vacuoles which project to give the cell a mulberry-like appearance. In florid infections, other organs and viscera are parasitized, particularly the liver and spleen.

In Africa the trypanosomal neural alterations are responsible for the clinical infection known as "sleeping sickness," whereas in Central and South America the trypanosomal infection manifests itself principally by a diffuse *myocarditis* (p. 687). The parasites localize within muscle cells of the myocardium to cause their distention and eventual rupture, changes accompanied by a heavy mononuclear leukocytic infiltration. The serous cavities of the body contain a cloudy transudate, and there is in some cases focal brain damage followed by glial proliferation somewhat reminiscent of that described in African sleeping sickness.

TOXOPLASMOSIS

Toxoplasmosis is a world-wide common disorder caused by an obligate intracellular protozoan, *Toxoplasma gondii.* The organism is round, ovoid or crescent-shaped and usually measures about 5×2.5 microns. It has a basophilic cytoplasm and a prominent nucleus. Transmission of this disease to man has only recently been clarified (Frenkel et al., 1970). The definitive host appears to be cats. Their excretion of oocysts provides a possible fecal-oral pathway of spread of the disease to man. Intermediate hosts such as cattle, sheep and pigs may likewise acquire the disease from contaminated grass and fodder bearing the oocysts. Man may then be infected by eating inadequately cooked meat. Carnivorism among animals may spread the disease widely to many species. Transplacental infection also occurs in man, inducing a congenital form of this disease.

Toxoplasma are capable of survival and replication within virtually any cell type encountered in the human host. The oocyst lodges in the bowel mucosa, germinates and releases organisms which are spread through the blood. In this dissemination, no organ or tissue is spared (Fig. 10–37). Nonetheless, the clinical manifestations span a wide range of severity, depending on natural resistance, acquired immunity, and the development of delayed hypersensitivity following exposure to the parasite. Thus, toxoplasmic infections range from asymptomatic to fatal. Acute generalized toxoplasmosis is usually manifested by

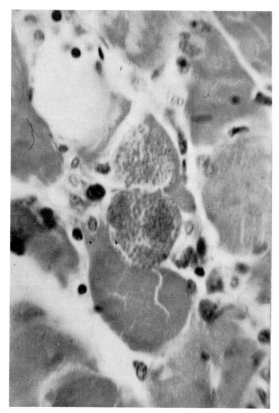

Figure 10–37. *Toxoplasmosis in parasitized skeletal muscle.*

a rash, involvement of the lungs, heart, skeletal muscles, liver, brain, retina and choroid. Parasitized cells are destroyed by the proliferation of trophozoites. An inflammatory infiltrate is found in these foci composed of macrophages and rare neutrophils. Reticuloendothelial hyperplasia and lymphadenopathy are prominent features of systemic toxoplasmosis. The changes in the lung take the form of an interstitial pneumonitis and are therefore quite similar to those seen in viral pneumonia. In the central nervous system, the basic lesion is a microglial nodule at sites of localization of the parasites.

Infants infected in utero tend to have subacute disease, probably because of passively transferred immunity. The major systems affected here are the brain, retina and choroid, once again with focal aggregations of mononuclear cells. Such lesions may eventually become fibrotic and calcified. The chorioretinitis, whether in infants or children, is usually bilateral and is made distinctive by the appearance of macular lesions in the retina. Diffuse myocardial lesions may cause cardiomegaly.

It is apparent that toxoplasmosis is a multisystem disorder with protean manifestations.

Among the major involvements are those of the brain, heart and lung, which can, indeed, lead to death. The diagnosis can be suspected often by the bilateral chorioretinitis, but the definitive diagnosis requires isolation of parasites (from blood, sputum, spinal fluid or diseased tissue) or the demonstration of elevated specific antibody titers.

DISEASES CAUSED BY HELMINTHS (WORMS)

Helminthic diseases are, relatively speaking, quite uncommon in industrialized nations but still are found in the Near and Far East, Africa, and Central and South America. In the United States, these conditions (with the possible exception of trichinosis) used to be localized principally to the southern regions. However, with the migratory movements of populations and with the popularity of travel, a significant change in the distribution of helminthic diseases is occurring in the United States. In a recent study by Birch and Anast (1957), it was shown that while the incidence of certain parasitic infections has remained relatively stable over the years, diseases caused by hookworm and whipworm and certain of the schistosome infections have increased remarkably in the northern cities. Only a brief survey of these disorders is given here, and for greater detail, reference should be made to Marcial-Rojas (1971).

TRICHINOSIS

Trichinosis is a common disease throughout the world contracted by eating meat containing viable cysts of *Trichinella spiralis*. The parasite principally localizes within the striated muscles and brain, and therefore classically evokes generalized muscular aches and pains, difficulty in respiration, and varying central nervous system derangements (Gould, 1945). However, the heart, lungs, liver and kidney, as well as other structures, are affected in severe infections. The disease is transmitted by the ingestion of inadequately cooked meat, principally pork, and despite our rather complete knowledge of methods for controlling this parasitic disease, it is still widely prevalent.

The parasite infects a wide variety of carnivores and herbivores. The chief reservoir for man is infected swine. About 5 per cent of pigs fed on uncooked garbage are infected in the United States. The larvae of the parasite encyst within the muscles of these infected animals and are ingested by man. After being released by the proteolytic digestion of the meat in the stomach, the larvae emerge and attach themselves to the mucosa of the duodenum, where, in active clinical cases, they can sometimes be found. These larvae mature into adult worms. After copulation, the female penetrates the wall of the duodenum down to and sometimes into the muscularis. About one week later, a host of larvae are produced that penetrate lymphatics or capillaries, and are drained to the lung and thence through the heart to the systemic circulation. In this fashion, the entire body is exposed. The larvae may then emerge from the capillaries to invade many sites. The striated muscles are the most suitable environment for their survival. *The heaviest infections are thus found in the diaphragm and in the gluteus, pectoral, deltoid, gastrocnemius and intercostal muscles. The extraocular muscles and muscles of the larynx may also be involved. The heart is also invaded.* It is of interest that the most active muscles in the body, depleted of glycogen, appear to be the most vulnerable. The serous cavities and central nervous system are additional favored sites of localization although no tissue is immune.

In the skeletal muscles, the larvae penetrate a muscle fiber and, in the early stages of the disease, destroy the involved cell and thus evoke an inflammatory reaction, characterized principally by lymphocytes and *eosinophils.* The adjacent cells may undergo hyaline coagulative degeneration or necrosis. These acute reactions are sometimes grossly visible as focal pale or hyperemic areas. As the disease becomes chronic, the focus becomes scarred, and in *voluntary muscles a cystic wall is deposited about the coiled larva* (Fig. 10–38). The wall of this cyst becomes calcified usually about one-half to two years after the invasion. It is highly significant that the encysted larvae remain viable for periods of up to 10 years or more. This chronic stage is sometimes grossly evident as foci of pale gray-white calcification.

The striated muscle fibers of the heart react somewhat differently. Here the acute inflammatory changes may be found during the early stages of the infection, along with a patchy but widely scattered interstitial myocarditis, *but the larvae do not become encysted.* Instead they undergo necrosis and therefore cannot be identified. The inflammatory pattern is fairly nonspecific save for the prominence of eosinophils and ultimately eventuates in fibrous scarring. Invasion of the central nervous system is usually reflected by a diffuse lymphocytic and mononuclear infiltration in the leptomeninges and by the development of focal gliosis in and about the small capillaries of the brain sub-

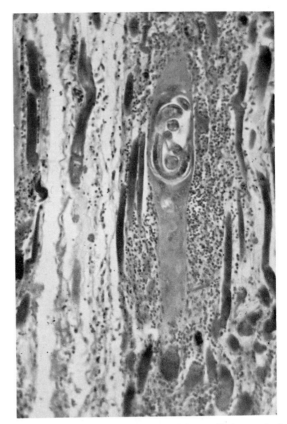

Figure 10–38. Trichinosis with a coiled encysted parasite within the skeletal muscle.

stance infiltrated with lymphocytes and eosinophils. Often, living or necrotic larvae can be identified within the inflammatory nodule. Focal inflammations have been described in the other sites mentioned, particularly in the lungs. In addition there may be fatty change of the liver cells and epithelial cells of the renal tubules, but it is probable that these alterations do not represent direct parasitic invasion. Conceivably these parenchymal alterations may be due to an accompanying malnutrition or deficiency state, perhaps potentiated or aggravated by the helminthic invasion.

In the majority of clinical cases, a history of the ingestion of improperly cooked pork products can be obtained. This exposure can be easily controlled. Trichinae are killed by cooking at a minimum temperature of 140° F. for at least 30 minutes per pound of meat. Freezing of the meat for 20 days at a temperature of 5° F. (minus 15° C.) will effectively destroy the trichinae. Unfortunately, about 30 per cent of the available meat supply in the United States is not under supervision. There is a widespread misconception that smoking and pickling of meats destroy the trichinae, and it is unfortunately such smoked and pickled meats that are frequently eaten in an inadequately cooked form.

The clinical symptoms of trichinosis are extremely varied and often the case has progressed beyond the acute stage at the time of discovery. The period of invasion of the intestinal mucosa is usually marked by vomiting and diarrhea, symptoms that suggest "food intoxication." During the hematogenous dissemination and the muscular invasion, widespread aches and pains and fever appear. Movement of the eyes and breathing and swallowing may be painful; patients often complain of backache and aching pain in the legs. Often the invasion of the lung evokes cough and dyspnea. The dyspnea is materially contributed to by the involvement of the muscles of respiration. The central nervous system invasion leads to headaches, disorientation, delirium and a variety of other signs and symptoms strongly suggestive of a diffuse encephalitis. Cardiac failure may appear when the myocardial injury is severe. Often, however, the patient only seeks attention some time later because of the persistent muscular aches and pains.

After the third week of the disease, precipitin, complement fixation and flocculation tests are positive except in overwhelming disease. A skin test is available. Two of the most helpful diagnostic features are: (1) muscle biopsy, best taken from the tendinous insertion of the deltoid or gastrocnemius muscles, and (2) an eosinophilia in the peripheral blood. This may be sufficiently striking to account for 70 per cent of the total circulating white count.

The mortality rate of this condition is low, but overwhelming infection may cause death when patients with severe involvement of the respiratory muscles develop intercurrent pulmonary bacterial infections.

STRONGYLOIDIASIS

Strongyloidiasis is a parasitic infection almost limited to the intestinal tract, caused by *Strongyloides stercoralis.* This thin, thread-like worm invades the body by penetration of the skin or buccal mucosa. On penetration, the larvae evoke a very scant local inflammatory reaction and then enter vessels to be carried to the lungs. They burrow out of the lung capillaries into the alveolar spaces, migrate up the respiratory tree, and are swallowed. By the time they reach the duodenum, they have achieved sexual maturity. The fertilized female burrows into the intestinal mucosa, usually at the level of the duodenum or jejunum, and here evokes its major damage. While attached to the duodenal mucosa, the female lays eggs which de-

velop into infective larvae. Passed with the stools, they may then infect new hosts or reinfect the original host, particularly in the perianal region. The stool-borne larvae may also pass through several free-living cycles in warm, moist soil so that they do not require a human host to complete their life cycle. The mature female is approximately 2 mm. in length and 25 to 75 microns in width. The smaller filariform stages usually average 400 × 15 microns.

The major anatomic changes are produced usually in the duodenum and jejunum, the skin at the site of entry, and the lungs through which the worms pass. The *mucosa of the affected bowel* is hyperemic, edematous and, in the more intense infections, has focal or confluent ulcerations. The parasites can be identified in the crypts of Lieberkühn and in the mucosa, and deposited eggs are sometimes present in the depths of these burrows (Fig. 10–39). The inflammatory reaction is quite variable, and only in the more severe instances is there a mixed leukocytic infiltration, characteristically containing many eosinophils. Much of this infiltration may be attributable to secondary infection. In the long chronicity of this intestinal infection, intestinal fibrosis may occur. The parasitic invasion only rarely extends below the muscularis mucosae. *At the skin site of entry,* a local inflammatory reac-

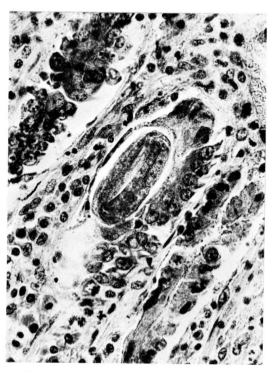

Figure 10–39. Strongyloidiasis in the duodenal mucosa with a central coiled parasite.

tion ensues, similar to that in the bowel. If larvae are trapped here, considerable fibrosis may ensue. Often the invasion of blood vessels is attended by a local petechial rash. Occasionally the parasites may, as they migrate out of the pulmonary vessels, evoke *focal minimal changes in the lungs in the form of intra-alveolar hemorrhages, and inflammatory infiltrations* that create small areas of pneumonic consolidation. Some of these larvae may invade the mucosa of the respiratory tree.

The clinical manifestations of this condition relate principally to the intestinal tract and lung. When the parasites emerge from the lung, they cause bronchial irritation, cough and mucous, bloody sputum. Often the parasites can be identified within the sputum. In the intestinal tract, they produce epigastric pain. Occasionally the parasites invade lower levels of the bowel, such as the ileum and colon, and give rise to abdominal cramps and diarrhea. Melena is a common accompaniment. As with most parasitic infections, there is a striking eosinophilia in the peripheral blood.

The final diagnosis rests upon the identification of the filariform larvae in the sputum or stools.

OXYURIASIS (ENTEROBIASIS)

Oxyuriasis is a world-wide, relatively insignificant parasitic infection almost completely limited to the appendix, ileum and cecum. The causative agent is *Enterobius vermicularis*, a pinworm that inhabits the intestinal tract of humans (Fig. 10–40). The females deposit their eggs about the anus and these eggs are then transferred to new hosts by fecal-oral contamination. Within the intestinal tract, the eggs mature and the worms attach themselves to the mucosa of the cecum, ileum and appendix. Here they may cause minimal inflammatory reactions, but sometimes when the parasite invades the superficial mucosa, it evokes a chronic granulomatous response characterized by abundant eosinophils (Symmers, 1950). A severe inflammatory reaction is rarely produced and pinworms are usually found incidentally in appendices removed for other causes. Infrequently, symptoms of appendicitis, or cramps and diarrhea, attend this parasitization. The mature worms about the anus may cause considerable pruritus and discomfort. Rarely these parasites may ascend the female genital tract to evoke endometritis, salpingitis and rarely peritonitis. The granulomatous reaction in these sites closely simulates tuberculosis. As found in tissue lesions, the adult worm approximates 10 mm. in length and about 0.5 mm. in width.

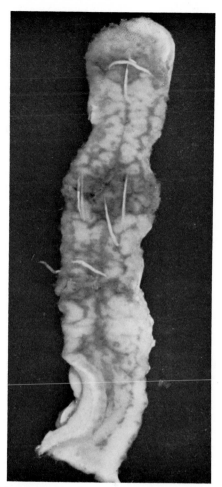

Figure 10–40. *Pinworms (oxyuriasis) in the appendix.*

FILARIASIS

Filariasis is a multipatterned, tropical parasitic infection caused by several forms of filaria. Each form of filariasis is caused by a specific parasite. In the usual usage of the term, reference is intended to Bancroft's filariasis, caused by the *Wuchereria bancrofti* The less common forms of filariasis are onchocerciasis, produced by *Onchocerca volvulus*, and loaiasis, caused by *Loa loa*.

Bancroft's filariasis is a chronic insidious disease that usually manifests itself by progressive lymphedema of the lower extremities and external genitalia. The infection is usually introduced by the bite of an infected mosquito (Culex, Aedes or Anopheles). These mosquitoes are themselves infected by biting persons with clinically active cases. The microfilaria, transmitted by the infected mosquito, penetrate deeply into the skin and permeate lymphatics and blood vessels. They are thus dispersed throughout the body and, by preference, localize in the lymph vessels and nodes, particularly about the external genitalia and in the groins. Here adult worms mature and the fertilized females discharge microfilariae. After a long period of latency that may last for months, the microfilariae reenter the blood vessels to be again available for infestation of the insect vector. The mature female filariae measure up to 100 mm. in length and 0.3 mm. in width. Mature males are about one-third this size. The microfilariae are much smaller, in the range of 200 × 100 microns.

The anatomic manifestations of filariasis stem from the localization of adult parasites in the lymph vessels and nodes. At these sites of localization, an inflammatory reaction ensues characterized by hyperplasia of the lymphatic endothelium and a perilymphatic infiltrate of eosinophils and other mononuclear leukocytes. In time, as the worms die and become necrotic, a surrounding fibroproliferative response evokes a small granuloma, complete with epithelioid and giant cells. The active inflammation is eventually replaced by scars that cause extensive obstruction of the lymphatics and retrograde sclerosis of the dependent lymph channels. Chronic lymphedema thus develops in the affected parts. This lymphedema leads to *elephantiasis* which is a late manifestation of cases that are chronically involved or have repeated infection. In the classic form with inguinal involvement, a brawny, tense edema involves the lower legs and genitalia (Fig. 10–41). With the persistence of this edema, subcutaneous fibrosis develops and is accompanied by marked thickening and hyperkeratosis of the overlying skin. As a consequence of the impairment of the blood supply, the skin is particularly vulnerable to trauma and infections, and these often complicate the anatomic lesions. Filariae may be found in dilated lymph vessels, in the centers of the focal granulomas, and in the lymphoid tissues in the areas of hel-

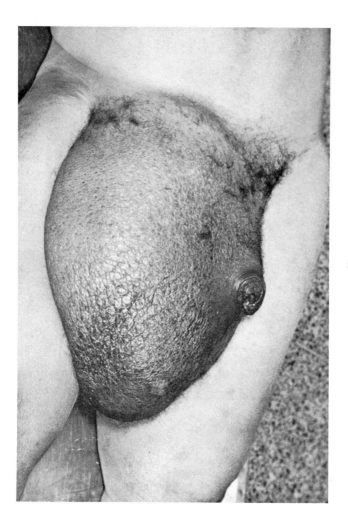

Figure 10–41. *Elephantiasis of the scrotum due to filariasis.*

minthic localization. Occasionally the worms die in situ and are calcified.

Onchocerciasis occurs in parts of Africa and in Guatemala and Mexico. It is transmitted by a Simulium species of small fly that serves as the vector from man to man. The African form is usually manifested by localization of the filariae in the subcutaneous tissues overlying bony protuberances, particularly in the lower extremities. The Central American form usually affects the scalp; however, many overlapping patterns are encountered. The localizations are followed by the development of small, subcutaneous, tumor-like, fibrous masses that serve as reservoirs of parasites (Fig. 10–42). Microfilariae escape from these tumors and migrate through the skin and subcutaneous tissues and frequently congregate in the corneal conjunctiva, eyeball and optic nerve, particularly in the form seen in Mexico. Thus, onchocerciasis may lead to disturbances in vision or total blindness.

Loaiasis is an African disease that is also distinctive in the localization of the filariae. The *Loa loa* is also known as the "eye-worm." This parasite lives in the subcutaneous tissues, but has a particular predilection for migrating through the skin and dermis across the temporal region, under the corneal epithelium, and thence across the bridge of the nose to cross the other eye. It may also migrate from these sites down the neck and through the subcutaneous tissues of the trunk. In its pathway, it sets up a transient inflammatory reaction but does not evoke the progressive fibrosis characteristic of Bancroft's filariasis.

ANCYLOSTOMIASIS (HOOKWORM DISEASE)

Hookworm disease is a clinical condition caused by infection with *Ancylostoma duodenale* or *Necator americanus.* These worms characteristically become attached to the intestinal mucosa, usually at the level of the duodenum, and principally cause an anemia. The disease is prevalent in both tropical and temperate climes. In the United States, it is encountered principally along the Atlantic seaboard and in the mining regions in and about Tennessee and Kentucky.

Larvae or eggs are deposited in soil. The filariform larvae that hatch from the eggs penetrate the skin, and then follow a pathway which is quite identical to that involved in strongyloidiasis. At the local site of skin penetration, a slight transient inflammatory reaction or a very intense, persistent "ground" itch ensues. The larvae then enter a capillary in the dermis and are carried to the lung. They then penetrate into the pulmonary alveoli, and migrate up the bronchi and trachea to be swallowed. In the small intestine, they develop into adults. Here the large parasites (approximately 10 × 0.1 to 0.4 mm.) attach themselves to villi, usually in the duodenum, by large gaping buccal cavities which suck in an intestinal villus. The worms secrete a toxic fluid which ruptures vessels within the villus, permitting them to suck blood continuously and thus obtain their oxygen and glucose requirements. At the same time, the mucosal lesion bleeds. It is estimated that a host may lose as much as 100 ml. of blood daily. Since the hookworm has a life span of several years, heavy infestation may account for considerable loss of blood. The female hookworm lays thousands of eggs per day which, deposited in soil, may develop to produce infective stages for a new host.

The anatomic lesions stem from the local invasion of the intestinal mucosa, the passage through the lungs and the chronic blood loss. The wall of

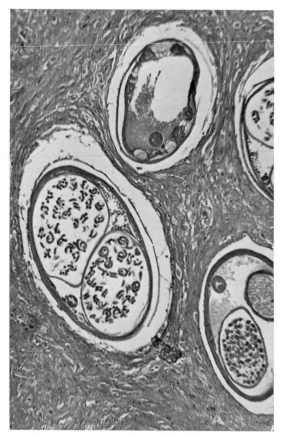

Figure 10–42. *Onchocerciasis* (Onchocerca volvulus) *with gravid filaria enclosed in a subcutaneous fibrous nodule.*

the jejunum is thickened by edema, principally localized to the submucosa. The parasites are often readily visualized in situ. Surrounding these parasites, there is mononuclear and eosinophilic infiltration. Often there is ulceration and even frank gangrene of the mucosal epithelium. Inflammatory changes are found in the lymphatics of the mucosa and the regional nodes. Focal hemorrhages or inflammations are caused in the lungs. Classically, the patients are markedly anemic and have low serum iron levels because of the blood loss. The bone marrow may be hyperactive owing to a compensatory erythropoiesis. Almost always, other forms of worms, malnutrition and bacterial infections plague these individuals and collectively are responsible for considerable retardation of development, not only somatic but also sexual and mental. The diagnosis of this condition rests upon the identification of eggs in the stools.

ASCARIASIS

Ascariasis is a world-wide helminthic infection caused by a giant roundworm, *Ascaris lumbricoides.* The adult worm ranges from 15 to 30 cm. in length and 3 to 5 mm. in diameter. Eggs are deposited on the soil, and fecal contamination permits the parasite to be swallowed by a new host. The larvae develop in the duodenum or jejunum, penetrate the mucosa, enter the lymphatics or blood vessels, to be drained to the lungs, then emerge from the alveolar capillaries, migrate up the respiratory tree, to be swallowed into the intestinal tract. Unlike the larvae of the hookworms or Strongyloides, these larvae do considerable damage to the lung and often evoke a marked hemorrhagic and inflammatory reaction, which resembles a viral pneumonitis or an eosinophilic interstitial infiltrate referred to as *Loeffler's syndrome.* During the lung migration, the parasites may also produce apparent hypersensitivity reactions, which resemble bronchial asthma and diffuse peribronchitis and peribronchiolitis. In the intestinal tract, the worms cause a slight inflammatory reaction, characterized by a submucosal and mucosal infiltrate of lymphocytes, plasma cells and eosinophils. Occasionally, the organisms penetrate the intestinal wall and give rise to peritonitis. At other times, they may obstruct the biliary tract and excretory ducts of the pancreas. Occasionally, especially in children, the giant adult worms may become coiled upon themselves to produce partial or complete intestinal obstruction. The combination of malnutrition (so prevalent in those affected),

bacterial infections, and a heavy worm load may cause severe retardation of growth in children, accompanied by considerable mental retardation. The diagnosis is made by recovery of the eggs in the feces and sometimes by the isolation of fragments of the worm.

SCHISTOSOMIASIS

Schistosomiasis is a multiform, tropical, parasitic infection produced by the schistosomes or blood flukes. These principally involve the intestinal tract, urinary bladder and liver. Three species of schistosomes produce disease in man: *Schistosoma mansoni* (intestinal and visceral involvement), *S. japonicum* (intestinal and visceral involvement) and *S. haematobium* (bladder involvement). Schistosomes are not transmitted from man to man. Since the disease characteristically involves the intestines and the bladder, eggs escape in the feces and urine and, when deposited in fresh water, mature into larval forms that pass through a developmental period in snails and then emerge as infective cercariae. These cercarial forms become attached to man during swimming, wading or bathing. They penetrate the skin and enter peripheral capillaries, then drain to the lung and eventually squeeze through the alveolar capillaries to gain access to the systemic circulation. Only those which enter the mesenteric arteries and pass through the portal venous system survive. Within the portal blood, they develop into adolescent flukes and migrate against the flow out to the periphery of the portal venous drainage system. *S. japonicum* typically penetrates through the superior mesenteric venules and thus affects principally the small bowel. *S. mansoni* typically accumulates in the venules of the large bowel, and *S. haematobium* reaches the hemorrhoidal or pudendal veins through the inferior mesenteric vessels, and thence passes into the pelvic and vesical veins. *S. mansoni* and *S. japonicum* also drain in the direction of the portal flow to involve the liver.

The anatomic lesions of schistosomiasis can be divided into those of the bladder and intestine and those of the liver. In the *bladder and intestine,* the adult female deposits eggs within the small venules. Soon after larvae develop within the eggs and, when fully embryonated, these secrete active ferments that ooze through the external covering of the egg to injure the surrounding venule (Fig. 10–43). Thus weakened and subject to the obstructive effect of the eggs, the venules rupture, permitting escape of the embryos into the perivascular tissues of the small intestine, colon and bladder. Some of

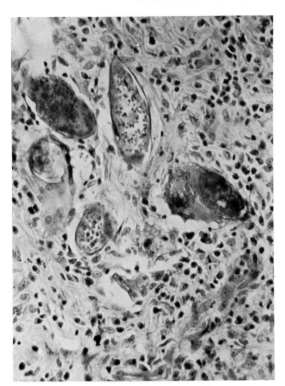

Figure 10-43. Vesical schistosomiasis with fully embryonated ova in the wall of urinary bladder.

these eggs erode through the mucosa of the bowel or bladder and are discharged in the excreta; others remain in the tissues. These mucosal perforations are responsible for the melena and hematuria associated with schistosomal infections.

The eggs excite an intense inflammatory reaction composed of an infiltrate of leukocytes, including eosinophils, accompanied by intense edema and hyperemia. When this reaction is close to the mucosal surface, there is extensive necrosis, ulceration and sloughing. In the deeper levels, the parasites evoke an intense inflammatory reaction (abscess formation) followed later by a chronic granulomatous proliferative response. Similar changes are found in the mesenteric lymph nodes, mesentery, and wherever the parasites are localized. *Following the chronic inflammatory reaction, there is often an intense inflammatory hyperplasia of the mucosa that may progress to the stage of forming polyps or carcinomas of the bladder and colon.* In the *liver,* the inflammatory reaction is at first an acute leukocytic infiltrate, then a chronic granulomatous response similar to that described in the bowel, followed in time by fibrous scarring. Often these scars as well as small white nodules of parasitic inflammatory reaction are visible in the liver parenchyma. These lesions do not create the diffuse fibrosis

of the more common types of cirrhosis but nonetheless may, in the aggregate, cause deformity of the liver and an increase in its consistency. Eggs and larvae, dead and viable, are found within these foci of reaction in all the sites of localization. The diagnosis of this condition is made by the demonstration of eggs and parasites in the feces and urine. The females average 20 mm. in length and 2 mm. in width. The eggs are ovoid in shape and are about 100×50 microns, although there is some variation between those of the different species.

CESTODIASIS (CESTODE OR TAPEWORM INFECTIONS)

Tapeworms are, in general, extremely large, flat worms that may achieve lengths of 10 to 20 feet. They are composed of thousands of rectangular proglottids that articulate with each other. Thirty or more species of tapeworms are responsible for human disease. Human tapeworm infections take one of two forms. (1) Those in which the mature worm is attached to the intestinal wall, producing so-called intestinal cestodiasis and (2) those in which the larval forms invade the organs of the body to produce so-called visceral and somatic cestodiasis. The first category will be discussed under the heading of intestinal cestodiasis. The visceral disorders discussed here are cysticercosis and echinococcosis.

Intestinal Cestodiasis. Among the many tapeworms, six in particular may cause intestinal disease in man: *Taenia saginata* (beef tapeworm), *T. solium* (pork tapeworm), *Hymenolepis nana* (dwarf tapeworm), *H. diminuta* (rat tapeworm), *Diphyllobothrium latum* (fish tapeworm) and *Echinococcus granulosus* (dog tapeworm). Disease caused by these parasites is world-wide in distribution and is usually contracted by the ingestion of undercooked meat or fish. The meat of these animals contains encysted eggs which, in the intestinal tract, mature into embryos that burrow onto the mucosa and at the same time attach themselves to the bowel wall by scolices which bear hooks. The mature worm then progressively develops to the extraordinary lengths mentioned above. Clinical manifestations may arise from: the number and mass of worms present, the trauma to the mucosa produced at the sites of intestinal attachment, and reactions to the metabolites of the worms. Thus, occasionally intestinal obstruction results. Abdominal pain and diarrhea, and indeed a syndrome closely resembling gallbladder disease comprise another possible symptom complex. Systemic manifestations including dizziness, restlessness and occasionally convulsions have been described. These are attributed to the production of toxic substances by the parasites. However, in some patients, tapeworms are present, manifested by the passage of proglottids in the stools, but no clinical signs or symptoms are evoked.

The diagnosis of intestinal cestodiasis is usually made by the finding of proglottids in the stools. Identification of the specific worm or worms involved depends upon the detailed examination of the proglottid, looking for distinctive morphologic features, detailed in Marcial-Rojas (1971). In some patients, the diagnosis is made by the identification of eggs in the stools and, rarely, by roentgenography (with contrast media) outlining the large tapeworms.

Cysticercosis. Cysticercosis is an infection in man produced by the ingestion usually of the cysts *(Cysticercus cellulosae)*, of the pork tapeworm, *T, solium.* Several isolated cases have been reported of similar infections by *T. saginata,* the beef tapeworm. The larvae, through one of the several pathways to be described, invade the wall of the small intestine and are hematogenously disseminated to all the tissues of the body with subsequent inflammatory reactions in the sites of localization. Man may swallow the cyst of *T. solium* by fecal contamination of food or by anus-to-mouth contamination, or the cysts may be regurgitated upward into the stomach in a patient who harbors the adult worms in the intestinal tract. When these cysts reach the upper levels of the small intestine, they hatch out the larval forms, which then penetrate the mucosa of the bowel and eventually permeate the mesenteric veins and lymphatics. They traverse the pulmonary capillaries and are thus carried to all the organs and tissues.

The cysticerci develop in any soft tissue, including the skin, subcutaneous tissues, muscles, heart, brain, liver, lungs and eyes. Each larva develops within the soft tissues into a small, thin, translucent cyst. The cyst evokes an inflammatory reaction, which is characterized by large numbers of eosinophils and polymorphonuclear neutrophils. The worms may eventually die in situ and excite a further inflammatory reaction, characterized by fibroblastic proliferation and giant cell and granuloma formation, eventuating in focal granulomas followed by calcifications. When these foci of inflammation occur in certain soft tissues of the body, they are without significance. However, when the heart valves, the orbit or the brain is invaded, important functional derangements may follow. The central nervous system manifestations usually take the form of jacksonian epilepsy. It is reported that about one in ten patients in Mexico who require brain surgery for the relief of epileptiform seizures is found to have cerebral cysticercosis.

Echinococcosis (Hydatid Disease). Echinococcosis, or hydatid disease, is caused by the larvae of the dog tapeworm, *Echinococcus granulosus.* The disease is characterized by the *development of Echinococcus cysts that sometimes achieve the massive diameter of 25 cm. or more.* Man, cattle, sheep, hogs and other mammals are the usual intermediate hosts of this dog tapeworm. The eggs of the worm are excreted in the feces of the infected dog. When these eggs are ingested by a vulnerable mammal, they hatch in the upper level of the small intestine, and the small embryos permeate the intestinal mucosa and enter the blood vessels and lymphatics to be distributed throughout the body. The organisms lodge in virtually any site, but there is a fairly standard pattern. *In man, over half of Echinococcus cysts are found in the liver. The other sites of localization in decreasing order of frequency are the lungs, bones and brain.* In these various organs, the embryos lodge within the capillaries and here incite an inflammatory reaction composed principally of mononuclear leukocytes and eosinophils. Many such embryos are destroyed, but the others develop into cysts.

The cysts begin at microscopic levels and progressively increase in size so that in five years or more they may have achieved the maximum diameter described (25 cm.). The cyst is filled with a relatively clear hydatid fluid. Enclosing this fluid there is an inner, nucleated, germinative layer and an outer, opaque, non-nucleated layer. *The outer nonnucleated layer is quite distinctive and has innumerable delicate laminations* as though made up of many layers of fine tissue paper. Outside this opaque layer, there is an inflammatory reaction on the part of the host which produces a layer of fibroblasts, giant cells, and mononuclear and eosinophilic infiltration. When these cysts have been present for about a half year, daughter cysts develop within them. These appear first as minute projections of the germinative layer which develop central vesicles and thus form tiny daughter cysts known as "brood capsules." Scolices of the head of the worm develop on the inner aspects of these brood capsules. These brood capsules may separate from the germinative layer to produce a fine sandlike precipitate within the hydatid fluid (Fig. 10–44).

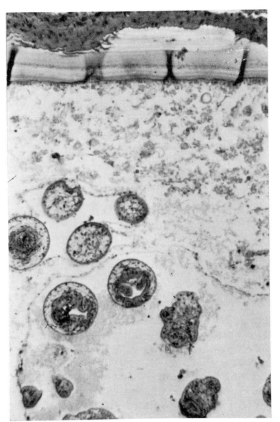

Figure 10-44. *Echinococcosis—the wall of the cyst with laminated outer layer and inner germinative layer, above. The cystic lumen contains many daughter "brood" capsules.*

This is the life cycle followed in the soft tissues, which permit the progressive enlargement of the cyst. It is therefore encountered characteristically in the liver or in other organs of the abdominal cavity. When the original implantation occurs in bone, it usually develops at the epiphyseal end. Fibrous adventitial encapsulation of the cyst does not occur, and the cyst, as it grows and develops increased pressure, permeates the spongy trabeculation of the bone to produce multiple diverticula. The intervening fragments of bone undergo pressure atrophy and frequently the bone cortex is eroded so that spontaneous fractures are not uncommon.

In a third pattern of localization known as the *alveolar hydatid,* found usually in Europe, the inflammatory response of the host does not produce a dense, enclosing, limiting membrane, nor is there a well developed, outer laminated wall to the cyst. As a consequence, the germinative layer penetrates the wall of the cyst and grows as protoplasmic masses into the surrounding soft tissue. This growth takes on the characteristics of an infiltrative malignancy, or perhaps is more closely akin to the insinuation of placental villi into the decidua of the uterus. These creeping masses of germinative epithelium produce multiple cystic cavities that create a sponge-like consistency to the affected tissue. There is a marked inflammatory reaction to this foreign parasitic tissue in the form of leukocytic infiltration with eosinophils, neutrophils and mononuclear cells; fibroblastic proliferation; giant cell formation; and inflammatory proliferation of the endothelial linings of the blood vessels in the local area. As a consequence, intravascular thromboses may lead to infarction of the tissues in these sites. In the course of time, the inflammatory response is transformed into a dense enclosing wall of fibrous, collagenous connective tissue. Prior to this fibrotic stage, this germinative epithelium may itself penetrate blood vessel walls and thus metastasize to other regions of the body. However, in these metastatic sites it usually does not develop into a characteristic hydatid cyst.

The clinical symptoms that stem from these conditions derive entirely from local destruction of tissues and the production of cystic masses. However, none of these clinical manifestations becomes apparent until years after the original infection. As a consequence, hydatid disease may manifest itself as a primary hepatic, pulmonary, central nervous system or osseous tumor. Impingement upon blood vessels may cause vascular thromboses and infarctions in these sites, bronchi may be eroded, pressure may be exerted upon vital centers in the brain, biliary tract obstruction may ensue, and hemorrhages are occasioned by the erosive action of these cysts. Infrequently a cyst may rupture, and the escape of hydatid fluid may evoke a massive anaphylactic reaction which is sometimes fatal.

TRICHURIASIS

Trichuriasis is a relatively insignificant infection of the cecum, appendix and colon caused by the *Trichuris trichiura,* also known as the whipworm. Infection by this round worm is contracted by the ingestion of food or water containing eggs. These foodstuffs are contaminated by the feces of a patient harboring the adult worms. In the ileocecal region where the adults mature and are localized, thousands of eggs are deposited in a day by a single worm. In the course of about three weeks, embryos hatch. They develop into mature whipworms in the gut, where the adults may cause minimal hyperemia and edema of the mucosa. Occasionally superficial ulcerations are produced, accompanied by the usual mononuclear and eosinophilic infiltration. Coiled worms may block the lumen of the appendix and produce symptoms of appendicitis. Clinically, these patients are usually asymptomatic but, when the infection is severe, it is accompanied by diarrhea and ill-defined abdominal pain. Many of these patients have a fairly profound anemia of obscure origin. Occasionally, as a secondary effect of the anemia, hypoxic, fatty changes may occur in the heart, liver and kidneys.

DISTOMIASIS

The distomes, like the schistosomes, are flatworms. Several species of distomes parasitize man, but only four are involved in major forms of disease in man: *Fasciolopsis buski* causes intestinal distomiasis, *Fasciola hepatica* and *Clonorchis sinensis* cause hepatic distomiasis and *Paragonimus westermani* produces pulmonary distomiasis.

Intestinal Distomiasis. The intestinal fluke, *Fasciolopsis buski, is the principal form of intestinal fluke which localizes within the mucosa of the small bowel and causes rather mild inflammatory ulcerations.* For the most part these infections are found in the South Pacific, Burma, India and China. Man is inhabited as only one stage of the life cycle of the intestinal fluke. The adult helminth, while attached to the intestinal mucosa, deposits eggs in the lumen. When these eggs contaminate fresh water, a larval form, the miracidium, hatches from each egg and invades an appropriate snail. Within this host, the larvae are transformed to cercariae, which upon leaving the snail become encysted upon water plants.

Man contracts the infection by the ingestion of these contaminated plants. The cysts are dissolved in the upper intestinal tract, and the larval forms emerge, mature into adult worms, and become attached to the mucosa of the small bowel by means of their suckers. At the local sites of involvement, a hemorrhagic inflammation ensues which is at first fairly nonspecific, although principally characterized by eosinophils. As these focal injuries progress, actual abscesses may develop in the mucosa, with considerable destruction of the intestinal mucosa. As a consequence of these anatomic lesions in the small bowel, the patients often have abdominal pain and diarrhea. When the infestation is very severe, a generalized, constitutional, febrile reaction appears attributable to absorption of toxic metabolites produced by the worms. Very infrequently, tangled masses of worms may produce acute intestinal ob-struction. The diagnosis is made by the identification of the characteristic eggs in the feces.

Hepatic Distomiasis. Hepatic distomiasis is a parasitic invasion of the bile ducts and liver parenchyma by liver flukes. *Fasciola hepatica,* also known as the "sheep liver fluke," is the principal offender and is found in all sheep-raising areas of the world. A close relative, *Clonorchis sinensis,* the Chinese liver fluke, is found only in the Far East. Both forms pass through essentially similar life cycles. In man, they inhabit principally the bile ducts of the liver. The eggs, when excreted into fresh water, develop into free-living miracidia. These are ingested by snails in which they develop into cercariae. From this point, the intermediate forms of *F. hepatica* encyst on blades of grass and are thus infective for man and sheep. The cercariae of *C. sinensis*, on the other hand, invade fish, and man becomes parasitized by the ingestion of improperly cooked food. Both forms of liver fluke mature in the upper intestinal tract and *invade the biliary passages of the liver of man. Here they induce a localized inflammatory reaction, as well as a striking hyperplasia of the bile duct epithelium. In some instances, bile duct carcinoma may evolve. As a consequence of these two changes, biliary obstruction often ensues.* In other instances, the worms may totally erode the bile duct walls and thus produce *parenchymal liver abscesses.* In the late stages of these infections, focal inflammatory scars may result, or when the biliary tract obstruction involves a duct of large size, *diffuse hepatic periportal fibrosis may create obstructive biliary cirrhosis.* Infrequently, these flukes may localize in other sites such as the abdominal wall, the brain, the orbit and the muscles of the neck.

The principal clinical manifestations of hepatic distomiasis are signs and symptoms suggesting cholecystitis, i.e., right upper quadrant pain, localized tenderness and sometimes jaundice and abdominal spasm. In heavy infections, fever, ascites and cachexia accompany these focalizing manifestations. The diagnosis is made by the identification of the appropriate eggs in the feces.

Pulmonary Distomiasis. Pulmonary distomiasis is caused by *Paragonimus westermani,* also known as the lung fluke. This infection is virtually limited to the Orient. This parasite specifically favors the lung as an optimal environment for its growth. Here eggs are deposited which are coughed up in the sputum. Those which enter fresh water develop into miracidia which enter appropriate snails for further development. After approximately 13 weeks within this host, cercariae emerge to invade crayfishes and crabs and are thus available for consumption by man.

The incompletely developed parasites penetrate the wall of the small intestine, enter the abdominal cavity, burrow through the diaphragm, and thus enter the lung. Here they localize principally near the smaller airways, where they develop into adults. However, in this migration some helminths remain in the abdomen, while others follow devious routes to the brain and other structures. In all their sites of localization, a focal inflammatory reaction ensues about the larval and adult forms. The inflammatory reaction again contains abundant numbers of eosinophils. Granulomatous formations may also develop. As a consequence, pulmonary abscesses, focal consolidations, necrotizing destruction of the bronchi or, in the later stages, patchy but widely distributed fibrous scarring may develop in the lungs. Sometimes these walled off inflammations create cysts that reach a diameter of 2 cm. and are classically filled with a brown, pasty exudate. The clinical diagnosis in a patient with the pulmonary involvement may often be made by the character of the coughed-up sputum and the identification of the eggs in this exudate.

INFLAMMATORY DISEASES OF UNKNOWN CAUSE

The diseases presented to this point have all had more or less well established etiologies. A very few diseases remain which are essentially inflammatory in nature, both from their clinical and anatomic characteristics, but are of somewhat obscure etiology. The two most important entities in this category are sarcoidosis and infectious mononucleosis.

SARCOIDOSIS (BOECK'S SARCOID, BESNIER-BOECK-SCHAUMANN DISEASE)

Of sarcoidosis it can truly be said that it is "an enigma wrapped in a mystery." Not only is its etiology unknown, but the basic characterization of this entity is in dispute. While the three major views of this condition disagree at many points, they all concur on the following definition. *"Sarcoidosis is a disease of unknown etiology characterized pathologically by epithelioid tubercles with inconspicuous or no necrosis, occurring in any organ or tissue and by the frequent presence of refractile or apparently calcified bodies in the giant cells of the tubercles"* (Third International Conference on Sarcoidosis, 1964).

Based on this histopathologic characterization, the first theory regarding the nature of sarcoidosis holds that it is an anergic or hypoergic form of tuberculosis. It is postulated that, in certain individuals, sensitization to the organism fails to develop and so caseation never appears in the tubercles.

The second concept of sarcoidosis focuses on the histopathologic reaction and defines the disease as any condition in which characteristic noncaseating tubercles are found in any organ or tissue of the body. In this view, sarcoidosis is not a discrete entity, but a congerie of entities sharing a common morphologic pattern. The granulomas are viewed as a response to indigestible residues which persist in the tissues, yielding noncaseating granulomas. Here the clinical symptomatology would be extremely varied and would depend on the nature of the injury inducing the granulomatous reaction. It should be noted, however, that hard, noncaseating tubercles are also encountered in leprosy, tertiary syphilis, fungus infections, berylliosis and in relation to a variety of forms of cancer. The proponents of this view are willing to dismiss these cases with known etiology as a "sarcoid reaction," and confine their definition only to cases of unknown etiology.

The third conception of sarcoidosis restricts this disease to a fairly well defined clinical syndrome that includes not only the characteristic histologic changes in tissues but also pulmonary lesions (patchy densities, fibrosis and emphysema), bilateral hilar adenopathy, uveoparotitis, osseous lesions, particularly in the short bones of the hands and feet, and the frequent occurrence of erythema nodosum of the skin. Hyperglobulinemia, mainly of the gamma fraction, but also of the alpha and beta fractions, and occasionally hypercalcemia and hypercalciuria are also usually present. In this view, sarcoidosis represents a well defined syndrome, albeit of unknown cause, that may produce definite clinical manifestations related to the sites of involvement mentioned earlier, but more often (three of four cases) is asymptomatic and is discovered only at autopsy.

Incidence. Sarcoidosis is an uncommon but not rare disorder with a peak incidence in the third to fifth decades. There are striking geographic differences in its frequency, not only from country to country, but also in ethnic groups living side by side. The highest rates are found in Sweden—64 cases per 100,000, based on x-ray studies. In contrast, Finland, a close neighbor, has a rate below 10 per 100,000 (Editorial, 1965). In New York City, the overall prevalence is said to be three per 100,000, but in blacks it is ten times more common than in whites.

Etiology and Pathogenesis. Common to all the conceptions mentioned above, is a non-caseating "hard tubercle" found in many organs of the body, principally the lungs, hilar lymph nodes and other locations within the lymphohematopoietic system (Fig. 10–45). Giant cells of either the foreign body or Langhans' type are commonly found. In addition, these tubercles classically contain laminated concretions composed of calcium and proteins known as Schaumann bodies. These are present in 80 to 90 per cent of the granulomas of sarcoidosis. In addition, stellate-shaped inclusions known as "asteroid bodies" are found in the giant cells in approximately 60 per cent of the granulomas (Fig. 10–46). Neither of these distinctive inclusions is diagnostic of sarcoid since both are occasionally identified in classic tuberculosis lesions.

The three conceptions of sarcoidosis relate to three theories of causation: (1) a microbiologic etiology, (2) a granulomatous response to any one of a number of possible substances which have in common persistance of some irritant within the tissues and (3) some form of altered immunologic response, possibly to a variety of antigenic stimuli. With respect to a microbiologic causation, the belief persists that sarcoidosis represents an unusual form of

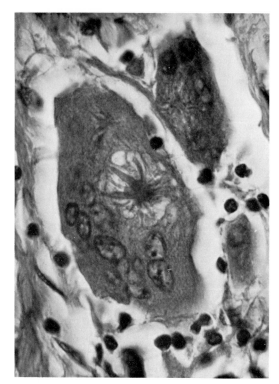

Figure 10–46. A characteristic asteroid within a giant cell.

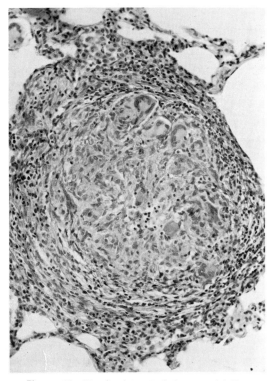

Figure 10–45. A characteristic sarcoid "noncaseating" granuloma with many giant cells.

tuberculosis. Phages capable of lysing *M. tuberculosis* have been isolated from sarcoid tissues, and so it is held that the bacteria are rapidly destroyed, accounting for the inability to identify these organisms in tissue lesions (Mankiewicz, 1964). Conceivably, these patients have developed a highly effective cell-mediated immunity to *M. tuberculosis* without the usual accompanying hypersensitivity to these organisms. Thus, one might get tubercle formation (granulomas) without the central caseation necrosis. However, most of the evidence indicates that, in terms of cell-mediated immunity, these patients are anergic although the humoral antibody system is intact and sometimes overactive. It is difficult to conceive of an effective cellular immunity against *M. tuberculosis* with deficient cell-mediated reactions to other antigens. Moreover, classic caseating tuberculosis is sometimes encountered in patients having other stigmata of sarcoidosis. Such a concurrence is generally interpreted as the coexistence of two diseases rather than a single disease presenting in two anatomic patterns. If these individuals can develop classic tuberculosis, how can sarcoidosis be an unusual response to *M. tuberculosis*? Recently, interest has turned to the herpes-like EB virus as the cause of this disease. In one study of 131 patients with sarcoidosis, all had high titers of antibodies against this virus (Hirshaut et al., 1970). However, approximately 75 per cent of controls had antibodies against the EBV, although in lower titers. It is difficult to wax enthusiastic about such a viral etiology because, at the present time, the EB virus is blamed for all manner of disease including Burkitt's lymphoma, nasopharyngeal carcinoma and infectious mononucleosis as well.

The possibility that sarcoidosis is simply a tissue response to any substance that persists as an inflammatory stimulus cannot be excluded. It is well known that granulomatous reactions can be evoked by complex carbohydrates, lipids, inert macromolecules and carrageenin, to name only some of the possible irritants. Possibly, then, the disorder referred to as sarcoidosis is merely a common morphologic response to a variety of irritants.

The third theory postulates some form of immunologic causation and, indeed, there are numerous immunologic hints surrounding sarcoidosis. The cell-mediated anergy characteristic of this disease certainly suggests an altered immune reactivity. Extracts of diseased tissue from a patient known to have sarcoidosis, when injected into the skin of a sarcoid subject, evoke a granulomatous response—the basis for the Kveim test. While such a granulomatous reaction has been interpreted as an expression of altered immunity, it has also been interpreted as demonstration of transmission of a microbiologic agent as yet unidentified (Mitchel and Rees, 1969). Cummings and Hudgins (1958) have pointed out the parallel between the geographic incidence of sarcoidosis throughout the world and the distribution of certain pine forests. These authors and others have pointed out that pine pollen has acid-fast staining qualities similar to those of the tubercle bacillus, and that it also contains acids closely related to those found in the waxy moiety of the tubercle bacillus. They, therefore, propose that sarcoidosis is a sensitivity reaction to a pollen antigen. It has further been possible to evoke granulomas in animals by the administration of pine pollen extract (Lindner et al., 1962). However, sarcoidosis appears to be more an urban than a rural disease, and it occurs in regions not having such trees. Thus, the etiology of this disorder remains unknown.

Morphology. In the large body of literature that has accumulated on this disease, pathologic involvement of virtually every organ in the body has been cited at one time or another (Freiman, 1948;

Longcope and Freiman, 1952). Only the more favored sites of localization are presented here.

Lymph Nodes. Lymph nodes are involved in the majority of cases. The most common group affected are those in the thorax, principally about the trachea and tracheobronchial bifurcation. The nodes are characteristically enlarged bilaterally, an enlargement that is demonstrable roentgenographically. The nodes appear soft, gray-red and nonmatted. Any other node in the body, particularly the cervicals, epitrochlears, preauriculars and postauriculars, may also be involved, and in addition the tonsils are affected in about one-quarter to one-third of the cases. Depending upon the stage of the infection, there may be no macroscopic alterations on cut section. In the more advanced, chronic stages of the disease, diffuse foci of fibrosis may be seen.

Histologically, the characteristic granuloma is a noncaseating "hard tubercle of epithelioid cells." In longstanding sarcoidosis, these granulomas undergo progressive collagenous fibrosis and ultimately are totally replaced by fibrous scars. It should be emphasized at this point that even in the stage of characteristic granuloma formation, the lesions are not pathognomonic of sarcoidosis. Other granulomas, such as the non-caseating lesion of tuberculosis, the lesion of berylliosis, foreign body and mycotic granulomas, and that of syphilis, are all histologically indistinguishable from the sarcoid nodule. Rarely, the granuloma of sarcoidosis has some central necrosis, making it virtually impossible to differentiate it from a tuberculous lesion. **As a teaching principle, when such necrosis is found, the diagnosis of sarcoidosis should not be made until tuberculosis has been clearly ruled out.**

Spleen. The spleen is affected in about three-quarters of the cases. When the process in this organ is widespread and marked, splenomegaly results and weights of over a kilogram have been recorded. However, the organ is usually unaffected grossly and the individual lesions cannot be seen. On occasion, these granulomas may coalesce to form small nodules which are barely visible macroscopically. The capsule is not involved. Histologically, the cellular proliferative granulomas or fibrosing or totally hyalinized lesions are dispersed throughout the splenic pulp.

Liver. The liver is affected slightly less often than the spleen. It may also be moderately enlarged and may contain scattered lesions throughout the substance, having no predilection for any specific localization within the liver lobule. It is to be remembered that when the liver or spleen is significantly enlarged in a clinical case suspected of being sarcoidosis, needle punch biopsy may permit the identification of one of the focal lesions.

Lung. The lung is a common site of involvement. Macroscopically, there is usually no demonstrable alteration, although at times the coalescence of granulomas may produce small nodules which are palpable or visible as 2 to 4 cm., noncaseating, noncavitated consolidations. Histologically, the lesions are distributed throughout the parenchyma, usually bilaterally, with some tendency to localize about blood vessels, bronchi and lymphatics. The wide distribution of the lesions in these organs suggests a hematogenous dissemination of some etiologic agent. While in occasional cases cellular proliferative granulomas are present, there appears to be a strong tendency for the lesions to heal in the lungs so that more often varying stages of fibrosis and hyalinization are found, often causing fairly diffuse parenchymal damage. There is, in fact a strong suspicion that in many cases of systemic sarcoidosis in which the lungs are not apparently involved at postmortem examination, previous lesions may have been present, but disappeared.

Bone. Bone marrow is an additional favored site of localization, but the exact incidence of this myeloid involvement is not clear. It is known that roentgenographic changes can be identified in about one-fifth of the cases of systemic involvement. The radiologically visible bone lesions have a particular tendency to involve short bones of the hands and feet. These lesions on roentgenograms produce small circumscribed areas of bone resorption within the marrow cavity or a diffuse reticulated pattern throughout the cavity with widening of the bony shafts and oftentimes new bone formation on the outer surfaces. Histologically, in these cases numerous characteristic sarcoid nodules are present in the marrow cavity.

Skin and Mucous Membranes. Skin lesions are encountered in about half of the cases. These are, in fact, the best known lesions of sarcoidosis and were the ones first described by Boeck. Sarcoidosis of the skin assumes a variety of macroscopic appearances, e.g., discrete subcutaneous nodules; focal, slightly elevated, erythematous plaques; or flat lesions that are slightly reddened, scaling, and resemble those of lupus. Occasionally, deeply situated nodules, resembling those of erythema nodosa, have also been described. Similar lesions may affect the mucous membranes of the oral cavity and have also been described in the larynx and upper respiratory tract. In all instances, sarcoid-like granulomas are found histologically in the sites of involvement.

Eye, Lacrimal and Salivary Glands. Involvement of the eye, the associated glands and the salivary glands is one of the most interesting features of sarcoidosis. This combination is seen in about one-fifth to one-half of the cases. The ocular involvement takes the form of iritis or iridocyclitis, either bilaterally or unilaterally. As a consequence of these inflammatory involvements, corneal opacities, glaucoma and total loss of vision may occur.

The posterior uveal tract is also affected, but less commonly, with resultant choroiditis, retinitis and optic nerve involvement. These ocular lesions are frequently accompanied by inflammations in the lacrimal gland with suppression of lacrimation. Bilateral sarcoidosis of the salivary glands, i.e., parotid, submaxillary and sublingual, completes **the combined uveoparotid involvement designated as Mikulicz's syndrome.**

Miscellaneous Sites. Sarcoid granulomas occasionally occur in the heart, kidneys and endocrine glands, particularly in the pituitary, as well as in the other tissues of the body.

Clinical Course. On the basis of the inconstant sites of localization of the tissue lesions, sarcoidosis is a protean clinical disease. As previously mentioned, approximately 75 per cent of cases are entirely asymptomatic and are only discovered incidentally at autopsy. In still other instances, the disease is discovered unexpectedly on a routine chest roentgenogram by the presence of bilateral hilar adenopathy. Occasionally, the pulmonary lesions and subsequent fibrosis produce patchy densities in the lung fields on x-ray. The symptomatic cases are sometimes first recognized by the appearance of skin lesions characteristic of erythema nodosa. At other times ophthalmologists recognize the loss of lacrimation and the associated iritis and uveitis as being sarcoid in origin. Splenomegaly, hepatomegaly or peripheral lymphadenopathy are other presentations of this condition. In the great majority of patients, however, there are no localizing systemic manifestations, and the patients come to medical attention because of mild fever, weakness, weight loss, joint pains and debilitation. Because of these variable and nondiagnostic clinical symptom complexes, the Kveim skin test is frequently of help in establishing a diagnosis. The presence of hyperglobulinemia, hypercalcemia or roentgenographic changes in the short bones of the hands and feet are helpful but not diagnostic features.

Sarcoidosis follows a fairly unpredictable course characterized by chronicity or by remissions that are sometimes spontaneous, sometimes initiated by steroid therapy and sometimes permanent. In only a few instances do the patients pursue a downhill course, usually to die of intercurrent infections or chronic cor pulmonale due to the diffuse lung fibrosis.

INFECTIOUS MONONUCLEOSIS (IM)

Infectious mononucleosis is a benign disease almost certainly of viral etiology characterized by fever, generalized lymphadenopathy, sore throat and the appearance in the blood of atypical lymphocytes (mononucleosis cells). It is also usually characterized by elevated levels of agglutinins to sheep red cells (Paul-Bunnell heterophil test). It has become increasingly apparent that IM affects not only the lymph nodes throughout the body but also commonly the spleen, liver and less often the heart, lungs, kidneys, hematopoietic system and central nervous system. Thus it may mimic many other disorders, particularly viral hepatitis.

Incidence. IM occurs principally in teenagers between the ages of 15 and 19 years. These patients tend to be in the upper socioeconomic classes and frequently are students in preparatory schools and colleges. World-wide in distribution, the disease usually occurs sporadically but sometimes appears in outbreaks, particularly in such closed communities as schools, military camps and other institutions.

Etiology. The evidence continues to accumulate that infectious mononucleosis is caused by the herpes-like Epstein-Barr virus (EBV). Almost all patients with IM develop high or rising titers to EBV during the course of their illnesses. Antibodies to EBV appear to protect against IM. In a study of freshmen at Yale University, only 24 per cent had antibodies to EBV (Evans, 1968). All subsequent cases of IM in this group of students occurred among those who were seronegative and none occurred among those who had already developed antibodies. The EB virus stimulates lymphocytes of patients with IM to proliferate into blastoid cells. Cultures of mononucleosis cells harbor the EB virus (Banatvala, 1970). Recently, it was shown that sera from eight patients with IM contained virus-specific IgM, and that this specific immunoglobulin was detectable for as long as the patient had persistent symptoms (Banatvala et al., 1972). IgM antibodies are presumptive evidence of an initial antigenic challenge, and therefore suggest a causal role for the EBV in the onset of this disease. Up to now it has not, however, been possible to isolate the virus from throat washings or to transmit the infection to subhuman primates. It is noteworthy, therefore, that a recent report presents strong evidence for the existence of EBV in throat washings of patients with IM (Gerber, 1972). Convincing as all this evidence may appear to be, doubters still contend that IM may merely be activating an unrelated latent EBV infection. At the present time, however, room for persistent doubt continues to narrow.

Morphology. Because the disease is almost invariably benign, anatomic studies have been confined largely to excised lymph nodes and liver biopsies, and to the rare patients who have died of rupture of the spleen or other complications (Kass and Robbins, 1950; Ziegler, 1944). The major alterations involve the peripheral blood, lymph nodes, spleen, liver, central nervous system and less significantly the heart, lungs and other organs.

The **peripheral blood** usually shows an absolute lymphocytosis with a total white cell count between 12,000 and 18,000, 95 per cent of which are lymphocytes. These are atypical lymphocytes, large, 12 to 16 microns in diameter, with an abundant, finely granular basophilic or acidophilic cytoplasm. The nucleus is variable in shape and may be round, ovoid, folded or bean shaped. The nuclear chromatin is usually finely divided but may be clumped. Nucleoli are usually absent. The most distinguishing feature of these atypical lymphocytes is small fenestrations or vacuolations in the cytoplasm. These abnormal cells are usually sufficiently distinctive to permit the diagnosis of infectious mononucleosis on peripheral blood smear or sometimes on histologic examination of tissue sections.

The **lymph nodes** are usually moderately enlarged throughout the body, principally in the posterior cervical, axillary and groin regions. Their histologic architecture is usually preserved but, in severe involvement, may become blurred by infiltrations of the atypical lymphocytes. Sometimes the follicles become extremely prominent due to hyperplasia of the atypical lymphocytes as well as native lymphoblasts and reticulum cells. When these atypical cells flood into the medullary portion, the nodal histology simulates the infiltrative pattern of leukemia, and the differentiation of this disease from leukemia rests upon the identification of the fenestrated lymphocytes characteristic of this disease. Involvement of the tonsils and lymphoidal tissue of the oropharynx is also common.

The **spleen** is usually enlarged two to three times and is often soft and fleshy with a hyperemic cut surface. When extremely soft, the trabecular markings and follicular structure may become indistinct. Histologically, there may either be prominence of the splenic follicles or the architecture may be blurred by the heavy accumulation of atypical lymphocytes. These cells sometimes infiltrate the trabeculae and the capsule and undoubtedly contribute in this way to easy rupture, a highly important clinical complication of this condition. Increased numbers of plasma cells are often present also.

The **liver** in most cases is affected as determined by such sensitive function tests as elevated serum levels of glutamic oxaloacetic transaminase (SGOT) and serum isocitric dehydrogenase (SICD). In a small series of 22 cases evaluated for liver involvement, all patients demonstrated abnormalities in the liver, either by function tests or liver biopsy (Nelson and Darragh, 1956). Despite such evidence of functional involvement, the liver is usually only mildly or moderately enlarged and is otherwise not unusual in its gross appearance. Histologically, there are three principal alterations: portal infiltrations consisting almost entirely of abnormal mononuclear cells, invasion of the sinusoids by the same cells, and areas of scattered parenchymal necrosis filled with mononuclear cells. These alterations may be extremely difficult if not impossible to differentiate from viral hepatitis.

The **central nervous system** is the seat of many nonspecific anatomic changes, i.e., congestion, edema and perivascular mononuclear infiltrates in the leptomeninges. Focal aggregates of mononuclear cells may occur in the perivascular area of the brain substance. Myelin degeneration and destruction of axis cylinders have been described in the peripheral nerves.

An interstitial "viral-type" pneumonitis has been observed in lungs, and atypical lymphocytes have been described in the heart and bone marrow to account for some of the altered function of these tissues.

Clinical Course. The diagnosis of this condition is difficult because it presents such varied clinical patterns. Final assessment must be based upon clinical, hematologic and serologic findings. Clinically, the disease often starts with a prodrome of chills, fever, malaise, sore throat and painful enlargement of the cervical nodes. A fairly severe pharyngitis and tonsillitis may become apparent, associated with a creamy exudate over these structures. Fine pinpoint petechiae in the palate are present at the height of the illness in somewhat less than half of the cases. On the basis of these findings, the common differential diagnosis involves a bacterial, principally streptococcal sore throat, but microbiologic study will fail to incriminate any specific agent. A fine macular skin rash resembling rubella develops in 10 to 15 per cent of the cases. Splenomegaly may give rise to left upper quadrant pain or discomfort. The hepatic enlargement may produce signs referable to the right upper quadrant and often is responsible for gastrointestinal complaints. The differential diagnosis in such cases is often infectious (viral) hepatitis. In other instances, the striking lymphocytosis associated with the lymphadenopathy raises the spectre of leukemia.

The hematologic findings, i.e., the elevated white count with a relative lymphocytosis and the recognition of the atypical lymphocytes, are crucial to the diagnosis.

In the classic case, abnormal levels of sheep red cell agglutinins are present in titers greater than 1 to 64 (the Paul-Bunnell heterophil test). These antibodies in infectious mononucleosis are not significantly absorbed by guinea pig kidneys, but are classically absorbed by beef erythrocytes producing a difference in the titers obtained in these two absorption tests. In addition and far more specific are the serodiagnostic procedures relating to the EBV discussed earlier.

The clinical course is usually one of progressive improvement after two to four weeks of febrile illness, but the intercurrence of hepatic involvement or myocarditis with its associated T wave abnormalities may prolong the illness. The many possible visceral involvements of infectious mononucleosis dictate the need for bed rest and conservatism in the management of these patients (Dunnet, 1963). Fatalities are rare and are almost invariably attributable to rupture of the spleen or to such intercurrent infections as pneumonia and meningitis. We come now to the final intriguing question of the relationship of IM to Burkitt's lymphoma (p. 757). Both are diseases of the lymphoreticular system and both have been attributed to the EBV. Dameshek (1969) speculated that in IM a wide variety of antibodies are produced which make the disease self-limited and benign. Could the lymphoma represent a disorder evoking less effective control mechanisms or, alternatively, might the virus initiate mutations in lymphocytes rendering them capable of uncontrolled growth into a lymphoma. Here the speculation must end.

INFECTIOUS LYMPHOCYTOSIS

Infectious lymphocytosis is a benign condition characterized by a striking relative and absolute lymphocytosis occurring in children usually who are completely asymptomatic. Its importance lies in the striking white cell counts that sometimes reach levels of over 100,000 per mm.^{3} with up to 90 per cent of the cells being adult small lymphocytes. It is obvious that such a peripheral white count would evoke suspicion of lymphatic leukemia. However, this entity of unknown etiology has a uniformly favorable outcome in the course of one to two weeks. It differs from infectious mononucleosis in many ways, principally in having adult mature lymphocytes in the peripheral smear and in having a negative Paul-Bunnell heterophil test.

Little is known of the anatomic changes in this condition because of the benign nature of the disease. Lymphadenopathy and splenomegaly are usually absent. The marrow on biopsy shows an increase in the number of mature lymphocytes. A few cases of lymph node biopsy have revealed reticuloendothelial proliferation, but in other instances no changes have been described (Barnes et al., 1949).

REFERENCES

Ash, J. E., and Spitz, S.: Pathology of Tropical Diseases. Philadelphia, W. B. Saunders Co., 1945.

Ashe, W. F., et al.: Weil's disease: complete review of American literature and abstract of world literature: 7 case reports. Medicine, *20*:145, 1941.

Baker, R. D.: Tissue changes in fungus disease. Arch. Path., *44*:459, 1947.

Banatvala, J. E.: Infectious mononucleosis: recent developments. Brit. J. Haemat., *19*:129, 1970.

Banatvala, J. E., et al.: Epstein-Barr virus specific IgM in infectious mononucleosis, Burkitt's lymphoma, and nasopharyngeal carcinoma. Lancet, *1*:1205, 1972.

Barnes, G. R., Jr., et al.: A clinical study of an institutional outbreak of acute infectious lymphocytosis. Amer. J. Med. Sci., *218*:646, 1949.

Birch, C. L., and Anast, B. P.: The changing distribution of helminthic diseases in the United States. J.A.M.A., *164*:121, 1957.

Bodian, D., and Horstmann, D. M.: In Horsfall, F. L., and Tamm, I. (eds.): Viral and Rickettsial Infections of Man. Philadelphia, J. B. Lippincott Co., 1965, p. 430.

Chanock, R. M.: Mycoplasma infections of man. New Eng. J. Med., *273*:1199, 1257, 1965.

Cheatham, W. J., et al.: Varicella: Report of two fatal cases with necropsy, virus isolation and serologic studies. Amer. J. Path., *32*:1015, 1956.

Clark, H. C.: The distribution and complications of amebic lesions in 186 post mortem examinations. Amer. J. Trop. Med., *5*:157, 1925.

Cole, H. N.: Lymphogranuloma inguinale. The fourth venereal disease. J.A.M.A., *101*:1065, 1933.

Councilman, W. T., et al.: The pathological anatomy and histology of variola. J. Med. Res., *6*:12, 1904.

Cummings, M. M., and Hudgins, P. C.: Chemical constituents of pine pollen and their possible relationship to sarcoidosis. Amer. J. Med. Sci., *236*:311, 1958.

Dameshek, W.: Speculations on the nature of infectious mononucleosis. In Carter, R. L., and Penman, H. G. (eds.): Infectious Mononucleosis. Oxford, Blackwell Scientific Publications, 1969, p. 225.

Davis, D. D., et al.: Microbiology. New York, Hoeber Medical Division, Harper & Row, 1968.

DeJongh, D. S., et al.: Postmortem bacteriology. Amer. J. Clin. Path., *49*:424, 1968.

Denton, J. F., and DiSalvo, A. F.: Isolation of B. dermatitidis from natural sites of Augusta, Georgia. Amer. J. Trop. Med., *13*:716, 1964.

Dunnet, W. N.: Infectious mononucleosis. Brit. Med. J., *1*:1187, 1963.

Editorial: Current thoughts on the epidemiology and etiology of sarcoidosis. Amer. J. Med., *39*:361, 1965.

Eliason, E. L., et al.: The *Clostridium welchii* and associated organisms. Surg. Gynec. Obstet., *64*:1005, 1937.

Evans, A. S.: Seroepidemiologic studies of infectious mononucleosis with EB virus. New Eng. J. Med., *279*:1121, 1968.

Felsen, J.: Acute and chronic bacillary dysentery. Amer. J. Path., *12*:395, 1936.

Fete, G. L.: Leprosy from the histologic point of view. Arch. Path., *35*:611, 1943.

Finland, M., et al.: Occurrence of serious bacterial infections since introduction of antibacterial agents. J.A.M.A., *170*:2188, 1959.

Freiman, D. G.: Sarcoidosis. New Eng. J. Med., *239*:664, 709, 743, 1948.

Frenkel, J. K.: Models for infectious diseases. Fed. Proc., *28*:179, 1969.

Frenkel, J. K., et al.: Toxoplasma gondii in cats: fecal stages identified as coccidian oocysts. Science, *167*:893, 1970.

Gerber, P.: Oral excretion of Epstein-Barr virus by healthy subjects and patients with infectious mononucleosis. Lancet, *2*:988, 1972.

Goodpasture, E. W., and House, J. J.: The pathologic anatomy of tularemia. Amer. J. Path., *4*:213, 1928.

Gould, S. E.: Trichinosis. Springfield, Ill., Charles C Thomas, 1945.

Grady, G. F., and Keusch, G. T.: Pathogenesis of bacterial diarrheas. New Eng. J. Med., *285*:831, 891, 1971.

Greaves, A. V.: Modern conceptions of the pathogenesis and morbid anatomy of malaria. Canad. Med. Ass. J., *54*:568, 1946.

Hart, P. D., et al.: The compromised host and infection. J. Infect. Dis., *120*:169, 1969.

Hirshaut, Y., et al.: Sarcoidosis: another disease associated with serologic evidence for herpes-like virus infection. New Eng. J. Med., *283*:502, 1970.

Horsfall, F. L., and Tamm, I.: Viral and Rickettsial Diseases of Man. 4th ed. Philadelphia, J. B. Lippincott Co., 1965.

Hyde, L., and Hyde, B.: Primary Friedländer pneumonia. Amer. J. Med. Sci., *205*:660, 1943.

International Sub-Committee of Virus Nomenclature: International Bulletin of Bacteriological Nomenclature and Toxonomy, *13*:217, 1963.

Jawetz, E., et al.: Review of Medical Microbiology. 9th ed. Los Altos, Calif., Lange Medical Publications, 1970.

Jeghers, H. J., et al.: Weil's disease: A report of a case with postmortem observations and review of recent literature. Arch. Path., *20*:447, 1935.

Joklik, W. K., and Merigan, T. C.: Concerning the mechanism of action of interferon. Proc. Nat. Acad. Sci., *56*:558, 1966.

Kass, E. H., and Robbins, S. L.: Severe hepatitis in infectious mononucleosis: report of a case with minimal clinical manifestations and death due to rupture of the spleen. Arch. Path., *50*:644, 1950.

Key, J. D., Jr., and Magee, W. E.: Fungal diseases in a general hospital: a study of eighty-eight patients. Amer. J. Clin. Path., *26*:1235, 1956.

Klainer, A. S., and Beisal, W. R.: Opportunistic infection: a review. Amer. J. Med. Sci., *258*:431, 1969.

Kurung, J.: Isolation and identification of pathogenic fungi from sputum. Am. Rev. Tuberc., *46*:365, 1942.

Lindner, A., et al.: Experimental granuloma formation with pine pollen. J. Exp. Med. Molec. Path., *1*:470, 1962.

Longcope, W. T., and Freiman, D. G.: A study of sarcoidosis: based on a combined investigation of 160 cases, including 30 autopsies from the Johns Hopkins Hospital and the Massachusetts General Hospital. Medicine, *31*:1, 1952.

Lurie, M. B.: Native and acquired resistance to tuberculosis. Amer. J. Med., *9*:591, 1950.

Lyons, C.: Bacteremic staphylococcal infection. Surg. Gynec. Obstet., *74*:41, 1942.

Mallory, F. B.: A histological study of typhoid fever. J. Exp. Med., *3*:611, 1898.

Mankiewicz, E.: The relationship of sarcoidosis to anonymous bacteria. Acta Med. Scand., Suppl. 425, *176*:68, 1964.

Marcial-Rojas, R. A.: Pathology of Protozoal and Helminthic Diseases. Baltimore, Williams and Wilkins Co., 1971.

Marcus, P. I., and Salb, J. M.: Molecular basis of interferon action: inhibition of viral RNA translation. Virology, *30*:502, 1966.

Marmion, B. P., et al.: A case of subacute rickettsial endocarditis: with a survey of cardiac patients for this infection. Brit. Med. J., *2*:1264, 1960.

Martland, H. S.: Fulminating meningococci infection with bilateral massive adrenal hemorrhage (the Waterhouse-Friderichsen syndrome). Arch. Path., *37*:147, 1944.

Martland, H. S.: The pathology of syphilis: with special reference to the development of luetic aortitis. Bull. N.Y. Acad. Med., *8*:451, 1932.

Merigan, T. C.: Interferons of mice and men. New Eng. J. Med., *276*:913, 1967.

Mitchel, R. S.: Control of tuberculosis. New Eng. J. Med., *276*:842, 905, 1967.

Mitchel, D. N., and Rees, R. J. W.: A transmissable agent from sarcoid tissue. Lancet, *2*:81, 1969.

Moulder, J. W.: The Psitticosis Group of Bacteria (CIBA Lectures in Microbial Biochemistry). New York, John Wiley and Sons, Inc., 1964.

National Health Education Committee: Fact on the Major Killing and Crippling Diseases in the United States Today. New York, 1966.

Neal, J. B., et al.: Meningitis due to the influenza bacillus of Pfeiffer (*Hemophilus influenzae*). J.A.M.A., *102*:513, 1934.

Nelson, R. S., and Darragh, J. H.: Infectious mononucleosis hepatitis, a clinical pathologic study. Amer. J. Med., *21*:26, 1956.

Novick, R. P.: Penicillinase plasmids of staphylococcus aureus. Fed. Proc., *26*:29, 1967.

Picchi, J., et al.: Q fever associated with granulomatous hepatitis. Ann. Intern. Med., *53*:1065, 1960.

Schipper, G. J.: Unusual pathogenicity of *Pasteurella multocida* isolated from the throats of common wild rats. Bull. Johns Hopkins Hosp., *81*:333, 1947.

Schwarz, J., and Muth, J.: Coccidiomycosis: a review. Amer. J. Med. Sci., *221*:89, 1951.

Sharp, W. B.: Pathology of undulant fever (brucellosis). Arch. Path., *18*:72, 1934.

Sheldon, W. H., and Heyman. A.: Studies on chancroid I. Observations of the histology with an evaluation of biopsy as a diagnostic procedure. Amer. J. Path., *22*:415, 1946.

Spaulding, W. B., and Hennessy, J. N.: Cat-scratch disease, a study of 83 cases. Amer. J. Med., *28*:504, 1960.

Spector, W. G.: The granulomatous inflammatory exudate. Int. Rev. Exp. Path., *8*:1, 1969.

Spink, W. W.: Family studies on brucellosis. Amer. J. Med. Sci., *227*:128, 1954.

Stuart, B. M., and Pullen, R. L.: Typhoid: clinical analyses of 360 cases. Arch. Intern. Med., *78*:629, 1946.

Symmers, W. St. C.: Pathology of oxyuriasis. Arch. Path., *50*:475, 1950.

Tamm, I., and Eggers, S. J.: Biochemistry of virus reproduction. Amer. J. Med., *38*:678, 1965.

Third International Conference on Sarcoidosis. Acta Med. Scand., Suppl. 425, 1964.

Thompson, J. G.: Weil's disease with myocarditis in South Africa. South American Med. J., *38*:696, 1964.

Trauger, D. A.: A note on tuberculosis epidemiology. Amer. Rev. Resp. Dis., *87*:582, 1963.

Warren, W. R.: Serum amylase and lipase in mumps. Amer. J. Med. Sci., *230*:161, 1955.

Watanabe, T.: Infective heredity of multiple drug resistance in bacteria. Bact. Rev., *27*:87, 1963.

Whittick, J. W.: Necropsy findings in a case of Q fever in Britain. Brit. Med. J., *1*:979, 1950.

Winship, P.: Pathologic changes in so-called cat scratch fever. Review of findings in lymph nodes of 29 patients and cutaneous lesions of two patients. Amer. J. Clin. Path., *23*:1012, 1953.

Wolbach, S. B.: The Pathology of the Rickettsial Diseases of Man, AAAS (monograph), 1948, pp. 118–125.

Wolleman, O. J., and Finland, M.: Pathology of staphylococcal pneumonia complicating clinical influenza. Amer. J. Path., *19*:23, 1943.

Wright, H. A., and MacGregor, A. R.: A case of meningitis due to *Bacterium monocytogenes*. J. Path. Bact., *48*:470, 1939.

Ziegler, E. E.: Infectious mononucleosis. Arch. Path., *37*:196, 1944.

Zimmerman, L. E., and Rappaport, H.: Occurrence of cryptococcosis in patients with malignant disease of the reticulo-endothelial system. Amer. J. Path., *24*:1050, 1954.

11

DEFICIENCY DISEASES

JOSEPH J. VITALE, M.D., Sc.D.*

PROTEIN-CALORIE	Vitamin E	Nicotinamide (niacinamide)
MALNUTRITION	Vitamin K	Folic acid
Marasmus	**Water-Soluble Vitamins**	B_{12} (cyanocobalamin)
Kwashiorkor	Vitamin C	B_6 (pyridoxine)
VITAMINS	Vitamin B	**MINERALS**
Fat-Soluble Vitamins	B_1 (thiamine)	**Iron**
Vitamin A	Riboflavin	**Zinc**
Vitamin D		

Most texts on the subject of nutrition usually begin with the observation that there are some 50 or 60 organic and inorganic substances which are indispensable to man and which are required in amounts ranging from microgram to gram quantities. These 50 or 60 essential nutrients include minerals, lipids or certain fatty acids, vitamins and specific amino acids. For man, the essential fatty acids are considered to be arachidonic, linoleic and linolenic. Eight amino acids are considered to be essential: tryptophan, lysine, phenylalanine, leucine, isoleucine, threonine, methionine and valine. Deficiency signs and symptoms, with or without alterations in the morphology of certain tissues, can be demonstrated for all of these essential nutrients in animals, but for man it has not been possible to associate unequivocally a disease state with all 50 or 60 of these substances.

Man usually meets his requirements for the essential nutrients by ingesting a variety of foods which include essentially four groups. The four are: (1) *Milk group*—cheese, ice cream and other milk-made foods can supply part of the milk. (2) *Meat group*—meats, fish, poultry, eggs or cheese, with dry beans, peas and nuts as alternatives. (3) *Vegetables and Fruits*—dark green or yellow vegetables, citrus fruit or tomatoes. (4) *Breads and Cereals*—enriched or whole grain; added milk improves nutritional values.

It should be stressed that an individual's requirement is dependent upon a host of variables acting singly, in combination or synergistically. Genetic make-up and environmental factors may result in a "no effect" of a diet low in an essential nutrient for one individual, whereas the same diet in another individual may result in overt disease.

Bascially, nutrients are required for growth and maintenance and all of the known metabolic functions associated with them. The requirement for the essential nutrients is relatively higher during growth, since they are needed not only for synthesis of new tissue but also for the maintenance of existing tissue. During growth, as well as in adult life, the daily requirements for each of the essential nutrients may be increased by a number of influences. For example, an individual with a chronic infection may have increased losses of essential nutrients. With fever, there is increased catabolism, decreased absorption and increased excretion of essential nutrients. Pregnancy obviously raises the requirements for essential nutrients. Thus, deficiency signs and symptoms can appear in the individual despite the intake of the recommended daily allowances set forth by the Food and Nutrition Board of the National Academy of Sciences and the National Research Council (1968).

Deficiency states may be primary (dietary inadequacy) or secondary (induced by some in-

---

*Professor of Pathology and Nutrition, Boston University School of Medicine.

475

fluence despite adequate intake). It is important to understand the underlying cause of deficiency signs and symptoms, since effective therapy will vary depending on whether it is primary or secondary.

Table 11–1 indicates situations in which the primary deficiency or the secondary induced deficiency states may occur.

Primary deficiency states are more important in so-called developing areas of the world (the United States included), but in affluent societies, deficiency states are more often secondary. Either as a result of ignorance, poverty or faddism, certain essential nutrients may be lacking in the diet, resulting in primary deficiency disease. Combinations of poverty with certain cultural taboos also will induce deficiency of a number of essential nutrients. When more than one nutritional deficiency exists, the patient may only present with the most limiting nutrient deficiency. For example, ingestion of a diet deficient in both thiamine and riboflavin would produce only those signs and symptoms associated with thiamine deficiency. One could easily *unmask* the riboflavin deficiency state by treating only with thiamine. The concept of an "unmasking" effect should not be confused with "induction" of a nutritional deficiency. Children subsisting on marginal diets low in protein may develop vitamin A deficiency or signs of some other fat-soluble vitamin deficiency if given adequate protein in the form of skim milk. The growth spurt which follows the feeding of protein could induce nutritional deficiencies unless adequate amounts of the other known essential nutrients are simultaneously provided.

In contrast, secondary deficiencies are usually the result of the several factors and combinations thereof listed in Table 11–1.

TABLE 11–1. ORIGINS OF PRIMARY AND SECONDARY DEFICIENCY STATES

---

1. Primary Deficiency

    Recommended Daily Allowances Not Met

        a. Ignorance
        b. Faddism
        c. Psychological
        d. Poverty

2. Secondary Deficiency (Induced)

    Recommended Daily Allowances Met
        a. Decreased or Defective Utilization, Imbalance, Reduced Intake
        b. Increased Utilization
        c. Increased loss
            (1) Malabsorption
            (2) Excretion

Brief examples of each of these situations follow:

1. *Decreased or defective utilization, imbalance and reduced intake* are exemplified by vomiting, diarrhea or faulty mastication which may result in decreased utilization of essential nutrients. Certain drugs may affect absorption (e.g., folic acid), while others may block uptake of a nutrient by organs (e.g., thioureas block iodine uptake by thyroid). Various nutrients in excess may block the absorption of other nutrients (imbalance). Avidin in uncooked egg whites binds biotin, resulting in a deficiency of that vitamin. A diseased organ may not be able to store efficiently an essential nutrient or to transform the nutrient into its metabolically active form (e.g., liver disease with decreased conversion of essential nutrients to coenzyme forms). Inborn errors of metabolism account for defective utilization (e.g., phenylalanine in phenylketonuria; tryptophan in Hartnup's disease). Surgical removal or diseases of certain areas of the gastrointestinal tract may lead to defective absorption of certain vitamins (e.g., with loss of the gastric intrinsic factor or resection of the ileum, there is decreased B_{12} absorption).

2. *Increased utilization* is seen in rapid rates of growth or recovery from disease. Requirements for many essential nutrients increase during pregnancy, lactation and with hypermetabolic diseases (hyperthyroidism).

3. *Increased loss* occurs with malabsorption and increased excretion of many nutrients in a number of clinical entities. Diuretics may increase the loss of certain electrolytes and vitamins (e.g., thiamine). Protein-losing enteropathies will increase the requirement for protein and other essential substances. Bleeding or excessive blood loss may increase the requirements for iron, folate and other nutrients. Burns, exudates and intestinal parasites all increase nutritional requirements.

For all species, including man, the first sign of any nutritional deficiency is loss of appetite and failure to grow. Additional, more specific manifestations will appear, depending on past dietary practices, the possible existence of infection and perhaps many other factors as well.

PROTEIN-CALORIE MALNUTRITION

The dietary protein requirement for infants is approximately 8 per cent of total calories. After the first year of life, it decreases to approximately 4 to 5 per cent of total calories.

These figures are based on proteins that have biologic values of 100 per cent. The biologic value (BV) of protein can be defined as the percentage of absorbed protein retained. A protein with a BV of 100 per cent implies that all of the protein (nitrogen) absorbed is retained. In turn, the amount retained is a function of the amino acid composition of the protein. High quality protein contains all of the essential amino acids in correct proportion; such protein would be 100 per cent retained and therefore would have a BV of 100 per cent. Proteins with low BV are poorly retained because they do not have all of the essential amino acids in the proper concentrations. Thus, in meeting protein requirements, the BV of the protein must be considered. Proteins with biologic values of less than approximately 60 per cent, for example, can never be ingested in sufficient amounts to meet protein requirements. It is possible, however, to combine two or more poor-quality proteins and have a mixture with a high or acceptable BV. Approximately 2.5 gm. of protein per kg. of body weight is the minimal requirement for infants, decreasing gradually to about 0.4 gm. per kg. of body weight in adults (Hegsted, 1957). However, as cited above, the Food and Nutrition Board has set higher limits. In diarrheal states, during infection and fever, etc., there may be increased catabolism and loss of proteins; thus, the requirements have built-in "safety factors." The total caloric requirement in infancy is usually stated as about 110 calories per kg. In adults, the daily requirement is about 2500 but may be higher depending on many factors including climate, stress and physical work.

MARASMUS AND KWASHIORKOR

Protein-calorie deficiency results in either marasmus or kwashiorkor, depending on the precise composition of the diet. *Marasmus is a state of malnutrition resulting from a deficiency of total calories.* Marasmus means "wasting away" and, in blunt terms, denotes starvation. In such deficient diets, the ratio of protein to calories may be normal (Fig. 11–1). *Kwashiorkor, on the other hand, results from a dietary deficiency of protein despite an adequate caloric intake* (Fig. 11–2). Kwashiorkor is the Ghanian term for second child. The syndrome was first described in infants displaced from the breast at a very early age by the birth of a second child. Obviously, diets inadequate in total calories with a disproportionate lack of protein will result in either marasmus or kwashiorkor, or in a mixed type, marasmus-kwashiorkor.

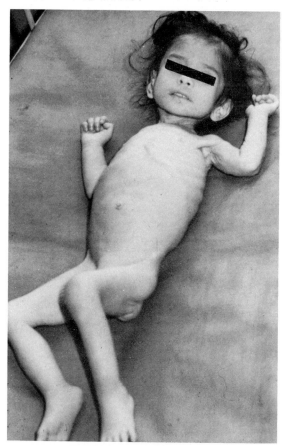

Figure 11–1. *Typical appearance of marasmus in a child two years and four months old (contrast with kwashiorkor, Fig. 11–2).*

The clinical manifestations of kwashiorkor (seen more often in children than adults) are varied, but include: growth failure, edema, hepatomegaly, anemia, hair changes and dermatoses. The child is often apathetic, anorexic, cries a great deal and is withdrawn and irritable. The edema may be generalized or it may be localized to the upper or lower extremities. There is always hypoalbuminemia and a decrease in the total serum protein, which does not always correlate well with the severity of the edema.

The skin lesions are pathognomonic when present but are not requisite for the diagnosis. Areas of depigmentation or hyperpigmentation or, in white infants, patches of dusky erythema lead to the characteristic "crazy pavement" appearance (Fig. 11–3). There is extensive desquamation in severe cases. The hair changes consist of pallor, straightening (if the normal hair is curly), fineness of texture and loose attachment of the roots, as evidenced by the ease with which the hair is pulled out. A

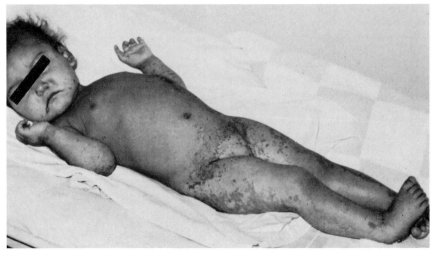

Figure 11-2. Kwashiorkor in a two-and-a-half year old girl. Note the cheilosis, dermatoses (arms, thighs) and edema (hands, legs and feet) with ascites.

"flag sign" may appear as alternating bands of light (depigmented) and dark areas in the hair, which in essence record alternating periods of good and bad nutrition. The liver is usually enlarged and fatty but never cirrhotic. The anemia may be of a mixed type, generally involving iron and folic acid deficiencies. Other signs may be present depending on the prior nutrition and adequacy of diet. For example, the extent to which manifestations of a deficiency of vitamin A or thiamine appear is a function of previous nutrition, dietary intake of these essential nutrients, infection and a host of other factors.

Marasmus and kwashiorkor, although different in many aspects, are related and perhaps represent the opposite ends of a disease spectrum with many intermediate expressions. The marasmic child may present many of the signs of kwashiorkor except for growth failure and edema. He is cachectic with little or no subcutaneous fat, appears alert and hungry and will eat ravenously if presented with food. The wasting is very apparent, and the child presents with more of a defect in weight than in height. Marasmus usually presents at an earlier age than kwashiorkor, and its pathogenesis has been usually attributed to early abrupt weaning and inadequate diet, followed by gastrointestinal infection and diarrhea. Epidemiologic studies would support the concept that some degree of marasmus usually precedes the clinical picture of kwashiorkor. Thus, marasmus, followed by a serious infection, may precipitate kwashiorkor. Indeed, usually after one treats the acute kwashiorkor patient, one finds a marasmic child beneath the edema.

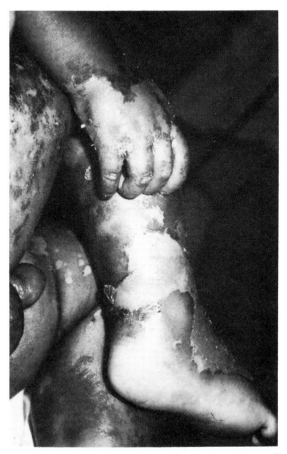

Figure 11-3. Dermatoses with marked edema of hands, legs and scrotum (kwashiorkor).

Morphology. The pathology of protein deficiency can be summarized quite simply: hypoplasia and atrophy.

Gastrointestinal Mucosa. The mucosa of the small bowel in kwashiorkor is atrophic, and in severe cases there is almost complete obliteration of the mucosal crypts and villus epithelial cells (Fig. 11—4). As a result, these patients lose many of the enzymes associated with the microvilli. Marked disaccharidase deficiencies occur, and therefore many of these children cannot be treated with milk because of the lactase deficiency. Curiously, there seems to be no absorptive defects other than the one associated with disaccharidase deficiency. There is usually no malabsorption of moderate levels of dietary fat and none of proteins. Recovery of the gastrointestinal changes in kwashiorkor can be achieved quite promptly by dietary means and with proper therapy for concomitant infections.

The Hematopoietic System. The anemia of protein-calorie marasmus is usually of the normochromic and normocytic type. However, after therapy with protein and other essential nutrients, associated deficiencies may be unmasked, such as a lack of folic acid or iron or both.

In kwashiorkor, the anemia is similarly normochromic and normocytic. The bone marrow is usually normocellular but the myeloid to erythroid ratio is above normal. Protein is apparently the only nutrient whose deficiency results in erythroid hypoplasia; it is referred to as erythroid atrophy to indicate that it is part of the general tissue wasting of protein deprivation (Ghitis and Vitale, 1963).

Liver. Fatty change is usually seen in protein malnutrition and is thought to be due to a decreased synthesis of the lipoproteins necessary for the mobilization of fat from the liver. There is no evidence that these children ever develop cirrhosis. With dietary therapy, there is a marked increase in the total serum lipids and in other fat soluble material, e.g., vitamin A. This increase in serum lipids is transient and reflects synthesis of those proteins required for fat transport.

In general, complete remission of all signs and symptoms of kwashiorkor can be achieved within four to six weeks with appropriate therapy. Infections of bacterial, fungal and viral origin are virtually inevitable in these malnourished infants and must be eradicated.

The literature is replete with studies on the relationship between protein malnutrition and mental retardation and/or performance. Suffice it to say that there is no clear evidence that protein-calorie malnutrition in the six-month or older child produces any irreversible damage to the brain. Perhaps fetal or neonatal malnutrition is more important in determining future performance than the protein malnutrition which occurs after the first six months of life. Protein-calorie malnutrition early in life or in infants of low birth weight may affect brain cell proliferation. It is during the last trimester and first six months of life that the marked proliferation of brain cells occurs which might be affected by the state of protein nutrition. There is evidence that social deprivation and the lack of proper stimuli early in life may have greater adverse effects on performance and motivation to learn than the state of nutrition. Tragically, the argument will continue to rage over whether protein-calorie malnutrition is a primary or a secondary factor in mental performance, while the number of malnourished children continues to increase.

It must be stressed that the child with protein-calorie malnutrition or the child with the "failure to thrive" syndrome may present with a number of signs and symptoms which can be

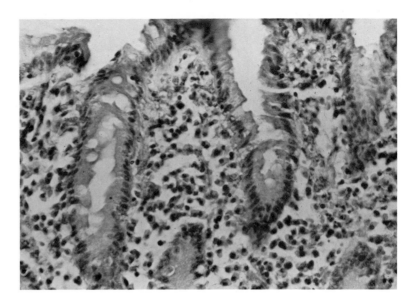

Figure 11–4. Small bowel biopsy from a child with marasmic kwashiorkor. Note marked villus atrophy and mild degree of lymphocytic infiltration.

mistaken for other diseases. This has resulted in improper therapy to the detriment of the child. Children with protein-calorie malnutrition have been improperly treated for such diseases as gluten enteropathy, hyperparathyroidism, tetany, gastroenteritis, Crohn's disease and even for such rare diseases as Hirschsprung's disease.

Usually there are other associated nutritional deficiencies accompanying the protein-calorie malnutrition. These include both the fat-soluble and water-soluble vitamins, as well as some of the minerals. A discussion of these follows.

VITAMINS

Vitamins are organic substances that, in minute amounts, take part usually as coenzymes in the complex biochemical reactions of the body. They do not enter significantly into the formation of cell structure and are not utilized as sources of energy. The discussion which follows will be limited to the role of vitamins in man.

FAT-SOLUBLE VITAMINS

The fat-soluble vitamins are in general less readily absorbed than the water-soluble vitamins. The various "interferences" previously listed tend to disturb the normal intake of these liposolubles more than that of the water-soluble vitamins. Most important among these are disturbances in pancreatic function and the large category of malabsorption syndromes. However, fat-soluble vitamins are generously stored, chiefly in the liver, and hence deficiency states only develop after protracted negative balances.

VITAMIN A (RETINOL—VITAMIN A₁, AND DEHYDRORETINOL—VITAMIN A₂)

(Deficiency states: night blindness, xerophthalmia, keratomalacia, epithelial keratinizing metaplasia, disturbances in bone growth)

NORMAL METABOLISM

Chemistry. Retinol is available to man in his diet in two forms: as the vitamin itself or as the provitamin precursors, the carotenes. The greater part of the usual dietary intake is in the form of carotenoids, of which 10 act as provitamins in varying degrees. The most important of these to man is beta carotene, consisting essentially of two linked vitamin A molecules. Vitamin A and the carotenes are not significantly soluble in water. Since they are fairly stable to heat, foods containing them retain their vitamin activity if cooked briefly.

Physiology. The absorption of the carotenoids can be influenced by a number of factors, including the levels of dietary fat and protein. Although beta carotene is the best source of vitamin A, its biologic activity is about half that of preformed vitamin A (retinol). Thus, in terms of meeting requirements, one needs approximately twice as much beta carotene as vitamin A.

In the lumen of the small intestine, vitamin A esters are hydrolyzed and packaged into micelles with the assistance of bile salts; alpha-tocopherol prevents destruction by oxidation. Carotene is converted into retinol and, together with preformed vitamin A, is esterified preferentially with palmitic acid. Retinyl palmitate is carried in chylomicrons via the lymphatic system through the thoracic duct to the blood stream and is stored in the liver. Stored retinyl ester is hydrolyzed by a liver enzyme; free retinol then travels via the blood stream to the tissues, where a metabolic requirement for the vitamin exists (Roels, 1970) (Wasserman and Corradino, 1971).

The vitamin A (retinol) requirement established by the Food and Nutrition Board varies according to age from 1500 I.U. for infants up to 4000 to 5000 I.U. (0.3 microgm. = 1 I.U.) for adults. The requirement during pregnancy and lactation is elevated to approximately 6000 to 8000 I.U. per day. The serum carotenoid levels for healthy adults in highly industrialized areas range from 90 to 220 microgm./100 ml. and, for vitamin A, range from 30 to 70 microgm./100 ml. Liver reserves of vitamin A in similar individuals vary from 25 to 200 microgm. per gm. of liver. *Vitamin A deficiency is usually secondary to malabsorption or other situations affecting fat absorption.* In vitamin A deficiency from whatever cause, both the carotenoid and vitamin A levels in plasma fall significantly and are sometimes used as one of the parameters for making the diagnosis of malabsorption.

Recent studies (Smith et al., 1970) have shown that retinol circulates in human plasma bound to a specific protein. This retinol-binding protein (RBP) has an alpha 1 mobility on electrophoresis and a molecular weight of approximately 21,000. In severe malnutrition where there is a reduction in total serum protein, the vitamin A levels may be low as a result of decreased production of RBP. With the administration of protein and recovery from malnutrition, serum levels of RBP rise, as do serum levels of vitamin A. Thus the serum vitamin A levels may be spuriously depressed and not accurately reflect body stores.

Vitamin A tolerance curves are carried out by providing 0.22 gm. of vitamin A per kg. body weight and noting the rise in serum vitamin A. Normally, there is a 40 to 60 I.U. rise above the fasting level, whereas in cases of malabsorption or severe vitamin A deficiency, there is a "flat curve." Vitamin A palmitate and the water-soluble dispersible form in daily doses of 50,000 to 100,000 I.U., when given parenterally, produce very high blood levels which are maintained for about 48 hours. Continued treatment with vitamin A can be given via the oral route, provided there is no malabsorption, vomiting or diarrhea. Night blindness and conjunctival changes respond to 30,000 I.U. of vitamin A daily for two to three weeks, given as cod liver oil.

Notwithstanding that it has been over half a century since the original experiments were done which led to the discovery of this vitamin, *it is remarkable that we do not understand any other metabolic role of vitamin A except for that in the visual cycle.* Indeed, it has been known for over 3000 years that vitamin A in the form of ox liver was a cure for night blindness. The human retina contains two distinct photoreceptor systems: the rods, which are responsible for vision in weak light, and the cones, which are responsive to light of high intensity and to colors. Retinol is the prosthetic group of photosensitive pigment in both photoreceptor systems. The major difference between the visual pigment in rods (rhodopsin) and that in cones (idopsin) is the nature of the protein bound to retinol. All of the reactions involved in the oxidation of retinol to retinal and stereochemical changes in the chain of the vitamin A molecule which occur in the visual process are known in some detail, and are discussed below. Wald (1968) first elucidated the vitamin A macromolecule interactions responsible for visual excitation, and was awarded the Nobel Prize for Medicine in 1967 for these discoveries.

PATHOLOGY

Basis of Deficiency State. Avitaminosis A may occur as a primary deficiency due to an inadequate diet. However, for reasons already stated, the tissue reserves are of such magnitude as to make simple deficiency states extremely unlikely. In a study conducted in England on 16 volunteers with diets containing not more than a trace of vitamin A for nine months, the plasma level fell from an initial average of 88 I.U. to 74 I.U. per 100 cc. of plasma, not a significantly low level. More commonly, avitaminosis A occurs as a conditioned deficiency from disorders affecting fat absorption, such as biliary tract disease, pancreatic disease, sprue and severe intestinal disease. Inadequate reserves in patients with severe liver disease may also lead to depleted vitamin A levels. These conditioning influences may act not only by depleting the body stores, but also by inhibiting its mobilization from depot sites, and by depressing the vitamin-carrying capacity of plasma.

Disease States. These include night blindness (hemeralopia or nyctalopia); epithelial metaplasia, including xerophthalmia; keratomalacia and follicular dermatitis; and disturbed bone growth (Mason, 1954).

Night Blindness. Night blindness (impaired vision in subdued light) is usually due to vitamin A deficiency, though it also may be due to other causes. Vitamin A in its aldehyde form, known as retinal, and a protein called opsin are the structural constituents of the photosensitive pigment of the rod cells of the retina called rhodopsin or visual purple. It is the action of light causing an isomerization of this pigment that is responsible for initiation of the nervous impulse to the optic nerve which results in visual acuity in subdued light. The pigment is broken down to opsin and a stereoisomer of retinal in this reaction. In the dark, through a series of well elucidated steps, the correct geometric form of retinal is reconstituted and combines spontaneously with opsin to form rhodopsin once again so that the cycle can be repeated. However, during visual activity some of the retinal becomes an inactive isomer, and so is permanently lost. Thus, a constantly available source of additional vitamin A is necessary to maintain adequate levels of visual purple. A similar, though less well understood situation exists for cone vision in bright light. Here also a vitamin A aldehyde is combined with a specific protein to form iodopsin.

Epithelial Metaplasia. In some as yet unknown fashion, vitamin A is necessary for the maintenance of the specialized epithelial surfaces of the body, e.g., the mucous membranes of the eyes; the mucosa of the respiratory, gastrointestinal and genitourinary tracts; the lining epithelia of gland ducts; and the ducts of skin appendages. Wolbach and Bessey (1942) have characterized the general nature of these epithelial changes resulting from vitamin A deficiency as "atrophy of the epithelium concerned, reparative proliferation of the basal cells and growth and differentiation of the new products into a stratified keratinizing epithelium." From this description, it is apparent that in the sites mentioned the normal epithelium, whatever its type, is replaced by inappropriate keratinized, stratified squamous epithelium. If the epithelium is normally stratified and keratinized as is the skin, it becomes excessively keratinized. The nonkeratinized, stratified squamous mucosa, such as is found in the conjunctiva, cornea and vagina, becomes keratinized. When the epithelium is more specialized, e.g., the columnar epithelium of the respiratory tract, cuboidal epithelium that lines ducts, or transitional epithelium of the urinary tract, the changes take the form of atrophy of the normal mucosal surface and eventual replacement of it by stratified squamous, keratinized epithelium (Fig. 11—5).

In the eye, the scleral and corneal mucous membrane becomes keratinized. The goblet mucous cells in these surfaces disappear and, along with this change, the lining of the ducts of the tear glands is replaced by keratinized, stratified squamous epithelium. The keratin debris plugs the ducts. The normal moist, mucosal surfaces become dry, granular and roughened, resembling skin (**xerophthalmia**). The keratin debris accumulates in whitish plaques (Bitot's spots). These modifications lead to significant irritation in the orbit. Visual acuity is impaired by the keratinization and thickening of the corneal mucosa. This surface may ulcerate and lead to softening and opacity of the cornea with secondary infection. As the corneal involvement progresses, vascularization and infiltration by inflammatory cells hasten the softening and sometimes lead to frank perforation. These corneal changes are referred to as **keratomalacia.**

In the respiratory tract, including the nose, nasopharynx and sinuses, the normal columnar **ciliated epithelium is replaced by nonciliated, stratified squamous epithelium,** which seriously impairs the normal defensive function of the mucosa. The presumed sequence of changes is, first, atrophy of the specialized epithelial cells, then metaplasia of the basal elements to squamous epithelial cells, with growth of these cells to form keratinized epithelium. Ciliary action is thus lost and the normal secretions are suppressed. The desquamated keratin debris acts as foreign bodies, producing irritation which predisposes to superimposed infections. The epithelial changes in the nose provide a source of diagnostic scrapings, which may reveal keratinized scales in place of the usual cells, an aid in the diagnosis of this avitaminosis.

In the urinary tract, particularly in the renal pelvis and bladder, **the keratin debris may serve as a nidus for the formation of urinary tract stones,** which further predispose to inflammatory changes and infections.

Changes in the skin have been described by some and denied by others, since it is postulated that the skin is normally keratinized and hence cannot be subject to squamous metaplasia. The alterations mentioned include hyperplasia and hyperkeratinization of the epidermis, and plugging of the hair shafts and sebaceous gland ducts by piled up masses of keratin, which produces numerous minute papules and gives a rough, sandpaper-like texture to the skin. This condition is known as **follicular or papular hyperkeratosis or dermatosis.** Similarly, plugging of the ducts of the salivary glands and pancreas may give rise to significant digestive disturbances.

Disturbed Bone Growth. Wolbach (1937) has shown retardation of normal bone growth in avitaminotic young, growing animals. Conversely, large doses of vitamin A so stimulated bone growth that development normally requiring a year occurred within a few weeks. Epiphyseal bone formation appears to be the specific process affected. The increased growth rate is accompanied by bone resorption and an increased fragility. At the present time, no well defined retardation changes have been established in infants, possibly because comparable severe deficiency states are extremely unlikely in children receiving either mother's or cow's milk. The skeletal alterations in animals may lead to changes in the central nervous system, presumably because, in instances of retarded bone growth, the brain and cord grow faster than the skull and spinal canal and are compressed by their bony confinements. Once again, the human counterpart has not yet been described.

Although profound changes have been described in the dentition of vitamin A deficient animals, corroboration of these observations in man has not yet been made.

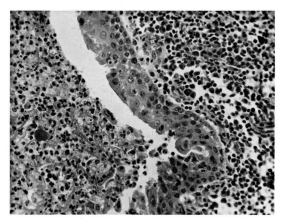

Figure 11—5. Squamous metaplasia of the epithelial lining of a duct in the pancreas.

The clinical manifestations of vitamin A deficiency include night blindness, keratomalacia and a papular dermatitis, frequently accompanied by diseases of the respiratory tract incident to the keratinized metaplasia of the epithelial surfaces of these organs. Impairment of visual acuity in dim light is usually the first demonstrable change. The changes in the conjunctival mucosa of the eye offer considerable support to the appropriate diagnosis.

Toxicity. Excesses of vitamin A may produce both acute and chronic toxicity. The acute toxicity of hypervitaminosis A was accurately described hundreds of years ago when early Arctic explorers noted the development of headaches, dizziness, vomiting and diarrhea soon after the ingestion of polar bear liver, an exceptionally rich source of vitamin A. Skin desquamation has followed. The same syndrome has since been encountered in infants given an entire ampule of vitamin A concentrate containing 350,000 units (Braun, 1962). In these infants, sudden striking elevations of intracranial pressure have been noted to the point that bulging of the fontanelles has occurred. Skin desquamation soon followed. These manifestations rapidly clear in a few days after overdosage has been stopped, and no permanent sequelae have been noted.

Chronic toxicity is more difficult to detect and has not been widely appreciated as a hazard by the medical profession (Jeghers and Marraro, 1956). It has most often been encountered in young adults given large doses (up to 600,000 units daily) for acne or to prevent colds. The manifestations are most protean and include bone pain, loss of hair, skin desquamation, anorexia, hepatomegaly and headaches with chronically increased intracranial pressure leading to hydrocephalus. These unfortunates have even been submitted to neurologic surgery, while others have been put into whole body casts for relief of the skeletal complaints. More often, the dominant symptoms have related either to the skin with pruritus, hyperkeratosis and varying degrees of alopecia, or to the skeletal system with painful swellings along the bones associated with radiologic evidence of new bone formation and cortical bone thickening. A few patients have developed a bleeding diathesis relieved by vitamin K.

Experimentally, congenital anomalies can be induced in the offspring of pregnant rats, an observation worth remembering in the indiscriminate use of vitamin supplementation during pregnancy.

VITAMIN D

(Deficiency states: rickets and osteomalacia)

NORMAL METABOLISM

Chemistry. Of the forms of vitamin D that exist in nature, the two most important to man are vitamin D_2 (ergocalciferol), found principally in food, and vitamin D_3 (cholecalciferol), produced in the skin by irradiation of 7-dehydrocholesterol. Both forms undergo similar metabolic transformations in the liver; vitamin D_2 is converted to 25-hydroxyergocalciferol and D_3, to 25-hydroxycholecalciferol. The efficiency of conversion of D_2 to its more active form is significantly less than that of D_3. Therefore, D_3 is the more potent of the two forms.

The main circulating form of vitamin D is 25-hydroxycholecalciferol (25-HCC). Several metabolites of 25-HCC are now known to exist, the most important of them being 1,25-dihydroxycholecalciferol (1,25-DHCC). This compound is currently thought to be the final active metabolite of vitamin D_3. It acts more rapidly than 25-HCC in stimulating intestinal calcium absorption and in mobilizing skeletal calcium. The sole site of hydroxylation of 25-HCC to 1,25-DHCC is the kidney, and its production of 1,25-DHCC is controlled by both parathyroid hormone and circulating levels of 25-HCC. Parathyroid hormone (p. 1346) suppresses the conversion of 25-HCC to 1,25-DHCC and enhances the formation of 21,25-DHCC, less active in calcium absorption and probably favoring bone resorption, osteoporosis and osteomalacia. 21,25-DHCC is very effective in mobilizing bone but is not effective in intestinal calcium transport. However, 25,26-DHCC, another metabolite of vitamin D, is very effective in enhancing calcium transport across the gut but is not active in mobilization of bone calcium (Raisz, 1972) (Wasserman and Taylor, 1972) (DeLuca, 1969, 1971).

Physiology. The precise role of vitamin D in mineralization of bone matrix is still incompletely understood. However, in recent years a great deal has been learned regarding the complex interrelations between vitamin D, its various metabolites and parathyroid hormone and their action in calcium metabolism. *Most likely the failure of bony calcification in vitamin D deficiency states is due to a failure of supply of calcium and phosphate to the bone.* Vitamin D does not seem to participate directly in the calcification process. Along with PTH and perhaps calcitonin, the principal role of vitamin D and its metabolites is to regulate calcium and phosphorus metabolism and thus permit normal mineralization of bone.

A number of factors are involved in the maintenance of normal serum and tissue calcium levels and bone calcification. In animals fed low calcium diets, there is a greater conversion of 25-HCC to 1,25-DHCC. In contrast, when animals are fed high calcium diets, 25-HCC is converted to 21,25-DHCC. Parathyroid hormone also participates in regulation of the serum calcium levels. One action of parathyroid hormone (PTH) may be to change vitamin D metabolism by altering the intracellular calcium level in the kidney. PTH facilitates the uptake of calcium by the kidney cell. Assuming that the calcium concentration in the kidney cell triggers the conversion of 25-HCC to either 1,25-DHCC or 21,25-DHCC and that PTH facilitates calcium entry into the kidney cell, then a drop in serum calcium would lower intracellular levels and favor the formation of 1,25-HCC, whereas an increase above "normal" would favor the formation of the inactive form, 21,25-DHCC. In addition to these actions, PTH may also have a direct effect on the kidney's metabolism of vitamin D.

Another major role of vitamin D is the facilitation of calcium absorption in the gut. *Vitamin D, perhaps in conjunction with PTH, controls the synthesis of a calcium-binding protein (CaBP) found in the cells of the small intestine.* This CaBP facilitates transport of calcium across the epithelial cell in an ATP requiring system (DeLuca, 1969).

The vitamin D requirement set forth by the Food and Nutrition board is 400 I.U. per day for all ages and sexes. Absorption of the various forms of vitamin D occurs in the intestinal tract. Bile salts and especially the salts of deoxycholic acid are particularly necessary. Any hepatobiliary disorder impairs the absorption of this vitamin. Impaired absorption of fat also lowers the intestinal uptake of this fat-soluble vitamin so that pancreatic disease, sprue or celiac disease, and other causes of poor absorption of fat may lead to a conditioned deficiency. These malabsorption syndromes are perhaps the most important causes of avitaminosis D in the western world.

As with vitamin A, the liver is the chief storage depot, but significant amounts are also found in the skin and the brain with smaller quantities in the lungs, spleen and bones. Even large doses are totally retained and stored and exert an antirachitic effect for long periods.

For a thorough understanding of the disease states produced by vitamin D deficiency, normal osteogenesis and the role of vitamin D should be outlined briefly. Bone is formed by two totally distinct processes, membranous bone formation and endochondral bone formation. In *membranous bone formation*, osteoid matrix is formed within connective tissue by specialized mesenchymal cells. This osteoid is then converted into bone by the mineralization of the matrix through the action of osteoblasts. Bone is thus formed without the intermediary development of cartilage. Such bones are the cranium, the mandible and a portion of the clavicle. Appositional growth along the shafts of long bones is accomplished by this type of growth pattern, and accounts for the expansion in diameter with increase in length. In the state of vitamin D deficiency, with inadequate phosphate and calcium and impaired deposition of these minerals into the osteoid matrix, insufficient mineralization occurs and results in excessive osteoid and the creation of a soft, yielding, easily deformed bone.

The second pathway, *endochondral bone formation*, occurs in all other bones of the skeletal system. The stages of this complex bone growth can be followed best by description of the sequence of events occurring at the epiphyseal plate in one of the long bones. Continuous growth of the epiphyseal cartilage produces expansion of the cartilaginous plate, both toward the shaft (diaphysis) of the bone and toward the distal end of the bone. At the same time, the cartilaginous growth on the diaphyseal side undergoes constant resorption and replacement, a process that has been likened by Wolbach to "a constantly retreating" line with progressive lengthening of the bone.

The resorptive changes along the diaphyseal surface of the cartilaginous plate comprise the crux of endochondral bone formation. At the line of junction between the cartilage and bone, the most superficial older cartilaginous cells grow larger and line up to form vertical columns of cells oriented in the long axis of the bone, separated by spicules of matrix that form a "picket fence" palisade. The most peripheral of these cartilage cells undergo degeneration and create long, separated, parallel fingers of cartilaginous matrix that appear to project into the osetochondral junction. Lime salts are deposited in the cartilaginous spicules (*provisional calcification*), and simultaneously capillaries and osteoblasts grow between the spicules. Osteoid tissue formed by the osteoblasts first layers the spicules of cartilage and then replaces them as they undergo resorption. The deposition of calcium and phosphate into the osteoid tissue creates bone. The newly formed spicules of bone, however, do not represent the final architecture, since there is continuous remodeling as the lines of weight-bearing and stress are modified by growth. Even in adult life, reworking and reshaping of bone maintains a constant bone reformation and necessitates continual adequate levels of calcium, phosphate and vitamin D.

There is, with avitaminosis D, a failure of bone

mineralization, but no failure of osteoid formation (Lamm and Neuman, 1958). Normal bone is primarily composed of the minerals calcium and phosphate, along with substantial amounts of OH^-, $CO_3^=$ and citrate. Trace amounts of other ions, such as Na^+, Mg^{++} and Fl^-, are also present. The mineral salts of bone are arranged into crystalline structures of ultramicroscopic size closely resembling hydroxyapatite with extremely large surface areas per volume. There is believed to be a wide variability in the mineral content of these crystals. The spaces between the crystals are filled with organic matrix, water and solid constituents not included within the crystalline structure. The collagen fibers of the matrix serve as reinforcing strands and, when conditions are appropriate, probably act as seed crystals in the initiation of crystal formation. The electron microscope shows the crystals lying within the organic matrix, water and solid constitu-pattern around the collagen fibers.

While the bone appears to be very rigid and static, at the microscopic level it is in a state of constant flux. This is particularly true of those crystals with exposed surfaces. These comprise the *labile* portion of bone. Mineral exchange is relatively slow where there are no exposed surfaces, and this portion of bone is therefore termed *stable*. About the crystalline surfaces is found the important *surface hydration shell*, which contains ions in equilibrium with both the surrounding medium and the adjacent crystals. The noncrystalline components of bone, in contrast, remain relatively constant, although water is displaced by the formation of new crystals. According to our present understanding, such displacement of water may occur up to the point where there is just sufficient water left for the diffusion of new material into the bone structure. Even so, at that point the diffusion and exchange of ions are very slow so that bone is mobilized only with great difficulty.

The *mineralization of the matrix is controlled by both humoral and local conditions. Humoral conditions* include the supply and transport of the necessary minerals to the proper loci. The principal ions involved in bone formation, namely calcium and phosphate, must be present in sufficient amounts so that the surrounding medium is supersaturated with respect to the bone mineral, yet not to the degree at which spontaneous precipitation would occur. The values of these concentrations are not known since the solubility product of calcium and phosphate has never been adequately calculated. *Local influences* determine the precise loci of mineralization and thus prevent random calcification of tissues. Enzymes, particu-

larly alkaline phosphatases, are believed to play an important role in this local control, most probably as destroyers of an inhibitor substance and releasers of chemically active phosphate radicals from organic complexes. The supersaturated solution must be seeded, followed by precipitation of the minerals and crystal formation. It has been mentioned that collagen is believed to be the substance that acts as the seed crystal, but other poorly defined substances, possibly the mucopolysaccharides of the ground substance, may also be necessary. The act of crystallization is not a simple precipitation, but rather comprises an orderly stepwise addition of ions from the hydration shell to the developing stable structure.

There is much dispute as to whether the hydration shell and the extracellular fluid are in equilibrium. The surface crystals are exposed to their hydration shells, which in turn are in contact with the extracellular fluid. Some postulate a gradient which maintains a differential between the pH at the surface of the crystal and that of the circulating fluids. They propose that the production of acid by the bone cells keeps the pH at the surface of the crystal lower than that of the extracellular fluid. The lower pH is thought to be essential for the solubilization of the mineral phase and for the movement of ions from bone to blood and vice versa.

It is obvious that both the formation and the mobilization of the mineral phase of bone involve many complexities. How is such a delicate process regulated? Of the many contributing factors involving bone formation, only a few will be cited.

Until the epiphyses close, growth hormone of the anterior lobe of the pituitary is essential for growth in the length of long bones. With hypophysectomy, there is a cessation of growth of the epiphyseal disk as proliferation of the cartilage ceases. Administration of growth hormone before final closure will cause a prompt renewal in bone development. There is no understanding of the biochemical action of this hormone.

A deficiency of thyroid hormone will lead to cretinism, a condition in which there is a general retardation of skeletal development and growth. The alterations generally resemble those of the hypophysectomized animal. Androgens also play a role in bony development. Animals castrated at birth do not have a normal bone development.

A number of factors are known to have effects upon the matrix of bone and thus on bone formation. Corticosteroids affect the matrix of bone, but the effect is believed to be nonspecific and secondary to the systemic regulatory functions of the adrenal steroids. Experimental fractures in animals heal slowly when glucocorticoids are administered. This is believed to be due to a depression of osteoblastic activity. It is well known that with Cushing's syndrome there are skeletal changes, including osteoporosis, yet the biochemical pathway is ill defined.

Vitamin A is necessary in rats for growth and maturation of epiphyseal cells. Thus, endochondral bone formation is defective with vitamin A deficiency. Remodeling of existing bone also fails with avitaminosis A.

Vitamin C is known to have an important role in the formation and maintenance of bone. Suffice it here to say that with scurvy there is a decrease in the production of collagen and bone matrix. Thus, though the calcification process is not affected, the bone is abnormal.

PATHOLOGY

Basis of Deficiency State. The development of rickets or osteomalacia is not merely a function of simple mineral or vitamin D deficiency. Many clinical studies indicate clearly that for obscure reasons there is a marked individual susceptibility to the disease, i.e., constitutional susceptibility. The rate of growth and age of a child materially affect his susceptibility to rickets. After the second year of life, the incidence is greatly reduced. It is of interest that in severely malnourished children, there is a considerable diminution in the need for the antirachitic factors, since their growth is retarded. Sunlight is an important factor in the prevention of rickets. In tropical climates, there is virtually no need for vitamin D from exogenous sources since sufficient protection is derived from the irradiation of the skin precursors. Moreover, it must be remembered that a deficiency of calcium or phosphate in the diet may lead to changes identical with rickets or vitamin D induced osteomalacia.

Disease States. Simple exogenous deficiencies are somewhat uncommon in the United States at present because of the widespread use of vitamin D fortified food. Deficiencies are still found, however, in low economic levels, and conditioned deficiencies may be encountered secondary to hepatobiliary disease, with the use of certain drugs, in kidney disease and in patients with parathyroid disease. Effective therapy in any of these situations may be accomplished by first correcting the primary defect and, secondly, by the administration of vitamin D. In hepatobiliary disease, there is inadequate absorption of the fat-soluble vitamins in the gut. There is an increased incidence of rickets and osteomalacia in epileptics being treated with anticonvulsant drugs. Anticonvulsant drugs apparently not only inhibit the conversion, in the liver, of vitamin D to 25-HCC, the initial biologically active form of vitamin D, but they also enhance vitamin D conversion to inactive metabolites (Hahn et al., 1972). Thus, patients on anticonvulsant therapy should be provided with supplemental vitamin D (Editorial, 1972).

Since the kidney is the sole site for the conversion of 25-HCC to 1,25-DHCC, it would seem obvious that the diseased kidney may be limited in this capacity. Patients with chronic and severe renal disease often develop signs and symptoms of vitamin D deficiency. The administration of physiologic doses of vitamin D does not improve the "vitamin D deficiency" state, but pharmacologic doses may. Brickman et al. (1972), studying vitamin D metabolism in patients with renal failure, demonstrated that the administration of 100 units (2.7 microgm.) of 1,25-DHCC daily for 6 to 10 days was effective in raising the serum calcium and phosphorus levels, increasing the absorption of calcium from 30 to 220 per cent and decreasing fecal calcium by 25 to 70 per cent. In contrast, 40,000 units (1 mg.) of vitamin D was ineffective. However, to be effective, the 1,25-DHCC had to be provided parenterally. In chronic renal disease, the oral administration of high doses of 25-HCC is more effective than that of vitamin D_2 or D_3, but it may also be more toxic.

Hyperparathyroidism induces bone disease, demineralization of bone, hypercalcemia and elevated serum alkaline phosphatase activity. How it exerts these effects is still somewhat unclear, but present evidence suggests that it increases the requirement for vitamin D. The oral administration of large doses of vitamin D_3 will counteract the effects of hyperparathyroidism on bone (Woodhouse et al., 1971). It is possible that the increased levels of PTH channel the renal metabolism of vitamin D into the jurisdiction of the metabolites most active in bone resorption. This effect of increased levels of PTH can be corrected by large doses of vitamin D_3 which would suggest a block in one of the metabolic pathways of vitamin D beyond the level of 25-HCC (Galante et al., 1972).

Deficiency States: Rickets (In Children), Osteomalacia (In Adults). The gross anatomic changes are more meaningful with an understanding of the underlying microscopic alterations. Many of the histologic changes in rickets and osteomalacia can be surmised from the discussion of normal osteogenesis. The basic alteration can then be characterized as **failure of mineralization of osteoid matrix with a consequent excess of osteoid tissue in the bones** (Kramer and Kanof, 1954).

The essential changes will be listed first and then described in somewhat greater detail.

1. Failure of deposition of calcium into the cartilage; failure of provisional calcification.

2. Failure of the cartilage cells to mature and disintegrate or be destroyed, with resultant overgrowth of cartilage.

3. Persistence of distorted irregular masses of cartilage, many of which project into the marrow cavity.

4. Deposition of osteoid matrix on cartilaginous remnants with formation of a disorderly, totally disrupted osteochondral junction.

5. Abnormal overgrowth of capillaries and fibroblasts into the disorganized zone.

6. Bending, compression and microfracture of soft, weakly supported osteoid and cartilaginous tissue with resultant skeletal deformities.

Although there is still some controversy as to the first deviation from normal in endochondral bone, it is generally believed that failure of mineralization of the palisade of cartilage matrix is the fundamental defect. The cartilage cells that have aligned themselves between the fingerlike projections of matrix fail to degenerate or are not invaded properly by capillary fibroblasts. As a result, the continued growth leads to an excess of cartilage. The epiphysis becomes widened, and large irregular, tongue-like processes of cartilage extend toward the shaft of the bone. In the plane of section, many of these cartilaginous projections may appear as large plates or islands of cartilage totally detached from the adjacent epiphysis. The osteochondral junction, which is normally quite regularly aligned, becomes completely jagged and disorderly. About and between the cartilaginous masses and spicules, osteoid matrix is produced by the normally functioning osteoblasts, but the matrix does not become mineralized and therefore accumulates in excess. Accompanying increased vascularization and fibrosis are present in the affected area (Fig. 11–6). Some calcification may be present in the scattered osteoid spicules in a spotty fashion, possibly related to varying levels of vitamin D deficiency, but in the florid advanced cases, mineralization is notably markedly deficient or quite absent. This zone of disorderly osteoid matrix and cartilage, known as the metaphysis, is soft, and may become distorted under the stress of weight-bearing. The entire metaphyseal area supported only by soft osteoid tissue and cartilage may become compressed with consequent widening and mushrooming of the external diameter of the bone. The bone may bend, or the epiphysis be displaced out of line so that it is no longer at right angles to the long axis of the bone. These displacements and microscopic

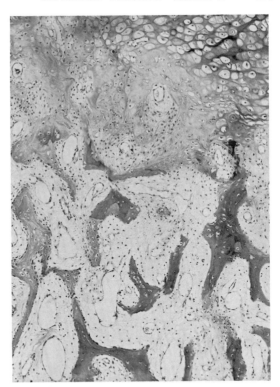

Figure 11–6. *A detail of a rachitic costochondral junction. The palisade of cartilage is lost. Some of the trabeculae are old, well formed bone, but the paler ones consist of unmineralized osteoid tissue.*

fractures cause further disarray of the rachitic zone and lead to hemorrhages, hemosiderosis and fibrosis.

In the areas of membranous bone, there is a failure of mineralization of newly formed osteoid tissue with accompanying increased fibrosis and vascularization. In the adult, cartilaginous bone growth has ceased, and therefore osteomalacia is reflected in changes similar to those that occur in membranous bone formation. In the appositional growth in the diameter of the bones, the newly formed osteoid matrix produced by osteoblasts is not mineralized. In addition, in the constant reworking of bone, mineralized bone is replaced by osteoid matrix so that even previously well formed bone becomes softer and more fragile and therefore susceptible to fracture and deformity.

Gross anatomic lesions are almost totally confined to the skeletal system and result from the formation of weak, poorly mineralized bone. The degree of deformity depends upon the severity of the rachitic process, its duration, the rate of growth of the individual and the stresses and tensions to which the bones are subject. Age is a particularly important factor, not only with respect to the growth rate, but also insofar as it conditions the type of stress. Obviously, the very young infant lying in bed is subject to different pressures and stresses than the child of two or three years who is already walking. During infancy, the nonambulatory child places greatest stress upon the head and chest. The softened occipital bones may become flattened and the cranium can be buckled inward by pressure but, with release of the pressure, elastic recoil snaps the bones back into their original positions. This clinical sign is known as **craniotabes**. It is best elicited in the frontal regions where there is greatest curvature of the skull. An excess of osteoid tissue produces **frontal bossing** and a **squared appearance to the head**. The chest becomes markedly deformed because of the overgrowth of cartilage and osteoid tissue at the costochondral junction, giving rise to the "**rachitic rosary**." The weakened metaphyseal area here is subject to the stress of gravity and the pull of the respiratory muscles and thus becomes progressively depressed. Along with this depression, the sternum and anterior portion of the rib cage tend to protrude and create the **pigeon-breast deformity**. The diaphragm causes a sharp depression that girdles the thoracic cavity at the lower margin of the rib cage **(Harrison's groove)**. In the young infant, the pelvis may become deformed by the stress of gravity.

When the child begins to ambulate, in addition to these deformities, changes occur in the vertebral column, pelvis and long bones. Commonly, a sharp forward curvature of the lumbar spine develops (lumbar lordosis). This lordosis may further accentuate the pelvic deformity. Support of the body weight leads to deformities in the long leg bones, and since frequently these children tend to sit and support themselves with their hands rather than stand, deformities occur in the long bones of the upper extremities as well. It should be emphasized here that the skeletal alterations described represent a florid, far advanced case and that suboptimal or varying levels of vitamin D intake may modify the derangements to the point at which alterations are so subtle as to escape detection.

Osteomalacia is extremely difficult to identify in the adult, since bony growth is already completed and marked deformities rarely develop. Osteomalacia is usually discovered as an increased radiolucency of bones or as an increased vulnerability to fractures (p. 1443).

Toxicity. Large excesses of vitamin D are well tolerated. Extreme overdosage (in the range of 1000 times the normal intake) causes hypercalcemia and consequent hypercalciuria. The high calcium levels are probably attributable to increased absorption of calcium from the intestinal tract as well as to mobilization of skeletal calcium (Follis, 1956). As a consequence of the increased levels of calcium in the blood, metastatic calcifications may occur and the hypercalciuria predisposes to the for-

mation of renal stones (p. 1138). Sufficient renal damage may occur to cause renal failure. The mobilization of skeletal calcium leads to the generalized bone disease known as osteoporosis (p. 1442). In addition to these morphologic alterations, there are many nonspecific complaints such as nausea, vomiting, diarrhea and signs of general toxicity.

VITAMIN E (ALPHA-TOCOPHEROL)

NORMAL METABOLISM

Chemistry. A group of fat-soluble tocopherols all have vitamin E activity. Four closely related chemical homologues are identified as alpha-, beta-, gamma- and delta-tocopherols. The alpha-tocopherol is the most active form biologically. All have been isolated in pure form, and all have been synthesized.

The tissue content of vitamin E varies widely, with the highest concentrations in the pituitary, testes and adrenals. The concentration in plasma in normal adults ranges between 0.8 and 1.4 mg. per 100 ml. However, in infancy and in premature infants these levels may fall to 0.04 to 0.4 mg. per 100 ml.

A primary vitamin E deficiency has never been established in man although it has been almost half a century since the original description of vitamin E deficiency in rats was first noted (Evans and Bishop, 1923). However, in 1968 the Food and Nutrition Board of the National Research Council established a requirement for vitamin E (alpha-tocopherol) of 25 to 30 mg. daily. These figures are based on the studies of Horwitt et al. (1961) who demonstrated that human subjects existing on a diet low in vitamin E for a period of five years developed, as would be expected, low plasma vitamin E levels and, using the hydrogen peroxide in vitro test, increased red cell hemolysis (Rose and Gyorgy, 1949). These studies of Horwitt et al. (1961) suggest that the requirement for vitamin E varies from 5 mg. per day in those on diets low in polyunsaturated fatty acids (PUFA) to 30 mg. in those on diets high in PUFA (60 gm. of corn oil daily).

Physiology. *It is generally accepted that the major function of vitamin E in metabolism is that of an antioxidant* (Wasserman and Taylor, 1972). It has been shown in experimental animals that the amount of vitamin E required in the diet to prevent signs of a deficiency depends on: (1) the amount of dietary PUFA, especially linoleic acid and (2) the presence of other natural or synthetic fat-soluble antioxidants in the diet as well as in the animal. Apparently, each gram of dietary PUFA increases the daily requirement of vitamin E by about 0.6 mg. Thus, it is easy to produce vitamin E deficiency in animals fed diets high in polyunsaturated fatty acids. Human studies yield the same findings.

A variety of anatomic and functional alterations have been described in vitamin E deficient rats, rabbits, guinea pigs and dogs. Depending on the species, vitamin E deficiency has been shown to produce changes in nerve tissue, in the erythron, in muscle and in the reproductive organs. Vitamin E is necessary for full development of the embryo. In its absence, conception and beginning embryogenesis may occur, but are promptly followed by resorption of the fetus. Fertilization does take place, however, indicating that vitamin E has no effect in supporting ovulation or reproductive ability in the female. Vitamin E appears to be necessary for the normal activity of the germinal epithelium of the male rat and guinea pig but not of the rabbit or mouse. In its absence, the spermatogonia and spermatocytes degenerate, with consequent loss of fertility. *There is no evidence, however, that vitamin E plays any role in sterility in man*

Peroxidation and pigmentation of fat occurs in animals fed vitamin E deficient diets high in polyunsaturated fatty acids. The pigmentation of the adipose tissue is the consequence of the formation of two products: one is a fat-soluble yellow pigment having yellow-green fluorescence while the other is dark brown and insoluble in both fat solvents and water. It has been suggested that the insoluble pigment, termed *ceroid*, is produced by polymerization of polyunsaturated fatty acid peroxides with lipoproteins.

In animals fed vitamin E deficient diets, there is a decrease in respiration of liver homogenates and in mitochondrial systems. It has been suggested that vitamin E may be an active participant as a cofactor in electron transfer catalysis. The decline in cellular respiration in vitamin E deficiency does not appear to affect the major components of the citric acid cycle or the transfer of electrons, but rather the mechanisms which couple oxidation and the transfer of electrons. Conceivably, vitamin E bridges the oxidative components of the citric acid cycle substrates with the coenzyme Q (Co Q) reductase system. Another possibility is that vitamin E plays some role in stabilizing membranes and/or membrane-bound NAD.

There appears to be a rather complex interrelationship between selenium and vitamin E. A number of the deficiency signs associated with low vitamin E intake can be prevented or mitigated by selenium or other antioxidants. Certain signs and symptoms which are produced in animals fed diets low in vitamin E and selenium can be corrected by either or both nutrients, depending on the experimental model and target organ. Animals fed a diet deficient in vitamin E and selenium develop hepatic necrosis with ultrastructural and enzymic alterations of the hepatocytic plasma membrane. While both vitamin E and selenium may act as antioxidants in preventing such damage to cell membranes, they may also behave as membrane stabilizers, unrelated to their antioxidant properties. The recent study by Machado et al. (1971) demonstrated that morphologic deterioration of the hepatocytic plasma membrane was accompanied by a progressive and significant decrease in the activity of those enzyme systems involved in the transport of electrolytes across cell membranes. Additional evidence is accumulating that the metabolic role of vitamin E may be more than merely an antioxidant (Rotruck et al., 1972).

PATHOLOGY

Disease States. *Save for some studies in premature infants, there is no clear evidence that vitamin E plays any important etiologic role in any clinical or hematologic disorder of man.* In recent years, it has been observed that infants of low birth weight placed on artificial formulas may develop edema, reticulocytosis, thrombocytosis, decreased erythrocyte survival time and some form of hemolytic anemia associated with low serum vitamin E levels. These formulas contained a low ratio of vitamin E to polyunsaturated fatty acids and, when these infants were supplemented with vitamin E, the signs and symptoms attributed to the vitamin E deficiency were corrected (Balsley and Speckmann, 1971) (Wasserman and Taylor, 1972).

It has been reported that vitamin E deficiency may cause megaloblastic anemia in children with protein-calorie malnutrition, although the control aspects of these studies have been questioned (Majaj et al., 1963) (Baker et al., 1968) (Leonard and Losowsky, 1971). However, Nair et al. (1971) recently reported that in four patients with symptoms of porphyria, the administration of vitamin E decreased the urinary excretion of aminolevulinic acid, porphobilinogen, coproporphyrins and uroporphyrins to normal levels. Vitamin E levels, initially low in whole blood, returned to normal concomitant with clinical improvement. Of interest was the additional finding that the coproporphyria associated with chronic alcoholism was not affected by vitamin E administration.

In blood, vitamin E is transported with the beta lipoproteins. Thus in patients with abetalipoproteinemia, serum vitamin E levels are low, and there is decreased red cell survival (using the H_2O_2 in vitro test). No other clinical manifestations are apparent in such patients. Vitamin E administration returns the plasma levels to normal and corrects the hemolytic component.

VITAMIN K

(Deficiency state: hypoprothrombinemia)

NORMAL METABOLISM

Chemistry. The first observations on the role of vitamin K in the economy of animals and man were made by Dam in 1929. He showed that chicks fed diets low in fat developed hemorrhages and impaired blood clotting. In 1935, it became clear that there was a fat-soluble nutrient which was apparently responsible for preventing the hemorrhages in normal well fed animals and which was designated K by Dam (1966). It is now known that vitamin K plays an important role in the formation and biosynthesis of prothrombin (factor II) and other blood clotting factors (factors VII, IX and X).

Vitamin K exists in three forms. Two occur naturally—vitamin K_1 (phylloquinone) and vitamin K_2 (menaquinone). Vitamin K_3 (menadione) is a synthetic product (2-methyl-1, 2-naphthoquinone) which has the basic structure of the naturally occurring vitamins. Green plants are high in vitamin K_1, whereas animal tissues and metabolic products of intestinal bacteria and other microorganisms are high in vitamin K_2. All three forms are biologically active but vary in potency depending upon various factors including structural side chains and animal species.

Synthesis of K_2 by the intestinal bacterial flora is the most important source of the vitamin in the body. It is absorbed in the small bowel, for the most part, in the jejunum. *Vitamin K deficiency occurs when there are significant alterations in the intestinal flora or defects in fat absorption* With obstructive biliary disease, the deficient flow of bile into the intestine leads to inadequate absorption of the fat-soluble vitamins. Diseases of the pancreas also affect vitamin K absorption secondary to defects in lipid absorption. Menadione, K_3, is water-soluble and presumably would be less affected than either K_1, or K_2 which are fat-soluble. The highest concentrations of this nutrient are found in the liver, followed by the gastrointestinal tract, skeletal muscle and plasma.

The exact action of vitamin K in the synthesis of the blood clotting factors is not well understood. It was thought that vitamin K was involved in oxidative phosphorylation, but a number of studies indicate that a deficiency of vitamin K does not lead to uncoupling of oxidative phosphorylation. Moreover, the ATP levels in livers of vitamin K deficient rats remain normal. Currently, the evidence points toward an effect in transforming a precursor protein to the final product. Several studies have indicated that in vitamin K deficiency or in the presence of vitamin K antagonists, a plasma protein (which has been labeled PIVKA or Protein Induced by Vitamin K Absence or Antagonist) accumulates. Recently, abnormal prothrombin and abnormal factor IX have been detected in the blood of individuals with vitamin K deficiencies or in those who have been treated with anticoagulants. It has been suggested that these abnormal forms might represent PIVKA or the precursor proteins. With the administration of vitamin K or the removal of vitamin K antagonists, there is a marked decline in this precursor protein and restoration of prothrombin and other blood clotting factors to normal levels. It is possible that this precursor protein is similar to the "modified thrombin zymogen" suggested by Tishkoff et al. (1968), or it may be the preprothrombin suggested by Seegers (1967). Thus, the current data suggest that *vitamin K acts at the postribosomal level and perhaps transforms a precursor protein to the final product either by altering the configuration of the precursor or by attachment of other essential components such as carbohydrate to it* (Wasserman and Taylor, 1972) (Wasserman and Corradino, 1971).

PATHOLOGY

Basis of Deficiency State. Simple primary deficiency from inadequate dietary intake is extremely rare. There is very little information concerning the average human intake of vitamin K. Moreover, little is known about vitamin K requirements. It has been difficult, therefore, to establish a daily recommended allowance, but Frick et al. (1967) showed that approximately 0.03 mg. of vitamin K per kg. of body weight, given intravenously, was required to obtain normal blood clotting in vitamin K depleted human adults. In clinical practice, a deficiency of vitamin K results from (1) inadequate intake (rare) of vitamin K, (2) failure of absorption from the intestine, (3) lack of bacterial synthesis, (4) inadequate vitamin reserves in the newborn due to low vitamin K stores in the mother and (5) administration of vitamin K antagonists. Thus, hypovitaminosis K almost invariably represents a conditioned deficiency resulting from coexistent disease, particularly obstructive biliary disease with a deficient flow of bile into the intestines and inadequate absorption of this fat-soluble vitamin. Any other intestinal disturbance associated with malabsorption of fat, such as has been cited in the discussion of vitamins A and D, may likewise result in inadequate absorption of this vitamin. Intestinal disorders producing hypermotility, vomiting or impaired absorption, for example, severe ulcerative colitis, will result in vitamin K deficiency. If the normal colonic bacterial flora is destroyed by the use of antibacterial drugs or by a colectomy, a deficiency may result.

Hypoprothrombinemia may be seen in the newborn. When the mother's stores of vitamin K are small, the neonatal reserve is small. After birth, the slender reserves in these infants are utilized, and this leads to inadequate prothrombin formation. These low levels do not begin to rise until approximately 4 to 7 days after birth, presumably concurrent with the establishment of the intestinal flora in the colon of the infant and the synthesis of more vitamin K. However, other factors may enter into the neonatal deficiency.

Recent studies have indicated that breast-fed infants, in contrast to those fed cows' milk, may be more prone to vitamin K deficiency and hemorrhagic disease. Recently, Keenan et al. (1971) made comparisons of prothrombin times in infants: (1) fed cows' milk, (2) fed breast milk, (3) fed bottled human milk and (4) fed only sterile water. The infants fed cows' milk had lower prothrombin times (higher prothrombin levels) than the other groups. Cows' milk, then, is superior to breast milk in maintaining a normal prothrombin time. Cows' milk may also favorably influence the intestinal flora and the endogenous synthesis of vitamin K. However, the authors concluded that the dietary supply was more important than the effect of the cows' milk on the intestinal flora. Sutherland et al. (1967) similarly documented that, without vitamin K administration or supplementation, the incidence of bleeding episodes was significantly greater in breast-fed infants than in those fed a formula containing cows' milk. Moreover, in the newborn full-term infant, the liver does not begin to produce bile until a few days after birth. All fats are poorly absorbed, therefore, including vitamin K. Moreover, in the premature infant, the incompletely developed liver is not maximally effective in the synthesis of prothrombin and related clotting factors. Postnatal absorption is further hindered because of gastrointestinal hypomotility and poorly established pancreatic function during the early days of life. Thus, in the infant, antibiotic therapy which alters the intestinal flora, diarrhea, malabsorption and the diet (breast milk vs. cow's milk) may all contribute to a serious deficiency of vitamin K. For the newborn infant, it has been suggested that a single dose of 1 mg. of vitamin K_1 immediately after birth is adequate to prevent a hemorrhagic diathesis.

Disease States: Hypoprothrombinemia-Hemorrhagic Diathesis. Historically, hypoprothrombinemia and its resultant defective clotting were at one time considered to be due to deficiency of a single blood factor, prothrombin. It has now become clear that hypoprothrombinemia is, in reality, a deficiency of four closely related factors: prothrombin and factors VII, IX and X. In vitamin K deficiency, there is insufficient formation of all four factors. The usual Quick one-stage prothrombin test measures the adequacy of all four, and thus, in usual clinical practice, the term hypoprothrombinemia does not indicate whether only one or all four factors are deficient. An isolated deficiency of only one of these related factors will produce a lowered prothrombin level (prolonged prothrombin time), and this result is loosely interpreted by the all-inclusive term of prothrombin deficiency or hypoprothrombinemia.

In addition to a deficiency of these factors, when hemorrhages occur in a vitamin K deficiency, it must be assumed that some cause exists for damage to vessel walls and initiation of bleeding. Trauma, obvious or apparently trivial, is the most likely basis for such vascular injury. Common sites for these hemorrhages are operative wounds, particularly those incurred in the surgical relief of obstructive jaundice with its associated malabsorption of vitamin K. Petechial bleeding may also occur into the skin, mucous membranes (particularly in the intestinal tract), serosal surfaces, and in any other organ or cavity of the body. When the levels of prothrombin are severely depressed, the hemorrhages may assume major proportions. When they affect vital structures, such as the brain, they may cause death. Moderate deficiencies of vitamin K do not have untoward effects, and to produce a hemorrhagic diathesis the hypoprothrombinemia must be severe, the critical level commonly being placed at a value of 20 per cent of the normal prothrombin time. Dicumarol, a widely used clinical anticoagulant, appears to counteract the effect of vitamin K to produce lowered levels of all four factors.

WATER-SOLUBLE VITAMINS

The water-soluble vitamins are rapidly and readily absorbed from the alimentary canal. Disease, if it is to impair the uptake of these nutrients, must be severe. However, the storage of certain of the B compounds is scant and deficiencies may develop with brief periods of inadequate intake or absorption.

VITAMIN C

(Deficiency state: scurvy)

NORMAL METABOLISM

Chemistry. Vitamin C (*l*-ascorbic acid) is a water soluble, six-carbon compound closely related to glucose. It has been isolated in crystalline form and has likewise been synthesized. It readily gives off two hydrogen ions to assume an oxidative form known as dehydroascorbic acid, but it can be reversibly reduced. In fact its physiologic activity may be related to this reduction-oxidation potential. Usual methods of cooking markedly reduce the vitamin C content of foods by aqueous extraction of this water-soluble element and by degradative oxidation hastened by the cooking temperature.

The guinea pig, monkey and man must rely totally upon exogenous sources for this vitamin. The mouse, rat, rabbit and dog, on the other hand, are capable of synthesizing it from precursors. As mentioned earlier, however, increased needs for essential nutrients, including ascorbic acid, may arise. For example, in rats with wounds, supplementation of the diet with vitamin C hastens healing. Similar evidence exists for man.

Physiology. Vitamin C as a water-soluble product is rapidly absorbed from the small intestine. It passes directly into the portal blood and thence to the body at large. It is stored in many tissues and appears to attain concentrations in the various organs in direct proportion to their metabolic activity. Thus, it is found in the following organs in decreasing order of concentration: pituitary, adrenal cortex, corpus luteum and thymus. Smaller but significant amounts are found in almost all the viscera, such as the kidneys, heart and lungs. The known metabolic products of vitamin C in man are oxalate, ascorbic acid and dehydroascorbic acid.

Many functions have been ascribed to this compound. It is necessary for the normal metabolism of phenylalanine, tyrosine and dihydroxyphenylalanine (dopa). It has also been demonstrated to be of importance in maintaining the succinic dehydrogenase activity of skeletal muscle in infants. In the same way, a drop in alkaline phosphatase activity of the plasma, bone and other tissues has been noted in deficient animals. The large amounts of vitamin C in the adrenal cortex raise the question of whether it may be important in the formation of adrenal steroids.

Most importantly, vitamin C is essential for the formation of collagen, ground substance, osteoid, dentine and intercellular cement substance. Its exact role in the formation of most of these products is still somewhat obscure, but much is known about its function in the production of collagen. Man as well as animals are dependent upon an exogenous source of vitamin C, and have a deficient production of collagen when there are depleted levels of this nutrient in the tissues. This lack of collagen becomes evident in the delay of wound healing and in the low tensile strength of the resultant scar (Edwards and Dunphy, 1958).

Vitamin C is necessary for the hydroxylation of proline to hydroxyproline and of lysine to hydroxylysine within the fibroblast. Precisely where and how this nutrient acts is uncertain. A deficiency of it may block hydroxylation after the amino acids have been incorporated into the polypeptide chain of the almost complete collagen molecules. Alternatively, vitamin C may be required for the synthesis of specific transfer RNA necessary for the delivery and incorporation of hydroxylated proline into the collagen polypeptide. Any defect in hydroxylation results in impaired fibrillation of collagen. Aerobic metabolism is required for this hydroxylation since anaerobic conditions or inhibitors of aerobic metabolism completely prevent the formation of hydroxyproline, hydroxylysine and collagen. Without vitamin C the hydroxyl groups cannot be added, and the procollagen may not fibrillate (p. 100).

Vitamin C deficiency, or scurvy, is also associated with degenerative changes in the endoplasmic reticulum of the fibroblast (Ross and Benditt, 1965). There is disintegration of endoplasmic reticulum and the formation of large vacuolated structures. Ribosomes are shed from their membranous attachments. These changes can be reversed promptly by the administration of vitamin C. Complete reversal of these changes can occur within 24 hours, and recognizable collagen fibrils appear in the extracellular space within 12 hours. It is not clear whether this rapid response to vitamin C is due to increased synthesis of procollagen, to hydroxylation of stored intracellular precursor of collagen, and/or to repair of fibroblast structure.

In summary, ascorbic acid is vital for collagen formation at several points, i.e., the preservation and maturation of fibroblasts and the incorporation of hydroxyproline and hydroxylysine (Gould, 1966). Much more controversial is a postulated role for vitamin C in the maintenance of collagen. There is some evidence that already formed collagen is slowly resorbed in the scorbutic animal, but this action is not unequivocally established.

Much less is known about the function of vitamin C in the production of ground substance. It appears that ascorbic acid may be involved in the sulfation of the acid mucopolysaccharides of the ground substance. Whether this defect in sulfation has a secondary effect on collagen formation is not clear. It is generally accepted that collagen fiber formation is an essentially extracellular precipitation of soluble proteins elaborated by the fibroblasts and possibly other mesenchymal cells. Thus fibrogenesis occurs within ground substance and, while it is possible that the appropriate ground substance must be important, the evidence bearing on this question is scanty. As mentioned earlier, ascorbic acid is vital to the formation of the osteoid matrix produced by the osteoblast and the elaboration of cement substance required to maintain the integrity of capillary walls. Little is known, in reality, about the defect in formation of cement substance. Conceivably, defective formation of normal connective tissue involving ground substance and collagen rather than inadequacy of cement substance may underlie the easy rupture of capillaries in scorbutic patients, producing the well known hemorrhagic diathesis in this disorder.

PATHOLOGY

Basis of Deficiency State. Contrasting with the fat-soluble vitamins already discussed, a deficiency of vitamin C almost inevitably indicates an improper dietary intake, since it is rapidly and readily absorbed and thus little affected by intestinal derangements. Moreover, since this vitamin is widely distributed in fruits and vegetables and normal body stores can sustain long periods of deprivation, the dietary deprivation must be prolonged and severe to create a deficiency state. In a noteworthy experiment conducted upon himself, Dr. J. H. Crandon, along with his colleagues (1940), demonstrated that on a rigidly restricted diet the plasma level of ascorbic acid fell progressively but did not reach undetectable levels until 41 days of dietary restriction. The vitamin C content in white blood cells, however, did not reach undetectable levels until 120 days.

Initially, Dr. Crandon experienced increasing fatigue and decreased exercise tolerance. Within approximately six months, perifollicular hemorrhages and failure of wound healing were noted.

In a recent study by Hodges et al. (1971), vitamin C deficiency was induced in normal healthy adult volunteers. These studies also demonstrated perifollicular hemorrhages occurring within 49 to 90 days. This is in contrast to the British Medical Research Council Study (Bartley et al., 1953) in which perifollicular hemorrhages were not noted in some subjects until 182 days and, in others, only after 238 days. The differences in the time of onset of signs of vitamin C deficiency among these studies may have been due to differences in the dietary levels of vitamin C. The experimental vitamin C deficient diet of the British group may have contained trace amounts of ascorbic acid, sufficient to delay the onset of manifestations of a deficiency state.

Petechial perifollicular hemorrhages were the first manifestation to appear and were followed by ecchymoses, coiled hairs, gum changes, hyperkeratosis, congested hair follicles, dyspnea, arthralgia, joint effusions, neuropathy and anemia in varying degrees. One of the interesting clinical observations made in the study of Hodges et al. (1971) was the appearance of Sjögren's (Sicca) syndrome, one of the diffuse connective tissue disorders. All subjects in the study developed one or more of the component features of this syndrome, and two men developed the complete syndrome.

The first signs of scurvy may appear when the plasma ascorbic acid level falls below the normal level of 1 mg. per 100 ml. to perhaps 0.25 mg. per 100 ml. The vitamin C pool size in the adult male is about 1.5 gm. and decreases to approximately one-third this amount when signs of scurvy appear. The minimal amount of ascorbic acid necessary to prevent or cure scurvy appears to be slightly less than 10 mg. daily. However, the daily administration of larger amounts will result in more rapid disappearance of symptoms and signs of scurvy and more prompt replacement of the body pool. Since vitamin C is readily absorbed from the gastrointestinal tract, it need not be given parenterally. Massive oral doses will suffice. Curiously, the Food and Nutrition Board recommends a daily intake of over 60 mg. per day whereas the British take a more realistic view and recommend a daily intake of approximately 15 to 20 mg. of vitamin C per day.

Recently, Linus Pauling (1970) made the claim that high doses of vitamin C, up to 1 gm. per day, will prevent common colds. The majority of the scientific community awaits proof of this claim. Ironically, Crandon, on a vitamin C deficient diet, wrote of himself: "There was almost complete freedom from respiratory infections throughout the experimental period, covering the months of October to May. Only two very transient and mild attacks of coryza were noted, each lasting but about a few days. In previous winters, it has not been uncommon for the subject to suffer from frequent, severe upper respiratory infection" (Crandon et al., 1940). Avitaminosis C has no apparent effect on humoral antibody formation. Hodges et al. (1971) found the antibody response to thyroid antigen at the height of clinical scurvy to be normal. However, it must be admitted that cellular immunity is more likely to be important in viral respiratory infections. There are concerns that high vitamin C intake may be hazardous to health (Goldsmith, 1971) (Beaton and Whalen, 1971) (Rhead and Schrauzer, 1971) (Ginter, 1971). Massive doses of vitamin C may produce increased urinary excretion of oxalates, and oxaluria favors the formation of kidney and bladder oxalate stones. Moreover, there is some evidence that susceptible individuals who habitually ingest large amounts of ascorbic acid may, under normal circumstances, become scorbutic. Abnormally high vitamin C intake may increase the requirement for vitamin C. Thus, scurvy may become more common if the current practice of massive vitamin C intake, particularly by pregnant women, continues. It should be noted, however, that a single large dose of ascorbic acid or perhaps similar dosages even for several days, weeks or months are not likely to be injurious by any criteria.

Disease States (Scurvy). Prolonged vitamin C deficiency gives rise to "subclinical scurvy," followed later by the full-blown picture. Even on severely restricted diets, considerable time may be required for the transition from the latent to the manifest disease. Scurvy is much more prevalent in the spring and fall for somewhat obscure reasons. Two peak age incidences are encountered. The first is seen when children subsist largely on unsupplemented processed formulas between the ages of six months and two years, and the second, in the very aged with restricted, bizarre diets.

Almost all the anatomic and clinical features of scurvy can be derived from an understanding of the normal function of ascorbic acid. Scorbutus is characterized, then, by failure of formation of collagen, osteoid, dentine and intercellular cement substances (Wolbach, 1937). As a result of these defects, the major anatomic alterations affect wound healing, bone formation and the integrity of blood vessels with a resultant hemorrhagic diathesis. Anemia is often present, possibly related to the excessive hemorrhages.

Wound Healing. The **failure of formation of collagen** is most evident in the repair of wounds. In the experiment by Crandon et al. (1940), after 182 days of dietary restriction, wound healing was markedly impaired, and the tensile strength of the scar diminished. Yet after 100 days of this scorbutic diet, a wound showed completely normal healing, indicating once again the large reserve of vitamin C in the body. Along with the deficiency of collagen, as might be anticipated, hemorrhages into the tissues were prominent.

Histologically, fibroblastic proliferation is evident in the reparative phase of wound healing. However, this granulation tissue differs from normal in that it contains an abundant amorphous, granular ground substance deficient in collagen. The reparative process results then in a loose, cellular connective tissue relatively devoid of collagen. Hemorrhages are prone to occur in these areas due to the lack of intercellular cement substance between the endothelial cells of newly formed capillaries. In the same way, walling off of infections is inadequate in scorbutic individuals, and abscess formations fail to show the usual collagenous connective tissue-enclosing barrier so that the infection is poorly delimited for long periods of time.

Bone Formation. It is apparent from the previous discussion of normal osteogenesis that the formation of the protein-mucoprotein osteoid matrix of bone is vital for normal bone development and growth. **In scurvy, the primary deficiency is in the formation of osteoid matrix, not in the mineralization or calcification such as occurs in rickets.** As a consequence, membranous bone growth and endochondral bone formation are severely disrupted. The total disorganization of the epiphyseal line of growth parallels that found in rickets. The palisade of cartilage cells is formed as usual and is provisionally calcified but, in the scorbutic state, the osteoblasts are incapable of forming bone matrix. Resorption of the cartilaginous matrix then fails or slows and, as a consequence, there is an overgrowth or persistence of cartilage with downgrowth of long spicules and projection of cartilaginous masses and plates into the marrow shaft, producing a change quite similar to that seen in rickets (Fig. 11–7). The usual formation of new osteoid matrix on the degenerating spicules is absent, and the persistent cartilage becomes patchily or completely calcified.

On microscopic inspection, it should then be evident that the failure is one not of mineralization but of osteoid formation (Fig. 11–8). Fibroblasts proliferate in this scorbutic zone and form a loose, disorganized connective tissue, but no collagen is formed. Thus, structural strength is markedly decreased, and the stress of weight-bearing or muscle tension may produce actual dislocation of the epiph-

appears in noncontrolled experiments, is generally more severe and involves more systems than one sees in experimental scurvy. One can only speculate that the difference is related to other nutritional deficiencies or other factors such as associated infectious diseases and diarrhea.

Formation of Teeth. In experimental animals, striking changes occur in teeth. The clinical counterpart of these changes in infants and adults is less clearly defined and is described in Chapter 20 (p. 879). Resorption of the alveolar bone causes the teeth to loosen, fall out or become displaced out of line.

Gingivitis. Swelling, hemorrhages and secondary marginal infections of the gingival margins are common in severely scorbutic patients. The deficiency of vitamin C does not of itself cause the inflammation, but rather impairs the normal defensive responses of the mucous membranes. Thus, the massive gingival enlargement so characteristic of scurvy results from the combined effects of lack of vitamin C and nonspecific inflammation.

Hemorrhagic Diathesis. Hemorrhages comprise one of the most striking clinical and anatomic manifestations of scurvy. These hemorrhages

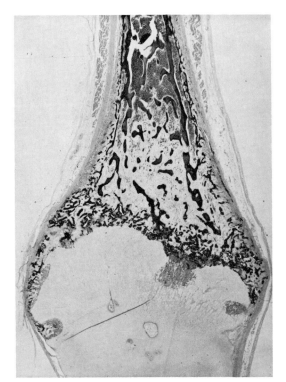

Figure 11–7. A longitudinal section of a scorbutic costochondral junction with widening of the epiphyseal cartilage and projection of masses of cartilage into the adjacent bone.

ysis. The soft, poorly formed bone is subject to compression and distortion, because virtually all the stability of this area rests upon calcified, cartilaginous matrix, which is totally inadequate as a substitute for normal bone. The poorly formed capillaries in the area rupture easily, particularly when stress on the bone causes unusual tensions or fractures. Massive red blood cell extravasation may therefore occur in the epiphyseal area. With the deficiencies in cement substance and collagen, **the periosteum is loosely attached and extensive subperiosteal hematomas are common.** At a later stage blood pigment, derived from such hemorrhage, is deposited within macrophages and fibroblasts in these areas. In those cases in which the deficiency is not extreme, some osteoid tissue may be formed, but it is inadequate in amount, and the structural strength of the bone remains below normal.

In the classic clinical case of scurvy, many of the skeletal deformities and alterations are due to the superimposed hemorrhages and fractures. In experimental animals, far less disorganization is observed when the extremity is protected from stress or trauma by plaster casts. It is thus apparent that the severity of the anatomic changes depends upon factors other than the simple vitamin C deficiency. Moreover, scurvy, as it presents naturally and as it

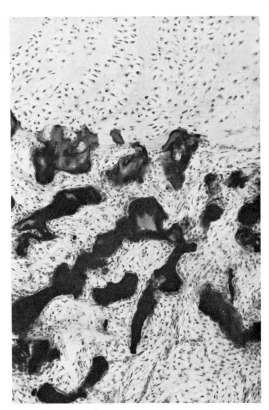

Figure 11–8. A detail of a scorbutic costochondral junction. The orderly palisade is totally destroyed. There is dense mineralization of the spicules present but no evidence of newly formed osteoid.

are predicated upon deficiency of intercellular cement substance or connective tissue support which weakens the cohesion of the endothelial cells in the capillary walls to the point that the minor trauma of usual daily life causes rupture of these vessels and extensive hemorrhage. Histologically, these vessels may appear to be entirely normal, for the alterations are beyond the range of microscopic visualization. Although hemorrhages can occur into any tissue or organ of the body, favored sites are the subperiosteum and subcutaneous tissues (producing petechiae or large ecchymoses) and into the joints of the lower extremities (presumably because of the stresses involved in standing, walking and lying down) (Fig. 11–9).

Hemorrhages into the gingivae may occur, but carefully controlled studies indicate that this extravasation is largely due to poor oral hygiene and areas of localized infection rather than to any intrinsic vascular disease (Fig. 11–10). Hemorrhages into the conjunctivae, eyeballs, brain, kidneys and joints are also encountered. Nosebleeds, hematuria and melena may occur likewise on the basis of capillary fragility. This weakening of the capillary wall is especially evident when venous pressures are increased, as occurs in the ordinary recording of blood pressure. Showers of petechiae occur distal to the blood pressure cuff (the basis of the vaulable diagnostic tourniquet test). It should be noted, however, that other conditions, such as leukemia and certain of the bleeding dyscrasias, may produce similar capillary bleeding.

From the anatomic lesions it is possible to anticipate to a considerable extent the clinical features of scorbutus. Because the tissues and bones of infants are in a state of active growth, infantile scurvy differs in some degree from the adult form. The deficiency state usually occurs in bottle-fed babies, and first becomes manifest by a series of vague, insidious symptoms of loss of appetite, weight loss, list-

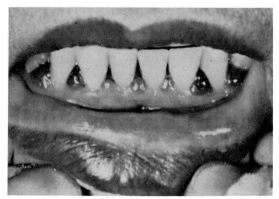

Figure 11–10. *Scorbutic hemorrhagic sponginess of the interdental gingival papillae.*

lessness, irritability and pallor reflecting the anemia. Development is retarded. Soon, as the deficiency becomes more marked, the child becomes more irritable and tends to lie quietly to spare unnecessary activity, with legs characteristically flexed onto the abdomen or in the frog position, relieving tension on the muscles, tendons and fasciae. The first definitive findings may be those of gingival sponginess and a hemorrhagic diathesis (Fig.11–10), causing petechiae or ecchymotic hemorrhages into the skin. Nosebleeds, melena, bleeding into the joints and muscles, and subperiosteal hemorrhages (manifested by sudden painful swelling of a joint or an extremity) also occur. Changes in the teeth and skeletal system occur only as late manifestations.

The scorbutic patient is classically anemic, and the anemia is usually normocytic and normochromic. The cause of this anemia is still controversial. A large contributing factor is undoubtedly the tendency to hemorrhage with resultant loss of blood, but most of the iron pigment is retained since the bleeding is internal, and synthesis of hemoglobin and red cells should not be impaired. In some cases, the anemia may not be the result of vitamin C deficiency per se, but rather it may be due to concomitant or induced nutritional deficiencies, e.g., folic acid. Under these circumstances, the anemia is macrocytic and hyperchromic and responds promptly to folic acid therapy.

Recent evidence implies that certain nondietary environmental factors play a permissive role in the development of vitamin C deficiency. A recent study suggests that smokers have a much lower level of vitamin C in whole blood than do nonsmokers. This difference did not seem to be related to vitamin C intake but rather to a difference in the metabolism of vitamin C in smokers (Pelletier, 1970).

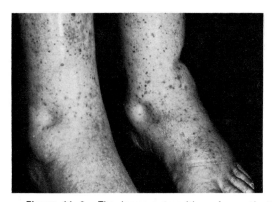

Figure 11–9. *The lower extremities of a patient with marked malnutrition, nutritional edema and petechial hemorrhages related to low levels of vitamin C.*

Low levels of ascorbic acid have been noted in the blood of patients with rheumatoid arthritis, and a recent study implicates aspirin as the cause (Sahud and Cohen, 1971). In vitro, it was demonstrated that aspirin blocks the uptake of ascorbic acid by blood platelets. Thus, patients with rheumatoid arthritis receiving high doses of aspirin should be administered supplemental ascorbic acid. This caution is supported by the fact that guinea pigs maintained in a semiscorbutic state bleed much more readily when challenged with aspirin than do control animals.

Paradoxically, there is some evidence that scurvy or subclinical scurvy may have some beneficial effects. A number of observations imply that the metabolism of ascorbic acid and iron are interrelated. The suggestion has been made that scurvy, which is common in the Bantu people of South Africa, may in fact protect these individuals from hemochromatosis. Lipschitz et al. (1971) proposed that patients such as the Bantus, who have hemosiderosis with concomitant vitamin C deficiency, never develop hemochromatosis because the excess iron is distributed in the reticuloendothelial cells, whereas in hemochromotosis not associated with vitamin C deficiency, iron is found in parenchymal cells.

The clinical diagnosis of scurvy rests on the features just cited with characteristic x-ray findings of the disturbed bone formation, low plasma levels of vitamin C, urinary excretion measurements following administration of vitamin C (saturation test), increased capillary fragility and a history of dietary deficiency.

VITAMIN B COMPLEX

The vitamin B complex comprises an ever growing group of essential nutrients that are chemically unrelated, but have in common a tendency to occur together in certain foodstuffs. Liver, yeast, milk and leafy green vegetables are in general abundant sources of these substances. *Biologically they divide themselves into two large groups: those involved in the intracellular metabolism of carbohydrates, fats and proteins and those related to blood cell production.* The former group includes nicotinamide, riboflavin, thiamine, pantothenic acid and biotin. These are often referred to as the "energy releasing vitamins." They serve as coenzymes and as hydrogen or electron acceptors and transfer agents in the host of oxidation-reduction reactions involved in the secondary metabolism of fats, carbohydrates and proteins. The energy releasing reactions provide the basis for the synthesis of the high energy bonds in ATP, vital for the metabolic activity of cells. So it is

that a deficiency of the B vitamins will tend to be manifest in tissues with a high level of metabolic activity and high turnover rate of cellular structure. Stomatitis, gastritis, hematologic disorders and involvement of the nervous system (normally totally dependent on carbohydrate for its energy needs) run through the clinical syndromes that comprise the vitamin B deficiencies.

The B vitamins that have important roles in blood formation are often designated "the hematopoietic vitamins" and include vitamin B₁₂ (cobalamin) and folic acid. As will be seen, deficiencies of these essential nutrients lead to a spectrum of macrocytic anemias including the important pernicious anemia.

VITAMIN B₁ (THIAMINE)

(Deficiency state: beriberi)

NORMAL METABOLISM

Chemistry. Free thiamine is a basic substance made up of a substituted pyrimidine and a substituted thiazole ring which are connected by a methylene bridge. It is usually prepared in the form of its ester, thiamine hydrochloride, which is a water-soluble salt, resistant to heat in acid solution. In its crystalline form it is very stable. It is available from natural sources in pure form and has been synthesized. In the body it exists as thiamine pyrophosphate, the biologically active form, also known as cocarboxylase. In the ordinary process of preparation of food, much of the thiamine is extracted because of its solubility in water.

Physiology. As a water-soluble vitamin, thiamine is readily and rapidly absorbed through the upper intestinal tract. Absorption is unaffected by most intestinal disorders except those which produce severe anorexia and vomiting or marked gastrointestinal hypermotility. Entering the circulating blood, it is available to all body cells and appears to be chiefly stored in the muscles, liver, heart, kidneys and brain, although other organs also contain trace amounts. The total storage is *not* great, since there is a constant *daily need* for this vitamin, and relatively short periods of deprivation may lead to significant deficiency states. The brain appears to be able to conserve its resources better than other tissues.

It is principally and readily excreted by the kidneys. Thiamine as the cocarboxylase participates in the oxidation of alpha-keto acids. More specifically it serves in the transfer of aldehydic groups in the oxidative decarboxylation of pyruvate and alpha-keto glutarate. If this step is blocked by a deficiency of thiamine, pyruvate accumulates. It is postulated that pyruvate is toxic and may impair the function of neurons. Nerve fibers may also be affected because thiamine is necessary for the synthesis of acetylcholine. Alternatively, it must not be forgotten that nervous tissue is heavily dependent on carbohydrate for its energy requirements so that thiamine deficiency must not be considered merely as a pyruvate poisoning.

Still another possibility must be considered: the pyruvate toxicity might exert its effect indirectly by causing anorexia, inanition and secondary imbalances that lead to famine edema (wet beriberi) and cardiac disturbances (beriberi heart disease). Thiamine pyrophosphate may also aid in the synthesis of fat using pyruvic acid intermediates. So it is obvious that this vitamin serves as a coenzyme in many roles and in various tissues but always at the cellular level.

The recommended daily allowance for infants, children (one to eight years) and adults is approximately 0.2 to 0.4, 0.5 to 1.0 and 1.2 to 1.4 mg., respectively. An additional 0.2 to 0.5 mg. daily is recommended during pregnancy and lactation.

PATHOLOGY

Basis of Deficiency State. Because this vitamin is readily absorbed, conditioned deficiencies are quite uncommon, although they occur in severe gastrointestinal disease and in hyperthyroidism or other states which produce increased demands. The low body stores and the relatively small amounts available in food potentiate the development of simple exogenous deficiencies. These are widespread in the Orient, and are also encountered in the United States, usually in the lower income groups, in food faddists, and particularly in chronic alcoholics with restricted dietary habits, in whom there may also be some malabsorption of dietary thiamine.

Disease States (Beriberi). Beriberi in Singhalese means "weakness." If an individual with thiamine deficiency is asked to stand from a squatting position, he may fall on his face unless assisted. Such patients will exhibit extreme calf tenderness. Beriberi has been divided into three syndromes on the basis of the most prominent presenting clinical features: **dry beriberi**, signs and symptoms chiefly localized to the neuromuscular system; **wet beriberi**, neuromuscular complaints associated with edema; and **cardiac beriberi**, presenting chiefly as cardiac decompensation. Usually, however, the three forms overlap in part or in whole. The ana-tomic changes in all three clinical forms are, for the most part, confined to the heart and nervous system (Vedder, 1938).

Heart. The changes may be slight or absent, even in cases which are otherwise consistent with the diagnosis of cardiac beriberi. In better defined examples, particularly those of acute onset, the heart is characteristically dilated and flabby, and may be somewhat paler than normal. The dilatation may affect all chambers or, at times, one side more than the other; right-sided dilatation more often predominates. No endocardial or valvular alterations are produced. Intersitital edema is the most consistent finding. Although microscopic changes such as hydropic degeneration, fatty change and marked swelling of myocardial fibers have been described quite consistently in animal experiments, similar lesions in man are rare and inconstant. The acute myocardial necrosis encountered in animals is rarely present in clinical cases.

In man, gross and microscopic lesions in the heart in beriberi are not pathognomonic, and are useful only in confirming the clinical diagnosis. The genesis of these cardiac changes is unclear. Dilatation of the peripheral arterioles and capillaries occurs in thiamine deficiency with a consequent increased blood flow from the arterial to the venous side of the circulation. Possibly this heightened blood flow throws an increased load on the right side of the heart, followed by cardiac failure and, in some instances, dilatation of the entire heart. This concept is entirely speculative, as there has been very little careful microscopic study of well documented clinical cases of beriberi uncomplicated by other deficiencies.

Nervous Tissues. Here again, there is a paucity of critical information. For the most part, the changes affect the peripheral nerves, motor and sensory, the spinal cord and the brain stem. In the peripheral nerves, there is fatty degeneration of the myelin sheaths. This usually begins in the sciatic nerve and its branches, but may ascend so as to involve the spinal cord and, in time, other peripheral nerves. In severe cases, the polyneuropathy frequently takes the form of an ascending symmetrical peripheral neuropathy. In far advanced deficiency states, degenerative changes involve not only the myelin sheaths but also the axon process, which may become fragmented. Histologically, these peripheral cord and nerve lesions are, however, not different from those found in other conditions such as diabetes, pernicious anemia and pellagra. Moreover, it has been pointed out that many of the so-called cases of beriberi in which these lesions are present probably represent multivitamin deficiencies so that observed alterations cannot be ascribed with certainty to thiamine insufficiency alone.

Congestion and edema of the brain have been described as the result of a lack of thiamine. In the medulla and pons, cerebellum and dorsal root ganglia, neuronal degenerative changes, such as chromatolysis, and alterations in the size and staining characteristics of the nuclei have been observed, but are not established as due to a specific B_1 deficiency.

One type of brain involvement encountered in this deficiency state deserves special mention as a distinct clinical entity, i.e., **Wernicke's disease.** In this disorder, focal degenerations and hemorrhages usually occur in a symmetrical distribution in the paramedian and paraventricular nuclei of the thalamus and hypothalamus, in the mammillary bodies and about the nuclei of origin of the cranial nerves supplying the extraocular muscles. In the involved areas, the ganglion cells show the degenerative changes already described, and vessels may show dilatation or rupture with focal or ring petechial hemorrhages. This disorder is almost invariably encountered in alcoholics, but it is not restricted to these patients. Virtually identical changes have been produced in pigeons on experimental diets deficient in thiamine hydrochloride. However, because in these experimental diets all other possible deficiencies were not carefully controlled, there is still some doubt as to the specificity of these changes with respect to vitamin B_1. Nonetheless, in clinical practice, striking therapeutic response follows the administration of vitamin B_1 to these patients.

The previously described anatomic changes provide a reasonable basis for the various clinical syndromes included under the designation of beriberi. Cases with predominantly myocardial involvement usually come to clinical attention because of signs and symptoms of cardiac failure, already referred to as cardiac beriberi. Heart failure due to vitamin B_1 deficiency differs from that caused by many other forms of heart disease and is known as high output failure. It is characterized by peripheral dilatation, a ruddy, warm, dry skin, as well as a decreased circulation time and a normal to slightly increased venous pressure. The decrease in circulation time in the presence of a failing circulatory system is an uncommon clinical combination, arising out of the peripheral vasodilation; it should raise a suspicion of this deficiency state. In some cases, striking peripheral edema is present, which usually affects the lower extremities, but may also affect the trunk, face and body cavities. This edema is usually attributed to cardiac decompensation, as no other plausible mechanism has been found.

Motor and sensory peripheral nerve lesions marked by such neuromuscular findings as numbness and tingling of the legs, sensory disturbances of the affected parts, tenderness of the calf muscles, atrophy and weakness of muscles of the extremities with depression and loss of reflexes may dominate in some cases of thiamine deficiency and produce so-called dry beriberi. These neuromuscular changes are frequently accompanied by marked loss of appetite, weakness and malaise.

When the neuromuscular syndrome is accompanied by edema, it is termed wet beriberi. In either instance, an element of cardiac failure may be present.

Wernicke's syndrome is quite distinctive. The classic case presents the triad of confusion, ataxia and ophthalmoplegia, as well as clinical findings undoubtedly related to the degenerative lesions in the central nervous system. Anorexia, personality changes, weight loss and debility are often present in all these forms of vitamin B_1 deficiency. The clinical diagnosis is best substantiated by the therapeutic response to thiamine.

Toxicity. Although transient mild symptoms such as dizziness and flushing may be produced in certain individuals upon the administration of thiamine hydrochloride, massive doses have been given without untoward effects.

RIBOFLAVIN

(Deficiency states: cheilosis, glossitis, dermatitis and ocular lesions)

NORMAL METABOLISM

Chemistry. Riboflavin is a slightly water-soluble, yellow pigment insoluble in fat solvents, required for normal intracellular respiration. It is composed of a combination of D-ribose, and isoalloxazine. Under ultraviolet rays, it exhibits a characteristic green fluorescence. This aids in its identification in tissue sections. It is inactivated by light, but is thermostable. When phosphorylated, it yields riboflavin 5-phosphate, an essential component of the flavoprotein coenzymes. These coenzymes serve as important hydrogen acceptors in the oxidative degradation of short-chain fatty acids as well as in other synthetic reactions. Riboflavin is widely distributed in nature in both plant and animal foods as riboflavin or riboflavin phosphate or as a constituent of the flavoproteins.

Physiology. Riboflavin is rapidly absorbed from the upper intestinal tract, and is almost immediately phosphorylated into its active form. It may at times be phosphorylated prior to absorption. As a constituent of all cells, it is stored throughout the body, but the exact amount of this storage is not known. The liver is probably one of the most important sites for the storage of this vitamin. From experimental studies, which require as long as four or five months to produce signs of apparent clinical deficiency, it appears that the stores must be quite large. It has been indicated previously that, in its phosphorylated form, riboflavin is an important respiratory enzyme which is not poisoned by carbon monoxide or cyanide compounds. Riboflavin aids in the transfer of oxygen from the plasma to the substrate of tissue cells and in hydrogen transport. Since this vitamin cannot be synthesized by man or animals, it is obvious that the oxidative metabolism of all animal cells depends upon adequate sources of this nutrient. The recommended daily allowance ranges from 0.4 mg. for infants to 1.5 mg. for adults and 1.8 to 2.0 mg. during pregnancy and lactation.

PATHOLOGY

Basis of Deficiency State. As with most of the water-soluble vitamins, the majority of clinical cases of ariboflavinosis fall into the category of simple or primary deficiencies in which the dietary intake is inadequate. While this is not common in this country, it is extremely prevalent in the Orient and in other areas where living conditions are poor. In the United States, it is most often encountered as a dietary deficiency in alcoholics and in residents of the poorer backward areas. Conditioned deficiencies may occur and, for the most part, follow the pattern of those described under thiamine, i.e., severe gastrointestinal disease with either marked vomiting or hypermotility of the alimentary tract. Disorders associated with the excretion of large volumes of urine may increase the daily loss of this vitamin and produce a deficiency state.

Disease States. Riboflavin deficiency, or ariboflavinosis, in man is associated with changes at the angles of the mouth known as cheilosis or cheilitis, glossitis and also ocular and skin changes. While no one of these findings is specific, in the aggregate they are highly suggestive of ariboflavinosis.

Cheilosis. Cheilosis, or as it is sometimes called, cheilitis, is usually the first and most characteristic sign of this deficiency state. However, it must not be assumed that cheilosis is an invariable or pathognomonic manifestation of ariboflavinosis. Identical lesions are found in aged individuals with poor dentition who are not vitamin deficient. There is little doubt that in most instances these oral lesions are nonspecific. However, it is fair to state that riboflavin deficiency is a well recognized cause of cheilitis. It begins as areas of pallor at the angles of the mouth, with first a hyperkeratosis of the epidermis and a dermal inflammatory infiltrate.

Cracks or fissures radiate from the corners of the mouth. These tend to become secondarily infected, and produce a macerated, bleeding, inflammatory, fissured lesion. In far advanced cases, the lesions occur not only on the skin surfaces but also in the oral mucous membrane at the angles of the mouth and along the vermilion border of the lips. The involvement is usually bilateral, but is occasionally unilateral.

Glossitis. The tongue may take on a so-called magenta hue, strongly resembling the red-blue coloration of cyanosis. Presumably this alteration reflects atrophy of the mucosa of the tongue (Fig. 11–11).

Ocular Lesions. The eye changes may be classified as superficial interstitial keratitis. In the earlier stages, the superficial layers of the cornea are invaded by capillaries. Interstitial inflammatory infiltration and exudation follow to produce opacities and even ulcerations of the corneal surface. The lesion usually affects both eyes, but in certain instances it may be unilateral. Conjunctivitis is a common accompaniment.

Dermatitis. A greasy, scaling dermatitis occurs over the nasolabial folds and may extend into a butterfly distribution to involve the cheeks and skin about the ears. Scrotal and vulvar lesions are common. In the well defined cases, atrophy of the skin may develop. It is to be emphasized that the histologic changes are not in themselves distinctive or pathognomonic of ariboflavinosis. It is their distribution which suggests the diagnosis.

Toxicity. Few critical studies are available on the possible toxicity of this element, but available data indicate that relatively large doses are tolerated without untoward effects.

NICOTINAMIDE (NIACINAMIDE)

(Deficiency state: pellagra)

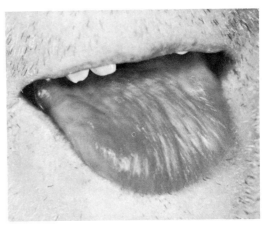

Figure 11–11. The glazed, shiny, atrophic tongue of riboflavin deficiency.

NORMAL METABOLISM

Chemistry. As the functional component of the two important coenzymes, codehydrogenase I NAD and codehydrogenase II NADP, nicotinamide plays an essential role in the electron transport involved in cellular respiratory reactions. It is widely distributed in most food substances, and is particularly abundant in liver, yeast, whole grain cereals, beef, pork, fruits and most vegetables. It has also been shown that mammalian tissues can synthesize nicotinic acid from tryptophan, but only when there is no concomitant deficiency or pyridoxine, riboflavin or thiamine.

Physiology. Niacinamide is absorbed in the upper intestinal tract. The various manifestations produced in animals and man by a deficiency of this nutrient do not appear to be readily explainable on the basis of its known biochemical activities, and this raises the possibility that it may have other metabolic activities as well. One of the related functions of this vitamin may be concerned with pigment metabolism. Patients and animals suffering from a deficiency of this vitamin show increased excretion of certain porphyrins and indican. The administration of nicotinamide or nicotinic acid to pellagrins rapidly corrects this defect.

The recommended daily allowance ranges from 5 mg. equivalents in infancy to about 18 in adults. Sixty milligrams of tryptophan may serve as the equivalent of 1 mg. of niacin.

PATHOLOGY

Basis of Deficiency State. Despite the advances in knowledge in nutrition, there is still a considerable endemic incidence of this avitaminosis. In the poverty-stricken areas of the world, the deficiency is probably due to simple inadequate intake of niacin. Conditioned deficiencies may develop from other clinical problems, such as chronic alcoholism, gastrointestinal distrubances, bizarre dietary habits, increased demands of pregnancy, lactation, hyperthyroidism, infections and other stressful situations. Deficiency of niacin produces the clinical entity of pellagra in humans and black tongue in dogs. It has been shown that dogs maintained on a cornmeal diet deficient in niacin and proteins develop classic signs of black tongue, while other animals fed similar niacin-deficient diets, but given a more adequate protein intake, fail to develop the tongue changes. These observations point out that, in some way, adequate levels of tryptophan may compensate for a deficient intake of niacin but not for a total niacin lack.

Disease States. The term pellagra, strictly speaking, refers to rough skin. The clinical syndrome, however, is classically identified by most clinicians by the three D's — **dermatitis, diarrhea** and **dementia.**

The dermatitis occurs on the body symmetrically and, while it may affect any region, tends to be most severe in areas of exposure to chronic irritation or sunlight, such as the face, dorsa of the hands, wrists, elbows, knees and in the inframammary and perineal folds. The margins of these areas of involvement are usually sharply demarcated from normal skin, and this provides one of the more important differential features from other types of dermatitis. The changes consist at first of redness and thickening of the skin with hyperkeratosis and scaling (Fig. 11–12). These early alterations are followed by increased vascularization and chronic inflammation with edema of the subepithelial dermal connective tissue, followed eventually by desquamation of the epidermis. With these regressive changes, areas of depigmentation and increased pigmentation may develop so that at this stage a variegated dermatitis is present with brown scaly areas alternating with areas of depigmented, shiny, atrophic skin. With chronicity, the skin may become markedly thickened by subcutaneous fibrosis and scarring. Lesions similar to these may occur in mucous membranes, particularly the oral cavity. In the mouth, the early stages are marked by vascular congestion and edema of the tongue and later by atrophy of the mucous membrane and ulceration so that the tongue becomes red, swollen and beefy, changes which are reminiscent of the black tongue found in animals.

The diarrhea exhibited by patients with pellagra is presumed to be due largely to mucous membrane lesions which have the same anatomic pattern as the changes in the skin. In experimental animals, it has been observed that the first histologic alterations represent vascularization, edema and inflammation of the submucosal connective tissue of the intestinal lining, which lead to atrophic mucosal

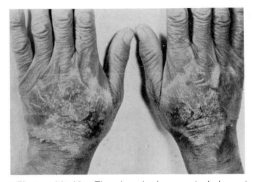

Figure 11–12. The sharply demarcated characteristic scaling dermatitis of pellagra.

glandular changes and eventual atrophy and ulceration of the overlying mucous membrane. These lesions may be found throughout all levels of the intestine, but are most prominent in the esophagus, stomach and colon.

The **dementia** is based upon degeneration of the ganglion cells of the brain, accompanied by degeneration of the tracts of the spinal cord. These spinal cord lesions bear a close resemblance to alterations in the posterior columns observed in pernicious anemia, and raise the question of whether or not a deficiency of another factor in the B complex, such as B_{12}, may also be implicated in the development of this specific lesion in pellagrins. Macrocytic anemia may appear in some cases.

Some of the most dominant complaints of these patients are persistent fatigability and weakness, which have been misinterpreted as malingering or neurosis. Although the skin manifestations eventually appear, they may at times be delayed until significant involvement of the intestinal tract or central nervous system has already developed.

Toxicity. The parenteral administration of niacinamide quite commonly produces transient peripheral vasodilation, burning sensations in the mouth, nausea and abdominal cramps. Nicotinamide by mouth does not produce these symptoms. No persistent ill effects have been described from the administration of doses well in excess of the therapeutic range.

FOLIC ACID

(Deficiency state: megaloblastic anemia)

NORMAL METABOLISM

Chemistry. Folacin (folic acid, folate) or pteroylglutamic acid (PGA) is a synthetic product not usually found in nature. It is usually conjugated with two or six molecules of glutamic acid which are linked at the gamma-carbon positions. The physiologically active form is a reduction product, tetrahydrofolic acid (THF). Pteroylpolyglutamates, the natural forms found in food, are presumably modified during absorption to yield mainly a reduced pteroylglutamate (THF). Where in the process of absorption the reduction occurs is not clear. Folates are most likely absorbed passively since their concentration in the normal diet far exceeds that in serum or blood. The present evidence strongly suggests that the major form of serum folate is the N5 methyl-THF.

The form that folate takes in the red cell may be different from that found in the liver, serum or other tissues. Evidence has been presented that, in red cells, folate is predominantly a polyglutamate or conjugated derivative of N5 methyl-THF. The serum folate level ranges from 3 to 16 nanogm. per ml. in well nourished people; the concentration in red blood cells is many times higher.

There are five known coenzyme forms of folacin, and their major role is in the transfer of one-carbon units to appropriate metabolites in the synthesis of DNA, RNA, methionine and serine. Perhaps the two reactions which contribute most to the one-carbon pool are those involving conversion of serine to glycine, and of histidine to glutamic acid. In the serine to glycine reaction, THF is methylated to N5, 10 methylene-THF. This form is essential for DNA synthesis. Formiminoglutamic acid (FIGLU), an intermediate in the conversion of histidine to glutamic acid, loses its formimino group ($-CH=NH$) to THF, resulting in the formation of glutamic acid and N5 formimino-THF. In folate deficiency or impaired utilization, urinary FIGLU is increased.

Another coenzyme form, N5,10 methenyl-THF, can be derived either from formimino-THF or N5,10 methylene-THF. Formate arising from the metabolism of choline to glycine or from tryptophan reacts with THF to form still another coenzyme form, N10 formyl-THF. In the biosynthesis of methionine, N5 methyl-THF is the coenzyme form, and in this reaction, which appears to require vitamin B_{12} as a cofactor, the methyl group is used to methylate homocysteine, forming methionine. THF is thus regenerated in this reaction and is now available to "pick up" additional one-carbon units for synthesis of DNA and RNA.

Physiology. The preponderance of evidence suggests that folate deficiency is extremely difficult to produce in animals unless: a folic acid antagonist is administered, vitamin C deficiency is induced, or a high level of methionine is added to a diet already deficient in folic acid. Dietary folic acid deficiency may be equally difficult to produce in man. From studies in human subjects, the daily requirement for folic acid is of the order of 10 to 50 microgm. However, it should be remembered that such studies were carried out using the synthetic product, pteroylglutamic acid, not the polyglutamate form found in food. This may account in part for the recommended daily allowance of folic acid set forth by the Food and Nutrition Board of 400 microgm. Higher allowances may be necessary during pregnancy and lactation. Human volunteers fed low folate diets for periods of up to eight months developed no signs of folate deficiency notwithstanding serum levels of less than 1 nanogm. per ml.

The serum folate level may not be predictive of folate deficiency. Indeed, there is still some question as to whether man, like the rat, may not derive enough folate from bacterial synthesis (intestinal flora) to meet daily requirements. Further, FIGLU may also be of little value in diagnosing dietary folate deficiency, since this compound is found in excessive amounts after histidine loading in patients with vitamin B$_{12}$ deficiency, in neoplastic disease, thyrotoxicosis or iron deficiency (Vitale, 1966).

PATHOLOGY

Basis of Deficiency State. Folacin deficiency, from whatever cause, appears to result in megaloblastic dysplasia of cells principally in the bone marrow and gastrointestinal tract, macrocytic anemia and perhaps glossitis. It remains to be proved that folacin deficiency does, in fact, produce morphologic changes in the gastrointestinal tract. Quite the contrary, morphologic changes of the small bowel may precipitate folate deficiency. It may well be that dietary folate deficiency is not a major problem but that, instead, secondary folate deficiency (induced) may be the more serious world health problem. Secondary folate deficiency may result from failure to absorb circulating enterohepatic or dietary folate, increased urinary excretion of THF, increased destruction of folate, interference in the synthesis and/or activation of enzymes necessary for proper folate utilization, or the production of antifolates. Folate deficiency signs may also appear in neoplasia, thyrotoxicosis, iron deficiency, pregnancy, myeloproliferative diseases, and hemolytic diseases for reasons which are not entirely clear.

Disease States: Megaloblastic Anemia. Megaloblastic anemia may occur in sprue or in other diarrheal and malabsorption states. It has been demonstrated that 25 microgm. of PGA per day effects a remission of this megaloblastosis in a high percentage of patients despite their daily intake of approximately 1000 to 1300 microgm. of dietary folate. Conceivably, such patients have a defect in the production and/or secretion of enzyme(s) necessary for splitting of glutamic acid residues from dietary polyglutamates or folacin (Bernstein et al., 1970). Another possible explanation of folate deficiency in malabsorption syndromes may involve the enterohepatic circulation of folacin. Baker et al. (1965) studied the excretion of folic acid in the bile of eight fasting persons and, in all cases, folate activity of the duodenal fluid was higher than that of serum. Thus, the sprue patient may deplete himself of folate by inefficient reabsorption of folate secreted into the gastrointestinal tract.

There are still other disease entities in which folate metabolism may be altered. The megaloblastic anemia seen in alcoholics has usually been attributed to poor dietary habits and low folate intakes. However, Sullivan and Herbert (1964) studied alcoholic patients with low serum folate levels and with megaloblastosis. Three patients were treated with folacin but, if these patients were also given whisky, the bone marrow again became megaloblastic despite normal serum folate levels. The effect of alcohol, however, could be overcome by giving large amounts of folate. The mechanism by which ethanol produces megaloblastosis is not clear, but the effect may be mediated by aberrations in the enzyme system(s) concerned with folate metabolism or one-carbon transfers.

Megaloblastosis may also be present in certain malignant syndromes. It has been argued that active cell proliferation may increase the need for folacin, but this theory has been questioned by some investigators.

A number of drugs—anticonvulsants, antimalarials and oral contraceptives—can induce folate deficiency disease (Roe, 1971). These same agents may also adversely affect vitamin B$_{12}$ metabolism although the evidence for such an action is not as clear-cut as it is for folate. Thus, when long-term therapy with any of these drugs is employed, it is necessary to supplement the intake of both vitamin B$_{12}$ and folate. If folate alone is administered, a deficiency of B$_{12}$ may result. Conversely, folate increases the metabolism of various anticonvulsant drugs and so inactivates them more rapidly (Baylis et al., 1971). Thus, in patients receiving folate therapy and anticonvulsants, an increased frequency of seizures may be observed. It is now clear that the seizures are not attributable to folate and/or folate deficiency but rather to the action of folate on the metabolism of these anticonvulsants.

Certain vitamin B$_{12}$ deficiency findings may be attributed to a defect in folate utilization. The anemia of B$_{12}$ deficiency may be corrected by large doses of folic acid (greater than 400 microgm. per day) but the neurologic lesions of B$_{12}$ deficiency can be precipitated in such cases.

Toxicity. Large pharmacologic doses of folic acid have not been associated with any untoward effects (Moir et al., 1971) (Hellstrom, 1971).

VITAMIN B$_{12}$ (CYANOCOBALAMIN)

(Deficiency state: pernicious anemia)

NORMAL METABOLISM

Chemistry. Of all the vitamins, B_{12} is the largest (molecular weight of about 1500) and probably the most complicated in structure and metabolism. The isolation of the crystalline cobalt-containing vitamin occurred some 20 years after the discovery in 1926 that pernicious anemia could be treated with whole liver. The term cobalamin refers to vitamin B_{12} minus the cyanide group. There are two major components of the B_{12} molecule, one resembling a porphyrin and the other a nucleotide. The porphyrin-like complex has four reduced pyrrole rings linked with cobalt.

Physiology. B_{12} is synthesized only by certain microorganisms and its presence anywhere, including food, can be traced to microorganisms growing in soil, water, intestine, sewage and rumen. Its absorption is dependent on intrinsic factor. *A deficiency of intrinsic factor leads to a vitamin B_{12} deficiency as is detailed on p. 715.*

Vitamin B_{12} is absorbed in the ileum. Once the B_{12} enters the mucosal epithelial cell, it is transferred to the blood and is carried principally via the portal system to the liver where the greater portion is retained. In the blood, B_{12} is conjugated to two proteins, an alpha and a beta globulin, referred to as transcobalamins I and II, respectively. In serum, the concentration in normal man may vary considerably from 100 to 900 picogm. (1×10^{-12} gm.) per ml.

Approximately 1 microgm. of B_{12} per day has been suggested as the minimum recommended allowance. This amount was based on the observation that it would maintain many patients with pernicious anemia in remission. However, the remission may be incomplete and, to adequately restore liver reserves, blood levels and the normal morphology of red cells, larger amounts of vitamin B_{12} are required. About 10 to 20 per cent of dietary B_{12} is absorbed, and thus the recommended daily dietary intake for normal man should be 10 to 15 microgm. Good sources are liver, kidney, fish and meat products.

One of three coenzyme forms, dimethylbenzimidazolylcobamide, has been found in bacteria, animals and man and is required for optimum activity of methyl malonyl coenzyme A isomerase. Vitamin B_{12} is also intimately linked to folate metabolism (Vitale, 1966) (Vitale and Hegsted, 1969) (Iseri et al., 1972), and a deficiency of B_{12} is reflected in aberrations in DNA and RNA synthesis. The results of several studies utilizing animals, bacteria and human beings support the generally accepted view that *vitamin B_{12} is an essential cofactor for the enzyme system(s) involved in the transfer of the methyl group of N5 methyl-THF to homocysteine.* As a result, some investigators believe that in B_{12} deficiency there is an accumulation of N5 methyl-THF. Others believe that THF (the unmethylated form) "piles up." In either case, B_{12} deficiency results in many of the disturbances noted in folate deficiency, apparently by making THF "unavailable" for the "pickup" of one-carbon units for the synthesis of DNA and RNA (see Folic Acid, p. 502).

PATHOLOGY

Basis of Deficiency State. Primary deficiency of vitamin B_{12} is rare but can occur in pure vegetarians who eat no animal meat or dairy products. However, even in such individuals, the time required to produce all of the hematologic and neurologic signs of B_{12} deficiency may be several months or years. Most of the B_{12} deficiency states are induced, and the mechanisms include (1) inadequate production of intrinsic factor (autoimmune response and gastrectomy); (2) competition for B_{12} or interference with intrinsic factor function (bacterial overgrowth, fish tapeworm, blind-loop syndromes, etc.); (3) impaired absorption—general or selective malabsorption syndromes, ileal disease or resection; and (4) loss—defective binding by tissue, liver and serum proteins.

Disease States: Megaloblastic Anemia and Neurologic Disease (Pernicious Anemia). A deficiency of vitamin B_{12}, however induced, produces hematologic and neurologic changes. However, signs and symptoms may not appear until body stores are largely depleted. These anatomic changes are discussed in detail on p. 716.

Toxicity. Large daily doses of vitamin B_{12} (1000 microgm. or more) have been given without untoward effects.

PYRIDOXINE (B_6)

NORMAL METABOLISM

Chemistry. There are three naturally occurring substances for which the term pyridoxine is used: pyridoxine, pyridoxal and pyridoxamine. All are equally active metabolically. All three forms are converted by appropriate tissues or organisms to the active coenzyme form, pyridoxal-5^1-phosphate whose major function is related to amino acid or protein metabolism. The following are known metabolic processes in which pyridoxine is involved: (1) transamination; (2) amino acid decarboxylation; (3) formation of melanin; (4) metabolism of tryptophan; and (5) transmethylation of methionine. Pyridoxine also acts as a cofactor in porphyrin biosynthesis, in phosphorylase activity, in the metabolism of unsaturated fatty acids and cholesterol, in the maintenance of the integrity of neuronal tissue and in antibody production.

Physiology. Not very much is known about pyridoxine absorption. It is found principally in the extracellular fluid, and very little is stored. Most foods are rich in pyridoxine, and a primary deficiency is most unlikely. Any excess intake of pyridoxine is excreted in the urine as pyridoxic acid, a metabolically inactive product. In blood, the levels of pyridoxine range from 2 to 8 microgm. per ml. Leukocyte concentrations are relatively high, varying from 1 to 2 microgm. per ml.; nerve tissue, 0.5 microgm. per gm.; liver, 6 to 9 microgm. per gm.

The human requirement has not been definitely established. However, infants receiving less than 50 microgm. of B_6 per liter of milk developed convulsive seizures which were ameliorated by providing B_6. Human milk contains approximately 120 microgm. per liter. With a B_6 deficiency, xanthurenic acid, an intermediate in tryptophan metabolism, is excreted in abnormally large amounts after a tryptophan load test (0.54 gm. per kg. of body weight of DL-tryptophan). Based on such a test, the requirement for infants has been placed between 200 to 400 microgm. of B_6 per day. The average diet provides 2200 to 3000 microgm. of B_6 per day.

PATHOLOGY

Basis of Deficiency State. Primary pyridoxine deficiency has not been observed in man, but deficiency signs and symptoms have been observed secondary to the administration of pyridoxine antagonists or various drugs, to malabsorption and, under certain conditions, to excessive alcohol ingestion.

Disease States. The feeding of a pyridoxine antagonist, 4-deoxypyridoxine, produced the following signs and symptoms in human subjects: seborrheic dermatitis and erythema (around the nasolabial folds, eyebrows and cheeks); glossitis, cheilosis, angular stomatitis, blepharitis, peripheral neuropathy and lymphopenia.

Vitamin B_6 deficiency signs have been reported in patients receiving isonicotinic acid hydrazide for the treatment of tuberculosis, in those receiving oral contraceptives, in patients receiving antihypertensive drugs, and in patients with Parkinson's disease being treated with L-dopa (Roe, 1971) (McLaren, 1969).

About 100 cases of so-called pyridoxine-responsive anemia have been reported. These patients usually develop hemochromatosis with marked hyperferremia, and the response to B_6 is almost always transient. It is interesting that in animals, B_6 deficiency results in an iron deficiency type of anemia although the animals have hyperferremia.

In recent years, some evidence has been presented that oxaluria can be mitigated and the development of renal calculi blocked by the administration of pyridoxine and magnesium oxide to patients who persistently form renal stones (Gershoff and Prien, 1967). Pyridoxine deficiency in the rat and cat results in increased urinary excretion of oxalate and formation of calcium oxalate stones. The pathology associated with these lesions in animals has been well described (McCombs and Gershoff, 1972).

Toxicity. No toxicity to B_6 administration has been reported.

MINERALS

A number of minerals are essential for the maintenance of health. Some, such as iron, are present in large amounts, but others, for example cobalt, fall into the category of trace elements. Most have been or will be discussed in connection with the major function of the specific mineral. Cobalt is of major importance in vitamin B_{12} deficiency and is discussed in relationship to this vitamin. Selenium is of principal importance in connection with vitamin E. Here it is only necessary to consider the nutritional aspects of iron and zinc.

IRON

As a cause of deficiency disease on a global basis, iron is probably no less important a nutrient than protein. Around the world, the most common form of anemia is that resulting from iron deficiency. In a recent nutrition survey in the United States, the most prevalent nutritional deficiency observed was related to iron lack. In most instances, the iron lack results from a combination of a primary dietary deficiency and chronic blood loss.

The body's rigorous conservation of iron was described in detail on p. 50 (Harris and Kellermeyer, 1970). Here our attention is focused on the nutritional aspects of iron deficiency.

Iron is found in food mainly in the ferric form, bound to proteins, amino acids and organic acids, or in the form of heme-iron complexed to protein. Before being absorbed, it must be chemically reduced and/or split from its complex. Only about 10 per cent of ingested iron is absorbed, and normal iron absorption requires gastric acid juices. Gastrectomy leads to malabsorption of iron. Ascorbic acid assists in the absorption of iron as an antioxidant maintaining the iron in the ferrous state. Iron deficiency may arise despite adequate dietary intake. In the advanced years of life, there is impaired absorption of iron. In some part, this may be related to impaired gastric acid secretion, but it may have more mysterious origins.

Whatever the cause, a lack of iron leads to an iron deficiency anemia, discussed on p. 719. It is, however, important to emphasize that iron deficiency, even in the absence of anemia, may compromise the individual's performance and ability to work. In time, however, the iron lack will lead to a microcytic, hypochromic anemia. However, before such manifest iron deficiency anemia becomes evident, a transient phase of normochromic, normocytic anemia may occur, reflecting slight reduction in the total body iron pool. In the clinical consideration of hypochromic, microcytic anemia, it is necessary to appreciate that in chronic infection, lead poisoning, rheumatoid arthritis, vitamin B$_6$ deficiency and thalassemia, the peripheral blood smear can mimic that seen in iron deficiency despite normal serum iron levels. Generally, the clinical signs produced by all of these systemic diseases should permit their differentiation from iron lack anemia.

There is recent evidence that iron deficiency may affect the utilization of folic acid. It has been repeatedly pointed out that, with severe iron deficiency anemia, there is a defect in folate utilization resulting in red cell abnormalities characteristic not only of iron deficiency but also folate deficiency as well (Vitale et al., 1966) (Velez et al., 1966) (Chanarin, 1969). A deficiency of iron may also have effects on enzymes involved in the transfer of one-carbon units. Formimino glutamic acid is excreted in excessive amounts in many patients with iron deficiency, implying that in some way the iron is involved in the function of enzymes concerned with one-carbon transfers. These observations are contrary to standard concepts that iron-containing enzymes are inviolate even in the presence of severe iron depletion. Decreased concentrations of certain iron-containing enzymes have been noted in severely iron-depleted individuals but, to date, no clinical consequences of these enzyme deficiencies have been observed. Arbeter et al. (1971) have shown decreased phagocytic activity of neutrophils in patients with iron deficiency anemia. This functional alteration was associated with a decrease in activity of myeloperoxidase (an iron-containing enzyme) in the neutrophils. A lack of iron has also been shown to produce gastric erosions in experimental animals, and it has been suggested that similar changes may occur in individuals with chronic and/or severe iron deficiency (Cowan et al., 1966). In regions of the world where iron deficiency is prevalent, intestinalization of the stomach associated with achlorhydria and achylia has been observed in an increased frequency (Fig. 11–13). Such abnormal gastric morphology and function have been associated with an increased incidence of gastric cancer (Velez and Vitale, 1971). It is evident, therefore, that iron deficiency may have far more wide-ranging implications than the production of only an anemia.

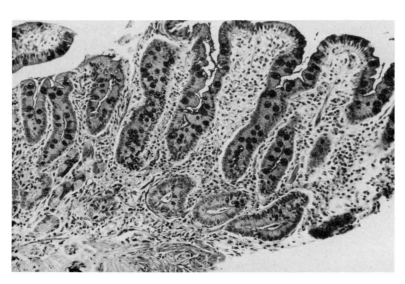

Figure 11–13. *Gastric biopsy of a 17-year-old boy with moderate to severe iron deficiency anemia of long duration. There is intestinalization of the gastric mucosa with achlorhydria and achylia. Appearance of specimen resembles that of colon or small bowel as seen in tropical sprue. The mucosal epithelial cells contain dark mucin globules characteristic of colonic mucosa (PAS stain).*

ZINC (Zn)

In recent years, zinc has evoked a great deal of interest among surgeons since it has reportedly been used successfully to enhance wound healing. Other studies have also related low serum zinc levels to poor gonad maturation and function, dwarfism, anemia, liver disease and cancer. Possibly, zinc may have a more important role in clinical medicine than was previously suspected.

Zinc is a trace metal widely distributed in food, and the average intake is estimated to be between 10 and 15 mg. per day. Meat, fish, eggs, whole grains and legumes are rich in zinc. Cows' milk provides 3 to 5 mg. per liter and galvanized cans are equally good sources of zinc in liquid foods, particularly if they are acidic. Oysters, also, are particularly rich in zinc. Not much is known about zinc metabolism except that calcium and phytates may inhibit absorption while EDTA facilitates zinc absorption. The site of zinc absorption appears to be in the distal end of the small bowel. Normal plasma levels range from 90 to 120 microgm. bound to albumin and, to a lesser extent, to globulins. The total body zinc content is approximately 2 gm. in a 70 kg. man. Muscle is the main storehouse of zinc, accounting for more than half of the total body zinc. A number of enzymes contain zinc, including carbonic anhydrase, carboxypeptidase, alcohol dehydrogenase, glutamic dehydrogenase, several of the isozymes of alkaline phosphatase, tryptophan desmolase, malic dehydrogenase and lactic acid dehydrogenase. Zinc deficiency may be associated with decreased activity of these enzymes but the evidence is not clear. The pathology of zinc deficiency is not well documented. There is some evidence that the oral administration of zinc sulfate (200 mg. three times daily) significantly increases the rate of wound healing and of the healing of decubitus ulcers (Hallbook and Lanner, 1972). In man, zinc deficiency has been associated with stunted physical growth, stunted growth of external genitalia and disappearance of pubic, axillary and facial hair (Prasad et al., 1967) (Sandstead, 1968) (Halsted et al., 1968). Zinc deficiency has also been implicated in the pathogenesis of alcoholic cirrhosis.

REFERENCES

Arbeter, A., et al.: Nutrition and infection. Fed. Proc., 30:1421, 1971.

Baker, S. J., et al.: Excretion of folic acid in bile. Lancet, 1:685, 1965.

Baker, S. J., et al.: Failure of vitamin E therapy in the treatment of anemia of protein calorie malnutrition. Blood, 32:717, 1968.

Balsley, M., and Speckmann, E. W.: A new look at vitamin E in clinical medicine. J. Oklahoma State Med. Ass., 64:482, 1971.

Bartley, W., et al.: Vitamin C Requirements of Human Adults. Medical Research Council Special Report Series No. 280. London, H. M. Stationery Office, 1953.

Baylis, E. M., et al.: Influence of folic acid on blood-phenytoin levels. Lancet, 1:62, 1971.

Beaton, G. H., and Whalen, S.: Vitamin C in the common cold. Canad. Med. Ass. J., 105:355, 1971.

Bernstein, L. H., et al.: The absorbtion and malabsorption of folic acid and its polyglutamates. Amer. J. Med., 48:570, 1970.

Braun, I. G.: Vitamin A. Excess, deficiency, requirements, metabolism and misuse. Pediat. Clin. N. Amer., 9:935, 1962.

Brickman, A. S., et al.: Action of 1,25-dihydroxycholecalciferol, a potent, kidney-produced metabolite of vitamin D, in uremic man. New Eng. J. Med., 287:891, 1972.

Chanarin, I.: Megaloblastic Anemias. Oxford and Edinburgh, Blackwell Scientific Publications, 1969.

Cowan, B., et al.: The gastric mucosa in anemia in Punjabis. Gut, 7:234, 1966.

Crandon, J. H., et al.: Experimental human scurvy. New Eng. J. Med., 223:353, 1940.

Dam, H.: International symposium on recent advances in research on vitamins K and related quinones. Vitamins Hormones, 24:295, 1966.

DeLuca, H. F.: Metabolism and function of vitamin D. In Deluca, H. F., and Suttie, J. W. (eds.): The Fat Soluble Vitamins. Madison, Wis., University of Wisconsin Press, 1969.

DeLuca, H. F.: Vitamin D: a new look at an old vitamin. Nutr. Rev., 29:179, 1971.

Editorial: Anticonvulsant osteomalacia. Lancet, 2:805, 1972.

Edwards, L. C., and Dunphy, J. E.: Wound healing. New Eng. J. Med., 259:224, 275, 1958.

Evans, H. M., and Bishop, K. S.: The production of sterility with nutritional regimes adequate for growth and its cure with other foodstuffs. J. Metab. Res., 3:233, 1923.

Food and Nutrition Board of the National Research Council: Recommended dietary allowances: a report. Publication, No. 1694. 7th rev. ed. Washington, D.C., National Academy of Science, 1968.

Follis, E. H.: Hypervitaminosis D. Amer. J. Clin. Path., 26:400, 1956.

Frick, P. G., et al.: Dose response and minimal daily requirement for vitamin K in man. J. Appl. Physiol., 23:387, 1967.

Galante, L., et al.: Effect of parathyroid extract on vitamin D metabolism. Lancet, 1:985, 1972.

Gershoff, S. N., and Prien, E. L.: Effect of daily MgO and pyridoxine administration to patients with recurring calcium oxalate kidney stones. Amer. J. Clin., Nutr., 20:393, 1967.

Ghitis, J. J., and Vitale, J. J.: Anemias of protein calorie malnutrition. Postgrad. Med., 34:300, 1963.

Ginter, E.: Vitamin C deficiency and gallstone formation. Lancet, 2:1198, 1971.

Goldsmith, G. A.: Common cold: prevention and treatment with ascorbic acid not effective. J.A.M.A., 216:337, 1971.

Gould, B. S.: Collagen Biosynthesis in Wound Healing. Proceedings of a Workshop. National Academy of Science. U.S.A. National Research Council. 1966, p. 99.

Hahn, T. J., et al.: Effect of chronic anticonvulsant therapy on serum 25-hydroxycalciferol levels in adults. New Eng. J. Med., 287:900, 1972.

Hallbook, T., and Lanner, E.: Serum-zinc and healing of venous leg ulcers. Lancet, 1:780, 1972.

Halsted, J. A., et al.: Plasma zinc concentration in liver diseases. Comparison with normal controls and certain other chronic diseases. Gastroenterology, 54:1098, 1968.

Harris, J. W., Kellermeyer, R. W.: The Red Cell. Cambridge, Mass., Harvard University Press, 1970.

Hegsted, D. M.: Theoretical estimates of protein requirements of children. J. Amer. Diet. Ass., 33:225, 1957.

Hellstrom, L.: Lack of toxicity of folic acid given in pharmacological doses to healthy volunteers. Lancet, 1:59, 1971.

Hodges, R. E., et al.: Clinical manifestations of ascorbic acid deficiency in man. Amer. J. Clin. Nutr., 24:432, 1971.

Horwitt, M. K., et al.: Polyunsaturated lipids and tocopherol requirements. J. Amer. Diet. Ass., 38:231, 1961.

Iseri, O. A., et al.: Vitamin B_{12} and methionine metabolism in the buffalo rat liver and hepatoma. Lab. Invest., 27:226, 1972.

Jeghers, H., and Marraro, H.: Hypervitaminosis A, its broadening spectrum. Amer. J. Clin. Nutr., 4:603, 1956.

Keenan, W. J., et al.: Role of feeding and vitamin K in hypo-prothrombinemia of the newborn. Amer. J. Dis. Child., *121*:271, 1971.

Kramer, B., and Kanof, A.: Pathology in human beings of vitamin D deficiency. In Sebrel, W. H., Jr., and Harris, R. H. (eds.): The Vitamins. Vol. 2. New York, Academic Press, Inc., 1954, p. 232.

Lamm, M., and Neuman, W. F.: On the role of vitamin D in calcification. Arch. Path., *66*:204, 1958.

Leonard, P. J., and Losowsky, M. S.: Effect of alpha-tocopherol administration on red cell survival in vitamin E deficient human subjects. Amer. J. Clin. Nutr., *24*:388, 1971.

Lipschitz, D. A., et al.: The role of ascorbic acid in the metabolism of storage iron. Brit. J. Haemat., *20*:155, 1971.

Machado, E. A., et al.: Studies on dietary hepatic necrosis. II. Ultrastructural and enzymatic alterations of the hepatocytic plasma membrane. Lab. Invest., *24*:13, 1971.

Majaj, A. S., et al.: Vitamin E responsive megaloblastic anemia in infants with protein calorie malnutrition. Amer. J. Clin. Nutr., *12*:374, 1963.

Mason, K. E.: Effects of vitamin A deficiency in human beings. In Sebrel, W. H., Jr., and Harris, R. H. (eds.): The Vitamins. Vol. 1. New York, Academic Press, Inc., 1954, p. 137.

McCombs, H. L., and Gershoff, S. N.: Effects of vitamin B_6 deficiency on the rat kidney. Lab. Invest., *26*:515, 1972.

McLaren, D. S.: The vitamins. In Bondy, P. K. (ed.): Diseases of Metabolism. Philadelphia, W. B. Saunders Co., 1969.

Moir, A. T. B., et al.: Lack of effect of folic acid administration on cerebral metabolism. Lancet, *2*:798, 1971.

Nair, P. P., et al.: Vitamin E and porphyrin metabolism in man. Arch. Intern. Med., *128*:413, 1971.

Pauling, L.: Vitamin C and the Common Cold. San Francisco, W. H. Freeman and Co., 1970.

Pelletier, O.: Vitamin C status of cigarette smokers and non smokers. Amer. J. Clin. Nutr., *23*:520, 1970.

Prasad, A. S., et al.: Studies on zinc deficiency: changes in trace elements and enzyme activities in tissues of zinc-deficient rats. J. Clin. Invest., *46*:549, 1967.

Raisz, L. G.: A confusion of vitamin D's. New Eng. J. Med., *287*:926, 1972.

Rhead, W. J., and Schrauzer, G. N.: Risks of long term ascorbic acid overdosage. Nutr. Rev., *29*:262, 1971.

Roe, D. A.: Drug induced deficiency of B vitamins. New York J. Med., *1*:2770, 1971.

Roels, O. A.: Vitamin A. Physiology. J.A.M.A., *214*:1097, 1970.

Rose, C. S., and Gyorgy, P.: Tocopherol and hemolysis in vivo and in vitro. Ann. N. Y. Acad. Sci., *52*:231, 1949.

Ross, R., and Benditt, E. P.: Wound healing and collagen formation. J. Cell Biol., *27*:83, 1965.

Rotruck J. T., et al.: Prevention of oxidative damage to rat erythrocytes by dietary selenium. J. Nutr., *102*:689, 1972.

Sahud, M. A., and Cohen, R. J.: Effect of aspirin ingestion on ascorbic acid levels in rheumatoid arthritis. Lancet, *1*:937, 1971.

Sandstead, H. H.: Zinc, a metal to grow on. Nutr. Today, (March):12, 1968.

Seegers, W. H.: Blood Clotting Enzymology. New York, Academic Press, Inc., 1967.

Smith, F. R., et al.: Radio immunoassay of human plasma retinol-binding protein. J. Clin. Invest., *49*:1754, 1970.

Sullivan, L. W., and Herbert, V.: Suppression of hematopoiesis by ethanol. J. Clin. Invest., *43*:2048, 1964.

Sutherland, J. M., et al.: Hemorrhagic disease of the newborn. Amer. J. Dis. Child., *113*:524, 1967.

Tishkoff, G. H., et al.: Preparation of highly purified prothrombin complex. J. Biol. Chem., *243*:4151, 1968.

Vedder, E. B.: The pathology of beriberi. J.A.M.A., *110*:893, 1938.

Velez, H., and Vitale, J. J.: Personal communication, 1971.

Velez, H., et al.: Folic acid deficiency secondary to iron deficiency in man. Amer. J. Clin. Nitr., *19*:27, 1966.

Vitale, J. J.: Present knowledge of folacin, Nutr. Rev., *24*:289, 1966.

Vitale, J. J., and Hegsted, D. M.: Effects of dietary methionine and vitamin B_{12} deficiency on folate metabolism. Brit. J. Haemat., *17*:467, 1966.

Vitale, J. J., et al.: Secondary folate deficiency induced in the rat by dietary iron deficiency. J. Nutr., *88*:315, 1966.

Wald, G.: The molecular basis of visual excitation. Nature, *219*:800, 1968.

Wasserman, R. H., and Corradino, R. A.: Metabolic role of vitamins A and D. Ann. Rev. Biochem., *40*:501, 1971.

Wasserman, R. H., and Taylor, A. N.: Metabolic roles of fat-soluble vitamins D, E and K. Ann. Rev. Biochem., *41*:179, 1972.

Wolbach, S. B.: The pathologic changes resulting from vitamin deficiency. J.A.M.A., *108*:9, 1937.

Wolbach, S. B., and Bessey, O. A.: Tissue changes in vitamin deficiencies. Physiol. Rev., *22*:233, 1942.

Woodhouse, N. J. Y., et al.: Vitamin D deficiency and primary hyperparathyroidism. Lancet, *2*:283, 1971.

12

ENVIRONMENTAL PATHOLOGY

The term environmental disease applies to disorders emanating from air, soil and water pollution as well as those diseases resulting from drug abuse and the many toxic chemicals and potentially injurious physical agents (including radiation) to be found in man's environment. While such diseases collectively constitute only a small fraction of clinical disorders, they have a disproportionate importance because all are theoretically preventable. To fail to recognize an infant as having lead poisoning is to permit him to return to a crib covered with a lead-based paint on which he has been cheerfully and dangerously chewing. Speaking on this problem of preventable diseases and the failure of physicians to be more active in their control, Rothschild (1970) levels the charge: "It should be clear to all who call themselves health professionals that if you are not part of the solution, you are part of the problem!"

Man's mindless destruction of his environment has greatly expanded both the range and frequency of environmental diseases (Epstein, 1972). Despite our belated recognition of the meaning of ecology, the deteriorating environment continues its downward spiral, unchecked as yet by adequate measures. To quote

Kotin (1971), "The well-being of man is crucially linked to his physical environment. By benefit or threat, it specifically plays a predominant role in man's health. Many adverse effects are of long standing, but rapid technological change, accumulation of contaminants and waste products, increasing population as well as increasing per capita consumption, and progressive concentration of people in urban centers have greatly magnified the threats and complicated the problems of keeping adverse effects down to acceptable limits." The socio-economic problems of population control, food supply and water pollution are staggeringly important and impinge heavily on the health of man, but they are better treated by others expert in these fields. Here we shall deal only with the environmental disorders of the individual.

AIR POLLUTION—PNEUMOCONIOSES

At one time, diseases caused by the inhalation of vapors, smokes and dust were largely

509

encountered in those working in certain hazardous occupations, such as the coal miner, the asbestos fabricator and the quarry worker. In this smoggy day, air contaminants predispose to or provoke respiratory ailments in the general population, particularly in those living in industrialized urban centers. Some will recall Donora, Pennsylvania and London in the recent past with their frightening epidemics of respiratory deaths. The nature of the dangerous pollutants, their tolerable limits and their injury-producing pathways are poorly understood. To be found in city air are variable mixtures of industrial wastes and residues of the combustion of fuels such as coal and gasoline. The ever-changing distribution of sulphur and carbon oxides, organic residues containing tars and aldehydes (some of which may be potentially carcinogenic) and the vaporized metals and acids emitted by industry and gasoline engines makes the problem of identifying specific dangerous pollutants enormously complex. It is sobering to learn that the use of gasoline additives in North America is said to be responsible for the discharge in motor exhaust of more than 200,000 tons of lead per year (U.S. Public Health Service, 1966). It is generally believed that this "atmospheric soup" acts by exacerbating preexisting respiratory diseases such as chronic bronchitis (p. 802) and emphysema (p. 792) rather than by inducing a specific new entity. However, the possible carcinogenic potential of these pollutants demands careful investigation.

Much better defined are the pneumoconioses of occupational origin caused by the inhalation of mineral or organic dusts; 31 specific forms have been described (Spencer, 1968). *Important determinants in the causation of a pneumoconiosis are: (1) the concentration of the pollutant in the air, (2) its size and shape, (3) its chemical nature and solubility and (4) the duration of exposure.* The particle concentration required to produce disease with injurious agents is truly incredible. It is estimated that a man may work for his entire life in an environment containing 5×10^6 particles of quartz (silica) per cubic foot of air without developing silicosis, but 100×10^6 particles in the same volume of air would almost certainly induce the disease. These data indicate not only the amazing concentration of pollutant to which one may be exposed with apparent safety, but also the relatively narrow range between safety and danger.

Particle size is an important consideration since, in general, dusts or pollutants must be small enough to be carried in the inspired air into the bronchoalveolar unit in order to cause disease. The most dangerous particles are below 3 to 5 microns in diameter. Above this

dimension, approximately 90 per cent are trapped in the mucus of the nasopharyngobronchial tree (Green, 1970). Below this size, they are carried in the tidal air volume into the lower respiratory passages and possibly into the alveoli. When the concentration is not overwhelming, particles between 0.5 and perhaps 5 microns in diameter may penetrate to the smaller bronchioles and alveoli. Most are trapped and cleared (90 per cent) by mucociliary activity, but those that remain are potentially injurious. Considerable concern was expressed a few years ago about the possible injurious actions of inhaled aerosolized toiletries such as hair sprays. Studies, however, have demonstrated that in most instances the vinyl copolymers are too large to reach the distal respiratory unit (Brunner, 1963). Once within the alveoli, all foreign substances of particulate nature can only be cleared by phagocytic pulmonary macrophages. The defensive pulmonary mechanisms, however, can be overwhelmed by excessive concentrations. It is relevant in this connection to point out that concurrent cigarette smoking or other adverse influences such as ethanol may virtually wipe out the macrophage response and reduce this defensive mechanism to helplessness. Green and Carolin (1967) have shown, for example, that the phagocytic capacity of rabbit alveolar macrophages for bacteria can be reduced to near zero by exposing these cells to the gas phase of cigarette smoke. The effect occurs within minutes of exposure of the macrophages.

Still unknown is the manner in which inhaled dusts cause tissue reactions. Do the particles directly penetrate the alveolar walls and there, because of their chemical toxicity or physical structure, induce tissue injury or, instead, are they first phagocytized by macrophages causing release of injurious lysosomal enzymes as these cells are killed? Also to be considered is the possibility that the damage is mediated by a hypersensitivity reaction. Any of these mechanisms might be operational in the production of disease, perhaps one being more important than the other in specific disorders, as will become clear in the following discussion of a few of the more important pneumoconioses.

ANTHRACOSIS

Pulmonary anthracosis—the accumulation of dust pigments in the lungs—is the identifying morphologic hallmark of urban life. It is present, to some degree, in the lungs of virtually every adult city dweller. The anthracotic pigments lie within the macrophages in the alveolar spaces in and about parenchymal and subpleural lymphatic channels and in the draining lymph nodes. Other than causing blackening of the tissues, the process in the usual city dweller is innocuous and causes no respiratory dysfunction. Neither does such pigmentation predispose to respiratory infections. However, studies of coal miners indicate that more extreme deposits of coal dust may cause significant disease (Naeye, 1970). In these workers, the marked anthracosis is called "miner's lungs" or "black lungs." The pulmonary scars in these coal miners were attributed to concurrent exposure to silica, but it has become clear that coal dust alone may cause "simple pneumoconiosis" or, at more extreme levels, the disabling "progressive massive fibrosis." The simple pneumoconiosis usually involves the upper more than the lower lobes and takes the form of "coal macules" in the centers of secondary pulmonary lobules. These macules comprise aggregates of anthracosis-laden macrophages about terminal and respiratory bronchioles, accompanied by a mild fibroblastic reaction. The lymphatic channels about the bronchioles are simultaneously overloaded. As these accumulations progress, they induce a fibroblastic reaction which encroaches on the lobular arterioles, narrowing their lumina. In time, the vascular insufficiency worsens, and areas of heavily pigment-laden, dense fibrosis appear. Sometimes the centers of these scars consist of massive collections of coal dust that literally flow out on being sectioned. In many cases, coal dust-laden phagocytes are found layering the alveolar septa. Overgrowth of the alveolar lining epithelium incorporates these phagocytes into the septal wall, but a new layer of phagocytes may then become attached and, in this fashion, the alveolar space is progressively encroached upon by the ever-widening alveolar walls. Subsequently, emphysema of both the panlobular and centrilobular types is almost an inevitable concomitant (p. 792) (Ishikawa et al., 1969).

The extreme anthracosis in "miner's lungs" predisposes to other forms of respiratory disease such as chronic bronchitis and bacterial infections. But even in the absence of such complications the progressive massive fibrosis causes marked respiratory difficulty and frequently results in premature death. Wyatt (1971) contends that "the risk of death among coal miners has been nearly twice that of the general population and higher than that of any other occupational group in the United States. Mixed anthracosilicotic patterns are encountered in hard coal miners.

SILICOSIS

Dusts of silica (silicon dioxide) in the free state, in crystalline form such as quartz dust, or in the amorphous colloidal state as in diatomaceous earth may all cause silicosis. These dusts are encountered in many industries, particularly in the mining of gold, iron and coal, in stonework, quarrying, sandcasting, grinding and polishing of metals and stone, manufacture of pottery and ceramics, and sandblasting.

Important in the pathogenesis of silicosis are the quantity and duration of the exposure as well as the mechanism by which silica exerts its injurious effect. As was mentioned, particles larger than 5 microns in diameter rarely cause disease since they do not reach the bronchoalveolar units. Those most dangerous are in the range of 0.5 to 3 microns in diameter. Mention has already been made of the enormous concentrations of siliceous dust necessary to induce disease (p. 510). The time exposure required for the development of this disease obviously depends on the intensity of the exposure but, in most instances, ranges from 10 to 15 years. No well substantiated cases have been observed with exposure of under two years, however heavy the contamination.

Controversy has existed for years over how silica particles cause cell and tissue injury. Direct mechanical trauma resulting from the physical characteristics of the particle and chemical toxicity from the formation of silicic acid have largely been invalidated as mechanisms of tissue injury. Instead, Allison et al. (1965) propose that injury is mediated by destruction of phagocytic macrophages. Once within the alveoli, the silica particles are phagocytized by macrophages. The phagocytic vacuole bearing the silica particle then fuses with lysosomes to release powerful lytic enzymes into the vacuole. However, a fine layer of silicic acid present on the surface of the silica particle reacts with the bounding membrane of the vacuole, increasing its permeability, and so lysosomal enzymes diffuse into the cytoplasm of the macrophage and cause its death. The release of enzymes and necrotic cell products including phospholipids from the destroyed macrophages injures the adjacent pulmonary parenchymal cells and exerts a strong fibrogenic influence. The silica particles, released from their now dead captors, are once again phagocytized by other macrophages to continue the chain reaction. Still not excluded, however, is the possibility that the toxic action of silica is exerted by its acting as an antigen or, more correctly, as a hapten. Immune globulins have been identified in the silicotic pulmonary lesions of man, and rabbits injected with quartz particles coated with homologous serum protein develop antibodies to the silica-protein complex (Scheel et al., 1954).

Morphology. In the early stages of this disease, there may only be minute nodules which impart a fine, sand-like texture to the lung parenchyma. Microscopy will disclose that these are distributed along subpleural, peribronchiolar and perivascular lymphatics. With progression, the individual nodules increase in size, and some coalesce to become visible to the naked eye. This parenchymal involvement tends to be located in the upper lobes and about the hilar regions but, in severe cases, the involvement is widespread. With advancement, the gray to black nodules become progressively larger, stony hard and, in far advanced cases, large areas of the lungs may be converted to massive scars with only small intervening patches of compressed emphysematous lung parenchyma. The tracheobronchial lymph nodes draining the lung exhibit a similar progression of nodularity and eventual fibrosis. Anthracotic pigmentation which is almost invariably present, particularly in miners of "hard coal," imparts the blackness to the scarred areas. Especially striking is the development of dense fibrous obliterative adhesions between the pleural surfaces which render it extremely difficult to remove the lungs from the thorax. This morphologic pattern may be markedly modified by tuberculosis which often (up to 80 per cent) coexists in these vulnerable lungs.

The early microscopic lesions of silicosis are rarely encountered in man. From animal experimentation, it has been shown that the first reaction to silica particles is the accumulation of pulmonary macrophages within the alveolar spaces. Phagocytosis of the particulate material leads, as has been indicated, to the death of many cells and the onset of a fibroblastic reaction in the particular focus. Some of the macrophages swell and assume an epithelioid appearance. The addition of multinucleate giant cells converts the focus into a granuloma that closely resembles a hard tubercle (p. 412). With the passage of time, the granuloma becomes progressively more fibrotic and is eventually converted into an acellular nodule of concentric layers of hyaline-appearing connective tissue. Contiguous nodules may be enclosed within enveloping collagenous layers and, in this fashion, the fibrotic process extends (Fig. 12—1). Scattered infiltrates of lymphocytes and plasma cells and trapped masses of anthracotic pigment are usually present in the scarred areas. The lung parenchyma is thus encroached upon and, in time, large areas of the lung may be replaced by the advancing disease. Important in the differentiation of silicosis from other forms of fibrosing granulomas is the polari-

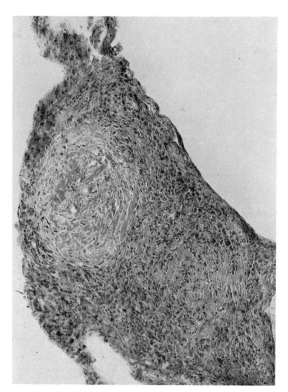

Figure 12–1. Silicosis. Several still discernible fibrous nodules are now fused together by scarring of the intervening parenchyma.

scopic demonstration of birefringent particles of silica within the fine, cleft-like spaces between the collagenous lamellae of the silicotic nodules. Similar histologic findings are found in the affected tracheobronchial nodes. The identification of coexistent tuberculosis may be difficult unless unmistakable caseation is present in the granulomatous foci or acid-fast bacilli can be identified.

Clinical Course. Clinical manifestations appear only when the pulmonary changes are well advanced. For many years during its evolution, silicosis is asymptomatic and is often discovered on routine chest film by the characteristic "snowstorm" appearance imparted by the focal fibrosing granulomas. Eventually, the progressive scarring leads to dyspnea on exertion, associated with a marked decrease in lung compliance and in gas diffusion. Usually these respiratory difficulties are mild at the outset but, over the course of years, the relentless progression of the pulmonary fibrosis eventually causes incapacitating dyspnea and orthopnea. Classically, these patients are afebrile and have no systemic manifestations of an infection. The appearance of fever or rapid worsening of the patient's condition should raise the suspicion of superimposed tuberculosis. In most cases, the slow progression spans decades and, while the pulmonary lesions cripple, they do not kill. However, in some patients, death is caused by ventilatory insufficiency or by the development of cor pulmonale and cardiac failure incident to the right heart strain. Superimposed tuberculosis, as would be anticipated, is a grave complication.

ASBESTOSIS

Asbestos is a complex silicate occurring in a variety of chemical combinations and physical forms. Asbestos, after being mined, must be crushed to extract the fibers from the dust. Regrettably, the fibers, having the desired unique characteristics of heat resistance and tensile strength, are far more dangerous than the amorphous dust. In 1935, it is estimated that about 500,000 tons of asbestos were mined in the Western world, but in 1965 this figure had skyrocketed to 5,000,000 tons. Paradoxically, those engaged in quarrying the mineral rarely contract the disease. While they are theoretically exposed to high concentrations of airborne contamination, the danger has long been recognized and such workers are protected by adequate safeguards. In contrast, those who fabricate the asbestos into heat-resistant boards, brake lining and tiles and those employed in the installation of asbestos insulation are often exposed to seemingly low levels of air contamination and so do not take adequate precautions. A recent report underscores this hazard (Murphy et al., 1971). In a survey of 101 shipyard workers engaged in installing asbestos insulation, 38 per cent were found to have asbestosis. Of particular interest is the fact that these workers were exposed to concentrations of approximately 5 million particles of asbestos per cubic foot of air, long considered to be the threshold value or the safe upper limit of airborne contamination.

The onset of the disease after exposure is quite variable. While some have developed pulmonary lesions as soon as one to two years after working with asbestos products, most develop no manifestations until 20 to 30 years later.

Morphology. Because of the large fiber size (on the order of 50 microns in length and a half micron in diameter), inhaled fibers generally settle out within the bronchi, bronchioles and respiratory bronchioles. Here they excite, within the walls of the airways, a histiocytic and giant cell reaction leading to the formation of granulomas. In the course of time, these granulomas undergo fibrosis, and the scarring extends into the adjacent alveoli to produce parenchymal nodular scars and thickening of alveolar walls. Only the smallest particles reach the alveoli to elicit a similar reaction in the septal walls. Because most clinical cases come to attention in the late fibrotic stage of this disease, it is rare to identify well defined granulomas. However, even the sclerosed granulomas are made distinctive by the presence of so-called "asbestos bodies" within the dense fibrous scar. These appear as elongated beaded or segmented bodies with rounded drumstick ends produced by encrustation of protein and iron salts on the native fibers (Fig. 12–2). With time these fibers fragment. Asbestos bodies may also be found lying along alveolar septa and in the fibrous thickened alveolar walls. Such air spaces as remain are often distended, distorted, emphysematous and sometimes have hyperplastic thickening of their lining epithelium.

As might be anticipated from the microscopic findings, the lungs grossly have nodular and confluent scars. The lower lobes are most severely affected. A characteristic and almost invariable alteration is the development of dense, fibrous thickening of both the parietal and visceral pleura of the lung with an associated obliterative fibrous pleuritis. Superimposed bacterial infections in the form of chronic bronchiectasis (p. 806) or tuberculosis are common complications. The tracheobronchial nodes are usually spared, presumably because the large fibers are not easily phagocytized and so are not carried through lymphatics.

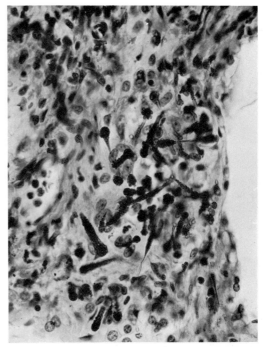

Figure 12–2. Asbestosis of the lung in high power detail to demonstrate the pathognomonic "asbestos bodies."

Clinical Course. The clinical manifestations of asbestosis are very much like those of silicosis. For long years, asbestosis may be completely latent, but once symptoms begin to appear, they tend to worsen more rapidly than is the case with silicosis. Progressive respiratory insufficiency leading to death within one year of onset of symptoms is sometimes encountered.

There has been great controversy in the literature over two aspects of this disorder: (1) the true prevalence of asbestosis and (2) its relationship to the production of cancer in the lungs. Anjilvel and Thurlbeck (1966) made the surprising observation that asbestos bodies could be found in the fluid of lung macerates in 48 per cent of adult males autopsied in Montreal. Recently, however, Gross et al. (1969) cast doubt on this observation. They contended that particles indistinguishable from the so-called asbestos bodies can be produced by encrustation of other forms of fibers and so these apparently distinctive structures lack specificity. Equally in doubt is the frequency of the induction of pulmonary cancers by asbestos. It has been reported that bronchogenic carcinoma occurs in about 14 per cent of all cases of asbestosis, usually developing about 16 to 18 years after the exposure to asbestos (Telischi and Rubenstone, 1961). Pleural mesotheliomas are also associated with asbestosis and were the cause of death in 5 per cent of 325 patients with this pneumoconiosis in contrast to the 0.01 per cent incidence of this rare neoplasm in the population at large (Belleau and Gaensler, 1968). To further confuse the issue, a five-year epidemiologic survey of 20 million Canadians revealed a prevalence of one mesothelioma per million population (McDonald et al., 1970). It would appear that with this low prevalence of mesotheliomas, asbestosis is either a much rarer form of pneumoconiosis than some of the above data would indicate or, alternatively, it does not carry a high cancer risk. The best reconciliation of these seeming conflicts might be that the finding of asbestos bodies in lung juice should not be equated with pneumoconiosis but, when a bona fide disease uncommonly develops, it creates a well defined predisposition to cancer.

BERYLLIOSIS

Beryllium dusts and vapors are highly dangerous and cause both pulmonary and systemic lesions. With its high tensile strength and resistance to fatigue, this metal is widely used in alloys and in the construction of instruments and fabrications for the aerospace industry. Recognition of the hazard involved in the handling of this metal came after World War II. Beryllium was then used as a phosphor in fluorescent lights, and accidental breakage of these tubes led to episodic but heavy exposures. This use of beryllium has been discontinued, a practice which undoubtedly contributes to the declining incidence of berylliosis. Those at greatest risk now are engaged in extracting the metal from its ores and in the preparation of its alloys and instruments. Berylliosis has also been encountered in those who live close to plants emitting vapors, dusts or smoke containing this metal. For reasons that are not clear, there is a striking individual susceptibility to berylliosis since less than 2 per cent of those exposed develop untoward reactions. The pneumoconiosis tends to be more frequent in those who have returned to their hazardous occupation after some period of absence. This observation, together with the finding that patients with berylliosis often have a positive skin test for this metal, raises the possibility that hypersensitization may play some role in the toxicity of this metal.

Finely divided metallic beryllium, beryllium oxide and its acid salts are all apparently capable of inducing toxic reactions. Depending on the solubility of the form of beryllium and its concentration in the inspired air, two forms of pneumoconiosis occur, acute and chronic berylliosis, the latter much more commonly.

Acute berylliosis is usually due to exposure to the soluble acid salts of beryllium. It is manifested by the sudden onset of cough, respiratory distress, fever and weakness. The ventilatory embarrassment may lead to death within weeks, but this is not common. The lungs in these patients are congested, edematous and heavy. The histologic reaction is essentially that of an acute chemical pneumonitis with congestion and neutrophilic infiltration of the septal walls and filling of the alveoli by fibrin, red cells and neutrophils, creating a virtually bronchopneumonic pattern. In the course of days, this alveolar exudate is largely replaced by macrophages and lymphocytes, sometimes still enmeshed in fibrin. The alveolar septa are widened by the edema and the interstitial leukocytic infiltrate. With progression, the intra-alveolar exudate organizes and, at the same time, septal fibrosis develops, accounting for a gas diffusion block, the usual precipitating cause of death. In those less severely affected, the acute pneumonitis may resolve and leave no residuals. **In acute berylliosis, granulomas are not formed** as they are in the chronic form of this disease.

Chronic berylliosis is better known as **beryllium granulomatosis** because it is characterized by the formation of focal granulomata which strongly resemble those of sarcoidosis and tuberculosis. These are distributed, often in vast numbers, in the interstitial tissue of the subpleura and septa and about blood vessels and bronchi. The beryllium granuloma may contain Langhans' type or foreign body type giant cells. Often these giant cells partially or completely enclose large (50 microns) basophilic lamellated calcific concretions known as Schaumann bodies or star-shaped acidophilic asteroids. These distinctive inclusions are more characteristic of sarcoidosis than berylliosis and can also be found in other diseases (Freiman and Hardy, 1970). Most of the granulomata are noncaseating and resemble "hard tubercles" but some may contain necrotic centers. In time, the fibrosing reaction in and about the granulomata leads to an interstitial widespread fibrosing chronic pneumonitis. The lungs are heavy, traversed by gray-white scars and contain areas of dense fibrosis with intervening areas of abnormally dilated emphysematous alveoli. The fibrosing reaction obliterates alveoli and traps small air-containing spaces which develop hyperplastic alveolar lining epithelium. The pleural surfaces are often thickened and fibrotic but usually not adherent to the chest wall. There is usually a fairly dense lymphocytic infiltrate about the granulomas as well as within the dense fibrous scars. Freiman and Hardy (1970) point out that cases with intense inflammatory infiltrates and well developed "sarcoid-like" granulomata tend to have a better prognosis. The tracheobronchial nodes share in the granulomatous and fibrotic reactions. While the constellation of the above findings is usually highly suggestive, in the absence of a well defined occupational exposure, it may be necessary to chemically identify the beryllium in the lung. Often, beryllium is also present in the urine, but this finding is so inconstant as to render a negative test unreliable. Unlike asbestosis, chronic berylliosis does not seem to predispose to lung cancer (Hardy, 1961).

Accompanying the chronic pulmonary lesions may be granulomatous involvement of the liver, kidney, spleen, lymph nodes and skin. Indeed, chronic persistent ulcerations of the skin may develop at sites of scratches or injuries where beryllium has been introduced.

Clinically, the granulomatosis is far more insidious than the acute pneumonitis. The time between exposure and appearance of symptoms ranges from weeks to decades. Often the exposure is quite brief, such as the inhalation of beryllium dust following the breakage of a single fluorescent lamp. Cough, dyspnea and respiratory distress slowly develop over the course of months to years. These manifestations are indistinguishable from those produced by other chronic lung diseases including the other forms of pneumoconiosis.

OTHER PNEUMOCONIOSES

As mentioned earlier, there are a great variety of pneumoconioses. Some are caused by organic and inorganic dusts. *Farmer's lung* is a form of pulmonary hypersensitivity to a variety of airborne plant antigens, as well as possibly spores and molds growing on stored grains, hay and wood. The onset of this condition is usually quite acute, within hours to days following a heavy exposure. The lesions take the form of an acute to chronic interstitial pneumonitis with alveolar exudate and occasionally granuloma formations (Seal et al., 1968). *Byssinosis* is a form of pneumoconiosis produced by the inhalation of airborne fibers of cotton, linen and hemp. Here the pulmonary changes are principally those of chronic bronchitis and emphysema. The clinical disorder has many features of asthma. Histamine liberators in the dust have been implicated in the causation of the respiratory difficulties and, indeed, many of the acute manifestations can be alleviated by antihistaminics (Nicholls et al., 1967). For details on the many other possible pneumoconioses, reference should be made to the excellent monograph by Spencer (1968).

CHEMICAL INJURIES

Chemical agents, including drugs, are responsible for a considerable number of deaths each year. In the United States in 1967, approximately 5000 suicides were committed with chemical agents. More tragic were the approximately 2000 accidental deaths which occurred, mostly in children, from the ingestion of drugs and chemicals, some seemingly as innocuous as aspirin. Any chemical or drug in sufficient quantity is capable of causing injury (Fig. 12–3). Even glucose and salt are injurious to cells in high concentrations, but some are highly toxic, such as the poisons. Table 12–1, derived from the Vital Statistics of the United States (1967), indicates the most commonly used methods of suicide. Alcohol is not included as a listed cause of poisoning in this table but is often so classified by medicolegal experts. Indeed, alcohol abuse generally accounts for as many deaths as all other chemical agents collectively.

In contrast to the agents used to commit

TABLE 12–1. CHEMICAL CAUSES OF SUICIDE, 1967—UNITED STATES*

Chemical Causes of Suicide	No. of Deaths	Total No. of Deaths
I. Suicide from poisoning by analgesic and soporific substances collectively		2689
By morphine and other opium derivatives	6	
By barbituric acid and derivatives	1694	
By salicylates	87	
By others	902	
II. Suicide from poisoning by other solid and liquid substances		656
By strychnine	42	
By phenol compounds	5	
By lye and potash	49	
By mercury and its compounds	8	
By arsenic and its compounds	46	
By fluorides	15	
By all other unspecified agents	491	
III. Suicide from poisoning by gases collectively		2202
By motor vehicle exhaust gas	2049	
By other motor exhaust gas	1	
By carbon monoxide	141	
By other poisonous gases	11	
IV. Suicide from poisoning by gases in domestic use		148

*Data derived from U.S. Vital Statistics, 1967, Vol. II. Mortality, Section 1.

suicide, deaths from accidental poisoning most commonly result when children or drunken adults take an overdose of some common drug. Leading the list as causes of fatal acci-

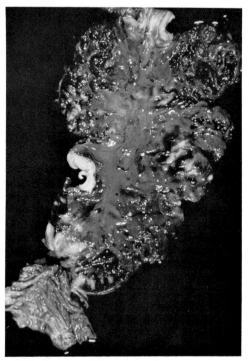

Figure 12–3. A large coagulum of blood and mucin is present on the surface of the stomach in a suicide accomplished by the ingestion of lye.

dental poisoning are barbituric acid and derivatives (approximately 20 per cent), other sedatives, analgesic and soporific drugs (approximately 18 per cent), aspirin and other salicylates (approximately 10 per cent), morphine and other opium derivatives (6 per cent), followed by a long list of agents such as corrosive acids and alkalis, lead, arsenic, household bleaches, detergents, ammonia, kerosene and virtually every other "forbidden" household product within reach of "little hands" (McCarthy, 1967).

Yet another category of fatal chemical injury is drug abuse, not limited to the narcotic addict only but too widely encountered, as is well known, among those searching for "kicks." Here a relatively small group of drugs are involved which have in common profound effects on the central nervous system. The subject of drug abuse is treated in a later section (p. 528).

GENERAL PRINCIPLES GOVERNING CHEMICAL INJURY

The injurious effect of a chemical (drug) upon the body is governed by three variables: (1) the vulnerability of individual tissues, (2) the mode of action of the product and (3) its pathways of absorption, metabolism and excretion—all of which affect the concentration in specific tissues.

Tissues and cells vary widely in their sus-

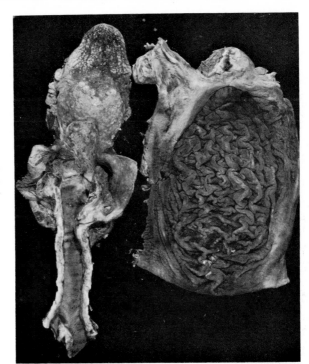

Figure 12–4. The action of swallowed sulfuric acid is demonstrated by the discoloration and corrosion of the anterior portion of the tongue and the intense discoloration of the gastric mucosa.

ceptibility to specific chemicals and drugs. In some instances, there are hints as to why there is such selectivity. Lead, for example, exerts its principal effect on the central nervous system, the hematopoietic system and the kidney. It impairs heme synthesis and also apparently acts as a poison of respiratory enzymes involved in electron transport, as will become clear in the following discussion (p. 524). The latter action might explain its central nervous system effect since ganglion cells are so totally reliant on aerobic respiration. However, why should the kidneys be more vulnerable to such respiratory damage than, for example, the mucosal cells lining the intestinal tract? Carbon tetrachloride, whose action was discussed on p. 28, affects principally the liver and kidneys. Yet its mode of action appears to be principally peroxidation of lipids affecting cellular membranes and particularly the rough endoplasmic reticulum with impairment of protein synthesis. Theoretically, then, CCl_4 should have widespread effects on all cells in the body, but such is not the case. The basis for selective injurious effect is thus often not clear.

Chemicals and drugs may act either locally or systemically after absorption. Corrosive agents such as strong acids and alkalis exert chiefly local effects, and poisonings with these agents are usually readily evident by the obvious signs of damage to the tongue, lips and oral cavity (Fig. 12–4). On the other hand, most agents act systemically only after absorp-

tion. Barbiturates create no local injury in the intestinal tract but act as depressants of the central nervous system. Carbon monoxide has only a trivial effect on the lungs when inhaled but acts as a systemic asphyxiant, blocking oxygen carriage by hemoglobin. A few agents, such as the phenols, have both local and systemic actions.

Little elaboration is required on the importance of the concentration of the drug or chemical. All exert their injurious effect only when their tolerated threshold level is exceeded and this level is highly specific for each agent. The levels achieved are a function of the amount taken in, its rate of metabolism, possible storage in the body and its rate of excretion. For example, lead is excreted extremely slowly, and so small doses may accumulate over the span of months. Barbiturate, on the other hand, is fairly rapidly metabolized and is not cumulative. Because the patterns of tissue damage are quite fixed for each agent, they provide important clues to the specific agent implicated.

NONTHERAPEUTIC AGENTS

ETHYL ALCOHOL

Many would object to the citation of ethyl alcohol as a poison but it is so categorized by many states. Without entering into this philosophic debate, all would agree that alcohol is a central nervous system depressant, that an overdose can be fatal and that alcoholism is often involved in fatal car accidents. In the U.S., for example, drunken drivers are responsible for more than 50 per cent of fatal car accidents. Its widespread use and abuse implicate it in more deaths in privileged societies than all other poisons and drugs together. Three clinical syndromes of alcoholism are identified: (1) drunkenness, (2) acute alcoholism and (3) chronic alcoholism. The last mentioned is not considered here since it involves many complex issues such as protein malnutrition, vitamin deficiency and enhanced susceptibility to bacterial infections which make it impossible to attribute the functional and organic derangements to mere chronic poisoning. Some of these issues are considered in the discussion of the cirrhosis associated with alcohol abuse (p. 1025).

The deleterious effects of drunkenness and acute alcoholism are dependent on blood alcohol levels and so its metabolism must be understood. Following ingestion, about 90 per cent of the alcohol is absorbed in the stomach and small intestines within one hour. About 5 per cent of the absorbed alcohol is excreted through the skin, lungs and kidneys. Approximately 95 per cent is catabolized in the liver into acetate, some of which enters the Kreb cycle and may be converted into carbohydrates and fat. The greatest part, however, is ultimately degraded to CO_2 and water. Two enzyme systems are involved in its catabolism. Liver cells possess a zinc-containing enzyme, hepatic alcohol dehydrogenase, which catalyzes the initial oxidation of ethanol to acetaldehyde. The activity of alcohol dehydrogenase is NAD dependent. Thereafter, the acetaldehyde is converted to acetyl coenzyme A, requiring the activity of an aldehyde dehydrogenase and adequate stores of NAD. The rate-limiting step in this pathway of ethanol metabolism appears to be the availability of hepatic NAD, not the levels of dehydrogenase (Mendelson, 1970). The second pathway of metabolism of alcohol involves the microsomal oxidase system, presumably identical with that involved in the metabolism of such drugs as barbiturates. This microsomal system, localized in the smooth endoplasmic reticulum of hepatic cells, is also NAD-NADPH dependent. It converts ethanol to acetaldehyde as does the dehydrogenase system.

The systemic effects of alcohol are most directly related to the blood levels developed which, in turn, depend on the quantity of alcohol ingested and its rate of metabolism. Later we shall see that another factor, tolerance, also modifies the effect of alcohol on the brain. To put the problem in perspective, blood alcohol levels of 100 to 150 mg. per 100 ml. of blood are considered intoxicating levels. The fatal threshold level of alcohol for some individuals is on the order of 500 + mg. per 100 ml. Fortunately, it is difficult to achieve such fatal levels, because stupor usually intervenes. It should be "sobering" to realize that in the fasting individual of average size, four or five 1-ounce drinks of beverage whiskey consumed in a short period of time on an empty stomach will induce a blood alcohol level of 100 + mg. per 100 ml. It is metabolized at the rate of about 15 mg. per 100 ml. per hour, but this rate is quite variable. Food in the gastrointestinal tract slows the rate of absorption which is also significantly modified by body size and perhaps by acquired tolerance.

Most controversial are the issues of whether there is considerable variation among individuals in the rate of metabolism of alcohol and whether prolonged use will lead to an increased rate of metabolism and hence tolerance. A number of studies have indicated that the rate of ethanol metabolism is only slightly greater in alcoholics than in nonalcoholics. Morphologic and biochemical evidence of *induction* of the microsomal oxidase system has been demonstrated in man by the repeated administration of alcohol to "normal" volunteers (Rubin and Lieber, 1971). While there is then some adaptive response to chronic exposure to this substance, it is nonetheless sharply limited in its capacity to handle large amounts (Mendelson, 1968). Indeed, sufficiently high blood alcohol levels will inhibit the metabolic enzyme systems and so produce a downward spiral. But the level of tolerance seen in alcoholics is greater than can be explained merely by an increased rate of metabolism. As Mendelson (1970) has said: "Although enhanced rates of ethanol metabolism have been demonstrated to occur in man after prolonged drinking, this enhanced metabolic rate cannot explain the considerable degree of tolerance for alcohol shown by alcoholics who may have very high blood ethanol levels and continue to perform cognitive and perceptual motor tasks reasonably well." Despite all efforts, the nature of this tolerance still evades us and has been vaguely attributed to adaptation of the central nervous system neurons to increased levels of ethanol (Newman, 1941) (Mello and Mendelson, 1970).

Alcohol acts as a central nervous system depressant or inhibitor; it affects first the cerebral cortex and then progressively the lower centers. The stimulation commonly ascribed to alcohol is due in reality to the depressant effect of this substance upon the cortical inhibitory controls. With sufficiently high blood levels, the vital centers in the medullary region are depressed and respiratory arrest may follow. The morphologic effects of acute alcoholism are quite insignificant and are confined to cerebral edema with congestion of the meningeal and superficial cortical vessels. The findings in the remainder of the body are inconstant and nonspecific (Wright, 1941).

Not considered here are the important social and psychologic problems of alcohol dependence and withdrawal manifestations since these are more properly the concern of the internist and psychiatrist. For further details on these concerns, reference might be made to the excellent review by Mendelson (1970).

METHYL ALCOHOL

Methyl alcohol may be absorbed either by the accidental or suicidal ingestion of the liquid alcohol or by the inhalation of alcoholic fumes in industry. Relatively trivial local injuries are produced at the sites of absorption. When ingested, methyl alcohol causes patchy edema and hemorrhages in the stomach. On inhalation, edema and hemorrhage occur into the lung tissues, chiefly in the subpleural regions. However, methyl alcohol exerts its prime toxic effect after absorption by its oxidation to formaldehyde and formic acid, both of which are more toxic than the parent substance. These derivative substances cause degeneration of the receptor cells of the retina with associated degeneration of the optic disc and nerve. A proposed mechanism for this selective toxicity is as follows. The eye is dependent upon a constantly available source of ATP for the synthesis of rhodopsin. It is now thought that the formaldehyde and formic acid derived from methyl alcohol inhibit retinal hexokinase, thus depressing glucose metabolism and the synthesis of ATP (Kaplan, 1962). While methanol and its derivatives once absorbed are widely distributed in the body, proportional to the water content of the various tissues, it is hypothesized that it exerts its principal effect on the retina due to the high water content of the eye (Keeney and Mellinkoff, 1951). Swelling of the brain and brain stem may also occur, accompanied by marked congestion of the cerebral vessels. Degenerative changes may develop in the cortical nerve cells with exposure to large doses if sufficient time elapses before death. The central nervous system and retinal damage accounts for the major clinical features of the poisoning—variable degrees of central nervous system depression to frank coma and visual impair-

ment—which sometimes eventuates in total blindness. Both the eye and brain changes are reversible, and recovery is possible with effective treatment and cessation of exposure.

CARBON MONOXIDE

Carbon monoxide is a nonirritating, inert gas, without color, taste or odor, produced by the imperfect oxidation of combustible carbon-containing material. It is probably responsible for a major proportion of all suicidal and accidental deaths. Inhalation of a 1 per cent concentration may prove fatal within 10 to 20 minutes, depending upon the degree of physical activity and the respiratory rate of the individual. Some concept of the apparent insignificance of this fatal level can be gained from the fact that ordinary illuminating gas contains approximately 16 per cent of carbon monoxide, while the exhaust from automobile motors contains approximately 7 per cent. Indeed, it has been estimated that the exhaust from an average car in a small closed garage could reach lethal levels within 5 minutes. Since the absorption of this agent may be cumulative, toxic effects depend upon the total exposure, i.e., the concentration in the inspired air and the duration of exposure. Levels of gas in the inspired air lower than 1 per cent may cause slowly developing, delayed damage and eventuate in death days after removal from further exposure.

Carbon monoxide acts as a system asphyxiant. Its affinity for hemoglobin is 200 to 300 times greater than that of oxygen. The formation of a relatively stable carboxyhemoglobin destroys the oxygen-carrying capacity of hemoglobin. Symptoms related to a systemic hypoxia begin to appear when the hemoglobin is 20 to 30 per cent saturated with carbon monoxide. When the hemoglobin is 60 to 70 per cent saturated, unconsciousness and death are likely. Lower levels may produce such mental confusion as to render the victim incapable of helping himself (Polson and Tattersall, 1969). Once carboxyhemoglobin is formed, the body rids itself of it only in the usual course of the breakdown of the affected red cells and their replacement by newly formed normal erythrocytes. The hypoxia most profoundly affects the central nervous system.

Acute Poisoning. In acute, fatal cases, the blood appears a bright cherry red and produces marked hyperemia of all the tissues. Striking hyperemia, edema and diffuse punctate hemorrhages throughout the cerebral hemispheres are frequent. Degeneration of the cortical and nuclear ganglion cells may be widespread or may take the form of patchy, asymmetrical lesions. The most common finding is symmetrical degeneration of the basal ganglia, particularly the lenticular nuclei (Dutra, 1952). Rarely, in the acute case, the muscle cells of the myocardium, the hepatic cells and the epithelial cells of the proximal convoluted tubules of the kidneys suffer from hypoxic fatty damage. Death usually ensues too rapidly in acute monoxide poisoning to permit the full development of these visceral lesions.

In fatal exposure, the brain lesions lead to the insidious onset of loss of consciousness, progressing into deep coma and death. When the exposure has not been too great and the tissue hypoxia not too profound, complete recovery is possible without residual defects. However, central nervous system residuals, such as impairment of memory, vision, hearing and speech, may remain in some of the recovered acute cases (Dalgaard, 1962).

Chronic Poisoning. Chronic poisoning may result from prolonged inhalation of relatively low levels of monoxide gas. This low-grade hypoxia insidiously gives rise to degenerative changes in the central nervous system that resemble those described in the acute form, but are less severe. Hypoxic degenerative fatty changes in the kidney, liver and heart are much more common in chronic intoxication than in acute. Clinically, in addition to the insidious onset of disturbances in brain function, these chronically exposed patients may suffer from renal, hepatic or cardiac failure that eventuates in death days or weeks after the last exposure. However, chronic poisoning is usually nonfatal, and complete recovery is the rule. It is to be emphasized that the tissue lesions of monoxide poisoning are not pathognomonic, but merely reflect nonspecific severe anoxemia.

PHENOL GROUP

The phenol group of organic corrosives includes phenol and cresol. *Both these compounds act as local corrosives and as systemic poisons.* These compounds may be absorbed through the skin, lungs or intestinal routes. When spilled upon the skin, they cause immediate necrosis of tissues and large chemical burns which ulcerate and become superficially infected. When these compounds are ingested either accidentally or with suicidal intent, immediate coagulation of the mucosa of the upper alimentary tract occurs, followed by sloughing necrosis. Through any pathway, these compounds may be absorbed systemically and cause central nervous system depression with vascular collapse associated with a dusky cyanosis. Necrosis of the renal and hepat-

ic cells may develop in the course of 24 to 48 hours. Chronic intoxications from the repeated absorption of small doses are extremely rare. The phenols are dangerous poisons, happily rarely encountered. Cases are on record, for example, of a nurse in an operating room spilling a bottle of carbolic acid on herself, being immediately treated, and yet absorbing a fatal dose of the phenol through the skin in a matter of minutes of exposure.

BENZENE (BENZOL)

Benzene is a coal and crude coal tar derivative which is highly volatile and is used as a solvent, particularly in the rubber and leather industries, as well as in the preparation of paints, paint removers, fabric cleaning compounds and cigarette lighter fluids. Poisoning may occur either from the inhalation of fumes in industry or from the accidental ingestion of the fluid. *Poisoning from benzene is a product of three factors: the degree of individual susceptibility, the duration of exposure and the concentration of fumes.* Individual susceptibility appears to be the most variable of these three influences. Identical exposure of two individuals may yield total resistance in one and sudden death in the other. The cause of this difference is believed to be due to the degree of activity of the detoxifying mechanism of the body. Benzene can be eliminated directly via the lungs; however, most benzene is converted to phenol and then sulfated. The level of enzymic activity of the sulfating mechanism in the liver is directly proportional to the degree of individual resistance. Toxicity depends on the absorption of amounts greater than can be excreted or metabolized with resultant accumulation of the toxic compound in the body.

Acute Poisoning. Death has been reported after the ingestion of 1 ounce of benzene or after the short-term inhalation of vaporous fumes in concentrations of approximately 20,000 parts per 1,000,000 of air. These acute cases are clinically manifest by flushing, cyanosis, dizziness, fever, convulsions and all degrees of agitation up to frank delirium. Death is usually preceded by a period of coma. At autopsy, such cases are characterized by irritative reactions in the respiratory passages, gastrointestinal tract and brain, i.e., excessive mucinous secretions within the trachea, bronchi and bronchioles; hemorrhages into the pulmonary tissue; excessive mucin secretion and hemorrhages into the mucosa of the stomach and intestines; and edema and congestion of the brain with subarachnoid hemorrhages.

Chronic Poisoning. Fumes in concentrations of approximately 100 to 200 parts per 1,000,000 of air have been known to cause damage. The *toxicity* in such cases appears insidiously and usually first *becomes manifest by marked abnormalities in the peripheral blood*, such as elevation or depression of the red and white cell counts and depression of the platelet counts (Deichman et al., 1963). The most sensitive indices of benzene toxicity in the blood are a slight eosinophilia, a decrease in the relative number of polymorphonuclear leukocytes, or the appearance of immature white or red cells in the peripheral blood (p. 776).

It is apparent from these very variable blood findings that no single hematologic pattern is evoked. Rarely, cases with marked elevations of the red cells (polycythemia) and the development of frank leukemia have been described. Morphologically, the bone marrow, spleen, liver and lymph nodes are primarily affected. The marrow may be of normal or increased cellularity, particularly in those cases manifesting polycythemia and leukemia, but most often it is of markedly decreased cellularity (hypocellular), sometimes to the extreme of almost acellularity (Mallory et al., 1939). The spleen may be normal in size, but is sometimes enlarged up to weights of over 1000 gm. Foci of hematopoiesis are usually present in the spleen and vary in prominence, depending upon the degree of marrow destruction. Cases with severe marrow hypofunction usually manifest the most marked degrees of splenic hematopoiesis. Phagocytosis of partially destroyed red cells in the endothelial cells of the splenic sinuses and hemosiderin deposits may also reflect the abnormal destruction of red cells caused by this agent. In more severe cases, the liver may show central necrosis and, in the majority of instances, contains foci of erythropoiesis similar to those described in the spleen. The lymph nodes are usually not markedly enlarged, but may demonstrate hematopoietic foci in severe cases.

Consequent to the marked abnormalities in blood formation, these patients usually develop many forms of bacterial infection, particularly bronchopneumonia, which is the usual precipitating cause of death. Rare patients may die of bleeding tendencies induced by the thrombocytopenia or from widespread leukemic infiltrations.

KEROSENE

Kerosene is one of the most frequent forms of accidental poisoning in children. It is usually encountered in children living in rural areas and among lower income groups where homes are heated by kerosene stoves. The victims generally range in age from one to six years. Presumably they mistake the colorless liquid for water or they are enticed into tasting the pink or blue fluid created by the introduction of dyes into the kerosene. Although ingested, the major clinical manifestations of this poisoning result from inhalation of the agent with the induction of a fulminant bronchopneumonic process having the characteristics of a lipid pneumonia (p. 826). Kerosene is also a narcotic and produces drowsiness and somnolence so that the onward progression of the respiratory symptoms in the sleeping unobserved child may pass unnoticed until too late.

CHLORINATED HYDROCARBONS

Chloroform and particularly carbon tetrachloride have become increasingly important causes of accidental and intentional poisoning. These products are often used both in the home and in industry as components of cleaning fluids and degreasing agents. There is marked individual susceptibility to both agents, so that similar levels of exposure may produce widely differing injuries. Alcoholism appears to heighten individual vulnerability. Chloroform and carbon tetrachloride both induce central necrosis of the liver but, in addition, carbon tetrachloride also causes intensive renal tubular necrosis, principally of the distal convoluted and collecting tubules, sometimes also involving the proximal convoluted tubules. In both organs, the early cytologic changes consist of fatty change of affected cells, soon followed by coagulative necrosis. The pathogenesis of these cell injuries was discussed earlier on p. 28. When the poisoning is severe, the entire lobule and virtually the total liver are destroyed. If the patient survives, many of these changes are completely reversible and adequate liver function may be restored.

With carbon tetrachloride, the renal tubular changes may be sufficiently severe to produce signs of renal insufficiency, occasioned by necrosis and sloughing of the epithelial cells into the tubular lumina. Granular casts, red cell casts and hemoglobin casts are often found within these tubules. Here again, if the damage is not too extensive, epithelial regeneration may virtually restore normal structure and function. Quite recently, the clinical diagnosis of these intoxications has been made easier by the demonstration that it is possible to identify these solvents in the breath long after exposure (Stewart et al., 1965).

CYANIDE

Cyanide is a highly toxic respiratory poison lethal to man in amounts less than 0.1 gm. It was once the favorite of those bent on suicide and homicide, but has now been displaced by carbon monoxide and barbiturates which offer "more pleasant" ways of dying. Poisoning may result from the inhalation of hydrocyanic gas or from the ingestion of compounds of cyanide, usually potassium cyanide. These substances are rapidly absorbed and may cause death within minutes. Once absorbed, all cyanide compounds are rapidly converted in the body to *hydrogen cyanide, which has an extreme toxicity for cytochrome oxidase.* However, the poison is not cumulative and is detoxified in the body to thiocyanate. Injurious levels depend, therefore, on rates of absorption and detoxification. Cyanide poisoning causes tissue anoxia at the *intracellular level.*

Acute Poisoning. Acute fatal poisonings are characterized by petechiae in the skin, mucous membranes and serosal membranes of the body (Gettler and St. George, 1934). It is not clear whether these petechial lesions result from generalized vascular injury alone or from the combination of systemic hypoxia and the severe convulsive seizures which accompany the poisoning. All the tissues of the body characteristically exude a pungent, bitter, almond-like odor. When the poison is taken orally, edema, hemorrhage and necrosis of the gastric mucosa may result. In acute poisonings, the brain may show minimal to slight edema with petechial hemorrhages. Because poisoned cells cannot use oxygen, the blood is fully oxygenated, imparting to it and the tissues a cherry red color reminiscent of carbon monoxide poisoning. The symptoms of acute cyanide poisoning are rarely observed, since death usually ensues within 10 minutes. It is said to be preceded characteristically by severe clonic convulsive seizures.

Chronic Poisoning. Cyanide poisoning may occur from chronic, prolonged absorption of small amounts of poison over the course of days to weeks. The tissue hypoxia under these circumstances is progressive but not immediately fatal. Slowly developing changes affect the brain, liver and kidneys. Grossly, the brain may be entirely normal but, on microscopic section, degeneration of ganglion cells is usually evident, sometimes to the point at which these cells become totally necrotic and disappear and are said to have dropped out. Hypoxic fatty change of the renal convoluted tubular epithelial cells and centrilobular fatty change of the liver may also be identified.

Clinically, progressive disturbance of cerebral function in the chronic form leads to the development of unconsciousness and frank coma. When the patient survives for a sufficient time, symptoms of impaired liver and renal function may become manifest.

MERCURY

Mercury poisoning, its major manifestations and once common occupational setting have been hallowed by Lewis Carroll in his enduring phrase, "mad as a hatter." This metal was once used in the silvering of mirrors and the production of felt hats, and workers often developed toxic mental changes, called madness. Mercuric chloride was also once a favored agent among suicides. It is still used in industry in photo engraving and tool hardening. Certain insecticides and fungicides contain mercury, creating household hazards. Today mercury poisoning is rare but merits brief consideration because of the recent flurry of excitement occasioned by the finding of mercury contamination in tinned tuna fish. The background of this concern relates to an outbreak of mercury poisoning in Japan about 10 years ago traced back to the fish diet of the victims. As a consequence, all Japanese canned fish became suspect, principally tuna which was indeed found to contain small amounts of mercury. Subsequently, it was determined that a factory had heavily contaminated a fairly localized body of coastal water where most of those poisoned had obtained their daily sustenance. However, mercury was once used in antifouling paints on ships, and extremely small amounts are present in waters throughout the world. Thus the Japanese tragedy called attention to a global problem. At the present time, the minute quantities encountered in fish are not considered significant because, in small doses, mercury does not accumulate in the body. It is excreted through the kidneys, colon, bile, sweat and saliva. However, significant daily increments could lead to the buildup of toxic levels.

Mercury compounds are protein precipitants and are thus capable of inactivating enzymes, particularly the cytochrome oxidases involved in cellular respiration. In addition, mercury may complex with sulfhydryl and phosphoryl groups and so damage cellular membranes. Mercuric compounds are more toxic than mercurous. Toxicity may result from the inhalation of mercury vapors or the absorption of inorganic or organic compounds through the skin or intestinal tract. There is much current controversy over the issue of whether poisoning from inorganic compounds produces a disease different from that caused by organic compounds (Bidstrup, 1964). *Organic mercury poisoning* has been said to be a more serious disease developing suddenly, causing ataxia, dysarthria and constricted visual fields. *Inorganic compounds* more often produce slowly developing chronic disease, characterized by dermatitis, gingivitis, loosening of the teeth, stomatitis, gastroenteritis, renal tubular damage, neurologic changes including tremor, deafness, aphasia and often the personality changes so characteristic of "Alice's hatter" (loss of memory, loss of attention span and emotional instability). Others deny that inorganic and organic mercury poisoning produce distinctive syndromes and contend that there is much overlap (Kark et al., 1971).

The anatomic changes of *chronic mercury poisoning* are found in those sites exposed to the highest concentration of this metal, i.e. the oral cavity, stomach, kidneys and colon (Troen et al., 1951). In the oral cavity, mercury is eliminated through the salivary glands and causes excessive salivation. It deposits on the gingival margins to produce a gingivitis and gingival discoloration closely resembling the "lead line." Loosening of the teeth results. When ingested, the compounds may cause focal to massive confluent necrosis of the gastric epithelium (the point of entry). Excreted through the urine, it produces damage to the proximal convoluted tubular cells (pathway of excretion) manifested by disruption of the endoplasmic reticulum, mitochondrial swelling, plasma membrane breaks and the appearance of eosinophilic droplets within the cytoplasm. Almost invariably, some cells are killed and undergo necrosis (Gritzka and Trump, 1968).

The eosinophilic droplets are attributable to the heavy proteinuria with resorption of the protein by the tubular epithelial cells (Oliver et al., 1954) (Fig. 12–5). The proteinuria may be sufficiently heavy to induce the nephrotic syndrome (p. 1107). Although the glomeruli may appear undamaged, basement membrane thickening may be seen with the electron microscope and this injury undoubtedly induces the heavy proteinuria. Calcifications in injured cells may appear within days of the tubular injury. The colonic mucosa may exhibit focal necroses and ulcerations resembling those described in the stomach (an additional pathway of excretion). Despite the neurologic changes in chronic mercury poisoning, there are no reports available on the pathologic findings in the brain.

In *acute mercury poisoning*, the morphologic changes may include those described for the chronic form of this disease but, more often, they are confined to the brain. These include scattered foci of atrophy throughout the cerebral cortex, atrophy of the occipital lobes producing enlargement of the occipital horns of the lateral ventricles, atrophy of the cerebellar folia, as well as other changes (Takeuchi et al., 1962).

Before closing this discussion of mercury, it is comforting to know that metallic mercury such as is commonly used in clinical thermometers is without hazard. Indeed, the liquid metal was once used in the treatment of obstinate constipation where its specific gravity and the laws of gravity combined to create a potent therapeutic modality.

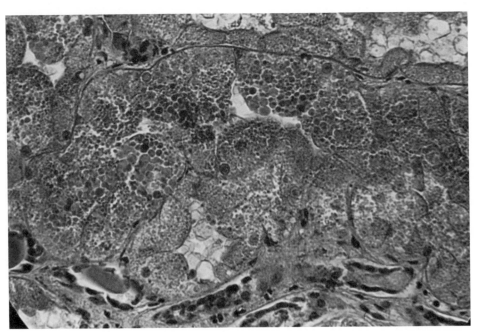

Figure 12–5. *Coagulative necrosis of the epithelial cells in the proximal convoluted tubules following suicide by the ingestion of mercury. The large eosinophilic droplets of resorbed protein are evident.*

LEAD

Lead poisoning (plumbism) is a prime example of a current environmental disease. Most cases of plumbism result from the progressive absorption and storage of small amounts of lead until toxic levels eventually accumulate in the body. Sometimes the exposure is massive and the poisoning develops suddenly. Two forms of plumbism are thus encountered—an acute as well as a chronic disorder. The acute form usually follows ingestion of lead salts with suicidal intent or industrial heavy exposure to lead vapors or organic forms of lead, and spray painting with lead-based paints (Campbell and Williams, 1968). The chronic form of the disease is most often encountered in children who chew on furniture covered with a lead-base paint. Chronic poisoning may also follow lead-battery burning, the use of improperly fired ceramic mugs lined with a lead-containing glaze, contaminated drinking water particularly in old homes having lead pipes, and the copious consumption of moonshine prepared in lead-containing stills. The problem of chronic exposure is compounded by the lead vapors resulting from the combustion of gasoline containing antiknock additives such as tetraethyl lead. These exhausts contaminate not only the air but eventually also the soil and thus water supplies and foods. As mentioned earlier, it is estimated that 200,000 tons of lead are added to the environment annually in North America by motor exhaust. As a consequence of this almost ubiquitous contamination, the average adult harbors about 150 to 400 mg. of body lead and has blood levels which average 25 microgm. per 100 ml. (Goyer, 1971). Levels of only 80 microgm. per 100 ml. in the blood may be productive of clinical symptoms.

Many variables in the absorption, storage and excretion of lead modify the blood levels and therefore the toxicity and acuteness of the poisoning. Lead absorbed from the gastrointestinal tract passes to the liver and is excreted back into the duodenum through the bile. Some is reabsorbed but some is excreted in the feces. When absorbed from the respiratory tract, it rapidly enters the circulation where it produces its full effect. After absorption, some is excreted from the blood through the kidneys at a fairly slow rate which may be adequate to prevent toxic effects if the rate of absorption is low. At the same time, the lead in the blood is carried to the bones where much is stored and is thus also removed from the blood. Obviously, the ultimate blood level achieved depends on the rate of absorption counterbalanced by the rates of storage and excretion.

Lead intoxication produces changes principally in three organ systems: the hematopoietic system, the central nervous system and the kidneys. Both acute and chronic lead poisoning induce an anemia. The anemia results from inadequate hemoglobin synthesis as well as abnormal hemolysis of red cells. The former effect has been localized to impairment in an early step in heme synthesis involving the enzyme delta-amino levulinic acid (ALA) dehydratase. Patients with lead poisoning excrete large amounts of the delta-ALA, and elevated levels of this metabolite in the urine may be the first clue to a developing chronic lead poisoning. The basis for the abnormal hemolysis is less clear. It has been proposed that lead salts coat red cells and render their membranous envelopes liable to rupture. *Characteristic of lead poisoning is stippling of red cells* (a coarse basophilic granulation best demonstrated by modifications of the methylene blue stain). It should be emphasized that stippling is not diagnostic of lead poisoning since it may be encountered under other circumstances. However, until proved otherwise, it should imply plumbism.

In the central nervous system, both the brain and peripheral nerves are affected. Lead encephalopathy is most prominent in acute poisonings but may also occur in chronic intoxication. Widespread degeneration of the cortical and ganglionic neurons is accompanied by diffuse edema of the gray and white matter (Fig. 12–6). Involvement of the brain is usually manifested by ataxia, convulsions or a reduced level of consciousness. The peripheral nerves most

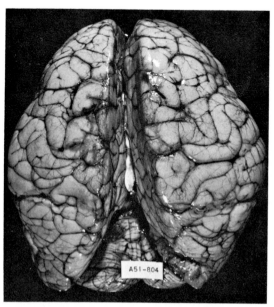

Figure 12–6. *Cerebral edema in lead poisoning. The gyri are flattened and widened and the sulci are narrowed and relatively inapparent.*

often injured are the motor nerves supplying the most actively used muscles of the body. The morphologic change takes the form of myelin degeneration of the axis cylinders. Thus the extensor muscles of the wrist and fingers are ordinarily the first and most severely involved, producing the characteristic "wrist and finger drop." Paralysis of the peroneal muscles of the leg may cause "foot drop."

The renal lesions generally cause less obvious manifestations than those resulting from involvement of the blood and central nervous system. However, patients with lead poisoning may have proximal tubular dysfunction manifested by aminoaciduria, glycosuria and hyperphosphaturia comprising the Fanconi syndrome. The basis for these tubular dysfunctions is not entirely clear but it has been shown in the experimental animal that lead salts damage mitochondrial respiration, possibly because lead inhibits a dehydrogenase essential to pyruvic acid metabolism and electron transport (Goyer and Krall, 1969). Why this action should be selective for the renal tubular cells and not affect other cells is obscure. A characteristic finding in chronic plumbism is the development of intranuclear acid-fast inclusions within the proximal renal tubular lining cells and hepatocytes. It has been speculated that these inclusions may result from resorption of lead from the blood or urine which is then bound to protein to produce the inclusion body, thus in effect removing lead from the circulation. Whatever their interpretation, the identification of such inclusions is a useful morphologic hallmark of lead poisoning.

Other alterations may be encountered in chronic plumbism. The local formation and precipitation of lead sulfide upon the gingival mucosa creates the so-called "*lead line.*" This pigmentation is closely simulated by mercury and bismuth poisoning as well as by inflammatory discoloration of the gingival tissue in chronic gingivitis. Patients with chronic lead poisoning often have crises of severe abdominal colic of uncertain etiology. The deposit of lead in the epiphyseal ends of the bones in children produces characteristic radiodensities (Fig. 12–7). These sites of deposit presumably reflect the more intense vascularization of these growing ends of bone with consequent greater transfer of lead from the blood.

In some large part, lead poisoning is a preventable disease, especially that encountered in children. Laws prohibiting the use of lead paint and lead in gasoline would go a long way toward controlling this "silent epidemic" (Rothschild, 1970).

ARSENIC

Arsenic poisoning, once a favorite pastime of the Borgias, is today happily uncommon. The various arsenical salts, oxides and arsene gas are all highly dangerous. Arsenicals are used in fruit sprays, weed killers, insecticides, rat poisons and, indeed, in a number of industrial processes. Acute poisonings, usually suicidal or homicidal, are rarely encountered, but chronic poisonings by long exposure to arsenical dusts, arsene gas in industry, or to foods bearing a coating of arsenic-containing plant sprays still account for occasional deaths. The mode of action of arsenic in causing cellular injury is still obscure. It is, however, known that arsenic binds with sulfhydryl (SH) groups. Hence in chronic poisoning, the hair, nails and surface squames of the skin accumulate detectable amounts. It is likely, therefore, that arsenic may inactivate other SH-containing enzymes and so constitute an inhibitor of respiratory enzymes. The resultant clinical syndromes take one of three forms: fulminating poisoning, acute poisoning and chronic poisoning, obviously depending on the dose-rate absorbed modified by its elimination in the urine and feces.

Fulminating Poisoning. Massive doses of arsenic are rapidly absorbed and kill within an hour or two. The patients usually die in profound shock, seemingly triggered by peripheral vasodilatation and extreme reduction in the effective circulating blood volume. Arsenic,

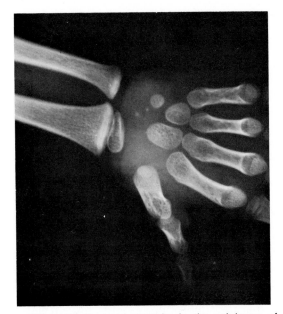

Figure 12–7. *Lead deposits in the epiphyses of the wrist have caused a marked increase in their radiodensity so that they are as radiopaque as the cortical bone.*

however, may also act as a depressant on the central nervous system and hence paralyze vasomotor control.

Acute Poisoning. The morphologic changes and clinical signs and symptoms depend upon the duration of survival. With the ingestion of large doses, death may ensue within 24 hours unaccompanied by any striking morphologic lesions. Death appears to be due to the depressant effect of the compound upon the central nervous system. With less severe poisonings, *the major anatomic changes are found after the first day in the vascular system, brain, gastrointestinal tract and skin.* Generalized visceral hyperemia develops with petechial hemorrhages in the serous membranes and skin; the latter changes are caused by necrotizing damage to capillary walls. With survival for 2 or 3 days, intestinal lesions are encountered chiefly in the stomach in the form of congestion and edema, replaced soon with petechial hemorrhages and foci of dark red-black coagulation necrosis. Sloughing of these necrotic areas produces ulcerations that may be dispersed or may coalesce to form large, denuded, raw surfaces. Similar lesions may become evident in the remainder of the intestinal tract. Lesions may also appear in the brain in the course of 2 to 3 days. These take the form of widespread petechial hemorrhages, apparently due to necrosis of the capillary walls, together with marked diffuse cerebral edema. Thromboses may occur in these injured vessels and give rise to focal areas of infarction within the brain substance. When patients with high toxic doses survive 4 to 5 days, fatty changes in the parenchymal cells of the kidneys and liver may occur, accompanied sometimes by fatty change of the myocardium.

The clinical signs and symptoms of arsenic poisoning depend largely upon the size of the ingested dose and the duration of the survival of the victim. In its most violent form, there is the rapid onset of vascular collapse and central nervous system depression, followed by coma and death within hours. In less acute forms, the presenting signs and symptoms may be marked vomiting followed by severe, persistent, watery diarrhea. Central nervous system depression and vascular collapse may follow. The petechial hemorrhages become evident in the skin at this time. The anatomic changes in the kidneys and liver rarely create prominent clinical problems, although in certain patients damage to the heart may produce late-developing cardiac decompensation.

Chronic Poisoning. The major changes involve the gastrointestinal tract, nervous system and skin. These alterations resemble somewhat those of the acute form but are less severe in degree. Vascular lesions and petechial hemorrhages are not prominent. In the intestinal tract, congestion, edema and small superficial ulcerations may develop in the stomach and small intestine. The changes in the nervous system appear to be most prominent in the peripheral nerves, with myelin degeneration and destruction of axis cylinders. Brain lesions are uncommon. Focal or large confluent areas of dark brown-black pigmentation occur in those skin areas which are normally most deeply pigmented. The palms of the hands and soles of the feet develop thickening of the keratin layer of the skin. In the chronically exposed, such as the arsenic eaters of India and Syria, these skin lesions have progressed occasionally to the formation of frank epithelial carcinomas (Cannon, 1936). The kidneys and liver may also suffer damage similar to that encountered in acute intoxication.

The clinical characteristics of chronic poisoning differ from those in the acute form. At the onset, generalized weakness and malaise appear insidiously, followed by muscular weakness of the hands and feet. Some cases develop frank paralysis and anesthesia in areas of neural involvement. Rather commonly, severe, persistent diarrhea reflects the intestinal pathology. Frequently, the diagnosis is first suspected by the characteristic pigmentary changes in the skin. When the source of intoxication is discovered and further exposure stopped, complete recovery is the rule with appropriate therapy.

THERAPEUTIC AGENTS

SALICYLATES

The most common cause of accidental poisoning in children results from their gaining access to methyl salicylate (oil of Wintergreen) or aspirin. The fatal dose of these agents is very variable, but fatalities have been reported in infants with the ingestion, at one time, of 2 to 4 gm. of aspirin. Methyl salicylate is even more toxic, and as little as 5 ml. may be fatal in the infant. Fifteen grams of aspirin in one dose is fatal for adults. High blood levels of salicylate act as a stimulant to the respiratory center. Characteristic, then, of the victim is a striking increase in the rate of breathing (hyperpnea). As a consequence, carbon dioxide is blown off through the lungs and the pH of the plasma rises to produce a respiratory alkalosis. Thereafter, a chain of metabolic adjustments ensues such as an increased urine output with excretion of bicarbonate, a shift of potassium into cells causing hypokalemia and an increased metabolism of fats which may lead to a ketosis and, in time, to a metabolic acidosis. The syndrome is further complicated by the almost invariable concurrence of severe vomiting (related to the aspirin-induced gastritis) with its additional losses of fluid and electrolytes. Fatalities, when they occur, are probably related to the serious losses of water and shifts in electrolytes, the most threatening of which is the falling level of blood potassium.

Morphologically, salicylism induces only a few changes. Hemorrhagic ulcerative gastroenteritis is the most prominent finding. In addition, salicylates inhibit platelet aggregation and may therefore block the homeostatic role of platelets in maintaining the integrity of the vascular endothelium. As a consequence, petechiae sometimes appear in the skin but are more prominent in the serosal surfaces and meninges.

Because the salicylates are strong irritants of the gastric mucosa, the victim is often spared by the prompt vomiting which follows overdosage. When seen early, most of these children can be saved by gastric lavage, hemodialysis and effective control of the blood pH and serum electrolytes.

PHENACETIN

Phenacetin is a widely used and abused analgesic implicated in the causation of chronic interstitial nephritis, a potentially fatal renal disease. It is available throughout the world in a number of proprietary preparations which generally also contain one or more of the following drugs: aspirin, caffeine, aminopyrine and phenazones. Because of these shotgun mixtures, it has been difficult to determine which of the components is responsible for the renal changes but some believe that the clinical evidence strongly points to phenacetin as the common denominator (Bell, 1969). Virtually all reported cases of analgesic nephropathy occur in patients who have taken phenacetin compounds over the span of many months to years, sometimes to total amounts over 50 kilos. Such abuse is particularly frequent in Europe, principally in the Scandinavian countries, where phenacetin-containing preparations have been in vogue for headaches and all manner of mild aches and pains.

The clinical consequences of phenacetin abuse include, in addition to the renal disease, anemia and gastrointestinal lesions. The chronic interstitial nephritis closely resembles the chronic pyelonephritis of diabetics, complete with renal papillary necrosis (p. 270).

The genesis of the papillary necrosis is poorly understood but there is some suspicion that a metabolite of phenacetin, N-acetyl-p-aminophenol, is concentrated in the renal papillae and may here induce cellular necrosis through pathways still not understood (Bleumle and Goldberg, 1968). Anemia is found in approximately 80 per cent of patients having a history of chronic phenacetin ingestion. The anemia is in part hemolytic but may also result from impaired synthesis of hemoglobin since methemoglobin and sulfhemoglobin are sometimes found in the red cells of these patients. The gastric lesions closely resemble the hemorrhagic ulcerative gastritis induced by the salicylates and may indeed be related to the almost invariable presence of aspirin in the phenacetin preparations. In this connection, it should be pointed out that analgesic nephropathy has also been attributed to aspirin abuse alone and the precise cause of the renal disease remains in dispute (Murray et al., 1971) (p. 1125).

BARBITURATES

An overdose of barbiturates has long been in vogue as a method of suicide. Accidental poisoning is also encountered, particularly in children and in adults who unknowingly take excessive amounts of these drugs. There is a wide range of individual susceptibility to barbiturates, and relatively small amounts may induce dangerous blood levels in some. Furthermore, alcohol and the barbiturates produce additive depressant effects on the central nervous system, and so the combination is dangerous. Both agents are metabolized in the liver cell by microsomal enzyme systems and, while the body will adapt to the continued exposure to barbiturates and to some extent to alcohol, the latter, in sufficient amounts, may damage the liver cell and render it unable to metabolize barbiturates. Similarly, any liver disease impairs the metabolism of barbiturate and permits it to reach toxic levels in the blood even after relatively moderate doses. And finally, there is the controversial issue of "barbiturate automatism." This refers to patients who have been taking barbiturates on a regular schedule and forget their having had a recent dose, and so take additional medication until they build up toxic levels. Many deny the existence of automatism and imply that such actions are volitional.

It is difficult to set a specific lethal threshold for the barbiturates because of the many factors which influence their pharmacodynamics. The short-acting barbiturates, such as seconal, are in general more toxic than the long-acting, such as phenobarbital. Even in the absence of the predisposing influences mentioned above, as little as 3 gm. of the short-acting barbiturates or 5 gm. of the long-acting agents may be potentially fatal in the normal adult. Contrariwise, recovery of an attempted suicide has been reported after an overdose as large as 30 gm. of phenobarbital.

The barbiturates act principally on the central nervous system and at first cause depression of the cortical ganglion cells. At higher drug levels, the basal ganglia and medulla are affected, resulting in paralysis of the vital control centers, particularly those involving respiration. The systemic hypoxia in turn may cause vasomotor collapse and shock. The depressed respiration and vasomotor changes predispose to bronchopneumonia which often comprises the final blow. In addition, skin and blood vessel lesions may also develop in these patients, perhaps as a consequence of the development of hypersensitization to the drug. The commonest form of skin lesions are large bullous vesicles seen in 5 to 10 per cent of the patients. These are so typical of this drug as to be referred to as "barbiturate blisters." In some patients, these bullous lesions are generalized, creating the pattern known as exfoliative dermatitis (p. 1388). In other instances, the skin changes take the form of an itching maculopapular rash—so-called dermatitis medicamentosa (p. 1385). Occasionally, widespread hypersensitivity angiitis develops, closely resembling polyarteritis nodosa (p. 236). Other more inconstant anatomic changes are sometimes encountered, including hypoxic injury to the kidney tubular epithelium. Despite its depressant action on the brain, in many cases the neuronal changes are exceedingly scanty or take the form of nonspecific hypoxic injury; and so, even in fatal cases, the diagnosis of this form of poisoning rests largely upon chemical identification of the drug in body fluids and tissues (Baker, 1960).

DRUG ABUSE

Any of the now more than 10,000 drug products available on the market has the potential of being harmful, but here we are concerned with the small group of dangerous drugs now all too commonly abused which have a profound effect on the central nervous system. These can be divided into depressants (principally heroin and the barbiturates), stimulants (principally cocaine and the amphetamines), and hallucinogens (principally mescaline, lysergic acid diethylamide—LSD, and marihuana) (Froede, 1972). Despite the widespread legal and illegal use of these agents, there is a surprising paucity of "hard, clean" data on their effects on tissues and organs as distinct from their possible psychologic and social implications. Most of the available information relates to the "hard" drugs, principally heroin and LSD, and there is virtually none at the present time on the untoward anatomic effects of marihuana (if any).

The problem of establishing the consequences of a given agent has been enormously complex. Most addicts take or have taken a variety of drugs. Weird and exotic mixtures and combinations of drugs are "shot," sniffed and swallowed in the search for a new experience. Many cutting agents, such as talc and quinine, are blended with heroin, for example, and these introduce their own hazards. The very frequent contamination of the injectate with cotton fibers, bacteria and heaven knows what else adds new dimensions to the injury-producing potential of drug addiction. Nonetheless, improved toxicologic methods which permit the determination of the blood levels of specific drugs such as heroin have made it possible to connect certain tissue changes with specific agents. A well defined pathology of drug abuse has emerged.

Drug abuse is the leading cause of death in New York City in the age range of 15 to 35 years. Although the specific number of deaths directly attributable to drug abuse is somewhat uncertain, data derived from the medical examiner's office in New York City give some idea of the growing menace of addiction. Between 1918 and 1939, drugs were responsible for approximately 50 deaths per year. In 1960, the annual number of deaths climbed to 199 and five years later, to 306. But in 1969, drug abuse deaths had skyrocketed to 1016 (Baden, 1971). Before the "older generation" assumes too shocked an attitude toward these doleful numbers, the problem should be set in perspective by noting that alcohol alone, and its attendant car accidents, is probably responsible for twice as many deaths as all of the dangerous drugs together. Compilations of mortality data are somehow remote. In more personal terms, the data available indicate that narcotic addicts have roughly a one out of 200 (or 0.5 per cent) chance of dying during a given year merely as a result of being an addict. Approximately two-thirds of these deaths are caused by direct drug toxicity. The remaining one-third are attributable to homicide, suicide and accidents related to the use of drugs. But even this tragic mortality tells not the whole story, for drug addiction also results in a very significant morbidity.

The pathogenesis of drug-related lesions involves four distinctive mechanisms: (1) the direct toxic action of the agent, (2) the effect of possible contaminants, (3) hypersensitivity reactions to the drug and its contaminants and (4) diseases contracted in the course of the use of drugs. By considering each of these mechanisms, the major pathology of drug abuse can be reasonably well covered.

The direct toxicity of heroin has been well established (Louria et al., 1967). Chronic users of this agent have been found to have quite distinctive changes in their lungs and liver, considered to be directly attributable to the drug. Alterations in the central nervous system are observed which are probably related to the hypoxia caused by the pulmonary changes. The pulmonary lesions are believed by Siegel (1972) to be sufficiently distinctive to merit being called "narcotic lung." In fatalities caused by heroin, marked but patchy pulmonary congestion and edema have been found, made distinctive by focal atelectasis, emphysema, hemorrhages, aspiration of gastric juices and mononuclear cell accumulations within the alveoli and alveolar walls (Fig. 12–8). In those who have died 12 to 24 hours after the onset of their pulmonary pathology, fibrinous and neutrophilic exudates are often found in the alveoli representing the development of a bronchopneumonic process. The anatomic evidence that heroin produces striking and

sometimes fatal changes in the lungs seems well established.

Diffuse necrotizing angiitis, virtually indistinguishable from polyarteritis nodosa, has also been attributed by Citron et al. (1970) to direct drug toxicity. They suggest that the lesions are not of hypersensitivity origin and implicate either amphetamines or LSD. The possibility that marihuana may induce similar vascular lesions has also been raised (Nabas, 1971).

Another instance of toxic effect, admittedly far more controversial, concerns the possible mutagenic effect of LSD. The literature on this subject is quite vehement in support of and in denial of an association between the chronic use of this agent and the development of chromosomal abnormalities. This subject is discussed more fully on p. 176.

Contaminants and agents used to "cut" the strength of some drugs may themselves be productive of disease. Many of the addictive drugs, such as morphine, heroin and methadone, are mixed with a variety of filler materials, the most common being magnesium silicate (talc), quinine and cornstarch (Fig. 12–9A and B). In other instances, after dissolving tablets such as morphine or heroin in water, the addict filters it through a cotton pledge and thereby fills the filtrate with small cotton fibers. "Mainlining" these concoctions (intravascular injection) introduces all manner of particulate material into the blood which lodges in the microcirculation and evokes foreign body granulomata. As might be anticipated, the lungs are the major filters and so often develop a diffuse granulomatosis. Talc is the worst offender and can often be identified within foreign body giant cells in granulomata as doubly refractile crystalline bodies (Hopkins and Taylor, 1970). Similar granulomata may be found in perivascular locations in the liver, spleen and lymph nodes (Fig. 12–10). Even widely scattered granulomata in most instances are probably not productive of either morbidity or mortality. Rarely, however, widespread granulomatosis has been implicated as a cause of altered pulmonary function, secondary cor pulmonale and even death (Karliner et al., 1969) (Bainborough and Jericho, 1970).

Hypersensitivity reactions to drugs are thought to be the cause of some of the lesions encountered in addicts. In heroin addicts, the liver is sometimes enlarged (up to 2000 gm.) and grossly congested. The gallbladder may be distended and tensely filled with a thick mucoid bile. But perhaps most distinctive is a striking enlargement of the portahepatic and peripancreatic lymph nodes which may achieve a tenfold increase in size. This curious

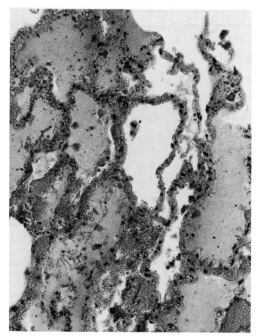

Figure 12–8. *The lung of a heroin addict with patchy edema and atelectasis. Many of the alveolar spaces are filled with a proteinous fluid.*

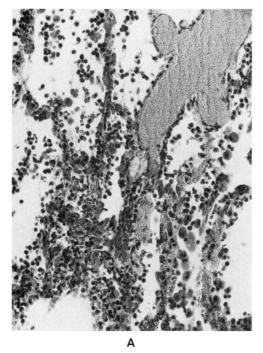
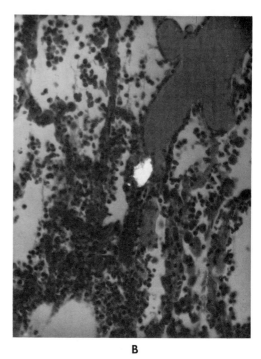

A   B

Figure 12–9. The lung of a heroin addict. The alveoli contain many desquamated mononuclear cells. A large congested vessel is seen at the upper right, and immediately below it is a small collection of crystalline material seen better under polarizing light (B) as doubly refractile deposits of talc.

lymphadenopathy is of obscure nature but has been attributed to some immunologic reaction to a product produced by the degradation and metabolism of heroin in the liver (Edland, 1972). As mentioned earlier, the angiitis ob-

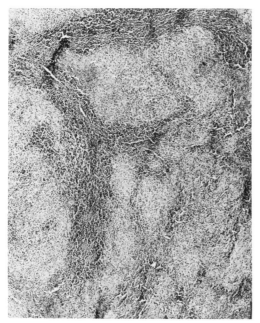

Figure 12–10. The spleen of a heroin addict with numerous granulomata containing doubly refractile particles (visible in polarized light) of talc.

served in addicts might result from drug toxicity, but many of the morphologic vascular changes resemble those found in hypersensitivity diseases such as systemic lupus erythematosus and so an immunologic origin for these vascular lesions cannot be excluded as yet (Lignelli and Buchheit, 1971) (Helpern, 1971). Fulminating reactions to intravenously administered heroin, which are of such an acute nature as to suggest an anaphylaxis-like reaction, sometimes befall addicts (Werner, 1969). Coroners repeatedly report finding the needle still in place within the vein of the dead victim.

The greatest threat to the addict comes with the use of "the needle." The transmission of viral hepatitis has become virtually epidemic in many urban centers. Edland (1972) reports the following data from the New York State Department of Health: in 1960, of 41 cases of serum hepatitis reported, approximately 83 per cent were felt to be transfusion associated and only 17 per cent, drug associated. In 1969, there were a total of 171 cases reported, of which 22 per cent were related to transfusions and 77 per cent, to drug addiction. In these two years, the number of cases occurring in people over the age of 30 was about the same (approximately 30 each year) and almost all were transfusion associated. In striking contrast, the incidence of hepatitis in the 15 to 25-year-old group in 1960 was five cases as compared with 126 in 1969. The hepatic changes are identical with those of viral hepatitis (p. 1004), and here it is only necessary to point out that in over 50 per cent of the cases, the hepatitis resulted in either death or extensive liver damage with postnecrotic scarring.

Addiction is now largely responsible for the resurgent prevalence of tetanus (Cherubin, 1967) (Louria et al., 1967). Addicts are by no means immune to all forms of microbiologic infections and, indeed, develop more than their share of bacterial endocarditis, skin infections (abscesses from "popping" of drugs), lung abscesses, bronchopneumonia, tuberculosis and septic thrombophlebitis to cite some of the more common problems.

The central nervous system is not spared in drug addiction, but it is likely that the changes result from hypoxia, bacteremias and involvement of the brain in the systemic necrotizing angiitides (Solitare, 1972) (Adelman and Aronson, 1969). The hypoxia is generally attributable to the pulmonary changes described in heroin addiction and the depression of the respiratory centers encountered in barbiturate overdosage. To date, no neuropathologic changes characteristic of the addictive state have been found. The cerebral edema, necroses or fatty change of the neurons seen in addicts are entirely compatible with hypoxic injury. Notwithstanding, the experimental administration of morphine to laboratory animals has revealed similar neuronal changes as early as one and one-half days after the administration of the drug, raising the possibility of a more direct causal relationship (Horning, 1934). It is worth pointing out that, despite all of the profound psychologic potentials of these mind-manipulating agents, no distinctive neurologic lesions have been identified which can be related to these psychologic effects. Despite the reported occurrences of marihuana- and LSD-induced psychoses, no anatomic changes in the CNS have yet been identified in the brains of these individuals.

The citation of anatomic changes associated with drug addiction might be extended to include a variety of neuropathies and myopathies as well as certain mutagenic hazards encountered in the occasional case. But without detailing these unusual complications, it should be evident that the addict's search for a "new experience" or a "new world" sometimes leads him to "the other world."

GENERAL SUMMARY OF THE CLINICAL AND MORPHOLOGIC REACTIONS TO POISONS

Poisonings are not common in usual clinical and pathologic practice, and it is therefore difficult to maintain a familiarity with the pertinent data relating to each poison. Moreover, each agent causes fairly specific patterns of injury, and thus the sum total of detailed knowledge required assumes large proportions. It is therefore desirable to provide certain generalizations about poisonings, in which the usual toxic agents are separated into large groups based upon common modes of toxic action. Some chemical agents are violent tissue poisons and exert a profound effect on any organ or structure contacted. Others only act systemically and then exert their principal effect on vulnerable organ sites. The pathologist and the clinician can thus, to a certain extent, categorize the nature of the poisoning by the pattern of damage. These basic patterns will be considered under the headings of local and systemic changes.

LOCAL CHANGES

Many poisons produce injury immediately upon contact with tissue at their sites of entrance. The corrosive agents, which include both organic and inorganic acids and alkalis, are prime examples of such chemicals. Acids spilled or thrown upon the skin may produce extensive areas of necrosis with sloughing and deep ulceration. Taken by mouth, they cause violent damage to the intestinal tract, affecting the oral cavity, laryngopharynx, esophagus and stomach. These cases are readily identified anatomically by the violent corrosive destruction of the tissues contacted by the chemical, appearing within minutes to hours after exposure. Clinically, they are also manifest by the rapid appearance of chemical burns of the skin and oral cavity, as well as by the almost immediate development of violent nausea, vomiting and hematemesis following the ingestion of the corrosive. Such clinical findings at least suggest a locally destructive poison. Appropriate preventive and supportive therapeutic measures can be instituted while the precise identity of the chemical is being explored both by careful historic review of the patient's recent actions and by the chemical analyses of the skin surface or gastric washings. Absorption of these locally acting agents such as the phenols may also give rise to systemic effects, but in general these are usually far less striking than the contact injuries described.

SYSTEMIC CHANGES

Most poisons exert their effect only after absorption into the blood. Most of the heavy metals, alcohol, barbiturates and opium alkaloids act in this fashion. Once absorbed, they produce widespread damage, but in general the organs chiefly affected are the central nervous system, the liver and kidneys. Other tissues are less commonly involved, such as the blood, the heart and the peripheral nerves. By establishing the pattern of organ involvement, it is possible sometimes to suspect the causative poison.

In the *central nervous system*, the effects of poisons tend to take one of two forms. Widespread degeneration of the ganglion cells accompanied by cerebral edema is usually caused by asphyxiants, such as carbon monoxide and the cyanides. Focal areas of softening of the cerebral cortex, thalamic region and medullary centers, presumably on a hypoxic basis, may accompany the widespread neuronal damage. On the other hand, many poisons produce fatal outcomes without creating clearly defined morphologic alterations. These drugs (such as the barbiturates and heroin) exert chiefly a functional depressant effect, which affects first the cerebral cortex and then descends to involve the vital centers of respiration and circulation. Death in these cases is usually due to respiratory arrest. Occasionally, the profound systemic hypoxia caused by respiratory depression may give rise to changes in the brain resembling those described in the asphyxiants. However, the cerebral changes in the depressant agents are usually entirely inconstant and nonspecific. These respiratory depressants may induce hypoxic changes in other viscera such as the liver, kidneys and heart.

On the basis of these central nervous system derangements, it can be postulated that patients who present findings chiefly referable to brain dysfunction, such as stupor, listlessness, respiratory depression or coma, are most likely to have absorbed an agent causing functional depression (barbiturates, morphine and heroin) or an agent leading to hypoxic damage to neurons (carbon monoxide and cyanides). Moreover, it is sometimes possible to ascertain further, even in the fairly early stages, the pattern of brain dysfunction and thus provisionally suspect the specific agent involved. The barbiturates and heroin cause cortical depression first, while monoxide and cyanide tend to affect first the lower brain centers. However, ultimately the precise identification of the specific agent depends upon chemical or toxicologic analysis of tissues or body fluids.

The *liver* is commonly affected in poisonings, since it acts as one of the principal detoxifying centers of the body. It is affected by a wide variety of agents including the heavy metals, corrosives, many of the organic solvents and chemicals leading to systemic hypoxia. The liver damage in most cases follows a fairly standard anatomic pattern. In the mildest or early cases, the change may represent simply swelling of the hepatic cells. In the more severe injuries fatty change occurs, which may show a characteristic zonal distribution affecting the center of the lobule in phosphorus poisoning. If the patient survives long enough, or in cases of chronic toxicity, extensive destruction and necrosis may give rise to a condition referred to as diffuse hepatic necrosis or acute yellow atrophy. Such extensive damage, however, is not usually encountered in patients who die within the first 24 hours.

Clinical symptoms and signs referable to hepatic damage may then be caused by poisoning by any one of a number of toxic agents. If the hepatic changes appear early and are accompanied by significant cerebral findings, hypoxia can be assumed to be an unlikely cause, since the brain is much more vulnerable to this disturbance than the liver. The absence of local skin and gastric findings militates against corrosives. By this form of reasoning, it may be possible to rule out the less likely etiologic agents and thereby simplify the task of ascertaining the precise cause.

The *kidneys* similarly are particularly sensitive to a variety of agents such as mercury, bismuth and organic solvents as well as to hypoxia. The most vulnerable portion of the kidney structure is the proximal convoluted tubules, which undergo swelling, fatty change or frank necrosis, depending upon the severity of the attack and the duration of the exposure. In more severe intoxications, the distal convoluted tubules may also be affected. The glomeruli and collecting tubules appear to be remarkably resistant to most poisons.

The sites of secondary involvement in these poisonings are the blood, peripheral nerves and heart. The changes in the blood usually take the form of increased hemolysis, such as is produced by lead poisoning, or the development of a modified hemoglobin complex produced, for example, by carbon monoxide. The alterations in the peripheral nerves usually consist of myelin degeneration, such as is seen in chronic lead poisoning. The heart reacts to most poisons by the development, first, of swelling of the cardiac muscle fibers followed by fatty changes. This may be encountered with the heavy metals and in severe hypoxic states.

From these comments, it is evident that in the performance of postmortem examinations in suspected cases of systemic poisoning, primary attention should be directed to the brain, liver and kidneys, followed by examination of the peripheral nerves, blood and heart. Although alterations may occur in other organs or tissues, they are not found with sufficient frequency to be of diagnostic help. An extremely important and not to be forgotten part of the medicolegal examination in cases of poisoning is the collection of body fluids for chemical and toxicologic analysis.

PHYSICAL INJURIES

The many forms of physical energy that may give rise to injury can be classified into four groups: mechanical violence, changes in atmospheric pressure, changes in temperature and electromagnetic energy. Of the physical agents, mechanical violence exemplified by the everyday occurrence of auto accidents is the most frequent cause of injury encountered in clinical practice. Much detail on mechanical injuries is unnecessary in general pathology, since only rarely do such cases necessitate pathologic study save for legal purposes. Changes in atmospheric pressure and temperature are relatively uncommon causes of injury and can be considered with some brevity. Radiation injuries, on the other hand, have assumed frightening importance as potential causes of widespread destruction.

MECHANICAL VIOLENCE

Injury from mechanical violence may occur whenever a mass hits the body, the body collides with a stationary mass or, as sometimes occurs, both body and mass are in movement at the moment of impact. Several categories of tissue injury or wounds may result which can be grouped broadly into sites: (1) soft tissue injuries, (2) bone injuries and (3) head injuries. Injuries of the bones (p. 1440) and of the head (p. 1525) involve specialized problems best considered in the chapters dealing with these structures. The soft tissue injuries fall principally into the realm of surgery and involve no special problems in anatomic pathology, and can thus be dismissed in a consideration of this type. The possible systemic reactions to trauma are presented in the consideration of shock (p. 345).

CHANGES IN TEMPERATURE

As a homeothermic animal, man must maintain his internal temperature within the narrow range of 88° to 113° F., and even this upper limit can be tolerated only very briefly. However, it is by no means certain that the lower temperature cited represents an absolute limit, since at the present time our knowledge of the reactions of the body tissues to cold is being rapidly expanded by the use of hypothermia as a potential clinical tool in surgery.

Since abnormally high and low temperatures produce different patterns of tissue damage and have different pathogenic mechanisms, they are discussed separately.

ABNORMALLY LOW TEMPERATURES

Pathogenesis of Injury. The precise mechanism by which chilling or freezing of tissues causes injury is still unknown. Three possibilities are suggested, all of which may act conjointly (Friedman, 1945). (1) The metabolism of cells may be slowed or blocked by the lowering of their temperature to the point at which inhibition or suppression of vital metabolic activities results in cell damage or death. (2) Freezing temperatures may crystallize the water content of cells. (3) Chilling produces vasoconstriction at first, followed by paralysis of vasomotor control with attendant vasodilatation and increased permeability, in turn producing exudation of serum and plasma. When the injury is sufficiently severe, intravascular clotting occurs and results in anoxic changes and even infarction necrosis of the tissues affected (Friedman and Kritzler, 1947).

Anatomic Alterations. Low temperatures have both local and systemic effects on the body.

Local Reactions. Nonfreezing and freezing temperatures produce similar forms of local injury which differ only in severity. *Immersion or trench foot* results from exposure to long-continued, nonfreezing temperatures. The most important causes of tissue damage in these instances are vasoconstriction and tissue ischemia. When the tissue is first chilled, it appears either pale gray and waxen or has a blotchy mottled cyanosis. The later developing vasodilatation in vessels already injured results in exudation of large amounts of fluid, producing severe swelling and large bullae or vesicles. Thrombosis may then occur, and the ischemia may lead to frank necrosis with gangrene of the affected part. When the chilling reaches freezing temperatures, death of the cells is more certain, but similar mechanisms are operable. Injury to the nerve fibers in the local area may accompany either the nonfreezing or freezing hypothermia, giving rise to sensory and motor disturbances.

Systemic Reactions. When the entire body is exposed to low temperature, there is at first marked vasoconstriction of the skin vessels and, as a result, the skin becomes extremely pale. As the hypothermia continues, marked peripheral vasodilatation and hyperemia develop. Cooling of the peripheral blood soon causes depression of the temperature in the vital organs, particularly the brain, though the usual mechanism of death appears to be circulatory failure. Sudden acute chilling may cause death within a relatively short time without apparent alteration of the bodily tissues. Under these circumstances, there may be no pathognomonic anatomic changes demonstrable at the time of postmortem examination. With more slowly developing, protracted hypothermia, the anatomic changes are usually limited to the superficial tissues and extremities and resemble those described in the local reactions.

THERMAL BURNS

When thermal burn injury causes, as it does, approximately 9000 deaths annually in the United States, it is obviously a problem of considerable clinical magnitude. This problem is further highlighted by the fact that a large proportion of the fatalities occur among children and young adults. The risk of death after extensive thermal burns is roughly proportional to the percentage of total body surface involved. In general, involvement of over 20 per cent of the total body surface is considered as an extensive burn having possible lethal significance. The depth of the burn injury is also contributory to the outcome. The older terminology of first, second and third degree burns has now been replaced by the division into "partial" or "full thickness" burns. This distinction has clinicopathologic significance since a full thickness burn implies destruction of the dermal appendages from which reepithelialization occurs. A full thickness burn is, therefore, not capable of self repair and must be grafted. While at one time it was thought that the clinical problem of burns related to the immediate care of the area of tissue destruction, it is now apparent that the later developing systemic ramifications are, in fact, more important.

The *immediate effects* of burns relate not only to the outright coagulation of tissue but also to microcirculatory changes. These vascular alterations may be due directly to the heat but, unquestionably, are also chemically mediated by such vasoactive compounds as histamine and bradykinin. Increased vascular permeability is marked, permitting massive loss of water and proteins into the site of injury, sometimes with sufficient depletion of blood volume to cause shock and even death. With improved fluid replacement therapy in the last decade, most of the patients without antece-

dent cardiovascular, renal or pulmonary disease now survive the immediate postburn period (days 1 to 5). Patients exposed to noxious fumes arising from the combustion of materials such as mattress fillings have striking pulmonary transudation and exudation that may in itself lead to an early death.

The *late systemic effects* of burns are of far greater importance than the immediate problems just mentioned. These are of greater diversity and complexity than was formerly appreciated.

Sepsis resulting from burn wound infection is probably the single most important cause of death in the seriously burned patient. In a recent study, it was concluded that 74 per cent of fatalities died with a significant degree of burn wound infection (Teplitz, 1969). Studies on both man and animals indicate that the burn wound is generally sterile for a period of approximately 24 hours after injury. Bacteria then contaminate the surface and rapidly proliferate to staggering numbers in the range of 100,000 to hundreds of millions of bacteria per square centimeter of burn wound injury. These bacteria progressively invade the deeper layers to eventually reach the subjacent viable tissue. Though staphylococci and streptococci have been chief offenders in the past, the gram-negative bacilli, predominantly *P. aeruginosa, P. vulgaris* and *A. aerogenes* in order of decreasing importance, have now become the major clinical problem. These bacteria *known as the gram-negative rods* liberate products which of themselves are capable of producing endotoxic shock but, in addition, there is direct invasion of the viable subjacent tissue that leads to massive infection of the subcutaneous fat as well as to penetration of the blood vessel walls to produce bacteremias.

Not only is the burn area itself colonized by bacteria but the entire skin surface of the patient harbors organisms that have the distressing potential of producing infections at venipuncture sites, septic phlebitis in veins used for fluid replacement therapy, and infections in and around tracheostomies.

Pathologic changes are commonly found in the lungs of fatally burned patients. *Severe pulmonary edema* is present in approximately 30 per cent of patients dying within either the immediate resuscitative or postresuscitative periods. The pulmonary edema has been described on p. 349 as "shock lungs." Loss of albumin from the burn wound may lead to hypoalbuminemia with decreased plasma osmotic pressure further favoring pulmonary edema. The possible role of direct injury to the pulmonary vascular bed by the inhalation of fumes is difficult to evaluate but has unquestionably contributed to the mortality of patients trapped in enclosed spaces. In addition to the edema, secondary infections with the production of bronchopneumonia, intra-alveolar hemorrhages and atelectasis are also frequently found.

Acute *gastroduodenal stress ulcers* are found in about half the patients dying of burn injuries. Although Curling originally described duodenal ulcers in burned patients, more recent studies have shown that gastric ulcers are more common. These ulcers are classically multiple, most apt to occur in the body or fundus of the stomach, and histologically have only a sparse inflammatory reaction without the granulation tissue or fibrosis seen in the base of the typical peptic ulcer. The etiology of these acute stress ulcers remains obscure, although high circulating levels of steroids and gastric microcirculatory alterations have been proposed. While most of these ulcers occur as a terminal event, in a few cases perforation has been the primary cause of death. More often, they produce massive gastrointestinal bleeding that complicates the management of these patients.

Many other organs are affected in the fatally burned patient. Shock kidneys (acute tubular necrosis or hemoglobinuric nephrosis) are found in approximately 10 per cent of these patients. Although some implicate destruction of red cells in the burn wound in the pathogenesis of these renal lesions, the preponderance of evidence suggests that circulatory insufficiency and renal ischemia are more important. The adrenal glands usually exhibit all of the changes encountered in shock (p. 1300). There is no good evidence that there is any adrenal insufficiency as a significant pathogenetic factor in burn fatalities. Fatty changes in the liver, focal necroses and central congestion are frequently present but are rarely of sufficient magnitude to constitute clinical problems. Occasionally, minimal myocardial focal necroses are seen attributable either to circulatory insufficiency or conceivably to bacterial invasion of the myocardium, but these rarely evoke clinical manifestations.

CHANGES IN ATMOSPHERIC PRESSURE

The direction of the pressure change (in general, the body withstands increases of pressure better than decreases), the magnitude of the change and the rate of change all modify the extent, nature and severity of the tissue damage. For example, sudden violent increases in pressure cause trauma by compression of the thorax and abdomen while the following negative wave of pressure results in explosive rupture of the respiratory tree or hollow viscera. The same pressure changes, applied slowly, might be without effect.

Changes in atmospheric pressure cause injuries in one of three ways: (1) Sudden increases or decreases of pressure may produce mechanical damage—blast injury. (2) With sudden decrease in pressure, free gaseous bubbles may be released in the blood and act as emboli referred to as caisson disease (p. 337). (3) In low atmospheric pressures, lowered oxygen tension in the inspired air causes systemic hypoxia as is seen in high altitude reactions.

BLAST INJURY

Blast injury is incurred from sudden violent changes in pressure as in an explosion. The forces may be transmitted by air (air blast) or by water (immersion blast). These two forms of injury differ in several respects. In air blast, compressive waves impinge against the body, usually from one direction, followed by a sudden wave of decreased pressure exerting a negative pressure effect. By pressure on the surface of the body, collapse of the thorax, rupture of solid viscera and widespread hemorrhage may result. The compressive wave may also enter the body orifices, particularly the respiratory passages, and exert its direct effect upon the lungs. The lungs thus sustain multiple hemorrhages associated with rupture of alveolar walls or massive lacerations. Visceral infarctions due to mysteriously developing gaseous emboli have been noted in animals experimentally exposed to blast injury.

In immersion blast, the pressure is applied to the body from all sides, tending to force the body up out of water. Persons floating in an erect position are lifted slightly, if at all, and thus sustain severe injuries to the lower half of the body, while individuals floating horizontally on the surface may simply be tossed out of the water virtually unharmed. The positive pressure in immersion blast compresses the abdomen, and causes lacerations of the diaphragm and compressive rupture of the hollow viscera of the intestines as well as solid organs, i.e. spleen, kidneys and liver. The wave of compression may enter the anal orifice and produce an explosive effect on the large bowel. Rupture of the intestines may also occur from sudden expansion of the abdominal contents during the ensuing negative phase of pressure.

HIGH ALTITUDE REACTIONS

At altitudes above 15,000 feet and certainly above 20,000 feet, there is a physiologically significant decrease in available oxygen. Unless artificial supplies are available, severe systemic hypoxia may result, causing loss of consciousness, circulatory or respiratory collapse, and death. Long-term exposure to moderate elevations in altitude evokes systemic changes which compensate for the reduced oxygen tension in the inspired air. Such adaptations are observed in individuals living in mountainous areas and are chiefly characterized by an increased red cell formation (compensatory polycythemia). In this way, although the oxygen saturation of hemoglobin is reduced, the total supply of available oxygen is normal.

ELECTRICAL INJURIES

The passage of an electrical current through the body may be without effect or may cause tissue injury or sudden death, depending on the size of the current and its pathway. Electrical energy injures or kills by one of two methods. First, the conduction of an electrical current through the body produces interruption of neural conduction, for example, the normal rhythmic cardiac and respiratory impulses from the medulla (the mechanism of death in electrocution), and at the same time causes ionization of protoplasmic elements with injury or destruction of cells. Second, the transformation of electrical energy into heat causes burns.

With respect to the first mechanism, body tissues in general are good conductors of electricity and, when placed in the pathway of an electric current, transmit this current to some point of exit in contact with the ground. In the course of this passage, the maximal local injuries are usually produced at the skin sites of entry and exit, since the skin has the highest resistance to the flow of electrical energy. Once having entered the body, the current tends to flow in all directions and passes in a broad front through the cross sectional areas that intervene between its entrance and exit points. The high potentials thus dispersed may cause little damage except possibly for their action upon neuroregulatory mechanisms. It is for this reason that currents passing through the brain or the left side of the body and heart are more dangerous than pathways that bypass such vital organs.

Much of the damage caused by electrical energy is due to the production of heat. The amount of heat produced is influenced by many factors: (1) the duration of the exposure (heat production is cumulative), (2) the resistance of the tissues and (3) the intensity (amperage) of the current. The skin is the tissue of highest resistance in the body and, therefore, other factors being equal, develops the highest levels of heat. Dry skin and thick skin are more resistant than moist or thin skin and thus generate more heat. The surface area making up the contact with the electrical current also modifies the total amount of heat developed within cells. It has already been indicated that, when the contact surfaces are large, dispersion of the energy load lowers the heat generation to which individual cells are exposed. A similar potential applied in a concentrated focus might produce serious damage. It is this principle which permits the passage of high electrical potentials through broad cross sectional areas of the body without causing morphologic alterations.

The morphologic effects of the passage of an electrical current vary from superficial skin burns to deep visceral lesions. With high intensity current, linear arborizing burns known as "lightning marks" appear on the skin. Usually burn marks will be found at the points of entry and exit of the current. Low intensity currents, especially when there is a good contact surface as with moist skin or through water, may cause no skin reaction and yet be of sufficient intensity to produce death by disturbing the cardiac or pulmonary rhythmic impulses. The internal morphologic effects are varied and depend on the voltage and amperage of the current. Lightning may cause sufficient heat and production of steam to explode solid organs and even fracture bones. Focal hemorrhages from rupture of small vessels may be seen in the brain. Sometimes death is preceded by violent convulsions related to the passage of the current through the nervous system.

RADIANT ENERGY

Radiant energy when used in the treatment of cancer can be lifesaving but, on the other hand, it can be terrifyingly destructive as was graphically documented at Hiroshima and Nagasaki (Key, 1971). The use of radiant energy for treatment of disease has become commonplace in clinical practice and, indeed, has spawned the emergence of such specialties as nuclear medicine and radiobiology devoted solely to the clinical applications of radiant energy.

The effect of radiation on cells at the physicochemical level is largely ionization of the individual molecules and atoms of the cell. Ionization is brought about by the transfer of the energy possessed by the radiation to the target matter, inducing the displacement of electrons from atoms and/or molecules. Radiation may also cause excitation or increase in the energy of an electron in an atom or molecule, but such excitation does not appear to be as potent a mechanism for producing physicochemical change within the cell (Lea, 1962). To understand the biologic effects of radiation, some of the basic concepts of the nature of radiant energy will be presented, followed by a consideration of its pathologic effect on cells and tissues.

FORMS OF RADIANT ENERGY

The spectrum of radiation includes two distinctive forms of energy propagation, the first consisting of electromagnetic radiation propagated by wave motion, the other comprising fast-moving particles (alpha and beta), neutrons and protons.

Electromagnetic radiation comprises a broad range of wave-propagated energy which includes electrical, radio, infrared, visible and ultraviolet rays and, of particular interest here, roentgen (x) and gamma rays. X-rays and gamma rays are quite similar in their interactions, but differ in their origin. The former are machine generated while gamma rays are emitted by the spontaneous decay of radioactive nuclides such as naturally occurring radium and uranium and the man-made radioisotopes. Both x-rays and gamma rays are very energetic, extremely penetrating and ambiguously partake of the characteristics of both waves and particles. They can exhibit wave characteristics such as diffraction, but their energy is delivered in packets. The energy in each of these packets is spoken of as a quantum. The range penetration of x-rays depends on the voltage capacity of the x-ray machine but, in general, at least more than one set of ion pairs is produced by electromagnetic radiation before its energy is dispelled.

Particulate radiation consists of particles of definite mass and charge which are given off by both naturally occurring and artifically produced radioactive elements, processes of fission as in atomic reactions, particle accelerators and may also be derived from the interaction of electromagnetic radiation with other matter. As far as radiobiology is concerned, the most important particulate radiation includes beta particles, better known as electrons, alpha particles, protons and neutrons. Many other forms of high energy particles such as muons, pions and other heavy ions have now been recognized but, at the present time, are not extensively used in medical practice (Rosen, 1971).

The electron, as is well known, has a negative charge and a relatively small mass. Electrons are involved in electrical, chemical and atomic processes and, indeed, primarily or secondarily, participate in all radiation energy transfers within cells and tissues. When an electron comes into close proximity to another electron orbiting about a nucleus, the repulsion of the two like charges may dislodge the electron from its orbit, thus creating secondary particulate radiation. Since electrons are very light, they are easily deflected by collisions and thus pursue an erratic path. Although the total distance traveled and the number of interactions may be great, forward motion in a straight line is very short.

Alpha particles, the stripped nuclei of the helium atoms, have a charge of + 2 and an atomic weight of 4. Because they have a greater mass than electrons, they travel much slower and have a shorter course. However, because of its greater charge, an alpha particle will be involved in far more interactions per unit of path length than an electron. The positively charged alpha particle ionizes atoms by attraction of the negatively charged orbiting electrons. Because of its very low penetrability and the protection afforded the skin by the layer of keratin, alpha radiation from radioactive elements does not present any serious external hazard but can be harmful internally if ingested or inhaled as in nuclear fallout. In nuclear fission, however, this hazard is minimal compared to the external threat from gamma radiation.

The proton is much like the alpha particle but is smaller. It represents the nucleus of a hydrogen atom with a mass of 1 and a positive charge. Protons are not normally emitted by radioactive substances but, when produced in high energy accelerators, may be transformed to high energy radiation capable of great penetration and destructiveness.

The neutron has a relative mass equal to that of the hydrogen nucleus, but it is without charge. As mentioned, neutrons and protons comprise the nucleus of an atom. Neutrons may be produced by atomic fission and as secondary forms of particulate radiation when alpha particles or electromagnetic photons interact with other matter.

MECHANISMS OF ACTION

It is somewhat anticlimactic to admit that, although we know that radiation causes ionization of matter, we still do not understand precisely how radiant energy exerts its biologic effect on the cell. Two proposals have been made: (1) the "*target theory*" also known as the "direct hit," "quantum hit" or "direct action" theory and (2) the "*indirect action*" theory.

The "*target theory*" proposes that radiant

energy acts by direct hits on target molecules within the cell. It is possible that a single hit might ionize and inactivate a single vital compound or a substance, thus damaging or even killing the cell. Equally possible is the requirement that multiple targets must be hit or a single target must be hit more than once. The cumulative evidence suggests that DNA is the most vulnerable target of radiation and, more specifically, the linkage and bonds within the DNA molecule (Hutchinson, 1966). However, the macromolecules within membranes and other cytoplasmic constituents are also damaged by radiation.

The *"indirect theory"* proposes that radiant energy exerts its effect by producing free "hot" radicals such as peroxides within cells that secondarily interact with and damage specific targets. Since water is a major constituent of cells, it is postulated that ionizing radiation may release ionized H^+ and OH^- which are very unstable as well as other unstable intermediates such as HO_2 and H_2O_2 (Bacq and Alexander, 1961). Because these primary radicals are so highly unstable, they react very rapidly with themselves and other solutes in the solution. The consequent chain of chemical reactions is known as the "secondary chemical reaction." In this sequential manner, according to the "indirect theory" a crucial biochemical change is believed to take place, causing cell damage or death.

The transfer of energy to a target atom or molecule from the incident source of radiant energy occurs within microfractions of a second, yet its biologic effect may not become apparent for minutes or even decades. *Radiation therefore has a latency* (Rugh, 1968). During this latent period, it must be assumed (although poorly understood) that sequential reactions are occurring which ultimately exert a detectable functional or morphologic effect. Both "direct" and "indirect" actions of radiation could start such a chain reaction, but the "indirect theory" would relate better to its latent effect.

The concept of *linear energy transfer (LET) is of critical importance in the transfer of radiant energy to the incident target.* LET defines the amount of energy transferred per unit path length and involves such considerations as mass, charge and velocity. The LET value of a form of radiation indicates the likelihood of its having an effect within a target area. Alpha particles, for example, because of their large mass and high charge have a much higher LET potential than beta particles of the same energy. Gamma rays have a relatively low LET because of their penetrability, thus dissipating their energy over a long distance.

Equally important to the understanding of the biologic effect of radiant energy is its ability to penetrate tissues. *The penetration of radiant energy depends largely on the energy and nature of the radiation and is equally dependent on the nature of the target matter* which constitutes the collision course of the radiation. The penetrance of the several forms of radiation varies widely. As alluded to earlier, alpha particles are more sluggish and penetrate less deeply through the skin than the lighter, lower charge electrons of the same energy. The penetrability of electromagnetic radiation depends largely on its energy. Much deeper penetration is achieved by 100 kV. generated roentgen rays than by that produced by 10 kV. machines. Gamma radiation derived from cobalt bombs, for example, may be as deeply penetrating as that produced by supervoltage x-radiation (Tessmer, 1971). The various cells and tissues of the body also differ in their capacity to resist penetration by radiant energy. The outer keratinous shell of man is an excellent albeit not impermeable radiation shield. Once penetrated, however, the subcutaneous tissues offer far less resistance to penetration. With respect to living matter, penetration is a function of the number of interactions between the radiant energy and target matter which eventually absorbs all of the energy in the radiation. Penetration ceases once all energy has been dissipated.

QUANTITATION OF RADIATION

The biologic effect of radiation is largely dependent on the total dosages and the rate of its delivery and absorption. Later we shall discuss the variable sensitivity of the differing cells and tissues in the body to radiation, but here it should be emphasized that all living matter can be destroyed by sufficiently high doses of radiant energy delivered over a short period of time. Many victims of the atomic bombs in Japan within 500 meters of the hypocenter were apparently killed instantaneously by the intensive radiation since they were found dead without evidence of mechanical trauma or burns wherever they happened to have been at that instant. *Critical, then, to the biologic effects of radiation are dosage and rate of delivery.*

The *quantitation of radiation* is expressed in several kinds of units for the various forms of radiant energy. X-rays or gamma rays are measured in roentgens (R). A roentgen unit is a measure of the ionization produced by electromagnetic radiation in air, defined as the quantity of radiation required to induce in 1 cc. of air an emission equivalent to 1 electrostatic unit of charge. Roentgens deal with air exposure, but it is obvious that more important is the quantity absorbed. The rad (r) comprises the quantity of radiation based upon the absorption of 100 ergs of energy per gm. of target tissue. For example, one roentgen will lead to the absorption of about 87 ergs per gm. of tissue. Radioactive elements are quantitated in curies. A curie is defined as the quantity of any radionuclide which suffers 3.7×10^{10} disintegrations per second. Two additional terms are applied to radioisotopes. The half-life of a radioactive compound designates the time span during which half of the atoms decay. The specific activity of a radioisotope indicates the relative or proportionate number of radioactive atoms in a given substance.

The time span over which a given dose of radiation is absorbed plays an important role in determining its biologic action and involves the controversial issue of cumulative effect. At one time it was believed that radiant energy was cumulative and fractional doses had an additive effect. At very low dose rates, this concept is basically correct, but much depends on the time interval between doses and the latent biologic effect of the radiation. The ionizing action of radiant energy is virtually instantaneous, but the consequences of such ionization may be apparent at once or only after some long delay. At relatively low dose rates, both normal and tumorous cells may recover from their radiant injury and repair within the time span between exposures (Russell et al., 1958). If cellular recovery is not complete at the time of delivery of the second dose of radiation, there is some additive effect. While, then, divided doses may have some cumulative effect, the total impact of the radiant energy is not as great as would have been achieved by delivery of one single dose equivalent to the sum of the divided doses. Indeed, there is some evidence that fractional doses of radiation accelerate repair of cells and that some acquired resistance or adaptation may occur within exposed but still vital cells. Conceivably, more resistant clones may replace the former vulnerable cells. In any event, it is clear that the rate of absorption of radiant energy materially modifies its total effect. Notwithstanding, it is frequently necessary to use divided dosages in the radiotherapy of cancer and other diseases in the belief that the normal cells and tissues which are simultaneously unavoidably exposed will recover and repair more rapidly than the cancer cells.

BIOLOGIC EFFECTS OF RADIATION

This consideration of radiobiology is divided into three parts: (1) general effects of radiation on all cells and tissues, (2) changes in certain specific organ systems induced by radiation and (3) total body irradiation.

General Effects on Cells and Tissues. Radiant energy produces a number of morphologic effects on all cells and tissues of the body, but none are unique. Any of the changes encountered in irradiated cells may also be seen in other forms of injury such as those caused by microbiologic or toxic agents, heat, cold and ischemic injury. Indeed, some drugs such as the alkylating agents so closely mimic the effect of radiation that they are referred to as radiomimetic. The vulnerability or radiosensitivity of the many specialized forms of cells and tissues in the body varies widely. In general, *cells are sensitive to radiant energy in direct proportion to their reproductive or mitotic activity and in inverse proportion to their level of specialization* (Anderson Hospital and Tumor Institute, 1965). The same generalization applies to cancers. The more rapidly growing and undifferentiated the neoplasm, the more likely it will be radiosensitive. In general, tumors arising from radiosensitive tissues are themselves radiosensitive. The relative radiosensitivities of cells and associated cancers are given in Table 12–2 modified from Rubin and Casarett (1968).

While Table 12–2 provides some useful generalizations regarding the relative radiosensitivity of cells and their cancers, there are many strange exceptions which defy understanding. For example, lymphocytes are exquisitely radiosensitive. While some are rapidly dividing, others are long-lived, perhaps for the lifetime of man; but as far as we now know, all are vulnerable to relatively low levels of radiation. The seminoma, which is believed to arise ultimately from germ cells, is radiosensitive as the table indicates, but the embryonal carcinoma which also arises from germ cells is radioresistant. Other factors may play a role here, and perhaps the immune response (more evident in the case of the seminoma) cooperates to enhance the lethal effect of radiation. Normal colonic epithelium is very radiosensitive, but the adenocarcinomas taking origin from such cells are less so. These exceptions underscore the necessity for conservatism in prognosticating the possible effectiveness of radiotherapy in the treatment of a specific tumor in the individual patient. To quote from Rubin and Casarett (1968), "The variation in tumor response to irradiation is one of the most perplexing aspects of radiotherapeutics. The entire spectrum, from radiosensitivity to radioresistance, is encountered not only among different histopathologic types of tumors, but also in similar malignant processes

TABLE 12–2. RADIOSENSITIVITY OF SPECIALIZED CELLS
AND THEIR TUMORS

Radio-sensitivity	Normal Cells	Tumors
High	Lymphoid, hematopoietic (marrow), germ cells, intestinal epithelium, ovarian follicular cells	Leukemia—lymphoma, seminoma, dysgerminoma, granulosa cell carcinoma
Fairly high	Epidermal epithelium, adnexal structures (hair follicles, sebaceous glands), oropharyngeal stratified epithelium, urinary bladder epithelium, esophageal epithelium, gastric gland epithelium, ureteral epithelium	Squamous cell carcinoma of skin, oropharyngeal, esophageal, cervical and bladder epithelium, adenocarcinoma of gastric epithelium
Medium	Connective tissue, glia, endothelium, growing cartilage or bone	Endothelio- and angiosarcomas, astrocytomas, the vasculature and connective tissue elements of all tumors
Fairly low	Mature cartilage or bone cells, mucous or serous gland epithelium, pulmonary epithelium, renal epithelium, hepatic epithelium, pancreatic epithelium, pituitary epithelium, thyroid epithelium, adrenal epithelium, nasopharyngeal nonstratified epithelium	Liposarcoma, chondrosarcoma, osteogenic sarcoma, adenocarcinoma of: breast epithelium hepatic epithelium renal epithelium pancreatic epithelium thyroid epithelium adrenal gland epithelium colon epithelium, squamous cell cancer of the lung
Low	Muscle cells, ganglion cells	Rhabdomyosarcoma, leiomyosarcoma, ganglioneuroma

Adapted from Rubin, R., and Casarett, G. W.: Clinical Radiation Pathology. Philadelphia, W. B. Saunders Co., 1968, p. 903.

in different hosts and occasionally in the same host."

All cells can be affected by radiant energy and, indeed, all living matter can be killed by radiation. The more radioresistant the cell, the greater the amount of radiation required to produce the effect. The changes involve both the cytoplasm and the nucleus. During the initial response to radiant injury, there is cellular swelling, cytoplasmic vacuolization and alterations in plasma membranes. Mitochondria enlarge, assume distorted shapes, and some are disrupted. These mitochondrial changes may be secondary to other metabolic dislocations, since many observations suggest that mitochondria themselves are relatively radioresistant (Tsinga and Casarett, 1965). The endoplasmic reticulum is also affected, but lysosomes appear to be more resistant and are often increased in number (Ghidoni, 1967). The nuclear changes are marked and include nuclear swelling, vacuolation, focal disappearance of the nuclear membrane and, in severely affected cells, nuclear pyknosis or lysis. Following radiation injury, cells often assume bizarre sizes and shapes, sometimes with the formation of giant cells containing an extremely bizarre

pleomorphic nucleus or more than one nucleus. Such nuclear pleomorphism and cellular distortion may persist for years after the radiation exposure.

DNA is thought to be the most vulnerable macromolecule within the cell. The basic effect of radiant energy is inhibition of DNA synthesis and interference with, and/or delay of, the mitotic process. One fundamental target that has been proposed is the synthesis of mRNA and the production of vital enzymes such as thymidine kinase and DNA polymerase so that normal synthesis of DNA is prevented and vital metabolic pathways are blocked or altered, leading to death of cells. For this reason, dividing cells are more susceptible to radiation injury. All phases of the cell generation cycle can be affected by radiation, but the G_2 phase (just prior to mitosis) and the S (synthetic) phase are more vulnerable than the M and G_1 phases. It follows, therefore, that slowly dividing cells are less radiosensitive, probably because they have a longer time to recover from the radiation injury before they go into mitosis. It hardly need be reiterated that any and all of these effects are dose-rate dependent.

A wide range of chromosomal and chromatid mutations is induced by radiation, including deletions, breaks, translocations, interadherence of chromosomes, fragmentation and, indeed, all forms of abnormal chromosome morphology (Amarose et al., 1967). The mitotic spindle often becomes disorderly or even chaotic. Polyploidy and aneuploidy may be encountered. As is well known, radiation injury has the potential of inducing neoplasia with all of its attendant karyotypic abnormalities (p. 138). It should be evident that the constellation of cellular pleomorphism, giant cell formation, conformation changes in nuclei and mitotic figures creates a more than passing similarity between radiation-injured cells and cancer cells, a problem that plagues the pathologist when evaluating postirradiation tissues for the possible persistence of tumor cells. It should be noted that none of these mitotic and chromosomal mutations are diagnostic of radiation since they can be produced also by radiomimetic chemicals such as the nitrogen mustards and other alkylating agents.

Vascular changes are prominent in all irradiated tissues (dose-rate dependent), be they normal or neoplastic. As was pointed out earlier, endothelial cells are only moderately radioresponsive but, with the intensive therapy administered to tumors, radiational changes are almost always seen in the vasculature of the neoplasm itself and in the normal tissues interposed between the source of the radiation and the neoplasm. During the immediate postirradiation period, vessels may show only dilatation accounting for the erythema of the skin seen so often in radiotherapy. Later or with higher dosages, a variety of regressive changes appear including endothelial cell swelling, vacuolation or even dissolution with total necrosis of the walls of small vessels (such as capillaries and venules). Affected vessels may rupture, yielding hemorrhages or, alternatively, they may thrombose. For reasons unknown, these vascular changes are peculiarly spotty in their distribution along the course of a vessel and so, in the same tissue section, some channels are affected and others spared. In some part, the cancericidal effectiveness of radiation is attributable to such vascular damage. At a later stage, endothelial cell proliferation and collagenous hyalinization with thickening of the media are seen in irradiated vessels, resulting in marked narrowing or even obliteration of the vascular lumina.

Organ System Involvements. The effects of radiation on certain specific organs and systems are worthy of special citation either because of the particular vulnerability of the organ or its frequent involvement.

The *skin* is in the pathway of all intentionally or accidentally delivered external radiation. The changes encountered range from mild postirradiation (2 to 3 days) erythema to late-appearing cancers. Depending on the dose-rate and penetrability of the radiant energy, one may observe postirradiation (two to three weeks) edema and epithelial desquamation (four to six weeks). These changes are followed by blotchy, increased pigmentation or depigmentation, hyperkeratosis, epilation (one to two months) skin atrophy, dermal and subcutaneous fibrosis and, in some instances, telangiectases and ulcerations (one-half to five years). Histologically, the epidermal cells may show any of the general cytologic alterations described previously (p. 540) while the underlying dermis exhibits the characteristic radiation-induced vascular changes accompanied by hyaline collagenization of connective tissue and basophilic degeneration of elastic fibers. The atrophy, depigmentation and telangiectasia commonly persist for decades. Rarely, ulcerating squamous cell cancers appear many years later, sometimes as long as 56 years later (Cade, 1957).

The *hematopoietic and lymphoid systems* are extremely susceptible to radiant injury. With high dose levels, severe lymphopenia may appear within hours of radiation, along with shrinkage of the lymph nodes and the spleen. Radiation directly destroys lymphocytes, both those in the circulating blood and in the tissues (nodes, spleen, thymus, gut) and causes all of the cytologic disorganizations already described. Regeneration is prompt, however, from viable precursors, with restoration of the normal lymphocyte complement of the blood within weeks to months. The circulating granulocyte count may at first rise but begins to fall toward the end of the first week. Levels near zero may be reached during the second week. If the patient survives, recovery of the normal granulocyte counts may require two to three months. Platelets are similarly affected, with the nadir of the count occurring somewhat later than that of the granulocytes, while recovery is similarly delayed. The hematopoietic cells in the bone marrow are also quite sensitive to radiant energy, including the red cell precursors. The marrow may become virtually acellular weeks after heavy exposure and contain only varying numbers of disintegrated cells. Erythrocytes are radioresistant, but anemia may appear after two to three weeks and be persistent for months because of marrow damage. Obviously, the severity of the blood and marrow depletion and its clinical significance depend on the dosage of the radiation and the extent of marrow damage. Whole body irradiation may be lethal. Localized exposure may have no effect on the circulating blood counts. The neutropenia and thrombocytopenia are responsible for increased susceptibility to infections and bleeding diatheses in the post-irradiation period. If the patient survives these hazards and the hypoxic injury resulting from the anemia, regeneration from primitive precursors may yield complete recovery.

Studies of the survivors of the atomic bombs have unmistakably demonstrated the leukemogenic effect of radiation (Anderson, 1971). The incidence of all forms of leukemia (save possibly chronic lymphocytic leukemia) in the long-term survivors of the bombings at Nagasaki and Hiroshima has been increased ten to fifty-fold above that of the control population. For some mysterious reason, chronic lymphocytic leukemia has always been rare among the Japanese. Children exposed in utero also have developed a higher incidence of leukemia. This leukemogenic effect, as would be expected, is dose-related inasmuch as those nearest the hypocenters bore the brunt of these disorders (Hollingsworth, 1960) (Brill et al., 1962).

The *gonads* in both the male and female, particularly the germ cells, are highly vulnerable to radiation injury, and sterility is a frequent residual of such damage. In the testis, spermatogonia then spermatocytes, spermatids and spermatozoa are radiosensitive in the order given. The cytologic changes to be observed are those already described (p. 540) but, as late residuals, there may be total atrophy and fibrosis with hyalinization of the testicular tubules. Sertoli cells and interstitial cells are radioresistant. Within the ovary, the germ cells and even more so the follicular granulosal cells are vulnerable. Indeed, for given dosages of the same form of radiation, sterility is more frequent in the female than in the male, principally because of radiation destruction of the ovarian follicles. Cessation of menses and menopausal changes may be temporary or permanent, depending on the dosage of radiation. In passing, it should be noted that the uterus and cervix are quite radioresistant and hence permit the installation of radioactive elements into the uterine cavity for the treatment of endometrial carcinomas.

The *lungs*, because of their rich vascularization, are vulnerable to radiation injury, and shortness of breath, coughing and even acute fatal respiratory insufficiency may appear within weeks to months following sufficient exposure of large segments of the lung fields. During the acute phase, the endothelial cell changes described in the blood vessels are seen in the alveolar capillaries. The increased vascular permeability may lead to marked pulmonary congestion, edema, fibrin exudation, the formation of hyaline membranes and even total filling of the air spaces by a rich proteinous and cellular debris, creating changes very similar to those of bacterial pneumonia. Later changes include fibrosis of the alveolar walls and the described vascular wall thickening and luminal obliteration. The resultant respiratory dysfunction may be crippling or fatal since the "radiation pneumonitis" creates a profound alveolocapillary block. Bronchogenic carcinomas have followed the prolonged inhalation of radioactive dusts by those working in uranium mines.

The *gastrointestinal tract* is so radiosensitive that it is frequently affected in all forms of deep radiation. Soon after exposure, patients often have loss of appetite, nausea and vomiting, and many develop severe diarrhea for a period of days. As might be expected, the intestinal epithelium is very vulnerable because of its high turnover rate, and all forms of nuclear and cellular pleomorphism along with mitotic abnormalities are seen in mucosal cells in the postirradiation period. Mucosal edema, hyperemia and ulcerations may appear, accompanied by vascular and connective tissue changes in the submucosa. Later effects comprise mucosal and submucosal atrophy and fibrosis, accompanied sometimes by similar atrophy and fibrosis of the muscularis. These changes may indeed cause intestinal and esophageal strictures or even complete obstruction.

Nervous tissue is in general relatively radioresistant, but sufficiently high doses may damage astrocytes and cause late-appearing injury to neurons (Zeman, 1968). However, functional changes may appear during the immediate postirradiation period even though no morphologic changes are visible in the neurons. Necrosis of the brain and spinal cord has been reported following high dosages of radiation, presumably due to involvement of the small blood vessels. Unlike adult nervous tissue, embryonic nerve cells and glial cells are radiosensitive, and relatively small doses in animals have caused severe damage to the developing central nervous system. Indeed, children of the Japanese survivors of the atomic bombs, exposed in utero, have shown an increased incidence of microcephaly and mental retardation (Troup, 1971).

Ultimately, all organs and cells are vulnerable to sufficiently high levels of radiant energy but those not already mentioned are relatively radioresistant, for example, the thyroid, parathyroid, pituitary and adrenal glands, the liver, mature bone and cartilage. Growing bone and cartilage are, however, relatively radiosensitive and development has been stunted in survivors of the atomic bomb who were exposed during childhood (Troup, 1971). The kidneys are moderately radiosensitive and, indeed, sometimes develop so-called radiation nephritis, following sufficient exposure.

Total Body Radiation. Exposure of large areas of the body to even very small doses of radiation may have devastating effects and, in many instances, may be lethal. Such exposure is sometimes assumed as a calculated risk in the treatment of leukemia or in the attempt to suppress immune responsiveness in patients about to receive an organ transplant. More often, the exposure is not anticipated, resulting from some reactor or nuclear weapon accident. Shielding, such as clothing, has some protective effect and was, indeed, responsible for limiting the injuries of the Marshall Islanders and others similarly exposed to accidental fallout radiation (Conard and Hicking, 1965). The effects of such radiant energy are determined by the effectiveness of the shielding, the quantity of radiation and its rate of delivery. As little as 100 rads of radiant energy in total body exposure delivered in one dose may be followed by nausea, vomiting and alterations in the peripheral blood. To place this dose level in context, it must be appreciated that doses of 4000 rads or more are often used in carefully shielded patients in the radiotherapy of tumors. Warren (1961) has provided an excellent summary of the significance of various levels of whole body exposure (Table 12–3). The lethal range for man begins at about 500 rads of total body radiation, but is quite certain at 1000 rads. In this range, exposure is followed shortly by nausea, vomiting, diarrhea, loss of appetite, fever and thirst. Bloody diarrhea may appear early. Sometimes there is an interval during which the manifestations abate only to be followed by the recurrence of fever, malaise, diarrhea, accompanied by marked depression of all circulating blood cells.

These fatal radiation syndromes have been divided into three patterns: (1) bone marrow syndrome, (2) intestinal syndrome and (3) central nervous system syndrome (Rubin and Casarett, 1968). The bone marrow syndrome, appearing at 100+ rads, is, as could be anticipated, dominated by marked depression of lymphocytes, platelets and neutrophils in the circulating blood, reflecting an aplastic bone marrow. It usually appears within three weeks to two months. In most of these cases, bleeding problems or infections precipitate death.

TABLE 12–3. LEVELS OF WHOLE BODY EXPOSURE TO RADIATION

Dosage (rads)	Effect
0.001	2½ days natural background radiation
0.01	No detectable effect
1	No detectable effect
10	Barely detectable qualitative changes in lymphocytes
100	Mild acute radiation sickness in some; slight diminution in blood cell counts; possible nausea and vomiting; possible transient reflex changes
1000	Depression of blood cell and platelet formation; damage to gastrointestinal mucosa; severe acute radiation sickness; death within 30 days
10,000	Immediate disorientation or coma; death within hours
100,000	Death of some microorganisms
1,000,000	Death of some bacteria
10,000,000	Death of all living organisms; some denaturation of proteins

From Warren, S.: The Pathology of Ionizing Radiation. Springfield, Ill., Charles C Thomas, 1961. Courtesy of Charles C Thomas, Publisher.

Currently, blood transfusion and bone marrow transplantation save many of these patients. The intestinal syndrome induced by 500 to 1000 rads is characterized by nausea, vomiting and severe diarrhea. It appears days to weeks following the exposure. Loss of fluids, electrolyte disturbances and circulatory collapse precipitate the death here. The central nervous system syndrome only appears when the exposure is at the level of 2000 to 5000 rads. But with this level of exposure, it may become clinically manifest within hours, long before any hematopoietic or intestinal symptoms appear. It is characterized by convulsions and death within hours to days, usually due to lethal damage to the neurons.

Even when the total body radiation is not fatal, late manifestations may appear in the form of irreversible aplastic anemia, cataract formation in the lens of the eye, developmental and mental defects in children and an increased incidence of leukemic, thyroid and sometimes multiple cancers in various organs (Steer, 1971) (Beebe et al., 1962). The oncogenic effects of radiation were discussed on p. 134.

It is important for the physician, in his use

of this extremely valuable diagnostic and therapeutic tool, to be aware of the injury-producing potential of radiant energy and its possible long latent effects. In few areas of medicine is the old dictim more applicable—be sure that the treatment is not more dangerous than the disease.

REFERENCES

Adelman, L. S., and Aronson, S. M.: The neuropathological complications of narcotics addiction. Bull. N.Y. Acad. Med., 45:225, 1969.

Allison, A. C., et al.: Observations on the cytotoxic action of silica on macrophages. In Davies, C. N. (ed.): Inhaled Particles and Vapors. Oxford, Pergamon Press, 1965, p. 121.

Amarose, A. P., et al.: Residual chromosomal alterations in female cancer patients after irradiation. J. Exp. Molec. Path., 7:58, 1967.

Anderson Hospital and Tumor Institute: Cellular Radiation Biology. Eighteenth Symposium on Fundamental Cancer Research, Houston, 1964. Baltimore, Williams and Wilkins Co., 1965.

Anderson, R. E.: Leukemic and related disorders. Hum. Path., 2:515, 1971.

Anjilvel, L., and Thurlbeck, W. M.: The incidence of asbestos bodies in the lungs at random necropsies in Montreal. Canad. Med. Ass. J., 95:1179, 1966.

Bacq, Z. M., and Alexander, P.: Fundamentals of Radiobiology. New York, Pergamon Press, 1961.

Baden, M. M.: Narcotic abuse: a medical examiner's view. In Wecht, C. H. (ed.): Legal Medicine Annual. New York, Appleton-Century-Crofts, 1971.

Bainborough, A. R., and Jericho, K. W. F.: Cor pulmonale secondary to talc granuloma in the lungs of a drug addict. Canad. Med. Ass. J., 103:1297, 1970.

Baker, A. B.: Histologic changes in the brains of dogs after long-term barbiturate intoxication. Arch. Path., 70:208, 1960.

Beebe, G. W., et al.: Studies of the mortality of A bomb survivors. Radiat. Res., 16:253, 1962.

Bell, D.: Analgesic nephropathy: clinical course after withdrawal of phenacetin. Brit. Med. J., 3:378, 1969.

Belleau, R., and Gaensler, E. A.: Mesothelioma and asbestosis. Respiration, 25:67, 1968.

Bidstrup, P. L.: Toxicity of Mercury and its Compounds. Amsterdam, Elsevier Publishing Co., 1964.

Bleumle, L. W., and Goldberg, M.: Renal accumulation of salicylate and phenacetin: possible mechanisms in the nephropathy of analgesic abuse. J. Clin. Invest., 47:2507, 1968.

Brill, A. B., et al.: Leukemia in man following exposure to ionizing radiation. A summary of the findings in Hiroshima and Nagasaki and a comparison with other human experience. Ann. Intern. Med., 56:590, 1962.

Brunner, M. J.: Pulmonary disease and hair spray polymers: a disputed relationship. J.A.M.A., 184:851, 1963.

Cade, S.: Radiation induced cancer in man. Brit. J. Radiol., 30:393, 1957.

Campbell, A. M. G., and Williams, E. R.: Chronic lead intoxication mimicking motor neuron disease. Brit. Med. J., 5:582, 1968.

Cannon, A. G.: Chronic arsenical poisoning. New York J. Med., 36:219, 1936.

Cherubin, C. E.: The medical sequelae of narcotic addiction. Ann. Intern. Med., 67:23, 1967.

Citron, B. P., et al.: Necrotizing angiitis in drug addicts. New Eng. J. Med., 283:1003, 1970.

Conard, R. A., and Hicking, A.: Medical findings in Marshallese people exposed to fallout radiation. J.A.M.A., 192:457, 1965.

Dalgaard, J. B.: Post-mortem findings in carbon monoxide deaths. Acta Path. Microbiol. Scand., Suppl., 154:186, 1962.

Deichman, W. B., et al.: The hematopoietic tissue toxicity of benzene vapors. Toxic. Appl. Pharmacol., 5:201, 1963.

Dutra, F. R.: Cerebral residua of acute carbon monoxide poisoning. Amer. J. Clin. Path., 22:925, 1952.

Edland, J. F.: Liver disease in heroin addicts. Hum. Path., 2:75, 1972.

Epstein, S. S.: Environmental pathology. Amer. J. Path., 66:352, 1972.

Freiman, D. G., and Hardy, H. L.: Beryllium disease. The relation of pulmonary pathology to clinical course and prognosis based on a study of 130 cases from the U.S. Beryllium Case Registry. Hum. Path., 1:25, 1970.

Friedman, N. B.: The pathology of trench foot. Amer. J. Path., 21:387, 1945.

Friedman, N. B., and Kritzler, R. A.: The pathology of high altitude frostbite. Amer. J. Path., 23:173, 1947.

Froede, R.: Drugs of abuse: legal and illegal. Hum. Path., 3:23, 1972.

Gettler, A. O., and St. George, A. V.: Cyanide poisoning. Amer. J. Clin. Path., 4:429, 1934.

Ghidoni, J. J.: Light and electron microscopic study of primate liver 36–48 hours after high doses of 32 million electronvolt protons. Lab. Invest., 16:268, 1967.

Goyer, R. A.: Lead toxicity: a problem in environmental pathology. Amer. J. Path., 64:167, 1971.

Goyer, R. A., and Krall, R. C.: Ultrastructural transformation in mitochondria isolated from kidneys of normal and lead intoxicated rats. J. Cell Biol., 41:393, 1969.

Green, G. M.: In defense of the lung. Amer. Rev. Resp. Dis., 102:691, 1970

Grenn, G. M., and Carolin, D.: The depressant effect of cigarette smoke on the in vitro antibacterial activity of alveolar macrophages. New Eng. J. Med., 276:422, 1967.

Gritzka, T. L., and Trump, B. F.: Renal tubular lesions caused by mercuric chloride. Electron microscopic observations: degeneration of the pars recta. Amer. J. Path., 52:1225, 1968.

Gross, P., et al.: Pulmonary ferriginous bodies in city dwellers. Arch. Environ. Health, 19:186, 1969.

Hardy, H. L.: Beryllium disease: a continuing diagnostic problem. Amer. J. Med. Sci., 242:150, 1961.

Helpern, M.: Angiitis in drug abusers. New Eng. J. Med., 284:113, 1971.

Hollingsworth, J. W.: Delayed radiation effects in survivors of the atomic bombings. A summary of the findings of the atomic bomb casualty commission. 1947–59. New Eng. J. Med., 263:481, 1960.

Hopkins, G. B., and Taylor, D. E.: Pulmonary talc granulomatosis. Amer. Rev. Resp. Dis., 101:101, 1970.

Horning, E. S.: Cytopathological studies of morphine poisoning and chronic morphinism in the albino rat with reference to subsequent lecithin treatment. Amer. J. Path., 10:219, 1934.

Hutchinson, F.: The molecular basis for radiation effects on cells. Cancer Res., 26:2045, 1966.

Ishikawa, S., et al.: The "emphysema profile" in two midwestern cities in North America. Arch. Environ. Health, 18:660, 1969.

Kaplan, K.: Methyl alcohol poisoning. Amer. J. Med. Sci., 244:170, 1962.

Kark, R. A. P., et al.: Mercury poisoning and its treatment with n-acetyl-d, 1-penicillamine. New Eng. J. Med., 285:10, 1971.

Karliner, J. S., et al.: Lung function after pulmonary edema associated with heroin overdose. Arch. Intern. Med., 124:350, 1969.

Keeney, A. H., and Mellinkoff, S. M.: Methyl alcohol poisoning. Ann. Intern. Med., 34:331, 1951.

Key, C. R.: Studies of the acute effects of the atomic bombs. Hum. Path., 2:475, 1971.

Kotin, P.: Pathology of environmentally induced diseases. Amer. J. Path., 64:165, 1971.

Lea, D. E.: Actions of Radiations on Living Cells. Cambridge, Mass., Cambridge University Press, 1962.

Lignelli, G., and Buchheit, W. A.: Angiitis in drug abusers. New Eng. J. Med., 284:112, 1971.

Louria, D. B., et al.: The major medical complications of heroin addiction. Ann. Intern. Med., 67:1, 1967.

McCarthy, M. A.: Selected types of poisoning as causes of accidental death, U.S., 1964. Public Health Rep., 82:1025, 1967.

McDonald, A. D., et al.: Epidemiology of primary malignant mesothelial tumors in Canada. Cancer, 26:914, 1970.

Mallory, T. B., et al.: Chronic exposure to benzene (benzol): the pathologic results. J. Indust. Hyg. Toxic., 21:355, 1939.

Mello, N. K., and Mendelson, J. H.: Experimentally induced intoxication in alcoholics: a comparison between programmed and spontaneous drinking. J. Pharmacol. Exp. Ther., 173:101, 1970.

Mendelson, J. H.: Biologic concomitants of alcoholism. New Eng. J. Med., *283*:24, 71, 1970.

Mendelson, J. H.: Ethanol-1-C^{14} metabolism in alcoholics and nonalcoholics. Science, *159*:319, 1968.

Murphy, R. L. H., Jr., et al.: Effects of low concentrations of asbestos: chemical, environmental, radiologic and epidemiologic observations in shipyard pipe coverers and controls. New Eng. J. Med., *285*:1271, 1971.

Murray, R. M., et al.: Analgesic nephropathy: clinical syndrome and prognosis. Brit. Med. J., *1*:479, 1971.

Nabas, G. G.: Cannabis arteritis. New Eng. J. Med., *284*:113, 1971.

Naeye, R. L.: Pulmonary disease in Appalachian soft coal workers. Amer. J. Path., *59*:104a, 1970.

Newman, H. W.: Acquired tolerance to ethyl alcohol. Quart. J. Stud. Alcohol, *2*:453, 1941.

Nicholls, P. J., et al.: Histamine release by compound 48/80 and textile dusts from lung tissue in vitro. In Davies, C. N. (ed.): Inhaled Particles and Vapours. Vol. 2. Oxford, Pergamon Press, 1967, p. 69.

Oliver, J., et al.: Cellular mechanism of protein metabolism in the newborn. I. The structural aspects of proteinuria, tubular absorption, droplet formation and the disposal of proteins. J. Exp. Med., *99*:589, 1954.

Polson, C. J., and Tattersall, R. N.: Clinical Toxicology. Philadelphia, J. B. Lippincott Co., 1969, p. 578.

Rosen, L.: Relevance of particle accelerators to national goals. Science, *173*:490, 1971.

Rothschild, E. O.: Lead poisoning: the silent epidemic. New Eng. J. Med., *283*:704, 1970.

Rubin, E., and Lieber, C. S.: Alcoholism, alcohol and drugs. Science, *172*:1097, 1971.

Rubin, P., and Casarett, G. W.: Clinical Radiation Pathology. Philadelphia, W. B. Saunders Co., 1968, pp. 850, 894 and 903.

Rugh, R.: Damage to cells by ionizing radiation. Atompraxis, *14*:13, 1968.

Russell, W. L., et al.: Radiation dose rate and mutation frequency. Science, *128*:1546, 1958.

Scheel, L. D., et al.: Toxicity of silica. II. Characteristics of protein films adsorbed by quartz. Arch. Indust. Hyg., *9*:29, 1954.

Seal, R. M. E., et al.: The pathology of acute and chronic stages of farmer's lung. Thorax, *23*:469, 1968.

Siegel, H.: Human pulmonary pathology associated with narcotic and other addictive drugs. Hum. Path., *2*:55, 1972.

Solitare, G. B.: Neuropathologic aspects of drug dependency (narcotic addiction). Hum. Path., *2*:85, 1972.

Spencer, H.: Pathology of the Lung. Oxford and London, Pergamon Press, 1968, p. 376.

Steer, A.: Symposium: the delayed consequences of exposure to ionizing radiation. Pathology studies at the Atomic Bomb Casualty Commission, Hiroshima and Nagasaki, 1945–1970—"Other tumors." Hum. Path., *2*:541, 1971.

Stewart, R. D., et al.: Diagnosis of solvent poisoning. J.A.M.A., *193*:115, 1965.

Takeuchi, P., et al.: A pathological study of Minamata disease in Japan. Acta Neuropath. (Berlin), *2*:40, 1962.

Telischi, M., and Rubenstone, H. I.: Pulmonary asbestosis. Arch. Path., *27*:234, 1961.

Teplitz, C.: Pathology of burns. In Artz, C. P., and Moncrief, J. A. (eds.): Treatment of Burns. 2nd ed. Philadelphia, W. B. Saunders Co., 1969.

Tessmer, C. F.: Radiation effects in skin. In Berdjis, C. C. (ed.): Pathology of Irradiation. Baltimore, Williams and Wilkins Co., 1971, p. 146.

Troen, P., et al.: Mercuric chloride poisoning. New Eng. J. Med., *244*:459, 1951.

Troup, G. M.: Symposium: the delayed consequences of exposure to ionizing radiation. Pathology studies at the Atomic Bomb Casualty Commission, Hiroshima and Nagasaki, 1945–1970. II. Growth and development. Hum. Path., *2*:493, 1971.

Tsinga, E., and Casarett, G. W.: Mitochondria and radiation sensitivity of cells. U.S. Atomic Energy Commission Report UR-666, 1965.

U.S. Public Health Service: Symposium on environmental lead contamination. Publication No. 1440, March, 1966.

Warren, S.: The Pathology of Ionizing Radiation. Springfield, Ill., Charles C Thomas, 1961.

Werner, A.: Near fatal hyperacute reaction to intravenously administered heroin. J.A.M.A., *207*:2277, 1969.

Wright, A. W.: General pathology and some special complications of alcoholism. Arch. Path., *32*:670, 1941.

Wyatt, J. P.: Occupational lung diseases and inferential relationships to general population hazards. Amer. J. Path., *64*:197, 1971.

Zeman, W.: Introduction to neuropathology related to physical forces. In Minckler, J (ed.): Pathology of the Nervous System. Vol. 1. New York, McGraw-Hill, 1968, p. 862.

13

DISEASES OF INFANCY AND CHILDHOOD

Children are not merely "little people" nor are their disorders merely variants of the diseases of adult life. The single most hazardous time of life is unquestionably the neonatal period. Never again is the individual confronted with more dramatic challenges than in the transition from dependent intrauterine existence to independent postnatal life. From the moment the umbilical cord is severed, the circulation through the heart is radically rerouted. Respiratory function must take over the role of oxygenation of the blood. Maintenance of body temperature and other homeostatic constants must now be borne alone by the fledgling organism. Most of the disorders of the neonatal period (first four weeks of life) and the first year of life are encountered only in the young, and others, only in newborns; and so, justifiably, pediatrics and pediatric pathology have become specialties unto themselves.

SURVEY OF PEDIATRIC DISEASES

It is difficult to believe that in the United States in 1967, considering all ages from birth to senility, "certain diseases of early infancy" comprise the fifth leading cause of death, superseded only by cardiovascular disease, cancer, accidents and pulmonary infections, in that order. The causes of death in the first year

of life are listed in Table 13–1. This table further indicates that "certain diseases of early infancy," which embrace a heterogeny of conditions, account for over half of all deaths in those under the age of one. Paradoxically, over the course of years, with improvement in the medical care of the mother and child, congenital malformations and postnatal asphyxia have risen in importance as causes of death. Years ago, many of these newborns would have represented intrauterine fetal deaths or stillborns. The precipitous drop in the total death rate from all causes (2067) in the first year of life to 71 in the age group 1 to 4 years documents the hazards of the early days of life. Indeed, the mortality rate for the second to 12th month of the first year of life is less than half that for the first month alone. Attention should also be drawn to the category "other accidents" (not related to motor vehicles), a tragic wastage of life and potential. The data given apply to a so-called "economically privileged" society. In other areas such as regions of Asia, Africa, India and South America, the prime causes of infant and childhood mortality in the twentieth century are still infectious (including parasitic) and nutritional disorders, a commentary on our so-called civilization. With this overview, we can now consider some of the specific pediatric disorders.

TABLE 13–1. CAUSES OF DEATH IN INFANCY AND CHILDHOOD*

Causes	Under 1 year	1–4 years	5–14 years
Total deaths	2067	71.1	37.5
Certain diseases of early infancy	1364	0.1	0.0
Immaturity	374		
Postnatal asphyxia and atelectasis	363		
Ill-defined diseases peculiar to early infancy, including nutritional maladjustment	290		
Birth injuries	186		
Pneumonia of newborn	63		
Hemolytic disease of newborn	34		
Hemorrhagic disease of newborn	15		
Other diseases	39		
Congenital malformations	329	10	2
Respiratory infections	204	12	2
Gastritis, duodenitis, enteritis and colitis, except diarrhea of newborn	29	2	0.2
Meningitis and meningococcal infections	24	3	0.5
Other infective and parasitic diseases	18	2	0.8
Major cardiovascular-renal diseases	16	2	7
Malignant neoplasms including neoplasms of lymphatic and hematopoietic tissues	6	8	7
Motor vehicle accidents	9	11	9
Other accidents	68	21	9

Rates per 100,000 population in specified group.

*Adapted from Vital Statistics of the United States, 1967. Vol. II. Mortality, Part A. U.S. Dept. of H.E.W. Public Service and Mental Health Administration. National Center for Health Statistics.

PREMATURITY

Prematurity is difficult to define in precise terms. It might be supposed that the premature infant is one born prior to full term when the period of gestation is known. However, many full-term infants suffer from nutritional and other disturbances and are extremely small and immature, with the same constitutional inadequacies as the infant born prior to term. The most useful definition, then, is: *infants are considered premature when they weigh at birth less than 2500 gm. (5 pounds 8 ounces) irrespective of the length of the gestation.* The mortality rate in this group of low-birth-weight infants is exceedingly high. It has been estimated that about 90 per cent of the infant mortality in the United States occurs in the less than 10 per cent of infants born with birth weights of less than 2500 gms. Even the survivors in about one-third of the instances have significant intellectual and motor handicaps.

At one time, deaths in the low-birth-weight group were usually attributed to prematurity or immaturity. Currently, with better methods of managing such disadvantaged infants, immaturity is not considered a justifiable cause of death in infants weighing more than 1000 gm. at birth. "Death due to prematurity" is justified for those having birth weights of 500 gm. or less because here the physiologic and anatomic immaturity is so extreme as to be incapable of sustaining independent life. Those in the 500 to 1000 gm. range of birth weights have a chance of surviving but have serious handicaps. Respiratory motions are feeble, and so expansion of the lungs is incomplete. Hypoxia, respiratory distress and secondary pulmonary infections account for a large fraction of the deaths in this group. Intracranial hemorrhages, particularly intraventricular hemorrhages, are additional important causes of death in the low-birth-weight group. The skull in the premature lacks the rigidity of the fully developed skull; the brain substance is incompletely developed and has little innate structural strength—both predisposing to traumatic rupture of delicate vessels at the time of birth.

The indiscriminate use of the term prematurity as a cause of death obscures the important concept that in many instances specific, remediable causes underlie the fatalities among these vulnerable infants. Infections, hypoxia (whatever the cause) and fluid and electrolyte imbalances, to name only a few of the once often fatal disturbances, are now readily controlled in most instances. Similarly, many of the specific neonatal diseases, formerly frequently fatal, have been brought at least partially under control. And so the ill premature infant who weighs over 1000 gm. may be restored to health with appropriate diagnosis and treatment. Nonetheless, since prematurity causes the death of very low-weight infants and significantly biases the probable outcome of others, it is appropriate to consider the features of immaturity of the more vital organs.

IMMATURITY OF THE LUNGS

During the first half of fetal life, the development of the lungs consists essentially of the formation of a system of branching tubes from the foregut that eventually give rise to the trachea, bronchi and bronchioles. The alveoli only begin to differentiate at approximately the seventh month of gestation. They are at first imperfectly formed, with thick walls and large amounts of inter- and intralobular connective tissue. The vascularization is buried within this connective tissue and is not in immediate contact with the alveolar spaces (Fig. 13–1). The alveolar lining epithelium at this time is cuboidal and not anatomically suited to effecting the rapid transfer of oxygen to the blood. Progressive maturation of the lungs produces thinning of the alveolar lining cells, expansion of the alveolar spaces and disap-

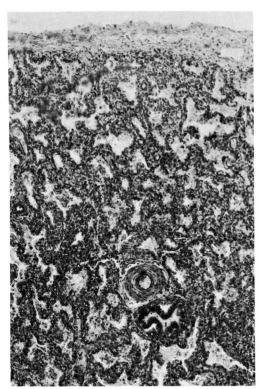

Figure 13–1. *Immaturity of the lung from a six-month fetus. The septa are thick and cellular and the alveolar spaces are small.*

pearance of the abundant interalveolar mesenchyme. With these changes, the alveolar capillaries come into intimate contact with alveolar spaces. However, even at full term, the alveoli are small, the septa are considerably thicker than in the adult, and the connective tissue stroma enclosing the alveolar capillaries is more abundant than in later life.

In the stillborn infant, then, the lungs are grossly unexpanded, red and meaty, and usually sink when immersed in water. The alveolar spaces are incompletely expanded and usually contain pink proteinous precipitate and amniotic debris.

This native histologic pattern is rarely encountered in the premature live-born since respiration, artificial resuscitation and abnormal respiratory efforts all modify the original state. Respiration dilates the alveoli, and abnormal respiratory efforts may cause marked distention of scattered alveoli. Many of the alveoli may be filled with amniotic fluid and its contents, i.e., squamous epithelial cells, lanugo hairs, mucus and proteinous debris. The significance of this fluid in the lungs of the newborn is controversial and will be discussed more fully later (p. 553). These lungs may float when immersed in water, but this test is not in-

fallible. Despite the fact that infants may have breathed prior to death, the very weak respiratory muscles and shallow respiration with little exchange of air or resorption of the contained air may cause the lungs to sink when placed in water. Contrariwise, bacterial growth may produce gas that will create buoyancy in the lungs. The "floating test" is, therefore, not a critical index of postnatal respiration.

The immature lung, then, is poorly suited to carry out ventilatory function and is furthermore extremely vulnerable to superimposed infections. Respiratory distress and hypoxia are, therefore, the most common mechanisms of death in low-weight premature infants.

IMMATURITY OF THE KIDNEYS

In addition to immaturity of the lungs, the premature infant will also have incomplete development of the kidneys. Grossly, fetal lobulations are usually readily visible on the cortical surface. The most striking changes are found on histologic examination of the subcapsular glomeruli. These structures have an organoid, glandular appearance imparted by persistence of cuboidal cells in the parietal and visceral layers of Bowman's capsule (Fig. 13–2). The abundance of these cells frequently

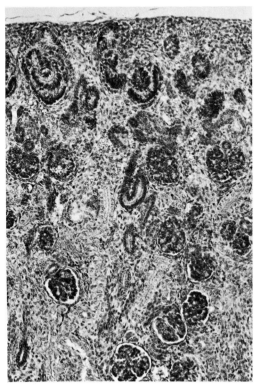

Figure 13–2. *Immaturity of the glomeruli. The epithelium of Bowman's capsule is cuboidal and masks the underlying vascular tuft.*

masks the underlying vascularization of the glomerulus. Despite the underdevelopment of these subcapsular glomeruli, the deeper glomeruli may be well formed with thin pavement epithelial cells and, in the premature infant, renal function is usually adequate to permit survival.

IMMATURITY OF THE BRAIN

The brain is also incompletely developed in the premature. The surface is relatively smooth and devoid of the typical convolutions found in the cerebral hemispheres of the adult. The brain substance is soft, gelatinous and easily torn, and the definition between white and gray matter is somewhat ill defined. This lack of separation is in large part attributable to poorly developed myelination of the nerve fibers. Notwithstanding this underdevelopment, to the best of our present knowledge, the vital brain centers are sufficiently developed even in the very premature infant to sustain normal central nervous system function. However, the homeostasis is not perfect, and the premature has difficulty in maintaining a constant normal level of temperature and has poor vasomotor control, irregular respirations, muscular inertia and feeble sweating. None of these difficulties is incompatible with survival.

IMMATURITY OF THE GASTROINTESTINAL TRACT

The premature infant displays some digestive disturbances, particularly in the handling of fats. On this account, deficiencies of the fat-soluble vitamins are occasionally encountered. These digestive disturbances are entirely functional and temporary, and the gastrointestinal tract is usually anatomically normal and apparently well developed.

IMMATURITY OF THE LIVER

The liver, although large relative to the size of the premature infant, suffers from lack of physiologic maturity. Some of this increase in size is due to persistence of extramedullary hematopoiesis in this organ. Many or most of the functions of the liver are marginally adequate to carry out the demands placed upon them. Almost all newborns and particularly those with low birth weight have a transient period of physiologic jaundice within the first postnatal week. This jaundice stems from both breakdown of fetal red cells and inadequacy of the biliary excretory function of liver cells. Deficiencies of bilirubin glycuronyl transferase, hydroxylating enzymes, protein synthetic capacity, to name only a few hepatic systems, all characterize the immature liver.

APGAR SCORE

The Apgar score devised by Dr. Virginia Apgar represents a clinically useful method of evaluating the physiologic condition and responsiveness of the newborn infant and hence its chances of survival. Table 13–2 indicates the five parameters to be scored and how they are quantitated (Apgar, 1953). The newborn infant may be evaluated at 1 minute or at 5 minutes. A total score of 10 indicates an infant in the best possible condition. The correlation between the Apgar score and the mortality during the first 28 days of life is very impressive. Infants with a 5-minute Apgar score of 0 to 1 have a 50 per cent mortality within the first month of life. This drops to 20 per cent with a score of 4 and to almost 0 per cent when the score is 7 or better (Drage and Berendes, 1966). The birth weight significantly modifies the Apgar score, as would be expected, and the outlook for survival. When infants having scores between 0 and 3 were segregated into groups based on birth weight, the following

TABLE 13–2. EVALUATION OF THE NEWBORN INFANT

Sign	0	1	2
Heart rate	Absent	Below 100	Over 100
Respiratory effort	Absent	Slow, irregular	Good, crying
Muscle tone	Limp	Some flexion of extremities	Active motion
Response to catheter in nostril (tested after oropharynx is clear)	No response	Grimace	Cough or sneeze
Color	Blue, pale	Body pink, extremities blue	Completely pink

Sixty seconds after the complete birth of the infant (disregarding the cord and placenta) the five objective signs above are evaluated and each is given a score of 0, 1 or 2. A total score of 10 indicates an infant in the best possible condition.

Modified from Virginia Apgar: A proposal for a new method of evaluation of the newborn infant. Cur. Res. Anesth. Analg., *32*:260, 1953.

results were obtained: with a birth weight of under 2001 gm., the mortality within the first 28 days of life was almost 80 per cent; with a birth weight of between 2001 and 2500 gm. the mortality rate was 30 per cent; and with a birth weight of 2501 gm. and over, the mortality rate was 15 per cent.

BIRTH INJURIES

Birth injuries constitute an important cause of death in the premature and full-term infant as well as in children during the first year of life. These injuries may affect any part or any region of the body, but most commonly involve the head, skeletal system, liver, adrenals and peripheral nerves. Considering the violent expulsive forces to which the fragile fetus is exposed, it is quite surprising that birth injuries are so relatively uncommon. It is important to stress that while some birth injuries are avoidable, even with optimal obstetric care, some are unavoidable. If the process of birth were not laborious to mother and infant, why would it have been termed "labor?"

HEAD

Caput succedaneum and *cephalhematoma* are so common even in normal uncomplicated births as to hardly merit the designation of birth injury. When the head is the presenting part, some portion of the scalp is exposed in the progressively dilating cervical os. As the fetus is subjected to the compressive forces of labor, fluid tends to accumulate in the small area of the scalp that presents in the cervical os and is not exposed to the increased uterine pressures. *The progressive accumulation of interstitial fluid in the soft tissues of the scalp gives rise to a usually circular area of edema, congestion and swelling called a caput succedaneum.* When the presenting part of the fetus is not the head, similar edema may involve whatever region presents in the cervical os, so that the swelling may occur on the buttocks in a breech presentation or on the face in a face presentation.

Hemorrhage may occur into these areas of edema and, when it involves the scalp, produces a cephalhematoma. Usually the blood accumulates between the outer table of the calvarial bone and the pericranial or periosteal membrane. The swelling does not cross the cranial sutures and is therefore distinct from a caput succedaneum, which occurs more superficially in the soft tissues of the scalp. Both forms of injury are of little clinical significance and are only of importance insofar as they must be differentiated from skull fractures with attendant hemorrhage and edema. In approximately 25 per cent of cephalhematomas, there is an underlying skull fracture.

The skull bones may be fractured or may override each other, particularly when there is some disturbance in the ordinary mechanism of labor. Precipitate or sudden delivery with incomplete molding of the head, overenthusiastic use of forceps, and prolonged intense labor with disproportion between the size of the fetal head and birth canal are some of the common circumstances that surround the occurrence of these skull injuries. Most often the fractures are linear, cause no symptoms and require no treatment. Depressed fractures (buckling inward of an area) are more serious and require correction.

Intracranial hemorrhage is probably the most common important birth injury. These hemorrhages are generally thought to be related to excessive molding of the head or sudden pressure changes in its shape as it is subject to the pressure of forceps or sudden precipitate expulsion. Prolonged labor, anoxia, hemorrhagic disorders or an intracranial vascular anomaly are important predispositions. The hemorrhage may arise in tears in the dura, particularly in the falx cerebri and tentorium cerebelli; the dural sinuses may be stretched beyond their elastic limit and rupture; the substance of the brain may be torn or bruised leading to intraventricular hemorrhages or bleeding into the brain substance; or vessels that traverse the subdural space may be ruptured. Whatever their origin, intracranial hemorrhages are of great importance, since they cause sudden increases in intracranial pressure, damage to the brain substance, herniation of the medulla or base of the brain into the foramen magnum and serious, frequently fatal, depression of function of the vital medullary centers.

SKELETAL SYSTEM

The bones most frequently fractured at birth are the clavicles and the long bones of the extremities. These injuries are usually readily recognized soon after birth and are amenable to surgical correction without significant sequelae.

LIVER

In the infant, the disproportionately large liver is vulnerable to abnormal stresses placed upon the abdomen, particularly during delivery of the head in breech presentations. Rupture of the liver may cause serious, sometimes fatal, intraperitoneal hemorrhage. Fortunately, this type of injury is uncommon.

ADRENALS

Hemorrhage into the medulla of the adrenals is a not uncommon finding in stillborns and premature infants dying soon after birth. Presumably, the sources of this hemorrhage are the relatively large, thin-walled venous sinuses of the medulla of the gland. The basic factors that initiate such hemorrhage are still obscure. Hypoxia with direct injury to the thin-walled medullary sinusoids and trauma over the adrenals have been assumed to be most important. Not infrequently, petechial hemorrhages in the serosal membranes of the body cavities accompany the adrenal hemorrhages, further implicating systemic hypoxia.

CONGENITAL MALFORMATIONS

Congenital malformations may be described as gross structural defects present at birth. There has been some difficulty with the interpretation of the term "structural." To some it has implied malformations visible to the naked eye or recognzed by conventional clinical instruments. To others it has also included microscopic changes as well as metabolic defects such as are seen in the inborn errors of metabolism. Here the term is used in the limited sense of teratologic abnormalities in structure on a gross morphologic level. In various surveys, the incidence of congenital malformations in live-born infants ranges from about 1 to 3 per cent (Ivy, 1957) (Stevenson et al., 1950).

In a real sense, malformations found in live-born infants represent the less serious developmental failures in embryogenesis since they are compatible with live birth. It has been estimated that perhaps 20 per cent of fertilized ova are blighted from the outset. Less severe anomalies that are still incompatible with fetal survival terminate in spontaneous abortion. Chromosomal abnormalities have been identified in from 2 to 45 per cent of such abortuses (the mean being approximately 20 per cent) (World Health Organization, 1970). As one descends the scale of severity of anomalies, a level is reached which permits more prolonged intrauterine survival, but often then causes stillbirth, or possibly permits live-birth despite the handicaps imposed by the anomaly.

It is ironic that comparisons of old and new statistics suggest that congenital malformations have become more frequent recently (McIntosh et al., 1954) (Malpas, 1937). This increase could be due to the elimination of other fatal diseases imparting greater importance to congenital malformations or possibly to better diagnostic procedures that uncover more of these anomalies. There is a strong likelihood, however, that better prenatal care and nutrition permit survival to birth of infants who formerly might have died in utero. Whatever the reason, congenital malformations constitute major causes of mortality in infants under one year of age as is indicated in the table on p. 547.

These teratologic defects take many diverse forms, and some will be mentioned in the discussion of their causation (Fig. 13–3). It is neither feasible nor necessary to describe each since the more important are presented in the chapters concerned with disorders of individual organs and systems. It suffices here to say that every organ and tissue in the body has, at one time or another, been the site of a developmental failure.

Pathogenesis.   The causation of congenital malformations is a subject of intense interest particularly to parents who have borne one malformed child. The question always arises: Does the developmental failure represent a hereditary trait likely to effect subsequent offspring? Although it is frequently impossible to answer such a question, a few facts are known: *Malformations can be divided into four categories (1) those associated with chromosomal aberrations, (2) those arising in gene mutations, (3) those which are non-genetic and result from teratologic environmental factors and (4) a group resulting from a combination of both genetic and environmental influences.*

The subject of chromosomal aberrations and their possible causes was discussed previously in the chapter on genetics (p. 174). There it was pointed out that a number of well defined developmental syndromes arise in karyotypic aberrations involving the autosomes (Down's syndrome or trisomy 22, Ed-

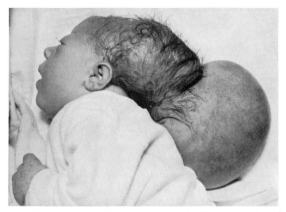

Figure 13–3.   *Meningomyelocele. A common form of malformation caused by incomplete closure of the vertebral column and herniation of the dura and cord substance.*

wards' syndrome or trisomy 18, and Patau's syndrome or trisomy 13). Aberrations of the sex chromosomes are also responsible for malformations as in the Klinefelter's, Turner's and intersex syndromes. The autosomal aberrations result in far more devastating malformations than those which are sex-linked. Congenital malformations other than these have been reported in association with chromosomal abnormalities. The great preponderance of these anomalies associated with visible changes in the karyotype arise as defects in gametogenesis and so are not familial. Subsequent siblings are not likely to suffer a similar fate. There are, however, rare forms of isolated teratologic defects related to transmissible chromosomal abnormalities and, of course, these are passed from one generation to the next, constituting familial disorders.

Malformations associated with gene mutations abound. Those related to dominant genes include achondroplasia, multiple exostoses, osteogenesis imperfecta, polydactyly, syndactyly (fusion or webbing of fingers or toes), arachnodactyly (spider-like fingers as in Marfan's syndrome), and facial clefts. Malformations related to recessive modes of inheritance include some forms of infantile polycystic kidneys, anomalies associated with the storage diseases (p. 295), and the Laurence-Moon-Biedl syndrome. Some malformations have variable modes of inheritance, e.g., dominant in some families, recessive in others and sex-linked in still others. Into this category fall a large array of malformations involving the digits such as brachydactyly, polydactyly and syndactyly. *Almost all of these developmental failures associated with gene mutations are hereditary and are therefore familial* (Warkany and Kalter, 1961).

The subject of environmental teratogens must be approached cautiously. It has been exceedingly difficult to determine whether environmental influences such as viral infections, drugs and radiation to which the mother may have been exposed during pregnancy lead to developmental failures by inducing alterations in the genome of the gametes or zygote or by epigenetic mechanisms in the micro-environment of the fertilized ovum or early embryo. Notwithstanding, certain influences are believed to exert their effect without altering the genome. *Best established as an environmental cause of congenital malformations is rubella infection during pregnancy.* The usual associated malformations consist of cardiac defects, deformities of the eye (especially cataract), microcephaly with deafness, mental retardation as well as dental defects. The likelihood of such mal-

formation and the severity of the teratologic changes vary according to the time of the maternal infection. Defective liveborn children are encountered in 23.4 per cent of pregnancies when rubella is contracted in the first month of pregnancy, 21.3 per cent in the second month and 10.4 per cent in the third month. Infections in the last two trimesters of pregnancy do not apparently damage the fetus (Siegel and Greenberg, 1960). The significance of the timing of the infection is not only quantitative but qualitative as well. Heart and eye defects predominate when rubella occurs in the first or second months and hearing defects when rubella is contracted in the second and third months of pregnancy (Swan and Tostevin, 1946). Karyotypic abnormalities have not been demonstrated in the leukocytes of these malformed children, but this of course does not exclude the possibility of gene mutation—a possibility that is not given serious credence at the present time. The recognition that rubella produces congenital malformations aroused great interest in other infectious diseases during pregnancy. The collective evidence indicates that no etiologic importance can be ascribed to mumps, chickenpox and poliomyelitis, but some suspicion remains with measles and cytomegalic inclusion disease.

The role of drugs or chemicals as teratogens involves again the issue of whether they act as environmental influences or mutagens. The best evidence for environmental action derives from the well documented association between cretinism (p. 1324) in the infant and iodine deficiency in the pregnant mother. Malformed infants born of mothers who had taken thalidomide during pregnancy further document the effect of environment on embryogenesis. No karyotypic alterations have been identified in these infants born with so-called "seal" extremities (phocomelia). But once again, gene mutations cannot be totally excluded. Similarly, radiation, a well known mutagen, may act by direct damage to cells without altering their genetic apparatus. In the studies of infants born after their mothers had been exposed to the atomic bombs, malformations such as microcephaly and anomalies of the central nervous system were encountered in the absence of evidence of genetic damage (Neel and Schull, 1956).

Some congenital malformations are the consequence of both genetic and environmental influences. Into this category fall such anomalies as cleft lip, cleft palate, club foot, congenital dislocation of the hip, hypertrophic pyloric stenosis, anencephaly, spina bifida and renal aplasia.

After considering all of these possible causations of teratology, we must recognize that some structural defects arise mysteriously, making it clear that much is still unknown. Cases are on record of monozygotic twins of whom only one has congenital defects. Theoretically, such twins are identical in genetic endowment and were exposed to the same environmental influences, but variation in vascular supply to the embryo, mechanical factors in utero, slight differences in intrauterine position or other changes in the immediate environment of the developing embryo may have contributed to the malformation. It is important, in closing, to stress that malformations generally occur multiply. The finding of one should raise suspicion of the existence of others that are possibly visceral and not immediately apparent. The infant born with extra digits may well have mental retardation and other abnormalities comprising the Laurence-Moon-Biedl syndrome. But it must be cautioned that polydactylism may occur as the sole anomaly. Congenital malformations, then, may be sporadic or familial, trivial or fatal, important clues to other abnormalities or solitary defects.

RESPIRATORY DISTRESS SYNDROME IN THE NEWBORN

The most common and most urgent emergency in the delivery room is respiratory distress in the newborn. It may be the consequence of central nervous system failure, inadequacy of the function of the muscles of respiration, or may be due to anomalies of the lungs. All of these problems may coexist, as in the premature infant, and one may lead to the other. Similarly, the full-term infant who suffers brain injury during birth, with damage to the respiratory centers, suffers from inadequate respiration and incomplete expansion of the pulmonary alveoli. Here our attention is focused on the pulmonary lesions underlying the respiratory distress syndrome, particularly aspiration of amniotic contents, atelectasis neonatorum, hyaline membrane disease and congenital alveolar dysplasia. It may be very difficult to distinguish among these syndromes clinically, but each has distinctive morphologic features which will be described.

ASPIRATION OF AMNIOTIC CONTENTS

Many premature and full-term infants die an asphyxial death and, at autopsy, disclose large amounts of amniotic contents in the air spaces of their lungs (Farber and Sweet, 1931). While there is still doubt, it is generally be-

lieved that respiratory movements begin early in gestation, probably during the first trimester of pregnancy. These movements, at first somewhat intermittent and irregular, become more regular by the time of birth. There is still no agreement whether the alveoli are thus filled with amniotic fluid or whether this activity produces a mere tidal flow within the trachea and bronchi. However, since the respiratory passages are completely open, it is reasonable to assume that the alveoli must contain some fluid during intrauterine existence. Possibly some of it is a transudate from the blood but, in all probability, it is mixed with amniotic contents. Since in the full-term infant dying of other causes within the first few days of life, the lungs do not contain large amounts of amniotic debris, it can be argued that this foreign material within the alveoli must be either resorbed or expelled at birth. When, however, the birth has been associated with some asphyxia (immaturity of the infant or depressed respirations caused by maternal sedation or anesthesia) or when some functional or anatomic abnormality in the fetus provokes abnormally active respiratory motions, excessive amounts of amniotic fluid may be drawn into the lungs. This is most likely to occur in premature infants who already suffer from respiratory deficits.

Whatever the setting, amniotic fluid and debris within the alveoli block normal ventilatory function and so may contribute significantly to the causation of death. So-called aspiration of amniotic contents is recognized histologically by the presence in the alveoli of large amounts of amniotic debris, i.e., amorphous proteinous precipitates, desquamated keratotic squames, mucus, lanugo hairs and particulate lipid material representing the vernix caseosa.

ATELECTASIS NEONATORUM

Atelectasis (nonexpansion of the lungs) neonatorum is one of the major causes of hypoxia and death in infants dying within the first days to weeks of postnatal life. The atelectasis may result from failure of expansion of the lungs following birth, *primary atelectasis*, or from resorption of the contained air following initial expansion of the lungs, *secondary atelectasis*.

Primary atelectasis implies that adequate respiration has never been established. It is not a primary disease, and causes must be sought for its existence. It is characteristic of prematures in whom the respiratory centers in the brain and muscles of respiration are poorly developed and whose respiratory motions are feeble. Intrauterine anoxia resulting from retroplacental hemorrhage, premature separation of the placenta, kinking of the umbilical cord, or twisting of the cord around the neck of the infant may all cause respiratory failure and atelectasis. Even in full-term infants, brain damage may depress the function of the respiratory centers to cause feeble respiration and inadequate expansion of the alveoli.

The lungs at autopsy are collapsed, red-blue, noncrepitant and are flabby and rubbery. Characteristically, these lungs fail to float when immersed in water. Histologically, the alveoli resemble the native fetal lung. The alveolar spaces are uniformly small, have a crumpled appearance and are surrounded by thick septal walls. A prominent cuboidal epithelium lines the alveolar sacs, and often there is a granular proteinaceous precipitate mixed with amniotic debris within the air spaces.

Secondary atelectasis can only occur in infants who have established respiration and subsequently die usually during the first few days or weeks of postnatal life. In these infants, the respiratory movements may have been inadequate from the outset, and the lungs may never have become entirely inflated. When further complications such as aspiration of secretions or blood during the passage through the birth canal, depression of the respiration of the child due to heavy sedation of the mother, or postnatal infections are superimposed on these partially collapsed lungs, complete atelectasis may develop.

In contrast to primary atelectasis, the lungs in the secondary form are unevenly affected and have alternating areas of collapsed and aerated parenchyma. The pleural surface is thus mottled, being red-blue in the depressed areas and pale pink to gray in the crepitant areas. Usually the subcrepitant areas are most prominent in the basal regions where there is the poorest respiratory excursion. The histologic changes are those described under the primary form alternating with areas of adjacent hyperinflation, sometimes called compensatory emphysema.

Both primary and secondary atelectasis impose a critical burden upon the already fragile respiration in the newborn, particularly in the premature group. Both forms of atelectasis must be considered as emergencies requiring immediate attention because not only do they cause severe respiratory distress, but they are prime soils for bacterial invasion. In the well developed infant, both forms of atelectasis are remediable disorders.

CONGENITAL ALVEOLAR OR PULMONARY DYSPLASIA

Congenital alveolar dysplasia is a rare condition encountered in premature or full-term infants who manifest respiratory difficulties from birth. Anomalous development of the lungs fails to produce well developed alveolar spaces, best characterized as too few alveoli and too much interstitial tissue. The pleural surfaces are smooth and glistening, but the lungs are large, red-blue, meaty and subcrepitant. On microscopic examination, the dominant feature is that of an abundant, loose mesenchymal tissue, resembling the primitive mesenchyme from which the lungs are derived. Small abortive alveoli lined by cuboidal epithelium are scattered through this vascularized connective tissue. The bronchi and bronchioles are usually well developed. Histologically, the lungs of these infants resemble those of the fetus of four to five months' gestation.

The inadequate development of the lungs does not permit life for more than a few days, and usually these infants die of profound respiratory distress or of some superimposed pulmonary infection.

HYALINE MEMBRANE DISEASE (HMD)

HMD, also known as the "idiopathic respiratory distress syndrome," is the most common cause of respiratory failure in the newborn. *It is usually encountered in premature infants, almost always after a brief period of air breathing.* In the classic case, soon after birth the low-weight infant becomes hypotensive, extremely dyspneic, tachypneic and cyanotic with poor breath sounds and an expiratory grunt. In the past, most have died a hypoxic death, but with respirator positive-pressure assistance, the disease may run its natural clinical course of 3 to 5 days followed by complete recovery.

Incidence. Recent studies indicate that our concepts of the clinical setting in which HMD is encountered require revision. It had always been postulated that the disease was associated with the triad of prematurity, maternal diabetes and caesarian section birth. Clearly, prematurity is a major predisposition and, in general, the lower the birth weight, the greater the danger. The incidence of HMD in prematurity ranges between 10 and 50 per cent, depending upon the distribution of birth weights in the population studied. For mysterious reasons, infants under 1000 gm. appear to be less vulnerable than those in the 1000 to 2000 gm. range. Currently, it is believed that maternal diabetes is *not* necessarily a predisposing factor, except insofar as it leads to premature delivery (Gellis and Hsia, 1959). Likewise, HMD does not appear to be related to delivery by caesarian section, but rather to the indications for caesarian section, namely fetal distress, premature separation of the placenta and other emergencies requiring immediate caesarian section often before full term. If only elective caesarian sections are considered, the risk is not significantly greater than with normal, spontaneous vaginal delivery.

Morphology. While acidophilic membranes lying free within the alveoli or along the alveolar walls are still the most reliable criteria for the anatomic diagnosis of this condition, many other pulmonary changes are present which are probably more important in causing the disturbed pulmonary function. The lungs are solid, airless, heavier than normal and usually sink in water (Lauweryns, 1965). Histologically, there is widespread atelectasis alternating with isolated, overdistended alveoli or alveolar ducts. When lung sections are taken immediately after death, much more even aeration is present. A prominent feature is intense vascular engorgement, principally in the alveolar capillaries, accompanied by pulmonary arteriolar constriction. The congestion often leads to micropulmonary alveolar hemorrhages. The pulmonary lymphatics are usually distended, tortuous and engorged with fibrinous fluid (Lauweryns et al., 1968). The hyaline membranes previously mentioned are randomly scattered either lying within alveoli or within the terminal alveolar ducts (Fig. 13–4). At one time, the membranes were thought to represent inspissated amniotic secretions, but it has been clearly shown that they are largely made up of fibrin and cell debris chiefly derived from necrotic alveolar lining pneumocytes (Gitlin and Craig, 1956).

The available evidence now suggests the following sequence of events: pulmonary anoxia leads to increased permeability of the alveolar capillaries with the transudation or exudation of fibrin. Concomitantly, there is hypoxic injury to the pulmonary alveolar epithelium and the necrotic cell debris is trapped in the fibrin coagulum. Thus, in places the hyaline membrane may cover vital or necrotic alveolar lining cells, or the membrane may lie directly apposed to the lamina propria of the alveolar wall when all the underlying lining cells have sloughed. Sometimes the alveolar epithelium proliferates over the surface of the membrane to essentially incorporate it within the alveolar septum. In the course of time, the membrane may separate to lie free within the air space. Here it may undergo partial digestion or phagocytosis by macrophages (Barter, 1966). Later it will be seen that a deficiency of pulmonary surfactant is thought to be important

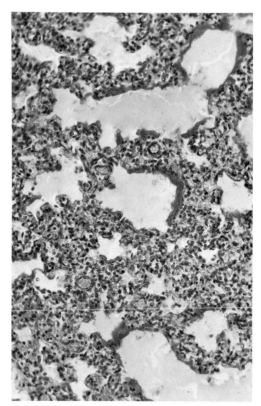

Figure 13–4. Hyaline membrane disease. There is alternating atelectasis and emphysema of the alveoli, and many air spaces are filled with fluid and lined by thick hyaline membranes.

in the genesis of this condition. Concentric lamellar bodies within type II pneumocytes are considered to be the morphologic expression of the secretion of pulmonary surfactant. One would anticipate a deficiency of these lamellar bodies in a child suffering from a lack of pulmonary surfactant, but surprisingly they are usually present, though in decreased number, in the lungs. So there is a suspicion that in the immature infant destined to develop HMD, these configurations and pulmonary surfactant are largely absent, but that in the subsequent days during the course of the disease, active synthesis takes place (Balis, 1966).

Pathogenesis. Because the primary cause of HMD is still unknown, a plethora of hypotheses have sprung up. The major ones might be listed as follows: (1) *pulmonary vasoconstriction at the level of the small arteries and arterioles leading to pulmonary hypoperfusion; (2) deficiency of surfactant; (3) increased alveolar wall permeability with fibrin exudation ; (4) deficiency of fibrinolysin; and (5) amniotic fluid aspiration.* All of these theories may be valid and indeed may be interrelated. After examining some of the data in support of each, a unifying concept will be presented indicating their interplay.

A number of observations support the concept of *increased pulmonary vascular resistance and pulmonary hypoperfusion,* including hemodynamic studies, morphologic evidence of arteriolar and small artery vasoconstriction and the frequent demonstration that these infants have an abnormally patent ductus arteriosus. During fetal life, most of the venous blood passes from the venous to the arterial circulation through the foramen ovale and ductus arteriosus, bypassing the lung. At birth, with the onset of breathing, pulmonary vascular resistance is normally reduced, resulting in an increase in pulmonary blood flow which raises the pressure in the left atrium and so closes the foramen ovale. At the same time, the ductus arteriosus constricts and begins to close. In HMD with high pulmonary vascular resistance, the ductus remains patent and the high right atrial pressure produces a shunt from right to left, thereby bypassing the lungs and adding to the general hypoxia.

Pulmonary surfactant activity has repeatedly been observed to be decreased in HMD (Rufer, 1968). Several lines of evidence indicate that in normal human embryos, surfactant begins to be produced by type II alveolar cells at about 23 weeks of gestation. It is possible to follow the fetal production of surfactant by analysis of the amniotic fluid obtained during pregnancy. By such studies, it has been shown that the titer of surfactant rises abruptly at 30 to 35 weeks of gestation (Clemento et al., 1972). Thus the premature infant may not have reached the stage of development permitting synthesis of adequate amounts of surfactant. Why infants should vary over a five-week time span in the onset of such synthesis is unknown but, in HMD, it is proposed that there is insufficient elaboration of surfactant to permit normal expansion of alveoli, thus leading to widespread atelectasis. Perhaps it is the "late bloomers" who are destined to develop HMD. In any event, with the deficiency of surfactant, the alveoli cannot be maintained fully inflated, and the disturbed air pressure relationships within the alveoli predispose to alveolar capillary congestion as well as transudation and exudation of plasma fluids and proteins. However, even if there were a deficiency of surfactant, other factors must play a role since the administration of aerosolized surfactant does not significantly improve blood-gas exchange or prolong survival in these infants.

Increased capillary wall permeability is attested to by the appearance of fibrin exudates within the alveolar spaces, by the abundant evidence indicating increased lymphatic drainage from the lungs and the frequent presence of edema fluid within the alveolar spaces (Lauweryns, 1970).

A deficiency of fibrinolysin might contribute to the causation of this disaster insofar as normal mechanisms for the removal of fibrin exudate would be impaired. Low circulating titers of plasminogen can be demonstrated in some premature infants with HMD. However, the administration of fibrinolytic preparations has not improved the outcome in these affected infants, and other evidence of abnormal clotting or disseminated intravascular coagulation to be anticipated with a significant deficiency of fibrinolysin is rarely present.

Despite the fact that the membranes in the lungs are not considered to be derived from *aspirated amniotic contents,* it is still likely that such aspiration may worsen or contribute to the pathophysiology of HMD. It has repeatedly been observed that the second-born of twins is frequently more severely affected, suggesting that perinatal asphyxia and perhaps aspiration of amniotic fluid play some role.

Nelson (1970) has offered yet another proposal which embodies many of the above mentioned theories of causation. He proposes that the disease be looked upon essentially as a manifestation of shock in the newborn. In support of his thesis, he points out that most infants are hypotensive at birth (some investigators say because they are deprived of the placental blood volume—the so-called placental transfusion). The systemic circulatory insufficiency leads to generalized hypoxia and acidosis. Reflex mechanisms are called into play which induce pulmonary vasoconstriction as well as vasoconstriction of other vascular beds, thereby shunting blood to the vital organs, e.g., the brain and heart. In the face of prematurity and deficient surfactant, the pulmonary hypoperfusion logically leads to *congestive atelectasis* and increased exudation of plasma proteins. Defective fibrinolytic mechanisms and aspiration of amniotic contents contribute to the problem. While, then, many influences might contribute to the pathophysiology, the basic process might be circulatory insufficiency having its greatest impact on the lungs in these premature, predisposed infants.

Clinical Course. It is difficult to express a prognosis for this disease since respiratory distress in the newborn has many causes which are difficult to differentiate in the living patient, and so one can never be certain of survival figures for any one of the individual entities. If an infant has respiratory distress and survives, was it caused by HMD, atelectasis or perhaps aspiration of amniotic contents?

Moreover, other factors contribute to the mortality such as the possible coexistence of birth injury, general immaturity and low birth weight as well as pulmonary dysplasia and secondary infections. Nonetheless, with mechanical positive pressure ventilation and/or other supportive measures, the mortality for the respiratory distress syndrome in newborns has been reduced to 30 to 50 per cent (Daily et al., 1971) (Vidyasagar and Chernick, 1971). Surviving infants are generally free of sequellae, but a few may have some residual neurologic damage.

ERYTHROBLASTOSIS FETALIS—HEMOLYTIC DISEASE OF THE NEWBORN

When the fetus inherits red cell antigenic determinants from the father that are not present in the mother, the "foreign" antigens may evoke a maternal immune reaction leading to hemolytic disease in the infant. For such to occur, the fetal red cell antigens must gain access to the maternal circulation and, in turn, the antibodies evoked in the mother must traverse the placental barrier to enter the fetus. While any of the numerous red cell antigenic systems might theoretically be involved in such cross immunization, the only antigens sufficiently strong to induce clinically significant immunologic disease are the ABO and certain of the Rh antigens. The resultant hemolytic reaction may cause either death of the fetus, usually in the third trimester of pregnancy, or severe, sometimes fatal, disease in the newborn. Thus, *erythroblastosis fetalis may be defined as a hemolytic disease in the newborn caused by blood group incompatibility between mother and child.*

Incidence. The incidence of this condition depends upon chance red cell antigenic differences between mother and infant (Mollison, 1967). While Rh incompatibility is much less common than ABO incompatibility, it generally poses a greater antigenic challenge, induces stronger immunologic reactions and hence causes more severe hemolytic disease. Rh incompatibility is therefore generally more life threatening. Almost always, ABO incompatibility occurs with a group O mother and an infant having A or B or, of course, both red cell antigens. The probability of this concurrence has been estimated to be 1 in 30 to 180 births. However, in only one in five of such instances is the immunologic reaction strong enough to induce hemolytic disease in the infant. The Rh system possesses somewhat more than 25 blood antigens. Practically, however,

the strong Rh antigens may be divided into three sets: C and its allele c, D and its allele d, and E and its allele e. These are inherited as linked sets, and so the genotype of an individual might be CDE-cde. Such an infant would be Rh-positive. Alternatively, the genotype might be cde-cde, representing an Rh-negative infant. The problem is further simplified by the fact that the strongest antigen responsible for most cases of severe hemolytic disease in the newborn is D. About 15 per cent of white women and men are Rh-negative (d/d). Thus, while there is approximately a 12 per cent chance (85 per cent of 15 per cent) of the mating of an Rh-positive man with an Rh-negative woman, only about 5 per cent of Rh-negative mothers have babies with hemolytic disease. This lower than expected incidence is due to many factors. About 55 per cent of Rh-positive fathers are heterozygous for the D antigen and so may have Rh-negative children. More important is the titer of antibody produced by the mother, and the capacity of Rh-negative women to form antibodies is quite variable. Sensitization to a clinically significant degree rarely occurs with the first pregnancy, and small family size reduces the general incidence of erythroblastosis fetalis. Fortunately, mismatched transfusions have been virtually eliminated as causes of prior sensitization. However, once prior sensitization has occurred in an earlier pregnancy, subsequent Rh-positive fetuses are at high risk.

Pathogenesis. If the maternal antibodies are the agents of the immunologic hemolysis in the infant, why does the disease usually become manifest in the third trimester of pregnancy or immediately after birth? Moreover, since O mothers normally possess agglutinins to A and B antigens, why do these not cause fetal death early in pregnancy? With regard to the last mentioned issue, naturally occuring agglutinins belong to the 19S IgM class and are too large to cross the placenta. Thus, in both the ABO and Rh systems, it is necessary to predicate entry of fetal red cells into the maternal circulation, evoking antibodies capable of traversing the placental barrier. It is well known that the epithelium covering placental villi atrophies in the late stages of pregnancy. The naked villi are more vulnerable to microtrauma, permitting red cells to escape and enter the maternal circulation. Hence the infusion of red cells into the mother occurs usually at the very late stages of pregnancy or possibly even during the onset of labor. The antibodies so evoked, whether triggered by ABO or Rh antigens, are of the 7S IgG class, and so freely pass the placental barrier to enter the fetal circulation.

The titer of antibody, its rate of production, and the ability of the fetus to increase its red cell production to compensate for the hemolysis combine to determine the outcome. Significant fetal disease is rarely encountered with maternal titers of IgG antibodies of less than 1:8. There is, however, no perfect correlation between the severity of the fetal disease and the antibody titer. The most important clue to potential disease is a positive direct Coombs' test on fetal cord blood. The severity of the hemolytic reaction can be monitored by the serum bilirubin levels in the infant. In affected infants, these levels rise rapidly postnatally and may reach extremely high levels (over 20 mg. per 100 ml.) in the first 3 days of life. In the premature or low-birth-weight infant, the bilirubin excretory capacity may not have achieved its full capacity, further contributing to the hyperbilirubinemias. The unconjugated bilirubin is water-insoluble and has an affinity for lipids. It may therefore localize in the lipids of the brain where it can produce, as will be seen, serious damage.

Morphology. The anatomic findings in erythroblastosis fetalis vary with the severity of the hemolytic process (Lindsay, 1950). Stillborn infants are characteristically markedly anemic and have manifestations of edema and congestive failure. Live-born children may succumb promptly or within the next several weeks or recover completely, usually aided by therapy which must sometimes be quite heroic. Most immediate postnatal deaths are the consequence of severe hemolysis and consequent circulatory failure. In those that survive longer, the erythroblastosis fetalis manifests itself in several ways which are arbitrarily divided into three syndromes. In its mildest form, the child may be only slightly anemic and may survive without further complication, the so-called **congenital anemia of the newborn.** With more severe hemolysis, the anemia and pallor are accompanied by obvious jaundice, the **icterus gravis** syndrome. Edema resulting from circulatory failure frequently accompanies the jaundice, and is sometimes so severe as to merit the designation of anasarca. This pattern is known as **hydrops fetalis.** In all three syndromes, the liver and spleen are enlarged, depending upon the severity of the hemolytic process and the compensatory extramedullary erythropoiesis.

The most serious threat in erythroblastosis is central nervous system damage known as **kernicterus.** In jaundiced cases, the unconjugated indirect bilirubin appears to be particularly toxic to the brain, probably affecting oxidative metabolism of brain tissue. The brain is enlarged, edematous and, when sectioned, has a bright yellow pigmentation (kernicterus) particularly in the basal ganglia, thalamus, cerebellum, cerebral gray matter and spinal cord. This pigmentation is evanescent and fades within 24 hours despite prompt fixation. It is therefore necessary to section the brain immediately in suspected cases to establish the diagnosis. It is worth noting that such pigmentation of the brain is not limited exclusively to erythroblastosis fetalis, since it has also been described in milder form in infants with severe physiologic jaundice of the newborn. This bile pigmentation of the brain is of considerable theoretical interest because, in the adult, some blood-brain barrier blocks the passage of bilirubin into the spinal fluid and substance of the brain even when there is severe jaundice. The systemic hypoxia caused by the extreme hemolysis may play some role in rendering this barrier abnormally permeable in these infants.

Histologically, the diagnosis of erythroblastosis fetalis depends upon the identification of abnormally increased erythropoietic activity in the infant. The red cell series in the marrow is hyperactive, and extramedullary hematopoiesis is almost invariably present in the liver, spleen and possibly in other tissues, such as the lymph nodes, kidneys, lungs and even the heart (Fig. 13–5). This hematopoietic activity is sufficiently striking to account for increased numbers of reticulocytes, normoblasts and erythroblasts in the circulating blood (Fig. 13–6). The larger of these immature blood cells tend to become trapped in the pulmonary

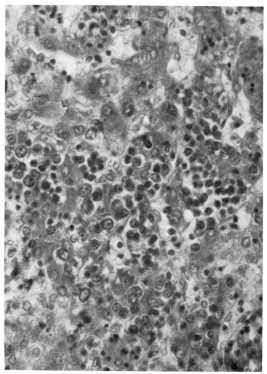

Figure 13–5. *Liver in erythroblastosis fetalis with a focus of extramedullary hematopoiesis.*

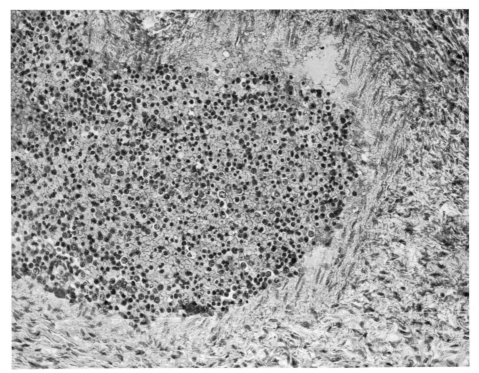

Figure 13-6. *A large pulmonary vessel in an erythroblastotic infant, loaded with nucleated red cell forms.*

capillaries and account for the diagnostic value of examination of the lung in this disease. Evidence of subcutaneous and visceral edema is present in the hydrops syndrome along with fluid in the peritoneal, pleural and pericardial cavities. The histologic changes in the central nervous system are not too well documented, but consist principally of bile pigmentation of nerve fibers and cells with degeneration of ganglion cells. In the more severe cases, there is periportal fibrosis and ductular bile stasis in the liver along with the extramedullary hematopoiesis.

Placental alterations may be virtually diagnostic. If the infant is not edematous, the placenta is normal in size. When edema is present in the fetus, the placenta is usually larger and heavier than normal, and essentially exhibits considerable edema in the form of enlargement of the cotyledons and individual villi. Immature forms of the red cell series can be seen in the fetal blood vessels. The stroma in the villi is spread apart to create a loose connective tissue which often contains large, round to polygonal, pink, epithelium-like, lipid-laden **Hofbauer cells** (Fig. 13–7). The Langhans' cells of the chorionic epithelium are unusually persistent. Rarely, foci of extramedullary hematopoiesis may be evident in the stroma of the villi. Cardiac hypertrophy, when present, probably reflects some element of hypoxia and failure. Unexplained is the occasional hyperplasia of the islets of Langerhans.

Clinical Course. The clinical patterns of erythroblastosis vary, as has already been indicated, from stillbirth to the mildest degrees of anemia in an otherwise healthy child. Infants with clinically significant disease fall into one of the three overlapping but somewhat distinctive syndromes: (1) congenital anemia of the newborn, (2) icterus gravis possibly with kernicterus and (3) fetal hydrops with the highest mortality, almost invariably associated with cardiac failure, jaundice, anemia and kernicterus. In general, kernicterus is not encountered until the serum bilirubin levels exceed 20 mg. per 100 ml. However, the size of the baby, the rapidity of the rise of serum bilirubin and the infant's general state of health all contribute to the development of kernicterus. It has been postulated that even lower levels of serum bilirubin may induce more subtle evidences of motor and mental retardation (Boggs et al., 1967).

The possible development of hemolytic disease in the newborn must be suspected in any Rh-negative or O mother when the father possesses antigens "foreign" to the mother. Under such circumstances, maternal antibodies are monitored in the third trimester of pregnancy, the Coombs' test is performed on fetal cord blood, and infant serum bilirubin levels are followed throughout the first days of

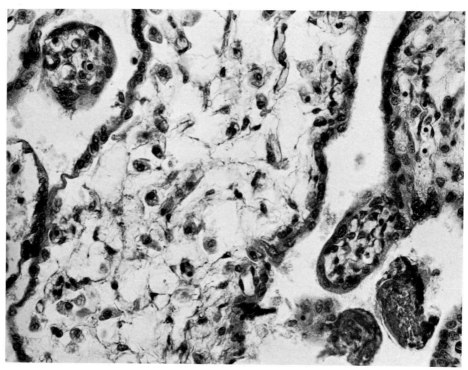

Figure 13–7. *A high power detail of a placental villus to demonstrate the edema and round to oval Hofbauer cells.*

postnatal life. Since severe erythroblastosis is readily treated by exchange transfusions, early recognition of the disorder is imperative. In appropriate cases, amniotic fluid analysis for elevated bilirubin levels will give evidence, prior to birth, of possible trouble. Much more important than treating affected infants is the prevention of this disease, and erythroblastosis of Rh origin is a gratifying example of a disease that has been virtually conquered. It has been found that Rh sensitization in the mother can be prevented or at least reduced by the prompt postnatal (within 72 hours) administration of human Rh (anti-D) immunoglobulins (Rhogam) to the mother. How this anti-Rh antibody prevents or lowers sensitization is still not clear. Among the several theories, two are favored. The antibody might either lyse the fetal red cells or merely coat them and favor their sequestration in the RE system, particularly the liver, thus clearing the blood of the immunogenic antigens (Mollison, 1962). Alternatively, the passively administered anti-D globulins might suppress an immune reaction in the mother, perhaps by binding to the antigenic determinants on the fetal red cells, thus lowering or blocking their immunogenicity (Schiff, 1969). Whatever the mechanism, with this form of treatment, sensitization of Rh-negative mothers has been remarkably re-

duced, and so subsequent clinically significant hemolytic reactions in their infants have also been reduced. Such therapy cannot reduce the incidence of ABO incompatibility but, as mentioned, it is happily in most cases a less serious clinical problem.

CYSTIC FIBROSIS

Cystic fibrosis is a systemic hereditary disease of children, adolescents and young adults in which there is dysfunction of all or many of the exocrine glands, leading to the elaboration of viscid mucus and a high salt concentration in sweat. It is not only one of the most common disorders of childhood but is also one of the most enigmatic in terms of its causation. Clearly the designation cystic fibrosis is a misnomer. It harkens back several decades to a time when cystic and fibrotic changes in the pancreas were considered to be the major manifestations of this condition. Thus the term "fibrocystic disease of the pancreas" also persists in the literature. Then the widespread defect in mucus secretion was dignified by the synonym "mucoviscidosis." Further study made it evident that an invariable and diagnostic characteristic of this disorder is the secretion of abnormally high levels of electrolytes, principally salt, in the sweat (the basis for the sweat test). Thus it has become clear that the disorder is systemic, affecting all exocrine glands including those elaborating mucin.

Incidence. There is general agreement that the mode of inheritance of cystic fibrosis is autosomal recessive (Di Sant Agnese and Talamo, 1967). Homozygotes have the classic disease, but heterozygotes are asymptomatic and express no detectable phenotypic change. It is apparent, then, that diseased infants must have carrier or affected parents. From the evidence that when one child has cystic fibrosis, siblings have a 25 per cent chance of also being affected, it would appear that a single mutant gene of large affect is involved. The distribution of this hereditary trait in the general population is widespread. Several surveys indicate that the incidence of the fully expressed disease is about one in 1500 to 2000 live births. In various pediatric clinical centers, cystic fibrosis is found in 2 to 4 per cent of autopsies. There are striking racial differences in the distribution of the trait. It is predominantly a disease of the white race and is encountered much less frequently in blacks, principally those in the United States. Only rare cases have been identified in native African blacks. It is equally rare in those of Oriental or Mongolian descent.

Pathogenesis. Not only is the cause of this disease unknown, but even the primary site of attack is uncertain. Any theory of causation must explain why so many varied exocrine glands are affected, some elaborating mucin, others serous secretion, and still others producing sweat of an abnormal composition. Why is the glandular involvement so unpredictable in the individual patient, with severe pancreatic damage in certain individuals while in others this gland is spared? And finally, why is the disease severe in some and relatively mild in others? *The five most widely debated theories might be categorized as: (1) abnormality of mucus secretion, (2) autonomic dysfunction, (3) some humoral abnormality, (4) ion transport dysfunction and (5) abnormal calcium metabolism in exocrine glands.*

The secretion of an abnormal mucus is clearly one of the basic defects in cystic fibrosis. The mucus is more viscid and obstructs pancreatic ducts, bronchioles and salivary gland ducts, and so damages these organs. The increased viscosity of the mucin has been attributed to increased fucose and decreased sialic acid levels in the glycoproteins (Gische et al., 1959). In addition, it has recently been shown that fibroblasts derived from these patients elaborate increased amounts of mucopolysaccharides and thus have abnormally intense metachromatic staining (Danes, 1969). Interestingly, fibroblasts from heterozygotes behave exactly

as do those from homozygotes. The precise significance of these cell culture observations is not clear nor is the similarity of the fibroblasts derived from homozygotes and heterozygotes, but some abnormality in secretion is vaguely suggested.

Autonomic dysfunction would be a rational method of explaining a disorder involving such a wide variety of exocrine glands. Hyperactivity of the autonomic nervous system might explain the increased parotid secretory rate in patients with cystic fibrosis. It could also explain increased secretion of sweat. However, no structural abnormality has been identified in the autonomic nervous system and the disease cannot be mimicked by the chronic administration of parasympathomimetic drugs. The evidence of autonomic dysfunction is at best, then, meager.

Some *humoral abnormality* has been recently proposed by Spock et al. (1967) who demonstrated a serum factor in patients with cystic fibrosis, which disorganizes the ciliary rhythm in explants of respiratory epithelium. This serum factor appears within the macroglobulin fraction, and conceivably it might act by altering transport of electrolytes across the cell membrane, thereby predisposing to not only abnormal ciliary action but also abnormal secretion of mucus and sweat. Interestingly, the existence of the serum factor was confirmed by another investigator who noted that serum from patients with cystic fibrosis impaired ciliary activity of oyster gills (Bowman et al., 1969).

The *ion transport dysfunction theory* focuses on the sweat electrolyte abnormality which is present in virtually all patients with cystic fibrosis. The high concentrations of sodium chloride in the sweat are thought to be the result of failure of reabsorption of sodium chloride by the ducts of the sweat glands. Indeed, it has been noted that saliva or sweat from patients with cystic fibrosis, when introduced into the parotid glands of rats, inhibits sodium reabsorption. It has not been possible to isolate the precise substance having this inhibitory effect, but Mangos and McSherry (1967) were able to extract from serum a small polypeptide capable of not only inhibiting sodium reabsorption but also disorganizing the ciliary beat in the bioassay system (Spock, 1969).

The most recent theory relates the abnormalities in mucus and sweat to *excess secretion of calcium* by the exocrine glands (Gibson et al., 1971). Here it is postulated that the increased secretion of calcium into the mucus somehow makes it hyperpermeable to water, and so water is excessively reabsorbed, resulting in a viscid mucus. At the same time, the increased amounts of calcium in the sweat lead to increased reabsorption of water and, therefore, to a relative excess of sodium chloride. Still to be explained, however, is how calcium affects the permeability of mucus and exerts its action on the sweat ducts.

It is clear that each of the various theories has its own particular focus and no one attempts to present a unifying overview. It can be more truly said of this disease than of most that all is confusion with regard to its genesis.

Morphology. The anatomic changes are highly variable and depend on which glands are affected and on the severity of this involvement. In some infants, the disease is quite mild, does not seriously disturb their growth and development, and they readily survive into adolescence or adult life. In others, the pancreatic involvement is severe and impairs intestinal absorption because of the pancreatic achylia, and so malabsorption, inanition and stunted development not only seriously hamper life but shorten survival. In others, the mucus secretion defect leads to obstruction of bronchi and bronchioles and crippling fatal pulmonary infections. Thus, cystic fibrosis may be compatible with long life or may cause death in infancy.

Pancreatic abnormalities are present in approximately 80 per cent of patients. In the milder cases, there may be only accumulations of mucus in the small ducts with some dilatation of the exocrine glands. In more advanced cases, the ducts are totally plugged, causing atrophy of the exocrine glands and progressive fibrosis (Fig. 13–8). Because many of these children are being kept alive by appropriate therapy, the advance of the disease sometimes leads to total atrophy of the exocrine portion of the pancreas, leaving only the islets within a fibrofatty stroma. The total loss of pancreatic exocrine secretion impairs fat absorption, and so avitaminosis A may contribute to squamous metaplasia of the lining epithelium of the ducts in the pancreas which are already injured by the inspissated mucus secretions. In part because of the absence of the pancreatic amylases and in part owing to the deranged gastrointestinal mucus secretions, thick tenacious plugs of viscid mucus may be found in the small intestine of infants. Sometimes these cause small bowel obstruction known as **meconium ileus.**

The **liver involvement** follows the same basic pattern. Bile canaliculi are plugged by mucinous material. When this is of long duration, progressive bile duct proliferation and portal fibrosis appear along with a periportal mononuclear cell infiltration. Thus biliary cirrhosis with its diffuse hepatic nodularity may develop in the longer surviving cases. Such severe hepatic involvement is encoun-

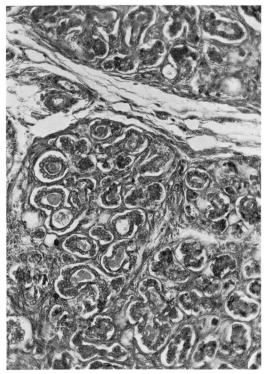

Figure 13–8. Cystic fibrosis of pancreas. The ducts are dilated and plugged with mucin, and the parenchymal glands are totally atrophic and replaced by fibrous tissue.

tered in only approximately 2 per cent of the patients, although minor hepatic changes are found in as many as 25 per cent.

The **salivary glands** are frequently involved with histologic changes similar to those described in the pancreas, i.e., progressive dilatation of ducts, squamous metaplasia of the lining epithelium and glandular atrophy followed by fibrosis.

The **pulmonary changes** are the most serious complications of this disease. These stem from the viscous mucus secretions of the submucosal glands of the respiratory tree as well as from the secondary metaplastic epithelial changes resulting from the deficiency of vitamin A. Grossly, the lungs may be emphysematous or atelectatic, depending on whether the mucus plugs cause subtotal or total obstruction of the respiratory passages. The bronchioles are often distended with thick mucus and the normal columnar cells are transformed into squamous epithelium. Superimposed infections give rise to severe chronic bronchitis and bronchiectasis (p. 806). In many instances, lung abscesses develop. It is of interest that in over 90 per cent of these patients, *Staphylococcus aureus* is the causative agent. With current effective therapy against this organism, increasing numbers of these pulmonary infections are now being caused by *Pseudomonas* *aeruginosa.* A variety of other morphologic changes may be present secondary to the malabsorption as will be evident from the following discussion.

Clinical Course. Few childhood diseases are as protean as cystic fibrosis in clinical manifestations. The symptomatology may range from mild to severe, from onset at birth to first becoming evident years later, and from syndromes which present essentially as cardio-pulmonary disease to those which present as intestinal obstruction or as prolapse of the rectum due to chronic constipation. In the classic case, the disorder is discovered in a child between the second and 12th month of life who comes to attention because of malodorous stea-torrhea and recurrent chronic pulmonary infections (Prior, 1961). Severely affected newborns may fail to regain their birth weight. In others, (approximately 5 to 10 per cent) the meconium ileus produces intestinal obstruction and, indeed, such may occur in utero and lead to perforation of the gut. The pancreatic insufficiency induces a malabsorption syndrome manifested principally as inanition, fat intolerance, steatorrhea and deficient absorption of the fat-soluble vitamins A, D and K (p. 946). Avitaminosis K may in turn lead to bleeding tendencies. In almost all instances, if the infant or child survives long enough, chronic cough, obstructive pulmonary disease and persistent pulmonary infections develop and are responsible for approximately 80 to 90 per cent of deaths. As previously mentioned, the causative organisms are predominantly *Staphylococcus aureus* and *Pseudomonas aeruginosa.*

At least three of the four following criteria are required for the diagnosis of cystic fibrosis: (1) increase in electrolyte concentration of sweat, (2) deficiency or absence of pancreatic enzymes in duodenal drainage, (3) chronic pulmonary disease usually with the isolation of the specific organisms mentioned and (4) a family history of the disorder.

It is difficult to express a prognosis for a disease which spans such a wide range of severity. In years past, about half of the infants died before the age of 10, three-quarters before 20 years of age, and almost all by 30 years of age. More effective and intensive therapy, better diagnosis and better control of respiratory complications have improved this outlook as is indicated by the report of Shwachman et al. (1970). He divided his 130 patients into three groups: (1) those diagnosed prior to the development of symptoms, (2) those with mild symptoms, and (3) those diagnosed during hospitalization for management of severe disease. Over the 20-year period of the study, approximately 25 per cent of those in groups 1

and 2 and 33 per cent of those in group 3 had died. Among the 101 survivors, 14 were in excellent health, 71 had mild disease and 12 had moderately or severely advanced disease with a poor prognosis. Over all, the calculated survival rate for all 130 patients at age 20 was 77 per cent. These data indicate that, although cystic fibrosis is indeed a grave disease, with optimal medical management, the large majority of patients will survive into adult life.

CYTOMEGALIC INCLUSION DISEASE (CID)

This viral infection caused by the DNA cytomegalovirus is characterized morphologically by the appearance of large intranuclear and smaller intracytoplasmic inclusion bodies in strikingly enlarged cells (epithelial and mesenchymal) of many viscera. The infection may be acquired in utero or at any time postnatally even into adult life. CID thus may cause still-birth or appear as a systemic disorder in the newborn or any time thereafter. Sophisticated techniques for identification of this disease have made it apparent that the cytomegalovirus is widespread, and as many as 81 per cent of certain populations over the age of 35 either harbor the virus or have been exposed to it, but only a small fraction ever develop the disease (Rowe et al., 1956) (Stern and Elek, 1965). Thus, CID offers an example of a host-parasite relationship where the clinical disease only emerges in those who are particularly susceptible. In most of these instances, the causative agent had probably been harbored by the host before birth or for many years. So CID is principally encountered in infants, particularly in prematures, who have not yet developed any immunologic resistance and in those rendered vulnerable by debilitating disease (diabetes mellitus, cancer, leukemia, lymphoma), immunosuppressive therapy and malnutrition (Fine, 1970).

Morphology. The congenital and infantile forms of the disease tend to be severe and widespread. The organs most often affected in order of frequency are the salivary glands, kidneys, liver, lungs, pancreas, thyroid, adrenals and brain. In most viscera, the gross changes are minimal and consist chiefly of edema and slight enlargement of the affected organ. Randomly scattered throughout these organs are markedly enlarged cells, often with a diameter of 40 microns or more, possessing large pleomorphic nuclei harboring an intracellular acidophilic inclusion. The inclusion may have a diameter in excess of 15 microns, and characteristically it is surrounded by a cleared halo demarcating it from the nuclear membrane. Ultrastructural studies have shown that the inclusion is composed of a net-like mass of finely granular, fairly dense chromatin material in which virus particles are scattered (Anzil et al., 1970). Small basophilic inclusions are found in the cytoplasm, and these have also been observed to contain or be composed of virions (Fig. 13–9). Usually cells so affected remain vital and evoke no inflammatory reaction, but on occasion they die and the necrotic debris evokes a leukocytic response. Thus focal necroses may be encountered within the salivary glands, liver, adrenals and kidneys. When the liver is heavily attacked, the focal necroses may add up to a diffuse hepatitis. In the lungs, the disease takes the form of an interstitial pneumonitis accompanied by the characteristic intracellular inclusions in the alveolar lining cells. The brain, when affected, may bear the brunt of the disease. Two types of lesions are seen: focal acute inflammatory changes with innumerable inclusion-bearing giant cells distributed principally in a narrow band in the subependymal and subpial tissue, and necrotic lesions irregularly scattered in the cerebrum. In some stillborns, these lesions are accompanied by marked gliosis and microcephaly. Frequently the chronic foci of injury become calcified. The ganglion cells within and about the areas of focal damage show all ranges of injury from chromatolysis to frank necrosis. The bone marrow may also be involved and contain hematopoietic cells with typical inclusions as well as focal areas of cell necrosis.

In the debilitated adult, CID may represent a newly acquired infection or activation of a long-harbored commensal. While the disease may be systemic in distribution in the severely debilitated adult, it is more often limited to an interstitial pneumonitis, perhaps with widely scattered cytomegalic cells in other viscera.

Clinical Course. The clinical manifestations of CID reflect the severity of involvement of specific organs. Usually signs and symptoms are referable to the liver, hematopoietic and central nervous systems. Hepatomegaly and splenomegaly are the result of excessive extramedullary hematopoiesis With severe hepatic involvement seen most often in the congenital and infantile forms, icterus appears and the clinical picture resembles a diffuse hepatitis. These infants also usually have anemia and thrombocytopenia with a hemorrhagic diathesis resulting from depletion of platelets. A wide range of neurologic symptoms may be present, resembling an infectious meningitis in some and, in others, focal brain damage or a diffuse encephalopathy. Severely affected infants who survive may have mental retardation.

The diagnosis depends on: (1) the isolation of the cytomegalovirus from urine, blood, saliva or tissue; (2) the demonstration of complement fixing antibodies in the blood; and (3) the identification of characteristic cytomegalic cells containing inclusions in either tissue biopsies or shed renal tubular cells in the urine. It should be cautioned that patients may excrete virus in the urine without having classic cytomegalic inclusion disease (Birnbaum et al., 1969). After an infection, patients may also continue to excrete virus in their urine for months and even years.

The prognosis of cytomegalic inclusion disease of infancy is grave. Congenitally acquired CID with systemic manifestations is usually fatal although, as was pointed out, clinically inapparent infections undoubtedly exist. Disease that becomes apparent some time after birth is still very serious and many infants die. Survivors have a high likelihood of suffering mental and/or motor retardation (Berenberg and Namkervis, 1970). In older children and adults, the disease is only rarely fatal and then only when some serious illness has predisposed to the viral infection. In these circumstances, CID perhaps acts only as the final straw.

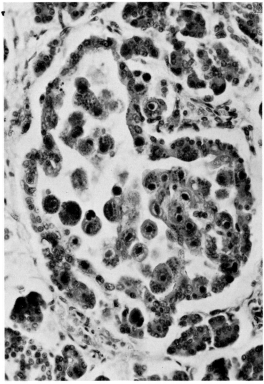

Figure 13–9. Cytomegalic inclusion disease. A nest of affected cells in the pancreas with striking intranuclear inclusions and smaller cytoplasmic granules.

PHENYLKETONURIA (PKU)

PKU is an inborn error of metabolism characterized principally by elevated serum levels of phenylalanine and progressive mental retardation. The mode of inheritance is autosomal recessive, and only homozygotes express the metabolic defect. It is an uncommon entity, having an incidence of about one in ten to 20,000 births. Variants of PKU have been identified characterized by elevated levels of serum phenylalanine without mental retardation (Blaskovics and Nelson, 1971). Whether these variants conceivably represent partially manifesting heterozygotes who have a less severe metabolic block is unclear. *The underlying basis for the metabolic derangement is a hereditary deficiency of phenylalanine hydroxylase required for the conversion of phenylalanine to tyrosine.* As a consequence, phenylalanine builds up in the blood to high levels (in the classic case, usually above 25 mg. per 100 ml.). Serum tyrosine levels are normal or decreased, and abnormal metabolites of phenylalanine are excreted in the urine, principally phenylpyruvic acid and orthohydroxyphenylacetic acid. Screening procedures for this disorder are based on the detection of phenylpyruvic acid in the urine, employing either the ferric chloride test or the bacteria inhibition assay of Guthrie and Sosi (1963).

Infants suffering from a lack of phenylalanine hydroxylase are born apparently normal and have at birth little or no elevation of their serum phenylalanine levels. Similarly, the urine may contain no detectable metabolites. Usually, however, within two weeks to three months, the serum levels of phenylalanine rise, and these infants begin to excrete phenylpyruvic acid and show signs of brain damage in the form of abnormal EEG's and seizures. Characteristically, they develop a musty or vinegary odor resulting from the excessive production of phenylacetic acid. Eczema of the skin may develop. Progressively thereafter, the neurologic deficit worsens, seizures become more frequent and severe, there is delay in motor development and, usually by the end of the first year, moderate to severe retardation with schizoid tendencies become apparent. The phenylalaninemia may rise to levels of 100 mg. per 100 ml. Because of their deranged tyrosine metabolism, these infants synthesize little or no melanin, and so frequently have unusually fair skin, blond hair and blue eyes, even when the parents have very dark complexions.

The histologic findings in the brain are variable and nonspecific. Usually the brain is decreased in weight. Demyelination or defective development of myelin produces spongy, focal lesions of the white matter (Malamud, 1966). With progression of the disorder, these defects become more evident, the demyelination more widespread and the spongy foci more obvious (Salguero et al., 1968).

How the metabolic defect induces these anatomic changes is still mysterious. Perry et al. (1970) reported recently that *serum* glutamine concentrations were subnormal in phenylketonuric patients with severe intellectual impairment but, by contrast, were essentially normal in two untreated phenylketonuric subjects with *normal* intellect. It was implied that the deficiency of glutamine *in the brain* impaired normal myelination. Subsequently, McKean and Peterson (1970) pointed out that in the cerebrospinal-fluid compartment and in cerebral white matter the glutamine levels were *not* depressed but the phenylalanine concentrations in the cerebrospinal fluid were abnormally high, even exceeding those found in the blood. They postulated that the high levels of phenylalanine competitively interfered with the active uptake of other amino acids by the brain, and further suggested that, in the patients destined to develop brain damage, transport mechanisms responsible for the flux of phenylalanine between blood and cerebrospinal fluid were impaired. At the present time, it is not certain that elevated blood or brain phenylalanine levels are responsible for the mental retardation and, indeed, the possibility that abnormal levels of other plasma amino acids may play a role cannot be excluded (Efron et al., 1969).

Despite the fact that the precise pathophysiology of PKU is still obscure, there is abundant evidence that the advance of the disease and mental retardation can be prevented by placing infants on diets which meet their protein needs and, at the same time, lower the serum phenylalanine levels (Forssman et al., 1967). Some infants, as they grow older, develop alternate metabolic pathways since return to normal diet is not followed by hyperphenylalaninemia. This potentially devastating disease can be detected soon after birth by measurement of the concentration of phenylalanine in the serum and by tests for its metabolites in the urine. However, it should be stressed that these abnormalities may not be present immediately after birth and may not become manifest for 4 days to one or two weeks. Moreover, it should also be stressed that all patients with elevated phenylalanine levels will not necessarily develop mental retardation and may represent one of the variants free of the predisposition to brain damage.

GALACTOSEMIA (GALACTOSE INTOLERANCE)

Galactosemia is an inborn error of metabolism arising out of a hereditary deficiency of a specific enzyme, galactose-1-phosphate uridyl transferase, necessary for the normal metabolism of galactose. When this enzyme is missing, abnormal elevations of galactose in the blood follow and in time cause serious, sometimes fatal, physical and mental defects in the infant. The mode of inheritance is autosomal recessive, fully expressed in the homozygote while the heterozygote is clinically normal.

Infants appear normal at birth but, soon after milk feeding has been instituted, develop listlessness, vomiting, diarrhea and failure to thrive. Jaundice appears early and may seem to be a continuation of the neonatal physiologic jaundice. Soon thereafter, hepatomegaly, splenomegaly and cataracts (opacification of the lens of the eye) develop along with signs of hepatic failure. The liver damage may induce a prothrombin deficiency and a hemorrhagic tendency, along with lowered glucose levels and attendant hypoglycemic symptoms. The downward course of the disease may be quite rapid and may lead to death from inanition, secondary infections or hepatic failure.

The liver bears the brunt of the damage in these infants, although other organs such as the brain, kidney and eyes are also affected. The early hepatomegaly is due largely to fatty change but, in time, cirrhosis supervenes. Microscopically, there is extensive fat throughout the liver lobule as well as bile stasis, both within ductules at the periphery of the lobule and within biliary canaliculi. Often liver cells are arranged in a rosette-like fashion about the bile plugs. With progression of the disease, a delicate fibrosis appears first in the periportal regions and eventually extends to produce scars bridging adjacent portal tracts. These liver changes have a remarkable resemblance to those found in patients with the cirrhosis of alcohol abuse. Occasionally, in addition to fat the liver cells contain an excess of glycogen.

Nonspecific but definite alterations appear in the central nervous system. Loss of nerve cells, gliosis and edema are particularly prevalent in the dentate nuclei of the cerebellum and the olivary nuclei of the medulla. There is similar gliosis in the cerebral cortex and white matter, but only occasional damage in the basal ganglia (Smetana and Olen, 1962).

The correlation of the clinical and morphologic findings with the metabolic defect is not entirely obvious at the present time. This much is known. Lactose is composed of the two monosaccharides, galactose and glucose. Normally, after being split in the intestinal tract, the galactose is absorbed and then is converted to glucose by three enzymic reactions as shown at the bottom of this page. The hereditary deficiency of galactose-1-phosphate uridyl transferase blocks reaction (2), and as a consequence galactose levels rise in the blood. At the same time galactosuria appears accompanied by generalized amino aciduria resulting from damaged renal tubular reabsorption. It is not clear whether the brain lesions are directly related to the elevated galactose levels or to other metabolic problems encountered in these infants such as the low blood glucose levels. Neither is the mechanism of injury to the lens understood.

The diagnosis is readily established by a variety of tests. The transferase is normally found in liver, leukocytes and erythrocytes, and sensitive enzyme assays permit identification of the enzyme lack in these cells. Heterozygotes having a less severe deficiency of the transferase can also be detected by the sensitive enzyme assays. The elevated galactose levels in the blood and the galactosuria are less specific but are valuable clues to the existence of the enzyme defect. In this connection, it should be pointed out that variants of galactosemia other than the lack of transferase exist, such as a hereditary deficiency of galactokinase. These variants mimic the transferase syndrome by inducing hypergalactosemia, but they are in general less severe and rarely cause mental deterioration (Hsia, 1967).

Early recognition of this disorder permits institution of a life-saving dietary regimen. When milk is withdrawn from the diet early and is replaced by a galactose-free product, the infant is spared all clinical and morphologic changes. If the dietary measures are not instituted early enough, the cataracts, once developed, are irreversible and require surgical ex-

(Reaction 1) $$\text{Galactose} + \text{ATP} \xrightarrow{\text{Galactokinase}} \text{Galactose-1-phosphate} + \text{ADP}$$

(Reaction 2) $$\begin{array}{c}\text{Galactose-1-phosphate} \\ + \\ \text{UDP-glucose}\end{array} \xrightarrow[]{\begin{array}{c}\text{Galactose-1-phosphate}\\ \text{uridyl transferase}\end{array}} \text{UDP-galactose} + \text{glucose-1-phosphate}$$

(Reaction 3) $$\text{UDP-galactose} \xrightarrow[]{\text{UDP-galactose-4-epimerase}} \text{UDP-glucose}$$

cision. The hepatomegaly is, however, reversible if cirrhosis has not already developed. Still unknown is whether early mental symptoms will clear on such a therapeutic regimen. Once the mental deterioration has become advanced, however, it is beyond recall.

ALKAPTONURIA WITH OCHRONOSIS

Alkaptonuria is an inborn error of phenylalanine-tyrosine metabolism characterized by the accumulation in the body and excretion in the urine of homogentisic acid. It is another of the hereditary "missing enzyme" syndromes having an autosomal recessive mode of inheritance in which homozygotes are incapable of synthesizing the enzyme, homogentisic oxidase. Phenylalanine and tyrosine are normally transformed, by successive steps, to homogentisic acid which is then further degraded to malonyl acetoacetate. When the oxidase is lacking, the homogentisic acid cannot be catabolized and so accumulates in the body and is excreted in the urine. On standing, urine from affected patients becomes black owing to oxidation and polymerization of the homogentisic acid. Although this metabolic defect usually becomes manifest in infancy, for reasons that are not clear, it may not become evident until the second or third decade of life. The slow accumulation of homogentisic acid in cartilage, connective tissue and tendons results in their developing a blue-black pigmentation seen most prominently in the ears, nose and cheeks. Articular cartilages are similarly pigmented. There is some evidence that the pigment accumulates in these sites because it binds to collagen. *It is the blue-black pigmentation of these sites which is referred to as ochronosis.* While the ochronosis produces some unusual cosmetic effects, its principal significance lies in its predisposing to severe degenerative arthritis, encountered in about half of the older patients with alkaptonuria. The arthritic disease is not related in intensity to the pigmentation of the cartilage, nor is it understood how the pigmentation predisposes to such cartilaginous injury. The metabolic defect is otherwise without consequence and, while it is not life-threatening, the arthritis may become crippling. It is unfortunately impossible to devise a life-sustaining diet free of both tyrosine and phenylalanine, and so there is no effective treatment for this disorder.

TUMORS OF INFANCY AND CHILDHOOD

Tumors are generally considered to be lesions that occur only in later life, and it is therefore surprising and important to note that *malignant tumors are a major cause of disease and death in infancy and childhood.* In addition, benign tumors are common in children, some of which may arise as congenital defects.

The definition of neoplasia in the infant and young child is somewhat difficult. Displaced cells and masses of tissue may be present from birth that are apparently normal in appearance histologically, but nonetheless grow at approximately the same rate as the growth of the infant. Should such lesions be construed as new growths or simply as congenital malformations that enlarge along with the child? In recognition of these intergrades between normal tissue growth and true neoplastic growth, several special categories of tumorous lesions have been created.

Choristomas. The term choristoma has been applied to microscopically normal tissues that are present in abnormal locations. A synonym for such a lesion is an *aberrant rest* or *heterotopic tissue.* These were described on p. 128.

Hamartomas. The term hamartoma designates an *excessive focal overgrowth of mature normal cells and tissues in an organ or tissue composed of identical cellular elements.* Accordingly, disorganized masses of lymphocytes, reticuloendothelial cells, sinuses, blood vessels and occasional lymphoid follicles may be found as apparent tumors within the spleen. All these elements are normally indigenous to this organ, but the disorganization, the overgrowth and the encapsulation clearly indicate the anomalous status of such masses. Disorganized masses of hepatic cells, blood vessels, bile ducts and connective tissue in the liver create an additional hamartoma (Fig. 13–10). Hamartomas may occur in any organ in the body, but are most common in the spleen, liver, kidneys, lungs and pancreas.

Neoplasms. Between the ages of one and 14, cancer is the third leading cause of death. Five forms are of preponderant importance: leukemia-lymphoma (30 to 50 per cent), brain tumors (20 to 25 per cent), neuroblastomas (approximately 5 per cent), Wilms' tumors (approximately 5 per cent) and bone tumors (approximately 5 per cent). All of these cancers will be described in the chapters dealing with the pathology of specific organs and systems. Our purpose here is merely to point out certain features which differentiate cancers arising in early life from those of later life. Some are hereditary in origin, for example, the retinoblastoma transmitted as an autosomal dominant trait. Chronic myelogenous leukemia is quite common in children with Down's syndrome (p. 187). The frequency of malignant lymphomas is in-

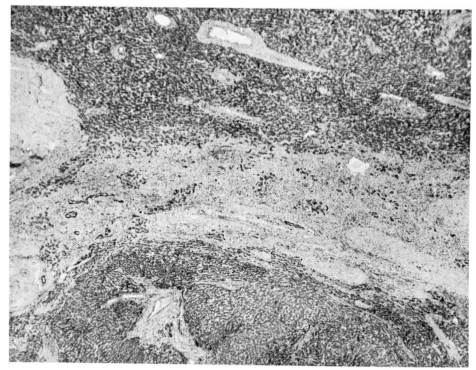

Figure 13–10. Hamartoma of liver. The broad band of fibrous tissue separates normal liver substance above from virtually identical-appearing hamartomatous parenchyma below.

creased also in certain genetically determined immunologic deficiency states. Some cancers in early life appear to arise in embryonic rests of cells. Thus extragonadal malignant teratomas arising in the pelvis and sacrococcygeal region are more common in children than in adults. The rapid growth of the infant and child involving active cellular proliferation may account in some part for their predisposition to mesenchymal soft tissue sarcomas and sarcomas of bone. Therapeutic irradiation of the child has more grave potential than an equivalent exposure of the adult. As is pointed out on p. 1340, irradiation of the head, neck and chest in infancy has been shown to lead to an increased frequency of thyroid cancer, sometimes several decades later. Thus, ironically, the use of radiation as a therapeutic measure for one form of cancer in childhood has been followed by the appearance of another form of cancer, presumably related to the radiation exposure. For example, curative radiotherapy of retinoblastomas has been followed by osteogenic sarcomas arising in areas exposed to the radiant energy.

An additional feature which differentiates childhood cancers from those of later life is their general tendency to grow rapidly, sometimes to enormous size without producing significant anemia, weight loss or cachexia. Often a palpable mass in the abdomen is the first clinical indication of a Wilms' tumor of the kidney or a neuroblastoma arising in the adrenal medulla. Many of these neoplasms are fortunately radioresponsive or can be effectively controlled or even destroyed by combined radiation, drugs and immunologic therapy. However, the dangers of radiotherapy in the infant and child have already been pointed out. It is a maxim in clinical practice that if metastasis or recurrence has not occurred after removal of a tumor in a period of time equivalent to the age of the patient plus nine months, the probability of cure is very high.

Benign tumors are much more common in early life than are cancers. Many indeed may be congenital, and may remain undetected only to appear after a period of years as they grow along with the child. The most common are hamartomas, hemangiomas, lymphangiomas and nevi. Hemangiomas arise most often in the skin. Whether they should be called true tumors is a controversial issue, and some prefer to consider them as congenital malformations. In either event, they are usually of little significance save for the disfigurement they produce. Lymphangiomas are, however, much more serious problems. They may be present at birth or appear at any time during childhood—principally in the neck and

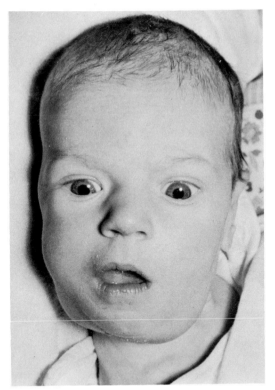

Figure 13–11. An infant with a submandibular lymphangioma causing irregular swellings beneath the chin and in the right buccal region.

axillary regions (Fig. 13–11). Less commonly, they are encountered in retroperitoneal or mesenteric locations as well as in viscera. While they are described more completely on p. 631, here it should be pointed out that although they are rarely malignant, they tend to insinuate themselves into tissue spaces and between cleavage planes and, since they grow along with the child, constitute difficult management problems. Surgical enucleation can be curative, but it is often exceedingly difficult to resect the insinuated ramifications, and so recurrences are common. Regrettably, with each recurrence, more rapid growth ensues, sometimes leading to malignant transformation. Nevi are another form of extremely common benign tumor (? congenital malformation) of infancy and childhood. Commonly referred to as "moles," they may occur on any part of the skin as pale brown to black pigmented lesions. Described in more detail on p. 1400, it is only necessary to point out that in infancy and childhood these nevi are almost invariably benign. However, at the time of puberty, certain types begin to grow more rapidly and may become melanocarcinomas. In general, the risk of such malignant transformation is small, militating

against any policy of attempted removal of all nevi in the child. It is, however, necessary to be aware of those sites known to be most ominous and not to ignore lesions which undergo rapid increase in size or consistency in the child at puberty. The occurrence and nature of other forms of neoplasia in this age group will be cited along with the consideration of these lesions in adults.

In concluding this chapter, it must be apparent that we have only skimmed the surface of the large catalogue of pediatric diseases. The disorders presented, however, are among the most common and important, and rightfully belong within the scope of general medical knowledge. As stated at the outset, the major disorders of infancy and childhood are peculiar to the age group. Only a few, such as cytomegalic inclusion disease, also affect adults and then they usually present quite different morphologic and clinical features. The disorders of childhood and those of adults differ more than the child and the adult themselves.

REFERENCES

Anzil, A. P., et al.: Cerebral form of generalized cytomegaly of early infancy. Light and electron microscopic findings. Virchow. Arch. Path. Anat., *351*:233, 1970.

Apgar, V.: A proposal for a new method of evaluation of the newborn infant. Curr. Res. Anesth. Analg., *32*:260, 1953.

Balis, J. U.: Maturation of postnatal human lung and the idiopathic respiratory distress syndrome. Lab. Invest., *15*:530, 1966.

Barter, R. A.: Pulmonary hyaline membrane, late results of injury to the lung lining. Arch. Dis. Child., *41*:489, 1966.

Berenberg, W., and Namkervis, G.: Long-term follow up of cytomegalic inclusion disease of infancy. Pediatrics, *46*:403, 1970.

Birnbaum, G., et al.: Cytomegalovirus infections in newborn infants. J. Pediat., *75*:789, 1969.

Blaskovics, M. E., and Nelson, T. L.: Phenylketonuria and its variations: a review of recent developments. Calif. Med., *115*:42, 1971.

Boggs, T. R., et al.: Correlation of neonatal serum total bilirubin concentration on developmental status at age eight months. J. Pediat., *71*:553, 1967.

Bowman, B. H., et al.: Oyster ciliary inhibition by cystic fibrosis factor. Science, *164*:325, 1969.

Clemento, J. A., et al.: Assessment of the risk of the respiratory distress syndrome by a rapid test for surfactant in amniotic fluid. New Eng. J. Med., *286*:1077, 1972.

Daily, W. J. R., et al.: Mechanical ventilation of newborn infants. Anesthesiology, *34*:132, 1971.

Danes, B. S.: Cell cultures and genetic disease. Hosp. Pract., *4*:88, 1969.

Di Sant Agnese, P. A., and Talamo, R. C.: Pathogenesis and physiopathology of cystic fibrosis of the pancreas. New Eng. J. Med., *277*:1287, 1344, 1399, 1967.

Drage, J. S., and Berendes, H.: Apgar scores and outcome of the newborn. Pediat. Clin. N. Amer., *13*:635, 1966.

Efron, M. I., et al.: Effect of elevated plasma phenylalanine levels on other amino acids in phenylketonuric and normal subjects. J. Pediat., *74*:399, 1969.

Farber, S. L., and Sweet, L. K.: Amniotic sac contents in the lungs of infants. Amer. J. Dis. Child., *42*:1372, 1931.

Fine, R. N.: Cytomegalovirus in children, postrenal transplantation. Amer. J. Dis. Child., *120*:197, 1970.

Forssman, N. H., et al.: Histological and chemical studies of a case of phenylketonuria with long survival. J. Ment. Defic. Res., *11*:194, 1967.

Gellis, S. S., and Hsia, D. Y.: The infant of the diabetic mother. Amer. J. Dis. Child., 97:1, 1959.

Gibson, L. E., et al.: Relating mucus, calcium and sweat in a new concept of cystic fibrosis. Pediatrics, 48:659, 1971.

Gische, Z., et al.: Composition of mucoprotein fractions from duodenal fluid of patients with cystic fibrosis and from controls. Pediatrics, 24:74, 1959.

Gitlin, D., and Craig, J. M.: Nature of the hyaline membrane in asphyxia of the newborn. Pediatrics, 17:64, 1956.

Guthrie, R., and Sosi, A.: A simple phenylalanine method for detecting phenylketonuria in large populations of newborn infants. Pediatrics, 32:338, 1963.

Hsia, D. Y-Y.: Clinical variants of galactosemia. Metabolism, 16:419, 1967.

Ivy, R. H.: Congenital anomalies: as recorded on birth certificates in Division of Vital Statistics of Pennsylvania Department of Health for the period 1951–1955 inclusive. Plas. Reconstr. Surg., 20:400, 1957.

Lauweryns, J. M.: Hyaline membrane disease: a pathological study of 55 infants. Arch. Dis. Child., 40:618, 1965.

Lauweryns, J. M.: Hyaline membrane disease in newborn infants. Macroscopic, radiographic and light and electron microscopic studies. Hum. Path., 1:175, 1970.

Lauweryns, J. M., et al.: Pulmonary lymphatics in neonatal hyaline membrane disease. Pediatrics, 41:917, 1968.

Lindsay, S.: Hemolytic disease of the newborn infant (erythroblastosis fetalis). J. Pediatrics, 37:582, 1950.

Malamud, N.: Neuropathology of phenylketonuria. J. Neuropath. Exp. Neurol., 25:254, 1966.

Malpas, P.: Incidence of human malformations and significance of changes in maternal environment in their causation. J. Obstet. Gynaec. Brit. Comm., 44:434, 1937.

Mangos, J. A., and McSherry, N. R.: Sodium transport: inhibitory factor in sweat of patients with cystic fibrosis. Science, 158:135, 1967.

McIntosh, R., et al.: Incidence of congenital malformation: study of 5964 pregnancies. Pediatrics, 14:505, 1954.

McKean, C. M., and Peterson, N. A.: Glutamine in the phenylketonuric central nervous system. New Eng. J. Med., 283:1364, 1970.

Mollison, P. L.: Blood Transfusion in Clinical Medicine, 4th ed. Oxford, Blackwell Scientific Publications, 1967, p. 697.

Mollison, P. L.: The reticuloendothelial system and red cell destruction. Proc. Roy. Soc. Med., 55:915, 1962.

Neel, J. V., and Schull, W. J.: The effect of exposure to the atomic bombs on pregnancy termination in Hiroshima and Nagasaki. Washington D.C., National Academy of Science, National Research Council. Government Printing Office Publication No. 461, 1956, p. 216.

Nelson, N. M.: On the etiology of hyaline membrane disease. Pediat. Clin. N. Amer., 17:943, 1970.

Perry, T. L., et al.: Glutamine depletion in phenylketonuria. New Eng. J. Med., 282:761, 1970.

Prior, J. A.: Diffuse exocrinopathy (cystic fibrosis). Ohio Med. J., 57:1121, 1961.

Rowe, W. P., et al.: Cytopathogenic agent resembling human salivary gland virus recovered from tissue cultures of human adenoids. Proc. Soc. Exp. Biol. Med., 92:418, 1956.

Rufer, R.: The influence of surface active substances on alveolar mechanics in the respiratory distress syndrome. Respiration, 25:441, 1968.

Salguero, I. F., et al.: Neuropathologic observations in phenylketonuria. Trans. Amer. Neurol. Ass., 93:274, 1968.

Schiff, P.: The immunology of Rh-haemolytic disease. A review. Med. J. Aust., 2:915, 1969.

Shwachman, H., et al.: Studies in cystic fibrosis. Report of 130 patients diagnosed under 3 months of age over a 20 year period at the Children's Hospital Medical Center, Boston, Mass. Pediatrics, 46:335, 1970.

Siegel, M., and Greenberg, M.: Fetal death, malformation and prematurity after maternal rubella. Results of prospective study 1949–1958. New Eng. J. Med., 262:389, 1960.

Smetana, H. F., and Olen, E.: Hereditary galactose disease. Amer. J. Clin. Path., 38:3, 1962.

Spock, A.: Cystic fibrosis: current theories concerning the pathogenesis. Minn. Med., 52:1429, 1969.

Spock, A., et al.: Abnormal serum factor in patients with cystic fibrosis of the pancreas. Pediat. Res., 1:173, 1967.

Stern, H., and Elek, S. D.: The incidence of infection with cytomegalovirus in a normal population. A serological study in greater London. J. Hygiene, 63:79, 1965.

Stevenson, S. S., et al.: 677 congenitally malformed infants and associated gestational characteristics. I. General considerations. Pediatrics, 6:37, 1950.

Swan, C., and Tostevin, A. L.: Congenital abnormalities in infants following infectious diseases during pregnancy with special reference to rubella: third series of cases. Med. J. Aust., 1:645, 1946.

Vidyasagar, D., and Chernick, V.: Continuous positive transpulmonary pressure in hyaline membrane disease: a simple device. Pediatrics, 48:296, 1971.

Warkany, J., and Kalter, H.: Congenital malformations. New Eng. J. Med., 265:993, 1046, 1961.

World Health Organization: Five years of research on human genetics. W.H.O. Chron., 24:248, 1970.

14

DISEASES OF AGING

Theories of Aging
Morphologic Changes of Aging
   Cellular and extracellular
      alterations

Alterations in organs
   Skin
   Heart
   Aorta

RE and lymphoid systems
Neoplasms
**Clinical Implications of
Senescence**

No one needs to be told that geriatrics, the diagnosis and treatment of diseases of aged individuals, is a medical speciality of great importance destined to become even more important in the years to come. The number of individuals in the population over the age of 65 is on the increase in the United States, both in absolute and relative terms (Fig. 14–1). In the foreseeable future, it is inevitable that more than 10 per cent of the total population of the United States will be 65 years of age or over. The provision of adequate socioeconomic and medical care for them constitutes one of the major problems of our day. Advances in medical care have already significantly extended the mean life span, but it is interesting

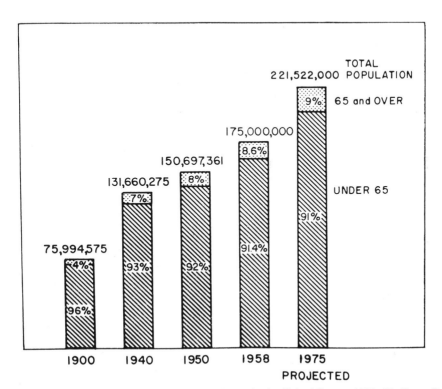

Figure 14–1. *Population increase in people 65 and over in the United States, 1900–75. (From Patterns of Incidence of Certain Diseases Throughout the World—Opportunities for Research Through Epidemiology. Washington, D.C., U.S. Government Printing Office, 1959.)*

that the maximum life span has remained about the same since antiquity.

Aging and senescence begin in fact at the moment the ovum is fertilized. For the purposes of this discussion, aging may be defined as those changes in structure and function that (1) occur usually following the attainment of reproductive maturity; (2) result in a decreased ability to adapt to or overcome environmental or internal challenges; and (3) result in an increased probability of death with time (Mildvan and Strehler, 1960). This definition includes the four cardinal criteria of the phenomenon of aging: (1) universality, (2) progressiveness (and irreversibility), (3) intrinsicality (property of the organism) and (4) deleteriousness. Senescence is obviously closely related to aging, but whereas aging emphasizes all transitions in time, senescence emphasizes the quality of the transitions and the accumulation of the deleterious ones. While the biologic processes of aging occur on the cellular and tissue levels throughout life and even before birth (if changes in the placenta and the involution of fetal structures are included), gerontology and geriatrics are concerned with the period when the deleterious factors of aging manifest themselves in the decline of functional capacity and in an increased mortality rate. It must be realized, however, that decline in function proceeds at differing rates in the various organs and tissues. For example, for visual and auditory acuity, muscle activity, endocrine function and connective tissue elasticity, it may be demonstrated to begin in the third decade of life. Geriatrics is concerned principally with the later periods generally referred to as senescence and with the threat of death evoked by every illness.

Aging and senescence are the consequences of two separate sets of influences: constitutional (genetic) and environmental. In man and free-living animals, it is virtually impossible to separate or identify the effects of these two sets. In lower animals with highly inbred strains, some interesting observations on environmental factors have been made. It has been shown that the rate of aging can be slowed by (1) dietary restriction, (2) lowering of the body temperature, (3) administration of antioxidants and (4) attempts to thwart autoimmune mechanisms. In the classic studies of McKay et al. (1939) on underfeeding rats, it was shown that the maximum age could be doubled. These animals grew at a substantially lower rate and continued this slow increment long after the control animals had ceased to grow. It is noteworthy that this prolongation of life span was associated with a delayed onset of tumors, chronic diseases related to senescence

and, moreover, the tail collagen of these growth-retarded rats was found to be "young" in response to heat shrinkage. As will be seen, collagen is one of the tissue components that is most vulnerable to aging changes. No parallel studies have been done of species closer to man, but they would certainly appear to be desirable. A partial parallelism might add many youthful years to life but, as Strehler (1967) cautions, "an 'average' life span of 70 years is probably preferable to a 'mean' life span of 85!" Lowering of body temperature in fish has paradoxically increased growth and increased longevity (Liu and Walford, 1970). However, in contrast, homeothermic rats maintained at low ambient temperature have a considerable decrease in life span (Johnson et al., 1963). These contradictory results are best explained by the accelerated metabolic activity in the cooled homeotherms required to maintain body temperature and are therefore consistent with Pearl's (1928) "rate of living theory" to the effect that the duration of life is inversely proportional to the rate of energy expenditure. Antioxidants such as vitamin E prolong the life span of mice to a small degree (Harman, 1969). As is discussed later, oxygen-free radicals are considered to be one of the causes of aging changes in cells, and so vitamin E might serve in the role of antioxidant. Mice raised in a germ-free environment and rats splenectomized early in life had longer mean life spans (Gordon et al., 1966) (Albright et al., 1969). Both of these interventions were interpreted as blocking the immune mechanisms and hence autoimmunity.

THEORIES OF AGING

No one would deny that the rate of aging varies among individuals and certainly among ethnic groups. Lawton (1965), in a discussion of the historic developments in the biologic aspects of aging, calls attention to a Thomas Parr who reputedly committed a sexual offense at 102, married with "complete marital bliss" at 120 and died in 1639 at the age of 152. Aside from this remarkable creature, evidence abounds in the form of the spry and mentally acute octogenarians contrasting sharply with the frail "empty shells" of those much younger. The ethnic contrasts are often more vivid, as witness the wizened, worn faces and bodies of many young members of native tribes living under primitive conditions. Such facts of life make clear that the rate of aging is variable whether it be due to genetic programs or environmental influence. Innumerable theories have been offered in explanation of these facts. None satisfactorily copes with all observed data, and all are highly speculative. Some of the more important theories dealing with both genetic and environmental influences are presented here.

Cross-Linkage Theory. This theory proposes that aging is caused by increasing cross-linkage of protein and nucleic acid molecules (Bjorksten, 1968). In effect, it is suggested that over the span of years, cross-links between atoms and molecules accumulate, altering the chemical behavior and biochemical efficiency of the original molecules. Such cross-linkage is thought to be particularly important in the aging of collagen and DNA.

Collagen Theory. In essence, this theory holds that collagen, accounting for about 40 per cent of a human's total protein, tends both to increase in amount and to cross-link slowly but progressively with age (Carpenter and Loynd, 1968). The cross-links cause the collagen fibers to shrink with age, and the combination of increase in amount and contraction is postulated as a cause of anoxic injury to tissues and organs. While this theory has been challenged by many, it does provide a specific mechanism for one of the symptoms of age—wrinkling of the skin.

Free Radical Theory. This conception is essentially an explanation of the manner by which cross-linkages develop. It holds that free radicals within the organism cause the production of molecular cross-linkages. Its chief support derives from the studies employing antioxidants which both decrease the density of free radicals and prolong life in mice (Harman, 1962).

Waste-Product Theory. It has long been assumed, but without substantial proof, that aging represents the progressive accumulation of metabolic waste products. Attempts have been made to identify such waste products in the blood which might inhibit growth and metabolism of cells, but without success. It is known that lipofuscin accumulates with age and, indeed, has been called the "wear and tear" pigment. In some aged individuals, it may constitute as much as 30 per cent of the weight of heart muscle (Strehler et al., 1959). There is, however, no proof that the lipofuscin interferes with function. Perhaps, however, other more subtle metabolic waste products are important in this connection; but this is purely speculation.

Genetic-Mutation Theory of Aging. Aging might be an extension of the processes of differentiation. Certainly, the senescence of ovaries at the time of menopause is the consequence of in-built programs residing either in the genes or in genetic expression. There is good evidence that the genome significantly

conditions life span. On the average, identical twins have a mean difference in their life spans of three years, whereas fraternal twins have a mean difference of six years (Powell et al., 1966). It is generally proposed that, with aging, errors in replication, transcription and translation of DNA increase. These errors could be the consequence of cross-linking of DNA molecules, random mutations, loss of certain species of transfer RNA, and increased formation of DNA-histone complexes, thereby inactivating it. These represent mechanisms by which cell metabolism and viability could be impaired (Goldstein, 1971). Szilard (1959) has formalized this concept of genetic-mutation aging by proposing that genes are exposed throughout life to what he calls "aging hits" and these occur with a constant probability per unit of time. The accumulation of hits and the progressive inactivation of genes eventually lead to a critical point where further hits may cause death. Consistent with this theory is the increase in chromosomal breaks and aneuploidy with advancing age. Further support comes from the correlation of the frequency of demonstrable chromosomal aberrations in strains of rats with decreased life spans as compared to rats with longer life spans (Curtis, 1966).

Autoimmune Theory. This theory is based on the concept that, with advancing age, mutations give rise to forbidden clones that react against self and thus degrade and eventually destroy the organism (Walford, 1969). A striking increase in spontaneously occurring autoantibodies has been demonstrated in clinically normal older persons (Walford, 1969). Such autoimmune diseases as rheumatoid arthritis, chronic thyroiditis and pernicious anemia are more common in the last half of life than in the first. Obviously, however, not all elderly people acquire immunologic diseases, and so this conception of aging may not have universality.

A number of other theories exist such as those which view aging as a progressive response to stress or relate it to the metabolic rate or, alternatively, to gradual loss of the nervous system's control over the organism's cells; and while theories abound, well established facts are scant. In the last analysis, the causes of aging are still mysterious.

SOME MORPHOLOGIC CHANGES OF AGING

All aged individuals invariably have a variety of morphologic changes acquired over the span of decades. The separation of those changes due to the residuals of disease and the virtually omnipresent atherosclerosis from those related only to aging is difficult if not impossible. Ultimately, every aged individual dies as a result of some disease. "Death due to senile change" is extremely rare. In old age, the lethal threshold falls until even the most trivial intercurrent "stress" causes death. Thus, at postmortem examination, there is never the opportunity to view senescence devoid of complicating causes of tissue and cell injury. Despite these difficulties, certain changes have been ascribed to aging since they are seen as a common background against which the diseases and vascular insufficiency have asserted their special alterations. These aging changes are discussed at the level of cells (and tissues) and at the level of organs.

CELLULAR AND EXTRACELLULAR ALTERATIONS

A host of changes have been seen at the cellular level. These involve the nucleus and cytoplasm with its contained organelles. In senescence, the number of parenchymal cells declines, cell size and staining properties become more irregular and binuclear cells become more frequent (Tauchi, 1962). The more differentiated the cell, the more aging changes are evident. Thus the neuron in the young individual is characterized by a diffusely basophilic cytoplasm, conspicuous organelles and a well defined, only focally basophilic nucleus, contrasting sharply with "senile" neurons having scanty Nissl substance, a nucleus distorted by variable irregular clumps of dense chromatin and a cytoplasm simplified by loss of organelles, including mitochondria. Liver cells show variation in size and shape with age. The number of binuclear forms increases. The nuclear outline becomes somewhat irregular, along with clumped basophilia of the chromatin within the nucleus (Kleinfeld et al., 1956). The changes are even more evident at the level of the electron microscope, and swelling vacuolization and disruption of the cristae of the mitochondria have been seen in neurons (Bondareff, 1964). Perhaps the most striking change in "senile" cells is the progressive accumulation of lipofuscin pigment. This is seen principally in the liver, heart and nervous system (Strehler and Mildvan, 1962). In addition to the above morphologic observations, the incidence of visible chromosomal aberrations as well as the incidence of cells with an excess or deficiency of chromosomes increases with age (Curtis and Crowley, 1963).

Aging is also associated with biochemical alterations in cells. A qualitative decline in the activity, and alteration of nucleotides of RNA, has been correlated with aging. Paralleling this is an apparent increase in histone-DNA binding. It is believed that when histone complexes to DNA, the genetic material is inactivated, and so there is some evidence that senescence is characterized by progressive loss of genetic programs (von Hahn, 1964/65).

Collagen, as mentioned previously, undergoes age-related changes. With the passage of time, collagen becomes increasingly rigid and inflexible. The sclerotic connective tissue impedes mobility and the nutrition of parenchymal cells. The rigidity of collagen mainly due to increased cross-linking is accompanied by a decrease in its water content and a change in its molecular arrangement that leads to increased thermal contractility and decreased solubility. Whether such changes are justifiably considered deteriorative or maturational is semantic, but certainly the aged individual lacks the litheness and suppleness of the young. Some of the most consistent associations with aging are: the spinous ligaments become more unyielding, and the intervertebral discs shrink. This specialized field has been extensively reviewed (Gross, 1961; Kohn, 1963; Sinex, 1964).

Elastin, too, suffers a patchy kind of degradation in senile animals (Piez, 1968). In addition, there is an increase of elastin fibers in aging connective tissue in general, particularly in the dermis, endocardium and most prominently in the entire arterial system. In addition to this quantitative change, the elastic fibers have an increased basophilia and are altered qualitatively so that they appear matted, smudged and twisted. Such alterations are particularly well seen in the senile elastosis of the skin discussed below

ALTERATIONS IN ORGANS

Skin. Senile keratosis and senile atrophy of the skin combined with characteristic wrinkling will be briefly mentioned in another chapter (p. 1374). In aging of the skin, atrophy and some disorientation of the layers of the epidermis occur but, in addition, changes develop in the dermis and appendages. In aged individuals, about 72 to 79 per cent by weight of the human dermis is composed of collagen with the aging changes described above. There is a concomitant increase of thick and twisted elastic fibers in the dermis (Rasmussen et al., 1965) (Montagna, 1965). Such elastosis is more marked in the exposed portions of the skin where large areas of the dermis show basophilic staining of the elastic fibers when stained with orcein or other methods for elastica (Fig. 14–2). While there has been some question

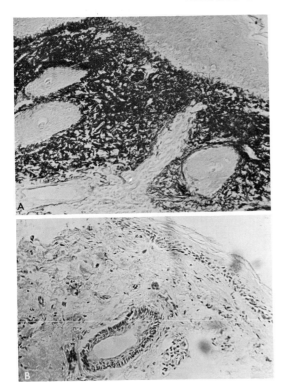

Figure 14–2. A, *Senile elastosis of dermis.* × *160. Stained with Gomori's aldehyde-fuchsin.* B, *The same area as at A, but treated with elastase before staining with aldehyde-fuchsin.*

about the nature of this smudged basophilic substance and some have held that it is collagenous in origin, by chemical and histochemical methods it has been shown at least in greater part to be identical with true elastin (Shushan, 1964). A relationship between these elastotic changes and cutaneous carcinoma has been postulated (Gillman et al., 1955).

The eccrine sweat glands show involution and partial fibrosis, and there is a decrease in the number of the surrounding nerve fibrils. However, the decreased secretion of sebum in senescence is not explained by atrophy of the sebaceous glands alone but is also due to hormonal dysfunction (Montagna, 1965).

Graying of hair is not caused by depigmentation of existing hair but by replacement of new hair follicles which, over the course of years, contain progressively less melanin pigment. The mechanism of formation of melanin pigment was explained elsewhere, so it suffices here to say that, with age, hair follicles contain progressively smaller amounts of dopa-oxidase and tyrosinase, both required in melanin synthesis (Fitzpatrick et al., 1965). There may or may not be a decrease in the number of melanocytes. It is interesting to note that aging of melanin-forming systems occurs at different rates in various organs. There is no "aging" of the retinal pigment epithelium. Melanin pigment is gradually reduced in the substantia nigra but remains constant in amount in the leptomeninges (Fitzpatrick et al., 1965).

In the aging exposed skin, spotty proliferation of melanocytes at the epidermal-dermal junction is the histologic basis for the well known senile lentigo.

Heart. A clear separation of aging changes from those due to disease is more difficult in the heart than in other organs. This is mainly due to the almost universally present coronary atherosclerosis which, having developed over many decades, produces cardiac changes in the great majority of persons living through senescence. There are, however, a few cases in which the coronary arteries have remained free of atherosclerosis. Probably as a result of natural processes of selection, a considerable percentage of persons surviving into the eighth decade of life belong in this category. This is reflected in autopsy data in which atherosclerosis of the coronary arteries is found to be less prevalent in those dying during the eighth decade of life than in the preceding decade. The decline in the prevalence of coronary heart disease after 75 years of age is also evident from clinical data. According to a report of the U. S. Department of Health, Education and Welfare, the peak prevalence of arteriosclerotic heart disease (17 per cent) occurs in the 65 to 74-year-old group and then decreases to 12.4 per cent in the 75 to 79-year-old group.

If one excludes coronary atheromatosis, high blood pressure and hearts containing stigmata of chronic rheumatic or other inflammatory disease, one should theoretically be able then to identify the changes related to aging. In such selected hearts, there is no significant weight variation between the young adult and the senescent (Reiner et al., 1959). However, age-related changes are present in the various tissues of the heart. According to some, interstitial fibrous tissue is increased in the atrial myocardium, accompanied by an infiltration of adipose tissue. This may also be seen frequently in the wall of the right ventricle (McMillan and Lev, 1962). Others, however, have denied the increase in fibrous tissue and contend that there is a constant ratio between the connective tissue and the muscle mass in the human myocardium that is independent of age and weight of the heart. They hold that any increase of supportive tissue is the result of hypoxia resulting from alterations in the vascular supply, perhaps at the level of the finer circulation.

The muscle fibers gradually increase in thickness until maturity but then remain constant. The progressive accumulation of lipofuscin in the aging myocardium has long been recognized by pathologists and, as mentioned, may account for 30 per cent of the tissue weight.

The endocardium in senescence is thickened, especially in the atria, and is rich in fibers taking the stain for elastic tissue. Similar changes can be seen in the mitral and tricuspid leaflets, but these age changes are difficult to differentiate from healed rheumatic lesions (Fig. 14–3) (Angrist, 1964) (Ungar and Ben-Ishay, 1965).

Thickening of the intimal layer of the intramyocardial branches of the coronary arteries begins in the third decade of life and is accompanied by progressive elastification of the media. These alterations appear to be independent of atherosclerotic and hypertensive disease and therefore represent a true age change (Fig. 14–4).

Aorta. With advancing age, the aorta becomes wider and more tortuous (Fig. 14–5) (Ben-Ishay et al., 1962). The changes are paralleled by a progressive loss of elasticity. However, despite the progressive dilatation, the thickness of the intima and the media increases until about 45 to 50 years, and then remains constant. Only during the ninth decade does the media begin to decrease in thickness. This thinning is produced by elimination of elastic fibers and atrophy of muscle elements accompanied by some collagenization (Fig. 14–6) (Movat et al., 1958). A thorough discussion of the morphologic, biochemical and histochemical changes in the aortic wall re-

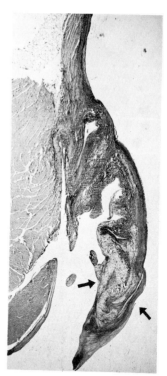

Figure 14–3. Mitral valve of 66-year-old female showing diffuse thickening and abundant elastosis extending into endocardium of the atrium (arrows). × 6. Aldehyde-fuchsin.

lated to aging can be found in the monograph edited by Lansing (1959).

All these senile changes are accentuated by concurrent atherosclerosis, but they are clearly related to age and are present in equal intensity in ethnic groups both prone and resistant to atherosclerosis.

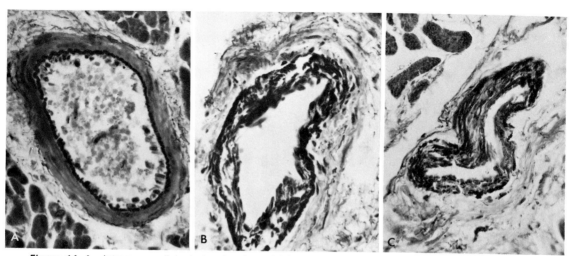

Figure 14–4. Intramyocardial arteries showing, with increasing age, progressive elastification at first of intima and later also of the media. A, Age 19; B, age 41; C, age 71. The three cases were free of rheumatic or ischemic heart disease.

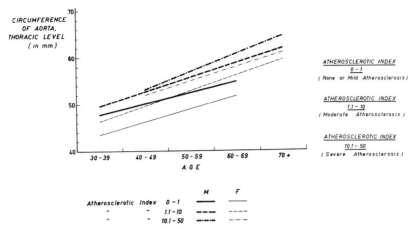

Figure 14–5. *Age-dependent enlargement of the aorta, related to the degree of atherosclerosis. (From Ben-Ishay, Z., et al.: Atherosclerosis and aging of the aorta in the adult Jewish population of Israel. Amer. J. Cardiol., 10:407, 1962.)*

RE and Lymphoid Systems. Separate mention of these systems is indicated, despite the scarcity of findings, first, because of the well known decreased resistance of the aged to infections, and second, because an autoimmune reaction has been suggested as one possible cause of aging itself (Blumenthal and Berns, 1964). Indeed, flagging defense mechanisms in senescence may explain the frequency of fatal, often staphylococcal bronchopneumonia, a pulmonary disorder only seen as often in infancy and childhood when the defenses are as yet poorly developed. Often

these bronchopneumonias follow viral infections, particularly influenza (McKeown, 1965).

Variations with age of the mass of lymphoid tissue in the body are difficult to determine, except for the spleen, but the lymphoid mass apparently reaches its maximum development at about puberty. At this time there is rapid involution of the thymus. The average weight of the spleen increases until about 30 years of age and then slowly falls throughout life. The decrease in weight becomes well marked by the sixth and seventh decades of life (Marshall, 1961). This decrease in splenic

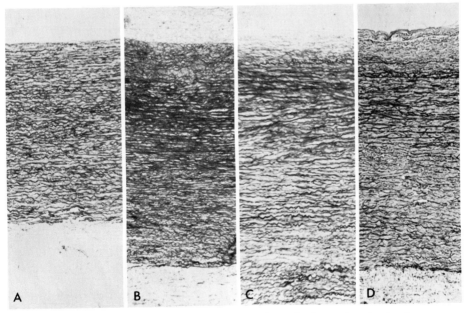

Figure 14–6. *Thoracic aorta at different ages in areas free of atherosclerosis showing progressive disarrangement of elastic fibers and their replacement by collagen. The thickness of media increases until middle age. A, Age 15; B, age 25; C, age 56; D, age 70.*

weight is accompanied by progressive involution of the malpighian bodies of the spleen. These involutional alterations may in fact begin in the third decade. There is concomitant hyaline thickening of the follicular arteries throughout life that occasionally can be seen as early as the second decade of life. The nature of this vascular hyalin has not been chemically identified. This change, often described as arteriosclerosis, is not related to either hypertension or arterial lesions in the systemic vessels.

Despite the general atrophy of the spleen, increased numbers of plasma cells have been noted in it in persons above 70 years of age, and this observation has been correlated with increased levels of serum globulins in advanced life (Haferkamp, 1964).

A lead connecting aging to an immunologic reaction has been the common finding of amyloidosis in aged patients. The pathogenesis of amyloid was discussed on p. 282 where it was pointed out that amyloid might result from some accentuated or deranged immunologic reaction. Accordingly, it has been suggested that senile amyloid may be the result of autosensitization to the progressive endogenous disintegration of cells throughout life (Blumenthal and Berns, 1964).

Senile amyloidosis in the heart as an aging lesion is more frequent in persons over 55 years of age and becomes increasingly prevalent with each subsequent decade of life. Similarly, hyalin or amyloid can be demonstrated in the islets of Langerhans in a large majority of persons aged 60 to 90, independent of the presence of diabetes (Ehrlich and Ratner, 1961). Primary isolated amyloidosis has been known for many years to occur in the peripheral and autonomic nervous system. Only recently have improved methods of identification of amyloid made it possible to corroborate older reports of the deposit of this substance in senile and presenile deterioration of the brain (Schwartz et al., 1965). These central nervous system changes have recently been classified into three groups: senile plaque formation, meningovascular amyloidosis with or without systemic amyloidosis, and so-called "senile cerebral amyloidosis" (Haberland, 1964). However, it is by no means clear that amyloid results from an antigen-antibody reaction, and any association between senile amyloid and an autoimmune causation for aging is tenuous at best (Marshall, 1961).

NEOPLASMS

The relationship between advancing years and an increased frequency of cancer is well known. Indeed, in most nonselected postmortem studies in general hospitals, cancer accounts for about one death in five. Quite often, these autopsies on individuals over the age of 50 disclose a considerable number of unrecognized tumors, both benign and malignant, and a remarkable number of multiple primary neoplasms (Mulligan, 1959) (Delarue et al., 1931) (McKeown, 1965). This prevalence of neoplasia in senescence is difficult to explain, but attempts were made in the earlier discussion of carcinogenesis. Age-related mutations and loss of repressor control mechanisms are two of the possible pathways mentioned (Kohn, 1963). Alternatively, it is conceivable that over the course of years the cumulative exposure to carcinogenic agents such as aromatic hydrocarbons or radiant energy might eventually induce the formation of a tumor (Failla, 1958). While the explanations are hypothetical, the increased prevalence of cancer in senescence is not.

CLINICAL IMPLICATIONS OF SENESCENCE

The medical and economic care of aged individuals has become one of the major areas of concern of privileged countries. For reasons already discussed, the disproportionate increase in the percentage of the population over age 65 imposes upon physicians need for greater concern with geriatrics.

The use of age 65 as the lower age limit of senescence, although generally accepted by society and law, is obviously without meaning medically. Aging, as has been noted, begins with fertilization of the ovum, and it is commonplace knowledge that individuals age at greatly varying rates. Senescence then is better defined as beginning when there are loss of vigor, the previously described changes in the skin, slowed activity of the musculoskeletal system and the onset of obvious deterioration of mental function.

It is necessary to emphasize that the aged patient rarely dies with a single disease. The long list of anatomic diagnoses compiled after each postmortem attests to this fact. This multiplicity of pathologic changes in one individual creates serious problems in clinical diagnosis, matched only by the difficulty in clinical evaluation of the infant in the first months of life. Moreover, the senile patient often has confusingly atypical symptomatology of such well characterized diseases as thyrotoxicosis, appendicitis, peptic ulcer, pneumonia and diabetes mellitus (Stieglitz, 1954) (Geill, 1960) (Krieger-Lassen, 1962). While arteriosclerosis, hypertension and cancer constitute the major killers in senescence, almost invariably there is a host of associated findings in the individual patient. Usually these associated lesions contribute little or nothing to the cause of death, and all too often they are casually dismissed by the physician as "incidental findings." But in many instances they are more than incidental and, indeed, may make the last years of life miserable for the patient. It is impossible to cite all the specific diseases that are particularly associated with advanced age, but a few examples will be cited here.

Chronic osteoarthritis is often taken for granted as an inevitable concomitant of age. Although this skeletal disorder rarely comprises a direct cause of death, it often contributes to the fatality by predisposing to decreased mobility of the patient, increased frequency of phlebothrombosis and embolism, or induces accident proneness with its associated soft tissue and skeletal injuries that often initiate the downhill course to death. Osteoarthropathy of the knee joint is reported to be present in 48 per cent of individuals in the fourth decade of life and in virtually 100 per cent of patients during the ninth decade.

The *gastrointestinal tract* often harbors a variety of lesions in aged individuals, including senescent decay of the teeth and their surrounding structures, atrophy of the salivary glands, atrophic gastritis and polyps of the colon. Often completely unanticipated peptic ulcers are encountered. Cholecystitis and cholelithiasis are found as an apparent surprise in a number of cases. Diverticulosis of the colon is present in 5 to 10 per cent of the population over the age of 65. While any of these disorders may be of little clinical significance in the individual case, they may contribute significantly to the burden of life in the late years, impairing the capacity to eat and enjoy food as well as giving origin to a host of gastrointestinal complaints.

Chronic renal disease is an almost inevitable finding in autopsies on senescent individuals. The two most common lesions are pyelonephritis and benign nephrosclerosis.

Benign prostatic hyperplasia and cystocele, often associated with cystitis, frequency, nocturia and dysuria, are virtual hallmarks of the late years.

Senile changes in the lung, arteriosclerotic alterations in the heart and legs and varicose formations in the lower legs make the cardiovascular and respiratory systems a prominent source of infirmity in the age group under consideration.

While somewhat outside the scope of our present consideration, it is nonetheless worthwhile to mention the changed tolerance to drugs of aged individuals, evidenced by delayed or incomplete absorption or excretion of administered medications (Stieglitz, 1954).

The disorders just mentioned are obviously only a random sampling of the problems of senescence. However, it is clear, because of the prevalence of certain diseases and the atypical symptomatology characteristic of advanced life, that geriatrics is destined to become as important and as specialized an area of medicine as pediatrics.

REFERENCES

Albright, J. F., et al.: Presence of life shortening factors in spleens of aged mice of long life span and extension of life expectancy by splenectomy. Exp. Geront., 4:267, 1969.

Angrist, A.: Aging heart valves and a unitary pathological hypothesis for aging. J. Geront., 19:135, 1964.

Ben-Ishay, Z., et al.: Atherosclerosis and aging of the aorta in the adult Jewish population of Israel. An anatomic study. Amer. J. Cardiol., 10:407, 1962.

Bjorksten, J.: The cross-linkage theory of aging. J. Amer. Geriat. Soc., 16:408, 1968.

Blumenthal, H. T., and Berns, A. W.: Autoimmunity and aging. In Strehler, B. L. (ed): Advances in Gerontological Research. Vol. 1. New York, Academic Press, 1964.

Bondareff, W.: Histophysiology of the aging nervous systems. Advances Geriat. Res., 1:1, 1964.

Carpenter, E. G., and Loynd, J. A.,: An integrated theory of aging. J. Amer. Geriat. Soc., 16:1307, 1968.

Curtis, H. J.: Biological Mechanisms of Aging. Springfield, Ill., Charles C Thomas, 1966.

Curtis, H., and Crowley, C.: Chromosome aberrations in liver cells in relation to the somatic mutation theory of aging. Radiol. Ther. Res., 19:337, 1963.

Delarue, J., et al.: Le cancre chez le vieillard. Bull. Cancer., 48:17, 1931.

Ehrlich, J. C., and Ratner, I. M.: Amyloidosis of the islets of Langerhans. A restudy of islet hyalin in diabetic and non-diabetic individuals. Amer. J. Path., 38:49, 1961.

Failla, G.: The aging process and cancerogenesis. Ann. N. Y. Acad. Sci., 71:1124, 1958.

Fitzpatrick, T. B., et al.: Age changes in the human melanocyte system. In Montagna, W. (ed): Advances in Biology of Skin. Vol. VI. Oxford, Pergamon Press, 1965, p.35.

Geill, T.: Old age, disease and death. Excerpta Med. (XX), 3:447, 1960.

Gillman, T., et al.: Abnormal elastic fibers. Appearance in cutaneous carcinoma, irradiation injuries and arterial and other degenerative connective tissue lesions in man. Arch. Path., 59:733, 1955.

Goldstein, S.: The biology of aging. New Eng. J. Med., 285:1120, 1971.

Gordon, H. A., et al.: Aging in germ-free mice: life tables and lesions observed at natural death. J. Geront., 21:380, 1966.

Gross, J.: Aging of connective tissue: the extracellular components. In Bourne, G. H. (ed): Structural Aspects of Aging. London, Pitman, 1961.

Haberland, C.: Primary systemic amyloidosis: cerebral involvement and senile plaque formation. J. Neuropath. Exp. Neurol., 23:135, 1964.

Haferkamp, O.: Immunology and immunochemistry of old age. In Hanse, P. F. (ed.): Age with a Future. Copenhagen, Munksgaard, 1964.

Harman, D.: Prolongation of life: a role of three radical reactions in aging. J. Amer. Geriat. Soc., 17:721, 1969.

Harman, D.: Role of free radicals in mutation, cancer, aging and the maintenance of life. Radiat. Res., 16:753, 1962.

Johnson, H. D., et al.: Effects of 48° F. (8.9 C) and 83° F. (28.4 C) on longevity and pathology of male rats. J. Geront., 18:29, 1963.

Kleinfeld, R. G., et al.: Electron microscopy of intranuclear inclusions found in human and rat liver parenchymal cells. J. Biophys. Biochem. Cytol., 2:435, 1956.

Kohn, R. R.: Human aging and disease. J. Chron. Dis., 16:5, 1963.

Krieger-Lassen, H.: Geriatric problems in surgery. A clinical review with a statistical survey of mortality rates as related to age. J. Geront., 17:167, 1962.

Lansing, A. I.: Elastic tissue. In Lansing, A. I. (ed.): The Arterial Wall. Baltimore, Williams & Wilkins Co., 1959.

Lawton, A. H.: The historical developments in the biologic aspects of aging and the aged. Gerontologist, 5:25, 1965.

Liu, R. K., and Walford, R. L.: Observation on the life spans of several species of annual fishes and of the world's smallest fishes. Exp. Geront., 5:241, 1970.

Marshall, A. H. E.: Aging changes in lymphoid and myeloid tissues. In Bourne, G. H. (ed.): Structural Aspects of Aging. London, Pitman, 1961.

McKay, D. M., et al.: Retarded growth, life span, ultimate body size and age changes in the albino rat after feeding diet restricted in calories. J. Nutr., 18:1, 1939.

McKeown, F.: Pathology of the Aged. London, Butterworth, 1965.

McMillan, J. B., and Lev, M.: The aging heart. IV. The myocardium and epicardium. In Shock, N. W. (ed.): Biological Aspects of Aging. New York, Columbia University Press, 1962, p. 163.

Mildvan, A. S., and Strehler, B. L.: A critique of theories of mortality. In Strehler, B. L. (ed.): The Biology of Aging. Publication No. 6. Washington, D.C., American Institute of Biological Sciences, 1960, p. 309.

Montagna, W. (ed.): Advances in Biology of Skin. Vol. VI, Aging. Oxford, Pergamon Press, 1965.

Movat, H. Z., et al.: The diffuse intimal thickening of the human aorta with aging. Amer. J. Path., 34:1023, 1958.

Mulligan, R. M.: Geriatric cancer. Cancer, 12:970, 1959.

Pearl, R.: The Rate of Living. Being an Account of Some Experimental Studies on the Biology of Life Duration. New York, Alfred A. Knopf, 1928.

Piez, K. A.: Cross-linking of collagen and elastin. Ann. Rev. Biochem., 37:547, 1968.

Powell, K. E., et al.: Cellular aspects of aging: a review. Illinois Med. J., 130:613, 1966.

Rasmussen, D. M., et al.: Effect of aging on human dermis: studies of thermal shrinkage and tension. In Montagna, W. (ed.): Advances in Biology of Skin. Vol. VI. Oxford, Pergamon Press, 1965, p. 151.

Reiner, L., et al.: The weight of the human heart. I. "Normal" cases. Arch. Path., 68:58, 1959.

Schwartz, P., et al.: Fluorescence microscopy demonstration of cerebro-vascular and pancreatic insular amyloid in presenile and senile states. J. Amer. Geriat. Soc., 13:199, 1965.

Shushan, S.: Studies on elastic tissue. Ph.D. thesis, Jerusalem, 1964.

Sinex, F. M.: Cross-linkage and aging. In Strehler, B. L. (ed.): Advances in Gerontological Research. Vol. I. New York, Academic Press, 1964.

Stieglitz, E. J. (ed.): Geriatric Medicine. Medical Care of Later Maturity. Philadelphia, J. B. Lippincott Co., 1954.

Strehler, B. L.: Environmental factors in aging and mortality. Environ. Res., 1:46, 1967.

Strehler, B. L., and Mildvan, A. S.: Studies in the chemical properties of lipofuscin age pigment. In Shock, N. W. (ed.): Biological Aspects of Aging. New York, Columbia University Press, 1962.

Strehler, B. L., et al.: Rate and magnitude of age pigment accumulation in the human myocardium. J. Geront., 14:430, 1959.

Szilard, L.: On the nature of the aging process. Proc. Nat. Acad. Sci., U.S.A., 45:30, 1959.

Tauchi, H.: Mechanism of senile atrophy: histopathological micrometrical and electron microscopical studies. In Shock, N. W. (ed.): Biological Aspects of Aging. New York, Columbia University Press, 1962, p. 157.

Ungar, H., and Ben-Ishay, Z.: Rheumatic and age changes of the heart in Israel. Israel J. Med. Sci., 1:50, 1965.

von Hahn, H. P.: Age-related alterations in the structure of DNA. II. The role of histones. Gerontologia, 10:174, 1964/65.

Walford, R. L.: The Immunologic Theory of Aging. Copenhagen, Ejner Munksgaard, 1969.

15

BLOOD VESSELS

NORMAL

Some of the distinctive anatomic and functional aspects of vessels are of considerable significance to an understanding of the diseases that affect these structures. Based upon their size and certain histologic features, arteries are divided into three categories: (1) large or elastic arteries, which include the aorta, (2) medium-sized or muscular arteries, also referred to as distributing arteries and (3) small arteries (usually under 2 mm. in diameter) and arterioles that course, for the most part, within the substance of tissues and organs. All arteries characteristically possess three coats—a tunica intima, a tunica media and a tunica adventitia—most clearly distinguished in the larger vessels. As the vessels diminish in caliber, the three separable coats become progressively more indistinct and eventually disappear as identifiable layers in the arterioles.

The *large elastic arteries* of the body include the aorta and its major branches: innominate, subclavian, beginning of the common carotid, and the origins of the pulmonary arteries. The tunica intima of these vessels is composed of a smooth layer of thin endothelial cells based upon a delicate membrane that penetrates between the subendothelial connective tissue and underlying smooth muscle cells. At birth, the tunica intima is quite thin. Throughout life, the intima thickens by the progressive accumulation of mucopolysaccharide ground substance. So-called myointimal cells appear

581

somewhat mysteriously in the ground substance and contribute to the intimal thickening by the synthesis of collagen and elastic fibrils. As will be seen later, these myointimal cells are major participants in the lesions of atherosclerosis. The outer limit of the tunica intima is demarcated by a poorly defined zone of longitudinally dispersed elastic fibers that create a thick felting of elastic tissue. These fibers are not compacted into a discrete internal membrane in vessels of this caliber, and are poorly separated from the elastic fibers contained within the media.

The *tunica media,* or muscular layer, is rich in elastic tissue in the large arteries, hence their designation as elastic arteries. The elastic fibers of the media are disposed in fairly compact layers separated by alternating layers of fibromuscular tissue. Condensation of the elastic tissue at the outer limit of the media produces a poorly defined external elastic membrane. The Verhoeff elastic tissue stain is of considerable value in pathology, since the elastic fibers are sensitive to injury and their disappearance is frequently one of the first indications of some abnormality.

The *tunica adventitia* is a poorly defined layer of investing connective tissue in which elastic and nerve fibers and small, thin-walled nutrient vessels, the vasa vasorum, are dispersed. These nutrient vessels are derived from exiting arterial branches at points where they pass through the adventitia of the main vessel. The vasa course back into the wall of the artery and can usually be identified in the outer third of the media. They ramify into minute, poorly defined channels in the inner layers and, according to many investigators, completely fail to enter the intima. Arterial walls in general are poorly vascularized. Such thin-walled capillaries as may be present would be subject to the full thrust of the systolic blood pressure in the major vessel and would probably collapse under such stress. The inner layer, then, depends largely on direct imbibition for its nutritional needs. The thin-walled nutrient vessels depend for their support on the surrounding adventitia and media. Diseases such as idiopathic medial necrosis, which injure these supporting elements, predispose to rupture of the vasa vasorum.

The elastic content of the media of these large vessels provides great resilience, and their rebound following systole aids in the forward propulsion of the blood. In the aging process, the elastic fibers deteriorate and are replaced by fibrous tissue. With this loss of elasticity, these vessels expand less readily under the increased pressure of systole and thus cause some elevation of the systolic blood pressure in older age groups. The loss of elasticity further predisposes to stretching and elongation and accounts for the progressive development of tortuosity in these arteries in the older age groups.

The *muscular arteries of medium size,* the distributing arteries, are the "named" vessels that distribute the blood to organs and tissues, such as the renal, superior mesenteric, popliteal, radial and ulnar arteries. The three coats are still well defined in these vessels and are derived by gradual transition from the layers in the larger elastic arteries. The inner limit of the intima is clearly defined by a compact, wavy internal elastic membrane. Normally this membrane is a single discrete layer; occasionally two layers may be present, but in general reduplication or fibrillation denotes an increased formation of elastic tissue incident to such abnormal stress as hypertension.

The *tunica media* is largely made up of circular or spiral smooth muscle cells arranged in concentric layers. Fine elastic fibers are dispersed through the media. These are visualized only with elastic tissue stains. The muscular character of the media makes it appear distinctly red in contrast to the yellow color of the media of elastic arteries. The outer limit of the media is marked by a well defined external elastic membrane that is usually somewhat less well developed and delineated than the internal membrane (Fig. 15–1). Some fibrillation and lamination may be evident in this external

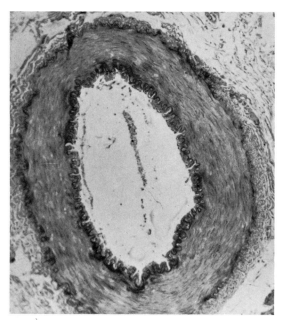

Figure 15–1. *A normal muscular artery with clearly defined internal and external elastic membranes.*

membrane. As these distributing arteries decrease in caliber, the external and then the internal elastic membranes become progressively thinner and less well defined. The tunica adventitia resembles that present in the large vessels, but contains a more abundant neural innervation, reflecting the role these vessels play in the autonomic regulation of blood flow. The vasa vasorum in arteries of medium size are usually extremely small and difficult to visualize histologically.

Small arteries are usually distinct from the muscular arteries not only in their size, but also in the progressive loss first of the clearly defined external elastic membrane and then their internal elastic membrane so that, at the prearteriole level, the definition between the three coats is virtually lost. The tunica adventitia is of relatively greater thickness in these small vessels and approximately equals that of the tunica media. As the vessels approach the order of arterioles, the wall comprises an endothelial lining based upon a scant subendothelial connective tissue, a layer of muscular media and an investment of collagenous adventitia (Fig. 15–2). Altogether the thickness of the wall is usually about equal to the diameter of the lumen of the vessel. The arterioles are richly supplied by nervous connections with the autonomic nervous system, and these vessels constitute the major point of autonomic control of vascular flow. In this role, the small arteries and the arterioles bear the brunt of elevations of blood pressure and respond to these abnormal stresses by marked alterations in their structure, to be detailed.

The differentiation of these three types of arteries is of considerable importance in pathology, since each class of vessel tends to have its own pattern of pathologic lesions. Thus, it will be shown that in the various types of arteriosclerosis, atheromatosis is most typical of the elastic and muscular arteries, medial calcific sclerosis occurs in the muscular arteries and, in the small arteries and arterioles, arteriosclerosis takes the form of diffuse thickening of the vascular wall by proliferation of endothelial cells and fibromuscular tissue. Moreover, in order to interpret the increases or decreases in elastic tissue encountered in hypertension, one must first know the normal base line in the particular vessel involved.

Veins in general are thin-walled vessels with relatively large lumina. The three separable coats as seen in the arteries are not well defined. The tunica intima is composed largely of an endothelial lining based upon a scant connective tissue layer. Internal elastic membranes delimiting the inner extent of the tunica intima can be well identified only in the largest veins, such as the venae cavae, portal vein and major pulmonary veins. The media is poorly developed and is only prominent in the largest veins, and at best is unevenly distributed and provides very inadequate support in the thinned-out areas. Veins are thus predisposed to abnormal irregular dilatation, compression and easy penetration by tumors and inflammatory processes. The adventitia is composed of a thin layer of investing connective tissue. Valves, essentially endothelial folds, are found in many veins, particularly those in the extremities. These valves break the column of blood and reduce the hydrodynamic load in the propulsion of blood back toward the heart. The competence and function of these valves depend, however, upon the normal integrity of the vein wall.

The *lymphatics* are extremely thin-walled structures, difficult to identify in tissue sections because of their tendency to collapse under ordinary tissue pressures. Clear identification depends upon the recognition of thin-walled, endothelium-lined channels devoid of blood cells. The major lymphatics, however, possess a thin supporting muscular wall, as well as valves. Histologically, therefore, it is sometimes difficult to distinguish these major trunks from blood vessels.

While the major function of the lymphatics is as a protective drainage system, they also constitute an important pathway for the dissemination of disease by the conduction of bacteria and tumor cells to distant sites. The important role which the lymphatics also play in the normal return of interstitial tissue fluid to the blood must not be overlooked and has been referred to previously (p. 60). Obstruction of these channels causes lymphedema.

PATHOLOGY

Although vessels are secondarily affected by lesions in adjacent structures, primary vascular disease is the major concern of the present chapter. In general, all types of vascular diseases are significant because they may (1) weaken the walls of vessels and lead to dilatation or rupture, (2) narrow the lumina of vessels and produce ischemia or (3) damage the endothelial lining and provoke intravascular thrombosis.

The most important primary vascular diseases affect the arteries and, of these, the most prevalent and clinically significant is atherosclerosis. In the course of time, this disorder affects virtually every individual to some degree.

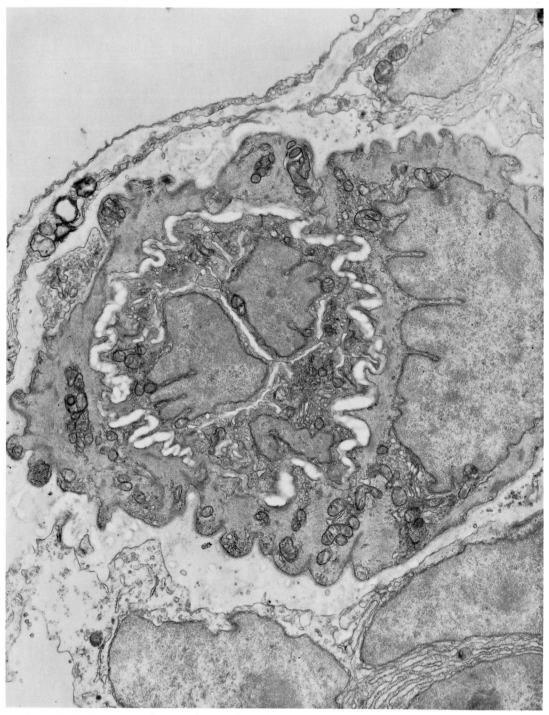

Figure 15–2. *Low power electron micrograph of contracted arteriole. Wavy translucent ribbon of internal elastic membrane encloses three endothelial cells. One smooth muscle cell is on right.*

The other arterial diseases are very much less common but, in the individual instance, may be responsible for considerable disability and even death. Certain of the venous disorders, such as varicose veins, are also very commonly encountered in clinical practice, in a frequency that almost approaches that of atherosclerosis. In general, however, these diseases of veins are more noteworthy for the disability they produce than for their importance as causes of death. This should not imply, however, that venous diseases are unimportant. Many are disabling to the point of crippling, and certain disorders, such as phlebothrombosis, may lead to death by embolism. Diseases of arteries, veins and lymphatics will be considered separately. Tumors of these vessels, however, will be considered as a group, since these neoplasms are for the most part quite similar clinically and anatomically, irrespective of their origin in an artery, vein or lymphatic.

ARTERIES

CONGENITAL ANOMALIES

It is quite surprising that the development of the far-flung complicated branching and anastomosing system of blood vessels and lymphatics eventuates so consistently in a fairly standard or normal anatomic pattern. It is, therefore, not unanticipated that many aberrations from the classic pattern may be found. Most of these anomalies in the course and the distribution of arteries are of importance only in surgical operative technique, where the recognition of the deviation is important to the surgical dissection. Occasionally, however, these minor anomalies have a greater significance in potentiating or even preventing disease. For example, a double renal arterial supply may prevent infarction of a kidney when one of the vessels is occluded by a thrombus or embolus. On the other hand, by crossing anterior to the ureter, the aberrant renal vessel may compress the ureter and obstruct the outflow of urine and eventually cause serious renal disease (hydronephrosis). In a somewhat analogous fashion, maldevelopment of a major coronary branch may predispose the myocardium to infarction. In addition, among these diverse and, for the most part, unimportant vascular anomalies, two remain that merit brief consideration.

CONGENITAL OR "BERRY" ANEURYSM

Developmental weaknesses in the cerebral vessels in and about the circle of Willis frequently yield to the sustained thrust of the blood pressure and form small, saccular, aneurysmal outpouchings (berry aneurysms). These aneurysms almost invariably occur at the bifurcations or branchings of the cerebral vessels, and are almost never found in other vessels. The musculature of these cerebral arteries not only is poorly developed throughout, but is particularly deficient at these points of branching, and the integrity of these vessels is mainly dependent upon their internal elastic membrane. Hydrodynamic studies have shown that maximal pressure is exerted in vessels at points of bifurcation. The prolonged stress at these points tends to cause degeneration of the elastic membrane which further weakens the wall at these sites, thus explaining the localization of these "berry" aneurysms. These aneurysms are incidental findings in about 1 to 2 per cent of routine postmortems on adults of both sexes. They are somewhat more common in advanced age and it is assumed that they progressively balloon out over the course of years, particularly in the presence of hypertension. *They are most common in the anterior half of the circle of Willis and in the internal carotids, the anterior and middle cerebrals, and the anterior and posterior communicating arteries.* The other intracranial vessels are affected less frequently. In about half of the cases, multiple aneurysms are found.

The aneurysms are usually saccular or spherical dilatations, up to 1.5 cm. in diameter, which tend to lie in the Y formed by branching vessels. Rarely they reach the relatively large size of 5 to 6 cm. in diameter. They communicate with the artery through small to large mouths, which sometimes have the diameter of the sac itself. Frequently the walls are calcified and occasionally the aneurysmal sac is filled with thrombus. Death may be caused by rupture leading to subarachnoid hemorrhage or sometimes penetrating hemorrhages into the brain substance. Aneurysmal dilatations of the cerebral vessels closely simulating berry aneurysms may result from the vascular weakening produced by atherosclerosis, syphilis or nonspecific arteritis incident to bacterial meningitis.

ARTERIOVENOUS FISTULA OR ANEURYSM

Abnormal communications between arteries and accompanying veins may arise as developmental defects, from rupture of an arterial aneurysm into the adjacent vein, from penetrating injuries that pierce the wall of artery and vein and produce an artificial communication, and from inflammatory necrosis of adjacent vessels. The communication, therefore, is in only certain instances developmental in origin. The connection between artery and vein may consist of a well formed vessel or a vascular channel formed by the canalization of a thrombus, or may be mediated through an aneurysmal sac. Such lesions are extremely rare and are usually small. They are of some clinical significance, since they short-circuit blood from the arterial to the venous side and throw an increased burden upon the right side of the heart, predisposing to cardiac failure. Sometimes the very tortuous mass of vessels that presumably represents an arteriovenous aneurysm is designated as a *cirsoid aneurysm.*

Interestingly, small arteriovenous aneurysms are believed to be very common in the lungs, to the point of being almost a normal detail. These are so small that they are without hemodynamic significance in the normal pulmonary flow.

ARTERIOSCLEROSIS

Arteriosclerosis literally means "hardening of the arteries," but more accurately it refers to a group of processes which have in common thickening and loss of elasticity of arterial walls. Three distinctive morphologic variants are included within the term arteriosclerosis: *atherosclerosis,* characterized by the formation of atheromata (focal intimal plaques), *Mönckeberg's medial calcific sclerosis,* characterized by calcification of the media of muscular arteries, and *arteriolosclerosis,* marked by proliferative fibromuscular or endothelial thickening of the walls of small arteries and arterioles. These three forms are relatively easily distinguished by their morphologic appearance. More than one pattern can be identified in the same individual in different vessels or even in the same vessel. In fact, atherosclerosis and Mönckeberg's medial sclerosis often occur together, particularly in the arteries of the legs of aged individuals. Because atherosclerosis is so overwhelmingly the most common and important form of arteriosclerosis, the terms are generally used interchangeably unless otherwise specified.

ATHEROSCLEROSIS (AS)

Among the killers in the Western world, atherosclerosis is overwhelmingly in first place. Global in distribution, in economically developed societies it has steadily climbed in incidence to reach alarming epidemic proportions. The vascular involvement in its evolution re-mains silently submerged for some long time only to surface when it has reached the stage of producing arterial insufficiency. Although any artery may be affected, the aorta and the coronary and cerebral systems are the prime targets, and so myocardial infarcts (heart attacks) and cerebral infarcts (strokes) are the two major consequences of this disease. Myocardial infarcts (MI) alone account for 20 per cent of all deaths in the United States, almost entirely attributable to atherosclerosis. The principal victims are men in the prime of their productive lives. This vascular disorder also causes a variety of other less calamitous events including progressive renal insufficiency, so-called arteriosclerotic heart disease, gangrene of the legs, mesenteric occlusion and progressive ischemic encephalopathy, adding to its toll. AS with its consequences is probably the major contributor to the United States' doleful world rank of 24th in life expectancy for men. Its variable severity among nations, individuals, social and ethnic groups is evidence that AS is not an inevitable consequence of life. Understanding why some individuals have only mild disease while others are severely affected and discovering the cause of this rampant disorder are two of the most urgently sought goals of medicine today.

Definitions. AS is a slow, progressive disease which starts almost at birth and is characterized by the formation of ever more atheromata in the aorta and in medium and large arteries.

The basic lesion—the atheroma—consists of a raised focal fibrofatty plaque within the intima, having a core of lipid (mainly cholesterol, usually complexed to proteins, and cholesterol esters) and a covering fibrous cap. These atheromata are sparsely distributed at first but, as the disease advances, they become more and more numerous and sometimes literally cover the entire intimal surface of severely affected arteries. As the plaques increase in size by accumulating lipid and fibrous scar, they progressively encroach on the lumen of the artery as well as on the subjacent media. Consequently, atheromata compromise arterial blood flow and weaken affected arteries, possibly resulting in aneurysms. Many eventually undergo a variety of complications—e.g., (1) calcification, (2) internal hemorrhages, (3) ulceration through the endothelial surface with discharge of embolic debris into the blood stream and (4) overlying thrombus formation on the surface of the (usually ulcerated) plaque. In the progression of this vascular disease, no symptoms may be produced for 20 to 40 years or longer and, unless the lesions precipitate clinical manifestations by virtue of organ injury, they may remain undiscovered until postmortem examination. In the absence of such organ injury, AS can be recognized during life only by radio-angiography or, in some cases, by visualization of the deposits of calcium in the advanced atheromata.

Epidemiology and Incidence. Epidemiologic and incidence data deserve close attention because the variable occurrence and severity of this disease among individuals and groups provide important clues to its pathogenesis. Epidemiologic data are largely expressed in terms of *number of deaths caused by coronary heart disease* since the arterial lesions are almost impossible to detect until they provoke "atherosclerotic events" (morbidity or mortality related to the existence of atherosclerosis). In 1937, in the United States there was a total of 1,450,427 deaths, and only 204,570 (14 per cent) were caused by cardiovascular disease. In 1967, there were 1,851,323 total deaths in the United States and, among these, 1,002,111 (54 per cent) were caused by cardiovascular disease (almost all related to atherosclerosis). The enormous increase in this problem over the span of 30 years amply justifies the term epidemic. The death rate from CHD (almost entirely atherosclerotic) in the United States in 1967 was approximately 350. In contrast, it was about 150 in Sweden, Italy and Switzerland. Only Finland had a higher death rate than the United States (World Health Organization, 1970*b*). The comparative data become even more striking when specific age groups are considered. In Denmark, Norway and Sweden, the mortality rate for men under the age of 55 is less than half that for the same age group in the United States (Department of Health, Education and Welfare, 1971). For men between the ages of 35 and 64, the death rate in Japan is 64 compared to 400 for the United States, a sixfold difference. Japanese who migrate to the United States and adopt the life style and diet of their new home acquire the predisposition to atherosclerosis of the resident American population. The suggestion is strong that differences in diet, life style and personal habits may be important in the pathogenesis and progression of this disease.

Age, sex and family background condition the severity of atherosclerosis in the individual, as do a group of so-called "*risk factors*," i.e., dietary intake of lipids and serum lipid levels, obesity, hypertension, cigarette smoking, personality structure, underlying metabolic disease and physical exercise.

Age is the dominant influence on the development of clinically significant AS. It is now well documented that primordial aortic fatty streaking begins in infancy in all populations. In a recent study in the United States, 43 per cent of infants one to 12 months of age had such lesions and, in children over the age of one year, aortic fatty streaking was universal (Schwartz et al., 1967). As will be seen, such early aortic lesions may not be the antecedents of the more ominous lesions in adults. However, coronary artery fatty streaks, very likely the progenitors of progressive atheromata, usually begin to appear in vulnerable populations by age 10. Thereafter, atheromata generally increase in size, become more widely distributed, develop more complications and cause more arterial narrowing with each passing decade (Eggen and Solberg, 1968). Among 300 American soldiers killed in the Korean War (average age, 22 years), potentially significant coronary atherosclerosis was found in 77 per cent (Enos, 1955). The death rate from CHD rises with each decade up to age 75 and then declines slightly. It seems reasonable to ascribe this decline to natural selection whereby survival beyond the age of 75 occurs only if severe AS is not present. It is evident, then, that some degree of AS is universal in predisposed populations.

There are striking *sex differences* in the incidence and severity of atherosclerosis. The use of the term incidence for a disease that is universal is somewhat paradoxical, but is intended to indicate the rate of diagnosis of disease sufficiently advanced to be a potential source of organ injury. Women in active reproductive life are sheltered from the development of advanced atheromatosis. Consequently, the death rate from CHD is far greater in males than in females during the first half of life. Indeed, myocardial infarction is rare in the premenopausal woman unless she is predisposed to atherosclerosis by multiple risk factors. Even in the age group of 45 to 54, the mortality rate of white males is five times that of white females. After menopause, the severity of AS in women approaches that of men but, even at advanced ages in the absence of high-risk factors, women have somewhat less atherosclerosis than men.

Some families suffer an increased frequency of fatal heart attacks at an early age, presumably indicating *familial predisposition*. Whether this proneness is genetic in origin or is due to common environmental influences is uncertain since members of a family may share similar diets, modes of life and social habits as well as genes. Nonetheless, there is good evidence that constitutional factors predispose to AS. In a recent survey, it was found that first degree relatives of female index patients (having had a heart attack) had a sevenfold increased risk of fatal CHD as compared to the general population. For relatives of male index patients, however, the risk was only approximately doubled (Slack and Evans, 1966). Familial forms of hyperlipoproteinemia exist which have a well documented association with premature AS. Such inborn errors of metabolism underlie some (but by no means all) of the familial predisposition to this disease.

Many "*risk factors*" accentuate the progression of AS and increase the frequency of CHD. Four are considered of major importance: (1) dietary intake of fats and serum lipid levels, (2) obesity, (3) hypertension and (4) cigarette smoking. *The largest body of evidence points toward the dietary intake of lipids and serum lipid levels as the predominant factors which increase the risk of AS* (Keys, 1957) (Jolliffe, 1959). High saturated fat intake, high levels of cholesterol in the diet, hypercholesterolemia, hypertriglyceridemia and hyperlipoproteinemia have all been correlated with the severity of AS and the incidence of CHD (Kannel et al., 1964) (Truett et al., 1967) (Kannel, 1971c). With few exceptions, populations consuming large quantities of saturated fats and cholesterol have relatively high serum levels of cholesterol and beta lipoproteins and a high mortality from CHD. In the Framingham study, the incidence of CHD in men aged 45 to 54, with serum cholesterol levels of 220 to 249 mg. per 100 ml. (not generally regarded as unusually high), was 48 per cent higher than in those with serum cholesterol levels under 220 mg. per 100 ml. (Kannel, 1971c). The correlations of CHD with serum beta lipoproteins and total serum lipids are virtually as good, as will be discussed presently. Still a very vexed issue is which of the lipid fractions is most important.

Obesity and total caloric intake are correlated with an increased risk of dying from the clinical complications of AS. The correlation is closest in those who are extremely obese (beyond a single standard deviation from the mean optimal weight). It must be recognized, however, that obese individuals tend to have more severe hyperlipidemia, hypertension and diabetes mellitus. Excess carbohydrates contribute not only to obesity but also to hyperlipidemia through converging metabolic pathways. That the obesity is actually more closely correlated with CHD than with acceleration of AS suggests that the cardiac workload imposed by the obesity in the presence of atherosclerotic narrowing of coronary arteries may be the dominant influence.

Hypertension is a major risk factor; the higher the blood pressure, the greater the risk.

The impact of hypertension depends somewhat upon the serum lipid levels. Even modest elevations of blood pressure can become ominous in the presence of marked hypercholesterolemia, and severe hypertension can be dangerous even with normal lipid levels. Conversely, high serum cholesterol levels are less hazardous with normal blood pressure. In this connection, it should be noted that AS is uncommon in the pulmonary circulation where extremely low arterial pressures prevail even though these vessels are bathed in the same lipid-laden blood. Only when pulmonary hypertension supervenes does the pulmonary circulation develop AS. Hypertension is particularly significant as a risk factor for strokes, and even moderate reductions in the blood pressure have been shown to significantly lower the incidence of strokes.

There is a clear-cut association between *cigarette smoking* and susceptibility to CHD (Strong et al., 1969). According to the Surgeon General's report on smoking, "cigarette smoking males have a higher coronary heart disease death rate and are inclined to have more coronary atherosclerosis than non-smoking males. This death rate may on the average be 70 per cent greater and, in some, even 200 per cent greater or more in the presence of other known 'risk factors' for coronary heart disease. Female cigarette smokers also have higher coronary heart disease death rates than do non-smoking females, although not as high as those for males. In general, death rates from this disease increase with amounts smoked" (Department of Health, Education and Welfare, 1967). Cessation of cigarette smoking is followed by a reduction in the risk of dying from CHD, but it requires 10 or more years for the risk to return to that of nonsmokers (Kahn, 1966). Interestingly, among Japanese with their low incidence of CHD, cigarette smoking does not appear to have a significant influence on the incidence of the disease, suggesting perhaps, that in those whose diets are low in saturated fats and who have low serum lipid levels, cigarette smoking has little effect.

Metabolic derangements, particularly those producing hypercholesterolemia, lead to premature and accelerated AS. Thus diabetes mellitus, hypothyroidism and the nephrotic syndrome are all characterized by premature rampant AS. Similarly, inborn errors of lipid metabolism such as familial hypercholesterolemia (type II A hyperlipoproteinemia) and familial hyperlipidemia (type III hyperlipoproteinemia) are characterized by premature florid AS often accompanied by xanthomatosis.

A host of other influences have been identified which increase the severity of AS, but the data are less unequivocal than for the major risk factors cited above. An aggressive, achievement-oriented personality and a stressful life are associated with an increased risk of CHD and a predisposition to AS (Morris and Gardner, 1969). Obviously these influences are more prevalent in urban life and in industrialized nations. The role of physical activity in protecting against fatal ischemic heart disease and possibly coronary atherosclerosis is somewhat controversial (Dawber et al., 1966). It appears that sedentary men are more susceptible to sudden death from heart attack than are physically active men. In one study, the least active men, about 15 per cent of the participating males, had about three times the risk of the 15 per cent most active physically (Kannel, 1971a). That physical activity acts directly on the development of atheromatosis is unclear. Instead, its prime effect may be to promote collateral circulation in the heart in persons with a poor coronary circulation and thus reduce the incidence of fatal CHD (Morris et al., 1966). Additional factors vaguely correlated with enhanced risk include emotional stress, increased pulse rate, softness of drinking water and elevated levels of serum uric acid.

Each of the major risk factors contributes individually to the possible development of clinically significant AS, but *multiple factors* exert a greater than additive effect. In the Framingham study of 2000 men between the ages of 30 and 59, 270 were considered to be at low risk because they had blood pressures below 140/90, serum cholesterols less than 193 mg. per 100 ml. and normal electrocardiograms. Over a 10-year period, the development of clinical heart disease in this favorable group was only one-seventh of that in the total group of 2000 men, which of course included this favorable group. Among the men with only slightly higher blood pressure (up to 160/95) and slightly higher blood cholesterol levels (up to 250 mg. per 100 ml.), neither of which are regarded as markedly abnormal, the incidence of clinical CHD was 4.5 times greater than in the low-risk group. Stated in another way, when three risk factors were present, the rate of heart attacks was seven times greater than when there were none; when two risk factors were present, the risk was increased fourfold; and with one risk factor, the increase was twofold. For this disease of unknown etiology, these studies of epidemiology and individual susceptibility have the great importance of pointing out possible interventions that might substantially slow the progression of AS and reduce the risk of fatal heart attacks.

Morphology. The pathogenesis of this disease is better understood with some knowledge of its morphology. There is general agreement about most of the macroscopic features of AS, but much disagreement about the nature of the "early lesion" and ultrastructural details. The arteries most commonly affected are the coronary and cerebral arteries and the aorta with its major divisions, i.e., the innominate, common carotid and iliac arteries. However, any artery of large or medium size and occasionally even smaller arteries may be involved. The fine distal ramifications are usually spared. The pulmonary arteries may also be affected but generally only when there is pulmonary hypertension. Although it is a matter of some dispute, most investigators believe that the first visible "early" lesion is a barely elevated fatty dot or streak. This streak is best visualized morphologically by staining the opened artery with Sudan IV, coloring the lesion bright orange. Some researchers, however, contend that the earliest lesion is a focal area of edema appearing somewhat like a tiny blister, while others suggest that the early lesion is a thin layer of deposited surface thrombus (Haust, 1971). In any event, there is good agreement that whatever the initial changes, fatty streaks appear in the aorta of all children older than one year, regardless of race, sex or environment. At this early age, the lesions are localized in the aortic valve ring region, the area of the ductus scar, and just distal to the intercostal ostia. These **aortic** fatty streaks in infancy are probably not the progenitors of the more significant atheromata of later life. In the adult, atheromata rarely occur in the aortic valve ring region, even in patients having advanced AS. Moreover, in populations having relatively little atherosclerosis, aortic fatty streaking in childhood is just as common as in those prone to advanced disease. The extent of aortic intimal surface covered by fatty streaks increases with age from about 10 per cent in the first decade to 30 to 50 per cent in the third decade. By this age, the fatty streaks have disappeared in the valve ring region and are present in the posterior wall of the thoracic aorta and throughout the abdominal aorta, the sites prone to the development of the advanced lesions.

Coronary artery fatty streaking is first observed at about 15 years of age in all populations but, in the predisposed, streaks increase in number and severity with every passing decade. The streaking is most abundant in the proximal segment, i.e., within the first 2 cm. from the coronary artery orifices. These fatty streaks correspond to the later developing, more advanced atheromata and are, therefore, a better predictor of clinically significant coronary artery lesions to come. The extent and severity of fatty streaks in the cerebral arteries are similar up to age 34 in populations that vary widely in predisposition to cerebrovascular disease, but beyond this age they are more numerous and advanced in populations with a high incidence of cerebrovascular disease.

As early fatty streaks evolve into the atheromata of the clinically significant form of the disease, they enlarge and become raised into characteristic yellow subintimal plaques which encroach on the vascular lumen (Figs. 15–3 and 15–4). They vary in size from one to several centimeters in diameter and are round, ovoid or map-like in contour. On section, they have a central collection of soft, granular, greasy material. The overlying endothelium is intact. With further progression, they not only enlarge but also bulge more into the lumen. Some remain soft, pulpy and yellow, while others assume a yellow-white cast and still others become firm, white, fibrous plaques. As will be seen, these changes are induced by progressive fibrous replacement of the soft, yellow, lipid centers.

As fibrofatty atheromata further evolve in the progression of severe AS, they undergo a variety of alterations producing what are referred to as **"complicated lesions."** (1) Hemorrhage into an atheroma may cause sudden ballooning of the plaque. (2) Fissures or cracks may appear in the endothelial covering but, more often, the atheroma ulcerates and sheds much of its endothelial covering. (3) Ulcerated atheromata may discharge their debris into the bloodstream to produce microemboli (cholesterol emboli). (4) Superimposed thrombosis, the most feared complication, may occur on fissured or more often ulcerated lesions (Figs. 15–5 and 15–6). (5) Almost always, atheromata in advanced disease undergo patchy or massive calcification which occurs whether the atheromata are ulcerated or nonulcerated. In severe atherosclerotic disease, small arteries are converted to virtual pipestems and the aorta may assume an eggshell brittleness. (6) Although atherosclerosis is basically an intimal disease, in severe cases it injures the underlying media and may produce sufficient weakness to permit aneurysmal dilatation. This is discussed more fully on p. 615.

The causes of fissuring and ulceration are poorly understood. Undoubtedly the thin, intimal-endothelial covering of the atheroma is precariously vital at best. Mechanical stress on such weakened areas may suffice to explain the fissuring. Alternatively, hemorrhages into the atheroma may cause sudden increase of tension on the thinned-out cap, rupturing it. A small fissure might appear first and permit blood from the lumen of the artery to dissect into the plaque, ultimately rupturing it (Constantinides, 1965). In the capacious aorta, thrombi overlying atheromata are limited to mural masses which cover the ulcerated surface. When AS is florid, the thrombi may coalesce to form large masses many centimeters in length. However, the rapidly moving bloodstream in the center of the aorta usually prevents total occlusion of the lumen.

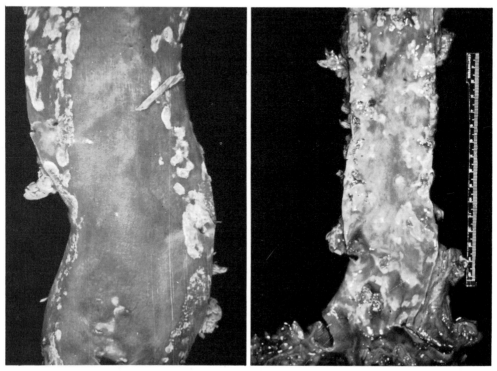

Fig. 15–3   Fig. 15–4

Figure 15–3. Atherosclerosis. An early stage with widely scattered, barely elevated intimal plaques.
Figure 15–4. Atherosclerosis. More extensive lesions with deformity of the endothelial surface.

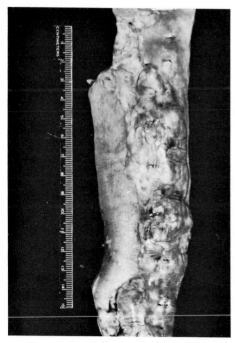

Fig. 15-5

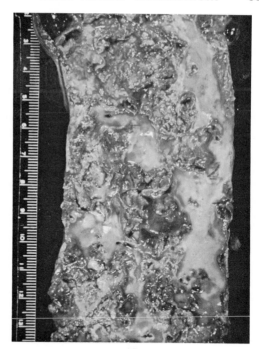

Fig. 15-6

Figure 15-5. Atherosclerosis. A more advanced stage with coalescence of atheromas and deformity of endothelial surface.

Figure 15-6. Mural thrombosis on underlying atherosclerosis.

In smaller arteries, particularly those in the brain and heart, the thrombosis is almost always occlusive and may be the ultimate event causing strokes and myocardial infarction, respectively.

While AS is a universal disease, "complicated lesions" are seen only in those with extremely advanced disease. In predisposed individuals and populations, the entire abdominal aorta may become virtually "one continuous, complicated lesion." The thoracic aorta including the arch is usually less severely affected and, remarkably, in the absence of intercurrent syphilitic aortitis, the root of the aorta (first 4 to 6 cm.) is almost always totally spared even in those with advanced abdominal aortic disease. While all atheromatosis is "bad," it is the "complicated lesions," particularly superimposed thrombosis, which gives to this disease its grave clinical significance (McGill et al., 1963).

The chronologic microscopic evolution of the atheroma, from its origin to its advanced stage, has been the subject of an enormous amount of detailed study (Geer et al., 1961) (Geer and McGill, 1967) (Ghidone and O'Neal, 1967). There is good agreement that all atheromata begin as intimal lesions which, as they enlarge, may affect the subjacent media. The intima, it will be recalled, is bounded on its luminal surface by a covering of endothelium and deeply by the internal, elastic membrane in arteries and by the musculoelastic media in the aorta. In the infant, the intimal layer is narrow and con-

tains a scant amount of mucopolysaccharide ground substance, bearing scattered collagen and elastic fibrils and occasional smooth muscle cells, all of which increase in amount over the span of the next three decades such that the intima progressively thickens. Significantly, this intimal thickening is most marked in the coronary arteries, the abdominal segment of the aorta, the iliac and femoral arteries and sites of branching from large arteries, the precise locations where AS is most commonly found later in life. Indeed, the intimal thickening in the coronary arteries is greatest in the proximal portions bearing the brunt of atherosclerotic disease. Special attention should be called to the intimal smooth muscle cells. They are capable of synthesizing collagen and elastic fibers, and they become laden with lipids in the developing atheroma. They thus have the potential of both fibroblasts and macrophages, and therefore have been called multipotential mesenchymal cells or, alternatively, myointimal cells (Getz et al., 1969).

Most investigators believe that the "early lesion," representing the origin of the fully developed atheroma, consists of accumulation of lipids in the intima. The lipid appears first within myointimal cells either in the immediate subendothelial area or deeper in the intima. Often such lipid-laden cells — lipophages, also called foam cells — are accompanied by microscopic droplets of lipid which are not enclosed within cells but lie along the elastic fibers in the depth of the intima (Figs. 15-7 and

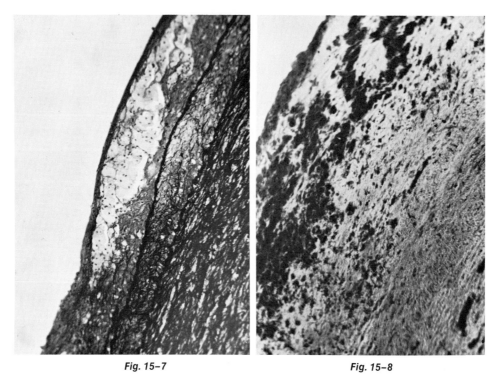

Fig. 15–7   Fig. 15–8

Figure 15–7. Atherosclerosis—a subintimal collection of foam cells or lipophages.
Figure 15–8. Atherosclerosis—a Sudan IV fat stain of the same vessel. The lipid deposits appear intensely black.

15–8). Electron microscopy also discloses in such early lesions lipid-bearing pinocytotic vesicles in the endothelial cells. Several features of these early lesions are in some dispute. One issue involves the nature of the lipid-laden cells; specifically at issue is whether all are of smooth muscle origin. Several investigators have proposed that at least some are macrophages or mononuclear cells derived from the blood (Cookson, 1971). Another basic question is whether the lipid deposition is secondary to some prior alteration in the arterial intima, such as local injury, focal enzyme loss or the focal insudation (permeation) of plasma proteins or edema fluid (More and Haust, 1961). Others have suggested that platelet aggregation or a microscopic coating of thrombus may be the "initial" change in atherogenesis (Haust, 1971). Moss and Benditt (1970) raise yet another possibility. They point out that spontaneous plaques in the chicken are composed largely of aggregates of somewhat modified smooth muscle cells containing no demonstrable lipid. Significance is attributed to this change because electron microscopic studies on human atheromata reveal that smooth muscle cells are prominent in early lesions (Geer, 1965). By analogy, then, the question is raised whether the initial alteration is the focal aggregation of such myointimal cells rather than deposition of intimal lipid. The "initial lesion" con-

troversy has not been resolved, but no matter what comprises the earliest change, lipid accumulation soon dominates the developing atheroma.

The progressive accumulation of lipids, principally cholesterol (probably in the form of lipoproteins) and cholesterol esters within myointimal cells, leads to focal clusters of large, ballooned-out "foam cells" so characteristic of advanced atheromatosis. Various constituents of the plasma, principally albumin and fibrin, have also been demonstrated within these fatty atheromata (Haust, 1968). At this stage, the atheroma is likely to have bulged into the lumen of the vessel. With progression, a fibrous cap accumulates over the luminal surface. The stimulus for such fibroplasia is mysterious, and is attributed to the death of lipid-laden cells with release of irritant lipid. Such fibroplasia may enclose the atheroma on all sides, leaving a central fatty mass containing intact foam cells as well as lipid-laden debris rich in spicules of crystallized cholesterol. Some lesions are entirely converted to solid fibrous plaques (Fig. 15–9). The margins of such fibrous or fibrofatty atheromata usually become vascularized, and sometimes fresh hemorrhages or, later, hemosiderin granules are found within the atheroma (Fig. 15–10). The other complications such as rupture of the atheroma through the intimal surface, superimposed thrombosis and the

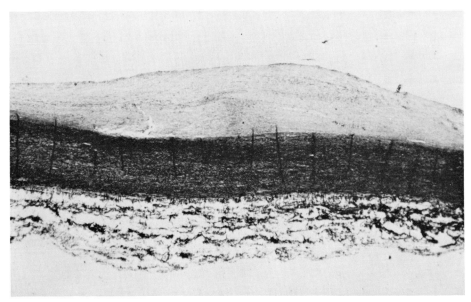

Figure 15–9. *A cross section of a fibrous plaque lying within the intima above the black-staining elastic media of the aorta.*

progressive deposition of granules or clumped masses of basophilic calcium may now ensue.

Large atheromata impinge on and damage the subjacent media. The internal elastic membrane is frayed or destroyed and the underlying media undergoes considerable pressure atrophy and fi-

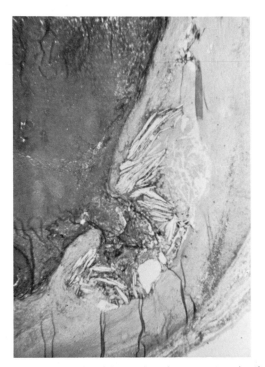

Figure 15–10. *Atherosclerosis—a ruptured atheroma surrounded by crystalline clefts and filled with hemorrhage that extends into the vessel lumen to form a thrombus.*

brosis. In the aorta, there may be loss of elastic fibers in the media as well. These changes are accompanied by adventitial fibrosis and lymphocytic cuffing about the vasa vasorum. Although primarily an intimal disease, AS is, therefore, capable of causing significant medial damage and aneurysms (Fig. 15–11).

Having discussed the range of atheromatous lesions, a few words should be said about their possible regression. Almost as an article of faith, without conclusive data, it is believed that the fatty streak and possibly the beginning fatty atheroma may regress before they become fibrotic if predisposing risk factors abate. Most of this belief derives from the study of matched groups of animals. Both groups were maintained on an atherogenic diet until lesions appeared. Then the experimental group was placed on a nonatherogenic diet for a period of months to years, and the severity of the atheromatosis in the two groups was compared. It was obviously impossible in the individual animal to be certain of the extent of the atheromatosis at the point in time when the atherogenic diet was discontinued. Despite these uncertainties, regression has been reported in cholesterol-fed rabbits after a period of maintenance on a cholesterol-free diet (Anitschkow, 1933). Recently, some regression of atheromatosis has been reported in a similar study on subhuman primates (Armstrong et al., 1970). In support of these animal studies, it will be recalled that in infancy fatty streaks appear within the first decade in the aortic valve ring region, but neither fatty streaks nor atheromatosis are seen in this site in the adult in the absence of intercurrent aortic disease such as syphilitic aortitis (Fig. 15–12). So it must be assumed that these early lesions re-

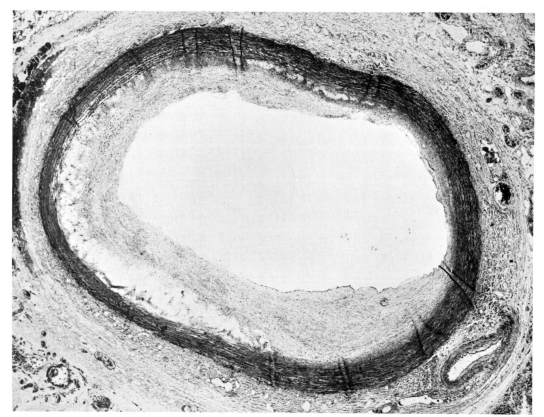

Figure 15–11. *Atherosclerosis. Eccentric fibrous thickening of the intima with a deeply situated atheroma in the lower left field encroaching on the media. The black stained elastica is thinned in this region.*

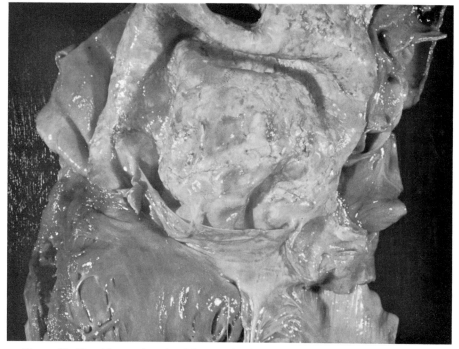

Figure 15–12. *Atherosclerosis of the proximal aorta superimposed on luetic aortitis.*

gressed, although such fatty streaking may not be equatable with developing atheromata. There is general agreement, again without definitive proof, that once the atheroma has reached the stage of fibrosis or has become "complicated," no regression is possible. Since this stage of advancement is generally reached early in adult life, it is obvious that any intervention which attempts to prevent the development of potentially serious atheromatosis in man must be instituted virtually during childhood. However, it may still be possible to prevent the progression of atheromata and the formation of new plaques by interventions later in life.

Pathogenesis. The subject of atherogenesis is a veritable multisided battleground where investigator after investigator makes a seeming breakthrough, only to be repulsed by conflicting evidence. The literature is abundant and contradictory, and only an overview, hopefully balanced, can be presented here. For more detailed authoritative information, reference should be made to: Cowdry (1967), Constantinides (1965), Miras et al. (1969), Raab (1966), Brest and Moyer (1967), and Sandler and Bourne (1963). We can begin by acknowledging that the cause or etiology of AS is still unknown. In the absence of such knowledge, one can only attempt to characterize the pathogenesis of this disease. Wissler and his colleagues have ably presented the dimensions of the problem in their statement: "Atherosclerosis is a complex process which may be regarded as dynamic interaction among (a) the structural and metabolic properties of the arterial wall, (b) the components of the blood and (c) the hemodynamic forces" (Getz et al., 1969). Before considering the many proposals which follow, it is necessary to recognize that any concept of pathogenesis must take into consideration the following well established observations.

1. Among members of all populations, irrespective of environment, AS begins to develop at a very early age, probably in infancy.

2. The severity of AS increases with age, and virtually 100 per cent of both males and females in predisposed populations have at least some atherosclerosis at death.

3. There is great variation in the severity of this disorder among individuals of comparable age.

4. Over all, women suffer less from atherosclerosis and coronary heart disease than men and are particularly sheltered prior to menopause.

5. There are striking national differences in the severity of atherosclerotic vascular disease.

6. There is a clear association between the development and severity of the disorder and elevated blood lipids, principally cholesterol, triglycerides and beta lipoproteins.

7. By a variety of interventions which generally have in common elevations of blood lipids, models of this disease can be produced in many laboratory animals including subhuman primates.

8. There is substantial evidence that a number of risk factors accelerate the development of AS and increase the incidence of CHD.

No single theory of pathogenesis copes adequately with all of these established observations. The numerous postulations can be segregated into four general categories dealing with: (1) filtration (principally of lipids); (2) altered structure or metabolism of arterial wall; (3) intimal stress and injury; and (4) thrombogenesis or encrustation.

While there is some argument as to the nature of the *initial* step, it is clear that the fully developed atheroma is marked principally by the intimal accumulation of lipid. The largest body of evidence supports the view that excessive *filtration of lipids or lipoproteins*, derived from the serum, is the basic cause of atheromatosis (Newman and Zilversmit, 1962) (Jensen, 1967) (Watts, 1971). Consonant with this proposition are the following observations: (1) Lipids and lipoproteins normally filter into the arterial wall and are there metabolized or returned to the vascular lumen—the so-called "lipid flux." (2) Measures that increase levels of serum lipids will produce AS in animals. (3) There is a clear association between serum lipid levels (principally cholesterol but, as will be seen, other lipid fractions as well) and the development of AS and CHD. (4) Patients with familial hyperlipoproteinemia develop premature AS and often suffer fatal heart attacks at an early age. (5) Many of the risk factors, such as hypertension and cigarette smoking, which accelerate AS have greatest effect when there is elevation of serum lipid levels. However, which particular lipid fraction or transport form is most important remains a subject of fervent dispute. Among the voluminous published studies, serum cholesterol, triglycerides, phospholipids, nonesterified fatty acids and various serum lipoproteins have each been accorded primary significance in atherogenesis. However, the writing most heavily incriminates cholesterol, the cholesterol-rich beta lipoproteins and the triglyceride-rich pre-beta lipoproteins (Kannel, 1971b) (Watts, 1971).

As is well known, all lipids in plasma circulate in combination with protein (Schumaker and Adams, 1969). The free fatty acids are bound to albumin. The other lipids are complexed with proteins, forming the lipoproteins. Electrophoresis and ultracentrifugation are the principal methods for both separation and identification of the lipoproteins. With these techniques, four major families are identified: (1) chylomicra having the lowest density, (2) very low-density lipoproteins now called pre-beta lipoproteins, (3) low-density lipoproteins now called beta lipoproteins and (4) high-density lipoproteins now called alpha lipoproteins. Other less common families also exist. With respect to the problem of atherogenesis, there is almost complete agreement that the high-density alpha lipoproteins are not implicated. The remaining three categories are characterized in some greater detail in Table 15–1.

It is evident that each of the implicated categories of lipoproteins contains cholesterol and triglycerides in varying relative amounts. Within the recent past, it has become evident that all clinical hyperlipidemia can be resolved into several quite distinctive lipoprotein profiles. Fredrickson et al. (1967) described five patterns, but subsequently his type II was again subdivided, creating six types of hyperlipoproteinemia schematized in Table 15–2 (World Health Organization, 1970a). Each of these types of hyperlipoproteinemia is, in part, genetically conditioned and, in part, induced by environmental influences, but IIA and III are almost completely genetically conditioned. A few additional words about each. Type I is characterized principally by hypertriglyceridemia, related to high levels of circulating chylomicra. Since chylomicra represent dietary fat in transit to the tissues, the hyperlipidemia here can be ameliorated by reducing the fat intake. Type IIA is characterized principally by a great excess of cholesterol and includes cases that in the past have been called familial hypercholesterolemia. This pattern responds poorly to dietary measures which would be a low-animal-fat, low-cholesterol regimen. The risk of CHD in these patients is significantly elevated. Type IIB is well named as overin-

dulgence hyperlipidemia. Here both cholesterol and triglycerides are elevated, but dietary control of both lipids and carbohydrates in most cases will bring about substantial improvement in the blood lipid levels. Since this is a common pattern and these individuals are at high risk, this form of hyperlipoproteinemia is responsible for a significant portion of all CHD deaths. Type III closely resembles type IIB save that the former is quite rare and is largely genetic in origin. In type III, both cholesterol and triglyceride levels are elevated, and patients with this inborn error of metabolism are at high risk of CHD. The type IV hyperlipoproteinemia is essentially a hypertriglyceridemia related to excessive carbohydrate intake. The cholesterol levels are relatively normal or only slightly elevated, and these patients are benefited by dietary restriction of carbohydrates rather than by reduction of fat intake. As a common pattern, type IV contributes significantly to the total deaths from CHD. Type V appears to be a composite of types I and IV where contributions are made by hereditary influences as well as by exogenous dietary excesses. These patients are often uncontrolled diabetics or alcoholics. Elevated levels of chylomicra and pre-beta lipoproteins are encountered in this form of hyperlipoproteinemia, producing some slight elevation of cholesterol levels with marked elevation of triglyceride levels (Lehmann and Lynes, 1972). Types IIB and IV are not only the most common patterns encountered in the population, but also carry significantly elevated risks of CHD.

We may now return to the lipid filtration theory of atherogenesis. Among the various lipids and lipoproteins, *the fraction most incriminated in the production of AS on the basis of our current knowledge seems to be cholesterol, although its lipoprotein transport form may actually comprise the critical feature.* A large body of epidemiologic, clinical and experimental evidence points in this direction (Frantz and Moore, 1969). Serum cholesterol concentrations above 200 mg. per 100 ml. are rarely found in animals or in

TABLE 15–1. MAJOR PLASMA LIPOPROTEINS

	Chylomicrons	Pre-Beta Lipoproteins (VLDL)	Beta Lipoproteins (LDL)
Density	0.94	0.98	1.03
Sf class	10,000	20–400	0–20
Greatest molecular diameter	5000	700	350
Per cent composition			
Protein	2	10	21
Phospholipid	7	22	22
Cholesterol (including esters)	10	20	50
Glycerides	80	55	10

TABLE 15-2. HYPERLIPOPROTEINEMIA

Type	Familiar Name	Prevalence	Lipoprotein Abnormality	Cholesterol Level	Triglyceride Level	Cause	Coronary Disease Risk
Normal			None: beta > alpha > pre-beta chylomicra absent	<220 mg. per 100 ml.	<150 mg. per 100 ml.	Moderation in all things	
I	Exogenous or dietary hypertriglyceri-demia	Rare	Chylomicra present	+ or normal	+++	Dietary fat not cleared from plasma	+
IIA	Hypercholesterol-emia (familial)	Moderately common	Beta lipoprotein raised	++	Normal	? Hereditary met-abolic defect	+++
IIB	Overindulgence hy-perlipidemia	Common	Beta and pre-beta raised	+ to ++	+ to ++	Long-term dietary excess ? + hereditary element occa-sionally	+++
III	Familial hyperlipide-mia	Rare	Broad beta present	++	++	Hereditary meta-bolic defect	+++
IV	Endogenous hyper-triglyceridemia	Common	Pre-beta raised	+	++	Excessive intake of carbohydrates	++
V	Mixed (types I and IV) endogenous-exogenous hyper-triglyceridemia	Fairly common	Chylomicra pres-ent and pre-beta raised	+	+++	? Metabolic defect	+

From World Health Organization: Classification of hyperlipidaemias and hyperproteinaemias. Bull. W.H.O., *43*:891, 1970.

humans except where man lives within an af-fluent society, and CHD is rare in animal and human populations with serum cholesterol levels below 200 mg. per 100 ml. (Kannel et al., 1961). Even in animals with relatively high serum cholesterol levels, the cholesterol is present mostly in the form of alpha lipopro-teins which are not atherogenic. As was pointed out earlier, numerous epidemiologic surveys have shown that the incidence of CHD parallels the level of serum cholesterol (Keys, 1970). But perhaps most incriminating are the numerous animal studies in which reasonable facsimiles of human AS are induced by choles-terol feeding, although other interventions such as suppression of thyroid function are sometimes required (Wissler and Vesselino-vitch, 1968). It is further clear that atheromata are rich in cholesterol and cholesterol esters. Most of the evidence suggests that this choles-terol finds its way from the plasma into the ar-terial wall (Adams et al., 1964) (Dayton and Hashimoto, 1970). However, as will be dis-cussed presently, it is not clear that all of the lipid within the atheroma enters by filtra-tion.

All that has been said of cholesterol could equally well apply to the beta lipoproteins which are, of course, rich in cholesterol, and to the pre-beta lipoproteins which also contain some cholesterol. Any atherogenic diet in ani-mals based on the feeding of cholesterol inevi-

tably produces elevations of both the beta and pre-beta lipoproteins. Lipoproteins immuno-logically identical to those in the plasma have been reported in atheromata (Walton and Wil-liamson, 1968). Beta lipoproteins labeled in the plasma have been traced into human ath-erosclerotic plaques (Hollander, 1967). In-deed, one of the major problems plaguing the experimentalist in this field is the inability to el-evate one serum lipid fraction by an ath-erogenic diet without simultaneously affecting the others (Brown, 1969). So the question must be asked, is it merely the level of cholesterol or is it the physicochemical configuration of the lipid or the relative levels of the various lipid-lipoprotein fractions which is most ath-erogenic? Conceivably the cholesterol accumu-lation might be a secondary phenomenon rather than the actual origin of the atheroma.

The quality rather than the quantity of dietary fat may be important. Populations con-suming largely vegetable and fish oils have low levels of atherosclerosis. These oils contain higher proportions of unsaturated fatty acids and, indeed, an intake of such lipid results in lowering of plasma cholesterol (also phospho-lipids and glycerides) even when the total die-tary intake of lipids and cholesterol remains high. In the rat, short-term feeding of unsatu-rated fatty acids appears to have delayed the development of atheromata in animals on ath-erogenic diets (Scott et al., 1964).

A high carbohydrate dietary intake has also been associated with accelerated AS and CHD and, indeed, underlies the type IV hyperlipoproteinemia (Yudkin and Morland, 1967). A reduction in carbohydrate intake lowers pre-beta lipoproteins as well as serum triglycerides, and it has been argued that there is a better correlation between plasma lipids and dietary carbohydrates than with dietary lipids (Yudkin, 1967 to 1968). The plethora of proposals attests to the fact that none is entirely convincing.

Assuming that plasma lipids are involved in atherogenesis, how do they filter into or in some way gain access to the intima? Here again we find great controversy. Electron micrographs have disclosed in endothelial cells overlying atheromatous lesions, vesicles and invaginations of the plasma membrane interpreted to be pinocytosis of plasma lipids (Buck, 1958). Increased porosity of the endothelial cell layer related to injury to the endothelium might predispose to filtration of macromolecules as will be discussed later. Transport in blood monocyte-macrophages has also been proposed as has dissociation of the lipoprotein complexes at the endothelial barrier permitting only the freed cholesterol to pass into the arterial wall (Dayton and Hashimoto, 1970). Patently, the problem of how lipids enter or filter into the arterial wall remains unresolved.

Altered metabolism of the arterial wall might be the cause of AS, or at least contribute significantly to its genesis. All of the cholesterol in atheromata cannot be accounted for by filtration alone. It is clear that arterial tissue can synthesize cholesterol (Chobanian, 1968). Increased biosynthesis of phospholipids, fatty acids and sterols has been documented in arteries already developing atheromata (Geer and McGill, 1967). In addition, many observations suggest that atherogenesis may be the result of impaired catabolism or mobilization of lipids in arterial walls. Uncoupling of oxidative phosphorylation occurs with aging and in arteries already developing atheromata (Patelski et al., 1968). Lipase and esterase activity are diminished in the aortas of animals on atherogenic diets. Watts (1971) has stressed local loss of ATPase activity in atheromatous lesions and postulates the following sequence. "Loss of ATPase and oxidative enzymes indicates a disturbance of energy metabolism. Metabolic removal of lipids (he lays greatest emphasis on beta lipoproteins) then would fail, leading to foam cell alteration." In essence, this concept proposes that atherogenesis results from a disturbance of the balance between beta lipoproteins perfusing the wall and the capacity of the

cells to metabolize the lipids carried by these proteins. Other researchers have said the same of cholesterol, triglycerides and other lipoproteins. This general proposal fits other observations suggesting local changes in mucopolysaccharide ground substance (principally glycosaminoglycans) as the alteration which leads to lipid accumulation. It is suggested that complexing of these macromolecules with protein within the intima could alter intimal permeability and favor sequestration or pooling of lipid (Berenson, 1971). All of these metabolic impairments might favor the intimal accumulation of lipids either by increased endogenous synthesis or by slowed or impaired catabolism or mobilization of filtered lipids. Building on this general theory, Caro and his colleagues (1971) have recently offered an ingenious explanation of how reduced mobilization of lipids leads to atheroma formation. They point to the tendency for lesions to form at turbulent branch points and at sites where flow rate is reduced, such as in the abdominal aorta. Could the concentration of endogenously synthesized cholesterol build up to higher levels at these locations because the lower shear force of the blood coursing over the endothelial surface failed to carry away the cholesterol as it diffused to the surface? In any event, it is clear that there are myriad notions relating atherogenesis to altered arterial wall metabolism.

Some form of arterial or, more specifically, intimal injury may underlie the genesis of atheromata. Consistently over the years, certain investigations have pointed to damaged endothelium or intima as necessary prerequisites for excessive filtration of plasma lipids or lipoproteins. It will be recalled that one pattern of early lesion was characterized as small, gray, gelatinous or edematous elevations. These have long been attributed by More and Haust (1961) to focal endothelial injury and the development of intimal edema. They have also demonstrated exudation or, as they prefer to call it, insudation of fibrin within these edematous areas and have raised the question of whether degeneration of the fibrin contributes to the local lipid accumulation. It is argued that hypertension contributes to atherogenesis by stress injury of arteries. Hypertension and hyperlipidemia are a potent combination in the development of atherosclerotic plaques in the experimental animal. Moreover, hypertension and "normal" concentrations of lipids in the blood, over an appropriate length of time, will also produce lesions (Freis, 1969). Atheromata are prone to develop where the jet lesion of a patent ductus arteriosus impinges, proximal to a coarctation and at sites of turbulence such as about the mouths of arterial branches. Atheromata also tend to develop along the posterior wall of the aorta fixed to the prevertebral fascia where it is caught between the hammer of the arterial pulse and the anvil of the skeletal system. Atherosclerosis in the pulmonary arteries is strongly associated with pulmonary hypertension and is rarely seen in its absence. In rabbits on an atherogenic diet, when a segment of the inferior vena cava and the aorta are exchanged, the transplanted portion of the inferior vena cava develops AS, but the segment of aorta now incorporated in the venous system fails to develop lesions. Both transplants are obviously exposed to the same blood lipids, but the pressure relationships are reversed. Increased arterial wall tension has been shown to increase the permeability of the endothelium (Glagov, 1965). Intimal thickening almost always precedes atherogenesis, and it is argued that thickening of the intima renders it relatively hypoxic since it only receives blood supply by imbibition from the lumen of the artery. It will be remembered that the vasa vasorum which nourish the arterial walls permeate from the adventitial side and only penetrate as far as the outer third of the media. Thus the inner portion of the media and thickened intima may always be relatively hypoxic and vulnerable to further reduction in oxygen tension. In the experimental animal, low levels of oxygen saturation increase the atherogenic potential of dietary regimens.

Constantinides (1968) has placed great emphasis on some form of subtle injury, with opening of interendothelial cell junctions, as the requisite prelude to atherogenesis. Such injury was inducible by lowered plasma osmolarity, extremes of pH, anoxia, cyanide and by infusions of vasoactive amines (Constantinides, 1969). Others have also pointed to increased aortic permeability as the first step in atherogenesis (Klynstra and Bottcher, 1970). In this context, it has been proposed that an autoimmune reaction first injures the endothelial lining of blood vessels, predisposing to lipid filtration (Burch, 1964). It is of interest that severe atheromatosis has been described in allotransplanted human hearts within a short span of months, providing some support to the contention that vascular injury, in this instance an immune reaction, potentiates this disease. The issue of intimal injury remains only as a plausible theory, largely because no clear pathogenetic mechanism for such injury in AS has yet been identified. Nonetheless, it may well contribute because the presence of such large molecules as fibrin and lipoproteins within the arterial wall implies some form of increased endothelial permeability, perhaps on the basis of arterial injury (More and Haust, 1957). Conceivably, arterial wall injury constitutes the initiating event which permits excessive filtration into the arterial wall. Equally valid is the possibility that the arterial injury impairs efflux or catabolism of endogenously synthesized lipids.

The encrustation or thrombogenic hypothesis of atherogenesis was first proposed over 100 years ago and still persists as a viable, albeit not widely held, conception. It is based on two fundamental arguments: first, if a mural thrombus forms on the surface of an artery and persists, it will in the course of time be covered by a new endothelium to become, in effect, a thickened intimal plaque; second, having thus been incorporated, the thrombotic material will undergo degenerative changes obscuring its origins and making it no longer distinguishable from the necrotic debris characteristic of the centers of advanced atheromata (Duguid, 1946, 1948). It is important to stress that, without doubt, arterial thrombi occur as a complication of advanced atherosclerotic lesions and are often the significant event leading to tissue infarction and clinical disease. However, the thrombogenic theory raises the issue of whether intimal lesions may begin as surface encrustations of thrombus.

There are two major difficulties in relating the thrombogenic hypothesis to the early stages of atherogenesis: (1) What initiates thrombus formation on the endothelial surface? (2) How can we explain the rich lipid content of the atheroma if it is derived from thrombotic debris? With respect to the first issue, it may be necessary to postulate, as mentioned earlier, some form of subtle endothelial injury. Fry (1968) has shown structural changes in endothelial cells at sites of turbulence and in locations exposed to high shear rates of blood flow. Certainly, hypertension might be a contributory factor. Other still obscure injurious influences may exist as have been cited earlier. Alternatively, some imbalance between the continuing formation of fibrin in the circulation and its removal by fibrinolysis might potentiate thrombus formation. As was discussed in Chapter 9, the maintenance of the fluidity of the blood is at best a precarious balance. Alimentary lipidemia and diets high in animal fats have been shown to inhibit fibrinolytic activity of the blood (Greig, 1956). They also enhance thrombosis as do stress, tobacco smoking and diets of saturated long-chain fatty acids. One might therefore postulate the following sequence: Subtle endothelial injury might lead to a surface film of fibrin which might then permit the adherence of platelets. Vasoactive amines released from platelets might then increase endothelial permeability, possibly exposing subendothelial tissue as a further stimulus to platelet aggregation. Thereafter, the thrombotic sequence would ensue abetted by influences inhibiting fibrinolysis.

The second issue, namely, the lipid content of advanced atheromas, has been addressed largely by animal experiments. When fibrin or whole blood clot is injected intravenously into rabbits, the emboli which lodge in the pulmonary arteries are subsequently organized with the formation of localized fibroelastic thickenings, but the lipid content therein is inconspicuous (Thomas et al., 1956). However, when the injected fragments are rich in platelets, a fibrofatty plaque more closely resembling the atheroma appears (Hand and Chandler, 1962). The content of lipids can be increased when the animal is first made hyperlipemic. Furthermore, it is possible that in the course of the organization of the thrombus the endothelial disruption might potentiate the filtration of lipid. All of this evidence merely points to possibilities, and the viability of the thrombogenic hypothesis is based more on plausibility than on documented observations in man (French, 1971). There is, nonetheless, good evidence that thrombi contribute significantly to the development of complicated lesions and occlusion of vessels in the advanced stages of atherosclerosis, and there is considerable probability that mural thrombi may also lead to growth of plaques.

Any increased tendency to thrombosis, then, may have grave consequences in the individual already suffering from atherosclerosis. Many studies have shown that coagulation and fibrinolytic factors are altered in patients with atherosclerosis, ischemic heart disease and stroke. Elevations of plasma fibrinogen and the plasma procoagulants, factors V, VII, VIII, IX and X, have been reported including shortening of several standard clotting time tests, such as the prothrombin time and the partial thromboplastin time (Ettinger et al., 1969) (Penick and Roberts, 1964). Hyperlipidemia and long-chain saturated fatty acids enhance platelet adhesiveness, further compounding the risk (Mustard and Packham, 1970). *The control of this thrombotic diathesis may be as important in reducing the clinical impact of atherosclerotic disease as the control of atherogenesis.*

Having discussed the major theories of atherogenesis, it is apparent that no single proposition is consonant with all of the established observations. For example, the basis for the protection afforded the premenopausal female, apparently by ovarian function, is still unexplained. It may well be that *atherosclerosis is a disease of multifactorial origin.* In some individuals, perhaps, extreme levels of hyperlipidemia and filtration are dominant, while in others deranged metabolism of the arterial wall or endothelial injury may potentiate atherogenesis despite little filtration of lipids. Perhaps the cumulative effects of multiple factors are involved. One could propose intimal injury followed by platelet adhesion with release of vasoactive amines increasing intimal permeability, leading to greater filtration of lipids or lipoproteins. This would in turn derange the arterial wall metabolism which might then further compound the intimal injury and lead to a vicious cycle. Perhaps, then, there is no single cause of atherosclerosis, and there is some truth in all of the theories of atherogenesis.

Clinical Significance. The clinical manifestations of atherosclerosis are as varied as the vessels affected and the extent of the atheromatous change. The lesions themselves do not cause symptoms or signs. They cause clinical disease only by (1) narrowing the vascular lumina to cause ischemic atrophy, (2) sudden occlusion of the lumen by superimposed thrombosis or hemorrhage into an atheroma producing frank infarction, (3) providing a site for thrombosis and then embolism or (4) weakening the wall of a vessel followed possibly by aneurysm formation or rupture. Although theoretically any organ or tissue in the body may be so involved, symptomatic atherosclerotic disease is most often localized to the heart, brain, kidneys, lower extremities and small intestine. The importance of such vascular disease was amply documented by some of the epidemiologic data cited earlier in this discussion. It will be further documented throughout the remaining chapters of the book since vascular disease comprises a significant part of all organ and system pathology.

Given the fact that AS and CHD are virtually epidemic in affluent populations, methods of possible control are understandably major concerns of these groups. A number of clinical trials of prevention of AS and CHD have been instituted. All make the assumption that five factors capable of alteration are of cardinal importance: diets high in cholesterol and saturated fat, hypercholesterolemia, obesity, hypertension and cigarette smoking. It should be emphasized, however, that some aspects of this assumption are still heatedly disputed. Some researchers are not convinced of the role of hyperlipidemia in atherogenesis.

Others argue that reduction of dietary cholesterol intake is of little consequence in the light of endogenous synthesis of this sterol, and still others are more concerned with the roles of physical inactivity, stress of living, thrombogenesis and the content of polyunsaturated fat in the diet. Increasing the proportion of polyunsaturated fatty acids in the diet has been a matter of controversy but, nonetheless, has been shown on fairly good evidence to lower serum cholesterol levels even when the cholesterol intake is maintained constant. Despite this contention, most of the trials are based on modifications of the diet. Some have also attempted to control hypertension, weight and smoking while adding physical exercise to the regimen. The specific modifications of the diet among the many trials are too numerous to detail. In general, they take the form of lowering the total caloric intake, lowering fat intake, restricting carbohydrate intake and substituting polyunsaturated fats for saturated fats. Lowering of serum cholesterol levels is one of the principal goals of all of these regimens. The end point in all of these trials is an attempt to demonstrate reduction in mortality from CHD. Some are primary prevention trials, i.e., employing experimental subjects apparently free of previous "atherosclerotic events"; others are secondary prevention trials in which men with previous manifestations of atherosclerotic disease were placed on a modified regimen in hope of reducing subsequent events. At the time of this writing, although the results are modestly encouraging, no clear mandate has been achieved (Dayton and Pearce, 1969).

In the Dayton and Pearce (1969) secondary prevention study of middle-aged and elderly men living in a veterans' home, the major intervention was the substitution of highly unsaturated fat in the form of vegetable oils for saturated fat. The total dietary fat was kept at usual levels. Among 422 men in the control group, there were 27 sudden deaths due to CHD, while in the experimental group of 424 men, there were only 18. Other manifestations of atherosclerotic disease such as cerebral infarcts and ruptured aneurysms were proportionally reduced. However, amputation for gangrene was as frequent in the experimental as in the control group. It could be argued that all of the individuals were adult at the time of institution of the regimen and undoubtedly already suffered from AS too advanced to reasonably expect improvement in prognosis.

In a primary prevention trial of men aged 40 to 59 who were free of clinical coronary disease or other life-limiting illness, Stamler (1971) reports even more dramatic results, namely a 40 per cent reduction in the coronary death rate for all men in the program, including the dropouts, while for men remaining active in the program, the rate was 75 per cent lower. These results should be interpreted with the caution that the sample size in all groups was small, the experimental subjects were highly motivated volunteers, and the control population was not randomly assigned (Intersociety Commission for Heart Disease Resources, 1970). In this study, total calories were restricted, diets were moderate in total fat and carbohydrate, low in saturated fat, low in cholesterol and simple sugars and moderate in polyunsaturates and salt. Antihypertensive drugs were employed when necessary; physical exercise was encouraged, and about half of the volunteers in the experimental group stopped cigarette smoking during the seven years of the trial. In yet another quite recent study of mental patients (institutionalized) on a cholesterol-lowering diet only, approximately a 50 per cent reduction in mortality from CHD was achieved (Miettinen et al., 1972).

Thus, although the cause of AS remains unknown, the early clinical prevention trials point to the evils which accompany affluence and to the wisdom of moderation in living habits, particularly dietary habits.

MÖNCKEBERG'S MEDIAL CALCIFIC SCLEROSIS (MEDIAL CALCINOSIS)

Medial sclerosis is characterized by ring-like calcifications within the media of medium to small arteries of muscular type. Although Mönckeberg's medial calcific sclerosis may occur together with atherosclerosis in the same individual or even in the same vessel, *the two disorders are totally distinct anatomically, clinically and presumably etiologically.* The vessels most severely affected are the femoral, tibial, radial and ulnar arteries and the arterial supply of the genital tract in both sexes. The coronary arteries are likewise subject to medial calcinosis. Both sexes are affected indiscriminately. This disorder is rare in individuals under 50 years of age. Its genesis is still obscure, but according to prevailing concepts, medial calcification is related to prolonged vasotonic influences, a belief based largely upon animal experimental work. In animals, analogous medial calcifications can be produced by the prolonged intravascular infusion of such vasoconstrictors as epinephrine and nicotine.

The disorder is characterized by ring-like or plate calcifications within the wall of a vessel that create a "gooseneck lamp" nodularity on palpation. Sometimes the patchy deposits coalesce to create a more solid calcification that converts the vessel into a rigid calcific tube. It should be particularly noted that **these medial lesions do not encroach on the vessel lumen.** The endothelium may be ridged or deformed, but it remains intact. The calcification is not associated with any inflammatory reaction, and the intima and adventitia are largely unaffected. Commonly, bone and even marrow may form within the calcific plaques. Frequently, coexistent atheromata complicate the histologic changes (Fig. 15–13).

This disorder is of relatively little clinical significance. It accounts for roentgenographic densities in the vessels of the extremities in aged individuals, but it is to be remembered that the lesions are *not* productive of narrowing or occlusion of vascular lumina (Silbert et al., 1953).

ARTERIOLOSCLEROSIS

Included under this heading are two entities: hyaline arteriolosclerosis and hyperplastic arteriolosclerosis. Although both lesions are clearly related to elevations of blood pressure, other etiologies may also be involved.

Hyaline arteriolosclerosis is most often encountered in aged patients having moderate elevations of systolic blood pressure (in the range of 160 to 180 mm. Hg). This form of essential or benign hypertension is not usually associated with significant elevation of the diastolic pressure. Hyaline arteriolosclerosis is also commonly encountered in diabetics, and while most have concomitant hypertension, some are normotensive.

Whatever the clinical setting, the vascular lesion comprises a homogeneous, pink, hyaline thickening of the walls of arterioles with loss of underlying structural detail and with narrowing of the lumen of the vessel (Fig. 15–14). Under the electron microscope, irregular thickening of the basement membrane can be visualized, produced apparently by deposition of increased amounts of PAS-positive material similar to basement membrane. Often smooth muscle cells are trapped within these deposits (Weiner et al., 1965). In the diabetic, plasma proteins, principally immunoglobulins, have been identified in the hyalinized walls of these arterioles. The interpretation of these plasma proteins is controversial, as is discussed below. Intimal and medial

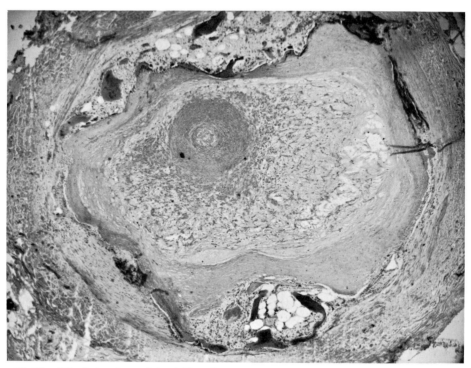

Figure 15–13. *Mönckeberg's medial calcific sclerosis and atherosclerosis. The vessel lumen is markedly narrowed by the intimal atherosclerosis. Dark, medial, calcific deposits with bone and bone marrow formation indicate the presence of Mönckeberg's sclerosis.*

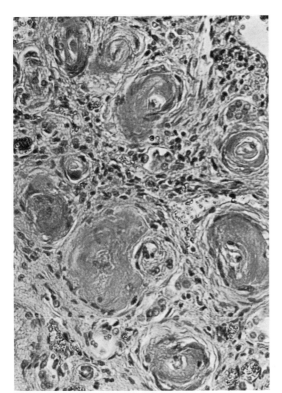

Figure 15--14. Hyaline arteriolosclerosis of numerous small vessels in the kidney. Patient had prolonged moderate hypertension.

collagenization adds to the hyaline change of the arteriolar walls.

This form of arteriolosclerosis is best seen in the kidneys, but is also encountered in other arterioles throughout the body (pancreas, gallbladder, adrenals, mesentery). It is generally believed that it reflects the chronic stress of moderate elevations of blood pressure. In normotensive diabetics, the hyaline thickening may be due to the deposition of plasma proteins secondary to either an immune reaction or increased permeability of the arteriolar walls. However, other studies have reported that the hyalin is the same in both diabetics and hypertensive nondiabetics (Fisher et al., 1966). Whatever the pathogenesis, the narrowing of the arteriolar lumina causes impairment of the blood supply to affected organs, particularly well exemplified in the kidneys. Thus, *hyaline arteriolosclerosis is a major morphologic characteristic of benign nephrosclerosis* where the arteriolar narrowing causes diffuse renal ischemia and symmetrical contraction of the kidneys (p. 1130).

Hyperplastic arteriolosclerosis is generally related to more acute or severe elevations of

blood pressure, and is therefore characteristic of malignant hypertension (diastolic pressures usually over 110 mm. Hg).

This form of arteriolar disease is identified with the light microscope by onionskin concentric laminated thickening of the walls of arterioles with progressive narrowing of the lumina (Fig. 15—15). Under the electron microscope, these reduplicated cells appear to be derived from myointimal cells (Spiro et al., 1965). The basement membrane is likewise thickened and reduplicated. Frequently but not invariably, these hyperplastic changes are accompanied by deposits of fibrinoid and acute necrosis of the vessel walls referred to as **necrotizing arteriolitis** (Fig. 15—16). The significance of the fibrinoid is uncertain, but might be due to increased permeability of the arteriolar intima permitting excessive diffusion of plasma proteins. Some mysterious form of primary arteriolitis is hypothesized, resulting in insudation of fibrinogen into the vascular walls (Linton et al., 1969). An immunologic reaction has been suggested as the etiology of the arteriolitis because complement as well as gamma globulins have been described in the arteriolar walls by Paronetto (1965). However, the nature of the antigenic challenge, if such exists, is certainly a

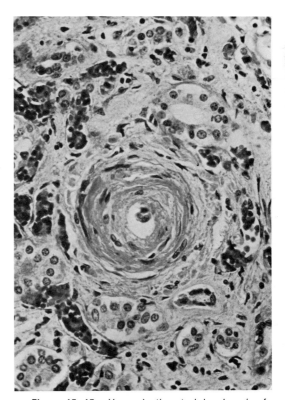

Figure 15--15. Hyperplastic arteriolosclerosis of a small vessel in kidney. Patient was young man who died with blood pressure 310/160.

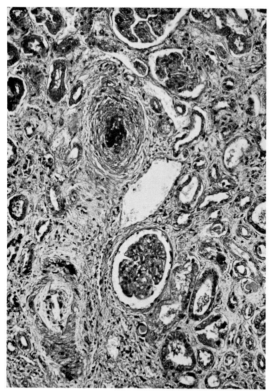

Figure 15–16. *A hyperplastic arteriole in the kidney with fibrinoid necrosis of the intimal layer. Patient died of renal failure secondary to malignant hypertension.*

puzzle and at the present time it is best to admit that the genesis of these arteriolar lesions remains unknown.

This pattern of hyperplastic arteriolosclerosis is almost never seen unless the patient has malignant hypertension. When present, *it may produce severe renal ischemic damage known as malignant nephrosclerosis* (p. 1132). The arterioles in other tissues throughout the body are also affected, favored sites being the periadrenal fat, gallbladder wall, peripancreatic and intestinal arterioles. Why these vessels should show more pronounced change than others is not clear.

Not infrequently, the two forms of arteriolosclerosis coexist in the same vessel, a condition facetiously referred to as "*benignant.*" When present, these changes are interpreted to imply a period of slow moderate elevation of blood pressure followed by a phase of rapidly mounting hypertension. Such occurs when a malignant phase of hypertension becomes superimposed on preexistent, mild, essential hypertension. While it is generally believed that the hypertension precedes and, indeed, produces the arteriolar lesions, still not excluded are other possible etiologies for the arteriolar narrowing which might then lead to hypertension by causing renal ischemia.

PULMONARY VASCULAR SCLEROSIS

This designation refers to the vascular changes associated with pulmonary hypertension. They take the form of atheromata within the larger arteries and hyperplastic proliferative thickening of the small arteries and arterioles (arteriolosclerosis). Further discussion of these lesions is found on p. 789.

INFLAMMATORY DISEASES

Arteritis is encountered in a great diversity of diseases and clinical settings. In some instances such as polyarteritis nodosa, the inflammatory involvement of the arteries is the fundamental basis of the disorder. In most cases, however, the arteritis is secondary to or only one component of some underlying disease as, for example, in systemic lupus erythematosus and the other connective tissue diseases. In fact, necrotizing arteritis is a hallmark of most immunologic disorders (Fig. 15–17). The consideration of these forms of arteritis was presented on p. 236. Here additional forms of arteritis will be discussed, e.g., nonspecific arteritis, giant cell arteritis, Takayasu's arteritis, and thromboangiitis obliterans (Buerger's disease).

NONSPECIFIC ARTERITIS

Nonspecific arteritis is produced when an artery is injured by bacterial toxins, direct bacterial invasion, mechanical trauma, radiant energy, chemical toxins, or any form of vasculotoxin. Most instances are caused by the direct invasion of bacteria from a neighboring infection. These lesions are most often associated with necrotizing inflammations and are frequently encountered in ulcerative colitis, in bacterial pneumonia, adjacent to caseous tuberculous reactions, in the neighborhood of abscesses and in the superficial cerebral vessels in cases of meningitis. Much less commonly, they arise from the hematogenous spread of bacteria. This hematogenous pathway presumably accounts for the seeding of the aortic wall in cases of septicemia or bacterial vegetative endocarditis. The resultant inflammation in this circumstance is specifically designated as *bacterial endaortitis.* Such lesions may cause rupture or produce weakening of the aortic walls with the formation of a *mycotic aneurysm.*

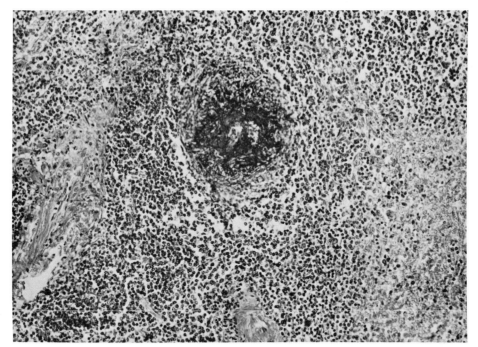

Figure 15–17. *Acute necrotizing arteritis in the spleen in a patient with a fulminating penicillin sensitivity reaction.*

The vascular inflammation is completely nonspecific in character with edema, fibrin precipitation and leukocytic infiltration in the affected arterial wall. Exudate may layer the endothelial surface and predispose to intravascular thrombosis or even rupture of the artery. The inflammatory involvement usually extends into the perivascular tissues. If the inflammatory reaction is prolonged, fibroblastic scarring may eventually cause narrowing and sometimes total obliteration of the vascular lumen.

Clinically, nonspecific arteritis is important on several counts. By inducing thrombosis, it adds an element of infarction to tissues that are already the seat of inflammatory reaction. It may, therefore, materially worsen the initial infection. For example, in bacterial meningitis, inflammation of the superficial vessels of the brain may predispose to vascular thromboses with subsequent infarction of the brain substance and extension of the subarachnoid infection into the brain tissue. In tuberculous meningitis, it is the vascular involvement that leads to the most serious sequelae. While such arterial lesions undoubtedly occur commonly in any type of inflammatory disease, they usually involve small rather than large arteries, and are therefore of little consequence except in the occasional case.

GIANT CELL ARTERITIS (TEMPORAL ARTERITIS, CRANIAL ARTERITIS)

Temporal arteritis is a focal granulomatous inflammation of arteries of medium and small size that affects principally the cranial vessels, especially the temporal arteries in older individuals (Meneely and Bigelow, 1953). In the more severe expressions of this disorder, lesions have been found in arteries throughout the body and, in some cases, the aortic arch has been involved to produce so-called giant cell aortitis (Hunder et al., 1967). For obscure reasons, occasionally granulomatous lesions are found throughout skeletal muscles, usually in relationship to the vasculature, giving rise to the concept that this form of arteritis is best designated as *polymyalgia arteritica* (Hamrin et al., 1968). Both sexes are equally susceptible and most patients are over 50 years of age. In contrast, polyarteritis nodosa, which bears strong morphologic resemblance to disseminated giant cell arteritis, and Takayasu's disease, which is the common cause of the aortic arch syndrome, both tend to affect much younger individuals.

Etiology and Pathogenesis. The cause of this disease remains a puzzle. The morphologic alterations seem to suggest some peculiar degenerative change in elastica and, accordingly, some immunologic reaction against these fibrils has been proposed. Some support for such a conception is provided by the finding in some patients of elevated gamma globulins and by the striking response that is sometimes achieved by corticosteroid treatment. In addition, the recognition of systemic patterns of this disease with prominent involvement of muscles has raised the issue as to whether this disorder may be a form of rheumatoid arthritis with rheumatoid arteritis (having a more firmly established immune basis). The absence of serologic evidence of rheumatoid arthritis in almost all cases of giant cell arteritis argues against the identity of rheumatoid disease and giant cell arteritis. The granulomatous nature of the inflammtory response obviously led to the suspicion of an infectious etiology. However, no microbiologic agent has ever been isolated from affected vessels and so the puzzle persists.

Morphology. As indicated earlier, any artery, including the aorta, may be affected. The temporal arteries are involved in from 40 to 70 per cent of patients, and may have morphologic changes in the absence of clinical evidence of tenderness or ocular manifestations. Conversely, almost half of all patients having manifestations of temporal arteritis, such as headache, tenderness over the artery, visual loss and facial pain, will have systemic involvement and the syndrome of polymyalgia rheumatica. But negative temporal artery biopsies have been reported in patients having such classic manifestations of this disease, and it must be assumed that the lesions were focal and were missed on biopsy. Affected arteries develop nodular enlargements which may be palpable in superficial situations such as the temple. Sometimes the overlying skin is erythematous and edematous.

The histologic changes are quite variable and fall into three general patterns: (1) granulomatous lesions replete with giant cells, localized principally in the region of the internal elastic membrane; (2) nonspecific white cell infiltration (neutrophils and occasional lymphocytes and eosinophils) throughout the arterial wall; and (3) intimal fibrosis, usually with an intact, internal elastic lamina (Bevan et al., 1968) (Fig. 15–18). The relationship of these three patterns to each other is unclear. At one time, it was thought that the initial histologic change is degeneration and fragmentation of the internal elastic membrane. It was proposed that the fragmented fibers then excited a chronic inflammatory reaction characterized chiefly by large numbers of lymphocytes, macrophages and prominent foreign body giant cells. Strangely, the giant cells are almost invariably the Langhans variety with peripherally placed nuclei. More recently, it has been suggested that the initial pathologic change is progressive alteration in the smooth muscle of the media with secondary destruction of elastic fibers (Reinecke and Kuwabara, 1969). Such changes might excite the diffuse acute inflammatory infiltrate without giant cell reaction, not too dissimilar to the alterations of polyarteritis nodosa. It would be logical to assume that this pattern might

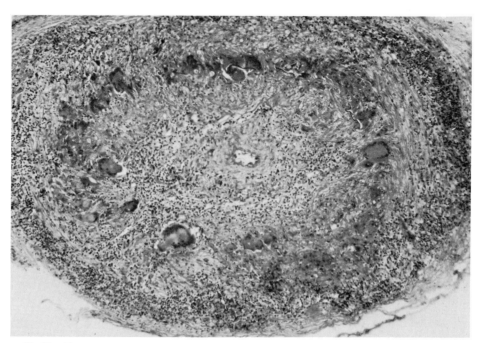

Figure 15–18. *Temporal giant cell arteritis. The circumferential giant cells mark the location of the degenerated internal elastic membrane.*

represent the initial acute phase of the disease, followed in time by secondary alterations in elastic fibers, leading to the granulomatous pattern. Moreover, the intimal fibrosis might represent the burned-out stage of the disease. Tempting as such speculation might be, such a sequence has not been established and so remains hypothetical. Thrombus formation commonly occurs in affected vessels, and may be followed by either obliteration of the lumen or organization and recanalization.

Clinical Course. The disease may be insidious and vague in onset or may be heralded by the sudden onset of headache and visual impairment. Most often, the illness begins with general symptoms of weight loss, malaise, fever, anorexia and nausea, followed by generalized muscular aching and stiffness in the shoulders and hips, manifestations that suggest a flu-like syndrome. Such an onset would be characterized as polymyalgia rheumatica. In those with a more acute onset, there is often prominent local symptomatology overlying the temporal arteries, including severe throbbing pain along the course of the artery, tenderness, swelling and redness in the overlying skin and acute visual loss to the point of total blindness. Ischemic optic neuritis may soon appear in such patients. Indeed, in some instances, the progressive development of blindness is the only manifestation of the vascular disease. Involvement of visceral vessels may give rise to manifestations of myocardial ischemia, gastrointestinal disturbances or neurologic derangements. Those with involvement of the aortic arch may develop symptomatology identical to that of Takayasu's or aortic arch syndrome.

The diagnosis of this condition, as must be apparent, is treacherous. Biopsy may be diagnostic, but may be entirely negative in otherwise characteristic clinical syndromes. Careful palpation of arteries in the hope of identifying a focal area of tenderness or nodularity is most important in securing an appropriate biopsy. As mentioned, however, histologic changes may be present in clinically normal vessels. In the absence of morphologic confirmation, it may be necessary to institute therapy on clinical grounds alone. In some instances, the disease is of acute and almost calamitous onset and corticosteroid therapy must be instituted promptly to prevent visual impairment. More often, however, giant cell arteritis pursues a more indolent, benign course which, in many instances, leads eventually to a complete and permanent remission. In a small proportion of cases with widespread systemic involvement, the course is progressively downhill to a fatal outcome.

TAKAYASU'S SYNDROME (AORTIC ARCH SYNDROME, PULSELESS DISEASE)

A partial list of the descriptive terms, in addition to those indicated, by which this rare disorder has been known includes primary aortitis, aortitis syndrome, giant cell arteritis of the aorta and nonsyphilitic aortitis. The multiplicity of terms indicates the state of confusion about the precise nature of this entity, if indeed it is an entity. Perhaps the major problem is the lack of clearly defined limits separating Takayasu's syndrome from other forms of aortic involvement. Syphilis and atherosclerosis undoubtedly account for at least 95 per cent of the involvements of the aortic arch and thoracic aorta. Giant cell arteritis involving the aorta makes a small further contribution to such involvements (p. 605) (Hunder et al., 1967). Nonetheless, there are occasional instances of thickening of the wall of the aortic arch, with narrowing of this segment of the aorta and the mouths of its branches, which cannot be clearly ascribed to any of these disorders. To these cases, diagnosed by a process of exclusion, the designation aortic arch syndrome is applied, and some, perhaps all, conform to the curious disorder first described by Takayasu in 1908. He brought to attention a clinical syndrome characterized principally by ocular disturbances and marked weakening of the pulses in the upper extremities, related to fibrous thickening of the aortic arch with narrowing to virtual obliteration of the origins of the great vessels arising in the arch (Judge et al., 1962). A significant number of well studied cases have since been reported from Japan, Korea, South Africa, Thailand, Sweden and England, with surprisingly few examples from Western countries. The illness is seen predominantly in the 10- to 50-year-old age group, and 90 per cent of these patients are under the age of 30. There is a striking female predilection in the range of 80 to 90 per cent.

Etiology and Pathogenesis. Perhaps the major problem confounding the search for the cause of Takayasu's arteritis has been the confusion about the fundamental issue: Is it a specific entity or is it a wastebasket for all forms of aortic involvement not clearly ascribable to well defined entities? Conceivably, there might be multiple etiologies leading to aortic thickening. Nasu (1963) called attention to a positive tuberculin test and often overt tuberculosis in a large proportion of his cases. However, neither tubercle bacilli nor other microorganisms have been identified in the lesions. Circulating antiartery antibodies have been identified in some cases, raising the possibility of an immunologic causation, but obviously these antibodies could represent a secondary response to some primary form of arterial injury. Other features suggest a relationship to the connective tissue diseases of presumed immunologic etiology, such as the predilection for younger females, occasional positive tests for the rheumatoid and LE cell factors and hyperglobulinemia. The apparent effectiveness of corticosteroids in inducing remissions lends an additional bit of weight to a possible immunologic origin. But at the present time, the disorder is best considered as idiopathic.

Morphology. Although classically, Takayasu's arteritis involves the aortic arch, in 32 per cent of the cases, it also affects the remainder of the aorta and its branches and, in 12 per cent, it is limited to the descending thoracic and abdominal aorta (Nakao et al., 1967). In some instances, the lesions are focal or multifocal in origin and do not involve entire segments of the aorta (Restrepo et al., 1969). Whether focal or diffuse, the gross morphologic changes comprise, in most cases, irregular thickening of the aortic wall with intimal wrinkling. When the aortic arch is involved, the orifices of the major arteries to the upper portion of the body may be markedly narrowed or even obliterated, accounting for the designation pulseless disease. In approximately 50 per cent of aortic arch involvements, the pulmonary artery is also affected. Histologically, the early changes appear to begin at the junction of the adventitia and media, and consist of an adventitial mononuclear infiltrate with perivascular cuffing of the vasa vasorum. These changes are similar to those of syphilitic aortitis. However, unlike the luetic lesion, the adventitial changes are accompanied by a diffuse polymorphonuclear infiltration and later a mononuclear infiltration in the media. In some cases, granulomatous changes appear within the media, replete with Langhans' giant cells and central caseating necrosis, producing more than a casual similarity to tuberculosis. In other instances, the medial reaction contains numerous giant cells, raising the strong possibility that such cases in reality are instances of giant cell arteritis. In the course of time, the inflammatory changes permeate the wall of the artery and lead to striking intimal thickening. Later stages show focal or diffuse loss of musculoelastic tissue, with extensive fibrosis of the media and marked acellular collagenous thickening of the intima. The fibrosing reaction thickens the wall of the aorta three- or fourfold, and extends into the proximal segments of the aortic branches, reducing their lumina to tiny, slit-like orifices. Thrombosis may be superimposed on this process and may, indeed, totally obliterate the lumina of the aortic branches.

Clinical Course. The salient clinical features include weakening of the pulses of the upper extremities, a marked drop in blood pressure in the upper extremities, often accompanied by elevation in the pressure in the lower extremities (sometimes inappropriately referred to as "reversed coarctation"), ocular disturbances such as visual defects, retinal hemorrhages, iris atrophy and total blindness as well as various neurologic deficits, ranging from syncope, dizziness, focal weaknesses, and paresthesias to complete hemiparesis. All of these clinical manifestations reflect arterial insufficiency to the head and upper extremities. But in about 66 per cent of these patients, these vascular manifestations are preceded by a long prodrome of nonspecific malaise, low-grade fever, weight loss and nausea lasting for a period of weeks to months. Occasionally, polyarthralgia, arthritis, stiffness of the shoulder muscles, dyspnea and palpitations are additional manifestations encountered in these patients. Severe hypertension is not infrequent and may well be due to involvement of the mouths of the renal arteries. The narrowing of the aortic arch sometimes leads to bizarre bypass channels, and a so-called "coronary steal syndrome" has been described in which the coronary circulation becomes diverted through new collateral anastomotic channels to the area below the obstruction of the aorta. The most common cause of death is either heart failure or unexplained sudden death. The latter, in some instances, is probably related to rupture of aortic aneurysms in patients with hypertension. The course of the disease is quite variable, and if the patient survives the first year or two of illness, the fibrotic quiescent stage may ensue and permit long survival, albeit with distressing neurologic and visual impairments.

THROMBOANGIITIS OBLITERANS (BUERGER'S DISEASE)

At the turn of the last century, Buerger described an apparently distinctive disease characterized by segmental, thrombosing, obliterative, acute and chronic inflammation of arteries and veins that occurred almost exclusively in men who were cigarette smokers. He attributed the disease to some infectious agent which he could not isolate but was able to transmit by transplantation of thrombus from acutely affected vessels. About 10 years ago, the specificity of this entity came under severe challenge. Fisher (1957), and later Wessler and his colleagues (1960), contended that the lesions described by Buerger were not distinctive and were in fact indistinguishable from atherosclerosis, systemic embolization, or peripheral arterial or venous thrombosis. For a short time this opinion prevailed and Buerger's disease as an entity came into disrepute.

However, several carefully reasoned and documented studies have since appeared, bolstering the original concept of the specificity of thromboangiitis obliterans as an entity quite distinct from atherosclerosis or its consequences. To quote from one of the most convincing of these reports, "Regardless of whether one accepts Buerger's disease as an entity, one cannot question the existence of a clinical syndrome which can with historic justice be termed the Buerger syndrome: occlusive peripheral vascular disease that occurs almost exclusively in men. It begins before 35 years in most and before 20 years in some. In many it affects the arms as well as the legs; it occurs almost solely in tobacco smokers; it demonstrates an intimate relationship of remission and relapse to cessation or resumption of smoking and it manifests excruciating pain out of proportion to that found in other forms of peripheral vascular disease. In many it is associated with migratory thrombophlebitis, but it is not associated with diabetes mellitus, hypercholesterolemia or heart disease which might be the source of emboli" (McKusick et al., 1962). In a provocative article entitled "Buerger's Disease Revisited," Wessler (1969) recently again reiterated: "My personal conjecture is that the term Buerger's syndrome is presently used as an umbrella for the occasional patient with peripheral arterial thrombosis the cause of which is unknown." Because the controversy continues, at the present time the entity cannot be discarded.

Etiology. Despite the fact that Buerger proposed an infectious agent as the etiology of this arterial disorder, to date, none has been identified. The relationship of this disorder to cigarette smoking is one of the many controversial features of the disease. Most patients are heavy smokers, and most are benefited when they stop smoking. This issue is discussed more fully later. The striking male preponderance further suggests a possible influence of male sex hormones or the absence of female sex hormones, but here again no clearly defined mechanisms can be outlined.

Morphology. The lesions are sharply segmental and usually involve arteries of small and medium size. Only rarely are larger arteries affected. It should be noted that, in contrast to atherosclerosis, Buerger's disease predominantly affects the medium and small arteries and only occasionally the larger arteries. Both upper and lower extremities are affected in thromboangiitis, in contrast to atherosclerosis which usually spares the upper extremities. Thromboangiitis has also been de-

scribed in the heart, lungs, brain, gastrointestinal tract and male genitalia. **After the arterial involvement, the accompanying veins and adjacent nerves are often secondarily affected, leading to progressive fibrous encasement of these three structures.** The affected segment of vessel tends to be firm and indurated, but is not aneurysmally dilated. It often contains an organized recanalized thrombus that is not macroscopically different from that found in atherosclerosis.

Only relatively few early lesions have been available for study because most of the pathologic specimens have been obtained from extremities amputated after a long chronic course of the disease. The acute involvements of either artery or vein are characterized by polymorphonuclear infiltration of all coats of the vessel wall, together with mural or occlusive thrombosis of the lumen. **Small microabscesses within the thrombus create a pattern quite distinct from the bland thrombosis of atherosclerosis.** These abscesses have a central focus of polymorphonuclear leukocytes surrounded by a fibroblastic, epithelioid cell, granulomatous enclosing wall which often contains Langhans' type giant cells (Fig. 15–19). In time, the thrombus undergoes organization and recanalization and the small microabscesses are replaced by fibrosing granulomas. Although the inflammatory reaction permeates the entire thickness of the vessel wall, the basic underlying architecture is still preserved. The consequence of this anatomic involvement is virtual total occlusion of the affected vessel until recanalization establishes new channels. Because this is a remitting, relapsing disease, it is possible to find lesions within the same vessel or different vessels at different stages of chronicity. This pattern may be encountered in either arteries or veins. When both are simultaneously involved, the accompanying nerve often gets trapped in the fibrous reaction.

Clinical Course. The anatomic changes have many etiologic and clinical implications. The impression cannot be escaped that Buerger's disease begins in young males as an inflammatory process within the thrombus rather than within the arterial wall. Usually there is no atherosclerosis in the vessels having the sharply segmental occlusions of Buerger's disease. It is true, of course, that over the years of recurrence of Buerger's disease, atherosclerosis may develop in such vessels and may therefore make differentiation of Buerger's disease from atherosclerosis difficult. The involvement of the upper extremities such as occurs in thromboangiitis obliterans would be distinctly unusual in atherosclerosis.

Whatever the outcome of the controversy, it is clear that these patients suffer from vascular insufficiency often leading to gangrene of the extremities. Severe pain is common in the

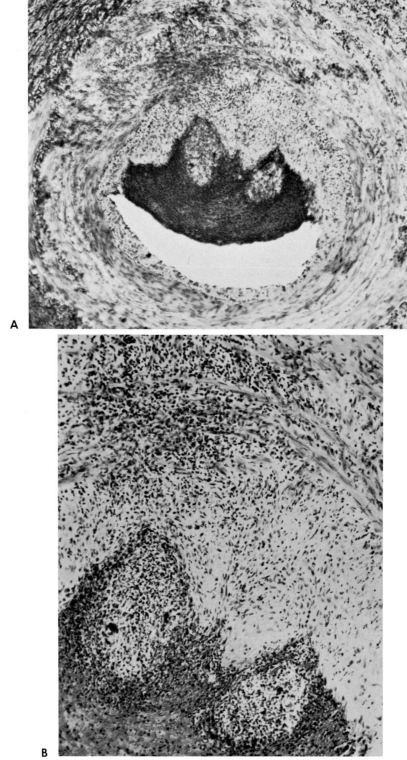

Figure 15–19. A, *Thromboangiitis obliterans. A partially occluded vein containing an organizing thrombus.* B, *High power detail of* A. *The vessel wall is above. Two microabscesses (containing giant cells) are evident in the margin of the thrombus.*

affected parts, in contrast to the relative painlessness of atherosclerotic occlusion. Most students of this disease believe that abstinence from tobacco, particularly cigarette smoking, is mandatory in these patients (Schatz et al., 1966). There is, however, some disagreement about this as well, and indeed the disease has been reported among patients who do not smoke at all. Thus the one-to-one relationship between smoking and disease onset and progression is still disputed.

SYPHILITIC VASCULITIS

Syphilitic vascular involvement may take one of many forms. During the tertiary stage of syphilis, aortitis and aneurysm formation may develop, but this complication has become increasingly rare as a consequence of the improved control and treatment of this disease. A much more rare form of aortitis is known as *gummatous aortitis.* Here gummas exactly resembling those described in other tissues sometimes develop within the wall of the aorta, usually in the ascending portion of the arch. These focal lesions create small, raised, rubbery subendothelial plaques or are found only as microscopic foci of gummatous necrosis within the wall of the aorta.

Small vessel lesions *(obliterative endarteritis)* may also occur in syphilis. This may develop in any stage of acquired or congenital lues. This vasculitis consists of an *adventitial inflammation, which is classically characterized by lymphocytic and plasma cell perivascular cuffing.* The inflammation often produces a highly vascularized connective tissue, which extends into the wall of the vessel and narrows or even obliterates the lumen, creating the obliterative endarteritis. Although spirochetes must be present, they are extremely scant and are difficult to find even with silver impregnation techniques.

Syphilitic aortitis with dilatation of the aortic valve ring is important as a cause of heart disease (p. 616). Syphilitic vasculitis in the small vessels of the meninges may cause serious brain damage.

RHEUMATOID AORTITIS AND ARTERITIS

It is now a well established fact that rheumatoid arthritis is a connective tissue disease of apparent immunologic origin, which affects not only joints but also any other organ or structure in the body. The cardiovascular system is affected as one of the major secondary targets of this disorder. Aortitis and arteritis of small and medium-sized arteries and cardiac lesions are well documented features of this wide-ranging entity. Because the joints are the primary targets, this disease, along with its cardiovascular features, is discussed on p. 1466.

RHEUMATIC ARTERITIS

In acute rheumatic fever, arteries and veins are sometimes the site of an acute vasculitis. The reaction comprises an acute fibrinoid necrosis accompanied by a polymorphonuclear exudate. It closely resembles the changes of hypersensitivity angiitis and polyarteritis nodosa, but sometimes is distinctive because it may remain localized to the intima. Only rarely does the necrosis extend through the media to involve the adventitia. Such rheumatic vasculitis is usually an inconspicuous component of the acute rheumatic attack. Tissue damage in affected parts is rarely observed.

SUMMARY OF THE NECROTIZING ANGIITIDES

It must be apparent that there is a wide variety of acute inflammatory vascular involvements. Their morphologic similarities are an obvious source of confusion. Table 15–3 on the following page provides some salient and distinguishing characteristics of the major forms of necrotizing angiitis, including some of the prototype lesions discussed in Chapter 7.

OTHER VASCULAR DISORDERS

RAYNAUD'S DISEASE

Raynaud's *disease* is a functional vasospasm causing trophic changes or even frank gangrene in the affected part. It affects most commonly the tip of the nose, fingers, hands and feet, i.e., the extreme periphery (acral parts) of the vascular system. It should not be confused with Raynaud's *phenomenon.* This syndrome refers to any cause of arterial insufficiency in the acral parts and is most often caused by organic arterial occlusion (arteriosclerosis, thrombosis, embolism, SLE, scleroderma). Of the 66 cases of Raynaud's phenomenon reported by de Takats and Fowler (1962), only 7 were due to the vasospastic Raynaud's disease.

Raynaud's disease is characterized by *episodic, symmetrical vasoconstriction of the small arteries and arterioles of the extremities,* usually the hands, with resultant variable pallor and hyperemia. In longstanding, chronic cases, trophic changes develop with atrophy of the skin, subcutaneous tissues and muscles. When the process continues sufficiently long, ulcerations

TABLE 15-3. THE CHARACTERISTICS OF SYSTEMIC NECROTIZING ANGIITIDES

Necrotizing Angiitides	Vessels Involved	Organ or Tissues Affected	Principal Morphologic Features	Immunoglobulins and Complement in Lesions	White Cell Reaction
Polyarteritis nodosa	Muscular arteries	Gastrointestinal tract, mesentery, liver, gallbladder, kidney, pancreas, lung, muscles, other sites	Lesions of varying ages; all layers of vessels with acute fibrinoid necrosis and extensive periarterial inflammation	Frequent	Neutrophils and numerous eosinophils
Hypersensitivity angiitis (Arthus lesion)	Small venules, capillaries, arterioles	All organs and tissues (skin, muscles, heart, kidneys, lungs)	Acute necrotizing vasculitis with fibrinoid necrosis of entire wall; often thrombosis of lumen	Frequent	Neutrophils
Giant cell arteritis	Muscular arteries	Usually temporal, ophthalmic and cranial arteries; may be systemic	Disruption of elastic lamina with most intense reaction in intimal medial layers; later permeates; giant cells engulf elastic fiber fragments; occasionally thrombosis of lumen	Infrequent	Neutrophils rare, lymphocytes, histiocytes and occasionally plasma cells
Wegener's granulomatosis	Small arteries, arterioles	Lungs, kidneys, upper respiratory tract; occasionally systemic	Acute necrotizing vasculitis with fibrinoid necrosis of vessel wall; often proximate to granulomas in tissues	Negative	Neutrophils, occasionally eosinophils, histiocytes
Systemic lupus erythematosus	Arterioles and capillaries	Kidneys, skin, heart muscles, nerves; may be widespread	Same as hypersensitivity reaction	Frequent	Neutrophils
	Splenic arterioles	Spleen	Onionskinning		
Buerger's disease	Arteries, veins, nerves	Extremities, viscera uncommonly	Thrombosis with microabscesses; acute inflammation permeates wall artery, but preserves underlying architecture	Negative	Neutrophils
Rheumatoid arteritis	Muscular arteries	Mostly extremities, viscera uncommonly	Adventitial neutrophil and mononuclear reaction sometimes permeates wall	Negative	Neutrophils and monocytes
Rheumatic arteritis			Indistinguishable from hypersensitivity angiitis		

or even frank ischemic gangrene may develop. The *lower extremities are seldom involved,* a strong differential point from other organic occlusive diseases. The disease preponderantly affects *young females* below 40 to 50 years of age, but males are involved in about one-fifth of the cases. This sex distribution further differentiates this condition from Buerger's disease and arteriosclerosis. Cold weather appears to aggravate the vasospasm and accentuate the progression of ischemic changes. The etiology is completely obscure and is postulated to be related to some form of hyperlability of the autonomic innervation of the affected vessels. Studies of the arterial supply in the involved areas usually reveal essentially normal vessels. Several reports have cited suggestive intimal thickening and endothelial proliferation, but it is generally believed that these changes reflect the state of spasm of the vessel rather than true organic changes.

ACROCYANOSIS

Acrocyanosis is a somewhat less significant disorder which manifests itself chiefly by coolness and cyanosis of the fingertips and toes associated with sensory disturbances, such as paresthesias, numbness and tingling. Since this disorder rarely causes sufficient tissue destruction to require surgery, there has been little opportunity for morphologic study. Acrocyanosis may, however, precede the development of the condition known as morphea, one of the variants of scleroderma (p. 242). The atrophy of skin and muscles and replacement fibrosis lead to anatomic alterations which are characteristic of systemic scleroderma. On this ground, it may reasonably be questioned whether acrocyanosis is a distinct disorder or merely a prodrome or abortive form of acrosclerosis. The main condition to be differentiated is Raynaud's disease.

IDIOPATHIC CYSTIC MEDIAL NECROSIS (MEDIONECROSIS)

This mysterious disorder is characterized by focal but widespread destruction of the musculoelastic media of the aorta. Less commonly, the coronary arteries and major branches of the aorta may also be similarly affected. It is usually discovered as a chance finding at postmortem in patients who were entirely free of related symptomatology. However, it may have grave importance since it weakens the aortic wall and predisposes to rupture of vasa vasorum and intimal tears, followed by hemorrhage within the media, which cleaves the laminar planes only to eventually burst out in a massive hemorrhage. Thus arise the frequently fatal calamitous dissecting aneurysms (p. 617).

Etiology and Pathogenesis. For many years, dating back to the time of Erdheim, the focal medial defects were thought to be the consequence of hypoxic medial damage related to narrowing of the vasa vasorum. It is well known that patients with dissecting aneurysms and medionecrosis are usually hypertensive and might logically have hyperplastic arteriolosclerosis of the vasa vasorum. However, despite the fact that most of these patients are indeed hypertensive, significant narrowing of the vasa vasorum can only rarely be documented in association with the medionecrosis. Nonetheless, focal medial lesions are frequently found in the aorta proximal to a congenital coarctation where severe local hypertension exists. Conceivably, elevated levels of blood pressure, by increasing the expansile thrust on the aorta, might compress the thin-walled vasa vasorum and thus lead to hypoxia without inducing visible structural changes in the walls of these small vessels.

An alternative explanation for the focal medial lesions has been proposed in the form of some metabolic defect in the synthesis or maintenance of the ground substance, collagen and elastic fibers of the tunica media. Marfan's syndrome is a hereditary disorder characterized by defective formation of elastic tissue. These patients have a variety of structural defects involving the suspensory ligaments of the lens and the capsules of joints, but principally, from the standpoint of our interest, almost invariably have medionecrosis of the aorta. It has in fact been suggested that medionecrosis is simply a forme fruste of Marfan's syndrome. The metabolic defect might also be due to exogenous influences. Foods rich in beta aminopropionitriles derange, in the laboratory animal, the normal synthesis of collagen and elastic fibers and lead to the experimental syndrome known as lathyrism (Bornstein, 1970) (Tanzer, 1965). Rats, for example, fed on sweet pea meal rich in proprionitriles often develop a variety of structural defects but also medionecrosis and sometimes die of dissecting aneurysms. The compounds in some manner interfere with intramolecular cross linkages in collagen and thus render it both abnormally soluble and deficient in tensile strength (Page and Benditt, 1972). Turkeys also acquire medionecrosis when treated with estrogens, and it is of interest that dissecting aneurysms are more common in women during pregnancy. Experimental copper deficiency also leads to medionecrosis, possibly by impairing the action of copper-dependent enzymes in the aortic media. Paralleling this experimental finding, it has been observed that patients having Wilson's disease (a metabolic disorder characterized by an excess accumulation of copper), treated with a copper chelating agent such as penicillamine, sometimes develop medionecrosis (Walshe, 1968). But all of these pathogenetic observations are "grasping at straws" and, at the present, the disorder is best considered as idiopathic.

Morphology. As mentioned, medionecrosis is primarily a disorder of the aorta but may also affect the coronary arteries and major branches of the aorta (Brody et al., 1965). In the absence of dissection, lesions may be discovered as incidental microscopic findings. On occasion, the weakened aorta is slightly dilated, but rarely to the extent justifying the term aneurysmal dilatation. The characteristic microscopic lesion is that of focal separation of the elastic and fibromuscular elements of the tunica media by small cleft-like or cystic spaces filled with ground substance (Gore and Seiwert, 1952). In the individual foci, the normal laminar pattern of the aortic wall is destroyed and is replaced by a poorly delimited area of increased, slightly basophilic, amorphous material resembling the ground substance of connective tissue (Fig. 15—20). These foci are referred to as cystic, but there are no well defined enclosing walls or sharp delineations. The lesions are haphazardly distributed throughout the thickness of the media. In some cases, there is no obvious increase of mucopolysaccharide ground substance, only apparent disappearance of muscle fibers and condensation of poorly formed elastic fibers (Rottino, 1939). Whether these histologic variations have some differing etiologies is unknown. The alterations are subtle in character and extent, and are readily missed on superficial inspection of routine tissue stains. For this reason, elastic tissue stains are desirable to highlight focal areas of apparent destruction or separation of the normal lamellae of the medial wall. Occasionally, a slight inflammatory reaction surrounds these areas of necrosis but, in most cases, the lesions are devoid of significant vascularization, white cell infiltration or surrounding fibrosis.

Medionecrosis of itself is without clinical significance, but it is an anatomic alteration of considerable gravity because it predisposes to dissecting aneurysms.

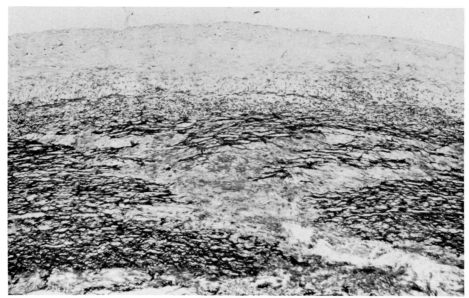

Figure 15–20. *Idiopathic medial necrosis. The large defect in the laminar pattern of the aortic wall is highlighted by the elastic tissue stain.*

AORTIC ANEURYSMS

One of the most striking results of all forms of vascular disease is the formation of an aneurysm. An aneurysm is a localized abnormal dilatation of any vessel. Aneurysms may occur in any artery or vein of the body, but they are most common and most significant in the aorta. Aortic aneurysms produce serious clinical disease and often cause death by rupture. Several of the vascular diseases presented rather commonly give rise to aortic aneurysms. The description of these lesions has been deferred until now so that the various forms can be considered as a group and the differential features can be more sharply outlined.

Aneurysms may be classified by their location, their etiology or their gross appearance. *According to location,* an aneurysm should be listed as arterial or venous, the specific vessel affected, as, for example, the splenic artery or popliteal vein, and when possible further localized to the precise site in the affected vessel, namely, the transverse portion of the arch of the aorta, the descending thoracic aorta or the lower abdominal aorta. *With respect to etiology,* aneurysms may be classified by indicating, when known, the specific nature of the vascular damage that leads to the aneurysmal dilatation. Virtually any of the diseases discussed may, under special circumstances, predispose to aneurysmal dilatation of arteries or veins; however, the *three most important causes are:* arteriosclerosis, syphilis and cystic medionecrosis. These disorders are responsible for almost all aortic aneurysms. Less commonly, aneurysms of smaller vessels are caused by polyarteritis nodosa, trauma such as leads to an arteriovenous aneurysm, congenital defects such as produce the berry aneurysms, and nonspecific inflammations that significantly weaken vascular walls and cause so-called *mycotic aneurysms.*

The *classification of aneurysms by gross appearance* attempts to characterize the macroscopic shape and size of the aneurysmal dilatation. A *berry* aneurysm refers to a small, spherical dilatation rarely exceeding a diameter of 1 to 1.5 cm. A *saccular* aneurysm might be described as a giant berry aneurysm. These dilatations are usually essentially spherical. They vary in size up to huge structures 15 to 20 cm. in diameter. In their more usual distribution, saccular aneurysms are frequently 5 to 10 cm. in diameter. The aneurysmal sac is connected to the vessel lumen by a mouth varying in size, which may virtually have the same diameter as the aneurysmal dilatation. Characteristically, these aneurysms are partially or completely filled by thrombus. Usually the thrombus is laid down in progressive layers and is thus clearly laminated *(lines of Zahn).* In many, the oldest region is adjacent to the vessel wall and the freshest accretion is on the surface. At other times, the thrombus may be poorly attached to the vessel wall and, by the contraction of the blood clot, may produce a thin, cleft-like space between the clot and the vessel into which fresh blood seeps so that the oldest portion of the thrombus is in contact with the flow of blood.

A *fusiform* aneurysm is one in which there is gradual, progressive dilatation of the vessel lumen. These aneurysms then take on a spindle shape, and the aneurysmal lumen is in direct continuity with the vascular lumen. Frequently these fusiform dilatations are eccentric so that one aspect of the wall is more severely affected. The fusiform aneurysm varies in diameter up to 20 cm. and is very variable in length, many involving the entire ascending and transverse portions of the aortic arch, while others may extend over large segments of the abdominal aorta. Infrequently, the fusiform dilatation is extremely long and produces a length of expanded vessel of fairly uniform diameter referred to as *cylindroid.* This anatomic variant is merely a deviation from the more usual fusiform dilatation.

On the basis of these classifications, it is possible to characterize an aneurysm fairly specifically as, for example, a congenital berry aneurysm of the anterior cerebral artery or an arteriosclerotic fusiform aneurysm of the lower abdominal aorta.

Attention may now be turned to a more detailed consideration of the three most important types of aneurysms, i.e., arteriosclerotic, syphilitic and dissecting aneurysms of the aorta.

ARTERIOSCLEROTIC (ATHEROSCLEROTIC) ANEURYSMS

With the falling incidence of tertiary syphilis, arteriosclerotic aneurysms have become the most common form. They rarely develop before the age of 50 and are much more common in males, in the ratio of 5 to 1 (Crane, 1955). They usually occur in the abdominal aorta or common iliacs, but rarely they affect the arch and thoracic aorta (Figs. 15–21 and 15–22). Luetic aneurysms are extemely *infrequent* in the abdominal aorta, and in the series reported by Crane, 97 per cent of abdominal aneurysms were arteriosclerotic in origin. As a general principle, *all fusiform, cylindroid or saccular aneurysms of the abdominal aorta should be considered as arteriosclerotic until proved otherwise.*

Arteriosclerotic aneurysms are usually positioned below the renal arteries and above the bifurcation of the aorta. They are usually fusiform or cylindroid. The saccular pattern is distinctly less common. Not infrequently, these aortic aneurysms are accompanied by smaller fusiform or saccular dilatations of the iliac arteries. The genesis of these aneurysms is severe atherosclerosis with extension of the atheromas into the media. There is consequent destruction of the fibromuscular-elastic supporting layer of the aorta. With this severe atherosclerosis, it is very common to find atheromatous ulcers within the aneurysm, covered by mural thrombi. Sometimes the entire aneurysmal dilatation is filled with thrombus. Such mural thrombi are

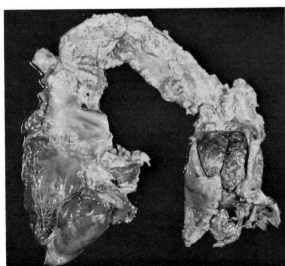

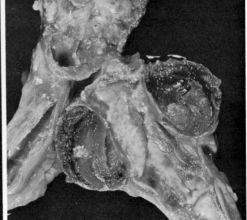

Fig. 15–21

Fig. 15–22

Figure 15–21. Arteriosclerotic aneurysm of the abdominal aorta with mural thrombosis.

Figure 15–22. Arteriosclerotic saccular aneurysm of the common iliac artery filled with laminated thrombus.

prime sites for the formation of emboli that almost invariably lodge in the vessels of the lower extremity.

Occasionally the aneurysm may affect the take-offs of the renal, superior and inferior mesenteric arteries, either by producing direct pressure on these vessels or by narrowing or occlusion of their ostia with mural thrombi. In the same way, the thrombus may impinge upon the common iliac arteries. These aneurysms give rise to clinical symptoms by varied secondary effects: (1) rupture into the peritoneal cavity or retroperitoneal tissues with massive or fatal hemorrhage, (2) impingement upon an adjacent structure, as compression of a ureter or erosion of the vertebrae, (3) occlusion of a vessel from either direct pressure or mural thrombus formation, particularly the vertebral branches that supply the spinal cord, (4) embolism from the mural thrombus and (5) presentation as an abdominal mass that simulates a tumor.

All writers agree that large arteriosclerotic aneurysms materially shorten longevity. Most fatalities are caused by rupture. It has been shown that this danger of rupture is directly related to the size of the aneurysm. Those patients having aneurysms less than 6 cm. in diameter rarely died of rupture, whereas 80 per cent of those with aneurysms 7 cm. or more in diameter suffered fatal rupture. On this basis, there is a growing conviction that large aneurysms should be replaced with prosthetic grafts when discovered.

SYPHILITIC ANEURYSMS

Syphilitic aneurysms are almost always confined to the thoracic aorta and usually involve the arch. While the ascending and transverse portions of the arch are favored sites, many times the dilatation extends proximally to the level of the aortic valve and distally to the level of the diaphragm. Very few occur below the diaphragm and above the level of the renal arteries. Since arteriosclerotic aneurysms are uncommon in this location, at least *90 per cent of thoracic aneurysms are attributable to syphilis.*

These aneurysms vary in gross appearance to encompass the saccular, fusiform and cylindroid types (Figs. 15–23 and 15–24). Many times the aneurysmal masses achieve the diameter of 15 to 20 cm. or become even larger. The development of these aneurysms is based upon the medial destruction characteristic of tertiary luetic aortitis. As was pointed out, atherosclerosis almost invariably develops in the thoracic aorta in the presence of syphi-

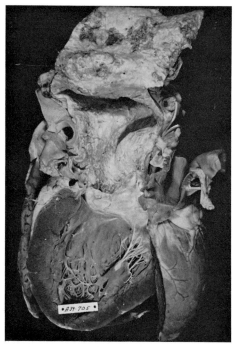

Fig. 15–23

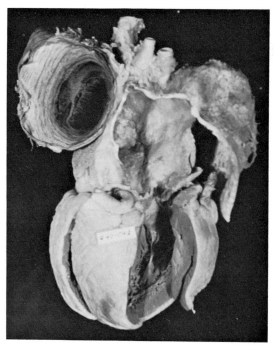

Fig. 15–24

Figure 15–23. *Advanced atherosclerosis superimposed on luetic aortitis. The ascending arch is widened and thrown into irregular folds by the aneurysmal dilatation.*

Figure 15–24. *A saccular syphilitic aneurysm of the ascending arch of aorta filled with laminated blood clot.*

litic involvement, and unquestionably such severe atherosclerosis contributes materially to further weakening of the aortic wall. Over the course of time, these expansile, pulsating masses cause erosion of ribs and vertebral bodies. Older textbooks contain many illustrations of syphilitic aneurysms that have eroded through the thoracic cage to assume a subcutaneous position. Such extreme cases are only rarely encountered today. In many instances, death has been precipitated in these cases by dramatic external rupture. Alternatively, these aneurysms may erode into contiguous structures, and death may be caused by sudden rupture into the pericardial sac, pleural cavities, bronchi, trachea or esophagus.

Clinically, luetic aneurysms tend to occur in a somewhat younger age group than the arteriosclerotic, and are not infrequently discovered in persons 40 years of age or even younger. Males are affected about two to three times more often than females. Luetic aneurysms are much more prone to be associated with striking clinical manifestations than the arteriosclerotic abdominal aneurysm. Within the confined space of the thoracic cage, these enlargements give rise to signs and symptoms referable to: (1) encroachment upon the thoracic structures, (2) respiratory difficulties due to encroachment on the lungs and airway, (3) difficulty in swallowing due to compression of the esophagus, (4) persistent brassy cough due to irritation or pressure on the recurrent laryngeal nerves, (5) pain caused by erosion of bone—ribs and vertebral bodies, and (6) cardiac disease as the aneurysm leads to dilatation of the aortic valve or narrowing of the coronary ostia. Most patients with luetic aneurysms die of cardiac decompensation secondary to the cardiac involvement described. The next most common cause of death is fatal hemorrhage due to rupture into the mediastinum, pleural cavities, pericardium, respiratory passages, esophagus, or externally. Surgical replacement of the incompetent aortic valve or the aneurysmal dilatation now offers a new prognosis for these patients.

DISSECTING ANEURYSMS

The third and least common form of aortic aneurysm is the dissecting aneurysm. Most but not all instances occur in aortas previously weakened by idiopathic cystic medial necrosis (p. 612). These aneurysms differ from the luetic and atherosclerotic in that they are *not* usually associated with marked dilatation of the aorta, but instead are characterized by hemorrhagic cleavage of the laminar planes of the aortic media which dissects for variable distances, sometimes affecting the entire length of the aorta. Dissecting aneurysms most commonly occur in the 40 to 60 year age group, with a striking male predilection: about 6 to 1 (Layman and Wang, 1968) (Osmundson, 1971). Isolated cases have been reported in infants and in the extremely aged. As mentioned earlier, females appear to be particularly vulnerable during pregnancy. Hypertension is an almost invariable antecedent and may well play an important role in initiating the intramural hemorrhage.

It is most widely believed that rupture of vasa vasorum within the media initiates the hemorrhage (Burchell, 1955) (Hirst et al., 1958). It is postulated that foci of medionecrosis envelop the vasa vasorum. Since these vessels are extremely thin-walled, the loss of external support renders them highly vulnerable to rupture under the direct systolic thrust of the aortic blood pressure. From this origin, the blood dissects along the laminar planes of the aortic media proximally and distally. According to this concept, the intramural hemorrhage then commonly, but *not invariably,* ruptures through the inner layers of the media and intima to reenter the lumen of the aorta. These intimal ruptures usually occur proximally but may also take place distally. Hypertension, a common clinical finding in these patients, further favors the likelihood of intimal rupture.

On the other hand, certain writers favor the belief that *the weakened aortic wall undergoes abnormal dilatation with stretching and consequent tearing of the intima.* The blood then enters the media and dissects through long tracts of aorta and, in some instances, reruptures once again into the aortic lumen and produces a second intimal tear far removed from the proximal defect. Intimal tears in the ascending portion of the thoracic arch are found in about 90 per cent of dissecting aneurysms. Distal defects are found in a smaller number of these cases. However, approximately *5 per cent of dissecting aneurysms do not have an intimal tear,* and considerable weight is placed upon this observation to support the view that the hemorrhage is initiated by ruptured vasa vasorum.

The dissecting aneurysm is characterized anatomically by long hemorrhagic dissections within the media of the aorta. This hemorrhage occurs quite characteristically between the *middle and outer thirds* of the media (Fig. 15–25). While the aorta may be abnormally widened, the lumen is rarely the site of true aneurysmal dilatation, such as has been described in the luetic and arteriosclerotic aneurysms. The dissection usually begins in the

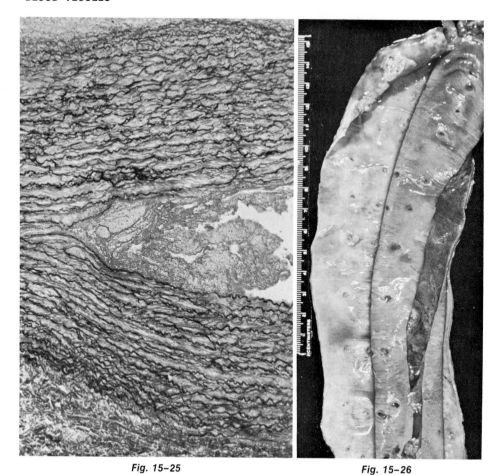

Fig. 15-25   **Fig. 15-26**

Figure 15-25. *Dissecting aneurysm of aorta. The advancing dissection is cleaving the laminar planes of the media.*

Figure 15-26. *Dissecting aneurysm of the aorta viewed from the adventitia. The adventitia and outer layer of the media have been folded back to demonstrate the cleavage.*

ascending portion of the arch and extends proximally toward the heart, as well as distally along the aorta (Fig. 15-26). The extent of the dissection is quite variable, but not infrequently the entire aorta is traversed, with extension into the iliac and femoral arteries.

Many times the dissection extends into the great vessels of the neck and, in other instances, into the coronary, renal, mesenteric and iliac arteries (Fig. 15-27). The extravasation may completely encircle the aorta or may extend along one circumscribed segment of the circumference. Infrequently the dissection is very short, and the extravasation almost directly penetrates the entire thickness of the aorta to cause immediate rupture. *The proximal intimal tears are usually found within 5 to 10 cm. of the aortic valve.* These tears are usually transverse or oblique, 4 to 5 cm. in length, and have sharp, clean but jagged margins (Fig. 15-28). Some are oriented in the long axis of the ves-

sel. The second tear, when found, is well removed from the initial defect, and usually is situated at the point of the farthest dissection of the hemorrhage. The amount of clotted or fluid blood found within the dissection is very variable. It may consist of only a thin layer that has simply cleaved the cystic media, apparently against little resistance or, on the other hand, may be considerably more massive to produce apparent, saccular, fusiform dilatations of the outer layers of media and adventitia. These large accumulations probably result from an initial dissection that meets with resistance to further extension and causes local ballooning of the weakened external layers. Eventually, *in almost all these dissections, external hemorrhage occurs into the periadventitial tissues or into surrounding structures or cavities.*

At postmortem examination, the most common precipitating cause of death is rupture of the dissection into any of the three body cavities, i.e., pericardial, pleural or peritoneal. Perhaps most often such rupture occurs by dissection back toward the heart with escape of blood into the pericardial sac. In certain instances, patients may survive for a period of days, weeks or even months, but usually death occurs within the first few days. Quite rarely, cases are discovered in which a new vascular channel has apparently been formed within the media of the aortic wall that connects the proximal and distal intimal tear. It is assumed that in these *double-barreled aortas*, the two intimal tears have permitted the establishment of a through-and-through blood flow and thus averted a fatal extra-aortic hemorrhage. In the course of time, such false channels may become endothelialized and, indeed, become involved by atherosclerosis. Infrequently, such favored and unusual patients die of completely unrelated causes.

DeBakey and his associates (1965) have divided these aneurysms into three groups on the basis of the extent of the dissection. Type I begins in the ascending aorta and extends distally for a distance. Type II includes those cases where the dissection is confined only to the ascending aorta. Type III comprises those instances where the dissection begins distal to the subclavian artery. The prognosis and clinical significance of these three types, as will be seen, differ significantly.

The clinical manifestations of a dissecting aneurysm derive from: (1) the dissection itself and (2) problems consequent to occlusion of the arteries arising from the aorta. The classic features related to the dissection are the sudden onset of excruciating pain, usually beginning in the anterior chest, radiating to the back and moving downward as the dissection progresses. The intensity of this pain is readily confused with that of acute myocardial infarction. Helpful in this differentiation is the fact that, although patients with acute dissection may appear to be in shock, they generally have normal or elevated systemic arterial pressures in counterdistinction to the hypotension usually associated with myocardial infarction. The localization of the pain is related to the site of initiation of the intra-aortic hematoma and thus differs among the three types described by DeBakey et al. (1965). It is often episodic and recurrent as bouts of advancing dissection occur. About 15 per cent of patients with acute aortic dissection have no pain in the chest, back or abdomen. These patients may present with the sudden onset of congestive heart failure associated with aortic valvular incompetence resulting from aneurysmal dilatation of the

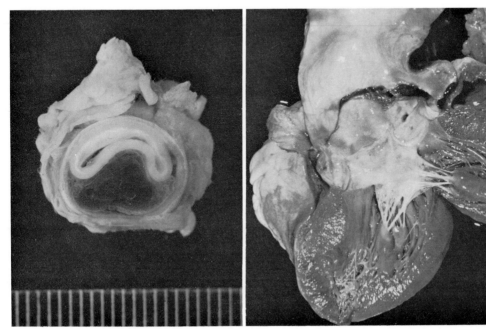

Fig. 15–27

Fig. 15–28

Figure 15–27. *A cross section of the common carotid with extension of a dissecting aneurysm and collapse of the vessel lumen.*

Figure 15–28. *The irregular jagged transverse tear in the intima in a dissecting aneurysm.*

aortic valve ring. Such a presentation is characteristic of type I. Sometimes a murmur is audible over the back and interscapular region, caused by the turbulence of the blood flow over the proximal intimal tear.

The involvement of the origins of the aortic branches produces a multitude of seemingly bizarre findings. Most striking is the development of inequality of the pulses and blood pressures between the right and left arms or between the arms and legs. Compression of the small vertebral branches may cause sensory and motor changes in the lower half of the body. Involvement of the renal arteries may produce findings referable to the kidneys, such as costovertebral angle pain, hematuria or even oliguria and complete anuria. Rarely, a myocardial infarction results from dissection into and about a coronary artery. Occasionally, small hemorrhagic leaks may cause manifestations of pericarditis or pleuritis (Hume and Porter, 1963). Death from a dissecting aneurysm is most often the result of rupture into the pericardial, pleural or peritoneal sacs, or sometimes into the retroperitoneal tissues.

The antemortem diagnosis of dissecting aneurysm and the differentiation of the three types are based largely on contrast medium aortography which usually shows enlargement of the aortic shadow, compression of the true lumen, filling of the false lumen and increased thickness of the aortic wall. With such contrast methods, it is usually possible to determine where the dissection begins and how far it extends. The prognosis for patients with dissecting aneurysms has markedly improved in the recent past. At one time, the disease was almost invariably fatal and, according to a review by Hirst et al. (1958), 3 per cent of the patients died immediately, 21 per cent within 24 hours, 60 per cent within two weeks and 90 per cent within three months. Two major advances in treatment have been achieved. DeBakey and his associates (1965) have reported an operative mortality rate of 21 per cent in a series of 179 patients. If the patients survived plication of the aortic wall, many had a long survival. More recently, however, acute aortic dissection has been treated by intensive antihypertensive medical therapy. With this regimen, about 10 per cent die within the first 24 hours, an additional 10 per cent within the first year and the total mortality at the end of three years is only 40 per cent (Palmer and Wheat, 1967) (Wheat et al., 1969). The type III dissections have a much better prognosis than type I. Patients with the type III lesion have a threefold better chance of survival than those with the type I.

While the three most important aneurysms have been described in detail, it

should be reiterated in conclusion that any of the vascular diseases cited in the previous chapter may produce aneurysmal dilatations in any vessel of the body, and all aneurysms wherever they may occur have the grave clinical potentials of causing compression, erosion and infarction of structures, as well as massive, sometimes fatal, hemorrhage.

VEINS

Although diseases of veins are extremely common clinical problems, only comparatively few entities are responsible for this high incidence. Varicose veins and phlebothrombosis together account for at least 90 per cent of clinical venous disease. In general, the diseases of veins are of clinical significance on two accounts. First, the majority of these disorders predispose to intravascular thrombosis and potential embolism, and since the systemic veins are most often affected, pulmonary embolism and infarction are the potential serious sequelae. Second, intravascular thrombosis, narrowing or abnormal dilatation of veins with subsequent incompetence of the venous valves all cause venous stasis. A fairly constant clinical pattern follows, with passive congestion of the affected area accompanied often by dusky cyanosis and edema. In many cases, venous drainage is restored by the opening of collateral bypasses. Often, however, the collateral channels create new clinical problems well exemplified by the production of varices in the esophagus when the portal vein is obstructed. The possibility of rupture of the esophageal varices is of far greater clinical importance than the underlying cause of the portal vein obstruction. On these two scores, diseases of veins take on great clinical significance.

VARICOSE VEINS

Varicose veins are abnormally dilated, tortuous veins produced by prolonged, increased intraluminal pressure. While any vein in the body may be affected, the superficial veins of the leg are the preponderant site of involvement. Two special types of varicosities are productive of important clinical problems. Portal hypertension (usually due to cirrhosis of the liver) leads to venous bypasses in the esophageal and hemorrhoidal veins. Varices may develop in these vessels.

Incidence. Varicose veins in the legs are common. It is estimated that 10 to 20 per cent of the general population eventually develop this disorder in the course of life. It is much more common in the age groups over 50, in which the incidence may reach a figure of 50 per cent of individuals. Over the age of 30, females are affected four times more commonly than males, a reflection of the venous stasis in the lower legs caused by pregnancy. In younger individuals there is no striking sex preponderance.

Pathogenesis. The many factors that predispose to the development of varicosities can be grouped into two categories: those that relate to the support of the vein wall, and those that relate to the production of increased venous pressures within the veins. Veins are frail structures which depend for their integrity upon a thin media and the support of surrounding structures. A familial tendency toward the development of varicosities is postulated to be due to heredoconstitutional defective development of the walls of veins. Obese persons have a greater tendency to develop varicosities, probably because of the poor tissue support offered by the large accumulations of subcutaneous fat. The increase in the incidence of varicose veins with age is at least in part attributable to the loss of tissue tone, atrophy of muscles and senile degenerative changes within the wall of the veins. Dilatation of veins has the additional important consequence of rendering the venous valves incompetent, thereby greatly increasing the head of pressure in the lengthy dependent veins of the lower extremities. The increase in luminal pressure leads to further dilatation and a vicious cycle.

The most important influence on intraluminal venous blood pressure is posture. When the legs are dependent for long periods of time, venous pressures in these sites are markedly elevated (the increase has been measured to be ten times the normal). Therefore occupations that require long periods of standing and long rides frequently lead to marked venous stasis and pedal edema, even in normal individuals with essentially normal veins (*simple orthostatic edema*). Any condition that compresses or obstructs veins may cause marked increases of venous pressure distally so that pregnancy, intravascular thrombosis, tumor masses that compress or narrow veins, encircling garters, and compressive circumferential surgical dressings or casts all promote the development of varicosities.

Varicose veins occur principally in the superficial veins of the body, especially those of the lower extremities. The superficial veins are peculiarly susceptible because of their relatively inadequate external support. The lower extremities are most commonly affected because, in the erect position, these vessels are subject to the greatest increases of pressure. Several deep plexuses are also frequently involved i.e., the esophageal and periesophageal veins, the hemorrhoidal veins, and the periovarian, periuterine and periprostatic plexuses. However, any vein may be affected if some local cause for venous obstruction exists. The affected veins are dilated, tortuous and elongated. The dilatation is asymmetrical and irregular, causing nodular swellings, fusiform enlargements and even aneurysmal distentions. Accompanying this asymmetrical dilatation, there is marked variation in the thickness of the wall with thinning at the points of maximal dilatation. When the disease is longstanding, however, compensatory hypertrophy of the medial muscle and fibrosis of the wall may produce a thick, opaque vessel wall.

Intraluminal thrombosis and valvular deformities (thickening, rolling and shortening of the cusps) are frequently discovered when these vessels are opened. These valvular changes contribute materially to venous stasis and further the development of varicosities and edema. Microscopically, the changes are quite minimal and consist of variation in the thickness of the wall of the vein caused by the dilatation on the one hand, and by hypertrophy of the smooth muscle and subintimal fibrosis on the other hand. Frequently, there is degeneration of the elastic tissue in the major veins and spotty calcifications within the media (**phlebosclerosis**). When thrombosis has occurred, additional alterations may be found which will be detailed in the consideration of **phlebothrombosis**.

Clinical Course. Varicose dilatation of veins renders the valves incompetent and leads to venous stasis, congestion, edema and thrombosis. In the usual site of involvement, namely, the legs, the distention of the veins is often painful, but most patients have no symptoms until marked venous stasis and edema develop. *Some of the most disabling sequelae are the development of persistent edema in the extremity and trophic changes in the skin which lead to stasis dermatitis and ulcerations* (Fig. 15–29). Because of the impaired circulation, the tissues of the affected part are extremely vulnerable to injury. Wounds and infections heal slowly or tend to become chronic *varicose ulcers*. Although varicose veins frequently thrombose, embolization to the lungs is *uncommon* from these superficial small vessels.

Varicosities in the internal plexuses, such as occur in the esophagus and anus in portal hypertension, are responsible for clinically significant disease which will be considered under the discussion of these organs.

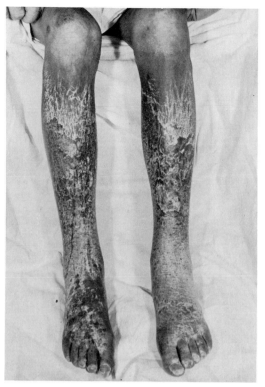

Figure 15–29. *Stasis dermatitis in varicose veins of the lower extremity.*

PHLEBOTHROMBOSIS AND THROMBOPHLEBITIS

According to current thought, phlebothrombosis and thrombophlebitis are two designations for a single entity. In the past, thrombophlebitis was conceived of as some mysterious primary phlebitis which, in turn, led to thrombosis. It was theorized that thrombophlebitis induced firmly attached intravascular thrombi which were less likely to embolize than the noninflammatory, hence less firmly attached, thrombi in phlebothrombosis. Considerable importance was attached, therefore, to the differentiation of thrombophlebitis from phlebothrombosis. However, faith in the reality of a primary phlebitis of unknown cause has slowly ebbed as more has been learned of the sequence of events which induce and then follow thrombosis (p. 330). Within a few hours after a vein develops a thrombus, an inflammatory reaction is seen within the wall, thus constituting a form of phlebitis, albeit usually not very severe. The entire conception of a mysterious primary thrombophlebitis has thus largely been discarded.

Secondary phlebitis and consequent thrombosis may, however, be caused by direct local injury to veins, either by bacterial invasion from a neighboring infection or by mechanical trauma, burns and other types of vascular injury. Such a sequence is, however, uncommon and can account for only a small fraction of venous thrombi.

The factors that predispose to venous thrombosis and the settings in which it is most often encountered have already been considered in the general discussion of thrombosis (p. 325). It need simply be reemphasized now that cardiac failure (particularly that associated with slowed venous return), neoplasia, pregnancy, the postoperative state and prolonged bed rest or immobilization are probably the five most important clinical settings predisposing to venous thrombosis. Phlebothrombosis is also commonly encountered in superficial varicose veins of the lower extremity. While such lesions are painful and sometimes somewhat disabling, they do not have the significance of the thromboses within the deep veins, as they rarely are the origin of emboli.

Some concept of the frequency with which the veins of the body develop thromboses can be gained from the analysis of 861 clinical cases at the Mayo Clinic (Barker et al., 1940, 1941).

Small saphenous veins and deep veins of the calf	486
Iliofemoral vein	254
Great saphenous veins	155
Superficial veins and varices of leg	14
Veins of arms	7
Other veins	23

It is clearly evident that the veins of the leg account for over 90 per cent of the cases, and that the lower leg is preponderantly affected. Specific mention should be made of the periprostatic plexus in the male and the pelvic veins in the female as additional moderately common sites for the appearance of thrombi. The large veins in the skull and the dural sinuses are possible sites of thrombosis when these channels become inflamed by bacterial infections of the meninges, middle ears or mastoids. Inflammatory diseases in these locations are in close physical and vascular continuity with the dural sinuses and provide ready pathways for the spread of infection. Similarly, infections in the abdominal cavity, such as peritonitis, acute appendicitis, acute salpingitis and pelvic abscesses, may lead to acute inflammation of the portal vein (pylephlebitis) or its tributaries.

Thrombosed veins usually appear distended when filled with fresh, red-blue or old, granular, gray-brown thrombi. Soon after the thrombosis develops, abacterial nonspecific inflammatory changes appear in the affected segment of vein. When the thrombus remains in situ for a few days, organization and recanalization occur. In only a few cases can a true bacterial thrombophlebitis be identified, usually when bacteremic seeding of the thrombus supervenes. Such a diagnosis requires demonstration of a bacterial basis for the inflammation.

Clinical Course.

These venous disorders tend, on the whole, to arise insidiously and to produce in the early stages few, if any, signs or symptoms. When symptoms do occur, they are referable either to the local venous stasis or to embolism from the dislodged thrombus. The local manifestations consist of edema distal to the occluded vein, dusky cyanosis and dilatation of superficial veins. Sometimes local heat, tenderness, redness, swelling and pain occur. However, even these signs may be absent, for when the patient is bedridden and the leg remains elevated, edema and congestion may be minimal or totally absent. Usually, however, in overt cases pain can be elicited by pressure over affected veins. In involvement of the lower extremities, squeezing the calf muscles or forced dorsiflexion of the foot evokes "Homans' sign" (p. 332). Because of the insidiousness of such vascular disease, it is necessary to examine vulnerable bedridden patients daily for the presence of Homans' sign or other indications of venous occlusion.

Not infrequently, the local process remains entirely silent and the first manifestation of the venous disorder is the development of an embolic episode. Indeed, pulmonary embolism is one of the most common clinical problems, particularly in hospitalized patients. Various series have indicated a gross incidence of pulmonary emboli in 6 to 8 per cent of hospital populations. Moreover, the embolism played a significant role in the cause of death in about 5 per cent of all autopsies, or in about two-thirds of the instances where it was found (Hume et al., 1970). It is of significance that clinical signs attributable to venous thrombosis of the lower extremities were present in only 10 to 20 per cent of this group.

The gravity of the possible consequence of phlebothrombosis strongly influences the management of all cardiac, postpartal and postoperative cases (p. 332). All such patients are urged to move about constantly in bed, perform muscle exercises to stimulate the venous flow in the legs and become ambulatory as soon as is clinically feasible. In particularly vulnerable individuals, such as those with varicose veins and in the older age groups, anticoagulant therapy may be administered when long-term bed rest is mandatory. Many surgeons even favor prophylactic ligation of the deep femoral or iliac veins in recognition of the potential hazard of venous thrombosis. It should be recognized, however, that while most venous thromboses occur in the legs, a small percentage arise in other sites such as have been mentioned, and therefore iliac or femoral ligation will not preclude, in all instances, the possibility of a serious pulmonary complication.

In addition to the problem of thromboembolism, bacterial infection of a thrombus is a source of bacteremia and septic emboli. In the dural sinuses, such intravascular infections may spread to cause meningitis or abscess formations in the contiguous regions of the brain. Phlebitis of the portal veins may seed the liver with bacteria and produce multiple liver abscesses.

PHLEGMASIA ALBA DOLENS AND MIGRATORY PHLEBITIS

There are two special variants of primary phlebothrombosis, both of obscure nature. One is known as phlegmasia alba dolens (milk leg) and the other as migratory phlebitis. *Phlegmasia alba dolens* (painful white leg) refers to iliofemoral venous thrombosis occurring usually in pregnant women in the third trimester or immediately following delivery. Because of its association with pregnancy, this condition has also been called "*milk leg.*" Classically, marked painful swelling of the lower extremity results, but experimental evidence suggests that venous stasis alone does not produce such severe edema. It is postulated that the thrombus initiates a secondary phlebitis and the perivenous inflammatory response induces lymphatic blockage as well (Haller and Mays, 1963). The predisposition to thrombosis here is attributed to the stasis of flow caused by the pressure of the gravid uterus and to the development of a hypercoagulable state during pregnancy. An increase in both the number and adhesiveness of platelets, accompanied by an increase of fibrinogen and factors VIII and VI, as well as some inhibition of the normal fibrinolytic mechanisms, has been documented in pregnant women (Shaper et al., 1968).

Migratory thrombophlebitis is the term given to the appearance of venous thrombi, often multiple, which classically disappear at one site only to reappear elsewhere. This curious disorder is usually encountered in patients having a deep-seated visceral cancer. This association was brought to the attention of the medical world by Trousseau, who ironically developed migratory phlebitis himself as the first manifestation of his fatal pancreatic cancer. With considerable justice, then, migratory thrombophlebitis in patients having cancer is referred to as *Trousseau's sign*. Although pancreatic cancer appears to more regularly induce this venous disorder, it may also be encountered with cancer of any other viscus in the body, for example, in the lung, stomach, colon or kidney. The basis of this predisposition to thrombosis is somewhat uncertain, but has been attributed to released necrotic products of the tumor which have thromboplastic properties. It is undoubtedly also predisposed to by a number of additional influences including confinement to bed, surgical interventions, the usually advanced age of the patient, and by other hypercoagulable alterations encountered in these mortally ill individuals (Sise et al., 1962).

PHLEBOSCLEROSIS

Phlebosclerosis refers to a not very significant primary thickening and hardening of the walls of veins. The inferior vena cava and the iliac, popliteal and portal veins are the prime sites of involvement. This condition is somewhat analogous to atherosclerosis of the arteries. It consists essentially of fibrous intimal proliferation and hypertrophy of the medial musculature. Frequently calcium and lipids are deposited in the areas of fibrosis with obliteration of the underlying architecture of the wall of the vein. As a consequence, the veins are thickened and contracted and have a ropy consistency on external palpation. When the condition is far advanced, the lumina may be narrowed and obstructive venopathy may result.

OBSTRUCTION OF SUPERIOR VENA CAVA (SUPERIOR VENA CAVAL SYNDROME)

Although obstruction of the superior vena cava is an uncommon condition, it is of such clinical importance when present that it merits separate consideration. The vena cava is usually obstructed by neoplasms which compress or invade the vein. The most common tumors that do this are primary bronchogenic carcinoma and primary tumors of lymph nodes, lymphomas, arising in the mediastinal lymphoid tissue. There are other less common causes for vena caval obstruction, such as aortic aneurysms, carcinoma of the esophagus, or any type of metastasis appropriately located close to the superior vena cava.

The venous obstruction produces a fairly distinctive symptom complex, referred to as the superior vena caval syndrome. It is manifested by marked dilatation of the veins of the head and neck with dusky cyanosis of the head, neck and arms. In the course of time, dilated, subcutaneous, collateral patterns become evident in the upper portion of the body. Because commonly the pulmonary vessels are also compressed along with the superior vena cava, severe respiratory distress may develop. The superior vena caval syndrome requires active treatment to prevent its progression.

OBSTRUCTION OF INFERIOR VENA CAVA (INFERIOR VENA CAVAL SYNDROME)

Obstruction to the inferior vena cava may be caused by the same processes that affect the superior vena cava. The two most common mechanisms that lead to inferior vena caval obstruction are propagation of a clot upward from the femoral and iliac veins and neoplasms. The neoplasms may cause external compression of the inferior vena cava, may permeate the walls from without, such as occurs with lymphomatous involvement of the para-aortic nodes, or may directly extend into the inferior vena cava by progressive advancing growth within one of the caval tributaries. This last circumstance is particularly well exemplified by the renal cell carcinoma, which has a striking tendency to invade the renal vein and extend in continuity up the renal vein into the inferior vena cava, often inducing total thrombotic occlusion of this vessel. Less common causes of caval obstruction are external pressure of aneurysms of the abdominal aorta, inflammatory reactions in and around the inferior vena cava and extension of a hepatic vein thrombosis into the inferior vena cava.

As would be anticipated, obstruction to the inferior vena cava induces marked edema of the legs, distention of the superficial veins of the lower abdomen that serve as bypasses and, when the thrombus extends up to the renal veins, a nephrotic-like syndrome which resembles that produced by renal vein thrombosis.

OBSTRUCTION OF HEPATIC VEIN (BUDD-CHIARI SYNDROME)

When obstruction to the hepatic vein produces symptoms, it is known as the Budd-Chiari syndrome. Occlusion of the hepatic vein in two-thirds of cases occurs apparently spontaneously without obvious cause. An endophlebitis is proposed but is often difficult to document. The remaining one-third of the patients have a great variety of apparent causes such as polycythemia vera and neoplasms that extend up the inferior vena cava into the drainage junction of the hepatic vein. Cancers within the liver may directly permeate the hepatic veins to cause obstruction. An additional important pathogenetic mechanism for hepatic vein obstruction is cirrhosis of the liver with or without superimposed carcinoma of the liver. Rare causes are abscesses or parasitic disease within the liver, mediastinal tumors that narrow the inferior vena cava, and inflammatory processes in the subdiaphragmatic region that affect the venous outflow of the liver.

The resultant venous obstruction may arise either acutely or subacutely. In the former instance, the patient has the manifestations of an apparent acute abdomen accompanied by rapid enlargement of the liver and ascites. When the thrombosis occurs more slowly, hepatomegaly, ascites and jaundice appear insidiously. Further details on this derangement are available on page 999).

LYMPHATICS

Because of their widespread distribution and important role as drainage channels, involvement of the lymphatics is almost inevitable in all inflammations and whenever tumors metastasize through these vessels. In the majority of these instances, the lymphatic lesions are so small and focal as to have no significance. However, in some instances these secondary lesions represent serious complications that sometimes overshadow the primary disease. These important secondary processes and a few rare lymphatic disorders are presented here.

SECONDARY LYMPHATIC DISORDERS

LYMPHANGITIS

Bacterial infections may spread into and through the lymphatics to create acute inflammatory involvements in these channels. The most common etiologic agents are the group A beta hemolytic streptococci, although any virulent pathogen may be responsible for an acute lymphangitis. Anatomically, the affected lymphatics are dilated and filled with an acute leukocytic exudate, chiefly neutrophils and histiocytes. The inflammation usually extends through the wall into the perilymphatic tissues. Sometimes the surrounding reaction is so extensive as to convert the process into a cellulitis or into multiple focal abscesses. The lymph nodes of drainage are almost inevitably in-

volved, with changes characteristic of acute lymphadenitis.

Clinically, lymphangitis is recognized by painful subcutaneous red streaks that extend along the course of lymphatics with painful enlargement of the regional lymph nodes. If the lymph nodes fail to block the spread of the bacteria, the infective material may eventually drain into the venous system and initiate a bacteremia or septicemia. In rare instances, these inflammatory processes may persist for days or weeks and become transformed into chronic lymphangitis with eventual thrombosis of the lymphatics and fibrous replacement of the entire structure.

SECONDARY LYMPHEDEMA

Any occlusion of lymphatic vessels is followed by the abnormal accumulation of interstitial fluid in the affected part, referred to as *lymphedema*. The commonest causes of such lymphatic blockage are (1) spread of malignant tumors with obstruction of either the lymphatic channels or the nodes of drainage; (2) radical surgical procedures with removal of regional groups of lymph nodes, for example, the axillary dissection of radical mastectomy; (3) postradiation fibrosis; (4) filariasis; and (5) postinflammatory thrombosis and scarring of lymphatic channels. The morphologic changes within the lymphatics consist of dilatation proximal to the points of obstruction, accompanied by increases of interstitial fluid. Persistence of the edema leads to an increase of interstitial fibrous tissue, most evident subcutaneously. Enlargement of the affected part, "peau d'orange" appearance of the skin, skin ulcers and brawny induration are sequelae to such lymphedema.

PRIMARY LYMPHATIC DISORDERS

LYMPHEDEMA PRAECOX

Lymphedema praecox is an extremely uncommon condition affecting chiefly females between the ages of 10 and 25, characterized by the progressive onset of edema in one or both feet. In the usual case, the edema begins around the age of puberty. The edema may remain localized to the feet or ankles or, with increasing severity of the condition, progress up the extremity into the lower trunk or other regions of the body. The edema is unremitting and slowly accumulates throughout life. The progressive enlargement of the extremity causes disability but rarely additional complications. The etiology is entirely obscure. Anatomically, such patients have only moderate dilatation of the subcutaneous lymphatic channels and increased interstitial fluid, replaced in longstanding cases by fibrosis. The involved extremity may increase to many times its normal size, and the skin may become thickened and resemble orange peel. In some cases, ulcerations develop in the affected skin areas.

MILROY'S DISEASE (HEREDOFAMILIAL CONGENITAL LYMPHEDEMA)

The term Milroy's disease should be limited to those cases of lymphedema which are present from birth and appear in sufficiently large numbers of blood relatives to indicate a mendelian hereditary trait. The condition is presumed to be caused by faulty development of lymphatic channels, possibly with poor structural strength, permitting abnormal dilatation and incompetence of the lymphatic valves. The stasis of lymph accounts for the progressive accumulation of increased amounts of interstitial fluid and edema. In classic Milroy's disease, the lower extremities are the major site of involvement and frequently the only site.

When other areas of the trunk or face are involved, there is considerable controversy whether the term Milroy's disease should be extended to include these variants. Cases are on record, however, in which other regions have been affected from birth, and these presumably belong in the heredofamilial category. Sometimes these cases have bizarre distributions of the edema with involvement of only one area of the anterior abdominal wall, or one or both of the orbital regions, without evidence of disease in the lower extremities. The external genitalia and the upper extremities are additional uncommon sites of localization. The anatomic changes in all these variants of Milroy's disease are identical with those described in lymphedema praecox. Because the disease persists from infancy, replacement fibrosis occurs in the edematous regions, causing permanent enlargement and deformity of the affected parts. The fibroedematous skin areas are very susceptible to trauma, infections and ulcerations.

SIMPLE CONGENITAL LYMPHEDEMA

This disorder is distinguished from Milroy's disease by the fact that it affects only one member of the family, but it is present from birth. The anatomic distribution, histologic findings and clinical significance are identical.

TUMORS

Neoplasms of blood vessels and of lymphatic channels can be described together because, in both instances, the histogenetic origin of these tumors is the endothelial lining cell. These tumors present many complexities, both in classification and significance. The following discussion will present the theoretical considerations for this complexity and a relatively simplified classification that provides reasonably clear-cut distinctions between the lesions in each category.

Most of the confusion with respect to tumors of vessels centers on two points: (1) Are small vascular lesions, so commonly found in infants at birth, true tumors or merely anomalous hamartomas? (2) How does one differentiate tumorous vascular proliferation from non-neoplastic vasoproliferations such as are encountered in inflammatory states and in association with other types of tumors? First, with respect to *the hamartomatous nature of certain benign vascular lesions*, 70 per cent of benign, focal, well differentiated vascular lesions, so-called angiomas and lymphangiomas, are present from birth. These grow slowly and perhaps only commensurately with the growth of the infant and child. There is, then, considerable question whether they are true neoplasms, or merely congenital anomalies not having the significance of new growths. In either event, it will be shown that the lesions are generally of little clinical significance, and their true nature is largely of academic interest.

The *differentiation of vascular neoplasms from vasoproliferative lesions* is sometimes very difficult. Granulation tissue, it will be remembered, consists in part of actively budding, growing capillaries. Such granulation tissue may appear as a mass of blood vessels having an active fibroblastic stroma. In the same way, in any type of malignancy, the nutrient blood supply proliferates along with the parenchymal, neoplastic cells. Sometimes this vascularization is so abundant that it may appear to represent a part of the true neoplasm rather than merely a supporting element. No clear definition between these vasoformative processes and true vascular neoplasms can be outlined. *If the blood vessel proliferation is accompanied by a significant inflammatory reaction and by ulceration of the overlying skin,* it would at least suggest that the vasoformation is inflammatory rather than neoplastic. By contrast, many vascular neoplasms grow beneath an intact epithelium free of inflammatory change. Careful evaluation of the regularity of the endothelial cells and the vascular sinusoids may also provide a clue to whether the lesions are due to controlled growth of mature, well formed blood vessels or are uncontrolled neoplastic proliferations with presumably more cellular and vascular atypicality.

Vascular neoplasms are divided into benign and malignant on the basis of two major anatomic characteristics: the degree to which the neoplasm is composed of well formed vascular channels, and the abundance and regularity of the endothelial cell proliferation. In general, benign neoplasms are made up largely of well formed vascular channels with a very insignificant amount of regular endothelial cell proliferation, while on the opposite end of the spectrum, the frankly malignant tumors are largely solidly cellular and anaplastic and reproduce scant numbers of only abortive vascular channels (Geschickter, 1935).

TELANGIECTASIS

The term telangiectasis designates a group of abnormally prominent capillaries, venules and arterioles that create small focal red lesions, usually in the skin and mucous membranes of the body. These dilatations probably represent congenital anomalies or acquired exaggerations of preexisting vessels, and are therefore not true neoplasms. They are included, however, under the category of tumors since they appear as small tumor-like masses that require differentiation from true neoplasms. There are two special types of telangiectasia.

SPIDER TELANGIECTASIA

The spider telangiectasis consists of a focal minute network of subcutaneous small arteries or arterioles arranged in a radial fashion about a central core. They are usually found on the upper parts of the body, particularly the face, neck and upper chest, and are most common in pregnant women or in patients with liver disease, particularly cirrhosis of the liver. It is believed that the hyperestrinism found in these two conditions in some way evokes these vascular changes. Grossly, the lesions are minute areas of redness, 2 to 5 mm. in diameter, which on close inspection have the spider-like radiations described. Histologically, only abnormally dilated vessels are found. Because these are composed of arterial vessels, they frequently pulsate, a useful diagnostic feature. They are chiefly of significance as an aid to the diagnosis of an underlying cirrhosis of the liver.

HEREDITARY HEMORRHAGIC TELANGIECTASIA (OSLER-WEBER-RENDU DISEASE).

This entity is characterized by multiple small aneurysmal telangiectases distributed over the skin and mucous membranes of the body, present from birth and apparently of hereditary origin. It is an extremely uncommon disorder, transmitted as a *dominant mendelian trait by either the male or the female, and affects both sexes equally.*

Grossly, the lesions are found directly beneath the skin in any region of the body or directly beneath the mucosal surfaces of the oral cavity, lips, alimentary tract, respiratory tract and urinary tract, as well as in the liver, brain and spleen. The individual lesions are usually small, less than 5 mm. in diameter, but coalescent lesions may produce red-blue masses up to several centimeters in diameter. Microscopically, the lesions consist of thin-walled, dilated capillary and venular channels, usually filled with fluid blood. The walls of these channels are composed of only a single layer of endothelial cells based upon a delicate connective tissue. In one plane of section, the numerous branching vessels produce a honeycombed mass sharply delimited but not encapsulated from the surrounding tissue.

Clinically, Osler-Weber-Rendu disease is principally characterized by hemorrhages that arise from the rupture of the many superficially located lesions. Nosebleeds and bleeding into the intestinal, urinary or respiratory tract are common clinical manifestations. This hemorrhagic tendency appears to become more pronounced with increasing age, and most patients require medical attention only in middle to late adult life. The diagnosis should be suspected when widely scattered telangiectases are found on the skin or mucous membrane of the lips and oral cavity. Usually these hemorrhages are readily controlled, and patients with this condition have a normal life expectancy. Occasionally massive bleeding may prove fatal.

STURGE-WEBER DISEASE (ENCEPHALOTRIGEMINAL ANGIOMATOSIS)

This is an extremely uncommon congenital disorder attributed to faulty development of certain mesodermal and ectodermal elements. It is characterized by venous angiomatous masses in the leptomeninges over the cortex and by ipsilateral port-wine nevi of the face (p. 1409) and is often associated with mental retardation and radiopacities in the skull. Here again, in this condition one finds developmental defects in the blood vessels associated with much more serious developmental defects in internal organs, in this instance, the central nervous system. The importance of this entity lies, then, in the recognition that a large vascular malformation in the face may well be more than a coincidence in a child who exhibits some evidence of mental deficiency (Peterman et al., 1958).

ANGIOMA

Angiomas are benign lesions of either blood vessel *(hemangioma)* or lymphatic *(lymphangioma)* origin that faithfully create well formed vascular channels. Usually present from birth, they may represent congenital hamartomas or benign neoplasms arising in a congenital defect. Although they are present in the newborn, at this early stage they may be so small as to be inapparent. On this basis, most investigators consider these lesions as hamartomas that grow along with bodily development. However, there is no certainty that these lesions cannot arise spontaneously as true neoplasms in children or adults. With growth, these masses become grossly visible and may reach several centimeters in diameter or become even larger. In many instances, they cease to enlarge at maturity and enter a period of apparent dormancy. Careful studies have disclosed that the vascular lumina of these lesions are connected with the surrounding blood vessels or lymphatics through a solitary afferent and efferent channel. This interesting observation helps to explain why spontaneous or induced thrombosis of the vascular connections may lead to thrombosis of the entire lesion with consequent organization and apparent obliteration of the tumor. Several variants of angiomas are distinguished.

HEMANGIOMA

Capillary Hemangioma. Capillary hemangiomas are so designated because *they are composed of blood vessels that, for the most part, conform to the caliber of normal capillaries.* Although any organ or tissue may be involved, they usually occur in the skin, subcutaneous tissues, and the mucous membranes of the oral cavity and lips. They may also occur in internal viscera, such as the liver, spleen and kidneys. They are, for the most part, small lesions which vary from a few millimeters up to several centimeters in diameter. Characteristically, they are bright red to blue and on a level with the surface of the skin or slightly elevated. Occasionally, pedunculated lesions are formed attached by a broad to slender stalk (Fig. 15–30). The covering epithelium is usually intact, but in exposed positions, traumatic ulceration of the overlying epithelium may create a weeping, oozing lesion that bleeds on slightest trauma. Uncommonly, capillary hemangiomas may take the form of large, flat,

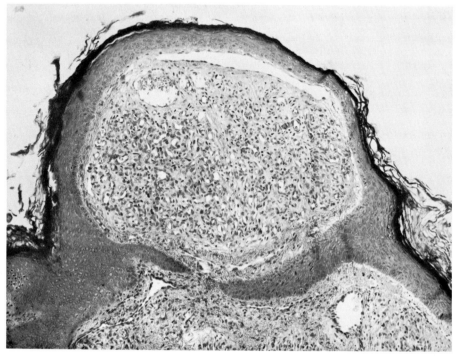

Figure 15–30. *Capillary hemangioma of the skin.*

map-like, red-blue discolorations that cover large areas of the face or upper parts of the body referred to in this pattern as *"port-wine stains"* or inappropriately as "port-wine nevi."

On section, the red-blue lesions are usually *well defined but unencapsulated.* Small, finger-like projections may extend into surrounding tissue spaces and planes of cleavage. This form of growth may create the appearance of invasiveness, but clinical experience has shown that this pattern of growth is produced by extension along planes of least resistance rather than malignant aggressiveness. Frequently, many channels are thrombosed and areas may have undergone fibrous organization. Histologically, the lesions are sharply circumscribed from the surrounding tissue, but are not encapsulated. They are made up of closely packed aggregations of thin-walled capillaries, separated by scant connective tissue stroma. The channels are lined by normal endothelial cells and are usually filled with fluid blood. Many times, the lumina are partially or completely thrombosed and organized. Rupture of vessels causes further scarring and also accounts for the hemosiderin pigment found in occasional instances.

Clinically, these lesions are probably hamartomatous developmental defects and are of little significance except insofar as they require differentiation from more important neoplasms. These lesions may ulcerate and become secondarily infected, bleed or cause cosmetic defects. Transformation into malignant tumors, if it occurs at all, is extremely rare.

Cavernous Hemangioma. Cavernous hemangiomas are distinguished by the formation of *large, cavernous, vascular channels.* Frequently, numerous small, capillary-like lumina are dispersed among the cavernous channels, and there is in reality no sharp line of distinction between the capillary and cavernous forms. The term cavernous hemangioma should be reserved for those lesions which are preponderantly composed of vascular channels considerably larger than those of capillary size. These hemangiomas often occur on the skin and mucosal surfaces of the body, but are also found in many viscera, particularly the liver, spleen, pancreas, and occasionally in the brain. In one rare entity, *Lindau-von Hippel disease,* cavernous hemangiomas occur within the cerebellum or brain stem and eye grounds, along with similar angiomatous lesions or cystic neoplasms in the pancreas and liver.

Grossly, the usual cavernous hemangioma is a red-blue, soft, spongy mass 1 to 2 cm. in diameter. On section, the lesions are sharply defined and compressible and exude blood. Quite rarely, giant forms occur that affect large subcutaneous areas of the face, extremities or other regions of the body. Histologically, the mass is sharply defined, but not encapsulated, and made up of large, cavernous, vascular spaces, partly or completely filled with fluid blood separated by a scant connective tissue stroma (Fig. 15–31). Intravascular thrombosis or rupture of channels may modify the histologic appearance.

In most situations, the tumors or hamartomas are of little clinical significance although, when present in the brain, they are potential sources of increased intracranial pressure or hemorrhage. Malignant transformation of the cavernous hemangioma is an extremely rare occurrence.

Sclerosing Hemangioma (Dermatofibroma, Histiocytoma). Sclerosing hemangiomas are believed by some to be capillary hemangiomas that become transformed from a highly vascularized lesion to a solidly cellular tumor by the progressive proliferation of endothelial cells and connective tissue stroma. This histologic transformation is presumed to occur over the course of many years and, therefore, while these lesions are believed to arise at birth, the sclerosing pattern does not become well defined until young to middle adult life. Others deny the vascular

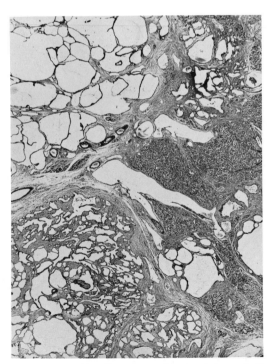

Figure 15–31. *Cavernous hemangioma of the liver.*

origin of these lesions and refer to them as *dermatofibromas* or *histiocytomas*. The lesions have the same distribution as the capillary hemangiomas and are usually the same size. With the cellular proliferation, the vascular channels are compressed or obliterated, and the tumor loses its red-blue color and becomes pale gray to yellow-tan. They most often lie within the dermal and subcutaneous fibrous tissue, but sometimes are slightly elevated or even pedunculated. Nonetheless, they are totally covered by epithelium. On section, they are solid, somewhat poorly delimited lesions that usually contain bright yellow areas due to the accumulation of lipids.

The histologic pattern on first impression is that of a cellular tumor composed of tightly whorled and interlacing bundles of spindle cells (Fig. 15–32). Vascular channels may be inapparent until close inspection discloses that the central cores of the tight concentric whorls contain almost totally obliterated vascular channels. *The identification of these partly obliterated lumina is requisite for the diagnosis.* In some areas, the tumors may be quite collagenous, while in other areas old hemorrhage, hemosiderin pigment and large foreign body type giant cells may be present. One of the distinctive features of the sclerosing hemangioma is scattered or nested macrophages that have a foamy, granular cytoplasm (lipophages). Presumably, these cells have imbibed lipid debris derived from the breakdown of blood. While the margins of this lesion are usually distinct from the surrounding tissue, *no true encapsulation exists* and pseudopod-like extensions may project into adjacent tissue spaces and cleavage planes. Usually there is no significant variability in nuclear or cell size or shape, and there is no significant mitotic activity.

The sclerosing hemangioma is a relatively insignificant lesion that is chiefly of interest because its firm consistency arouses the suspicion that it may represent some more serious type of new growth. Second, as projecting lesions they may become ulcerated or infected, or bleed.

LYMPHANGIOMA

Lymphangiomas are the analogues in the lymphatic system of the hemangiomas of blood vessels. These tumors are also believed to arise as congenital rests or hamartomas and, as such, are present at birth, but may be so small as to be missed. Growth occurs along with the development of the infant and produces lesions that become macroscopically visible. Both sexes are affected equally.

Simple (Capillary) Lymphangioma. These masses are composed of small lymphatic channels. They tend to occur subcutaneously in the head and neck region, as well as in the axilla. Rarely, they are found in the trunk, within internal organs or in the connective tissue in and about the abdominal or thoracic cavities.

On body surfaces, they are slightly elevated or sometimes pedunculated lesions, 1 to 2 cm. in diameter. They may occur as flat, subcutaneous or submucosal masses. In internal structures, they are sharply circumscribed, compressible, gray to pink lesions. Histologically, they are composed of a network of endothelium-lined lymph spaces that can *be differentiated from capillary channels only by the absence of blood cells.* Sometimes the lining cells hypertrophy and become cuboidal, and take on the appearance of glandular epithelium. A scant fibrous tissue stroma, which occasionally contains aggregates of lymphocytes or small lymphoid nests, separates the small channels. In addition, fat or muscle cells or hemangiomatous portions may be present (hemangiolymphangioma). It must be assumed that these extraneous components are trapped elements or are indicative of a mixed origin. These tumors are completely benign clinically and usually of little significance. They thus represent the lymphatic analogue of capillary hemangiomas.

Small lesions raise the problem of the differentiation of true lymphangiomas from abnormal dilatations of lymphatics (*lymphangiectasis*), a differentiation that is largely of academic interest alone.

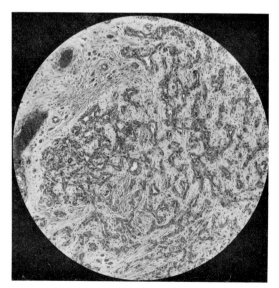

Figure 15–32. *Sclerosing capillary hemangioma with considerable fibrous ingrowth.*

Cavernous Lymphangioma (Cystic Hygroma).

These benign lymphatic tumors are composed of cavernous lymphatic spaces and, therefore, are analogous to the cavernous hemangioma. They almost invariably occur in the neck or axilla and only occasionally retroperitoneally. Unlike the cavernous hemangioma, they are not necessarily limited to small lesions, but occasionally achieve considerable size, up to 15 cm. in diameter. Such large masses may fill the axilla or produce gross deformities in and about the neck. With the progressive dilatation of the lymphatic spaces, these tumors develop considerable expansile pressure and thus dissect along cleavage planes and simulate aggressive invasive growth. On section, they reveal a soft, compressible, sponge-like, red-pink tissue that freely exudes a watery fluid to reveal the underlying loose-textured pattern of the mass. On histologic examination, the tumors are made up of hugely dilated cystic spaces lined by endothelial cells and separated by a scant intervening connective tissue stroma. The stroma may harbor aggregates of lymphocytes, lymphatic tissue, and occasional islands of fat or muscle. The margins of the tumor are not discrete and these lesions are not encapsulated. The finger-like projections described in the gross may extend in and around contiguous normal structures. This growth potential creates a problem in their removal, and when bits of tumor are left in surgical resections, recurrence may be expected. Because of their large size, they may not only disfigure, but compress adjacent structures, such as blood vessels and even the trachea and esophagus. Malignant transformation rarely occurs.

GLOMANGIOMA

A glomangioma is usually a small, red-blue, benign tumor which arises from the cells of a glomus body. These lesions can be almost positively identified by their extreme painfulness. The normal glomus is a neuromyoarterial receptor which is sensitive to variations in temperature and regulates arteriolar flow. The glomus has an afferent artery, arteriovenous anastomosis and efferent veins. Surrounding the anastomosis, there is a collection of apparently specialized endothelial cells which differ from the usual type in that they are fairly plump, round to polygonal, and resemble epithelial cells. Sometimes these glomus cells are elongated and resemble smooth muscle cells. The nuclei of these cells are usually round and deeply chromatic, and vary little in their size and shape. Glomus bodies may be located anywhere in the skin, but are most com-

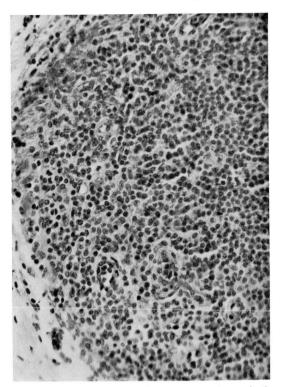

Figure 15–33. A medium power view of the margin of a glomus tumor, showing the great regularity of the glomus cells surrounding and obscuring the numerous small blood vessels.

monly found in the distal portion of the fingers and toes, especially under the nails. The glomangiomas follow this pattern of distribution.

Grossly, the lesions are usually under 1 cm. in diameter and many are *less* than 3 mm. in diameter. Tumors productive of significant pain have been described smaller than the head of a pin. When present in the skin, they are slightly elevated, rounded, red-blue, firm, exquisitely painful nodules. Under the nail, they appear as minute foci of fresh hemorrhage. Histologically, *two components are present: branching vascular channels* separated by a connective tissue stroma which contains the second element, *aggregates, nests and masses of the specialized glomus cells,* probably derived from pericytes. The individual cells are usually quite regular in size, with well defined cell membranes separating their scant cytoplasm. These neoplastic cells resemble, in all respects, normal glomus cells (Fig. 15–33). These cells may lie clustered around the vascular channels, but in other areas they are distributed through the fibrous stroma (Bailey, 1935). There is no definite encapsulation. Clinically, these tumors are readily recognized by the combination of their distinct color and their exquisite painfulness.

The slightest manipulation may trigger off severe paroxysms of pain, and even the preparatory motions of palpating the lesions evoke such attacks. Excision produces prompt relief.

HEMANGIOPERICYTOMA

A rare vascular tumor of relatively new delineation merits brief description—the hemangiopericytoma. This neoplasm may occur wherever there are capillaries, but most have been found in the superficial soft tissues (Stout, 1949). Most are small, but rarely they achieve a diameter of 8 cm. At first glance, they resemble the hemangioendothelioma with numerous capillary channels surrounded and enclosed within nests and masses of rounded endothelial cells. However, a hard look discloses that the endothelial cells are somewhat organoid and resemble the cells in the glomangioma. This has led to the discovery that these peculiar cells are in fact of pericyte origin. When silver impregnations are performed, it can be confirmed that these organoid cells are outside the basement membrane of the capillary and hence are not endothelial cells but rather pericytes.

These tumors at one time were thought to be always benign, but recent series disclose that as many as 50 per cent metastasize to lungs, bones and liver. Regional nodes are sometimes affected. It has become clear that these neoplasms are deceptively benign-appearing but, in fact, they are biologically aggressive (O'Brien and Brasfield, 1960). They must therefore be differentiated from the glomus tumor in which paroxysmal pain produces spectacular symptoms but benign behavior is characteristic.

CAROTID BODY TUMOR

A widespread misconception persists that carotid body tumors are chromaffin neoplasms similar to the pheochromocytoma of the adrenal medulla (p. 1316). It should be emphasized that the normal carotid body is a nonchromaffin, nonepinephrine-secreting structure, which functions as a chemoreceptor. There is abundant evidence that the carotid body is sensitive to changes in the pH, carbon dioxide and oxygen tensions of the circulating blood, and may be of major importance in the control of respiration. Tumors of this organ are also sometimes referred to as paragangliomas, a designation that only adds to the confusion, since the embryology of the carotid body is still open to dispute. These tumors are small, well encapsulated lesions, rarely over 5 cm. in diameter, that are intimately adherent to the bifurca-

tion of the common carotid artery. The attachment is sometimes so intense that it is impossible to establish a plane of cleavage between the vessel and the tumor. The cut surface is usually gray-red but is often discolored by hemorrhage, old blood or hemosiderin pigmentation.

Histologically, the characteristic pattern is that of nests or small aggregates of the epithelioid cells that comprise the normal carotid body. These nests are separated by a vascular stroma. Occasionally, the cells are much more spindled and resemble endothelial cells; at other times, the cells have an abundant pink, granular cytoplasm and are indistinguishable from epithelial cells. Similar tumors are sometimes found in the aortic body and in the glomus jugulare. Occasionally, multiple discrete tumors appear simultaneously in any of the structures providing origin for these neoplasms. Although a few cases have been recorded as malignant with metastases, these are open to some question and, on the whole, these neoplasms may be considered as almost invariably benign.

In spite of their location, studies indicate that these tumors probably do not produce a "carotid sinus syndrome" any more frequently than is encountered in patients without neoplasms. For the most part, these lesions are called to clinical attention because of a palpable mass or because of an increasing awareness on the part of the patient of the transmitted arterial pulse.

HEMANGIOENDOTHELIOMA

A hemangioendothelioma is a true neoplasm of vascular origin composed predominantly of masses of endothelial cells growing in and about vascular channels. In the progressive spectrum of vascular tumors, the *hemangioendothelioma represents an intergrade between the well differentiated hemangiomas and the frankly anaplastic, totally cellular hemangioendotheliosarcomas.* Certain writers use the term hemangioendothelioma to refer to a malignant endothelial tumor. This usage is confusing and inappropriate, since the malignant counterpart should properly be referred to as a sarcoma. The hemangioendothelioma follows the pattern of distribution of the hemangiomas and is most frequently encountered in the skin, but may affect viscera, particularly the spleen and liver.

Grossly, the tumor has the appearance of a well demarcated, pale gray to gray-red, firm mass which varies in size usually up to 4 to 5 cm., but is sometimes larger. Histologically, vascular channels are evident, but the domi-

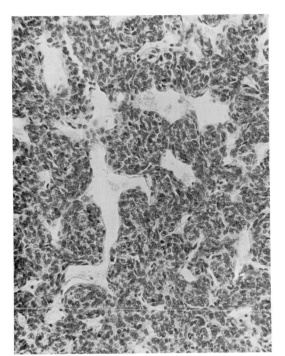

Figure 15–34. *Hemangioendothelioma. The increased cellularity differentiates this lesion from the cavernous hemangioma.*

nant feature consists of masses and sheets of typical spindled endothelial cells, which may grow in whorls or undifferentiated sheets. There is little evidence of variability in nuclear or cell size. Occasionally, plump, somewhat larger cells are encountered, producing a slight pleomorphism to the cell pattern. Mitotic figures, if present, are of the normal variety and scant in number. The margins of these tumors are clearly defined but unencapsulated. Frank anaplasia is not present within the present usage of the term hemangioendothelioma (Fig. 15–34).

Clinically, the tumor is of chief importance in its differentiation from other more ominous growths. Although these lesions are benign and are cured by local removal, malignant behavior occurs in a small percentage of cases, possibly because of difficulty in differentiating these tumors from endotheliosarcomas. These lesions sometimes present considerable difficulty in classification and, to this particular tumor, Ewing's statement may well be applied: "Tumors are not always benign or malignant."

HEMANGIOENDOTHELIOSARCOMA (ANGIOSARCOMA)

As the name indicates, this tumor is a malignant neoplasm of vascular origin, charac-terized by masses of endothelial cells displaying the cellular atypicality and anaplasia found in all malignancies. It occurs in both sexes at all ages, somewhat more commonly in the young. It may be found anywhere in the body, most often in the skin, liver, spleen, lungs, bones, and occasionally retroperitoneally. Grossly, as a malignant tumor, it is usually a large, fleshy mass of pale gray-white, soft, encephaloid tissue, sometimes up to 15 to 20 cm. in diameter. The margins are not well defined because of its invasiveness, and they blend imperceptibly with surrounding structures. Areas of central softening, necrosis and hemorrhage are frequent. Occasionally, smaller lesions are found (3 to 4 cm. in diameter) which appear deceptively benign with apparent sharp demarcation.

Microscopically, *all degrees of differentiation of these tumors may be found,* from those that are largely vascular with plump, anaplastic but recognizable endothelial cells to tumors that are quite undifferentiated and produce no definite blood vessels and are markedly atypical. In this more malignant variant, pleomorphism, tumor giant cells and mitoses are characteristic (Fig. 15–35). These sarcomas may be similar in their cytologic detail to fibrosarcomas and leiomyosarcomas. It is therefore sometimes difficult to determine in these spindle cell sarcomas the exact cell or tissue of origin, and careful scrutiny of the better differentiated areas is necessary to identify the endothelial and vascular or-

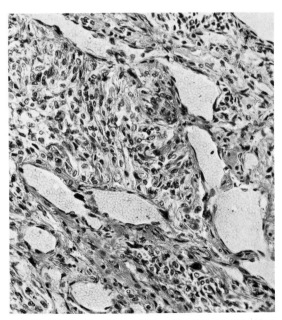

Figure 15–35. *Hemangioendotheliosarcoma of low malignancy and only moderate anaplasia.*

igin. Frequently helpful is the finding of somewhat atypical endothelial cells apparently lining a vascular channel or producing piled-up masses of cells apparently invading the lumen of a vessel. Also of aid is the phosphotungstic acid-hematoxylin stain (PTAH). With this special stain, the fibrils so characteristic of fibrous tissue and smooth muscle are, classically, absent.

Clinically, this tumor has all the usual significance of a malignancy with local invasion and distant metastatic spread. The pathways of dissemination are characteristically through the blood, but lymphatic spread may also occur. Some patients survive only weeks to months, whereas others may live for many years.

KAPOSI'S SARCOMA (MULTIPLE IDIOPATHIC, HEMORRHAGIC SARCOMATOSIS)

This dermatologic condition of extremely obscure nature is characterized by the appearance of multicentric, red-blue, violaceous tumor masses over the skin and sometimes in the internal viscera. There is much confusion about this disorder, particularly with respect to its genesis. Early cases of Kaposi's sarcoma have been described with multiple disseminated skin lesions resembling either benign capillary hemangiomas or chronic inflammatory foci. In the course of time, repeated biopsies have disclosed a progressive, increased cellularity in these multicentric areas, eventuating in markedly cellular, spindle cell lesions having many of the characteristics of a fibrosarcoma or of an endotheliosarcoma (Tedeschi, 1958) (Fig. 15–36). In this stage, visceral involvements are encountered which are either additional multicentric primary foci or metastatic nodules. With this late, full-blown stage, therefore, the designation of sarcomatosis is well merited. While this curious condition eventuates in frank malignancy of probable endothelial origin, through its long life history it presents as a dermatologic disorder and is therefore more appropriately considered in the chapter on skin (p. 1416).

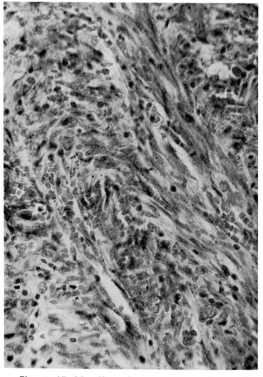

Figure 15–36. Kaposi's sarcoma. A medium power view of the highly cellular, vascular spindle cell sarcoma.

REFERENCES

Adams, C. W. M., et al.: Autoradiographic evidence for the outward transport of $_3$H-cholesterol through rat and rabbit aortic wall. J. Path. Bact., 87:297, 1964.

Antischkow, N.: Experimental arteriosclerosis in animals. In Cowdry, E. V. (ed.): Arteriosclerosis: A Survey of the Problem. New York, The Macmillan Co., 1933, p. 271.

Armstrong, M. L., et al.: Regression of coronary atheromatosis in Rhesus monkeys. Circ. Res., 27:59, 1970.

Bailey, O. T.: The cutaneous glomus and its tumors – glomangiomas. Amer. J. Path., 11:915, 1935.

Barker, F. W., et al.: A statistical study of post-operative venous thrombosis and pulmonary embolism. I. Incidence in various types of operation. II. Predisposing factors. Proc. Staff Meet. Mayo Clin., 15:769, 1940; 16:1, 17, 33, 1941.

Berenson, G. S.: Carbohydrate macromolecules and atherosclerosis. Hum. Path., 2:57, 1971.

Bevan, A. T., et al.: Clinical and biopsy findings in temporal arteritis. Ann. Rheum. Dis., 27:271, 1968.

Bornstein, P.: The cross linking of collagen and elastin and its inhibition in osteolathyrism. Amer. J. Path., 49:429, 1970.

Brest, A. N., and Moyer, J. H. (eds.): Atherosclerotic Vascular Disease (A Hahnemann Symposium). New York, Appleton-Century-Crofts, 1967, p. 8.

Brody, G. L., et al.: Dissecting aneurysms of the coronary artery. New Eng. J. Med., 273:1, 1965.

Brown, D. F.: Blood lipids and lipoproteins in atherogenesis. Amer. J. Med., 46:691, 1969.

Buck, R. C.: The fine structure of the aortic endothelial lesions in experimental cholesterol atherosclerosis of rabbits. Amer. J. Path., 34:897, 1958.

Burch, P. R. J.: Cardiovascular diseases: new etiological considerations. Amer. Heart J., 67:139, 1964.

Burchell, H. B.: Aortic dissection (dissecting hematoma; dissecting aneurysm of the aorta). Circulation, 12:1068, 1955.

Caro, C. G., et al.: Atheroma and arterial wall shear. Observation, correlation and proposal of a shear dependent mass transfer mechanism for atherogenesis. Proc. Roy. Soc. London (Biol.), 177:109, 1971.

Chobanian, A. V.: Sterol synthesis in the human arterial intima. J. Clin. Invest., 47:595, 1968.

Constantinides, P.: Experimental Atherosclerosis. Amsterdam, London, New York, Elsevier Publishing Co., 1965, p. 1.

Constantinides, P.: Lipid deposition in injured arteries. Electron microscopic study. Arch. Path., 85:280, 1968.

Constantinides, P.: Ultrastructural injury of arterial endothelium.

I. Effects of pH osmolarity, anoxia and temperature. II. Effects of vasoactive amines. Arch. Path., 88:99, 106, 1969.

Cookson, F. B.: The origin of foam cells in atherosclerosis. Brit. J. Exp. Path., 52:62, 1971.

Cowdry, E. V.: Arteriosclerosis. 2nd ed. Springfield, Ill., Charles C Thomas, 1967.

Crane, C.: Arteriosclerotic aneurysms of the abdominal aorta: some pathologic and clinical correlations. New Eng. J. Med., 253:954, 1955.

Dawber, T. R., et al.: Vital capacity, physical activity and coronary heart disease. In Raab, W. (ed.): Prevention of Ischemic Heart Disease: Principles and Practice. Springfield, Ill., Charles C Thomas, 1966.

Dayton, S., and Hashimoto, S.: Recent advances in molecular pathology: a review. Cholesterol flux and metabolism in arterial tissue and in atheromata. Exp. Molec. Path., 13:253, 1970.

Dayton, S., and Pearce, M. L.: Prevention of coronary heart disease and other complications of atherosclerosis by modified diet. Amer. J. Med., 46:751, 1969.

DeBakey, M. E., et al.: Surgical management of dissecting aneurysms of the aorta. J. Thorac. Cardiovasc. Surg., 49:130, 1965.

Department of Health, Education and Welfare: The health consequences of smoking. A public health service review. Public Health Service Publication No. 1696, Washington, D.C., U.S. Govt. Printing Office, 1967, p. 25.

Department of Health, Education and Welfare: United States, Vol. I, Publication No. (NIH) 72-137, June, 1971.

de Takats, G., and Fowler, E. F.: Raynaud's phenomenon. J.A.M.A., 179:1, 1962.

Duguid, J. B.: Thrombosis as a factor in atherosclerosis. J. Path. Bact., 60:57, 1948.

Duguid, J. B.: Thrombosis as a factor in the pathogenesis of coronary atherosclerosis. J. Path. Bact., 58:207, 1946.

Eggen, D. A., and Solberg, L. A.: Variation of atherosclerosis with age. Lab. Invest., 18:571, 1968.

Enos, W. F.: Pathogenesis of coronary disease in American soldiers killed in Korea. J.A.M.A., 158:1912, 1955.

Ettinger, M. G., et al.: Stroke: United States and Japan. Blood coagulation studies. Geriatrics, 24:116, 1969.

Fisher, C. M.: Cerebral thromboangiitis obliterans. Medicine, 36:169, 1957.

Fisher, E. R., et al.: Ultrastructural studies in hypertension. I. Comparison of renal vascular and juxtaglomerular cell alterations in essential and renal hypertension in man. Lab. Invest., 15:1409, 1966.

Frantz, I. D., Jr., and Moore, R. B.: The sterol hypothesis in atherogenesis. Amer. J. Med., 46:684, 1969.

Fredrickson, D. S., et al.: Fat transport in lipoproteins. An integrated approach to mechanisms and disorders. New Eng. J. Med., 276:34, 94, 148, 215, 273, 1967.

Freis, E. D.: Hypertension and atherosclerosis. Amer. J. Med., 46:735, 1969.

French, J. E.: Atherogenesis and thrombosis. Seminars Hemat., 8:84, 1971.

Fry, D. L.: Acute vascular endothelial changes associated with increased blood velocity gradients. Cir. Res., 22:165, 1968.

Geer, J. C.: Fine structure of human aortic intimal thickening and fatty streaks. Lab. Invest., 14:1764, 1965.

Geer, J. C., and McGill, H. C., Jr.: The Evolution of the Fatty Streak. Atherosclerotic Vascular Disease (a Hahnemann Symposium). New York, Appleton-Century-Crofts, 1967, p. 8.

Geer, J. C., et al.: The fine structure of the human atherosclerotic lesion. Amer. J. Path., 31:263, 1961.

Geschickter, C. F.: Tumors of blood vessels. Amer. J. Cancer, 23:568, 1935.

Getz, G. S., et al.: A dynamic pathology of atherosclerosis. Amer. J. Med., 46:657, 1969.

Ghidone, J. J., and O'Neal, R. M.: Recent advances in molecular pathology. A recent review of ultrastructure of human atheromas. J. Exp. Molec. Path., 7:378, 1967.

Glagov, F.: Hemodynamic factors in localization of atherosclerosis. Acta Cardiol., Suppl., 11:311, 1965.

Gore, I., and Seiwert, V. J.: Dissecting aneurysm of the aorta. Pathologic aspects and analysis of 85 fatal cases. Arch. Path., 53:121, 1952.

Greig, H. B. W.: Inhibition of fibrinolysis by alimentary lipemia. Lancet, 2:16, 1956.

Haller, J. A., and Mays, T.: Experimental studies on iliofemoral venous thrombosis. Amer. Surg., 29:567, 1963.

Hamrin, B., et al.: Polymyalgia arteritica, further clinical and histopathological study with a report of six autopsy cases. Ann. Rheum. Dis., 27:397, 1968.

Hand, R. A., and Chandler, A. B.: Atherosclerotic metamorphosis of autologous pulmonary thrombo-emboli in the rabbit. Amer. J. Path., 40:469, 1962.

Haust, M. D.: Electron microscopic and immuno-histochemical studies of fatty streaks in human aorta. In Miras, G. J., Howard, A. N., and Paoletti, R. (eds.): Progress in Biochemical Pharmacology, Vol. 4. Basel, New York, S. Karger, 1968, p. 429.

Haust, M. D.: The morphogenesis and fate of potential and early atherosclerotic lesions in man. Hum. Path., 2:1, 1971.

Hirst, A. E., et al.: Dissecting aneurysms of the aorta: a review of 505 cases. Medicine, 37:217, 1958.

Hollander, W.: Recent advances in experimental and molecular pathology. Influx synthesis and transport of arterial lipoproteins in atherosclerosis. Exp. Molec. Path., 7:248, 1967.

Hume, D. M., and Porter, R. R.: Acute dissecting aneurysm. Surgery, 55:122, 1963.

Hume, M., et al.: Venous Thrombosis and Pulmonary Embolism. Cambridge, Mass., Harvard University Press, 1970, p. 9.

Hunder, G. G., et al.: Giant cell arteritis producing an aortic arch syndrome. Ann. Intern. Med., 66:578, 1967.

Intersociety Commission for Heart Disease Resources: Atherosclerosis study group and epidemiology study group: primary prevention of the atherosclerotic diseases. Circulation, 42:A55, 1970.

Jensen, J.: The kinetics of the in vitro cholesterol uptake at the endothelial cell surface of the rabbit aorta. Biochim. Biophys. Acta, 135:544, 1967.

Jolliffe, N.: Fats, cholesterol and coronary heart disease. A review of recent progress. Circulation, 20:109, 1959.

Judge, R. D., et al.: Takayasu's arteritis and the aortic arch syndrome. Amer. J. Med., 32:379, 1962.

Kahn, H. A.: The Dorn study of smoking and mortality among U.S. veterans: report on 8½ yrs. of observation. Nat. Cancer Inst. Monogr., 19:1, 1966.

Kannel, W. B.: The disease of living. Nutr. Today, 6:2, 1971a.

Kannel, W. B.: Lipid profile and the potential coronary victim. Amer. J. Clin. Nutr., 24:1074, 1971b.

Kannel, W. B.: Serum lipid precursors of coronary heart disease. Hum. Path., 2:109, 1971c.

Kannel, W. B., et al.: Factors of risk in the development of coronary heart disease. Six year follow up experiences. Ann. Intern. Med., 55:33, 1961.

Kannel, W. B., et al.: Risk factors in coronary heart disease. An evaluation of several serum lipids as predictors of coronary heart disease. The Framingham study. Ann. Intern. Med., 61:888, 1964.

Keys, A.: Coronary heart disease in seven countries. Circulation, Suppl. 1, 41:1, 1970.

Keys, A.: Diet and the epidemiology of coronary heart disease. J.A.M.A., 164:1912, 1957.

Klynstra, F. B., and Bottcher, C. J. F.: Permeability patterns in pig aorta. Atherosclerosis, 11:451, 1970.

Layman, T. E., and Wang, Y.: Idiopathic cystic medionecrosis and aneurysmal dilatation of the ascending aorta. Med. Clin. N. Amer., 42:1145, 1968.

Lehmann, H., and Lynes, J. G.: Hyperlipoproteinaemia classification: the optimum routine electrophoretic system and its relevance to treatment. Lancet, 1:557, 1972.

Linton, A. L., et al.: Microangiopathic hemolytic anemia and the pathogenesis of malignant hypertension. Lancet, 1:1277, 1969.

McGill, H. C., Jr., et al.: Natural history of human atherosclerosis lesions. In Sandler, M., and Bourne, G. H. (eds.): Atherosclerosis and Its Origins. New York and London. Academic Press, 1963, p. 39.

McKusick, V. A., et al.: Buerger's disease: a distinct clinical and pathologic entity. J.A.M.A., 181:5, 1962.

Meneely, J. K., and Bigelow, N. H.: Temporal arteritis. A critical evaluation of this disorder and a report of 3 cases. Amer. J. Med., *14*:46, 1953.

Miettinen, M., et al.: Effect of cholesterol-lowering diet on mortality from coronary heart-disease and other causes. Lancet, *2*:7782, 1972.

Miras, C. H., et al. (eds.): Progress in Biochemical Pharmacology. Recent Advances in Atherosclerosis. Vol. 4. Basel, New York. S. Karger, 1969.

More, R. H., and Haust, M. D.: Atherogenesis and plasma constituents. Amer. J. Path., *38*:527, 1961.

More, R. H., and Haust, M. D.: Encrustation and permeation of blood proteins in the genesis of arteriosclerosis. Amer. J. Path., *33*:593, 1957.

Morris, J. N., and Gardner, M. J.: Epidemiology of ischemic heart disease. Amer. J. Med., *46*:674, 1969.

Morris, J. N., et al.: Incidence and prediction of ischaemic heart disease in London businessmen. Lancet, *2*:553, 1966.

Moss, N. S., and Benditt, E. P.: The ultrastructure of spontaneous and experimentally induced arterial lesions. Lab. Invest., *23*:231, 1970.

Mustard, J. F., and Packham, M. A.: Factors influencing platelet function: adhesion, release and aggregation. Pharmacol. Rev., *22*:97, 1970.

Nakao, K., et al.: Takayasu's arteritis. Clinical reports of 84 cases and immunological study of 7 cases. Circulation, *35*:1141, 1967.

Nasu, T.: Pathology of pulseless disease. Angiology, *14*:225, 1963.

Newman, H. A. I., and Zilversmit, D. B.: Quantitative aspects of cholesterol blocks in rabbit atheromatous lesions. J. Biol. Chem., *237*:2078, 1962.

O'Brien, P., and Brasfield, R. D.: Hemangiopericytoma. Cancer, *22*:453, 1960.

Osmundson, P. J.: Acute aortic dissection. Postgrad. Med., *49*:132, 1971.

Page, R. C., and Benditt, E. P.: Diseases of connective and vascular tissues. IV. The molecular basis for lathyrism. Lab. Invest., *26*:22, 1972.

Palmer, R. F., and Wheat, M. W., Jr.: Treatment of dissecting aneurysms of the aorta. Ann. Thorac. Surg., *4*:38, 1967.

Paronetto, F.: Immunocytochemical observations on the vascular necrosis and renal glomerular lesions of malignant nephrosclerosis. Amer. J. Path., *46*:901, 1965.

Patelski, J., et al.: Changes in phospholipase A, lipase and cholesterol esterase activity in the aorta in experimental atherosclerosis in the rabbit and rat. J. Atheroscler. Res., *8*:221, 1968.

Penick, G. D., and Roberts, H. R.: Intravascular clotting: focal and systemic. Int. Rev. Exp. Path., *3*:269, 1964.

Peterman, A. F., et al.: Encephalotrigeminal angiomatosis (Sturge-Weber disease). J.A.M.A., *167*:2169, 1958.

Raab, W. (ed.): Prevention of Ischemic Heart Disease: Principles and Practice. Springfield, Ill., Charles C Thomas, 1966.

Reinecke, R. D., and Kuwabara, T.: Temporal arteritis. Arch. Ophthal., *82*:446, 1969.

Restrepo, C., et al.: Non-syphilitic aortitis. Arch. Path., *87*:1, 1969.

Rottino, A.: Medial degeneration of the aorta as seen in 12 cases of dissecting aneurysm. Arch. Path., *28*:1, 1939.

Sandler, M., and Bourne, G. H. (eds.): Atherosclerosis and its Origins. New York and London, Academic Press, 1963, p. 39.

Schatz, I. G., et al.: Thromboangiitis obliterans. Brit. Heart J., *28*:84, 1966.

Schumaker, V. N., and Adams, G. H.: Circulating lipoproteins. Ann. Rev. Biochem., *38*:113, 1969.

Schwartz, C. J., et al.: Gross aortic sudanophilia and hemosiderin deposition. A study on infants, children and young adults. Arch. Path., *83*:325, 1967.

Scott, R. F., et al.: Short term feeding of unsaturated vs. saturated fat in the production of atherosclerosis in the rat. Exp. Molec. Path., *3*:421, 1964.

Shaper, A. G., et al.: The platelet count. Platelet adhesiveness and aggregation and the mechanism of fibrinolytic inhibition in pregnancy and the puerperium. J. Obstet. Gynaec. Brit. Comm., *75*:433, 1968.

Silbert, S., et al.: Mönckeberg's arteriosclerosis. J.A.M.A., *151*:1176, 1953.

Sise, H. S., et al.: On the nature of hypercoagulability. Amer. J. Med., *33*:667, 1962.

Slack, J., and Evans, E. A.: The increased risk of death from ischaemic heart disease in first degree relatives of 121 men and 96 women with ischaemic heart disease. J. Med. Genet., *3*:239, 1966.

Spiro, D., et al.: The cellular pathology of experimental hypertension. I. Hyperplastic arteriosclerosis. Amer. J. Path., *47*:19, 1965.

Stamler, J.: Acute myocardial infarction: progress in primary prevention. Brit. Heart J., Suppl., *33*:145, 1971.

Stout, A. P.: Hemangiopericytoma: a study of 25 new cases. Cancer, *2*:1027, 1949.

Strong, J. P., et al.: On the associations of cigarette smoking with coronary and aortic atherosclerosis. J. Atheroscler. Res., *10*:303, 1969.

Tanzer, M. L.: Experimental lathyrism. Int. Rev. Connect. Tissue Res., *3*:91, 1965.

Tedeschi, C. G.: Some considerations concerning the nature of the so-called sarcoma of Kaposi. Arch. Path., *66*:656, 1958.

Thomas, W. A., et al.: Thrombo-embolism, pulmonary arteriosclerosis and fatty meals. Arch. Path., *61*:380, 1956.

Truett, J. J., et al.: A multivariate analysis of the risk of coronary heart disease in Framingham. J. Chron. Dis., *20*:511, 1967.

Walshe, J. M.: Toxic reactions to penicillamine in patients with Wilson's disease. Postgrad. Med. J., Suppl.: 6, 1968.

Walton, K. W., and Williamson, N.: Histological and immunofluorescent studies on the evolution of the human atherosclerotic plaque. J. Atheroscler. Res., *8*:599, 1968.

Watts, H. F.: Basic aspects of the pathogenesis of atherosclerosis. Hum. Path., *2*:31, 1971.

Weiner, J., et al.: The cellular pathology of experimental hypertension. II. Arteriolar hyalinosis and fibrinoid change. Amer. J. Path., *47*:457, 1965.

Wessler, S.: Buerger's disease revisited. Surg. Clin. N. Amer., *49*:703, 1969.

Wessler, S., et al.: A critical evaluation of thromboangiitis obliterans. The case against Buerger's disease. New Eng. J. Med., *262*:1149, 1960.

Wheat, M. W., Jr., et al.: Acute dissecting aneurysms of the aorta. Treatment and results in 64 patients. J. Thorac. Cardiovasc. Surg., *58*:344, 1969.

Wissler, R. W., and Vesselinovitch, D.: Experimental models of human atherosclerosis. Ann. N.Y. Acad. Sci., *149*:907, 1968.

World Health Organization: Classification of hyperlipidaemias and hyperproteinaemias. Bull. W.H.O., *43*:891, 1970*a*.

World Health Organization: Vital statistics and cause of death. World Health Statistics Annual 1967, *1*:1970*b*.

Yudkin, J.: Sugar and coronary thrombosis. Postgrad. Med., *44*:67, 1967–68.

Yudkin, J., and Morland, J.: Sugar intake and myocardial infarction. Amer. J. Clin. Nutr., *20*:503, 1967.

16

HEART

This chapter opens with the two ends of the cardiac spectrum, certain normal aspects of cardiac embryogenesis and morphology and a brief review of congestive heart failure, the final destination of most pathways of serious cardiac disease.

NORMAL

Embryology. Normally, by the fourth week of embryonic life, the paired primitive aortic arches have fused to form a single vascular channel with four distinct dilatations known as (1) the sinus venosus, which receives the venous return and later becomes the superior vena cava and coronary sinus, (2) the atrium, (3) the ventricle and (4) the bulbus, which is continuous with the ventral aorta, later forming the pulmonary and aortic conuses. The channel elongates and bends to form an S shape. The bulbus and the ventricle create the top half of the letter S, and the atrium and sinus venosus, the lower. In the process of bending and twisting, the atrium and sinus assume the cephalic position, which they occupy in the normal adult heart, and the ventricle and the bulbus are positioned below.

Between the fifth and eighth weeks of fetal life, the atrium and the ventricle become separated by a transverse septum into two independent chambers. Each of these major chambers is divided into a left and right side by a longitudinal septum. Thus, the four-chambered adult heart develops. The primitive atrioventricular valves and semilunar valves form soon afterward. The bulbus becomes the primitive truncus arteriosus, which is then divided by a septum into the aorta and pulmonary artery. By the end of the second month of pregnancy, there is a four-chambered heart with well developed valves connected to the vascular system by venous and arterial trunks identical to those found in the adult. *Since the development of the heart is complete by the end of the eighth week of pregnancy, adverse influences, such as maternal rubella, which are capable of affecting fetal heart development are dangerous only during the first two months of pregnancy.*

Anatomy. Determination of the size of the heart is of great importance in both clinical and pathologic practice. In the female, the normal weight is generally stated as 250 to 300 gm., and in the male, 300 to 350 gm. Allowance must be made for height and skeletal structure. Since the heart may stop in systole or diastole or may have undergone dilatation prior to death, certain dimensions are also of importance. Normally the thickness of the right ventricle is 3 to 5 mm., and the left ventricle, 1.3 to 1.5 cm. Ventricular thicknesses that fall above these levels indicate hypertrophy and enlargement; measurements below these normal ranges would imply dilatation. However, these measurements must be interpreted with reference to heart weight, as cardiac dilatation may produce falsely low ventricular measurements.

Ring circumference may supply information about valve size. Approximate normal values for the ring circumferences are:

Tricuspid valve	12.0 cm.
Pulmonic valve	8.5 cm.
Mitral valve	10.0 cm.
Aortic valve	7.5 cm.

In some circumstances, measurement of the valve ring does not adequately express the degree of valvular deformity. In rheumatic heart disease, for example, fusion of the leaflets may produce funnel-shaped or buttonhole stenoses without affecting the ring's circumference. The orifice should therefore be measured when stenosing valvular disease is present. Estimating functional capacity of a valve from its anatomic structure is frequently difficult and inaccurate, despite such measurements. Slight dilatation of the heart may disappear after death to make a previously incompetent valve appear normal. Inapparent scarring or narrowings may have caused murmurs of stenosis.

A few comments on certain special features of the gross anatomy may be useful. On gross inspection, the valve leaflets should be delicate, translucent and without apparent vascularity. When vascularization occurs here, it implies the prior existence of some inflammatory stimulus. All act as loose flap valves which balloon out under the impact of the regurgitant blood. They are apposed or come in contact with each other at a line of closure marked by a linear thickening most evident in the semilunar leaflets. The centers of each of these linear thickenings are occupied usually by small fibrous nodules, the corpora arantii. Round to oval fenestrations, 1 to 3 mm. in diameter, frequently occur in the semilunar cusps, close to the commissures. The normal chordae tendineae are thin cords which originate from the papillary muscles and divide progressively into fine, delicate, hair-like strands which insert into the free margins of the atrioventricular leaflets. Thickening of these chordae is one of the conspicuous features of rheumatic endocarditis.

Normally, the pericardium contains up to 30 ml. of clear fluid. As a serosal membrane, it reacts to inflammatory and neoplastic diseases in the same fashion as do the linings of the pleural and peritoneal cavities.

The usual manner in which the heart is opened is indicated in Figure 16–1. These incisions essentially follow the course of the blood and create two anterior flaps which can be lifted to expose the underlying valves without disturbing their relationships.

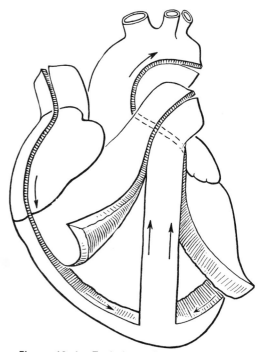

Figure 16–1. *Technique of opening heart. Arrows indicate directions of cuts.*

Histologically, the epicardium and parietal pericardium are usual mesothelium applied to an underlying fibrofatty tissue. The internal structure of the myocardial fiber differs from the skeletal striated muscle fiber only in its branching characteristics and central nuclei. At the point where branching fibers meet, there is an intercalated disc separating individual fibers. The myofibrils in the heart muscle cell are traversed by the usual A bands and I bands found in skeletal muscle, the I band having the characteristic centrally located Z line. A sarcomere is that portion of the cell contained between two Z lines. The myocardial fiber is especially rich in mitochondria, reflecting the high oxidative metabolic level of these cells. In the normal heart, the nuclei are fairly uniform in size and bear a fairly constant relationship to the mass of the individual cells. Significant disturbance in this nuclear-cytoplasmic ratio suggests some underlying derangement such as atrophy, hypertrophy or previous inflammatory disease. The Purkinje system lying subendocardially in the myocardium can often be differentiated by its vacuolated appearance due to a high content of cytoplasmic glycogen. Grossly or microscopically, the endocardium itself is so thin as to be virtually inapparent.

Blood Supply to the Heart. *Functionally, the right and left coronaries behave as end arteries, although anatomically there are numerous intercoronary anastomoses in most normal hearts.* It will be recalled that the ostia of the coronary arteries lie within the sinuses of Valsalva behind the aortic valve leaflets. Thus, these ostia are virtually closed by the valve leaflets during systole, and filling occurs during diastole. Knowledge of the area of supply of the three major coronary trunks helps to explain the correlation between vascular occlusions and myocardial infarctions. The left anterior descending branch supplies most of the apex of the heart, the medial half of the anterior surface of the left ventricle, the contiguous third of the anterior wall of the right ventricle and the anterior two-thirds of the interventricular septum. The right coronary artery supplies the remainder of the anterior surface of the right ventricle, the posterior aspect of the right ventricle, the adjacent half of the posterior wall of the left ventricle and the posterior third of the interventricular septum. To the left circumflex branch is left only a small portion of the lateral aspect of the left ventricle, anteriorly and posteriorly. Thus, *occlusions of the right as well as the left coronary artery cause left ventricular damage.* The atria are supplied by branches from the arteries on the corresponding side. At the cellular level, individual muscle fibers are almost uniformly accompanied by individual capillaries. This distribution may be important in hypertrophied hearts where it is postulated that enlarged fibers may become so thick as to outgrow their blood supply.

It is now amply documented that *in all or virtually all human hearts, there are numerous intercoronary anastomotic channels of the order of 40+ microns in diameter.* In the normal heart, little blood courses through these channels because the blood pressure on both ends of a channel is the same and there is no flow gradient. However, when one trunk is slowly narrowed, a pressure gradient develops, blood flows from the high to the low pressure system and simultaneously the channels slowly enlarge. Thus, these anastomoses may play a role in supporting the blood flow to deprived areas of the myocardium, depending on the rate of development of the narrowing in the major trunk and the extent of the enlargement of the anastomoses.

CONGESTIVE HEART FAILURE (CHF)

The consequence of most serious forms of heart disease is frequently congestive heart failure, also known as cardiac failure or cardiac decompensation. It would seem logical, therefore, to consider this clinical syndrome at the outset. CHF has been defined as "the pathologic state in which an abnormality of myocardial function is responsible for the failure of the heart to pump blood at a rate commensurate with the requirements of the metabolizing tissues" (Braunwald et al., 1967). *CHF occurs either because of a decreased myocardial capacity to contract or because an increased pressure-volume load is imposed on the heart.* Whether caused by primary damage to the heart muscle or secondary to chronic excessive workload as in severe valvular heart disease, the ultimate basis of all heart failure is defective myocardial contraction. Commonly, both an increased load and diminished contractility are operative. The immediate hemodynamic consequences are diminished cardiac stroke volume (sometimes called forward failure) and damming back of blood in the venous system (so-called backward failure).

Compensatory mechanisms come into play whenever failure begins to develop. Cardiac dilatation (Frank-Starling mechanism) and cardiac hypertrophy may compensate for decreased myocardial contractility and increased mechanical loads since the enlarged muscle mass in the hypertrophied heart provides a greater contractile capacity (Pool and Braunwald, 1968). Other mechanisms support this cardiac adaptation, such as an increased end-diastolic volume with increased stroke volume and expansion of the blood volume through renal retention of salt and water. The adrenal output of catecholamines is increased, further enhancing cardiac output. But at some point in time, cardiac decompensation sets in as the compensatory mechanisms are overloaded and, indeed, come to constitute an added burden on an organ already taxed to its limit. The myocardial hypertrophy itself may become detrimental, possibly because diffusion of oxygen in the hypertrophied heart is impaired as the distance between the capillaries increases commensurate with the hypertrophy of the myocardial fibers (Bing et al., 1968). Alternatively, it has been proposed that an increased rate of turnover of proteins in the hypertrophied heart leads to augmented wear and tear and subsequent failure (Meerson, 1962). There is, however, considerable evidence that both of these explanations are simplistic and, indeed, the ultimate basis for the failure of the myocardial cell is still obscure. Certainly it is a well documented clinical observation that patients with hypertrophied hearts may remain compensated for years only to decompensate at some point in time, without an apparent "new event" to precipitate the failure.

Considerable attention has been directed to the question of whether myocardial failure ultimately results from a defect in the production of energy, its conservation or its utilization. Disturbed mitochondrial function has been reported by some investigators and denied by others. An abnormality of excitation-contraction coupling has been proposed and refuted. Alterations in the contractile proteins, actomyosin and myosin, have been questioned. Derangements have been suspected in the sarcoplasmic reticulum through which calcium ions flow during the delivery of the electrochemical impulse for contraction. All of these studies are too lengthy to be detailed here and are well reviewed (Braunwald et al., 1967) (Bing et al., 1968). In last analysis, at the present time the basis for myocardial cell failure in CHF remains a mystery.

Before turning to the morphologic changes encountered in CHF, it is well to point out that the syndrome of heart failure must be distinguished from states of circulatory insufficiency in which myocardial function is not primarily impaired. The most clear-cut example of circulatory insufficiency is hemorrhagic (hypovolemic) shock which is a state of profound circulatory insufficiency not initiated by myocardial dysfunction, although the myocardium may become secondarily involved. Moreover, circulatory congestion may arise because of abnormal salt and water retention in the absence of serious disturbance of myocardial function such as is seen in chronic renal failure. Again, the increased blood volume imposes a burden on the heart which may in time lead to myocardial dysfunction. In any event, it is clear that circulatory derangements may arise from extracardiac sources and impose deficits (hypoxia and congestion) similar to those induced by CHF.

The significant morphologic changes encountered in CHF are all away from the heart and are produced by the secondary effects of the failing circulation upon the organs supplied by the heart. In other words, it is impossible from morphologic examination of the heart to differentiate the damaged but compensated heart from one that has decompensated. Cardiac hypertrophy and dilatation, along with the changes of the underlying cardiac disease, are present but are not themselves pathognomonic of CHF. Ultrastructural studies have yielded a variety of suggestive alterations, for example, changes in sarcomere length, subtle changes in mitochondria, and others, but again these changes are not diagnostic of the decompensated myocardial cell.

Although the heart is a single organ, to some extent it acts as two distinct anatomic and functional units. Under various pathologic stresses, one side or, rarely, even one chamber may fail before the other(s) so that, from the clinical standpoint, left-sided and right-sided failure may occur separately. However, since the vascular system is a closed circuit, failure of one side cannot exist for long without eventually producing excessive strain upon the other, terminating in total heart failure. The clearest understanding of the pathologic physiology is derived from considering failure of each side separately.

LEFT-SIDED HEART FAILURE

As will be discussed, left-sided heart failure is most often caused by (1) coronary heart disease, (2) hypertension and (3) aortic and mitral valvular diseases (rheumatic heart disease, calcific aortic stenosis, congenital heart disease, bacterial endocarditis and syphilitic heart disease). Except with obstruction at the mitral valve, the left ventricle is usually dilated, sometimes quite massively. With mitral stenosis, the dilatation is confined to the left atrium. The distant effects of left-sided failure are manifested most prominently in the lungs, although the function of the kidneys and brain may also be markedly impaired.

Lungs. With the progressive damming of blood within the pulmonary circulation, pressure in the pulmonary veins mounts and is ultimately transmitted to the capillaries. Normally, hydrostatic pressure in the capillaries ranges between 6 and 9 mm. Hg. With increases to 25 or 30 mm. Hg., congestion followed by frank edema occurs. The lung is particularly vulnerable to the development of edema, because its loose honeycomb structure exerts no significant tissue pressure against the escape of fluids. At first, the transudate is limited to perivascular "cuffing." Later, there is thickening of the alveolar walls as fluid accumulates within them. Finally, the transudate overflows into the alveoli *(pulmonary edema)* (p. 321) (p. 786). Not infrequently, transudate accumulates within the pleural space, producing a gross pleural effusion.

These anatomic changes produce striking clinical manifestations. Dyspnea on exertion is usually the earliest complaint of patients in left-sided heart failure. Later, shortness of breath is present even at rest. The pathogenesis of this dyspnea might simply be ascribed to inadequate oxygenation of the blood flowing through the functionally impaired lungs. However, numerous studies indicate that the probable explanation is much more complex and in all likelihood involves hypoxemia of the respiratory center and carotid sinus, but more importantly, encroachment on the vital capacity of the lungs produced by the congestive vascular distention. Cyanosis may be present because of the impaired oxygenation of the blood, but it is usually minimal in left-sided failure. A characteristic and therefore highly important symptom of left-sided failure is *paroxysmal nocturnal dyspnea,* the sudden onset of respiratory distress which wakes the patient from sleep. The pathogenesis of this phenomenon is not completely understood, but several factors may be operative. With recumbency, there is decreased venous pressure in the dependent portions of the body, hence gradual resorption of tissue edema. The movement of fluid from the interstitium back into the vascular space produces an augmented blood volume, which in turn is reflected in an increase in pulmonary congestion. Moreover, there is less functional pulmonary reserve in the recumbent position than in the erect posture, because the resting position of the diaphragm is higher, encroaching on the vital capacity of the lungs. It is also possible that during sleep the irritability of the central nervous system is depressed and may permit the accumulation of edema fluid without evoking such normal defense mechanisms as coughing. As failure becomes more advanced, the patient becomes unable to sleep at all in the recumbent position—i.e., he becomes *orthopneic*—and must prop himself up with pillows. Cough is a common accompaniment of left-sided failure and, in severe cases, may raise frothy, blood-tinged sputum.

Kidneys. The hemodynamic derangements occurring with left-sided heart failure may markedly affect the kidneys. Decreased blood flow to the renal arteries, along with venous congestion, lead to sludging within the kidney, with consequent hypoxia and a reduction in arteriolar pulse pressure and glomerular filtration rate (GFR). Plasma renin and angiotensin levels are elevated. As the glomerular filtration rate falls, renal retention of salt and water occurs. Increased tubular reabsorption contributes to the sodium retention. Teleologically, this may be looked upon as the response of the kidneys to what they interpret as hypovolemia. Salt and water retention is further enhanced by the augmented secretion of adrenal mineralocorticoids, particularly aldosterone. The elaboration of these steroids may represent a nonspecific stress response, as well as be a result of hemodynamic alterations, especially as they affect the kidneys. The consequent increase in total blood volume eventually adds considerably to the load upon the heart and contributes to the generalized edema. With severe disturbances in renal blood flow, impaired excretion of nitrogenous products may cause azotemia, known as *prerenal azotemia.*

Brain. Cerebral hypoxia may give rise to many symptoms, such as irritability, loss of attention span and restlessness, and may even progress to stupor and coma. These symptoms, however, are almost invariably encountered only in far advanced congestive heart failure.

RIGHT-SIDED HEART FAILURE

Right-sided heart failure occurs in relatively pure form in only a few diseases. Usually it is combined with left-sided failure, because any increase in pressure in the pulmonary circulation incident to left-sided failure must inevitably produce an increased burden on the right side of the heart. The causes of right-sided failure, then, must include all those which create left heart failure, particularly lesions such as mitral stenosis, which produce great increases in the pulmonary pressure.

Fairly *pure* right-sided failure most often

occurs with *cor pulmonale*, i.e., right ventricular strain produced by intrinsic disease of the lungs or pulmonary vasculature. In these cases, the right ventricle is burdened by increased resistance within the pulmonary circuit. Dilatation of the heart is confined to the right ventricle and atrium. Other and less common causes of right-sided heart failure include myocardial infarction of the right ventricle and diffuse myocarditis, which appears to affect the right ventricle more often than the left for reasons to be presented later. Rarely, right-sided failure is caused by tricuspid or pulmonic valvular lesions. Clinically, constrictive pericarditis simulates right-sided failure by the damming of blood back into the systemic venous system, although the right ventricle itself may be normal.

The major morphologic and clinical effects of right-sided failure differ from those of left-sided failure in that pulmonary congestion is minimal, while engorgement of the systemic and portal systems is more pronounced. It should be remembered, however, that in both instances the twin problems of systemic venous congestion and impaired cardiac output remain qualitatively the same. The major organs affected by right-sided heart failure are the liver, spleen, kidneys, subcutaneous tissues, brain, and entire portal area of venous drainage.

Liver. The liver is usually slightly increased in size and weight and on sectioning displays a prominent "nutmeg" pattern (Fig. 16–2). This descriptive term refers to congestive red accentuation of the center of the liver lobules surrounded by the paler, sometimes fatty, peripheral regions of the liver lobule. There may be some widening of the space of Disse microscopically, as well as enlargement and congestion of the central veins and central portions of the vascular sinusoids. The liver cells in the central region may become somewhat atrophic as a result of the pressure of the distended vascular sinusoids. Together, these changes are called *chronic passive congestion* (CPC) of the liver. If the congestive failure is severe and rapidly developing, the passive congestion may lead to rupture of the sinusoids, with actual necrosis of the liver cells, producing *central hemorrhagic necrosis*. If the patient does not die of the usually severe cardiac failure, in time the central areas become fibrotic, creating so-called *cardiac sclerosis*, also known as *cardiac cirrhosis*.

Spleen. Splenic congestion produces a larger, heavier organ which is tense and cyanotic. On section, blood freely exudes and the tissue collapses so that the capsule becomes wrinkled. Microscopically, there may be marked

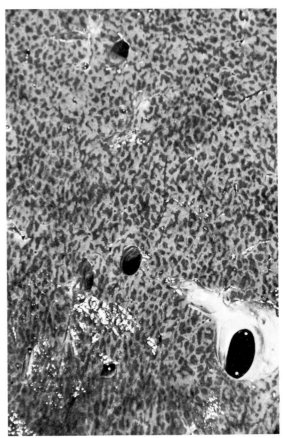

Figure 16–2. *A close-up view of the transected surface of the liver with marked chronic passive congestion — the so-called nutmeg pattern.*

sinusoidal dilatation, accompanied by areas of recent hemorrhage and possibly deposits of hemosiderin pigment. With longstanding congestion, the enlarged spleen may achieve weights of 500 to 600 gm. (normal, ±150 gm.), and the longstanding edema may produce fibrous thickening of the sinusoidal walls. The areas of previous hemorrhage are now transformed to hemosiderin deposits, to create the firm, meaty organ characteristic of *congestive splenomegaly*.

Kidneys. Congestion and hypoxia of the kidneys are more marked with right-sided heart failure than with left, leading to greater fluid retention and more pronounced prerenal azotemia.

Subcutaneous Tissues. Some degree of peripheral edema of dependent portions of the body occurs regularly. Indeed, ankle edema may be considered a hallmark of CHF. In severe or longstanding cases, edema may be quite massive and generalized, a condition termed *anasarca*. Of probable significance in the perpetuation of edema is the diminished clearing of plasma aldosterone by the congested liver. This contributes to the elevated levels of this hormone (Genest et al., 1968).

Brain. Symptoms essentially identical with those described in left-sided failure may occur, representing venous congestion and hypoxia of the central nervous system.

Portal System of Drainage. Splenic congestion has already been described. In addition, abnormal accumulations of transudate in the peritoneal cavity may give rise to ascites. Congestion of the gut may cause intestinal disturbances.

In summary, right-sided heart failure presents essentially as a venous congestive syndrome, with hepatic and splenic enlargement, peripheral edema and ascites. In contrast to left-sided failure, respiratory symptoms may be absent or quite insignificant. *It is to be emphasized at this point that although the consideration of heart failure has been divided into two functional units, in the usual case of frank chronic cardiac decompensation, these early stages have already passed, and the patient presents with the picture of full-blown CHF, encompassing the clinical syndromes of both right and left heart failure.*

MAJOR TYPES OF HEART DISEASE

Heart disease is today the most important cause of morbidity and mortality in all industrialized nations. In the United States, disorders of the heart caused approximately 38 per cent of all deaths and so were responsible for the deaths of 721,268 individuals in 1967. The five categories of fatal heart disease codified in the United States Vital Statistics in that year were:

Coronary heart disease	573,153 deaths
Endocarditis and myocarditis	52,679 deaths
Hypertensive heart disease	49,975 deaths
Rheumatic heart disease	14,176 deaths
Other	31,267 deaths

The prevalence of cardiac disease has steadily mounted in the United States. In 1900, the death rate from heart disease was 165 per 100,000 population. In 1955, the figure had risen to almost 500 and in 1964, to approximately 520. In some part, these data reflect the ever larger proportion of the aged in the population but, in larger part, they result from the alarming increase in the prevalence of coronary heart disease. Alone it accounts for about 31 per cent of the total mortality in the United

States or approximately four-fifths of all cardiac deaths. Children are regrettably all too liberally represented among the deaths from rheumatic heart disease and congenital heart disease (included in the "other" category).

Marked shifts have occurred over the past few years in the relative importance of various forms of heart disease. Seven types of cardiac disease now dominate clinical practice:

1. Coronary heart disease (80 per cent of all cardiac deaths).
2. Hypertensive heart disease (9 per cent).
3. Rheumatic heart disease (2 to 3 per cent).
4. Congenital heart disease (approximately 2 per cent).
5. Bacterial endocarditis (approximately 1 to 2 per cent).
6. Syphilitic heart disease (approximately 1 per cent).
7. Cor pulmonale (approximately 1 per cent).
8. Other (approximately 5 per cent).

It is obvious that coronary heart disease has commanding preeminence. In contrast, rheumatic heart disease and bacterial endocarditis have become much less frequent since the advent of effective antibacterial therapy. Syphilitic heart disease, too, has fallen in frequency, but not as significantly as the other two entities just mentioned. Hypertensive heart disease also has fallen in importance with the availability of improved methods of control of elevated blood pressure. Despite the gains in some of these categories, the losses in the form of the near epidemic proportions of coronary heart disease have yielded a net increase in the overall prevalence of cardiac disease.

Because of their importance, each of the seven major types of heart disease will be discussed individually, followed by a general discussion of the other forms. In the later general discussion, the diseases will be categorized according to whether they affect primarily the epicardium, the myocardium or the endocardium. Such a division is, to some extent, arbitrary as many cardiac diseases affect more than one layer of the heart.

CORONARY HEART DISEASE (CHD)

The term coronary heart disease is the generic designation for three types of cardiac disease all resulting from insufficient coronary artery blood flow. CHD, also called ischemic heart disease, has been defined by the World Health Organization (1957) as "the cardiac disability, acute and chronic, arising from reduction or arrest of blood supply to the myocardium in association with disease processes in the coronary arterial system." In 95 per cent or more of such cases, the insufficiency is due to atherosclerotic narrowing of the coronary arteries with or without superimposed thrombosis. The rare causes of coronary insufficiency include syphilitic aortitis with narrowing of the coronary ostia; dissecting aneurysms extending back into the coronary vessels; rheumatic, temporal arteritis, and polyarteritis nodosa involving coronary arteries; embolic occlusions and direct trauma to the heart inducing coronary thrombosis. *Depending upon the rate of the development of the arterial narrowing and its ultimate severity, the cardiac ischemia may induce only asymptomatic diffuse atrophic fibrotic changes in the myocardium, often associated with valvular deformities, or acute crises of chest pain with or without infarction of the myocardium.* Thus three distinctive, albeit overlapping, forms of coronary heart disease are recognized:

1. *Arteriosclerotic heart disease* (ASHD) evolves from slow, progressive narrowing of the coronary arteries occurring over the span of years. The dependent myocardium is slowly deprived of an adequate arterial supply and so undergoes atrophy with individual fiber necrosis, leading to diffuse small areas of scattered fibrosis. The heart valves, particularly on the left side, may simultaneously become thickened, fibrotic and calcified. Patients with ASHD may have no evidence of cardiac disease until the cardiac damage is advanced and heart failure develops, but they are at high risk of developing crises of anginal pain or a myocardial infarct.

2. *Myocardial infarction* is the catastrophic, frequently fatal form of CHD, usually resulting from precipitous reduction or arrest of a significant portion of the coronary flow. Almost always, severe atherosclerotic narrowing, often associated with total thrombotic occlusion, is present in one or more of the major coronary arterial trunks.

3. *Angina pectoris* is a symptom complex consisting of severe paroxysmal chest pain resulting from transient ischemia that precariously falls short of inducing ischemic necrosis of the myocardium. Underlying such episodic pain, there is almost always marked coronary atherosclerosis, and frequently such patients have the other features of arteriosclerotic heart disease. However, by definition, myocardial infarction is not present.

Obviously, there is much overlap among these three patterns of CHD. Very commonly, the patient with ASHD suffers repeated attacks of anginal pain only to succumb eventually to a myocardial infarction. Conversely, the patient who recovers from a myocardial infarct may well suffer from chronic cardiac insufficiency characteristic of decompensated ASHD.

PATHOGENESIS OF CHD

Coronary heart disease implies an imbalance between the coronary arterial supply to the myocardium and its metabolic needs. The balance involves three factors: (1) the adequacy of the coronary arterial flow, (2) the metabolic demands of the myocardium and (3) the oxygen content of the blood.

To a large degree, the pathogenesis of CHD is the pathogenesis of atherosclerosis of the coronary arteries (p. 595) (Fig. 16–3). Other forms of coronary vascular disease are the exception as previously noted. Several features of coronary atherosclerosis deserve special mention. The atheromatous involvement usually affects all three major trunks of the coronary system, frequently but not necessarily in equal measure. Only uncommonly is a single trunk severely narrowed while the others are spared. Generally, multiple stenoses are found among the three trunks. As indicated in the earlier discussion of atherosclerosis (p. 589), the proximal segments (first 5 cm.) tend to bear the most severe lesions although, in the right coronary artery, they may be distributed more distally. It is important to appreciate that a coronary artery may still carry sufficient blood to the myocardium until the original lumen is decreased by 70 to 75 per cent or more. Only this level of narrowing causes a greater resistence to flow than that imposed by the myocardial capillary bed itself (Roberts, 1971). Lesser luminal reductions are therefore without functional significance. In the great majority of all forms of CHD, the atheromata are complicated—i.e., fibrotic, calcified or ulcerated—and sometimes the lumen is totally occluded, usually by superimposed throm-

---

Figure 16–3. A, *An angiogram of the opened heart with the* normal *coronary arteries filled with radiopaque mass. On the right is the horizontal main right coronary artery with small descending twigs. On the left is visualized the major left descending ramus and the horizontal major left circumflex ramus. Between these two are several large accessory branches. The vessels show progressively diminishing lumina with no irregular narrowings or obstructions. B, An angiogram of an opened heart with severely narrowed and occluded atherosclerotic coronaries. The right coronary artery fails to fill over much of its length. The twigs of this vessel are filled by retrograde anastomotic collaterals. There is uneven narrowing and tortuosity of the left descending ramus and left circumflex ramus. Compare with A.*

See illustration on opposite page.

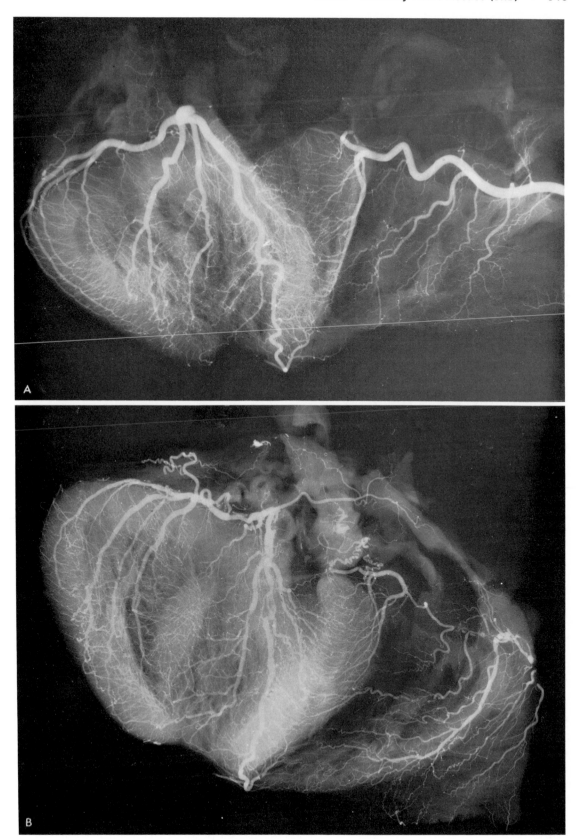

Figure 16–3. *See legend on opposite page.*

bosis. Total occlusion of a coronary artery may be present without resulting in myocardial infarction and, conversely, myocardial infarction may be found without total occlusion of any of the coronary trunks. This complex relationship of coronary thrombosis and myocardial infarction is discussed later (p. 649). When one of the trunks is totally obstructed and no myocardial infarction is found, it is assumed that the intercoronary anastomotic channels were capable of supplying adequate blood flow to maintain the viability of the dependent myocardium. However, the mere existence of anastomotic collaterals does not necessarily protect against acute myocardial infarction. A recent in vivo coronary arteriographic study showed acute myocardial infarction to be as common in a group of patients with demonstrable collateral vessels as in those without such anastomotic channels (Helfant et al., 1971). The important determinants are: (1) the rate of development of the arterial narrowing; when it occurs slowly, the enlargement of the collateral channels permits functionally significant levels of flow and (2) the coronary perfusion pressure.

Alterations in the cardiovascular hemodynamics are also important in reducing coronary flow, particularly since they are almost always imposed on arteries already narrowed by omnipresent atherosclerosis. Stenosis of the aortic valve impairs coronary filling, either because the valvular fibrosis and calcification extend to the coronary ostia or because the stenosed rigid valve cannot completely close during diastole and the resultant regurgitation reduces the diastolic pressures to below that necessary for adequate coronary filling. Syphilitic involvement of the aortic valve and aorta is particularly important because the mouths of the coronary arteries are often narrowed by the inflammatory process. Moreover, in luetic aortitis, the aortic valve ring stretches, elongating and narrowing the valvular leaflets. As the leaflets narrow, the coronary ostia are exposed. Thus, the full forward thrust of the systolic flow passes directly across the ostia, inducing a negative pressure within the origins of the coronary arteries. The aortic valvular dilatation simultaneously produces a valvular insufficiency which likewise leads to a fall in the diastolic pressure, further hampering coronary filling. The same obtains for aortic regurgitation in rheumatic heart disease. Severe hypotension such as is encountered in hypovolemic states (shock) is a particularly grave threat in the aged atherosclerotic patient with marginal coronary flow and, not infrequently, an acute myocardial infarction occurs during or immediately following surgery.

Myocardial ischemia is a relative term involving supply and demand. The metabolic needs of the myocardium are high and it is extremely sensitive to hypoxia. Increased myocardial demands such as occur during exercise, pregnancy, hyperthyroidism and other hypermetabolic disorders may lead to myocardial fiber injury or death when coronary flow is already reduced. The older person who drops dead while shoveling snow or who suffers a heart attack during an emotional crisis provides tragic testimony to the role of increased myocardial demand.

The oxygen content of the arterial flow obviously is one of the factors in the equation. Thus, any disorder which diminishes the oxygen-carrying capacity of the blood may unhinge the balance between demand and supply. Anemia with lowering of the hemoglobin concentration of the blood, reduction of the blood pO_2 in pulmonary disease, abnormal right-left shunting of blood and abnormalities in hemoglobin dissociation (release of oxygen) render reduced levels of arterial flow even more threatening.

ARTERIOSCLEROTIC HEART DISEASE (ASHD)

Arteriosclerotic heart disease is characterized anatomically by atherosclerosis of the coronary arteries with consequent ischemic atrophy and fibrosis of the myocardium. These changes are usually, but not invariably, accompanied by degenerative fibrocalcific damage to the heart valves. The other causes of coronary arterial narrowing previously mentioned may produce similar myocardial and valvular alterations, but are extremely rare and should be specifically designated; for example, syphilitic coronary ostial narrowing with myocardial fibrosis.

Here we should bring up the controversial and at least closely related entity known as senile heart disease or senile cardiomyopathy. It has been characterized as "disease of heart muscles due to the aging process exclusive of those myocardial changes which occur secondary to coronary arterial or other disease" (Burch and Giles, 1971). At autopsy, these individuals are almost invariably found to have some atherosclerosis of the coronary arteries, and so some consider the cardiac changes to be merely a form of ASHD. However, the atherosclerosis in such patients may be minimal. The possibility of past occult myocardial infections cannot be excluded as the etiology of the cardiac damage. Whether senile heart disease is a valid entity distinct from ASHD is still arguable, but it does raise the issue of the tendency to ascribe all cardiac failure in aged individuals to ASHD when other well defined forms of heart disease cannot be identified. This regrettable tendency leads to overdiagnosis of ASHD since other causes of cardiac failure may be found in the later decades of life. Indeed, there are forms of primary cardiomyopathy, including rheumatic myocarditis, which affect the aged as well as the young and which often are exceedingly difficult to diagnose. This admonition is of more than academic importance because some forms of myopathy are microbiologic or nutritional in origin and so are amenable to treatment. As emphasized in the preceding section, only when the narrowing of a coronary trunk reduces the lumen more than 70 per cent does it become functionally inadequate.

Morphology. The pathognomonic anatomic criteria of ASHD are the atherosclerotic involvement of the coronary arteries and diffuse myocardial fibrosis. Valvular deformities are frequent but not constant findings. The heart is usually smaller than normal, but may be of usual size. Occasionally it is enlarged but, in almost all such instances, long periods of cardiac decompensation underlie such cardiac hypertrophy or dilatation. Concomitant hypertension may also contribute to the enlargement (Clawson, 1939).

The coronary atherosclerotic involvement is usually diffuse, moderately severe and involves all three major trunks. Calcification may have converted the arteries into rigid pipestems which are resistant to transection. Although ulceration of these atheromas is frequent, superimposed thrombosis and total occlusion of a trunk is uncommon in the absence of myocardial infarction.

The myocardial fibrosis in ASHD may be difficult to detect on gross inspection. When severe, it appears as diffuse, patchy, gray-white streaking within the red-brown myocardium. Large, confluent areas of scarring probably represent old infarcts. The epicardial and endocardial surfaces are usually normal.

Valvular lesions, when present, usually involve only the left side of the heart. There may be only slight thickening of the leaflets. The chordae tendineae are rarely significanctly affected; cord-like thickenings are uncommon and usually denote concomitant rheumatic heart disease. There is often calcification of the mitral annulus, presenting in severe cases as nodular masses at the base of the mitral leaflets and encircling the valvular annulus. The aortic valve leaflets may also be thickened and often develop rounded calcific masses within the sinus of Valsalva. Similar calcifications may occur between the cusps of the aortic valve on the ventricular surface, producing intercommissural adhesions and obliteration of the demarcation between cusps. This form of **calcific aortic stenosis**

may resemble the healed calcified stage of rheumatic valvulitis, and it may not always be possible to identify with certainty the etiology of the aortic valvular damage (Fig. 16–4).

The distinctive microscopic features of ASHD are relatively few and consist of diffuse scarring of the myocardium. The fibrosis tends to occur perivascularly and in the preexistent fibrous septa (Fig. 16–5). Rarely, individual muscle fibers are separated by the increased fibrous tissue. The myocardial fibers themselves are frequently small and contain lipochrome ("wear and tear") pigment, producing so-called **"brown atrophy"** of the heart. **It is the coexistence of atherosclerotic involvement of the coronary arteries and the myocardial changes that delineates the diagnosis of arteriosclerotic heart disease,** even in the absence of well defined valvular changes.

Clinical Course. Compensated arteriosclerotic heart disease is completely asymptomatic and frequently is discovered only as an incidental finding at autopsy. Its presence usually becomes manifest by the insidious appearance of cardiac decompensation as the cardiac reserve is depleted grain by grain. Occasionally, the onset of CHF is more acute fol-

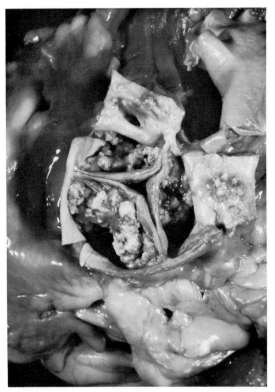

Figure 16–4. Calcific aortic stenosis. The granular masses of calcium are heaped up within the sinuses of Valsalva (view looking down at valve).

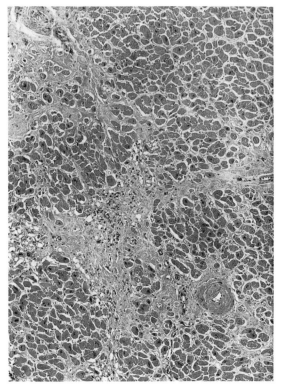

Figure 16–5. *Patchy fibrous scarring principally about blood vessels of the myocardium in arteriosclerotic heart disease.*

lowing a precipitating episode such as pneumonia or some other form of debilitating illness. Failure, when it becomes manifest, is initially left-sided due to the relatively greater demands on the left ventricle. The right ventricle appears to tolerate coronary insufficiency much better, perhaps because the transmural thebesian system is capable of sustaining the thinner ventricular wall. Ultimately, however, when left ventricular failure is present for a period of time, right-sided cardiac decompensation inevitably makes its appearance. The diagnosis of ASHD is established with near certainty when manifestations of angina pectoris or myocardial infarction appear. In the absence of such acute crises, the diagnosis is suspected when older individuals, in the absence of other forms of heart disease, develop aortic or mitral murmurs or electrocardiographic alterations indicative of myocardial damage. ASHD usually progresses slowly over the course of many years, leading ultimately to the development of cardiac decompensation. However, a serious cardiac arrhythmia or an infarction may supervene and cause death. More often, the patient dies of entirely unrelated causes before his ASHD becomes symptomatic.

ANGINA PECTORIS

Angina pectoris is a clinical syndrome characterized by paroxysmal attacks of chest pain, usually substernal or precordial, precipitated most often by effort and alleviated by rest. Because the pain is not associated with anatomic changes in the heart, i.e., myocardial infarction, angina pectoris is a clinical syndrome rather than an anatomic disorder. The diagnosis is only justified if there is no permanent electrocardiographic or anatomic evidence of myocardial damage related to the attack of pain. The pain is thought to arise from some sudden and transient imbalance between myocardial needs and coronary flow. Almost invariably, atherosclerosis of the coronary arteries, usually moderately severe, underlies such attacks. Infrequently, other disorders (p. 644) which are capable of reducing blood flow provoke anginal attacks.

Although it is tempting to postulate simply that increased myocardial metabolism outstrips the blood supply, the underlying precise mechanisms involved in such transient ischemia may be more complicated. Two proposals have been made: (1) paroxysmal spasm of the coronary arteries superimposed on coronary atherosclerotic narrowing and (2) occlusion of small branches rapidly compensated by collateral anastomotic flow, resulting in only temporary ischemia. Obviously, the two mechanisms are not mutually exclusive, and both may be operative either within the same individual or in different individuals. The concept of coronary spasm has been invoked because, on occasion, attacks of angina have appeared while the patient was at rest or when there appeared to be no basis for significant increased cardiac activity or metabolic needs. Indeed, transient, segmental spasm of the coronary arteries has been visualized in patients undergoing angiographic x-ray studies. Sometimes these spasms have evoked characteristic anginal pain, but often they have passed unnoted by the patient. Presumably, the severity of the spasm, its duration, the level of coronary reserve and the prior existence of enlarged anastomotic channels would determine whether the transient spastic narrowing induced anginal pain. The concept of vasospasm gains further support from the efficacy of such vasodilators as nitroglycerin in producing prompt relief of the pain.

The second postulated mechanism, invoking occlusion of a small branch of one of the main coronary trunks, stems from the studies of Blumgart and his colleagues (1940, 1941). These investigators pointed out the almost invariable presence of multiple small arterial occlusions (thromboses) at postmortem examination of patients who had suffered from angina pectoris. It was, of course, not possible to relate the development of the occlusions to the attacks. Nonetheless, it was postulated that the loss of blood supply due to blockage of a small arterial branch was the cause of a transient period of ischemia rapidly compensated by collateral flow. Both conceptions remain plausibilities, and the issue is still unsettled. It may be of further interest to point out that indeed we still do not know why myocardial ischemia should induce pain, usually referred to the chest, shoulder, left arm, neck or jaw; and, indeed, the neural pathways are still mysterious. While angina pectoris is not associated with myocardial necrosis, it has grave significance not only for the discomfort it creates, but because each attack carries the risk of a myocardial infarction or, at the very least, it indicates the existence of ASHD.

MYOCARDIAL INFARCTION (MI)

It is impossible to overstate the importance of myocardial infarction as a cause of disability and death. Although some epidemiologic data were given earlier (p. 587 and p. 643), it is relevant to note that in 1967 in the United States, coronary heart disease (CHD) was the most common cause of death and accounted for almost 600,000 deaths (approximately 31 per cent of all deaths), while in 1937 it occupied sixth place and was responsible for only 4.8 per cent of all mortality. Small wonder, then, that this disease is often spoken of as being epidemic in affluent societies. Cancer, no small problem itself, causes only half as many deaths. MI is responsbile for approximately two-thirds of CHD deaths. Alone, it causes about 20 to 25 per cent of all deaths in atherosclerosis-prone societies. Thus, MI assumes a grim and dominating place in medical practice.

Incidence. As indicated in the earlier consideration of atherosclerosis (p. 587), many considerations influence the risk of MI. Only the highlights will be briefly reiterated. The severity of coronary atherosclerosis and the frequency of myocardial infarction increase progressively with age, reaching a peak in the eighth decade of life. Males have a definite predisposition to MI, the overall ratio being about 2:1. This male vulnerability is most striking in the younger age groups, and the male-female ratio is still 5:1 between the ages of 45 and 54. It is often said that the prime targets for myocardial infarction are men at the height of their productive lives. MI is uncommon in women during their reproductive life unless they are predisposed by some of the risk factors discussed earlier (p. 587) (Kannel et al., 1961, 1964). Correlations have been drawn between MI and all of the following individual factors: excessive caloric intake, high dietary intake of fats (especially saturated animal fats), hyperlipidemia (particularly hypercholesterolemia), high serum levels of beta and pre-beta lipoproteins, hypertension, obesity, cigarette smoking, metabolic disorders leading to hypercholesterolemia (for example, diabetes mellitus, nephrosis and genetic lipidemias), physical inactivity, emotional and psychic stress, as well as other considerations presented in the earlier discussion. Among these many influences, four are known as "major risk factors": the serum lipid (cholesterol, beta and pre-beta lipoproteins) levels, obesity, hypertension and cigarette smoking. When three of these risk factors are present, the individual is rendered seven times more vulnerable to MI than those with none of these factors. With two major risk factors, vulnerability is increased fourfold, and with one major risk factor, twofold. Although blacks are more prone to hypertension than whites, their vulnerability to MI is much lower.

In descending rank order, Finland, the United States, New Zealand, Scotland, North Ireland, Australia, Canada, England and Wales have the highest death rates for coronary heart disease. In contrast, Sweden, Italy, Switzerland and Japan have the lowest death rates. For men between the ages of 35 and 64, the death rate in Japan is 64 compared to 400 for the United States. These differences are not thought to result from genetic predisposition, but rather relate to the environmental influences referred to as "risk" factors. In closing this consideration of incidence, it hardly needs to be stated that patients with angina or those who have survived a myocardial infarction are at particularly high risk.

Pathogenesis. Myocardial infarction results from sudden or relatively sudden arterial insufficiency. It may come as a surprise to learn that the pathogenesis of this arterial insufficiency has recently become a subject of some controversy. First the classic and conventional view will be presented, followed by the recent challenge. For many years, it has been held that total occlusion of one or more of the main coronary trunks, usually by a thrombus occurring at the site of a complicated atheroma, precipitated most myocardial infarcts. Ulceration or fracture of an atheromatous plaque or hemorrhage into a plaque were postulated as typical antecedents to such luminal thrombosis. Admittedly, other exotic bases of coronary artery occlusion exist, such as some form of arteritis of the coronary trunks, embolism and narrowing of the coronary ostia secondary to luetic aortitis; but these rare instances make no signifiant contribution to the prevalence of MI. *Hypercoagulability* of the blood would play an important role in this sequence. In support of the primary causal role of thromboses, whenever there is total occlusion of one or more of the main coronary trunks, a recent or old myocardial infarct can usually be demonstrated in the dependent myocardium. Rarely, total occlusions can be found in hearts having no infarction, explained on the basis of anastomotic circulation. However, myocardial infarction may occur in the absence of occlusive coronary disease and, indeed, in 15 to 20 per cent of infarcts, no occlusion can be found. As was discussed on p. 644, narrowing of coronary arteries down to marginal levels of adequacy predisposes to infarction whenever myocardial demands suddenly rise, oxygen transport in the blood falls or the patient suffers an acute severe hypotensive episode. *Thus, it was dogma for decades that coronary occlusion underlay infarction, and infarction usually implied occlusion,* although it could arise through other pathways.

Now we come to the recent controversy which has emerged. Roberts (1971) expresses it well: "The relationship of coronary thrombosis to myocardial necrosis needs reassessment: the evidence from systematic histologic study of the major coronary arteries in consecutive patients suggests that thrombi are more likely to be *the result* of acute myocardial infarction than the cause." In support of this contention, many recent surveys of acute myocardial infarcts have disclosed demonstrable coronary thrombosis in less than 50 per cent of the cases and, in one series, in only 29 per cent (Kagan et al., 1968) (Walston et al., 1970) (Ehrlich and Shinohara, 1964). These findings cannot be lightly attributed to technical errors (failure to find the thrombus) which might account for some small discrepancy but not for the absence of thrombosis in over half the cases. Furthermore, a provocative report suggested that the development of thrombosis is related to the duration of survival of the patient post infarction (Spain and Bradess, 1960). When the patient succumbed within the first hour following an MI, occlusions were found in only 16 per cent, which increased to 36 per cent in patients surviving one to eight hours, and to 54 per cent in patients who survived 24 hours or more before death. So the concept has emerged that myocardial necrosis is the primary event, followed in some patients by thrombosis of the coronary trunks. If such be the case, what

evoked the myocardial infarction? Here, recourse is made to principles discussed earlier: underlying marked atherosclerosis, sudden increase in myocardial demands, hypotension or reduced oxygen content of the blood may be all that is required to explain infarction. It is hypothesized, then, that atherosclerotic narrowing contributes to slowing or stagnation of coronary flow, and the development of ischemic myocardial necrosis and myocardial dysfunction triggers the postinfarction thrombosis. Logically, the thrombi would form at sites of most severe narrowing where there would be greatest turbulence. Another explanation has also been offered, e.g., platelet aggregation in the microcirculation. Could rupture of an atheromatous plaque release sufficent collagen, ADP or other aggregating factors to trigger massive platelet aggregation in the watershed of a large coronary trunk which would thus produce ischemic necrosis and secondarily lead to thrombosis? The lively issue of the precise pathogenesis of MI remains unresolved, but it has more than theoretical implications. The classic view would hold that thrombotic tendencies are of great importance in causing infarction and so efforts must be directed toward control of the clotting risk. The "heretics" would dismiss hypercoagulability and the causal role of thrombosis.

Whatever the sequence of events leading to the infarction, it is clear that the muscle cells undergo ischemic necrosis. The intracellular changes encountered in such cell death have been intensively studied in experimental models (Jennings, 1969). Within 8 to 10 seconds after placing a ligature about a main coronary trunk in dogs, the affected myocardium becomes cyanotic and, within the first minute, the injured myocardium ceases to contract and often bulges with each systole. In such animals, the myocardial cell injury is reversible when the occlusion is maintained for less than 20 or 30 minutes. Indeed, the cardiac surgeon often induces cardiac asystole without perfusing the coronary arteries for this length of time with apparent complete safety. It must be appreciated that in this clinical situation the heart is at rest. Irreversible cell injury begins to appear in the dog in a few cells when coronary flow is obstructed in a main trunk for 30 minutes, but the complete extent of the ischemic necrosis only becomes evident by one to two hours. However, when myocardial blood flow is cut off by inducing *microcirculatory blockade* such as can be effected by platelet aggregation in the capillary beds, irreversible ischemic damage appears within 5 minutes (Robbins, 1972). It appears that in the ligated main trunk models, anastomoses contribute some blood flow to the involved myocardium, albeit not sufficient to prevent the ultimate development of ischemic necrosis. Moreoever, in induced cardiac asystole, the heart escapes injury because of the reduced metabolic needs.

The myocardium is almost completely dependent on aerobic metabolism. Reduction in blood supply induces local hypoxia and, at the same time, the myocardium becomes deficient in exogenous substrates such as glucose, amino acids and fatty acids. End products of metabolism accumulate. Intracellular levels of ATP, NAD and the cytochromes are reduced. Anaerobic glycolysis then becomes the principal source of energy, and lactic acid accumulates. Enzymic function is inhibited as the intracellular pH falls. The almost immediate cessation of contractile function after coronary artery ligature is probably not due to simple depletion of energy sources since ATP is still present in such cells. Rather, it may be due to the effect of the increased intracellular acidity on the ability of calcium ions to activate contraction. Intracellular water and electrolyte homeostasis is deranged, and the cells lose potassium and magnesium. At the same time, enzymes such as the lactic dehydrogenases (LDH), glutamic oxaloacetic acid transaminase (GOT) and creatine phosphokinase (CPK) leak out (Jennings et al., 1957, 1964). These metabolic and biochemical changes are accompanied by a host of histologic and ultrastructural changes to be detailed below.

Morphology. Despite the controversy about which comes first—thrombotic occlusion or infarction—total occlusion of a coronary artery will be found in the majority of cases. In most instances, the occlusion is caused by a thrombus located at a severely stenotic, complicated atheromatous lesion. In a few instances, hemorrhage into an atheroma may have caused sudden bulging to complete the occlusive process and, even more rarely, an ulcerated plaque may have discharged its debris to plug a distal stenosis. The distribution of these occlusions varies among many series reported, but in the author's experience, 80 per cent of the obstructive lesions are found in either the left anterior descending trunk or the right coronary artery, about equally divided. Most of the occlusions are found in the first 5 to 6 cm. of these major trunks. Frequently, more than one occlusive lesion, perhaps of different ages, can be demonstrated in the patient with one or several myocardial infarctions. Sometimes the multiple blockages produce only a single infarct, and it must be assumed that anastomotic circulation was adequate at the time of the earlier occlusion to maintain the viability of the dependent myocardium, but eventually the second occlusion rendered

this auxiliary network inadequate. Thus, it is possible for a recent occlusion of the right coronary artery to cause an infarction in the area of distribution of the left anterior descending. Presumably, marked narrowing of the left anterior descending led to the development of collateral circulation from the right coronary artery. Subsequent occlusion, then, of the right coronary, resulted in infarction of that area of the myocardium whose marginal viability was sustained by collateral circulation. Such a phenomenon is referred to as **paradoxic infarction** where the final causative vascular event occurs in one major trunk while the ischemic necrosis appears in an area normally dependent upon another trunk. For the many reasons already given, no occlusion may be encountered in hearts having a myocardial infarct.

Whatever the coronary trunk affected, the infarct almost invariably occurs in the left ventricle or interventricular septum. Even when the right coronary is obstructed, the infarct appears in the posterior wall of the left ventricle and posterior region of the interventricular septum. It is proposed that the thicker-walled left ventricle carrying the brunt of the cardiac workload is more dependent on blood supply than the thinner-walled right ventricle which may receive sufficient oxygen and nutrition through the thebesian system and by imbibition. For this reason, atrial infarcts are very uncommon. In about 5 per cent of left ventricular infarcts, the right ventricle and/or the atria are also affected. Right ventricular infarcts are more frequent in the presence of cardiac hypertrophy involving the right ventricle or congestive failure. In most instances of myocardial infarction, particularly when the infarct exceeds 3 to 4 cm. in diameter, it extends throughout the thickness of the myocardium to involve the contiguous epicardium and endocardium. Small infarcts, however, may be confined to the central muscle mass. Rarely, small lesions are localized to the subendocardial zone, in which case they are termed **Zahn's infarcts.** Infarcts usually have an irregular perimeter, dictated by the pattern of the interdigitating vascular supply.

Depending upon the length of survival of the patient, the ischemic area undergoes a progressive sequence of macroscopic changes (Mallory et al., 1939). Because of the earlier consideration of the time required for biochemical reactions to effect morphologic changes, it should come as no surprise that myocardial infarcts **less than 12 hours old** are virtually inapparent on gross examination. A slight pallor may be present. By **18 to 24 hours,** the area is usually more clearly anemic and gray-brown, contrasting with the surrounding normal red-brown myocardium. The consistency is still unaltered. Between the **second and fourth days,** the necrotic focus becomes more sharply defined with a hyperemic border. The central portion is distinctly yellow-brown and soft, due to the onset of fatty

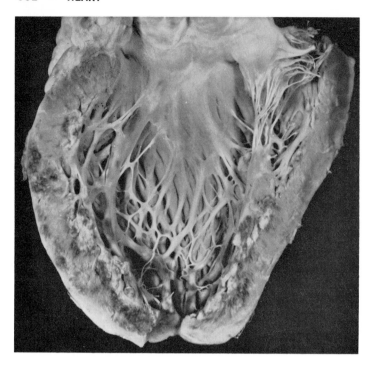

Figure 16–6. Myocardial infarction. An infarct of approximately one week's duration. The necrotic muscle is pale and is rimmed by darker increased vascularization.

change. Between the **fourth and tenth days,** the infarct is easily distinguished and varies from yellow-gray to bright yellow with the progression of fatty change. The central necrotic tissue is maximally soft and often contains areas of hemorrhage. The margins are intensely red and highly vascularized (Fig. 16–6). Becoming grossly apparent at approximately the **tenth day,** there is progressive replacement of the necrotic muscle by the ingrowth of fibrous, vascularized scar tissue. In most instances, this scarring is well advanced by the end of the sixth week, but the time required for total replacement depends upon the size of the original infarct. In many hearts, infarcts of varying ages may be identified. These may represent repeated infarctions, or perhaps are due to the centrifugal expansion of a central older focus, a process known as **progressive infarction.**

There are many complications associated with myocardial infarcts. A **fibrinous** or **fibrino-hemorrhagic pericarditis** usually develops about the second or third day. This may be localized to the region overlying the necrotic area or it may be generalized, in which case it is speculated to be of autoimmune origin. With healing of the infarct, the pericarditis usually resolves, but occasionally it organizes to produce permanent **fibrous adhesions.** Involvement of the ventricular endocardium often results in dense fibrous thickening as well as in **mural thrombosis,** which produces a risk of **peripheral embolism** (Fig. 16–7). Rupture of the infarct may occur, most often toward the end of the first week or in the beginning of the second, when

the ischemic focus is maximally soft. However, with excessive activity, such as occurs in psychotic patients, rupture may occur within a day of infarction or, in other instances, it may occur as late as the end of the second week. Most ruptures lead to massive pericardial hemorrhage and **cardiac tamponade.** Rupture of the interventricular septum produces a left to right shunt. With large infarcts, the consequent tough fibrous scar may undergo progressive

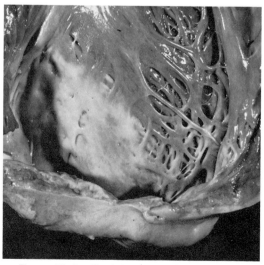

Figure 16–7. Healed myocardial infarction. The myocardium of the apical region is thinned and pale gray. The subendocardial fibrosis is apparent as pale gray thickening of the endocardium.

ballooning in the course of months to years, eventually to produce a **ventricular aneurysm.** Mural thrombosis is common in such aneurysms.

Under the light microscope, the coagulative necrosis of the irreversibly injured cells is not detectable with usual tissue stains for the first six to 12 hours. Glycogen depletion (using the PAS stain) and histochemical methods to detect loss of oxidases and dehydrogenases may disclose alterations earlier (one to two hours). Soon thereafter, the myocardial fibers undergo coagulation necrosis, usually accompanied by some interstitial edema, fresh hemorrhage and scant marginal neutrophilic exudation. During the subsequent days, the neutrophilic exudation increases, the dead fibers become more distinctly coagulated, nuclei become pyknotic or disappear, the cross striations become indistinct and the cytoplasm becomes filled with finely dispersed fat droplets (Fig. 16—8). Removal of the necrotic cytoplasm occurs both by catalysis initiated by release of lysosomal enzymes and phagocytosis by scavenger macrophages. Fibrovascular ingrowth becomes evident in the margins toward the end of the first week, and usually completely replaces the area of necrosis by six weeks although, in very large infarcts, central islands of persistent necrotic muscle may be present even months after the acute event (Figs. 16—9 and 16—10). Although the infarct may

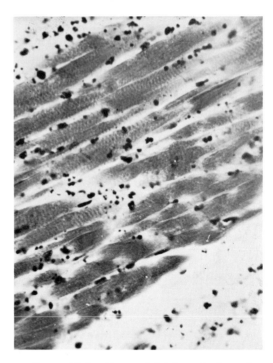

Figure 16-8. Myocardial infarct 3 days of age. The muscle fibers are still reasonably intact and cross striations are apparent.

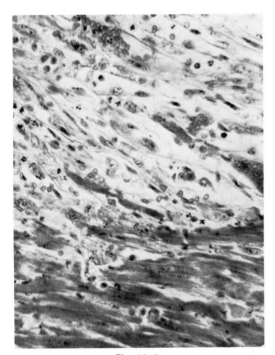

Fig. 16-9

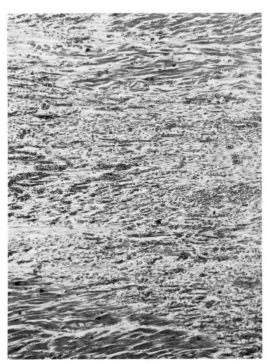

Fig. 16-10

Figure 16-9. Myocardial infarct 10 days of age. The margin of the infarct shows loss of sarcoplasm of fibers and ingrowth of fibroblasts.

Figure 16-10. Myocardial infarct of approximately two week's duration with marked vascularization, resorption of necrotic muscle cells and beginning cellular fibrous replacement.

appear to have traversed the entire thickness of the left ventricle or interventricular septum, there is usually a very narrow zone of preserved subendocardial and subepicardial muscle. Presumably, these cells are maintained by imbibition.

As is well known, cell death occurs some long time before the changes become sufficiently advanced to become apparent under the light microscope. Great effort has been made to establish histochemical or ultrastructural parameters of early cell death in the hope of being able to clearly document myocardial infarction in the patient who dies suddenly and shortly after an acute attack (Shnitka and Nachlas, 1963) (Fine et al., 1966) (Morales and Fine, 1966). By electron microscopy, ultrastructural alterations can be seen following 60 minutes of ischemia. Some of these changes are relaxation of myofibrils, the appearance of prominent I bands, swelling of mitochondria and decrease in the matrix density of the mitochondria (Jennings et al., 1969). Irreversibly injured cells leak potassium, and depleted levels of this electrolyte in areas of infarction have been proposed as being useful in identifying the early (one hour) infarct (Zugibe et al., 1966). But despite all of these sophisticated techniques, the problem of identifying the very early infarct is still not solved.

Clinical Course. The onset of an MI is usually marked by sudden, devastating, crushing substernal or precordial pain which often radiates to the left shoulder, arm or jaw. In most instances, the pain is accompanied by anxiety, faintness, sweating, dizziness, nausea and vomiting. Uncommonly, the infarct occurs silently or is considered by the patient to be indigestion. All too frequently (in about 20 to 25 per cent of all acute attacks), sudden death is the first clinical manifestation of acute myocardial infarction. Here sudden death is defined as that which occurs within an estimated 24 hours of the onset of acute symptoms and signs. Those who survive the onset of the acute attack usually suffer a drop in blood pressure, sometimes to shock levels. Electrical disturbances appear almost at once and are so common that they can hardly be considered as complications, but rather as part of the symptom complex. They take the form of disturbances in rate, rhythm or conduction. The most frequent arrhythmias are ventricular and atrial extrasystoles, sinus tachycardia and sinus bradycardia. The most lethal, probably accounting for most of the sudden deaths, are complete heart block, ventricular fibrillation and sinus tachycardia (Jewitt et al., 1969). Even in the absence of arrhythmias, about two-thirds of acutely infarcted patients develop acute myocardial failure and pulmonary edema (Lown et al., 1969). In about 10 per

cent of these patients, the acute myocardial failure is so profound as to constitute cardiogenic shock. When this supervenes, the outlook is particularly grave and approximately 70 to 90 per cent of such patients die despite all efforts to reverse it. The combination of pulmonary edema and shock comprises a true therapeutic nightmare since the administration of fluid or blood for the hypotension only worsens the pulmonary problem.

The diagnosis of acute myocardial infarction can often be made as soon as the patient is seen. The patient is likely to be sweaty, ashen gray, laboring for breath, anxious and obviously gravely ill. However, in most instances, laboratory evidence is necessary to confirm or establish the diagnosis. In the early course, elevation of serum levels of myocardial enzymes may be expected. Classically, SGOT and LDH levels rise to a peak in 12 to 24 hours. While the SGOT soon falls, the LDH may remain elevated for 7 to 10 days. However, hepatocellular disease and pulmonary infarctions, both of which constitute possible differential diagnoses in a patient with chest pain, also cause elevation of the same enzymes. Most cardiologists, therefore, prefer quantitation of creatine phosphokinase (CPK). Elevated levels of this enzyme are encountered earlier (six to eight hours) and promptly fall to normal within 48 hours. CPK also has greater specificity since it is only found in cardiac and skeletal muscles, and it is highly unlikely that skeletal muscle disease could mimic the symptom complex of myocardial infarction. Electrocardiographic changes are even more definitive than serum enzymes. Classically, there is first elevation of the ST segment within 24 hours, followed by the development of abnormal Q waves and inversion of the T waves. Moreover, as the acute infarct evolves over the span of days and weeks, the changing electrocardiographic patterns document the presence of an acute and later healing infarct. A variety of nonspecific clinical findings are also present in the acutely infarcted patient such as leukocytosis, elevated C-reactive proteins and an increased erythrocyte sedimentation rate. An enormous array of more sophisticated techniques are also employed such as coronary arteriography, vector cardiography, determinations of lactic acid levels in the venous effluent of the coronary sinus and others. Diagnostic methods are not lacking; only effective methods of prevention and cure are.

The major complications of myocardial infarction include, as mentioned in the presentation of the morphologic changes: (1) rupture of the infarct, (2) thromboembolism possibly arising from mural thrombi or from thrombosis in the deep veins of the legs, presumably secondary to bed rest and circulatory stasis, (3) development of a ventricular aneurysm in the late healed stages of the process and (4) fibrinous pericarditis which usually occurs early and is not generally of great clinical significance.

It is surprisingly difficult to obtain a longitudinal overview of the ability of these patients to survive at different stages in the progress of their disease. As stated, about 20 per cent of all MI's end in sudden death (Paul, 1971). Most of these deaths occur at home or in the ambulance and so are not included in hospital data (Kuller, 1969). In those who reach the hospital and receive optimal clinical care, the death rate for the first week of the disease is of the order of 10 to 15 per cent. Thereafter, about 6 or 7 per cent die during the subsequent 28 days. Among those who survive for a month, the mortality remains about 5 per cent per year for the next five years and then gradually falls to control rates. In general, the mortality for an acute attack is in the range of 30 to 40 per cent. The early deaths are usually due to electrical failures, and these represent perhaps the most tragic aspect of this disease. These sudden deaths are more common in younger patients, and many might have been saved by the effective therapy now available for preventing or controlling arrhythmias. Thereafter, cardiogenic shock and cardiac decompensation along with rupture of the heart are the major causes of death in the first week. Subsequently, cardiac decompensation and embolization underlie most of the fatalities. Unpredictable, but often fatal, is the sudden extension of the acute infarct or a new infarct with the attendant risks of arrhythmia, cardiac decompensation and power failure. The challenges for the future are not only to control atherosclerosis and thus lessen the incidence of this devastating disease, but also to devise means of promptly reaching these patients after infarction so as to control the electrical failures that contribute so heavily to sudden death. Some of the efforts made to reduce the incidence of severe coronary atherosclerosis and, therefore, myocardial infarction were discussed on p. 601. It suffices here to say that in a recent study of mental patients (institutionalized), a cholesterol-lowering diet effected approximately a 50 per cent reduction in the mortality from myocardial infarction in both males and females (Miettinen et al., 1972).

HYPERTENSIVE HEART DISEASE

Hypertensive heart disease is characterized anatomically by marked left ventricular hypertrophy, resulting from sustained systemic hypertension. Hypertension is here defined as an elevation of blood pressure above 90 mm. Hg diastolic, or 140 mm. Hg systolic. The myocardial hypertrophy may maintain cardiac compensation for many years, even in the presence of the increased workload occasioned by the hypertension, but eventually 30 to 40 per cent of these patients succumb to cardiac complications. It is one of the most common and most important forms of heart disease, and it is estimated that close to 100,000 deaths are caused annually by heart failure due to hypertension. However, this mortality rate must be interpreted with the knowledge that hypertension, while affecting the myocardium, also predisposes to the development of coronary atherosclerosis. Thus, about half of the deaths are directly attributable to hypertensive heart disease, and the other half, to hypertension-aggravated coronary heart disease.

Incidence. The incidence of hypertension reported in the literature varies widely, presumably because different levels of blood pressure have been selected as the upper limits of normal, and because the methods of obtaining the data also differ. Perera (1948) states that hypertension is found in about 5 per cent of the adult population. In individuals over the age of 50, this incidence might be increased to about 25 to 30 per cent.

While it is known that hypertension is most common in middle or later life, it may also occur in youth and even infancy. Females are affected about twice as often as males, but females tolerate elevations of blood pressure much more blandly than males without developing heart or vascular damage. Heredity occupies an important place as one of the predisposing factors. About 46 per cent of the offspring have hypertension if both parents are hypertensive, while only 3 per cent of the offspring of normotensives have elevated levels of blood pressure. Race and climate are also of some importance. Hypertension is somewhat more common in blacks in the United States than among the white population. Hypertension is also less common and less severe in tropical and semitropical climates. Environmental conditions, possibly those that impose stress, materially affect the incidence of hypertension, as illustrated by the lower incidence of hypertension in Chinese people living in their own country as compared with the Chinese living in the United States. It has repeatedly been demonstrated that elevated blood pressures are more common in the overweight, and that reduction in weight is accompanied by a lowering of the blood pressure.

Etiology and Pathogenesis. The theoretical considerations of the etiology and pathogenesis of hypertension are considered under the discussion of the kidney (p. 1128). Nevertheless, it is pertinent at this time to consider the effect of sustained hypertension upon the heart.

The blood pressure can only be elevated when the peripheral arterial resistance to the flow of blood is increased. The increased peripheral resistance must be due either to widespread vasoconstriction of the peripheral vascular bed, principally the arterioles and small arteries, or to diffuse organic vascular disease. Both mechanisms are involved in most cases of systemic hypertension. The heart, then, must maintain a normal cardiac output against this increased peripheral resistance, and can only accomplish this augmented workload by an increased expenditure of energy, accomplished by physiologic stretching of its muscle fibers, followed by hypertrophy. From recent surveys, it appears as though the level of hypertension, rather than the duration, is the major factor in the development of the cardiac hypertrophy. *As long as the cardiac reserve is not exhausted and the hypertrophy maintains a normal cardiac output, compensation may exist.* Eventually, however, the cardiac reserve is exhausted and

dilatation of the failing heart ushers in decompensation. The factors that determine when the hypertrophied heart will decompensate are still mysterious, but some consideration of this enigma was given on p. 640. In this particular setting, the augmenting effect of elevated levels of blood pressure on the advance of coronary atherosclerosis undoubtedly contributes to the ultimate onset of cardiac failure.

The principal morphologic evidences of hypertensive heart disease are left ventricular thickening with accompanying increases in size and weight of the heart (Fig. 16–11). It should be noted that **the anatomic diagnosis of hypertensive heart disease can be made only in the absence of other cardiac abnormalities, such as valvular lesions, congenital abnormalities and diseases of the aorta, which of themselves may be productive of increased cardiac workload** and consequent myocardial hypertrophy. Such abnormalities make the anatomic diagnosis of hypertensive heart disease impossible, although, admittedly, concomitant hypertension may have contributed to the myocardial hypertrophy.

During the stages of compensated hypertensive heart disease, the hypertrophy principally affects the left ventricle. The hypertrophy may thicken the left ventricular wall to more than 2.5 cm. and

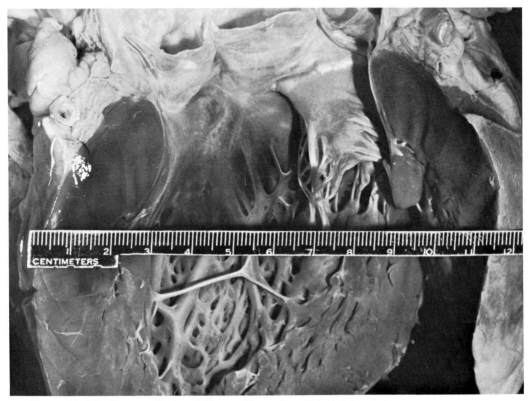

Figure 16–11. Hypertensive heart disease. The myocardial thickness is increased to 2 to 2.5 cm.

increase the total weight of the heart to 500 to 700 gm. Thickening of the left ventricular wall occurs at the expense of the volume of the left ventricular chamber, and is referred to as **concentric hypertrophy.**

With the onset of decompensation, dilatation of the left ventricle occurs, and the overall dimensions of the heart may be considerably enlarged. It may be only at this time that cardiac enlargement is sufficiently prominent to be demonstrable on x-ray or clinical examination. The stretching of the heart wall decreases the thickness of the myocardium and may thus mask the preexistent thickening. Incomplete emptying of the failing left ventricle throws an increased burden through the atria and pulmonary circulation onto the right side of the heart, with resultant hypertrophy and dilatation of all cardiac chambers. Valvular deformities and pathologic involvement of the epicardium and endocardium are absent. Although coronary atherosclerosis is not an intrinsic feature of hypertensive heart disease, it is frequently found in such hearts because of the causal relationship mentioned previously.

There are no microscopic characteristics of hypertensive heart disease, and microscopic examination of the myocardium is largely of value in ruling out other forms of myocardial disease that may produce cardiac failure and hypertrophy. Although the muscle fibers must have increased in size, they often do not appear abnormally large on simple microscopic examination. Electron microscopy has disclosed increased numbers and enlargement of mitochondria and increased numbers of myofibrils (Pelosi and Agliati, 1968). The coronary circulation may be entirely normal, but is commonly the seat of atherosclerosis. Occasionally, the arteriolar walls are thickened as a reflection of the hypertension.

Increasing awareness of a large group of rare cardiopathies that cause cardiac hypertrophy has compounded the difficulty in making a diagnosis of hypertensive heart disease. These conditions, some familial, others nutritional and still others of unknown causation, may all produce cardiac enlargement without apparent hypertension. They are discussed more fully on page 689.

Clinical Course. Compensated hypertensive heart disease is asymptomatic and consists merely of cardiac enlargement without signs or symptoms of circulatory insufficiency. The patient, however, may have other symptoms of hypertension, such as palpitation, headaches and poorly defined asthenia. Abnormalities of the retinal vessels and eye grounds known as hypertensive retinopathy may appear. These ocular changes are associated with extremely severe hypertension.

Symptoms of cardiac decompensation predominantly reflect left ventricular failure.

The clinical manifestations stem chiefly from pulmonary congestion and edema caused by the venous stasis in the lungs. These consist of dyspnea, paroxysmal nocturnal dyspnea, orthopnea, cough and hemoptysis. Concomitant coronary atherosclerosis may complicate the clinical picture by producing signs and symptoms referable to coronary vascular insufficiency. The diagnosis of this condition is based on the finding of systemic hypertension and clinical, roentgenologic or electrocardiographic evidence of cardiomegaly. Other causes for the cardiac enlargement must be ruled out.

The course of hypertensive heart disease is quite variable. When the hypertension is of moderate severity, the heart disease may be well tolerated for decades. With severe hypertension, decompensation is usually followed by death within a year.

It should be made clear at this point that heart disease is only one of the ways in which hypertension kills. In the milder form of "essential" hypertension (p. 1128), about 25 per cent die of heart failure; 15 per cent, of cerebrovascular accidents; and a few, of renal failure. Most die of unrelated causes. With malignant hypertension (p. 1130), most die of renal failure, but a few, of cerebral hemorrhage or cardiac failure. Potent and effective antihypertension therapy is now available and promises dramatic control of hypertension and its sequelae.

RHEUMATIC HEART DISEASE (RHD)

Rheumatic fever (RF) is a systemic nonsuppurative inflammatory disease apparently caused by an immunologic reaction to an infection with group A beta hemolytic streptococci. Classically, the disease occurs in acute febrile attacks spaced by remissions lasting from months to years or even decades. The joints, tendons, fascial sheaths, serosal membranes, skin, respiratory system and vessels may all be affected in variable combinations, but it is the heart which bears the brunt of the attack and suffers the most disabling, often irreversible, damage. Thus, rheumatic fever is principally of importance because it may lead to rheumatic heart disease. The involvement of the other sites is generally benign and reversible.

Morphologically, RF is characterized by focal inflammatory lesions located usually within the connective tissue of the affected organs. In the heart, the lesions are particularly distinctive and are referred to as Aschoff bodies. *The Aschoff body comprises a localized area of inflammation having a central deposit of amorphous fibrinoid material surrounded by an inflammatory infiltrate of mesenchymal cells* (Fig. 16–12). For many years, rheumatic fever was considered to be a hypersensitivity "collagen disease," along with rheumatoid arthritis and systemic lupus erythematosus. However, it is now apparent that collagen itself is not the prime target of attack in any of these diseases, and so they are all now referred to more generally as "connective tissue diseases." There is much justification for such a categorization in the case of rheumatic fever because recent evidence indicates that connective tissue mucopolysaccharides appear to be one of the antigenic targets of the immunologic response, but more important targets are cardiac and smooth muscle cells.

Incidence. The incidence of RF has undergone a gratifying decline as the result of prevention and prompt treatment of streptococcal infections with antibacterial drugs. Nonetheless, it continues to be a major cause of heart disease, particularly in children. Many factors influence the development of this disease, such as age, heredity and socioeconomic conditions. It rarely affects children under four years of age (Glancy et al., 1969). About 90 per cent of patients have their first attack between the ages of five and 15 years, but adults, even of advanced years, are still vulnerable to primary and recurrent attacks. Some genetic predisposition to rheumatic fever is suspected but not well established. This disease occurs in only 3 per cent of persons with untreated group A streptococcal pharyngitis. But among those with a history of a previous attack, the disease recurs in about 50 per cent following subsequent streptococcal infection, suggesting some peculiar individual predisposition. Familial clustering of the disease is also common, but this is more likely related to exposure of family groups to a common causative agent. Indeed, rheumatic fever is particularly prevalent among those living under crowded, inadequate conditions, presumably reflecting cross infections and poor medical care (Gordis et al., 1969). For this reason, nonwhites have a higher incidence of rheumatic infections than whites, but no inherent racial susceptibility has been identified.

Evidence of the decline in the incidence and in the morbidity and mortality rates of RF over the past several decades in the United States comes from several sources. Among college freshmen, rheumatic heart disease or a history of rheumatic fever declined over the years, 1956 to 1965, from a prevalence rate of 17 per 1000 students to 11. Over the 40-year time span, 1920 to 1960, the death rate from this disease between the ages of five and 25 fell nearly 90 per cent. But rheumatic fever and rheumatic heart disease are not disappearing medical problems because in 1967 they were still responsible for over 14,000 deaths in the United States. Although it is predominantly a disease of childhood, because of its long chronicity and occasional onset in advanced life, RF is also a cause of cardiac disease and death in the aged.

Etiology and Pathogenesis. While strong, the evidence for a causal relationship between beta hemolytic streptococcal infections and acute rheumatic fever is not irrefutable. Usually the attack develops from one to four weeks following a pharyngitis. Any strain of the group A streptococci may be involved. It should be noted, however, that almost half of the patients fail to provide a history of antecedent acute infection and have negative throat cultures at the time they seek medical attention. This phenomenon might be explained as an asymptomatic and subclinical streptococcal infection because serologic evidence of streptococcal infection can be found in well over 95 per cent of these patients (Stollerman and

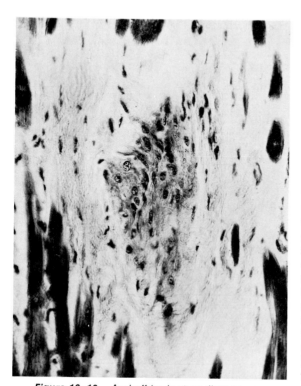

Figure 16–12. Aschoff body at medium power.

Pearce, 1968). Elevated titers of antistreptolysin O (ASO) are present in about 85 per cent of patients, and most of the remainder have significant titers of antistreptokinase, antidesoxyribonuclease, antihyaluronidase or antibodies to one of the other streptococcal enzymes. Further evidence of the streptococcal relationship has been provided by the remarkable effectiveness of prophylactic regimens of penicillin or one of its derivatives in preventing not only streptococcal infections but also attacks of rheumatic fever. However, reports still appear suggesting that other bacterial or viral infections may incite attacks of rheumatic fever. Burch and his colleagues (1970), in a tightly reasoned critique, point out that viruses are much more common causes of pharyngitis than streptococci, can themselves cause valvular lesions in animals, and may well underlie the cardiac pathology in almost half of the patients who have negative throat cultures for streptococci. Moreover, nonspecific rises of the ASO titer have been shown to occur with nonstreptococcal infections. The precise etiology of rheumatic fever must continue to remain an open question but, for the present, streptococcal infections are most strongly implicated.

Another bothersome problem in the pathogenesis of this disease is that the precise mechanism by which streptococcal infections (if they are etiologic) evoke rheumatic fever is still not known. Five proposals have been made: (1) persistence of streptococci, (2) the development of L-forms of streptococci, (3) injury resulting from streptococcal products, (4) an abnormal hypersensitivity reaction to the streptococci and (5) antibodies to streptococci cross reacting with the tissues of the host. The first three proposals are insufficiently documented or accepted to merit further discussion, but are reviewed in a recent paper (Joorabchi, 1969). With regard to the last two, there is abundant evidence in support of an immunologic reaction. The latent period between the pharyngitis (? streptococcal infection) and the onset of acute RF fits well. Acute RF has many morphologic resemblances with other forms of immunologic disease such as systemic lupus erythematosus and rheumatoid arthritis. But the problem remains of whether rheumatic fever is the result of an abnormal or perhaps excessive immune reaction against streptococcal antigens (thus likening the disease somewhat to poststreptococcal glomerulonephritis) or, instead, results from antigenic overlaps between streptococci and the tissues of the host. In the latter circumstance, antibodies against the shared antigens would induce the tissue lesions. *The weight of ev-* *idence at the present time suggests that antibodies against streptococci cross react with myocardial fibers, smooth muscle cells in arterial walls and connective tissue glycoproteins to induce the characteristic morphologic changes.* Antibodies to heart muscle have been demonstrated in the sera of up to 77 per cent of patients with acute rheumatic fever, in approximately 15 per cent of those with inactive rheumatic heart disease and in 0 to 4 per cent of healthy controls (Kaplan et al., 1961) (Kaplan and Frengley, 1969). Immunoglobulins and complement, principally localized in the sarcolemma of cardiac myofibers and in the walls of blood vessels, have been found by immunofluorescent techniques in the myocardium of children dying of fulminant rheumatic carditis (Kaplan et al., 1964). The injection into rabbits of cell walls of streptococci isolated from rheumatic fever patients yields antibodies which can be localized by immunofluorescent techniques in the sarcolemma of myocardial fibers and the smooth muscle of the walls of blood vessels, the precise locations in which gamma globulins have been found in patients (Kaplan and Meyeserian, 1962). Cross reactions have also been demonstrated between the antigens derived from human heart muscle and the cell membrane of all group A streptococcal strains tested (Zabriskie et al., 1964). The antibodies against group A streptococci also cross react with structural glycoproteins derived from heart valves of man, providing a possible explanation for the attack in RF of not only the myocardium but also the endocardium, cardiac valves and extracardiac sites.

Despite all this immunologic evidence, dilemmas remain. The deposits of immunoglobulins and complement are usually not solely concentrated in the Aschoff bodies, long thought to be the focal points of injury in active rheumatic involvement. The glycoproteins that are cross reactive with streptococcal antibodies are distributed throughout the body, and if such be the case, why the focal and selective distribution of Aschoff bodies in rheumatic fever? Other questions could be raised, but it will suffice that the genesis of this disease is still not completely understood.

Morphology. The pathognomonic focal inflammatory lesion of rheumatic fever is the Aschoff body. Aschoff bodies are classically found in the heart, but somewhat less distinctive variants are also encountered in the synovia of joints, in and about joint capsules, tendons and fascia and, less often, in serosal membranes and subcutaneous tissues. Aschoff bodies proceed through three phases: (1) exudative, (2) proliferative and (3) healed. Only

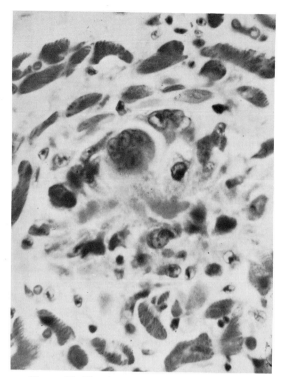

Figure 16-13. Aschoff body at high power detail to illustrate the multinucleate giant cell and central "fibrinoid necrosis."

the proliferative phase is diagnostic of RF. In the early exudative phase, the central fibrinoid focus within the connective tissue of the heart is surrounded by white cells, chiefly neutrophils and scattered lymphocytes, plasma cells and histiocytes. The collagen fibers in this focus may appear swollen and ragged, but this is attributable to their **being layered by proteinous deposits** rather than to injury. As mentioned earlier, immunoglobulins in active rheumatic fever are found principally in the sarcolemma of muscle cells and are not abundant, if present at all, in the centers of these Aschoff bodies. This enigma remains unexplained. In the distinctive proliferative phase which follows, the central focus is surrounded by a rim of mononuclear white cells, fibroblasts, large modified mesenchymal cells known as Anitschkow myocytes and an occasional multinucleate Aschoff giant cell (Fig. 16–13). Anitschkow myocytes are also known as "caterpillar cells" because the chromatin is disposed in the center of the nucleus in the form of a slender, wavy ribbon that resembles an attenuated body with innumerable fine leg-like projections. The origin of these cells is controversial, but most investigators consider them to be altered fibroblasts rather than modified muscle cells (Wagner and Siew, 1970). The giant cells classically have one, two or several folded multilobate nuclei with prominent "owl-eyed" nucleoli. **Fully developed Aschoff bodies**

having all the features just described are **morphologic hallmarks of RF.** The late healed phase evolves by progressive fibrosis and hyalinization of the focus of inflammation. Only a scattering of lymphocytes with occasional plasma cells and histiocytes may persist as the last remnants of the earlier focus of cellularity.

The significance and genesis of the Aschoff body are among the more intriguing puzzles in pathology. For some long time, it was believed that the exudative and proliferative stages denoted clinical activity of the disease. With the advent of cardiac surgery and the availability of biopsies of auricular appendages, exudative and proliferative Aschoff bodies were found in the hearts of 40 to 50 per cent of rheumatic patients undergoing repair of chronic stenosing valvular deformities. These patients had been meticulously screened by all available clinical techniques and were judged to have quiescent disease. Two interpretations are possible: the proliferative phase of the Aschoff body might persist as a focus long after clinical signs of activity have disappeared; alternatively, rheumatic fever might constitute a latent disorder which smolders over the span of years. Aschoff bodies might then be present in the absence of acute attacks. We can go no further in attempting to explain the significance of the Aschoff body. The localization of Aschoff bodies is equally inscrutable. When found in the heart, they are largely distributed in perivascular, subendocardial and subepicardial connective tissue. Curiously they are rarely found within the mass of closely packed myocardial cells, as might be expected if the antigenic targets of the streptococcal antibodies are the sarcolemma or plasma membranes of muscle cells and connective tissue glycoproteins. Murphy (1960) has demonstrated smooth muscle fibers in the endocardium and valve leaflets. Conceivably, then, the reaction producing valvular and connective tissue localizations might focus on the smooth muscle cells or on the glycoproteins. Perhaps the extracardiac lesions represent other targets attacked by the cross reacting antibodies. Here the matter must rest.

Rheumatic carditis develops with the initial attack in about half of the cases. Any of the three layers of the heart—epicardium, myocardium or endocardium—may be involved singly or in combination. Most often, all three layers are affected simultaneously (pancarditis) (Clawson, 1940). Depending on the stage of the disease, the heart may exhibit the features of acute rheumatic carditis, chronic or so-called healed rheumatic carditis or, in some cases, chronic carditis with superimposed active carditis when the patient has experienced recurrent attacks.

During the acute stage, the pericarditis takes the form of a diffuse, nonspecific fibrinous or serofibrinous inflammatory reaction described previously (p. 80) as a "bread and butter" pericarditis (Figs.

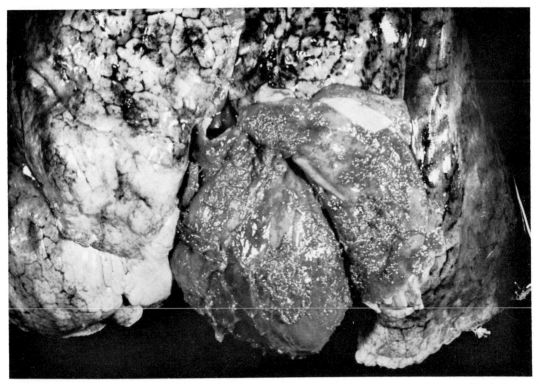

Figure 16-14. *Acute rheumatic fibrinous pericarditis. The pericardial sac has been opened with the heart still attached to the lungs.*

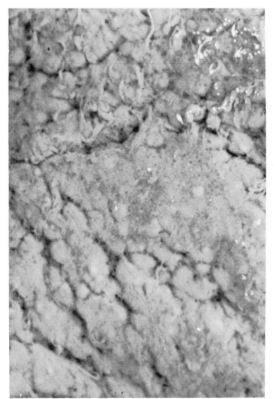

Figure 16-15. *A close-up of the shaggy pericardial fibrinoid exudate to illustrate the "bread and butter" quality of the exudate.*

16—14 and 16—15). As with all fibrinous exudations, the pericarditis may either resolve or become organized, usually resulting in only delicate violin-string adhesions or plaque-like thickenings of the pericardial surfaces that do not impair cardiac function. Aschoff bodies may be seen in the subserosal fibrofatty tissue in fulminant cases.

Myocardial involvement with Aschoff bodies localized principally in the connective tissue stroma of the myocardium is responsible for most of the deaths during the acute, active phase of the disease. The myocarditis may be inapparent on gross inspection, save possibly for some dilatation, pallor and flabbiness of the heart muscle. The extent of the myocardial involvement becomes evident only on histologic examination with the identification of Aschoff bodies. Later, as mentioned, the Aschoff bodies become fibrosed and are virtually inapparent since the scarring blends in with the surrounding connective tissue background. Rarely, in extremely florid instances, the myocardial involvement takes the form of diffuse or patchy increases in ground substance associated with a prominent neutrophilic infiltration in perivascular and subepicardial areas. It would be quite impossible to establish the identity of such changes without the recognition of occasional, widely scattered, characteristic Aschoff bodies. While myocarditis may exist alone, it is usually accompanied by endocarditis.

Endocardial involvement is the most ominous aspect of rheumatic fever and causes most of the deaths, usually long after the acute disease has subsided. While any valve may be affected, the mitral valve alone is affected in nearly 50 per cent of the cases, and the mitral and aortic valves together in almost 50 per cent of the cases. Trivalvular involvement which includes the tricuspid valve and solitary involvement of the aortic valve are encountered only rarely (Morrow et al., 1968). The pulmonary valve is uncommonly affected either alone or in combination. Early, the acutely affected valves are red, swollen and thickened. This is usually most marked toward the free margins of the cusps. These changes may be accompanied by a precipitate of fibrin or extrusion of ground substance which produces tiny (1 to 2 mm.) friable vegetations (**verrucae**) along the lines of closure of the leaflets (Fig. 16–16). These verrucae appear as irregular warty projections, and probably result from the precipitate of fibrin at sites of erosion or ulceration of inflamed endocardial surfaces along the lines of closure where the leaflets impinge upon each other. They occur on the surfaces exposed to the forward flow of blood and are distributed either along the entire line of closure or in small clusters with uninvolved intervening areas. At the commissures, they may cause interadherence of leaflets. Similar verrucae may sometimes be seen along the chordae tendineae. Histologic examination of these lesions may be nonspecific, revealing only precipitation of fibrinoid with an underlying, nonspecific, leukocytic infiltrate. However, plump fibroblasts and cells resembling the Anitschkow myocytes are occasionally found rimming the base of the vegetation. Recognizable Aschoff bodies are rarely present in these acute valvular lesions.

It is believed, but not definitely established, that acute rheumatic valvulitis may resolve without residuals but, in most instances, it leads to fibrous scarring and permanent deformity. As organization of the endocardial inflammation takes place, the valvular leaflets become thickened, fibrotic, shortened and blunted (Fig. 16–17). Fibrous bridging across the valvular commissures often produces a rigid **"fish mouth" or "button hole" stenotic deformity of the mitral valve** (Fig. 16–18). The chordae tendineae simultaneously become thickened, fused and shortened. When the tricuspid valve is involved, the changes resemble those of the mitral, but they are almost never as marked. In the aortic valve, the fibrosis also produces interadherence and stenoses as well as prominent nodular calcifications in the sinuses of Valsalva behind the leaflets. These aortic valve morphologic alterations are also encountered in aortic stenosis from other causes. With a tight mitral stenosis, the left atrium, and sometimes the right as well, progressively dilate. Often thrombi form within the auricular appendages. The mural endocardium in the left atrium may develop map-like thickenings called **McCallum's plaques.** These are thought to represent subendocardial aggregations of Aschoff bodies accompanied by pooling of ground substance. In time, these plaques may undergo fibrosis, leaving only an irregular area of endocardial wrinkling. It is to be emphasized that in the late healed stage of endocarditis, histologic changes are generally nonspecific since all Aschoff bodies may have disappeared. The recognition of healed rheumatic valvulitis is, therefore, more dependent on characteristic gross appearances than on histologic changes. Because the disease is characterized by recurrent attacks, acute rheumatic changes may be superimposed on those of healed carditis.

Rheumatic arthritis appears during the early stages of acute attacks in about 75 per cent of patients. Relatively few observations are available on these joints since they generally resolve and leave few sequelae. Early the synovial membranes are thickened, red, granular and sometimes ulcerated. Histologically, increased amounts of ground sub-

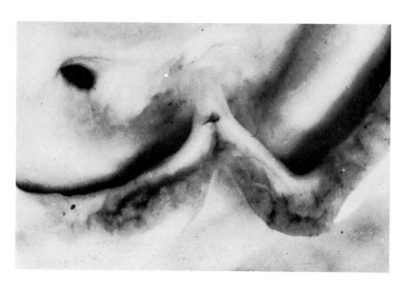

Figure 16–16. Acute rheumatic aortic valvulitis with rows of fibrinous vegetations along the lines of closure of the valve leaflets.

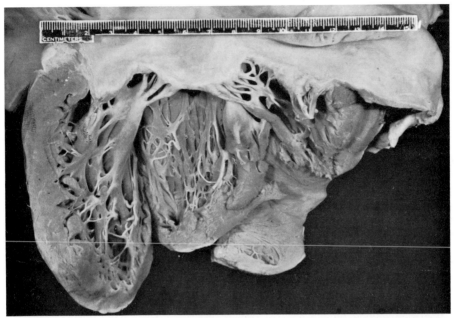

Fig. 16–17

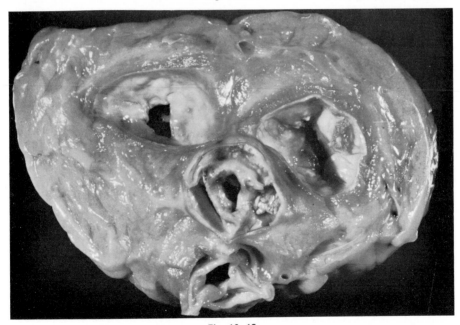

Fig. 16–18

Figure 16–17. *Healed mitral rheumatic valvulitis illustrating the fibrous thickening of the leaflets and the fusion, thickening and shortening of the chordae tendineae.*

Figure 16–18. *Healed trivalvular rheumatic valvulitis as viewed from above with the atria cut off. The aortic valve is in the mid-center field, the mitral in the upper right and the tricuspid in the upper left. All three valves are stenotic, fibrosed and markedly deformed.*

stance, focal deposits of fibrinoid and lesions resembling Aschoff bodies may be seen in the synovial membranes and occasionally in the tendons, joints and periarticular tissues. In rare cases, the underlying articular cartilage is exposed, and such cases may explain the rare finding of fibrous bridging across the joint space long after the acute phase has subsided. There is a strong suspicion, however, that such permanent joint damage may be the result of rheumatoid arthritis, and that the original diagnosis of rheumatic fever was in error. Typically, the arthritis of rheumatic fever is benign, transient and leaves no residual damage.

Skin lesions are encountered during the acute phase of the attack in a minority of patients. They take the form of **subcutaneous nodules** or a rash known as **erythema multiforme or marginatum.** The nodules are most often located overlying the extensor tendons of the extremities at the wrist, elbows, ankles and knees. They may occur singly or multiply. They vary in size from 1 to 4 cm. in diameter and are sharply circumscribed, freely movable, painless masses. Often there is redness of the overlying skin. Histologically, they appear as giant Aschoff bodies with a large central mass of fibrinoid enclosed within a rim of plump fibroblasts, lymphocytes, histiocytes and cells resembling Anitschkow myocytes. Aschoff giant cells are exceedingly uncommon. The erythematous lesions comprise large macules or papules which occur largely on the trunk. They are presumed to result from some hypersensitivity reaction related to the underlying systemic disease and are described more completely on p. 1419.

Rheumatic arteritis has been described in the coronary, renal, mesenteric and cerebral arteries as well as in the aorta and pulmonary vessels during the height of an attack. The morphologic alterations are characteristic of hypersensitivity angiitis and were described on p. 220 (Fig. 16–19).

Rheumatic pneumonitis is a rare complication of the acute disease which closely resembles a viral pneumonitis, both in its clinical manifestations as well as in its morphologic changes. The alveolar septa are thickened, edematous and infiltrated by mononuclear leukocytes and rare neutrophils. The air spaces often contain proteinous precipitate and fibrin which sometimes is layered on the alveolar walls to produce hyaline membranes. These histologic changes account for the fact that the lungs are firmer and heavier than normal, with poorly defined areas of congestion and increased consistency. Aschoff-like bodies have been described in the lungs, but they are not of the classic cardiac variety. More common than the acute pneumonitis are the changes of marked pulmonary congestion and edema seen in patients having a tight mitral stenosis for years. The stenosis first induces marked left atrial dilatation which in time leads to chronic, long-standing severe congestion of the lungs described on p. 321.

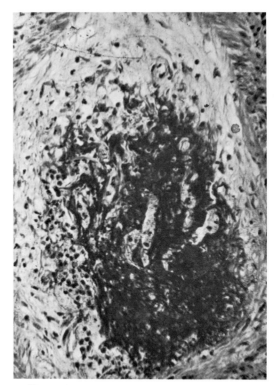

Figure 16–19. *Acute rheumatic vasculitis with extensive fibrinoid deposits and leukocytic infiltration.*

Clinical Course. Classically, the acute attack of rheumatic fever follows a streptococcal infection, usually a pharyngitis, after an interval of one to four weeks. The onset may be quite abrupt, with fever, tachycardia and painful swollen joints, or it may be exceedingly subtle and insidious in the form of vague malaise and mild fever. There are no specific symptoms or signs pathognomonic of rheumatic fever, and the diagnosis usually rests on the concurrence of two or more suggestive findings referred to as "Jones' criteria." These are set forth in Table 16–1. It is generally held that a diagnosis of rheumatic fever can be made when at least two of the major or one major and two minor criteria are exhibited by the patient. It is important to emphasize that the designation "major" relates to specificity and not to frequency of the manifestation. About three-quarters of these patients have acute arthritis characteristically migratory in nature. As the pain and swelling subside in one joint, others become involved. About half of the patients develop signs of cardiac involvement during the acute attack resulting from myocarditis or fibrinous pericarditis. The development of endocarditis is

TABLE 16–1. JONES' CRITERIA (REVISED) FOR GUIDANCE IN THE DIAGNOSIS OF RHEUMATIC FEVER*

Major Manifestations	Minor Manifestations
Carditis	*Clinical*
	Previous rheumatic fever or
Polyarthritis	rheumatic heart disease
	Arthralgia
Chorea	Fever
Erythema Marginatum	*Laboratory*
	Acute phase reactions
Subcutaneous Nodules	Erythrocyte sedimentation
	rate, C-reactive protein,
	leukocytosis
	Prolonged PR interval

Supporting Evidence of Streptococcal Infection

Increased titer of streptococcal antibodies
  ASO (antistreptolysin O)
  Other antibodies
Positive throat culture for group A streptococcus
Recent scarlet fever

*The presence of two major criteria, or of one major and two minor criteria, indicates a high probability of the presence of rheumatic fever. Evidence of a preceding streptococcal infection greatly strengthens the possibility of acute rheumatic fever. Its absence should make the diagnosis doubtful (except in Sydenham's chorea or longstanding carditis).

These criteria, originally proposed by T. Duckett Jones in 1944, were revised by the Council on Rheumatic Fever and Congenital Heart Disease of the American Heart Association.

From Stollerman, G. H., et al.: Committee report: Jones' criteria (revised) for guidance in the diagnosis of rheumatic fever. Circulation, 32:664, 1965. Revised, 1967. By permission of The American Heart Association, Inc. © 1967.

difficult to detect during the initial acute attack. Chorea (rapid, jerky, involuntary movements of the arms and legs), which occurs up to several months after the acute attack, is a third major manifestation of rheumatic fever. The skin changes generally appear long after the acute attack during the chronic phase of the disease. While the "minor manifestations" and supporting evidence of streptococcal infection are less specific, they must frequently be relied upon to establish a diagnosis. Because patients with a first attack of rheumatic fever are vulnerable to recurrences, a history of rheumatic fever should be weighed heavily when entertaining the diagnosis.

The most feared aspect of rheumatic fever is the development of carditis. In general, the younger the patient, the more likely the involvement of the heart. During the initial acute attack, it is the myocarditis that is most threat-ening, causing arrhythmias and other conduction disturbances. Atrial fibrillation is particularly common and is often associated with the development of auricular thrombi which are potential sources of emboli (Fig. 16–20). Cardiac dilatation may develop and produce murmurs of insufficiency, principally of the mitral valve. Such a murmur often disappears following the acute attack if the valve itself has not been damaged. On the whole, the prognosis of the primary attack is generally good, and only 1 per cent of patients die of fulminant rheumatic fever.

The long-term outlook for patients after an initial attack depends largely on whether carditis has occurred and on its severity. In the absence of cardiac involvement and recurrent attacks, the patient might be entirely free from residuals for the rest of a normal life. Most of such patients are now placed on continuous prophylactic antibacterial therapy which has been shown to be remarkably effective in preventing exacerbations of the disease (Quie and Ayoub, 1968). When carditis has occurred, the outlook depends on the severity of the valvular deformity. Such individuals may have little cardiac dysfunction and only a persistent murmur. However, some patients show progressive worsening of their cardiac status, presumably because of slowly progressive stenosing fibrosis of affected valves. This phenomenon is poorly understood, but has been attributed to subclinical activity of the disease. Women have a greater tendency for such progressive valvular scarring and are thus more vulnerable to longstanding mitral stenosis (Stollerman and Pearce, 1968). But even those who have suffered severe aortic or mitral valvular stenosis can now be greatly benefited by valvular surgery or prosthetic replacement of damaged valves. Without surgery and with mild stenosis of the mitral valve, the 10-year survival is in the order of 80 per cent. However, if the initial mitral damage is severe, the 10-year survival is low. Death is usually the consequence of progressive intractable congestive failure. Some patients die of superimposed complications. The damaged valves may become bacterially infected, giving rise to bacterial endocarditis. Embolization from mural thrombi within the atrial appendages may cause fatal infarctions of the brain or kidneys. Recurrent acute attacks rapidly worsen the prognosis. It should not be forgotten that recurrent or primary attacks may occur even in the advanced years of life, and so the prophylaxis against recurrent streptococcal infections must be maintained for the life of the patient.

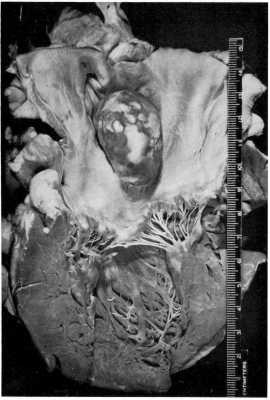

Figure 16–20. A well organized atrial mural thrombus in a heart with inactive rheumatic myocarditis.

CONGENITAL HEART DISEASE

Anomalous development of the heart continues to be an important cause of cardiac disease, representing the most common form of heart disease among children under the age of four. These anomalies either interfere with the normal streamlined flow of blood through the chambers, or produce shunts and abnormal pathways of flow. Often the resultant turbulence creates dramatic heart murmurs. When the anomaly permits blood to be shunted from the right to the left side of the heart (i.e., toward the systemic circulation), short-circuiting the lungs, the admixture of poorly oxygenated blood with that in the arterial circulation induces cyanosis, usually from birth. In contrast, when blood is shunted from left to right, a larger than normal volume reaches the lungs, but there is initially no cyanosis. However, in time, pulmonary hypertension ensues and sufficiently raises the pressure on the right side of the heart to produce a right to left shunt and, with such reversal of

flow, the late appearance of cyanosis, often termed *cyanose tardive.*

The exact incidence of the various forms of congenital heart disease varies among studies, depending on the population surveyed and the diagnostic methods employed. In autopsy series, the more severe and complicated forms will be represented excessively. In clinical series, some of the milder forms are likely to be missed unless sophisticated hemodynamic, angiographic and catheterization procedures are employed. Recognizing these difficulties, several fairly large studies have yielded the following approximate distribution (Storstein et al., 1964) (Nadas, 1963) (Hansen and Warburg, 1961).

	Per Cent
Acyanotic Shunt (Left-Right)	
Patent ductus arteriosus	12 to 20
Atrial septal defect	12 to 20
Ventricular septal defect (Roger's disease)	15 to 20
Cyanotic Shunt (Right-Left)	
Tetrology of Fallot	8 to 15
Eisenmenger complex (variant of the tetralogy of Fallot)	5
Transposition of great vessels	2 to 3
No Shunt	
Coarctation of the aorta	5 to 7
Aortic stenosis	4 to 5

Many other less common forms of congenital anomaly exist and can be found in the references cited. Attention should be called to the fact that the great preponderance of all forms of congenital heart disease fall into the acyanotic or cyanose tardive category and so may not be obvious at birth.

Etiology. Genetic and environmental influences contribute to the causation of congenital heart disease. For some forms, heredity plays a dominant and possibly total role. In certain families, atrial septal defects appear to be transmitted by autosomal dominant modes. Hereditary transmission is less clearly defined but is suspected in ventricular septal defects, pulmonary stenosis and tetralogy of Fallot. But in most forms of congenital heart disease, both heredity and the environment contribute and, in some instances, environmental influences are preponderant. German measles (rubella) during the first trimester of pregnancy is a well recognized cause of cardiac anomaly (p. 552). Other forms of viral infection during the first trimester of pregnancy have been less clearly implicated. Drugs such as thalidomide, taken during the fifth to eighth week of pregnancy, may contribute to anomalous development of the heart. All such environmental influences can only have effect on the developing heart when the fetus is exposed during the first two months of gestation. Indeed, most congenital anomalies originate during the fifth to eighth week of fetal life, the interval in which the definitive structure of the heart is being established. In this short span of time, the atria and ventricles separate, all valves form and the primitive truncus arteriosus is divided into the aorta and pulmonary artery. Development of the fetal heart is complete by the ninth week, and so environmental influences can no longer induce anomalous development of the heart.

VENTRICULAR SEPTAL DEFECTS (ROGER'S DISEASE)

This form of anomalous development of the heart is the most common cardiac anomaly. It represents approximately 15 to 20 per cent of all cases of congenital heart disease. Because it produces prominent clinical features, such as a loud systolic murmur and thrill, it is easily diagnosed and is the most readily identified form of congenital heart disease. Depending upon the size of the defect, the life expectancy may be normal or materially reduced. Patients with large uncorrected defects die in infancy, but if the opening is small there may be little disability. While ventricular defects may occur as isolated anomalies, they are often associated with other malformations such as the tetralogy of Fallot.

Between the fifth to eighth week of fetal life, the common ventricular chamber is divided into a right and left side by the formation of an interventricular septum. A large muscular wall grows upward, from what will be the apex of the heart, toward the atrioventricular partition. The posterior portion of this septum usually fuses adequately, but the anterior portion may not. An anterior defect is left which normally is closed by the downgrowth of a membranous septum which fuses to the already developed muscular partition. When this membranous septum fails to completely fuse with the muscular portion, the patency of the interventricular septum continues. The membranous segment of the interventricular wall originates as a downgrowth from the partition which divides the bulbus arteriosus into the pulmonary artery and aorta. For this reason, interventricular septal defects are commonly associated with anomalous development of these two major vessels and their semilunar valves.

The interventricular defect may be only a minute probe patency, or may be several centimeters in diameter. Commonly, the margins of the patency are somewhat thickened by the turbulence of the blood flow through the opening (Fig. 16–21). Right ventricular enlargement develops since the flow of blood is almost invariably from left to right. Areas of endocardial thickening, **jet lesions**, may develop in the right ventricle, at the point where the jet stream impinges upon the lining of the right ventricular chamber. With progressive overload of the right side of the heart, pulmonary hypertension and pulmonary vascular sclerosis may cause reversal of flow through the ventricular defect and cyanosis may appear. This congenital anomaly, then, is responsible for **tardive cyanosis**.

Since most of these defects are small, the most characteristic physical sign is a loud systolic murmur, sometimes referred to as a *machinery murmur, commonly accompanied by a thrill*. In those patients who succumb as a result of this form of anomaly, right-sided heart failure is the most common cause of death. The second most frequent cause of death is superimposed vegetative endocarditis on the margins of the defect or on the right ventricular endocardial jet lesions. Brain abscesses and paradoxical emboli are unusual terminal events. Surgical closure of these defects is now accomplished with relative ease, totally transforming the outlook for these patients.

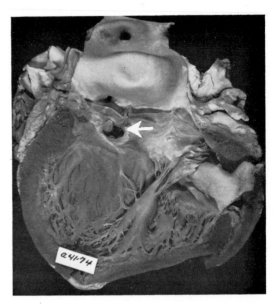

Figure 16–21. A ventricular septal defect with fibrous thickening of the margins of the patency. (arrow)

Mention should be made of the possibility of complete failure of interventricular septal development, creating a common ventricle. This condition is referred to as *cor triloculare biatriatum* or, if the atrial septum is also missing, *cor biloculare*.

ATRIAL SEPTAL DEFECTS

At approximately the fourth week of fetal life, the membranous septum primum grows downward from the posterior wall of the common atrial chamber, dividing it into right and left sides. The base of this membrane, which attaches to the atrioventricular partition, is incomplete and leaves an opening, the *ostium primum*. Subsequently, a second defect appears in this membrane in its superior portion, known as the *ostium secundum*. By the seventh week of life, a second septum grows upward, slightly to the right of the primary membrane. In the ordinary course of events, this second membrane closes the ostium primum, and usually closes the ostium secundum. However, since this secondary membrane is itself not complete, it creates an aperture known as the foramen ovale. This foramen ovale is juxtaposed to a more or less intact region of the first septum, and a flap-like covering to the foramen ovale is thereby formed. As long as the blood pressure on the right side of the heart remains greater than that on the left, as obtains during fetal life, flow occurs through this foramen ovale. However, because of the reversal of the pressure relationships at birth, this flap is held closed, preventing regurgitation from the left to right atrium. In this connection it should be remembered that after birth, the systemic blood pressure is six to eight times greater than that in the pulmonary circulation. After birth, usually within the first three months of life, the primary septum fuses to the margins of the foramen ovale but, in rare instances, a year or two elapses before fusion. In many instances, slit-like oblique defects persist through which small probes can be passed. These defects, however, are of only anatomic interest since functionally the thin membrane serves as a competent flap valve.

Large defects create a left to right atrial shunt. This classic form of interatrial defect occurs high in the atrial septum. Other defects may occur in relation to the low-situated ostium primum. Communications between the atria may be found in almost any site in the interatrial septum. In the most extreme cases, the entire membrane is absent and the heart may exist essentially as a three-chambered structure (**cor triloculare biventriculare**).

The clinical gravity of the atrial defect is entirely dependent upon the volume of blood flowing through it. Persistent flow from left to right produces a chronic right-sided overload, leading to cardiac enlargement, chiefly of the right side of the heart, with pulmonary hypertension and pulmonary artery dilatation. Loud systolic murmurs accompany these physiologic derangements. As long as the pressure on the left side of the heart is greater than on the right, cyanosis does not appear. It is only in the late stages when the pulmonic hypertension exceeds the systemic blood pressure that reversal of flow occurs and right-sided venous blood is introduced through the septal defect, into the left atrium with consequent cyanosis.

The increased flow into the lungs produces, in time, congestion of the lungs, and, in longstanding cases, *pulmonary vascular sclerosis* (p. 789). Cyanosis does not develop until late in the course (*tardive cyanosis*). The clinical significance and prognosis of these cases are shaped by the coexistence of associated developmental anomalies and the functional patency of the defect, to be discussed next.

ATRIAL SEPTAL DEFECTS WITH MITRAL STENOSIS (LUTEMBACHER'S DISEASE)

The combination of an atrial septal defect with mitral stenosis is known as Lutembacher's disease. This combination is found in perhaps 5 per cent of the cases with significant atrial defects. The mitral stenosis may be due either to a congenital anomalous development of the valve or to acquired valvular disease, such as rheumatic heart disease. Lutembacher's disease occurs much more commonly in females and is found in any age group, since it is perfectly compatible with life. The septal defect is usually but not necessarily large, but may be very small. It is probable that many of these septal defects would be of no significance were it not for the increased left intra-atrial pressure occasioned by the mitral stenosis. This increase in pressure diverts blood from the left atrium into the right atrium and results in a more marked overload of the right side of the heart than in simple interatrial defects. In these cases, the predominant associated anatomic changes are those of dilatation of the left and right atria and hypertrophy of the right ventricle. The attendant pulmonary vascular congestion and sclerosis are also more severe.

The flow of blood is at first from left to right; cyanosis is not present, and in fact develops later than in uncomplicated cases of atrial defects because the mitral lesion increases the left-sided pressure and retards the reversal of flow.

The causes of death in this clinical condition and in uncomplicated atrial defects are usually (1) cardiac failure; (2) paradoxical embolism, in which emboli pass through the defect from the right to the left side; (3) bacterial endocarditis on the margins of the defect; (4) pulmonary hemorrhages incident to the pulmonary hypertension; (5) intercurrent systemic infections because of the constitutional inferiority of some of these patients; and (6) the development of brain abscesses. The precise genesis of these abscesses is still somewhat obscure, but it is hypothesized that minute septic emboli pass through the defect to reach the arterial circulation and thence lodge in the brain.

The prognosis in these forms of heart disease is, however, good and most patients live to adulthood. Interatrial defects and mitral stenosis are now both amenable to surgical therapy.

TRANSPOSITION OF THE GREAT VESSELS

Transposition of the great vessels may be either "corrected" or "uncorrected." In both, the aorta is in the anterior position usually occupied by the pulmonary artery. In the "corrected" transposition, the aorta emerges from a right-sided *arterial* ventricle and the pulmonary artery from the left-sided *venous* ventricle. Thus, except for the transposed positions of the chambers and vessels, the circulation in the "corrected" form is normal and could only be suspected from the unexpected location of an arterial cardiac catheter lying on the right or on the left with a venous insertion. It is of interest that the arterial ventricle often has a mirror-image tricuspid A-V valve and the venous ventricle contains a mirror image of the mitral valve. Ventricular septal defects or a patent ductus arteriosus often occur in such "corrected" transpositions and create functional abnormalities in the cardiac flow.

In "uncorrected" transposition, the great vessels are not only reversed in position, but the aorta takes origin from the venous ventricle and the pulmonary artery from the arterial ventricle. Survival is only possible by virtue of communications between the two circulations through septal defects, the foramen ovale, ductus arteriosus or other anomalous shunts.

TETRALOGY OF FALLOT

The four components are a high ventricular septal defect; a dextroposed aorta overriding the septal defect that receives blood from both the right and left ventricles; stenosis of the pulmonary valve, or so-called prepulmonic stenosis, which occurs in the pulmonary ventricular infundibulum below it; and hypertrophy of the right ventricle. This is the most common form of congenital heart disease associated with marked cyanosis from birth and clubbing of the fingers.

The embryogenesis of this combination of changes is closely tied up with the formation of the ventricular septum. The development of the interventricular septal defect has already been described. The membranous portion of the interventricular septum takes origin from the septum which divides the truncus arteriosus into the pulmonary artery and aorta. **Anomalous development of this septum, therefore, may give rise to anomalies which affect the aorta and the pulmonary artery, as well as the interventricular septum.** Malpositioning of this septum produces an overly large aorta and a narrow pulmonary artery with pulmonic or subpulmonic stenosis. In addition, excessive backward torsion of the entire truncus arteriosus swings the aorta to the right so that it is either totally dextroposed, communicating directly with the right ventricle, or overrides the division between the ventricles and receives blood from both the right and left sides. In the most severe forms of this anomaly, there is uncorrected transposition of the great vessels. Because of the pulmonary stenosis and the interventricular left to right septal defect, there is considerable increase in the blood pressure in the right side of the heart, which eventuates in right ventricular hypertrophy, the fourth component of the tetralogy (Fig. 16–22). **Thus the features of a tetralogy of Fallot are (1) transposition of the**

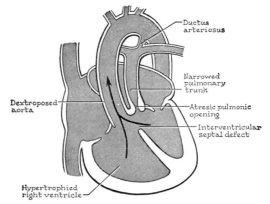

Figure 16–22. A diagram of the heart and major vessels showing the tetralogy of Fallot.

aorta, (2) pulmonic or subpulmonic stenosis, (3) interventricular septal defect and (4) right ventricular hypertrophy. When the pulmonic or prepulmonic stenosis is severe, **survival is only possible by virtue of persistent patency of the ductus arteriosus.** Blood may flow through this channel from the aorta into the pulmonary vascular bed and thus be oxygenated.

Clinically, these patients are severely cyanotic (morbus caeruleus), usually from birth. The flow of blood through the lungs is seriously reduced by the pulmonic lesions, and the aortic blood is derived from both right and left ventricles and is thus, in part, unoxygenated. The systemic hypoxia is reflected in polycythemia, clubbing of the fingers and retarded development with constitutional inferiority. Systolic murmurs occasioned by the pulmonary stenosis and ventricular septal defect, systolic thrills, and changes in the cardiac roentgenographic silhouette complete the characteristic clinical syndrome.

The prognosis in this condition is generally poor unless the deformities are amenable to surgical alleviation. Most patients succumb either in childhood or early adulthood, with an average life duration of about 12 years. Rare patients survive into middle life. The common causes of death are, as can be anticipated, right heart failure, bacterial endocarditis superimposed upon the cardiac anomalies, brain abscess and intercurrent respiratory infections in chronically debilitated patients. Various surgical procedures have now been developed for the closure of the septal defects and amelioration of the dextroposed aorta.

EISENMENGER COMPLEX

This combination of cardiac defects represents a variant of the tetralogy of Fallot in which pulmonic stenosis, or atresia, is not present. Some of these cases have pulmonary dilatation, despite the dextroposition of the aorta. This is a much rarer entity than the tetralogy of Fallot. The clinical signs and symptoms are much the same, but these patients, in general, have a better prognosis since a reasonably adequate pulmonary vascular flow exists. Some cyanosis is usual, nevertheless, because the right-sided aorta receives some unoxygenated blood from the right ventricle. The common causes of death are the same as those cited in the tetralogy of Fallot, but the mean age at death in this condition is 25 years as contrasted with 12 years for the tetralogy of Fallot.

PATENT DUCTUS ARTERIOSUS

Persistent patency of the ductus arteriosus may exist as a solitary lesion. More commonly, it is associated with other congenital anomalies, such as narrowing of the aorta, referred to as coarctation, pulmonary stenosis, the tetralogy of Fallot and, rarely, narrowing of the tricuspid valve, or tricuspid atresia. Because of its prominent clinical signs and symptoms, it is one of the more readily identified forms of congenital heart disease.

The sixth left aortic arch gives origin to the ductus. It connects the main, or left, pulmonary artery with the aorta below the origin of the left subclavian artery. In the fetus, blood from the right ventricle passes almost entirely through the patent ductus into the aorta, and only a small portion passes through the nonfunctioning lungs. Just prior to birth, considerably more passes through the pulmonary circulation. However, after birth, when the lungs assume their respiratory function and the pulmonary vessels expand, less and less is shunted through the ductus so that, in about 80 per cent of the cases, anatomic closure occurs by the third month of infantile life. The ductus, however, may persist in a small number of cases for as long as one to two years. When it persists beyond this period, it is abnormal. There is a striking sex preponderance in this anomaly, which occurs three times more commonly in females than in males.

There is no adequate explanation of the obliteration of the ductus after birth. Possibly with the fall in blood flow through the vessel, the normal muscular contractility of the wall causes progressive narrowing and eventual occlusion of the lumen and obliteration of the endothelial lining. It is also suggested that the high arterial oxygen saturation of the blood after birth stimulates endothelial and fibroblastic proliferation with eventual closure of the lumen. Mechanical turbulence of the blood flow through the ductus on both the pulmonary arterial and aortic sides has been ascribed importance in stimulating proliferation of the endothelium and subendothelial connective tissue to the point of obliteration of the patent channel.

The morphology of the ductus is quite variable. It may take the form of a distinct vessel with a length of 1 to 2 cm. and a diameter of 1 mm. to 1 cm. which bridges a gap between the aorta and the pulmonary arterial trunks. In other cases, the ductus may simply represent a fenestration between the apposed pulmonary and aortic trunks. Recognition of this variant is extremely important in the surgical correction of this defect, since it provides no vessel or channel which can be ligated.

Blood flows through the ductus from the aorta to the pulmonary artery and, for a long period of time, the patient is not cyanotic.

Surprisingly large volumes may pass through these defects (up to 75 per cent of the left ventricular output). The remainder of the body may thus be deprived of adequate circulation. When the effective volume output of the left side of the heart is reduced, left ventricular hypertrophy usually develops. Moreover, the increase in blood flow to the right side produces a right ventricular hypertrophy and, in longstanding cases, pulmonary hypertension, dilatation of the pulmonary vascular tree and pulmonary vascular sclerosis. Eventually the pulmonary hypertension leads to reversal of flow and cyanosis.

The most striking clinical feature of a persistent ductus arteriosus is a loud, prolonged systolic and diastolic murmur which has received many descriptive names, such as machinery-like, humming, sawing and train-in-tunnel. A systolic thrill usually accompanies the murmur. When the communication is large, the loss of aortic flow may lead to a low systolic and particularly a low diastolic pressure. This widening of the pulse pressure sometimes simulates certain of the features found in the regurgitation of luetic aortic valvulitis.

The prognosis in this condition depends upon the size of the communication. Patients with large defects may die of cardiac failure. Usually, there is a considerable reduction in the life span. The average survival is 40 years. This figure is subject to revision, since one of the more common causes of death is superimposed bacterial endarteritis in the ductus, which effective antibiotic therapy has done much to control. Moreover, at the present time, surgical ligation of this anomaly is a well established and highly successful procedure. When the defect is small, it may be completely asymptomatic and, untreated, permit a normal expectancy of life.

It is to be remembered, however, that in certain cases in which the patent ductus is complicated by other forms of congenital heart disease, the persistence of this communication is lifesaving. In the tetralogy of Fallot or marked pulmonary stenosis, blood flow to the lungs is possible only through the ductus, and obliteration of this channel may lead to death.

COARCTATION OF THE AORTA

Coarctation or narrowing of the aorta is a fairly common type of cardiac congenital anomaly in postmortem surveys. Of 1000 cases of congenital heart disease reviewed by Maude Abbott (1936) this occurred in 142. In more recent clinical surveys, the incidence appears to be much lower, approximately 6 per cent.

It is more common among males by a ratio of 4 to 1. Two forms of this defect (an infantile and an adult form) are recognized, but the distinction between them is not always clear cut.

The **infantile form** is characterized by a narrowing of the aorta which may be sufficient to obliterate the aortic lumen. This narrowing occurs in the root of the aorta proximal to the ductus arteriosus, which remains patent. Blood flows to the arterial system through the ductus, and hence survival is dependent upon the continued patency of the ductus which serves as a bypass.

Infants with this anomaly usually die soon after birth or within the first year of life unless surgical repair is accomplished. Friedberg (1966) relates the genesis of this defect to an alteration in the pathways by which the aorta receives blood. Normally some blood comes to the aorta directly from the ductus arteriosus and the remainder from the right heart by way of the foramen ovale. It is this latter flow which enters the left ventricle that supplies the root or isthmic segment of the aorta. In the development of infantile coarctation, most of the blood flow to the heart may for some unexplained reason be channeled through the ductus and, consequently, flow through the isthmic region is reduced. With this low pressure at the root of the aorta, the vessel fails to grow and expand normally and it remains a narrow channel or becomes entirely obliterated.

Adult coarctation involves a portion of the aorta distal to the ductus arteriosus. Narrowing is less severe and a much shorter segment of aorta is involved than in the infantile form. Almost invariably the ductus arteriosus is closed. The point of maximal constriction often appears as a prominent inner ring or an almost complete membrane. The lumen is usually about 5 mm. in diameter (Fig. 16–23).

Adult coarctation is believed by Friedberg (1966) to develop later in fetal life than the infantile type, and to be related to closure of the ductus arteriosus. Others hypothesize that the aortic narrowing is related to overgrowth of fibrous tissue and endothelial cells during obliteration of the ductus. Were this the case, however, one would anticipate cases of narrowing of the pulmonary artery at the point of origin of the ductus, a defect which has not been reported. Furthermore, the coexistence of anomalous bicuspid aortic valves in 40 per cent of the cases of adult coarctation supports the interpretation of this defect as a fetal develop-

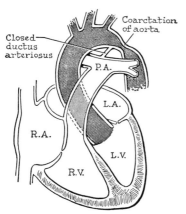

Figure 16–23. A diagram of the major vessels showing a postductal, or adult, form of coarctation of the aorta. The coarctation is distal to the closed ductus arteriosus (ligamentum arteriosum).

mental anomaly. Several macroscopic changes elsewhere in the vascular system are associated with these alterations in the aorta. Atherosclerosis and sometimes cystic medionecrosis and dissecting aneurysms tend to develop in this proximal segment. Eventually ventricular hypertrophy generally develops. Increased intra-aortic pressure proximal to the constriction may produce aneurysmal dilatation of this segment of the aorta or of the major arterial branches to the head and upper extremities which branch off before the constriction. Collateral circulation may develop from branches of the great vessels to the intercostal and internal mammary arteries. As their caliber increases, the vessels of this collateral circulation may become visible below the skin. Dilatation of the intercostal arteries may erode the lower margins of the ribs, producing characteristic notching on radiologic examination.

The adult form of coarctation of the aorta may be asymptomatic, and many times the disease remains undiscovered until fatal complications develop. When it is symptomatic, the major clinical findings relate to hypertension in the arterial system proximal to the constriction, and a drop in blood pressure distal to the narrowing. If the arterial supply to the brain is derived from the great vessels proximal to the constriction, headaches, dizziness, nosebleeds and nervousness reflect this hypertension in the brain. At the same time, weakness, coldness, pallor and numbness in the legs result from the diminished circulation in the lower half of the body. Perhaps the most important clinical finding is a significant difference between the blood pressure in the upper extremities, which is usually above normal, and the blood pressure in the lower extremities, which is markedly lower or may

even be unobtainable. A loud systolic murmur caused by the turbulent flow through the narrowing may be audible over the anterior chest, but more characteristically is maximal over the posterior chest in close proximity to the coarctation. The dilated, tortuous, collateral vessels and notching of the ribs provide strong confirmatory evidence.

The course and prognosis of the adult form depend upon the severity of the narrowing and the adequacy of the collateral circulation. Many patients survive into old age and die of other causes. In a large series, the mean duration of life, however, was about 40 years. Death is usually caused by one of four complications: (1) rupture of a dissecting aneurysm in the proximal aorta incident to the development of cystic medionecrosis (one-quarter of the cases) (p. 617); (2) bacterial invasion of the aorta (endarteritis) at the point of narrowing or at the point where the jet stream produced by the constriction impinges on the distal region of the aorta; (3) congestive heart failure due to the persistent hypertension; and (4) cerebral hemorrhages also related to the elevated blood pressure. Less commonly, vegetative endocarditis may become superimposed upon an associated anomalous bicuspid aortic valve. The natural course of this disease can now be totally modified by surgical measures which excise the point of narrowing and anastomose the severed ends of the aorta.

OTHER CONGENITAL CARDIAC DEFECTS

There are many other forms of congenital diseases, some having only academic interest. Others, however, are of clinical and functional significance, but will be treated briefly, since they are for the most part distinctly less common than those already mentioned.

Dextrocardia. True dextrocardia consists of a mirror-image transposition of the heart within the thoracic cavity. This cardiac shift may or may not be associated with complete transposition of all the viscera of the body, *situs inversus*. Both dextrocardia and the situs inversus are of clinical significance only insofar as they present a hazard to the novice studying physical diagnosis.

Congenital Valvular Defects. These anomalies have already been referred to in association with other developmental failures. They are, however, as a group quite common, many of them having no functional or clinical significance. Small *fenestrations*, oval or round defects 0.1 to 0.3 mm. in diameter, are commonly found in the semilunar cusps near the valvular commissures. Quite rarely these may be sufficiently large to produce some element of insufficiency. They are, however, for the most part of anatomic interest alone. Rarely the semilunar valves may have four leaflets. This abnormality is completely compatible with normal function. Congenital stenosis of any valve may occur. This is most common in the pulmonary valve, usually associated with a ventricular septal defect or the tetralogy of Fallot. Occasionally pulmonary stenosis exists as an isolated lesion. Narrowing of this orifice obviously impairs the flow of blood to the lungs, and is accompanied by many functional disturbances, such as overload of the right side of the heart, cyanosis and polycythemia. Congenital stenosis of the aortic valve occurs infrequently as an isolated lesion, but may produce a chain of sequelae similar to those described under coarctation of the aorta. Tricuspid or mitral stenosis as isolated lesions are extremely rare. The coexistence of mitral stenosis with an interatrial septal defect has already been described under Lutembacher's syndrome. The narrowing of any of these orifices may be minimal or extreme. When the valvular lumen is totally obliterated, the lesion is referred to as atresia.

Anomalies of the Coronary Artery. More than two coronary ostia are not infrequent. Usually the anomaly involves one vessel and consists of two ostia that merge almost immediately. These abnormalities are without functional significance. The coronary arteries may occupy unusual positions. These malpositions may simply affect the point of origin in the aorta, and have no significance. On the other hand, quite rarely one or both coronaries may take origin from the pulmonary artery, in which case serious clinical sequelae may follow since these vessels then transmit unoxygenated venous blood to the myocardium. Significant myocardial and endocardial ischemia may result and lead to progressive cardiac damage and eventual heart failure. In fact, the right-sided origin of a coronary artery is believed to comprise a possible basis for the development of endocardial fibroelastosis, to be discussed presently. Collateral anastomoses may develop under these circumstances and compensate for this abnormality.

Anomalous Bands and Cords. Anomalous bands or chordae may be present, chiefly in the ventricles. These may traverse the ventricular cavity and have little clinical significance except for the mysterious murmurs they cause. In the atrium, a network of thread-like strands may extend across the right atrial cavity or across the opening of the superior vena cava (Chiari's net). This is also usually of only incidental interest, but rarely these strands may initiate intravascular thrombosis or even become a locus for bacterial seeding.

Pericardial Defects. Quite commonly defects occur in the integrity of the parietal pericardium. Rarely, the entire parietal pericardium may be absent. These lesions are of importance only insofar as they create a common pleuropericardial space by which infections in the lungs have easy access to the epicardium of the heart. Rarely, collections of fluid in the pleural cavities may embarrass cardiac activity.

In conclusion, while the types of anomalies that may affect the heart are legion, most are rare and, therefore, of lesser clinical importance than the major anomalies first described.

BACTERIAL (VEGETATIVE) ENDOCARDITIS

Bacterial or, more properly, vegetative endocarditis, one of the most serious infections in man, is characterized by colonization of one or more of the heart valves by bacteria or other microbiologic agents, with the buildup of friable masses of organisms and blood clot producing so-called vegetations. The blood is continuously seeded with resultant metastatic dissemination of organisms to distant organs and tissues. Vegetative endocarditis accounts for about 1 per cent of cardiac disease, and it is surprising that despite the availability of antibacterial therapy, the frequency of this condition has not substantially diminished from preantibiotic times (Finland and Barnes, 1970). However, as will be seen, such therapy has substantially altered the distribution of the causative agents.

The time-honored division of vegetative endocarditis into acute and subacute forms has lost much of its meaning with the advent of antibacterial therapy. It was contended that acute bacterial endocarditis was a fulminant disease usually caused by highly virulent pathogens which attacked normal hearts with disastrous erosive destruction of the valves. In contrast, subacute bacterial endocarditis was conceived of as a milder variant caused by less pathogenic organisms such as *S. viridans* or enterococci infecting hearts which were the seat of preexisting disease such as rheumatic heart disease and congenital anomalies. However, it is now apparent that the virulence of the infecting organism, the resistance of the host, the existence of underlying cardiac disease and, most of all, the therapy all influence the severity and outcome of the infection and the survival of the patient (Lerner and Weinstein, 1966). Thus, in a resistant host or when appropriate therapy has been instituted promptly, a long subacute course may ensue or, indeed, the infection may be relatively mild and be rapidly controlled. The same organism in a host rendered more vulnerable by underlying cardiac disease, or when appropriate therapy has not been instituted soon enough, might produce an overwhelming infection, running a rapid acute course. The older concept that patients with previously damaged hearts tend to get infected with bacteria of lower virulence and thus generally have subacute bacterial endocarditis, while those with normal hearts develop more virulent infections, leading to acute bacterial endocarditis, is merely an expression of host-invader interaction. Damaged hearts are rendered vulnerable to organisms of relatively low virulence, but only aggressive organisms can implant on normal heart valves and in a more resistant host. In any event, the terms acute and subacute denote the course of the illness and have little morphologic significance. Much more important to the survival of the patient is the identification of the specific causative organism and the prompt institution of appropriate treatment.

The most important predisposing influence to bacterial endocarditis is preexistent cardiac disease. Rheumatic heart disease underlies about two-thirds of the cases; congenital heart disease (principally septal defects and bicuspid aortic valves), about a quarter; and the remaining small number includes normal hearts, arteriosclerotic heart disease and, rarely, syphilitic heart disease.

Etiology and Pathogenesis. The microbiologic flora of vegetative endocarditis has undergone substantial change in the antibacterial era. Organisms susceptible to therapy have markedly decreased in importance, while resistant organisms and all manner of fungi have grown in importance. In previous years, *Streptococcus viridans* and enterococci were the predominant cause of bacterial endocarditis. Today they account for 30 to 50 per cent of the cases. Table 16–2, drawn from a study of 337 patients between the years 1933 to 1965, indicates the frequencies of the causative organisms encountered in a population gathered from a large municipal hospital. These data indicate that *S. viridans* is still the most common cause of bacterial endocarditis. However, it accounted for only about 30 per cent of the cases. The next most common offender was *Staphylococcus aureus*, accounting for about 23 per cent. A number of other findings are of interest. Pneumococcal endocarditis has become rare, and the same may be said of gonococcal and meningococcal etiologies, probably attributable to the ready control of such infections by therapy. Similarly, *S. pyogenes* has also disappeared as a cause of this disease. Coincidentally, however, at the time potent antibacterial therapy came into wide use in the 1940's, the antibiotic-resistant organisms such as *S. aureus* and the gram-negative bacilli grew in importance. In many surveys, the incidence of staphylococcal endocarditis has increased from 9 per cent before the antibacterial era to about 20 to 30 per cent at the present time (Quinn, 1968). Most distressing is the evidence suggesting that these infections by resistant organisms are often hospital-acquired. Similarly, with their resistance to therapy, fungi such as *Candida albicans, Aspergillus fumigatus, Histoplasma capsulatum* and *Cryptococcus neoformans* have entered the ranks of the causative agents. Ultimately, however, any organism may and, indeed, has caused vegetative endocarditis and, in the vulnerable, particularly immunosuppressed host, agents once considered to be nonpathogenic have implanted on heart valves and induced sometimes fatal disease.

The usual routes of entry of the causative organisms are through: (1) dental infections and manipulations, (2) urinary tract instrumentation, (3) respiratory and skin infections, (4) peripartal sepsis, (5) infected burn wounds, (6) cardiac surgery and valvular prostheses, (7) infections associated with intravenous catheters and (8) the use of the "needle" by drug addicts. The last three have assumed great importance in recent years. As many as 10 to 15 per cent of cases of endocarditis have followed cardiotomy. Bacteria and fungi are almost inevitably implanted in the heart at the time of surgery and, in the presence of such "foreign bodies" as prosthetic heart valves, the hazards of infection, bacteremia and vegetative endocarditis are high. Intravenous catheters that remain in place for long periods of time comprise ideal avenues for the introduction of organisms into the blood. The use of the "needle" in drug addiction is an obvious source of infection and has resulted in vegetative endocarditis' becoming a major cause of death in these individuals (p. 531).

TABLE 16–2. ETIOLOGIC AGENTS OF BACTERIAL ENDOCARDITIS: BOSTON CITY HOSPITAL, 1933–1965 (12 SELECTED YEARS)*

| Organism | Patients per Year | | | | | | | | | | | | |
	1933	1934	1935	1941	1947	1951	1953	1955	1957	1961	1963	1964	Total
Pneumococcus	6	5	8	5	4	6	5[1]	0	4[1]	3[1]	1	3[2]	50[6]
Streptococcus pyogenes	3	4	3	5	0	0	2	0	1	2[1]	0	0	20[1]
Staphylococcus aureus	2	0	1	4	10[2]	13[1]	5	11	7	15[1]	7[1]	2	77[5]
S. viridans	6	5	11	9[2]	18[1]	16[8]	11[6]	2[2]	6[3]	3[2]	6[3]	5[4]	98[44]
Enterococcus	0	0	1	1	5	6	8	4	3	2	2[2]	3	35[2]
Staph. albus	0	0	2	0	3[2]	4[2]	10[6]	1	2	1[1]	6[3]	2[2]	31[16]
Gram-negative bacilli	0	0	1	0	6	9	14	8	2	1	5	3	49[0]
Miscellaneous	6	0	1	1	2	1	1	0	0	0	0	0	12[2]
Negative or not available	4	2	1	10	4[1]	1	1	0	2	1	0	2	28[1]
Total organisms (cases)	27	16	29	35	52	56	57	26	27	28	27	20	400[77]
Total patients	25	15	29	35[2]	43[17]	44[9]	38[12]	18[2]	22[4]	28[6]	23[9]	17[7]	337[68]

*Numbers in brackets indicate those who recovered.

From Finland, M., and Barnes, M. W.: Changing etiology of bacterial endocarditis in the antibacterial era. Ann. Intern. Med. 72:341, 1970.

Mention has already been made of the role of preexistent heart disease in increasing the vulnerability of the patient to infections on the heart valve. A few studies have suggested that vegetative endocarditis never begins with the direct implantation of organisms on valvular leaflets but, instead, requires first the development of small, bland, friable vegetations of fibrin and platelets designated as nonbacterial thrombotic endocarditis (p. 692). The existence of such prior changes must remain only a possibility since the fully evolved bacterial lesions destroy all evidence of the relatively trivial, tiny vegetations of thrombotic endocarditis.

Morphology. The anatomic changes in vegetative endocarditis are usually fairly spectacular and readily evident. The diagnostic finding is the friable, bulky bacterial vegetations on the heart valve (Fig. 16—24). These are often several centimeters in greatest dimension, but may be small and easily missed. They generally hang from the free margin of the leaflets as friable, irregular masses. These vegetations tend to occur singly or in a scattered few focal areas, but classically do not involve the entire free margins of the leaflets as do those in rheumatic fever. They are, moreover, significantly larger than the vegetations of rheumatic fever. Sometimes they cause perforation of the underlying valve leaflet or erosion of the chordae tendineae (Fig. 16—25). From this site of origin, they may extend to the surface of the leaflet, to the endocardium, or they may burrow beneath the valve to invade the ventricular wall or one of the great vessels leaving the heart.

In three-quarters of the cases, the mitral valve is affected (Wilson, 1963). The aortic valve is affected about as often, so that in many cases both valves are affected simultaneously. Valves of the right side of the heart are not affected in more than 15 per cent of all cases, the tricuspid somewhat more often than the pulmonic. Bacterial endocarditis may be superimposed upon a congenital deformity, in which case the vegetation develops at the site of the defect as around a patent ductus arteriosus.

The previous description refers to the appearance of the disease in its florid, active stage. More and more often, cases are now identified with heaped-up, calcified masses along the free margins of one of the valve leaflets, suggesting a preexistent vegetative endocarditis. Indeed, occasionally the history confirms this. It is, therefore, now appreciated that these vegetations may undergo progressive fibrosis and organization and eventually become calcified. Such a happy outcome is, however, not common since the disease when well developed is too often fatal.

Histologically, there is little to be seen save for the irregular, amorphous, tangled mass of fibrin strands, platelets and blood cell debris that, along with the masses of organisms, comprise the vegetation. The underlying leaflet shows the anticipated vascularization and nonspecific inflammatory response (Fig. 16—26). The bacteria may be extremely difficult to identify and are often deeply buried within the vegetation, an observation that explains the difficulty in controlling these infections by antibiotic therapy once they are well developed. An important part of the examination of these vegetations is the identification of the organism by direct smear and culture. While the tissue section morphology may provide a general clue to the type of organism, ultimately cultural identification is required.

A number of sequelae may ensue. Suppurative pericarditis may result from direct penetration of the heart wall or by lymphatic permeation. The burrowing infection may produce an interventricular septal defect. Erosion of the valve leaflets or of the chordae tendineae may cause sudden valvular insufficiency and acute cardiac decompensation. Seeding of the aorta may give rise to a bacterial endaortitis. The bacteremia may seed any organ in the body, but the kidney, spleen and brain are the most common sites of secondary infection. The myocardium itself may exhibit scattered metastatic abscesses. Seeding of the nail beds and of the skin may produce small petechial hemorrhages or even microabscesses. Acute splenitis or septic infarcts in the spleen are so commonplace as to be virtually a part of the disease. Similarly, septic infarctions which often become converted to abscesses occur in the kidneys and brain. Renal complications are encountered in 33 to 50 per cent of patients with vegetative endocarditis. The renal involvement takes many forms, including metastatic abscesses, infarctions (usually septic), focal glomerulitis, or glomerulonephritis (formerly called focal embolic glomerulonephritis) (p. 1100) and diffuse proliferative glomerulonephritis (p. 1093). Both forms of glomerulopathy are now considered to be immunologic in origin rather than due to direct embolization of bacteria.

Clinical Course. The two dominant clinical features of bacterial endocarditis are a prolonged septic febrile course and a changing cardiac murmur. The changing characteristic of the murmur is extremely important since it reflects the buildup and fragmentation of the valvular vegetations. Additional findings are splenomegaly, hematuria, due either to infarctions or to one of the renal complications mentioned, petechiae in the skin and evidence of embolic manifestations in the organs mentioned. While the disease may be suspected from such findings, for a definitive diagnosis the organisms should be isolated from blood culture. This may require numerous cultures

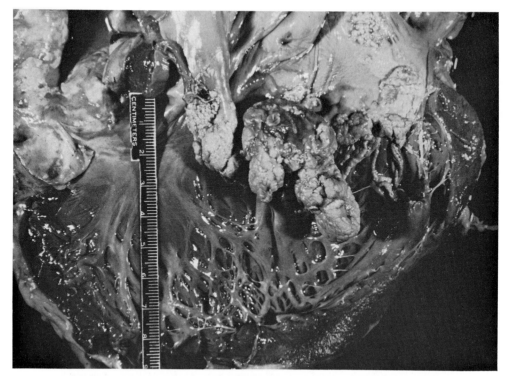

Fig. 16–24

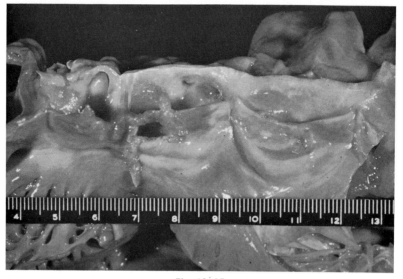

Fig. 16–25

Figure 16–24. *Vegetative bacterial endocarditis of the mitral valve with massive friable masses and extension of the vegetations to the atrial endocardium.*

Figure 16–25. *Vegetative endocarditis of the aortic valve with a through-and-through perforation of one of the cusps.*

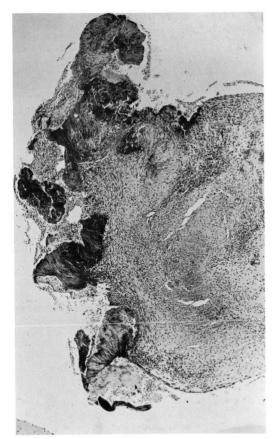

Figure 16–26. *A low power view of a bacterial vegetation illustrating the marked inflammatory infiltration. The black masses on the surface are bacteria in colony formation.*

since the bacteremic episodes may be transient and the organism may be one which is difficult to culture by usual techniques, as for example, microaerophilic streptococci or fungi.

Surprisingly, despite the wide availability of improved antibacterial drugs, there has been little change in the incidence of this disease and in the prognosis (Carpenter and Wallace, 1969). Table 16–2 indicates that over the past two decades, less than half of the patients have survived, although there is some slight improvement in the outlook recently. Death is usually due to uncontrolled infection, embolization, cardiac failure or renal insufficiency.

CALCIFIC AORTIC STENOSIS

Fibrosing stenosis and calcification of the aortic valve may occur in rheumatic fever, in healed bacterial endocarditis and in the late stages of arteriosclerotic heart disease. On occasion, marked calcific aortic stenosis is encountered in a heart free of stigmata of any of the disorders just mentioned. The thickened cusps are literally obliterated by dense, fibrous intercommissural adhesions which leave only a small valvular orifice, and the narrowed sinuses of Valsalva are filled with mound-like excrescences of calcium covered by a thin layer of endothelium. As a consequence, there is often marked left ventricular hypertrophy of a concentric nature, e.g., encroaching on the volume capacity of the chamber. The origin of such isolated aortic valvular disease has been argued for years. At one time, it was considered to be an expression of healed rheumatic heart disease affecting only the aortic valve, leaving no sequellae other than aortic valvular damage. However, in a study of 139 patients with anatomically isolated aortic valvular disease, a positive history of rheumatic fever was found in only 6 per cent of the patients (Roberts, 1970). Thus the pendulum has swung, and most investigators now believe that only in occasional instances is calcific aortic stenosis of rheumatic etiology. There is equally persuasive evidence against its representing healed vegetative endocarditis or a bizarre manifestation of degenerative arteriosclerotic damage to the heart. Currently in favor are the concepts that the calcific stenosing fibrosis represents the late sequellae of a congenitally deformed valve such as a bicuspid aortic valve or, in some instances, merely the consequence of damage to normal valves accumulated over the span of many decades. Indeed, most patients with this lesion are in the advanced years of life. Possibly those few instances where it occurs in a younger age group may comprise those patients with congenitally deformed valves (Roberts, 1970) (Edwards, 1962).

COR PULMONALE (PULMONARY HEART DISEASE)

Cor pulmonale refers to right ventricular hypertrophy, with or without cardiac failure, resulting from pulmonary hypertension arising in disease primary either within the pulmonary parenchyma or its vessels. Cor pulmonale is therefore the analogue of hypertensive heart disease and, accordingly, the right ventricle is primarily affected. It may thicken up to 1.5 cm. just as the left ventricle thickens with systemic hypertension. Excluded from this definition of cor pulmonale are those instances of right ventricular hypertrophy secondary to diseases in the heart, such as left to right anomalous shunts and mitral stenosis with its attendant marked pulmonary congestion and its effect on the pulmonary circulation (Neal et al., 1968). It should be noted that right ventricular hypertrophy often accompanies left ventricular hypertrophy, but such cardiac alterations are not included within the category of cor pulmonale.

The disorders most directly causing pulmonary hypertension are those affecting the pulmonary vasculature. Multiple or large pulmonary emboli are obvious sources of increased resistance to flow and pulmonary hypertension. Pulmonary vascular involvement is encountered in systemic polyarteritis nodosa and Wegener's granulomatosis. Intrapulmonary shunts between the systemic bronchial arteries and the pulmonary arterial system sometimes arise in chronic inflammatory processes in the lung, such as bronchiectases, lung abscesses and chronic pneumonitis imposing the systemic blood pressure on the pulmonary pressure. Rarely, the pulmonary vascular changes are idiopathic and are termed primary pulmonary vascular sclerosis (p. 789).

Any chronic lung disease may lead to cor pulmonale either by increasing pulmonary vascular resistance or by the induction of intrapulmonary vascular shunts. Included in this category are chronic obstructive pulmonary disease (chronic bronchitis and primary emphysema), the pneumoconioses, idiopathic interstitial fibrosis, bronchiectasis, extensive tuberculosis and sarcoidosis. Pulmonary or mediastinal tumors which compress the vessels constitute additional causes of this form of heart disease. It is important to recognize that, *in all of these pulmonary parenchymal disorders, the vasoconstrictive effects of hypoxemia and respiratory acidosis contribute significantly to the development of the pulmonary hypertension.*

Infrequently, cor pulmonale is caused by skeletal or neuromuscular derangements which interfere with pulmonary function such as severe kyphoscoliosis, poliomyelitis, the neuromuscular dystrophies and the Pickwickian syndrome. Presumably, these act by the induction of hypoxemia, acidosis and pulmonary vasoconstriction. The chronic hypoxemia, furthermore, leads to polycythemia, adding increased viscosity to the blood.

The pulmonary hypertension must usually be present for months to years before it induces right ventricular hypertrophy. During this long evolution, the cardiac changes evoke no symptoms until right-sided congestive heart failure ensues. Until then, the clinical manifestations are entirely those of the primary disorder. The diagnosis is made most often by radiography, cardiac catheterization and electrocardiography.

SYPHILITIC HEART DISEASE

World-wide measures for the prevention and control of syphilis have made syphilitic heart disease a somewhat rare entity. However, the increased incidence of syphilis within the past years may presage a return of this form of carditis to its former importance.

As a tertiary manifestation, luetic involvement of the heart usually does not become evident until 15 to 20 years after contracting the infection. These patients, therefore, usually range in age from 40 to 55 years. Males are more commonly affected than females in a ratio of approximately 3 to 1.

The pathogenesis of this condition involves an understanding of the various stages of syphilis already covered in Chapter 10. It is sufficient at this time to recall that from its primary site of entrance, the *Treponema pallidum* gains entrance to the venous circulation and is thus spread to the lungs. Here spirochetes are trapped in the lymphatic drainage and sometimes spread from the mediastinal nodes into the adventitia of the aorta. It is the involvement of the aortic media with destruction of the elastica and scarring of the musculature that causes the dilatation of the aortic valve ring and narrowing of the coronary ostia characteristic of luetic carditis (p. 378).

The microscopic lesions make the gross alterations more understandable and are presented first. The earliest adventitial changes comprise concentric, proliferative thickening of the walls of the vasa vasorum known as **obliterative endarteritis.** Characteristically, these vessels are surrounded by a collar of lymphocytes and plasma cells, predominantly the latter (Fig. 16–27). It is presumed that this narrowing of the nutrient arteries leads to ischemic destruction of the elastic tissue and smooth muscle of the media. Inflammatory vascularization and fibrous scarring follows (Fig. 16–28). These medial scars may bulge into the aortic intima (Fig. 16–29). Scars about the mouths of exiting vessels, particularly the intercostal and coronary arteries, may cause narrowing of these ostia leading perhaps to coronary insufficiency. With the loss of its musculo-elastic support, the aorta undergoes progressive stretching, and with it the aortic leaflets too become stretched.

On the basis of these microscopic changes, it can be deduced that the arch and thoracic portion of the aorta may become aneurysmally dilated. Such dilatation rarely extends below the diaphragm. The focal, medial and subendothelial scarring appears as pearly gray, elevated plaques, 1 to 3 cm. in diameter on the aortic surface. Because of the irregularity of the scarring and its contraction, longitudinal wrinkling or "tree barking" appears on the intimal surface. The coronary and intercostal ostia are often narrowed to pinpoints. Luetic aortitis predisposes to atherosclerosis so that even the root of the aorta becomes involved with atheromas. In

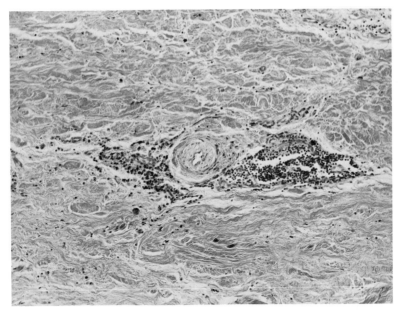

Fig. 16-27

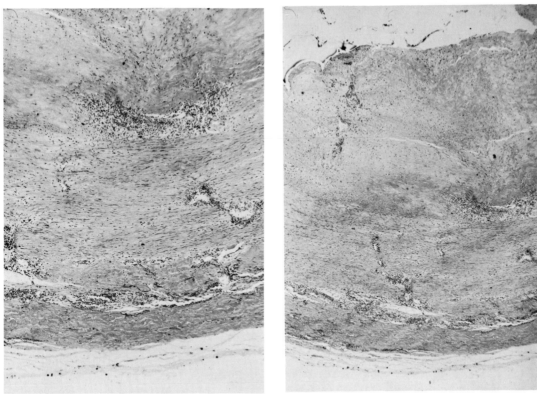

Fig. 16-28   Fig. 16-29

Figure 16-27. *Luetic aortitis. Obliterative endarteritis with narrowing of the lumen of the vasa vasorum accompanied by perivascular leukocytic infiltrate.*
Figure 16-28. *Luetic aortitis with scarring and vascularization of the media.*
Figure 16-29. *Luetic aortitis with medial damage and marked fibrous intimal thickening.*

fact, it is often the marked severity of the atherosclerosis in this region that provides the first clue to the existence of an underlying luetic disease. As a consequence of the dilatation of the aortic valve ring, the leaflets are stretched and narrowed and the commissures are widened. The free margins of the cusps roll down and become fibrotic and thickened (Fig. 16–30). The sinuses behind the leaflets become shallow to expose the coronary ostia. This is often referred to as a "high coronary take-off." A further consequence of dilatation of the valve ring is the development of aortic valvular insufficiency with consequent increased workload upon the left ventricle. Marked, sometimes extraordinary hypertrophy and dilatation of the left ventricle ensue with enlargements up to 1000 gm. **"cor bovinum."** The regurgitant aortic stream may cause endocardial thickenings where it impinges upon the mural endocardium of the left ventricle. These tend to assume a crescent shape with the concavity directed toward the regurgitant jet, reproducing on occasion miniature leaflets with shallow pockets (**pockets of Zahn**). Except possibly for some relative insufficiency of the mitral valve due to cardiac dilatation, the remainder of the heart is uninvolved.

Luetic aortitis is one of the feared forms of tertiary syphilis. While the carditis may remain asymptomatic for many years, aortic valvular insufficiency, coronary ostial narrowing, and aortic aneurysmal formation are all potentially fatal. The valvular insufficiency causes not only a loud aortic diastolic murmur, but consequent widening of the pulse pressure, the so-called bounding or Corrigan pulse. The wide pulse pressure may cause visible pulsations of the capillaries of the nail bed easily demonstrated by slight pressure over the fingernails. In time, the valvular insufficiency induces the cardiac enlargement mentioned. Occasionally, the thickening of the valvular cusps also produces a less pronounced systolic murmur. The coronary ostial involvement sometimes mimics atherosclerotic narrowing of the coronary arteries, with myocardial changes resembling those described in coronary artery insufficiency. Aneurysmal dilatation as a clinical disorder was discussed in Chapter 15. When luetic valvular insufficiency leads to cardiac decompensation, it is likely that death will ensue within one to three years (Webster et al., 1953).

Mention should be made here of the exceedingly rare entity of *congenital primary syphilitic myocarditis.* It sometimes takes the form of solitary or multiple gummas exactly resembling those that occur elsewhere in syphilis. In other instances, the myocarditis may be manifested as a diffuse interstitial inflammation composed of plasma cells, lymphocytes and histiocytes disposed particularly about the blood vessels, which themselves may be thickened by obliterative endarteritis.

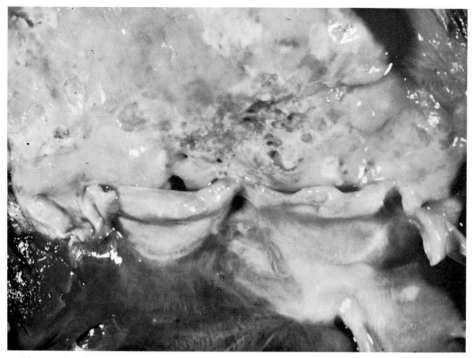

Figure 16–30. *Luetic involvement of the aorta and aortic valve. The opaque white plaques in the aorta are intimal scars. The valve leaflets are rolled and thickened.*

OTHER CARDIAC DISEASES CLASSIFIED BY ANATOMIC DIVISIONS

The major forms of heart disease which account for approximately 95 per cent of clinical cardiac problems have already been discussed. The remainder of the chapter will be oriented to the other forms of cardiac disease classified according to the anatomic division of the heart into its component layers, pericardium, myocardium and endocardium, each layer being given separate treatment. Sound basis exists for this approach, since, from the clinical standpoint, involvement of each one of these layers tends to produce signs and symptoms which are somewhat distinctive from those produced by disease of the other layers. For example, pericarditis, whatever its cause, may lead to a friction rub or to effusions which simulate enlargement of the heart, while all forms of myocarditis yield cardiac dilatation, electrocardiographic abnormalities and severe cardiac decompensation. By thus considering the disorders of each layer, a reasonable basis for clinical differential diagnosis is provided.

PERICARDIAL DISEASE

Pericardial lesions are almost always associated with, or secondary to, some disease, either in other portions of the heart, or in the surrounding structures. Rarely, pericardial involvements may occur as primary, isolated processes. There are only a relatively few anatomic forms of pericardial involvement.

ACCUMULATIONS OF FLUID IN THE PERICARDIAL SAC

Hydropericardium. Hydropericardium designates the accumulation of an excessive volume of serous transudate of low specific gravity in the pericardial cavity. Normally this sac contains between 30 and 50 cc. of thin, clear, straw-colored, translucent fluid. Under a variety of abnormal circumstances, transudations of up to a liter or more may collect, but volumes of over 500 cc. are distinctly uncommon.

Hydropericardium will occur in any generalized systemic disease that causes widespread edema or anasarca. It is, therefore, frequently encountered in cardiac failure, chronic renal disease, hypoproteinemic states and rarely in myxedema.

In hydropericardium, the serosal surfaces remain smooth and glistening, and the fluid is completely clear, watery or straw-colored and sterile. If the fluid persists for a long time, it may produce slight fibrous thickening and opacity of the pericardial surfaces. Neither adhesions nor obliteration of the pericardial sac occurs.

The clinical significance of this fluid depends upon the rate at which it accumulates. Rapid accumulation of several hundred cubic centimeters may be of much greater significance than the slow, gradual accumulation of larger quantities.

Hydropericardium must be differentiated from serous pericarditis—exudation of serous fluid. The fluid collections may be quite similar physically, but the serous effusion is inflammatory in origin, and is accompanied by histologic or bacteriologic evidence of inflammation.

Hemopericardium. The term hemopericardium should be limited to the accumulation of pure blood in the pericardial sac, and should be differentiated from hemorrhagic pericarditis, an inflammatory exudate containing blood mixed with pus.

Hemopericardium is almost invariably due to traumatic perforation of the heart, rupture of the heart wall secondary to myocardial infarction or rupture of the intrapericardial aorta. Quite rarely, it may follow penetration of a myocardial abscess or tumor. Less common causes of hemopericardium are rupture of the coronary arteries or laceration of these vessels by hypodermic needles used for intracardiac therapy. Hemorrhages in the bleeding diatheses, such as scurvy, leukemia or thrombocytopenia, are rare causes of this condition.

The blood that escapes because of rupture of the heart or aorta rapidly fills the sac under greatly increased pressure and produces cardiac tamponade (Fig. 16–31). As little as 200 to

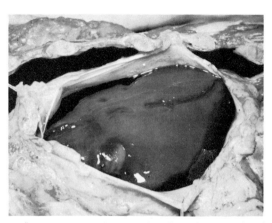

Figure 16–31. Hemopericardium. An opened pericardial sac in situ to expose the clotted blood that caused death after rupture of a myocardial infarct.

300 cc. may be sufficient to cause death. While intracardiac injections may cause leakage of blood, usually death is already imminent when such measures are attempted and, under these circumstances, only small amounts of blood-tinged fluid appear in the pericardial sac. Rarely, however, marked hemorrhage occurs, clearly emphasizing the hazard entailed in such therapy.

PERICARDITIS

Inflammations of the pericardium are also almost invariably secondary to myocardial or endocardial disease or lesions in other sites that extend to the pericardium either by continuity or through blood vessels or lymphatics. Primary pericarditis is a rarity. The various etiologic categories are presented in Table 16–3.

Acute Pericarditis. Acute pericarditis may be classified etiologically or anatomically. The former classification includes entities based upon the causative agent or disease such as those in Table 16–3.

These entities evoke a limited variety of inflammatory exudates which range from simple serous fluid to frank pus. It is therefore possible, on an anatomic basis, to classify pericarditis as:

1. Serous.
2. Serofibrinous.
3. Fibrinous.
4. Suppurative.
5. Hemorrhagic.

TABLE 16–3. CAUSES OF PERICARDITIS*

	Per Cent
1. Infectious pericarditis:	
Bacterial	16
Tuberculous	7
Viral	?
Mycotic and protozoan	?
2. Metabolic pericarditis:	
Uremic	17
Cholesterol	
Myxedematous (noninflammatory)	
3. Neoplastic pericarditis	8
4. Acute myocardial infarction	11
5. Traumatic pericarditis	3
6. Hypersensitivity pericarditis (either exogenous or endogenous antigens):	
Rheumatic fever	11
Other autoimmune diseases (SLE, rheumatoid arthritis, scleroderma, polyarteritis)	3
Serum sickness, drug reactions	
The postcardiotomy, postmyocardial infarction, and post-traumatic syndromes	
7. Idiopathic pericarditis	23

*From Sodeman, W. A., and Smith R. H.: Re-evaluation of the diagnostic criteria for acute pericarditis. Amer. J. Med. Sci., 235:692, 1958.

Combinations of these anatomic types are quite frequent and, in fact, are more usual than the pure forms just listed. In the present consideration, the anatomic classification will be followed, since it is impossible in many instances to determine from the pathologic examination the etiologic basis for the inflammatory response without other correlated data (Bloedorn, 1940). These morphologic subdivisions are of further importance since each yields, to some extent, distinctive clinical signs and symptoms.

Serous Pericarditis. Serous inflammatory effusions are characteristically produced by nonbacterial inflammations, such as rheumatic fever, diffuse lupus erythematosus, Concato's polyserositis, tumors and viral infections of the heart. Similar effusions are also frequently encountered in the early stages of any form of bacterial pericarditis. Occasionally, a tuberculous infection of the pericardial sac or infections in the tissues contiguous to the pericardium evoke an inflammatory exudation that is principally serous in the early stages. For example, a bacterial pleuritis may cause sufficient irritation of the parietal pericardial serosa to cause a sterile serous effusion. In time, however, infection may extend across the anatomic barrier and the serous exudate is transformed into a frank suppurative reaction.

An uncommon form of serous acute idiopathic pericarditis occurs as a primary disorder. It is a benign infection that spontaneously resolves in days to weeks. Coxsackie and ECHO viruses have been isolated from some cases, but many remain of unknown origin.

Morphologically, whatever the cause of serous pericarditis, there is an inflammatory reaction in the epi- and pericardial surfaces of polymorphonuclear leukocytes, lymphocytes and histiocytes. Sometimes bacterial organisms or malignant tumor cells may be identified in the fluid, thus providing an indication of the etiology. Usually the volume of fluid is not large and varies between 50 and 200 ml. Because it represents a purely exudative phenomenon, it occurs slowly and therefore rarely produces sufficient increase in pressure to encroach upon the cardiac function. The fluid resorbs when and if the underlying disease remits. Organization or fibrous adhesions rarely develop.

Fibrinous and Serofibrinous Pericarditis. These two anatomic forms are considered together because they represent essentially similar processes in which there is a more or less serous fluid mixed with a fibrinous exudate. This is the most frequent type of pericarditis. *Rheumatic fever is the most common cause of this form of exudation. The second most common* *cause is myocardial infarction.* Bacterial, viral and occasionally obscure myocardial inflammations may also produce similar changes. Uremia (renal failure) may evoke a serofibrinous or fibrinous inflammatory exudation in the pericardial cavity. Just as pneumonia or suppurative infections in the pleural cavities may produce serous pericarditis, in more severe cases they may cause the outpouring of fibrin. Mediastinitis must be placed in this same category. Rarely, a primary pericarditis is manifested by a fibrinous exudation.

The gross morphologic alterations have already been described on p. 660 (Fig. 16–32).

As is the case with all inflammatory exudates, *the fibrin may be digested with resolution of the exudate, or the fibrin may become organized.* Organization and fibrous interadherence result, sometimes with complete obliteration of the pericardial sac. This fibrosis yields a delicate, stringy type of adhesion, called adhesive pericarditis, which only rarely hampers or restricts cardiac action. In this fibrinous variety of pericarditis, the organization rarely extends to surrounding contiguous structures, such as the thoracic wall, diaphragm or lungs, and therefore results only in obliteration of the space. In some cases, organization merely produces plaque-like fibrous thickenings of the serosal membranes (Fig. 16–33).

From the clinical standpoint, *the development of a loud pericardial friction rub is the most striking characteristic of fibrinous pericarditis.* A collection of serous fluid may obliterate the rub by separating the two layers of the pericardium. Pain, systemic febrile reactions and signs suggestive of cardiac failure may accompany the pathognomonic friction rub.

Fibrinous or serofibrinous pericarditis rarely leads to serious sequelae.

Purulent or Suppurative Pericarditis. This form of pericardial inflammation almost invariably denotes the presence of bacterial, mycotic or parasitic invasion of the pericardial space by organisms. It is most frequent in young males (3 to 1) between 10 and 40 years old. These organisms invade the pericardial cavity by (1) direct extension from neighboring inflammations, such as an empyema of the pleural cavity, lobar pneumonia, mediastinal infections, or bacterial invasion from the myocardium through the epicardium, (2) seeding from the blood or (3) lymphatic extension. This last mechanism perhaps best explains the spread of tuberculous infections from the lungs to the mediastinal nodes and thence through the lymphatics into the pericardial space. Occasionally, however, adherence of a tuberculous lymph node to some portion of the pericardial sac provides a direct path. Quite rarely, a serosuppurative exudate may be produced by sterile inflammations, such as result from a myocardial infarction or uremia. Rarely, severe viral infections of the heart, such as influenza or poliomyelitis, may cause suppurative pericarditis.

Infrequently, suppurative pericarditis occurs as an isolated disease in the absence of

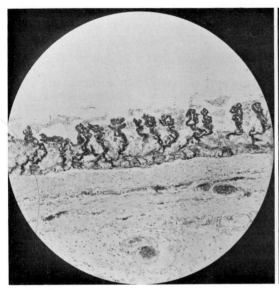
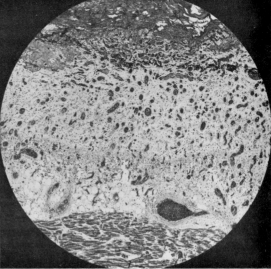

Fig. 16–32   Fig. 16–33

Figure 16–32. *Acute fibrinous pericarditis. The dark strands of fibrin are apparent on the epicardial surface.*
Figure 16–33. *Organizing fibrinous pericarditis. The myocardium is below; the amorphous material at the top is remaining fibrin.*

other infections or cardiac involvement– *primary pericarditis.* In certain of these instances, pericardial tap and bacterial culture have revealed bacteria that must be assumed to have been blood-borne and to have seeded the pericardium alone. Other cases have proved to be of viral etiology, particularly the Coxsackie and ECHO viruses, but usually these agents evoke a serous reaction.

On gross inspection, the suppurative pericardial fluid may consist of a thin, cloudy fluid, a frank, creamy pus or, in the case of tuberculosis, a thick, cheesy exudate characteristic of caseation necrosis. The volume of the exudate may vary from only a layer over the exposed surfaces to large volumes of pus, up to 500 cc. In the early stages, the exudate may be wiped off, exposing an underlying glistening surface, but soon the intense inflammatory reaction produces marked injection and granularity in the serosa.

On microscopic examination, intense inflammatory reaction characterizes the tissue changes. The reaction extends more deeply than that of the fibrinous variety, frequently involving the superficial regions of the myocardium. On the parietal surface, the inflammation may extend beyond the confines of the pericardial membrane into the surrounding mediastinal connective tissue, sometimes out into the pleural cavities and down onto the diaphragm to produce *mediastinopericarditis.* In the tuberculous variety of pericarditis, tubercles are characteristically present immediately beneath or above the serosal membranes.

The clinical findings are essentially the same as those present in fibrinous pericarditis, but while a friction rub may be present, it is not usually so prominent as in the fibrinous variety. On the other hand, the signs of systemic infection are more marked, for example, spiking temperatures, chills and fever.

Organization is the usual outcome of this inflammatory process with resolution being infrequent. Because of the greater intensity of the inflammatory response, the organization produces a rather dense interadherence of the epicardial and pericardial surfaces that may become calcified. *Mediastinopericarditis* or *concretio cordis,* having much greater clinical significance than simple adhesive pericarditis, may be the end result.

Hemorrhagic Pericarditis. Hemorrhagic pericarditis denotes an exudate composed of blood mixed with a fibrinous or suppurative effusion. It is most commonly caused by tuberculosis or by malignant neoplastic involvement of the pericardial space, but it may also be found in bacterial infections or in cases of pericarditis occurring in patients with some underlying bleeding diathesis. Hemorrhagic pericarditis must be differentiated from hemopericardium in which the fluid is purely blood of noninflammatory origin.

If the underlying cause is a tumor, neoplastic cells may be present in the effusion or in the pericardial or epicardial tissues. The clinical significance is that of a suppurative pericarditis, and resolution or organization with or without calcification is the eventual outcome.

Chronic or Healed Pericarditis. The term chronic pericarditis is a misnomer, since it refers in reality to a healed stage of one of the forms of pericardial inflammation already described. One pattern comprises the formation of pearly, thickened, nonadherent, epicardial plaques ("Soldier's plaque"). Alternatively, thin, delicate adhesions may develop which are termed diffuse or focal obliterative pericarditis according to their pattern. These rarely cause impairment of cardiac function but occur fairly frequently at autopsy and are often of obscure origin.

Two forms of healed pericarditis are of clinical importance: adhesive mediastinopericarditis and constrictive pericarditis.

Adhesive Mediastinopericarditis. This form of pericardial fibrosis usually follows a preexisting suppurative or tuberculous pericardial inflammation and is only a rare sequel to simple fibrinous exudate. As a result, it is *most commonly associated with bacterial infections or tuberculosis.* The pericardial sac is obliterated, and adherence of the external aspect of the parietal layer to surrounding structures produces a great strain upon cardiac function. With each systolic contraction, the heart is pulling not only against the parietal pericardium, but also against the attached surrounding structures. Systolic retractions of the rib cage and diaphragm, pulsus paradoxicus and a variety of other fairly pathognomonic findings may be observed clinically. *The increased workload causes cardiac hypertrophy and dilatation which may be quite massive in more severe cases.*

Constrictive Pericarditis. The formation of a dense, fibrous or fibrocalcific scar about the heart may result, as has been noted, from a preexisting suppurative or hemorrhagic pericarditis. Perhaps *the two most common causal agents which result in this type of damage are the pyogenic staphylococcus and the tubercle bacillus.* Fibrinous or serofibrinous inflammatory reactions rarely lead to this form of damage. In constrictive pericarditis, the pericardial space not only is obliterated, but is transformed into a dense layer of scar or calcification, many times 0.5 to 1.0 cm. thick, which resists dissection. In extreme cases, it appears as if the heart were enclosed within a plaster mold (*concretio cordis*). In less severe instances, only irregular calcific plates are produced.

Severe cardiac dysfunction results because the heart can no longer expand adequately during diastole. While the signs of cardiac failure may resemble those produced by mediastinopericarditis, the local findings in the heart are quite different. *Cardiac hypertrophy and dilatation cannot occur because of the dense enclosing scar* and, as a consequence, the heart is described as a small, quiet heart with reduced minute volume output and reduced pulse pressure. Constriction of the venae cavae during the fibrotic process may block the venous return to the right side of the heart.

This combination of findings, namely, constrictive pericarditis and compression of the venae cavae, is sometimes referred to as *Pick's disease.* It is to be emphasized that Pick's disease is not a specific entity, but rather a clinical syndrome resulting from a constrictive pericarditis. It is associated then with marked congestion of the liver, sometimes going on to congestive fibrosis in this organ (cardiac sclerosis or cardiac cirrhosis), splenomegaly and ascites.

TUMORS OF THE PERICARDIUM

Primary tumors of the pericardium are extremely rare. Among the benign group, lipomas and hemangiomas have been described. Other varieties may occur, such as fibromas, neuromas and myxomas, but they are medical curiosities. Primary malignancy in the pericardium implies an origin from either the mesothelial surfaces or the underlying fibrofatty tissue, with the resulting sarcoma resembling an analogous growth anywhere else in the body.

Secondary tumors affect the pericardial sac more commonly than primary tumors. These usually reach the pericardium through one of two channels, either direct extension from tumors in the other heart layers or organs in the chest, or metastatic spread of a distant malignancy. The most frequent tumors which directly invade the pericardium are lymphomas, which arise in the mediastinal or tracheobronchial lymph nodes, bronchogenic carcinoma of the lungs and carcinomas of the esophageal mucosa. Distant blood- or lymphatic-borne metastases may arise from malignancy in any organ of the body but, on the whole, metastatic as well as primary involvement of the pericardium is rare.

SEROUS ATROPHY OF PERICARDIAL FAT

While this form of atrophy affects all fat depots, it is particularly evident in the subepicardial and subpericardial fat. In any form of chronic inanition or malnutrition, the lipid vacuoles in the fat cells immediately subjacent to these serosal surfaces are resorbed. The cells then become filled with a thin, watery fluid. A pearly gray, wrinkled, loose, edematous opalescence is imparted to these surfaces, and on microscopic examination a thin, granular, proteinous precipitate is found within the preexisting fatty vacuoles. The entity is without intrinsic clinical significance, and is of interest only as an indicator of marked weight loss.

MYOCARDIAL DISEASE—CARDIOMYOPATHY

The term cardiomyopathy has come to have different meanings to the many writers on this subject. In its broadest interpretation, it has been defined as "an acute, subacute or chronic disorder of the heart muscle of unknown or obscure etiology, often with associated endocardial or sometimes with pericardial involvement, but not atherosclerotic in origin" (Goodwin, 1964). An alternative definition offers: "any dysfunction of the myocardium not attributable to coronary heart disease, valvular disease, hypertension or pulmonary heart disease" (Fejfar, 1968). So defined by exclusion, the cardiopathies obviously embrace a diverse and wide range of disorders. While many are of unknown or obscure etiology, some of the entities reasonably included under the designation cardiomyopathy are of fairly well defined etiology, such as the excessive deposits of glycogen in the glycogen-storage diseases (p. 296) and the myocardial alterations in beriberi heart disease (p. 497). Some attempt at further specificity is approached by dividing them into primary and secondary forms. In the primary cardiomyopathies, the myocardium is the sole or dominant site of injury and the myocardial involvement is not associated with generalized or systemic disease. Viral myocarditis, when the virus infection involves only the heart, is an example of a primary cardiomyopathy. Secondary cardiomyopathy, in contrast, refers to myocardial involvement as only one part of a generalized disorder, examples being rheumatic fever, the glycogen-storage disorders and systemic amyloidosis. A classification may also be based on pathologic and/or etiologic criteria as follows:

Hereditary	Familial cardiomyopathy, Marfan's syndrome, Hurler's disease (gargoylism), Friedreich's disease, progressive muscular dystrophy
Inflammatory	Microbiologic: bacterial, viral, mycotic, rickettsial, protozoal, Fiedler's (? giant cell) myocarditis
	Immunologic: rheumatic fever, rheumatoid arthritis, systemic lupus erythematosus, polyarteritis nodosa, systemic scleroderma, dermatomyositis, hypersensitivity reactions

Toxic (chemicals, drugs)	Emetine, chloroform, carbon tetrachloride, arsenic, phosphorus, bacterial toxins
Metabolic	Amyloidosis, hemochromatosis, potassium and magnesium depletion, glycogen-storage disorders
Nutritional	Alcoholic, beriberi heart disease
Endocrine	Thyroid and pituitary dysfunction
Idiopathic	Idiopathic cardiac hypertrophy, idiopathic cardiomyopathy, idiopathic hypertrophic subaortic stenosis, peripartal cardiomyopathy, endomyocardial fibrosis

Friedberg (1966), however, would reserve the term cardiomyopathy for the more insidious, often degenerative forms of myocardial damage, while the myocardiopathies of an inflammatory nature he terms myocarditis. Myocarditis, he points out, is usually of sudden onset and often produces acute cardiac failure. It is generally characterized by a prominent inflammatory reaction, with necrosis of isolated cells or small groups of myocardial fibers, and it tends to pursue a course of varying length. If the patient survives, it becomes quiescent, sometimes leaving behind little or no residual myocardial scarring. In contrast, in the cardiomyopathies, the myocardial alterations generally evoke little inflammatory reaction. Some are present from birth (as in the hereditary group), most run a protracted course, and many never remit. For long periods of time, they usually evoke no symptoms until, for mysterious reasons and apparently without provocation, cardiac failure insidiously sets in. Such a clear separation into myocarditis or cardiomyopathy is not always possible, and many cases must be classified arbitrarily. Recognizing these conceptual and nosologic difficulties, we shall here classify inflammatory myocarditis as a subgroup of the larger category of cardiomyopathies.

MYOCARDITIS (INFLAMMATORY CARDIOMYOPATHY)

In several studies, myocarditis was reported to be present in from 4 to 10 per cent of routine autopsies, but in many of these cases it was an incidental and chance finding (Wenger, 1968) (Saphir, 1941, 1942). Virtually every microbiologic agent and systemic immunologic disorder has, at one time or another, been the cause of an inflammatory myocarditis. In some instances, the myocarditis is secondary to a generalized disease, for example, in rheumatic fever; in other instances, it may be an isolated lesion and thus comprise a primary myocarditis.

Secondary myocarditis is far more common than primary, largely because rheumatic fever is the predominant cause of clinically significant inflammatory disease within the myocardium. Other causes of secondary myocarditis include the bacterial infections: diphtheria, typhoid fever, scarlet fever and penetration of infections from vegetative endocarditis. Viral disorders including influenza, poliomyelitis, mumps, measles, and infectious mononucleosis and especially those caused by the Coxsackie and ECHO viruses sometimes evoke inflammatory myocardial changes. Most rickettsial infections also induce some myocardial damage. Among the parasitic infections of principal importance are Chagas' disease, toxoplasmosis and trichinosis. The systemic connective tissue diseases such as SLE and scleroderma and generalized hypersensitivity reactions often involve the myocardium. The list of etiologies might be much longer.

Primary myocarditis is fortunately an uncommon clinical entity (Gore and Saphir, 1947). Among the more common causes are type B Coxsackie virus, ECHO viruses, *Toxoplasma gondii* and the trypanosomes of Chagas' disease. In addition, there are acute myocarditides of unknown etiology designated as Fiedler's myocarditis which may or may not be identical with the entity recently described as giant cell myocarditis. Both of these last mentioned forms of primary myocarditis are fortunately rare, but when present are often fatal.

An attempt will be made to present a survey of the morphologic changes seen in the various forms of myocarditis by dividing them into: (1) suppurative myocarditis, (2) interstitial myocarditis, (3) parenchymatous myocarditis and (4) miscellaneous forms of myocarditis.

Suppurative myocarditis may take the form of focal necroses or abscesses when caused by such pyogens as staphylococci, gram-negative bacilli, pneumococci and meningococci. Alternatively, it may represent a diffuse spreading infection with extensive neutrophilic exudation trekking through the interstitial connective tissue and between fibers, causing, at the same time, necrosis of small groups of muscle fibers. Such a pattern is characteristic of beta hemolytic streptococcal infections. With suppurative myocarditis, the abscesses may be visualized grossly or may only appear as minute yellow foci against the red-brown background of the myocardium. The spreading infections may be even more difficult to visualize and may be manifest only by some flabbiness of the myocardium associated with focal areas of gray-yellow pallor. In such acute forms of myocarditis, the heart is usually not enlarged, but is often dilated, principally on the right side.

Interstitial myocarditis is characteristic of

most viral involvements. Among the viruses, Coxsackie group B types 1 to 5 have been recognized as important causes of primary myocarditis and pericarditis. These affect principally children and young adults, males more often than females. In adults, the disease is relatively benign and self-limited, but when the virus is acquired as an intrauterine or neonatal infection, it may be fulminant and fatal (Blattner, 1968). The anatomic appearance of most forms of viral myocarditis is that of a diffuse interstitial inflammatory reaction throughout the heart. The individual myocardial fibers are separated by edema, and the intercellular and perivascular spaces are sprinkled with leukocytes, principally lymphocytes and macrophages (Fig. 16–34). There may be remarkably little myofiber necrosis. Rarely, in fulminant infections such as poliomyelitis, there are large numbers of granulocytes. When the disease has run its course, these acute changes are apparently reversible since, at some later date, no evidence of previous inflammatory changes are noted. However, occasional instances are encountered where diffuse interstitial fibrosis of uncertain etiology is present, and the possibility is raised of a prior viral infection.

Parenchymatous myocarditis refers to cases in which there is diffuse but spotty destruction of muscle cells. Such parenchymal injury is seen in diphtheria, typhoid fever, occasionally hemolytic streptococcal infections and is particularly characteristic of protozoan and parasitic

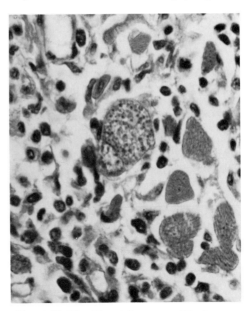

Figure 16–35. *Chagasic myocarditis. A myocardial fiber (center) is filled with parasites. Surrounding fibers have been destroyed and replaced by a leukocytic infiltrate.*

invasions. Involvement of the heart in trichinosis is described on p. 456, and in toxoplasmosis, on p. 455. Myocardial involvement is the most important aspect of Chagas' disease in approximately 80 per cent of patients. This trypanosomal infection, while uncommon in industrial nations, affects up to half of the population in endemic areas of South America. Patients may die during an acute attack (approximately 10 per cent) or they may enter a chronic phase lasting 10 or 20 years to develop progressive signs of cardiac insufficiency. In some instances, the cardiac damage develops without a history of an antecedent acute infection. In the fulminant forms of the disease, the flagellated trypanosomes leave the blood and invade RE cells, and smooth, skeletal and cardiac muscle cells. Within these cells, the protozoa are converted into aflagellate leishmanial forms which destroy cardiac muscle cells and produce so-called pseudocysts surrounded by a heavy infiltrate of granulocytes as well as occasional lymphocytes, monocytes and fibroblasts (Fig. 16–35). In this focus of necrosis, all myocardial fibers are destroyed. In the more chronic insidious forms of the disease, the inflammatory reaction tends to be more diffuse, with widespread interstitial mononuclear and eosinophilic infiltrations accompanied by necrosis of isolated muscle fibers; widespread fibrosis eventually ensues. Such hearts may be enlarged and dilated, and mural thrombi

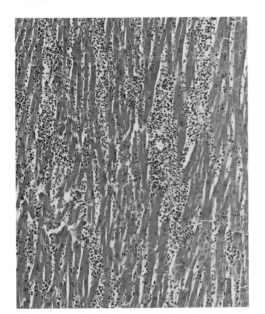

Figure 16–34. *Viral myocarditis. The myocardial fibers are separated by edema, and there is a diffuse interstitial, mononuclear leukocytic reaction.*

are frequent. Myocardial cells parasitized by the organisms are seen in the acute forms of the disease, but are difficult to identify in the chronic stages (Prata, 1968). The importance of Chagasic myocarditis is evident from the fact that it causes about 25 per cent of all deaths in persons between the ages of 25 and 44 in endemic areas (Fejfar, 1968).

Under the *miscellaneous* category of morphologic changes in myocarditis fall two specific entities: *Fiedler's myocarditis and giant cell myocarditis*, although these may be one and the same entity. *Fiedler's myocarditis* is a somewhat poorly defined clinicopathologic disorder, usually appearing as a primary or "isolated" myocarditis of acute onset which often rapidly leads to a fatal outcome. It is most common in young adults but has been reported at all ages. A variety of causative agents or mechanisms have been postulated, including viral infection, toxoplasmosis, immunologic reactions and perhaps hypersensitivity to drugs but, in last analysis, the cause is idiopathic. The anatomic changes as recorded in the literature are quite variable and raise the suspicion that more than one entity has been described as Fiedler's myocarditis. In some cases, there is a fairly diffuse interstitial inflammatory reaction characterized by edema, macrophages, eosinophils, lymphocytes and plasma cells, along with necrosis of isolated muscle fibers. At other times, the reaction is granulomatous with focal necroses of the myocardium. Occasionally, these lesions resemble tubercles or miliary granulomas with focal fibrosis and infiltrates of lymphocytes, plasma cells, macrophages and multinucleate giant cells. Grossly, the heart is usually dilated and hypertrophied, often strikingly so, and weights of 500 to 700 gm. are not uncommon. The histologic changes may not be evident to the naked eye or may appear as irregular, yellowish or gray streaks or dots. The pericardium and endocardium are not involved, but mural thrombi may be present in the ventricular chambers.

A condition quite similar to Fiedler's myocarditis has been reported in the literature under the name of *giant cell myocarditis* (Pyun et al., 1970). The anatomic changes in giant cell myocarditis are indistinguishable from or identical to those described in the granulomatous pattern of Fiedler's myocarditis, and it is entirely likely that we are dealing with the same entity under a different designation.

Immunologic reactions also induce a miscellany of anatomic forms of myocarditis. Those encountered in rheumatic fever and the so-called connective tissue diseases discussed in Chapter 7 need not be further detailed. But in addition to these well defined nosologic entities, hypersensitivity reactions, possibly to infectious agents or to drugs, sometimes induce myocardial changes. These take varied forms, ranging from acute arteritis with inflammatory changes, principally localized to the perivascular and connective tissue septa, to diffuse interstitial inflammation characterized by interfiber edema and mononuclear infiltrations admixed with eosinophils. Isolated myofiber necrosis may be present in rheumatoid heart disease, and there are often focal areas of myocardial necrosis and sometimes valvular thickenings (p. 694). Another form of immunologic reaction is encountered in cardiac transplantation, namely, that produced by histocompatibility rejection reactions. The changes are similar to those encountered in other forms of transplant rejection described on p. 211.

The clinical features associated with myocarditis depend on whether it is primary or secondary (i.e., overlaid by systemic manifestations) and on the severity of the myocardial damage. Only certain generalizations will be offered here. Often myocarditis is encountered at postmortem examination as an unexpected finding in patients who had no manifestations of cardiac disease. When cardiac signs are evoked, they take the form of (1) electrocardiographic changes including arrhythmias, (2) pain referable to the heart, (3) the rapid development of cardiac enlargement, (4) the rapid onset of congestive heart failure and (5) sometimes sudden death. Usually, the manifestations are predominantly those of right-sided congestive heart failure since the thinner-walled right ventricle expresses the myocardial injury earlier than the thicker left side of the heart. In general, in acute myocarditis the stage of maximal tissue injury is also the stage of maximal clinical evidence of myocardial disease in contrast to the cardiomyopathies which are far more insidious and latent. Important in arriving at a diagnosis of acute myocarditis is the exclusion of other well defined etiologic entities such as coronary heart disease and valvular heart disease. At best, the clinical diagnosis is difficult.

CARDIOMYOPATHY

The term cardiomyopathy, as used here, applies to those forms of myocardial disease, often of obscure etiology, characterized by the slow, insidious development of myocardial dysfunction and often intractable congestive heart failure. So used, the term cardiomyopathy excludes the more fulminant forms of myocardial disease just discussed under the heading of myocarditis. The cardiomyopathies can be divided into presumed etiologic categories as was done on p. 685. However, their causation is so uncertain that we shall simply divide them here into primary and secondary forms. The secondary patterns are seen in a diverse group of clinical settings as indicated in the previous classification. Most of these systemic disorders have been discussed elsewhere in this book. The primary cardiomyopathies are relatively few in number and are largely of unknown etiology. A few details of some of the more important forms follow.

Alcoholic cardiomyopathy is a form of cardiac disease related to the excessive consumption of alcohol, but it is still not clear that the alcohol is a direct myocardial toxin. There is, however, evidence that it is not a consequence of either thiamine deficiency or generalized malnutrition. Chronic alcoholism, even in patients who appear to be entirely well otherwise, results in the release of myocardial enzymes, suggesting a direct injurious effect on the myocardial fibers (Wendt et al., 1966). Alcoholic cardiomyopathy must further be differentiated from the *cardiomyopathy encountered in beer drinkers* which occurred in virtually epidemic form in Quebec and Omaha. This far more malignant disorder of acute onset and rapidly progressive CHF was traced to cobalt added to the beer to enhance its "head" (Symposium on Quebec beer drinkers' cardiomyopathy, 1967).

The prevalence of alcoholic cardiomyopathy is uncertain, but it has been estimated to account for about 3 per cent of all cases of heart disease admitted to veterans' or large municipal hospitals. It is almost entirely limited to the habitual heavy drinker. Anatomically, the heart shows mainly dilatation with slight hypertrophy of all cardiac chambers. The myocardium is pale and flabby. Occasional endocardial fibrotic patches and overlying thrombi may be present. On light microscopy, there may be little in the way of distinctive change. The usual findings are slight atrophy of myocardial cells and slight increase of interstitial tissue, but these are neither striking nor diagnostic. In contrast, electron microscopy will disclose widespread ultrastructural changes including loss or degeneration of contractile myofibrils, swollen mitochondria, cystic dilatation of the sarcoplasmic reticulum and increased numbers of liposomes (Sanders, 1970). A marked decrease in myocardial oxidative enzymes can also be demonstrated. The diagnosis depends on a history of habitual alcohol consumption and findings relative to widespread myocardial disease. Those who completely abstain from alcohol progressively improve and may later have no evidence of myocardial damage, but those who continue to drink pursue a course of progressively worsening CHF and about half will be dead in two to three years (Shanoff, 1972).

Idiopathic hypertrophy and *idiopathic cardiomyopathy* are the designations applied to a somewhat varied group of primary myopathies of unknown etiology which have in common only cardiac hypertrophy of mysterious origin and, eventually, progressive CHF. In some instances, the cardiac enlargement is present when the patient is first seen, and the possibility of a congenital origin cannot be excluded. However, other patients have apparently acquired the disease because previous examinations had not disclosed cardiac enlargement. A higher incidence of idiopathic hypertrophy has been found among those living in tropical climates. Some nutritional deficiency is suspected, and there is some evidence that protein calorie deficiency may cause myofiber atrophy and interstitial fibrosis which, in time, leads to failure and consequent hypertrophy of less affected muscle cells (Ramalingaswami, 1968). In other instances, past episodes of myocarditis or alcoholic myopathy might be the basis for the cardiac hypertrophy. Recently, immunoglobulins were demonstrated in the hearts of three patients apparently suffering from this disease (Das, 1971). The significance of these immunologic findings is unclear, and they might merely reflect a secondary response to previous myocardial damage (Kaplan and Frengley, 1969). It is entirely likely that multiple, diverse causations underlie the umbrella nonspecific designation—idiopathic hypertrophy.

The major pathologic findings are cardiac hypertrophy and mural fibrosis. The hypertrophy may be quite massive and may narrow the outflow tracts of either ventricle, obstruct the tricuspid valve or prevent proper closure of the mitral valve. Commonly there is some fibrosis of the myocardium which may be focal or diffuse. Electron microscopy has shown some sarcomeres with Z bands pulled wide apart while others were squashed together. Mural thrombi may be present in either or both ventricles, and occasionally there is patchy or diffuse endocardial fibrosis.

It is evident that the diagnosis of idiopathic hypertrophy is based largely on negative findings, e.g., the inability to establish any other basis for the cardiac hypertrophy and the absence of well defined nosologic entities. The clinical course is usually one of protracted cardiac failure, sometimes punctuated by pulmonary embolism arising in the right-sided ventricular mural thrombi. It is difficult to establish a prognosis for such a rag bag of disorders but, in general, the disease is resistant to therapy, and while many patients may live for decades with supportive treatment, in others, the course is slowly downhill with intractable CHF. In still others, sudden death is caused by arrhythmias or pulmonary embolization.

Peripartal cardiomyopathy is the term applied to primary myocardial disease mysteriously appearing in previously healthy women during the puerperium or, less frequently, in late pregnancy. It appears most commonly in the first two months after childbirth and manifests itself as the sudden onset of CHF. If the patient recovers, the failure may recur with successive pregnancies. The validity of this syndrome as a specific clinicopathologic entity is under challenge. Hudson (1970) states, "I do not believe that there is an underlying specific cardiomyopathy in such cases; many factors are concerned, for example toxemia, prolonged labor, shock and hemorrhage from sudden emptying of the gravid uterus, drugs such as oxytocin and ergometrine and noxious substances used as abortifacients." However, the occasional instances where cardiac failure develops when none of the adverse influences cited by Hudson are present would suggest that there may be such an entity as peripartal cardiomyopathy (Stuart, 1968). The anatomic findings are quite nonspecific and essentially disclose cardiac hypertrophy with focal or diffuse myocardial fibrosis, changes not dissimilar from those encountered in idiopathic hypertrophy described above.

Familial cardiomyopathy simply implies that a form of idiopathic cardiomyopathy has been encountered in family groups in such frequency as to suggest hereditary transmission of some genetic defect. In a recent report of 11 families, of 98 persons examined, 47 suffered from a cardiomyopathy (Kariv et al., 1971). Their mean age at the time of detection of the disease was 24 years, with a range of two to 61 years of age. There was no difference in incidence between the sexes. The pedigrees suggested transmission of an autosomal dominant mutant gene with high penetrance. The anatomic findings are not distinctive and comprise cardiac hypertrophy and dilatation affecting both right and left sides. The hypertrophy may be quite extreme and may cause obstruction to the ventricular outflow tracts as well as to the mitral and tricuspid valves. Mural thrombi are often present in the cardiac chambers, principally the ventricles. Histologically, the changes are again nonspecific, consisting largely of myocardial fibrosis, focal or diffuse, occasionally associated with individual fiber necrosis or larger areas of myocardial necrosis. No specific metabolic or biochemical

defect has been identified in the muscle fibers which might induce such changes, and the causation of the disease is totally obscure. Nonetheless, myocardial dysfunction and anatomic cardiac changes in young infants strongly suggest some influence present from birth. The diagnosis rests with the documentation of a cardiomyopathy and some familial background. Among the 47 cases identified in the study referred to earlier, 10 died during the follow-up period of seven years, and only 13 have remained asymptomatic and apparently entirely compensated.

The best example of *metabolic cardiomyopathy* is that found in association with abnormalities in the serum levels of potassium.

Hypokalemia affects the kidneys (p. 1113) and the skeletal muscles but is particularly damaging to the heart. The low serum levels of potassium may be brought about by: (1) an inadequate intake of potassium; (2) excessive loss as occurs in protracted vomiting, diarrhea or persistent diuresis; (3) adrenocortical hyperactivity (Cushing's syndrome, hyperaldosteronism); (4) shift of the electrolyte into cells as in some forms of periodic paralysis; and (5) the administration of adrenocorticoids. A variety of myocardial structural abnormalities have been observed in both experimental animals and man, including swelling of myocardial cells, loss of striations and a variety of regressive structural and ultrastructural alterations in fibers to the point of frank necrosis. The parenchymal changes may be accompanied by interstitial edema and, in some cases, interstitial fibrosis (Tucker et al., 1963) (Molnar et al., 1962). These cellular abnormalities have been attributed to alterations of membrane permeability induced by the electrolyte imbalance.

The low serum potassium greatly influences the resting potential across the myocardial cell membrane and these electrochemical effects, combined with the myocardial cell damage, result in serious conduction disturbances in the heart manifested by arrhythmias, characteristic electrocardiographic changes and sometimes cardiac arrest.

Hyperkalemia also causes cardiac changes. High serum levels can be induced by: (1) potassium infusions; (2) increased oral intake of potassium; (3) renal failure, especially in cases of acute tubular necrosis (ATN); (4) Addison's disease; (5) multiple transfusions of stored blood; (6) metabolic acidosis; and (7) sickle cell anemia. Hyperkalemia may also be encountered in the untreated stage of diabetic acidosis. Striking effects on cardiac rate (bradycardia) and rhythm (ventricular fibrillation or even cardiac standstill) are produced with distinctive electrocardiographic abnormalities.

Despite these clear-cut manifestations of myocardial injury, no well defined morphologic changes have been identified.

Endomyocardial fibrosis is an idiopathic form of myocardiopathy encountered principally or perhaps exclusively in Africa where it accounts for 10 to 15 per cent of the cardiac disease seen in hospitals (Davies, 1961). Occasional cases have been reported in temperate climes, but their etiologic identity is uncertain. Endomyocardial fibrosis closely resembles endocardial fibroelastosis described on p. 692. The latter entity shows no specific geographic distribution. The essential pathologic findings in endomyocardial fibrosis are cardiomegaly and thickening of the endocardium. The inflow tracts of the ventricles may show more endocardial fibrosis than the outflow tracts. The atria may be similarly affected, although usually to a lesser degree. The fibrosis converts the endocardium to a thick, tough, white layer which often involves the inner third of the myocardium (Shaper, 1968). The fibrosing process often enmeshes the chordae tendineae and even the cusps of adjacent valves and sometimes causes valvular insufficiency. In occasional cases, foci of necrosis of the myocardium are encountered and so it is assumed that much of the fibrosis represents scarring following active destruction of the inner layer of myocardium. Unlike endocardial fibroelastosis, in the African cardiomyopathy, there is very little elastic tissue within the collagenous fibrosis. Mural thrombosis is especially frequent in endomyocardial fibrosis and is found in all four chambers, principally in the left ventricle and right atrium. Embolization, therefore, is a common complication of this disease. The clinical findings and course are essentially similar to those of the other myopathies with the addition of the increased threat of embolization.

The clinical recognition and the differential diagnosis of the various cardiomyopathies are, at best, treacherous. It must be apparent that the cardiomyopathies represent an area of cardiology more characterized by semantic confusion, poorly defined entities and uncertain etiology than any other category of cardiac disease. The innumerable attempts to redefine and reclassify the cardiomyopathies have only led to a profusion of differing classifications and greater uncertainty. *Some clinical cardiologists have therefore admitted the large gaps in our knowledge and retreated to a pathophysiologic classification* which recognizes four hemodynamic patterns: (1) a pattern with virtually normal cardiac output, stroke volume and either normal or mildly elevated ventricular filling pressures; (2) a restrictive hemodynamic pattern characterized principally by elevated right and left ventricular filling pressures, reflecting a decreased compliance of the ventricle (this pattern resembles that seen in constrictive pericarditis); (3) an obstructive pattern with massive cardiac hypertrophy obstructing the left ventricular outflow tract and sometimes the right ventricular outflow, as well as the inflow tracts on both sides of the heart; and (4) a pattern characterized by biventricular failure manifested by a combination of low cardiac output, small stroke volume and a significant increase in both left and right atrial and ventricular end-diastolic pressures.

The pathophysiologic patterns do not conform to specific anatomic forms of cardiomyopathy as given before. The first pattern might be found in any early or mild form of myocardial involvement. Endomyocardial fibrosis and certain secondary forms of cardiomyopathy such as amyloidosis tend to produce restrictive hemodynamic patterns. In contrast, familial cardiomyopathy and idiopathic hypertrophy tend to produce obstructive hemodynamic syndromes. The congestive hemodynamic pattern is simply the end stage of many of the disorders mentioned before. One special type of obstructive syndrome has been designated as *idiopathic hypertrophic subaortic stenosis*. Cases so diagnosed are sometimes familial and sometimes sporadic (Morrow et al., 1968). Here we have a classic example of a pathophysiologic syndrome which has been confused with a specific disease. There is considerable clinical justification for the pathophysiologic categorizations because, for example, the obstructive myopathies are worsened by many of the commonly used cardiac drugs which increase myocardial contractility. Increase in the strength of the cardiac contraction sometimes simultaneously increases the obstruction to blood flow. Regrettably, it is impossible to further untangle this most interesting but confusing group of primary myocardial diseases.

ENDOCARDIAL DISEASE

While the myocardium is the vital component which maintains the volume output of the heart, it can perform adequately only with functioning valves. The most important pathologic entities that cause significant endocardial disease are rheumatic fever, disease incident to coronary arterial involvement, syphilitic heart disease, vegetative endocarditis, congenital heart disease and calcific aortic stenosis. There are only a few other lesions that significantly affect the endocardium.

NONBACTERIAL VERRUCOUS ENDOCARDITIS (LIBMAN-SACKS DISEASE)

In disseminated lupus erythematosus, mitral and tricuspid valvulitis is occasionally encountered. This form of endocardial involvement is one of the important components of this systemic immunologic disorder (Moschcowitz, 1946–47). The connective tissue of the valves may become the site of mucoid pooling, fibrinoid necrosis and subsequent collagenous fibrosis. Frequently, this type of inflammatory valvulitis leads to the formation of small vegetations on the valve leaflets that sometimes can be confused with the much larger, friable vegetations of vegetative endocarditis or with nonbacterial thrombotic endocarditis. The characteristics and significance of Libman-Sacks disease have already been discussed (p. 232).

NONBACTERIAL THROMBOTIC ENDOCARDITIS (MARANTIC ENDOCARDITIS)

This disorder is characterized by the precipitation of small masses of fibrin and other blood elements upon the valve leaflets, usually those of the left side of the heart. Small, 1 to 5 mm. vegetations are formed, which to a considerable extent resemble those of acute rheumatic endocarditis and Libman-Sacks disease. These vegetations may occur singly or multiply to form a small row along the line of closure of the leaflet. Less often, they occur at other sites on the leaflets and even on the pulmonic and tricuspid valves. In some instances, the affected leaflets have some form of previous damage, such as old inflammatory rheumatic changes or degenerative alterations due to vascular heart disease. Histologically, the vegetations are bland and there is no significant accompanying inflammatory reaction.

The significance and interpretation of these lesions is controversial. In most instances the patients with these valvular changes have died of some protracted debilitating disease, such as cancer, cardiac decompensation or some serious ailment. Accordingly, these vegetations have been interperted as occurring during the last days of life, and hence have been spoken of as *marantic endocarditis or endocardiosis*. However, recent studies propose that these lesions may occur prior to the agonal stages of life, and may be related to an increased tendency to clotting (the so-called hypercoagulable state) (MacDonald and Robbins, 1957). In these circumstances, the vegetations carry the potential of producing clinically significant emboli. As previously mentioned, some propose that this disease is an important subsoil for the development of bacterial endocarditis.

ENDOCARDIAL FIBROELASTOSIS

Endocardial fibroelastosis is an uncommon heart disease of obscure etiology characterized by focal or diffuse fibroelastic thickening of the mural endocardium. The disease occurs in infants, children and adults but is far more common in the first two years of life. There is no clearly defined sex preponderance or racial difference. It is, however, of considerable interest from the pathogenetic standpoint that cases have been reported in identical twins, triplets and in siblings, suggesting a possible heredo-familial transmission. Supporting such a genetic mechanism is the concurrence of congenital abnormalities elsewhere in the body, some in the heart. Some investigators state that such concomitant anomalies are rare, while others indicate a 75 per cent association. Cases associated with congenital anomalies are sometimes referred to as "secondary fibroelastosis," the remainder being called "primary fibroelastosis" (McCormick, 1958). In a series of 47 cases studied by Moller and his coworkers (1964), 23 were "primary" and, among the remaining "secondary" cases, 8 had associated aortic stenosis; 8, coarctation of the aorta; 3, anomalous origin of the left coronary artery from the pulmonary trunk; and 5, hypoplasia of the left ventricle.

The etiology and pathogenesis of this disorder remain unknown. Perhaps the earliest hypothesis is indicated by the historic name "fetal endocarditis." Since this endocardial lesion is sometimes encountered in stillborn fetuses, it is postulated that intrauterine infection of the endocardium leads to the dense fibrous scarring. This view, while not completely invalidated, is not generally held. Currently, five major hypotheses are offered: (1) intrauterine hypoxia, (2) abnormal differentiation of the bulbus cordis, (3) stress reaction, (4) a genetic metabolic defect of the myocardium and (5) inflammatory disease.

Hypoxia has received considerable acceptance as a possible cause. As pointed out earlier, in some cases the left coronary artery originates from the pulmonary artery, providing a plausible basis for hypoxic damage. In other cases, there is premature closure of the foramen ovale.

The concept of abnormal differentiation proposes that instead of the normal incorporation of the bulbus cordis into the ventricles, it overgrows to produce a markedly thickened fibrous layer that lines the cardiac chambers.

Many students of this disease have suggested that the endocardial lesion is a fibrosing reaction to cardiac dilatation and stress on the inner layers of the myocardium. The stress might occur in utero (accounting for the infantile cases) or might occur in later life. Moller and his group (1964) emphasize subtle mitral insufficiency as the source of the stress in the so-called "primary" form of the disease and point out the association of aortic valvular stenosis and coarctation of the aorta in many "secondary" cases.

On the grounds that the condition is often congenital, agreed to by most investigators, a genetic metabolic defect has been postulated. As previously mentioned, a definite familial pattern has been defined in a few cases (Kelley and Anderson, 1956). Without much supporting evidence, the proponents of this view represent the fibroelastosis as some inherited metabolic deficiency in the myocardial fiber causing weakness in the myocardium. Presumably, such weakness would lead to dilatation and to the fibrous thickenings that have been described above with the stress theory. It should be noted, however, that to date no metabolic defect or enzyme deficiency has been identified.

By electron microscopy, a thin layer of fibrin has been identified on the endocardial surface (Still and Boult, 1956). This finding has led to the suggestion that some inflammatory or necrotizing disorder of the subendocardial myocardium precedes and initiates the deposit of fibrin. But no clearly defined abnormality has been seen in the superficial myocardial cells.

Fibroelastosis of the endocardium appears as a diffuse or patchy opaque thickening of the mural endocardium, predominantly of the left ventricle. However, the left auricle, right ventricle and right auricle, in order of frequency, may also be involved (Fig. 16–36). The thickening appears as a pearly-white, diffuse lining, sometimes having a depth ten times normal. It is usually covered by an intact endocardium. Mural thrombi overlying the fibrotic endocardium are present in a small percentage of cases. The trabeculae carneae are often flattened. Almost invariably the heart is enlarged and dilated. The heart valves are affected in about half of the cases, principally the aortic and mitral valves. The valves on the right are rarely affected. The aortic valve involvement is usually most severe

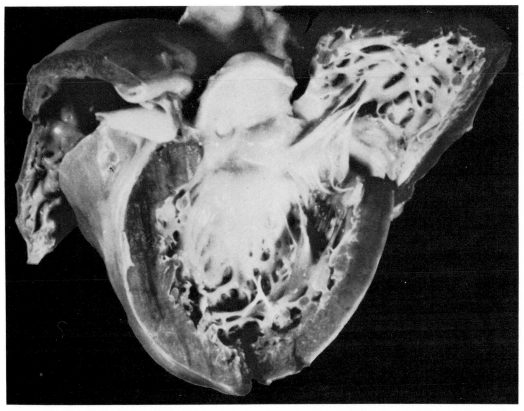

Figure 16–36. Marked fibroelastic thickening of the entire left ventricular lining with involvement of aortic valve in a 6-year-old who died of heart failure.

and takes the form of diffuse thickening, rigidity and nodularity of the cusps.

On histologic examination of these hearts, there is marked increase of collagenous and elastic fibers on the endocardial surface. The fibers generally run parallel to the surface. This fibrosis extends superficially into the immediate subjacent myocardium. Only occasionally are scattered lymphocytes present. A few cases have focal necroses in the myocardium immediately subjacent to the fibrotic endocardium, but it is not certain whether these necroses antedate the development of the endocardial thickening or, more likely, are a consequence of impaired vascular supply to the contiguous muslce fibers.

Superimposed upon this primary pattern of fibroelastosis are a variety of forms of cardiac and noncardiac congenital anomalies. As mentioned, some of these anomalies may have caused intrauterine anoxia. These include, among others, anomalous origin of the coronary arteries and coarctation of the aorta.

The significance of this lesion depends upon the extent of involvement. When focal, it may have no functional importance and permit normal longevity. When diffuse, it may be responsible for cardiac decompensation and death. In infants, the cardiac failure may be rapid, progressive and even fulminating. Usually, however, in older children and adults there are signs and symptoms of cardiac decompensation for months to years, and death is occasioned by emboli arising in the mural thrombi or by chronic cardiac failure and its superimposed complications.

RHEUMATOID HEART DISEASE

Of recent date, increasing attention has been drawn to cardiac lesions in patients having rheumatoid arthritis. These heart involvements are, however, uncommon and in a large series of 100 patients with generalized arthritis, only five instances of recognizable rheumatoid lesions were found in the heart (Cruickshank, 1958). Those with more florid active rheumatoid arthritis yield a higher incidence of cardiac lesions (up to 50 per cent) so that it seems probable that the more active the arthritis, the greater the likelihood of carditis. The major problem in identifying rheumatoid heart disease is its differentiation from rheumatic heart disease. In the 100 patients cited, a variety of additional cardiac lesions were found. Some were characteristic of rheumatic heart disease, but the majority consisted of nonspecific valvular thickenings, myocardial inflammations and old pericarditis. Much confusion stems from the inclusion of these rheu-

matic and nonspecific alterations under the heading of rheumatoid disease.

The diagnostic features of rheumatoid heart disease consist of rheumatoid granulomas in the mitral and aortic rings and in the myocardium. Infrequently, the tricuspid valve is affected. These granulomas comprise a central focus of fibrinoid necrosis surrounded by a collar of radial, palisaded fibroblasts, accompanied by a diffuse nonspecific chronic inflammation (Figs. 16–37 and 16–38). Plasma cells are prominent in this infiltrate. Infrequently, these foci of active inflammation in the valve leaflets give rise to nonbacterial vegetations considerably larger than those seen in active rheumatic heart disease. As these granulomas persist and become chronic, they cause fibrosis, thickening and calcification of the affected valve leaflets and occasionally the attached chordae tendineae, changes that may well simulate old rheumatic heart disease. The lesions in the myocardium lead to focal and interstitial fibrosis. Aortic valvular dilatation may occur, particularly in those instances having rheumatoid lesions within the aorta itself, described on p. 611.

As for the clinical significance of these lesions, little is known except that they may produce murmurs and occasionally disturbances in the conduction system. It does not seem unreasonable, however, that in some instances the involvement may be sufficiently severe to cause cardiac failure.

CARCINOID SYNDROME

Of the many bizarre syndromes in medicine, the carcinoid syndrome is one of the most fascinating. The association of peculiar flushing of the skin, transient attacks of cyanosis, diarrhea, bronchoconstrictive episodes resembling asthma and cardiac disease, with a carcinoid tumor that has metastasized to the liver, for a long time defied the human imagination. Although all these features had been identified in patients with these tumors, it did not seem reasonable that all these manifestations could be related. Subsequently, it was shown that the argentaffinoma elaborates into the circulation 5-hydroxytryptamine (5-HT) and other kinins which are capable of inducing the bronchoconstrictive and vasomotor attacks described, and it also became clear that in some mysterious way these patients develop fibrous stenosis of the valves of the right side of the heart. The left-sided valves are not affected. The pathogenesis of these valvular changes is still totally unknown. The products from the tumor must drain through the venous system into the right heart and then through the lungs. It is of inter-

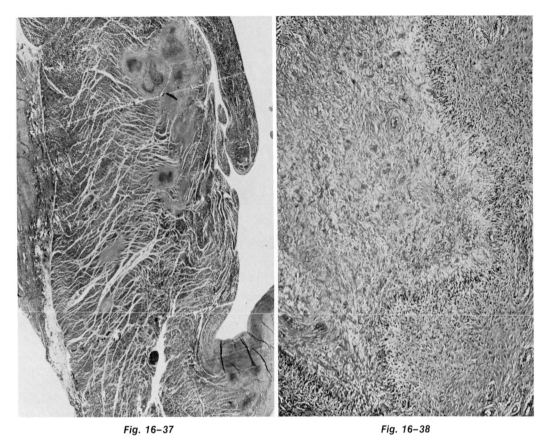

Fig. 16–37   Fig. 16–38

Figure 16–37. *Rheumatoid heart disease. Low power scan of the left ventricular wall studded with focal areas of necrosis (see Fig. 16–38).*

Figure 16–38. *A high power detail of a rheumatoid granuloma with the collar of palisaded reactive cells about the focus of necrosis.*

est that in a single passage through the lung, the 5-HT is almost totally inactivated by a monoamine oxidase present in pulmonary tissue. This would suggest some basis for the development of the right-sided lesions and the absence of left-sided lesions. However, it has been impossible to induce similar lesions in experimental animals by the administration of high levels of 5-HT or to demonstrate any fibroplastic effect of this substance. The origin, therefore, of the valvular stenosis remains obscure. (For further details, reference may be made to the more complete discussion of this subject on p. 942.)

TUMORS OF THE HEART

Primary tumors of the heart are extremely rare but are of great clinical interest since they are more often benign than malignant and are often attached by slender stalks that make them amenable to surgical removal. They are, however, very difficult to diagnose clinically because of their rarity and because they often

present as a mysterious cause of cardiac decompensation (Goldberg and Steinberg, 1955). However, with present-day techniques of cardiac catheterization and cardioangiography, they can frequently be diagnosed clinically, permitting lifesaving surgical removal. Some idea of their frequency can be obtained by the incidence of primary and malignant cardiac tumors in necropsy series ranging from 1 in 2000 to 1 in 10,000 autopsies. Secondary tumors are 10 to 20 times more common (Somer and Loth, 1960).

PRIMARY TUMORS—BENIGN

The most common primary tumor of the heart is the myxoma (Fig. 16–39). It should be stressed, however, that some do not consider this a true neoplasm, but rather an organized mural clot. These usually occur as globular or polypoid masses, arising from the endocardial surface that project into the cardiac chambers, most often in the left atrium or auricle. Some are sessile, but many are attached

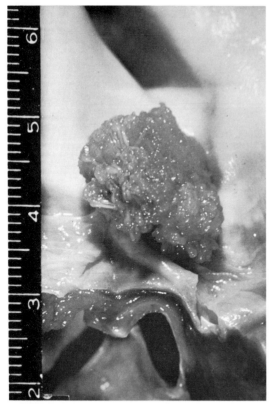

Figure 16–39. *Myxoma of the heart attached to the wall of the left atrium.*

by only a slender stalk, permitting them to move freely in the blood, sometimes to act as ball-valve obstructions to the heart valves. They are usually covered by a thin, glistening endothelial layer and have a semitranslucent, yellow-gray, gelatinous transected surface. Microscopically, they are composed of an abundant acellular ground substance in which is found widely separated spindle or stellate cells resembling fibroblasts or myxoma cells. Scattered within the ground substance are occasional smooth muscle cells. Vessels of varying size are also present, some well developed, others having large cavernous lumina. The vascular components and the variety of cell types led to the concept that these lesions are organizing thrombi. However, a recent electron microscopic study suggests instead that these tumors are true neoplasms arising in multipotential mesenchymal cells capable of differentiating along all of the cell lines mentioned (Ferrans and Roberts, 1973).

Rhabdomyomas have also been described in the heart (Straus and Merliss, 1945). Here again there is considerable evidence that these represent multipotential overgrowths in which the striated muscle fibers of the heart predominate. Other less frequent forms of be-

nign neoplasms have been described, such as fibromas, lymphomas and angiomas.

SARCOMAS

Primary malignancies of the heart are far less common than benign tumors. The most frequent patterns are a variety of poorly differentiated "spindle cell" tumors and lymphosarcomas (Whorton, 1949). Rhabdomyosarcomas are also reported as primary in the heart, but there is some question as to whether all are actually of striated muscle cell origin. Many may not even have arisen in the heart because, in the reported cases, other sites of involvement were present that could conceivably represent the primary lesions.

SECONDARY TUMORS

Metastatic involvement of the heart may occur in any widely disseminated malignancy. A great many of these secondary lesions result from spread of bronchogenic carcinomas and lymphomas arising in the mediastinal nodes. However, there are many undoubted instances of blood- or lymphatic-borne metastases from carcinoma of the kidney, stomach, lungs, breast and melanocarcinoma. Only rarely is the secondary involvement of the heart important except in those instances when the metastases evoke pericardial hemorrhagic effusions that produce cardiac tamponade.

REFERENCES

Abbott, M. E. S.: Atlas of Congenital Cardiac Disease. New York, American Heart Assoc., 1936.

Bing, R. J., et al.: What is cardiac failure? Amer. J. Cardiol., 22:2, 1968.

Blattner, R. J.: Myopericarditis associated with Coxsackie virus infections. J. Pediat., 73:932, 1968.

Bloedorn, W. A.: The recognition and treatment of the various forms of pericarditis. Med. Ann. D.C., 2:422, 1940.

Blumgart, H. L., et al.: Angina pectoris, coronary failure and acute myocardial infarction. The role of coronary occlusions and collateral circulation. J.A.M.A., 116:91, 1941.

Blumgart, H. L., et al.: Studies on the relation of angina pectoris, coronary thrombosis and myocardial infarction to the pathologic findings (with particular reference to the significance of collateral circulation). Amer. Heart J., 19:1, 1940.

Braunwald, E., et al.: Mechanisms of contraction of the normal and failing heart. New Eng. J. Med., 277:794, 910, 962, 1967.

Burch, G., and Giles, T.: Senile cardiomyopathy. J. Chronic Dis., 24:1, 1971.

Burch, G. E., et al.: Pathogenesis of "rheumatic" heart disease: critique and theory. Amer. Heart J., 80:556, 1970.

Carpenter, C. C., and Wallace, C. K.: Bacterial endocarditis: current concepts. John Hopkins Med. J., 124:339, 1969.

Clawson, B. J.: Coronary sclerosis: an analysis of 928 cases. Amer. Heart J., 17:387, 1939.

Clawson, B. J.: Rheumatic heart disease: an analysis of 796 cases. Amer. Heart J., 20:454, 1940.

Cruickshank, B.: Heart lesions in rheumatoid disease. J. Path. Bact., 76:223, 1958.

Das, S. K.: Immunoglobulin binding in cardiomyopathic hearts. Circulation, *44*:612, 1971.

Davies, J. N. P.: The heart of Africa. Cardiac pathology in the population of Uganda. Lab. Invest., *10*:205, 1961.

Edwards, J. E.: On the etiology of calcific aortic stenosis. Circulation, *26*:817, 1962.

Ehrlich, J. C., and Shinohara, Y.: Low incidence of coronary thrombosis in myocardial infarction. Arch. Path., *78*:432, 1964.

Fejfar, Z.: Cardiomyopathy: an international problem. Cardiologica (Basel), *52*:9, 1968.

Ferrans, V. J., and Roberts, W. C.: Structural features of cardiac myxomas, histology, histochemistry and electron microscopy. Hum. Path., *4*:111, 1973.

Fine, G., et al.: Experimental myocardial infarction. A histochemical study. Arch. Path., *82*:4, 1966.

Finland, M., and Barnes, M. W.: Changing etiology of bacterial endocarditis in the antibacterial era. Ann. Intern. Med., *72*:341, 1970.

Friedberg, C. K.: Diseases of the Heart. Philadelphia and London, W. B. Saunders Co., 1966, p. 992.

Genest, J., et al.: Endocrine factors in congestive heart failure. Amer. J. Cardiol., *22*:35, 1968.

Glancy, D. L., et al.: Fatal acute rheumatic fever in childhood despite corticosteroid therapy. Amer. Heart J., *77*:534, 1969.

Goldberg, H., and Steinberg, I.: Primary tumors of the heart. Circulation, *11*:963, 1955.

Goodwin, J. F.: Cardiac function in primary myocardial disorders. Brit. Med. J., *1*:1527, 1964.

Gordis, L., et al.: Studies in the epidemiology and preventability of rheumatic fever. II. Socioeconomic factors and the incidence of acute attacks. J. Chronic Dis., *21*:655, 1969.

Gore, I., and Saphir, O.: Myocarditis: a classification of 1402 cases. Amer. Heart J., *34*:827, 1947.

Hansen, A. T., and Warburg, G. E.: Congenital heart disease in a clinical material. Acta Chir. Scand., Suppl., *283*:107, 1961.

Helfant, R. H., et al.: Functional importance of the human coronary collateral circulation. New Eng. J. Med., *284*:1277, 1971.

Hudson, R. E. B.: The cardiomyopathies: order from chaos. Amer. J. Cardiol., *25*:73, 1970.

Jennings, R. B.: Symposium on the pre-hospital stage of acute myocardial infarction. II. Early phase of myocardial ischemic injury and infarction. Amer. J. Cardiol., *24*:753, 1969.

Jennings, R. B., et al.: Electrolyte alterations in acute myocardial ischemic injury. Circ. Res., *14*:260, 1964.

Jennings, R. B., et al.: Enzymatic changes in acute myocardial ischemic injury. Arch. Path., *64*:10, 1957.

Jennings, R. B., et al.: Ischemic injury of myocardium. Ann. N.Y. Acad. Sci., *156*:61, 1969.

Jewitt, D. E., et al.: Incidence and management of supraventricular arrhythmias after myocardial infarction. Amer. Heart J., *77*:290, 1969.

Joorabchi, B.: Pathogenesis of rheumatic fever. Clin. Pediat., *8*:405, 1969.

Kagan, A., et al.: Coronary artery thrombosis and the acute attack of coronary heart disease. Lancet, *2*:1199, 1968.

Kannel, W. B., et al.: Factors of risk in the development of coronary heart disease. Six year follow-up experiences. Ann. Intern. Med., *55*:33, 1961.

Kannel, W. B., et al.: Risk factors in coronary heart disease. An evaluation of several serum lipids as predictors of coronary heart disease. The Framingham study. Ann. Intern. Med., *61*:888, 1964.

Kaplan, M. H., and Frengley, J. D.: Autoimmunity to the heart in cardiac disease. Current concepts of the relation of autoimmunity to rheumatic fever, postcardiotomy and postinfarction syndrome and cardiomyopathies. Amer. J. Cardiol., *24*:429, 1969.

Kaplan, M. H., and Meyeserian, M.: Immunologic cross reaction between group based streptococcal cells and human heart tissue. Lancet, *1*:706, 1962.

Kaplan, M. H., et al.: Immunologic studies of heart tissue. IV. Serologic reactions with human heart tissue as revealed by immunofluorescent methods, isoimmune, Wasserman and autoimmune reactions. J. Exp. Med., *113*:17, 1961.

Kaplan, M. H., et al.: Presence of bound immunoglobulins and complement in the myocardium in acute rheumatic fever. Association with cardiac failure. New Eng. J. Med., *271*:637, 1964.

Kariv, I., et al.: Familial cardiomyopathy. Amer. J. Cardiol., *28*:693, 1971.

Kelley, J., and Anderson, D. H.: Congenital endocardial fibroelastosis associated with cardiac malformations, including a report of familial instances. Pediatrics, *18*:539, 1956.

Kuller, L.: Sudden death in arteriosclerotic heart disease: the case for preventative medicine. Amer. J. Cardiol., *24*:617, 1969.

Lerner, P. I., and Weinstein, L.: Infective endocarditis in the antibiotic era. New Eng. J. Med., *274*:199, 259, 323, 1966.

Lown, B., et al.: Coronary and precoronary pain. Amer. J. Med., *46*:705, 1969.

MacDonald, R. A., and Robbins, S. L.: The significance of non-bacterial thrombotic endocarditis: an autopsy and clinical study of 78 cases. Ann. Intern. Med., *46*:255, 1957.

Mallory, G. K., et al.: The speed of healing of myocardial infarction. Amer. Heart J., *18*:747, 1939.

McCormick, W. F.: Endocardial fibroelastosis. A summary of the literature and a review of 24 new cases. South. Med. J., *51*:1232, 1958.

Meerson, F. C.: Compensatory hyperfunction of the heart and cardiac insufficiency. Circ. Res., *10*:250, 1962.

Miettinen, M., et al.: Effect of cholesterol-lowering diet on mortality from coronary heart-disease and other causes. Lancet, *2*:7782, 1972.

Moller, J. H., et al.: Endocardial fibroelastosis, a clinical and anatomic study of 47 patients with emphasis on its relationship to mitral insufficiency. Circulation, *30*:759, 1964.

Molnar, Z., et al.: Cardiac changes in the potassium-depleted rat. Arch. Path., *74*:339, 1962.

Morales, A. R., and Fine, G.: Early human myocardial infarction. A histochemical study. Arch. Path., *82*:9, 1966.

Morrow, A. G., et al.: Obstruction to left ventricular outflow: current concepts of management and operative treatment. Ann. Intern. Med., *69*:1255, 1968.

Moschcowitz, E.: Essays on the biology of disease: Libman-Sacks disease. J. Mount Sinai Hosp. N.Y., *13*:143, 1946–1947.

Murphy, G. E.: Nature of rheumatic heart disease. Medicine (Balt.), *39*:289, 1960.

Nadas, A. S.: Pediatric Cardiology. Philadelphia and London, W. B. Saunders Co., 1963, p. 792.

Neal, R. W., et al.: A pathophysiological classification of cor pulmonale: with general remarks on therapy. Mod. Conc. Cardiovasc. Dis., *38*:107, 1968.

Paul, O.: Myocardial infarction and sudden death. Hosp. Pract., *6*:91, 1971.

Pelosi, G., and Agliati, G.: The heart muscle in functional overload and hypoxia. A biochemical and ultrastructural study. Lab. Invest., *18*:86, 1968.

Perera, G. A.: Diagnosis and natural history of hypertensive vascular disease. Amer. J. Med., *4*:416, 1948.

Pool, P. E., and Braunwald, E.: Fundamental mechanisms in congestive heart failure. Amer. J. Cardiol., *22*:7, 1968.

Prata, A.: Chagas' heart disease. Cardiologica (Basel), *52*:57, 1968.

Pyun, K. S., et al.: Giant cell myocarditis. Light and electron microscopic study. Arch. Path., *90*:181, 1970.

Quie, P. G., and Ayoub, E. M.: Rheumatic fever. Postgrad. Med., *44*:73, 1968.

Quinn, E. I.: Bacterial endocarditis. Postgrad. Med., *44*:82, 1968.

Ramalingaswami, V.: Nutrition and the heart. Cardiologia (Basel), *52*:57, 1968.

Robbins, S. L.: Personal observation, 1972.

Roberts, W. C.: Anatomically isolated aortic valvular disease. The case against its being of rheumatic etiology. Amer. J. Med., *49*:151, 1970.

Roberts, W. C.: The pathology of acute myocardial infarction. Hosp. Pract., *6*:89, 1971.

Sanders, M. G.: Alcoholic cardiomyopathy. A critical review. Quart. J. Stud. Alcohol, *31*:324, 1970.

Saphir, O.: Myocarditis: general reviews with an analysis of 240 cases. Arch. Path., *32*:1000, 1941; *33*:88, 1942.

Shanoff, H. M.: Alcoholic cardiomyopathy. An introductory review. Canad. Med. Ass. J., *106*:55, 1972.

Shaper, A. G.: Endomyocardial fibrosis. Cardiologia (Basel), *52*:20, 1968.

Shnitka, T. K., and Nachlas, M. M.: Histochemical alterations in ischemic heart muscle and early myocardial infarction. Amer. J. Path., *42*:507, 1963.

Sodeman, W. A., and Smith, R. H.: Re-evaluation of the diagnostic criteria for acute pericarditis. Amer. J. Med. Sci., *235*:672, 1958.

Somer, S. K., and Loth, E. S.: Primary lymphosarcoma of the heart. Review of the literature and report of 3 cases. Cancer, *13*:449, 1960.

Spain, E. M., and Bradess, V. A.: Relationship of coronary thrombosis to atherosclerosis and ischemic heart disease. Amer. J. Med. Sci., *240*:701, 1960.

Still, W. J. S., and Boult, E. H.: Pathogenesis of endocardial fibroelastosis. Lancet, 2:117, 1956.

Stollerman, G. H., and Pearce, I. A.: Changing epidemiology of rheumatic fever and acute glomerulonephritis. Advances Intern. Med., *14*:201, 1968.

Stollerman, G. H., et al.: Committee report: Jones' criteria (revised) for guidance in the diagnosis of rheumatic fever. Circulation, *32*:664, 1965.

Storstein, O., et al.: Congenital heart disease in a clinical material. Acta Med. Scand., *176*:195, 1964.

Straus, R., and Merliss, R.: Primary tumors of the heart. Arch. Path., *39*:74, 1945.

Stuart, K. L.: Peripartal cardiomyopathy. Cardiologia (Basel), *52*:44, 1968.

Symposium on Quebec beer drinkers' cardiomyopathy. Canad. Med. Ass. J., *97*:881, 1967.

Tucker, V. L., et al.: Cardiac necrosis accompanying potassium deficiency and administration of corticosteroids. Circ. Res., *13*:420, 1963.

Wagner, B. M., and Siew, S.: Studies in rheumatic fever. Significance of the human Anitschkow cell. Hum. Path., *1*:45, 1970.

Walston, A., et al.: Acute coronary occlusion and the "power failure" syndrome. Amer. Heart J., *79*:613, 1970.

Webster, B., et al.: Studies in cardiovascular syphilis. The natural history of syphilitic aortic insufficiency. Amer. Heart J., *46*:117, 1953.

Wendt, V. E., et al.: Acute effects of alcohol on the human myocardium. Amer. J. Cardiol., *17*:804, 1966.

Wenger, N. K.: Infectious myocarditis. Postgrad. Med., *44*:105, 1968.

White, P. D.: Changes in relative prevalence of various types of heart disease in New England. J.A.M.A., *152*:303, 1953.

Whorton, C. M.: Primary malignant tumors of the heart. Cancer, 2:145, 1949.

Wilson, L. M.: Pathology of fatal bacterial endocarditis before and since the introduction of antibiotics. Ann. Intern. Med., *58*:84, 1963.

World Health Organization: Technical report. Series No. 117. Geneva, 1957.

Zabriskie, J. B., et al.: An immunological relationship between streptococcal membranes and human heart tissue. Fed. Proc., *23*:343, 1964.

Zugibe, F. T., et al.: Determination of myocardial alterations of autopsy in the absence of gross and microscopic changes. Arch. Path., *8*:409, 1966.

17

BLOOD AND BONE MARROW

NORMAL

Without attempting to review completely normal hematopoiesis, it is pertinent to review certain aspects which are essential to an understanding of diseases of blood.

DEVELOPMENT OF BLOOD CELLS

In the human embryo, the first recognizable blood cells are formed in blood islands of the yolk sac. These cells develop from primitive forms which are also identified as stem cells (hemohistioblasts or hemocytoblasts) in adult marrows. During the second month of intrauterine life, the major hematopoietic effort is taken over by the liver and, in the fifth month, by the spleen. The splenic activity pro-gressively subsides during the last three months of fetal life. However, small foci of blood formation persist in the liver until birth. Myeloid (marrow) formation of blood commences in the fifth month of fetal life. The myeloid foci appear first in the centers of the bone marrow cavities and expand to occupy the entire marrow space by the time of birth. Until puberty, virtually the entire skeleton remains active in hematopoiesis. After puberty, this dispersed hematopoiesis progressively contracts so that, in the adult, only the skull, vertebrae, ribs, sternum, innominate bones and the proximal thirds of the humerus and femur retain active red marrow. The factors that govern this contraction are not well understood, but it is attributed to the lower temperature of the marrow cavities in the periphery of the body.

699

Several important clinical implications stem from this development. Marrow aspirations for the evaluation of normal hematopoiesis are futile if taken from the distal two-thirds of the femur or humerus. In disorders that evoke an increased formation of blood, the hematopoietic activity reverts toward the fetal pattern. Thus, in chronic anemias, the fatty marrow in the distal humerus and femur may become active and, if the need is protracted and severe, extramedullary foci may reappear in the spleen and the liver. The expansion of hematopoiesis occurs in the reverse order of contraction.

CELLS OF THE BONE MARROW AND THEIR ORIGINS

When subjected to fixatives and tissue-staining methods, the cells of bone marrow and peripheral blood differ in appearance from those in air-dried, Giemsa-stained smears. It is well to become familiar with the morphology of individual cell types within tissue sections since the diagnosis of blood disorders often depends on this procedure. Figure 17–1A provides such a view of the maturation of the erythrocyte. The granulocyte series is depicted in Figure 17–1B, the lymphocytes in Figure 17–1C and the monocytes in Figure 17–1D. It should be noted particularly that, in all series, the most immature form is represented by the stem cell or, in the case of the lymphocyte series, by a very close relative (a primitive mesenchymal stem cell). Because this cell is so little differentiated, it has a similar appearance in each series. It can be fairly easily identified in tissue sections because it has abundant basophilic cytoplasm and a relatively large nucleus measuring at least two-thirds the diameter of the cell. The nucleoli are particularly prominent, which suggests that this cell is active in protein synthesis. Now a few details regarding each line of development will be given.

Erythropoiesis. In the erythrocytic maturation series depicted in Figure 17–1A, number 1 represents the stem cell. It is apparent that the evolution of the mature erythrocyte from the stem cell represents a continuum of subtle morphologic changes. Several levels are singled out for specific names, but there are no absolute criteria to identify these levels. In the series indicated, number 2 might be termed a proerythroblast; 3, an erythroblast;

and 4, normoblasts. Note the rather fuzzy "bearded" margins of the erythroblast, a somewhat distinctive feature that helps to differentiate these cells from the other blast forms encountered in the bone marrow. The normoblasts show the progressive accumulation of hemoglobin as they become more acidophilic. Both normal and abnormal crenated erythrocytes are shown, one containing a fragment of unextruded pyknotic nucleus.

Usually, erythrocytes develop through this sequence of three mitotic divisions within 4 days. Most of the available evidence suggests that when a cell divides mitotically, one of the daughter cells usually retains its primitive characteristics and remains the progenitor of similar cells while the other daughter cell progressively matures in the manner illustrated. Isotopic labeling of iron has shown that most of the iron required for hemoglobin synthesis is taken in at the proerythroblast or early erythroblast level. Division of this cell's ancestors halves the iron content each time, leaving at the completion of the sequence sufficient iron for the synthesis of the normal hemoglobin content in the mature erythrocyte. Mitotic division occurs to the level of the normoblast. By this geometric progression, normoblasts are the most abundant cells of the erythropoietic series found in normal bone marrow.

The maintenance of the normal red cell mass is one of the most delicately balanced processes in the body. With an average cell life span of 120 days, a significant portion of the total mass of red cells must be replaced daily. An enormous amount of work has documented the existence of an exquisitely sensitive feedback mechanism mediated by the humoral factor erythropoietin. Exact amounts of erythropoietin must be elaborated "to regulate production by the marrow of just enough erythrocytes each day to compensate for those destroyed yesterday" (Gurney, 1966). The nature and origin of erythropoietin are still in some dispute. Despite some conflicting evidence, erythropoietin appears to be a protein or polypeptide having a molecular weight in the range of 60 to 70,000. Most recent studies indicate that the kidneys elaborate a renal factor called renal erythropoietic factor (REF) which behaves as an enzyme and acts upon some substrate in normal plasma to produce an erythropoietic stimulating factor (ESF) (Gordon et al., 1967). The stimulus for the

---

Figure 17–1. A, *Maturation of erythrocytes from their stem cell precursor. Several abnormal crenated erythrocytes are included.* B, *Maturation of granulocytes from their stem cell precursor. The mature neutrophil and eosinophil are depicted.* C, *Maturation of lymphocytes from their mesenchymal precursor.* D, *Maturation of monocytes from their mesenchymal or stem cell precursor. Phloxine-methylene blue stain.*

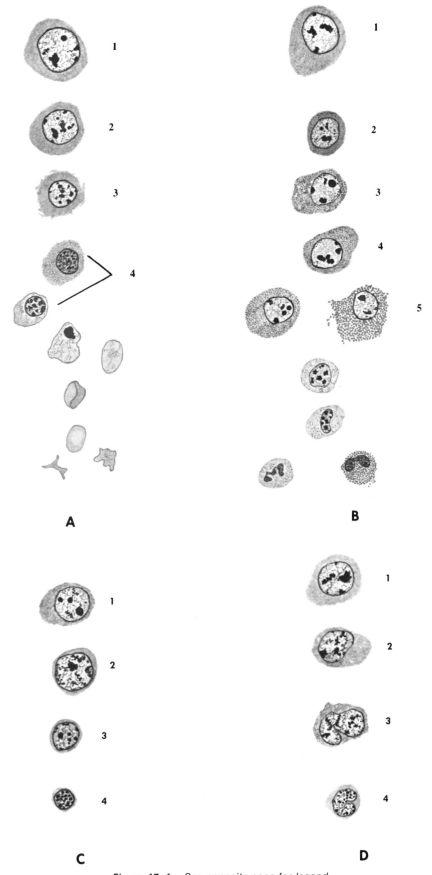

Figure 17–1. *See opposite page for legend.*

production of ESF appears to be reduction in the oxygen tension or oxygen-carrying capacity of the blood. Indeed, increased amounts of erythropoietin can be shown as a compensatory response in a variety of anemias. Erythropoietin appears to stimulate the differentiation of primitive stem cells into red cell precursors. More specifically, in hematopoietic tissues the administration of erythropoietin will increase the synthesis of DNA and RNA, as well as the enzymes involved in active cell proliferation and maturation (Hodgson, 1967).

Sometimes there is inappropriate elaboration of erythropoietin, resulting in the production of abnormal numbers of red cells (erythrocytosis). Elevated levels of erythropoietin have been reported in a few cases of spontaneously occurring polycythemia and in polycythemic patients with a wide variety of tumors (renal cell carcinomas, sarcomas and adenomas; renal tuberculosis; polycystic kidney disease; bronchogenic carcinoma; hepatoma; uterine leiomyomas; pheochromocytoma and some cerebellar vascular tumors). Although in some cases the tumor itself may have produced the erythropoietin, it has not been possible to rule out an indirect effect of tumor upon kidney. In either case, removal of the tumor has been followed by remission of the polycythemia.

Leukopoiesis. Leukopoiesis refers to the formation of white cells. Classically it is divided into three distinct lines, granulocytic, lymphocytic and monocytic. In the granulocytic series in Figure 17–1*B*, it is evident that cell 2, the myeloblast, is smaller than the stem cell and is, indeed, smaller than its descendants, the promyelocytes, indicated at level 3. Often present in the cytoplasm of myeloblasts are Auer rods (Fig. 17–2). Identification of these inclusions helps to confirm that certain immature cells in leukemic patients are actually of myeloid origin. Cell 4 represents a promyelocyte. It shows the beginning accumulation of specific granules, well developed in the succeeding more mature myelocytes (5). Nothing need be said about the maturation of the lymphocytes (Fig. 17–1*C*) and monocytes (Fig. 17–1*D*) because, as depicted, they mature primarily by decrease in size, basophilia and nuclear/cytoplasmic ratio as they divide to eventually give rise to the circulating forms.

Cell recognition is so important that certain generalizations should be reiterated. The more primitive the cell, the greater its size and the more basophilic its cytoplasm. As indicated in Figure 17–1, the most primitive stem cell or mesenchymal precursor has a basophilic cytoplasm which rarely contains discernible gran-

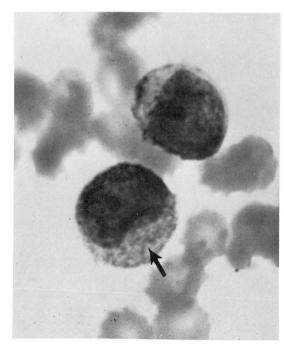

Figure 17–2. *Myeloblasts in peripheral blood in a patient with myelogenous leukemia. Lower cell contains Auer rods indicated by arrow.*

ules. This basophilia of the cytoplasm is presumably due to the rich content of RNA, an attribute of active protein synthesis. Such cells have relatively large nuclei, occupying over half the cell. It is also obvious from the illustrations that it is extremely difficult to distinguish the "blast" forms one from another. Most helpful is the tendency for the erythroblast to have a somewhat fuzzy "bearded" margin, separating it from the more clearly marginated "blasts" of white cell formation. Recourse must often be made to presumptive identification of "blasts" by the "company they keep," since in general they will be positioned close to their more mature descendants. In the normal marrow, the proportion of nucleated myeloid cells to nucleated red cells is in the range of 4 to 1. Obviously, increases or decreases at certain stages of erythropoiesis alter this ratio. A considerable portion of all marrow cavities is occupied by fat, the proportion varying from one bone to the other. In the adult, even the active hematopoietic marrow of the vertebrae is about half fat. As increased activity occurs, this fat is replaced. *Diseases of the blood and bone marrow are characterized not only by abnormalities in individual cells but also by alterations in their relative or absolute numbers and in their distribution throughout the body.*

ANEMIAS

Despite the daily use of the term, there is no general agreement upon the definition of anemia. It has been defined in two ways: (1) as a reduction in the concentration of hemoglobin in the peripheral blood and (2) as a reduction in the total hemoglobin-red cell mass. While in general both phenomena occur together, there are occasional instances where an increase in blood volume by dilution reduces the hemoglobin concentration although red cell mass is not affected. Conversely, immediately following acute hemorrhage, the hemoglobin concentration is not lowered until the blood volume is restored by hemodilution. Yet the hemoglobin-red cell mass is decreased and the reduced blood volume impairs tissue oxygenation. Despite these unusual examples, anemia here will be defined as a reduction in hemoglobin concentration in the circulating blood. It is far easier in clinical practice to derive this value than red cell mass. With rare exception, low hemoglobin concentration implies impaired tissue oxygenation which is the major functional deficit imposed by anemia.

Ultimately all anemias are caused by one of the following mechanisms:

1. Increased loss of red cells.
   a. Hemorrhage.
2. Increased rate of red cell destruction.
   a. Hemolytic anemias.
3. Decreased production of red cells.
   a. Nutritional deficiencies.
   b. Bone marrow suppression or replacement—marrow failure.

Although this classification is somewhat simplistic, it has virtue from a morphologic standpoint. In general, those *anemias which result from increased losses or destruction of red cells are associated with hypercellular and functionally hyperactive bone marrow.* Often there is an increase in the size of the "erythron" (the combined mass of mature and immature cells comprising the entire erythrocytic series). In contrast, *the anemias resulting from decreased production of red cells have, in general, hypoactive marrows.* However, it should be cautioned that hypoactivity is not inconsistent with hypercellularity. In pernicious anemia, for example, the marrow is generally hypercellular; but due to the deficiency of an essential nutrient, there is a maturational arrest in erythropoiesis, and the marrow fails to put out normal numbers of mature erythrocytes. Anemias resulting from bone marrow suppression or replacement secondary to metastatic cancer, radiant injury or some systemic infection are sometimes marked by fairly specific anatomic lesions in the marrow, such as infiltrative elements or marrow destruction. Bone marrow biopsies verify that, in the anemic patient, the marrow may be acellular, hypocellular or hypercellular. The hypercellular marrow may reflect maximum output of red cells, as in the patient with a hemolytic anemia or, conversely, may express some block in output, as occurs with pernicious anemia. The marrow biopsy is usually most helpful in diagnosing the patient with anemia due to marrow failure, since often the basis for the marrow suppression can be identified within the biopsy specimen.

CHARACTERISTICS OF ANEMIA

Morphology of Anemia. The pattern and severity of tissue changes depend, to a considerable extent, upon the suddenness and quantity of the blood loss and the duration of the anemia. With sudden severe hemorrhage, red cells and circulating blood volume are lost proportionally, with the possible development of shock and its attendant clinical and morphologic changes (p. 345). When the blood loss is slow, when red cell destruction outpaces production, or when some other impairment of red cell formation leads to an anemia, the resultant tissue hypoxia is characteristically reflected in certain morphologic alterations.

The skin is pale and usually becomes thin and inelastic as the epidermis and dermis atrophy. Frequently, the nails become brittle and lose their normal convexity to assume a concave shape (spoon-shaped). Cells that are particularly vulnerable to hypoxia may undergo fatty change or even ischemic necrosis. Such damage is most frequently encountered in the muscle cells of the myocardium, the epithelial cells of the proximal convoluted tubules of the kidney, the centrilobular hepatic cells and the sensitive ganglion cells of the cortex and basal ganglia (p. 26).

In addition to these changes that result from hypoxia, hemosiderosis is commonly found in patients with anemia. This increased iron deposition is due either to excessive destruction of red cells by abnormal mechanisms or to the accumulation of unused dietary or therapeutically administered iron. Thalassemia is a condition in which a block in iron utilization accounts, at least in part, for the severe hemosiderosis, and the diffuse iron pigmentation that follows repeated transfusions exemplifies the hemosiderosis of therapeutic origin. These iron deposits follow the pattern already described as systemic hemosiderosis (p. 276) and are most prominent in the reticuloendothelial cells. If the hemosiderosis is severe, it may affect other organs and tissues, particularly the heart and glandular structures, to produce so-called exogenous hemochromatosis (p. 278).

The increased demand for erythropoiesis in anemia causes the fatty marrow to become active and red (expansion of the erythron) if the marrow is capable of response. In some anemic states, such as aplastic anemia, the marrow cannot react. When the need is great, extramedullary hematopoiesis ensues, reverting to the fetal patterns of blood formation.

Clinical Features of Anemia.

Attendant on the deranged physiology and morphologic alterations described, patients with anemia present many nonspecific clinical signs and symptoms. Classically these patients are pale and many have the deformity of the nails described. Weakness, malaise and easy fatigability are common complaints. The lowered oxygen content of the circulating blood leads to dyspnea on mild exertion. Cyanosis is not an attribute of anemia because only unoxygenated hemoglobin produces the dusky blue coloration. Indeed, the severely anemic patient may not survive cyanosis, since approximately 5 gm. of reduced hemoglobin is required to induce cyanosis. If the fatty changes in the myocardium are sufficiently severe, cardiac failure may develop and compound the respiratory difficulty caused by reduced oxygen transport. Occasionally, the myocardial hypoxia manifests itself by angina pectoris, particularly when a preexisting vascular disease has already rendered the myocardium partially ischemic. With acute blood loss, renal dysfunction may arise from vasoconstriction of the afferent arterioles of the glomeruli, as blood is diverted to more vital structures. Oliguria and anuria may develop in the shock kidney. Central nervous system damage may be evidenced by headache, dimness of vision and faintness. Splenomegaly and hepatomegaly sometimes can be found in patients with increased hematopoiesis in these organs. However, the most characteristic features of the anemia become evident only with the laboratory studies of the peripheral blood.

ANEMIAS OF INCREASED BLOOD LOSS—HYPERACTIVE BONE MARROW

ACUTE BLOOD LOSS ANEMIA

The clinical and morphologic reactions to blood loss depend upon the rate of hemorrhage and whether the blood is lost externally or internally. With acute blood loss, the alterations reflect principally the loss of blood volume rather than the loss of hemoglobin. Shock and death may follow. If the patient survives, the blood volume is rapidly restored by shift of water from the interstitial fluid compartment. Hemodilution, which begins at once, reaches its full effect within 48 to 72 hours. Plasma proteins and then, only slowly, erythrocytes are progressively replaced. There is some expansion of the erythron, principally by an increase in the numbers of erythroblasts and normoblasts, but only rarely is the expansion sufficient to convert the inactive fatty marrow into functional marrow. When the blood is lost internally, as into the peritoneal cavity, the iron can be recaptured, but if the blood is lost externally, the adequacy of the red cell recovery may be hampered by iron deficiency.

CHRONIC BLOOD LOSS ANEMIA

When the loss of blood is so insidious that it does not affect the blood volume but only the hemoglobin level, it is referred to as chronic blood loss anemia. Implied is an imbalance between the productive capacity of the marrow and the loss of red cells. Since the marrow is capable of prodigious expansion of its production, such an imbalance almost invariably stems from deficient iron reserves. Therefore, this anemia is better called *iron deficiency anemia*. Iron deficiency may result from a number of causes, and is discussed later (p. 719).

ANEMIAS OF INCREASED BLOOD DESTRUCTION (HEMOLYTIC ANEMIAS)—HYPERACTIVE BONE MARROW

The hemolytic anemias have three cardinal characteristics: (1) reduction in the survival time of the erythrocyte, (2) retention of the destroyed red cells and their iron within the body, principally within the reticuloendothelial system, and (3) functionally hyperactive bone marrows. Since there is no loss of iron from the body, there is no inability to synthesize more hemoglobin. As a consequence, these anemias are almost invariably characterized morphologically by expansion of the erythron and by marked erythropoietic hyperactivity of the bone marrow.

The survival time of the red cell may be shortened by defects inherent within the red cell (intracorpuscular), by abnormal mechanisms external to the red cells (extracorpuscular) or by combinations of these two. Based on these mechanisms, the more important disorders can be simply classified:

1. Intracorpuscular abnormalities:
   a. Hereditary spherocytosis.
   b. Sickle cell anemia, hemoglobin S disease.
   c. Thalassemia.

d. Other hemoglobinopathies (sickle cell-hemoglobin C disease, sickle cell-hemoglobin D disease, etc.).

e. Paroxysmal nocturnal hemoglobinuria.

2. Extracorpuscular abnormalities:
   a. Erythroblastosis fetalis.
   b. Autoimmune hemolytic disease.
   c. Acquired hemolytic anemia due to toxic, bacterial and physical agents.
   d. Microangiopathic hemolytic anemia.

3. Combinations of intracorpuscular and extracorpuscular abnormalities:
   a. Primaquine-sensitive hemolytic anemia (glucose-6-phosphate dehydrogenase deficiency).
   b. Favism (glucose-6-phosphate dehydrogenase deficiency).
   c. Hemolytic disease in lead poisoning, burns and in association with the vitamin B deficiency anemias.

Almost all the important intracorpuscular defects are based on hereditary errors in the synthesis of red cell stroma, hemoglobin production or intracellular metabolism. By contrast, the anemias of extracorpuscular origin are acquired, some by toxic or mechanical injury and others by the development of abnormal immune mechanisms.

Since excessive red cell destruction is the common denominator of all hemolytic anemias, whatever the cause, the clinical and morphologic changes in this group of disorders have more similarities than differences. The hemolytic process results in either intravascular or extravascular destruction of red cells. When the destruction is intravascular and massive, hemoglobinemia and hemoglobinuria may result. Excretion of this pigment sometimes leads to hemoglobinuric nephrosis (acute tubular necrosis). In addition, increased conversion of the heme pigment to bilirubin leads to the development of jaundice. Since this jaundice is due to unconjugated pigment, it is of the acholuric variety. As a further consequence of the excessive formation of bilirubin, gallstones (pigment stones) are liable to develop in these patients. In hereditary spherocytosis, for example, cholelithiasis has been reported in 50 to 85 per cent of adults and also has been found in children under 10 years of age. In the hemolytic anemias, the erythrocyte usually has a normal volume, although its shape may be distorted, as will be seen. The mean corpuscular hemoglobin concentration is also usually normal, but there are some exceptions.

The diseases characterized by extravascular red cell destruction are marked by hyperactivity of the reticuloendothelial system. The increased destruction of red cells in the reticuloendothelial system leads to accumulation of excessive amounts of hemoglobin and hemosiderin in these phagocytic cells. Sometimes phagocytosis of still recognizable inferior or damaged cells is seen. Since the spleen plays a major role in this red cell destruction, it is commonly enlarged and, as will be seen in the discussion of hereditary spherocytosis, is sometimes quite massive in size.

In all hemolytic diseases, there is expansion of the erythron due to the increased erythropoietic activity. Reactivation of previously fatty areas commonly occurs and sometimes is accompanied by extramedullary hematopoiesis in the liver and spleen. Within these areas of increased erythropoietic activity, the dominant cell is the normoblast (Fig. 17–3).

Before discussing individually some of the common hemolytic syndromes, it may be helpful to briefly review the pathophysiology of hemolytic disease. For our purposes, consider the mature red cell to have three components: (1) hemoglobin, (2)

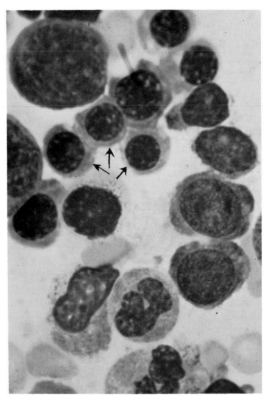

Figure 17–3. *Marrow smear from one of the hemolytic anemias illustrating a large stem cell* (upper left), *erythroblasts* (lower right) *and numerous normoblasts with round, darkly chromatic nuclei* (arrows).

membrane and (3) an energy-producing and anti-oxidant system required for the preservation of the function of (1) and (2). The preservation of the erythrocyte is critically dependent on the prevention of oxidation of either heme or globin. Oxidation precipitates hemoglobin into insoluble inclusions which may damage the membrane or, in some way, render the red cell vulnerable to premature destruction either by phagocytes in the marrow itself or by reticuloendothelial cells throughout the body. Thus it is possible in pathophysiologic terms to divide the hemolytic anemias into three categories: (1) those resulting from membrane disturbances, (2) those resulting from the synthesis of abnormal hemoglobin and (3) those arising in defects in metabolism of the red cell.

Membrane disturbances are characteristic of spherocytosis and paroxysmal nocturnal hemoglobinuria. Disorders of hemoglobin synthesis underlie thalassemia, and the hemoglobin precipitates into large inclusions which impinge on the membrane and lead to engulfment by phagocytic cells. Oxidant drugs will precipitate even normal hemoglobin and lead to hemolytic disease. Abnormal oxidative metabolism of the red cell characterizes two hereditary disorders of erythrocytes: glucose-6-phosphate dehydrogenase (G6PD) deficiency and pyruvate kinase (PK) deficiency. The former is far more common and will be discussed later, but it will suffice here to point out that G6PD is required in the normal glycolytic pathway involved in the production of reduced NAD. Such oxidative metabolism is devoted largely to preservation of the thiol (SH groups) in hemoglobin and membrane proteins. With a G6PD deficiency. NADP is not produced and membrane proteins and globin are oxidized, rendering the cells susceptible to destruction (Nathan and Segel, 1971). In addition to these intracorpuscular defects which lead to hemolytic disease, disorders of the vasculature or plasma factors may cause red cell destruction. Red cells can be physically damaged when they are driven against roughened areas of the endothelium or through abnormally small lumina such as are encountered in hypertensive arteriolosclerosis or against shearing objects such as artificial heart valves. Such are the circumstances which lead to microangiopathic hemolytic anemia. Red cell antibodies either cause cells to be lysed by binding complement or render them abnormally permeable. Spherocytes which result from the increased permeability are trapped in the reticuloendothelial system and destroyed. Against this background, we can now turn to some individual entities.

HEREDITARY SPHEROCYTOSIS (CONGENITAL HEMOLYTIC ANEMIA)

Hereditary spherocytosis is characterized principally by erythrocytes in which an inherent metabolic defect of the envelope causes the cell to assume a spheroid shape. This defect leads to excessive osmotic fragility, resulting in increased hemolysis, anemia and jaundice. The spleen, which appears to play a major role in the increased destruction, is enlarged and, when removed, abolishes the abnormal hemolytic process although the red cell abnormality persists.

Hereditary spherocytosis is transmitted to both sexes as a single mendelian dominant. All races are affected, although most cases occur in whites, particularly in those of northern European stock. Despite the fact that the defect in the red cells is present from birth, the disease may not be recognized until later life.

Pathogenesis. The salient features of the pathophysiology of hereditary spherocytosis are: (1) the existence of an intracorpuscular defect, probably membranous and (2) the fact that the spleen is required for the excessive destruction of red cells. The nature of the intracorpuscular defect is somewhat obscure, but it appears that the membrane permits influx of excess sodium and requires continual high-energy expenditure to maintain a balanced efflux. Biochemical abnormalities in the membrane have been identified. There is a loss involving all lipids proportional to their concentration in the membrane (Reed and Swisher, 1966). This symmetrical loss suggests that small fragments of the membrane are shed, resulting in a decrease in surface area relative to volume. This loss of surface might make the cells smaller in volume, less distensible and account for some increased osmotic fragility. But simple overdistention alone cannot account for the genesis of this disease since splenectomy abolishes the abnormal hemolysis. Following splenectomy, the erythrocyte survival time returns to normal or nearly normal ranges despite the persistence of the membranous defect. Thus it is proposed that the distended erythrocyte is trapped or sequestered in the splenic circulation where the falling pH eventually slows glycolysis and synthesis of ATP essential for the "sodium pump" (Jacob, 1968, 1969). Why such sequestration should occur only in the spleen and not in other reticuloendothelial organs remains a mystery. The therapy of this disease is apparent, i.e., splenectomy.

Morphology. Perhaps the most outstanding morphologic feature of this disease is the spheroidal shape of the red cell, apparent on smears as a lack of their central zone of pallor. In addition to the general features of all hemolytic anemias previously detailed (p. 704), certain alterations are fairly distinctive. Massive splenic enlargement is more characteristic of hereditary spherocytosis than of the other forms of hemolytic anemia. Weights of over 1000 gm. are not uncommon. This enlargement is due to striking congestion of the cords of Billroth, leaving the splenic sinuses virtually empty. Hypertrophy of the sinusoidal lining cells or of the reticular cord cells is sometimes present, and phagocytized erythrocytes are frequently found within these cells. Occasionally these cells, active in red cell destruction become multinucleate and assume giant forms. Hemosiderosis is prominent in the longstanding cases. Despite these rather characteristic microscopic features, the macroscopic appearance of the spleen is not distinctive, save for its size and congestion.

Because the anemia with this disease is often quite severe, there is considerable expansion of the erythropoietically active marrow (Fig. 17–4). In certain cases, this may cause resorption of the inner layers of the cortical bone with new appositional growth on the outer layers. An irregular nubbly subperiosteal outer layer may be formed, particularly on the vault of the skull, which results in perpendicular rays of radiodensity resembling a crew haircut.

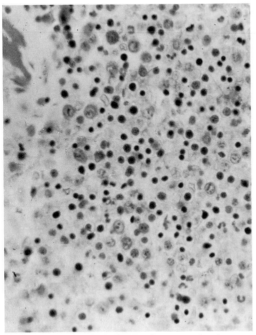

Figure 17–4. *Hereditary spherocytosis—bone marrow. A high power detail of the normoblastic hypercellularity represented by almost all the dark round nuclei visible.*

The production of white cells and platelets is usually unaffected, except during a "crisis" when all lines of development may be depressed. Cholelithiasis (pigment stones) occurs in from 50 to 85 per cent of the cases, and sometimes these stones obstruct the common bile duct, resulting in an obstructive as well as hemolytic jaundice.

Clinical Course. The severity of the disease varies greatly from one patient to another. In some, it manifests soon after birth but in most, not until adult life. In some, the anemia is so mild as to be asymptomatic; in others, the anemia is quite severe and is often accompanied by "hemolytic crises." These acute episodes are characterized by the sudden onset of a wave of massive hemolysis accompanied by fever, abdominal pain, nausea, vomiting, low blood pressure, tachycardia and even shock. Occasionally these hemolytic episodes are associated with apparent aplasia of the bone marrow which, for obscure reasons, suddenly ceases to produce red cells, white cells and platelets. During active hemolysis, the patients classically become jaundiced. Leg ulcers appear in a few cases presumably because the abnormal shape of the red cells causes increased sludging in the peripheral circulation.

The most constant features in all patients are some degree of anemia and splenomegaly. The anemia is usually moderate with red cell counts between 3,000,000 and 3,500,000 per mm.³ During crises these counts may drop to 1,000,000 or less. The mean corpuscular volume (MCV) and mean corpuscular hemoglobin concentration (MCHC) are usually within normal limits, but the red cells on smear lack their central zone of pallor. The osmotic fragility is increased. Save during an aplastic "crisis," the peripheral white cell and platelet counts are normal. Such hematologic findings with a familial history are virtually diagnostic of this disorder.

Commonly this disease follows a long chronic course, and many patients survive to old age. Death, however, may occur during the acute crises from blood destruction or may be caused by such intercurrent complications as biliary tract disease associated with the development of pigment stones. Hereditary spherocytosis can be cured by removal of the spleen.

SICKLE CELL DISEASE

Sickle cell anemia is the classic prototype of a hereditary hemoglobinopathy resulting from a point mutation in the genetic code such that a single amino acid is substituted for another in one of the polypeptide chains of hemoglobin. As a consequence, hemoglobin

S is formed instead of the normal hemoglobin A. Of this disease, Pauling (1971) recently wrote:

> Sickle cell anemia is the first disease to become thoroughly understood; the first disease for which a clear and complete explanation of the manifestations could be formulated. This understanding of the nature of the disease has led . . . to the development of a method of controlling the crisis of the disease. Sickle cell anemia thus has become the first disease for which there is a known molecular basis for pathogenesis, a molecular basis for diagnosis and a molecular basis for treatment.

Incidence and Genetics.

The tendency toward sickling is dependent on both the relative quantity of Hb-S in erythrocytes and the level of O_2 tension in their microenvironment. Red cells with 100 per cent of Hb-S will sickle at physiologic O_2 tensions but, with reduction of the level of Hb-S (and therefore higher levels of Hb-A), progressively lower levels of O_2 tensions are required to induce sickling. The genetic determinant for the production of hemoglobin S is allelic with that determining the production of hemoglobin A. The mutation appears to be expressed as an autosomal incomplete dominant. *Heterozygotes with one normal allele and one abnormal allele produce both hemoglobin S and hemoglobin A and only manifest the sickle cell trait.* Erythrocytes of such individuals contain from 20 to 40 per cent of hemoglobin S, but the red cells are not misshapen under normal living conditions. Rarely, a patient with the trait suffers in vivo sickling when there is some basis for marked systemic hypoxia, such as flying at high altitudes in nonpressurized cabins, respiratory depression as in deep anesthesia, or severe respiratory disease with extreme oxygen unsaturation. The sickle cell trait produces no clinical disorder and is compatible with a normal life span. *Homozygotes can form no Hb-A and so have the full-blown anemia. Erythrocytes from such individuals contain approximately 80 to 100 per cent of hemoglobin S; sickling is present at all times, and small reductions in blood O_2 levels induce sickling crises.* In the United States, hemoglobin S is virtually limited to blacks among whom there is an incidence of about 8 per cent. However, only about one in 40 is homozygous and so has the disease. Hb-S is present in almost half of the members of certain African tribes but is also found in many of Mediterranean origin.

Some patients may inherit more than one genetic mutation and therefore produce not only hemoglobin S but hemoglobin C, D or one of the many other abnormal hemoglobins. These patients may or may not have sufficient hemoglobin S to induce either the trait or the anemia since the abnormal sickle form depends upon the quantity of hemoglobin S present in the erythrocyte. If sufficient hemoglobin S is present to induce sickling, these complex disorders may be designated sickle cell hemoglobin C disease or sickle cell hemoglobin D disease, entities that can be diagnosed only by electrophoretic or biochemical identification of the abnormal hemoglobins.

Pathogenesis.

As is well known, each of the four heme groups in the normal hemoglobin A molecule is associated with a polypeptide chain. The chains are of two kinds: the alpha chains, each of which contains 141 amino acid residues; and the beta chains, 146 residues. The unravelling of the genetic and biochemical origins of sickle cell disease is a monument to the work of many and the genius of a few. Over 20 years ago, Pauling and his co-workers (1949) suggested that the abnormal "sickling behavior" might be due to the presence of a chemically different type of hemoglobin molecule which, on deoxygenation, would aggregate into rods and deform the erythrocyte. Subsequently, Perutz and Mitchison (1950) documented that deoxygenated hemoglobin S had a much lower solubility than deoxygenated hemoglobin A. This property led to crystallization of the hemoglobin S in the erythrocyte. Six years later, Ingram (1956) showed that hemoglobin S was the result of a genetically determined abnormality in which valine was substituted for glutamic acid in the sixth amino acid from the C-amino terminus of the beta polypeptide. Murayama (1966) recently postulated precision scale molecular models to explain the effect of sickle cell hemoglobin on the erythrocyte. He proposed that the substitution of valine for glutamic acid in the two beta chains permitted the formation of an intramolecular hydrophobic bond between the two substituted valines, creating a stereoconfigurational alteration which permits molecular stacking and the formation of filamentous stacks. Electron microscopy has since demonstrated such filaments (or, as they are sometimes called, crystalline cables or tubules) within the red cell (White and Heagan, 1970). These cables or filaments are aligned in situ and distort the thin membranous envelope of the red cell (Gabuzda, 1971). The concept of molecular stacking further ingeniously explained the relationship between sickling and deoxygenation. This proposed that in the deoxygenated state, the beta chains complement adjacent alpha chains within the hemoglobin molecule as do a lock and key, and so can stack. With oxygenation, slight but critical conformational changes occur, which block molecule-to-molecule matching and stacking is prevented. It appears that this serious disease results from a mutation in the triplet code for a single amino acid in a large molecule having hundreds of amino acids.

The hemoglobin molecular stacks are the basis for what has long been recognized under the polarizing microscope as "birefringent tactoids." The birefringence is imparted by the rigidity of these molecular stacks or cables and by their tendency toward parallel alignment. However, how such sickling leads to red cell destruction is still somewhat uncertain. Mechanical stresses imposed on the rigidly deformed cell reasonably might lead to fragmentation during circulatory stresses. Alternatively, it is well known that the sickle forms tend to sludge, favoring sequestration in the sinusoids of the spleen. So stagnated, these erythrocytes are soon depleted of energy-dependent homeostatic mechanisms.

As cited earlier, the tendency for sickling and the severity of the red cell deformity are dependent upon both the amount of hemoglobin S in the red cell and the oxygen tension in its microenvironment. Obviously, patients could not survive if all of their cells were simultaneously sickled. It has been shown that even in homozygotes the proportion of sickled cells in vivo varies from approximately 10 to 30 per cent in venous blood. However, in tissues where large amounts of oxygen are extracted from the blood or when oxygen tensions are reduced, the number of sickled forms may increase sharply (Figs. 17–5 and 17–6). Moreover, such a sickling crisis begins a vicious cycle. Sickling of the cells leads to sludging, and the viscosity of the blood increases. The mechanical fragility of the cells increases. The fragmented and sickled forms further slow the flow of blood. More oxygen is thus taken from the red cells in the slowed passage through the tissues and more cells go into the sickled form. The consequent circulatory stasis, tissue hypoxia, and sickle cell thrombi account, in large part, for many of the morphologic and clinical manifestations common in persons having sickle cell disease.

Morphology. The anatomic alterations are based upon the following three characteristics of

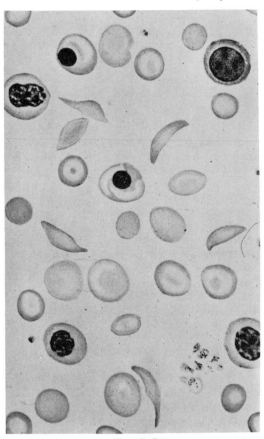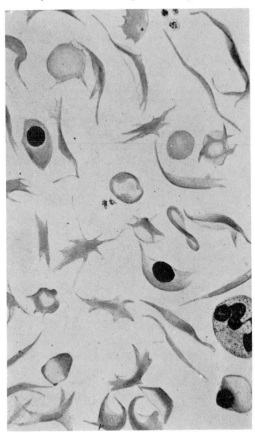

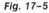

Fig. 17–5 Fig. 17–6

Figure 17–5. *In vivo sickling in a patient with sickle cell anemia (compare with Figure 17–6). (Drawing through the courtesy of Edith Piotti, Harvard Medical School.)*

Figure 17–6. *In vitro sickle cell preparation from same blood as illustrated in Figure 17–5 to highlight the augmentation of sickling induced by low oxygen tension.*

sickle cell anemia: increased destruction of the sickled red cells with the development of anemia, increased release of hemoglobin and formation of bilirubin, and capillary stasis and thrombosis (Diggs and Ching, 1934). Sickling of the red cells may be identified in tissue sections, particularly those fixed in formalin, because under these conditions anaerobiosis develops before complete fixation. However, sickling may not be evident when the section is quickly fixed. The consequence of the increased red cell destruction and anemia have already been detailed in the general consideration of all hemolytic anemias. Briefly, these involve pallor of the skin, systemic hemosiderosis and fatty changes in the heart, liver and tubules of the kidney. Rarely, the erythrostasis in the liver leads to so-called sickle cell cirrhosis. These changes are particularly prominent in patients with sickle cell anemia because of the usual severity of the anemia. The bone marrow is hyperplastic, with activation of fatty marrow. This increased activity is principally at the level of normoblasts, but there may be an increase in the more primitive forms as well. The white cells and megakaryocytes are unaffected. The expansion of the marrow may lead to resorption of bone, with secondary new bone formation to produce the roentgenographic appearance in the skull of the "crew haircut." Extramedullary hematopoiesis may appear in the spleen, liver and rarely in other sites.

In children, during the early phase of the disease, the spleen is commonly enlarged up to 500 gm. Histologically, there is marked congestion of the red pulp, sometimes most prominent in the cords of Billroth, creating large lakes of red cells, sickled and jammed together. Sometimes the sinuses are equally congested but, at other times, they are empty (Fig. 17–7). This erythrostasis in the spleen may lead to thrombosis and infarction or at least to marked tissue hypoxia. Sometimes the resulting focal fibrous scars contain deposits of hemosiderin and calcium, so-called Gandy-Gamna bodies. Continued scarring over the course of years causes progressive shrinkage of the spleen so that, in long-standing adult cases, only a small nubbin of fibrous tissue may be left; this is called **autosplenectomy.** Infarctions secondary to red cell sludging and anoxia may occur also in the liver, brain, kidney and bone marrow.

Thrombotic occlusions have also been described in the pulmonary vessels, and many patients have cor pulmonale. Vascular stagnation in the subcutaneous tissue leads to leg ulcers in approximately 50 per cent of the adult patients but is rare in children. The increased release of hemoglobin leads to pigment gallstones in some patients and all patients develop hyperbilirubinemia during periods of active hemolysis.

Clinical Course.
Sickle cell disease does not become apparent until the second or third year of life as the fetal hemoglobin (hemoglobin F) is gradually replaced by hemoglobin S

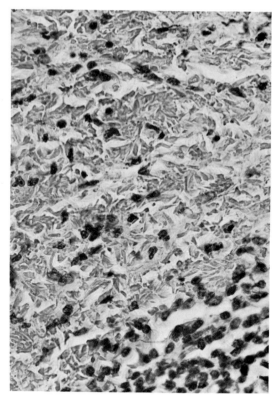

Figure 17–7. Spleen—sickle cell anemia. The congested red pulp jammed with sickled erythrocytes.

rather than by the normal hemoglobin A. From this time, the disorder tends to run a chronic, persistent course, punctuated by crises. During intercritical periods, the patients may manifest only weakness and fatigability. Cardiac murmurs or cardiac abnormalities may appear related to hypoxic injury to the myocardium. Some have renal manifestations related to erythrostasis within the kidney and disruption of the countercurrent mechanism. Splenomegaly sometimes found in children resolves by autosplenectomy, and it has been said that when splenomegaly is present in the adult, the diagnosis of sickle cell anemia should be ruled out. Abnormal liver function may occur secondary to hypoxic fatty change or, more rarely, due to the eventual development of cirrhosis.

Superimposed on this background are the critical attacks which induce a variety of symptom complexes, sometimes bizarre, depending on the particular organ or organs most severely affected by the hypoxia and/or red cell thrombi. Vaso-occlusive episodes may induce painful crises related to a particular organ, commonly the spleen or one of the bones in the skeletal system. Leg ulcers are one of the worst problems. Headaches, stiff neck, convulsions, hemiplegia or coma may develop as a consequence of hypoxia and thromboses in the central nervous system. In addition to the crises of pain, patients may suffer attacks of active hemolysis or aplastic crises where, for unknown reasons, the bone marrow ceases to function. Hepatic crises also occur, manifested by an intensification of the usual level of jaundice, related presumably to sequestration of sickled cells in hepatic sinusoids.

In the usual case, the red cell count and hemoglobin level are reduced to about half. The anemia is usually normocytic and normochromic, but the stained blood smear will usually indicate, in the frank anemia, at least some sickle forms. When these smears are examined under conditions that favor lower oxygen tensions, sickling becomes prominent. In addition, marked anisocytosis and poikilocytosis are often present. Mechanical fragility is normal when the cells are not sickled, but as they assume the abnormal shape it is increased. The ultimate criterion of the presence of sickle cell disease is the electrophoretic demonstration of hemoglobin S.

The prognosis of sickle cell anemia has undergone remarkable change with the development of therapeutic strategies to achieve desickling of erythrocytes in the living patient. Reasoning that the attack must be directed against the hydrophobic bonds implicated by Murayama as being essential for sickling, investigators are now evaluating glucose-urea solutions and other agents such as potassium cyanate which block the intramolecular bonding (Nalbandian and Evans, 1971). The use of these forms of therapy is so recent that we have no idea yet as to their effect on the long-term outlook for these patients. Formerly, most patients died within the first three decades of life, usually from thrombosis of a major vessel in some vital structure or from central nervous system damage.

THALASSEMIA (TH)

Correctly speaking, this topic is the thalassemic syndromes, a group of entities characterized by varying degrees of hemolytic anemia ranging from essentially asymptomatic compensated hemolytic anemia to a severe, fatal form that causes death in childhood. *The common denominator is a partial or complete depression in the formation of one of the globin chains of hemoglobin.* In addition, among individuals with symptomatic anemia, there is ineffective erythropoiesis and rapid destruction of newly released erythrocytes which bear inclusions of precipitated unstable globin chains resulting from unbalanced globin synthesis (Nathan, 1972).

Incidence. These hereditary disorders are encountered mostly in people whose ancestors originated from the northeastern shores of the Mediterranean, hence the designation "thalassemia." The distribution of the disease, however, also includes a wide band extending from northern Africa and southern Europe to the Philippines and random cases in the United States and the British Isles.

The range of clinical severity of the various syndromes depends upon the zygosity of the patient and on whether the mutation affects the alpha or beta chains of globin. Most of the genetic evidence suggests a single autosomal, incomplete dominant mode of transmission. *Heterozygotes may be entirely asymptomatic and are described as having thalassemia minor. Persons with thalassemia major, the severe form of the disease, are homozygous.* With defective beta chain synthesis, known as beta thalassemia, the production of hemoglobin A ($\alpha_2\beta_2$) is slowed and partially replaced by hemoglobins not requiring beta chains, namely, hemoglobin F ($\alpha_2\gamma_2$) and hemoglobin A$_2$ ($\alpha_2\delta_2$). Alpha thalassemia is due to decreased production of alpha chains: all hemoglobins are affected, including hemoglobins A, F and A$_2$. Homozygosity for alpha thalassemia almost invariably leads to an accumulation of unmatched gamma chains which results in a useless respiratory pigment known as hemoglobin Barts. This hemoglobin gives up little oxygen to the tissues at physiologic partial pressures of oxygen, and so the fetus dies of hypoxia. Thus, alpha thalassemia is extremely rare. *The unqualified term thalassemia major, then, generally applies to the common variant of homozygous beta thalassemia.*

Pathogenesis. In beta thalassemia, decreased amounts of hemoglobin collect in the maturing red cell, resulting in hypochromic, microcytic erythrocytes. Current evidence suggests that *the inherited defect slows the rate of synthesis of the globin chains in hemoglobin A.* There appears to be a decrease or alteration of messenger RNA which in some way slows or inhibits initiation of beta chain synthesis. An excess of alpha chains are synthesized, and the excess precipitates to form the inclusion bodies seen in these abnormal erythrocytes (Marks and Bank, 1971). The spleen interacts with the inclusion-containing thalassemic red cells, destroying some and deforming others into "tear drop" shapes (Wennberg and Weiss, 1968). It is thought that the globin aggregates alter membrane permeability, possibly by mechanical damage or possibly by combining with membrane sulfhydryl groups, rendering such cells vulnerable to sequestration and destruction in the spleen (Weatherall et al., 1969). With splenic sequestration, the intracellular glycolytic metabolism impairs the antioxidant capacity of the red cell and so renders it susceptible to destruction. Ineffective erythropoiesis has been attributed to the development of large insoluble inclusions of alpha chains in the majority of bone marrow erythroid precursors in these patients (Fessas, 1963).

Morphology. The major morphologic alterations, in addition to those characteristic of all hemolytic processes, involve the bone marrow and spleen (Whipple and Bradford, 1936). The bone marrow is markedly hyperplastic, with expansion of the erythron to the fetal level. All the fatty marrow may thus be reactivated. The dominant change is in the red cell series, with a striking shift toward the primitive forms all the way back to the erythroblasts and stem cells (Fig. 17–8). The expansion of the marrow leads to thinning of the cortical bone. New bone formation on the external aspect reflects the rarefaction occurring within the medullary cavity. These changes may be found not only in the skull, as described in hereditary spherocytosis (p. 706), but may also affect the face and long bones (Fig. 17–9).

Splenomegaly produced by marked extramedullary hematopoiesis may be extreme, with weights of up to 1000 to 1500 gm. Similar extramedullary foci may be present in the liver. There is little evidence of erythrophagocytosis in the RE system. Slowed erythropoiesis reduces utilization of iron; most patients have variable amounts of hemosiderosis, some quite extreme. The etiology of such pigmentation is difficult to determine since many of these patients have received numerous trans-

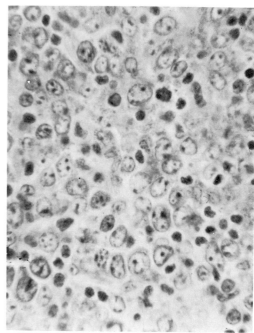

Figure 17–8. Thalassemia—bone marrow. A high power detail of the primitive erythroblasts and stem cells in the profound erythropoietic hyperactivity.

fusions necessary to sustain life. Rare cases have been reported in which severe myocardial hemosiderosis, associated with the systemic hemosiderosis, has caused cardiac failure and death.

Clinical Course. Beta thalassemia major, the homozygous pattern, usually becomes manifest very early in life, as hemoglobin F

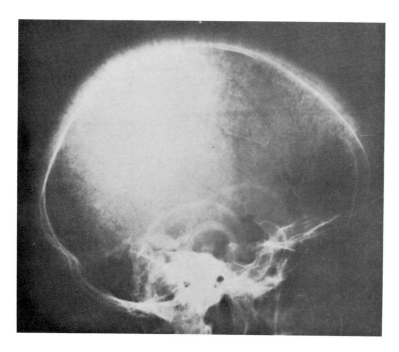

Figure 17–9. Thalassemia. X-ray of the skull to show new bone formation on outer table producing the perpendicular radiations characterized as a "crew haircut."

cannot be replaced by normal hemoglobin A. The disease always becomes apparent within the first decade. These children fail to develop normally and are retarded from birth. A few patients with this homozygous pattern have survived into adult life. Almost invariably, splenomegaly is present and may be so extreme as to cause a protuberant abdomen in the child. The skeletal changes described may be evident on x-ray. Occasionally, these children develop a mongoloid facies induced by the new bone formation involving the skull and facial bones (Silver, 1952).

From the laboratory standpoint, thalassemia major is characterized by a severe microcytic, hypochromic anemia, with erythrocyte counts down to 1,000,000 per mm.[3] The MCV is often reduced to 60 cubic microns, with an accompanying decrease in the MCH. Stained smears of the peripheral blood show a variety of abnormal forms, including target cells, poikilocytosis, anisocytosis and stippled cells. In addition, nucleated red cells are frequently present, reflecting the release of immature forms from the marrow. The leukocyte count is often elevated, reflecting the general marrow hyperactivity, and immature forms may be released into the peripheral blood. The platelet count is generally normal. As a reflection of the hemolytic process, there is elevation of the indirect reacting bilirubin in the serum and an increased excretion of urobilinogen. Elevation of the serum iron is quite characteristic, suggesting deficient utilization. Interestingly, in both thalassemia major and minor, osmotic fragility is reduced, not increased.

Thalassemia minor is usually asymptomatic. These patients are sometimes discovered during the investigation of a mild anemia. Occasionally, fairly significant hypochromic microcytosis is present. Splenomegaly is sometimes present but is usually not pronounced.

The prognosis in beta thalassemia appears to be related to the age of the patient when the anemia first becomes manifest. Infants and children with thalassemia major rarely survive into adult life and are only sustained by repeated transfusions. In the heterozygous pattern, a normal life expectancy may be anticipated.

PAROXYSMAL NOCTURNAL HEMOGLOBINURIA

This rare disorder is characterized by paroxysms of intravascular hemolysis and hemoglobinuria occurring most frequently during or immediately after sleep. It affects both sexes of all ages but is most common during the third and fourth decades. An intracorpuscular red cell defect which markedly shortens the cells' life span has been demonstrated in some of these patients. However, the nature of this defect is not clear. The hemolysis is triggered and accentuated when the pH of the serum is reduced below 7.0. Perhaps this explains the increased hemolysis during sleep when there may be carbon dioxide retention. Other defects have been identified, such as reduction of the acetylcholine esterase content of the stroma of the red cells and depletion of the -SH groups. In neither case, however, can the defect be related clearly to the increased hemolysis. No abnormal antibodies have been identified, and the osmotic fragility is normal.

Most often, this condition is benign and self-limited, but occasionally massive hemolysis may lead to death. Hemoglobinuria (hypoxic nephrosis) potentially may develop during the course of the acute crises and, with recurrent episodes, hemosiderin is deposited in the renal tubules (Fig. 17–10). The disease is

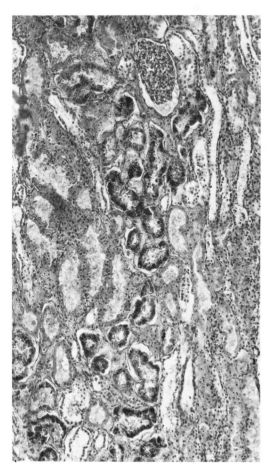

Figure 17–10. *Paroxysmal hemoglobinuria. The dark renal tubules are heavily laden with hemosiderin in a 37-year-old patient with multiple recurrent hemolytic episodes.*

a constant threat to these patients because bacterial infection, drugs and even menstruation may precipitate hemolytic crises.

AUTOIMMUNE HEMOLYTIC ANEMIA

Autoimmune hemolytic anemia is characterized by antibody-mediated destruction of red cells. It may occur as a primary disorder (idiopathic autoimmune hemolytic anemia) or secondary to some underlying disease such as lymphoma, leukemia, systemic lupus erythematosus, viral infections and sarcoidosis. Both the primary and secondary forms are related to the appearance of circulating immunoglobulins directed against red cell antigens. The nature and pathogenesis of these anemias were discussed on p. 226, and the morphologic changes common to all forms of hemolytic anemia, on p. 704.

MICROANGIOPATHIC HEMOLYTIC ANEMIA

This term identifies a hemolytic process seen in a wide variety of disorders that have in common microcirculatory lesions which damage and destroy erythrocytes. Most of the evidence suggests that the hemolysis results from mechanical damage to erythrocytes as they squeeze through abnormally narrowed channels or impinge upon obstacles in their course. Other than immediate rupture, a wide variety of erythrocytic abnormalities are produced and are recognized in the peripheral blood film as "burr cells," "helmet cells," and "triangle cells," as well as fragments of erythrocytes and schistocytes. This form of anemia is encountered in disseminated intravascular coagulation (DIC), thrombotic thrombocytopenic purpura (TTP), the hemolytic-uremia syndrome, malignant hypertension, renal cortical necrosis, systemic lupus erythematosus, metastatic adenocarcinoma, and in patients who have malfunctioning prosthetic heart valves or who have been maintained on mechanical cardiac assist or bypass pumps for long periods of time (Brain, 1970). The common denominator is the presence of some vascular lesion or mechanical appliance predisposing erythrocytes to injury. In DIC, the microthrombi constitute the point of impaction. In malignant hypertension, it is the markedly narrowed arterioles. In systemic lupus erythematosus, it is the necrotizing arteritis and arteriolitis. And where prosthetic heart valves and pumping machines are employed, the appliance is responsible.

In most of these settings, the hemolysis is only a minor part of the major clinical problem, and rarely do these patients have the morphologic changes encountered in the more chronic hemolytic diseases discussed earlier.

OTHER HEMOLYTIC DISEASES

In addition to the types already described, there are many other forms of hemolytic anemia arising from either intracorpuscular defects or extracorpuscular influences. Within this miscellaneous category is a large group of so-called enzyme-deficient hemolytic anemias. All are examples of "inborn errors" in which the erythrocyte lacks a specific enzyme necessary for its maintenance and survival (Valentine, 1970) (Keitt, 1971). The prototype is the so-called primaquine-sensitive anemia resulting from a deficiency of G6PD. It was pointed out on p. 706 that the erythrocyte is critically dependent on energy sources for its survival and, with a deficiency of G6PD, the human red cell is deprived of the energy normally made available by the metabolism of glucose via the oxidative hexose monophosphate shunt. A bewildering array of other enzyme deficiencies have been identified which affect the Embden-Meyerhof pathway and nonglycolytic metabolic pathways. Further details on these disorders are available in the references just cited.

Also included in the group of miscellaneous hemolytic disorders are the anemias caused by extracorpuscular mechanisms, including those associated with drug ingestion, heavy metals, toxins of bacterial origin and such physical agents as thermal injury and ionizing radiation. Some of these agents, such as certain drugs, act as haptens to evoke antibodies which induce hemolytic reactions. Others, such as lead, directly injure membranes and render the red cell vulnerable to hemolysis. While the pathophysiologic mechanisms vary, all induce hemolysis which, if persistent or recurrent, may lead eventually to the morphologic changes common to this category of anemias.

ANEMIAS DUE TO DECREASED RED CELL PRODUCTION

Daily in man, slightly less than 1 per cent of all red cells become obsolescent and are destroyed. Unless the marrow production can keep up with this constant drain, anemia results. Decreased production of red cells is encountered whenever there is a deficiency of some vital substrate or when the marrow is suppressed or is replaced by some space-occupying lesion. Although the bone marrow is functionally hypoactive in all such settings, it may be very cellular, as will be documented in the discussion of pernicious anemia.

VITAMIN B₁₂ DEFICIENCY

The major effect of a deficiency of vitamin B_{12} (cobalamin) is delayed DNA synthesis in all proliferating cell systems throughout the body (Beck, 1968). Principally affected are the bone marrow, tongue, buccal mucosa and alimentary tract. The precise role of this vitamin in DNA synthesis is still somewhat obscure. In vitro, vitamin B_{12} is required for the conversion of methyl-malonyl CoA to succinyl CoA and of homocysteine to methionine. Like folic acid, B_{12} participates in one-carbon transfers and may share with folate a final common pathway. Because the conversion of methylmalonyl CoA to succinyl CoA is blocked, increased levels of the former substance are excreted in the urine in avitaminotic patients, providing one of the most sensitive and early laboratory tests for vitamin B_{12} deficiency.

A deficiency of cobalamin may arise in a number of ways:
1. Dietary deficiency of animal protein.
2. Gastric defect—intrinsic factor deficiency.
   a. Pernicious anemia, acquired or congenital.
   b. Total gastrectomy or severe gastritis.
3. Intestinal malabsorption.
   a. Parasites or bacterial overgrowth—tapeworm, intestinal diverticulosis, intestinal "blind loops."
   b. Resection or extensive inflammation of distal ileum.
   c. Congenital receptor deficiency.
   d. Sprue, steatorrhea or other malabsorption states.

Common to all of these B_{12} deficiencies are: (1) erythropoietic megaloblastosis of the marrow, related to impaired DNA synthesis, (2) ineffective erythropoiesis, (3) macrocytosis and hyperchromia of the red cells, (4) a hemolytic component probably arising from some obscure intracorpuscular defect, (5) mild jaundice and (6) elevated serum iron levels. These features will be discussed in greater detail in the consideration of pernicious anemia, the most important of the B_{12} deficiency states.

PERNICIOUS ANEMIA (PA)
(ADDISONIAN ANEMIA)

Among the cobalamin deficiency syndromes, pernicious anemia caused by a lack of intrinsic factor in the stomach is by far the most common and the most important. In addition to the erythropoietic megaloblastosis and hyperchromic macrocytosis of the circulating red cells, it is characterized by prominent gastrointestinal and neurologic manifestations (i.e., combined system disease). *A gastric defect in the elaboration of intrinsic factor (IF) blocks the normal absorption of B_{12} (formerly known as the extrinsic factor).* The defect may appear as a congenital inability to elaborate intrinsic factor, and so pernicious anemia may develop in the infant or young child (McIntyre et al., 1965). This lack of intrinsic factor appears to be a specific synthetic defect not related to any underlying gastritis or, indeed, to any detectable gastric lesion. Frequently, these children exhibit minimal to no diminished secretion of hydrochloric acid or pepsin (Lillibridge et al., 1967). Far more commonly, PA presents itself in elderly adults as an acquired disease. In this age group, pernicious anemia is characterized by a diffuse atrophic gastritis in which the hydrochloric acid content and the volume of gastric secretion as well as the elaboration of pepsin and the critical production of intrinsic factor are all diminished. Save for the differences in the gastric pathology, the childhood and adult forms of this anemia manifest similar morphologic changes. Likewise, both forms show a familial incidence. Against this background, we can now turn to the consideration of the more common form of the disease in adults.

Incidence. The disease is one of middle to later life and affects about 0.1 per cent of the population. Males and females are affected equally and, while it has been described in blacks, it is more common in whites, particularly those of Scandinavian descent. A genetic background for pernicious anemia has long been recognized. Relatives of patients have a greater incidence of PA than the general population of the same age. Furthermore, relatives without overt PA more frequently exhibit achlorhydric gastritis and diminished ability to absorb oral test doses of vitamin B_{12} than do age-matched controls (Whittingham et al., 1969). The recent report of pernicious anemia in one adult identical twin but not the other strongly suggests that the genetic component determines a predisposition which becomes manifest only under appropriate environmental conditions (Balcerzak et al., 1968).

Pathogenesis. The pathogenesis of PA is the pathogenesis of the severe atrophic gastritis, resulting in inadequate elaboration of intrinsic factor (IF). The lack of IF must be quite profound because it probably requires no more than 1 per cent of the stomach's normal IF secretory capacity for absorption of adequate amounts of cobalamin. Normally, three steps are involved: (1) As the vitamin is released during digestion of animal proteins, it is tightly bound to intrinsic factor. Only small amounts of IF are necessary, but this small requirement is mandatory for absorption of

B_{12}. (2) The IF-B_{12} complex is transported to the distal ileum. This complex partially protects the vitamin from competitive absorption by the intestinal flora. (3) The complex splits at the plasma membrane of the epithelial cells of the distal ileum and, by some energy-requiring process, the B_{12} is transported to the interior of the epithelial cells. The IF is left behind and is briefly available to complex with more B_{12}. The adsorption of the IF-B_{12} complex to the ileal mucosa can occur only when the pH of the intestinal contents is above 6.5 and calcium or magnesium ions are present. Following incorporation within the mucosal epithelial cell, B_{12} is transferred to the blood where it is bound to a protein and transported to the sites of DNA synthesis throughout the body.

There is substantial evidence that, *in the adult form of the disease, the lack of IF is secondary to a severe atrophic chronic gastritis in which destruction of parietal cells results from an autoimmune reaction against antigens in the gastric mucosa* (Castle, 1970). The diffuse atrophy of the stomach is regularly associated with an intense infiltration of lymphocytes, histiocytes and plasma cells into the gastric mucosa. Complement fixing serum antibodies directed against the cytoplasm of normal gastric parietal cells can be demonstrated in up to 90 per cent of patients with PA (Irvine, 1965). Identical antibodies are found in the serum of about one-third of the blood relatives of patients and in approximately a similar proportion of patients with primary myxedema or Hashimoto's goiter, other diseases of presumed autoimmune origin (Doniach and Roitt, 1964). Moreover, clinical pernicious anemia occurs in about 12 per cent of patients with Hashimoto's thyroiditis, suggesting some systemic predisposition, in these patients, to the emergence of reactions against "self." However, it should be noted that antiparietal cell antibodies can be demonstrated in many persons having no clinical or laboratory evidence of pernicious anemia. Indeed, the incidence of achlorhydria, chronic gastritis and parietal cell antibodies rises steadily in the general population after middle age.

Of more *specific etiologic importance are anti-intrinsic factor antibodies in patients with PA.* These are seldom found in any other form of gastritis not associated with the hematologic disorder. These IF antibodies are of two kinds: "blocking" antibodies which prevent IF from complexing with B_{12} and "precipitating" antibodies which react with IF either before or after its combination with the vitamin. "Blocking" or "precipitating" antibodies to IF can be demonstrated in most patients with PA (Carmel and Herbert, 1966). Histo-

logic evidence is supporting: the lymphoid and plasma cell infiltration in the atrophic gastritis is very likely the site of a humoral or cell-mediated autoimmune reaction.

Thus, it would seem that *a genetically determined defect in immunologic tolerance for antigens present in the stomach predisposes these patients to PA* likening this disorder to Hashimoto's thyroiditis (Roitt and Doniach, 1969). What initiates such an autoimmune reaction is still mysterious. Does the genetic influence act at the level of the immunocyte? Alternatively, could it be that either programmed premature degeneration of gastric cells or some subclinical chronic infection alters the antigenic properties of the parietal cells? Such possibilities have not been excluded.

Morphology. Actively replicating cells such as those in the gastric and small intestinal mucosa and bone marrow cannot synthesize DNA and divide properly. They develop a variety of morphologic changes, principal among which is increase in nuclear and cellular size. Erythropoiesis is deranged, and erythroblasts transform to megaloblasts. There is failure of production of sufficient numbers of normoblasts to maintain the normal level of red cells in the peripheral blood. Such red cells as are produced are abnormally large (macrocytic). Neutrophils are similarly enlarged as described below. In addition, for obscure reasons some abnormal hemolysis augments the anemia.

The full-blown morphologic alterations of untreated pernicious anemia are rarely encountered today because parenteral liver extracts with high vitamin B_{12} content are almost invariably administered to patients with all forms of anemia. However, since the untreated case presents the classic alterations, it will be described indicating, where pertinent, the effects of therapy. **The major specific changes are found in the bone marrow, alimentary tract and central nervous system. Widespread nonspecific alterations are incident to the generalized tissue hypoxia and abnormal hemolysis of blood.**

The bone marrow of untreated pernicious anemia is soft, red, jelly-like and extremely hypercellular. It extends into the areas formerly occupied by fatty marrow. Sometimes this expansion extends to extramedullary hematopoiesis in the spleen and liver. Histologically, there is marked erythropoietic hypercellularity in which the erythroid elements sometimes equal or even outnumber the myeloid elements. **The most striking characteristic is the appearance of nests of the specific megaloblasts** (Peabody, 1927) (Fig. 17–11). These cells are different from normal erythroblasts in that megaloblasts are larger and have a delicate, finely reticulated nuclear chromatin and a stringy basophilic cytoplasm. Occasionally, the cytoplasm stains

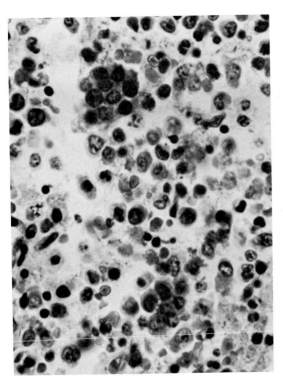

Figure 17–11. Pernicious anemia. Two nests of darkly stained megaloblasts in the bone marrow.

slightly pink and is described as polychromatophilic. These cells may account for 10 to 25 per cent of all nucleated forms in the marrow. Normoblasts are, by comparison, few in number, and there is a notable dearth of maturing red cells, suggesting a maturational arrest at the megaloblastic level. The red cells formed by the megaloblasts are characteristically macrocytic. They appear hyperchromic because of their large size, but in reality the mean corpuscular hemoglobin concentration (MCHC) is normal. There may be a relative increase in the number of leukopoietic elements, but more striking is the presence of mature large polymorphonuclear leukocytes, the "macropolys." These cells characteristically have large nuclei, sometimes with six to seven individual lobes (Fig. 17–12). Megakaryocytes are not significantly altered.

With antipernicious anemia therapy or spontaneous remission, the megaloblasts, macrocytes and macropolys disappear. Normal maturation and erythropoiesis reappear and are reflected in a great increase in the number of normoblasts and their descendants.

In the **alimentary system,** abnormalities are regularly found in the tongue and stomach. The tongue is shiny, glazed and "beefy" **(atrophic glossitis).** The changes in the stomachs of adults are those of atrophic gastritis (p. 914) manifested by thinning of the gastric mucosa. These atrophic changes are usually completely **absent** from juve-

nile patients with pernicious anemia. In the atrophic stomach, the submucosal vessels are readily visible and so produce a shiny red mucosal surface. The most characteristic histologic alteration is the atrophy of the gastric glands affecting both chief cells and parietal cells. The parietal cells virtually completely disappear, as one would expect if these cells are, indeed, the target of an immune reaction. The glandular lining epithelium is metaplastically replaced by mucus-secreting goblet cells that resemble the lining of the large intestine, a change referred to as **"intestinalization."** Some of the cells as well as their nuclei may increase to double the normal size. Presumably, these enlargements reflect the megaloid alterations discussed earlier. As will be seen, patients with pernicious anemia have a higher incidence of gastric cancer. It may be that these cellular alterations underlie a predisposition to malignancy (Magnus, 1958) (Payne, 1961).

Although parenteral administration of vitamin B_{12} will correct the bone marrow changes in pernicious anemia, the gastric atrophy and achlorhydria persist unaffected. This exception is entirely compatible with the thesis that the gastric changes are autoimmune in origin and are the cause and not the effect of the deficiency of B_{12}.

Central nervous system lesions are found in approximately three-quarters of all cases of fulminant pernicious anemia. **The principal alterations involve the spinal cord where there is myelin degeneration of the dorsal and lateral tracts.** Less frequently, degenerative changes occur

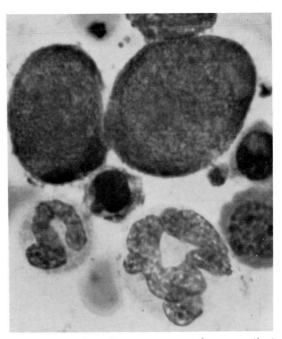

Figure 17–12. A marrow smear from a patient with pernicious anemia. Two megaloblasts are seen above and a "macropoly" below.

in the ganglia of the posterior roots and in the peripheral nerves (p. 1536). Degenerative myelin changes are evident rarely within the brain.

In addition to these fairly distinctive lesions, fatty degenerative changes in the heart, liver and kidneys may be present secondary to the systemic hypoxia. Because of the hemolytic tendency, hemosiderosis may be found in the liver, spleen and bone marrow and in other elements of the reticuloendothelial system, but the spleen and liver are not usually significantly enlarged. The skin in severe relapse has a peculiar lemon-yellow hue, not linearly related to the usually slightly elevated bilirubin levels in the plasma. In passing, it should be noted that megaloid nuclear changes sometimes are seen in the cervical cytology of female patients.

Clinical Course. Pernicious anemia is characteristically insidious in onset, so that by the time the patient seeks medical attention, the anemia is usually quite marked. The usual course is progressive but fluctuating, with spontaneous remissions followed by relapse. Presenting complaints are most often weakness and numbness or tingling in the extremities as a consequence of the spinal cord and peripheral nerve lesions. Many patients also have difficulty in walking, loss of vibratory sense, incoordination of movements, and even disturbed mentation. Sore tongue may result from the atrophic glossitis.

While the diagnosis may be suspected from these clinical findings, it can be substantiated only by laboratory tests. Megaloblastosis in the marrow and low serum levels of cobalamin establish the existence of a B_{12} deficiency. In the usual case, the serum B_{12} level is 100 picogm. or less (normal: 200 to 1000 picogm.). Gastric achlorhydria is virtually a requisite to confirm that the low B_{12} level is related to PA since, as was pointed out earlier, there are many causes of B_{12} deficiency (p. 715). The anacidity is persistent even after administration of histamine. When gastric acid is demonstrable, the diagnosis of pernicious anemia is tenuous. Red cell counts down to or less than 1,000,000 cells per mm.^{3} are not uncommon. The MCV and MCH are above normal due to the macrocytosis, and it follows that the hematocrit and hemoglobin are disproportionately high relative to the red count. However, the MCHC is not increased. On smear, the cells are variable in size and the many abnormally large macrocytes having the deep coloration of a high hemoglobin content account for the observed hyperchromia. With therapy, or in remission, the blood values and indices return toward normal and, with the resumption of erythropoiesis, large numbers of polychromatophilic erythrocytes, stippled red cells, reticu-

locytes and normoblasts appear in the circulating blood. The reticulocyte response to parenteral B_{12} therapy is a valuable diagnostic test for this anemia. Leukopenia and, more specifically, neutropenia are fairly constant. Large immature macropolys in the peripheral blood further substantiate the diagnosis. The platelets are generally decreased in number. In remission, these elements again reappear in normal numbers.

Certain complications may prove fatal. The exact incidence of gastric cancer is still controversial, but recent studies indicate that about 5 to 10 per cent of all patients with this anemia will develop such a carcinoma over the span of decades. Cardiac failure following fatty change of the myocardium and intercurrent infections are additional hazards. The recent dramatic improvements achieved by such anti-immune therapy as steroids provide a new dimension to the attack on this disease.

FOLIC-ACID DEFICIENCY ANEMIA

The anemia associated with a deficiency of folic acid is the often forgotten stepchild among the macrocytic, megaloblastic anemias. According to a recent report, folic-acid deficiency and vitamin B_{12} deficiency together account for more than 95 per cent of all megaloblastic anemias, the former being far more common than the latter (Sullivan, 1970). Folate deficiency is an extremely common cause of anemia in underprivileged societies; moreover, inadequate serum folate levels were found in 47 per cent of patients admitted to a municipal hospital in the United States (Leevy et al., 1965).

Pathogenesis. Folic acid, more precisely, pteroylglutamic acid (PGA), is present in small amounts in most foods, particularly green vegetables, citrus fruits and liver. The most common cause of a deficiency state is simply inadequate dietary intake. Thus, this form of anemia is widespread among malnourished populations. It is particularly encountered among alcoholics, both because of their nutritionally inadequate diets and because alcohol itself may suppress the response of the marrow to dietary folic acid. Pregnant women have a markedly increased dietary requirement for folic acid. Any one of the many malabsorption syndromes or persistent vomiting may lead to a deficient intake. PGA is absorbed probably by passive diffusion along the entire small intestine, largely from the upper jejunum. Hence, disease of this level of the small intestine is most likely to induce malabsorption of folic acid. Many drugs interfere with either the absorption or utilization of folic acid and thus produce an anemia, including (1) folate antagonists such as methotrexate, (2) purine analogues such as 6-mercaptopurine, (3) pyrimidine analogues such as 5-fluorouracil and (4) diphenylhydantoin and some of the oral contraceptives (Kahn, 1970).

A deficiency of PGA has somewhat the same cytologic effects as a deficiency of B_{12} because it too impairs DNA synthesis. PGA is biologically inactive, but it serves as a precursor to a number of coenzymes active throughout the body where single carbon atoms are transferred to or built into compounds. Thus, PGA and its coenzymes probably participate with vitamin B_{12} in donating methyl groups to homocysteine in the formation of methionine. As is the case with vitamin B_{12}, folic-acid derivatives are necessary for the synthesis of DNA. With a deficiency of folate, all actively dividing cell systems in the body are affected, principally the erythropoietic cells in the bone marrow. Here, too, the erythroblasts are transformed to megaloblasts and the erythrocytes to abnormally large macrocytes. The granulocytes are likewise affected and transform to "macropolys" with hypersegmented nuclei. In patients suffering from a severe deficiency of PGA, the production of leukocytes and platelets is impaired, resulting in leukopenia and thrombocytopenia. As iron utilization also is diminished, it progressively accumulates within RE cells and elevated levels of serum iron are observed.

Morphology. A deficiency of PGA is almost always accompanied by other avitaminoses and so it is difficult to be certain of changes related solely to folic-acid deprivation. As best we know, these alterations are limited to the bone marrow, peripheral blood and tongue. The evidence that folic-acid deficiency induces neurologic or psychiatric changes is controversial and has been well summarized by Harris and Kellermeyer (1970): "There is at present no compelling objective evidence that folic acid deficiency per se is causally related to neuropsychiatric changes...." The bone marrow changes, hematologic abnormalities and atrophic glossitis are identical with those described in pernicious anemia. However, not infrequently, these patients suffer from a concomitant lack of iron due to dietary inadequacies. This additional deficiency complicates the cytologic changes in both the bone marrow and the peripheral blood (Vitale et al., 1965). As with a B_{12} deficiency, nuclear enlargement and abnormalities are sometimes encountered in cervical mucosal cells, particularly during pregnancy when the requirements for folate are increased (Kitay and Wentz, 1969).

Clinical Course. In contrast to the patients suffering from a vitamin B_{12} deficiency, who for long years may appear pale rather than sick, most patients with folic-acid deficiency show considerable weight loss and are sick. The onset of the anemia is overshadowed by general weakness and malaise. The variety of clinical findings and the generally poor clinical condition reflect the multiple malnutritional deficiencies from which these patients usually suffer. Neurologic manifestations of thiamine deficiency are often present. Skin and perioral lesions characteristic of a deficiency of the B complex are common as is hepatomegaly, probably related to protein deficiency. Splenomegaly, attributable to either hepatic disease or intercurrent microbiologic infections, may be evident.

The differentiation of the anemia of folate deficiency from that of B_{12} deficiency requires direct assay of serum levels of folate and B_{12}. Normal serum folate levels are between 7 and 20 nanogm. per ml., and levels below 4 are considered clinically significant. Unlike PA, the anemia of folic-acid deficiency is not associated with achlorhydria, providing another useful laboratory differential feature. However, the B_{12} deficiency states, other than that caused by the adult type pernicious anemia, may also have normal levels of gastric acid, so ultimately serum folate levels must be determined.

IRON DEFICIENCY ANEMIA

The deficiency of iron prevents the synthesis of adequate amounts of hemoglobin and results in an anemia characterized by the formation of small, poorly pigmented red cells, i.e., a hypochromic microcytosis. Stainable iron is not evident in the bone marrow. Iron deficiency anemia is without question the most common type of anemia encountered clinically. It occurs at all ages in both sexes and throughout the world.

Pathogenesis. *Iron deficiency anemia is usually merely the symptom of some underlying problem causing iron deficiency.* Remember from the earlier consideration of the metabolism of iron that the body closely conserves this element. The maintenance of normal levels and reserves of iron in the tissues is largely controlled by regulation of the absorption of iron. This balanced mechanism is more fully explained on page 273. It suffices for now to restate that the excretion of iron is fairly fixed at less than 1 mg. per day. Greater losses may occur through menstruation, pregnancy, lactation and exfoliation of the skin. Since large amounts of iron are contained in the ordinary diet within eggs, meat, liver and many vegetables, there is considerable excess iron that is not absorbed. However, with high losses of iron, increased amounts may be absorbed.

A negative iron balance can result from an inadequate absorption and/or from increased needs for iron beyond the capacity for increased absorption. Inadequate absorption of iron may occur with bizarre food habits, such as the avoidance of meats and vegetables, most frequently observed in this country among the very young who prefer a carbohydrate regimen, in the very old who live on "tea and toast" and in chronic alcoholics who drink their calories. Other causes of deficient intake were presented in the earlier discussion of this subject on p. 273. Intake may be sufficient but iron deficiency may still result from malabsorption such as occurs in sprue and celiac disease.

Physiologic losses or utilization in excess of the daily intake may account for a negative iron balance. The menstruating female loses twice as much iron annually as the male. It is estimated that a single pregnancy may account for as much as the normal annual loss of the male. Moreover, rapid growth produces increased demands on the iron stores due to increased needs for red cell, enzyme and tissue iron. This type of demand is particularly important in premature babies and infants who frequently have deficient iron stores at birth. The iron deficiency may be more severe in bottle-fed babies, since cow's milk is a poor source of iron.

The increased need for iron may be occasioned by pathologic losses. External bleeding is the most common cause of iron deficiency anemia. Since excessive physiologic losses of iron can occur only in women, an iron deficiency in the well fed (i.e., not malabsorbing) adult male can result only from pathologic losses (Strauss, 1948–49). A clinical maxim therefore states: "When an adult, reasonably well nourished male suffers from an iron deficiency anemia, look for the source of the blood loss."

Morphology. Knowledge of the pathology of simple iron deficiency anemia is limited by the fact that few patients die of this disorder alone. However, many patients die with variable degrees of iron deficiency anemia, some from related causes and others from disease independent of the anemia. Except under unusual circumstances, cases of iron deficiency anemia are mild, and there is insufficient depression of the hemoglobin level to cause fatty degenerative or atrophic changes in the susceptible organs. Hemosiderosis or stainable iron is notably absent since there is no increased internal destruction of blood and, in fact, all available iron stores are mobilized for hemoglobin synthesis. The skin and mucous membranes are pale. The nails may become spoon-shaped and have longitudinal ridges. There may be atrophy of the mucosa of the tongue (atrophic glossitis). The most constant anatomic alteration is an active marrow which is hyperplastic and is usually slightly but not markedly increased in volume. The moderate increase in the erythroid elements occurs dominantly at the level of the normoblasts and their maturation forms. This erythroid hyperactivity is roughly proportional to the degree of the anemia. Leukocytes and megakaryocytes are usually not affected. Extramedullary foci of hematopoiesis are uncommon although they may develop in severe cases. Hepatic and splenic changes are seldom present. In occasional cases, shelf-like epithelial partitions or horizontal ridges known as **esophageal webs** are found in the esophagus. It is also reported that there is a higher than normal incidence of esophageal carcinoma. It is not clear whether these alimentary tract lesions precede the development of anemia and possibly contribute to it by causing dysphagia of solid foods, such as meats, or whether the webs are in some obscure manner caused by the anemia.

Clinical Course. No one well defined clinical syndrome can be described because this disorder is encountered over such a wide span in age and is caused by such diverse conditions. Symptoms, when present, usually reflect the underlying cause of the anemia, e.g., alcoholism, pregnancy, malabsorption, etc. Anemia-related symptoms may be nonspecific: weakness, fatigability and pallor. Additional common complaints are gastrointestinal disturbances, which in fact may have been instrumental in producing the iron deficiency. Because of the atrophic glossitis, many patients have a sore tongue or difficulty in swallowing (Fig. 17–13). These oral manifestations in a patient with microcytic hypochromic iron deficiency anemia are referred to as the *Plummer-Vinson syndrome*.

Beyond these fairly nonspecific findings, the diagnosis ultimately rests upon the examination of the peripheral blood. The red cell count is depressed to moderate levels, usually averaging between 3,000,000 to 4,000,000 red cells per mm.[3] In severe cases, the count may be lower. The hemoglobin level is reduced below that commensurate with the RBC count because the cells are microcytic and hypochromic, reflecting the lowered MCH (Fig. 17–14) and MCHC. Usually the leukocytes and platelets are not affected.

The alert clinician who investigates an unexplained iron deficiency anemia occasionally discovers an occult infection or cancer and thereby saves a life.

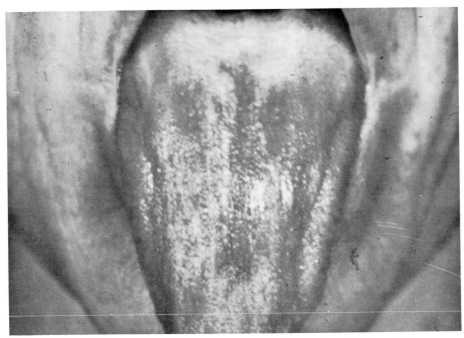

Figure 17–13. *The glazed atrophic mucosa of the tongue in a patient with iron deficiency anemia.*

ANEMIA OF BONE MARROW FAILURE (APLASTIC ANEMIA, PANCYTOPENIA)

Anemia is encountered in a wide variety of disorders in which there is neither excessive destruction of red cells nor any deficiency of

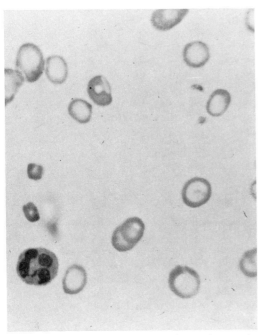

Figure 17–14. *Hypochromic microcytic anemia. A smear of the pale "thin" erythrocytes.*

known erythropoietic factors, and so the cause is attributed to bone marrow failure. Most often, all three lines are affected producing pancytopenia (Mohler and Leavell, 1958). In some patients, however, there is only anemia unassociated with a deficiency of white cells or platelets. Bone marrow failure is encountered in renal disease, liver disease, endocrine disturbances, advanced malignancy particularly with metastasis to the bone marrow, with chronic infections, and in certain hereditary disorders such as the Fanconi syndrome. Under the present heading, however, these forms of hematopoietic failure are excluded from discussion.

Pathogenesis. Here we are concerned with the aplastic anemia or pancytopenia which may occur mysteriously as an idiopathic disease or after exposure to a variety of drugs and chemicals. Most cases of aplastic anemia or pancytopenia are of unknown cause. Autoimmunity has been suggested, but circulating antibodies can only be demonstrated in a few instances, and usually these induce a hemolytic rather than an aplastic form of anemia (Harvard, 1962). Included in this category of idiopathic aplastic anemias are the rare cases associated with lesions of the thymus gland, particularly thymomas, where the pathogenetic mechanism is totally obscure (p. 1368). In some cases, the marrow failure is clearly related to exposure to such potent myelotoxins as radiant energy, benzene, nitrogen mustard, urethan and the wide variety of drugs now used in the treatment of leukemia. In many cases of leukemia, the possibility of marrow injury is a calculated risk assumed with the therapy to depress the abnormal proliferation of white cells. Marrow injury has also been associated with a heterogeneous group of drugs not considered to be directly myelotoxic. A listing by the American Medical Assocation cites the ten most common offenders among this group as chloramphenicol, phenylbutazone, chemical solvents, sulfonamides, insecticides, methylphenylethylhydantoin, gold, mepazine, chlorpromazine and oral hypoglycemic agents. With these agents, three variables are involved: severity of the depressant action on the marrow, quantity ingested and individual hypersensitivity to the agent. This last variable is the most important because, in some patients, rather trivial amounts may induce a significant hematopoietic depression. It has been observed that when a number of individuals have been exposed to identical levels of a particular substance, some escaped unharmed while others developed severe anemia or pancytopenia.

Morphology. Paradoxically, the bone marrow may be hypercellular, normocellular or hypocellular. Classically, the marrow is relatively acellular with an increase in the amount of fat. In some patients, hypercellularity is first encountered, followed by transformation to a hypocellular marrow. Regardless of the appearance of the marrow, there is failure of production or release of adequate numbers of mature elements. The failure may involve any one or a combination of the three main groups: red cells, white cells or platelets. Sometimes the more primitive myeloid cells persist, apparently failing to form the mature elements. At other times, only the white cell series or only the red cell series may be deficient. Some immaturity or depletion of megakaryocytes may be seen in cases involving a deficiency of platelets. Coincident with this depletion of hematopoietic cells, the marrow becomes diffusely albeit sparsely infiltrated with lymphocytes and plasma cells (Fig. 17–15). It is obvious from these variable marrow patterns that it is impossible, from examination of the bone marrow, to establish the adequacy of production of circulating blood cells. Only when the marrow precursors are notably absent can the diagnosis of marrow failure be made.

Extramedullary hematopoiesis may be found in severe cases, but it is usually not significant in amount, and splenomegaly and hepatomegaly are, at most, minimal. It seems paradoxical that ectopic foci appear in the presence of a mechanism that depresses marrow function. This phenomenon might be suggestive of an alteration incident only in the bony environment of normal hematopoiesis.

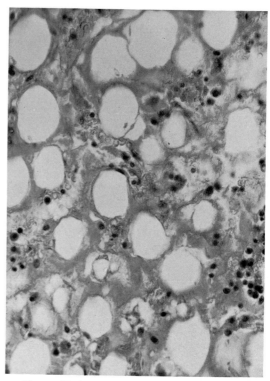

Figure 17–15. Pancytopenia—bone marrow. The bone marrow is hypocellular. Most of the nucleated forms present are lymphocytes and scattered plasma cells.

A number of morphologic changes may accompany these marrow failures. Fatty changes may result from the anemia. Also evident may be the pathology of bacterial infections or hemorrhagic diatheses secondary to the granulocytopenia or thrombocytopenia, respectively (p. 740). The toxic drug or agent may injure not only the bone marrow but also the liver, kidneys and other structures. Benzol, for example, may cause fatty changes in the liver and kidneys. In some of these anemias, for obscure reasons, there is a slightly increased hemolytic tendency and hemosiderosis may result.

Clinical Course. These forms of marrow failure may occur at any age and in both sexes. Usually the onset is gradual, but in some instances the disorder strikes with suddenness and great severity. The patients may first become aware of their disease by the progressive onset of weakness, fatigability and pallor. The thrombocytopenia may produce bleeding manifestations. At other times, the granulocytopenia is called to attention by repeated bacterial infections which are apparently more severe than would be anticipated in the normal individual.

The diagnosis rests largely upon the examination of the peripheral blood and the exclusion of other causes for the anemia or pancytopenia. In most patients, the red cells are normochromic and normocytic, but occasionally slight macrocytosis occurs. Signs of erythropoiesis such as polychromatophilia or reticulocytosis are characteristically absent. When pancytopenia is present, the white cell and platelet counts are also depressed. Sometimes the leukocytes drop to levels below 1000 per mm.[3] of blood and consist largely of lymphocytes.

Bone marrow biopsy can aid diagnosis when it discloses an aplastic or hypocellular marrow. It may also help to rule out other causes of depressed marrow function as metastatic cancer, leukemia, miliary tuberculosis or some underlying bone disease that has replaced the marrow space.

The prognosis in these disorders is quite unpredictable. If the toxic factor can be identified and further exposure avoided, the marrow production may be expected to recover. If idiopathic, the disease tends to be more prolonged and the outlook is less favorable. Some of these idiopathic cases spontaneously remit, but others deteriorate rapidly to death within months to a year.

OTHER FORMS OF MARROW FAILURE

Space-occupying lesions that destroy significant amounts of bone marrow must inevitably depress the productive capacity (Pisciotta, 1950). This form of marrow failure is referred to as *myelophthisic* anemia. As would be anticipated, all the formed elements of the blood are concomitantly affected. However, characteristically immature forms of the red and white cells appear in the peripheral blood, a phenomenon attributed to an "irritation effect." The most common cause of myelophthisic anemia is metastatic cancer arising from a primary lesion in the breast, lung, prostate, thyroid or adrenals (Fig. 17–16). Multiple myeloma, leukemia, osteosclerosis, the lymphomas and the reticuloendothelioses are less commonly implicated. Myelophthisic anemia has also been observed with myelofibrosis, a diffuse fibrosis of the marrow. Such cases are probably variants of the myeloproliferative syndrome. Occasionally, a patient with polycythemia will develop, over the course of years, myelofibrosis and myelophthisic anemia. Here again, the disorder is better considered as a variation of the myeloproliferative syndrome discussed on p. 738.

Diffuse liver disease, whether it be toxic, infectious or a form of cirrhosis, is for obscure reasons often associated with an anemia attributed to bone marrow failure. In most of these

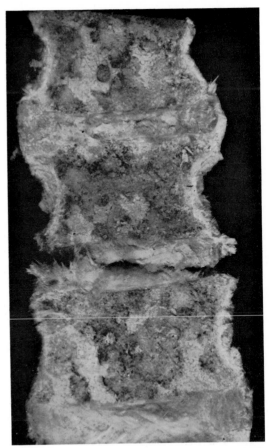

Figure 17–16. *Metastatic breast carcinoma in the vertebrae from a 53-year-old woman with marked myelophthisic anemia.*

instances, there is a pure erythropoietic depression; in about half the cases, the red cells are normocytic and, in the other half, the cells are macrocytic. Occasionally the red cell morphology is very much like that of pernicious anemia. Depression of the white cell count and platelets has been described, but is infrequent.

Renal diseases, acute and, more characteristically, chronic, sometimes produce severe anemia. Occasionally, a hemolytic type of anemia results with a shortened red cell life span but, in other cases, there is no increased hemolysis and the anemia appears to be purely one of bone marrow depression. In the great preponderance of these cases, no significant morphologic alteration can be detected in the bone marrow. The anemia is normocytic and normochromic. When the renal failure is acute and remits, marrow recovery follows.

Endocrine disorders, particularly those affecting the thyroid, pituitary and adrenal, may be associated with anemia. Myxedema stands out as the most important disorder in this category. In some of these cases, the anemia is normocytic, but in many it is macrocytic. Impaired absorption of vitamin B_{12} has been implicated in some cases of thyroid hypofunction which may produce, therefore, a pattern similar to that of pernicious anemia. Alternatively, it is possible that the decreased metabolic activity of the body secondarily slows marrow production. Supporting such a concept is the prompt recovery of marrow function following the administration of thyroid extract. Addison's disease (p. 1311) and hypofunction of the anterior lobe of the pituitary are sometimes associated with a normocytic anemia. The mechanisms here are obscure. In all these endocrine disorders, the bone marrow usually provides no morphologic clue to its physiologic hypoactivity.

Marrow failure has been recorded in rheumatoid arthritis and chronic infection, and although some obscure myelotoxic substance might be postulated, none has yet been identified.

POLYCYTHEMIA

Polycythemia refers to an increase in the concentration of red cells above the normal levels, usually with a corresponding increase in the hemoglobin level. Such an increase may be *relative*, when there is hemoconcentration, or *absolute*. *Relative polycythemia* is also known as erythrocytosis. *Absolute polycythemia*, while also characterized by an increase in the red cell count, is more precisely defined as an increase in the total red cell mass. It may occur as an idiopathic primary disorder, i.e., polycythemia vera, or as a secondary response to some disease or environmental influence inducing tissue hypoxia.

RELATIVE POLYCYTHEMIA (ERYTHROCYTOSIS)

Relative polycythemia results from loss of the fluid component of blood without a corresponding loss in the formed elements and is, therefore, a hemoconcentration phenomenon. Under these circumstances, there is a proportionate increase in the number of red cells, white cells and platelets. The causes of this condition include (1) deprivation of water, (2) loss of body fluids from vomiting, diarrhea and sweating, (3) loss of electrolytes with corresponding loss of body water, such as occurs with adrenal insufficiency, and (4) loss of plasma, as in shock. Since there is no absolute excess of cells, correction of reduced intravascular fluid volume is promptly followed by a return of the erythrocyte values to normal. There are no associated morphologic changes.

POLYCYTHEMIA VERA (PRIMARY POLYCYTHEMIA, VAQUEZ-OSLER DISEASE, ERYTHREMIA)

Polycythemia vera is an insidious disease of unknown cause, characterized by elevation of the total red cell mass sometimes to double the normal value. As a consequence, the red cell count and hemoglobin levels are elevated; frequently, the white cell and platelet counts are up as well. Males are affected somewhat more than females, most often between the ages of 40 and 60. The condition is more common in whites but occurs among blacks also.

Etiology and Pathogenesis. The cause of polycythemia is an increased production of red cells beyond the normal daily need (Pollycove et al., 1966). The erythrocytes have a nearly normal life span and, indeed, rather than being lengthened, there is some evidence that is it shortened. But the etiology of the excessive erythropoiesis is mysterious. It would be reasonable to suspect bone marrow hypoxia or increased levels of erythropoietin, but according to presently available techniques, neither condition is demonstrable in this disease (Adamson and Finch, 1968) (Hecht and Samuels, 1952). At the present time, the view is favored that polycythemia is akin to a neoplastic process affecting principally the erythropoietic precursors in the bone marrow. Presumably such cells, like all neoplastic cells, escape from physiologic controls and produce excessive numbers of erythrocytes. Several lines of evidence favor this hypothesis. There is growing documentation of two distinctive lines (clones) of erythropoietic cells in the marrow of these patients (Adamson and Finch, 1968) (Krantz, 1968). Presumably, one line is under physiologic control but the other is aberrant and uncontrolled. Additional support for the neoplastic theory comes from the very unpredictable course of this disease. In some patients, after a lapse of years to decades, markedly elevated white cell levels, leukemoid reactions, are encountered, and in others, frank leukemia develops, raising the question of whether the neoplastic influence spreads to the white cell series. More often, after a course of many years, these patients enter a phase of profound anemia usually associated with excessive proliferation of fibroblasts and myelofibrosis. This unpredictable course and variable transformation of polycythemia to leukemia, to anemia or to myelofibrosis has fostered the concept that *polycythemia vera might be merely one* *expression of a broader neoplastic myeloproliferative syndrome* which potentially might involve any of the marrow cell lines. In one patient, only red cells might be affected initially; in another, white cells; and in another, fibroblasts. During the evolution of any one disorder, unpredictable transformations might occur as the neoplastic influence shifts from the erythrocytic series, for example, to the granulocytic series. More details on the myeloproliferative syndrome follow on p. 738.

Whatever the underlying cause, a number of important alterations are encountered secondary to the increased red cell production. The expanded red cell mass induces hypervolemia, sometimes two- or threefold, which may in turn lead to hypertension. An increase in the viscosity of the blood not only places an added burden on the heart, but also impairs tissue perfusion. A thrombotic diathesis results from the increased viscosity and slowed flow. Along with the thrombotic diathesis, hemorrhagic tendencies paradoxically appear. This condition has been attributed to longstanding distention and engorgement of vessels such that elasticity is impaired and the vessels cannot vasoconstrict when injured. These secondary consequences are more important in producing clinical dysfunction than is the increased red cell mass per se.

Morphology. The major anatomic changes stem from the increase in red cell mass, the increase in total blood volume and the increase in the viscosity of the blood.

Plethoric congestion of all organs and tissues is characteristic of polycythemia vera. The major vessels are uniformly distended with a thick viscous blood which is usually not totally oxygenated. The liver is enlarged and frequently contains foci of myeloid metaplasia. The spleen is enlarged up to 250 to 350 gm. and is extremely firm and congested (Tinney et al., 1943). The splenic sinuses are packed with red cells as are all the vessels within the spleen. Hematopoiesis sometimes can be identified within the red pulp.

Consequent to the increased viscosity and vascular stasis, thromboses and infarctions are common, affecting most often the heart, brain, spleen and kidneys.

The active bone marrow is the primary site of alteration and is characteristically increased in size so that it floods into the fatty marrow. It has a soft, dark red succulence. Histologically, this is due to striking hyperplasia of all the erythropoietic forms while the intervening fat cells disappear. Normoblastic proliferation is usually predominant, but there is also some increase in both white cell and platelet formation. The expanding marrow may encroach upon the cancellous bone as well

as the cortical shafts. If the disease changes its course, the marrow pattern reflects this alteration and thus may become aplastic, fibrotic or even leukemic.

Hemorrhages occur in about one-third of the patients. These affect most often the gastrointestinal tract, oropharynx and brain. Sometimes these hemorrhages are spontaneous, but more often they follow some minor surgical procedure or trauma. Peptic ulceration has been described in about 20 per cent of these patients.

Clinical Course. The major clinical features of polycythemia vera stem from the increased blood volume, vascular stasis, thrombotic tendency, hemorrhagic diathesis and transmutation into anemia or leukemia. About 30 per cent of the patients die from some thrombotic complication, affecting usually the brain or the heart. An additional 10 to 15 per cent die from some hemorrhagic complication (Wasserman, 1954). The frequency of leukemic transformation has been overemphasized in the past. A recent large study pointed out that acute leukemia occurred in less than 1 per cent of patients managed with treatment other than radiation, but in 10 per cent of those who received radiotherapy (Modan and Lillienfeld, 1965). The implication is clear.

Classically, patients with polycythemia are plethoric or even cyanotic. Complaints such as headache, dizziness, gastrointestinal symptoms, hematemesis and melena are common. Splenic or renal infarction may produce abdominal pain. The bleeding tendency may manifest itself as skin purpura or ecchymoses. Hypertension is a consequence of the increased blood volume. Only when the abnormal increase in the number of red cells is discovered does the basis for these symptoms and signs become apparent, and so the diagnosis is usually made by laboratory studies. The red cell counts range from 6,000,000 to 10,000,000 with comparable elevations of the hemoglobin and hematocrit. The white cell count is also elevated, sometimes up to 80,000 cells per mm.[3] The alkaline phosphatase level of these granulocytes is classically above normal. After a long polycythemic phase, most patients become anemic and some, as cited above, eventually develop leukemia (Lawrence, 1969).

Another very rare entity should be mentioned here—*erythremic myelosis*, better known as *Di Guglielmo's disease*. In this condition, there is an apparent neoplastic proliferation of the erythroblasts in the marrow and flooding of the peripheral blood with these immature cells (Fig. 17–17). In contrast to polycythemia, the immature erythroblasts in Di Guglielmo's disease do not mature to yield increased numbers

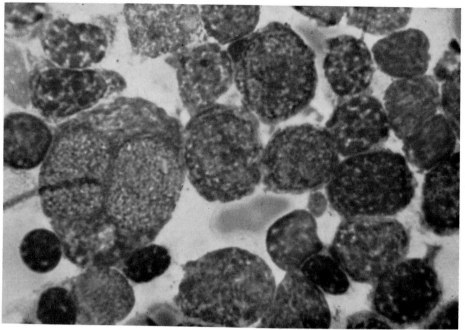

Figure 17–17. *A marrow smear from a patient with Di Guglielmo's disease, crowded with erythroblasts (one binucleate) and normoblasts.*

of normoblasts and red cells. The disease, therefore, is closely akin to leukemia and usually an anemia is present.

SECONDARY POLYCYTHEMIA

An increase in the concentration of circulating red cells may occur in any clinical circumstance involving tissue hypoxia or increased levels of erythropoietin formation. In the first category fall those individuals who live at very high altitudes, such as inhabitants of the Andes in South America and the Himalayas in India. Cardiac lesions, such as right to left shunts, which result in oxygen unsaturation of the arterial blood, lead to polycythemia. Diseases of the lung are also obvious causes of arterial oxygen unsaturation. Within this category are emphysema, diffuse pulmonary fibrosis, arteriovenous pulmonary fistulas and alveolocapillary blocks of whatever cause.

Secondary polycythemia is encountered in a growing number of clinical disorders involving excess formation of erythropoietin. Here the oxygen saturation is normal and the cause of the elevated levels of erythropoietin is obscure. Included among these disorders are cancer of the kidney, renal tuberculosis, renal adenoma, polycystic kidney disease, carcinoma of the lung or liver, ovarian tumors, uterine leiomyomas, pheochromocytoma and cerebellar vascular tumors.

As expected, removal of the implicated tumor or control of the underlying disease is followed promptly by a reversion of the blood count to normal.

In contrast to polycythemia vera, the erythrocytosis in the secondary form is usually not accompanied by any significant elevation in white cell or platelet counts. Moreover, the red cell counts are not usually as markedly elevated as in the primary form of this disease.

DISORDERS OF WHITE CELLS

Abnormal decreases and increases in number may affect the white cells as well as the red cells. Conditions involving decreased numbers of granulocytic white blood cells are termed agranulocytoses. Those characterized by abnormal increases of white blood cells comprise the large and very important category of leukemias.

AGRANULOCYTOSIS (GRANULOCYTOPENIA)

Reduction in the number of granulocytes in the peripheral blood is the principal characteristic of granulocytopenia. This disorder, then, is the analogue of aplastic anemia. The lymphocytes are not affected, and so a relative lymphocytosis reflects the loss of circulating granulocytes. The disease affects both sexes at any age, with a slight preponderance in females.

Pathogenesis. In general, the pathogenesis of agranulocytosis follows the same pattern as that of pancytopenia or aplastic anemia. Certain cases arise mysteriously without apparent cause and may, in fact, be a variant of pancytopenia such that only the production of white cells is affected. A larger fraction of the cases follows exposure to certain drugs now known to potentially depress granulocyte production. In most cases, the mechanism of action of the drug is unknown but, in the case of aminopyrine, there is some evidence that hypersensitivity is involved. It has been shown that relatively small doses of aminopyrine may cause the rapid disappearance of circulating granulocytes from the peripheral blood. Blood taken from such individuals suffering from severe granulocytopenia produces a reduction in circulating granulocytes in the normal recipient, strongly suggesting the presence of agglutinins against leukocytes (Moeschlin and Wagner, 1952). No such immunologic reaction can be demonstrated with any of the other drugs that have produced agranulocytosis. In these cases, there is a direct relationship between the dosage level of the drug and the severity of the white cell depression, implying a direct toxicity proportional to the serum level of the injurious agent. The drugs that have produced such toxic depression are too numerous to list completely, but the more important ones are some of the antihistaminics, e.g., phenothiazine; some of the antibacterial agents, such as sulfonamides, chloramphenicol, streptomycin and certain of the tetracyclines; and the antithyroid agent thiouracil. Also implicated are aminopyrine, as mentioned, and chlorpromazine. Nitrophenol and some of the gold preparations are capable of inducing depression of the granulocytes. Many of these drugs have in common a benzene ring, but the significance of this observation is unclear.

While we speak easily of drug toxicity as the cause of the marrow depression in granulocytopenia, there is no clear idea of the mechanism by which these agents act. Do they block mitotic activity or instead induce maturation arrest? Alternatively, do they destroy circulating granulocytes and so deplete the formed elements in the peripheral blood, eventually leading to exhaustion of the bone marrow? These questions remain unanswered.

Morphology. The major anatomic alterations in granulocytopenia involve the bone marrow. Early in the course of the disease, the bone marrow may be hyperplastic with increased numbers of immature white cell precursors, chiefly stem cells, myeloblasts and myelocytes. Presumably this early proliferative stage reflects the initial shock effect of the toxic or hypersensitivity reaction. In the course of 2 to 3 days, **the bone marrow becomes progressively hypocellular as the number of leukopoietic elements dwindles. The polymorphonuclear leukocytes and the myelocytes are principally affected.** In certain cases, however, the more mature white cells persist and the immature myeloid cells disappear. In these instances, when the early forms are scant, soon thereafter the more mature white cells of necessity disappear. Erythropoiesis and megakaryocytes usually remain at normal levels. Occasionally increased numbers of plasma cells and lymphocytes are found in the marrow, particularly as the marrow becomes acellular.

Infections are the second characteristic feature of agranulocytosis (Darling et al., 1936). Ulcerating necrotizing lesions of the gingiva, floor of the mouth, buccal mucosa, pharynx or anywhere within the oral cavity (agranulocytic angina) are quite characteristic of agranulocytosis (Fig. 17–18). These ulcers are typically deep, undermined, and covered by gray to green-black necrotic membranes from which numbers of bacteria or fungi can be isolated. Similar ulcerations may occur in the skin, vagina, anus or gastrointestinal tract, but these sites are much less frequently involved. Severe necrotizing infections are also encountered, but less prominently, in the lungs, urinary tract and kidneys. All

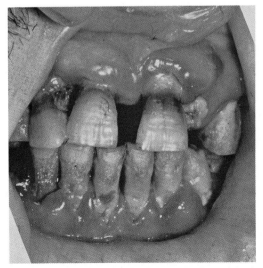

Figure 17–18. Granulocytopenia. The gingival margins have chronic suppurative necrotizing infection due to the loss of protective white cells in the circulation.

these sites of infection are characterized by massive growth of bacteria (or other agents) with relatively poor leukocytic response. In many instances, the bacteria grow in colony formation (botryomycosis) as though they were cultured on nutrient media. The regional lymph nodes draining these infections are enlarged and inflamed. The spleen and liver are rarely enlarged.

Clinical Course. Granulocytopenia tends to follow a fairly characteristic clinical pattern (Battle, 1950). The initial symptoms of this disorder are often malaise, chills and fever, followed in sequence by marked weakness and fatigability, symptoms which stem from the severe infections characteristic of this disorder. In severe granulocytopenia with virtual absence of neutrophils, these infections may become so overwhelming as to cause death within a few days. Less extreme depression of the marrow may appear insidiously and come to light only during the investigation of frequent and persistent minor infections.

Characteristically, the total white count is reduced to 1000 cells per mm.³ of blood and, in certain instances, to levels as low as 200 to 300 cells. Usually there is no associated anemia, save that caused by the infections, nor is there thrombocytopenia.

The prognosis is very unpredictable. Before the advent of antibiotics, the mortality caused by secondary infections ranged between 70 and 90 per cent. At present the antibiotics allow a much better prognosis since, in many instances, the adverse effects of the toxic drug are discovered early, and the depression of white cells eventually remits. The idiopathic form, too, may spontaneously remit, or it may progressively worsen, leading to death.

At times, granulocytopenia may be due to excessive splenic destruction of neutrophils, a process known as *splenic neutropenia*, a form of hypersplenism (p. 772). The differentiation of these cases from granulocytopenia of marrow origin is a difficult problem requiring marrow, splenic, and blood studies, and frequently the problem is not resolved until splenectomy is performed.

One interesting variant of granulocytopenia, *cyclic neutropenia*, deserves mention. This is a very rare, obscure disorder characterized by the cyclic disappearance of the neutrophils from the circulation at approximately three-week intervals. It occurs in both males and females. It does not bear any constant relationship to the menstrual cycle in females. No immunologic reaction has been demonstrated, and the nature of this condition is a complete mystery. Cases well studied with serial bone marrow biopsies have disclosed cyclic arrest in the production of the granulocytes, which is timed with the disappearance of these cells from the circulating blood.

LEUKEMIA

Leukemia may best be considered as a neoplasm of the white blood cells and is so classified in the *International Lists of Causes of Death*. It is characterized chiefly by: the appearance of abnormal, immature white cells in the circulating blood; diffuse and almost total replacement of the bone marrow with the leukemic cells; and widespread infiltrates of the liver, spleen and other tissues, analogous to metastatic dissemination of a solid tissue cancer. Usually the peripheral white cell count is markedly elevated, sometimes to levels of, or higher than, 1,000,000 per mm.³ of blood. In some instances, particularly in the acute leukemias, fewer than normal numbers of leukocytes are present in the circulation. This variation is referred to as *aleukemic or leukopenic leukemia*. However, even in these cases, some of the white cells in the blood are immature and abnormal, and the infiltration of the various organs and tissues resembles that found in the more typical case. Unless the term aleukemic is appended, the usual form of leukemia with elevation of the peripheral count is implied.

Leukemia may be classified on the basis of (1) type of cell involved in the disorder, i.e., granulocytic or myelogenous, lymphocytic or lymphatic, and monocytic; (2) the level of the peripheral white count, i.e., leukemic or aleukemic; and (3) the progression of the clinical course, i.e., acute or chronic. Unless otherwise designated, myelogenous leukemia refers to the neutrophilic series. The other myelogenous patterns, such as eosinophilic and basophilic, are always specifically designated. In theory, therefore, there should be the categories of acute and chronic myelogenous, lymphocytic and monocytic leukemia (Fig. 17-19). The three forms of acute leukemia and chronic myelogenous and lymphatic leukemia are well recognized entities. But most cases of chronic monocytic leukemia are mixed myelo-monocytic. Apparently here immature cells in the marrow simultaneously differentiate along myelogenous and monocytic lines. When pure monocytic leukemia appears, it is usually of nonmarrow histiocytic origin, and these forms are sometimes identified as histiocytic leukemia (still a form of monocytic leukemia) (Fig. 17-20.) Occasionally, a very fulminating leukemia is encountered associated with extremely immature forms in the blood. These abnormal cells may be so undif-

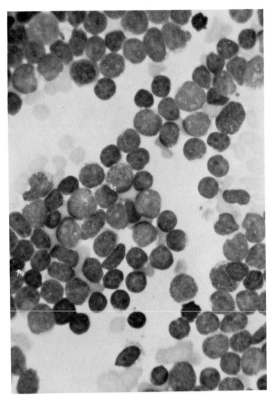

Figure 17–19. *A peripheral blood smear in a patient with chronic lymphatic leukemia, crowded with mature and slightly immature lymphocytes. (WBC 120,000—92 per cent lymphocytes.)*

cytic leukemia, and the reticulum cell sarcoma gives rise to a histiocytic (monocytic) leukemia. In the same way, the solid masses of plasma cells that constitute the plasmacytoma or multiple myeloma sometimes give rise to a plasmacytic leukemia.

Incidence. Today leukemia accounts for about 4 per cent of all cancer deaths. All ages and both sexes are affected, males slightly more often than females. In general, acute leukemia is encountered in childhood and the chronic forms in later life. However, acute myelogenous leukemia (AML) may occur at any age, whereas acute lymphatic leukemia (ALL) is largely confined to children. In the very recent past, the overall prevalence of leukemia among different age groups has undergone some striking changes. During the two decades following World War II, there was a steep rise in its incidence, accounting for about a five to sixfold increase both in the United States and in England and Wales (Scott, 1957). Within the past decade in the United States, the United Kingdom and New Zealand,

ferentiated as to deserve the designation *stem cell leukemia.*

In general, *the chronic forms of leukemia have the highest white counts and the circulating white cells tend to be of the more mature variety. In contrast, the acute leukemias may have only moderate elevation of the white cell count (30,000 to 100,000 cells per mm.³), but the cells are more likely to be of the primitive "blast" form.*

The biologic behavior of leukemia is quite unpredictable. Diseases that have run a chronic smoldering course for a long period of time may suddenly release showers of very immature "blast" forms in the peripheral blood and assume the appearance of an acute leukemia. These episodes are commonly referred to as "blast crises." At this time, the prognosis becomes that of the acute fulminating pattern of leukemia. Still other patients begin with a lymphoma (a neoplasm of lymphoid tissue) and, in the course of their disease, begin to exhibit leukemic patterns in the blood (p. 753). Almost always in these cases, the type of leukemia will correspond to the histogenetic pattern of the lymphoma. Thus the lymphocytic lymphoma would be expected to yield a lympho-

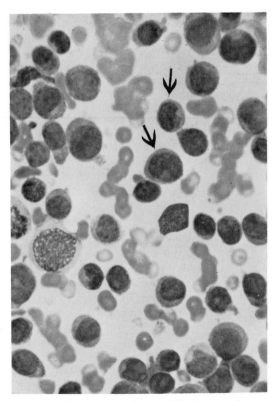

Figure 17–20. *A peripheral blood smear in a patient with acute monocytic leukemia. Many of the leukocytes are monocytes and earlier blast forms, and several classic monocytic reniform indented nuclei are visible in the upper center (arrows). (WBC 46,000—42 per cent monocytes and monoblasts.)*

the childhood rate has begun to fall. That of the middle years of life has held steady. However, the rise has continued in the older age group although there is evidence of some slowing of this rate of climb (Gunz, 1969). The rise in the prevalence of leukemia following World War II raises an interesting question: Was the increase due merely to better case finding or were environmental factors involved? Obviously one thinks of the atomic bombs and the effects of ionizing radiation, as will be discussed presently.

The relative frequency of the various types of leukemia differs among reported series. Wintrobe (1967) indicates the following general distribution:

Chronic lymphatic leukemia	28.6%
Chronic myelogenous leukemia	26.6%
Acute lymphatic leukemia	20.0%
Acute myelogenous leukemia	16.9%
Acute monocytic leukemia	7.8%

It is apparent that this listing does not include chronic monocytic leukemia which is almost always of the myelomonocytic form.

Etiology and Pathogenesis. Turning first to the subject of pathogenesis, it is generally held that leukemia is a form of cancer, implying that it represents an excessive uncontrolled proliferation of white cells affecting one of the various leukocytic stem lines. The other possibility, however, has not been ruled out, i.e., prolongation of the life of leukemic cells permitting their abnormal accumulation over the span of time. In fact, a number of investigators have demonstrated a prolonged life for these leukemic cells (Galbraith, 1966) (Athens et al., 1968). Isotopic labeling techniques have shown that their residence time in the blood and marrow as well is prolonged. One of the basic defects in such cells might be their loss of programmed differentiation, and in this regard the lymphocytes in chronic lymphatic leukemia lack immunocompetence (Cronkhite, 1968) (Dameshek, 1967). Bearing on this problem of "proliferation" versus "accumulation" is another controversy as to whether leukemia is due to a mutation in a stem cell(s) with consequent overgrowth of this "bad seed" (clonal theory) or whether the cellular abnormality affects all cells and is imposed by external and possibly reversible influences. The "bad seed" theory would fit best with excessive proliferation; the "environmental influence" conception could be compatible with prolonged intravascular life. This controversy is more than academic. If leukemia arose in an abnormal clone, present attempts to totally destroy all leukemic marrow cells by therapy would be

reasonable. If the external influence theory were correct, such therapy would be of no avail unless the environmental causes were controlled. Numerous studies have attempted to confirm the clonal theory with mixed results (Greenberg et al., 1971) (Sandberg et al., 1971) (Ichikawa, 1970). Relevant to this discussion is the well known Philadelphia chromosome found in the precursors of erythrocytes, neutrophils and megakaryocytes in almost all cases of chronic myelogenous leukemia (p. 138). Here it would be most reasonable to postulate a stem line mutation with the subsequent evolution of the leukemia from this "bad seed." However, from the study of solid tissue cancers, it is well known that such external agents as chemical carcinogens, viruses and radiation all impose chromosomal abnormalities in their induction of cancers (Sandberg and Hossfeld, 1970). There is, on the other hand, a considerable body of evidence that external influences are at work in the production of leukemia as will be discussed presently, but here a single relevent case report might be cited. Fialkow et al. (1971) noted the recurrence of lymphoblastic (acute lymphatic) leukemia in a girl who had been treated by whole body irradiation followed by a marrow transplant from her brother. The recurrent leukemic cells lacked the Barr body or sex chromatin and were presumably derived from the transplanted cells donated by her brother. Here the leukemia reappeared, notably as a population of cells totally different from the pretreatment population, suggesting external influences.

The cause of leukemia is shrouded in the mystery of the origin of all neoplasia. As with solid tissue cancers, four sets of influences are thought to be important: (1) ionizing radiation, (2) viruses, (3) chemicals and (4) genetic predisposition.

Ionizing radiation and leukemogenesis have been discussed earlier on p. 134. To recapitulate briefly, the evidence for this association has been drawn largely from the study of survivors of the atomic bombs. About two years after these events, the rising incidence of leukemia, principally of the myelogenous forms, reached virtually epidemic levels (Bizzozero et al., 1966). There was a linear correlation between incidence and dosage as calculated by distances from the hypocenter of the blast. This evidence has been supported by data showing an increased incidence (once again dose related) of leukemia in men receiving large doses of radiation for symptoms of arthritis of the spine (Court-Brown and Doll, 1957). Furthermore, it has been noted that, until recently, physicians experienced twice the incidence of leukemia found in the general population, largely due to a six to ninefold increase in frequency among radiologists. This occupational hazard has been largely controlled by rigorous safety measures. There is then abundant evidence for the leukemogenic hazards of radiation.

Viruses as causative agents of leukemia in man is one of the primary topics in medicine today. It has long been known that viruses cause leukosis in chickens, a disease having many similarities with mammalian leukemia. Gross in 1951 was the first to report the induction of leukemia in mammals when he transmitted the disease to newborn susceptible mice by a cell-free filtrate now known to have contained virus particles. Leukemogenic viruses have also been found in rats, cattle, pigs and cats. Daily one anticipates the report of the isolation of a similar agent in man (Dmochowski, 1971). Despite a mounting body of suggestive evidence, there is no final proof of a viral etiology for any form of leukemia in man. Electron microscopy has disclosed cytoplasmic RNA virus C-particles in leukemic cells derived from some patients (11 of 48) (Dmochowski, 1971) with both myelogenous and lymphatic leukemia (Awano et al., 1970). A variety of viruses have been isolated from leukemic cells (Grace, 1967). Many clusters of leukemia cases have been reported, suggesting cross transmission of an infective agent (Heath and Hasterlik, 1963). But perhaps most exciting has been the recent evidence relating to "reverse transcriptase." All of the animal leukemogenic viruses are RNA viruses. Spiegelman et al. (1970) have documented the presence of RNA-directed DNA polymerase (reverse transcriptase — see p. 129) in leukemic cells derived from animals. Recall that the reverse transcriptase provides the mechanism by which RNA viruses are able to modify the genome of transformed cells, in this case leukemic cells. Of significance to our discussion is the recent identification of this same enzyme in some human leukemic cells, which strongly suggests the possible presence of RNA viruses (Gallo et al., 1970). However, the identical viral agents isolated from leukemia patients also have been found in normal individuals. The viral particles in leukemic cells might merely be "passengers." Herpes virus now has been found in so many neoplastic settings that doubt is cast as to its causative significance in all settings. Notwithstanding, the last word on the subject of viruses and leukemia in man is yet to be written.

Chemical agents and leukemogenesis can be treated with brevity. Toxic exposure to benzol, such as occurs to those employed in chemical, dry cleaning and other industries, has been associated with an increased frequency of leukemia as well as other forms of blood dyscrasias. These leukemias are almost always granulocytic (myelogenous). But overall, this occupational hazard makes a trivial contribution to the prevalence of this disease.

Genetic predisposition to leukemia appears likely on the basis of some increased frequency of these diseases in certain families and especially among certain close relatives such as identical twins. This prevalance is more than can be explained by chance alone (Gunz, 1966). Supporting some genetic influence are the well known relationships between trisomy of chromosome 21 (Down's syndrome, p. 187) and acute leukemia and that between the changes in chromosome 22 (the Philadelphia chromosome, p. 138) and chronic myelogenous leukemia. These observations make it seem likely that, here and perhaps in other instances, some genetically determined chromosome imbalance may predispose to leukemogenesis. Indeed, the less than 10 per cent of patients with chronic myelogenous leukemia who do not have the Philadelphia chromosome comprise an atypical group in other respects as well. Usually they are males over the age of 65 years who have short survival times and relatively low white cell counts. While the leukemic cells in the Philadelphia "positive" cases almost always have an abnormally low content of alkaline phosphatase, in the Ph "negative" cases, the cells often have normal levels of alkaline phosphatase. It is entirely possible that this small fraction represents a different disease manifested by a myelogenous leukemic overgrowth.

In last analysis, despite all of these data pointing to environmental causation and genetic predisposition, in the great preponderance of leukemic cases, no substantial evidence of a known or presumed causation can be identified. Thus, for leukemia, its etiology and pathogenesis is the proverbial iceberg, the great bulk of which is hidden. Indeed, we have no evidence that all forms of leukemia arise through similar pathways, and it is not at all unlikely that the various forms of leukemia have totally different origins and comprise different diseases.

Morphology. Although the various forms of leukemia differ in the specific types of cells involved, all tend to produce certain basic morphologic alterations that can be considered a general anatomic pattern of leukemia. **These alterations can be conveniently divided into primary changes directly related to the abnormal numbers of white cells and secondary changes that stem from the destructive effects of the cellular infiltrates and overgrowths as they seed various organs and tissues.** The leukemias are principally characterized by abnormal flooding or infiltration of the bone marrow, lymph nodes, spleen, liver and kidney. Any other tissue of the body may be involved, but with less frequency and usually less severely than the organs just cited. Leukemic cells more or less resemble their normal counterparts in the marrow or lymph nodes, save perhaps for a greater tendency to immaturity and the possible development of some anaplastic atypicality in individual scattered cells.

The **bone marrow** in the full-blown case has a muddy red-brown to gray-white color as the normal hematopoiesis is overrun by masses of white cells. The marrow replacement begins focally but, as the disease progresses, becomes generalized to affect all the normally active red marrow. It sometimes extends into areas of previously fatty marrow (Figs. 17—21 and 17—22). As the disease advances, the native marrow cells are progressively replaced. These neoplastic cells encroach upon and erode the cancellous and cortical bone. All the bones of the skeletal system are affected, but the process is usually first evident and most florid in the vertebral bodies, sternum, ribs and pelvis. Sometimes the bony infiltrates in myelogenous leukemia become tumorous masses called **chloromas**. These may arise within the bone or subperiosteally in any portion of the skeleton, but more often they affect the skull. The tumors are a distinctive evanescent green when first examined but rapidly fade as the pigment of uncertain type oxidizes. The color can be restored by the use of such reducing agents as hydrogen peroxide and hyposulfite. As variants of the myelogenous infiltrates, these tumors are interesting but have no specific clinical significance.

The **lymph nodes** throughout the body usually are enlarged in all forms of leukemia. There is, however, a marked difference in the degree of enlargement in various forms. Since lymphatic leukemia presumably arises within lymphoid foci in both the bone marrow and the lymph nodes, it is responsible for the most striking degrees of lymphadenopathy (4 to 5 cm. in diameter) (Fig. 17—23). The nodal enlargement of myelogenous leukemia is much less prominent and, in monocytic leukemia, lymphadenopathy is of only moderate to minimal severity. In all the leukemias, involved lymph nodes characteristically remain discrete, rubbery and homogeneous, features that distinguish these enlargements from the matted, sometimes soft, fluctuance of inflammatory involvement. The cut section is soft and gray-white, and tends to bulge above the level of the capsule. When the enlargement is extreme, areas of hemorrhage or infarction may appear. All nodes in the body are not uniformly affected, and the distribution of lymphadenopathy is quite variable from one case to another.

On histologic examination, the nodes are partially or completely flooded by the neoplastic cell type to an extent that is roughly proportional to the

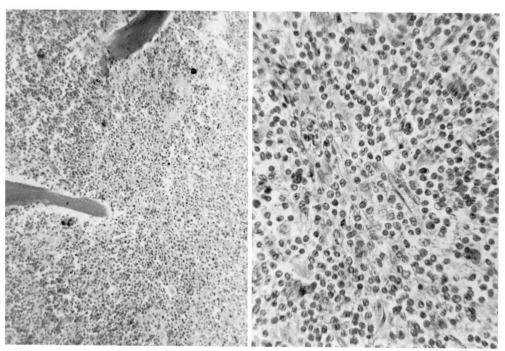

Fig. 17–21   Fig. 17–22

Figure 17–21. Chronic lymphatic leukemia. Low power view of marrow flooded by uniform leukemic cells.
Figure 17–22. Lymphatic leukemia. Medium power view of same bone marrow as in Figure 17–21 to illustrate monotony of lymphocytes.

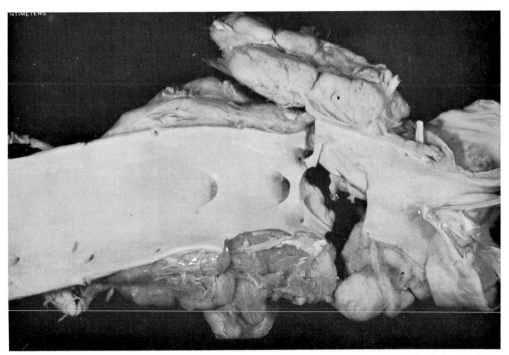

Figure 17—23. Periaortic lymph node enlargement in a child with chronic lymphatic leukemia.

enlargement of the node and the stage of advancement of the leukemia. Eventually the sinuses are flooded and all structures, including the germinal follicles, are obliterated. The leukemic cells may invade the capsule of the node and flood out into the surrounding tissues. Such total flooding of nodes is quite characteristic of lymphatic leukemia, less so of myelogenous leukemia, and least prominent in monocytic leukemia.

The **spleen** is enlarged to a variable degree in almost all instances. Myelogenous leukemia produces the most striking splenomegaly; splenic weights of 5000 gm. or more are not unusual. Such spleens may virtually fill the whole abdominal cavity and extend into the pelvis. Infarcts due to leukemic infiltration and obstruction of vessels are frequent in chronic myelogenous leukemia. In lymphatic leukemias, the spleen rarely exceeds 2500 gm. in weight. In monocytic leukemia, it is uncommon for the spleen to exceed 1000 gm. In all instances, the capsule becomes somewhat thickened. Frequently fibrous adhesions develop to surrounding structures.

On section, the splenic substance is usually more firm than normal and has a muddy gray appearance. In the extreme splenomegalies, the normal splenic follicles become indistinct and the tissue assumes a homogeneous appearance. Such a complete obliteration, however, is not likely in the minimal involvements of monocytic leukemia. Histologically, the leukemic infiltrations of the spleen follow the patterns described in the lymph nodes.

They vary from focal to diffuse involvement to progressive obliteration of the underlying architecture in the areas affected.

The **liver** is commonly enlarged in all forms of leukemia but not to the same degree as the spleen. Hepatomegaly tends to be somewhat more striking in lymphatic leukemia than in the other forms, but rarely does the liver weight exceed 2500 gm. Hepatic involvement is usually diffuse in nature and, therefore, does not cause any striking alterations in the cut surface. Occasionally, however, patchy aggregates about portal areas may cause a diffuse, fine mottling that is visible on gross inspection (Fig. 17—24). Massive foci of infiltration of gray-white tissue sometimes appear that closely resemble metastatic patterns of other forms of cancer. The hepatic infiltrates tend to follow certain microscopic patterns which are somewhat distinctive for each form of leukemia. The infiltrates of myelogenous leukemia are not well defined and are present throughout the lobule (Fig. 17—25). Some aggregates of cells may be found in the portal triads but, in addition, cells are dispersed along the liver cords subjacent to the vascular sinusoidal walls. The infiltrates are characteristically localized to the portal areas in lymphatic leukemia (Fig. 17—26). The central regions of the liver lobule are relatively spared in this dyscrasia. The hepatic infiltrates of monocytic leukemia are least prominent and are very often absent. When present, they tend to follow the pattern described in myelogenous leukemia.

In addition to these organ involvements, leuke-

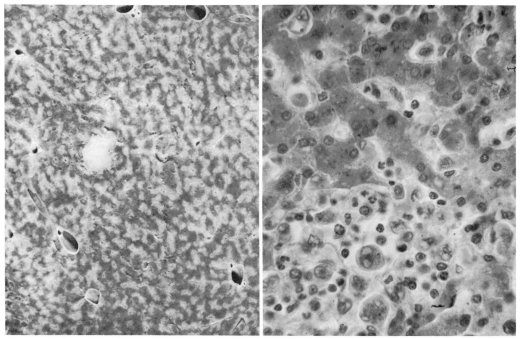

Fig. 17–24   Fig. 17–25

Figure 17–24. Chronic lymphatic leukemia in the liver. A close-up of the cut surface of the liver to illustrate unusually prominent leukemic infiltration producing a fine regular mottling.

Figure 17–25. Acute myelogenous leukemia in the liver. A microscopic detail to illustrate scattered "polys" through the sinusoids.

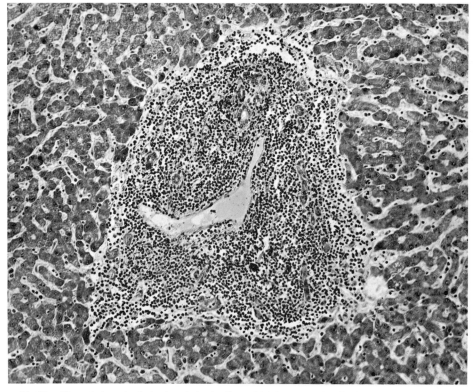

Figure 17–26. Chronic lymphatic leukemia in the liver. A high power detail of a periportal infiltrate. (Reprinted through courtesy of Oxford University Press; from Jackson, H., Jr., and Parker, F., Jr.: Hodgkin's Disease and Allied Disorders.)

mic infiltrates are frequently found in the kidneys, adrenals, thyroid, myocardium and in many other tissues of the body. In all these sites, the infiltrates begin as small perivascular aggregates that progressively diffuse through the stroma of the affected organ. As the cells accumulate in sufficient number, they may compress and destroy adjacent parenchymal structures. When the infiltrates become large enough, they may produce macroscopically visible, pale gray areas of infiltration. However, these infiltrates are usually different from ordinary metastases. They tend to be less sharply circumscribed and are more diffusely infiltrated so that they do not wipe out the underlying architecture as completely as do the metastases of other types of cancer (Fig. 17–27).

Special mention should be made of the leukemic infiltrates of the skin and mucous membranes of the gingiva. On occasion, abnormal cells accumulate in the dermal and subcutaneous connective tissue (leukemia cutis). These cause variable forms of elevated to flat, pale to red skin macules or papules. Infiltrates in the gingiva are particularly characteristic of monocytic leukemia. These patients have swelling and hypertrophy of the gingival margins, and frequently the soft involved tissues freely ooze blood or become secondarily bacterially infected, forming superficial necrotic ulcerations.

Numerous ultrastructural and immunologic studies have been made of leukemic cells. For example, it has been demonstrated that the lymphocytes in lymphatic leukemia are less responsive to phytohemagglutinin blast transformation than normal cells (Oppenheim et al., 1965) (Schrek, 1967). This finding is consonant with the observation that leukemic cells are deficient in protecting patients against microbiologic invasion. A variety of ultrastructural deviations from the norm have been identified. They involve nuclei, nucleoli, endoplasmic reticulum, mitochondria, Golgi complexes and ribosomes (Schumacher et al., 1970). However, none of these ultrastructural deviations provide diagnostic hallmarks of leukemia. As mentioned earlier, viral particles have been observed in numerous instances but are frequently absent. In general, these "harder looks" at the leukemic cell have not provided new insights.

Secondary Changes. By secondary changes are meant those lesions that stem from the destructive, erosive effects of the aggressive leukemic infiltrates. Anemia and thrombocytopenia are characteristic secondary consequences of the leukemic involvement of the bone marrow. The anemia is myelophthisic in nature and may become quite profound and lead to systemic and local tissue hypoxia. A hemorrhagic diathesis results from the thrombocytopenia, and abnormal bleeding is one of the most characteristic manifestations of all forms of leukemia. Purpura and ecchymoses may occur in the skin with or without leukemic infiltrates. Hemorrhages into the gingivae and hemorrhagic foci in the urinary bladder, the mucosa of the renal pelves and calyces, the serosal membranes lining the body cavities, and the serosal coverings of the viscera, particularly of the heart and lungs, are standard features in the advanced leukemic. Not uncommonly, intraparenchymal hematomas develop, most frequently in the brain. Many times, this widespread hemorrhagic tendency is the most obvious anatomic finding at postmortem in these cases.

Although the total white cell count is usually elevated in leukemia, the circulating abnormal white cells have little defensive capacity, resulting in an enhanced susceptibility to bacterial infection. The morphologic changes of these infections may be found in any organ or site in the body but are particularly common in the oral cavity, skin, lungs, kidneys, urinary bladder and colon. The bacterial infections of leukemia resemble, to a great extent, those found in granulocytopenia, since both have in common a deficiency of functioning leukocytes.

The leukemic proliferation in the bone marrow

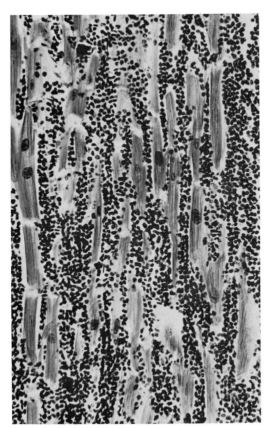

Figure 17–27. Chronic lymphatic leukemia infiltrates in the heart muscle. (Reprinted through the courtesy of the Oxford University Press; from Jackson, H., Jr., and Parker, F., Jr.: Hodgkin's Disease and Allied Disorders.)

causes expansion of the marrow spaces, encroachment upon the cancellous and cortical bone, and resultant osteoporosis with increased radiolucency. The infiltrates within other tissues and organs remain confined to the interstitial connective tissue for the most part. The parenchymal elements are thus spread apart but are not usually severely damaged. For this reason, hepatic, renal or cardiac failure is extremely uncommon in these cases. Only rarely does enlargement of the portahepatic nodes encroach sufficiently upon the extra-hepatic biliary ducts to cause obstructive jaundice.

Special Features of the Various Types of Leukemia. The leukemic cells in acute myelogenous leukemia usually span the range of myeloblasts to metamyelocytes. Usually there is some small proportion of mature granulocytes. The cells of chronic myeloid leukemia range from myelocytes to mature granulocytes. In most cases of chronic myeloid leukemia, the neutrophils have very low levels of alkaline phosphatase (Pedersen and Hayhoe, 1971). The significance of this finding is unclear, but it has been related to the loss of part of the Philadelphia chromosome, implying that a specific gene regulating alkaline phosphatase activity has been deleted from the number 22 autosome. In this connection, a high leukocyte alkaline phosphatase activity has been observed in neutrophils in patients with Down's syndrome (trisomy 21) (Alter et al., 1962). Whatever its meaning, the low enzyme content of the neutrophils is a very helpful finding in the differentiation of true leukemia from the sometimes abnormally high granulocyte counts encountered in leukemoid reactions and extreme levels of leukocytosis. The lymphatic leukemias span the range from immature blasts to quite mature small lymphocytes, depending on the acuteness or chronicity of the leukemia. In the chronic monomyeloid leukemias, some cells have the appearance of monocytes while others show differentiation toward granulocytic precursors. On the other hand, in the acute pure monocytic leukemias, the cells have the appearance of monoblasts with some forms showing maturation toward the adult monocyte. Obviously, the foregoing are broad generalizations, and there are many exceptions. Indeed, the course of the disease in any form of leukemia may change with successful suppressive therapy or may suddenly worsen with the development of acute blast crises.

Clinical Course. The clinical manifestations are somewhat different in the acute and chronic leukemias (Kirschbaum and Preuss, 1943) (Lynch, 1954) (Southam et al., 1951). The acute leukemias usually show a fairly abrupt onset and become manifest by the appearance of fever, progressive prostration, weakness and malaise. In the course of a few weeks to months, hemorrhagic manifestations and bacterial infections punctuate the course and emphasize the existence of some serious disorder. Usually the lymphadenopathy, splenomegaly and hepatomegaly are not sufficiently well advanced in these acute leukemias to arouse the patient's attention or to contribute significantly to the clinical problem. In children, the striking neoplastic proliferations in the bone marrow may give rise to bone and joint pain.

Chronic leukemia is much more insidious in onset and is usually ushered in by progressive weakness and weight loss or the sudden appearance of a peripheral lymph node or lymph nodes. Usually the weakness and malaise have been noted for some time before the patient seeks medical attention. Commonly, the profound anemia at this time causes considerable exertional dyspnea. In some cases, the patient first becomes aware of a heavy dragging sensation in the abdomen produced by the splenomegaly. At other times, the enlarged spleen and liver are detected as abdominal masses. For these reasons, the patients seek medical attention. Not uncommonly, however, the existence of the leukemia is discovered in the course of a medical examination for other reasons. By the time the patient comes to medical attention, generalized lymphadenopathy, splenomegaly and hepatomegaly are usually present. Anemia, bleeding diathesis and recurrent or persistent infections are frequent accompaniments.

Many times, hemorrhages from the bleeding diathesis are the presenting and dominant manifestations of leukemia. These patients may have sudden hematemeses, profuse nosebleeds (epistaxis), massive melena or, at other times, persistent hematuria. The disease sometimes comes to light because of unusual bleeding from the gums. Other patients may say, "I bruise very easily."

In the usual case of leukemia, the markedly elevated white count, the abnormal circulating immature forms and the derangement in the differential count provide sufficient data to establish the diagnosis. Variable degrees of anemia and often marked thrombocytopenia are usual accompaniments. It was pointed out that in many of these cases there may be some difficulty in establishing the specific type of leukemia, particularly when the disease is acute and the peripheral blood contains only blast forms. In most instances, however, sufficient numbers of mature cells are present to suggest the presumptive nature of their more immature precursors. When the counts are not markedly elevated, or when the leukemia is of the aleukemic variety, there may be more difficulty in establishing the diagnosis from the peripheral blood.

One of the most difficult types of leukemia

to identify is the monocytic variety. Remember that splenomegaly, hepatomegaly and lymph node enlargement are not prominent in this disease. Frequently, the white counts are not markedly elevated and anemia and thrombocytopenia may not be profound. The predilection to gingival infiltration in this disease makes this site a possible source of diagnostic histologic material.

In most cases of leukemia, the course is progressively downhill although therapy may induce remarkable remissions lasting from months to years in some patients. A few generalizations can be made but, for further details, reference must be made to the literature (Wiernik and Serpick, 1970) (Cutler et al., 1967) (Szippin et al., 1971). On the average, the prognosis in the acute forms of leukemia is less favorable than in the chronic forms. Less than 10 per cent of such patients may be expected to survive for longer than 24 months. With acute leukemia, the length of survival is inversely related to the patient's age, and the longest survivals are encountered in those under age 10. In chronic leukemia, the outlook is somewhat less bleak, and combinations of radiation and chemotherapy have sometimes held the disease in check for years. Death may result from superimposed bacterial infections, progressive inanition, hemorrhages (particularly into the brain), massive external bleeding as into the gastrointestinal tract, or cardiac or renal failure occasioned by the hypoxic damage. Perhaps the most common terminal event is an infection, usually preceded by a "blast crisis" in which normal white cells disappear and the circulating blood is literally flooded with immature "blast" forms of white cells. At the same time, the hemoglobin concentration, the hematocrit and platelet count precipitously fall, often triggering massive fatal hemorrhages. Such a sequence is particularly characteristic of chronic myeloid leukemia (Gardikas et al., 1971).

Unusual Types of Leukemia. *Eosinophilic myelogenous leukemia* is a special variant of the usual myelogenous leukemia. The complete maturation of the granulocytes to produce eosinophilic granules within the white cells implies that most of these cases conform to the pattern of chronic leukemia. In all other respects, they resemble the usual myelogenous leukemia.

Stem cell leukemia is the name applied to those extremely acute fulminating dyscrasias in which there is complete reversion of the neoplastic cells to the most primitive type found in the bone marrow. This variant is extremely uncommon, and usually pursues a ful-

minating, progressive course to death within weeks to several months.

Histiocytic leukemia is a rare form which is related to monocytic leukemia. In the earlier discussion of the origin of the white cells, it was indicated that, at least according to one view, the monocyte is derived from the bone marrow and from precursors identical with or closely related to the precursors of the granulocytes. Support for the bone marrow origin of the monocyte is derived from the fact that it contains oxidase granules along with the other granulocytes. On this basis, monocytic leukemia (sometimes called Nägeli type) occurs occasionally in a mixed mono-myeloid pattern in which hybrid cells are encountered that have some of the characteristics of each of the parent types. A cell that is morphologically similar to the monocyte and is oxidase-negative is sometimes encountered in the circulating blood in inflammatory and leukemic states. This cell is apparently identical with the macrophages of inflammatory infiltrates and is called a histiocyte. These histiocytes are derived either from mesenchymal tissue cells or directly from reticuloendothelial cells throughout the reticuloendothelial system (Belding et al., 1955). They are thus presumably closely related to or identical with tissue macrophages. Histiocytes are normally not present in the circulating blood. However, in histiocytic leukemia (sometimes called the Schilling type), it is postulated that neoplastic proliferation accounts for their flooding into the peripheral blood to produce a leukemia that is anatomically quite similar to the monocytic variant. Further support for this separation of histiocytic leukemia from monocytic leukemia is derived from those cases of reticulum cell sarcoma that eventually develop a leukemic component in the form of a reticulum cell (histiocytic) and not a monocytic leukemia (p. 754).

Plasma cell leukemia has already been mentioned as occurring in association with neoplastic proliferation of plasma cells in the bone (multiple myeloma) and in soft tissues (plasmacytoma) (p. 249). (Fig. 17–28). Currently, these related plasma cell proliferations are interpreted as a systemic neoplasia of plasma cells that at one time manifests itself principally with bone lesions, at other times begins presumably in soft tissues, and at still other times is associated with leukemic invasion of the blood. These plasma cell dyscrasias tend to arise in the advanced years of life and cause death within two to three years. Presumably because of the patient's rapid demise, the full complement of morphologic alterations in-

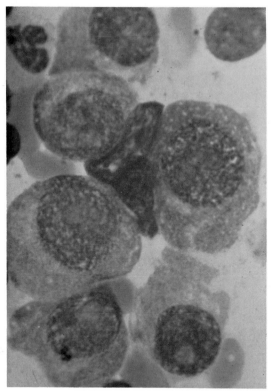

Figure 17–28. *A marrow smear from a patient with plasmacytoma of bone illustrating fairly mature plasma cells apparently compressing and distorting an unidentifiable nucleus.*

volving the bones, visceral organs and blood is seen only in rare instances.

MYELOPROLIFERATIVE SYNDROME

Reference has already been made (p. 724) to the transmutable nature of polycythemia vera in its evolution over the span of decades. In some patients, for example, the marrow becomes fibrotic and anemia supervenes. Others may develop chronic granulocytic (myelogenous) leukemia. In a rare case, the polycythemia may be replaced by leukemic flooding of the bone marrow and peripheral blood with erythroblasts, thus transforming the disease to erythroleukemia or Di Guglielmo's syndrome. In explanation of these and other possible changeovers, Dameshek (1970) proposed the concept of *the myeloproliferative syndrome*. He postulated that in some patients the bone marrow—specifically one or more of its stem lines—might become abnormally active or virtually neoplastic, and the particular stem line principally affected might change with time. Theoretically, the abnormal proliferation might initially involve the erythrocytic, granulocytic, megakaryocytic or fibroblastic populations within the marrow. If the erythrocytic line predominated, presumably the patient would have polycythemia vera or, conceivably, erythroleukemia. Granulocytic overgrowth would lead to chronic myelogenous leukemia. Excessive overgrowth of megakaryocytes might lead to so-called megakaryocytic leukemia. Moreover, it was proposed that one of the end stages of the various expressions of the myeloproliferative syndrome was myelofibrosis resulting in anemia and, along with it, extramedullary myeloid metaplasia. Other changeovers might occur in the course of the disease, but generally in the direction of more serious disease, for example, polycythemia to leukemia, but not the reverse. An overview of the ramifications of the myeloproliferative syndrome is provided in Table 17–1. Such a conception provides a satisfying explanation of the polycythemic patient who later becomes anemic and develops extramedullary myeloid metaplasia. It would further provide an understanding of the development of chronic granulocytic leukemia late in the course of polycythemia vera.

It must be emphasized that the myeloproliferative syndrome is not a specific disease but rather a concept which appears to fit observed clinical phenomena. It would seem that the bone marrow reacts to some mysterious stimulus by abnormal proliferation of one or more of its cell populations. There is a suggestion that abnormal regenerative activity may lead to loss of control and the myeloproliferative syndrome. Myelofibrosis with extramedullary myeloid metaplasia has been observed in benzol workers as well as in those exposed to excessive doses of radiation. Conceivably, bone

TABLE 17–1. MYELOPROLIFERATIVE SYNDROME

Proliferating Elements	Clinical Entities
Erythroid	Polycythemia vera Erythroleukemia (Di Guglielmo's syndrome)
Granulocytic	Chronic granulocytic leukemia
Megakaryocytic	Megakaryocytic myelosis Megakaryocytic leukemia
Reticular cells with fibers (fibroblasts)	Myelofibrosis (including myeloid metaplasia and agnogenic myeloid metaplasia)

marrow damage might have been incurred, followed by regeneration which went beyond normal feedback controls.

Several aspects of the myeloproliferative syndrome deserve notice. In many patients, the proliferation simultaneously affects more than one of the marrow populations. Thus in a patient with polycythemia vera, there is simultaneous abnormal proliferation of white cells, which accounts for the abnormally high white counts in these patients. At the same time, megakaryocytic proliferation may give rise to excessively high platelet counts. In almost all of its expressions, the myeloproliferative syndrome is characterized by a marked increase in dysplastic megakaryocytopoiesis throughout the marrow, comprising one of the major hallmarks of this syndrome. When chronic granulocytic leukemia supervenes in the course of polycythemia vera, the granulocytes often lack the Philadelphia chromosome so characteristic of the usual forms of chronic granulocytic leukemia. Moreover, in chronic granulocytic (myelogenous) leukemia associated with the Philadelphia chromosome, the alkaline phosphatase level of the leukemic granulocytes is significantly depressed. But in the chronic granulocytic leukemia associated with the myeloproliferative syndrome, the alkaline phosphatase content of the leukocytes is either normal or elevated. As mentioned earlier, this subset of this form of leukemia appears to represent a different disease or a distinct variant.

The myelofibrotic expression of the myeloproliferative syndrome is also interesting. In this variant, extramedullary hematopoiesis appears in the spleen, liver, lymph nodes and even in other tissues of the body. The splenomegaly may achieve weights up to 3000 gm. At one time, this entity was called *agnogenic (idiopathic) myeloid metaplasia of the spleen*. The splenic changes were considered the primary lesion in this disorder. Today the myelofibrosis is thought to be primary and the splenic metaplasia a compensatory reaction. In any event, we are faced in this syndrome with the paradox of extramedullary myeloid hematopoiesis while myeloid hematopoiesis is progressively choked off by the development of marrow fibrosis. Characteristic of such extramedullary hematopoiesis is prominent, dysplastic megakaryocytopoiesis. Also, immature white and red cell elements are released from these sites, accounting for the appearance of normoblasts, erythroblasts, myelocytes and, occasionally, myeloblasts in the circulating blood. In this situation, there is once again the strong inference that the causative influence affects only the bone marrow, permitting extramyeloid sites to flourish so extensively as to release immature marrow cells into the circulation. Whatever its nature, the concept of a myeloproliferative syndrome is important since it dictates the need to carefully follow all patients having one of these related entities since, at any point in time, and without warning, the clinical course may be dramatically altered and, along with it, the prognosis for survival.

HEMORRHAGIC DIATHESES

It is logical at this point to consider all of the significant hemorrhagic disorders, whether they be related to platelet abnormalities or not. All have in common a tendency to either spontaneous bleeding or excessive bleeding following trauma. Spontaneous bleeding usually takes the form of numerous small hemorrhages (purpura) into the skin, mucous membranes, internal organs or other tissues. Excessive bleeding following trauma may be triggered by such trivial provocations as bumping into the corner of a table or taking a misstep, followed by massive bleeding into the knee joint.

Ultimately, the causes of all hemorrhagic diatheses may be divided into: (1) increased fragility of vessels; (2) platelet deficiency or dysfunction; (3) derangements in the hemostatic mechanism; and (4) combinations of (2) and (3) as in disseminated intravascular coagulation.

Increased fragility of the vessels is characterized by: (a) the apparently spontaneous appearance of purpura, (b) a positive tourniquet (capillary resistance) test and (c) normal platelet count, bleeding time and coagulation time. These disorders are also known as the nonthrombocytopenic purpuras, and the most important entity in this category is the *allergic purpura of Henoch-Schönlein*.

Deficiencies of platelets (thrombocytopenia) are characterized by (a) spontaneous purpura as well as excessive bleeding following even minor trauma, (b) a positive tourniquet test and (c) a reduced platelet count, prolonged bleeding time, but normal coagulation time. The positive tourniquet test reflects the well known important role of platelets in maintaining the normal integrity of the vascular channels. Deficiencies of platelets may be both qualitative as well as quantitative. The most important quantitative deficiency is known as primary idiopathic thrombocytopenic purpura. Qualitative defects in platelet function are encountered in uremia, Glanzmann's thrombasthenia, after aspirin ingestion and in von Willebrand's disease.

Derangements in hemostasis are encountered in a wide variety of hereditary and acquired disorders affecting one or more of the specific clotting factors discussed previously (p. 316). These hemostatic disorders are characterized by (a) spontaneous purpura and excessive bleeding following even minor trauma, (b) normal tourniquet test usually and (c) normal platelet count, normal bleeding time, but prolonged coagulation time. Most of the famous "bleeders" of history and the numerous patients who suffer prolonged and excessive hemorrhage following dental procedures or trivial trauma fall into this category.

Disseminated intravascular coagulation (DIC) is characterized by widespread intravascular clotting in the microcirculation throughout the body, which consumes both platelets and the clotting factors. Thus, it is also referred to as *consumption coagulopathy*. It occurs as a complication of a wide variety of clinical diseases. The widespread clotting and consequent depletion of the vital components of the hemostatic mechanism induces a hemorrhagic diathesis. Hence, DIC presents laboratory and clinical features of both thrombocytopenia and a coagulation disorder. Against this overview, we can turn to a more detailed discussion of the more important hemorrhagic diatheses.

HEMORRHAGIC DISORDERS RELATED TO INCREASED VASCULAR FRAGILITY

Increased capillary fragility has many causes. Perhaps the most important is hypersensitivity. Experimental studies have shown that a nonthrombocytopenic purpura related to increased vascular fragility can be produced in animals by the administration of antisera developed against vascular endothelium (Clark and Jacobs, 1950). Henoch-Schönlein purpura of man is thought to have an immunologic origin. Hypersensitivity reactions to bacteria or food products are thought in some way to induce damage to vessels of microcirculatory size. Supporting such a view is the morphologic similarity between the microcirculatory vascular lesions in *Henoch-Schönlein purpura* and those seen in some of the "connective tissue" diseases of presumed immunologic nature (Norkin and Wiener, 1960) (Panner, 1962). Skin biopsies taken during the height of this hemorrhagic disease in man have disclosed mononuclear perivascular cellular infiltrates in the dermis associated with thrombi in these small dermal vessels, changes reminiscent of those encountered in experimentally induced vascular hyperfragility.

Increased vascular fragility is encountered in many infections, particularly scarlet fever, vegetative bacterial endocarditis, meningococcemia, typhoid fever, smallpox, malaria, rickettsial infections and, indeed, in many bacteremic states. A variety of chemicals and drugs have been observed to induce increased vascular fragility: principally phenacetin, aspirin, bismuth, mercury, arsenic and snake venoms. Remember from the earlier discussion that important manifestations of avitaminosis C are increased capillary fragility with purpura, subperiosteal hemorrhages, and hemorrhages into the growing epiphyses in children. The differentiation of increased capillary fragility as a cause of hemorrhagic diatheses from the bleeding tendencies related to derangements in platelets and the hemostatic mechanism requires the laboratory studies previously mentioned (p. 739).

HEMORRHAGIC DIATHESES RELATED TO PLATELET ABNORMALITIES— THROMBOCYTOPENIAS

Marked reduction in the number of circulating platelets (thrombocytopenia) is the most common cause of generalized bleeding. The depletion of platelets generally has to be quite extreme, to levels on the order of 10,000 to 20,000 platelets per mm.[3] (normal range 150,000 to 350,000 per mm.[3]), before the hemorrhagic tendency becomes clinically evident. Very rarely, despite a normal platelet count, bleeding tendencies are related to deranged platelet function such as is seen following aspirin ingestion, in uremia and in von Willebrand's disease. The many causes of thrombocytopenia are categorized in Table 17–2.

From the clinical standpoint, platelet deficiency syndromes are divided into primary (also known as idiopathic) thrombocytopenic purpura and secondary (symptomatic) thrombocytopenia in which there is an apparent or overt cause for the decrease in the number of platelets.

PRIMARY OR IDIOPATHIC THROMBOCYTOPENIC PURPURA (ITP)

ITP is a primary thrombocytopenia which occurs most frequently in children and young adults and is quite uncommon late in life. Although its etiology is still unknown, there is substantial evidence that the great majority of

TABLE 17-2. CAUSES OF THROMBOCYTOPENIA

Decreased Production

1. Bone marrow replacement by leukemia, fibrosis, osteosclerosis and metastatic cancer
2. Bone marrow aplasia: idiopathic, drug induced, ionizing radiation, chemotherapeutic agents used in treatment of cancer
3. Drugs: thiazides, estrogens
4. Deficiency diseases: B_{12}, folic acid, kwashiorkor, chronic iron deficiency
5. Hereditary: Hegglin's anomaly
6. Idiopathic

Increased Destruction

1. Due to antibodies: idiopathic or primary thrombocytopenia, neonatal thrombocytopenia, immunologic reactions triggered by drugs, chemicals and foods, connective tissue diseases, some lymphomas and carcinomas
2. Postinfectious: rubella, varicella, mumps and after pertussis vaccination
3. Bacteremia and viremia
4. Splenomegaly
5. Massive hemangioma
6. Extensive burns, heat stroke
7. Postpartum thrombocytopenia
8. Disseminated intravascular coagulation

cases result from antibodies directed against platelets. An antiplatelet IgG has been isolated from the serum of these patients. The administration of this antibody to normal recipients is followed by a prompt reduction in the level of circulating platelets. The antibody does not directly lyse platelets, but rather renders them abnormally sticky and thereby more readily trapped in the spleen. Thus the spleen plays a pivotal role in ITP and, in many patients, splenectomy is followed by remarkable improvement. These 7S gamma globulins are capable of crossing the placental barrier and account for the neonatal thrombocytopenia (first four to 12 weeks after birth) encountered in children born of mothers with ITP. A small number of these primary thrombocytopenias are not of immunologic origin and are thought to result from marrow aplasia or hypoplasia (Harrington, 1971).

The immunologic response in ITP appears mysteriously and may best be considered as a form of autoimmunity directed against platelet antigens. It is no surprise then that ITP often develops in the course of systemic lupus erythematosus, and certainly in some patients the first manifestation of SLE is the insidious appearance of thrombocytopenia (Rabinovitz and Dameshek, 1960). While the deficiency of platelets obviously impairs hemostasis, increased capillary fragility may contribute to the bleeding diathesis in this disease. As is well known, platelets are involved in maintaining the integrity of blood vessels, and the countless trivial traumas of daily life may give rise to abnormal bleeding when there are insufficient platelets to plug the minute vascular injuries.

Morphology. The principal morphologic lesions of thrombocytopenic purpura are found in the spleen and bone marrow (Nickerson and Sunderland, 1937). The secondary changes related to the bleeding diathesis may be found in any tissue or structure in the body.

The **spleen** may be larger than normal, but is otherwise grossly within normal limits. Histologically, there is congestion of the sinusoids and some hyperactivity and enlargement of the splenic follicles, manifested by increased mitotic and phagocytic activity of the reticulum cells. There is a scattered neutrophilic and eosinophilic infiltrate within the pulp and, in many instances, megakaryocytes are found within the sinuses and sinusoidal walls. However, in many cases of thrombocytopenic purpura, the splenic findings are not distinctive, and in all instances can hardly be considered as pathognomonic of this disorder. Abnormal masses of agglutinated platelets or evidence of unusual phagocytic activity within the reticuloendothelial cells of the splenic sinuses is conspicuously absent, findings that might be anticipated in this condition.

The alterations in the **bone marrow** are equally disappointing. Most often the bone marrow appears quite normal and contains the usual numbers and types of the erythropoietic and leukopoietic cells. Moreover, the megakaryocytes appear entirely normal. An increased number of megakaryocytes has been reported. Some may be apparently immature with large, nonlobulated, single nuclei. However, these findings are not invariable and are of doubtful significance.

The secondary changes relate to the hemorrhages that are dispersed throughout the body. The skin, serosal linings of the body cavities, epicardium and endocardium, lungs, and the mucosal lining of the urinary tract are favorite sites for such petechial and ecchymotic hemorrhage (Fig. 17–29). Hemorrhages are also prone to occur in the brain, joint spaces, nasopharynx and gastrointestinal tract.

The clinical manifestations of this disease are quite variable. Occasionally, the disease begins with a sudden shower of petechial hemorrhages into the skin without apparent antecedent injury or disease. More frequently, there is a long history of easy bruising, nosebleeds, bleeding from the gums and extensive hemorrhages into soft tissues from relatively minor trauma. Also, the disease may become manifest first by the appearance of melena, hematuria or excessive menstrual flow. Subarachnoid hemorrhages and intracerebral

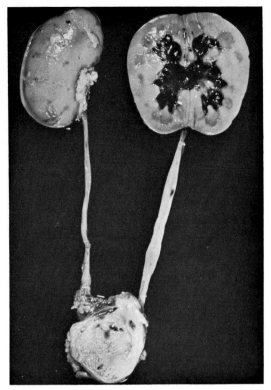

Figure 17–29. Thrombocytopenic purpura. The urinary tract with intrapelvic hemorrhages in the kidneys and focal mucosal hemorrhages in the urinary bladder.

hemorrhages are serious consequences of thrombocytopenic purpura.

The diagnosis can be only suspected in any case characterized by spontaneous or excessive hemorrhages, and must be confirmed by the demonstration of thrombocytopenia usually unaccompanied by either anemia or leukopenia. The prolongation of the bleeding time and the normal or relatively normal clotting time confirm the presence of thrombocytopenia. *A diagnosis of primary thrombocytopenia, however, should be made only after all the possible overt causes for platelet deficiencies, such as were listed in Table 17–2, have been ruled out.* As might be expected in an immune disorder, steroids will sometimes provide effective control of the excessive platelet destruction. Splenectomy is also beneficial, particularly in adults having chronic relapsing disease. Approximately 75 per cent of such patients will be permanently cured by splenectomy.

SECONDARY THROMBOCYTOPENIA

When there is a significant depression in the peripheral platelet count associated with a well defined underlying cause, the thrombocytopenia is termed secondary. Secondary thrombocytopenia is encountered in a wide variety of clinical circumstances as was indicated in Table 17–2.

In the peripheral blood, platelets have a normal life span of 8 to 10 days. It is apparent that for normal platelet levels to be maintained, up to 10 per cent of the circulating platelets must be replaced daily. Any mechanism that impairs the capacity of the megakaryocytes to maintain this fantastic level of productivity would lead shortly to a thrombocytopenia. Space-occupying lesions of the bone marrow are among the more important of these mechanisms. Included here are metastatic cancer, the reticuloendothelioses, leukemia, marrow fibrosis and osteosclerosis. It is not certain whether these diseases literally crowd the megakaryocytes out of the bone marrow or whether they utilize so much of the available nutrition as to deprive the megakaryocytes of needed substrate. Radiant energy, such as x-rays, is capable of destroying platelet production. Cases of secondary thrombocytopenia have been described in patients with the hypersplenic syndrome (p. 772). It is assumed here that stasis and sequestration of platelets lead to their intrasplenic destruction. In similar fashion, thrombocytopenia has been described in hemangioma—endotheliomas where there is trapping of blood in the vascular spaces of the neoplasm.

Chemical agents have long been known to induce thrombocytopenia, but the mechanism of their action is uncertain. Many agents such as ristocetin, benzol, nitrogen mustard, urethan and the antimetabolites probably act by direct toxicity on the bone marrow. However, for an even larger group of chemical agents, immunologic mechanisms are now thought to be important. In many instances, the amount of exposure to the drug is extremely small and insufficient to account for direct toxicity. Antibodies developed against the drug, bacteria or food antigens may fix to the platelets and, by binding complement, lyse the platelets. These antibodies have been shown to be capable of causing lysis of platelets in the test tube and so the spleen is not directly involved in the platelet destruction. Other causes of thrombocytopenia are hypothermia and heat stroke, but in neither case is the pathogenetic mechanism understood.

THROMBOTIC THROMBOCYTOPENIC PURPURA (TTP)

This very unusual disease was first described by Moschowitz in 1925. *It is characterized by thrombocytopenic purpura, hemolytic anemia, a variety of neurologic disturbances and renal dis-*

ease. Widespread thrombi are found in the arterioles, capillaries and venules. It seems possible that this disorder is merely one expression of the more general syndrome of disseminated intravascular coagulation (DIC) discussed below. However, in TTP, the female to male ratio of 2 to 1 and the fact that this disease rarely occurs in patients over the age of 40 suggest that it may be a disorder distinctly separate from the DIC complex. Vascular lesions at the site of the thrombi, reminiscent of immunologic injury, have been described in some cases, and recent reports suggest that viruses or Bartonella-like organisms may be the inciting cause of the immune response. In many respects, the disease resembles the Schwartzman reaction encountered in animals. The neurologic and renal manifestations may reflect merely ischemic injury secondary to the microthrombi, and the anemia might well conform to that of the microangiopathic hemolytic anemia discussed on p. 714 (Taub et al., 1964).

HEMORRHAGIC DIATHESES RELATED TO ABNORMALITIES IN CLOTTING FACTORS

At one time or another, a deficiency of virtually every one of the known clotting factors has been reported as the cause of a bleeding disorder. In some instances, this deficiency is hereditary and presumably represents inheritance of a mutant gene blocking the synthesis of the specific coagulation factor. In other instances, the deficiency is acquired. Most important among these heterogeneous disorders are the hereditary deficiencies of factors VIII, IX and von Willebrand's disease and the acquired hypoprothrombinemias and hypofibrinogenemias.

FACTOR VIII DEFICIENCY (HEMOPHILIA A, CLASSIC HEMOPHILIA)

A deficiency of factor VIII (antihemophilic globulin, AHG) is almost always a hereditary disorder transmitted as an X-linked recessive trait. The disease is, therefore, largely limited to males, but may appear in homozygous females. Consistent with the Lyon hypothesis, occasional female heterozygotes may also have a complete deficiency of factor VIII when the normal X is inactivated in those cells responsible for synthesis of coagulation factors. In about 10 per cent of males, factor VIII is present in normal amounts but, for some reason, is functionally inadequate. This subset has been designated hemophilia A+ while the pure deficiency state is referred to as

hemophilia A−. In the latter group, bleeding manifestations become apparent only when the depletion of factor VIII is quite profound. Purpura is usually uncommon and these patients have a negative tourniquet test since they have no inadequacy of platelet numbers or function. The bleeding tendency in hemophilia is usually expressed as excessive hemorrhage following any form of significant trauma. Classically, the hemorrhagic tendency first becomes evident following injury or some operative procedure, often dental. Occasionally, these patients suffer apparently spontaneous hemorrhages into the subcutaneous, submucosal, retroperitoneal, periarticular and other tissues. However, in many instances, these apparently spontaneous "bleeds" follow sudden movements, exertion or other plausible bases for microtrauma to the affected site. Hemorrhages into the brain are again an important cause of death. At one time, about 50 per cent of severely affected patients died before the age of five years. However, the recent use of transfusions of factor VIII have substantially improved the prognosis (Edson, 1970). With such therapy, hemophiliacs may now survive into adult life and rear children, which may account for some increased frequency of this disorder in recent years. The outlook for survival and the severity of the hemorrhagic tendency are both roughly related to the level of the deficiency of the antihemophilic globulin.

FACTOR IX DEFICIENCY (HEMOPHILIA B, CHRISTMAS FACTOR)

Factor IX (plasma thromboplastin component, PTC) deficiency can be briefly characterized as a milder form of the classic hemophilia A. The interesting designation Christmas disease has no festive connotation, but rather refers to the name of the original patient identified with this disorder. It too is inherited as an X-linked recessive trait and has been identified in two forms: hemophilia B+ where factor IX is not absent but rather functionally abnormal, and hemophilia B− characterized by an absolute deficiency of the specific factor (Twomey et al., 1969). Christmas disease or factor IX deficiency can be differentiated from factor VIII deficiency only by identification and characterization of the specific deficient factor.

VON WILLEBRAND'S DISEASE

Von Willebrand's disease is a bleeding disorder characterized by a deficiency of factor VIII as well as ineffective platelet function. The platelet count is normal, but the platelets appear to lack normal adhesiveness, and so these patients have both a prolonged coagulation time and a prolonged bleeding time. Patients suffering from this rare disorder exhibit tendencies toward purpuric hemorrhages throughout the body as well as excessive bleeding following trauma. The hematologic defect is transmitted as an autosomal dominant, and therefore is encountered in both sexes. Females are at particular risk because they almost invariably have severe menorrhagia (Strauss and Bloom, 1965).

HYPOPROTHROMBINEMIA

Normal prothrombin levels or "prothrombin times," as measured by the usual clinical tests, depend on normal levels of factors II, V, VII and X. *A deficiency of any one of these factors will be expressed as hypoprothrombinemia.* Although hereditary deficiencies of one or more of these factors have been described, much more common is acquired hypoprothrombinemia. The most common cause of this deficiency is hepatic or biliary tract disease. The mechanism in chronic hepatocellular disease is inadequate synthesis of one or more of the involved coagulation factors. Biliary tract disease produces its effect more indirectly. The fat-soluble vitamin K is apparently necessary for the synthesis of prothrombin, factor VII and factor X. Under normal circumstances, vitamin K is synthesized by bacteria in the intestinal tract and, in the presence of bile salts, is then absorbed in the gastrointestinal tract. Bile salts are critical, and the absorptive functions of the bowel must be adequate. Thus, deficiencies of vitamin K with resultant hypoprothrombinemia may result from any one of the following: (1) severe hepatobiliary disease, especially when there is obstruction to the outflow of bile, (2) malabsorption from any cause, (3) alteration in the normal bacterial flora, resulting from the prolonged use of broad spectrum antibiotics, (4) inadequate dietary intake of vitamin K (rare) and (5) inadequate vitamin K reserves in the newborn as a result of marginal levels in the mother. Among these many possible causes, *biliary tract disease, particularly obstructive jaundice, is the most important basis for hypoprothrombinemia.*

A significant bleeding diathesis develops only when there is fairly profound depression of the prothrombin levels. Remember that dicumarol serves as a commonly used clinical anticoagulant because it is an antagonist of vitamin K. Only when the prothrombin levels are markedly diminished by such anticoagulation do they lead to serious bleeding in the patient. Common sites for these hemorrhages are

operative wounds, particularly those incurred in the surgical relief of obstructive jaundice, petechial and ecchymotic hemorrhages into the skin and mucous membranes, abnormal bleeding into the genitourinary and gastrointestinal tracts and, occasionally, hemorrhages into vital organs such as the brain.

DEFIBRINATION SYNDROME (AFIBRINOGENEMIA OR HYPOFIBRINOGENEMIA)

A deficiency of fibrinogen in the circulating blood may be due to either inadequate synthesis of this protein or to abnormal destruction or loss of it. A rare cause of inadequate synthesis is the so-called congenital or constitutional hypo- or afibrinogenemia (Gitlin and Borges, 1953). Here the defect appears to reside in some inherited inability to synthesize this protein, and thus there is no fibrinogen to convert to fibrin. Defective formation also may be encountered in protein deficiencies and in severe liver disease, but usually in the latter instance there is an accompanying hypoprothrombinemia.

Deficiencies due to fibrinogen destruction are encountered in leukemia, metastatic disease of the bone and bacterial infection. These disorders are thought to cause depletion of fibrinogen by the formation of fibrinolysin. Such depletion has been well documented in prostatic carcinoma and in certain of the bacterial infections. Such enhanced fibrinolysis as a primary event is much more rare than secondary fibrinolysis which follows some primary clotting disorder (Merskey et al., 1967). In all likelihood, disseminated intravascular coagulation is the most common setting in which defibrination occurs. The bleeding tendency in all these conditions resembles that of hemophilia, but usually it is not so severe or serious.

DISSEMINATED INTRAVASCULAR COAGULATION (DIC, CONSUMPTION COAGULOPATHY, SECONDARY FIBRINOLYSIS)

In a wide range of clinical settings, fibrin thrombi form in the microcirculation throughout the body. Such disseminated intravascular coagulation is not a primary disease but rather a secondary complication of some underlying disorder which seriously deranges normal hemostasis. It is best considered as the human counterpart of the Schwartzman reaction in animals. In the Schwartzman reaction, widespread intravascular coagulation can be induced by appropriately spaced multiple injections of bacterial endotoxin or by a single injection of endotoxin following reticuloendothelial blockade (Brodsky and Siegel, 1970). *In DIC, widespread intravascular coagulation induces: (1) a deficiency of clotting factors, primarily of fibrinogen; (2) thrombocytopenia; (3) the appearance of circulating anticoagulants; (4) excessive fibrinolysis and (5) an abnormal bleeding tendency* (Bachmann, 1969). Thus we have the apparent paradox of a coagulation disorder giving rise to a hemorrhagic diathesis. The term "consumption coagulopathy" explains this apparent paradox insofar as the rapid consumption of coagulation factors, including platelets, induces a deficiency of these in the circulation and, at the same time, the fibrinolytic system is activated, further contributing to the bleeding tendency (Kwaan, 1972). In all probability, DIC is a more important cause of pathologic bleeding than all of the congenital coagulation disorders previously discussed.

Etiology and Pathogenesis. The term DIC does not imply a distinct pathologic entity, but rather describes a pathophysiologic reaction to a variety of underlying disorders (Colman and Rodriguez-Erdmann, 1970). McKay (1965) has stated this in another way by defining DIC as an intermediary mechanism of disease. The many diseases which trigger its appearance are associated with one or more of the following derangements:

1. Release of tissue thromboplastin activating the extrinsic clotting mechanism.
2. Activation of the intrinsic clotting mechanism.
3. Depletion of normally present inhibitors of blood coagulation.
4. Impairment of the clearance mechanisms in the reticuloendothelial system and liver for activated clotting factors.
5. Significant slowing of blood flow.

Among these possible pathogenetic mechanisms, activation of either the extrinsic or intrinsic clotting systems is probably the most common and important influence. A list of clinical conditions associated with disseminated intravascular coagulation follows. These are divided into categories indicating, to the extent possible, the presumed pathogenetic mechanism involved (Table 17–3).

In some of these clinical settings, DIC appears in the course of the disease and constitutes a serious complication which often leads to death. However, in others, the DIC may be the fundamental mediator of the disease. In this latter category are such entities as toxemia of pregnancy, shock, hemolytic-uremic syndrome and malignant hypertension. Conceivably, in toxemia of pregnancy small fragments of placenta gain access to the maternal circula-

TABLE 17–3. CLINICAL CONDITIONS ASSOCIATED WITH DISSEMINATED INTRAVASCULAR COAGULATION

Procoagulants from Tissues (Tissue Thromboplastins)
   Premature separation of the placenta (abruptio placentae)
   Retained dead fetus
   Amniotic fluid embolism
   Carcinomatosis
   Burns
   Acute leukemia

Procoagulants from Red Blood Cells (Massive Hemolysis)
   Incompatible transfusion
   Malaria
   Paroxysmal nocturnal hemoglobinuria
   Extracorporeal circulation

Procoagulants from Other Sources
   Bacterial infections
   Gram-negative septicemia (*E. coli*, meningococci)
   Viral infections
   Snake bite
   Acute pancreatitis (trypsin)
   Fat embolism
   Hyperlipemia (free fatty acids, chylomicrons)

Damage to Endothelial Cells
   Rocky mountain spotted fever
   Heat stroke
   Immunologic injury (SLE, proliferative glomerulonephritis)

Vascular Stasis
   Shock
   Catecholamines
   Cyanotic congenital heart disease
   Massive pulmonary embolism
   Giant hemangioma (Kasabach-Merritt syndrome)

Mixed or Unknown Causes
   Neonatal deaths
   Hemolytic-uremic syndrome
   Rejection of homotransplant (local DIC)
   Hyaline membrane disease (local DIC)
   Toxemia of pregnancy
   Malignant hypertension

tion and initiate microvascular coagulation. The subsequent small vessel obstructions induce tissue damage in the kidneys, liver and elsewhere. In the same way, endothelial cell injury related to the hypoperfusion of shock might trigger DIC and lead to the full-blown manifestations of irreversible shock. Endotoxic shock may, in fact, be an expression of the development of the Schwartzman reaction in man (Hardaway, 1966).

Whatever the clinical setting, DIC has three consequences: (1) the widespread formation of microthrombi within the capillary and small vascular channels produces ischemia to tissue and organs, (2) the microthrombi constitute a pathogenetic mechanism for hemolysis of red blood cells to produce microangiopathic hemolytic anemia and (3) a bleeding diathesis may eventuate. In addition to consumption of coagulants and activation of fibrinolysis, anticoagulants appear in DIC and contribute to the bleeding tendency. The fibrinolysis cleaves the deposited fibrin polymers to yield fibrin split products (FSP), some of which are powerful anticoagulants and interfere with the clotting of fibrinogen by thrombin (Deykin, 1970). So it is apparent that DIC is an extremely complex syndrome representing a massive disarray of the hemostatic mechanism in which simultaneously there may be evidence of accelerated coagulation, activation of the fibrinolytic system, a thrombotic diathesis and a bleeding diathesis.

Morphology. In general, thrombi are found in the following sites in order of decreasing frequency: kidneys, skin, lungs, testes, heart, adrenals, central nervous system, spleen and various endocrine glands. However, no tissue is spared. Renal thrombi are most abundant in the glomerular capillaries. They may evoke only reactive swelling of the endothelial cells or sometimes an acute focal glomerulitis replete with an infiltration of neutrophils. The consequent renal ischemia may induce only focal tubular cell necrosis, but in severe cases microinfarcts or even total renal cortical necrosis eventuates (p. 1135). The changes in the lungs take the form of fibrin thrombi within alveolar capillaries, hyaline membrane formation (p. 554), diffuse pulmonary edema, and occasionally thromboses within larger vessels. In the central nervous system, microinfarcts may be caused by the fibrin thrombi occasionally complicated by simultaneous fresh hemorrhage. Such changes are the basis for the bizarre neurologic signs and symptoms sometimes observed in this syndrome. Microthrombi may appear in the myocardium, but only rarely are they associated with infarction. The manifestations of DIC in the endocrine glands are of considerable interest. In meningococcemia, the massive adrenal hemorrhages of the Waterhouse-Friderichsen syndrome (p. 1312) are probably related to fibrin thrombi within the microcirculation of the adrenal cortex. Similarly, Sheehan's postpartum pituitary necrosis (p. 1358) may be one of the expressions of DIC. In toxemia of pregnancy (p. 1255), the placenta exhibits widespread microthrombi, providing a plausible explanation for the premature atrophy of the cytotrophoblast and syncytiotrophoblast encountered in this condition.

The bleeding manifestations of DIC are not dissimilar from those encountered in the hereditary and acquired disorders affecting the hemostatic mechanism discussed above.

Clinical Course. As is evident from the previous discussion, DIC usually appears in the course of some underlying disorder. The onset may be fulminating as in endotoxic shock or amniotic fluid embolism, or it may be insidious and chronic as in cases of carcinomatosis or retention of a dead fetus (Brodsky and Siegel, 1970). Overall, about 50 per cent of individuals with DIC are obstetric patients having complications of pregnancy. In this setting, the disorder tends to be reversible with delivery of the fetus. About 33 per cent of the patients have carcinomatosis. The remaining cases are associated with the very varied entities previously listed. The myriad manifestations may be slight or climactic and depend on whether circulatory obstruction or bleeding tendencies predominate and where the intravascular coagulation strikes. It is almost impossible to detail all the potential clinical presentations, but a few common patterns may be cited. Respiratory symptoms such as dyspnea, cyanosis and extreme respiratory difficulty may predominate. Neurologic signs and symptoms represent another pattern including convulsions and coma. Renal changes such as oliguria and acute renal failure may dominate. Circulatory failure and shock may appear suddenly or develop progressively. Hemorrhagic problems may dominate as in the obstetric patient who suffers massive vaginal bleeding during or immediately after delivery. But in all instances, the signs and symptoms may change during the course of the disease as thrombotic manifestations are replaced by hemorrhagic complications or vice versa. Accurate clinical observation and sophisticated laboratory studies are necessary for the diagnosis. It is usually necessary to monitor the following parameters: fibrinogen, platelets, factors V and VIII, prothrombin time, soluble fibrin monomer complexes and fibrinolytic activity (Nalbandian et al., 1971).

The prognosis is highly variable and depends, to a considerable extent, on the underlying disorder. In some cases such as obstetric disorders, this secondary complication tends to be self-limited. In others, it can be controlled with prompt and effective treatment aimed at control of the excessive clotting tendency and concomitant bleeding diathesis. However, often DIC pursues a fulminating downward course and thus constitutes the terminal event in the patient's chronic disease.

REFERENCES

Adamson, J. W., and Finch, C. A.: Erythropoietin and polycythemias. Ann. N.Y. Acad. Sci., *149*:560, 1968.

Alter, A., et al.: Leukocyte alkaline phosphatase in mongolism: a possible chromosome marker. J. Clin. Invest., *41*:1341, 1962.

Athens, J. W., et al.: The kinetics of neutrophilic granulocytes in chronic myelocytic leukaemia: a review. In Zarafonetis, C. J. D. (ed.): Proceedings of the International Conference on Leukaemia-Lymphoma. Philadelphia, Lea and Febiger, 1968, p. 219.

Awano, I., et al.: Viruses in human cancer and leukemia. Tohoku J. Exp. Med., 102:233, 1970.

Bachmann, F.: Disseminated intravascular coagulation. D. M., December:3, 1969.

Balcerzak, S. P., et al.: Discordant occurrence of pernicious anemia in identical twins. Blood, 32:701, 1968.

Battle, J. D.: The diagnosis and treatment of acute agranulocytosis. Cleveland Clin. Quart., 17:38, 1950.

Beck, W. S.: Deoxyribonucleotide synthesis and the role of vitamin B_{12} in the erythropoiesis. Vitamins Hormones, 26:413, 1968.

Belding, H. W., et al.: Histiocytic and monocytic leukemia: a clinical hematological and pathologic differentiation. Cancer, 8:237, 1955.

Bizzozero, O. J., et al.: Radiation-related leukemia in Hiroshima and Nagasaki 1946–1964. I. Distribution, incidence and appearance time. New Eng. J. Med., 274:1095, 1966.

Brain, M. C.: Microangiopathic hemolytic anemia. Ann. Rev. Med., 21:133, 1970.

Brodsky, I., and Siegel, N. H.: The diagnosis and treatment of disseminated intravascular coagulation. Med. Clin. N. Amer., 54:555, 1970.

Carmel, R., and Herbert, V.: Presence of "precipitating" or "blocking" antibody to intrinsic factor in gastric juice or serum of nearly all pernicious anemia patients. Clin. Res., 14:482, 1966.

Castle, W. B.: Current concepts of pernicious anemia. Amer. J. Med., 48:541, 1970.

Clark, W. G., and Jacobs, E.: Experimental non-thrombocytopenic vascular purpura: a review of the Japanese literature with preliminary confirmatory report. Blood, 5:320, 1950.

Colman, R. W., and Rodriguez-Erdmann, F.: Terminology of intravascular coagulation. New Eng. J. Med., 282:99, 1970.

Court-Brown, W. M., and Doll, R.: Leukaemia and Aplastic Anaemia in Patients Irradiated for Ankylosing Spondylitis. London, H. M. Stationery Office, 1957.

Cronkhite, E. P.: Kinetics of leukemic cell proliferation. In Dameshek, W., and Dutcher, R. M. (eds.): Perspectives in Leukemia. New York, Grune and Stratton Inc., 1968, p. 158.

Cutler, S. J., et al.: Ten thousand cases of leukemia 1940–1962. J. Nat. Cancer Inst., 39:993, 1967.

Dameshek, W.: Chronic lymphocytic leukemia: an accumulative disease of immunologically incompetent lymphocytes. Blood, 29:566, 1967.

Dameshek, W.: The myeloproliferative disorders. In Clark, W. J. (ed.): Myeloproliferative Disorders of Animals and Man. Washington, D.C., U.S. Atomic Energy Commission, 1970, p. 413.

Darling, R. C., et al.: The pathological changes in the bone marrow in agranulocytosis. Amer. J. Path., 12:1, 1936.

Deykin, D.: The clinical challenge of disseminated intravascular coagulation. New Eng. J. Med., 283:636, 1970.

Diggs, L. W., and Ching, R. E.: Pathology of sickle cell anemia. Southern Med. J., 27:839, 1934.

Dmochowski, L.: Current status of the relationship of viruses to leukemia, lymphoma and solid tumors. In Leukemia-Lymphoma, 14th Annual Clinical Conference on Cancer, 1969. Chicago, Ill., Year Book Medical Publishers, 1971, p. 37.

Doniach, D., and Roitt, I. M.: An evaluation of gastric and thyroid autoimmunity in relation to hematologic disorders. Seminars Hemat., 1:313, 1964.

Edson, J. R.: Hemophilia, von Willebrand's disease and related conditions: a spectrum of laboratory and clinical disorders. Hum. Path., 1:387, 1970.

Fessas, P.: Inclusions of hemoglobin in erythroblasts and erythrocytes of thalassemia. Blood, 21:21, 1963.

Fialkow, P. J., et al.: Leukaemic transformation of ingrafted human marrow cells in vivo. Lancet, 1:251, 1971.

Gabuzda, T. G.: Sickle cell disease. Delaware Med. J., 43:124, 1971.

Galbraith, T. R.: Studies on the longevity, sequestration and release of the leukocytes in chronic myelogenous leukemia. Canad. Med. Ass. J., 95:11, 1966.

Gallo, R. C., et al.: RNA dependent DNA polymerase of human acute leukemic cells. Nature (London), 228:927, 1970.

Gardikas, C., et al.: Some data concerning the onset of the acute myeloblastic crises in chronic myeloid leukaemia. Acta Haemat., 46:201, 1971.

Gitlin, D., and Borges, W. H.: Studies on the metabolism of fibrinogen in two patients with congenital afibrinogenemia. Blood, 8:679, 1953.

Gordon, A. S., et al.: The kidney and erythropoiesis. Seminars Hemat., 4:337, 1967.

Grace, J. T., Jr.: Formal discussion: hematopoietic cell cultures and associated herpes-type viruses. Canad. Res., 27:2494, 1967.

Greenberg, P. L., et al.: Granulopoiesis in acute myeloid leukemia and preleukemia. New Eng. J. Med., 284:1225, 1971.

Gross, L.: "Spontaneous" leukemia developing in C3H mice following inoculation in infancy with AK leukemic extracts of AK embryos. Proc. Soc. Exp. Biol., 76:27, 1951.

Gunz, F. W.: The changing aspects of leukaemia. Med. J. Aust., 1:526, 1969.

Gunz, F. W.: Genetic factors in the genesis of leukaemia. In Proceedings of the 11th Congress of the International Society of Haematology. Sydney, 1966, p. 183.

Gurney, C. W.: Erythropoietin and erythropoiesis. Arch. Intern. Med., 65:377, 1966.

Hardaway, R. M.: Syndrome of Disseminated Intravascular Coagulation with Special Reference to Shock and Hemorrhage. Springfield, Ill., Charles C Thomas, 1966.

Harrington, W. J.: Differential diagnosis and management of thrombocytopenias. Med. Times, 99:53, 1971.

Harris, J. W., and Kellermeyer, R. W.: The Red Cell. Production, Metabolism, Destruction, Normal and Abnormal. Cambridge, Mass., Harvard University Press, 1970, p. 393.

Harvard, C. W. H.: An investigation of refractory anemia. Quart. J. Med., 31:21, 1962.

Heath, C. W., Jr., and Hasterlik, R. J.: Leukemia among children in a suburban community. Amer. J. Med., 34:796, 1963.

Hecht, H. H., and Samuels, A. J.: Observations on the oxygen content of sternal bone marrow with reference to polycythemic states. Fed. Proc., 11:68, 1952.

Hodgson, G.: Synthesis of RNA and DNA at various intervals after erythropoietin injection in transfused mice. Proc. Soc. Exp. Biol. Med., 124:1045, 1967.

Ichikawa, Y.: Further studies on the differentiation of a cell line of myeloid leukemia. J. Cell Physiol., 76:175, 1970.

Ingram, V. M.: A specific chemical difference between the globins of normal and human sickle cell anemia hemoglobin. Nature (London), 178:792, 1956.

Irvine, W. J.: Immunologic aspects of pernicious anemia. New Eng. J. Med., 273:432, 1965.

Jacob, H. S.: The defective red blood cell in hereditary spherocytosis. Ann. Rev. Med., 20:41, 1969.

Jacob, H. S.: Dysfunction of the red blood cell membrane in hereditary spherocytosis. Brit. J. Haemat., 14:99, 1968.

Kahn, S. B.: Recent advances in the nutritional anemias. Med. Clin. N. Amer., 54:631, 1970.

Keitt, A. S.: Enzyme-deficient hemolytic anemias. Mechanisms, diagnosis and treatment. Mod. Treatm., 8:402, 1971.

Kirschbaum, J. D., and Preuss, F. S.: Leukemia: a clinical and pathologic study of 123 fatal cases in a series of 14,400 necropsies. Arch. Intern. Med., 71:777, 1943.

Kitay, D. Z., and Wentz, W. B.: Cervical cytology and folic acid deficiency of pregnancy. Amer. J. Obstet. Gynec., 104:931, 1969.

Krantz, S. B.: Application of the in vitro erythropoietin system to the study of human bone marrow disease: polycythemia vera. Ann. N.Y. Acad. Sci., 149:430, 1968.

Kwaan, H. C.: Disseminated intravascular coagulation. Med. Clin. N. Amer., 46:177, 1972.

Lawrence, J. H.: Leukemia in polycythemia, relationship to splenic myeloid metaplasia and therapeutic radiation dose. Medicine, 70:763, 1969.

Leevy, C. M., et al.: Incidence and significance of hypovitaminemia in a randomly selected municipal hospital population. Amer. J. Clin. Nutr., 17:259, 1965.

Lillibridge, C. B., et al.: Childhood pernicious anemia: gastrointestinal secretory, histological and electron microscopic aspects Gastroenterology, 52:792, 1967.

Lynch, M. J.: Monocytic leukemia. Canad. Med. Ass. J., 70:620, 1954.

Magnus, H. A.: A reassessment of the gastric lesion in pernicious anemia. J. Clin. Path. (London), 11:289, 1958.

Marks, P. A., and Bank, A.: Molecular pathology of thalassemia syndromes. Fed. Proc., *30*:977, 1971.

McIntyre, O. R., et al.: Pernicious anemia in childhood. New Eng. J. Med., *272*:981, 1965.

McKay, D. G.: Disseminated Intravascular Coagulation. An Intermediary Mechanism of Disease. New York, Hoeber Medical Division, Harper & Row, 1965.

Merskey, C., et al.: The defibrination syndrome, clinical features and laboratory diagnosis. Brit. J. Haemat., *13*:528, 1967.

Modan, B., and Lillienfeld, A. M.: Polycythemia and leukemia: the role of radiation treatment. Medicine, *44*:305, 1965.

Moeschlin, S., and Wagner, K.: Agranulocytosis due to the occurrence of leukocyte-agglutinins (pyramidon and cold agglutinins). Acta Haemat., *8*:29, 1952.

Mohler, D., and Leavell, B. S.: Aplastic anemia. Analysis of 50 cases. Ann. Intern. Med., *49*:326, 1958.

Murayama, M.: Molecular mechanism of red cell "sickling." Science, *153*:145, 1966.

Nalbandian, R. M., and Evans, T. N.: Sickle cell disease. A molecular approach to pathogenesis, diagnosis and treatment. Mich. Med., *70*:411, 1971.

Nalbandian, R. M., et al.: Consumption coagulopathy: practical principles of diagnosis and management. Hum. Path., *2*:377, 1971.

Nathan, D. G.: Thalassemia. New Eng. J. Med., *286*:586, 1972.

Nathan, D. G., and Segel, G. B.: Pathophysiology of common hemolytic syndromes. Postgrad. Med., *50*:179, 1971.

Nickerson, D. A., and Sunderland, D. A.: The histopathology of idiopathic thrombocytopenic purpura. Amer. J. Path., *13*:463, 1937.

Norkin, S., and Wiener, J.: Henoch-Schönlein syndrome. Amer. J. Clin. Path., *33*:55, 1960.

Oppenheim, J. J., et al.: III. Immunologic and cytologic studies of chronic lymphatic leukemia cells. Blood, *26*:121, 1965.

Panner, B.: Nephritis of Schönlein-Henoch syndrome. Arch. Path., *74*:230, 1962.

Pauling, L.: Foreword. In Nalbandian, R. M. (ed.): Molecular Aspects of Sickle Cell Hemoglobin. Clinical Applications. Springfield, Ill., Charles C Thomas, 1971.

Pauling, L., et al.: Sickle cell anemia: a molecular disease. Science, *110*:543, 1949.

Payne, R. W.: Pernicious anemia and gastric cancer in England and Wales. Brit. Med. J., *1*:1807, 1961.

Peabody, F. W.: The pathology of the bone marrow in pernicious anemia. Amer. J. Path., *3*:179, 1927.

Pedersen, B., and Hayhoe, F. G. J.: Cellular changes in chronic myeloid leukemia. Brit. J. Haemat., *21*:251, 1971.

Perutz, M. F., and Mitchison, J. M.: State of haemoglobin in sickle cell anaemia. Nature (London), *166*:677, 1950.

Pisciotta, A. V.: Clinical and pathologic effects of space-occupying lesions in the bone marrow. Amer. J. Clin. Path., *20*:915, 1950.

Pollycove, M., et al.: Classification and evolution of patterns of erythropoiesis in polycythemia vera as studied by iron kinetics. Blood, *28*:807, 1966.

Rabinovitz, Y., and Dameshek, W.: Systemic lupus erythematosus after (idiopathic) thrombocytopenic purpura. A review. Ann. Intern. Med., *52*:1, 1960.

Reed, C. F., and Swisher, S. N.: Erythrocyte lipid loss in hereditary spherocytosis. J. Clin. Invest., *45*:777, 1966.

Roitt, I., and Doniach, D.: Gastric autoimmunity. In Miescher, P. A., and Mueller-Eberhard, H. J. (eds.): Textbook of Immunopathology. New York, Grune and Stratton, 1969, p. 534.

Sandburg, A. A., and Hossfeld, D. K.: Chromosomal abnormalities in human neoplasia. Ann. Rev. Med., *21*:379, 1970.

Sandberg, A. A., et al.: Chromosomes and causation of human cancer and leukemia. Cancer, *27*:176, 1971.

Schrek, R.: Effect of phytohemagglutinin on lymphocytes from patients with chronic lymphocytic leukemia. Arch. Path., *83*:58, 1967.

Schumacher, H. R., et al.: The lymphocyte of chronic lymphatic leukemia. I. Electron microscopy: onset. Cancer, *26*:895, 1970.

Scott, R. B.: Leukaemia. Lancet, *1*:1053, 1162, 1957.

Silver, H. K.: Mediterranean anemia. Calif. Med., *76*:162, 1952.

Southam, C. M., et al.: A study of the natural history of acute leukemia with special reference to the duration of the disease and the occurrence of remissions. Cancer, *4*:39, 1951.

Spiegelman, S., et al.: RNA directed DNA polymerase in oncogenic RNA viruses. Nature (London), *227*:1029, 1970.

Strauss, H. S., and Bloom, G. E.: von Willebrand's disease. New Eng. J. Med., *273*:171, 1965.

Strauss, M. B.: Hypochromic anemia. Amer. Pract., *3*:65, 1948–1949.

Sullivan, L. W.: Differential diagnosis and management of the patient with megaloblastic anemia. Amer. J. Med., *48*:609, 1970.

Szippin, C., et al.: Variation and survival among patients with acute lymphocytic leukemia. Blood, *37*:59, 1971.

Taub, R. N., et al.: Intravascular coagulation, the Schwartzman reaction and the pathogenesis of thrombotic (thrombocytopenic) purpura. Blood, *24*:775, 1964.

Tinney, W. S., et al.: The liver and spleen in polycythemia vera. Proc. Staff Meeting Mayo Clin., *18*:46, 1943.

Twomey, J. J., et al.: Studies on the inheritance and nature of hemophilia B_m. Amer. J. Med., *46*:372, 1969.

Valentine, W. N.: The hereditary hemolytic anemias associated with erythrocyte enzyme deficiencies. Advances Intern. Med., *16*:303, 1970.

Vitale, J. J., et al.: Folic metabolism and iron deficiency. Lancet, *2*:393, 1965.

Wasserman, L. R.: Polycythemia vera: its course and treatment: relation to myeloid metaplasia and leukemia. Bull. N.Y. Acad. Med., *30*:343, 1954.

Weatherall, D. G., et al.: The pattern of disordered hemoglobin synthesis in homozygous and heterozygous beta thalassemia. Brit. J. Haemat., *16*:251, 1969.

Wennberg, E., and Weiss, L.: Splenic erythroclasia: an electron microscopic study of hemoglobin H disease. Blood, *31*:778, 1968.

Whipple, G. H., and Bradford, W. L.: Mediterranean disease: thalassemia (erythroblastic anemia of Cooley). J. Pediat., *9*:279, 1936.

White, J. G., and Heagan, B.: The fine structure of cell free sickled hemoglobin. Amer. J. Path., *58*:1, 1970.

Whittingham, S., et al.: The genetic factor in pernicious anaemia. A family study of patients with gastritis. Lancet, *1*:951, 1969.

Wiernik, P. H., and Serpick, A. A.: Factors affecting remission and survival in adult, acute, non-lymphocytic leukemia. Medicine, *49*:505, 1970.

Wintrobe, M. M.: Clinical Hematology. Philadelphia, Lea and Febiger, 1967, p. 985.

18

LYMPH NODES
AND SPLEEN

LYMPH NODES

NORMAL

Lymph nodes are widely distributed throughout the body, and lymphoid tissue is the main component of the spleen, tonsils, adenoids, thymus and Peyer's patches in the intestine. Lymphoid aggregates are also widely distributed in the bone marrow, lungs, gastric and appendiceal mucosa, and other tissues.

Lymph nodes, in general, are discrete structures, ovoid in shape, that vary from a few millimeters to 1 to 2 cm. in length. Their consistency is soft and their cut surface is gray-white. They are surrounded by a capsule composed of connective tissue and a few elastic fibrils. The capsule is perforated at various points by afferent lymphatics which empty into the peripheral sinus subjacent to the capsule. Branches of the sinus extend into the nodes and terminate at the hilus, where the efferent lymphatics emerge. All lymphatics are lined by reticuloendothelial cells. Situated in the cortex or peripheral portion of the node are spherical aggregates of lymphoid tissue, the so-called primary follicles or germinal centers. These are composed of lymphocytes, lymphoblasts, histiocytes and rare reticular stem cells supported by strands of delicate reticulin. The histiocyte is two to three times the size of the lymphocyte, has an amphophilic cytoplasm,

and has a round to bean-shaped nucleus with finely divided chromatin. In the normal germinal follicle, the lymphocytes and lymphoblasts outnumber the histiocytes. The relative proportion of these follicular cells in disease states depends somewhat on the varying conditions of the body. In some diseases, the majority of the cells are young lymphocytes; in other conditions, the predominant cells are histiocytes, many of which may contain phagocytized nuclear debris. In the subcapsular zone there are lymphocytes, and extending into the central part or medulla of the nodes are the medullary cords, composed of adult lymphocytes and reticular cells. The distribution of the B and T lymphocytes in this lymphoid population was described on p. 195. In addition, fibroblasts and plasma cells are found in these cords, as is an occasional granulocyte. The supporting structure throughout a lymph node is, for the most part, a delicate reticulin of fibroblastic origin which connects peripherally with the capsule. Each node's blood supply is furnished by arteries which enter at the hilus and by veins which leave at the same site. The lymph nodes are part of the reticuloendothelial system.

The morphologic description of the lymph node just given is highly idealized and falsely static. In reality, lymph nodes are among the most labile structures in the body. Relatively large at birth, they undergo progressive atrophy throughout life. Their size and morphology is modified by stress, thyroid and adrenal function, as well as immune responses. As secondary lines of defense, they are constantly responding to stimuli, even in the absence of clinical disease. Trivial injuries and infections effect subtle changes in lymph node histology. More significant bacterial infections inevitably produce enlargement of nodes and sometimes leave residual scarring. For this reason, in the adult, the lymph nodes are almost never "normal" since they usually bear the scars of previous encounters. Notably, such previous events render the inguinal nodes particularly inappropriate for evaluative biopsies. Except in the child, it is difficult to find a "normal" node and, frequently, in histologic evaluations, it is necessary to distinguish changes secondary to past experience from those related to present disease.

PATHOLOGY

Although rarely the site of primary disease (significant exceptions being the important proliferative disorders, i.e., lymphomas and Hodgkin's disease), lymph nodes act as defensive barriers and are secondarily involved in virtually all systemic infections and in many neoplastic disorders arising elsewhere. The infections that lead to lymphadenitis are so numerous and varied that it is impossible to detail each since such description would comprise a virtual catalogue of all systemic microbiologic diseases. Moreover, in most instances, the lymphadenitis is of a banal variety and is entirely nonspecific, designated acute or chronic nonspecific lymphadenitis.

The specific node or nodes that are affected in various microbiologic diseases depend, to a considerable extent, upon the location of the infection, the nature of the invading organism and the severity of the disease. An infection of the hand involves first the nodes about the elbow and then those in the axilla. If the causative organism is of relatively low virulence, the lymphadenitis may remain localized to the arm and axilla. If the infection is more severe, these barriers may be overwhelmed and the inflammatory reaction may spread to nodes in the neck and the mediastinum—the secondary chains in the pathway of lymphatic drainage. On the other hand, many biologic diseases are characterized by bacteremias or viremias, and others are associated with the elaboration of powerful exotoxins circulated through the blood. In these diseases, there is a generalized lymphadenitis and possibly splenitis irrespective of the location of the primary infection.

Metastases to nodes are a much more common clinical problem than are primary tumors. However, lymph nodes are the site of primary disease in the important proliferative disorders—the lymphomas and Hodgkin's disease. The following discussion will deal principally with nodal inflammations, lymphomas and Hodgkin's disease.

INFLAMMATION

ACUTE NONSPECIFIC LYMPHADENITIS

These nonspecific nodal inflammations take one of two patterns: (1) suppuration in nodes that drain infections caused by pyogenic organisms, and (2) diffuse reticuloendothelial hyperplasia, edema and leukocytic infiltration in diseases caused by nonpyogenic biologic agents, for example, the spirochetes, rickettsiae and viruses. Acutely inflamed lymph nodes, whatever the nature of the infection, usually show congestion and edema and an increased number of leukocytes, especially neutrophils. These cells are found in the sinuses and may distend them. The cells lining the sinuses become hypertrophied and cuboidal and often undergo hyperplasia. The inflammatory reaction may extend into the extrasinusoidal tissues. The germinal centers often show increased numbers of histiocytes containing phagocytized cellular debris (Fig. 18–1). When the inflammation is caused by nonpyogenic organisms, the inflammatory changes may be limited to these. However, when caused by the common pyogens, abscesses may develop in the follicles or lymphoid pulp. Macroscopically, the nodes in both types of histologic reaction become swollen, gray-red and engorged. Abscess formation modifies the appearance. Perinodal tissues may become secondarily involved in the permeation of the inflammatory response.

Acutely inflamed nodes are most commonly seen in the cervical region in association with infections of the teeth or tonsils or in the axillary or inguinal regions secondary to infections of the extremities. Similarly acute lymphadenitis is found in the nodes draining an acute appendicitis, acute enteritis or any other acute infection. Generalized lymphadenopathy is characteristic of the secondary stage of syphilis, viral infections and bacteremic or exotoxic diseases.

Clinically, nodes with acute lymphadenitis are enlarged because of the cellular infiltration

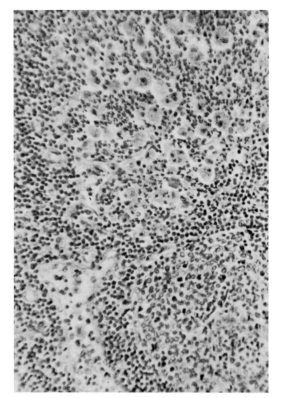

Figure 18–1. Acute lymphadenitis. High power detail of germinal centers with large histiocytic cells showing phagocytic activity.

active, containing either increased numbers of immature lymphocytes, many of which show mitoses, or increased numbers of histiocytes (Fig. 18–2). These latter cells characteristically contain phagocytized cellular debris and bacteria. There is also frequently an increased number of lymphocytes and free histiocytes in the sinus, giving rise to the picture known as "sinus catarrh." Hyperplasia of the sinusoidal lining cells is a usual accompaniment, and commonly a plasma cell infiltration in the lymphoid cords occurs. In the course of the infection, the nodes frequently become extensively scarred with fibrous replacement of focal areas or large tracts of the follicles and lymphoidal pulp. As a rule, such scarring renders them unsatisfactory for biopsy specimens. Nodes with chronic lymphadenitis are moderately to markedly enlarged and, on cut section, have an increased consistency imparted by the fibrous scarring.

Characteristically, these nodes are not tender because they are not under increased

and edema. As a consequence of the distention of the capsule, they are tender to touch. When abscess formation is extensive, they become fluctuant. The overlying skin is frequently red, and sometimes the penetration of the infection to the skin surface produces draining sinuses, particularly where the nodes have suppurative necrosis. If the infection has not caused extensive destruction of the nodal tissues, control of the infection is followed by resolution of the inflammatory changes, and the nodes progressively shrink and resume their former gross and microscopic appearance. On the other hand, scarring follows the more severe destructive diseases and the nodes become more firm to palpation.

CHRONIC NONSPECIFIC LYMPHADENITIS

In association with chronic infections, such as those that are prone to occur in the teeth or tonsils, the regional nodes are usually affected.

Microscopically, the germinal centers of the node with chronic lymphadenitis are enlarged and

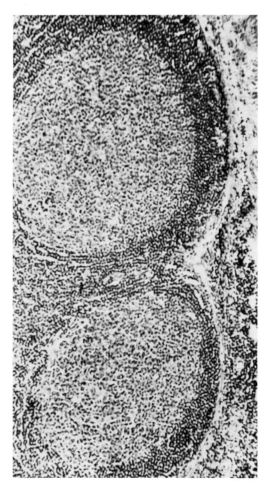

Figure 18–2. Chronic lymphadenitis, demonstrating the marked enlargement and prominence of the germinal follicles.

pressure. Chronic lymphadenitis is particularly characteristic of inguinal and axillary nodes. The inguinal nodes are a relatively small group which drain extremely large areas of the torso and the lower extremities; they bear a heavy burden consequent to infections anywhere in these regions. For this reason, inguinal nodes are particularly inappropriate as biopsy specimens for the study of hematologic and lymphomatous disorders. The same may be said of the axillary nodes. In contrast, the nodes of the cervical region drain relatively small areas. However, infections are so common and persistent in the oral pharynx that cervical nodes are sometimes involved in longstanding, chronic lymphadenitis.

Mention should be made here of the *changes encountered in immunologic reactions.* The lymph nodes undergo enlargement and histologic alterations virtually indistinguishable from the chronic reactive lymphadenitis described above. Often, there is striking hyperplasia of the nodal follicles. In cell-mediated responses, increased numbers of blast cells are seen in the deeper T-cell region of the node, while in humoral reactions the parafollicular B zones contain increased numbers of plasma cells.

DERMATOPATHIC LYMPHADENITIS (LIPOMELANOTIC RETICULOENDOTHELIOSIS)

Dermatopathic lymphadenitis is the name given to a *peculiar but nonspecific chronic lymphadenitis that occurs in nodes draining the sites of chronic dermatologic diseases.* Such lymph node involvement is commonly associated with eczema, psoriasis, exfoliative dermatitis, neurodermatitis and seborrheic dermatitis. The nodes are usually moderately enlarged and are characterized by the following features: (1) histiocyte or reticular cell hyperplasia in the germinal follicles, (2) hyperplasia of the reticuloendothelial sinusoidal cells, (3) accumulation of melanin and, less prominently, hemosiderin within the phagocytic cells of the node, and (4) the appearance of finely divided lipid granules in these phagocytic cells. Often the reticuloendothelial proliferation produces large sheets of cells. Because of these prominent histologic features, this condition is also known by the more descriptive term of *lipomelanotic reticuloendotheliosis.* The genesis of these histologic changes appears to lie in the persistent drainage of superficial, chronic, inflammatory lesions of the skin with the breakdown of epithelial cells releasing both melanin pigment and fatty debris. This condition is of little clinical significance and is important chiefly as an ana-

tomic lesion that should not be confused with lymphomatous involvements of the nodes.

LYMPHOMA

The designation lymphoma refers to a group of neoplastic disorders, primary in lymphoid tissue, arising in the various cell types native to lymphoid tissue, i.e., lymphocytes, histiocytes and their common precursors, the reticular stem cells (Rappaport, 1966). Although they appear to have all the attributes of cancers, there are reasons for suspecting that certain, or possibly all, forms are not true neoplasms but rather excessive cellular proliferations in response to some inflammatory or immunologic stimulus. Thus, their very nature is uncertain, an issue which will be amplified in the subsequent discussion. Because of this unresolved controversy, some investigators prefer to call these growths *lymphoproliferative* or *immunoproliferative disorders* (Lukes and Parker, 1971). British and European writers prefer the noncommittal terms *reticuloses* or *reticuloendothelioses.* Even the designation "lymphoma" is something of a misnomer, since whatever their basic nature, all behave like malignant processes which, when untreated, progressively spread to contiguous lymphoid tissues and eventually disseminate to the viscera, particularly the liver, spleen and lungs. Perhaps more appropriately, they might have been termed lymphosarcomas, but regrettably this term was once applied to a specific pattern of lymphoma, and so continued use of this term would only add to the confusion.

The classification of the various forms of lymphoma underscores these conceptual and nosologic difficulties. Hodgkin's disease is a particularly good case in point. For many years, it was considered a form of lymphoma and, indeed, it is still so considered by many. However, it has many striking differences from the other forms of lymphoma which are composed essentially of one neoplastic cell type. In contrast, Hodgkin's disease presents with a variety of histologic patterns. In one, the enlarged lymph nodes are composed predominantly of lymphocytes. In another, termed the mixed cellularity pattern, a variety of cells are found, including lymphocytes, histiocytes, neutrophils, eosinophils and plasma cells, and the pattern is reminiscent of an inflammatory process. In still another pattern, the nodes are almost totally fibrotic, and in yet another variant, the nodes are composed almost solely of highly anaplastic tumorous reticular cells. Early in the course of any individual's disease, the nodes might show the lymphocytic or mixed cellular patterns and later the disease might transform to the anaplastic reticular pattern. Because of the range of morphology—the possibility of transformation always to more malignant-appearing forms—and for other reasons as well, there is a strong suspicion that Hodgkin's disease may begin as an inflammatory or immunoproliferative disorder which, in time, converts to a true neoplasm (p. 760. Thus there is a growing preference to consider Hodgkin's disease not as a form of lymphoma but rather as some reactive process which in its inception is inflammatory, only later becoming neoplastic. More is involved than semantics here. Merely to designate Hodgkin's disease as a form of lymphoma tends to obscure the possibility that it may not be a true neoplasm but, instead, may have a specific remediable cause. We cannot resolve this issue but will here consider Hodgkin's disease separately as a distinct entity and will not include it in the discussion of lymphoma.

Classification of Lymphomas. A lymphoma may be composed of lymphocytes, histiocytes or reticular stem cells. In some instances, the nodal overgrowth is complete—a *diffuse*, monotonous proliferation of a single cell type but, in other instances, low power microscopic examination discloses only *nodular* collections of neoplastic cells. For many years, the nodular pattern which appeared to reproduce large lymphoid follicles was construed as a neoplasm taking origin from the follicles of the lymph node, and so was designated "follicular lymphoma" or "giant follicle lymphoma." The concept implied that two cell types, i.e., the lymphoblast (or lymphocyte) and the histiocyte, native to the follicle, had simultaneously become neoplastic. *Current interpretations of the nodular pattern propose that any one of the malignant lymphomas may occur in either a nodular or diffuse form* (Sheehan and Rappaport, 1970). Presumably, all lymphomas begin in multicentric focal aggregates of neoplastic cells within a single node or a cluster of nodes. As these lesions evolve, the nodules enlarge, coalescing to create the diffuse form. The nodular pattern is now interpreted as an early stage of the diffuse involvement and not as a specific form of lymphoma derived from follicles. Based on this view, the following classification of lymphoma by Gall and Rappaport (1958) has the virtues of simplicity, wide current usage and proven clinical relevance.

For clarity and emphasis we shall underscore the concept that theoretically any one of the histogenetic types of lymphoma may occur in the nodular or diffuse pattern. In actual practice, the nodular pattern is encountered most frequently in the lymphocytic (PD),

CLASSIFICATION OF MALIGNANT LYMPHOMA (MAY OCCUR AS NODULAR OR DIFFUSE)

Lymphocytic, well differentiated (WD)
Lymphocytic, poorly differentiated (PD)
Stem Cell (including Burkitt's lymphoma)
Histiocytic
? Mixed Cell Type

mixed and histiocytic lymphoma patterns. It is quite rare in the lymphocytic lymphoma (WD). Perhaps, then, all lymphomas do not begin with the nodular pattern. Most of those that begin as nodular lesions progress to the diffuse form, but a few never convert and in fact may spread to viscera to eventually kill the patient (Butler, 1970).

The mixed cell type (included here with certain doubt) refers to those lymphomas in which two types of neoplastic cells, i.e., poorly differentiated lymphocytic forms and histiocytic forms, appear to proliferate simultaneously. Some researchers, however, consider such a mixed cell lymphoma to be a poorly differentiated lymphocytic lymphoma, or perhaps a stem cell lymphoma, which has proliferated along its two possible lines of differentiation, i.e., lymphocytic and histiocytic. The designation histiocytic lymphoma replaces the older term reticulum cell sarcoma. Missing from this classification, for reasons already given, are the giant follicle lymphoma and Hodgkin's disease. Also omitted is the older designation lymphosarcoma, since there is no agreement as to precisely what is meant by this term. Burkitt's lymphoma is a special variant of the stem cell lymphoma which is sufficiently distinctive to merit separate consideration.

Here we should bring up *the relationship between lymphomas and leukemia*. Both conditions may be considered as variable expressions of the same basic disorder. Typically, *lymphomas* involve solid tissues, e.g., nodes, spleen, liver, and few if any neoplastic cells spill into the blood. Their spread has the attributes of solid tissue cancers. The *leukemias*, by contrast, diffusely and uniformly involve the marrow, flood into the blood in the early stages of the disease, and subsequently permeate lymph nodes throughout the body as well as the spleen, liver and, in time, virtually all the other organs. It would appear almost as though the lymphocytic, histiocytic and stem cell leukemias were composed of noncohesive cells which arise in marrow lymphoid tissues, overflow into the blood and then seed other sites in the body. In some patients, lymphomatous involvement of nodes for a period of time is followed in the evolution of the disease by the development of leukemic dissemination. *Most cases of leukemia arise as primary systemic disorders without evolving from the lymphomatous state and, conversely, most lymphomas are not associated with leukemic blood-borne dissemination.* With some exceptions, as noted in Table 18–1, the cell types of leukemias and lymphomas are usually identical or at least closely related.

Incidence.   The lymphomas may occur at any age but have a peak incidence in the sixth decade. Males are affected about twice as often as females and whites more than nonwhites. Burkitt's lymphoma is something of an exception (as is discussed below) and is seen principally in native children in central Africa.

Collectively, the lymphomas and their related leukemias accounted for about 10 per cent of deaths from cancer in the United States in 1967 (Vital Statistics of the United States, 1967).

Etiology.   A host of viral agents including the Gross, Graffi, Moloney and Rauscher viruses have been shown to produce lymphomatous diseases in a variety of experimental animals (Dmochowski, 1970). There is a growing body of evidence, but no definite proof, that lymphomas in man are also caused by viruses. The distribution of the Burkitt lymphoma through central Africa in a geographic belt having high median temperatures, heavy rainfall and abundant mosquitoes suggests insect transmission of a viral agent. Presumably, children are principally affected because they have not developed prior immunologic resistance to the infectious agent (Burkitt, 1968). As discussed previously (p. 130), a herpes type virus known as the Epstein-Barr virus (EBV) has been isolated from cultured Burkitt's lymphoma cells. Viral C-particles have been identified by electron microscopy, and immunofluorescent tests have disclosed viral capsid antigens as well as viral specific cell membrane antigens in cultured Burkitt's lymphoma cells (Henle et al., 1970) (Klein et al., 1969). These patients also have significantly higher titers of antibodies to these antigens than are found in control populations. Elevated titers of antibodies to the EBV also have been identified in patients with lymphocytic lymphoma (Johansson, 1971). In addition, C-type viral particles have been seen in the cells of various forms of lymphoma (Dmochowski, 1970). However, despite all of this evidence, there is no proof that viral particles or their antibodies have any causal significance. The viruses might merely be "passengers."

Recently, another theory of possible causation has aroused great interest. It has been observed that *patients suffering from some form of immune deficiency or autoimmune disease have an increased incidence of lymphoma, as well as a higher incidence of cancer in general* (Hoover and Fraumeni, 1973). The same has been observed in mice having spontaneous autoimmune disease (Mellors, 1966). Fudenberg (1971) has postulated that, in patients having immune deficiencies, "forbidden clones" may emerge which cannot be destroyed because of the inadequacies of immune surveillance. On the one hand these clones may induce autoimmune disease or, on the other hand, through progressive mutations, may emerge as uncontrolled neoplastic clones. Consonant with such a theory is the now well documented increased incidence of lymphomas in transplantation patients receiving long-term immunosuppressive therapy (Penn et al., 1969).

The viral and immune deficiency theories may be related. In the earlier discussion of neoplasia (p. 140), it was indicated that there is a growing body of evidence that potentially oncogenic C-type RNA viruses are widely present in animals and man. Evidence for their presence is the identification of so-called "viral oncogenes" inserted into the genome of the mammalian cells by the virus-directed "reverse transcriptase." If such oncogenic viruses were indeed widely present, it would be logical to assume that an immune deficiency would potentiate the expression of the oncogene to thus produce a neoplasm, possibly a lymphoma. Seductive as such a concept may be, it is still in the realm of speculation.

Morphology.   All of the lymphomas are characterized by lymphadenopathy and, as the disease advances, splenomegaly, hepatomegaly and eventually involvement of other viscera. At first only one or a single chain of nodes is involved. In an analysis of a large series of cases, the cervical chain (either side) was the primary site of involvement in approximately 30 to 40 per cent of the cases, the axillary nodes, in approximately 20 per cent of the cases, followed in order by the inguinal, femoral, iliac and mediastinal nodes (Banfi et al., 1968). Involvement of the oropharyngeal lymphoid tissue is rela-

TABLE 18–1.   RELATIONSHIPS OF
LYMPHOMAS AND LEUKEMIAS

Lymphoma (Diffuse or Nodular)	Leukemia
Lymphocytic, WD	Chronic lymphatic
Lymphocytic, PD	Rare (? Leukosarcoma cell)
Histiocytic	Monocytic (Schilling)
	Histiocytic
Stem Cell	Stem cell
	Undifferentiated acute lymphatic

tively uncommon in the lymphocytic lymphomas but occurs eventually in approximately 50 per cent of the histiocytic lymphomas. In all forms of lymphoma, affected nodes are variably enlarged, sometimes up to massive size (10 cm. in diameter). They are generally soft and fleshy and are usually discrete without adherence to surrounding structures. On cut surfaces, the nodular forms may present foci of nodularity barely apparent to the naked eye. Nodes with diffuse disease are homogeneously gray and have the appearance of fish flesh (Fig. 18–3). Necrosis, hemorrhage and foci of cystic softening are uncommon. With advance of the disease, the tumorous tissue may permeate the capsule of the node and extend into the pericapsular tissues to produce interadherence and matted, nodular tumorous masses. Such a gross appearance is characteristic of the diffuse patterns of lymphoma. Lymphomatous spread to the spleen, liver or other viscera may be inapparent macroscopically, may only produce hepatosplenomegaly without grossly visible lesions but, on occasion, may yield small to moderate-sized tumorous nodules resembling metastases.

Microscopically, in the well advanced diffuse patterns, the normal architecture of the lymph nodes is totally flooded by a monotonous sea of neoplastic cells (Fig. 18–4). Often microscopic permeation and penetration into the pericapsular fibrofatty tissue is evident even in those nodes which appear discrete and unattached to surrounding structures on gross inspection. Permeation of blood vessel walls, usually of veins, is sometimes found particularly in the histiocytic form. When the nodular pattern is present, discrete focal aggregates of lymphomatous cells are found, separated by compressed native architecture (Fig. 18–5). Silver impregnation stains may highlight the collar-like compression of the native reticular architecture as the expanding nodular aggregates of lymphomatous cells push the stroma of the node ahead of them (Fig. 18–6).

Diagnosis of the specific type of lymphoma rests with the cytologic identification of the particular form of neoplastic cell.

Lymphocytic Lymphoma, Well Differentiated. In the diffuse pattern, the node is flooded by a monotony of uniform, small lymphocytes exactly resembling those encountered in inflammatory infiltrates (Fig. 18–7). No other cell types are present, save perhaps for a few persistent native cells not totally obscured by the lymphomatous replacement. Such cytology would be indistinguishable from that of chronic lymphatic leukemia

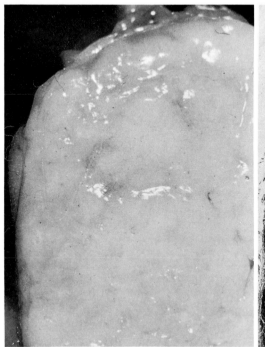

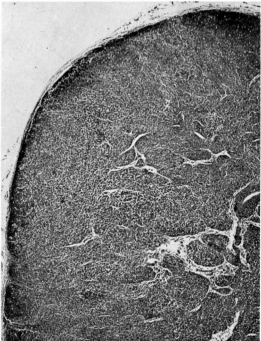

Fig. 18–3   Fig. 18–4

Figure 18–3. Lymphocytic lymphoma (diffuse). The nodal architecture is entirely replaced by lymphomatous involvement. (Reprinted through the courtesy of Oxford University Press. From Jackson, H. J., Jr., and Parker, F., Jr.: Hodgkin's Disease and Allied Disorders. Figures 18–5, 18–7, 18–8, 18–10, 18–11, 18–15, 18–16, 18–17 from the same source.)

Figure 18–4. Lymphocytic lymphoma (well differentiated) diffuse. The entire node is flooded by a monotony of well differentiated lymphocytes.

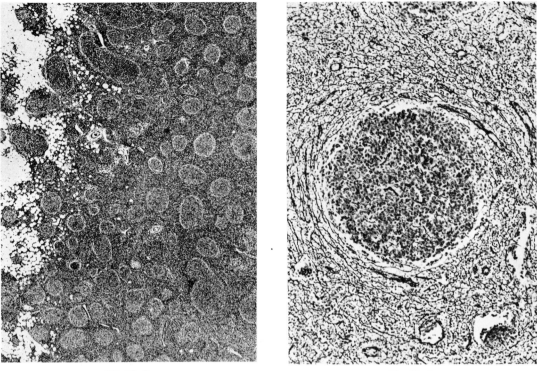

Fig. 18–5   *Fig. 18–6*

Figure 18–5. *Lymphocytic lymphoma (poorly differentiated) nodular pattern.*
Figure 18–6. *Lymphocytic lymphoma (poorly differentiated) nodular pattern. The silver impregnation stain highlights the collar-like compression of the fibrillar native reticular framework produced by the expansile growth of the lymphomatous nodule.*

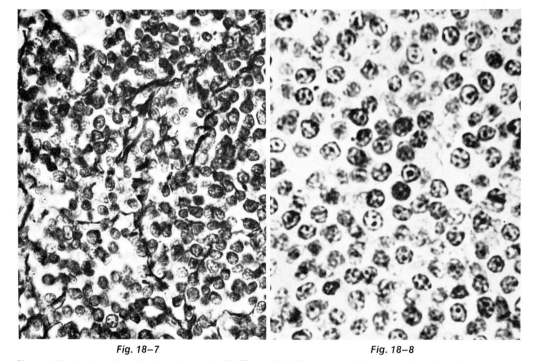

Fig. 18–7   *Fig. 18–8*

Figure 18–7. *Lymphocytic lymphoma (well differentiated) composed of mature lymphocytes.*
Figure 18–8. *Lymphocytic lymphoma (poorly differentiated). The cells are larger than mature lymphocytes with larger, more vesicular nuclei containing nucleoli.*

with well developed infiltration of the nodes. In the nodular pattern, aggregates of lymphocytes produce pseudofollicles separated by compressed but preserved native lymph node structure. As mentioned, in time, such nodularity is lost if the disease evolves into the diffuse form.

Lymphocytic Lymphoma, Poorly Differentiated. The cellular aggregation here is composed of small to medium to large-sized lymphocytes, many of which resemble lymphoblasts. In the medium-sized cells, the nuclei are characteristically somewhat irregular and often have sharp cleavages giving them an apparent lobulated conformation. In the larger blast-like cells, the nucleochromatin is less dense and small nucleoli may be present. These nuclei are rimmed by a variable amount of cytoplasm, never abundant and more or less characteristic of all lymphocytic forms (Fig. 18–8). Here again, the pattern may be either diffuse or nodular.

Stem Cell (Including Burkitt's) Lymphoma. As the term indicates, the lesions in this disorder consist of masses of primitive, reticular stem cells. These cells have a size approaching that of the large lymphocyte or lymphoblast and contain round to oval, remarkably uniform nuclei with finely divided chromatin and small nucleoli. In some cells, the nucleoli are prominent, but in many they are quite indistinct. The cytoplasm is somewhat more abundant than in the cells of the lymphocytic lymphomas, and in the usual H & E stain, it is pale gray. With the Feulgen stain, the cytoplasm is strongly pyroninophilic, indicating an abundance of RNA. These cells tend to be somewhat cohesive and lie in poorly defined clusters even in the diffuse form of the lymphoma. One of the most distinctive histologic features in some stem cell lymphomas are scattered, large histiocytes having an abundant pale cytoplasm which often contains phagocytized debris. Against the darker background of the stem cells, these large, pale cells create a so-called "starry sky" appearance (Fig. 18–9). These histiocytes are probably benign reactive cells responding to some inflammatory or antigenic challenge, but their presence carries a poor prognosis (Oels et al., 1968). **This starry sky pattern of stem cell lymphoma was initially considered characteristic of Burkitt's lymphoma (described below), but additional study has indicated that it may occur in any form of stem cell lymphoma** (Bennett et al., 1969). Only rarely is the stem cell lymphoma nodular.

Histiocytic Lymphoma. Formerly designated by the term **reticulum cell sarcoma**, these lesions are composed of histiocytes (macrophages) which vary from poorly differentiated forms with scanty cytoplasm to better differentiated cells with abundant cytoplasm. Sometimes these cells form almost giant cells. The nuclei are characteristically extremely variable in size and shape. Some are round

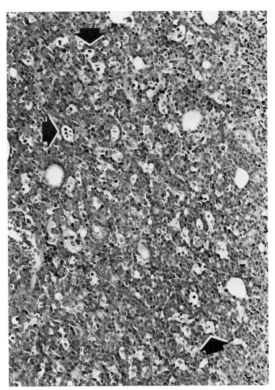

Figure 18–9. Stem cell lymphoma (Burkitt's). The background is composed of lymphocytes. The arrows indicate pale histiocytes containing phagocytic debris. The large clear vacuoles are artefacts.

to oval while others are bean-shaped, and still others are extremely pleomorphic with apparent pseudopods (Fig. 18–10). Not infrequently, two or even three nuclei are found within a single cell which thus comes to strongly resemble the Reed-Sternberg cell of Hodgkin's disease (p. 760). Phagocytized debris is sometimes present within the cytoplasm. Often these cells stimulate the native fibroblastic stroma to produce increased amounts of reticulin, apparent only in special silver impregnations. The increase in reticulin may create an elaborate background network separating and enclosing individual lymphoma cells (Fig. 18–11). Low power microscopy is most helpful in differentiating this form of lymphoma from the others since, whether diffuse or nodular, the histiocytic lymphoma tends to present greater variation in the shape and size of cells than the monotony seen in the other forms of lymphoma already described.

Clinical Course. All lymphomas tend to produce similar clinical manifestations depending largely on the stage of advancement of the disease. Most patients come to attention, presumably early in the evolution of their disease, because of the mysterious appearance of a painless enlarged node or group

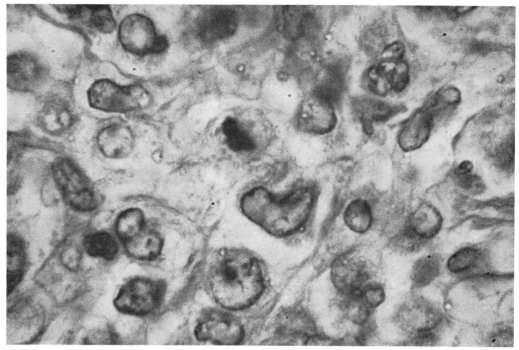

Figure 18-10. *Histiocytic lymphoma (reticulum cell sarcoma). A high power detail of pleomorphism of cells with formation of apparent pseudopods best seen in the nuclei.*

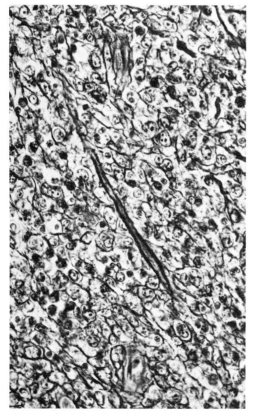

Figure 18-11. *Histiocytic lymphoma (reticulum cell sarcoma). A silver impregnation stain to outline abundant reticulin strands laid down between cells.*

of nodes, usually in the cervical region. No constitutional signs such as weakness, fever, weight loss or anemia are present. Indeed, *nodal enlargement in the absence of an apparent cause in an otherwise healthy patient most favors the diagnosis of lymphoma.* Sometimes the disease comes to attention in the investigation of an enlarged mediastinal node(s) discovered on routine chest film. In other instances, it presents as inguinal adenopathy which is at first attributed to some inflammatory reaction until the progressive enlargement reaches an ominous size. In all of these settings, biopsy of the node is required for diagnosis.

In about one-quarter of the patients, involvement of deep-seated nodes remains occult until splenomegaly or hepatomegaly becomes evident. In such patients the disease is usually more advanced, and weakness, weight loss, fever and anemia are often present. Infrequently, lymphomas arise in the lymphoid tissue of the gut and first become manifest because of gastrointestinal symptoms or the production of a malabsorption syndrome (p. 946). With the advance of the disease, the lymphadenopathy becomes more widespread, splenohepatomegaly more marked, and osteolytic bone lesions may appear, with resultant pain and pathologic fractures (Fig. 18-12). In the course of the dissemination, any organ or system may be involved, e.g., enlargement of the kidneys with urinary abnormalities, varied

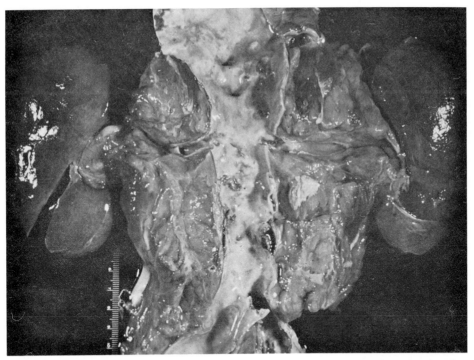

Figure 18–12. *Histiocytic lymphoma (reticulum cell sarcoma) primary in retroperitoneal periaortic nodes.*

neurologic manifestations from central or peripheral nervous system involvement.

The prognosis depends mainly on two considerations: (1) the specific form of lymphoma (the cytologic pattern and whether diffuse or nodular) and (2) the extent of involvement at the time of initial diagnosis. A widely used system (staging) has been developed for expressing the extent of spread of the disease. This method was originally devised for Hodgkin's disease but has subsequently been revised and adopted for all lymphomas (Rosenberg, 1966).

CLINICAL STAGES OF HODGKIN'S DISEASE (ADOPTED FOR ALL LYMPHOMAS)

I. Disease limited to one anatomic region.
II. Disease in two or three regions on the same side of the diaphragm.
III. Disease on both sides of the diaphragm but limited to lymph nodes, spleen and Waldeyer's ring (oropharyngeal lymphoid tissue).
IV. Involvement of organs such as bone marrow, lung, liver, gastrointestinal tract and other viscera in addition to lymph nodes, spleen or Waldeyer's ring.

From Rosenberg, S. A.: Report of the Committee on the staging of Hodgkin's disease. Cancer Res., 26:1310, 1966.

All stages are further subclassified as A or B: A refers to patients without systemic symptoms; B denotes documented evidence of fe-ver, night sweats or pruritus. Several generalizations may be made regarding staging. Most lymphomas begin in a single region and then progressively become generalized. The appearance of leukemia markedly worsens the outlook and occurs in about 7 per cent of patients with lymphoma (Jacobs, 1968). Some of these relationships are presented in Table 18–2. Overall, the five-year survival is in the order of 30 to 50 per cent, but rapidly changing therapeutic modalities involving principally larger dosages of radiotherapy and chemotherapy are continually improving this outlook. Ten- and 15-year remissions are now achieved in some cases, but whether these are complete cures awaits proof.

Burkitt's Lymphoma. Although morphologically a stem cell lymphoma, Burkitt's lym-

TABLE 18–2. CLINICAL BEHAVIOR OF LYMPHOMA

	Likelihood of Leukemia
Slowly Progressive	
Lymphocytic lymphoma, WD	+++
Nodular patterns (all types)	
Moderately Progressive	
Lymphocytic lymphoma, PD	++
Rapidly Progressive	
Histiocytic lymphoma	+
Stem cell lymphoma	++

phoma merits separate consideration because it has a number of distinctive features. First described by Burkitt in African children in 1958, the disease has now been identified throughout the world, most often in children. In Africa, most patients are between the ages of two and 14 years; the median age is five years. Unlike the usual forms of lymphoma, it most often manifests as an enlarged destructive lesion in the alveolar processes of either the maxilla or mandible. Occasionally, it presents as an abdominal mass or with involvement of the ovary, thyroid or kidney. Wherever it arises, it tends to grow in a localized area, eroding and destroying contiguous structures without involving distant nodes, the liver or spleen (Burkitt, 1968). Rarely if ever do these patients develop leukemia. Untreated, the disease is rapidly progressive and causes death within a year to 18 months.

The most exciting aspect of Burkitt's lymphoma is the growing body of evidence that it is caused by the Epstein-Barr virus as discussed on p. 754. Patients with Burkitt's develop immune responses in the form of humoral antibodies and cell-mediated, delayed hypersensitivity reactions against both the EBV and tumor-specific antigens. Those individuals with good immune responses derive remarkable benefit from chemotherapy and show prolonged remissions and sometimes cures. It is hypothesized that the chemotherapy so blunts the vitality of the lymphomatous cells that the immune response is able to control or sometimes destroy them.

HODGKIN'S DISEASE

The argument as to whether Hodgkin's disease should be considered a form of lymphoma was presented earlier (p. 752) and is academic so long as one does not lose sight of the still mysterious nature of this disorder. Indeed, the more we learn about this unique malady, the greater the number of uncertainties raised. Its clinical and morphologic characteristics simultaneously implicate an inflammatory and a neoplastic disease. There are reasons for believing that *Hodgkin's disease may begin as an inflammatory disorder and, in the course of time, transform to a neoplastic state resembling in its potential the other lymphomas.* Before discussing other uncertainties, we should begin with the well established facts generally agreed upon.

Hodgkin's disease may take one of many morphologic patterns which seemingly have little in common with each other. *The one common denominator among all forms is the presence of a somewhat distinctive histiocytic tumor giant cell*

known as the Reed-Sternberg (RS) cell. Identification of this cell is essential for the histologic diagnosis of Hodgkin's disease although, as will be seen later, the RS cell is extremely pleomorphic, difficult to specifically characterize, and is simulated by other forms of giant cells. *Classically, it is a large, multinucleated cell, most often binucleated (or bilobed) with the two halves often appearing as mirror images of each other (Fig. 18–13). The nucleus is enclosed within an abundant amphophilic cytoplasm. Prominent within the nuclei are large, "owl-eyed" nucleoli generally surrounded by a clear halo.* The nucleoli are classically acidophilic or, at the least, amphophilic and react strongly with RNA stains. Giant cells having all the characteristics of the multinucleate cell just described are sometimes found which contain only a single nucleus replete with large nucleolus. While such cells may be biologic variants of the RS cell, they are not diagnostic of Hodgkin's disease. Other cells, uninucleate or multinucleate, may not have a nucleolus; these too are nondiagnostic. One additional variant, the so-called *lacunar cell,* is encountered primarily within one of the distinctive patterns of this disorder, specifically, nodular sclerosing Hodgkin's disease. The lacunar Reed-Sternberg cell generally has a single nucleus lying within an extremely palestaining cytoplasm bordered by a sharply defined cell membrane. The nucleus thus appears to sit within a lacuna (Fig. 18–14). There

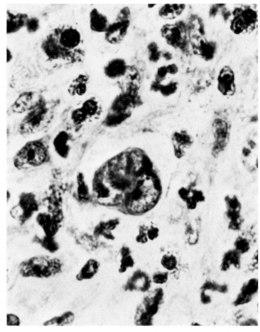

Figure 18–13. *Reed-Sternberg giant cell in Hodgkin's disease.*

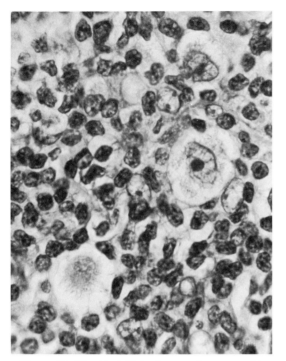

Figure 18–14. Hodgkin's disease—lacunar cells.

are reasons for believing that the multilobate and multinucleate giant cells with their huge nucleoli are obsolescent cells suffering all manner of polyploidy and chromosomal deletions which render them nonviable, dying cells. Thus the many biologic variants described above, although less diagnostic, may be the critical proliferating viable cells responsible for the perpetuation of the disease.

It is somewhat anticlimactic to report that cells closely simulating or identical with RS cells have been identified in conditions other than Hodgkin's disease. Lukes et al. (1969) have reported Reed-Sternberg-like cells in infectious mononucleosis, and Rappaport and his colleagues (1971) have observed cells resembling the Sternberg-Reed cell in solid tissue cancers, mycosis fungoides, lymphomas, and in other conditions as well (Strum et al., 1970). Thus, to quote Rappaport and his colleagues (1971), "we believe that a definitive diagnosis of Hodgkin's disease cannot be rendered in the absence of Sternberg-Reed cells, but that the diagnosis depends upon the total histologic picture." Thus, we are faced with the dilemma that a histologic diagnosis of Hodgkin's disease cannot be made without identifying Reed-Sternberg cells, but Reed-Sternberg cells cannot be identified unless they are present in Hodgkin's disease. Recognizing this difficulty, we can turn to the classification and morphology of the various patterns of Hodgkin's disease, an understanding of which facilitates the

consideration of the etiology and pathogenesis.

Classification and Morphology. Over the past many decades, there have been innumerable attempts to divide the range of histologic patterns of Hodgkin's disease into categories which express the probable clinical course and prognosis to be anticipated. A time-honored classification (still used) is that of Jackson and Parker (1947). For reasons which will become clear in the discussion that follows, Lukes and his colleagues more recently reclassified the various histologic patterns which were subsequently again revised by a nomenclature committee (Lukes and Butler, 1966) (Lukes et al., 1966a) (Lukes et al., 1966b). The disease has not changed; only our view of it has. It serves no purpose to describe in detail the morphologic picture of all of the older categories. Table 18–3 presents a comparison of these three classifications and, in general, the relationship of the older categories to those most widely used at present.

The major justifications for the reclassification of Hodgkin's disease are: (1) a new conception of the significance of the lymphocytic and histiocytic components in Hodgkin's disease and (2) recognition of the nodular sclerosis variant and its far more favorable prognosis. At the time of the Jackson and Parker classification in 1947, little was known of cell-mediated immunity and the important role of lymphocytes and histiocytes in such responses. Based on this knowledge, experts in the field of Hodgkin's disease have become convinced that the presence of such cells implies an active

TABLE 18–3. COMPARISON OF CLASSIFICATIONS OF HODGKIN'S DISEASE*

Jackson and Parker (1947)	Lukes et al. (1966b)	Revision of Nomenclature Committee (Lukes 1966a)
Paragranuloma	Lymphocytic and/or Histiocytic a. Nodular b. Diffuse	Lymphocyte predominance
	Nodular sclerosis	Nodular sclerosis
Granuloma	Mixed	Mixed cellularity
	Diffuse fibrosis	
Sarcoma	Reticular	Lymphocyte depletion

*From Butler, J. J.: Histopathology of malignant lymphomas and Hodgkin's disease. In Leukemia-Lymphoma, A Collection of Papers Presented at the Fourteenth Annual Clinical Conference on Cancer, 1969, at the University of Texas, M. D. Anderson Hospital and Tumor Institute at Houston, Houston, Texas. Chicago, Ill., Year Book Medical Publishers, Inc., 1970, p. 135. Copyright © by Year Book Medical Publishers. Used by permission.

host defense and a more favorable prognosis. Conversely, those patterns of Hodgkin's disease depleted of lymphocytes and histiocytes are now thought to be more ominous since these hosts are either unable or have failed to respond immunologically to their disease.

Lymphocyte Predominance. This designation now embraces the paragranuloma pattern of Jackson and Parker (1947) and the subsequent lymphocytic and/or histiocytic nodular and diffuse patterns. In many series of cases, approximately 20 per cent of the patients present with this form. Cytologically, these nodes are replaced by nodules or a diffuse infiltrate of mixtures of lymphocytes and histiocytes. Most commonly, the node presents a monotonous sea of lymphocytes closely resembling lymphocytic lymphoma, WD or chronic lymphatic leukemia. Scattered histiocytes may be present in this background of lymphocytes. The critical diagnostic feature of this pattern is the generally infrequent and widely scattered RS cells (Fig. 18–15). They often lack the large "owl-eyed" nucleoli which make these giant cells distinctive. Recall that without their identification, however, the diagnosis of Hodgkin's disease cannot be made.

Mixed Cellularity. This variant, which represents about 25 per cent of the patients in any large collection of cases, includes the granuloma category of Jackson and Parker (1947). Here the appearance of the lymph node most resembles an inflammatory reactive process and contains a mixed population of lymphocytes, histiocytes, neutrophils, eosinophils and plasma cells (Fig. 18–16). Often there are areas of apparent inflammatory necrosis and varying degrees of fibrosis, particularly in proximity to the necrotic foci (Fig. 18–17). Eosinophils are often abundant and, in fact, may be present in sheets. Classic RS cells are usually plentiful. Lymphocytes are much less numerous than in the lymphocyte predominance form.

Lymphocyte Depletion. This pattern, which accounts for less than 20 per cent of the usual distribution of cases, corresponds to Hodgkin's sarcoma (as defined by Jackson and Parker) as well as to some of their more fibrotic variants of Hodgkin's granuloma. It also embraces the diffuse fibrosis and reticular patterns of Lukes. The range of morphology is quite broad and includes nodes which are largely or completely replaced by disorderly masses of connective tissue harboring only infrequent RS cells as well as a variant composed of large, pleomorphic anaplastic uni-

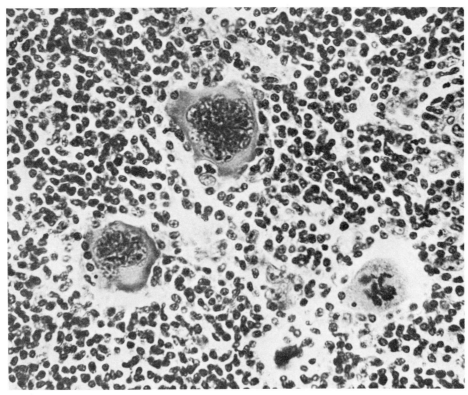

Figure 18–15. *Hodgkin's disease—lymphocyte predominance. Multinucleate Reed-Sternberg cells are unusually numerous in the field.*

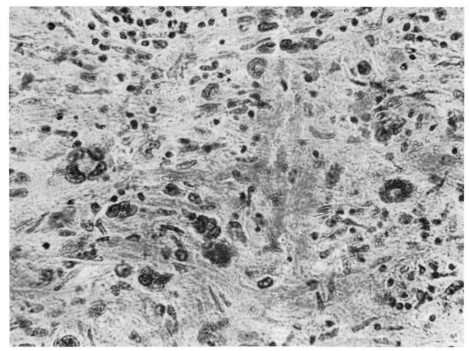

Figure 18–16. *The original case of Hodgkin's disease on which the first anatomic diagnosis was established. This pattern would now be called mixed cellularity.*

nuclear and multinuclear undifferentiated histiocytes. Some of the cells have the appearance of anaplastic variants of the RS cell and some conform to the classic prototype (Fig. 18–18). Significant in both the diffuse fibrosis and reticular patterns is the paucity or complete absence of lymphocytes. Similarly, eosinophils, plasma cells and areas of necrosis are absent. For a time, this category was divided into diffuse fibrosis and reticular variants, but it soon be-

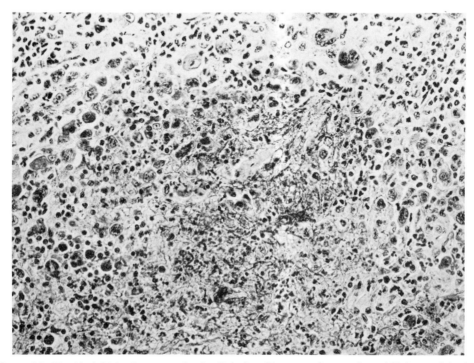

Figure 18–17. *Hodgkin's disease—mixed cellularity with areas of necrosis and fibrin precipitation.*

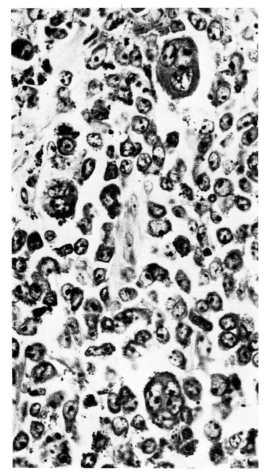

Figure 18–18. *Hodgkin's disease—lymphocyte depletion. The cellularity is composed almost entirely of anaplastic reticular forms with two large Reed-Sternberg cells above and below.*

came apparent that both pursued a similar rapidly downhill clinical course that justified their being lumped together into the category lymphocyte depletion.

Nodular Sclerosis. This newly defined category, which includes approximately 35 to 40 per cent of patients, is made distinctive by two features: (1) birefringent bands of collagen which extend into the node from the capsule, segregating and enclosing nodules of abnormal lymphoid tissue and (2) the tendency for the Reed-Sternberg cells to assume the lacunar morphology described on p. 760. Classically, the collagen bands are well defined and made of parallel arrays of fibers which are doubly refractile under polarized light (Fig. 18–19). In some cases, the fibrosis is abundant, leaving only suggestive islands of lymphoid tissue. Within these lymphoidal nodules, the pattern may take the form of lymphocyte predominance, mixed cellularity, or, at times, may be

composed almost entirely of lacunar cells. The delineation of this pattern of Hodgkin's disease may be quite treacherous since recent reports indicate that, in some patients, the collagen is scant and the diagnosis rests on the numerous lacunar cells. In other cases, the birefringent collagen is abundant, but lacunar cells are scant. Subsequent biopsies in these patients have disclosed the classic features of nodular sclerosis (Strum and Rappaport, 1971). It must be apparent that nodular sclerosis may, at times, be difficult to diagnose for all but the very expert (Rappaport et al., 1971).

Distribution of Lesions. At the outset, we should emphasize that the clinical staging of lymphoma discussed on p. 759 was in reality devised to provide a standardized nomenclature for the distribution and spread of Hodgkin's disease. An understanding of this clinical staging is crucial to the following discussion. In an analysis of 340 consecutive untreated cases of Hodgkin's disease, Kaplan (1968–69) found that when first seen, only 16 per cent were in stage I, 44 per cent in stage II, 26 per cent in stage III and 14 per cent in stage IV. In the great majority of cases in stage I, the unicentric focus of origin of the disease was in the lower cervical nodes or anterior superior mediastinum. The remaining stage I cases appeared

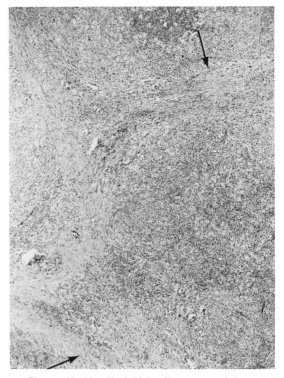

Figure 18–19. *Hodgkin's disease—nodular sclerosis. Bands of collagen traverse the node, isolating islands of lymphomatous tissue* (arrows).

to arise in either the axillary or inguinal nodes. There were no instances of primary Hodgkin's disease of the lungs, spleen or liver. More than half of the stage I cases arising in the superior mediastinum and adjacent lower cervical nodes turned out to be the nodular sclerosis variant. The remaining stage I cases were largely lymphocyte predominance. Almost always, the variants referred to as mixed cellularity and lymphocyte depletion were in stage III or IV when first diagnosed. In systemic spread, the disease may be found throughout all lymph nodes as well as in the spleen, liver, lungs, bones and in the pericardial, pleural and epidural spaces.

The gross appearance of involved nodes and viscera depends on the particular histologic variant. With lymphocyte predominance, the nodes have a soft uniform fish-flesh appearance and are not distinguishable from lymphoma. With mixed cellularity, foci of pale, opaque, yellow-white necrosis may be evident on the cut surface. With nodular sclerosis and the diffuse fibrotic patterns, involved nodes may be tough, gray-white and fibrous as would be expected. In such instances, groups of nodes are often firmly matted together. In the more aggressive forms, the disease may well have penetrated beyond the nodal capsules into the perinodal tissue. Involvement of spleen, liver, bone marrow and other solid organs usually takes the form of irregular, tumor-like nodules of tissue resembling that present in the nodes. At times the spleen is greatly enlarged and the liver moderately enlarged by these nodular masses which may coalesce to virtually replace the underlying native structure.

Clinical Course. The clinical features of Hodgkin's disease are a composite of those found in the lymphomas and in systemic infections. In individuals with focalized disease, the first manifestation may be the appearance of a painless, enlarged lymph node or nodes. Some of these patients and an even larger number of those with more diffuse disease suffer weight loss, weakness, fever, night sweats, pruritus, leukocytosis or leukopenia, eosinophilia and anemia. The febrile reaction classically takes the form of the so-called Pel-Ebstein fever characterized by temperature spikes at 2 to 3 day intervals separated by low-grade fever. This combination of fever, night sweats and weakness is highly reminiscent of an infection. With the advance of the disease, weight loss and weakness become more marked, splenomegaly, hepatomegaly and anemia more profound, and the patients next develop the cachexia common to all forms of cancer. One of the most characteristic features is the develop-

ment of anergy to antigens which normally elicit delayed cutaneous hypersensitivity (Aisenberg, 1962). In addition, a number of studies have suggested that the peripheral blood lymphocytes of patients with Hodgkin's disease are defective in their capacity to react to mitogenic stimulants and to undergo blast transformation (Hersh and Oppenheim, 1965). The significance of such immune unresponsiveness will be discussed soon.

The prognosis is strongly influenced by the dependent variables of the staging and the precise histologic variant involved. This relationship is shown in the following table drawn from data reported by Lukes and Butler (1966).

TABLE 18–4. RELATIONSHIP BETWEEN DEPENDENT VARIABLES OF STAGING AND HISTOLOGIC VARIANT IN HODGKIN'S DISEASE

Histologic Variant	Clinical Stage When First Seen (Approximate Percentages)		
	I	II	III
Lymphocyte predominance	70	20	10
Nodular sclerosis	40	40	20
Mixed	35	40	25
Lymphocyte depletion	15	35	50

Data from Lukes, R. J., and Butler, J. J.: The pathology and nomenclature of Hodgkin's disease. Cancer Res., 26:1063, 1966.

It is important to emphasize that, *in the individual patient, transformations may occur as the disease evolves. Patients having the lymphocyte predominance form of the disease may show, at subsequent biopsy, the mixed cellularity or lymphocyte depletion variants. Similarly, mixed cellularity may transform to lymphocyte depletion. The changes are always in the direction of more aggressive patterns of disease* and might be schematized as follows:

Lymphocyte predominance → Mixed cellularity → Lymphocyte depletion

On occasion, a group of nodes removed at one time may show several patterns simultaneously perhaps because they were caught in the process of change. Obviously, the prognosis is altered with each change in the form of the disease. It should be noted that *nodular sclerosis does not undergo transformation* and appears to be, in a sense, a different disease, as will soon be discussed.

Remarkable improvement has been achieved recently in the treatment of Hodgkin's disease with heavy doses of supervoltage radiation sometimes combined with chemotherapy, but success is largely limited by the stage of the disease. It is not unusual for cures to be achieved in patients with stage I and stage II disease and for remarkable control to be effected with more widely disseminated disease. Kaplan, (1968–69), one of the leading proponents of intensive radiotherapy, has reported recently almost 90 per cent five-year survival for stages I and II, 60 per cent five-year survival for stage III, and 35 per cent survival for stage IV. For all stages together, the five-year survival was 73 per cent. Accurate staging of the disease, then, is of paramount importance. It is now standard practice for such patients to have not only meticulous clinical examinations and extensive diagnostic radiography but in addition, bipedal lymphangiography and sometimes abdominal laparotomy to establish the possible presence of occult spread into the abdominal lymph nodes, spleen or liver.

Causation and Other Areas of Controversy. Much about Hodgkin's disease remains enigmatic as confirmed by the recent editorial entitled "Further in the Hodgkin Maze" (Editorial, 1971). What is the basic nature of the disorder—infectious or neoplastic? Do the many histologic variants represent biologic expressions of a single entity or more than one entity? Is the anergy primary to the development of the disease, or the consequence of destruction of lymphoid tissues? Does Hodgkin's disease begin in a single focus and then spread, or does the disease arise in multicentric foci? Other uncertainties might be cited, but the preceding represent the most important.

The basic nature of Hodgkin's disease remains a puzzle as mentioned earlier, since many features suggest an infectious process while others suggest neoplasia. Indicating an infectious disease are the clinical manifestations of fever, night sweats, leukocytosis, and the occasional patient who develops a peripheral eosinophilia. The mixed cellular variant of Hodgkin's disease with its predominance of eosinophils, neutrophils, plasma cells and occasional areas of necrosis more resembles an inflammatory disorder than a neoplasm. The fibrosing reaction in nodular sclerosis and the diffuse fibrosis of the lymphocyte depletion pattern would be compatible with a chronic inflammatory process. Countless infectious agents have been hailed as the etiology of Hodgkin's disease, but none of these propositions has withstood the test of time. More recently, enthusiasm waxed for the Epstein-Barr virus, but the excitement currently seems to be on the wane (Goldman and Aisenberg, 1970). Clusters of cases of Hodgkin's disease have been identified, one in a group of students in the same high school class (Vianna et al., 1971a). By painstaking and laborious efforts (interviewing 297 of 317 members of the class more than a decade after graduation), Davies (1972) has linked 40 cases of Hodgkin's to a clique, one or more of whom were exposed to friends with Hodgkin's disease. He feels so strongly about a transmissible agent that his recent study begins with the statement, "The long now outmoded controversy over whether Hodgkin's disease is infectious or neoplastic . . . ." However, no agent can be regularly isolated from involved nodes in this disease. Perhaps the agent may not be present in the typical nodal lesions but is held where intact lymphoid tissue may form a barrier. Possibly, only immune complexes producing an eosinophil response reach the nodes. In support of such speculation, it has been pointed out that the incidence of this disease is somewhat higher in those who have had a tonsillectomy or appendectomy, presumably providing breeches in the lymphoidal barrier (Vianna et al., 1971b).

On the other hand, there is a considerable amount of evidence that Hodgkin's disease is a neoplasm. Certainly its spread in the body conforms to that of a neoplasm. The cellular anaplasia encountered in the reticular variant of the lymphocyte depletion pattern justifies the older designation of Hodgkin's sarcoma and, in one case, a clone of hypotetraploid cells with distinctive marker chromosomes was identified (Seif and Spriggs, 1967). To reconcile these opposing points of view, *there is a widely held opinion that Hodgkin's disease starts as an inflammatory or infectious process which, in time, transforms to a true neoplasm.*

Yet another theory of causation of Hodgkin's disease suggests an immune disorder. The presence of anergy in these patients, the favorable prognosis for those variants containing numerous histiocytes and lymphocytes and, on the other hand, the ominous outlook in those forms depleted of lymphocytes are all consonant with an immune disorder. Speculation has been raised that the Reed-Sternberg cells are the neoplastic or antigenically altered components in Hodgkin's disease; and all other histologic features might represent a response to these "foreign agitators." In lymphocyte predominance, the host response theoretically would be strong and the disease kept in check, allowing for the favorable prognosis. If the Reed-Sternberg cells were not kept in check, other variants would successively appear, leading in time to the lymphocyte depletion pattern. Conceivably, some viral agent might be the mediator of the Reed-Sternberg cell neoplastic transformation, and the recruitment of the cell-mediated immune response against these invaders might, in time, lead to depletion or paralysis of this immune mechanism, providing an explanation for the anergy (graft vs.

host disease) (Order and Hellman, 1972). It suffices that, for the present, the nature and etiology of Hodgkin's disease remains an enigma.

Speculation recently has become intense about the possibility that the umbrella designation Hodgkin's disease embraces more than a single entity. Overall, males are affected nearly twice as often as females. The age incidence is bimodal with the first peak between the ages of 15 and 34 and the second over the age of 50 years. Nodular sclerosis, however, occurs predominantly in females and is heavily represented in the younger age peak. It tends to remain localized to the anterior superior mediastinum and lower cervical region and has, on the whole, a good prognosis. *It does not transform to the other variants.* Could it be a separate disease included under the term Hodgkin's disease only because it contains giant cells interpreted as Reed-Sternberg cells? The difficulty in the identification of these cells has already been described (p. 760). In a series of writings based on epidemiologic studies, MacMahon and his colleagues argue strongly for two etiologic entities (Newell, 1970) (Cole and MacMahon, 1968) (MacMahon, 1971). Again the issue remains unresolved.

The immunologic unresponsiveness of these patients has, for some long time, been considered a reflection of progressive destruction of the immune system by the disease. Studies of patients with stage I disease indicated that the incidence of immunologic hyporesponsiveness was far less than in those with advanced disease (Brown et al., 1967). However, recently an analysis of patients with stage I disease showed an extremely high incidence of anergy (Kaplan, 1968 to 1969). In the face of these discordant results, this problem remains unsolved. The cell-mediated anergy of this disease may not be merely the result of advanced lymphoidal destruction, but possibly may be crucial in the initiation of some form of immunologic causation.

The last controversy for consideration—namely, the issue of whether Hodgkin's disease begins in a unicentric focus or is multicentric from the very beginning—appears now to be resolved. By virtue of detailed lymphangiographic studies and the opportunity to follow patients with stage I to more advanced stages, the clear impression is gained that *the disease begins in one focus and then spreads via fairly predictable channels* (Kaplan, 1968–69). Thus, an origin in the anterior superior mediastinum would be expected to spread upward to the cervical region and through the lower mediastinum to below the diaphragm. Some of the so-called discontinuous or "skip" patterns of spread reported in the past might merely be examples of the inadequacy of earlier methods to detect minor degrees of involvement of deeply situated nodes and organs. With lymphangiography and exploratory laparotomy, these discontinuities have disappeared and now predictable patterns of spread can almost always be shown.

So we conclude this consideration of Hodgkin's disease with the unknown still outweighing the known.

SECONDARY TUMORS

Because of their widespread distribution and close lymphatic connections with the organs of the body, the nodes are commonly seeded by all forms of visceral cancer. Such metastatic spread occurs in both carcinomas and sarcomas but is more common with the former. The metastatic cells first proliferate in the sinuses and then eventually cause complete obliteration of the normal structure of the nodes. The metastasis usually resembles the primary tumor, but in some cases it is less well differentiated. If the primary is scirrhous, the secondary growth also tends to be scirrhous. In addition to metastases to the regional nodes, involvement of more distant nodes takes place as the disease progresses.

SPLEEN

NORMAL
PATHOLOGY
Congenital Anomalies
Inflammation
  Nonspecific acute splenitis
  Nonspecific subacute or
    chronic splenitis
  Specific forms of splenitis
    Tuberculosis
    Syphilis
    Typhoid fever

  Malaria
  Infectious mononucleosis
  Hyaline perisplenitis
Vascular Disease
  Acute congestion
  Chronic congestion
  Hypersplenism
  Infarcts
Hematologic Disorders
  Involving red cells
    Sickle cell anemia

    Hereditary spherocytosis
    Polycythemia vera
    Thalassemia
    Autoimmune hemolytic
      anemia
  Involving white cells
    Leukemias
    Agranulocytosis
  Involving platelets
    Thrombocytopenic purpura
      (idiopathic purpura,

Werlhof's disease)	Gaucher's disease	Primary
Involving more than one	Niemann-Pick disease	Benign
blood element	Hand-Schüller-Christian	Malignant
Myeloproliferative	complex	Secondary
syndrome (agnogenic	Diabetic lipoidosis	**Rupture of the Spleen**
myeloid metaplasia)	**Tumors**	**Interpretation of Splenomegaly**
Lipidoses		

NORMAL

The spleen is one of the so-called secondary lymphoid organs in contrast to the thymus (p. 195). It is active in blood formation during the initial part of fetal life. This function decreases so that at the fifth or sixth gestational month the spleen attains its adult character devoid of hematopoietic activity.

The spleen contains the largest amount of lymphoid tissue in the body. The organ is oval in shape and measures some 12 cm. in length, 7 cm. in width and 3 cm. in thickness. The average weight is 150 gm. Various pathologic conditions lead to marked variations in its size and weight. The spleen is bluish red and is surrounded by a slate gray, smooth, glistening capsule except at the hilus. Its consistency is firm, and its cut surface is red dotted with gray specks which are the malpighian corpuscles.

The splenic artery travels along the superior border of the pancreas, sometimes behind it, and is, therefore, vulnerable to pancreatic lesions. On entering the spleen, it immediately branches into the trabecular arteries which then enter the white pulp as central arteries. From here the arterial supply enters the red pulp. From this point on, there is considerable controversy. The age-old dispute centers about the question: is the circulation "open" or "closed"? Strangely, electron microscopists have not resolved this problem, but at least one careful study demonstrates an "open" circulation (Weiss, 1957).

To clarify this statement, it is necessary to give some of the details of the fine structure of the red pulp. It is made up of two principal elements, the splenic sinuses alternating with the splenic cords. The sinuses are long irregular channels lined by endothelial cells or flattened reticular cells. The recent electron microscopy study cited indicates pores or gaps between the lining cells, implying that the circulation is "open" and that the blood cells can freely leave the sinuses to enter the intervening cords, the so-called cords of Billroth. The basement membrane shared by the cord and the adjacent splenic sinuses is also perforated. Reticular cells with delicate processes sometimes bridge the cords of Billroth. Thus these highly phagocytic cells create an open meshwork of the cords. The blood that leaves the splenic sinuses

to enter the reticulated cords passes, as it were, through a complex filter. This type of circulation would suggest that foreign bodies above a certain size or of irregular shape might easily be trapped in the reticular net. Abnormal blood cells, for example, might easily be sequestered and destroyed by the actively phagocytic reticular cells. Confirming this impression, it has been demonstrated that granules with a diameter greater than 5 microns are largely retained while those of smaller size appear to pass.

The venous drainage of the sinuses and cords is not too well defined, but it is reasonable to assume that tributaries of the splenic veins connect with the sinuses of the red pulp. High resolution studies of the clearly defined veins indicate the usual normal architecture with an intact basement membrane and interlocking endothelial cells. From here, the splenic vein follows the course of the artery to join eventually with the superior mesenteric vein to form the portal vein. The so-called white pulp is composed principally of the malpighian corpuscles, while the red pulp constitutes the sinuses and intervening spaces. Extending from the capsule inward are the trabeculae containing blood vessels and lymphatics.

The aggregates of lymphoid tissue or malpighian corpuscles have the same structure as the follicles in the lymph nodes, but they differ in that the splenic follicles surround arteries so that on cross section each contains a central artery. These follicles are scattered throughout the organ and are not confined to the peripheral layer or cortex as in lymph nodes.

As a part of the reticuloendothelial system, the spleen plays an important role in the defense mechanism of the body and is also implicated in pigment and lipid metabolism. The spleen, however, is by no means essential to life for it can be removed with no ill effects upon the body as a whole, although certain abnormalities are produced in the circulating blood. Splenectomy may be followed by a temporary anemia and leukocytosis, an increase in the number of platelets and nucleated red cells as well as reticulocytes, and the appearance of Howell-Jolly bodies in the red cells.

The spleen has a poorly understood relationship to blood formation in the bone marrow.

When the normal activities of the bone marrow are interfered with, as occurs in replacement with tumor metastases and fibrosis, the spleen readily reverts to its embryonic function of blood formation. It is one of the sites of the removal of senescent red cells. Since it is one of the lymphoid organs, it supplies lymphocytes to the circulating blood and also takes part in immune reactions.

In animals, but to a questionable degree in man, the spleen has a reservoir function; i.e., in emergencies such as acute blood loss, large amounts of blood are liberated from the spleen into the general circulation.

PATHOLOGY

The spleen as the largest unit of the reticuloendothelial system is involved in all systemic inflammations, generalized hematopoietic disorders and many metabolic disturbances such as the lipoidoses. It is rarely the primary site of disease and, therefore, for correlation with clinical disease one must refer to underlying bases of splenic derangement.

CONGENITAL ANOMALIES

Complete absence of the spleen is rare and is usually associated with other congenital abnormalities. *Hypoplasia* is a more common finding.

Abnormal lobulations, either shallow or deep, are another form of anomaly. These must be distinguished from depressed healed infarcts.

Accessory spleens are common and have been encountered singly or multiply in one-fifth to one-third of all postmortems. They are usually small spherical structures which are histologically and functionally identical with the normal spleen, reacting to various stimuli in the same manner. They are usually situated in the gastrosplenic ligament or in the tail of the pancreas but are sometimes located in the omentum or mesenteries of the small or large intestine. Accessory spleens may have great clinical importance. In some hematologic disorders such as hereditary spherocytosis, thrombocytopenic purpura and hypersplenism, splenectomy is a standard method of treatment. If an accessory spleen is overlooked, the benefit from the removal of the definitive spleen is totally lost since the adverse influence of the splenic tissue, whatever it may be, is perpetuated by accessory spleniculi.

INFLAMMATION

NONSPECIFIC ACUTE SPLENITIS

Grossly, the spleen is enlarged (up to 200 to 400 gm.) and soft, and on section the pulp is often diffluent. The color of the cut surface varies from grayish red to deep red, and the malpighian corpuscles and trabeculae are usually obscured. These alterations are graphically designated by the term "tomato catsup" spleen.

Microscopically, the sinuses are engorged with blood and contain increased numbers of polymorphonuclear leukocytes and often also numerous macrophages, many of which may contain phagocytized red cells or pigment. The malpighian corpuscles may be hyperplastic or not affected. Hemorrhages may be seen in the pulp. This form of acute splenitis is often spoken of as **acute splenic tumor.**

The most common disease conditions producing acute splenitis are bacteremias as in vegatative endocarditis, but any other severe systemic inflammatory disorder, such as diphtheria, bacillary dysentery or pneumonia, may effect similar splenic changes. Acute splenitis may be induced by noninfectious disease and is encountered in any extensive tissue destruction of chemical or physical nature presumably because the spleen is active in resorption of necrotic cell products. In severe toxemic diseases, such as those caused by the group A hemolytic streptococcal infections, acute necrosis of the centers of the splenic follicles may occur. These reactions may or may not be accompanied by the diffuse pulp changes just described. Abscess formation may take place in pyemia or may be caused by septic emboli, especially those that arise in bacterial vegetations in the heart.

NONSPECIFIC SUBACUTE OR CHRONIC SPLENITIS

This condition is seen most commonly in certain specific diseases described in detail in the next section. The next most frequent cause is vegetative (bacterial) endocarditis.

The organ is enlarged, rarely up to 1000 gm., and is firm in consistency. The cut surface is gray, and infarcts are often present when the underlying cause is vegetative endocarditis. Microscopically, there are numerous macrophages and plasma cells in the sinuses and pulp spaces so that the architecture appears flooded and solid (Fig. 18–20). In addition, numerous polymorphonuclear leukocytes may be present. The littoral reticuloendothelial

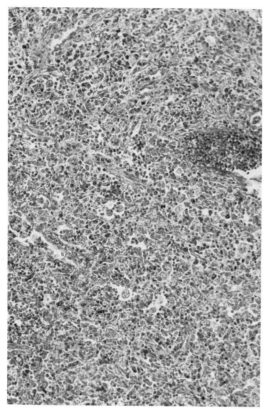

Figure 18–20. *Nonspecific chronic splenitis. A view of the spleen substance. The sinuses are filled with macrophages and other white cells so that the low power architecture is suffused with cells.*

cells are hypertrophic and cuboidal, and occasional cells may be found in mitotic activity. Very often these reticuloendothelial elements and the free macrophages in the sinuses contain phagocytized debris.

SPECIFIC FORMS OF SPLENITIS

While the following diseases have been described elsewhere as producing distinctive if not pathognomonic inflammatory reactions in all their sites of localization, certain ones will be described in this section because of the peculiarities of their lesions in the spleen. The specific infections which may affect the spleen are as follows: tuberculosis, syphilis, sarcoid, infectious mononucleosis, typhoid, brucellosis, malaria, kala-azar, histoplasmosis, torulosis, schistosomiasis, anthrax, actinomycosis, blastomycosis, echinococcosis and cysticercosis.

Tuberculosis. Miliary tubercles are almost always found in the spleen in generalized miliary tuberculosis. It was pointed out earlier that certain tissues favor the growth of tubercle bacilli and therefore are commonly involved in the hematogenous dissemination of miliary tuberculosis. The spleen is one such favorable soil. Although rare in adults, splenic involvement is common in children with pulmonary tuberculosis. The spleen is enlarged but usually does not exceed 500 to 600 gm. in weight (Fig. 18–21). Greater increases are uncommon. The tubercles are usually found in the malpighian corpuscles. Caseous, confluent tuberculosis is a more uncommon form of the disease. In the miliary form, the tubercular lesions are not evident grossly but, in the confluent variety, they are readily visible as yellow-white, irregular necroses.

Syphilis. The spleen is often enlarged in congenital lues, rarely more than twice normal. It is firm and microscopically shows an infiltration with lymphocytes and plasma cells and an increase in connective tissue. These alterations are entirely nondistinctive. Here and in acquired lues, gummas occur rarely. Splenomegaly in the tertiary stage is usually secondary to the congestive changes induced by luetic cirrhosis of the liver.

Typhoid Fever. The spleen is characteristically enlarged to the range of 250 to 500 gm. While focal necroses similar to those seen in other organs are present, the outstanding feature is the filling of the pulp with histiocytic cells containing numerous phagocytized red cells. The lining cells of the sinuses are hypertrophic and often display active phagocytosis of red cells and other cellular debris.

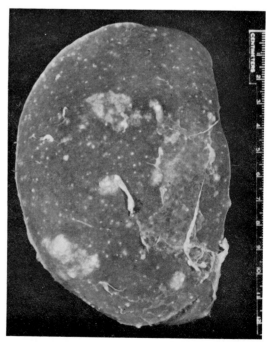

Figure 18–21. *Tuberculosis of spleen. The foci of pale white caseation are evident through the capsule.*

Malaria. In the acute stage the spleen is enlarged and soft. Microscopically, the parasites are seen in the pulp lying free, in red cells, or in reticulum cells. The lining reticuloendothelial cells are often stuffed with the parasites and malarial pigment. Focal necroses also occur. In the chronic stage the spleen is markedly enlarged, usually in the range of 1000 gm. but possibly up to 4000 gm. and is firm. The capsule is thickened and often adhesions to surrounding organs develop. Microscopically, there is a marked increase in connective tissue. With cure of the disease, the spleen shrinks. The histologic picture is characterized by scarring and masses of pigment in the reticular cells and sinus endothelial cells.

Infectious Mononucleosis. The spleen is enlarged in at least 50 per cent of the cases and is usually two to three times normal size. It is usually soft, fleshy and markedly hyperemic. The native architecture is blurred by the proliferation of typical and atypical lymphocytes that fill the sinuses, infiltrate the trabeculae and capsule, and produce an overall diffuse cellularity that suggests an infiltrative growth. The capsular infiltration is particularly significant because it tends to thin the capsule and thus predisposes this organ to rupture, one of the important complications of infectious mononucleosis (p. 470).

HYALINE PERISPLENITIS

Hyaline perisplenitis is an anatomic lesion of only academic interest. It is not associated with any clinical dysfunction. The lesion consists of marked collagenous thickening and "sugar coating" of the splenic capsule (Fig. 18–22). The involvement may be limited to a focal plaque or may totally envelop the spleen. The capsular fibrosis varies from one to many millimeters in thickness. Histologically, it consists only of dense, hyaline, collagenous, fibrous tissue that is limited to the capsule. The genesis of this lesion is totally obscure. It is postulated that it represents a healed, inflammatory perisplenitis. However, in most instances, no such infection can be identified anatomically or historically. Occasionally, these changes occur in patients who have longstanding ascites, and the hyaline perisplenitis is attributed to fibrosis of a chronic, capsular edema.

VASCULAR DISEASE

ACUTE CONGESTION

The spleen shows a mild degree of hyperemia during the process of digestion. A

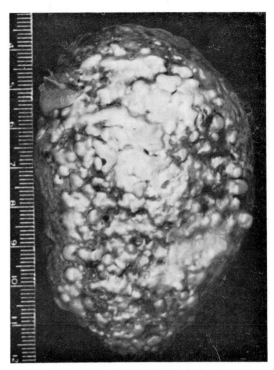

Figure 18–22. Hyaline perisplenitis.

more marked degree of active hyperemia is seen associated with various toxemias and acute infections. Grossly, the spleen is enlarged moderately, rarely over 250 gm. in weight, and is soft. Its cut surface is red. Microscopically, the sinuses are distended with red cells such that the distance between the malpighian corpuscles widens.

CHRONIC CONGESTION

Persistent or chronic venous congestion may cause enlargement of the spleen, a condition referred to as *congestive splenomegaly*. The venous congestion may be systemic in origin, may be caused by intrahepatic obstruction to portal venous drainage, or may be due to obstructive venous disorders in the portal or splenic veins. All these disorders ultimately lead to portal or splenic vein hypertension. *Systemic or central venous congestion* is encountered in cardiac decompensation involving the right side of the heart and therefore is found in any type of longstanding cardiac decompensation. It is particularly severe in tricuspid or pulmonic valvular disease and in chronic cor pulmonale. In systemic venous stasis there are accompanying congestive changes in the liver and intestines and frequently associated ascites and peripheral edema. Such systemic passive congestion produces only moderate enlargement of the spleen so that it rarely exceeds 500 gm. in weight.

The most common causes of striking congestive splenomegaly are the various forms of cirrhosis of the liver. The diffuse fibrous scarring of fatty nutritional cirrhosis and pigment cirrhosis evokes the most extreme enlargements. Less commonly the other forms of cirrhosis are implicated. In these conditions, there is sufficient impingement on the venous drainage through the liver to cause marked stasis within the portal system. At the same time, it is postulated that portohepatic artery shunts develop to further raise the portal and splenic vein pressures. Only infrequently does tumorous obstruction of the vasculature of the liver give rise to congestive changes in the spleen. It is therefore uncommon for diffuse metastatic seeding of the liver to produce significant portal hypertension. Primary hepatic carcinoma may be an exception when it invades the major hepatic vessels.

Congestive splenomegaly is also caused by obstruction to the extrahepatic portal vein or splenic vein. The venous obstruction may be due to *spontaneous portal vein thrombosis.* Such thrombosis is usually associated with some intrahepatic obstructive disease, or it may be initiated by inflammatory involvement of the portal vein *(pylephlebitis)* such as follows intraperitoneal infections. Thrombosis of the splenic vein itself may be initiated by the pressure of tumors in neighboring organs, for example, carcinoma of the stomach or pancreas. Less often, it occurs as a splenic thrombophlebitis resulting from suppurative peritonitis or as a bland thrombosis secondary to upper abdominal surgery or some disorder that predisposes to systemic venous thromboses.

Longstanding congestive splenomegaly produces marked enlargement of the spleen (1000 gm. or more); the organ is firm and becomes increasingly so the longer the duration of the congestion. The weight may reach 5000 gm. The capsule may be thickened and fibrous but is otherwise uninvolved. The cut surface has a meaty appearance and varies from gray-red to deep red depending upon the amount of fibrosis. Often the malpighian corpuscles are indistinct. Small gray to brown firm nodules scattered throughout the red pulp constitute the so-called **Gandy-Gamna** nodules described below. Microscopically, the pulp is suffused with red cells during the early phases but becomes increasingly more fibrous and cellular with time. The walls of the venous sinuses are thickened and cellular, and the space between them is filled with proliferated fibroblasts or reticuloendothelial cells (Fig. 18–23). Sometimes the sinuses are compressed by the sur-

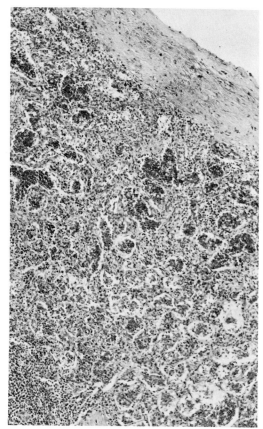

Figure 18–23. Congestive splenomegaly. The congestion of the sinuses, fibrosis and widening of the walls of the sinuses and the fibrosis of the capsule are the dominant features shown.

rounding cellularity. Foci of recent or old hemorrhage may be present with deposition of hemosiderin in histiocytes. It is the organization of these focal hemorrhages that give rise to the Gandy-Gamna nodules—foci of fibrosis containing deposits of iron and calcium salts encrusted on connective tissue and elastic fibers. The trabeculae are thickened and fibrous. In longstanding splenic congestion, foci of hematopoiesis appear, presumably as a response to the local vascular stasis and hypoxia.

HYPERSPLENISM

Hypersplenism is the term used to designate a symptom complex characterized by congestive splenomegaly, leukopenia and anemia (McMichael, 1934). For many years, this condition was referred to as *Banti's disease* and it was considered a primary hematologic disorder with secondary involvement of the spleen. Currently it is believed that the splenic enlargement is primary. The associated hematologic alterations, i.e., anemia, leukopenia, or thrombocytopenia, singly or in any combination, are attributed to excessive destruction of blood cells in the spleen — hence the designation "hypersplenism" (Dameshek, 1955) (Doan and Wright, 1946). The validation of this pathogenetic sequence for the hematologic change derives, in large part, from the clinical improvement that follows splenectomy.

The hypersplenic syndrome has been divided into primary and secondary types. Primary hypersplenism refers to increased splenic activity in the absence of known underlying cause for the increase in size or functional activity of the spleen. *Secondary hypersplenism* may occur in patients who have a recognized cause for the splenomegaly, such as leukemia, lymphoma, infectious diseases, congestive splenomegaly, or Felty's syndrome (a symptom complex comprising polyarthritis, fever, anemia, leukopenia and splenomegaly). However, even in these secondary patterns, the basis for the abnormal splenic hyperactivity is still not understood. In both the primary and secondary forms, the spleen is almost always enlarged, but a few investigators believe that splenomegaly is not a sine qua non, since they believe excessive activity may be associated with normal size.

Three mechanisms have been proposed to explain the increased destruction of the blood elements by the spleen. (1) Hyperplasia of reticuloendothelial elements might lead to increased sequestration and phagocytosis of the blood elements (Von Haam and Awny, 1948). In many patients, no morphologic evidence of increased phagocytic activity or sequestration is present, and hence other explanations are required. (2) The spleen might produce a hormone or circulating substance capable of depressing marrow function or of inhibiting maturation of marrow elements. Some experimental observations support this proposal. Palmer et al. (1953) were able to produce an experimental model of the hypersplenic syndrome in rats by administering methylcellulose to them. This macromolecular substance was phagocytized by the reticuloendothelial system and caused marked splenomegaly accompanied by anemia, leukopenia and thrombocytopenia. The administration of similar amounts of methylcellulose to previously splenectomized rats failed to produce the hematologic changes. Using this experimental model, Perez-Tamayo et al. (1960) demonstrated that the urine of these rats contained a substance which, when administered to normal rats, would produce thrombocytopenia and a delayed anemia. These results strongly suggested that a circulating substance

had been elaborated. The circulation of some inhibitory substance has also been demonstrated by parabiotic experiments. However, to date it has not been possible to identify similar circulating agents in patients. (3) The elaboration of antibodies against specific elements of the blood might explain their destruction. This pathogenesis was well documented in thrombocytopenia when Harrington and his coworkers (1951) demonstrated in vitro an antiplatelet factor from the plasma of patients with idiopathic thrombocytopenia. Leukoagglutinins also have been shown in certain patients with neutropenia and agranulocytosis. This conception of the hypersplenic syndrome likens the disorder to one of autoimmune origin in which, for obscure reasons, antibodies against self are produced in the spleen.

Whatever the underlying mechanism, the diagnosis of the hypersplenic syndrome can be established only by removal of the spleen followed by improvement in the hematologic derangement.

INFARCTS

Splenic infarcts are comparatively common lesions. Caused by occlusion of the major splenic artery or any of its branches, they are almost always due to emboli that arise in the heart. The spleen, along with kidneys and brain, ranks as one of the most frequent sites of localization of systemic emboli. The infarcts may be small or large, multiple or single, or sometimes involve the entire organ. Usually the infarcts are of the bland, anemic type. Septic infarcts are found in vegetative endocarditis of the valves of the left side of the heart. Much less often, infarcts in the spleen are caused by local thromboses, especially in leukemia, the myeloproliferative syndrome, sickle cell anemia, polyarteritis nodosa, Hodgkin's disease, and bacteremic diseases.

Infarcts are characteristically pale and wedge-shaped with their bases at the periphery where the capsule is often covered with fibrin (Fig. 18-24). Septic infarction modifies this appearance as frank suppurative necrosis develops. In the course of the healing of these splenic infarcts, large, depressed scars may occur. The uncommon pattern of scattered in situ thromboses is characterized as the "spotted spleen" or "fleckmilz." It is usually produced by acute infectious diseases which initiate acute vasculitis and thromboses of splenic vessels. In this condition, the splenic substance is dotted by minute infarctions that vary from 1 mm. up to 0.5 cm. in diameter.

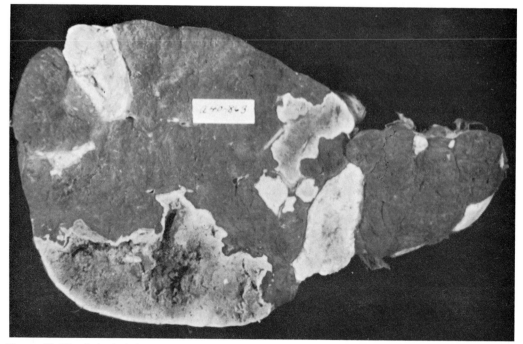

Figure 18–24. *Splenic infarcts. Multiple wedge-shaped lesions are present, the largest having developed cystic softening.*

Splenic infarcts are an important clinical consideration in older cardiac patients who suddenly complain of left upper quadrant pain. This clinical accident is a not unusual accompaniment of bacterial vegetative endocarditis. Occasionally in these cases, the fibrinous perisplenitis leads to friction rubs that can be heard in the left upper quadrant. The destruction of splenic substance is not critically significant and the major importance of these infarcts is their differentiation from other more serious intra-abdominal diseases that cause left upper quadrant pain, e.g., rupture of the spleen, perforation of the stomach or intestines, or rupture of an intra-abdominal aneurysm.

THE SPLEEN IN HEMATOLOGIC DISORDERS

DISORDERS INVOLVING RED CELLS

Sickle Cell Anemia. In the earlier stages of the disease seen in infants and children, the spleen is enlarged with marked congestion of the red pulp. Sinuses may be literally stuffed with sickled red cells. With the passage of time, the spleen undergoes progressive infarction and fibrosis and so decreases in size until, in adults, only a small mass of fibrous tissue may be found weighing less than 1 gm. *(autosplenectomy)* (Fig. 18–25). At this time fibrosis, hemo-

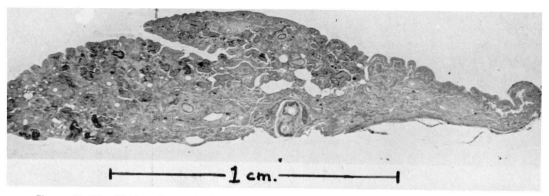

Figure 18–25. *Sickle cell anemia. A cross section of a totally fibrotic spleen, "autosplenectomy."*

siderin pigment and siderotic nodules are found within the red pulp, virtually replacing it and, at the same time, compressing the white pulp to the point of extinction.

It is generally believed that these changes result when sickled cells plug the vasculature of the splenic substance effectively producing ischemic destruction of the spleen. The lysis of the red cells releases the hemosiderin pigment found throughout the red pulp as well as in the siderotic (Gandy-Gamna) nodules.

Hereditary Spherocytosis (Congenital Hemolytic Jaundice). The spleen is enlarged and sometimes weighs over 1000 gm. The cut surface is purplish red and homogeneous. The characteristic microscopic picture is the presence of dilated and practically empty sinuses lined by hypertrophic endothelial cells (Thompson, 1932). There is a variable increase in iron pigment as well as iron encrustations in the trabeculae. Although similar anatomic alterations have been described in acquired hemolytic anemias, the spleen in these conditions is more often unremarkable save possibly for some increased hemosiderosis (p. 706).

Polycythemia Vera. The spleen is variably enlarged, rather firm, and blue-red in color. Commonly it weighs in the range of 250 to 350 gm. but rarely may be massively increased in size. Infarcts and thromboses are common. The follicles are small and the pulp congested. In some cases, foci of extramedullary myelopoiesis are present in the pulp.

Thalassemia. In the hereditary form of homozygous beta thalassemia, the spleen is enlarged in the range of 300 to 1000 gm. Grossly it appears dark red and congested. Microscopically, the principal alterations consist of variable degrees of sinusoidal congestion, hyperplasia of the reticuloendothelial cells and occasionally, foci of extramedullary hematopoiesis. Rarely, there is phagocytosis of red cells by the cells lining the sinusoids. This change, however, is not prominent and perhaps is more directly related to the number of transfusions the patient has received rather than to the underlying hematologic disorder. In occasional cases, hemosiderosis is present.

Autoimmune Hemolytic Anemia (AHA). Autoimmune hemolytic anemia (p. 226) may occur without underlying disease in the primary form, or it may be seen as a secondary disorder in patients already suffering from some disease of the reticuloendothelial or hematopoietic systems, such as lymphoma, leukemia, infectious mononucleosis and others. In the secondary form, the splenic changes are dominated by the underlying disease. In the warm antibody form, the spleen is variably enlarged. It appears congested but is otherwise not altered. On microscopic examination, the splenic follicles may be normal but sometimes are enlarged with active germinal centers. The red pulp is generally congested, sometimes with compression of the venous sinuses. In other cases, the sinuses contain small numbers of red cells. Particularly prominent are the hypertrophied lining cells of the sinuses, a change reminiscent of hereditary spherocytosis. That these enlarged cells often contain phagocytized red cells as well as hemosiderin pigment suggests that the spleen takes an active role in destroying erythrocytes.

DISORDERS INVOLVING WHITE CELLS

Leukemias. The leukemias produce some of the most striking forms of splenomegaly. Chronic myelogenous leukemia may be responsible for more extreme enlargement of the spleen than any other disease. Depending upon the duration of the disorder, the splenic weight usually ranges from 1000 to 3000 gm. Weights of 6000 to 8000 gm. are not rare. The organ is symmetrically enlarged, firm, has a thickened capsule and, on cut section, has a firm muddy, gray-red color. Characteristically, numerous small infarcts punctuate the cut surface and the splenic external appearance (Figs. 18–26 and 18–27). Histologically, the splenic architecture is nearly obliterated by a diffuse permeation of the leukemic cells of granulocytic origin. In acute myelogenous leukemia, the spleen may or may not be enlarged and is often remarkably negative save for scattered immature cells of the granulocytic series.

Chronic lymphatic leukemia is responsible for less severe degrees of splenic enlargement than chronic myelogenous leukemia. Rarely does the spleen exceed 2000 gm. in weight. The organ is symmetrically enlarged, has a thickened capsule and, on cross section, has the same gray-red, firm surface seen in myelogenous leukemia. Infarctions are uncommon, however. Diffuse infiltration with cells of the lymphatic type eventually causes total obscuration of the underlying architecture. In less advanced disease, follicles and sinuses may be discernible.

Monocytic leukemia causes only a mild degree of splenomegaly, rarely over 500 gm. in weight.

Agranulocytosis. The spleen is sometimes enlarged. Microscopically, there is congestion, and follicles are small and no polymorphonuclear leukocytes are present. In some cases small foci of necrosis are seen.

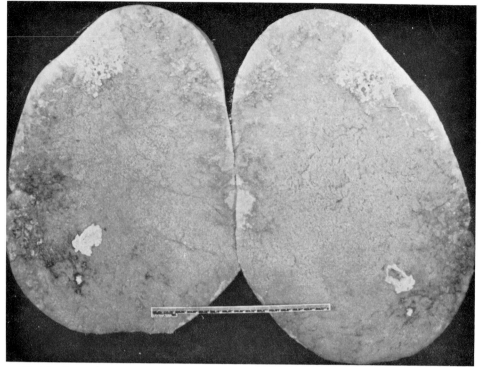

Figure 18–26. *Spleen in myelogenous leukemia. The massive enlargement dwarfs the 15 cm. rule. Numerous small infarcts are dispersed through the cut surface.*

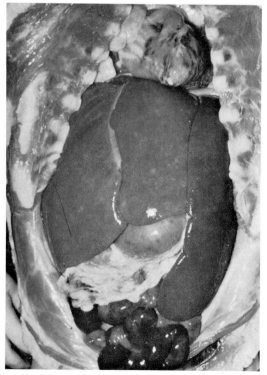

Figure 18–27. *The viscera in a child of 8 with chronic myelogenous leukemia. Note the massive hepatosplenomegaly, the pale leukemic infiltrates in the liver, and the hemorrhages in the subepicardial fat as manifestations of depression of platelet formation.*

DISORDERS INVOLVING PLATELETS

Thrombocytopenic Purpura (Idiopathic Purpura, Werlhof's Disease). The spleen is sometimes moderately enlarged in this condition and usually ranges between 150 and 250 gm. Macroscopically, it appears entirely normal. Histologically, the alterations are inconstant, subtle and, in any event, do not provide an anatomic basis for the abnormal destruction of platelets. The most constant microscopic features are active malpighian corpuscles, an abnormal number of eosinophils and megakaryocytes in the splenic pulp and, occasionally, focal areas of hemorrhage, presumably related to the bleeding diathesis (Nickerson and Sunderland, 1937).

DISORDERS INVOLVING MORE THAN ONE BLOOD ELEMENT

Myeloproliferative Syndrome (Agnogenic Myeloid Metaplasia, Chronic Nonleukemic Myelosis, Myelofibrosis). This entity is known by many names because, for some long time, it was thought to be a primary splenic disorder. At the present time, the view is favored that the splenic changes are a consequence of the myeloproliferative syndrome, principally the myelofibrotic variant (p. 738) (Ward and Block, 1970). Characteristically, the spleen shows striking extramedullary hematopoiesis along with dyspoietic megakaryocytosis. The following sequence is postulated: first, marrow hematopoiesis is suppressed or indeed replaced by extensive fibrosis of the marrow. The resultant anemia leads in time to compensatory extramedullary hematopoiesis affecting principally the spleen and, to a lesser degree, the liver. Along with such active extramedullary blood formation, immature white and red cells are sometimes released into the circulating blood, creating peripheral blood smears which may be confused with myelogenous leukemia.

The principal anatomic changes comprise striking extramedullary hematopoiesis. The principal site of such extramedullary hematopoiesis is the spleen, which is usually moderately to markedly enlarged, sometimes up to 4000 gm. (Fig. 18–28). The capsule is unaffected but occasionally shows underlying small infarcts. On section it is firm, red to gray and not dissimilar from that of myelogenous leukemia. However, the lymphoid follicles are usually preserved, implying that there has been no neoplastic obliteration of the native architecture. Histologically, there is usually orderly hematopoiesis in these extramedullary sites with relatively normal proportions of maturing red cells, white cells and platelets, but certain cases show a disproportional activity in any one of these three major lines.

The liver is also sometimes moderately enlarged with foci of extramedullary hematopoiesis. The lymph nodes are only rarely the site of blood formation and are usually not enlarged, an important feature since in the leukemias lymphadenopathy would classically be anticipated.

The bone marrow findings are extremely variable, ranging from hyper- to normo- to hypocellular marrows. The most common pattern is that of hypocellularity with secondary myelofibrosis. Notably absent in the marrow, as a differential point from leukemia, is any specific single cell line of neoplastic proliferation such as might be anticipated in myelogenous leukemia.

It is evident from the anatomic findings that patients with agnogenic myeloid metaplasia have extramedullary hematopoiesis as though there were primary marrow failure. Consequently, the various fetal sites of blood formation resume compensatory activity. Conceivably, certain atypical patterns of myelogenous leukemia might fit into this group wherein sufficient destruction of marrow elements by the leukemic cells might lead to the extramedullary hematopoiesis seen in myeloid metaplasia. The cases with myelofibrosis would also substantiate such a proposal.

Toxic injuries to bone marrow by such agents as infections, radiation and industrial solvents have been proposed as possible causes of this syndrome. Of the original ten cases described by Jackson et al. (1940), six patients had a history of exposure to industrial solvents. If toxic exposure were always the underlying cause, one would expect evidence of marrow injury in all cases, but as mentioned, hypercellular marrows are sometimes encountered.

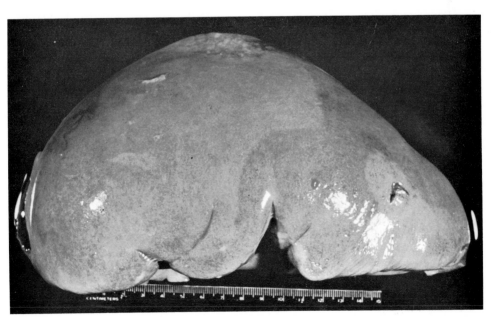

Figure 18–28. *Myeloproliferative syndrome. The organ is markedly enlarged and firm. The irregular shading of the capsule is artefact.*

It must be remembered in this connection that marrow hypercellularity is not necessarily associated with the production and release of adequate numbers of peripheral circulating blood cells. The finding of a polycythemic pattern in some patients, increased levels of platelets in others, and fairly striking elevations of the white count in still others supports the theory that agnogenic myeloid metaplasia is part of the myeloproliferative syndrome in which any one of the cell lines in the marrow may be involved. In the usual case, the principal derangement is proliferation of marrow stromal fibroblasts (Linman and Bethell, 1957).

LIPIDOSES

GAUCHER'S DISEASE

The spleen is enlarged, weighing sometimes as much as 8000 gm. and is firm in consistency. The color of the cut surface is grayish red with whitish streaks and flecks or nodules. The microscopic picture is characterized by large (20 to 80 microns) reticular cells or histiocytes, round or oval and often multinucleated, which fill the sinuses and pulp spaces and encroach on the follicles. The cells' cytoplasm which contains glucocerebroside has a characteristic crumpled tissue paper appearance (p. 299).

NIEMANN-PICK DISEASE

The spleen is enlarged and the cut surface is salmon colored. Microscopically, the histiocytic cells containing the lipid appear foamy and are situated mainly in the pulp spaces. The cells may contain one or two nuclei, but multinucleated cells as seen in Gaucher's disease are rare. The diameters of the cells vary from 20 to 40 microns (p. 300).

HAND-SCHÜLLER-CHRISTIAN COMPLEX

The typical granulomatous lesions of this disease are also found in the spleen and have the same characteristics as in other organs (p. 305).

DIABETIC LIPOIDOSIS

In untreated cases of diabetes, the pulp may be filled with large (up to 60 microns) histocytes filled with cholesterol or cholesterol esters. As a rule, the spleen is not greatly enlarged.

TUMORS

PRIMARY

In general, primary tumors, either benign or malignant, are rare.

Benign. The following types of benign tumors may arise in the spleen: fibromas, osteomas, chondromas, lymphangiomas and hemangiomas. The last-named two are the most common and are often cavernous in type. Undoubtedly, some of the hemangiomas are better classified as hamartomas rather than neoplasms.

Malignant. Any of the types of lymphomas or Hodgkin's disease primary in the lymph nodes (p. 752) may be primary in the spleen, and they have in this organ the same characteristics as in the lymph nodes. In addition to these lesions, hemangiosarcomas with metastases, especially to the liver, do occur (p. 633).

SECONDARY

The most common secondary tumors are sarcomas, principally the so-called malignant lymphoma group and Hodgkin's disease (Figs. 18–29 and 18–30).

Metastases of other types of tumors, especially carcinomas, are rare and usually occur only when generalized carcinomatosis has developed. An exception is widely disseminated melanocarcinoma that involves the spleen in about half the cases. The basis for the rarity of metastatic involvement is still obscure. Remember from the discussion of this problem in Chapter 4 that two general explanations are offered. First, there is the "unfavorable soil" hypothesis. Second, the theory propounded chiefly by Coman (1947) states that the thick-walled muscular arterioles of the splenic follicles trap tumor emboli and prevent them from reaching a more favorable lodgment in the capillary and sinusoidal beds of the spleen. A carcinoma may also spread to the spleen by retrograde growth through the splenic vein. In addition a carcinoma primary in one of the neighboring organs (stomach or intestine) can extend to and cover the splenic capsule with a layer of tumor tissue. Finally, retrograde metastases by way of the lymphatics may occur.

RUPTURE OF THE SPLEEN

Rupture of the spleen is usually caused by a crushing injury or a severe blow. Much less often, it is encountered in the apparent absence of trauma. This event is designated as spontaneous rupture although it is always said

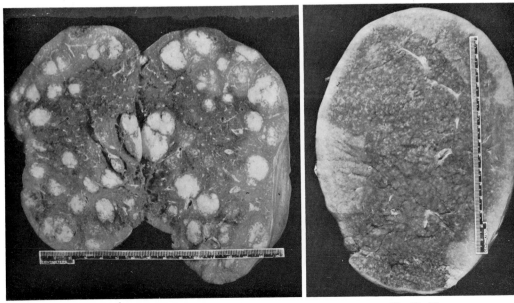

Fig. 18–29   **Fig. 18–30**

Figure 18–29. Histiocytic lymphoma (reticulum cell sarcoma) of the spleen in a case of generalized lymphomatous involvement of the mediastinal, abdominal and inguinal lymph nodes.

Figure 18–30. Lymphocytic lymphoma of the spleen. The enlarged pale follicles are evident on the cut surface.

that the normal spleen never ruptures spontaneously. In all instances of apparent nontraumatic rupture, some underlying condition should be suspected as the basis for the enlargement or weakening of this organ. Spontaneous rupture is encountered most often in infectious mononucleosis, malaria, typhoid fever, leukemia and in the other types of acute splenitis (Fig. 18–31). Rupture is usually followed by extensive, sometimes massive, intraperitoneal hemorrhage. The condition usually must be treated by prompt surgical removal of the

spleen to prevent death due to loss of blood and shock. In rare instances, clotting staunches the flow of blood. In some cases, following rupture, spleniculi may be found either localized or scattered throughout the peritoneal cavity; apparently they are transplants of splenic substance.

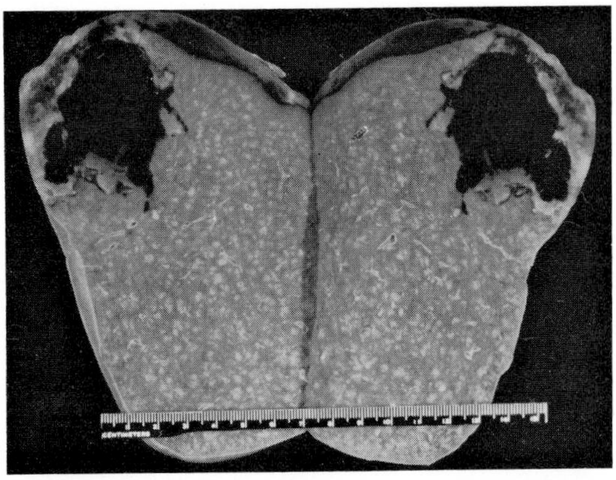

INTERPRETATION OF SPLENOMEGALY

Splenomegaly is a common clinical finding that demands an explanation whenever present. The enlargement of the spleen may be the predominant clinical feature in a patient, or it may occur as one of the manifestations in a much more complicated case having additional findings in other sites. Under all circumstances, it is necessary to carefully evaluate the splenomegaly with particular reference to its presumed etiology, its significance in the case as a whole, and its possible role in the production of the signs and symptoms manifested by the patient. An illustration may document these points more adequately.

A 65-year-old male in cardiac decompensation may have a clinically apparent splenomegaly. There is ample evidence to substantiate the existence of cardiac failure and generalized chronic passive congestion with slight enlargement of the liver, ascites, peripheral edema and perhaps findings of pulmo-

Figure 18–31. A large spontaneous hemorrhage into the spleen of a 27-year-old patient with infectious mononucleosis. The hematoma ruptured through the capsule and caused massive intraperitoneal hemorrhage

nary congestion and edema. However, in addition to these features, this patient also has the splenomegaly mentioned and enlarged mediastinal adenopathy that appears to be beyond the range of usual congestive or inflammatory changes. The combination of mediastinal adenopathy and splenomegaly suggests the possible existence of an underlying lymphoma or Hodgkin's disease. In this dilemma, the evaluation of the size of the spleen is of critical importance. If, for example, the spleen is only moderately enlarged and is calculated to be not more than two to three times normal size, such splenomegaly may be reasonably attributed to congestive enlargement. If, on the other hand, the spleen extends down to the level of the umbilicus and is calculated to have at least a twenty-fold increase in volume, such splenomegaly cannot be attributed to congestive splenomegaly of cardiac origin, and the possibility of an underlying lymphoma must be seriously entertained. Here a knowledge of the effects of various diseases on the spleen, particularly with respect to the usual degree of enlargement caused by these diseases, is fundamental to the evaluation of the clinical problem.

This example may make clear the necessity for an appreciation of the impact of various diseases on the spleen. Of particular importance is a knowledge of the usual limits of splenic enlargement caused by the various conditions described in this section. It would be quite erroneous to attribute enlargement of the spleen into the pelvis to acute splenitis and equally erroneous to accept as classic a case of hereditary spherocytosis without splenomegaly. A consideration of splenomegaly is presented, then, to aid in the interpretation of splenic enlargement in various diseases. These disorders will be divided into three grades of severity — massive, moderate and minimal enlargement.

DISORDERS THAT USUALLY CAUSE MASSIVE ENLARGEMENT OF THE SPLEEN (OVER 1000 gm.)

Chronic myelogenous leukemia
Chronic lymphatic leukemia — less massive than myelogenous form
Lymphomas — primary or secondary
Gaucher's disease
Myeloproliferative syndrome (myelofibrosis)
Primary tumors of spleen — extremely uncommon but both the benign and malignant forms may cause massive irregular splenomegaly
Malaria, kala-azar and other parasitic infestations, such as Echinococcus cyst
Congestive splenomegaly due to portal or splenic vein obstruction — an uncommon cause for massive enlargement; more usually causes moderate enlargement

CONDITIONS CAUSING MODERATE ENLARGEMENT (500 to 1000 gm.)

Chronic splenitis — particularly vegetative bacterial endocarditis
Tuberculosis, sarcoid, typhoid fever
Chronic congestive splenomegaly
Sickle cell anemia — in early stages of disease
Hereditary spherocytosis
Metastatic carcinoma or sarcoma
Infectious mononucleosis
Acute leukemias
Niemann-Pick disease
Hand-Schüller-Christian complex
Thalassemia
Autoimmune hemolytic anemia
Idiopathic thrombocytopenia
Hodgkin's disease

CONDITIONS CAUSING MINIMAL SPLENOMEGALY (USUALLY UNDER 500 gm.)

Acute splenitis
Acute splenic congestion
Miscellaneous acute febrile disorders, such as bacteremic states, systemic toxemias, systemic lupus erythematosus and intra-abdominal infections.

These categories are, of course, arbitrary and must be interpreted with considerable latitude. To imply that the spleen must always be massively enlarged in lymphomatous involvement would be erroneous. It should be equally obvious that massive enlargement of the spleen may be produced occasionally by sarcoidosis or secondary metastases to this organ. However, in the differential analysis of a clinical problem, the evaluation will be more often right than wrong by applying the previously cited categories to the interpretation of splenomegaly. In many instances, certain disorders can be excluded as plausible causes for the splenic involvement when the splenic size is inconsistent with the usual anatomic alterations found in this disease. Thus, when the lower pole of the spleen is below the iliac crest, the differential diagnosis should not start with a consideration of chronic splenitis due to some bacterial infection.

REFERENCES

Aisenberg, A. C.: Studies on delayed hypersensitivity in Hodgkin's disease. J. Clin. Invest., *41*:1964, 1962.
Banfi, A., et al.: Preferential sites of involvement and spread in malignant lymphomas. Europ. J. Cancer, *4*:319, 1968.
Bennett, J. M., et al.: Histopathological definition of Burkitt's tumor. Bull. W.H.O., *40*:601, 1969.
Brown, R. S., et al.: Hodgkin's disease. Immunologic, clinical, and histologic features of 50 untreated patients. Ann. Intern. Med., *67*:291, 1967.
Burkitt, D.: The African lymphoma: epidemiological and therapeutic aspects. In Zarafonetis, C. (ed.): Proceedings of the International Conference on Leukemia-Lymphoma. Philadelphia, Lea and Febiger, 1968, p. 321.

Butler, J. J.: Histopathology of malignant lymphomas and Hodgkin's disease in leukemia-lymphoma. 14th Annual Clinical Conference on Cancer, 1969. Chicago, Year Book Medical Publishers, Inc., 1970, p. 135.

Cole, P., and MacMahon, B.: Mortality from Hodgkin's disease in the United States. Lancet, 2:1371, 1968.

Coman, D. R.: Mechanism of invasiveness of cancer. Science. 105: 347, 1947.

Dameshek, W.: Hypersplenism. Bull. N.Y. Acad. Med., 31:113, 1955.

Davies, J. N. P.: Hodgkin's disease in the community. Hum. Path., 3:297, 1972.

Dmochowski, L.: Current status of the relationship of viruses to leukemia lymphoma and solid tumors in leukemia lymphoma. 14th Annual Clinical Conference on Cancer, 1969. Chicago, Year Book Medical Publishers, Inc., 1970, p. 37.

Doan, C., and Wright, C. S.: Primary, congenital, secondary and acquired splenic panhematopenia. Blood, 1:10, 1946.

Editorial: Further in the Hodgkin maze. Lancet, 1:1053, 1971.

Fudenberg, H. H.: Genetically determined immune deficiency as the predisposing cause of "autoimmunity" and lymphoid neoplasia. Amer. J. Med., 51:295, 1971.

Gall, E. A., and Rappaport, H.: Seminar on diseases of lymph nodes and spleen. In McDonald, J. R. (ed.): Proceedings of the 23rd Seminar of the American Society of Clinical Pathologists, New Orleans, 1958.

Goldman, J. M., and Aisenberg, A. C.: Incidence of antibody to EB virus, herpes simplex, and cytomegalovirus in Hodgkin's disease. Cancer, 26:327, 1970.

Harrington, W. J., et al.: Demonstration of a thrombocytopenic factor in the blood of patients with thrombocytopenic purpura. J. Lab. Clin. Med., 38:1, 1951.

Henle, W., et al.: Antibodies to Epstein-Barr virus in nasopharyngeal carcinoma, other head and neck neoplasms and control groups. J. Nat. Cancer Inst., 44:225, 1970.

Hersh, E. M., and Oppenheim, J. J.: Impaired in vitro lymphocyte transformation in Hodgkin's disease. New Eng. J. Med., 273:1006, 1965.

Hoover, R., and Fraumeni, J. F.: Risk of cancer in renal-transplant recipients. Lancet, 2:55, 1973.

Jackson, H., and Parker, F., Jr. (eds.): Hodgkin's Disease and Allied Disorders. New York, Oxford University Press, 1947.

Jackson, H., et al.: Agnogenic myeloid metaplasia. New Eng. J. Med., 222:985, 1940.

Jacobs, M.: Malignant lymphomas and their management. In Rentchnick, P. (ed.): Recent Results in Cancer Research Series. Vol. 18. New York, Springer-Verlag, 1968.

Johansson, B., et al.: Epstein-Barr virus (EBV)-associated antibody patterns in malignant lymphoma and leukemia. II. Chronic lymphocytic leukemia and lymphocytic lymphoma. Int. J. Cancer, 8:475, 1971.

Kaplan, H. S.: On the natural history, treatment and prognosis of Hodgkin's disease. Harvey Lectures, 64:215, 1968–69.

Klein, G., et al.: Relation between Epstein-Barr viral and cell membrane immunofluorescence in Burkitt tumour cells. III. Comparison of blocking of direct membrane immunofluorescence and anti-EBV reactivities of different sera. J. Exp. Med., 129:697, 1969.

Linman, J. W., and Bethell, F. H.: Agnogenic myeloid metaplasia, its natural history and present day managements. Amer. J. Med. Sc., 22:107, 1957.

Lukes, R. J., and Butler, J. J.: The pathology and nomenclature of Hodgkin's disease. Cancer Res., 26:1063, 1966.

Lukes, R. J., and Parker, J. W.: Disorders of the hematopoietic system. In Brunson, J. G., and Gall, E. A. (eds.): Concepts of Disease. New York, The Macmillan Co., 1971, p. 924.

Lukes, R. J. et al.: Hodgkin's disease: report of nomenclature committee. Cancer Res., 26:1311, 1966a.

Lukes R. J., et al.: Natural history of Hodgkin's disease as related to its pathologic picture. Cancer, 19:317, 1966b.

Lukes, R. J., et al.: Reed-Sternberg-like cells in infectious mononucleosis. Lancet, 2:1003, 1969.

MacMahon, B.: Epidemiology of Hodgkin's disease. Cancer Res., 27:416, 1971.

McMichael, J.: Pathology of hepatolienal fibrosis. J. Path. Bact., 39:481, 1934.

Mellors, R. C.: Autoimmune disease in NZB/B₁ mice. II. Autoimmunity and malignant lymphoma. Blood, 27:435, 1966.

Newell, G. R.: Age differences in the histology of Hodgkin's disease. J. Nat. Cancer Inst., 45:311, 1970.

Nickerson, D. A., and Sunderland, D. A.: The histopathology of idiopathic thrombocytopenic purpura. Amer. J. Path., 13:463, 1937.

Oels, H. C., et al.: Lymphoblastic lymphoma with histiocytic phagocytosis. Cancer, 21:368, 1968.

Order, S. E., and Hellman, S.: The pathogenesis of Hodgkin's disease. Lancet, 1:571, 1972.

Palmer, J. G., et al.: The experimental production of splenomegaly, anemia, and leukopenia in albino rats. Blood, 8:72, 1953.

Penn, W., et al.: Malignant lymphomas in transplantation patients. Transplant. Proc., 1:106, 1969.

Perez-Tamayo, R., et al.: Humoral factors in experimental hypersplenism. Blood, 16:1145, 1960.

Rappaport, H.: Tumors of Hematopoietic System. Washington, D.C., Armed Forces Institute of Pathology, 1966.

Rappaport, H, et al.: Report of the committee on histopathological criteria contributing to staging of Hodgkin's disease. Cancer Res., 31:1864, 1971.

Rosenberg, S. A.: Report of the committee on the staging of Hodgkin's disease. Cancer Res., 26:1310, 1966.

Seif, G. S. F., and Spriggs, A. I.: Chromosome changes in Hodgkin's disease. J. Nat. Cancer Inst., 39:557, 1967.

Sheehan, W. W., and Rappaport, H.: Morphological criteria in the classification of the malignant lymphomas. In Proceedings of the Sixth National Cancer Conference, American Cancer Society, Inc. and National Cancer Institute. Philadelphia, J. B. Lippincott Co., 1970, p. 59.

Strum, S. B., and Rappaport, H.: Interrelations of the histologic types of Hodgkin's disease. Arch. Path., 91:127, 1971.

Strum, S. B., et al.: Observation of cells resembling Sternberg-Reed cells in conditions other than Hodgkin's disease. Cancer, 26:176, 1970.

Thompson, W. P.: The splenic lesion in hemolytic jaundice. Bull. Johns Hopkins Hosp., 51:365, 1932.

Vianna, N. J., et al.: Extended epidemic of Hodgkin's disease in high school students. Lancet, 1:1209, 1971a.

Vianna, N. J., et al.: Tonsillectomy and Hodgkin's disease: the lymphoid tissue barrier. Lancet, 1:431, 1971b.

Von Haam, E., and Awny, A. Y.: Pathology of hypersplenism. Amer. J. Clin. Path., 18:313, 1948.

Ward, H. P., and Block, M. H.: Myeloid metaplasia, a reevaluation. In Clarke, W. J., Howard, E. B., and Hackett, P. L. (eds.): Myeloproliferative Disorders of Animals and Man. United States Atomic Energy Commission, 1970, p. 609.

Weiss, L.: Study of the structure of splenic sinuses in man and the albino rat with the light microscope and the electron microscope. J. Biophys. Biochem. Cytol., 3:599, 1957.

19

THE RESPIRATORY SYSTEM

LUNG

NORMAL

The lungs are ingeniously constructed to carry out their cardinal function, the exchange of gases between inspired air and the blood. The present consideration of the normal lung is confined to reemphasizing those features of the anatomy and function that are particularly pertinent to an understanding of the pathology of this organ.

The normal adult lung weighs approximately 300 to 400 gm. Sometimes forgotten is the surface presentation of the various lobes of the lungs. The two lower lobes present almost entirely on the posterior aspect of the thoracic cavity, while the upper lobes and right middle lobe present almost entirely on the anterior aspect. However, because the apical portions of the lower lobes are thin, pathologic processes throughout most of the upper lobes yield clinical signs that can be detected both anteriorly and posteriorly. The right middle lobe is separated from the posterior chest wall by a

782

thick mass of lower lobe. Disorders in the middle lobe, then, are reflected clinically chiefly by signs confined to the right anterior lower thorax.

The right main stem bronchus is more vertical and more directly in line with the trachea than the left. As a consequence, aspirated foreign material, such as vomitus, blood and foreign bodies, tends to enter the right lung rather than the left. In the normal state, the tracheal bifurcation creates an acute angle. Tumors may produce expansile masses within the tracheobronchial nodes situated in this angle which spread the bronchi apart to produce an obtuse angle, a bronchoscopic finding of occasional help. Progressive branching of the bronchi and the bronchioles eventually produces small terminal bronchioles less than 1 mm. in diameter, devoid of cartilaginous support. These terminal bronchioles further subdivide into air-carrying channels known as respiratory bronchioles which give off alveoli and then proceed into the alveolar ducts. Each alveolar duct serves a lobule, the functional unit of respiration which assumes great importance in the group of diseases known as emphysema. Each duct opens into two or three air spaces known as atria which, in turn, give off the terminal alveolar sacs more commonly called alveoli (Farber and Wilson, 1968). It is important to note that the alveoli open into these ducts and atria through large mouths. In the correct plane of section, therefore, all alveoli are open and have incomplete walls. This alveolar mouth is sometimes mistakenly interpreted as a defect caused by a rupture of an alveolar wall.

Of recent date, the division of the lung into bronchopulmonary segments has achieved considerable importance. These segments constitute functional and anatomic units. Each comprises one of the divisions of the major bronchi into the smaller order bronchi, bronchioles and ultimately the alveoli served by these airways. Each segment arises from an individual bronchial bud, and each has its own arterial and venous supply. The importance of this concept is that an inflammatory lesion in the major bronchus may drain into the subtended bronchopulmonary segment and spread the infection throughout this functional unit. In the same way, obstruction of the major bronchial division will cause disease in the subtended unit, but will theoretically leave the adjacent segments unaffected. It is not necessary to give the specific names here to each of these bronchopulmonary segments; suffice it to say that each of the well known lobes of the lungs has been divided into two or

four such units comprising a total of 18 bronchopulmonary segments.

Attention should be called to the double pulmonary arterial supply composed of the pulmonary and bronchial arteries. In the absence of significant cardiac failure, the bronchial arteries of aortic origin can sustain the vitality of the pulmonary parenchyma when the pulmonary arterial supply is shut off, as by emboli.

The passages of the respiratory tree (trachea, bronchi and bronchioles) are often considered to be rigid tubes. In fact, they are dependent on normal pressure relationships and the integrity of the surrounding lung parenchyma for the maintenance of their normal patency. Peribronchial or peribronchiolar fibrosis, destruction of alveolar walls, overexpansion or collapse of alveoli all secondarily lead to narrowing of the airways. Moreover, bronchi and bronchioles undergo striking changes in diameter during both normal and abnormal respiratory movements. With inspiration, bronchioles elongate and widen, and the posterior membranous portion of the trachea balloons out. With expiration, the reverse occurs and, in fact, the posterior membranous portion of the trachea and large bronchi collapses far into the lumen of the trachea. Forced, sudden expiration increases the intrathoracic pressure and this increased pressure further compresses the posterior membrane, narrowing the lumina of these airways to thin slits that emit the whistling sounds that can be produced even by normal individuals who violently exhale. Through this mechanism, even a small or partial obstruction in the airways may lead to forced expiration accomplished by increased intrathoracic pressure that further narrows the lumina of the respiratory tree. Thus, autopsy findings of only partial obstruction of the bronchus or trachea may be associated with striking changes in the distal lung substance that would suggest either complete or almost complete obstruction.

By fluoroscopic studies, the respiratory tree demonstrates wave-like peristaltic motions that help expel inhaled foreign material. Such motor activity is presumably dependent upon the well developed musculature of the trachea, bronchi and bronchioles. Inflammatory damage to these airways impairs this activity and further predisposes the lung to infection.

From the microscopic standpoint, it is well to remember that except for the vocal cords, which are covered by stratified squamous epithelium, the entire respiratory tree, including the larynx, trachea and bronchioles, is lined by pseudostratified, tall, columnar, ciliated epithelial cells, heavily admixed with mucus-secreting goblet cells. The mucinous secretion and cilia have important functions. The mucus moistens the inspired air and prevents drying of the delicate alveolar walls, and traps dust and particulate matter as well. The cilia aid in the removal of foreign material and contaminated mucus by constant beating wave-like motions that propel this material back into the larger bronchi and trachea where the cough reflex completes the expulsion. This ciliary action is of importance, since the upright position in man favors the drainage of foreign material, fluid and debris into the terminal alveoli. Numerous submucosal, branching, mucus-secreting glands are dispersed throughout the walls of the trachea, bronchi and bronchioles. These glands provide a plausible source for the development of adenocarcinomas of the lung.

The microscopic structure of the alveolar walls has now been well established by electron microscopy. An extremely rich intertwining network of anastomotic capillaries composes the most important element within the alveolar walls. These capillaries are supported by a delicate fibrous stroma enriched by elastic and reticulin fibers. The alveoli themselves are lined by a one-cell layer of epithelium (septal cells) attached to a basement membrane that separates them from the underlying endothelial cells of the capillaries. Two types of alveolar lining cells have been identified: flattened, plate-like, pavement *type 1* pneumocytes and rounded, granular *type 2* pneumocytes. The latter cells synthesize pulmonary surfactant, of importance in reducing the fluid tension at the fluid-air interface of the alveoli, thus facilitating their full expansion. Lamellar membranous bodies resembling myelin figures, thought to represent inclusions of this surfactant, are seen within these type 2 pneumocytes. For years, it was believed that septal cells were the origin of the omnipresent "dust cells" or macrophages found in alveolar spaces. Recent studies, however, indicate that the septal cells themselves are not phagocytic and that the free-lying macrophages are derived from blood monocytes. The alveolar walls are not solid, but are perforated by numerous pores (attributed to Kohn, but probably first described by Henle), which permit the passage of bacteria and exudate between adjacent alveoli. The entire lung substance including the walls of the alveoli is rich in elastic fibers which are, at least in part, responsible for contraction of the alveoli following normal inspiration.

The all-important respiratory function of the lungs can be divided into two aspects: *ventilation*, concerned with the movement of the air into the alveolar spaces, and *respiratory gas exchange*, involving the diffusion of oxygen and carbon dioxide across the alveolar capillary membrane.

Ventilation is largely a function of the respiratory muscles, particularly the diaphragm, and of the volumetric capacity of the lungs. It must be remembered that during a single quiet respiratory cycle approximately 500 cc. of air are moved in and out (tidal volume). However, the total lung capacity that reflects the maximum amount of air that can be moved in and out by forced inspiration and expiration is about 4000 cc. (vital capacity). Even after such forced expiration, there is a residual volume of about 1200 cc. that accounts for the normal buoyancy of pulmonary tissue when the lungs are floated in water. When there is abnormal collapse of the lungs (atelectasis), this residual volume may be sufficiently diminished to destroy this normal lung buoyancy. Disease states may impair normal ventilation by reducing the volume capacity of the lung or by obstructing the movement of air through the respiratory passages. Filling of the lung alveolar spaces by inflammatory exudate, such as occurs in various types of pneumonia, reduces the ventilatory capacity by lowering the vital capacity and tidal volume. Space-occupying fluid or tumors will also reduce ventilatory function. Compression of the lung by pleural fluid, exudate or thoracic deformities acts similarly. Lung ventilation may also be reduced by obstructive diseases, such as asthma, and neuromuscular disorders that weaken the muscles of respiration and therefore do not permit full expansion of the lungs.

Respiratory gas exchange is the second aspect of pulmonary function already mentioned. It is to a considerable part dependent upon the integrity of the alveolar wall and its capacity to permit the interchange of oxygen and carbon dioxide. Any disease that interposes edema fluid, fibrous tissue, exudate or neoplasm between the air spaces of the alveoli and the septal capillaries (alveolocapillary block) hampers respiratory exchange. Reduction in the rate of flow of blood through the lungs will also hamper such respiratory exchange.

A word about cyanosis is in order. It requires about 5 gm. of reduced hemoglobin per 100 ml. of blood to induce cyanosis. The cyanosis that is caused by deranged respiratory function can generally be alleviated by having the patient breathe 100 per cent oxygen, lowering the quantity of reduced circulating hemoglobin. In contrast, the cyanosis which is due to a right to left cardiovascular shunt is not affected by the level of oxygen in the inspired air. This difference forms the basis for an important clinical diagnostic test that helps distinguish cyanosis of pulmonary origin from that of abnormal arteriovenous shunts.

PATHOLOGY

It is impossible to overemphasize the importance of lung disease in the overall perspective of pathology and clinical medicine. Primary respiratory infections, such as bronchitis, bronchopneumonia and other forms of pneumonia, are commonplace in clinical and pathologic practice. In this day of cigarette smoking and air pollution, emphysema has become rampant, affecting large segments of the total population. Moreover, the lungs are secondarily involved in almost all forms of terminal disease, so that at autopsy some degree of pulmonary edema, atelectasis or bronchopneumonia, not to mention other possibilities, is found in virtually every postmortem. Malignancy of the lungs has risen steadily in incidence, until it is now the most common form of visceral malignancy in the male. Moreover, the lungs serve as a capillary filter of the venous drainage of the entire body, and as such are commonly involved in all forms of disease which invade the blood. In the present consideration of the lung, emphasis will be placed on primary diseases that affect this organ. Systemic disturbances which secondarily involve the lung will be largely omitted, since they receive consideration elsewhere as basic systemic processes. For example, certain forms of amyloidosis are known to affect the lung; but since this pulmonary involvement has already been cited in the discussion of amyloidosis, it can be omitted here.

CONGENITAL ANOMALIES

CYSTIC DISEASES OF THE LUNGS

Three conditions produce abnormally large air spaces in the lung parenchyma: (1) congenital bronchogenic cystic disease of the lung, (2) alveolar cysts and (3) bullous emphysema. Only the first two of these merit the designation of cystic disease. Bullous emphysema has a totally different pathogenesis and clinical significance and will be considered later under the emphysematous disorders of the lung (Cooke and Blades, 1952). There is, however, a growing clinical tendency to lump all three together under the term "*air space disorders.*"

Bronchogenic cysts are extremely uncommon. They are believed to arise in the em-

bryogenesis of the airways either as the result of pinching off of nests of epithelial cells or as the consequence of ballooning out of malformed bronchi under the continued thrust of the inspiratory pressures (Norris and Tyson, 1947). The latter form expands slowly over the course of years and may therefore not become clinically apparent until adult life. *These congenital malformations must be differentiated from the cystic dilatations that occur in the course of bronchiectasis* (p. 806).

Cystic lesions of congenital origin occur anywhere in the lungs as single or, on occasion, multiple cystic spaces varying in diameter from microscopic size to over 5 cm. in diameter. Often they are associated with congenital cystic disease of the liver, kidney and pancreas. They are usually adjacent to bronchi or bronchioles and may or may not have demonstrable connections. Histologically, they are lined by ciliated, mucus-secreting respiratory columnar epithelium, based upon a thin layer of connective tissue (Fig. 19–1). In the uncomplicated case, the cavities are either filled with mucinous secretion or, if there is an orifice draining the secretions, they may be filled with air. Infection of the secretions leads to suppuration often associated with progressive metaplasia of the lining epithelium or even total necrosis of the wall of the cysts to create a lung abscess.

Alveolar cysts are produced presumably by the progressive rupture of the alveolar walls to

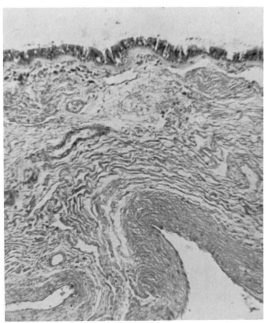

Figure 19–1. *Bronchogenic cyst of lung. A microscopic detail of the wall illustrating the respiratory lining epithelium.*

create large air spaces. It is not certain whether such alveolar rupture reflects some congenital developmental failure in the alveolar wall or whether inflammatory disease with fibrosis, aging and deterioration of the elastic and reticulin fibers predisposes to such rupture.

Alveolar cysts are more often multiple than are the bronchogenic cysts. Alveolar cysts tend to be located more or less centrally, most often in the upper lobes. This location contrasts with bullous emphysema, which is almost always peripheral. The walls of alveolar cysts are thin, fragile and poorly defined. These alveolar cysts vary in size from air spaces barely visible to the naked eye to some that virtually take up an entire lobe, giving rise to the descriptive term **"the vanishing lung syndrome."** Histologically, the linings are made up of compressed preexisting alveolar walls with some increased fibrous trabeculation composed in part of the perivascular fibrous tissue which is pushed ahead of the expanding air space. As would be expected, the surrounding lung substance is compressed and atelectatic. Rupture of these cysts into the pleural cavity may cause pneumothorax and collapse the lung. Less often, the increase in intrapleural pressure compresses and partially blocks the respiratory tree, causing progressive dilatation of the cyst. Under these circumstances, the cysts are blown up like a balloon with each inspiration.

Both bronchogenic and alveolar cysts are of clinical importance because (1) they may compress or displace sufficient lung volume to decrease the vital capacity and produce ventilatory insufficiency; (2) they are prime sites for the development of infection, which may then lead to the formation of lung abscesses, bronchopleural fistulas and sometimes empyema; (3) through the progressive cystic dilatation, vessels may be ruptured to cause hemorrhage and hemoptysis; and (4) rupture of the cysts into the pleural cavities may cause pneumothorax or dissection of air into connective tissue septa of the lung to produce interstitial pulmonary emphysema.

DISEASES OF VASCULAR ORIGIN

PULMONARY CONGESTION AND EDEMA

The general consideration of edema was given on p. 318. Pulmonary congestion and edema in particular was described on p. 321. Here it will suffice to recall the principal clinical settings in which pulmonary congestion and edema are encountered and briefly review the morphologic changes.

Heart failure, specifically left ventricular failure, leads to pulmonary congestion and edema by causing increased pulmonary venous pressure, sodium retention, hypervolemia and increased capillary permeability, secondary to hypoxic injury. Mitral stenosis in particular causes the most extreme forms of pulmonary congestion and edema, often designated as "mitral stenosis lung" (Parker and Weiss, 1936). Heavy wet lungs are also encountered in *shock,* in the early stages of pulmonary *bacterial, viral* and *mycotic infections,* in all cases of systemic edema such as is induced by *kidney disease* (especially the nephrotic syndrome) and in *hypersensitivity states* where the lungs are the target organs. Similar lung changes often develop in patients undergoing cardiac surgery who have been maintained on *extracorporeal cardiac pumps* for long periods of time. Why these mechanical assist devices cause pulmonary edema is still not clear, but sufficient hypoxia may result to cause death (Nahas et al., 1965). For obscure reasons, sudden *increases in cranial pressure* such as may follow cerebral strokes sometimes induce pulmonary edema.

Whatever the clinical setting, pulmonary congestion and edema create heavy wet subcrepitant lungs. The fluid tends to accumulate in the basal regions of the lower lobes. It is manifested by an intra-alveolar granular precipitate and widening of the alveolar septa (Fig. 19–2). Alveolar microhemorrhages and hemosiderin-laden macrophages (heart failure cells) generally appear in all longstanding cases, along with fibrosis of alveolar walls. In this manner, the wet soggy lungs become meaty and brown (brown induration). Changes such as these not only impair normal respiratory function but also predispose to infections, termed *hypostatic bronchopneumonia.* Thus bronchopneumonia often terminates long debilitating serious illness.

PULMONARY EMBOLISM, HEMORRHAGE AND INFARCTION

Occlusions of the pulmonary arteries by blood clot are almost always embolic in origin. In situ thromboses are rare and only develop in the presence of pulmonary hypertension and pulmonary atherosclerosis. However, thrombosis superimposed on a nonocclusive embolus may complete the arterial obstruction. The usual source of these emboli (thrombi in the deep veins of the leg) and the magnitude of the clinical problem were discussed on p. 335. There the awesome frequency of pulmonary embolism and infarction were emphasized. In a postmortem study, grossly recognizable pul-

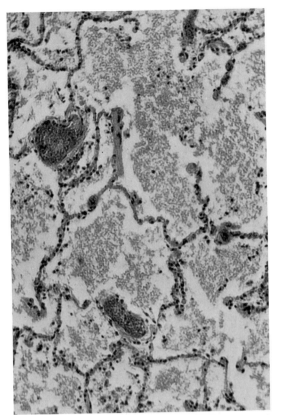

Figure 19-2. *Pulmonary edema. The granular precipitate within the alveolar spaces represents the solid constituents of the edema fluid.*

monary emboli were encountered in 6 to 8 per cent of the general population of hospital patients, rising to 25 to 30 per cent in those patients dying after severe burns, trauma or fractures (Hume et al., 1970). *Pulmonary embolism (with or without infarction) caused the death of approximately 3 to 5 per cent of all of the hospitalized patients and as many as 10 per cent of selected older groups* having advanced cancer, other chronic debilitating illnesses or some form of trauma (Sevitt and Gallagher, 1968).

Morphology. The morphologic consequences of embolic occlusion of the pulmonary arteries depend on the size of the embolic mass and the general state of the circulation (Fig. 19–3). Large emboli may impact in the main pulmonary artery or its major branches, or lodge astride the bifurcation as a **saddle embolus.** Sudden death often ensues owing to the block of blood flow through the lungs. The death may also be occasioned by acute dilatation of the right heart **(acute cor pulmonale).** In such sudden deaths, there may be no significant alterations in the lungs save perhaps for minimal hemorrhages in the alveoli. Smaller emboli travel out into the more peripheral vessels where they may or may not cause infarction. **In patients with an adequate cardiovascular circulation, the bronchial artery supply can sustain the lung parenchyma despite obstruction to the pulmonary arterial system. Under these circumstances hemor-**

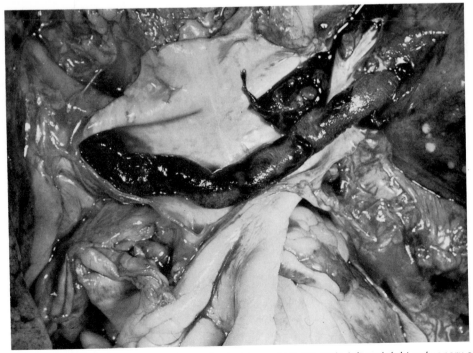

Figure 19-3. *A large embolus from the femoral vein lying astride the main left and right pulmonary arteries.*

rhages occur, but there is no infarction of the underlying lung parenchyma. These hemorrhages vary in size, up to 5 to 10 cm. in diameter, depending upon the magnitude of the occluded vessel. The hemorrhage may be central in the lung substance, but often extends to the periphery. While the underlying pulmonary architecture may be obscured by the suffusion of blood, hemorrhages are distinguished by the preservation of the native pulmonary substance. Resorption of the blood permits reconstitution of the preexisting architecture. Only rarely does organization of the hemorrhage yield fibrous scars.

Pulmonary emboli cause infarction when the circulation is already inadequate, namely, in patients with heart disease or those mortally ill with such conditions as advanced malignancy. It is for this reason that infarctions tend to be uncommon in the young. About three-quarters of all infarcts affect the lower lobes and, in over one-half of the cases, they occur multiply. They vary in size from lesions barely visible to the naked eye to massive involvement of large parts of an entire lobe. Characteristically, they extend to the periphery of the lung substance with the apex pointing toward the hilus of the lung (Castleman, 1940). The pulmonary infarct is classically hemorrhagic and appears as a raised red-blue area in the early stages. Often the apposed pleural surface is covered by a fibrinous exudate (Fig. 19–4). If the occluded vessel can be identified, it will be found near the apex of the infarcted area. The red cells begin to lyse within 48 hours, and the blue-red cyanotic appearance of the infarct fades, becomes paler and eventually red-brown as hemosiderin is produced. With the passage of time, fibrous replacement begins at the margins as a gray-white peripheral zone and eventually converts the entire infarct into a scar which is contracted below the level of the surrounding lung substance. Histologically, the diagnostic feature of pulmonary infarction is the ischemic necrosis of the lung substance within the area of hemorrhage (Fig. 19—5). Such necrosis affects not only the alveolar walls but the interstitial tissue, bronchioles and vessels. In the early stages of the lesion, the red cells that fill the alveoli are readily identified but, in the course of time, they disintegrate. The inflammatory reaction at the margins is entirely nondistinctive and represents organization of an area of necrotic tissue.

If the infarct is caused by an infected embolus arising in inflammatory disease of veins or in right-sided bacterial endocarditis, the infarct is modified by a more intense neutrophilic exudation and more intense inflammatory action. Such lesions are referred to as septic infarcts and, indeed, some are converted to abscesses.

Clinical Course. Pulmonary embolism and infarction are principally complications of

patients already suffering from some underlying disease. They are most commonly encountered in those with cardiac disease, cancer, any form of chronic debilitating illness or severe trauma. Aged patients, particularly those immobilized for long periods with fractures, are especially vulnerable. Younger women have an increased risk of suffering embolism to the lung and possibly infarction in late pregnancy, following delivery and with the use of "contraceptive pills" containing significant amounts of estrogens (p. 333).

The significance of pulmonary embolism depends upon the size of the occluded vessel, the number of emboli and the general status of the cardiovascular system. *Large emboli are one of the few causes of virtually instantaneous death.* If death occurs less suddenly, the clinical syndrome may mimic myocardial infarction with severe chest pain, acute dyspnea, shock, eleva-

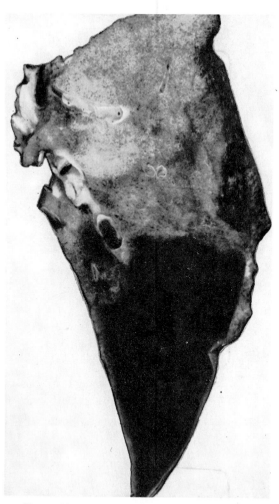

Figure 19–4. Cross section of a pulmonary infarct of several days' duration. The area of red-blue infarction appears densely black in the photograph.

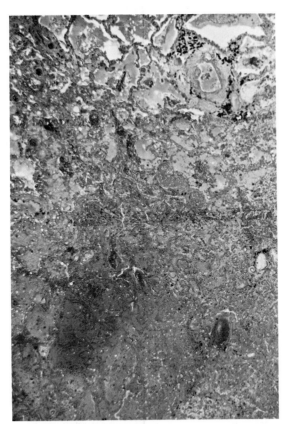

Figure 19–5. *Pulmonary infarction, showing junction of preserved parenchyma with an area of infarction necrosis. The alveolar spaces are suffused with blood.*

tion of temperature and increased levels of serum LDH (further mimicking myocardial infarction). Chest films and pulmonary angiography aid in this differential diagnosis. Among patients succumbing to massive embolism, 34 per cent die within one hour, another 35 per cent within 24 hours and an additional 27 per cent in 2 to 5 days (Fowler and Bollenger, 1954).

More often emboli are small. In those with a normal cardiovascular system, small emboli induce only transient chest pain and cough or possibly pulmonary hemorrhages without infarction. Only in the predisposed where the bronchial circulation itself is inadequate will they cause infarcts. Characteristically, such patients manifest dyspnea, tachypnea, fever, chest pain, cough and hemoptysis. An overlying fibrinous pleuritis may produce a pleural friction rub. In some patients, resorption of the lysed red cells in the infarct leads to transient episodes of jaundice (hyperbilirubinemia).

Emboli may be resolved if the patient survives the initial acute insult. The embolus will contract as do all blood clots; fibrinolytic activity may then further reduce its size, and remarkable resolution with total lysis of the clot may then follow. This happy outcome is seen in the relatively young, who are capable of surviving the initial blow (Soloff and Rodman, 1967) (Sabiston, 1968). When unresolved, multiple small emboli may, over the course of time, lead to pulmonary hypertension, pulmonary vascular sclerosis and chronic cor pulmonale. Perhaps the most important significance of the small embolus is that it often presages a larger one. The patient with a first pulmonary embolus has a 30 per cent chance of a second one and a 20 per cent chance that this second episode will be fatal.

Prevention of pulmonary embolism constitutes a major clinical problem for which there is no easy solution. Encouraging leg motion as well as isometric contraction of leg muscles while in bed, and early ambulation reduces the hazard of lower leg thrombosis. Anticoagulation may be indicated but will have no effect on already formed venous thrombi. A positive Homan's sign (p. 332) is a danger signal, but deep venous thromboses are often asymptomatic. The site of origin of the embolus is frequently unknown. It is sometimes necessary to resort to ligation of the inferior vena cava, no small procedure in an already seriously ill patient.

PULMONARY VASCULAR SCLEROSIS

This disorder is the analogue of atherosclerosis in the systemic circuit. It appears whenever there is pulmonary hypertension, whatever its cause, and therefore might be designated hypertensive pulmonary vascular disease. In most cases, the pulmonary hypertension results from known causes cited in the discussion of cor pulmonale (p. 677). Under such circumstances, the pulmonary vascular disease is referred to as *secondary pulmonary vascular sclerosis*. Infrequently, *primary pulmonary vascular sclerosis* is encountered in patients having no overt cause for their pulmonary hypertension. It has, in fact, been impossible to determine whether in this circumstance the pulmonary arterial changes are primary and induce the hypertension or the hypertension leads to the arterial disease. Obviously, the diagnosis of primary vascular sclerosis cannot be made until all secondary causes are excluded (Brill and Krygier, 1941).

Secondary pulmonary vascular sclerosis is encountered in both sexes and at all ages, principally in the elderly. While the primary form may also occur in either sex and at any age, it is most frequent in young women.

Pathogenesis. Since the causes of secondary pulmonary vascular sclerosis have already been considered (p. 677), we are here concerned with the pathogenesis of primary pulmonary hypertension. Four theories have been proposed, which is another way of saying the problem is still unsettled. The first postulates overactivity of the sympathetic autonomic system in which chronic vasoconstriction induces pulmonary hypertension and, in time, arterial thickening. In support of such a concept, it has been noted that a significant number of patients with so-called primary pulmonary vascular sclerosis suffer from vasospastic disorders of the systemic circulation, such as Raynaud's phenomenon (p. 611) (Walcott et al., 1970). The second theory proposes that multiple small pulmonary emboli are the cause of the pulmonary hypertension and, indeed, their organization and incorporation within the arterial walls may be the source of the atheromata encountered so often in this condition (O'Neal and Thomas, 1955). Possibly the organized blood clots arise as thrombi at sites of vascular injury (Blount, 1967). A third pos-

tulation suggests that the vascular lesions are primary and are the consequence of some hypersensitivity disease. Some slender support for this idea comes from the occasional patient with concomitant hypergammaglobulinemia and arthritis (Walcott et al., 1970). The fourth represents the pulmonary vascular lesions as being congenital in origin, perhaps resulting from anomalous development of the pulmonary vasculature.

Morphology. The vessel changes in both primary and secondary pulmonary vascular sclerosis are essentially similar and involve the entire arterial tree from the main pulmonary arteries down to the arterioles. In the main elastic arteries, the changes take the form of atheromatous deposits resembling atherosclerosis in the systemic arteries. They are rarely as marked, however, as those found in advanced cases of atherosclerosis of the systemic arteries and are not often calcified or ulcerated. The medium-sized muscular arteries have striking concentric medial hypertrophy (Fig. 19–6). In the milder cases, there are only intimal thickening and fibrosis and some adventitial fibrosis. In both me-

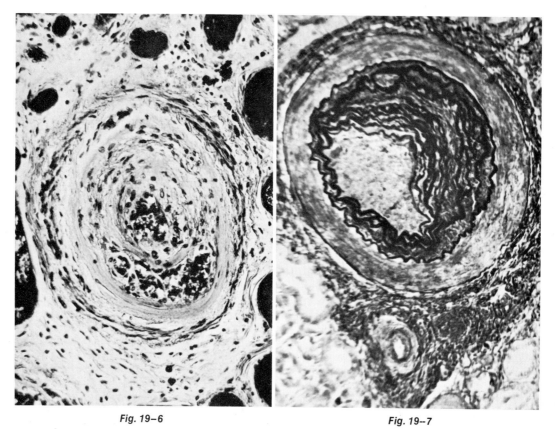

Fig. 19–6   Fig. 19–7

Figure 19–6. *Pulmonary vascular sclerosis. A histologic detail of a thickened artery to illustrate the "onion skinning."*

Figure 19–7. *Pulmonary vascular sclerosis with an elastic tissue stain showing the duplication of the internal elastic membrane.*

dium and small-sized arteries, the internal and external elastic membranes often undergo thickening and reduplication (Fig. 19—7). It is the arterioles that are most prominently affected, with striking increases in the thickness of the media sometimes narrowing the lumina to pinpoint channels. While these arterial changes are present in all forms of pulmonary vascular sclerosis, they are best developed in the primary form. Evidence of organized or organizing thrombi is common in both the primary and secondary forms of this vascular disease.

Clinical Course. Clinical signs and symptoms of both the primary and secondary forms of vascular sclerosis only become evident with advanced arterial disease. In the uncommon cases of primary disease, the presenting features are dyspnea and fatigue although, occasionally, syncopal attacks are the initial complaint. Some patients have chest pain of the anginal type and, indeed, develop severe respiratory distress and cyanosis. In the course of time, right ventricular hypertrophy and cor pulmonale develop. The prognosis is poor and death from decompensated cor pulmonale usually appears within two to eight years. On occasion, these patients pursue a fulminating course to death within months (Blount, 1967). The development of secondary pulmonary vascular sclerosis and the clinical manifestations of the pulmonary arterial lesions are usually masked by the underlying disorder responsible for the pulmonary hypertension.

ALTERATIONS IN THE EXPANSION OF THE LUNG

ATELECTASIS

Atelectasis refers either to incomplete expansion of the lungs or to the collapse of previously inflated lung substance. This disorder may be present at birth, may arise during the first days of postnatal life, or may occur anytime thereafter. Whenever it occurs, it is characterized by areas of relatively airless pulmonary parenchyma.

The term atelectasis should be applied only when the affected alveoli are normal structurally and therefore capable of reexpansion if the underlying cause can be removed.

Atelectasis Neonatorum. Atelectasis in the newborn is divided into primary and secondary forms. Synonymous with primary atelectasis is *congenital atelectasis*, implying that the lungs or some significant portion of them failed to expand at birth. The secondary form results when adequate inflation occurs but is followed soon thereafter by collapse. Congenital atelec-

tasis was discussed on p. 553. The secondary form of atelectasis neonatorum represents that encountered in the *respiratory distress syndrome* (p. 554).

Acquired Atelectasis. This form of the disease, encountered principally in adults, may be divided into *obstructive and compressive atelectasis.*

Pathogenesis. *Obstructive atelectasis* is the consequence of complete obstruction of an airway which, in time, leads to absorption of the oxygen trapped in the dependent alveoli, followed by their collapse. While some air may percolate through the pores of Kohn, it does not compensate for the airway blockage or prevent the collapse of the alveolar spaces. *Obstructive-absorptive collapse implies total blockage of the affected airway but continued blood flow through the affected alveolar walls.* The lung volume is diminished, and if a sufficient amount of parenchyma is affected, the mediastinum shifts toward the atelectatic lung.

Compressive atelectasis results whenever the pleural cavity is partially or completely filled by fluid exudate, tumor, blood clot or air (the last-mentioned comprising *pneumothorax*, p. 844). Similarly, abnormal elevation of the diaphragm such as follows peritonitis, subdiaphragmatic abscesses and abdominal carcinomatosis will induce basal atelectasis. With compressive atelectasis, the mediastinum shifts away from the affected lung.

Morphology. Acquired atelectasis may involve all lobes (massive collapse), which is usually incompatible with life. In the massive collapse that follows rupture of blebs or penetrating wounds of the chest cavity, the entire lung may be folded against the mediastinum as pneumothorax develops. Most often, it is not massive but lobar or segmental, bilaterally or unilaterally. In the most common pattern, caused by elevated diaphragms or the accumulation of fluid within the pleural cavities, it is basal and bilateral. The collapsed lung parenchyma is shrunken below the level of the surrounding normal lung substance and is red-blue, rubbery and subcrepitant with a wrinkled overlying pleura. In subtotal atelectasis of a portion of a lobe, the adjacent parenchyma often becomes overinflated, erroneously termed **"compensatory emphysema."** Histologically, the collapsed alveoli become slit-like, and the lung appears to have "too much tissue and too little air" (Fig. 19—8). There is no associated exudation unless superimposed infection has occurred. Congestion and dilatation of the septal vasculature are usually present owing to the loss of the compressive force of the air. Occasionally, segmental atelectasis of the basal portions of the upper lobes follows surgical operations, presumably

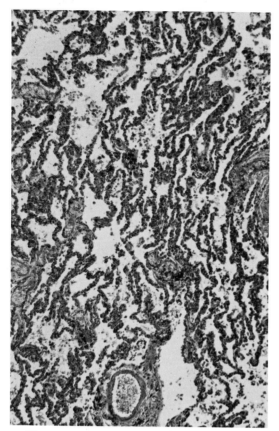

Figure 19–8. *Atelectasis. The alveoli are partially collapsed, producing slit-like spaces.*

because of obstructive secretions in the bronchi. These segmental lesions create horizontal linear radiographic shadows to which the descriptive term **"plate atelectasis"** is applied.

Clinical Course. From the knowledge that atelectasis is acquired either by obstruction of the airways or extrinsic compression of the lung substance, it is possible to deduce the clinical conditions in which it develops. The obstructive pattern is principally caused by excessive secretions or exudate within the second order and smaller bronchi and is therefore most often found in bronchial asthma, chronic bronchitis, bronchiectasis, postoperative states and with aspiration of foreign bodies. Surgical procedures in the oral cavity with aspiration of blood clots or tissue fragments are rare causes today of bronchial obstruction. Bronchial neoplasms are additional important causes of atelectasis, although in most instances they cause subtotal obstruction and produce emphysema. The comatose patient is particularly apt to collect secretions in his airways.

The compressive form of atelectasis is most commonly encountered in patients in cardiac failure who develop hydrothorax and in neoplastic effusions within the pleural cavities. It is also seen with rupture of a thoracic aneurysm causing hemothorax and in spontaneous or induced pneumothorax. Elevated diaphragms, as mentioned, are important causes of basal atelectasis, particularly in seriously ill postoperative patients. Their recumbent position with abdominal distention causing pressure against the diaphragm, their tendency to limit respiratory motions because of pain and their voluntary suppression of the cough reflex with resulting accumulation of secretions all contribute to the development of basal atelectasis and to serious respiratory embarrassment.

Atelectasis significantly reduces ventilatory functions and is therefore an important complication in the bedridden patient, particularly the elderly and in those recovering from surgery. Extensive atelectasis produces acute severe respiratory difficulty and, if bilateral as in massive collapse, may result in death. It is for this reason that tracheostomy is so often used as a means of "sucking out" the contained secretions in patients who, for one reason or another, are unable to successfully clear their bronchioles and bronchi and are thus prone to develop atelectasis.

Since the collapsed lung parenchyma can be reexpanded, atelectasis is a reversible disorder that should never be permitted to significantly contribute to a fatal outcome. Even if respiratory embarrassment is not marked, the atelectatic parenchyma is prone to develop superimposed infections such as bronchopneumonia, bronchiectasis and lung abscess.

EMPHYSEMA

There is no universally accepted definition of pulmonary emphysema. The American Thoracic Society and most American experts would define it as *a disease in which the air spaces distal to the terminal bronchioles are enlarged and their walls destroyed* (American Thoracic Society, 1962). Some American writers would modify this definition by referring to a "group of diseases" to acknowledge the fact that there are several distinctive morphologic patterns of emphysema. Enlargement of air spaces without destruction of septal walls is not designated emphysema, but rather hyperinflation of the lung. British colleagues generally do not demand tissue destruction in their conception of emphysema and recognize two large categories: (1) dilatation alone of air spaces and (2) dilatation with destruction of walls of air spaces (Fletcher, 1959).

Chaos is added to confusion when the

relationship of chronic bronchitis to emphysema is raised. It must be remembered that the definition of emphysema as used in America is an anatomic one. Most patients with clinically significant emphysema have an irreversible increase in resistance to air flow, and so emphysema clinically is often equated with "chronic obstructive pulmonary disease" (COPD). However, chronic bronchitis, a disease defined clinically as a persistent cough with the production of copious sputum, may also produce COPD. Many but not all patients with emphysema have chronic bronchitis. These interrelationships are best discussed by reference to the following diagram (Fig. 19–9). In the diagram, the shaded area of emphysema-bronchitis represents those individuals who are almost certain to have increased airway resistance and COPD. Those with anatomic emphysema alone may or may not have COPD, depending upon the severity of the pulmonary parenchymal changes. Those with chronic bronchitis alone also may not have COPD but may develop it with severe disease. To add to the complexity, there are rare patients who have both chronic bronchitis and emphysema without significant airway obstruction.

So the emphysema story is closely interwoven with chronic bronchitis. Emphysema is defined anatomically, chronic bronchitis clinically and COPD is a pathophysiologic syndrome. It is necessary to recognize, then, that among a series of patients with COPD, many and perhaps most will have only chronic bronchitis (since this is the commonest disease), some will have combined emphysema-chronic bronchitis, and some only emphysema.

Types of Emphysema. Although there are many classifications of emphysema, most investigators recognize three major forms: (1)

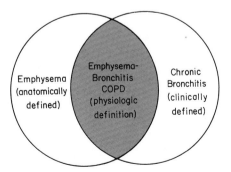

Figure 19–9. *Interrelationships of Chronic Bronchitis and Emphysema. (No quantitative distribution is implied by the demarcated areas.) (Adapted from Burrows, B., and Kettel, L. J.: Important considerations in emphysema-chronic bronchitis syndrome. Geriatrics, 24:72, 1969.)*

tractional or perifocal (paratractional, paracicatricial), (2) centrilobular (centriacinar) and (3) panlobular (panacinar). Additional categories have been established, such as compensatory, senile, focal and localized emphysema, but whether these represent true biologic variants of the disease is questionable, as will be discussed further below. In all forms of emphysema, the diagnostic features are to be found at the level of the pulmonary lobule (p. 783), the functional unit of the lung.

Tractional or *perifocal emphysema* occurs as a focal dilatation of air spaces with accompanying destruction of their walls involving part of or whole pulmonary lobules adjacent to areas of persistent atelectasis or scarring. The morphogenesis of the emphysematous changes probably involves a constellation of influences. The scarring and atelectasis collapse alveoli and thereby increase the elastic pull on the adjacent alveoli. The vascular supply to the distended air spaces is impaired by either distortion or damage to the microcirculation as it is trapped in the adjacent scars or compressed in the atelectatic areas. The small respiratory bronchioles are similarly narrowed or distorted, leading to partial obstruction. With such bronchiolar narrowing, air trapping may contribute to the distention of alveoli and, in turn, the distention further impedes blood supply. In this way, focal areas of lung substance become emphysematous. Such anatomic findings rarely cause symptoms because of the large pulmonary reserve.

In *centrilobular emphysema*, the septal destruction occurs centrally in the lobule while the alveoli in the periphery of the lobule are normal. It is important to recognize, then, that this anatomic definition is based upon the concept of the pulmonary lobule as the unit of lung substance. The affected alveoli may not always be strictly central but, in any event, in the centrilobular form of the disease a critical feature is the finding of both emphysematous and unaffected air spaces within the same lobule (Pratt and Kilburn, 1970) (Fig. 19–10). It is hardly necessary to point out that centrilobular emphysema is not limited to the central regions of the lung and, indeed, may occur in the apex, or randomly, but generally it is fairly diffuse and most marked basally.

In *panlobular emphysema*, the change is uniform over the whole lobule. Perhaps the term panacinar is more appropriate to indicate involvement of all alveoli or acini within the lobule. Generally, such panlobular emphysema is also diffuse throughout the lungs and generally it extends from the hilar region to the periphery of the lung (Pratt et al., 1963).

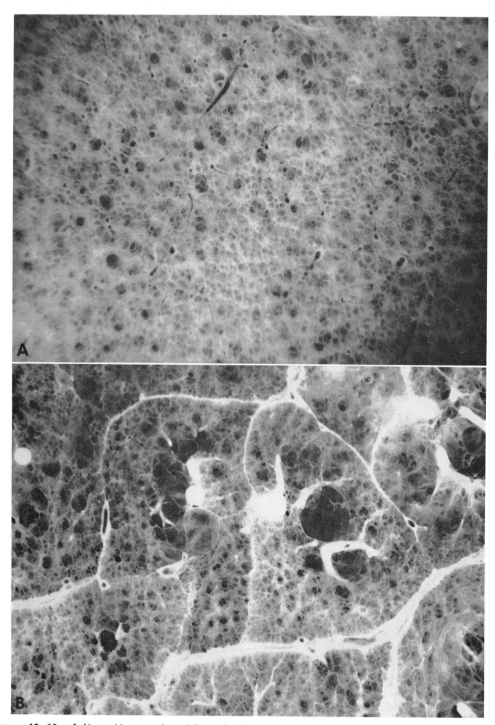

Figure 19–10. **A,** Normal lung as viewed through a dissecting microscope after fixation in inflation: magnification × 10. **B,** Centrilobular emphysema: magnification × 5.1. (The pulmonary arteries contain a barium-gelatin injection mass.) (From Bates and Christie: Respiratory Function in Disease.)

Now we come to the many other qualifying terms often applied to the basic disorder emphysema. *Compensatory* emphysema is sometimes used to designate dilatation of alveoli in response to loss of lung substance elsewhere. It is therefore a "first cousin" to tractional emphysema. It is best exemplified in the hyperexpansion of the residual lung parenchyma which follows surgical removal of a diseased lung or lobe. In most instances, this constitutes compensatory *hyperinflation* since there is no accompanying destruction of septal walls. However, any loss of lung substance increases the intrapulmonary negative pressure and therefore increases the pull on the residual lung substance. So it is possible that compensatory hyperinflation may, in time, lead to tractional emphysema.

Senile emphysema, referring to the somewhat voluminous lungs found so often in the aged, is another controversial entity. It was fashionable at one time to speak of "loss of elasticity" of lung substance with aging; careful analyses have failed to disclose any significant quantitative losses of elastic tissue, even in advanced age. Whether qualitative defects may arise in collagen or elastic fibers has not been ruled out (Ebert and Pierce, 1963). More likely, the lung alterations have a different causation. In the elderly, changes in the skeletal system, particularly the vertebral column, displace the rib cage upward and outward and increase the anteroposterior diameter of the chest (barrel chest). This increases the negative intrapleural pressure and the pull on the lungs, leading to a form of *compensatory hyperinflation.* In most instances, there is no destruction of lung substance and it is doubtful

whether the expanded lungs truly suffer from emphysematous changes. Certainly most of these patients suffer no respiratory deficit and have no COPD. A better designation would be senile hyperinflation. But, on occasion, a form of tractional emphysema may supervene, meriting the designation senile emphysema. Similar pulmonary changes are encountered with kyphosis or any other skeletal deformity which expands the chest cage.

Focal and localized emphysema simply refers to the gross distribution of the emphysematous change. In most instances, these represent random localized or focal distributions of centrilobular or tractional emphysema. Generally, relatively little lung substance is affected and the patients have no clinical manifestations because of the adequate pulmonary reserve. These designations, therefore, are useful insofar as they indicate anatomic lesions probably without clinical significance. In some instances, however, localized emphysematous lesions can occupy a volume as large as a whole lobe, producing reduction in the ventilatory efficiency of the remaining normal pulmonary tissue. Such patients may have expiratory air flow obstruction which is remarkably improved by successful removal or collapse of the localized process (Knudson and Gaensler, 1965).

Bullous emphysema merely refers to any form of emphysema that produces large subpleural blebs or bullae (Fig. 19–11). These cystic structures are not merely balloon-like cavities filled with trapped air; rather, they result from progressive destruction of septal walls, flooding over to encompass many contiguous pulmonary lobules. Most often, such bullae occur near the apex of the lung in relation to

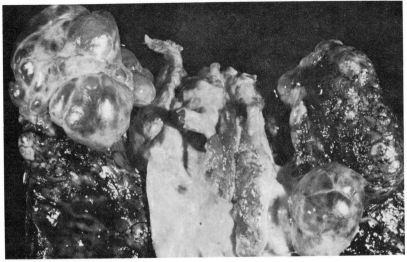

Figure 19–11. *Bullous emphysema with large apical and marginal subpleural bullae.*

old tubercular scarring and therefore comprise a form of tractional emphysema. Insufficient lung substance is affected to induce increased resistance to air flow but, on occasion, rupture of a bulla may give rise to pneumothorax.

Incidence. In considering the prevalence or incidence of emphysema, it must be remembered that, as defined here, it is an anatomic entity. Thurlbeck (1963), in one unselected postmortem study, reported that 50 per cent of patients had some degree of either panlobular or centrilobular emphysema. He considered the pulmonary disease to be responsible for the death of 6.5 per cent of these patients. Data on COPD may well include some cases of obstructive chronic bronchitis, combined chronic bronchitis and emphysema, as well as emphysema. Clinical studies suggest that chronic obstructive pulmonary disease is the most common form of pulmonary disease in man. Death rates from COPD are said to be doubling every five years, and today it is probably responsible for more deaths than carcinoma of the lung, ranking second only to heart disease (Markush, 1968) (Burrows and Kettel, 1969).

Both sexes are affected indiscriminately in the panlobular form, but men more often than women in the centrilobular pattern. Although emphysema does not become disabling until the fifth to eighth decades of life, it is well known clinically that ventilatory deficits may make their first appearance decades earlier in those destined to develop the full-blown disease (Burrows and Earle, 1969). Indeed, emphysematous changes were found in the lungs of teenagers dying of accidental causes, who had been exposed to environmental air pollution (Kleinerman et al., 1968). Certain genetic and familial predispositions have been identified as will be discussed below.

Pathogenesis. The following discussion relates to the two major forms of emphysema, centrilobular and panlobular. The origin of the tractional type has already been given. At the outset, it can be stated that the genesis of these two forms of emphysema is unknown, and therefore theories abound. Suprisingly, however, there is a lack of theories as to why some patients develop centrilobular emphysema and others, panlobular. While many frown on construing panlobular emphysema as merely an extension of centrilobular, some still hold to this view.

The question of whether chronic bronchitis (admittedly sometimes so mild as to not merit a clinical diagnosis) initiates the lesions in the air spaces or follows the development of emphysematous changes is a central controversial issue in the genesis of emphysema. First, the time-honored theory will be presented, followed by some of the conflicting evidence. The oldest hypothesis holds that chronic bronchitis induces partial obstruction of the airways, particularly in the respiratory bronchioles, which then leads to air trapping, progressive overdistention of alveoli and secondary damage to alveolar walls (Leopold and Gough, 1957) (McLean, 1958). Initiating influences might be air pollutants, particularly tobacco smoke. The latter is ascribed great causative importance. These irritants lead to increased mucus secretion in the walls of the bronchioles, eventual thickening of the mucosa of the bronchioles, narrowing of the lumina and thus increased resistance to air flow. As is well known, the bronchi and bronchioles expand during inspiration and are narrowed during expiration. Thus, with any superimposed narrowing or partial obstruction by excess mucinous secretions, there is a tendency for air trapping. The increased resistance to air flow leads to hypertrophy of the bronchiolar musculature, causing further narrowing. Secondary bacterial infection of the retained mucous secretions compounds the problem and induces an element of inflammatory fibrosis and narrowing of the air passages. Bronchial sequestration may occur, isolating the dependent pulmonary lobules and, in time, may lead to their total coalescence and to cyst formation. Allergic reactions to inhaled irritants or to endogenous bacteria may heighten the inflammatory response. The inflammatory disease further disturbs the blood supply to the bronchiolar walls as well as to the adjacent alveoli. As the bronchial and bronchiolar narrowing progresses, the increase in resistance to air flow further impairs expiratory emptying of the alveoli, and the patient must literally squeeze the air from his chest. In the normal state, expiration is a passive act, the air leaving the lungs because of elastic recoil. The increased expiratory effort further compresses the airways and adds to the expiratory obstruction. Air trapping and distention of the alveoli squeeze the septal capillaries, contributing to the loss of blood supply and destruction of the septae. Loss of these septal walls adds to the bronchial and bronchiolar narrowings since the normal pulmonary substance is elastic and tends to maintain the patency of the airways. Thus, a vicious cycle is created where partial obstruction leads to increased expiratory effort which, in turn, induces further obstruction (Farber and Wilson, 1968).

In support of this classic view, it is generally pointed out that emphysematous foci are often pigmented with carbon dust, particularly in centrilobular emphysema. Presumably, the coal dust and other noxious airborne particles (silicates, trace metals and organic residues) collect in the bronchioles and initiate the bronchiolitis, leading to the chain of events cited. Possibly toxic substances such as sulfur dioxide or nitrogen dioxide, adsorbed upon the particulate pigments, are concentrated in the sites of deposition (Boren, 1964).

Seductive as this classic theory may be, there is a substantial amount of evidence that the emphysematous changes in the septal walls may indeed be primary, albeit of mysterious origin, and in turn may lead to chronic bronchitis (Pratt and Kilburn, 1970). In some cases, no bronchitis can be found even on morphologic examination. Such instances are sometimes designated *primary emphysema*. Conversely, severe chronic bronchitis is not necessarily associated with emphysematous destruction (Simpson et al., 1963). If extension of the inflammation from the bronchioles to the adjacent septal walls played a role in the development of the destructive septal lesions, it is surprising that even electron microscopic examination of the septa (already partially disrupted) reveals no evidence of inflammatory disease (Reynolds, 1964). Indeed, the margins of the rents in the alveolar walls are covered by the septal epithelium with an intact subjacent basement membrane. Detailed examination of lungs with emphysema discloses many foci of pigmentation unrelated to injury of septal walls and, indeed, there is no relationship between severity of pigmentation and severity of the emphysema (Pratt, 1963). So the question has been raised: Does the destructive process in the septal walls deprive the bronchioles and bronchi of their tissue support, leading in turn to their narrowing, mucus retention, secondary infection and development of chronic bronchitis and bronchiolitis? What initiates such septal destruction is totally mysterious. While such a sequence of events provides a less satisfying theory of causation, some of the observations in support of it cannot be lightly dismissed.

Whatever the pathway, genetic factors contribute to the pathogenesis of emphysema. Laurell and Eriksson in 1963 called attention to a hereditary deficiency of the serum globulin alpha-1-antitrypsin in patients with severe diffuse panlobular emphysema. This pattern of emphysema tended to be bilateral and basilar in distribution and to occur in both sexes, principally in women at an early age. The mode of inheritance was postulated to be autosomal recessive. Nine codominant alleles and 17 different phenotypes have since been identified, creating a polymorphic spectrum of antitrypsin deficiency. It has been recommended, therefore, that this system be referred to as the *proteinase inhibitor system (Pi)*. Most homozygotes develop symptomatic COPD by age 40. Heterozygotes with the antitrypsin deficiency are also at increased risk (Falk and Briscoe, 1970). Recognition of this genetic influence makes clear why certain individuals develop emphysema with little provocation and others are much more resistant. Homozygotes may require little environmental input while heterozygotes will develop the disease only when exposed to significant environmental insults such as smoking (Mittman et al., 1971). However, not more than 10 per cent of all patients with emphysema are homozygous for alpha-1-antitrypsin deficiency (Lieberman, 1969). The heterozygous state has only been identified in approximately 9 to 14 per cent of two normal populations and 25.5 per cent of a series of patients with COPD, and so hereditary vulnerability cannot account for all cases of emphysema (Kueppers, 1969). Another genetic predisposition vaguely defined and unrelated to alpha-1-antitrypsin deficiency has also been reported, suggesting that still unidentified hereditary influences may be important (Larson et al., 1970). Significant as these gains may be in our understanding of this disease, we are still a long way from knowing its cause or, more likely, causes.

Morphology. Important criteria for the diagnosis and classification of the emphysemas are derived from the naked eye (or hand lens) examination of whole slices (Gough sections) of lungs fixed in inflation. Such slices, usually 2 mm. thick, permit identification of the coarsening of the native structure of the lung induced by emphysema, as well as its distribution throughout the lobes and the entire lung. The coarsening might also be called simplification of structure as air spaces coalesce, expand and lose their angularity. More detailed microscopic examination is necessary to visualize the abnormal fenestrations in the walls of the alveoli, complete destruction of septal walls and the distribution of damage within the pulmonary lobule. These septal changes are found in the walls of respiratory bronchioles, alveolar ducts and alveolar spaces. Enlargement of defects or coalescence of multiple adjacent ones can result in destruction of an entire septum, perhaps leaving only a strand of residual tissue, usually harboring a small blood vessel. In microscopic section, such a strand will appear as a "free-floating" island of tissue. With advance of the disease, adjacent alveoli fuse to produce even larger abnormal air spaces and possibly blebs or bullae. Often the respiratory bronchioles and vasculature of the lung are deformed and compressed by the emphysematous distortion of the air spaces and, as mentioned, there may or may not be evidence of bronchitis or bronchiolitis (p. 802) (Fig. 19–12).

The **differentiation of centrilobular from panlobular emphysema is made on the basis of the distribution of the septal destruction within the pulmonary lobule.** As mentioned, in centrilobular emphysema, the central air spaces are primarily involved and generally the peripheral alveoli in the lobule are spared and are essentially normal. In contrast, in panlobular emphysema, there is total involvement of the entire lobule. In both major forms of this disorder, there is remarkably little evidence of inflammatory change within the affected septa or air spaces.

The macroscopic appearance of emphysematous disease depends on the form of emphysema and its severity. Panlobular emphysema, when well developed, produces voluminous lungs, often overlapping the heart and hiding it when the anterior chest wall is removed. The pulmonary tissue is diffusely hypercrepitant and pillowy to palpation and

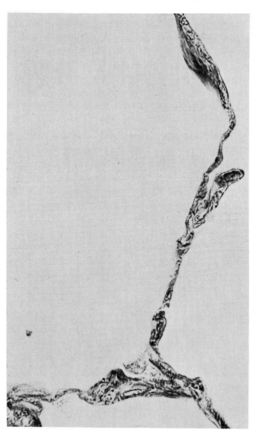

Figure 19–12. *Panlobular emphysema at high power detail, illustrating the avascularity of the septa—one basis for the marked cardiorespiratory complications of this disorder.*

the involvement usually extends out to the pleural surfaces (Fig. 19–13). The emphysematous lobes are uniformly pale owing to compression of the blood supply. Subpleural blebs or bullae may be present, but are often absent in this form of the disease. The macroscopic features of centrilobular emphysema are less impressive. The lungs may not appear particularly pale or voluminous unless the disease is well advanced. Generally, the upper two-thirds of the lungs are more severely affected. The lesions only become evident on sectioning of the lung since usually a narrow rim of subpleural lung parenchyma is spared. Large apical blebs or bullae are more characteristic of tractional emphysema, secondary to scarring. Tractional or perifocal emphysema is usually localized or focal and is seen as overdistended abnormal air spaces related to the sites of previous scarring or atelectasis.

Clinical Course. The clinical manifestations of emphysema do not appear until approximately one-third of the functioning pulmonary parenchyma is incapacitated. The panlobular form tends to be the most disabling because all alveoli are more or less affected. Considerable anatomic change may be present without producing clinical signs and symptoms. Dyspnea is usually the first symptom and it may appear with or without significant cough. In some patients, cough or wheezing is the chief complaint, easily confused with asthma. Typically, the dyspnea begins insidiously but is steadily progressive. Cough and expectoration are extremely variable and depend on the extent and severity of the associated bronchitis. Weight loss is common and may be so severe as to suggest a hidden malignant tumor. The physical findings are also variable. Classically, the patient is barrel-chested, dyspneic, with obviously prolonged expiration, and sits forward in his chair in a somewhat hunched-over position, attempting to squeeze the air out of his lungs with each expiratory effort. Classically, these unfortunates have a pinched face and breathe through pursed lips. All of these manifestations may be absent in those less severely affected. Hyperresonance related to the emphysematous changes may be present, but is unreliable as a diagnostic finding since it is also caused by simple hyperinflation without the destructive changes of emphysema. Similarly, chest films showing large, translucent lungs with low, flattened diaphragms are not diagnostic. *The only reliable and consistently present finding on physical examination is slowing of forced expiration.* A variety of other physiologic abnormalities can be demonstrated, as are detailed in the review by Burrows and Kettel (1969).

The differentiation of COPD originating

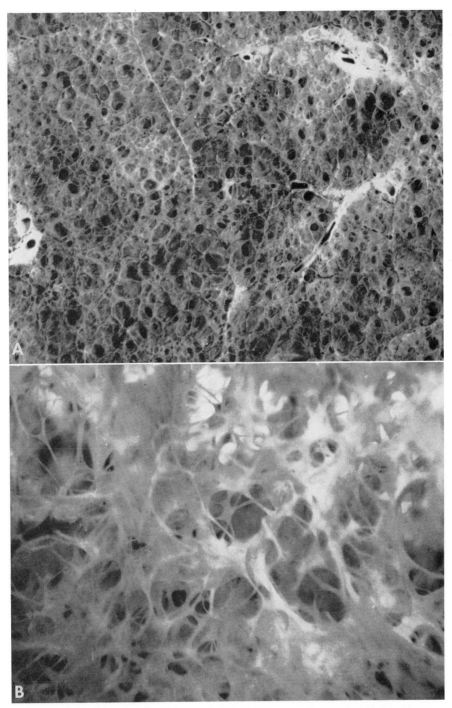

Figure 19–13. *A, Mild panlobular emphysema: magnification × 6. (Compare with normal lung structure, as shown in Figure 19–10A.) B, Severe panlobular emphysema: magnification × 10. (From Bates and Christie: Respiratory Function in Disease.) Compare with centrilobular pattern, p. 794.*

in chronic bronchitis from that due to emphysema is a difficult clinical problem requiring a variety of diagnostic procedures (Burrows et al., 1966). At the risk of oversimplification, with severe anatomic emphysema, cough is often slight, overdistention severe, diffusing capacity low and blood gases relatively normal. Such patients may overventilate and remain well oxygenated and, therefore, are euphoniously if somewhat ingloriously designated as "pink puffers." The patients with bronchial obstructive disease more often have a history of recurrent acute inflammatory episodes, persistent abundant purulent sputum, hypercapnia and severe hypoxemia, prompting the equally inglorious designation of "blue bloaters." A major hazard in severe emphysema, in addition to the respiratory difficulties, is the development of cor pulmonale and eventually congestive heart failure. Death of most of these patients is due to (1) right-sided heart failure, (2) respiratory acidosis and coma, and (3) massive collapse of the lungs secondary to pneumothorax. A surprising and still unexplained complication is peptic ulceration, found at autopsy in up to one-fifth of all patients with advanced disease.

INTERSTITIAL EMPHYSEMA

The entrance of air into the connective tissue stroma of the lung, mediastinum or subcutaneous tissue is designated as interstitial emphysema. Interstitial emphysema is totally distinct, both anatomically and clinically, from the forms of pulmonary emphysema previously described. Although in most instances alveolar tears in pulmonary emphysema provide the avenue of entrance of the air into the stroma of the lung, rarely, a wound of the chest that sucks air or a fractured rib that punctures the lung substance may underlie this disorder. Usually alveolar tears occur when there is a combination of coughing plus some bronchiolar obstruction, producing sharply increased pressures within the alveolar sacs. Children with whooping cough and bronchitis, adults with diphtheritic membranes, instances of obstruction to the airways (as by blood clots, tissue or foreign bodies) and individuals who suddenly inhale irritant gases are classic examples of how such tears may occur. Instrumentation of the airways, artificial resuscitation and positive pressure anesthesia are less common antecedents.

In all these circumstances, the tear is presumably widened by the dilatation of the full inhalatory effort, but as the lung collapses in expiration, the tear closes and blocks the escape of air. In this pump-like fashion, there is progressive accumulation of air that dissects through the fibrous connective tissue of the alveolar walls and into and along the fibrous septa of the lung to reach the mediastinum and thence possibly the subcutaneous tissues (Fig. 19–14). If the collection of air is small, it

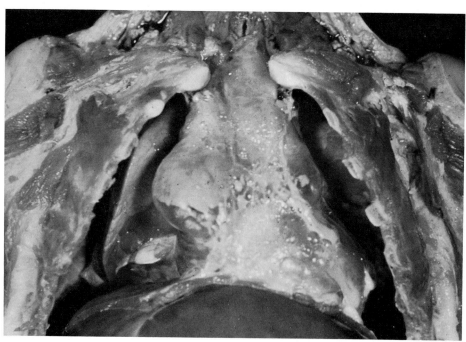

Figure 19–14. *Mediastinal emphysema. The air within the connective tissue produces the apparent "bubbles."*

usually has no clinical importance. However, extensive insufflation of the lung may encroach upon the small blood vessels to create a serious impairment of blood flow through the lungs. These patients may therefore have marked respiratory difficulty and severe cyanosis, occasionally terminating in death. When the interstitial air treks into the subcutaneous tissues, the patient may literally be blown up into an alarming, although usually harmless, "Michelin-tire-ad" with marked swelling of the head and neck and crackling crepitation all over the chest. In the majority of instances such air is resorbed promptly as soon as the point of entrance is sealed.

One pattern, *Hamman's syndrome*, deserves separation from the others. It comprises acute focal hyperinflation of a localized segment of lung that produces a tear in the lung substance and gives rise to interstitial emphysema. Usually there is no underlying clinically significant pulmonary emphysema. At the time of the tear, or because of the interstitial pressures within the lung, acute chest pain develops that may mimic a heart attack.

INFLAMMATIONS

ACUTE LARYNGOTRACHEOBRONCHITIS

Acute inflammations of the larynx and tracheobronchial tree are commonplace in industrialized nations because of the ever-present air pollutants. While these irritants alone rarely cause significant clinical disease, they render the mucosa of the airways vulnerable to microbiologic infections and allergic reactions. It is generally proposed that the air pollution causes mild degrees of inflammation which, in turn, weakens normal defense mechanisms and, at the same time, stimulates excessive mucinous secretions. The stage is thus set for bacterial or viral invasion. The agents most commonly involved are the *Staphylococcus aureus*, streptococci, *Haemophilus influenzae*, pneumococci and a variety of viruses including adenoviruses, influenza viruses and some of the ECHO group. Allergic reactions to pollens contribute to the inflammatory reaction. The mucinous secretions and inflammatory exudation lead to reflex coughing which, when persistent, may further traumatize and even denude the tracheal and bronchial mucosa.

The nature and extent of the morphologic changes depend, of course, on the severity of the inflammation. The lower portion of the trachea and major bronchi are principally involved. Early the affected mucosa is thickened, edematous and hypere-

mic. The surface is often layered by stringy mucus containing only a scant number of leukocytes. In severe disease, there is an intense inflammatory infiltrate in the respiratory mucosa, accompanied by mucopurulent exudation which harbors large numbers of viable and necrotic leukocytes as well as bacterial aggregates. Usually in the acute inflammations, there is no significant hyperplasia of the mucus glands and the mucosal layer is only mildly thickened. More intense inflammatory reactions may lead to ulcerative necrosis of focal areas, visible as irregular foci of red-green denudation (Fig. 19–15). As will be recalled, diphtheria (p. 390) produces an acute laryngotracheobronchitis, made distinctive by a gray to green, tough, fibrinous coagulum layering the mucosal surface designated as an inflammatory membrane or pseudomembrane. In those instances where allergic reactions are contributory, significant numbers of eosinophils may be present in the inflammatory exudate.

The clinical significance of these acute inflammations varies with the age of the patient and the etiology. Infants are, in general,

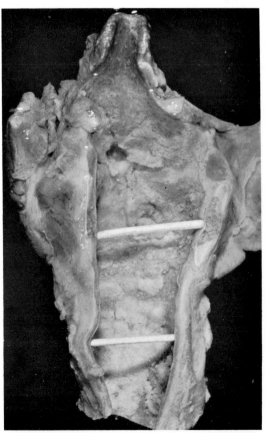

Figure 19–15. *Acute ulcerative laryngotracheobronchitis. The larynx and trachea have been opened posteriorly to demonstrate the extensive necrosis and exudation of the lining mucosa.*

more vulnerable than adults, probably because of their shorter and narrower tracheobronchial passages and the absence of mucus-secreting cells in their small bronchi or bronchioles. Secondary invasion by *H. influenzae* in this age group may induce a fulminating calamitous laryngotracheobronchitis leading, within the course of hours, to severe respiratory obstruction. Indeed, such inflammations may constitute medical emergencies requiring immediate tracheotomies and heroic therapeutic measures. The seriousness of diphtheria does not need emphasis. Save for these special instances, acute laryngotracheobronchitis is usually a mild illness characterized by a low-grade fever, malaise, hoarseness and productive cough. The disease is usually self-limited, particularly when further exposure to allergenic agents and air pollutants can be controlled. Recurrent acute attacks may, however, lead to chronic disease.

CHRONIC BRONCHITIS

This disorder, so common among habitual smokers and inhabitants of smog-laden cities, is not nearly so trivial as was once thought. When persistent for years, it may: (1) cause atypical metaplasia and dysplasia of the respiratory epithelium, providing a possible soil for cancerous transformation, (2) cause chronic obstructive disease (COPD) as discussed on p. 792, and (3) lead to cor pulmonale and heart failure. The widely accepted definition of chronic bronchitis is the clinical one—*chronic bronchitis is present in any patient who has persistent cough with sputum production for at least three months in at least two consecutive years* (American Thoracic Society, 1962). While both sexes and all ages may be affected, it is most frequent in middle-aged men. Seventeen per cent of all males and 8 per cent of females were considered to have chronic bronchitis in Great Britain in 1960 to 1961 (Editorial, 1961). The prevalence of this disease in the United States is not precisely known, but it is probably somewhat less common than in Great Britain.

Pathogenesis. Two sets of factors are important in the genesis of chronic bronchitis: (1) chronic irritation by inhaled substances and (2) microbiologic infections. Cigarette smoking remains the paramount etiologic influence (Thurlbeck and Angus, 1964). Heavy cigarette smoking alone will induce excessive mucus secretion, destroy the normal ciliary action of the respiratory epithelium and further cause squamous metaplasia and atypical dysplasia (Auerbach et al., 1962*a* and *b*). Other forms of atmospheric pollution have also been impli-

cated, principally sulfur dioxide and nitrogen dioxide (Kotin et al., 1963). The precise role of infections is less clear. It is generally felt that microbiologic invasion only occurs when preexisting chronic irritation and excessive mucus secretions lower normal defenses. Microbiologic cultures have, however, yielded inconstant findings ranging from reports that as many as 80 to 90 per cent of persons with chronic bronchitis are free of bacteria to those that describe the isolation of either pneumococci or *H. influenzae* in up to 80 to 90 per cent of cases (Buckley et al., 1957). Viruses, especially those of the respiratory syncytial group, undoubtedly also contribute but, once again, whether they are secondary passengers or primary causes is uncertain.

Morphology. The morphologic changes are most severe in the smaller bronchi and bronchioles, but may extend proximally to the bifurcation of the trachea. Hyperemia, swelling and bogginess of the mucous membranes are characteristic, frequently accompanied by excessive mucinous to mucopurulent secretions layering the epithelial surfaces. Sometimes heavy casts of secretion and pus fill the bronchi and bronchioles. **The critical morphologic feature is the thickness of the mucosal and submucosal gland layer** and, indeed, elaborate measurements have been made of the thickness of the bronchial mucus gland layer, correlating it with the severity and duration of the chronic bronchitis (Reid, 1960). Histologically, there is nothing unanticipated about the acute and chronic inflammatory response (Fig. 19–16). Occasionally, aggregates of lymphocytes are present within the subepithelial and deeper mucosal regions. The epithelium shows all degrees of reactive change, ranging from simple hyperplasia to squamous metaplasia and dysplasia. **Characteristic is the enlargement and hyperplasia of the mucus glands.** On occasion, the inflammatory reaction is accompanied by ulceration of the mucosal surface, sometimes followed by organization of the contained purulent secretion. In this manner, the lumina of the airways may be totally obliterated **(bronchiolitis fibrosa obliterans)** or polypoid masses of granulation tissue may markedly narrow the airway. In some cases, the bronchitis is associated with emphysema, as was discussed on p. 793.

The clinical sine qua non of chronic bronchitis is a persistent cough productive of copious sputum. For many years, no other respiratory functional impairment is present, but eventually dyspnea, on exertion, develops. With the passage of time, COPD may appear, accompanied by hypercapnia, hypoxemia and mild cyanosis. The differentiation of this form of obstructive lung disease from that associated with emphysema has already been discussed

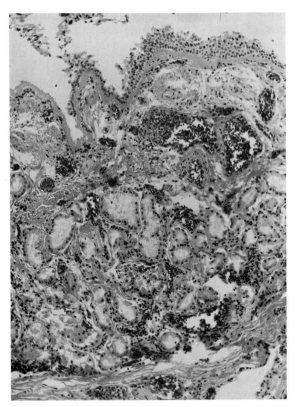

Figure 19–16. Chronic bronchitis. The lumen of the bronchus is above. Note slight desquamation of mucosal epithelial cells and marked thickening of the mucous gland layer (approximately twice normal). Vascular congestion is evident.

(p. 798). Longstanding severe chronic bronchitis commonly leads to cor pulmonale and possibly cardiac failure. Death may also result from further impairment of respiratory function incident to acute intercurrent bacterial infections.

BRONCHIAL ASTHMA

Asthma is a particularly distressing disease because those afflicted unpredictably experience disabling attacks of severe dyspnea and wheezing triggered by sudden episodes of bronchospasm. Between the attacks, early in the course of the disease, the patient may be virtually asymptomatic but, in time, chronic bronchitis or cor pulmonale often supervenes. Rarely, a state of unremitting attacks (*status asthmaticus*) proves fatal; usually such unfortunate patients have had a long history of asthma. In some cases, the attacks are triggered by exposure to an allergen to which the patient has previously been sensitized but, in others, no clear evidence of an allergic trigger can be identified.

Types and Pathogenesis. *Asthma is usually divided into two basic types: extrinsic and intrinsic, to which might be added a third mixed pattern where both extrinsic and intrinsic factors are operative. Extrinsic* or *atopic asthma* refers to the disease triggered by environmental antigens such as dusts, pollens, animal dander and foods, but potentially any antigen may be implicated. *Intrinsic asthma* refers to the disease in which the asthmatic attacks are not clearly related to exogenous allergens. A wide variety of stimuli appear to initiate attacks in these individuals, including relatively trivial respiratory infections, exercise, chilling and, in particular, emotional stress. In some patients, asthma appears to be a psychosomatic disease. There is a suspicion, however, that hidden allergens play some role, even in so-called intrinsic asthma. It is postulated that upper respiratory infections may sensitize patients to the microbial antigens harbored in their respiratory tracts. However, as will become clear, current theories of causation of intrinsic asthma lay less stress on allergic mechanisms than on autonomic nervous system imbalance. The form referred to as *mixed asthma* comprises the largest group of patients having components of both the intrinsic and extrinsic patterns. In many instances, patients with intrinsic asthma later develop the mixed type.

The identification of the reaginic immunoglobulin IgE by Ishizaka and Ishizaka (1967a) has unfolded the pathogenesis of atopic skin reactions as well as extrinsic asthma (a form of mucosal atopy). These workers showed that IgE was present in minute amounts in normal sera but was markedly elevated in the sera of patients with extrinsic asthma (Ishizaka and Ishizaka, 1967b). IgE-forming cells have been found in tonsils, adenoids, bronchial and peritoneal lymph nodes, skin and in the mucosa of the respiratory tract, stomach, small intestine and rectum. Following some antigenic stimulus evoking atopy, IgE is produced and fixes to human lymphocytes and tissue mast cells where it may persist for weeks. Thus sensitized, the particular organ or tissue harboring these mast cells becomes a "target" or "shock" organ on subsequent exposure to the specific antigen. A challenge dose of antigen then causes the release of vasoactive agents from the sensitized mast cells. Many chemical mediators, including histamine, bradykinin and slow-reacting substance (SRS), are activated, the last two perhaps as a result of the histamine-induced increased venular permeability (p. 68) (Grieco, 1970). Together these mediators cause contraction of smooth muscle, particularly that of the bronchi in the asthmatic. Presumably, histamine acts most rapidly, followed in turn by the slower-acting bradykinin and SRS.

The pathogenesis of intrinsic asthma is more obscure. There is good agreement on one fact: these patients do not have elevated levels of IgE (Berg and Johansson, 1969). Beyond this there is only speculation, the most common being that intrinsic asthma stems from some partial beta adrenergic blockade of the autonomic nervous system (Szentivanyi, 1968). Beta adrenergic stimulation causes relaxation of bronchial muscle. The beta blockage theory proposes that any stimulus such as psychic stress, exercise or chilling which activates the autonomic nervous system might trigger unopposed alpha adrenergic bronchoconstriction (Reed, 1968).

Yet another postulation is raised by Grieco (1970). Could asthma represent a disease that involves a lesion at the level of cyclic AMP in bronchial smooth muscle? The ultimate messenger of many hormones is the formation of cyclic AMP from ATP. Defective formation of cyclic AMP might block the normal release of catecholamines which help to maintain bronchodilation. Thus the asthmatic patient would be rendered vulnerable to attacks of bronchoconstriction. Although much has been learned about the origins of the asthmatic attacks in extrinsic asthma, the cause of intrinsic asthma is still highly speculative.

Morphology. The cardinal anatomic changes in asthma are found in the bronchi and bronchioles. Secondary changes such as hyperinflation of the al-

veoli or focal areas of atelectasis are frequent accompaniments, but the diagnosis rests with the demonstration of tenacious mucus plugs lying within bronchi and bronchioles that often completely occlude the lumina (Fig. 19–17). The walls of the bronchi may appear slightly thicker than usual, and sometimes there is denudation or sloughing of fragments of epithelium. In uncomplicated asthma, there is usually no significant suppuration within the bronchi and bronchioles. When marked infection supervenes, most investigators would prefer to designate the underlying disease as infective or suppurative bronchitis, implying that it is no longer asthma. Such patients with infective bronchitis may have a clinical syndrome somewhat like that of asthma, but the disease is no longer spasmodic, is no longer triggered by the same emotional and physical stresses and, in fact, represents a chronic obstructive pulmonary disorder quite distinct from asthma.

In the true case of asthma, there are many striking histologic changes such as the plugs of basophilic mucinous secretion lying within the bronchi. Classically, these secretions are PAS-positive and often contain "Curschmann's spirals," Charcot-Leyden crystals and numerous eosinophils. The underlying epithelium is edematous and has a striking inflammatory infiltrate, principally of eosinophils and lymphocytes (Fig. 19–18). There are thickening of the epithelial basement membrane and hypertrophy of the underlying smooth muscle (Fig. 19–19). The bronchial mucous glands sometimes are hyperplastic (Sanerkin, 1970). While the lungs often are overinflated, it is uncommon to find significant destruction of the alveolar septa or true emphysematous changes. If chronic bacterial infection has supervened as mentioned above, the changes

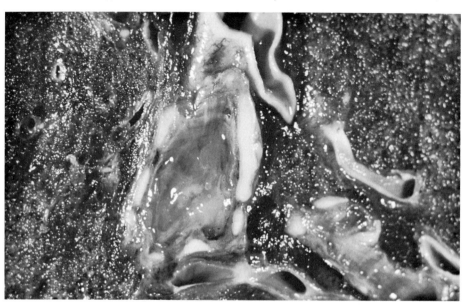

Figure 19–17. Bronchial asthma. A close-up of the transected bronchi. The largest is plugged with viscid mucus.

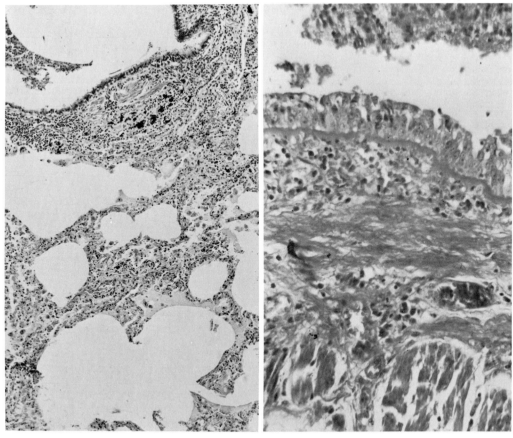

Fig. 19–18   Fig. 19–19

Figure 19–18. Bronchial asthma. Low power view of a distended bronchus (above) containing leukocyte-laden mucus and surrounded by a chronic inflammatory infiltrate. The alveoli are unevenly distended.

Figure 19–19. Bronchial asthma. A high power detail of the wall of a bronchus. Note the luminal mucus, (above) thickened basement membrane and hypertrophied muscle bundles at the bottom of the figure.

are those of inflammatory bronchitis and no longer comprise the disorder here defined as asthma.

Clinical Course. On the basis of the previously described changes, one can anticipate that an attack of asthma is characterized by the onset of respiratory difficulty with wheezing respiration, made particularly distinctive by prolongation of the expiratory phase. The victim labors to get air into his lungs and then cannot get it out, so that there is progressive hyperinflation of the lungs. The air gets trapped behind the mucus plugs. In the classic case, the acute attack lasts one to several hours and is followed by prolonged coughing with the raising of copious mucous secretions with considerable relief of the respiratory difficulty. In some patients, these symptoms persist at a low level all the time. In its most severe form, *status asthmaticus,* the severe acute paroxysm persists for days and even weeks and, under these circumstances, the ventilatory function

may be so impaired as to cause severe cyanosis and even death. The clinical diagnosis is aided by the demonstration of an elevated eosinophil count in the peripheral blood and the finding of eosinophils, Curschmann's spirals and Charcot-Leyden crystals in the sputum. The differentiation of extrinsic from intrinsic asthma has been rendered somewhat easier since discovery of the role of IgE in the former. The salient clinical characteristics of the two patterns is well summarized in Table 19–1 taken from Grieco (1970).

In the usual case, with intervals of freedom from respiratory difficulty, the disease is more discouraging and disabling than lethal. With appropriate therapy to relieve the attacks, these patients are able to maintain a productive life. However, in the more severe forms, the progressive hyperinflation may eventually produce emphysema. Superimposed bacterial infections may lead to chronic persistent bronchitis, bronchiectasis or pneu-

TABLE 19–1. CHARACTERISTICS OF EXTRINSIC AND INTRINSIC ASTHMA

Characteristics	Extrinsic	Intrinsic
Genetic influence	Present	Variable
Age of onset	<35	<5, >35
Hay fever	Frequent	Infrequent
Skin-sensitizing antibody	Usually present	Absent
Sputum	Eosinophils	Eosinophils PMN leukocytes Bacteria
Associated infection	Secondary	Primary
Intractable asthma	Uncommon	Common
Death	Rare	More frequent

From Grieco, M. C.: Current concepts of the pathogenesis and management of asthma. Bull. N.Y. Acad. Med., *46*:597, 1970.

monia that may ultimately cause death. In other cases, cor pulmonale and heart failure eventually develop.

BRONCHIECTASIS

Bronchiectasis is a chronic necrotizing infection of the bronchi and bronchioles leading to or associated with abnormal dilation of these airways. It is manifested clinically by cough, fever and the expectoration of copious amounts of foul-smelling, purulent sputum. It is rarely a primary pulmonary disorder, but usually develops as a sequel to some antecedent infection or obstructive disease within the lungs (Ogilvie, 1941). All ages and both sexes are affected, and it is quite common in childhood. In several series, more than half the patients had the onset of their disease before the age of 20 (Lindskog and Hubbell, 1955). The precise incidence of this disease is still unknown, but is reported to be present in up to 4 per cent of unselected autopsies. Because it may persist as a chronic, smoldering, latent infection without producing spectacular symptoms, it undoubtedly remains undiscovered in many individuals.

Etiology and Pathogenesis. It is still not certain whether bronchiectasis begins as an infection which causes necrosis and excavates the respiratory passages, or whether deranged respiratory physiology causes abnormal dilatation, poor drainage and secondary infection. Those who believe that infection is the primary change propose that antecedent pulmonary disease (asthma, bronchitis, tumors) or some foreign body causes partial or complete obstruction of the bronchi or bronchioles, and stasis provides the soil for infection. *Fibrocystic disease of the pancreas and avitaminosis A are important subsoils for the development of bronchiec-*

tasis, since in both of these entities there is squamous metaplasia of the normal respiratory epithelial mucosa, impairing normal defense mechanisms. Necrosis weakens the walls of these infected airways and dilatation ensues. When there is sufficient suppuration to cause total obstruction of the air passages, atelectasis develops in the surrounding pulmonary parenchyma and, with this collapse of the alveoli, there is further tendency to abnormal dilatation. The frequency, in these cases, of antecedent pulmonary and bronchiolar infections, such as pneumonia, tuberculosis, measles with respiratory involvement, whooping cough and influenza, supports this concept (Laurenzi, 1969). Many times, these antecedent infections are childhood diseases, thus explaining the occurrence of this disease in the young age group. Bronchiectasis in the ramifications of bronchi or bronchioles that are distal to tumors or foreign bodies further supports the obstructive, infective pathogenetic mechanism.

Chronic bacterial infections in the paranasal sinuses are present in these cases with such frequency that clinicians have coined the term "sinobronchial suppuration." Possibly the chronic, infective postnasal drip provides the source of bacterial contamination of the airways, that eventually leads to the establishment of persistent bronchiolar infection.

The specific nature of the infection does not appear to be important. Staphylococci, streptococci, pneumococci, *E. coli, H. influenzae, A. aerogenes* and airborne fungi are commonly isolated. In many cases, microaerophilic streptococci or bacteroides are identified, organisms that are capable of proliferating in the low oxygen tensions of the productive necrotizing inflammations. At one time, considerable emphasis was placed upon the frequent identification, in these infections, of fusiform bacilli and Vincent's spirochetes. While these organisms are commonly present, according to recent views they represent secondary saprophytes able to proliferate only in the presence of necrotic debris and, as such, are not primary etiologic factors. They may, however, contribute to the growth of more important pathogens by aiding in the proteolysis of necrotic tissue.

Those who postulate that deranged pulmonary function causes abnormal dilatation first, followed by infection, maintain that previous pulmonary disease destroys the normal support and function of the bronchi and bronchioles. The antecedent inflammation and its consequent scarring lead to persistent traction on the walls of the air passage. At the same time, the previous infection may have injured the elastic tissues and musculature of the walls of the bronchi, thus predisposing them to chronic dilatation. The atelectasis associated with many of these preceding lung infections aggravates the bronchiolar dilatation. The deranged, widened bronchi are thus rendered vulnerable to secondary infection, and the chain of exudation, necrosis and further obstruction follows. Congenitally malformed bronchi almost inevitably later develop bronchiectasis, supporting the concept of dilatation first, followed by infection.

Morphology. Bronchiectatic involvement of the lungs usually affects the lower lobes bilaterally, particularly those air passages which are most vertical. However, it is not uncommonly unilateral and segmental. Rarely, the bronchi of the upper and middle lobes are involved. When tumors or aspiration of foreign bodies lead to bronchiectasis, the involvement may be sharply localized to a single segment of the lungs. Usually the proximal segments of the respiratory passages, the first and second order bronchi, are unaffected and the most severe involvements are found in the third and fourth order bronchi and bronchioles. **The airways are dilated, sometimes up to four times the normal size.** These dilatations may produce long, tube-like enlargements (**cylindroid bronchiectasis**) or, in other cases, may cause **fusiform** or even sharply saccular distention (**saccular bronchiectasis**).

Characteristically, the bronchi and bronchioles are sufficiently dilated so that they can be followed, on gross examination, directly out to the pleural surfaces. By contrast, in the normal lung, the bronchioles cannot be followed by ordinary gross dissection beyond a point 2 to 3 cm. removed from the pleural surfaces. The lumina of the affected bronchi are characteristically filled with a suppurative, yellow-green, sometimes hemorrhagic exudate which, when removed, exposes a red-green or necrotic black, edematous, frequently ulcerated mucosa. Commonly the mucosa, when not ulcerated, is longitudinally wrinkled, suggesting that during life the air passages may have been considerably more dilated and that contraction at death caused wrinkling.

These anatomic changes are best brought out by sectioning the lung at right angles to the long axis of the affected airways. Under these circumstances, the bronchi and bronchioles appear abnormally prominent, thin-walled, dilated and filled with exudate. In more severe involvements, the dilatation may produce an almost cystic pattern to the cut surface of the lung, created by the widely dilated bronchioles and the compression of the intervening lung parenchyma (Fig. 19–20). Sometimes this honeycombed appearance causes confusion with bronchogenic congenital cysts of the lung. In the clinically significant cases, the lung parenchyma shows patchy emphysema and atelectasis, depending upon the degree of obstruction in the airways. When the infection extends to the pleura, as it often does, it evokes a fibrinous or suppurative pleuritis.

The histologic findings vary with the activity and chronicity of the disease. In the full-blown, active case, there is an intense acute and chronic inflammatory exudation within the walls of the bron-

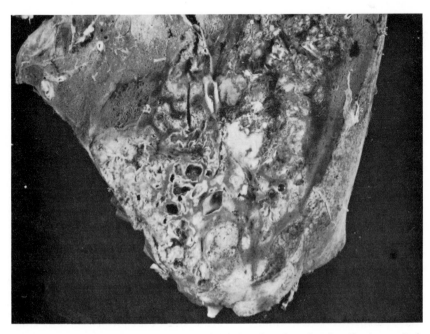

Figure 19–20. Bronchiectasis. The cut surface of the basal region showing the transected, markedly distended bronchioles.

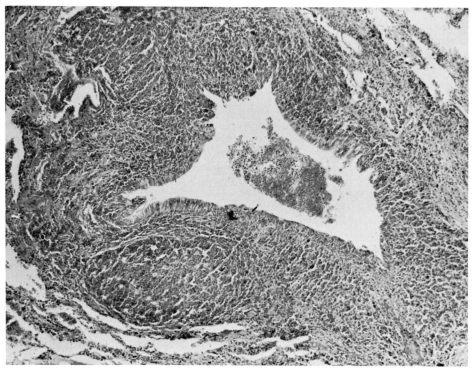

Figure 19–21. *Bronchiectasis. The bronchus is surrounded by an intense leukocytic infiltrate and the lining epithelium is eroded at 9 to 12 o'clock.*

chi and bronchioles, associated with desquamation of the lining epithelium and extensive areas of necrotizing ulceration (Fig. 19–21). The lumina of these affected airways contain large amounts of granular debris composed of necrotic inflammatory cells, respiratory mucosa and red cells. There may be pseudostratification of the columnar cells or squamous metaplasia of the remaining epithelium. In some instances, the necrosis may extend down to the smooth muscle and may even partly or completely destroy the bronchial or bronchiolar wall so that the infective process is in direct continuity with the lung parenchyma. In this instance, the process must be considered to have progressed to a lung abscess. Fibrosis of the bronchial and bronchiolar walls and peribronchiolar fibrosis develop in the more chronic cases. The scarring and chronic inflammation may extend into the surrounding alveoli and cause considerable deformity of the lung parenchyma.

When healing occurs, the inflammatory exudation subsides, and if the necrosis has not been too extensive, there may be complete regeneration of the lining epithelium. However, usually there has been so much injury that abnormal dilatation and scarring persist. In such healed cases, it may be impossible to distinguish preexistent bronchiectasis from bronchogenic congenital cysts. Often the epithelial regrowth takes the form of metaplastic squamous cells.

Clinical Course. The clinical manifestations are severe cough, expectoration of foul-smelling, sometimes bloody sputum and dyspnea and orthopnea in the severe cases. A systemic febrile reaction may occur when powerful pathogens are present. These symptoms are often episodic and are precipitated by upper respiratory infections or the introduction of new pathogenic agents. In the full-blown case, the cough is paroxysmal in nature. Exudate brought up into the sensitized areas of the main bronchi and trachea excites a violent paroxysm of coughing, which terminates in the raising of copious amounts of sputum. Such paroxysms are particularly frequent when the patient rises in the morning, and the changes in position lead to drainage of the collected pools of pus into the bronchi. In many instances, the chronic putrid suppuration produces a foul odor to the breath, which may be sufficiently offensive to make social outcasts of the sufferers. In the full-blown case, obstructive ventilatory insufficiency leads to marked dyspnea and cyanosis. Clubbing of the fingers sometimes develops in these patients.

The significance of bronchiectasis to the life span is still controversial. When the disease is acquired in adult life, it is compatible with fairly long survival. However, when the onset is in youth, it is probable that this disease materially shortens life. Few childhood bronchiectatics live beyond 40 years of age, unless adequately treated. These cases with an early onset usually develop one of several complications, such as lung abscesses, pneumonia or extension of the infection through the pleura to produce bronchopleural fistulas and exudative inflammation of the pleural cavity, known as empyema. In some cases, the infection causes acute vasculitis and small infected thrombi which break off and are carried to distant organs. The brain is frequently affected in this manner, producing metastatic abscesses or meningitis. When the disease is widespread in the lungs, chronic fibrosis may encroach on the pulmonary vascular bed and, in the course of years, may lead to the development of cor pulmonale. Amyloidosis is a further hazard in the case of long duration.

Bronchiectasis, parasinusitus and situs inversus (transposition of the viscera) constitute the triad of clinical findings known as *Kartagener's syndrome.*

BACTERIAL PNEUMONIA

Bacterial invasion of the lung parenchyma evokes exudative solidification (consolidation) of the lung parenchyma known as bacterial pneumonia. Many variables, such as the specific etiologic agent, the host reaction and the extent of involvment, determine the precise form of the pneumonia. Thus, classification may be made according to etiologic agent (for example, pneumococcic or staphylococcic pneumonia), according to the nature of the host reaction as suppurative, fibrinous, etc., or on the basis of the anatomic distribution of the disease as lobular (bronchopneumonia), lobar or interstitial pneumonia. The anatomic classification is often difficult to apply in the individual case since patterns often overlap considerably. The lobular involvement may become confluent to produce virtually total lobar consolidation; contrariwise, effective antibiotic therapy for any form of pneumonia may limit involvement to a subtotal consolidation. Moreover, the same organisms may produce lobular pneumonia in one patient, while in the more vulnerable individual a full-blown lobar involvement develops. Most important, from the clinical standpoint, is the identification of the causative agent and determination of the extent of the disease. Thus a patchy, lobular bronchopneumonia caused by an antibiotic-resistant staphylococcus may be infinitely more serious than a lobar pneumonia caused by the drug-sensitive pneumococci. Even with these difficulties, the time-honored anatomic classification still has the merit of presenting the span of the various severities of pneumonia encountered in clinical practice.

Bronchopneumonia (Lobular Pneumonia).
Patchy consolidation of the lung is the dominant characteristic of bronchopneumonia. This parenchymal infection usually represents an extension of a preexisting bronchitis or bronchiolitis. It is an extremely common disease that tends to occur in the more vulnerable two extremes of life, infancy and old age. In the young, there is little previous experience with pathogenic organisms, rendering these patients susceptible to organisms of even low virulence. Resistance likewise falls in the aged, particularly in those already suffering from some serious disorder. Bronchopneumonia thus frequently provides the period at the end of a long sentence of progressive heart failure or disseminated tumor. On this account, it is a common finding in postmortems.

Etiology. While virtually any pathogen may produce these lung infections, the common agents are staphylococci, streptococci, pneumococci, *H. influenzae, B. pyocyaneus* and the coliforms. Fungi (particularly Monilia, Aspergillus and Mucor) are sometimes the responsible agent, particularly in the predisposed vulnerable patient.

Pathogenesis. While bronchopneumonia may occur as a primary infection without antecedent disease, more frequently the soil is prepared by some previous infection or debilitating disorder. In children, whooping cough and measles are important antecedents. In the adult, chronic bronchitis, viral upper respiratory infections, cardiac disease, malnutrition, exposure, chronic alcoholism and disseminated cancer are the most important predispositions. Among these, the pulmonary edema of cardiac failure is preeminent. When the pneumonia is superimposed on such a substrate, it is designated as *hypostatic pneumonia.* The organisms, in all instances apparently gain access to the pulmonary parenchyma by passage down the airways to reach minute bronchioles and thence the surrounding alveoli. In the course of this passage, infections are set up in the bronchi and bronchioles that set the stage for the alveolar invasion.

Morphology. Bronchopneumonia comprises a nonspecific, suppurative inflammatory response in a loose alveolar tissue that offers little resistance to the accumulation of large amounts of exudate as well as free avenues of spread. The lobular consolidation may be patchily distributed through one lobe, but is more often multilobar and frequently bilateral and basal because of the tendency for secretions to gravitate into the lower lobes. While the consolidated foci tend to be distributed along the bronchial tree, this may only be apparent on microscopic examination. Often these consolidated areas are more easily palpated than visualized at postmortem examination. Well developed lesions are slightly elevated, dry, granular, gray-red to yellow and poorly delimited at their margins. They vary in size up to 3 to 4 cm. in diameter (Fig. 19—22). Confluence of these foci occurs in the more florid instances, producing the appearance of total lobar consolidation. When caused by such abscess producers as the staphylococci, central areas of necrosis often appear where slight pressure will express exudate from areas of abscess formation. The lung substance immediately surrounding areas of consolidation is usually slightly hyperemic and edematous, but the large intervening areas are generally normal. A fibrinous or suppurative pleuritis will develop if the inflammatory focus is in contact with the pleura; however, this is not common. With subsidence, the consolidation may resolve if there has been no abscess formation, or may become organized to leave residual foci of fibrosis.

Histologically, the reaction usually comprises a suppurative exudate that fills the bronchi, bronchioles and adjacent alveolar spaces (Figs. 19—23 and 19—24). Neutrophils are dominant in this exudation, and only small amounts of fibrin are usually present. Streptococcal bronchopneumonia in some instances produces some fibrinous reaction. Extravasated red cells are scanty. Generally it is

difficult to histologically identify the bacterial agents, except when the infection is highly virulent or the patient's resistance is extremely low and permits florid bacterial overgrowth.

This standard pattern of reaction may be modified by a number of variables. Any blood disorder that lowers the white count, such as leukemia, agranulocytosis or pancytopenia, or any disease that suppresses the immune response, such as hypo- or agammaglobulinemia, steroid therapy or immunosuppressive drugs, may render the patient particularly vulnerable to bacterial or mycotic growth, even those of low virulence, and permit virtual colony formation within the areas of exudation (**botryomycosis**). Extremely aggressive organisms or debilitation in the patient may lead to necrosis of the central regions of the lung lesions to produce the abscesses mentioned. Organization of the exudate may yield masses of fibrous tissue which constitute permanent residuals. Under happier circumstances, the exudate resolves, restoring the lung to its former state.

Particularly in infancy, but occasionally in adults, the bronchopneumonia may remain interstitial within the alveolar septa to produce an inflammatory reaction confined to the alveolar walls with little exudate in the air spaces. E. coli is the most common basis for such a reaction pattern in infancy, while the group B hemolytic streptococci are the most common causes in adults.

Clinical Course. The clinical signs and symptoms of lobular or bronchopneumonia

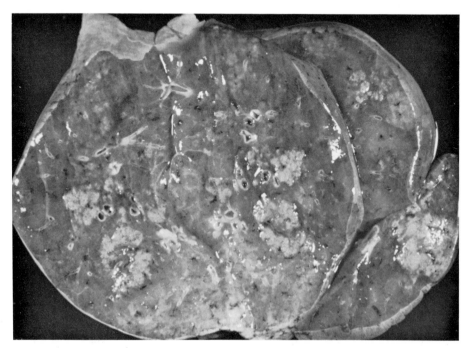

Figure 19–22. *Bronchopneumonia. The foci of consolidation appear pale and gray.*

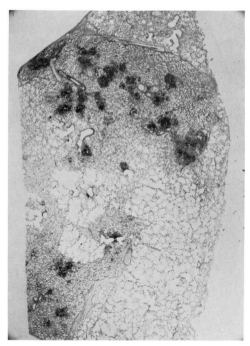 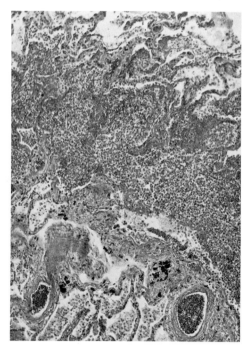

Fig. 19–23   Fig. 19–24

Figure 19–23 *Bronchopneumonia. A very low power view of a large histologic section to illustrate the patchiness of the inflammatory reaction.*

Figure 19–24. *Bronchopneumonia. A histologic detail of the exudative consolidation of the focus of inflammation.*

depend, as mentioned, upon the virulence of the invading agent and the extent of the pneumonic involvement. In the usually elderly person, there is a fever of 100 to 103° F., along with cough, expectoration and expiratory rales in one or more lobes. Often there is a previous history of confinement to bed, malnutrition, some underlying serious disorder or an upper respiratory infection (Ziskind and Saunders, 1953). Respiratory difficulty may be present, but is usually not prominent.

When the pneumonia is caused by antibiotic-sensitive organisms, the infection is readily controlled in patients not already mortally ill from some other cause.

The complications of bronchopneumonia are the formation of lung abscesses, spread to the pleural cavities producing empyema, spread to the pericardial cavity producing suppurative pericarditis, or the development of bacteremia with metastatic abscess formation in other organs and tissues in the body.

Lobar Pneumonia. *This is an acute bacterial infection of a large portion of a lobe or of an entire lobe, which tends to occur at any age, but is relatively uncommon in infancy and in late life.* Males are affected more often than females in the ratio of about 3 or 4 to 1. Of recent date, classic lobar pneumonia has been encountered very much

less often than in former years. Presumably, this lower incidence is attributable to the effectiveness with which antibiotics abort these infections and prevent the development of full-blown lobar consolidation.

Etiology. Approximately 90 to 95 per cent of all lobar pneumonias are caused by pneumococci. Most common are types I, III, VII and II, which altogether account for well over half of all cases. Type III causes a particularly virulent form of lobar pneumonia. However, not all lobar pneumonias are pneumococcal in origin. Occasionally, *H. klebsiella*, staphylococci, streptococci, *H. influenzae* and, currently in this day of antibiotic resistance, some of the gram-negatives, such as the pyocyaneus and Proteus bacilli, are also responsible for this lobar distribution of involvement, particularly in the vulnerable patient (Scott, 1952).

Pathogenesis. While lobar pneumonia may develop in a previously healthy individual, predisposing influences are often present, such as chilling, prolonged exposure and chronic alcoholism. The pathogenesis of a lobar distribution appears merely to be a function of the virulence of the organism and the vulnerability of the host. Heavy contamination by virulent pathogens may evoke this pattern in healthy adults, while organisms of lower virulence may accomplish the same in the predisposed.

The pathways by which the organisms gain access to the lung and cause the lobar distribution are controversial. Peribronchial and perivascular lymphatic dissemination and blood-borne spread are reasonably well ruled out. The probable route is through the respiratory passages. The wider distribution of this lobar form of pneumonic involvement may be attributed to the greater virulence of the organisms, and the more extensive exudation that leads to spread through the pores of Kohn. Moreover the copious mucoid encapsulation produced by the pneumococci protects the organisms against immediate phagocytosis and thus favors their spread.

Morphology. The histologic changes are presented first, since they make the gross alterations understandable.

Lobar pneumonia consists, in essence, of a widespread fibrinosuppurative consolidation of large areas and even whole lobes of the lung. In its evolution, the pneumonic involvement follows the basic pattern of all inflammations and begins with a serous exudation and accompanying vascular engorgement, followed by a fibrinocellular exudation, culminating ultimately in either resolution of the exudate or, less happily, in organization of the exudate.

Four stages of the inflammatory response have classically been described: congestion, red hepatization, gray hepatization and resolution. But present-day effective antibiotic therapy frequently telescopes or halts the progression so that often at autopsy the anatomic changes do not conform to the older classic stages.

The first **stage of congestion** represents the developing bacterial infection and is characterized by vascular engorgement, serous exudation and rapid proliferation of bacteria. The alveolar spaces thus contain, in addition to the proteinous edematous precipitate, scattered neutrophils and numerous bacteria, particularly when the causative organism is the pneumococcus. Occasionally macrophages are present. At this phase, there is no significant fibrin coagulum, and the underlying lung parenchyma is readily apparent.

The **stage of red hepatization** that follows is characterized by increasing numbers of neutrophils and the precipitation of fibrin to fill the alveolar spaces. The massive confluent exudation obscures the pulmonary architecture. Extravasation of red cells causes the coloration seen in the gross (Fig. 19–25). In many areas, the fibrin strands stream from one alveolus through the pores of Kohn into the adjacent alveolus. The white cells, while well preserved at this stage, contain engulfed bacteria.

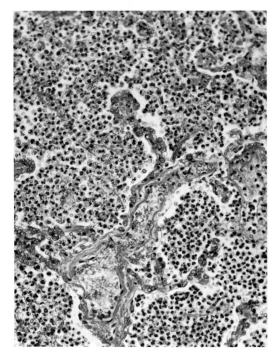

Figure 19-25. Lobar pneumonia. The stage of early red hepatization with congested septal capillaries and extensive white cell exudation into the alveoli. Fibrin nets have not yet formed.

An overlying fibrinous or fibrinosuppurative pleuritis is almost invariably present. Occasionally, when the total lobe has not been involved, the margin shows the features characteristic of the congestive stage.

The **stage of gray hepatization** follows with a continuing accumulation of fibrin associated with the progressive disintegration of inflammatory white cells and red cells. The fibrin now appears more clumped and amorphous. Classically, this exudate composed of deteriorating white cells, fibrin and red cells contracts somewhat to yield a clear zone adjacent to the alveolar walls disclosing the native architecture (Fig. 19–26). In the usual case, the alveolar septa are preserved. The pleural reaction of fibrin and white cells at this phase is more advanced. Sometimes, when the bacterial infection extends into the pleural cavity, the intrapleural suppuration produces what is known as **empyema**. It is the progressive disintegration of red cells and the persistence of fibrinosuppurative exudate that provide the basis for the gray hepatization.

The **final stage of resolution** follows in the great preponderance of cases with a favorable outcome. The consolidated exudate within the alveolar spaces undergoes progressive enzymic digestion to produce a granular, semifluid debris that is either resorbed or coughed up (Fig. 19–27). In such favorable cases, the normal lung parenchyma is restored to its normal state. The pleural reaction may simi-

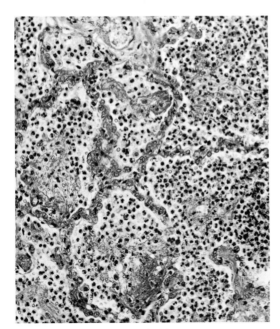

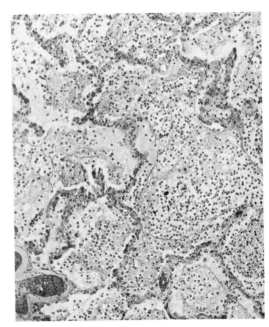

Fig. 19–26

Fig. 19–27

Figure 19–26. Lobar pneumonia. The stage of gray hepatization. The fibrin nets laden with leukocytes have contracted to yield the clear zones about the alveolar walls.

Figure 19–27. Resolving lobar pneumonia. The alveolar exudate has thinned out, the white cells are pyknotic and the alveolar walls again stand out.

larly resolve, but more often it undergoes organization, leaving fibrous thickening or permanent adhesions.

From these histologic changes, it is possible to deduce the gross anatomic features. Lobar pneumonia may involve one lobe completely or several lobes bilaterally or unilaterally. Classically, the entire lobe is involved, but often therapy limits the reaction to a portion of a lobe. The contiguous region of the adjacent lobe may show earlier phases of the inflammatory evolution than the primary site of involvement. In the initial stage of **congestion,** the affected lobe is heavy, red, boggy and subcrepitant and, on sectioning, yields a free ooze of a bloody serous fluid. The pleural surface may be dull, but does not have well developed exudation. With the onset of **red hepatization,** the lobe becomes heavier and assumes a "plaster cast" appearance of the thoracic cage, accurately reflecting the rib grooves and the diaphragmatic conformation. The cut surface at this stage is dry, granular and red, with a liver-like consistency, i.e., hepatization. The pleura is now layered with a well developed, granular, yellow fibrinous exudate (Fig. 19–28). The stage of **gray hepatization** evolves with progressive loss of redness. The now pale, gray-brown cut surface is still dry, granular and liver-like (Fig. 19–29), with persistence of the plaster cast appearance. The pleural reaction is still full-blown and sometimes is characterized by more overt suppuration to produce the empyema already mentioned. As **resolution** ensues, the lung again becomes wet, soggy and subcrepitant and again freely oozes a turbid exudation on cut section. By this time, the pleural exudate is less well defined, but often there appears the beginning fibrous shagginess of organization of the pleural reaction. Very frequently, there are interlobular adhesions at this stage, and occasionally loculated pockets of pus are found in the interlobular fissures.

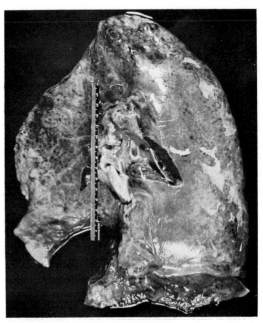

Figure 19–28. Lobar pneumonia. The stage of red hepatization. The lung is viewed from the external aspect to show the voluminous lower lobe, the "plaster cast" of the pleural cavity and the fibrinosuppurative pleuritis.

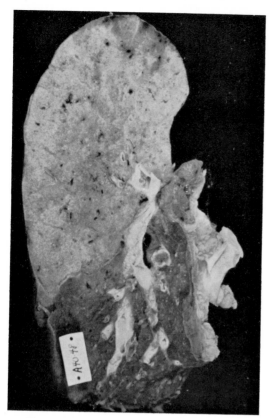

Figure 19–29. *Lobar pneumonia of the left upper lobe. The stage of gray hepatization with fairly sharp delimitation of the pneumonic process at the interlobar fissure.*

Many **complications** may supervene on this classic evolution. (1) The type III pneumococcus and the Klebsiella bacillus characteristically produce an **abundant mucinous secretion,** so that on cut section stringy, turbid exudate clings to the knife and is readily scraped off. (2) These same organisms and the staphylococci frequently cause **abscess formations,** producing foci of necrosis in the otherwise solidified lung substance. (3) **Organization of the exudate** may convert the lung into a carnaceous, solid tissue (Fig. 19–30). (4) **Bacteremic dissemination** to the heart valves, pericardium, peritoneum, brain, kidneys, spleen and joints may cause metastatic abscesses, meningitis or suppurative arthritis.

Clinical Course. In the classic pattern, the pneumococcus attacks otherwise healthy adults 30 to 50 years of age, while type III and *Klebsiella pneumoniae* occur most often in the elderly, the debilitated and chronic alcoholics. In all, the onset of the disease is sudden, with malaise, chills and fever. Cough appears with expectoration of at first a slightly turbid, watery sputum indicative of the stage of congestion, followed by a frankly purulent, hemor-

rhagic, so-called "rusty" sputum characteristic of the stage of red hepatization. The temperature elevation is very marked, frequently up to 103 to 104° F., and this elevation is usually maintained during the initial 4 to 7 days of the full-blown classic stages of consolidation if treatment is not instituted. Chills are characteristic and are sometimes so severe as to actually make the bed shake. These chills are presumed to represent episodes of bacteremia and hence mark the most favorable time to take blood cultures. If the causative organism is the type III pneumococcus or Klebsiella bacillus, the sputum has the same tenacious, mucinous quality as does the exudate in the lungs. Shortness of breath, dyspnea, orthopnea and cyanosis may appear when there has been considerable encroachment upon the vital capacity of the lung parenchyma. The fibrinosuppurative pleuritis is accompanied by pleuritic pain and pleural friction rub.

The physical findings vary with the stage of pneumonia. Within the first few days, limitation of breath sounds and fine crepitant rales herald the development of the stage of congestion. Two or three days after onset, more fully developed dullness, increased tactile and vocal fremitus and bronchial breath sounds reflect the solidification of the lung. At this stage, the fine crepitant rales often disappear. As resolu-

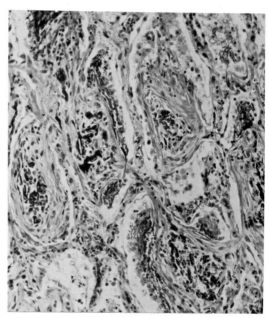

Figure 19–30. *Organization of lobar pneumonia. The alveolar spaces are virtually filled with connective tissue that can be seen in areas to be streaming through the pores of Kohn.*

tion occurs, moist rales reappear, the dullness diminishes and the bronchial breath sounds and tactile and vocal fremitus gradually subside.

This classic progressive symptom complex is, however, totally modified by the administration of antibiotics which alter the progression of the disease at any stage. Treated patients may be relatively afebrile with few clinical signs 48 to 72 hours after the initiation of antibiotics. For this reason, the classic "crisis" of lobar pneumonia, in which the temperature suddenly breaks and begins to fall, along with improvement in the patient's clinical condition, is now rarely encountered.

The identification of the organism and the determination of its antibiotic sensitivity are the keystones to appropriate therapy. Less than 10 per cent of patients with lobar pneumonia now succumb and, in most such instances, death may be attributed either to a complication such as empyema, meningitis, endocarditis or pericarditis or to some predisposing influence such as debility or chronic alcoholism.

PRIMARY ATYPICAL PNEUMONIA (PAP)

This term is applied to an acute febrile respiratory disease characterized by inflammatory changes in the lungs, largely confined to the septal walls. Because there is little intra-alveolar exudate, so typical of the bacterial and mycotic pneumonias, this interstitial pneumonitis has long been known by the incongruous designation "atypical pneumonia." In about half of the cases, no etiologic agent can be isolated. The largest group of known etiology are caused by *Mycoplasma pneumoniae*, also known as the Eaton agent (Armstrong, 1969). These pleuropneumonia-like organisms (PPLO) may represent protoplasts of streptococci since about 10 per cent of these patients have antistreptococcal MG agglutinins in their serum. Although *M. pneumoniae* is endemic, it may cause epidemics of PAP in populations living under crowded inadequate conditions. Viruses are the cause of the remaining cases of PAP of known etiology, including influenza types A and B, parainfluenza viruses, the respiratory syncytial viruses (RSV) and rhinoviruses. RSV is the most common cause of atypical pneumonia in infants. Other agents which have been isolated from cases of PAP include the Coxsackie and ECHO viruses, rickettsiae and, occasionally, the viruses of rubeola and varicella.

Any one of these agents may merely cause an upper respiratory infection recognized as the common cold, or a more severe lower respiratory infection, i.e., PAP. The circumstances which favor such extension of the infection are often mysterious, but include malnutrition, alcoholism and underlying debilitating illnesses.

Morphology. The viral and M. pneumoniae etiologies produce essentially similar morphologic patterns. Because the mild cases recover, our understanding of the anatomic changes is necessarily based upon the more severe, fatal expressions of these infections. The pneumonic involvement may be quite patchy or involve whole lobes bilaterally or unilaterally. The affected areas are red-blue, congested and subcrepitant. The weight of the lungs is usually moderately increased in the range of 800 gm. for each lung. On section, there is a slight ooze of red, frothy fluid, but since most of the reaction is interstitial, little of the inflammatory exudate escapes on transection of the lung substance. There is no obvious consolidation such as is encountered in lobar pneumonia. The pleura is smooth, and pleuritis or pleural effusions are infrequent.

The histologic pattern, too, depends on the severity of the disease. Predominant is the interstitial nature of the inflammatory reaction virtually localized within the walls of the alveoli (Parker et al., 1947). The alveolar septa are widened and edematous and usually have a mononuclear inflammatory infiltrate of lymphocytes, histiocytes and occasionally plasma cells. In very acute cases, neutrophils may also be present. In the fulminating cases of influenza, fibrin thrombi are found within the alveolar capillaries as well as small areas of necrosis of the alveolar walls associated with hemorrhage. In all forms of this atypical pneumonia, the alveoli are remarkably free of exudate and contain only a scattered pink precipitate of edema fluid in which are scattered occasional mononuclear cells. Fibrinous consolidation is conspicuously absent, except occasionally in the form of a pink, hyaline membrane lining the alveolar walls, apparently produced by transudation of fibrin through the walls of severely affected alveolar septa (Fig. 19–31). Sometimes the septal lining epithelium underlying the hyaline membrane is transformed by hypertrophy into cuboidal cells.

Superimposed bacterial infection modifies the histologic picture by causing ulcerative bronchitis and bronchiolitis. Spread of the bacterial invasion may yield the anatomic changes already described under bacterial pneumonia. Inasmuch as the inflammatory reaction in the uncomplicated case is interstitial in all but the most severe instances, it does not cause tissue necrosis. Subsidence of the disease is, in such cases, followed by reconstitution of the native architecture.

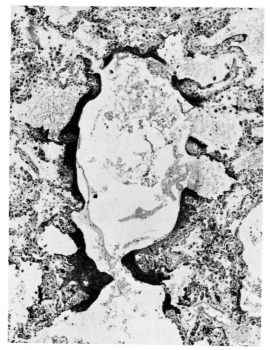

Figure 19–31. *Primary atypical (viral) pneumonia with prominent hyaline membranes and interstitial inflammatory infiltration.*

Clinical Course. As indicated, the clinical course is extremely varied. Many cases masquerade as severe upper respiratory infections or as "chest colds." Even the cases with well developed atypical pneumonia have few localizing symptoms. Cough may well be absent, and the major manifestations may consist only of fever, headache, muscle aches and pains in the legs. The cough, when present, is characteristically dry, hacking and unproductive of sputum because the inflammatory reaction is largely interstitial. The edema and exudation are both strategically located to cause an alveolocapillary block and thus evoke symptoms out of proportion to the scanty physical findings. Dullness, diminished breath sounds and rales may be virtually absent. One of the useful laboratory aids in differentiating the viral atypical pneumonia from the *M. pneumoniae* form of the disease is the cold agglutinin test which is positive with the Mycoplasma but usually negative in those pneumonias of viral origin. Isolation of the causative agent, whether viral or Eaton agent, is extremely difficult and requires fairly fastidious technical methods (Griffin and Crawford, 1965) (Forsyth et al., 1965).

The ordinary sporadic form of the disease is usually mild with a low mortality, below 1 per cent. However, primary atypical pneumonia may assume epidemic proportions with inten-sified severity and greater mortality, as was all too grimly documented in the highly fatal influenzal pandemics of 1915 and 1918.

The association of fever, respiratory disease that resembles PAP and mucocutaneous lesions (ulcers, bullae) in the nose, mouth, genitals or anus is designated as the *Stevens-Johnson syndrome*. The presence of cold agglutinins in these cases suggests an *M. pneumoniae* causation for this syndrome.

LUNG ABSCESS

The term pulmonary abscess describes a local suppurative process within the lung characterized by necrosis of lung tissue. While certain small differences exist between abscesses of the lung and those of other tissues, these pulmonary involvements essentially follow the pattern of abscesses in any tissue. Lung abscesses may develop at any age and are especially frequent in young adults. Oropharyngeal surgical procedures, sinobronchial infections, dental sepsis and bronchiectasis play important roles in their development. Males are affected somewhat more often than females.

Etiology and Pathogenesis. Although any pathogen, under appropriate circumstances, may produce an abscess, the commonly isolated organisms, are, in order of frequency, the *Streptococcus viridans*, *Staphylococcus aureus*, *Streptococcus hemolyticus*, pneumococci, some of the anaerobic streptococci, and a host of less common gram-negatives (Schweppe et al., 1961). Mixed infections occur very often because of the important causal role that inhalation of foreign material plays. The spirochetes and fusiform bacilli of Vincent's infection are often identified in these lesions, but their significance is as controversial here as it is in bronchiectasis. More likely, they are merely secondary saprophytic invaders. The causative organisms are introduced into their sites of focal destruction by the following mechanisms (Amberson, 1954): (1) *Aspiration of infective material.* This is particularly common in acute alcoholism, coma, anesthesia, sinusitis, gingivodental disease and debilitation in which the cough reflexes are depressed. Aspiration of gastric contents is particularly serious because the gastric acidity adds to the irritant role of the food particles and, in the course of aspiration, mouth organisms are inevitably introduced. (2) *Antecedent primary bacterial infection.* Post-pneumonic abscess formations are particularly associated with *Staphylococcus aureus*, *H. klebsiella* and the type III pneumococcus. Mycotic infections and bronchiectasis are additional antecedents to lung abscess formation. (3) *Septic embolism.* Infected emboli from thrombophlebitis in any portion of the systemic venous circulation or from vegetative bacterial endocarditis on the right side of the heart are trapped in the lung. (4) *Neoplasia.* Secondary infection is particularly common in the bronchopulmonary segment obstructed by a primary or secondary malignancy. This sequence is typical of bronchogenic carcinoma in which impaired drainage, distal atelectasis and aspiration of blood and tumor fragments all contribute to the development of sepsis. (5) *Miscellaneous.* Direct traumatic penetrations of the lungs, spread of infections from a neighboring organ, such as suppuration in the esophagus, spine, subphrenic space or pleural cavity, and hematogenous seeding of the lung by pyogenic organisms may all lead to lung abscess formation.

When all these causes are excluded, there are still many cases (25 per cent) in which no reasonable basis for the abscess formation can be identified. These are referred to as "*primary cryptogenic*" lung abscesses.

Morphology. Abscesses vary in diameter from a few millimeters to large cavities of 5 to 6 cm. Commonly, they are found in association with some of the antecedent pulmonary infections mentioned. They may affect any part of the lung and be single or multiple. The localization and number of abscesses are, in large part, dependent upon their mode of development. Pulmonary abscesses due to the aspiration of infective material are much more common on the right side than on the left, and are most often single. Presumably this is due, at least in part, to the more vertical course of the right bronchus. Abscesses which develop in the course of pneumonia or bronchiectasis are commonly multiple, basal and diffusely scattered. Septic emboli and pyemic abscesses, by the very haphazard nature of their genesis, are commonly multiple and may affect any region of the lungs (Fig. 19—32). Sometimes solitary pulmonary abscesses occur in the subapical and axillary portions of the upper lobes and the apical portion of the lower lobes, particularly on the right. This distribution appears to be in conflict with the presumed aspiration theory of their pathogenesis. However, for postoperative patients remaining recumbent for long periods of time, dependent portions of the lungs are not the bases.

Abscesses usually occur well out in the lung substance, close to or in contact with the pleura. They begin as a focus of hyperemia followed in time by central necrosis. At first the enclosing wall is poorly defined but, with time and progressive fibrosis, it becomes more discrete. Rupture through this containing wall may create grape-like multiloculations.

At the time of examination, the cavity may or

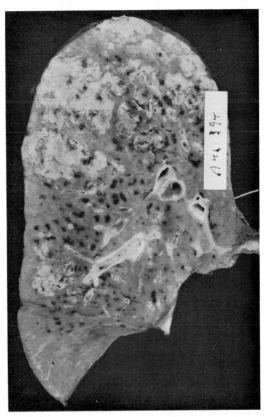

Figure 19–32. *Multiple pyemic abscesses of the lung, each surrounded by a wide rim of pale gray consolidation of the lung substance.*

may not be filled with suppurative debris, depending upon the presence or absence of a communication with one of the air passages. When such communications exist, the contained exudate may be partially drained to create an air-containing cavity. Superimposed saprophytic infections are prone to flourish within the already necrotic debris of the abscess cavity. These alter the appearance because their proteolytic action provides a favorable soil for the primary pathogen that then assumes an increased virulence to cause rapid spread of the infection. This sequence of events leads to large, fetid, green-black multilocular cavities with poor margination, designated as **gangrene of the lung.** The enhanced inflammations produce such rapid exudation and edema that the blood supply is compressed, adding an element of ischemic necrosis to the preexisting infection — hence the term gangrene. Occasionally, abscesses rupture into the pleural cavity to yield bronchopleural fistulas and empyema.

The histologic appearance of the abscess conforms to the standard pattern of nonspecific inflammatory reaction. The **cardinal histologic change is suppurative destruction of the lung**

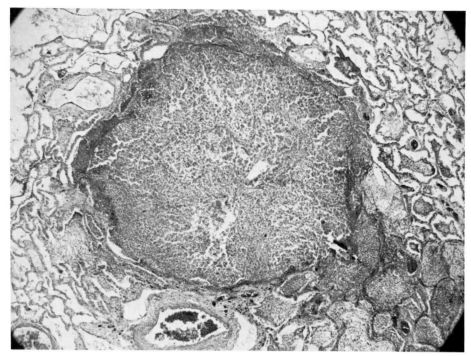

Figure 19–33. *A pyemic lung abscess with complete destruction of underlying parenchyma within the focus of involvement.*

parenchyma within the central area of cavitation (Fig. 19–33). In chronic cases, considerable fibroblastic proliferation produces a containing fibrous wall. There is often inflammatory pneumonic consolidation in the immediately adjacent alveoli. When gangrene supervenes, the affected necrotic parenchyma frequently persists for a period of time as shadowy outlines mimicking infarction necrosis. It is obvious that in the course of healing of such destructive lesions, permanent fibrous scarring must result.

Clinical Course. The manifestations of pulmonary abscesses are much like those of bronchiectasis and are characterized principally by cough, fever and copious amounts of foul-smelling purulent or sanguineous sputum. Characteristically, these patients have paroxysmal coughing as changes in position initiate sudden drainage of fluid exudate. At this time, a cupful of sputum may be raised, followed by marked relief of the cough and dyspnea. If the abscess is solitary, respiratory difficulty may be minimal. Clubbing of the fingers and toes, of uncertain pathogenesis, may appear within a few weeks after the onset of an abscess.

The diagnosis of this condition can only be suspected from the clinical findings and must be confirmed by roentgenography and bronchoscopy. Many times the fluid levels can be demonstrated by x-rays. Whenever an abscess is discovered, it is important to suspect an un-derlying carcinoma, since these are present 10 to 15 per cent of the time.

The course of pulmonary abscesses and their significance to the patient are quite variable. About one-quarter heal spontaneously and give rise to no sequelae. However, for the remainder, the outlook depends entirely upon the amount of lung tissue affected and the chronicity of the disease. If untreated, the process may extend to cause invalidism of the patient by virtue of the chronic suppuration and destruction of ventilatory function. While the span of life is undoubtedly shortened in such individuals, there are no valid figures which permit an exact estimate of this danger. Frequently, death is precipitated by extension of the infection into the pleural cavity or by the development of *brain abscesses* or *meningitis* from septic emboli. A rare patient may develop secondary amyloidosis.

PULMONARY TUBERCULOSIS

The general discussion of tuberculosis was presented on p. 411. Here our interest centers on the effects of this infection on the lungs. As the earlier discussion indicated, the overwhelming preponderance of tuberculous infections affect the lungs and, indeed, begin there. Pulmonary involvement is still the major cause of tuberculous morbidity and mortality.

It is the prevention and control of these pulmonary infections that have accounted for tuberculosis being the eighteenth leading cause of death in 1965 as compared with its being the leading cause of death in the United States in 1900 (National Health Education Committee, 1966). The death rate in the United States in 1965 from tuberculosis was 4.1 per 100,000 population as compared with a death rate of 200 in 1900. In the Netherlands, the death rate is approximately 3 per 100,000. Regrettably, in many parts of the world, underprivileged populations still suffer from death rates twenty-fold those of the Netherlands and other industrialized nations.

Despite this record of successful regional control, in some parts of the world tuberculosis ranks with malaria as a leading cause of death. It is still one of the most important infectious diseases in Western countries outranked perhaps only by pneumonia and renal infection and, in many of the closely crowded, disease-ridden urban slums in the United States, it is still the most important infection. It is estimated that for every death due to tuberculosis, there are 10 to 20 active infections. Thus, there is a large reservoir of this infection still to be found throughout the world. Since most tuberculous infections arise in or eventually involve the lungs, it is appropriate to consider these pulmonary changes in some detail.

Etiology and Pathogenesis. The various factors that condition the likelihood of developing tuberculosis and the influences that determine the severity and nature of the clinical infections have been presented in the basic consideration of this disease (p. 411). These considerations involve the natural and acquired resistance of the host, with particular emphasis on previous sensitization and acquired immunity, as well as the magnitude of the infective dose and virulence of the organisms. It was also pointed out that age and a variety of socioeconomic factors, such as nutrition, housing and crowding, are all relevant to the genesis of tuberculous infections. Intercurrent diseases, particularly diabetes mellitus and silicosis, materially predispose to tuberculosis.

Primary Pulmonary Tuberculosis. Save for the rare exception of intestinal (bovine) tuberculosis, and the even more uncommon skin, oropharyngeal and lymphoidal primaries, the lungs are the usual location of primary infections. Aspirated pathogenic tubercle bacilli implant on the alveolar walls. The droplet size capable of reaching the alveolar space has been intensively studied. Droplets larger than 15 microns in diameter are usually trapped in the upper respiratory passages and are then carried out by the normal mechanisms of the lung. It is therefore the minute, particulate, airborne contamination that produces the clinical infections.

Morphology. When first implanted in the lung parenchyma, the tubercle bacilli evoke a fairly nonspecific inflammatory reaction in the unsensitized individual. The subsequent macroscopic and microscopic alterations comprising the characteristic primary pulmonary infection have already been described as the **Ghon complex.** These can be summarized briefly. The usual site of localization of the parenchymal lesion is subpleural either just above or below the interlobar fissure between the upper and lower lobes. The focus of yellow-white caseation rarely exceeds 1 or 2 cm. in diameter. It is rarely cavitated and is classically well delimited from the surrounding substance. The regional nodes of drainage characteristically become enlarged and caseous (Fig. 19–34).

Histologically, there is an initial neutrophil aggregation that is transformed within 24 to 48 hours into a predominantly histiocytic response. During the ensuing week, there is a continued accumulation of histiocytes, some of which remain via-

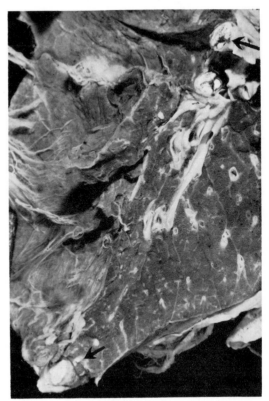

Figure 19–34. *Primary pulmonary tuberculosis. The parenchymal focus of white caseation is present in the lower left corner (arrow) and the caseated lymph nodes of drainage, in the upper right (arrow).*

ble while others undergo necrosis. During the interval, the development of sensitivity modifies the banal character of the exudate so that during the second week, the more characteristic tubercle develops, with central masses of histiocytes and possibly some caseation enclosed by a wall of epithelioid cells, lymphocytes, plasma cells and fibroblastic proliferation. Langhans' giant cells are frequently but not invariably present. Drainage to the regional tracheobronchial nodes produces a parallel series of changes in these sites.

The course and fate of this initial infection are extremely variable. Depending upon the factors of immunity, sensitization and aggressiveness of the invading agents, the initial tuberculous lesions may be largely proliferative or exudative in nature. The resistant host reacts with adequate phagocytic epithelioid cell response, fibroblastic walling off and eventual scarring. In the more vulnerable host, the lesions may be largely exudative in nature, i.e., with extensive inflammatory exudation, caseation and poor localization. In most instances, the primary complex is well controlled, tubercles are characterized by good defensive walling off and progressive scarring follows, accompanied usually by calcification. The same sequence may occur in the lymph nodes but, in general, the proliferative activity is less adequate in these sites and persistent foci of caseation may remain for months or years. In these nodes, then, viable microorganisms provide a site for endogenous reinfection later in life.

In a small percentage of infants and children, the primary infection is poorly tolerated, and an extensive exudative reaction leads to the confluence of many tubercles and the production of large areas of consolidation that may involve a segment or even a large proportion of the affected lobe to produce so-called *tuberculous pneumonia (pneumonia alba)*. When the exudation and caseation are extensive, dissemination may occur by erosion of a focus of caseation into a bronchus or bronchiole. Bacteria are thus spread to immediately contiguous segments of the lung. As this material is coughed up, higher levels of the respiratory tree are seeded by reaspiration of the material, and other lobes and the opposite lung may become secondarily infected. In this way, tuberculous infections are started in the trachea and larynx, and by the swallowing of the infective material, intestinal tuberculosis may develop (Auerbach, 1949). Through the lymphohematogenous routes, distant organs may be infected in the pattern already mentioned as *miliary tuberculosis* and *isolated organ tuberculous infection*. Primary tuberculosis, while usually a benign, self-limited disease, is nonetheless capable of progressive dissemination and spread

of infection to reproduce all the patterns of tuberculosis which are encountered in the adult reinfection types. However, even in these progressive cases, the infection may be halted at any stage, followed by fibrous encapsulation, scarring and calcification, leaving only fibrocalcific residues.

Reinfection, Adult or Secondary Pulmonary Tuberculosis. Most cases of adult or secondary pulmonary tuberculosis represent reactivation of an old, possibly subclinical infection (Trauger, 1963). The number of asymptomatically affected Americans is estimated to be of the order of 25 million (Mitchell, 1967). When secondary tuberculosis appears, it tends to produce more damage in the lungs than primary tuberculosis but, on the other hand, the risk of developing reactivated or secondary tuberculosis is much lower than the risk of acquiring a primary exposure. As was discussed earlier (p. 414), on initial contact with the tubercle bacillus, both hypersensitivity and some degree of partial immunity are acquired. The immunity establishes some resistance to reactivation of the disease and thus reduces the incidence of secondary tuberculosis. The hypersensitivity, however, leads to greater tissue destruction on account of the heightened inflammatory response. Therefore, this accentuated reaction only leads to walling off of the infected foci and localization of the infection after the caseating destruction has reached its height.

While most adult forms of pulmonary tuberculosis begin as apical lesions, the subsequent course of the infection is totally unpredictable and may lead to widespread exudative, proliferative, cavitated and calcified lesions throughout the lungs. Many attempts have been made to subdivide these anatomic lesions into categories based upon the nature and extent of the lesions. However, the disease refuses to follow these arbitrary subdivisions. It is therefore better to discuss the sequence of changes that comprise the full spectrum of pulmonary tuberculous lesions (Auerbach, 1936).

The **secondary pulmonary tuberculosis lesion** is almost invariably located in the apex of one or both lungs. It begins as a **small focus of consolidation, usually less than 3 cm. in diameter, located within 1 or 2 cm. of the apical pleura.** Less commonly, initial lesions may be located in other regions of the lung, particularly about the hilus. As reinfections, these lesions are usually associated with a considerable amount of proliferative response but, in the highly sensitized individual, exposed to a large number of virulent bacilli, considerable exudative consolidation may develop. The foci are fairly sharply circumscribed, firm, gray-white to yellow areas that have a greater or lesser component of central caseation and peripheral fibrous induration. In almost every case of reinfection tuberculosis, the regional nodes develop foci of similar tuberculous activity. In the favorable case, the initial parenchymal focus develops a small area of caseation necrosis that does not cavitate, because it fails to communicate with a bronchus or bronchiole. The subsequent course may be one of progressive fibrous encapsulation, leaving only fibrocalcific scars that depress and pucker the pleural surface and cause focal pleural adhesions. Sometimes these fibrocalcific scars become secondarily blackened by anthracotic pigment. In many instances a dense, collagenous, fibrous wall may totally enclose inspissated, cheesy, caseous debris that never resolves and remains as a granular lesion at postmortem examination.

Histologically, these lesions are characterized by both exudative and proliferative changes. At the outset, the inflammatory reaction consists largely of aggregates of monocytes and epithelioid cells, found within a coagulum of precipitated protein and fibrin within the alveolar spaces. However, at the time when most cases are available for tissue study, characteristic coalescent granulomas are present, composed of phagocytic and epithelioid cells surrounded by a zone of fibroblasts and lymphocytes that usually contains one or more charac-

teristic Langhans' giant cells. Some caseation is usually present in the centers of these tubercles, the amount being entirely dependent upon the sensitization of the patient and the virulence of the organisms (Fig. 19—35).

As the lesion progresses over weeks to months, more tubercles coalesce to create the confluent area of consolidation described in the gross. In the favorable case, over the course of the succeeding months, the proliferative fibrosis increases, the caseous debris is resolved to a variable extent and replaced by an ingrowth of fibroblasts, and eventually either the entire area is converted to a fibrocalcific scar, or the residual caseous debris becomes totally and heavily walled off by hyaline collagenous connective tissue. In these late lesions, the multinucleate giant cells tend to disappear. While tubercle bacilli can be demonstrated by appropriate methods in the early exudative and caseous phases, it is usually impossible to find them in the late fibrocalcific stages. However, it cannot be assumed that their absence in histologic sections is tantamount to their total destruction, since in many of these instances culture of the exudate or inoculation of this material into guinea pigs yields the organisms.

Later Progressive Pulmonary Tuberculosis. A variable, undetermined number of early lesions continue to progress over a period of months to years, to cause further pulmonary and even distant organ involvements.

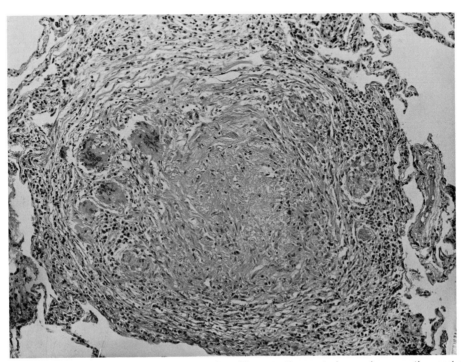

Figure 19—35. A characteristic tubercle in detail to illustrate the central granular caseation and epithelioid and giant cells.

Apical, fibrocaseous tuberculosis with cavitation fairly well describes the next stage of this disease. By erosion into a bronchiole, drainage of the caseous focus transforms it into a cavity. With this direct communication with an airway, growth and multiplication of the tubercle bacilli are favored by the increased oxygen tensions. At the same time, the local accumulations of inhibitory organic acids are drained and the significantly acid caseous material partially removed, further improving the environment for bacterial multiplication. Under these conditions, a ragged, irregular cavity is produced that may progressively increase in size, sometimes to occupy virtually the entire apex of the lung.

The cavity is lined by a yellow-gray caseous material, and is more or less walled off by fibrous tissue, depending upon the resistive mechanisms of the host and the age of the lesion (Fig. 19–36). Not uncommonly, thrombosed arteries may traverse these cavities to produce apparent fibrous bridging bands. This tendency for tuberculosis to incite thrombosis is a beneficial one, since it prevents the hematogenous dissemination of bacilli and the erosion of large vessels. On the other hand, many times thrombosis does not occur and this accounts for the hemoptysis associated with open cases. When such cavitation occurs in the apices, the pathways for further dissemination of the tuberculous infection are prepared. The infective material may now disseminate through the airways to other sites in the lung or upper respiratory tract. Spread may also occur to the lymph nodes, via the lymphatics and thence retrogressively through other lymphatics to other areas of the lung or to other organs. Miliary dissemination through the blood is a further hazard. In such progressive tuberculosis, pleural adhesions are almost inevitable, and may be only localized to the apices or may produce a generalized pleuritis and obliteration of the pleural cavity.

Advanced fibrocaseous tuberculosis with cavitation may affect one, many or all lobes of both lungs, in the form of isolated minute tubercles, confluent caseous foci or large areas of caseation necrosis. In some of the far advanced cases of pulmonary tuberculosis that have ended in death, postmortem examination reveals the lung converted to a mass of honeycombed cavities separated only by scant areas of scarring, compressed atelectatic, or compensatorily emphysematous lung parenchyma (Fig. 19–37). The degree of fibrous walling off and proliferative reaction depends, to a considerable extent, upon the chronicity of the disease and the defensive reaction to the advancing process. In many instances, the cavities coalesce to produce giant irregular spaces up to 10 and even 15 cm. in diameter. The intervening bands of barely recognizable parenchyma may contain areas of caseation necrosis, and it is indeed difficult to understand how the patient's respiratory function was sufficiently preserved to sustain life. In some of

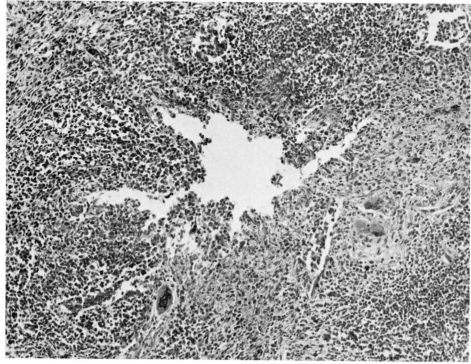

Figure 19–36. *Pulmonary tuberculosis, showing a characteristic microcavity with a granulomatous wall containing numerous giant cells.*

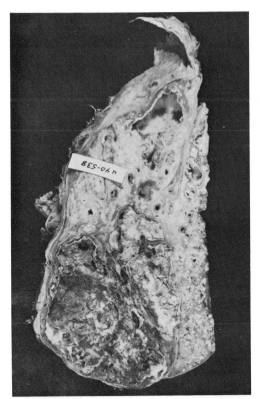

Figure 19–37. Far advanced cavitated pulmonary tuberculosis. The lung is honeycombed by cavities, the largest two appearing in the apical and basal regions.

these advanced cases, there is considerable scarring and calcification of the intervening areas, along with the advance of the lesions in other areas. All stages, then, of tuberculosis infection may be present, from the early tubercle to caseation necrosis to fibrocalcific scars.

In the forward advance of this disease, the pleura is inevitably involved and, depending upon the chronicity of the disease, serous pleural effusions, frank tuberculous empyema or massive obliterative fibrous pleuritis may be found. Usually, by the time the process has extended to multiple cavitations, the pleural reaction has reached the stage of dense fibrosis that virtually blocks the removal of the lungs from the chest cavity. In the course of extensive fibrocaseous tuberculosis, it is almost inevitable that tubercle bacilli become implanted on the mucosal linings of the air passages, and that **endobronchial and endotracheal tuberculosis** develop. These lesions may later become ulcerated to produce irregular, ragged, necrotic, mucosal ulcers. Accompanying the endobronchial tuberculosis, **laryngeal seeding and intestinal tuberculosis** are common. The incidence of laryngeal complications varies between 10 and 20 per cent, depending upon the stage of advancement of the pulmonary lesions. In minimal cases of apical tuberculosis,

laryngeal involvement is distinctly uncommon, and is probably of the order of 1 per cent. Intestinal tuberculosis is a much more frequent complication and is found in about 50 to 80 per cent of patients who die of far advanced disease.

Pulmonary tuberculosis may assume other patterns within the lungs. From the initial apical lesion, lymphatic dissemination may give rise to widespread miliary or small focal areas of exudative or proliferative tuberculous infection through one segment of the lung or through large areas of one or all lobes. Peribronchial lymphatic dissemination usually does not cause diffuse dissemination, but rather tends to be confined to one lung segment drained through one group of lymphatic channels. In these cases, the discrete yellow-white foci of consolidation are separated by apparently unaffected lung parenchyma, and are usually more easily felt than seen. It is to be remembered that individual tubercles are of microscopic size, and it is only when multiple tubercles coalesce or a single tubercle considerably enlarges that they become macroscopic. Such peribronchial lymphatic dissemination, of course, may coexist with other areas of fibrocaseous, confluent or cavitated tuberculosis.

Lymphohematogenous dissemination may give rise to miliary tuberculosis, confined only to the lungs or involving other organs as well. The distribution of the miliary lesions depends upon the pathways of dissemination. Tuberculous infection may drain via the lymphatics through the major lymphatic ducts into the right side of the heart, and thence spread into a diffuse, blood-borne pattern throughout the lungs **alone.** Since most of the bacilli are filtered out by the alveolar capillary bed, the infective material may not reach the arterial systemic circulation. However, usually such limitation to the lungs is not complete, and some bacilli pass through the capillaries to enter the systemic circulation and produce distant organ seedings. In other circumstances, a tuberculous focus may erode directly into a pulmonary **artery** and thence be spread only in the pattern of supply of this single vessel to produce a localized miliary dissemination within the alveolar parenchyma. On the other hand, extension into a pulmonary **vein** is likely to be followed by disseminated miliary tuberculosis throughout the body or isolated organ tuberculosis (p. 416).

In all instances of the miliary type of distribution, the individual focal lesions vary from one to several millimeters in diameter and are distinct, yellow-white, firm areas of consolidation that usually do not have grossly visible central caseation necrosis or cavitation at the time of examination (Fig. 19–38). Histologically, however, these present the characteristic pattern of individual or multiple confluent tubercles having microscopic central caseation. Similar gross and histologic lesions are found in other sites of seeding. It was pointed out

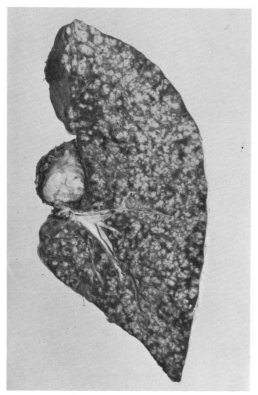

Figure 19–38. *Advanced miliary tuberculosis of the lung. The foci of caseation have coalesced to produce large nodules of consolidation.*

gestively cheesy material that converts the lung into a noncrepitant consolidated mass.

Histologically, the alveoli are filled with an exudate composed mostly of mononuclear phagocytes trapped within a large mass of granular, precipitated, fibrinoproteinous exudate. In the course of time, these areas may undergo total caseation necrosis with destruction of the underlying parenchyma, while in other areas recognizable or abortive tubercles may form and eventually yield confluent areas of fibrocaseous tuberculosis. Usually, however, with such overwhelming disease and low resistance, the patient does not survive to the stage of developing an adequate proliferative response. In the absence of well developed tubercles, it may indeed be difficult to establish on histologic grounds the tuberculous nature of the pneumonic process. However, numerous bacilli are usually present in such exudates, and acid-fast stains will disclose the indentity of the infection. Death, while usual, is not inevitable in such florid disease, and resolution of the exudate may occur with considerable restora-

earlier that certain organs, such as striated voluntary muscles, the heart, pancreas, testes, thyroid and stomach, are infrequent sites of miliary dissemination, while the liver, spleen, bone marrow, eye grounds, kidneys, adrenals, fallopian tubes, epididymides and meninges are more favorable soils. However, in any individual instance, the quantity and virulence of the infective material determine the likelihood and pattern of spread of such lesions. Although it is common to think of miliary dissemination as occurring from one single massive spillage of infective material into the blood, there is considerable evidence that such hematogenous dissemination may occur slowly and repeatedly over the course of weeks, months and even years.

In the highly susceptible, highly sensitized individual, the tuberculous infection may spread rapidly throughout large areas of lung parenchyma to produce a diffuse bronchopneumonia, or lobar exudative consolidation, at one time descriptively referred to as "galloping consumption" (Fig. 19–39). This anatomic pattern consists of a tuberculous **pneumonia alba** in which focal or confluent areas of lung parenchyma, sometimes involving total or multiple lobes, become completely filled with a gray-white, sug-

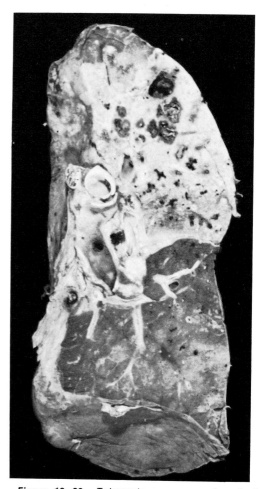

Figure 19–39. *Tuberculous pneumonia of the upper lobe viewed on the cut section of the lung.*

tion of previous architecture. Areas where the underlying structures have been destroyed become scarred, and fibrocalcific residues are therefore the rule. Inevitably, in tuberculous pneumonia, the infection extends into the pleural cavity.

In all cases of suspected tuberculous tissue changes, acid-fast smears, cultures and guinea pig inoculation to identify the bacilli should be employed before one makes a diagnosis of such clinical importance.

Clinical Course. The clinical course of pulmonary tuberculosis depends entirely upon the activity, extent and pattern of distribution of the tuberculous pulmonary infection. In the primary form, and the developmental stages of reinfection tuberculosis, the patient may be entirely asymptomatic. When sufficient lung parenchyma is affected in either of these instances, the first clinical manifestations are fever, malaise, weakness, night sweats, loss of appetite and loss of weight. These nonspecific constitutional reactions are believed to reflect a systemic toxemia of uncertain type, possibly related to the absorption of caseonecrotic debris. However, it should be emphasized that in many cases the anatomic lesions remain entirely silent and are only discovered after a considerable period of development in the course of routine screening chest x-rays. When bronchi are impinged upon or eroded, cough and productive sputum become prominent features. As the lung parenchyma is destroyed and vessels eroded, hemoptysis makes its appearance and is usually present in about half of all cases of pulmonary tuberculosis. Pleuritic pain (accentuated by deep breathing and coughing) appears as the infection extends to the pleural surface. In far advanced, terminal cases with the gradual progression of the tuberculous process and progressive destruction of lung parenchyma and ventilatory function, dyspnea, wheezing, and even cyanosis may occur. Hoarseness reflects laryngeal involvement, and gastrointestinal symptoms may arise secondary to intestinal lesions, but these are usually late manifestations.

This progressive course of clinical signs and symptoms may, of course, be halted at any stage when the advancement of the disease is checked and healing and resolution begin. On the other hand, the course may be punctuated by massive hemoptysis from erosion of a major vessel, by the appearance of a sudden, hectic, febrile illness as a manifestation of a diffuse miliary dissemination or by sudden central nervous system, renal or adrenal symptoms secondary to isolated organ involvements. Because tuberculosis is such a common disease and because it is so protean in its manifesta-

tions, it mimics many other disorders of inflammatory or neoplastic nature. Tuberculosis must be suspected in any form of febrile illness accompanied by clinical or radiographic signs of pulmonary lesions. It must be considered in the differential diagnosis of destructive disorders in any of the internal organs or bones of the body where it may present as a mass in the lungs, as a cause of bony defects, as a source of destructive erosion of the kidneys, or as the basis for superficial lymphadenopathy.

While the diagnosis can be suspected on the basis of clinical manifestations or x-rays, ultimately, the tubercle bacillus must be identified. Acid-fast smears as well as cultures and guinea pig inoculation of the sputum and gastric washings may be required. A negative tuberculin test is fairly strong evidence against the diagnosis, but it must be remembered that skin anergy is produced by all forms of severe illness, *including overwhelming tuberculosis* as well as measles, sarcoidosis, Hodgkin's disease, extreme old age, debility, steroids and other immunosuppressive treatment. Usually, such causes of anergy are readily evident. A positive tuberculin test, of course, does not indicate active disease since it merely denotes prior contact with the mycobacterium.

It is impossible to make meaningful generalities about the prognosis in tuberculosis since there are so many variables involved. The great majority of cases respond to present-day chemotherapeutic measures unless the disease is very advanced or intercurrent problems such as diabetes mellitus complicate the outlook. It should be recalled that amyloidosis may appear in longstanding chronic tuberculosis.

OTHER FORMS OF PULMONARY DISEASE

The lung is involved in a great variety of systemic diseases. Pneumonia is a common accompaniment of measles, tularemia, diphtheria and typhoid fever. Various forms of pneumonitis are the rule in systemic sarcoidosis, the mycotic infections and many others. Since these pulmonary involvements are only one feature of a systemic disease, it only remains to discuss here the few in which the pulmonary involvement is the primary or major problem in the disease.

PNEUMOCONIOSIS

This term designates a disease of the lungs caused by the inhalation of dust. Policard

(1962) defines it far more elegantly: "The conflict of living matter with the mineral world: the pneumoconioses."

The variety of clinically and anatomically described pneumoconioses appears to grow with each year. As environmental diseases, they have been covered in Chapter 12, with principal attention to anthracosis (p. 510), silicosis (p. 511), berylliosis (p. 514) and asbestosis (p. 513).

LIPID PNEUMONIA

Patchy or diffuse consolidation of the lung may be caused by the aspiration of a variety of oils. Aspiration of oil is usually encountered in infants and children who are forced to swallow cod liver oil against their resistance, or in small weak infants and in those with congenital malformations in whom the swallowing reflex may be deranged. In adults, lipid pneumonia usually follows the protracted use of mineral oil as a laxative or the use of oily nose drops or sprays. Even in the normal adult, oily nose drops may find their way into the respiratory tree during the course of the night. Rarely, cases of lipid pneumonia have been reported following the use of radiopaque oil for x-ray visualization of the respiratory tree. Under the circumstances in which these oily materials are aspirated, it can be anticipated that most cases of lipid pneumonia will be encountered in infants and young children, and in the debilitated and old.

The vegetable oils, commonly used in radiographic studies of the lungs, are the least irritating. In general, the more unsaturated the oil, the greater its toxicity. Some of the most reactive oils are those found in lard and peanuts, and chaulmoogra oils (Pinkerton, 1928). By contrast, corn and sesame oils are bland. Cod liver oil is not strongly irritant, but is most often implicated in lipid pneumonia in infants. Mineral oil is quite bland, but acts as an inert foreign body in tissues. When aspirated, even milk and cream are capable of evoking an inflammatory response.

Pathology. The extent of pneumonic reaction depends largely upon the quantity and chemical nature of the oil implicated. In general, the lesions are bilateral, but tend to affect the right lung more than the left because of the direct drainage path of the right main-stem bronchus. In individuals who are largely confined to bed, as in early infancy and in the very old, the dorsolateral portions of the upper lobes are the sites of drainage; in others, the basal regions are most often involved. The aspirated oil is emulsified once it reaches the alveoli, and the fine droplets are phagocytized by large numbers of

macrophages called out in response to this foreign material. In the early stages, the affected alveoli are partially or totally filled with aggregates of distended macrophages which contain large, clear, spherical, intracytoplasmic vacuoles (Fig. 19–40). Several such involved macrophages may coalesce to form a giant cell. Multiple vacuoles within a single macrophage impart a trabeculated pattern to the cytoplasm. Sometimes the coalescence of these vacuoles produces large, solitary, clear spaces which push the nucleus eccentrically and simulate a signet-ring cell. The alveolar septa characteristically show marked congestion, hyperemia and some widening, but remarkably little leukocytic reaction except in instances in which the oils are particularly irritant and necrotizing.

With progression of the lesion, fibroblasts invade the cellular lipid exudate and eventually organize the macrophagic inflammatory response (Russell et al., 1956). Multinucleate giant cells may develop within the alveolar organization. **Many times, the actively growing fibroblastic tissue and foreign body multinucleate giant cells form granulomas that resemble those found in tuberculosis and sarcoidosis.** This granulomatous pattern is particularly prone to occur when the involved oil is strongly irritant and destructive. Slow resorption of the oil with some resolution of the exudate may occur in certain cases, but usually permanent fi-

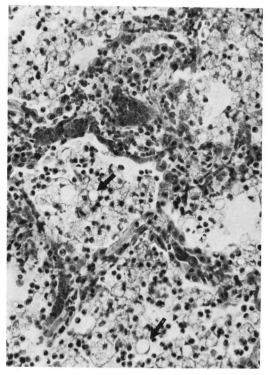

Figure 19–40. Lipid pneumonia. The alveoli contain the characteristic lipid-laden macrophages with large, clear cytoplasmic vacuoles (arrows).

brous scarring prevents the total resolution of this type of inflammatory reaction. The saturated vegetable oils and mineral oil may excite little fibrous reaction so that the organization is less prominent and the macrophages bearing the lipid remain in situ for long periods of time.

Identification of the involved oil is possible to some extent by the use of sudanophilic stains. Mineral oil stains yellow to orange with Sudan IV, but does not stain with osmic acid. Cod liver oil, on the other hand, gives a stronger red stain with Sudan IV and a black reaction with osmic acid.

On the basis of the histologic findings, it is possible to predict the gross appearance. Patchy foci (1 to 3 cm. in diameter) or segmental involvements vary from gray to bright yellow, and are dry and granular. The lesions are fairly sharply circumscribed and slightly elevated above the level of the cut lung surface (Fig. 19–41). The consistency of these foci is considerably more firm than in the usual bronchopneumonia and may even resemble neoplastic infiltration. Pleural reaction is rare. The anatomic diagnosis can only be suspected grossly and depends upon histologic examination for its verification.

Lipid pneumonia is chiefly of importance because of its frequent confusion with the caseous consolidation of tuberculosis or with neoplastic

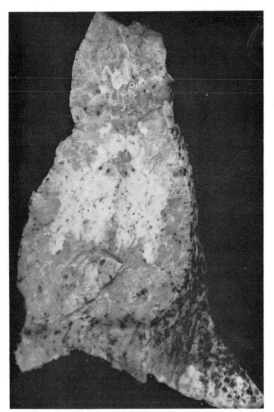

Figure 19–41. The focal irregular areas of lipid pneumonia are readily evident as pale areas.

infiltration. The anatomic diagnosis of lipid pneumonia further requires the differentiation of these lipid-laden macrophages from phagocytic macrophages laden with granular, fatty debris derived from any nonspecific inflammatory process. In both instances, the macrophages may be numerous and individually enlarged. However, in lipid pneumonia the vacuoles are clear, large and discrete, whereas in the fatty degeneration of tissue and exudative debris, the finely divided fat does not produce discrete vacuoles, but merely a pink, granular cytoplasm. Large giant cells and organization are more characteristic of lipid pneumonia.

Lipid pneumonia is an uncommon primary cause of clinical disease. It is usually discovered as an incidental finding at autopsy. However, symptomatic manifestations may be occasioned by superimposed bronchitis, bronchiolitis, bronchiectasis and bronchopneumonia. Presumably, if the areas affected become sufficiently extensive, embarrassment of pulmonary ventilatory function may lead to chronic respiratory symptoms and disability.

PULMONARY ALVEOLAR PROTEINOSIS

This entity, only recently described, is of unknown etiology and consequently of great interest. It causes a form of consolidation that mimics bacterial pneumonia. No specific clinical syndrome is produced. The original description of 27 cases included both males and females, most of whom were adults between 20 and 50 years of age. These patients, for the most part, presented a nonspecific, insidious onset of respiratory difficulty, cough and abundant sputum often containing chunks of gelatinous material. Many of the patients had symptoms lasting for years, and often there were repeated febrile illnesses that were considered to be attacks of pneumonia. In the original 27 cases, there were eight deaths due to progressive dyspnea, cyanosis and respiratory insufficiency (Rosen et al., 1958).

As the name indicates, this clinical symptomatology is due to a peculiar, homogeneous, granular precipitate within the alveoli, causing focal to confluent consolidation of large areas of the lungs (Fig. 19–42). On section, milky, turbid fluid exudes from these areas. As a consequence, there is a marked increase in the size and weight of the lung. In one of the cases, a weight of 3.5 kg. was recorded for one lung. The alveolar precipitate appears to be a granular proteinous material that is richly PAS-positive (presumably due to glycoproteins) and also contains finely divided lipid. The derivation of this material is uncertain but it may represent necrotic alveolar epithelial cells, particularly

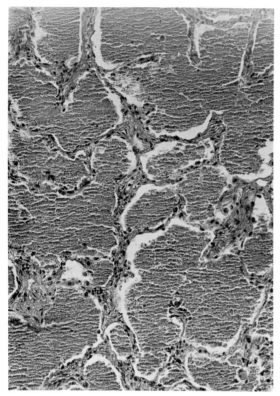

Figure 19–42. Pulmonary alveolar proteinosis. *The alveoli are filled with a dense amorphous protein-lipid granular precipitate.*

type 2 pneumocytes. Consonant with such a possibility, the involved alveoli are often lined by hypertrophic and hyperplastic pneumocytes, and focal areas of necrosis of these cells are seen with the light microscope. However, extracts of the lipid moiety of this alveolar precipitate have failed to reveal surfactant, a surprising finding if this material were truly derived from type 2 pneumocytes (Kuhn et al., 1966).

Within the amorphous alveolar precipitate, there are also occasionally concentric laminated bodies (possibly the surfactant) and long, needle-like crystalline spaces closely resembling cholesterol clefts. There is usually a surprising absence of any inflammatory reaction in the affected alveoli.

As mentioned, the etiology of this disorder is unknown and innumerable causations have been proposed. Suspicion persists that the lung changes are caused by some microbiologic agent but, to date, none has been reliably identified. Principal among these suspected agents are *Pneumocystis carinii* and Nocardia. Some patients suffering from this disease have an occupational exposure to irritating dusts and fumes. However, the large numbers of

similarly exposed individuals who do not have these lung changes militate against such a pathogenetic mechanism.

Other observations suggest that the alveolar deposit may reflect a deficiency of surfactant and consequent impairment of the normal alveolar clearing processes (Kuhn et al., 1966). The plethora of theories is documentary evidence that, to date, none has been firmly established.

GOODPASTURE'S SYNDROME

This uncommon but intriguing syndrome is characterized by the *simultaneous appearance of a form of proliferative, usually rapidly progressive glomerulonephritis and a necrotizing hemorrhagic interstitial pneumonitis.* The evidence is quite substantial that the renal and pulmonary lesions are the consequence of antibodies evoked by antigens common to the glomerular and pulmonary septal basement membranes (Poskitt, 1970). Most cases begin clinically with respiratory symptoms, principally hemoptysis and x-ray evidence of focal pulmonary consolidations. Very soon, manifestations of glomerulonephritis appear, leading to rapidly progressive renal failure. The common cause of death is uremia. While a few cases have been reported in females, there is a striking male preponderance in the ratio of 9 to 1 (Benoit et al., 1964). Most cases occur in the second or third decades of life.

In the classic case, the lungs are heavy and contain focal areas of red-brown apparent consolidation. Histologically, there are acute focal necroses of alveolar walls associated with intra-alveolar hemorrhages, fibrous thickening of the septa and hypertrophy of lining septal cells. Depending on the duration of the disease, there may be organization of the blood in the alveolar spaces. Often the alveoli contain hemosiderin-laden macrophages (Fig. 19–43). Immunofluorescent studies reveal linear deposits of immunoglobulins along the basement membranes of the septal walls in the areas of necrosis. Most of the immunoglobulins are IgG but trace amounts of IgM and IgA have also been identified (Koffler et al., 1969). The kidneys reveal the characteristic findings of proliferative or rapidly progressive glomerulonephritis, i.e., striking proliferation of glomerular mesangial, endothelial and epithelial cells, producing marked hypercellularity of the glomerular tufts (p. 1096). Prominent crescent formations fill Bowman's space when the renal involvement enters the phase of rapidly progressive glomerulonephritis. Immunofluorescence reveals linear deposits of immunoglobulins along the glomerular basement membranes similar to those seen

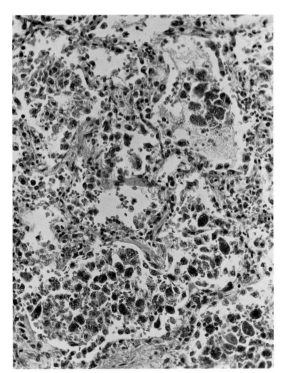

Figure 19–43. *The lung in Goodpasture's syndrome. The alveolar walls are thickened with focal areas of necrosis. The alveolar spaces contain hemosiderin-laden macrophages secondary to the intra-alveolar hemorrhages.*

in the lungs. As in the lung, most of these immunoglobulins are IgG mixed with trace amounts of IgM and IgA. Underlying the concurrence of renal and pulmonary lesions are elevated levels of immunoglobulins in the circulation, reactive against the glomerular and alveolar basement membranes.

The pulmonary and renal lesions characteristic of Goodpasture's syndrome have been produced in rats by injection of rabbit antirat lung serum (Hagadorn, 1969). These results have been confirmed by Willoughby and Dixon (1970). The trigger initiating this immune disorder in man is still obscure. One hypothesis proposes the development of autosensitization to normal glomerular basement membrane antigens, which then cross react with the alveolar basement membrane (Lerner and Dixon, 1968). It has been theorized that trace amounts of these antigens are normally excreted in the urine. Any mild injury to the kidney would bring immunocompetent lymphocytes to the kidney, which would thus be exposed to the mobilized antigens and so initiate an immune reaction. Alternatively, because most of the cases begin with pulmonary symptoms, it is suggested that a viral pneumonitis initiates the disease and exposes lung basement membrane to the immune system. Conceivably, cross reactivity of viral antigens with lung and glomerular basement membranes might be the pathogenetic mechanism.

Most cases reported to date have run a fairly acute course to death from renal failure, but it is not known how many less severe cases may have recovered. Steroids and immunosuppresive therapy have been of some benefit, but even more exciting are the reports of patients who have responded favorably to bilateral nephrectomy followed by long-term dialysis or renal transplantation (Pollak and Mendoza, 1971). Surprisingly, in the light of our present concepts of the immunogenetic basis of this disease, the pulmonary lesions have resolved following removal of the diseased kidneys.

IDIOPATHIC PULMONARY HEMOSIDEROSIS

This uncommon pulmonary disease of obscure nature usually presents with an insidious onset of productive cough, hemoptysis and weight loss associated with diffuse pulmonary infiltrations. While Goodpasture's syndrome is classically associated with glomerular disease, there is nonetheless a growing suspicion that pulmonary hemosiderosis is a variant of Goodpasture's syndrome. It, however, tends to occur in younger adults and children and shows no striking male preponderance.

The lungs are moderately increased in weight, with focal areas of consolidation that are usually red-brown to red. The cardinal histologic features of pulmonary hemosiderosis are reported as "striking degeneration, shedding and hyperplasia of alveolar epithelial cells and marked localized alveolar capillary dilatation" (Soergel and Sommers, 1962). In association with these epithelial cell changes, there are varying degrees of pulmonary interstitial fibrosis; hemorrhage into the alveolar spaces; hemosiderosis, both within the alveolar septa and in macrophages lying free within the pulmonary alveoli; and variable degrees of degeneration of alveolar interstitial and vascular elastic fibers (Fig. 19–44).

The etiology of this disorder is completely unknown, and while hypersensitivity is suspected, the many studies directed toward showing some immunologic derangement have all been unavailing. Because of prominence of alveolar-epithelial cell alterations in this condition, it has been postulated that the hemorrhages arise from some abnormality of alveolar epithelial cell growth and function. It

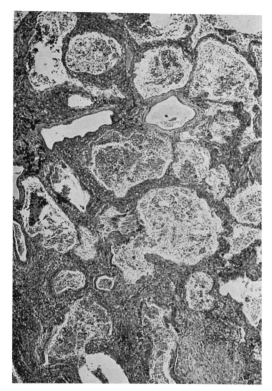

Figure 19–44. *Pulmonary hemosiderosis with interstitial fibrosis and red cells and red cell debris within alveoli. Considerable hemosiderin deposit is not readily seen in the black and white illustration.*

is postulated that the loss of these cells renders the underlying capillaries vulnerable to rupture and so hemorrhages result. In contrast to Goodpasture's syndrome, which appears to be highly fatal, idiopathic pulmonary hemosiderosis runs the gamut from mild to severe disease. Some cases have recurrent, not severe episodes of hemoptysis with intervening periods of good health. These patients may have a normal life span. Some develop progressive pulmonary fibrosis and run an erratic progressive course with advancing cardiac failure, while yet others may die acutely of massive pulmonary hemorrhage. Most patients follow a chronic remittent course over a period of years and then spontaneously or with treatment improve and have no further recurrences.

IDIOPATHIC INTERSTITIAL FIBROSIS (CHRONIC INTERSTITIAL PNEUMONIA, FIBROSING ALVEOLITIS, HAMMAN-RICH SYNDROME)

All of these terms refer to a poorly understood pulmonary disorder characterized histologically by a diffuse fibrosing interstitial pneu-

monitis (Hamman and Rich, 1944). It is by no means certain that the Hamman-Rich syndrome is a distinctive disorder and, indeed, similar changes may occur in the lung in the connective tissue diseases, particularly rheumatoid arthritis and scleroderma (Turner-Warwick and Doniach, 1965). The pulmonary lesion comprises edema of the alveolar walls accompanied by marked hyperplasia and hypertrophy of the alveolar lining cells, followed eventually by interstitial fibrosis and widening of the alveolar septa. Occasionally, necrotizing changes are found in the altered septal cells as well as in the bronchioles. A scant fibrinous exudate may accumulate in the alveolar spaces, sometimes layering the alveolar septa. The lower lung fields bilaterally are usually first affected, but ultimately the changes may spread to involve the entire lungs.

Males are affected more often than females, and although the disease may occur at any age, most patients are between 30 and 50 years of age.

As would be expected, patients exhibit varying degrees of respiratory difficulty and, in advanced cases, hypoxemia and cyanosis occur. The septal fibrosis, while histologically unimpressive, constitutes a significant physiologic alveolocapillary block. Cor pulmonale and cardiac failure may result. The prognosis in the individual case is unpredictable. In some patients, the disease remits spontaneously. In others, it is mild and permits long survival with some respiratory deficit but, in most cases, death occurs in about two years (Livingstone et al., 1964).

DESQUAMATIVE INTERSTITIAL PNEUMONITIS (DIP)

In 1965, Liebow et al., called attention to a distinctive pulmonary disease characterized anatomically by an interstitial fibrosing pneumonitis accompanied by aggregation of mononuclear cells within the alveoli, presumably desquamated from the alveolar walls. These patients usually present with the slow development of cough and dyspnea, eventually leading to marked respiratory embarassment, cyanosis and clubbing of the fingers. Classically, the radiologic picture is that of bilateral lower-lobe ground-glass infiltrates.

In well developed cases, the macroscopic lesions appear as patchy foci of induration and consolidation usually in the lower lobes bilaterally. Pleural adhesions may develop in relation to these lesions. Histologically, the earliest changes comprise edematous septal thickening, with dilatation of capillaries and infiltration of the septal walls by plasma cells, lymphocytes, histiocytes and occasional eosinophils. As the disease progresses, the edema is replaced by fibrosis and the infiltrate becomes predominantly one of plasma cells and lymphocytes. The fibrosis may cause marked thickening of the septal walls. The most striking finding is the accumulation, in the air spaces, of a large number of mononuclear cells (Fig. 19–45). Often, there is accompanying hyperplasia of the septal lining epithelial cells and desquamation of these cells into the air spaces. Nonetheless, electron microscopy strongly suggests that approximately 90 per cent of the desquamated cells are macrophages, many of which contain lipid vacuoles and PAS-positive granules. Some of these macrophages contain lamellar bodies within phagocytic vacuoles presumably derived from necrotic type II pneumocytes (Farr et al., 1970). Only the remaining 10 per cent of the cells may be identified as desquamated type II pneumocytes.

The causation of this disorder is unknown. It has been hypothesized that some immunologic, viral or toxic chemical injury occurs to the lung and induces the interstitial pneumonia and the alveolar epithelial proliferation. Although the basic nature of the disorder remains obscure, the patients are benefited by steroid therapy which often leads to clearing of the lungs. Whether persistent pulmonary fibrosis would be found at some later date despite such clinical improvement is not known.

LOEFFLER'S SYNDROME (PULMONARY EOSINOPHILIA)

In 1932, Loeffler described an apparently new syndrome characterized by transient pulmonary lesions, eosinophilia in the blood and a rather benign clinical course. In fact, in some of the reported cases, the lesions were discovered entirely incidentally at necropsy in patients who had died accidentally (Bayley et al., 1945). Roentgenograms are often quite striking, with shadows of varying size and shape in any of the lobes suggesting irregular intrapulmonary densities.

Gross inspection of these lungs discloses areas of increased consistency, varying from apparent interstitial foci of scarring to other areas of nodular consolidation, perhaps up to 5 cm. in diameter. The bronchi are often dilated and contain an abundant mucinous secretion. The histologic changes are quite varied and comprise the following: (1) foci of exudation into the alveolar spaces in the pattern of a bronchopneumonia; (2) a striking tendency toward organization of the pneumonic exudate; (3) areas of interstitial edema and septal thickening with an infiltration of lymphocytes and plasma cells, which may spill out into the adjacent alveolar spaces; (4) focal granulomatous lesions having central fibrinoid necrosis surrounded by a collar of characteristic fibroblasts and histiocytes suggestive of tuberculous granulomas or rheumatic lesions; (5) acute vascular lesions that vary from edema and thickening of the vessel walls to frank necrotizing arteritis suggesting changes seen in polyarteritis nodosa; and (6) bronchial alterations that are reminiscent of asthma, often with notable aggregations of eosinophils in the luminal secretion as well as in the walls of the bronchioles.

These histologic changes, it is obvious, are strongly reminiscent of the immunologic connective tissue diseases and suggest a hypersensitivity origin for this condition. However, no clear allergic basis has been identified, but neither has any microbiologic agent been isolated. The well recognized tendency for helminthic infections to produce marked eosinophilia has directed attention to this possibility.

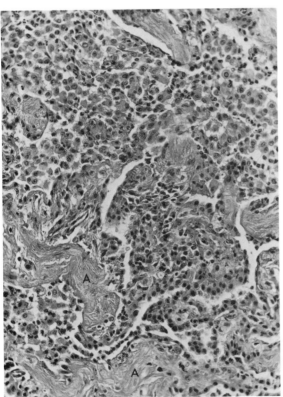

Figure 19–45. Desquamative interstitial pneumonitis. A high power detail of the lung to demonstrate fibrous thickening of alveolar walls (A) and the accumulation of large numbers of mononuclear cells within the alveolar spaces.

The Ascaris has been suspected, but no such parasitization has been regularly identified. Some similarity to eosinophilic granuloma has also been suggested, but the other manifestations of the Hand-Schüller-Christian complex are missing. The causation therefore remains unknown. The syndrome's manifestations generally clear spontaneously after a brief, self-limited course.

Other poorly understood and ill-defined disorders have been described associated with striking pulmonary eosinophilia, but not with increased eosinophil counts in the circulating blood. One has been called *chronic eosinophilic pneumonia*, characterized by focal areas of cellular consolidation of the lung substance distributed chiefly in the periphery of the lung fields. Prominent in these lesions are heavy aggregates of lymphocytes and eosinophils within both the septal walls and the alveolar spaces (Carrington, 1969). This rare entity is mentioned merely to indicate that there is a range of disorders in the lung associated with eosinophilia either in the lung substance or in the blood or sometimes in both.

WEGENER'S GRANULOMATOSIS

This rare disorder was considered previously with the hypersensitivity diseases (p. 247). It is characterized by *acute necrotizing lesions of the blood vessels and kidneys with particularly prominent involvement of the upper respiratory tract and lungs.* The focal necrotizing lesions, wherever they occur, resemble, to a considerable extent, tubercles with acute central necrosis, a resemblance that is heightened by the peripheral fibroblastic proliferation with accompanying Langhans' type or foreign type giant cells. In the lung, these foci often become confluent to produce areas of visible and palpable consolidation. Healing occurs by fibrosis, giving rise to permanent scars. For further details, reference should be made to the earlier discussion.

CYTOMEGALIC INCLUSION DISEASE

This is an uncommon *viral infection, principally of the young and the debilitated. It manifests itself by causing cellular and nuclear gigantism* along with intranuclear or intracytoplasmic inclusions in affected cells from which the disease derives its name. Many organs and tissues are affected by these random, scattered cellular alterations. The lungs often show a prominent interstitial pneumonitis. The cellular enlargement and inclusions are also found in the septal cells. The dramatic cellular inclu-sions and gigantism are also prominent in the kidney tubular cells, pancreas and salivary glands. The excretion of these affected renal tubular cells in the urine provides an important opportunity to establish the diagnosis. Further details are on page 563.

RHEUMATIC PNEUMONITIS

Rarely, in cases of rheumatic fever, patients develop signs and symptoms of pneumonic involvement. It is often difficult to determine whether this pneumonia is causally related to the rheumatic disease or is simply an intercurrent viral or bacterial infection. In the classic case, there is an interstitial pneumonitis virtually identical with a virus pneumonia but, superimposed upon this, there are extensive pulmonary edema and hemorrhages, as well as fibrinoid necrotizing changes in the alveolar walls and alveolar capillaries and acute vascular involvements typical of acute rheumatic angiitis (p. 611). There is also a prominent fibrinous exudation into the alveolar spaces sometimes followed by organization. These necrotizing vascular alterations suggest that the pulmonary lesion is not merely a viral pneumonitis. Increasing numbers of cases of rheumatic fever are being reported with pneumonitis, making it quite clear that the concurrence is more than coincidental (Scott et al., 1959). While in most cases the pneumonitis is not a major hazard, it has occasionally caused death (Massumi and Legier, 1965). When changes such as have been cited are found at postmortem, however, they must be interpreted with caution and conservatively should only be called rheumatic when accompanied by undoubted rheumatic fever.

TUMORS OF THE LUNG

Bronchogenic carcinoma is preeminent among the great variety of tumors that may arise in the lungs. In a review of 1218 primary malignancies of the lung, the following approximate distribution was found:

1. Bronchogenic carcinoma, 90 per cent.
2. Alveolar cell (terminal bronchiolar) carcinoma, 2 per cent.
3. Bronchial adenoma, 5 per cent.
4. Mesenchymal tumors, 1.4 per cent.
5. Miscellaneous, 1.5 per cent.

From this distribution, it is obvious that primary malignancy in the lung may be assumed to be bronchogenic until proved otherwise (Galofré et al., 1964).

BRONCHOGENIC CARCINOMA

In industrialized nations, public enemy number 1 among cancers is bronchogenic carcinoma. In males, it is indisputably the most common visceral malignancy and alone accounts for approximately 40 per cent of all cancer deaths in this sex. Females are affected far less frequently and, indeed, have a mortality rate from cancer of the lung one-sixth that of males.

Incidence. There is no longer any doubt that the rising incidence of bronchogenic carcinoma is real and not the spurious consequence of aging populations, better case finding and more accurate diagnosis. The annual number of deaths in the United States from cancer of the lung increased from 18,313 in 1950 to 45,838 in 1964. In the time span 1950–67, the death rate from cancer of the lung more than doubled for males, rising from 19.9 per 100,000 population to 42.5. In contrast, the death rate in females was 4.5 in 1950 and 7.5 in 1967 (United States Department of Health, Education and Welfare, 1966, 1967). Although the death rate for males is now awesome, it should not be overlooked that the death rate for females has also almost doubled in less than 20 years. These data on bronchogenic carcinoma must be viewed within the context of other forms of cancer. The death rate from cancer of the stomach and uterus has steadily fallen in the United States since 1950. There has been no appreciable change in the death rate for colorectal, prostatic, breast and pancreatic cancers over this time span. Only leukemia has become somewhat more common but, as compared with bronchogenic carcinoma, the increased prevalence has been trivial.

The disease occurs most often between the ages of 40 and 70 with a peak incidence in the sixth decade, but this lesion has appeared as early as the second decade of life.

Etiology. It is difficult to maintain a balanced position in the stormy controversy over the cause of bronchogenic carcinoma. On the one hand are found those who unwaveringly regard increased cigarette smoking as the sole reason for the increase in bronchogenic carcinoma; on the other side are those who regard other environmental factors as holding equal responsibility.

While the evidence indicting cigarette smoking as at least the major causal factor is well-nigh incontrovertible, there are still missing pieces in the jigsaw puzzle that bother many. Most of the fairly monumental documentation of the role of cigarette smoking may be found in two extremely thoughtful and thorough reports, the one from the Royal College of Physicians (1962) and the other a Public Health Service Review (United States Department of Health, Education and Welfare, 1968). The collected evidence is of three kinds: (1) statistical, (2) clinical and (3) experimental data on laboratory animals.

In 29 retrospective studies of patients who died of bronchogenic carcinoma compared with "controls," there was an invariable statistical association between cigarette smoking and lung cancer. For pipe smokers and cigar smokers, there was no statistically significant increase in incidence over control groups. In virtually all these reports, there was a direct correlation between the frequency of lung cancer and (1) the amount of daily smoking, (2) the tendency to inhale and (3) the duration of the smoking habit. Many analyses have demonstrated essentially the same findings. One of the most authoritative studies, by Hammond and Horn, of almost 200,000 men is summarized in Figure 19–46. To quote from their report, " . . . lung cancer showed an extremely high degree of association with cigarette smoking. The next highest association with cigarette smoking was for cancer of the following sites combined; lip, tongue, floor of mouth, pharynx, larynx, and esophagus. These are all sites directly exposed to cigarette smoke or material dissolved or condensed from cigarette smoke." Other statistical studies in the United States have shown that the increased risk of lung cancer is 4.9 to 15.9 times greater in cigarette smokers than in nonsmokers. The Royal College of Physicians reported on a careful survey of British doctors on the assumption that more objective data would be derived from such sources. Here the risk of developing lung cancer among smokers was twenty-fold greater than among nonsmoking physicians, with mortality ratios proportional to the amount of smoking.

The clinical studies have dealt largely with the changes in the lining epithelium of the respiratory tract in smokers and nonsmokers. In smokers, the epithelial changes observed are loss of ciliated cells, basal cell hyperplasia, squamous metaplasia and atypia of cells. Some patients had sufficient cytologic anaplasia to merit the diagnosis of carcinoma in situ. Auerbach and his colleagues (1957) attempted to quantitate the severity and frequency of these epithelial changes. They again showed a strong correlation between cellular abnormalities and the amount of smoking, particularly cigarette smoking. In their comparison of the bronchial epithelium in nonsmokers versus smokers (1962a), 0.9 per cent of the former group had atypical cells in the bronchial tree, whereas

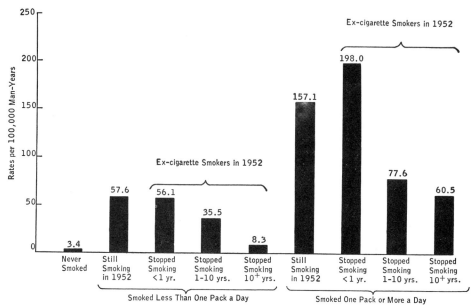

Figure 19–46. *Age-standardized death rates due to bronchogenic carcinoma in smokers and nonsmokers. (From Hammond, E. C., and Horn, D.: Smoking and death rates: report on forty-four months of follow-up of 187,783 men. I., II., J.A.M.A., 166:1159, 1294, 1958.)*

96.7 per cent of cigarette smokers had these changes. Other influences also were involved, such as age and urban living, but the dominant correlate was cigarette smoking (Auerbach, 1962*b*).

The experimental work has largely focused on attempts to induce cancer in experimental animals with extracts of tobacco smoke. To cite some of this evidence briefly, carcinogenic polycyclic hydrocarbons have been identified in cigarette smoke, but in minute amounts. It has been possible by protracted exposure of mice to induce skin tumors with these extracts (Wynder and Hoffman, 1966). There have been enormous efforts made to induce lung cancer in animals by exposing them to extracts of tobacco smoke, or tobacco smoke itself or combinations of tobacco smoke with air pollutants, viruses and other possible cocarcinogens, leading to the following conclusions: (1) to date, there is no carefully controlled good model of bronchogenic carcinoma in experimental animals produced by exposure to tobacco smoke alone, and (2) such experimental lung tumors as have been produced probably result from complex carcinogenic influences (Wynder and Hoffman, 1967).

Of recent date, a report has appeared of the induction of pulmonary neoplasms in dogs trained to smoke cigarettes for prolonged periods of time through tracheostomies (Hammond et al., 1970) (Auerbach et al., 1970). Among 86 dogs smoking filter tip and nonfilter cigarettes (approximately four to seven cigarettes a day) for at least 875 days, 12 invasive bronchioloalveolar tumors were found. But such lesions have no resemblance to the characteristic squamous cell carcinomas found in human smokers and similar lesions sometimes spontaneously arise in aged dogs. In addition, two dogs were found to have what were interpreted by the authors to be early invasive squamous cell carcinomas. In both cases, these lesions were neither grossly visible nor had they metastasized. Moreover, squamous metaplasia and dysplasia were also present, further complicating the interpretation of the ostensible cancerous changes. We must conclude that, at the present time, bronchogenic carcinomas have not been unequivocally induced in animals by exposure to cigarette smoke alone.

On the other side of the controversy, it has been pointed out that atmospheric pollutants have not been excluded as causative factors or at least as contributory factors (Kotin and Falk, 1959) (Clemo et al., 1955). Unquestionably we all "swim in a sea of carcinogens," and conceivably these play some role in the increased incidence of bronchogenic carcinoma today. It is pointed out in this regard that ore miners in Bohemia and Saxony extracting nickel, silver, cobalt, radium and uranium, some of them radioactive ores, suffer from a high incidence of pulmonary cancer, having a thirty-fold increased incidence over control populations in the same area. Industries using volatilized chromate and distillation products of coal have an incidence of lung cancer up to 15 times the attack rate in controls.

Genetic predisposition is known to be important with many forms of cancer, and several studies have shown this factor to possibly influence the frequency of bronchogenic carcinoma. Approximately 10 per cent of lung cancers occur among nonsmokers but, in this connection, it should be pointed out that most of these "nonsmoking cancers" are not of the common squamous cell variety found in smokers.

The pathogenetic argument need not be belabored further. While smoking, principally cigarette smoking, cannot be considered to be the proved solitary cause of bronchogenic carcinoma, the evidence is strong that it is a most important causal factor. This view has been well expressed in the final conclusions of the report on smoking and health by the Advisory Committee to the Surgeon General of the United States. They state: "(1) Cigarette smoking is causally related to lung cancer in men; the magnitude of the effect of cigarette smoking far outweighs all other factors. The data for women, though less extensive, point in the same direction. (2) The risk of developing lung cancer increases with duration of smoking and the number of cigarettes smoked per day and is diminished by discontinued smoking. (3) The risk of developing cancer of the lung for the combined group of pipe and cigar smokers is greater than in nonsmokers but much less than for cigarette smokers."

Morphology. Bronchogenic carcinomas arise most often in and about the hilus of the lung. About three-quarters of the lesions take origin from the lower trachea and first, second and third order bronchi. A small percentage have a more peripheral origin, but are still not located far out near the pleura. A very few primary carcinomas of the lung arise in the periphery of the lung substance from the alveolar septal cells or terminal bronchioles, but these are not classified as bronchogenic carcinoma and will be the subject of a later discussion.

In its development, **carcinoma of the lung begins as an area of in situ cytologic atypia which, over an unknown interval of time, then yields a small area of thickening or piling up of the bronchial mucosa.** With progression this small focus, usually less than 1 cm. in area, assumes the appearance of an irregular, warty excrescence that elevates or erodes the lining epithelium (Figs. 19–47 and 19–48). The tumor may then follow one of a variety of paths. It may continue to fungate into the bronchial lumen to produce an intraluminal mass. At other times, it rapidly penetrates the wall of the bronchus to infiltrate along the peribronchial tissue (Fig. 19–49) into the adjacent region of the carina or mediastinum. It may extend in this fashion into or about the pericardium. In other instances, the tumor grows along a broad front to produce a cauliflower intraparenchymal mass that appears to push lung substance ahead of it. Quite rarely, the tumor permeates the pulmonary parenchyma apparently with-

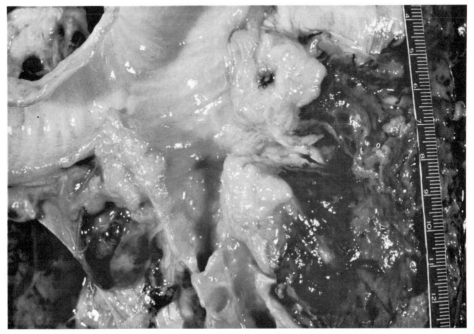

Figure 19–47. *The early stage of a bronchogenic carcinoma arising at the bifurcation of the trachea. The nodular neoplasm invades the wall of the trachea and the right main-stem bronchus at several points.*

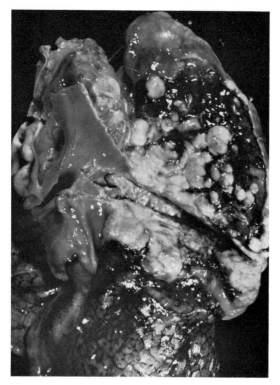

Figure 19–48. An invasive bronchogenic carcinoma with a piling up of tumor within the bronchial lumen.

out obliterating the native architecture to produce a form of pneumonic consolidation. In almost all patterns, the neoplastic tissue is gray-white and firm to hard. Especially when the tumors are bulky, focal areas of hemorrhage or necrosis may appear to produce yellow-white mottling and softening. Sometimes these necrotic foci cavitate. Extension may occur to the pleural surface and then within the pleural cavity.

Despite this variable behavior, certain characteristics remain uniform. **In all instances, a primary mucosal lesion may be found within the bronchus if sought for with sufficient diligence.** In most instances, spread to the tracheal, bronchial and mediastinal nodes can be found. The frequency of such nodal involvement varies slightly with the histologic pattern, but averages over 50 per cent (Reinhoff et al., 1965). The scalene nodes are affected in about half the cases, providing a valuable clinical means of diagnosing, by biopsy, these lesions.

More distant spread of bronchogenic carcinoma occurs through both lymphatic and hematogenous pathways. These tumors have a distressing habit of spreading widely throughout the body and often at a very early stage in their evolution. Often, the metastasis presents as the first manifestation of the underlying occult bronchogenic primary. Many craniotomies for brain tumor or explorations of a

bone tumor have been performed only to discover metastatic bronchogenic carcinoma. It is relevant to this discussion to note that a recent study proposes that it may require as long as nine years of growth for a squamous cell bronchogenic carcinoma to achieve a size of 2 cm. in diameter (Garland et al., 1963). It should be no surprise, therefore, that during this evolution the tumor may acquire the capacity for metastatic dissemination long before the primary site calls itself to clinical attention. While no organ or tissue is spared in the spread of these lesions, the adrenals, for obscure reasons, are involved in over half the cases. The liver (30 per cent), brain (20 per cent), bone (20 per cent) and the kidneys (15 per cent) are additional favorite sites of metastases.

Histologically, bronchogenic carcinomas are divided into three or four cell types in the following approximate distribution:

1. Squamous cell carcinoma, 70 per cent.
2. Adenocarcinoma, 10 per cent.
3. Undifferentiated carcinoma, 20 per cent.
   Large cell pattern, 10 per cent.
   Small cell pattern, 10 per cent.

Although some importance is attached to the histologic pattern in terms of curability, a considerable number of carcinomas grow in mixed patterns, making any classification arbitrary.

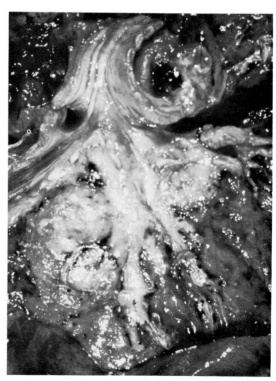

Figure 19–49. Bronchogenic carcinoma infiltrating the peribronchial lung substance.

Squamous cell carcinoma is found almost exclusively in men. It is the form most closely correlated with a smoking history, and it is the rising incidence of this lesion that accounts for the increased frequency of bronchogenic carcinoma. The microscopic features are familiar in the form of production of keratin and intercellular bridges in the well differentiated forms, but many less well differentiated squamous cell tumors are encountered which begin to merge with the undifferentiated large cell pattern. This tumor tends to metastasize locally and somewhat later than the other patterns, but its rate of growth in its site of origin is usually more rapid than the other types (Spratt et al., 1963). It has been estimated that it requires about four months for a squamous cell carcinoma to double its size or, from theoretical calculations, that it takes about nine years for these lesions to achieve a mass of 2 cm. in diameter.

The **adenocarcinoma** occurs about equally frequently in males and females and, therefore, does not show the striking male preponderance of the other histologic types. There is no clear correlation between the smoking history and the occurrence of this pattern of bronchogenic carcinoma and, indeed, in contrast to squamous cell carcinoma, there has been no significant increase in the frequency of this pattern over the recent past. The adenocarcinomas are usually more peripherally located and are characterized by the formation of glands with or without mucinous secretion. Occasionally, papillary growths are encountered resembling quite closely the bronchiolar carcinomas soon to be described, but the bronchogenic adenocarcinoma, unlike the bronchiolar lesions, obliterates the underlying native lung architecture, implying that it is much more aggressive and destructive. The time required for these lesions to double their volume is about seven months, and it has been suggested that it requires virtually 25 years for the adenocarcinoma to reach a size of 2 cm. Occasionally, this pattern arises in an area of scarring, suggesting that the local chronic inflammatory changes have triggered its development.

The **undifferentiated carcinomas** are, by default, those in which no squamous or adenomatous patterns can be defined. Some produce large anaplastic tumor cells bordering on giant cells, while others produce small closely packed "oat cells." Mitotic figures and tumor necrosis tend to be common in these lesions. There are no significant clinical differences in behavior between the small and large cell varieties, and often intergrades appear that defy clear-cut differentiation. Some of these undifferentiated tumors assume the appearance of a "spindle cell carcinoma" that mimics a sarcoma. These undifferentiated lesions are the most rapidly growing of all forms and have the poorest prognosis.

It is believed that all histogenetic patterns of bronchogenic carcinoma develop from one precursor, the multipotential basal resting or reserve cell of the bronchial epithelium. Presumably, under the irritant effect of such agents as tobacco smoke, atypical metaplasia provides a site of origin for the squamous cell tumors (Anderson, 1966). The reserve cells are also generally postulated as the site of origin of the adenocarcinoma, but the submucosal mucous glands cannot be excluded as an alternative possibility.

Secondary Pathology. These carcinomas cause many related anatomic changes in the lung substance distal to the point of bronchial involvement. **Partial obstruction may cause marked focal emphysema; total obstruction may lead to atelectasis.** The impaired drainage of the airways is a common cause for **severe suppurative or ulcerative bronchitis or bronchiectasis. Pulmonary abscesses** sometimes call attention to a silent carcinoma that has initiated the chronic suppuration. Compression or invasion of the superior vena cava may lead either to marked venous congestion or to the full-blown **superior vena caval syndrome.** Extension to the pericardial or pleural sacs may cause **pericarditis** or **pleuritis** with significant effusions.

Clinical Course. Lung cancer is one of the most insidious and aggressive neoplasms in the whole realm of oncology. In the usual case, it is discovered in a male in the sixth decade of life, whose symptoms are approximately of seven months' duration. The major presenting complaints are cough (75 per cent), weight loss (40 per cent), chest pain (40 per cent) and dyspnea (20 per cent). Not infrequently, the tumor is discovered by its secondary spread in the course of investigation of an apparent primary neoplasm elsewhere. Despite all efforts at early diagnosis by frequent radioscopic examination of the chest, the use of the Papanicolaou smears on sputum and bronchial washings, and the many improvements in thoracic surgery, the five-year survival rate is in the order of 7 per cent (James, 1966). In many large clinics, not more than 20 to 30 per cent of lung cancer patients have lesions sufficiently localized to even permit an attempt at resection. In general, the adenocarcinoma and squamous cell patterns tend to remain localized longer and have a slightly better prognosis than the undifferentiated cancers which usually are bulky invasive lesions by the time they are discovered. In a recent analysis of almost 4000 cases, the five-year survival of males was approximately 10 per cent with squamous cell carcinoma and adenocarcinoma, but only 3 per cent with undifferentiated lesions (Bignall and Martin, 1972). For mysterious reasons, women fared slightly worse than men and only about 5 per cent were alive at five years irrespective of the histologic pattern. Despite this discouraging outlook, it must never be forgotten that some patients have been cured by lobectomy or pneumonectomy, emphasizing the continued need for early diagnosis and adequate prompt therapy.

One of the most intriguing clinical aspects of bronchogenic carcinoma is the occasional undifferentiated tumor which elaborates humoral factors such as ACTH, ADH, gonadotrophins, parathormone, MSH and other less well characterized factors which lead to peripheral neuropathy, myopathy and pulmonary osteoarthropathy (p. 1447). Sufficient ACTH, for example, may be elaborated by these undifferentiated tumors to induce the full-blown Cushing's syndrome (Lipsett, 1965) (Azzopardi and Williams, 1968). It can only be speculated that, in such neoplasms, the genetic code for ACTH synthesis and the other hormones (normally repressed in all cells save those of the endocrine glands) becomes derepressed in the course of the carcinomatous transformation. There is much yet to be learned about the biology of these neoplasms, but most important is an understanding of their causation. Until we know more, cigarette smoking must stand indicted as at least a major villain in the piece.

ALVEOLAR CELL OR TERMINAL BRONCHIOLAR CARCINOMA OF THE LUNG

As the name implies, this rare form of cancer of the lung arises well out in the pulmonary parenchyma either from the lining cells of the alveoli or from the terminal bronchioles. It represents, in various series, from 1.5 to 5 per cent of all lung cancer. For many years, histologic changes indistinguishable from this form of cancer were also referred to as *pulmonary adenomatosis*. Adenomatosis in man was, moreover, very similar histologically to an apparently infectious disease of South African sheep known as *jagziekte*. It was conjectured that so-called adenomatosis in man might indeed represent an infectious disorder either transmitted from sheep or closely related to the disease of sheep. However, *increasing numbers of cases have been identified of so-called pulmonary adenomatosis in man with unmistakable evidence of cancerous behavior*, i.e., local invasion and metastatic dissemination. It was then postulated that adenomatosis might, in some instances, become transformed to a malignant tumor. However, numerous efforts have been made to identify an infectious agent in man without success. Also the many attempts to transmit cell-free extracts of the human bronchiolar or alveolar cell carcinoma back into sheep have been unavailing. Accordingly, it is now believed that while the disease of sheep and that of man have a histologic resemblance, they are quite distinct and, in man, there is no evidence of an infectious origin. Moreover, the validity of the entity known as adenomatosis in man has now been challenged and the changes are widely accepted as being a form of neoplasia.

Histologically, the terminal bronchiolar or alveolar cell carcinoma is characterized by distinctive tall, columnar to cuboidal epithelial cells which line up along alveolar septa and project into the alveolar spaces in numerous branching papillary formations (Fig. 19—50). The tumor cells often contain abundant mucinous secretion. Many times, the columnar cells desquamate into the alveolar spaces to virtually fill them and, in the more anaplastic lesions, masses of cytologically atypical epithelial cells fill the alveoli. Occasional large multinucleated giant cells are produced. The degree of anaplasia is quite variable, but most cases display good histogenetic differentiation toward the cells of

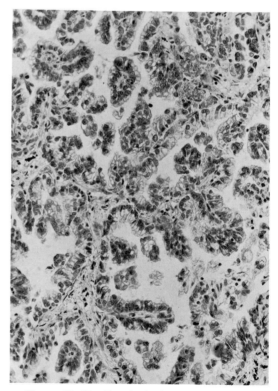

Figure 19–50. Terminal bronchiolar (alveolar) carcinoma with the characteristic tall columnar cell papillary growth characteristics.

origin, i.e., the septal cells or columnar cells that line the bronchioles. **One of the cardinal histologic features of this lesion is its tendency to preserve the native septal wall architecture** so that the tumorous infiltration behaves almost as an inflammatory exudate lining or filling the air spaces without destroying the underlying structure.

Macroscopically, the tumor almost always occurs in the peripheral portions of the lung either as a single nodule or, more often, as multiple diffuse nodules that sometimes coalesce to produce a pneumonia-like consolidation. Conspicuously absent are foci of mucosal origin of the neoplasm in the large bronchi or bronchioles. The parenchymal nodules have a mucinous gray translucence when secretion is present, and otherwise appear as solid gray-white areas, having a much sharper delineation from the surrounding lung parenchyma than pneumonia. However, the nodules are easily confused with pneumonia on casual inspection (Watson and Smith, 1951). Because the tumor does not involve major bronchi, atelectasis and emphysema are infrequent accompaniments. Metastases are not widely disseminated or large, nor do they occur early, but eventually appear in up to 45 per cent of cases. Presumably, these metastases develop only late in the more anaplastic variants (Decker, 1955).

Clinically, these tumors occur in patients of all ages from the second decade to advanced years of life. There is no striking sex preponderance as with bronchogenic carcinoma. The symptomatology, which usually appears late, is much like that of brochogenic carcinoma with cough, hemoptysis and pain as the major presenting findings. Despite the fact that these tumors are histologically more benign and appear to metastasize later, the overall five-year survival rate is about 5 per cent, certainly no improvement over that of other forms of primary lung cancer. In some part, this is due to the more silent nature of the early years of development.

BRONCHIAL ADENOMA

The term bronchial adenoma is something of a misnomer, since these tumors, although slowly growing, are frquently locally invasive and occasionally metastasize. On this account, they are better considered as *malignant neoplasms of low aggressiveness* (Goodner et al., 1961). They represent about 5 per cent of all primary tumors of the lung. Most patients with these lesions are under 40 years of age, and the incidence is approximately equal for both sexes.

Approximately 90 per cent of the adenomas are of the **argentaffinoma (carcinoid) type**, resembling lesions that occur within the gastrointes-

tinal tract (p. 942). The remainder produce a variety of patterns that are strangely reminiscent of tumors of the salivary glands. On this account, there is a strong suspicion that these patterns arise in the submucosal glands of the bronchi and thus have an origin similar to those of the salivary glands. Some of these variants are called **cylindroma** or **adenoid cystic carcinoma**. A very few have **a mucoepidermoid pattern**.

Histologically, the **carcinoid variety** is composed of nests, cords and masses of cells separated by a delicate fibrous stroma. In common with the lesions of the gastrointestinal tract, the individual cells are quite regular, have uniform round nuclei and infrequent mitoses (Fig. 19–51). However, unlike many of the lesions of the intestinal tract, these carcinoids rarely have argentaffine granules. Occasional carcinoid adenomas display variation in the size and shape of the cells and nuclei and, along with this pleomorphism, tend to demonstrate a more aggressive and more invasive behavior.

The **cylindromatous variants** reproduce the cords, strands and gland-like formations characteristic of the salivary gland tumors (p. 895). Often, these epithelial cells are separated by a fairly abundant hyalinized stroma in which there may be areas of myxoid transformation of the stroma or even bone formation. This cylindromatous pattern is of some clinical importance because it tends to be more malignant, having a three times greater likelihood of metastasis than the carcinoid pattern.

On gross examination, both types of tumors grow as finger-like or spherical polypoid masses that commonly project into the lumen of the

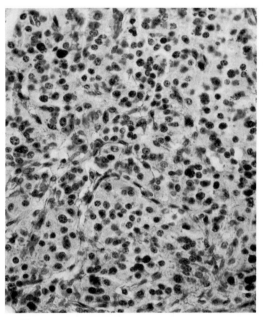

Figure 19–51. Bronchial adenoma of the "argentaffinoma type."

bronchus and are usually covered by an intact mucosa. They rarely exceed 3 to 4 cm. in diameter. Most are confined to the main stem bronchi. Others, however, produce little intraluminal mass, but instead penetrate the bronchial wall to fan out in the peribronchial tissue, producing the so-called "collar button" lesion. The parenchymal infiltration often forms a cohesive sphere apparently pushing the lung substance ahead of it (Fig. 19–52). This sharp line of delineation is more apparent than real since microscopic examination usually indicates local infiltration and no encapsulation.

The clinical manifestations of bronchial adenomas emanate from their intraluminal growth, their capacity to metastasize and the ability of some of these lesions to elaborate 5-hydroxytryptamine. Persistent cough, hemoptysis, impairment of the drainage of the respiratory passages with secondary infections, bronchiectasis, emphysema and atelectasis are all byproducts of the intraluminal growth of these lesions.

About 40 per cent of bronchial adenomas metastasize to regional nodes and cause enlargement of the hilar nodes. They may also metastasize to the liver to produce hepatomegaly. Of most interest, however, are those metastasizing lesions of the argentaffinoma pattern that are capable of producing the classic carcinoid syndrome, i.e., intermittent attacks of diarrhea, flushing and cyanosis (p. 943) (Editorial, 1960). It has, in fact, been possible to isolate 5-hydroxytryptamine from some lesions (Warner and Southern, 1958).

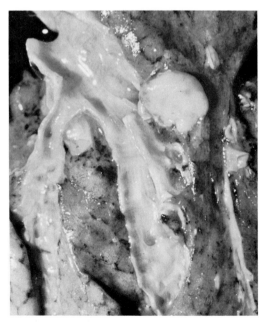

Figure 19–52. Bronchial adenoma growing as a spherical pale mass apparently external to the lumen of the bronchus. The mucosal primary is not seen.

Overall, most bronchial adenomas do not have secretory activity nor do they metastasize, but follow a relatively benign course for long periods of time and are therefore amenable to resection (Soutter et al., 1954).

SARCOMA

Large, bulky sarcomatous masses are found in the lung with great rarity. These have origin in the connective tissue framework of the lung, the smooth musculature of the bronchial walls or vessels, the cartilage in the bronchial walls and the lymphoid tissue which is dispersed throughout the lung parenchyma. The gross and microscopic growth features of these tumors resemble those of their counterparts in any other site.

MISCELLANEOUS TUMORS

The complex category of benign mesenchymal tumors, such as fibromas, lipomas and chondromas, may occur in the lung. They are rare.

The chondroma merits a brief description. It is usually discovered as an incidental, rounded focus of radiopacity on a routine chest plate, giving rise to what the roentgenologist calls a "coin lesion." These neoplasms are rarely over 3 to 4 cm. in diameter and are principally composed of mature hyaline cartilage. Occasionally, the cartilage contains cystic or cleft-like spaces and these may be lined by characteristic respiratory epithelium. At other times, there are admixtures of fibrous tissue, fat and blood vessels, making it clear that these lesions probably represent a *hamartoma* of the lung.

Dermoid and other teratogenous tumors may arise in the mediastinum and, in their expansile growth, compress or invade the lungs. These tumors presumably arise in sequestered nests of embryonic totipotential cells. Grossly and microscopically, these pleomorphic neoplasms resemble their ovarian counterparts. Primary lymphomas sometimes begin within the mediastinal and paratracheal nodes. None of the neoplasms have special qualities in these intrathoracic locations and do not require further description.

SECONDARY TUMORS OF THE LUNG

The lung is more often affected by metastatic growths than it is by primary neoplasms. Both carcinomas and sarcomas arising anywhere in the body may spread to the lungs via the blood or lymphatics or by direct continuity. As capillary filters, the lungs effectively screen out tumor emboli from the venous drainage of the body and further provide favorable conditions for the growth of these neoplastic seedlings. Growth of contiguous tumors into the lungs occurs most often with esophageal carcinomas and mediastinal lymphomas.

The pattern of metastatic growth within the lungs is quite variable. In the usual case, multiple discrete nodules are scattered throughout all lobes (Fig. 19–53). These discrete lesions are readily palpable and visualized on cut section and tend to occur in the periphery of the lung parenchyma, rather than in the central locations of the primary bronchogenic carcinoma.

As a second macroscopic variant, metastatic growths may confine themselves to peribronchiolar and perivascular tissue spaces, presumably when the tumor has extended to the lung through the lymphatics. Here the lung septa and connective tissue are diffusely infiltrated with the gray-white secondary neoplasm. Discrete masses may accompany this pattern of growth, but are not invariable. Least commonly, the metastatic tumor is totally inapparent on gross examination and only becomes evident on histologic section as a diffuse intralymphatic dissemination dispersed throughout the peribronchial and perivascular channels. In certain instances, the subpleural lymphatics may be outlined by the contained tumor, producing an anatomic pattern referred to as *lymphangitis carcinomatosa*. In a considerable number of these cases, the tumor may extend into adjacent veins.

Careful search for tumor emboli within pulmonary blood vessels should be made in all cases of neoplasia, since occasional nests and masses of neoplastic cells can be found lying within the thrombosed blood vessels. It has been reported that, in some of these cases, the organization of the clot blocks the growth of these tumor implants.

Occasionally, the tumor seems to fill the alveolar spaces while preserving the intervening septa, and thus produces a solidification without destruction of the lung parenchyma, resembling superficially the exudative pattern of bacterial pneumonia.

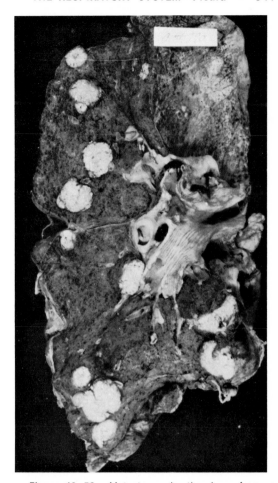

Figure 19–53. Metastases in the lung from a breast carcinoma in a 56-year-old woman.

The presence of lung metastases virtually precludes the possibility of definitive curative surgery at the primary site of the cancer. It is on this basis that routine chest x-rays are a requisite for any patient about to have operative removal of a primary neoplasm.

PLEURA

Pathologic involvement of the pleura is, with rare exception, a secondary complication of some underlying disease. The only primary disorders that are reasonably common are (1) primary intrapleural bacterial infections that imply seeding of this space as an isolated focus in the course of a transient bacteremia, and (2) a primary neoplasm of the pleura, a mesothelioma. However, even these conditions are very infrequent clinical occurrences. With these exceptions, pleural diseases usually follow some underlying disorder, most often pulmonary, and usually the pleural involvement is only an inconspicuous feature of the primary process.

These secondary infections are, however, extremely common, and pleural adhesions or other forms of pleural involvement are present in at least two-thirds of all postmortem cases. Occasionally, the secondary pleural disease assumes a dominant role in the clinical problem, as occurs in bacterial pneumonia with the development of empyema. The diseases of the pleura can be divided for convenience into inflammations, noninflammatory pleural collections and neoplasms.

INFLAMMATIONS

Inflammations of the pleura (pleuritis), depending upon their stage and causative agent, can be divided on the basis of the character of the resultant exudate into serous, fibrinous, serofibrinous, suppurative (empyema) and hemorrhagic pleuritis.

Serofibrinous. Serous, serofibrinous and fibrinous pleuritis are all caused by essentially the same processes. The amount of fibrinous component depends largely on the stage and severity of the inflammation. Fibrinous exudations generally reflect a later and more severe exudative reaction which, in an earlier developmental phase, might have presented as a serous or serofibrinous exudate.

The common causes of such pleuritis are inflammatory diseases within the lungs, such as tuberculosis, pneumonia, lung infarcts, lung abscess and bronchiectasis. Rheumatic fever, disseminated lupus erythematosus, uremia, the diffuse systemic infections caused either by bacteria or fungi, e.g., typhoid fever, tularemia, ornithosis, blastomycosis, coccidioidomycosis and a variety of other systemic disorders also cause serous or serofibrinous pleuritis. Occasionally, metastatic involvement of the pleura produces a pure serous or serofibrinous pleuritis. These fluids, then, may contain tumor cells that can be identified in sections of the sediment or by cytologic smear examination. Tuberculosis requires special emphasis. The pleura is almost invariably affected in this disease, and the pleural reaction in the early stages tends to remain as a serous or copious serofibrinous exudation, commonly designated as *pleurisy with effusion.*

It is frequently quite important to be able to differentiate a serous or serofibrinous exudate of inflammatory origin from a simple transudate of circulatory origin, particularly in older individuals suffering from cardiac decompensation, who may at the same time be suspected of pulmonary infections. In general, the serofibrinous and serous exudates consist of relatively clear, limpid, straw-colored fluid in which, occasionally, small strands of opaque,

yellow-white fibrin may be found floating. The specific gravity of these fluids tends, on the whole, to be greater than 1.016 to 1.020 and, frequently, by centrifugation, scattered lymphocytes, macrophages and a few polymorphonuclear neutrophils, as well as the ever-present mesothelial cells, can be found within the sediment. In contrast, the transudates are clear and watery fluids with a specific gravity less than 1.012. Only mesothelial cells are present in the sediment with possibly a few scattered lymphocytes.

In most instances of these forms of pleural involvement, the inflammatory reaction is only minimal, and the fluid exudate is resorbed with either resolution or organization of the fibrinous component. Since the exudative responses may sometimes cause the accumulation of up to several liters in each pleural cavity, they may be responsible for considerable encroachment upon lung space and give rise to respiratory distress. While the inflammatory process may be a minor part of the systemic or primary disease, the significance of large pleural effusions as a cause of respiratory difficulty cannot be overlooked. Moreover, these pleural effusions are ideal sites for bacterial and fungal growth and are, therefore, vulnerable to contamination, either by contiguous spread of organisms through the pleura, by seeding from the blood, or by the accidental introduction of organisms in the course of thoracentesis (withdrawal of fluid through a hypodermic needle).

Suppurative Pleuritis (Empyema). A frank, purulent pleural exudate usually implies bacterial or mycotic seeding of the pleural space. The empyema may affect one or both pleural spaces, and sometimes is walled off by fresh or old inflammatory adhesions into pockets or loculations. Most commonly, the contamination occurs by contiguous spread of organisms from intrapulmonary suppuration, but occasionally it occurs by lymphatic or hematogenous dissemination from a more distant infection. Rarely, suppurative infections below the diaphragm, such as the subdiaphragmatic or liver abscess, may extend by continuity through the diaphragm into the pleural spaces, more often on the right side.

Empyema is characterized by frank yellow-green creamy pus that may accumulate in large volumes (up to 500 to 1000 cc.), but usually in smaller amounts than the serous reactions described. The inflammatory reaction in the pleural membranes is commensurately greater than in the serofibrinous patterns, and the pleural exudate is characteristically made up of masses of polymorphonuclear neutrophils admixed with other leukocytes. While it may be difficult to visualize microorganisms on histologic preparations of the exudate, it should be possible to demonstrate them by cultural methods. Empyema may resolve, but this fortunate outcome is less common than organization of the exudate, with the formation of dense, tough fibrous adhesions that frequently totally obliterate the pleural space and make intact removal of the lungs at postmortem very difficult. Sometimes a thick, dense cartilaginous connective tissue layer is formed that envelops the lungs and seriously embarrasses pulmonary expansion. Calcification may occur in this scar tissue. Massive calcification is particularly characteristic of tuberculous empyema.

Hemorrhagic Pleuritis. True sanguineous inflammatory exudates must be differentiated from bloody or traumatic contamination of serous or serofibrinous exudates. The slight bleeding that often occurs in the course of withdrawal of the fluid is the most frequent cause of confusion. Hemorrhagic exudates are infrequent and are usually found only in hemorrhagic diatheses, rickettsial diseases and metastatic involvement of the pleural cavity. The sanguineous exudate must be differentiated from whole blood that may fill the pleural cavity when an aneurysm ruptures. When hemorrhagic pleuritis is encountered, careful search should be made for the presence of exfoliated tumor cells.

NONINFLAMMATORY PLEURAL COLLECTIONS

Hydrothorax. *Noninflammatory collections of serous fluid within the pleural cavities are called hydrothorax.* The fluid is clear and straw-colored, and has the other characteristics already mentioned. A variable volume may collect, ranging from amounts which simply fill the costophrenic angles (several hundred milliliters) up to massive accumulations that virtually fill the pleural cavities (in the range of 2 or 3 liters). Hydrothorax may be unilateral or bilateral, depending upon the underlying etiology. The most common cause of hydrothorax is cardiac failure and, for this reason, it is usually accompanied by pulmonary congestion and edema. In cardiac failure, the hydrothorax is usually, but not invariably, bilateral. The mechanism of unilateral hydrothorax in cardiac decompensation is quite obscure. It is also of considerable interest that in some instances these patients develop severe congestion and edema of the lungs with little hydrothorax, while in other cases the hydrothorax may be extreme with only little pulmonary involvement. Transudations may collect in any other systemic disease associated with generalized edema and are therefore frequently found in renal failure and in liver disease, particularly cirrhosis of the liver. In cirrhosis of the liver with ascites, it is generally believed that the fluid reaches the pleural cavity via transdiaphragmatic lymphatics.

An additional, obscure, but interesting cause for hydrothorax is a pelvic, usually ovarian, tumor. As first classically described by Meigs, a fibroma of the ovary was associated with ascites and right-sided hydrothorax (Meigs' syndrome). It is now appreciated that any type of ovarian tumor may cause this syndrome. The pathogenesis of the ascites is poorly understood and is theoretically attributed to pelvic congestion and lymphatic stasis. The hydrothorax is predicated upon transdiaphragmatic passage of ascitic fluid into the pleural cavity. Since the dome of the liver is closely applied to the right side of the diaphragm, capillarity draws the fluid from the right peritoneal gutter up under the right diaphragm, permitting it to pass through the lymphatic channels. Support for this concept has been produced by injection of India ink particles into the ascitic fluid, with the appearance of these particles in the thoracic cavity and their demonstration histologically within the transdiaphragmatic lymphatics.

In most instances, hydrothorax is not loculated, but occasionally in the presence of preexistent pleural adhesions, local collections may be found walled off by bridging fibrous tissue. Save for these localized collections, the fluid usually collects basally, when the patient is in an upright position, and causes compression and atelectasis of the inundated regions of the lung. When the fluid is removed, the underlying lung surface and parietal pleura are usually gray and glistening and, on histologic examination, there is no evidence of significant inflammatory reaction. Occasionally, when such fluid is present for a long time, it causes fibrous thickening and opacity of the pleural serosa, but rarely bridging adhesions. If the underlying cause is alleviated, hydrothorax may be resorbed, usually leaving behind no permanent alterations. Hydrothorax has the same significance as a serous pleural effusion insofar as it may encroach upon the thoracic space sufficiently to produce respiratory distress. In many instances, highly satisfying relief of respiratory distress is accomplished by the withdrawal of large pleural transudates.

Hemothorax. The escape of blood into the pleural cavity is known as hemothorax. It is almost invariably a fatal complication of a ruptured aortic aneurysm. Pure hemothorax is readily identifiable by the large clots that accompany the fluid component of the blood.

Since this calamity almost invariably leads to death within minutes to hours, it is uncommon to find any response within the pleural cavity. Rarely, leakage of smaller amounts may not prove fatal promptly, and provides a stimulus to organization and the development of pleural adhesions.

Chylothorax. Chylothorax designates an accumulation of milky fluid, usually of lymphatic origin, in the pleural cavity. Chyle is milky white because it contains finely emulsified fats. When it is allowed to stand, a creamy, fatty, supernatant layer separates. True chyle should be differentiated from turbid serous fluid, which does not contain fat and does not separate into an overlying layer of high fat content. Differentiation of chyle from turbid fluid can be made simply by dropping one of the sudanophilic dyes, such as scharlach R, into the suspected fluid and then examining the fluid under the microscope. The fine fat droplets take on the characteristic orange-red coloration of the stain. Chylothorax may be bilateral, but is more often confined to the left side. The volume of fluid is quite variable, but rarely assumes the massive proportions of hydrothorax.

Chylothorax is perhaps most often encountered in malignancies arising within the thoracic cavity, usually those of lymphomatous origin which often cause obstruction of the major lymphatic ducts. However, more distant cancers may metastasize via the lymphatics and grow within the right lymphatic or thoracic duct to produce obstruction. Presumably, in the presence of such obstruction, rupture of these ducts occurs, with the escape of the milky white chylous fluid. Less commonly chylothorax may accompany traumatic rupture or perforation of a lymphatic duct. Inflammatory causes are uncommon. Chylothorax is of importance chiefly as a suggestive feature of the presence of some malignancy in the body. However, as has been mentioned, it does not invariably have such significance.

Pneumothorax. Pneumothorax refers to air or gas in the pleural cavities. Pneumothorax may be spontaneous, traumatic or therapeutic. Spontaneous pneumothorax may complicate any form of pulmonary disease that causes rupture of an alveolus. An abscess cavity that communicates either directly with the pleural space or with the lung interstitial tissue may also lead to the escape of air. In the latter circumstance, the air may dissect through the lung substance or back through the mediastinum eventually to enter the pleural cavity. Pneumothorax is most commonly associated with emphysema, asthma and tuberculosis. Traumatic pneumothorax is usually caused by

some perforating injury to the chest wall, but sometimes the trauma pierces the lung to provide two avenues for the accumulation of air within the pleural spaces. Therapeutic pneumothorax was once a commonly practiced method of deflating the lung to favor the healing of tuberculous lesions. Such induced pneumothorax slowly subsides, however, because of absorption of the introduced air and requires constant replenishment. The same is true for spontaneous and traumatic pneumothorax, provided the original communication seals itself and blocks the further escape of air.

Of the various forms of pneumothorax, the one that attracts greatest clinical attention is so-called *spontaneous idiopathic pneumothorax.* This entity is encountered in relatively young people, appears to occur in the absence of demonstrable pulmonary pathology, and usually subsides spontaneously as the air is resorbed. Recurrent attacks are common and may be quite disabling, but nevertheless the etiology or basis for this condition remains totally unknown. Tuberculosis is often suspected as a latent disorder in these cases.

Pneumothorax can be identified anatomically only by careful opening of the thoracic cavity under water to detect the escape of gas or air bubbles. This technique is best performed by creating a pocket of a skin flap that can be filled with water before the thorax is opened. By puncturing the pleural cavity with some instrument under water, it is possible to note the escape of bubbles. Pneumothorax may have as much significance as a fluid collection within the lungs since it also causes compression, collapse and atelectasis of the lung, and may be responsible for marked respiratory distress. Occasionally, the lung collapse is very marked, when the defect acts as a flap valve and permits the entrance of air during inspiration but fails to permit its escape during expiration and thus effectively acts as a pump that creates tension pneumothorax. Not infrequently, pneumothorax may be accompanied by hydrothorax, serous effusion or purulent exudates, designated respectively as hydropneumothorax, seropneumothorax or pyopneumothorax.

TUMORS

The pleura may be involved in primary or secondary tumors. Secondary metastatic involvement is far more common than the primary tumors. Primary pleural tumors may be either benign or malignant. The benign forms take origin from the connective tissue, blood vessels, nerves and lymphatics of the subserosa. The only primary malignant tumor is designated as a mesothelioma, or sometimes as a pleural fibrosarcoma. These tumors have sarcomatous invasive growth characteristics and assume very varied histologic patterns partaking of the flat spindle-cell quality of the mesothelial cell or fibroblast, while in other areas they produce adenomatous and gland-like patterns in which the cells undergo hypertrophy and resemble epithelial cells. Primary mesotheliomas extend rapidly within the pleural cavities to produce multiple implants throughout the affected side and sometimes totally fill the pleural space with a gray-white, fleshy neoplastic tissue. Interestingly, many of these tumors have been associated with basal asbestosis, suggesting some possible causal relationship (p. 513).

The most common metastatic malignancies of the pleura arise from primary neoplasms of the lung and breast. Advanced mammary carcinomas frequently penetrate the thoracic wall directly to involve the parietal and then the visceral pleura. They may also reach these cavities through the lymphatics and, more rarely, the blood. In addition to these cancers, malignancy from any organ of the body may disseminate to the pleural spaces. Ovarian carcinomas are the major offenders, since the tumors tend to cause widespread serosal implants in both the abdominal and thoracic cavities.

For reemphasis, it should be pointed out that in most of these metastatic involvements, a serous or serosanguineous effusion follows that may contain desquamated neoplastic cells. For this reason, careful cytologic examination of the sediment is sometimes of considerable diagnostic value.

LARYNX

INFLAMMATIONS

There are only two reasonably common forms of disease of the larynx: inflammation and neoplasms. Inflammation of the larynx, laryngitis, usually occurs as a part of inflammatory disorders of the lungs and lower respiratory air passages. These have been discussed under the heading laryngotracheobronchitis. Occasionally, most often with heavy smokers, the larynx is affected alone without involvement of the lower air passages. However, the larynx may also be affected in many systemic infectious diseases, such as tuberculosis, syphilis, diphtheria and others, and it may also be secondarily involved in inflammations that begin in the oral cavity, such as streptococcal sore throat, thrush or any of the nonspecific bacterial disorders of the oral cavity or accompanying lymphoid structures. Laryngeal inflammation, while usually of trivial clinical significance, may at times be serious, particularly in infancy or childhood when the marked exudation or edema may cause laryngeal obstruction. The severe edema of allergic origin that may follow inhalation or ingestion of an allergen or that sometimes arises after a bee or insect bite may cause sudden alarming, but usually transitory, distress.

TUMORS OF THE LARYNX

Neoplasms of the larynx are, on the whole, uncommon. These tumors may be either benign or malignant, and the malignant forms are almost invariably squamous cell carcinomas.

Benign Neoplasms. The benign neoplasms run the gamut of every cell type found within this structure and, accordingly, include polyps and papillomas, chondromas and leiomyomas, corresponding to the native cellular structure of this organ. With the exception of the polyp and the papilloma, the benign tumors are extremely uncommon and follow the identical pattern of growth of these tumors situated anywhere in the body.

Polyps of the larynx are smooth, rounded, sessile or pedunculated nodules that rarely exceed 1 cm. in diameter, and occur most often on the true vocal cords. They are usually totally covered by epithelium that may become ulcerated when the nodules are exposed to the trauma of the opposing vocal cord. In fact, this strategic location raises the suspicion that these nodules may simply represent inflammatory overgrowths of tissue due to chronic irritation and that, therefore, polyps are not true neoplasms. In long-neglected cases, ulceration and superimposed bacterial infection may modify the macroscopic appearance. Microscopically, the polyp is composed largely of a core or stroma of connective tissue, varying from a loose myxomatous network to a dense, collagenous, hyaline scar-like mass. Usually, the nonulcerated and noninfected polyp has only scattered inflammatory white cells within the stroma. Frequently, the stroma is intensely vascularized and sometimes contains large, cavernous spaces that suggest the diagnosis of a hemangioma or angioma. The surface is covered with the stratified squamous epithelium indigenous to the vocal cord, but frequently, over the areas of contact with the opposite vocal cord, there is marked thickening of the epithelium with hyperkeratosis.

Polyps occur chiefly in adults and predominantly in males. There is much evidence to suggest chronic irritation as the etiologic basis for their development. They are more often found in heavy smokers or in individuals who impose great strain upon their larynx. Polyps are frequently found in singers and are sometimes designated as "singers' nodes." Because of their strategic location, they characteristically cause modification of the character of the voice and progressive hoarseness. It is not believed that they predispose to malignancy.

The *papilloma* is a true neoplasm that grows as a soft, succulent, raspberry-like, friable excrescence or nodule, usually upon the true vocal cords. These rarely exceed 1 cm. in diameter, are frequently ulcerated because of their fragility and bleed readily upon manipulation. As papillomas, they are composed of multiple finger-like projections that are barely discernible on gross inspection. On histologic inspection, these finger-like papillae are composed of a central core of fibrous tissue covered by fairly regular stratified squamous epithelium, which may show areas of hyperkeratosis. In many cases, protracted trauma to these masses produces marked epithelial atypicality and proliferation to the point at which the cellular changes begin to resemble the anaplasia of frank malignancy. It is therefore not uncommon to have great difficulty in distinguishing the benign papilloma from a malignant squamous cell carcinoma and, in fact, it is believed that these benign neoplasms have the potential of undergoing malignant transformation.

These lesions occur at any age and, while usually single in adults, may be multiple in children. In certain recorded cases of multiple papillomas in childhood, the lesions have regressed at puberty, suggesting a possible analogy with the spontaneous disappearance of warts on the skin (of known viral origin). A virus has been postulated as an etiologic agent for these laryngeal lesions but has not been confirmed. Alternatively, however, the association with childhood and disappearance at puberty point to an endocrine disturbance. These childhood tumors are responsible for progressive hoarseness and if large, encroachment upon the airway with respiratory difficulty.

Malignant transformation is rare in these lesions of childhood.

Malignant Tumors. While any type of malignancy, carcinomatous or sarcomatous, may arise in the larynx from the native cell population, all are extremely uncommon save for carcinomas arising in the surface epithelium. The carcinomas are usually found in adults beyond the fourth decade of life, and are considerably more common in males than in females, in the ratio of approximately 10 to 1. The basis for this sex relationship is not clear, but it is suspected that long continued irritation or trauma may play a role in their development. It is postulated that males working in industry and out of doors suffer from chronic laryngitis and throat irritation much more commonly than females. Supporting this contention is the oft-made observation that, in the areas of mucosa away from the cancer, the stratified squamous epithelium is thickened and hyperkeratotic and is the site of chronic inflammatory changes with metaplasia and dysplasia of the epithelial cells.

Most carcinomas of the larynx occur directly upon the vocal cords, but they may also occur above and below the cords, on the epiglottis, aryepiglottic folds and in the piriform sinuses. Those arising within the larynx are termed intrinsic, while those that extend or arise outside are designated as extrinsic. These

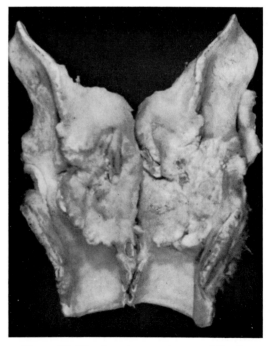

Figure 19–54. Invasive carcinoma of the larynx, transected to illustrate the intraluminal growth of the neoplasm.

malignancies follow the pattern of growth of all squamous carcinomas, and begin as in situ lesions that later yield pearly gray wrinkling and thickening of the epithelium to become plaque-like lesions which then ulcerate, fungate and extend centrifugally. They may, therefore, vary in size from small involvements less than 1 cm. in diameter to ulcerating, friable masses that involve large regions of the larynx, totally destroy one or both vocal cords and infiltrate widely into the perilaryngeal structures (Fig. 19–54). Histologically, 95 per cent are characteristically squamous cell carcinomas (Kirchner and Malkin, 1953). The rare adenocarcinomas are presumed to have origin in the bronchial mucus-secreting glands. The degree of anaplasia of the squamous cell pattern is quite variable, and very striking undifferentiation and anaplasia with massive tumor giant cells and multiple bizarre atypical mitotic figures are occasionally encountered in the more raidly growing lesions.

Clinically, these cases usually first become apparent by the onset of resistant, progressive hoarseness, followed possibly by pain, difficulty in swallowing, hemoptysis and eventually even by respiratory distress. Because the lesions are characteristically ulcerated, secondary infection may modify the clinical symptom complex by the appearance of fever and other systemic reactions to the inflammatory process. These neoplasms cause a high mortality and the five-year survival rate in a large series, despite all forms of therapy, is on the order of 25 to 30 per cent. Those intrinsic to the larynx tend to remain localized longer and have a better prognosis than the extrinsic lesions. The tumors kill by direct extension associated with ulceration, secondary bacterial infection and resultant debilitation, by widespread metastasis and by leading to secondary bacterial infections of the lower respiratory air passages and lungs, such as bronchopneumonia, lung abscess and bronchiectasis.

NASAL CAVITIES AND ACCESSORY AIR SINUSES

Inflammatory diseases are the most common disorders to affect the nose and accessory nasal sinuses. These inflammations are as frequent and as commonplace as the "common cold." Most of these inflammations are more discomforting than serious. However, occasionally persistent bacterial infections give rise to clinically significant disease and, in these instances, spread of the infection may lead to dangerous sequelae. Not to be forgotten is the occasional instance of inflammatory nasal disease which represents one facet of the systemic entity, Wegener's granulomatosis (p. 247). Tumors may arise in either the nasal cavity or the sinuses, but these are extremely infrequent. The familiar nasal "polyp" is not in reality a true neoplasm. These polyps represent focal accumulations of edema fluid accompanied by some hyperplasia of the submucosal connective tissue. As such, they are not neoplastic but rather inflammatory in nature.

RHINITIS

Rhinitis is the designation given to inflammation of the nasal cavities. These inflammations take varying clinical and anatomic forms and are sometimes divided into distinctive entities. However, these variants are closely interrelated and overlap sufficiently to be considered as differing expressions of a single entity. The etiology of rhinitis is based upon the interplay of viruses, bacteria and allergens. Acute rhinitis is almost invariably initiated by one of the many viruses now proved to cause upper respiratory infections. Several of the better studied adenoviruses (ARD, RI, APC) produce nasopharyngitis, pharyngotonsillitis and many other clinical variants that are all included under the category of the "common cold" or upper respiratory infection (p. 435).

These viral agents commonly evoke a profuse catarrhal discharge that is familiarly recognized as the beginning of a cold. In other instances, the acute rhinitis may be initiated by sensitivity reactions to one of a large group of allergens, perhaps most commonly the plant pollens. The mucinous discharge is virtually indistinguishable from that produced by the viruses. Bacterial infections commonly become superimposed upon either the viral or allergic acute phase. It is not clear whether such bacterial infection is initiated by the common micro-organisms that normally inhabit the nasal cavities or whether such infection is based upon the introduction of more pathogenic fresh contamination. In either case, staphylococci, streptococci, *H. influenzae* and pneumococci are commonly isolated. In the interplay of these various etiologic agents, it may well be that the catarrhal exudation evoked by viruses and allergens injures the normal protective ciliary action of the nasal mucosa and thus prepares the soil for the seeding of bacteria. Changes in temperature, exposure, inhalation of dust or chemical irritants and excessive dryness of the atmosphere may all contribute to this ciliary injury and thus predispose to rhinitis. Rarely, in the debilitated patient, such mycotic infections as moniliasis are encountered.

During the initial acute stages of the rhinitis, whether it is induced by viruses or allergy, the nasal mucosa is thickened, edematous and pale gray to red, depending upon the degree of hyperemia. The nasal cavities are narrowed. The turbinates are enlarged. The mucosal surfaces are covered by a thin watery to mucoid discharge which is relatively clear in the developmental stages. When such an acute reaction persists for a period of days, bacterial infection modifies the character of the discharge and produces an essentially mucopurulent to sometimes frankly suppurative exudate. The congestion, engorgement, edema and enlargement of the turbinates are heightened at this time. Focal enlargements of the mucosa give rise to nasal "polyps" which are merely inflammatory hypertrophic swellings, but not true neoplasms. In persistent suppurative exudations, superficial ulcerations or excoriations may appear.

Histologically, during the initial phases, the reaction is essentially one of extreme edema of the subepithelial connective tissue. The tissue takes on a loose myxomatous appearance and is sparsely infiltrated with neutrophils, lymphocytes, plasma cells and eosinophils. This edema is more marked in the polyps. The number of eosinophils is accentuated in some cases, presumably those of allergic origin. There is secretory hyperactivity of the mucus-secreting submucosal glands. In the stages of frank bacterial infection, the leukocytic infiltrate is considerably augmented and becomes predominantly neutrophilic. Hyperplasia or ulceration of the ciliated respiratory epithelium may develop and, in the more extreme cases, ulcerations may occur.

In long persistence of an acute suppurative rhinitis, fibrous scarring of the subepithelial connective tissue may occur. In some of these instances, the epithelium becomes atrophic, and foci of squamous metaplasia may develop. In these cases, the progressive submucosal fibrosis causes atrophy of the mucus-secreting glands. These histologic changes eventuate in a dry, glazed, shiny appearance to the nasal mucosa, with total loss of mucinous secretion, sometimes designated as *atrophic rhinitis* or *rhinitis sicca.*

The clinical manifestations of rhinitis are too familiar to bear repetition. The major significance of these usually insignificant disorders relates to their possible sequelae. The swelling of the nasal mucosa may obstruct the orifices of the accessory air sinuses and lead to sinusitis. The bacterially infected cases infrequently progress to osteomyelitis, cavernous sinus thrombophlebitis, epidural or subdural abscess, meningitis, or brain abscess. These complications, in the light of the great frequency of these nasal inflammations, are quite uncommon.

SINUSITIS

Inflammations of the nasal accessory sinuses are closely related to rhinitis. Almost invariably, acute inflammatory involvement of the nasal cavities precedes and leads to the infections and inflammations of the air sinuses by obstructing the drainage orifices of the sinuses. The etiologic considerations are therefore the same as those described in rhinitis.

The early acute phases of an acute sinusitis recapitulate the changes described in the nasal cavity. The edema of the lining epithelium may completely obstruct the drainage orifice of the sinus and, if the sinus fills up with mucus, lead to a *mucocele.* In the stages of secondary bacterial or mycotic infection, frank suppuration replaces the watery discharge. The accumulation of such pus is sometimes designated as an *empyema* of the sinus. The chronic bacterial infections may give rise to ulcerations, inflammatory metaplasia and progressive fibrosis of the subepithelial connective tissue to cause atrophic changes similar to those described in the nose.

Suppurative infections within the sinuses are of somewhat greater significance than those in the nose because of the close relationship of these structures to the cranial vault. The spread of these infections is more prone to produce osteomyelitis and the intracranial infections listed in the consideration of rhinitis.

TUMORS OF THE NASAL CAVITIES AND ACCESSORY AIR SINUSES

Tumors in these locations are extremely infrequent but may include the entire category of mesenchymal neoplasms derived from the blood vessels, connective tissues, nerve endings, lymphatics and lymphoid tissue, as well as new growths that arise from the epithelial lining. Since these tumors are identical with similar neoplasms arising from epithelium and mesenchyme described elsewhere, it is not necessary to treat them individually in this section. Brief mention may be made of two somewhat distinctive types. *Isolated plasmacytomas* may arise in the lymphoid structures adjacent to the nose and sinuses. These may protrude within these cavities as polypoid growths, varying from one to several centimeters in diameter, covered usually by an intact overlying mucosa. The histology is that of a malignant plasma cell tumor and is identical with that described in Chapter 7 (plasmacytoma) on page 248. However, it should be emphasized that the plasmacytomas here may occur as apparently *isolated* tumors unrelated to systemic plasma cell neoplasia.

Carcinomas in these locations take one of several histologic forms, i.e., squamous cell carcinoma, transitional cell carcinoma, lymphoepithelioma and adenocarcinoma. Squamous cell and adenocarcinomas are insidious malignancies that produce the characteristic ulcerating, fungating growth typical of these malignancies elsewhere. The *transitional cell carcinoma* is characterized histologically by strands and masses of polygonal to spindle cells growing within a fibrous stroma. The cell boundaries are poorly defined, and often the masses of cells take on the appearance of a syncytium. In many of these transitional growths, there is an abundant lymphoid infiltrate within the fibrous stroma, designated then as a *lymphoepithelioma*. All these malignancies progressively invade and destroy, spread to cervical nodes and, in late cases, metastasize to distant areas, i.e., lungs, pleural cavities, liver and remote chains of lymph nodes. As a group, these malignancies produce symptoms only when they are advanced to a stage at which curative resection is difficult, if not impossible, and the prognosis is poor.

An intriguing observation has recently come to light on nasopharyngeal carcinomas arising in the mucosal epithelial cells. These patients have been found to have high serum titers of antibodies against the Epstein-Barr virus (Henle et al., 1970). The levels of anti-EBV titers were equally elevated for all histologic patterns of nasopharyngeal carcinoma. In contrast, epithelial cancers arising in the head and neck produced no significant anti-EBV titers. The meaning of these findings is still obscure, but obviously raises the issue of the possible viral causation of nasal carcinomas.

REFERENCES

Amberson, J. B.: A clinical consideration of abscesses and cavities of the lung. Bull. Johns Hopkins Hosp., *94*:227, 1954.

American Thoracic Society: Chronic bronchitis, asthma and pulmonary emphysema. Statement by the committee on diagnostic standards for non-tuberculous respiratory disease. Amer. Rev. Resp. Dis., *85*:762, 1962.

Anderson, W. A. D.: Contributions of pathology to problems of human and experimental lung cancer. Amer. J. Clin. Path., *46*:3, 1966.

Armstrong, D.: Virus and mycoplasma respiratory infections. Advances Cardiopulm. Dis., *4*:175, 1969.

Auerbach, O.: The pathology and pathogenesis of pulmonary tuberculosis. Med. Clin. N. Amer., *20*:689, 1936.

Auerbach. O.: Tuberculosis of the trachea and major bronchi. Amer. Rev. Tuberc., *60*:604, 1949.

Auerbach, O., et al.: Bronchial epithelium in former smokers. New Eng. J. Med., *267*:119, 1962*a*.

Auerbach, O., et al.: Changes in bronchial epithelium in relation to sex, age, residence, smoking and pneumonia. New Eng. J. Med., *267*:111, 1962*b*.

Auerbach, O., et al.: Changes in the bronchial epithelium in relation to smoking and cancer of the lung. New Eng. J. Med., *256*:97, 1957.

Auerbach, O., et al.: Effects of cigarette smoking on dogs. II. Pulmonary neoplasms. Arch. Environ. Health (Chicago), *21*:754, 1970.

Azzopardi, J. G., and Williams, E. D.: Pathology of "non endocrine" tumors associated with Cushing's syndrome. Cancer, *222*:274, 1968.

Bayley, E. C., et al.: Loefflers syndrome: report of a case with pathologic examination of the lungs. Arch. Path., *40*:376, 1945.

Benoit, F. L., et al.: Goodpasture's syndrome. A clinical pathologic entity. Amer. J. Med., *37*:424, 1964.

Berg, T., and Johansson, S. G.: IgE concentrations in children with atopic diseases. A clinical study. Int. Arch. Allerg., *36*:219, 1969.

Bignall, J. R., and Martin, M.: Survival experience of women with bronchogenic carcinoma. Lancet, *2*:60, 1972.

Blount, S. G.: Primary pulmonary hypertension. Mod. Conc. Cardiovasc. Dis., *36*:67, 1967.

Boren, H. G.: Carbon as a carrier mechanism for irritant gas. Arch. Environ. Health, *8*:119, 1964.

Brill, I. C., and Krygier, J. J.: Primary pulmonary vascular sclerosis. Arch. Intern. Med., *68*:560, 1941.

Buckley, A. R., et al.: Adult chronic bronchitis: the infective factor and its treatment. Brit. Med. J., *2*:259, 1957.

Burrows, B., and Earle, R. H.: The course and prognosis of chronic obstructive lung disease. New Eng. J. Med., *280*:397, 1969.

Burrows, B., and Kettel, L. J.: Important considerations in emphysema-chronic bronchitis syndrome. Geriatrics, *24*:72, 1969.

Burrows, R., et al.: The emphysematous and bronchial types of chronic airways obstruction. Lancet, *1*:830, 1966.

Carrington, C. B.: Chronic eosinophilic pneumonia. New Eng. J. Med., *280*:787, 1969.

Castleman, B.: Healed pulmonary infacts. Arch. Path., *30*:130, 1940.

Clemo, G. R., et al.: The carcinogenic action of city smoke. Brit. J. Cancer, *9*:137, 1955.

Cooke, F. N., and Blades, B.: Cystic disease of the lungs. J. Thorac. Surg., *23*:546, 1952.

Decker, H. R.: Alveolar cell carcinoma of the lung (pulmonary adenomatosis): a study of 155 cases. J. Thorac. Surg., *30*:230, 1955.

Ebert, R. V., and Pierce, J. A.: Pathogenesis of pulmonary emphysema. Arch. Intern. Med., *111*:34, 1963.

Editorial: Argentaffinoma and bronchial adenoma. Lancet, *2*:355, 1960.

Editorial: Chronic bronchitis in Great Britain. A national survey carried out by the respiratory diseases study group of the College of General Practitioners. Brit. Med. J., *2*:973, 1961.

Falk, J. A., and Briscoe, W. A.: Chronic obstructive pulmonary disease and heterozygous alpha-1-antitrypsin deficiency. Ann. Intern. Med., 72:595, 1970.

Farber, S. M., and Wilson, R. H. L.: Chronic obstructive emphysema. Ciba Clin. Symp., 20:35, 1968.

Farr, G. H., et al.: Desquamative interstitial pneumonia: an electron microscope study. Amer. J. Path., 60:347, 1970.

Fletcher, C. M.: Terminology, definitions and classification of chronic pulmonary emphysema and related conditions. (Report of the conclusions of a Ciba guest symposium). Thorax, 11:286, 1959.

Forsyth, B. R., et al.: Etiology of primary atypical pneumonia in a military population. J.A.M.A., 191:364, 1965.

Fowler, E. F., and Bollenger, J. A.: Pulmonary embolism. Clinical study of 97 fatal cases. Surgery, 36:650, 1954.

Galofré, M., et al.: Pathologic classification and surgical treatment of bronchogenic carcinoma. Surg. Gynec. Obstet., 119:51, 1964.

Garland, L. H., et al.: The rate of growth and apparent duration of untreated primary bronchial carcinoma. Cancer, 16:694, 1963.

Goodner, J. T., et al.: The nonbenign nature of bronchial carcinoids and cylindromas. Cancer, 14:539, 1961.

Grieco, M. C.: Current concepts of the pathogenesis and management of asthma. Bull. N.Y. Acad. Med., 46:597, 1970.

Griffin, J. P., and Crawford, Y. E.: *Mycoplasma pneumoniae* in primary atypical pneumonia. J.A.M.A., 193:1011, 1965.

Hagadorn, J. E.: Immunopathologic studies of experimental model resembling Goodpasture's syndrome. Amer. J. Path., 57:17, 1969.

Hamman, L., and Rich, A. R.: Acute diffuse interstitial fibrosis of the lung. Bull. Johns Hopkins Hosp., 74:177, 1944.

Hammond, E. C., and Horn, D.: Smoking and death rates: report on forty-four months of follow-up of 187,783 men. I., II. J.A.M.A., 166:1159, 1294, 1958.

Hammond, E. C., et al.: Effects of cigarette smoking on dogs. I. Design of experiment, mortality and findings in lung parenchyma. Arch. Environ. Health (Chicago), 21:748, 1970.

Henle, W., et al.: Antibodies to Epstein-Barr virus in nasopharyngeal carcinoma, other head and neck neoplasms, and control groups. J. Nat. Cancer Inst., 44:225, 1970.

Hume, M., et al.: Venous Thrombosis and Pulmonary Embolism. Cambridge, Mass., Harvard University Press, 1970.

Ishizaka, K., and Ishizaka, T.: Characterization of human reaginic antibodies. Proceedings of the Sixth Congress of the International Association of Allergology. Montreal, November 5–11, 1967a.

Ishizaka, K., and Ishizaka, T.: Identification of IgE antibodies as a carrier of reaginic activity. J. Immun., 99:1187, 1967b.

James, A. G.: Cancer Prognosis Manual. New York, American Cancer Society, 1966.

Kirchner, J. A., and Malkin, J. S.: Cancer of the larynx: 30 year survey at New Haven Hospital. Arch. Otolaryng., 58:19, 1953.

Kleinerman, J., et al.: The occurrence and incidence of emphysematous lesions in man from 15–44 years of age. Amer. Rev. Resp. Dis., 98:152, 1968.

Knudson, R. J., and Gaensler, E. A.: Collective review: surgery for emphysema. Ann. Thorac. Surg., 1:332, 1965.

Koffler, D., et al.: Immunologic studies concerning the pulmonary lesions in Goodpasture's syndrome. Amer. J. Path., 54:293, 1969.

Kotin, P., and Falk, H. L.: The role and action of environmental agents in the pathogenesis of lung cancer. I. Air pollutants. Cancer, 12:147, 1959.

Kotin, P., et al.: Pulmonary Aspects of Air Pollution. Detroit, Fall Meeting of American College of Physicians, 1963.

Kueppers, F.: Obstructive lung disease and alpha-1-antitrypsin deficiency gene heterozygosity. Science, 165:899, 1969.

Kuhn, C., et al.: Pulmonary alveolar proteinosis: a study using enzyme histochemistry, electron microscopy, and surface tension measurement. Lab. Invest., 15:492, 1966.

Larson, R. K., et al.: Genetic and environmental determinants of chronic obstructive pulmonary disease. Ann. Intern. Med., 72:627, 1970.

Laurell, C. B., and Eriksson, S.: The electrophoretic alpha-1-globulin pattern of serum in alpha-1-antitrypsin deficiency. Scand. J. Clin. Lab. Invest., 15:132, 1963.

Laurenzi, G. A.: Suppurative disease of the lung. Advances Cardiopulm. Dis., 4:198, 1969.

Leopold, T. G., and Gough, J.: The centrilobular form of emphysema and its relation to chronic bronchitis. Thorax, 12:219, 1957.

Lerner, R. A., and Dixon, F. J.: The induction of acute glomerulonephritis in rabbits with soluble antigens isolated from normal homologous and autologous urine. J. Immun., 100:1277, 1968.

Lieberman, J.: Heterozygous and homozygous alpha-1-antitrypsin deficiency in patients with pulmonary emphysema. New Eng. J. Med., 281:279, 1969.

Liebow, A. A., et al.: Desquamative interstitial pneumonia. Amer. J. Med., 39:369, 1965.

Lindskog, G. E., and Hubbell, D. S.: An analysis of 215 cases of bronchiectasis. Surg. Gynec. Obstet., 100:643, 1955.

Lipsett, N. B.: Hormonal syndromes associated with cancer. Cancer Res., 25:1068, 1965.

Livingstone, I. L., et al.: Diffuse interstitial pulmonary fibrosis. Quart. J. Med., 33:71, 1964.

Markush, R. E.: National chronic respiratory disease mortality study. I. Prevalence and severity of death of chronic respiratory diseases in the United States, 1963. J. Chron. Dis., 21:129, 1968.

Massumi, R. A., and Legier, J. F.: Rheumatic pneumonitis. Circulation, 33:417, 1965.

McLean, K. H.: The pathogenesis of pulmonary emphysema. Amer. J. Med., 25:62, 1958.

Mitchell, R. S.: Control of tuberculosis. New Eng. J. Med., 276:842, 905, 1967.

Mittman, C., et al.: Smoking and chronic obstructive lung disease in alpha-1-antitrypsin deficiency. Chest, 60:214, 1971.

Nahas, R. A., et al.: Post-perfusion lung syndrome: role of circulatory exclusion. Lancet, 2:251, 1965.

National Health Education Committee: Facts on the major killing and crippling diseases in the United States today. New York, 1966.

Norris, R. F., and Tyson, R. M.: The pathogenesis of congenital polycystic lung and its correlation with polycystic disease of other epithelial organs. Amer. J. Path., 23:1075, 1947.

Ogilvie, A. G.: The natural history of bronchiectasis: a clinical, roentgenologic and pathologic study. Arch. Intern. Med., 68:395, 1941.

O'Neal, R. M., and Thomas, W. A.: The role of pulmonary hypertension and thromboembolism in the production of pulmonary arteriosclerosis. Circulation, 12:370, 1955.

Parker, F., Jr., and Weiss, S.: The nature and significance of the structural changes in the lungs in mitral stenosis. Amer. J. Path., 12:573, 1936.

Parker, F., Jr., et al.: Primary atypical pneumonia. Arch. Path., 44:581, 1947.

Pinkerton, H.: The reaction to oils and fats in the lung. Arch. Path., 5:380, 1928.

Policard, A.: The conflict of living matter with the mineral world: the pneumoconioses. Amer. J. Clin. Path., 15:394, 1962.

Pollak, V. E., and Mendoza, N.: Rapidly progressive glomerulonephritis. Med. Clin. N. Amer., 55:1397, 1971.

Poskitt, T. R.: Immunologic and electron microscopic studies in Goodpasture's syndrome. Amer. J. Med., 49:250, 1970.

Pratt, P. C.: The relationship between pigment deposits and lesions in normal and centrilobular emphysematous lungs. Amer. Rev. Resp. Dis., 87:245, 1963.

Pratt, P. C., and Kilburn, K. H.: A modern concept of the emphysemas based on correlations of structure and function. Hum. Path., 1:443, 1970.

Pratt, P. C., et al.: Correlation between post mortem pulmonary function and structure in panlobular emphysema. Lab. Invest., 11:177, 1963.

Reed, C. E.: Beta adrenergic blockade, bronchial asthma and atopy. J. Allerg., 42:238, 1968.

Reid, I.: Measurement of the bronchial mucus gland layer. A diagnostic yardstick in chronic bronchitis. Thorax, 15:132, 1960.

Reinhoff, W. F., et al.: Bronchogenic carcinoma: a study of cases studied at John Hopkins Hospital from 1933 to 1958. Ann. Surg., 161:674, 1965.

Reynolds, R. C.: Electron microscopy of destructive pulmonary emphysema. Med. Thorac., *22*:161, 1964.

Rosen, S. H., et al.: Pulmonary alveolar proteinosis. New Eng. J. Med., *258*:1123, 1958.

Royal College of Physicians: Smoking and Health. London, Pitman, 1962.

Russell, H. K., et al.: Lipoid pneumonia. New York J. Med., *56*:253, 1956.

Sabiston, D. C.: Pulmonary embolism. Surg., Gynec., Obstet., *126*:1075, 1968.

Sanerkin, N. G.: Causes and consequences of airways obstruction in bronchial asthma. Ann. Allerg., *28*:528, 1970.

Schweppe, H. I., et al.: Lung abscess, an analysis of the Massachusetts General Hospital cases from 1943 through 1956. New Eng. J. Med., *265*:1039, 1961.

Scott, R. F., et al.: Rheumatic pneumonitis: pathological features. Pediatrics, *54*:60, 1959.

Scott, W. F.: Bacterial pneumonia. S. Afr. Med. J., *26*:334, 358, 1952.

Sevitt, S., and Gallagher, N. G.: Venous thrombosis and pulmonary embolism: a clinico-pathological study in injured and burned patients. Brit. J. Surg., *55*:481, 1968.

Simpson, I., et al.: Severe irreversible airways obstruction without emphysema. Thorax, *18*:361, 1963.

Soergel, K. H., and Sommers, S. C.: Idiopathic pulmonary hemosiderosis and related syndromes. Amer. J. Med., *32*:499, 1962.

Soloff, L. A., and Rodman, T.: Acute pulmonary embolism. Amer. Heart J., *74*:710, 1967.

Soutter, L., et al.: A clinical survey of adenomas of the trachea and bronchus in a general hospital. J. Thorac. Surg., *28*:412, 1954.

Spratt, J. S., et al.: The frequency, distribution of rates of growth and the estimated duration of primary pulmonary carcinomas. Cancer, *16*:687, 1963.

Szentivanyi, A.: The beta adrenergic theory of the atopic abnormality in bronchial asthma. J. Allerg., *42*:203, 1968.

Thurlbeck, W. M.: The incidence of pulmonary emphysema. Amer. Rev. Resp. Dis., *87*:206, 1963.

Thurlbeck, W. M., and Angus, G. E.: A distribution curve for chronic bronchitis. Thorax, *19*:436, 1964.

Trauger, D. A.: A note on tuberculosis epidemiology. Amer. Rev. Resp. Dis., *87*:582, 1963.

Turner-Warwick, J., and Doniach, D.: Auto-antibody studies in interstitial pulmonary fibrosis. Brit. Med. J., *1*:886, 1965.

United States Department of Health, Education and Welfare: Diseases associated with smoking. National Center for Health Statistics; Vital and Health Statistics Series 20 No. 4, Public Health Service Publication No. 1000, Oct., 1966.

United States Department of Health, Education and Welfare: The health consequences of smoking. Public Health Service Review, 1967; Public Health Service Publication No. 1696, Jan., 1968.

United States Department of Health, Education and Welfare: Vital Statistics of the United States. Public Service and Mental Health Administration. National Center for Health Statistics, 1967.

Walcott, G., et al.: Primary pulmonary hypertension. Amer. J. Med., *49*:70, 1970.

Warner, R. R. P., and Southern, A. L.: Carcinoid syndrome and bronchial adenoma. Amer. J. Med., *14*:903, 1958.

Watson, W. L., and Smith, R. R.: Terminal bronchiolar or alveolar cell cancer of the lung. Report of 33 cases. J.A.M.A., *147*:7, 1951.

Willoughby, W. F., and Dixon, F. J.: Experimental hemorrhagic pneumonitis produced by heterologous anti-lung antibody. J. Immun., *104*:28, 1970.

Wynder, E. L., and Hoffman, D.: Current concepts of environmental cancer research. Med. Clin. N. Amer., *50*:631, 1966.

Wynder, E. L., and Hoffman, D.: Tobacco and tobacco smoke: studies in experimental carcinogenesis. New York, Academic Press, Inc., 1967.

Ziskind, M., and Saunders, M.: Acute suppurative bronchopneumonia. Amer. J. Med. Sci., *222*:81, 1953.

20

THE ORAL CAVITY

IRVING GLICKMAN, D.M.D.*

Revised by Violeta Arboleda Glickman, D.D.S., M.S.D., and
William C. Less, D.M.D.

---

*Deceased, 1972.

NORMAL

Tissues of the oral cavity are affected by the same basic pathologic processes as other areas of the body. However, in the oral cavity these pathologic processes produce unique clinical disease entities because the structures involved are peculiar to the area. Certain aspects of the normal structures warrant consideration here.

THE SALIVARY GLANDS AND SALIVA

The three major salivary glands are the parotid, submaxillary and sublingual. In addition, numerous minor salivary glands are found in the oral mucosa of the cheeks, lips, floor of the mouth, tongue and anterior faucial pillars. Secretions of the major and minor glands are serous or mucous or mixed.

Saliva serves as the culture medium and constant environment for oral microorganisms (Afonsky, 1961). It bathes the oral mucous membranes, teeth and gingiva and exerts some influence on the health and metabolism of these tissues. The flow and movement of saliva in the mouth exert a demulcent effect on the oral tissues, which may help to maintain the health of these tissues. Eating, talking and swallowing are impaired and difficult without the lubricant effects of saliva.

The composition of saliva (pH 6.2 to 7.4) is 99.5 per cent water and 0.5 per cent organic and inorganic solids. The principal organic components are glycoproteins. Other proteins, such as serum albumen and gammaglobulins, as well as carbohydrates are also present. The principal inorganic components are calcium, phosphorus, sodium, potassium and magnesium. Salivary enzymes, antibacterial factors, coagulation factors (VIII, IX, X, PTA), Hageman factor as well as vitamins (thiamine, riboflavin, niacin, pyridoxine, pantothenic acid, biotin, folic acid and B_{12}) are normally present in saliva (Dreizen and Hampton, 1969).

Many enzymes are normally present in saliva and are derived from the salivary glands, oral bacteria, leukocytes, oral tissues and ingested food (Chauncey, 1961). Some enzymes, such as amylase, aid in digestion, while others, such as hyaluronidase, lipase, beta glucuronidase, chondroitin sulfatase, amino acid decarboxylases, catalase, peroxidase, collagenase and neuraminidase, are increased in periodontal disease. The exact role of these enzymes in periodontal disease is under continuing investigation.

Oral tissues have a high resistance to exogenous infection, which is attributed in large measure to the contents and properties of saliva. The presence of lysozyme in saliva and its lytic effect on exogenous bacteria are significant. It is interesting to note that the normal oral bacterial flora are resistant to the normal salivary concentration of lysozyme, but most exogenous bacteria are susceptible. The presence of all forms of leukocytes, principally polymorphonuclear granulocytes, is another antibacterial factor. They are the source of many of the enzymes in saliva that destroy or inhibit the growth of exogenous bacteria.

The presence of antibodies in saliva has been known for some years, but interest has increased with the discovery of IgA as the main immunoglobulin in saliva. It is found in proportionately higher concentrations in saliva than in serum. IgA antibodies seem to be predominant in secretions that are rich in lysozyme as found in tears, tracheobronchial washings and colostrum. The IgA-lysozyme system represents a defense mechanism specifically associated with mucous membranes in the body, including the oral mucous membranes (Melcher and Bowen, 1969).

THE NORMAL ORAL FLORA

The oral microorganisms are predominantly indigenous parasites with little or no pathogenicity, but some are true pathogens. They may initiate oral disease or complicate disease caused by other factors. The microbial population is in symbiotic balance. It varies from time to time, with one or another group maintaining a relatively constant level. The percentage of similar organisms in different mouths varies. Invariably present are alpha and gamma streptococci, anaerobic streptococci, lactobacilli, gram-positive filaments, fusiform bacilli, vibrios, bacteroides, many forms of spirochetes, gram-positive and negative cocci, hemolytic streptococci, pneumococci, actinomycetes and yeasts of various types including Monilia.

TOOTH FORMATION

A review of tooth formation provides a useful background for an understanding of the various developmental dental anomalies and odontogenic tumors. The teeth are derived from ectoderm and mesoderm.

Teeth begin to develop about the sixth week of fetal life, with the formation of an epithelial structure called the dental lamina. At approximately the fifth uterine month, individual projections, which are the buds for the permanent dentition, develop from the dental lamina. The crown of the tooth is formed before root formation begins. *Dentine* formation precedes the formation of *enamel*, and exerts a stimulating effect upon the enamel-forming cells, just as close contact of the ameloblasts with the dental papilla is considered to be a stimulus for the differentiation of *odontoblasts* and the beginning of dentinogenesis. Surrounding the enamel organ and the dental papilla is a fibrous *dental sac*, which ultimately becomes the adult *periodontal* ligament which surrounds the root and the *dental follicle* which envelops the crown. For further details on tooth formation, see Sicher and Bhaskar (1972).

THE TEETH

The teeth consist of calcified tissues, the enamel, dentine and cementum, and a noncalcified, centrally located tissue, the pulp (Fig. 20–1). The *enamel* is the outer portion of the crown of the tooth. It is the hardest tissue in the body with an inorganic content in the neighborhood of 96 per cent, mainly acid calcium phosphate.

The *dentine* (70 per cent inorganic, 18 per cent organic) forms the inner portion of the crown and roots.

The *cementum* forms the outer covering of the roots. It is the most bone-like of the dental tissues (46 per cent inorganic, 22 per cent

organic) and consists of a calcified matrix with embedded collagen fibers.

The *pulp* is the soft connective tissue component of the tooth. It is contained in a continuous central enclosure in the dentine of the crown (pulp chamber) and root (pulp canal). A rich vascular and nerve supply and lymphatic drainage spread through the pulp from the foramen at the root apex. With age, the pulp undergoes painless regressive changes, such as fibrosis, reticular atrophy and calcification.

The *periapical area* is the region which immediately surrounds the root apex at the opening of the apical foramen. The pulp is continuous with the periodontal ligament, a fibrous connective tissue structure which attaches the tooth to the alveolar bone. Blood vessels pass from the periodontal ligament into the marrow spaces through vessel channels which perforate the alveolar bone. These provide pathways for the spread of infection from the pulp to the periodontal ligament into the alveolar bone and, less commonly, for hematogenous infections to involve the dental pulp. Throughout life, fibroblasts of the periodontal ligament differentiate to form cementum on the root and bone along the tooth socket.

THE ORAL MUCOSA AND SUPPORTING TISSUES

The oral mucosa consists of stratified squamous epithelium and underlying connective tissue. Based upon differences in structure, the oral mucosa is divisible into three zones as follows: the gingiva and the covering of the hard palate, which is termed the masticatory mucosa; the dorsum of the tongue, which is covered by specialized epithelium; and the lining of the remainder of the oral cavity with its thinner epithelium and compartively loose, vascular, underlying connective tissue. The *gingiva* warrants special mention because it is the most common site of oral mucous membrane disease. It is that part of the oral mucosa which covers the alveolar process and envelops the necks of the teeth to which it is attached. A V-shaped space approximately 1 to 2 mm. deep, outlined by the gingiva and the tooth surface in the area of attachment, is termed the *gingival sulcus*.

The *periodontium* is the term applied to the tissues which surround and support the teeth, namely, the gingiva, the periodontal ligament, the alveolar bone and the cementum. The tooth is attached to the jaw by collagen fibers of the periodontal ligament, which extend from the cementum of the root into the bone. For this reason, the cementum is included as one of the tissues of the periodontium. The periodon-

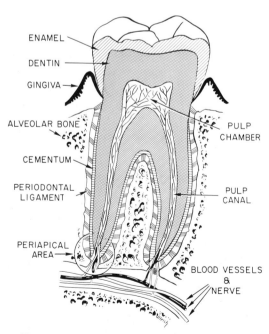

ENAMEL

DENTIN

GINGIVA

ALVEOLAR BONE

CEMENTUM

PERIODONTAL LIGAMENT

PERIAPICAL AREA

PULP CHAMBER

PULP CANAL

BLOOD VESSELS & NERVE

Figure 20–1. *Diagrammatic representation of the tooth structure and its supporting tissues.*

tal ligament is continuous with the connective tissue of the overlying gingiva and also communicates with the marrow spaces of the bone through blood vessels which pass through channels in the bone. The bone which forms the sockets in which the teeth are embedded is termed the *alveolar process (alveolar bone)*. It consists of cancellous trabeculae enclosed within dense peripheral cortical plates.

DENTAL (BACTERIAL) PLAQUE

Dental (bacterial) plaque when unstained is a nonvisible, soft, amorphous deposit which accumulates on the surfaces of teeth, dental restorations and all oral tissues. It tends to occur mostly on the gingival third of the teeth and subgingivally, particularly where there are surface cracks, defects and roughness. It is equally prevalent on the upper and lower teeth, but tends to affect the posterior teeth more than the anterior. It is readily revealed by disclosing solution of basic fuchsin which stains it bright red (Fig. 20–2). *It is the principal etiologic factor in the two most common chronic diseases of the oral cavity: caries and periodontal disease.*

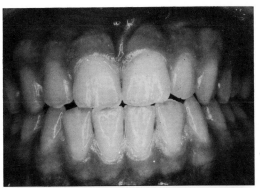

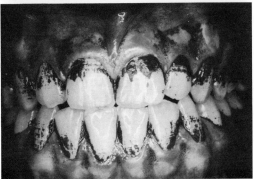

Figure 20–2. Above, *unstained teeth.* Below, *teeth stained with basic fuchsin disclosing solution, showing dental plaque as dark discoloration on teeth. (From Glickman, I.: Clinical Periodontology. 4th ed. Philadelphia, W. B. Saunders Co., 1972.)*

It is formed by adherence of a layer of bacteria to the tooth surface (Frank and Brendel, 1966). The organisms are attached to the tooth surface by an adhesive interbacterial matrix of glycoproteins (Selvig, 1969), or they adhere by virtue of an affinity of the hydroxyapatite of the enamel for the glycoprotein matrix. Dextrose is the major carbohydrate within the glycoproteins. Plaque grows by: (1) the proliferation of bacteria, (2) the addition of new bacteria to the surface of existing plaque and (3) the accumulation of bacterial products. Desquamated epithelial cells and leukocytes may adhere to already formed plaque, adding to its bulk.

The rate of formation of plaque is not related to the amount or frequency of food consumption. However, the consistency of the diet is of importance, and its formation is increased on soft diets and retarded on hard, chewy diets (Egelberg, 1965). It forms more rapidly during sleep than following meals (Leach, 1968). This may be related to the relative inactivity of the tongue, cheeks and lips or to a decrease in salivary flow during sleep.

The pathogenicity of plaque resides in its concentration of bacteria and their products (exotoxins, endotoxins and enzymes). It is believed that these products are capable of causing tissue damage but, it must be admitted, by mechanisms not well understood. Plaque develops very rapidly and, in fact, may appear within six hours after teeth are thoroughly cleaned (Eichel, 1970). As a practical consideration in the prevention of caries and periodontal disease, plaque should be thoroughly removed from the teeth upon arising (greatest accumulation during sleep) and approximately every six to eight hours during awake periods.

Efforts have been made to develop agents or enzymes which might digest or dissolve plaque before it accumulates in significant amount. In animal model systems where single species of dextran-producing bacteria *(S. mutans)* were employed as the cariogenic agent, the introduction of dextranase virtually prevented plaque and subsequent caries. Studies on humans thus far have not been conclusive. Plaque formation was reduced by such intervention but not prevented. It appears that plaque formation in humans involves a mixture of carbohydrate polymers of which dextran is important but not an exclusive component. Currently, a multiple enzyme approach is being investigated for humans (Mandel, 1972).

Dental plaque is the initial stage in the formation of calculus (tartar). All plaque does not become calculus, but all calculus begins as dental plaque. There is no consistent relationship between the age of plaque and its transformation into calculus (Oshrain et al., 1971).

DENTAL CALCULUS

Dental calculus (tartar) is an adherent calcified (or calcifying) mass that forms on the surface of teeth and dental prostheses. It forms above (supragingival) and below (subgingival) the gum margin.

The mineralization of dental plaque forms calculus. It consists of inorganic salts (calcium phosphate, calcium carbonate) and organic components (bacteria, desquamated cells and a mixture of polysaccharide-protein complexes).

Although calculus is not a normal feature of the oral environment, it is prevalent in most mouths. Principal locations are on the buccal (cheek side) of upper first molars and lingual (tongue side) of the lower incisors. These areas correlate with the duct openings of the major salivary glands, and it is thought that saliva is the source of minerals for calculus formation.

The role of calculus as the major etiologic agent in periodontal disease has shifted to its precursor, bacterial plaque. However, calculus remains important as an etiologic factor because it provides a fixed nidus for the continued accumulation of plaque (Glickman, 1972).

PATHOLOGY

Some oral diseases are caused by local factors and others represent oral manifestations of systemic disease. In many instances, there is a combination of local and systemic causation. The impact of oral disease upon the individual varies from the bacteremia caused by infection to the fatality of malignancy.

CONGENITAL MALFORMATIONS IN THE ORAL REGION

Clefts of the lip and palate are congenital malformations, sometimes hereditary, which may occur in many forms. They may be complete or incomplete (depending upon the extent of involvement), unilateral or bilateral or in the midline. Bilateral clefts may be symmetrical or asymmetrical. The following is a suggested classification (Pruzansky, 1953).

CLEFTS OF THE LIP (HARELIP)

When complete, these extend from the vermilion border through the alveolar ridge to the floor of the nose.

CLEFTS OF THE LIP AND PALATE

The complete unilateral cleft of the lip and palate forms a direct communication between the oral and nasal cavities on one side with the nasal septum attached to the palatal process of the other side. In complete bilateral clefts of the lip and palate, both nasal chambers communicate directly with the oral cavity. The palatal processes and the nasal turbinates are visible, and the nasal septum is in the midline and attached to the base of the skull. The premaxilla or intermaxillary segment protrudes anteriorly.

The *cleft palate* may involve only the soft palate or the soft and hard palates. Because midline fusion starts in the anterior region of the hard palate, clefts of the hard palate alone never occur. The outline of the cleft palate varies in shape and extent and, where a considerable portion of the hard palate is involved, the nasal chambers communicate directly with the oral cavity.

Congenital insufficiency of the palate is essentially a physiologic deficiency rather than an anatomic defect and refers to the condition in which the contact of the soft palate and posterior pharyngeal wall, which normally occurs in deglutition and phonation, cannot be achieved. Morphologic factors which might contribute to such functional impairment include abnormally short velum, anteroposterior deficiency in the hard palate or both the hard and soft palates, submucous clefts in the median line of the palatal process, the palatal aponeurosis or muscles of the velum.

Irregularity of the teeth, absence of the lateral incisor or the presence of supernumerary teeth, interference with feeding and swallowing, speech defects and psychologic disturbances complicate the occurrence of lip and palate clefts.

Extremely rare congenital anomalies of the jaws include agnathia (absence of the mandible or maxilla), micrognathia (pronounced underdevelopment of the mandible) and agenesis or failure in the formation of the condyle.

MEDIAN RHOMBOID GLOSSITIS

This is a developmental anomaly of the tongue in which the tuberculum impar persists in the midline in the posterior portion of the dorsum. It appears as an ovoid or angular, smooth, red, plaque-like area which is devoid of papillae. The incidence of median rhomboid glossitis is less than 1 per cent in the 5–18 age group; however, its presence in very young children is compatible with its supposed developmental etiology (Redman, 1970).

Other congenital anomalies of the tongue include the "bifid tongue" caused by failure in midline fusion, "scrotal tongue" in which there is an accentuated central furrow with lateral branches, microglossia, macroglossia and ankyloglossia (tongue tie).

FORDYCE GRANULES (FORDYCE'S DISEASE)

These are painless, pinpoint, yellow elevations which usually occur bilaterally in the posterior region of the buccal mucosa. They may be few or numerous. They are ectopic sebaceous glands which are extremely common and of no pathologic significance.

DISEASES OF THE TEETH AND DENTAL TISSUES

DEVELOPMENTAL ANOMALIES

The dentition and dental tissues are subject to a variety of developmental anomalies which are of interest but, for the most part, of little consequence as pathologic entities. *Anodontia*, missing teeth, may be complete or partial; the latter is the more common and tends to follow a hereditary pattern. Complete or almost complete anodontia occurs in *anhydric hereditary ectodermal dysplasia* in which tooth buds are absent throughout the jaws.

Gemination is the term applied when there is division of the tooth bud, resulting in a double or twin crown formed on a single root. *Fusion* is the joining of two teeth caused by a union of adjacent tooth germs.

Dilaceration is traumatically induced angular malformation of the portion of a root formed after an injury. If formation ceases as a result of trauma, a blunted root is the result. Shortened roots may also result from systemically induced inhibition in development in cretinism and rickets.

Supernumerary teeth develop when extra tooth buds differentiate from the dental lamina. These may be morphologically indistinguishable from normal teeth or may be dwarfed structures. They may interfere with eruption of adjacent teeth or may erupt without disturbing the normal arch form.

In infants, irradiation of the region of the developing teeth may produce the following defects: injury to the tooth germ so that the tooth does not form, dwarfing of the permanent teeth, premature completion of calcification and early eruption of the permanent teeth.

The following developmental defects create more serious problems.

Enamel Hypoplasia. Enamel hypoplasia is a defect in enamel formation. It may be caused by a variety of systemic disturbances which effect degenerative changes in the ameloblasts and thereby interfere with enamel formation. The hypoplastic defects vary in severity from isolated opaque spots in the enamel surface to horizontal defects with deeply pitted indentations which provide a kymographic recording of the period during which the systemic disturbance occurred. Toxemia and other severe disturbances during pregnancy affect enamel formation in utero. In infancy and childhood, exanthematous fevers, gastrointestinal disturbances, deficiencies of calcium, phosphorus or vitamin A and D can induce enamel hypoplasia (Sheldon et al., 1945). Enamel hypoplasia in deciduous teeth can occur as a manifestation of rubella infection of the mother during pregnancy (Guggenheimer et al., 1971).

There is some evidence that large doses of tetracyclines administered to children from ages one to 12 may cause enamel hypoplasia in some of the permanent teeth (Witkop and Wolf, 1963). Although the incidence of tooth decay is not increased in hypoplastic teeth, the destructive effect of the carious process is more severe.

Endogenous Discoloration. Pigments formed before or after birth may become incorporated in teeth in formation at the time and may permanently discolor them. Bile pigments in erythroblastosis fetalis cause bluish green to brown pigmentation. Uroporphyrin deposited in congenital porphyria produces pink to purplish brown discoloration. Administration of tetracyclines can cause permanent yellow to brown discoloration of the deciduous or permanent dentition. The drug is incorporated into the dentine and enamel during formation of the teeth. The deciduous teeth can be affected by maternal ingestion during the last trimester of pregnancy, and the permanent teeth are susceptible from birth to age 12 (Gardner, 1972).

After eruption, tooth surfaces are also discolored by exogenous staining by foods, chemicals and pigment-producing bacteria.

Mottled Enamel (Fluorosis). This is a specific type of enamel hypoplasia caused by *excessive* ingestion of fluoride. It occurs endemically in areas where the concentration of fluoride in the water exceeds one part per million. The incidence and severity of the mottling increase as the concentration of fluoride in the water rises. It occurs as discoloration and/or pitting of the teeth (Fig. 20–3). Degenerative changes in the ameloblasts in-

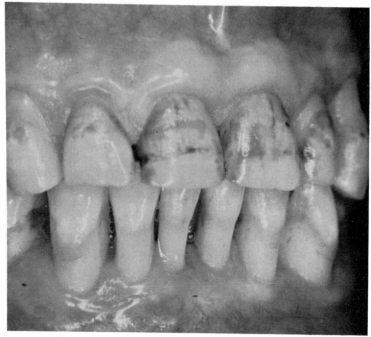

Figure 20–3. *Mottled enamel (fluorosis) showing discoloration and linear pitting of the teeth.*

duced by the systemic effect of the ingested fluoride are responsible for the enamel changes. It is of interest that enamel formed in "fluoride areas" is less soluble in acid and less susceptible to caries when the amount of ingested fluoride is not enough to produce mottling.

Congenital Syphilis. This infection sometimes results in dental deformities. Malformation of teeth in congenital syphilis results from degenerative changes in the ameloblasts and odontoblasts caused by syphilitic inflammatory changes in the developing tooth germ. The following may occur singly or together in congenital syphilis: the *hutchinsonian incisor* (smaller than normal with a pronounced taper and a notched incisal edge) and the "*mulberry molar*" (dwarfed crown with a "pinched" appearance).

Hereditary Developmental Disturbances. Several types of hereditary developmental disturbances affect all the teeth of the deciduous and permanent dentition. In *hereditary opalescent dentine (dentinogenesis imperfecta)*, the enamel is normal; the dentine is poorly formed, which causes the enamel to fracture away. The exposed dentine wears down rapidly, leaving small stumps (Fig. 20–4).

Hereditary amelogenesis imperfecta is an enamel defect which results in a thin hypoplastic enamel which wears away quickly, exposing the underlying dentine. It is inherited as a sex-linked dominant trait.

DENTAL CARIES

Ninety-five per cent of the population are affected by dental caries at some time in their lives. It is the principal cause of tooth loss up to the age of 35, after which it is exceeded by periodontal disease.

Dental caries is a localized, posteruptive, chronic destructive disease of calcified tissues of the teeth. The pattern of the lesion varies with the surface of the tooth involved. It is customary to distinguish between caries originating in pits and fissures, on smooth surfaces and on the cemental surface of exposed roots. There is evidence to suggest that the nature of the pathologic process may differ in each instance (World Health Organization, 1972).

The exact etiology of dental caries is not fully known; however, two essential features must exist to produce the disease: the presence of bacteria and that of fermentable carbohydrates. The microorganisms that are currently suspect are *Streptococcus mutans* and *S. sanguis*. The causative role of *S. mutans* has been confirmed by fulfilling Koch's Postulates in cases where nonhuman primates have been infected with this organism. Thus, dental caries is considered to be an infectious disease.

The most important fermentable carbohydrate in cariogenesis is sucrose. It is much more cariogenic than other sugars in both animals and man because of the ability of certain streptococci (*S. mutans*) to form tough in-

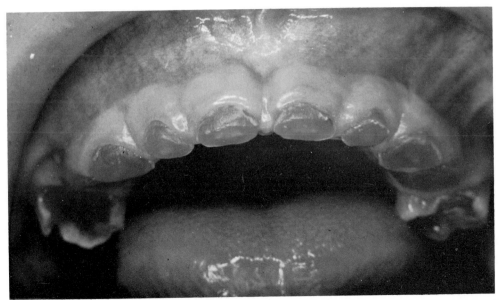

Figure 20–4. *Hereditary opalescent dentine (dentinogenesis imperfecta) in child showing teeth worn down to stained crown root stumps.*

soluble dextrans from it, and to ferment it into acid. Colonization of the tooth surface by cariogenic organisms is an essential precursor to demineralization of the underlying enamel. Dental (bacterial) plaque provides the "adhesive attachment" to the tooth (Gold, 1969).

The exact mode of action of the caries-pathogenic system is not fully known; however, the "acidogenic theory" is the most current and widely accepted. This theory maintains that the retention of fermentable carbohydrates and the concentration of acid-forming bacteria is especially great in plaque, and that this is the cause of the initial carious enamel decalcification. This is followed by enzymic lysis of the relatively sparse organic structure (Lura, 1969).

The susceptibility of the host is modified by a number of conditions such as the depth and shape of tooth crevices, spacing of teeth, rate of salivary flow and frequency of eating. The finding of decreased susceptibility to caries in people who lived in areas where fluoride was naturally present in their water supply has led to an exhaustive study of the use of fluorides for prevention of caries. The results of these epidemiologic studies are well known and have resulted in the use of fluorides (systemically and topically) to reduce susceptibility to caries. The use of one part per million of fluoride in drinking water (fluoridation) significantly reduces the caries rate throughout life if begun during the period of tooth formation (fetal life) and continued through age 12. Thereafter, additional bene-

fits can be achieved with topical application of stannous fluoride (Jenkins, 1971).

PULPITIS

Pulpitis is the inflammatory response of the dental pulp to a noxious irritant. Depending on the duration and severity of the irritant, the pulp may undergo acute or chronic inflammatory changes with varying degrees of degeneration which may terminate in necrosis, suppuration or gangrene. The early changes in pulpitis are reversible if the irritant is removed. The physical encasement of the pulp in a closed chamber causes increases in intrapulpal tissue pressure to be important in pulpal physiology and the progress of disease (Van Hassel, 1971). The inflammatory reaction and changes in intrapulpal tissue pressures result in pain (toothache—odontalgia). It is interesting to note that pain is the only response of the pulp to stimuli.

Caries are the principal cause of pulpitis. In advanced untreated cases, irreversible pulpal changes occur which result in necrosis. This necrotic pulp tissue can be removed by endodontic treatment (root-canal treatment), and the tooth retained. Other causes of pulpitis are tooth preparation, filling materials and attrition or erosion of the tooth surface (Langeland, 1972). Local irritants are the most common cause of pulpitis; however, systemically induced pulp changes do occur. Changes have been described in vitamin A and vitamin C deficiencies, hyper- and hypothyroidism, and protein deprivation (Glickman and Shklar, 1954). For a detailed review of the effect of systemic disease on the dental pulp, see Stanley (1972).

Pulpitis is important because it represents a stage in the sequence of events which begins on the tooth surface as caries and may develop into severe infection within the jaw with debilitating systemic sequelae. In isolated cases, such extending infections have been known to terminate fatally. The pathologic changes which may develop in the jaws from the extension of untreated pulpitis are described in the section which follows.

DISEASES OF THE JAWS

Because pathologic processes in the jaws result in changes in osseous tissue, the radiographic appearance is an important aspect of the individual diseases. Because isolated findings are incomplete, be they clinical, radiographic or microscopic, definitive diagnosis of osseous lesions of the jaws requires the integration of information derived from all sources.

The term "cyst" or "cystic" so commonly applied to discrete areas of radiolucency is frequently inaccurate. Such foci may be filled with granulation tissue, incompletely calcified bone, accumulation of giant cells, connective tissue, cartilage, blood derivatives or tumor cells or any combination of these elements. Although the center of such masses may become liquefied, they often lack the epithelial lining required by many oral pathologists before making a diagnosis of true cyst of the jaws.

PERIAPICAL DISEASE

The lesions which occur most commonly in the periapical area are the *granuloma*, the *alveolar abscess* and *the radicular cyst* (Fig. 20–5). These are inflammatory reactions to irritation from bacteria and bacterial products which extend from the pathologically involved pulp to the periodontal ligament and then spread into the surrounding alveolar bone. Less frequently, periapical disease results from trauma to the tooth, from drugs used in the treatment of the pulp or from the extension of infection from the gingiva.

The most common periapical lesion is the **granuloma.** This is a proliferating mass of chronic inflammatory tissue consisting of new blood vessels, proliferating connective tissue with a predominance of plasma cells along with lymphocytes, histiocytes

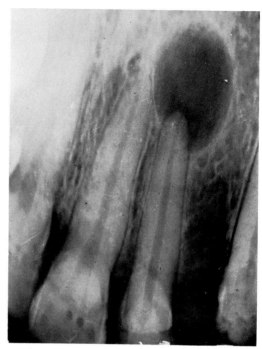

Figure 20–5. *Discrete area of radiolucency indicative of pathologic rarefaction of bone at the apex of the maxillary lateral incisor. This may be a granuloma, abscess or cyst. The thin white line surrounding the area is indicative of bone formation in response to the irritation from inflammation.*

and polymorphonuclear leukocytes. It is enclosed within a fibrous capsule which is an extension of the periodontal membrane of the involved tooth. The granuloma is a slowly expanding spherical lesion which causes resorption of the bone which it replaces, resulting in the radiographic appearance of a localized apical radiolucency.

The granuloma is a benign lesion which is generally symptom-free and exists unsuspected until detected by x-ray unless it becomes acutely inflamed. The granuloma may become transformed to a radicular cyst. Other possible modifications are central necrosis with suppuration and abscess formation or focal pathologic calcification. Root canal therapy, which entails removal of the involved pulp, is usually followed by resolution of the granuloma and its replacement by bone.

The *alveolar abscess* is a localized suppurative inflammation of the tissues in the periapical area. It generally occurs as a chronic response to low-grade infection or as secondary suppurative involvement of a granuloma. In some instances, it represents the chronic stage of an acute abscess. The alveolar abscess is a locally destructive lesion which may be symptom-free but which also may be attended by symptoms, such as a "gnawing feeling" in the area and sensitivity of the involved and sometimes adjacent teeth to percussion. There may be tenderness of the involved area to palpation and persistent lymphadenitis.

Microscopically, the lesion is one of chronic suppurative inflammation which may be walled off by a fibrous capsule or may destroy the capsule, with leukocytic involvement of the marrow spaces followed by necrosis of marrow and bone with bone resorption (Figs. 20–6 and 20–7). The suppurative inflammation may extend through the cancellous spaces and through the cortex, rupture the outer periosteum and appear in the oral cavity as a draining sinus ("gumboil").

In its early stage, the chronic abscess may produce no significant radiographic changes but, as the surrounding bone is destroyed, apical radiolucency is produced.

The acute alveolar abscess more often results from exacerbation of the chronic abscess, but it may occur as the initial lesion, depending upon the intensity of infection. The acute alveolar abscess causes throbbing pain, elevation of the tooth in its socket because of exudate in the periodontal ligament, swelling with distention and erythema of the skin,

regional adenitis and systemic complications, such as fever, leukocytosis, malaise and general debility. Possible sequelae include involvement of the maxillary sinus, cellulitis (p. 369), osteomyelitis, Ludwig's angina (p. 368), bacteremia and pyemia. In rare instances, cavernous sinus thrombosis and death have been reported.

Acute osteomyelitis of the jaws usually occurs in the mandible. Its most common cause is the direct extension of dental infection into the marrow spaces of the bone, generally secondary to trauma or from infection of a jaw fracture or occasionally from furunculosis of the skin. The bacteriology and anatomic and clinical features of osteomyelitis of the jaws are the same as in other bones as described in Chapter 31. The local and systemic symptoms are comparable to, but more severe than, the acute alveolar abscess. Establishment of drainage during the acute stages leads to a relatively painless, prolonged, chronic stage in which massive or focal bone necrosis, sequestration and tooth loss occur. In the early acute stage, there are no radiographic changes aside from the elevation of the teeth in their sockets. With the spread of the suppurative process and progressive bone necrosis, the radiograph presents a worm-eaten appearance followed by the formation of massive areas of radiolu-

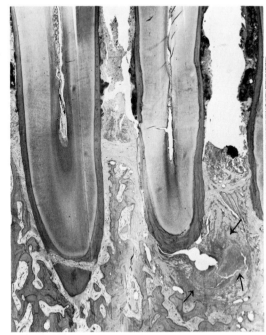

Fig. 20–6

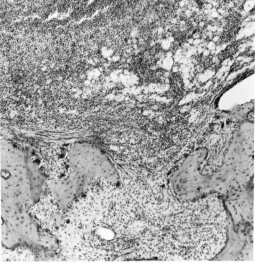

Fig. 20–7

Figure 20–6. *Mandibular anterior tooth with alveolar abscess at the apex (arrows). Unrelated but of interest is the fact that this is a case of extensive chronic destructive periodontal disease, showing reduction in the height of alveolar bone, periodontal pocket formation and calculus on the exposed roots.*

Figure 20–7. *Detailed study of alveolar abscess shown in Figure 20–6. Note purulent exudate replacing the marrow, and osteoclastic resorption of alveolar bone.*

cency. Complications and sequelae of osteomyelitis include paresthesia of the lip, fracture of the jaw, Ludwig's angina, sinusitis, pyemia and septicemia. In comparatively few instances, death has resulted following cavernous sinus thrombosis or pneumonia. Judiciously used, antibiotics alleviate the severity of osteomyelitis and its sequelae.

Therapeutic procedures which expose the jaws to irradiation from x-rays and radioactive substances also predispose the jaws to severe intractable osteomyelitis. Excessive irradiation leads to *osteoradionecrosis* in the absence of infection. Necrosis and sequestration of bone occur within several months after exposure and may be accompanied by deep-seated pain in the jaws and swelling and necrosis of the adjacent soft tissues. Or it may be a very slow, painless process with sequestration occurring after two or three years without notable clinical or radiographic signs. During this period, however, the bone is extremely susceptible to suppurative secondary infection which accentuates the necrotic process.

Extraction of teeth even several years after irradiation leads to extremely resistant and debilitating osteomyelitis. As preventive measures, exposure of the jaws during radiation therapy should be confined to a minimal area, and all teeth in the pathway of radiation should be extracted at least two weeks before treatment in order to permit healing of the tooth sockets. In the construction of artificial dentures following radiation therapy, extreme care must be exercised to avoid mucous membrane abrasion or ulceration which introduces the risk of infection of the underlying bone.

Chemicals, such as lead, bismuth, mercury, arsenic and phosphorus through industrial contact or in medicaments, may cause degenerative changes and even necrosis of the jaw bones and also increase the susceptibility to infection and osteomyelitis.

FOCAL INFECTION

It is relevant at this point to consider the controversial role of lesions in the jaws as possible foci of infection responsible for systemic disease. According to the concept of focal infection, a primary site of infection in one part of the body may serve as the focus from which infection emanates through the blood to other parts of the body. Although bacteria and their products are important causative factors in the production of periapical disease, all periapical lesions are not necessarily infected. Positive blood cultures, predominantly *Streptococcus viridans*, have been described in patients with varied degrees of dental caries and periodontal disease upon chewing and after scaling or extraction procedures.

The bacteremias are transient with most of the bacteria eliminated by the natural bodily defenses within 10 minutes. Transient bacteremias are usually unattended by clinical sequelae. However, in patients with rheumatic or congenital heart disease or with prosthetic valve replacements, bacteremia constitutes a real menace, since bacteria may lodge on the injured heart valve or prosthesis to establish a bacterial endocarditis. *Streptococcus viridans* is almost always the responsible organism (Wise et al., 1971) (Weinstein, 1972). Teeth should not be extracted in the hope of eliminating a systemic disease if there is no dental reason for removing them (Kaplan, 1971).

It should be stressed that when a focus of infection is suspected as the possible cause of a patient's complaint, the presence of periapical disease or periodontal disease does not necessarily indicate a relationship between the oral condition and the patient's problem.

CYSTS OF THE JAWS

Cysts of the jaws are saccular lesions lined with epithelium and contained within pathologically formed cavities in the bone. Cysts of the jaws are separated into two groups—odontogenic and nonodontogenic (fissural)—based upon their derivation.

Odontogenic Cysts. Odontogenic cysts arise from epithelium involved in tooth formation and include the *radicular cyst* and *follicular (including dentigerous) cysts*. Odontogenic cysts have a maximum incidence from age 30 to 60 and are twice as common in males. They occur mostly in the maxilla except for dentigerous cysts which occur more frequently in the mandible (Cabrini and Barros, 1970).

The *radicular cyst* arises from the apical granuloma. Follicular cysts arise from epithelium of the developing tooth. The radicular cyst is formed by the proliferation of epithelial cells within the granuloma. These cells are remnants of the epithelial structure involved in the formation of the root which subsequently undergoes disintegration. Many granulomas contain epithelial rests, but all granulomas which contain epithelial rests do not give rise to cysts.

The formation of a cyst from a granuloma entails the following process: proliferation of the epithelium stimulated by inflammation with the formation of a meshwork within the granuloma, degeneration and liquefaction of the central epithelium and connective tissue to form a cystic cavity, exudation from the inflamed peripheral connective tissue enlarging the central cavity, and continued proliferation of the epithelial cells forming an epithelial lining contained within a peripheral capsule. The connective tissue capsule generally presents some degree of chronic inflammation. Often the inflammatory process causes degeneration and ulceration of the epithelial lining (Fig. 20–8). Contained within the cystic cavity in varied proportions are some or all of the following: degenerated epithelial cells, cholesterol crystals, hemorrhage, blood pigments and pus.

Radicular cysts are benign, slowly enlarging lesions. They are usually symptom-free and expand at the expense of the surrounding bone, producing radiographically detectable cystic areas of radiolucency. Large cysts may distort the contour of the jaws, produce a thinning of the cortical plate or penetrate into the maxillary sinus or nasal cavity. Complete surgical removal is followed by an uneventful recovery.

Follicular cysts may occur where a tooth is missing or where a partially embedded or impacted tooth has been extracted. They develop from epithelium of the tooth follicle which was not completely removed. Follicular cysts are benign expanding lesions, which produce destruction of the bone and

appear radiographically as single radiolucent areas (monolocular) or as a large radiolucent area subdivided into smaller zones by intervening bony septa (multilocular). Follicular cysts are lined with stratified squamous epithelium and present the same microscopic features as the radicular cyst.

The *dentigerous cyst* is the most common follicular cyst. Characteristic of the dentigerous cyst is the fact that it occurs in relation to a partially erupted or totally embedded tooth, and at least the crown of the tooth to which the cyst is attached protrudes into the cystic cavity (Fig. 20–9). Follicular cysts may give rise to an ameloblastoma and, in extremely rare instances, may undergo malignant transformation.

Nonodontogenic Cysts (Fissural Cysts).
These are cysts formed from epithelial inclusions in the lines of fusion of the embryonic processes which form the jaws. *The nasopalatine or incisive canal cyst* develops in the incisive canal from the proliferation of epithelial inclusions retained within remnants of fetal nasopalatine ducts. These cysts occur in the midline between the roots of the maxillary central incisors, are usually symptom-free but occasionally attract the patient's attention because of a salty discharge into the oral cavity. The lumen is lined by epithelium which may be either stratified squamous or ciliated columnar, depending upon whether the cyst was derived from oral or respiratory epithelium. In some cases, both types of epithelium are present (Fig. 20–10).

Another cyst which occurs in the midline of the anterior maxilla is the comparatively uncommon *incisive papilla cyst*. It is a lesion of the soft tissue in the region of the incisors, does not involve the bone and may discharge salty fluid into the oral cavity.

Globulomaxillary cysts may develop from epithelial inclusions in the line of fusion of the globular and maxillary processes located between the roots of the maxillary lateral incisor and canine teeth. Recent studies question the origin of these cysts as being fissural, and instead suggest that they may be odontogenic in origin (Christ, 1970). These cysts characteristically wedge apart the roots of the aforementioned teeth, causing a change in the relationship of the tooth crowns (Fig. 20–11).

The median palatal cyst and median alveolar cyst occur in the midline of the palate in the posterior and anterior regions, respectively. The median palatal cyst is formed from epithelial inclusions in the line of fusion of the palatine processes. It results in a spherical cavitation in the posterior region of the hard palate

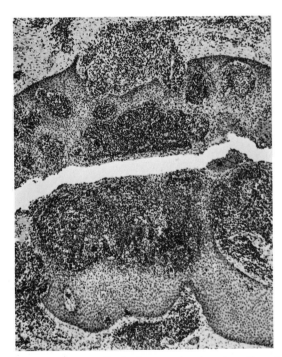

Figure 20–8. *Radicular cyst showing ulceration of stratified squamous epithelial lining, inflammation of the connective tissue capsule and purulent exudate in the central cavity.*

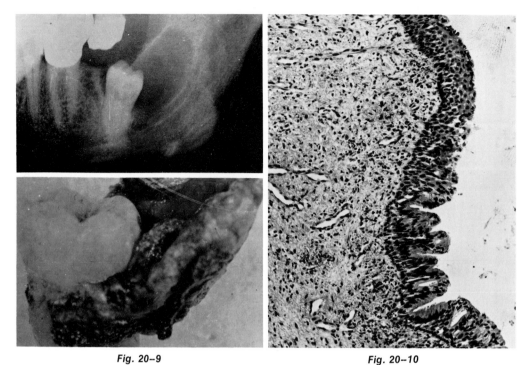

Fig. 20–9   **Fig. 20–10**

Figure 20–9. Above, *radiographic appearance of a dentigerous cyst enclosing crown of incompletely erupted mandibular third molar. Below, tooth shown in radiograph with cyst wall adherent to the tooth at the junction of the crown and root.*

Figure 20–10. *Incisive canal cyst showing both stratified squamous and columnar epithelial lining.*

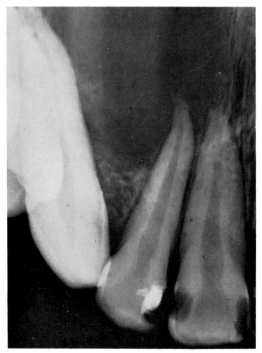

Figure 20–11. *Globulomaxillary cyst with characteristic wedging apart of the roots of the maxillary canine and lateral incisor.*

and occasionally causes a bulge in the roof of the mouth. The median alveolar cyst occurs between the roots of the central incisors, and is formed from epithelial inclusions in the line of fusion of the globular processes which form the premaxilla (Karmody and Gallagher, 1972). *Median mandibular cysts* may occur in the midline of the mandible but are extremely rare.

"Traumatic Cyst" of the Mandible. A lesion which should be discussed in connection with cysts of the jaws is the so-called "*traumatic,*" "*hemorrhagic*" or "*extravasation cyst*" of the mandible (Symposium, 1955). The prevalent theory is that this is a cavity in the bone which results from traumatically induced intramedullary hemorrhage which does not undergo normal organization and repair. Instead, the clot is encapsulated and gradually undergoes liquefaction. The fibrin of the clot is resorbed along with the bone which has undergone necrosis.

The cavity in the bone may be filled or partially filled with fluid or semifluid contents including fibrin, leukocytes and giant cells, or granulation tissue containing fragments of necrotic bone. A fibrous capsule may or may not be present and, in some instances, the cavity is empty.

These lesions are painless and appear as discrete, spherical, radiolucent areas which are frequently outlined by a reactive radiopaque margin. The latter is attributed to a bone formative reaction to the erosion of bone induced by the pressure in the stagnated blood and lymph channels at the periphery of the lesion. Explanations other than trauma have been suggested for the pathogenesis of these lesions, such as local disturbances in growth and development of bone, low-grade infection, marrow necrosis due to ischemia and tumors which have undergone degeneration. It is difficult to justify the designation of these lesions as "cysts." The absence of an epithelial lining sets them apart from true cysts of the jaws.

TUMORS OF THE JAWS

Tumors of the jaws may be derived from (1) tissues involved in tooth formation (odontogenic tumors), (2) other tissues and (3) salivary gland tissue (discussed in the section on Diseases of the Salivary Glands).

Odontogenic Tumors. A tumor derived from tissues involved in tooth formation is known as an odontoma (Bernier, 1960). Odontomas have been classified as "simple," derived from a single germ layer, or "composite," containing both ectodermal and mesodermal components. Odontomas may be either soft (noncalcified) or hard (calcified), depending upon the stage of tooth development and cellular differentiation at which tumor formation is initiated. With rare exception, they are benign central tumors and tend to occur in an area where tooth development has been disturbed and a tooth is absent. They may interfere with the eruption of adjacent teeth and are usually symptom-free and unsuspected until detected by x-ray. Pain may occur from encroachment upon a nerve.

Odontomas Derived from Ectoderm or Mesoderm (Simple). The *odontogenic fibroma* is a benign central tumor, usually of the mandible. It is an uncommon tumor, is generally painless and is detected by radiographic examination when it is revealed as an isolated spherical radiolucency which may be surrounded by a thin radiopaque line. When it occurs near the root of a tooth, it may be confused with a periapical lesion.

Microscopically, it is composed of stellate-shaped fibroblasts in a moderately fibrillar matrix. A few strands of epithelial cells of dental origin may be trapped in the tumor mass. Calcified dental tissue may be formed in this tumor, transforming it to a dentinoma or a cementoma. The malignant counterpart of this tumor, the odontogenic fibrosarcoma, has also been described.

The *cementoma* may occur as a single, more commonly multiple, spherical lesion, usually in the mandible, either attached to a tooth or as an isolated encapsulated mass. These are uncommon (24 in 10,000 cases) (Stafne, 1934), generally without symptoms and are detected by x-ray, but large lesions result in distortion of the jaw.

When attached to a root, they appear as a dense excrescence of interlacing trabeculae of cementum with sparse intervening connective tissue. They are surrounded by a fibrous extension from the periodontal membrane. These appear radiographically as a dense, solid, spherical radiopacity. The microscopic appearance of the isolated cementoma varies at different stages of development. It begins as a moderately cellular connective tissue mass within which cementum is formed. The cementum is arranged as trabeculae or spherical nodules along the border of which a layer of newly deposited cementum may be seen. These trabeculae and nodules coalesce as the intervening fibrous stroma is progressively diminished in amount until the mass is formed, for the most part, of cementum enclosed within a fibrous capsule.

The radiographic picture varies with the stage of development, from a discrete radiolucent area, to a mottled appearance with interspersed radiopacity, to an almost solid radiopacity, with clear-cut demarcation from the surrounding bone.

The *ameloblastoma (adamantinoma)* is a locally invasive, highly destructive tumor of the jaws which occurs most often in the mandible in the area of the molars and ramus. Ameloblastomas comprise approximately 1 per cent of the tumors which occur in and about the jaws (Small and Waldron, 1955). The most common extraoral location of the ameloblastoma is the pituitary; other sites are the tibia, upper lip and pharynx. The reported age range is seven to 82 years, with the highest incidence from 30 to 40 years. There is a slight predilection for females.

In its most common form, it consists of a meshwork of interlacing wide strands and islands of epithelial tumor cells in a moderately cellular connective tissue stroma (Fig. 20-12). The central portion of these structures consists of stellate-shaped cells which resemble the stellate reticulum of the enamel organ. The periphery is formed by a row of columnar or cuboidal cells similar to ameloblasts. Enamel formation, however, does not occur. Cystic degeneration of the epithelial cells and degeneration of the stroma give rise to microscopic cyst-like spaces in the tumor mass. Coalescence of the spaces

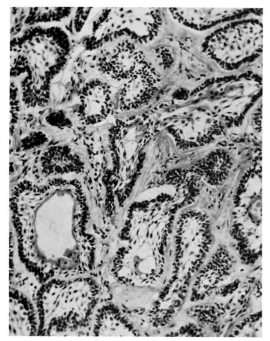

Figure 20–12. *Ameloblastoma showing islands of epithelium resembling the stellate reticulum of the enamel organ and an intervening connective tissue stroma. Small cysts are formed within the neoplastic epithelium.*

leads to gross cavitation and the transformation of the tumor from a solid to a cystic lesion. A connective tissue capsule may or may not be present.

Variations in the typical appearance include squamous metaplasia of the epithelium (acanthomatous ameloblastoma), prominence of numerous large, engorged capillaries (hemangioameloblastoma) and the adenoameloblastoma, characterized by odontogenic epithelium arranged in duct-like structures formed by cuboidal or columnar cells with basal or columnar cells surrounding spaces which are usually empty.

Different opinions attribute the origin of ameloblastoma to the epithelial rests of Malassez, the dental lamina, the outer enamel epithelium, the dental follicle around unerupted teeth, the oral epithelium or remnants of odontogenic epithelium in extraoral locations. Of considerable clinical importance is the fact that ameloblastomas occasionally develop from follicular cysts (Mehlisch et al., 1972).

The ameloblastoma starts as a central, solid, soft tissue mass which destroys the surrounding bone as it expands. With increase in size, the tumor undergoes degeneration and assumes a cystic structure. It appears radiographically as a discrete radiolucent area occasionally with peripheral bay-like projections or as a multilocular lesion consisting of a group of spherical radiolucent areas with intervening bony septa.

The ameloblastoma is at first painless and unsuspected and is detected by radiographic examination. However, pain and deformity of the jaw and face occur as the tumor enlarges. Less frequently, the tumor may rupture through the cortical plate and release its fluid content into the oral cavity. Large tumors replace a major portion of the maxilla and extend into the maxillary sinus and nasal cavity, or destroy the body of the mandible and part of the ramus, leading to pathologic fracture.

There is some question whether the ameloblastoma is a malignant tumor which can metastasize. An excellent review of this subject has been presented by Mehlisch (1972). Although instances of metastasis to the lungs, lymph glands, thorax and neck are claimed, it is the prevalent opinion that the ameloblastoma is a locally destructive benign tumor. In extremely rare instances, transformation of the tumor from ameloblastoma to carcinoma may occur, and presumably it is such cases which have metastasized. The ameloblastoma is usually radioresistant. Recurrence following incomplete surgical treatment is not uncommon.

Odontomas Derived from both Ectoderm and Mesoderm. The *composite odontoma* is derived from both ectoderm and mesoderm. It is usually calcified but may be noncalcified. The most frequent location is the molar region of either the mandible or maxilla, often in an area where a normal tooth has failed to form. Calcified odontomas (Figs. 20–13 and 20–14) are painless, may or may not cause a bulge in the contour of the jaw, may interfere with the eruption of teeth in the area and occasionally erupt into the oral cavity. They usually occur as separate central lesions but may be adherent to the surface of an otherwise normal tooth. Surgical removal is followed by uneventful recovery.

Benign Nonodontogenic Tumors. These tumors have recently been generalized in the category of fibro-osseous lesions. The characteristic finding is the replacement of normal bone architecture by a tissue composed of collagen fibers and fibroblasts and containing various amounts of calcified tissue. The lesions are all benign.

Some of the lesions included in this group are fibrous dysplasia, localized osteitis fibrosa cystica, fibrous osteoma, osseous dysplasia, ossifying fibroma, osteofibrosis, fibro-osteoma, periapical cementoma, cementifying fibroma, juvenile ossifying fibroma, osteoblastoma and osteoma (Waldron, 1970). The most common bony lesion of the jaws is the *exostosis*, which is a

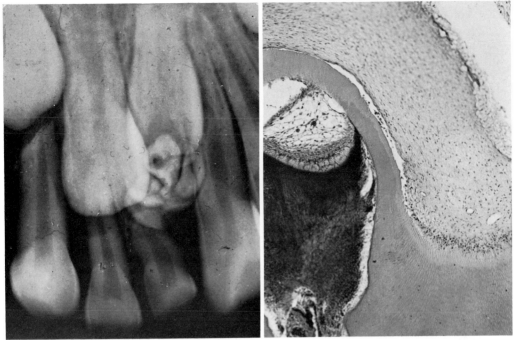

Fig. 20–13

Fig. 20–14

Figure 20–13. *Odontoma containing several miniature tooth-like structures and interfering with the eruption of the maxillary teeth.*

Figure 20–14. *Odontoma containing pulp, dentine and enamel.*

hyperplastic overgrowth of the bony surface rather than a true neoplasm. It occurs frequently on the posterior portion of the hard palate in the midline (torus palatinus), on the lingual surface of the mandible bilaterally in the premolar area (torus mandibularis) and infrequently at the genial tubercles. The exostosis may appear as a smooth bulging of the bone surface continuous with the adjacent area, or it may occur as a discrete, multilobular, spherical projection with a broad base that forms a nodular cluster. Exostoses are generally painless and slowly growing and present no problem unless the patient requires artificial dentures, in which case surgical removal may be necessary.

Osteoma is an uncommon tumor of the jaw. It occurs more often peripherally than as a central lesion. The mandibular condyle, the angle and inferior border of the mandible, the lateral surface of the mandible in the region of the mental foramen, the palate and the walls of the paranasal sinuses are the common locations. The osteoma is a hard, spherical, nodular, slowly growing, painless mass on the bone surface which may distort the face or occlude part of a sinus. It is usually a single lesion, but multiple osteomas do occur. When located within the jaw, it appears radiographically as a

dense, spherical, radiopaque zone demarcated from the surrounding trabeculae.

Ossifying fibroma and *fibro-osteoma* are terms often used interchangeably to connote a benign central tumor of the jaws which consists of fibrous connective tissue within which bone is formed. The ratio of fibroblasts to fibrillar stroma, the morphology of the cells and stroma, the degree of active bone formation and the proportion of the mass occupied by bone are all variable features which evolve as the tumor develops.

The bone is somewhat atypical and irregularly calcified and occupies a varying proportion of the overall mass. It may appear as sparse, newly formed trabeculae bordered by osteoid, a stage which some would refer to as an ossifying fibroma, or bone trabeculae may occupy the major portion of the mass, the fibro-osteoma stage. In the latter lesions, the bone presents multiple curvilinear markings and is devoid of osteoid at the margins. The metaplastic process whereby bone is formed is characteristic of the lesion. The connective tissue varies along with the bone formative activity. In areas of bone formation, the cells are large and elliptical or polyhedral in shape, and the matrix is densely collagenous. The fibrillar connective tissue assumes a granular and amorphous appearance, surrounding lacunar spaces containing deeply staining polyhedral cells. In zones of inactivity, the connective tissue cells are smaller and flattened, and the matrix is loosely fibrillar.

This is a benign lesion which is not usually encapsulated and does not undergo malignant transformation. It resembles fibrous dysplasia of the jaws to such a degree that it is considered by many to be the same condition. Growth of the lesion entails the slow replacement of the normal bone of the maxilla or mandible by connective tissue. With increase in size, there may be extreme destruction of the jaw and distortion in facial contour. The radiographic appearance is initially one of localized radiolucency but, as bone forms, radiopaque markings become apparent. Surgical removal leads to uneventful recovery. An excellent review of all the preceding tumors has been presented by Walker (1970).

Giant cell lesions occur both peripherally in the soft tissues of the gingiva and centrally in bone. The peripheral lesions are often referred to as "giant cell epulis." These represent inflammatory reactions to injury and hemorrhage, are not true neoplasms and hence are better designated as *giant cell reparative granulomas* (p. 1444) (Giansanti and Waldron, 1969).

Central giant cell reparative granulomas may occur within bone, again as reparative responses to hemorrhage (Figs. 20–15 and 20–16) and, in this location, require differentiation from the much more serious, centrally oc-

curring, aggressive true giant cell tumors of bone described on p. 1458. The differentiation of the central reparative granuloma from the giant cell tumor is difficult at all levels, clinically, radiographically and histologically (Leban et al., 1971). Both are usually unilateral solitary lesions but may appear bilaterally. The extent of bone destruction varies. The affected bone may be enlarged and deformed, but penetration of the cortical plate by the growing mass is uncommon. There may be involvement of the tissues surrounding the teeth, with resorption of tooth substance and loosening of the teeth. Radiographically, giant cell lesions appear as discrete areas of radiolucency, occasionally with scalloped margins, which may be subdivided by radiopaque demarcations. Histologically, both lesions have a spindle-cell stroma punctuated by multinucleate giant cells resembling osteoclasts, more so in the granulomas than in the tumors. The giant cells of the granuloma contain numerous (10 to 50) small nuclei in a large cell with abundant cytoplasm. The stromal fibroblasts in these reparative lesions are mature, uniform and display no anaplasia as would be expected in a reparative process.

In the giant cell tumor, the giant cells tend to bear a closer resemblance to the more anaplastic stromal cells and often have fewer and larger nuclei with more evidence of anaplastic qualities. Stated in another way, the giant cells of the tumor appear to be derived by syncytial fusion of the uninuclear stromal cells, although such an origin has not been proved.

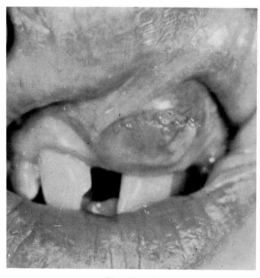

Fig. 20–15

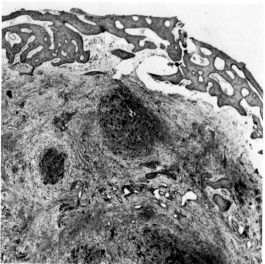

Fig. 20–16

Figure 20–15. *Bulbous expansion of the maxilla produced by a central giant cell lesion.*

Figure 20–16. *Multicentric foci of giant cells in central lesion shown in Figure 20–15. This lesion is a giant cell reparative granuloma.*

The giant cell tumor is more aggressive and invasive than the granulomatous lesion. The granulomatous lesion can be treated satisfactorily by curettage. The tumor requires surgical removal of the involved areas. Recurrence has been noted in occasional cases. Instances of metastasis to the lungs have been reported.

The chondroma and myxoma occur infrequently in the jaws. The *chondroma* may occur as a central lesion or as a peripheral, slowly growing, painless, firm, spherical mass which distorts the contour of the jaw and is covered by intact mucous membrane. The chondroma appears radiographically as an area of radiolucency with scattered, irregularly shaped, radiopaque markings where bone has been formed. Its anatomic features have been described elsewhere (p. 1456). Adequate surgical removal is followed by uneventful recovery. Cahn (1954) stresses the fact that the chondroma is an insidious tumor in that the radiograph is not a valid index of the extent to which it may have penetrated into the jaw. Misleading impressions from the radiograph are responsible for incomplete removal. This is followed by repeated recurrence or "reappearance" of the tumor and the likelihood of malignant transformation to chondrosarcoma with widespread metastasis and fatal termination.

Myxomas occur as central lesions which appear radiographically as radiolucent areas with an internal honeycombed, trabecular pattern. These tumors are derived from either osteogenic or odontogenic connective tissue cells or may represent degenerative transformation from a fibroma. Enlargement of the tumor results in distortion of the involved bone with extensive destruction and, in extreme cases, penetration into the oral cavity.

The *central fibroma, angioma* and *neurogenic tumors* (neurinoma, ganglioneuroma, neurofibroma and "amputation neuroma") are extremely rare benign jaw lesions.

Malignant Nonodontogenic Tumors. Primary malignant tumors are not common; however, they can occur anywhere in the jaws. These neoplasms are identical to those occurring elsewhere in the skeletal system. They include the following: osteogenic sarcoma, Ewing's tumor, multiple myeloma, malignant lymphoma (Burkitt's lymphoma), central fibrosarcoma, neurosarcoma and epidermoid carcinoma.

Malignant tumors of the oral cavity often invade the jaws, but *metastasis to the jaws* is uncommon. The mandible is more often affected than the maxilla. Carcinoma is the most common metastatic tumor seen in the jaws, arising in the prostate, the gastrointestinal tract, the breasts, lungs, cervix of the uterus and vagina. In the female, breast cancer is the tumor which most commonly metastasizes to the oral region (Bhaskar et al., 1971). Thyroid tumors, hypernephroma, malignant melanoma, lymphosarcoma, Ewing's tumor, chondrosarcoma and sympathicoblastoma have also been reported.

INVOLVEMENT OF THE JAWS IN SYSTEMIC DISEASES

Generalized Skeletal Disturbances. There are many systemic skeletal disturbances which involve the jaws and produce changes which must be differentiated from lesions of local origin. Although not routinely encountered, such involvement is significant in that it emphasizes the interrelationship of the jaws with the remainder of the osseous system. Radiographs of the jaw often lead to the first suspicion of the presence of a systemic skeletal disturbance. Descriptions of radiographic changes in the jaws in systemic skeletal disease often refer to the "absence of the lamina dura" as a significant finding. The lamina dura is a thin radiopaque line which is normally found in the radiograph around the roots of the teeth, conforming to their contour and separated from the roots by a thin shadow which represents the space occupied by the periodontal ligament. The lamina dura appears radiographically as a continuous radiopaque line, but it actually is a cribriform plate which forms the inner surface of the tooth socket and is perforated by numerous nutrient channels between the periodontal ligament and the bone. The absence of lamina dura in relation to all the teeth suggests the possibility of systemic bone disease. However, modification and even obliteration of the lamina dura in relation to individual teeth may be caused by angulation of the x-ray machine or a localized pathologic disturbance.

The jaws may be involved as part of polyostotic *Paget's disease* or as a monostotic form of the disease (Glickman and Glidden, 1942). In some instances, the mandible or maxilla or both are enlarged, while in others, the enlargement may be limited to a portion of the bone, or there may be no enlargement. Spaces develop between the teeth because of the enlargement and, in edentulous patients, difficulty is encountered in retaining artificial dentures. Impaired hearing resulting from slowly progressive deformity of the maxilla and nerve impingement is suggestive of Paget's disease. All the microscopic and radiographic changes characteristic of Paget's disease in other bones of the body may be duplicated in the jaws (see Chapter 31).

Fibrous dysplasia may affect the jaws with or without involvement of other bones (p. 1448). It may be symptomless or accompanied by local tenderness (Glickman, 1948). The contour of the individual bone may be normal or expanded. The radiographic appearance and extent of involvement vary. The lesions generally present an irregular area of radiolucency which may include stippled or mottled radiopaque markings or faint trabecular outlines (Fig. 20–17). Curettage and surgical excision are effective treatment measures.

When the jaws are involved in *Hand-Schüller-Christian* disease, the radiographic appearance is that of single or multiple discrete areas of radiolucency which represent zones in which the normal bone has been replaced by pads of granulation tissue and histiocytic cells characteristic of the disease. Increase in the size of the soft tissue pads causes loosening and exfoliation of the teeth. *Eosinophilic granuloma* may produce single or multiple lesions of the jaws without involvement of other areas of the skeletal system, or its occurrence in the jaws may represent an early stage in the course of Hand-Schüller-Christian or Letterer-Siwe disease. In all the aforementioned three conditions now thought to be variants of the same disease, there may be focal nodular masses or painful ulcerating lesions of the oral mucous membrane, which upon biopsy present pathognomonic microscopic features (p. 305). In *Gaucher's* disease, accumulations of large groups of lipid-laden reticular cells and histiocytes in the marrow spaces result in destruction of bone trabeculae with the formation of multiple radiolucent bony defects in the jaws (p. 299).

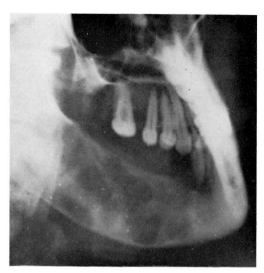

Figure 20–17. *Fibrous dysplasia showing multilocular radiolucency of the mandible.*

Changes in the jaws also occur in some of the comparatively rare bone diseases. *Leontiasis ossea* is a slowly progressive disease characterized by hyperostosis of the facial bones, the jaws and occasionally the skull. It is a disease of early age, sometimes seen at puberty. Microscopically, there is osteoclastic resorption and irregular deposition of new bone with a mosaic appearance resembling Paget's disease. The marrow may be replaced by dense fibrous connective tissue in which new bone is formed. The microscopic findings vary in different areas of the same patient. The bone changes result in gradual obliteration of the frontal sinuses with headaches, obstruction of the nasal airway, encroachment upon nerve foramina with neuralgia, compression of the optic nerve with disturbed vision and in some cases blindness, and enlargement of the jaws with malocclusion and difficulty in chewing and speech. The overall effect is production of marked facial deformity.

In *osteopetrosis (marble-bone disease Albers-Schönberg disease)*, the jaws may present diffuse radiopacity which obscures the outlines of the roots. Hyperostosis of the jaws has been described in *osteoporosis circumscripta cranii* (Rushton, 1956). Multiple fibro-osseous tumors in the jaws have been associated with *dyschondroplasia*, and hyperplastic callus formation was reported following tooth extraction in *osteogenesis imperfecta*. Deformity of the facial bones and radiolucent defects in the maxilla and mandible may appear as rare features of multiple neurofibromatosis. In *hereditary cleidocranial dysostosis*, development of the maxilla is impaired and the mandible appears to be in a protruded position, simulating prognathism. Retardation in the shedding of the deciduous teeth, failure in the eruption of permanent teeth, presence of supernumerary teeth and irregular alignment of the teeth are associated with the maxillary defect.

Endocrine Disturbances. Endocrine disturbances affect the jaws most strikingly during growth and development, but alterations may also occur in adults. In *hyperparathyroidism*, a disease usually seen in adults, radiographs of the jaws reveal generalized reduction in density with fine lace-like trabecular markings. The lamina dura may be absent throughout, and there may be cyst-like areas of radiolucency. Loss of lamina dura and giant cell tumors in the jaws are late signs of hyperparathyroid bone disease which, in itself, is uncommon. Complete loss of the lamina dura does not occur often, and there is a danger of attaching too much diagnostic significance to it. Other diseases in which it may occur are Paget's disease, fibrous dysplasia and osteomalacia. The roots may present an exaggerated tapered appearance, and the teeth may be mobile. The lace-like radiographic appearance results from thinning of the trabeculae by pronounced osteoclastic activity and the presence of incompletely calcified, newly formed trabeculae. The radiolucent cyst-like areas are produced by the replacement of bone by the so-called "brown tumors" characteristic of the disease (p. 1444).

Hyperparathyroidism secondary to renal insufficiency may result in osteitis fibrosa cystica in the jaws localized to areas of mechanical injury or infection. These appear as radiolucent foci of increased bone resorption, fibrous bone marrow and trabeculae of immature bone which may not calcify (Weinmann and Sicher, 1955).

In *cretinism (hypothyroidism)*, the cranium is disproportionately large, the jaws small, and tooth eruption is retarded. In *juvenile myxedema*, the formation of the jaws is disturbed, tooth eruption is retarded and root formation is impaired. In *hyperthyroid infants*, the alveolar bone appears somewhat rarefied. Osteoporosis of alveolar bone with fibrosis of the marrow accompanies the feeding of thyroid extract to experimental animals. In *dwarfism (hypopituitarism)*, the growth of the maxilla is arrested, with the mandible showing the greater change. Resorption of alveolar bone, with fibrosis of the marrow and the suggestion of a mosaic bone pattern, has been described in experimental animals with hypopituitarism.

Hyperpituitarism in adults results in acromegaly. Both the mandible and maxilla are increased in size. Disproportionate enlargement and anterior protrusion of the mandible are prominent and characteristic features which result from the following combination of changes: increase in vertical height of the ramus caused by activation of endochondral ossification in the condyle, resorption of bone producing an accentuated obtuse angle of the mandible, and apposition of bone in the area of the mental tuberosity. The increase in the height of the ramus creates a space between the mandible and maxilla, which is filled by appositional growth in the height of the alveolar processes and the eruption of the teeth. Spaces develop between the teeth in each arch, partly from pressure of the enlarged tongue and partly from wedging forces induced by contact of the teeth in function.

TEMPOROMANDIBULAR JOINT DISEASE

The temporomandibular joint is subject to the same disease processes as other joints in the body, modified somewhat by its unique anatomic and physiologic features. The diseases of the temporomandibular joint were reviewed in detail by Markowitz and Gerry (1950). However, special mention must be made here of the fact that malocclusion and functional disturbances of the dentition are common causes of trauma to the joint which may lead to stretching of the capsule, derangement of the disc relationships, osteoarthritis, subluxation and impaired joint movement.

Temporomandibular joint disorders are characterized by impaired function and pain. Impairment in function varies from slight to complete limitation of movement, with inability to open the jaws (trismus). The pain may be localized to the joint or may radiate to the masticatory muscles, particularly the temporal; it may be referred to other areas of the face, the occipital region, the tongue or the ear. Vertigo occurs in some cases. The pain may be constant or recurrent. Painless limitation of joint movement does occur, but infrequently. Temporomandibular joint disorders are more common in females than in males (3 to 1).

Patients who grind their teeth at night often complain of temporomandibular joint symptoms in the morning upon arising.

"Grating," "clicking" or "snapping" noises upon opening and closing the jaws may accompany the joint disorder or may precede it for months or years. The presence of such noises without symptoms is not always followed by joint disorders.

Tumors of the temporomandibular joint are rare. Osteoma (including tumor-like exostoses) is the most common in the condyle. Chondroma, chondrosarcoma, benign giant cell tumor, myxoma, ossifying fibroma and fibrosarcoma of the capsule have been reported.

DISEASES OF THE ORAL MUCOUS MEMBRANE

Inflammation is an almost constant feature of oral mucous membrane disease because local irritants, such as bacterial plaque, food debris and calculus, are so common. Most frequently, inflammation is the primary and only pathologic change. In other instances, it may be secondarily superimposed upon systemically predisposed tissues. In still others, the effects of a systemic disturbance upon the oral tissues are precipitated by local irritation and disappear when the local irritants are removed (Fig. 20–18).

Stomatitis is the designation for generalized inflammatory involvement of the oral mucosa.

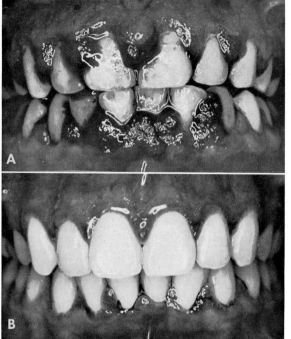

Figure 20–18. *Gingival response to local irritants in a patient with thrombocytopenia. A, Hemorrhagic enlargement of the gingiva induced by local irritation. B, Alleviation of the gingival condition following removal of local irritants.*

Gingivostomatitis is used when involvement of the gingiva is the predominant feature of a generalized inflammation of the oral mucosa.

PERIODONTAL DISEASE

The term periodontal disease refers to all disease processes to which the periodontium is subject, exclusive of pathologic changes in the area of the root apices (periapical diseases).

The periodontium refers to the tissues which surround and support the teeth, namely, the gingiva, the periodontal ligament, the alveolar bone and the cementum. That form of periodontal disease which consists of inflammation confined to the gingiva is called *gingivitis*. When the inflammation extends into the underlying supporting tissues and is accompanied by their destruction, the condition is called *periodontitis (pyorrhea)*. A chronic degenerative noninflammatory destruction of the periodontal tissues is called *periodontosis*.

Gingivitis. *Gingivitis* is by far the most common disease of the oral mucous membrane. There is some evidence of gingivitis in 85 to 95 per cent of 15-year-old children (Murray, 1969). It has also been reported that 99 per cent of the children between the ages of 11

and 17 have gingivitis (Sheiham, 1969). Gingivitis is inflammation of the gingiva. It may be acute, subacute, chronic or recurrent. *Chronic gingivitis* is the form in which it usually occurs. It is caused by irritation from bacteria, debris and a variety of other local factors such as food impaction and dental restorations. Bacteria normally present in the oral cavity proliferating within an adherent *plaque* on uncleansed tooth surfaces are the most common cause. All the gingivitis of early life does not necessarily develop into periodontitis but, with infrequent exceptions, periodontal disease that destroys adult dentition starts as gingivitis (Glickman, 1971). There are other less common forms of gingivitis caused by specific microorganisms or by local irritation aggravated by systemic conditions.

Chronic gingivitis is painless and noncontagious. It starts in the gingiva between the teeth and at the gingival margin around the teeth. The gingiva is swollen, discolored red or bluish red with a tendency to bleed when irritated by a toothbrush or coarse food.

Microscopically, the gingiva presents a dense inflammatory infiltrate, predominantly plasma cells with lymphocytes and scattered histiocytes. There are numerous engorged new blood vessels and varying degrees of fibroblastic activity and fibrosis. The inner surface adjacent to tooth may be ulcerated with suppuration.

Periodontitis (Pyorrhea). This is the principal dental disease of adults, accounting for the loss of nearly 80 per cent of the teeth after age 45. It results from the spread of inflammation from the gingiva into the bone, followed by bone destruction (Fig. 20–19), loosening of the teeth and their exfoliation if the process is not arrested by treatment. Suppuration of the inflamed gingiva is a common but not essential feature of the disease. Systemic conditions such as severe nutritional disturbances, endocrine imbalance and diabetes may aggravate the destruction produced by the spreading inflammation.

The periodontal pocket is an important clinical feature of periodontitis. Periodontal pockets are caused by inflammation which deepens the normal gingival sulcus. As periodontal pockets deepen, the underlying supporting structures are destroyed, the roots of the teeth are exposed to the oral cavity and the teeth loosen.

Microscopically, the connective tissue of the gingival wall of the periodontal pocket is formed by chronic granulation tissue. The epithelial lining is hyperplastic and infiltrated by edema, plasma cells

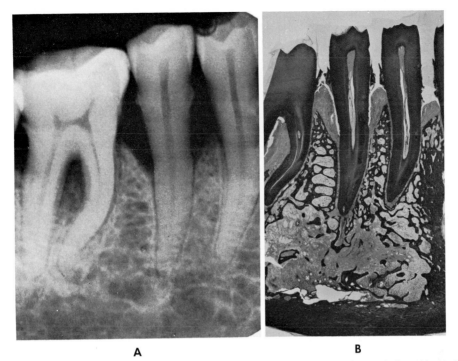

Figure 20–19. *Chronic destructive periodontal disease.* A, *Radiograph showing periodontal bone destruction.* B, *Section of jaw in radiograph shows calculus, periodontal pockets and bone destruction.*

and lymphocytes and a scattering of polymorphonuclear leukocytes. Ulceration and suppuration occur in the gingival wall. Calculus deposits adhere to the tooth surface wall of the pocket. Pus may be expressed from the pocket by digital pressure.

The underlying bone is not resorbed by the suppurative process, but the marrow spaces are replaced by chronic granulation tissue. There is pronounced osteoclastic activity along the bone margin adjacent to the inflammation but no bone necrosis.

Periodontitis is usually painless, but bleeding and foul taste may be present. As the disease advances, mastication is impaired because of looseness of the teeth and discomfort. The infected periodontal tissues are a potential source of bacteremia, which can be caused by chewing on loose teeth or by their extraction. Occasionally, acute abscesses (periodontal abscesses) are formed in periodontal pockets. These are painful and cause swelling of the surrounding area with regional lymphadenitis and toxic systemic symptoms in severe cases.

Periodontosis. The term periodontosis designates a chronic degenerative noninflammatory destruction of the periodontal tissues. It is not common, appears to follow a familial pattern and, although a systemic etiology is suspected, it has not thus far been demonstrated. It is characterized by severe, rapid destruction of the alveolar bone, with premature tooth loss. Periodontosis affects both males and females and is seen most frequently in the period between puberty and the age of 30.

Periodontosis also occurs as a feature of the Papillon-Lefevre syndrome (Gorlin et al., 1964) along with hyperkeratosis of the palms and soles and calcification of the dura.

Acute Necrotizing Ulcerative Gingivitis (Vincent's Infection; Trench Mouth). This is an acute necrotizing inflammation of the gingiva which produces the following characteristic lesions; marginal, punched-out, craterlike depressions of the interdental gingival papillae and gingival margin, covered with a gray pseudomembranous slough which is demarcated from the remainder of the gingiva. It occurs in relation to a single tooth or group of teeth or involves the gingiva throughout the mouth (Fig. 20–20). The inflammation is a response to nonspecific bacterial flora. This condition does not affect the mucous membrane of edentulous mouths.

Acute necrotizing ulcerative gingivitis is a painful condition which progressively destroys the gingiva and the underlying tissues. A fetid odor, increased salivation and spontaneous gingival hemorrhage or pronounced bleeding upon the slightest stimulation are characteristic clinical signs.

Diagnosis is based upon the clinical find-

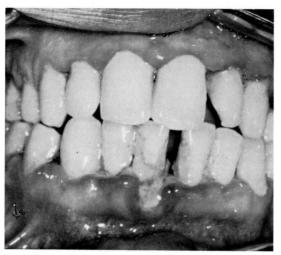

Figure 20–20. *Acute necrotizing ulcerative gingivitis with punched out, crater-like erosion of the gingiva and pseudomembranous covering.*

ings. The bacterial smear presents scattered bacteria, predominantly *Borrelia vincentii* and fusiform bacillus. However, it has not been established that the bacteria are the primary cause of the disease. The prevalent opinion is that acute necrotizing ulcerative gingivitis is not a specific spirochetal disease, but rather is caused by a complex of bacterial organisms requiring underlying tissue changes to facilitate destruction by the bacteria. Debilitating disease, psychogenic factors, nutritional deficiency and degenerative changes caused by local irritation are considered some of the factors capable of increasing susceptibility to destruction by bacteria. It has not been demonstrated that acute necrotizing ulcerative gingivitis is a contagious disease, and all attempts to transmit it from one human to another have failed.

MUCOUS MEMBRANE MANIFESTATIONS OF SYSTEMIC DISEASE

Diabetes. Dryness, burning and tenderness of the mouth, erythema of the oral mucosa, coated tongue, redness of the tongue, tendency toward periodontal abscess formation, pedunculated gingival polyps, swollen gingival papillae and chronic destructive periodontal disease with loosening of the teeth have all been described as oral changes either caused by or associated with diabetes. Clinical impressions linking oral mucous membrane disease with diabetes led to the designation "diabetic stomatitis." However, it has not been established that oral changes attributed to diabetes are actually caused by the diabetes per se

or by preexistent or coexistent metabolic disturbances or local factors.

Although susceptibility to more severe infection is increased in diabetes and healing of oral tissues is retarded (Glickman et al., 1966) inflammation in the oral cavity in diabetes is caused by local factors. Gingival biopsies in diabetic patients have disclosed microangiopathy similar to that found in the capillaries and arterioles of the skin (Keene, 1969). Periodontal disease is more severe than in nondiabetics. If local irritants are eliminated and oral hygiene is good, gingival disease can be avoided in diabetes. The erythema of the oral mucosa and tongue changes observed in some diabetic patients result from secondary nutritional deficiencies rather than from the diabetes per se.

Hematologic Disturbances. Changes in the oral cavity are often the earliest indication of the existence of a hematologic disturbance. However, the clinical oral findings are merely suggestive. They are not pathognomonic indices by which the specific nature of the blood disease can be determined, because much of the variation in clinical appearance is caused by locally induced inflammatory changes. Abnormal bleeding, from the gingiva or other areas of the oral mucosa, that is difficult to control is an important clinical sign suggesting a hematologic disorder.

Leukemia may be a significant factor in the causation of oral mucous membrane disease. Oral manifestations occur with greatest frequency in acute and subacute monocytic leukemia, less frequently in acute and subacute lymphatic and myelogenous leukemia and seldom in chronic leukemia.

It is important to understand that the oral changes generally attributed to leukemia result from a distorted response to local irritation rather than from the leukemia alone. Patients with acute or subacute leukemia may present no oral disease in the absence of local irritants, such as plaque, calculus, food debris, food impaction, ill-fitting bridges or injury from biting. In leukemia, the response to irritation in the oral cavity is altered so that the cellular component of the inflammatory exudate differs from that which occurs in nonleukemic individuals.

There is infiltration of immature leukemic cells and occasional mitotic figures indicative of ectopic hematopoiesis as well as a resultant degeneration of the gingival tissues (Fig. 20–21). The nature of the cells depends upon the type of leukemia. In some instances, there is superimposed acute inflammation with marginal necrosis and pseudo-

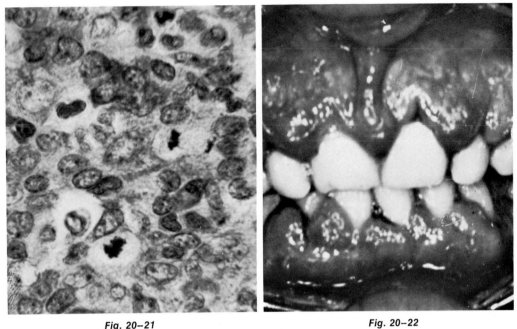

Fig. 20–21   *Fig. 20–22*

Figure 20–21. *Leukemic infiltration in gingival biopsy of patient with acute monocytic leukemia. Mitotic figures are indicative of ectopic hematopoiesis.*

Figure 20–22. *Diffuse enlargement of the gingiva in acute monocytic leukemia. Biopsy shown in Figure 20–21.*

membrane formation. Leukemic infiltration of the underlying alveolar bone and replacement of the normal marrow may also occur.

Although leukemia does not affect the prevalence of gingivitis, it does influence the severity of the inflammatory process. The inflamed gingiva differs from that of the non-leukemic individual in that it presents a cyanotic bluish red discoloration, is diffusely enlarged, markedly spongy and friable and bleeds upon slightest provocation or even spontaneously and persistently if the platelets are markedly reduced (Fig. 20–22). Infections are prone to progress in leukemics, with resultant painful necrosis of the gingiva. Ecchymosis occurs when the oral mucous membrane is traumatized.

In chronic leukemia, even in the presence of local irritation, the oral cavity usually presents no manifestations suggestive of hematologic disturbance. *Osteoporosis of alveolar bone, replacement of the marrow by leukemic cells and infiltration of the mucous glands have been reported as microscopic findings in chronic leukemia.*

The presence of leukemia is sometimes revealed by a gingival biopsy, but the gingival findings are merely suggestive and must be corroborated by hematologic study of the patient. The absence of leukemic involvement in a gingival biopsy does not rule out leukemia.

Soreness of the mouth and throat is often the patient's initial complaint in *infectious mononucleosis.* There is a diffuse erythema of the oral mucosa with petechiae in a few cases. The gingivae are swollen and reddened and bleed on slight provocation or even spontaneously. Cervical lymphadenitis accompanies the oral changes (p. 470).

In *agranulocytosis,* ulceration of the oral mucosa is characteristic, with isolated dark gray necrotic patches sharply demarcated from the surrounding mucosa due to the susceptibility of these patients to severe infections. The absence of a notable peripheral inflammatory reaction is a striking feature. Gingival hemorrhage, superimposed acute infection of the gingiva with a fetid odor and increased salivation are additional findings. *Microscopic changes in agranulocytosis include hemorrhage into the periodontal membrane and marrow, necrosis of the gingiva, osteoporosis of the alveolar bone and areas of bone necrosis (p. 726).*

Oral changes accompany *pernicious (macrocytic hyperchromic) anemia* in 75 per cent of the cases. The mucosa and lips are pale and yellowish and susceptible to ulceration by minor trauma. Marked pallor of the gingiva is a striking finding in pernicious anemia. The tongue is smooth, red and shiny because the fungiform and filiform papillae are atrophied. Swallowing is painful, the patients complain that the tongue feels raw, and there are sensations of burning and numbness (p. 715).

In *iron deficiency (microcytic hypochromic) anemia*, there is a notable ashen gray appearance of the oral mucosa. Atrophic tongue changes occur if the anemia is severe. A syndrome consisting of glossitis, ulceration of the oral mucosa and oropharynx, and dysphagia, known as the *Plummer-Vinson syndrome*, may develop in patients with chronic anemia. The vermilion border of the lips is very thin, the width of the mouth is narrowed and there is often angular cheilosis (Pindborg, 1968). It occurs mainly in females. Deficiencies in iron and vitamin B complex are responsible for this condition (p. 719). A predisposition to oral and pharyngeal carcinoma have been established.

In *sickle cell anemia*, the oral changes include generalized osteoporosis of the jaws, reported in about 80 per cent of the cases, with a peculiar stepladder alignment of the trabeculae of the interdental septa (Robinson and Sarnat, 1952) and pallor and yellowish discoloration of the oral mucosa (Mittleman et al., 1961) (p. 707).

In *thalassemia (Mediterranean anemia)*, the oral changes include pallor and cyanosis of the mucous membrane, malocclusion due to overgrowth of the alveolar ridge of the maxilla and an associated spreading of the teeth, with creation of large interproximal spaces (Cohen and Baty, 1945). Radiographic examination reveals generalized rarefaction of the jaws, with an alteration in trabecular pattern characterized by an irregularly arranged heterogeneous lattice with obliteration of the lamina dura in some areas (p. 711).

In *polycythemia*, the increase in circulating red blood cells produces either a reddish blue or bright red discoloration of the oral mucosa sometimes accompanied by abnormal gingival bleeding. Pinpoint or spider-like dilatation of the blood vessels of the oral mucosa is seen in the rare *Rendu-Osler-Weber disease (hereditary hemorrhagic telangiectasia)* (p. 627). Although the condition may be present in childhood, the blood vessels do not attain their full size until about the age of 35, when the telangiectases appear bright red or purple.

In the *Sturge-Weber* syndrome, there are telangiectases, vascular hyperplasia and enlargement of the gingiva with associated resorption of alveolar bone. In *thrombocytopenic purpura*, there is spontaneous bleeding from mucous membranes. Petechiae and hemorrhagic vesicles occur in the oral cavity, particularly in the palate and buccal mucosa. The gingiva is swollen, soft and friable. Bleeding occurs spontaneously or upon the slightest provocation and is difficult to control. Large hematomas occasionally result from extravasation of blood in areas where the buccal mucosa is traumatized by the teeth (p. 627). Special note should be made of the fact that the gingival changes represent an abnormal response to local irritation; the severity of the gingival condition is dramatically alleviated by removal of the local irritants (Fig. 20–18).

Hemophilia and *Christmas disease* are well known causes of excessive bleeding following any surgical procedure in the oral cavity.

Hormonal Disturbances. There are several types of gingival disturbances in which modification of the sex hormones is considered to be either the initiating or complicating factor.

Puberty is frequently accompanied by striking gingival changes in response to bacterial plaque or other local irritants which would ordinarily cause only moderate changes. Bluish red discoloration and enlargement of the gingiva with pitting on pressure comprise the clinical features which result from the underlying chronic inflammation with extensive exudation and edema and pronounced vascularity. The severity of involvement diminishes spontaneously as adulthood is approached but complete return to normal does not occur unless treatment is instituted. Although the prevalence and severity of gingival disease are increased in puberty, it should be understood that gingivitis is not a universal occurrence during this period; with proper care of the mouth, it can be prevented.

As a rule, the *menstrual cycle* is not accompanied by notable changes in the oral mucosa. However, patients are occasionally encountered with minor complaints, such as the periodic recurrence of "bleeding gums," or more distressing painful aphthae, herpetic vesicles or ulcers on the inner aspect of the lips, the tongue or the buccal mucosa, usually 2 or 3 days before menstruation. It has been reported that such lesions have disappeared during pregnancy and reappeared after delivery. In isolated cases, ulcerative vulvitis accompanies the oral lesions.

The reason for the disturbances in the oral cavity associated with the menstrual cycle is not understood. The tendency toward gingival bleeding may be explained on the basis of the periodic increased capillary fragility. Fastidious oral hygiene and the removal of local irritants which cause gingival inflammation usually suffice to curb the increased gingival bleeding. Systemic estrogenic therapy has been employed to prevent the appearance of the vesicles and ulcerated lesions.

Pregnancy itself does not cause gingivitis Gingivitis in pregnancy is caused by local irritants, just as it is in nonpregnant individuals. Pregnancy accentuates the gingival response to local irritants by increasing the vascularity of the gingiva. It thus produces a clinical picture different from that which occurs in nonpregnant individuals.

The effect of pregnancy upon the gingival response to local irritants is explained on a hormonal basis. There is a marked increase in estrogen and progesterone during pregnancy and a reduction after parturition. The severity of gingivitis varies with the hormonal levels in pregnancy (Hugoson, 1970). The aggravation of gingivitis has been attributed principally to the increased progesterone which produces dilatation and tortuosity of the gingival microvasculature, circulatory stasis and increased susceptibility to mechanical irritation—all of which favor leakage of fluid into perivascular tissues.

Pronounced vascularity is the most striking clinical feature. The gingiva is inflamed and varies in color from a bright red to a bluish red and there is an increased tendency to bleed. The gingival margin is edematous, shiny and somewhat friable, and sometimes presents a raspberry-like appearance. The gingival changes are usually painless unless complicated by acute infection, marginal ulceration and pseudomembrane formation. In some cases, the inflamed gingiva forms discrete tumor-like masses. Gingival enlargement in pregnancy is discussed on p. 886.

The microscopic changes in the gingiva in pregnancy are neither specific nor unique. Numerous engorged blood vessels are a prominent feature along with chronic inflammatory cellular infiltration, edema and epithelial hyperplasia.

Also increased in pregnancy are tooth mobility, pocket depth and gingival fluid. Clinical and laboratory studies discredit the notion that pregnancy increases the susceptibility to dental caries or that calcium is withdrawn from the teeth to satisfy the needs of the fetus.

Oral contraceptives aggravate the gingival response to local irritants in a manner similar to pregnancy (El-Ashry et al., 1970) and, in an extremely small number of patients, produce gingival changes comparable to those observed in pregnancy.

Menopausal gingivostomatitis (senile atrophic gingivostomatitis) is an uncommon condition which occurs during or after the menopause. It results from accentuation of the atrophy of the oral mucosa paralleling the change in the vagina which normally accompanies the diminution of ovarian secretion at this time. The patient complains of a dry burning sensation throughout the oral cavity, with extreme sensitivity to condiments. There is a diffuse erythema and shininess of the entire oral mucosa and, in severe cases, there is recurrent fissuring in the mucobuccal fold. *Microscopically, the epithelium is thinned and there is atrophy of the germinal and prickle cell layers; the connective tissue is inflamed.* In edentulous patients, even well fitting artificial dentures cause persistent soreness and pain. The atrophic epithelium offers little protection, and the patient cannot develop the adaptive epithelial thickening which ordinarily makes toleration of the denture possible. Estrogen administered systemically or in a topical ointment is often an effective palliative measure.

The signs and symptoms of menopausal gingivostomatitis are, in some degree, comparable to those of chronic desquamative gingivitis below. The prevailing opinion is that both these conditions arise from atrophy and diminished keratinization of the oral epithelium associated with a diminution in estrogen or a disturbance in its utilization. Signs and symptoms similar to those of menopausal gingivostomatitis occasionally occur following ovariectomy or sterilization by radiation in the treatment of malignant neoplasms.

Chronic Desquamative Gingivitis. Also known as gingivosis, this is an uncommon gingival disturbance which occurs in both sexes from the ages of 17 to 45 but is usually seen in females. In its mild form, it presents a painless diffuse erythema of the gingiva and the remainder of the oral mucosa. When severe, it is characterized by diffuse erythema plus scattered, irregularly shaped areas in which the gingiva is denuded and red. The intervening epithelium is friable and peels easily. There may be surface blisters which rupture, releasing an aqueous fluid. The severe disease is extremely painful. Coarse foods, temperature changes and condiments cannot be tolerated.

Microscopically, two types have been described (Glickman and Smulow, 1966). The lichenoid type is characterized by atrophic epithelium, subepithelial inflammation, destruction of the basement membrane junctional vesicles and separation of the epithelium. In the bullous type, the subepithelial connective tissue is replaced by edema, fibrin and leukocytes, and the formation of large subepithelial bullae which separate and elevate the overlying epithelium.

The most severe changes in chronic desquamative gingivitis are inflammatory and associated with local irritants. However, there is a continuing suspicion, as yet unsubstantiated, that it is primarily a systemically caused degenerative condition, and the inflammatory changes are secondary. This is the reason it is sometimes referred to as gingivosis. Hormonal imbalance, deficiency of estrogen in the female or testosterone in the male, and nutritional deficiency are suggested etiologic factors.

There is some question as to whether chronic desquamative gingivitis is (1) a single disease entity; (2) a variant of bullous and vesicular dermatologic disorders such as lichen planus, erythema multiforme or benign mucous membrane pemphigoid; or (3) a nonspecific gingival response to a variety of causes. Its origin may be systemic, but local irritants and the inflammation they produce account for many of its clinical and microscopic features. Treatment by removing local irritants, in addition to systemic corticosteroid therapy, is effective.

Childhood Diseases. Certain childhood diseases present specific alterations in the oral cavity. Among these are the communicable diseases. In *measles (rubeola),* Koplik's spots are pathognomonic and are found in 97 per cent of patients. These are seen 2 to 3 days before the rash appears. They occur most often on the buccal mucosa opposite the first molars or on the inner aspect of the lower lip, and appear as bluish white specks—pinpoint in size—surrounded by a bright red areola. They are best seen in daylight. At first only a few are present, but later they become numerous and coalesce. In addition to these specific lesions, measles may also be accompanied by erythema and edema of the gingiva and remainder of the oral mucosa, and by discrete bluish red discolored areas on the soft palate. In *chickenpox (varicella),* papillary eruptions and vesicles appear on the buccal mucosa. These rupture to form small ulcers (p. 432). Comparable but more extensive lesions are seen in *smallpox (variola)* (p. 430). Diffuse gray-red discoloration of the oral mucosa occurs in *scarlet fever* with the so-called "strawberry tongue" formed by a coated surface covering and underlying bright red discoloration with prominent papillae. In *diphtheria,* a gray, friable pseudomembrane is formed in the pharynx, which is usually accompanied by diffuse erythema of the oral mucosa.

Gingival disease, notably gingivitis and cyanosis of the mucous membrane and other oral symptoms, has been described in children with congenital heart disease (Kaner et al., 1946). These changes mirror the systemic cyanosis and tissue anoxia with increased vulnerability to infection.

Aging and the Cumulative Effects of Oral Disease. With time, chronic disease can produce many oral changes, and it is difficult to determine how much physiologic aging contributes to the total picture. Some contend that gingival recession, attrition and reduction in bone height in the aged result more from disease and factors in the oral environment than from physiologic aging. Although gingival recession, attrition and bone loss commonly occur with age, they are not present in all patients and vary considerably in the same age group.

In the aged, bone loss, pathologic migration of the teeth and loss of vertical dimension may be the results of periodontal disease and failure to replace missing teeth. In a study by Roper et al. (1972), age showed nonsignificant correlations with the presence of gingivitis and recession, the amount of accumulated debris and calculus and the depth of periodontal pockets.

Leukoplakia of the oral mucosa and staining of the teeth are common in aged individuals who are inveterate smokers. Wearing artificial dentures for years without rebasing, with a resultant reduction in vertical dimension, is a common cause of angular cheilosis in the aged.

Nutritional Disturbances. The effects of nutritional disturbances, either deficiencies or excesses, upon the developing and adult oral tissues have been extensively documented by animal experimentation and clinical studies (Schour and Massler, 1945; Spies, 1955). However, the evidence presents serious limitations of which one must be cognizant. The animal experiments deal for the most part with severe and sudden deprivation of nutrients which introduces the possibility of "stress" with hormonal changes which could effect tissue changes. Clinical studies in humans are hampered by such problems as the difficulty of assessing the harmful effects of local factors and determining the nature, duration and severity of the nutritional disturbances, or the extent to which the oral manifestations may be the result of coexistent systemic disturbances. Despite these limitations, there is little room for doubt that nutritional disturbances affect the development and maintenance of the oral tissues as well as their response to local environmental factors. The effects of deficiencies or excesses of specific nutrients upon developing teeth are reported in an excellent review referred to previously (Schour and Massler, 1945).

Attention has been directed to a relatively unexplored aspect of nutrition, namely, its effect upon the oral microorganisms. By its effect upon the oral bacteria, the composition of the diet may influence the relative distribution of types of organisms, their metabolic activity and their pathogenic potential, which in turn affect the occurrence and severity of oral disease. Loesche and Gibbons (1966) present an excellent analysis of this subject.

Specific changes in the oral mucosa are identified with deficiencies of the different components of *vitamin B complex* but, as a rule, more than one component is involved in deficiency disease (p. 497). Atrophic glossitis, angular cheilosis and gingivostomatitis occur in riboflavin deficiency (Fig. 20–23). Angular cheilosis is also produced by deficiency of *pyridoxine, nicotinic acid or calcium pantothenate.* Atrophic changes throughout the oral mucosa and angular cheilosis have also been identified with iron deficiency anemia. Reduction in the vertical dimension of the face from tooth loss or improperly constructed dentures results in a similar condition described as "pseudocheilosis."

In *nicotinic acid deficiency,* the tongue is "beefy red," glazed, painful, with "burning" (glossopyrosis) and atrophy of the fungiform and filiform papillae. Necrotizing inflammation of the gingiva has also been attributed to aniacinosis. Microscopic study of atrophic tongues caused by nutritional deficiencies in-

dicates an absence of the normal papillary projections in the epithelium and no evidence of normal keratinization or filiform papillae (Stein and Gold, 1955).

The presence of gingivitis and "bleeding gums" is popularly presumed to be indicative of *vitamin C deficiency.* In animals, acute vitamin C deficiency results in deficient formation of collagen, edema and microscopic hemorrhages in the gingiva and periodontal membrane, and osteoporosis of alveolar bone. However, vitamin C deficiency does not of itself cause gingivitis or bleeding gums in humans or animals. Nor will inflammation of the gingiva occur in vitamin C deficiency in the absence of local irritation. In *vitamin K deficiency,* gingival bleeding is the most common oral manifestation. It may cause excessive gingival bleeding after toothbrushing or chewing hard foods. Prothrombin levels below 20 per cent of normal are frequently accompanied by spontaneous bleeding from the gingival margins (Dreizen, 1971). Atrophy of the epithelium of the tongue and osteoporosis of the jaws have been described in animals with *protein deficiency.*

Pigmentations and Discolorations. There are many conditions in which change in the color of the oral mucous membrane is a prominent finding. Physiologic pigmentation *(melanosis)* of the oral mucosa occurs in blacks and many of the white groups. It represents an increased number of melanoblasts normally present in the basal layer of the epithelium in all individuals except albinos, regardless of whether the oral mucous membrane presents clinically detectable pigmentation. Melanotic patches also occur in the oral mucosa in hereditary intestinal multiple polyposis (Peutz-Jeghers syndrome).

Changes in the oral tissues may be caused by intoxication from metals, such as bismuth, silver, arsenic, mercury and lead, through industrial contact or ingestion in medicaments. This is different from tattooing produced by the accidental embedding of amalgam or other metal fragments.

Metallic intoxication results in ulceration of the mucous membrane and necrosis of the alveolar bone. Spotty discoloration of the oral mucosa and linear pigmentation of the marginal gingiva are prominent features. The latter has been referred to as a "bismuth" or "arsenic line" (black) (Fig. 20–24), "burtonian" or "lead line" (blue-gray) or "mercury line" (gray-violet). Silver (argyria) results in a violet marginal line, often accompanied by a diffuse bluish gray discoloration throughout the oral mucosa. The pigmentation along the inner aspect of

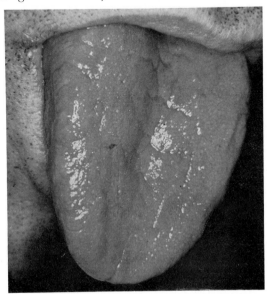

Figure 20–23. *Riboflavin deficiency with atrophic glossitis and angular cheilosis.*

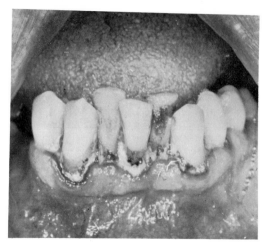

Figure 20–24. *Pigmentation of the gingiva caused by bismuth.*

the lips, the tongue, the cheek and the gingiva occurs only in areas subjected to local irritation or trauma. The pigmentation is caused by the deposition of metallic sulfides in the connective tissue. The increased capillary permeability in areas of inflammation permits perivascular infiltration of the tissues by the metal.

If inflammation is present, pigmentation occurs when the quantity of metal absorbed is insufficient to produce drug intoxication. All pigmentation disappears upon removal of local irritants or trauma responsible for the inflammation, even if contact with, or ingestion of, the metal is continued. Ulceration of the oral mucosa and necrosis of alveolar bone result from intoxication with other chemicals, such as benzine and phosphorus.

Other systemic conditions which may be accompanied by pigmentation of the oral mucosa are Addison's disease (brown or black patches in areas of local irritation); hemochromatosis (diffuse bronze discoloration); and the xanthomatous diseases (diffuse yellowish gray discoloration).

Hairy tongue is a brownish, elevated, mat-like discoloration of the dorsum of the tongue, usually in the posterior portion. Microscopically, it is formed by a dense accumulation of hypertrophied filiform papillae with a keratinized core and a brush-like bacteria-laden tuft. The etiology of hairy tongue is unknown. Debilitating systemic disease is considered a predisposing factor with infection secondary. Hairy tongue sometimes occurs following the oral use of oxidizing drugs.

Antibiotics may produce bluish black patches on the dorsum of the tongue. For an excellent review of oromucosal pigmentation, see Dummett and Barens (1971).

In *amyloidosis*, the color of the oral mucous membrane is not changed, but amyloid may be detected microscopically in the gingiva in 78 per cent of the cases. The amyloid is deposited extracellularly adjacent to the capillaries and appears as islands of hyalinized material which stain metachromatically with crystal violet (Meyer, 1950).

Total Body Radiation. Changes in the oral and pharyngeal mucosa have been described in individuals subjected to total body gamma ionizing radiation in the atomic detonations in Hiroshima and Nagasaki (Bernier, 1949). Hemorrhagic and necrotizing gingivitis with pseudomembrane formation, tonsillitis and pharyngitis occurred in some patients receiving lethal and sublethal dosages. The oral and pharyngeal lesions were attributed to leukopenia followed by local infection.

The microscopic changes in the oral mucosa were similar to those elsewhere in the gastrointestinal tract and included vacuolization of the epithelial cells, shrinkage of the nuclei, abnormal distribution of normally present melanin, almost complete absence of normal mitotic activity in the basal layer and extensive patches of necrosis in the stratum corneum. There were no changes in the collagen of the connective tissue, but there was perivascular infiltration of mononuclear cells in the papillary layer. Patchy necrosis of the tonsillar epithelium and eradication of the lymphoid elements were striking findings.

Gingival ulceration, bleeding, suppuration, periodontitis, denudation of roots and bone, and loosening and loss of teeth have been noted following treatment with external and internal radiation in patients with malignancies of the oral cavity and adjacent regions. Periodontal disease is a possible portal of entry for infection and the development of osteoradionecrosis following radiation therapy. For a complete review of the effects of radiation on the oral tissues, reference should be made to Rubin and Casarett (1968).

INFECTIONS OF THE ORAL MUCOUS MEMBRANE

Acute Herpetic Gingivostomatitis. Acute herpetic gingivostomatitis is an infection of the oral cavity caused by the herpes simplex virus (p. 433). It occurs most frequently in children and appears as a diffuse erythema of the gingiva and remainder of the oral mucous membrane. In its early stage, it is characterized by the presence of discrete, spherical, gray vesicles which may occur on the gingiva, labial and buccal mucosa, soft palate, pharynx, sublingual mucosa and tongue. After approximately 24 hours, the vesicles rupture and form small ulcers with a red, elevated, halo-like margin and yellow-gray central portion. The disease is accompanied by generalized "soreness" of the oral cavity. The ruptured vesicles are the focal sites of pain, and are particularly sensitive to touch, thermal changes and condiments. Cervical adenitis, fever and generalized malaise are common. The course of the disease is limited to 7 to 12 days.

Moniliasis (Thrush). Acute infection of the oral cavity with *Candida albicans* is the most common of the oral fungus diseases. Moniliasis is essentially a disease of infancy, although adults, particularly those who are debilitated or diabetic, may be affected (p. 448). In infants, epidemics may occur in nurseries from contaminated nipples, articles of clothing and bedding. There is also a significantly higher incidence in children born of mothers with monilial vaginitis. Moniliasis of the oral cavity is seen in immunosuppressed adults and in those on steroids over a long period. Usually these individuals were previously suffering from malnourishment or some debilitating illness. Moniliasis of oral mucosa as a result of antibiotic therapy alone is uncommon (Shklar, 1971).

Acute moniliasis produces multiple, white, adherent, curd-like patches irregularly distributed on the oral mucosa (Fig. 20–25). Removal of the patches exposes a raw bleeding surface. Inflammation and fissuring of the labial commissures and encrustations on the lip frequently accompany the intraoral lesions. When cultured, material from the lesion produces typical colonies of the fungus. Clinically,

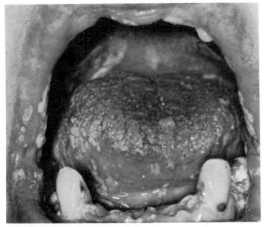

Figure 20–25. *Acute moniliasis with multiple, adherent, curd-like patches.*

thrush may simulate diphtheria, macerated epithelium of the buccal mucosa from chronic irritation (biting habit), leukoplakia and possibly lichen planus. These conditions are readily ruled out by laboratory procedures.

Chronic moniliasis is a rare type of *Candida albicans* infection resulting in a granulomatous lesion which begins in infancy or early childhood and may persist for several years. As the disease progresses, not only the oral mucosa is involved, but often the nails and the skin of the face and scalp are affected. Monilial granuloma manifests itself by a deep inflammatory reaction with the production of granulation tissue. Ultimate involvement of the lungs with multiple abscesses, often associated with kidney lesions, results in the death of the patient in a high percentage of cases.

Tuberculosis. Tuberculosis of the oral cavity is not common. It occurs secondary to pulmonary involvement; primary tuberculous oral lesions are extremely rare. The lesions appear as ulcerations on the tongue, gingiva or buccal mucosa. The lesions frequently start as small nodules representing multiple tubercles, set in a reddened surrounding area, which undergo ulceration. The ulcerations join to form a large patchy lesion with an irregular outline and covered by a grayish white slough. The lesions are characterized by considerable pain, and marked sialorrhea is generally present. Bacterial smears stained by the Ziehl-Neelsen method may show the acid-fast bacillus. This finding is not a consistent one. However, the characteristic granulomatous inflammatory picture is revealed by biopsy.

Actinomycosis. Actinomycosis is caused by the actinomycetes, microorganisms normally found in the oral flora. Approximately 90 per cent of all cases of actinomycosis are of the cervicofacial type and a large percentage of these follow tooth extraction (Rud, 1967). Invasion of the jaws leads to osteomyelitis. The tongue is occasionally the primary site of the disease. It starts as a deep-seated, painless nodule which grows slowly and eventually breaks through the mucosa discharging a yellowish purulent material. (For further details, refer to Chapter 10.)

Syphilis. Syphilis produces a variety of oral mucous membrane changes. Chancres occur on the lips and intraorally in the primary stage. The secondary stage is characterized by mucous patches and, less frequently, by macular lesions on the tongue. In tertiary syphilis, gummas may occur on the hard and soft palates and the tongue. Scar tissue formed in the healing of the gummatous lesions of the tongue produces a lobulated appearance (lingua lobulata). Interstitial glossitis (bald tongue) is more commonly identified with tertiary syphilis. The tongue is sclerosed, fibrosis replaces the musculature, and the surface is smooth and atrophic. Leukoplakia is a common secondary feature (p. 1398). Because the leukoplakic lesions may undergo malignant change, the incidence of carcinoma of the tongue in patients with syphilitic glossitis is high.

Noma (Cancrum Oris). Noma is a rare acute gangrenous disease which starts in the oral mucous membrane and penetrates rapidly into the underlying tissues and perforates the skin on the face (Fig. 20–26). Discoloration and sloughing of tissue, exfoliation of teeth and destruction of alveolar bone occur as the process progresses. Noma occurs more often in children than adults and, in all instances, is preceded by debilitating systemic disease. Microscopically, it appears as a nonspecific massive necrosis with remarkably sparse inflammatory reaction. It is initiated by anaerobic bacteria, among which are found fusospirochetal organisms, and terminates fatally.

Other, infrequently encountered, infections in the oral cavity include *histoplasmosis, herpes zoster molluscum contagiosum, verruca vulgaris, lymphogranuloma venereum, epizootic stomatitis (foot and mouth disease) and herpangina.*

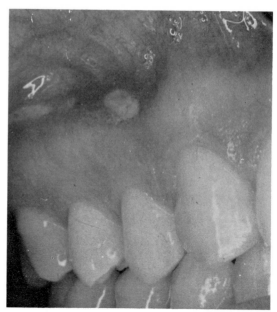

Figure 20–27. *Aphthous stomatitis showing typical ulcer with elevated margin.*

Aphthous Stomatitis (Canker Sore). Aphthous stomatitis, a common lesion of the oral cavity, is characterized by the appearance of depressed spherical ulcers. The ulcers consist of a saucer-like central portion which is red or grayish red with an elevated rim-like margin (Fig. 20–27). There is some question whether vesicle formation precedes the appearance of these ulcers and, in fact, forms the ulceration by rupture of the initial vesicle. The lesions may occur anywhere in the oral cavity, with the mucobuccal fold and the floor of the mouth common sites. Aphthous stomatitis is a painful condition characterized by single or multiple lesions. The duration of each lesion is usually 7 to 10 days. Aphthae may occur as occasional lesions at intervals which vary from months to years or may occur in acute episodes associated with gastrointestinal disturbances. Chronic recurrent aphthae is a perplexing condition in which one or more lesions in various stages are always present and the duration of involvement may extend over a period of years. The etiology of aphthous stomatitis is not known.

Herpes simplex virus was suspected of being the cause, but antibody and tissue culture studies discourage this opinion. Other factors suggested as causing or predisposing to aphthous stomatitis include psychosomatic, hormonal, allergic, hereditary, microbial, autoimmune and gastrointestinal disorders.

Aphthous stomatitis is a different clinical entity from acute herpetic gingivostomatitis. The ulcerations may appear the same in both

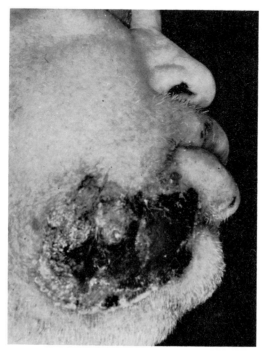

Figure 20–26. *Necrosis and discoloration of the face in noma.*

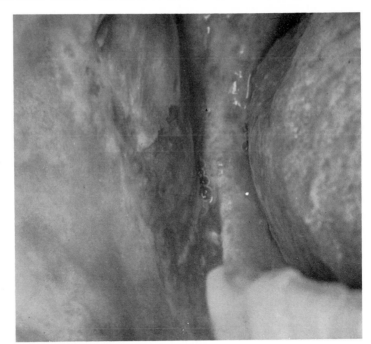

Figure 20–28. Lichen planus of the oral mucosa showing characteristic punctate and dendritic appearance.

conditions, but diffuse erythematous involvement of the gingiva and acute toxic systemic symptoms do not occur in aphthous stomatitis.

DERMATOLOGIC DISEASE

Manifestations of dermatologic disease frequently occur in the oral cavity (Figs. 20–28 and 20–29). Oral and skin lesions may occur together but occasionally the oral changes precede the skin lesions by several months or years. In cases of lichen planus, erythema multiforme and pyostomatitis vegetans, sometimes oral lesions are the only signs of the disease. For a detailed description of the clinical and microscopic features of the oral manifestations

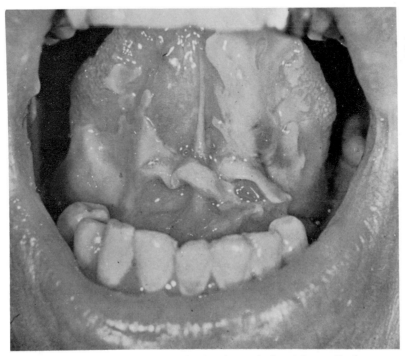

Figure 20–29. Pemphigus vulgaris showing typical vesicles on the tongue.

of the various dermatologic diseases, as well as their differential diagnosis and treatment, the reader is referred to the concise presentation in Glickman (1972).

Leukoplakia. Leukoplakia is a common and important oral condition. The term "leukoplakia" (white plaque) is a clinical one, descriptive of the whitish appearance produced by hyperkeratosis of the epithelium (Turesky et al., 1961). The significance of leukoplakia lies in the fact that, in some cases, it provides a favorable soil for the development of epidermoid carcinoma. The benign lesions cannot be differentiated from those undergoing malignant transformation except by microscopic examination.

Microscopically, leukoplakic areas present a thickening of the stratified squamous epithelium with varied degrees of hyperkeratosis. There may also be hyperplasia of the epithelium with extensions of rete pegs into the underlying connective tissue, which is usually inflamed (Fig. 20–30). Degeneration of epithelial cells in the basal layers results from infiltration by the inflammatory fluid and cellular exudate. Differentiation between benign lesions and those undergoing malignant change is based upon the presence of anaplastic changes in the epithelium.

Any area of the oral mucosa or lip may be affected. Common locations are the buccal mucosa in the third molar area and at the line of occlusion, the dorsal and ventral surfaces of the tongue and the palate. In the early stages the condition appears as grayish white, parchment-like streaks or irregularly shaped patches which are often bilateral. On the dorsum of the tongue, it may present diffuse involvement. Persistent lesions become thickened and hardened, usually with surface subdivisions which have a cobblestone appearance. Some lesions undergo fissuring and verrucous enlargement.

Leukoplakia occurs more often in males than females in a ratio of 9 to 1. Local irritation from rough tooth margins, trauma to the oral mucous membrane during chewing and thermal irritation from tobacco are believed to be causative local factors. Aside from the fact that leukoplakia frequently accompanies atrophy of the tongue in syphilis, its occurrence is not related to any other systemic disease. Differentiation from lichen planus is often a clinical problem. Biopsy is essential in the diagnosis of leukoplakia, particularly for the detection of malignant changes.

Smoker's Palate (Stomatitis Nicotina). This is a combination of leukoplakia of the palate and inflammation of the orifices of the mucous glands. The leukoplakia appears initially as a diffuse grayish overtone which may be slightly rippled or become hardened and leathery. Reddened, slightly elevated orifices

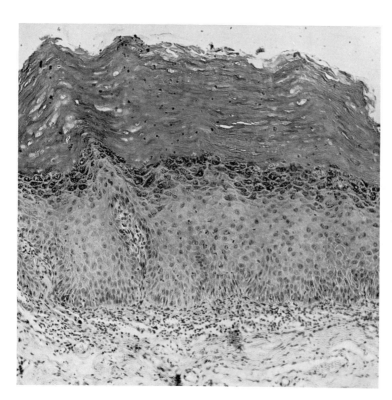

Figure 20–30. Leukoplakia showing thickening of the epithelium with prominent granular layer, pronounced hyperkeratosis and slight inflammation in the underlying connective tissue.

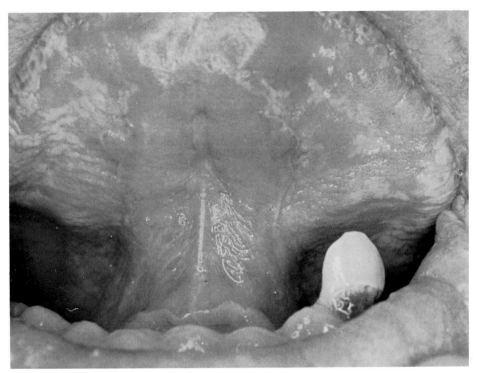

Figure 20–31. *White sponge nevus (white folded gingivostomatitis) showing diffuse involvement of the tongue and lips with minute surface folds.*

of the mucous glands protrude from the surface. Closure of mucous gland orifices leads to the formation of cysts.

White Sponge Nevus (White Folded Gingivostomatitis).
This is a benign, painless familial condition which may be present at birth or appear during childhood. It occurs in the oral cavity in males and females, with rectal and/or vaginal involvement. The surface of the oral mucosa is white, thickened and in minute folds with papillary projections (Fig. 20–31). Involvement may be patchy or generalized.

Microscopically, the epithelium is thickened and parakeratotic with vacuolization of cells and pyknotic nuclei. There is moderate plasma cell and lymphocytic infiltration of the underlying connective tissue.

TUMORS AND TUMOR-LIKE LESIONS OF THE MUCOUS MEMBRANE

Gingival Enlargement. Gingival enlargement is a common form of oral disease. It may be localized in relation to a single tooth or group of teeth or generalized throughout the mouth. As the gingiva increases in size, it covers portions of the crowns of the involved teeth and may interfere with chewing. When localized, it appears as a discrete tumor-like mass (Fig. 20–32). Microscopic study indicates that a variety of etiologic factors and pathologic processes may result in increase in the size of the gingiva. Gingival enlargement is therefore classified into the following groups based upon etiology and histopathology (Glickman, 1950): (1) inflammatory, (2) noninflammatory hyperplastic, (3) combined hyperplastic and inflammatory, (4) conditioned and (5) neoplastic.

Inflammatory gingival enlargement may result from chronic or acute inflammatory changes. The former is by far the more common cause. In chronic gingival enlargement, the increase in size results from fluid and cellular exudate new capillary formation and the proliferation of connective tissue and epithelium associated with the inflammation. Treatment consists of excision coupled with elimination of the responsible local irritants. Acute inflammatory enlargement is a painful, rapidly expanding lesion, which results from a localized acute suppurative process.

Noninflammatory gingival hyperplasia is most often seen in epileptic patients receiving diphenylhydantoin sodium (Dilantin) therapy (Glickman and Lewitus, 1941). It does not occur in every case. The reported incidence varies from 3 per cent to 62 per cent with the greater frequencies in younger patients. Its occurrence and severity are not necessarily re-

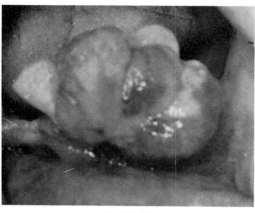

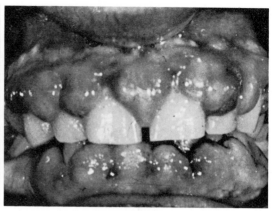

Fig. 20–32   **Fig. 20–33**

Figure 20–32. *Discrete tumor-like enlargement of the gingiva produced by chronic inflammatory response to local irritation.*

Figure 20–33. *Bulbous nodular enlargement of the gingiva resulting from hyperplasia in epileptic patient receiving Dilantin therapy.*

lated to the dosage or duration of drug therapy. The enlarged gingiva is mulberry-shaped, coral pink and firm with a minutely lobulated surface, painless, usually generalized throughout the mouth, and tends to be more severe in relation to the anterior teeth (Fig. 20–33). It does not occur in edentulous areas. The enlargement is produced by a hyperplasia of the epithelium with acanthosis and extension of rete pegs deep into the underlying connective tissue. The connective tissue is densely collagenous with numerous spherical or polyhedral fibroblasts and new blood vessels. Inflammatory involvement near the gingival surface adjacent to the teeth is a common finding. Removal of the enlarged gingiva is followed by recurrence as long as the drug therapy is continued. Spontaneous disappearance occurs within a month after the drug is discontinued.

Noninflammatory gingival hyperplasia also occurs under other circumstances. It is termed *"fibromatosis gingivae"* or "elephantiasis gingivae" and is extremely uncommon. The etiology is unknown, but hereditary, nutritional or hormonal causation has been suggested.

Combined gingival enlargement results when non-inflammatory gingival hyperplasia is complicated by locally induced inflammatory changes.

Conditioned gingival enlargement results when the systemic condition of the patient is such as to distort or exaggerate the usual gingival response to local irritation. Local irritation is necessary for the initiation of this type of enlargement. The systemic condition participates in determining the microscopic and clinical features. This type of gingival enlargement occurs in pregnancy, puberty, acute vitamin C deficiency and leukemia.

The *"pregnancy tumor"* occurs after the third month of pregnancy. The reported prevalence varies from 10 to 70 per cent. It appears as a bright red or dusky blue, mushroom-like mass on the gingiva which extrudes from between the teeth (Fig. 20–34). The surface is smooth and may present punctate red markings with ulceration at the base in some instances. The "pregnancy tumor" is not a neoplasm. It is a chronic inflammatory response to local irritation. The microscopic picture is consistent with a diagnosis of angiogranuloma. It consists of edematous chronic granulation tissue with a notable predominance of newly formed dilated capillaries (Fig. 20–35). The surface epithelium presents varying degrees of edema and degeneration and occasional areas of ulceration.

These lesions are painless unless they are secondarily infected. They may attain sufficient size to interfere with the occlusion and become traumatized. If it becomes necessary to remove them during pregnancy, the responsible local irritant must also be removed or else the lesion will recur. After delivery, the enlargement undergoes spontaneous reduction in size. Conditioned gingival enlargement also may occur during *puberty* in males and females. It represents an exaggerated chronic inflammatory response to local irritation.

Scorbutic gingival enlargement, considered a classic clinical sign of vitamin C deficiency, is not caused by the deficiency itself. It results from the conditioning effect of the deficiency upon the response of the gingiva to local irrita-

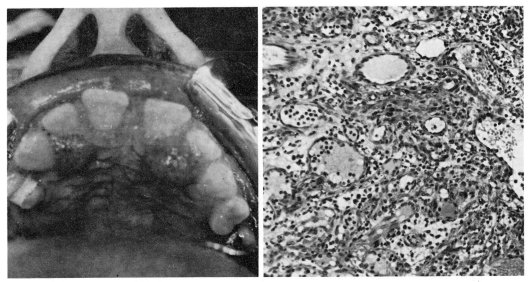

Fig. 20–34   Fig. 20–35

Figure 20–34. *Enlargement of the gingiva in pregnancy. Note discrete mushroom-like lesions on the palatal surface.*
Figure 20–35. *Biopsy of lesion shown in Figure 20–34, showing markedly vascular inflamed granulation tissue.*

tion. *Diminished fibroblastic activity caused by vitamin C deficiency inhibits the normal fibrosis whereby inflammation is ordinarily delimited.* Massive spongy gingival enlargement results from the spread of inflammation, which is complicated by the hemorrhages induced by the deficiency (Fig. 20–36). Enlargement of the gingiva does not occur in scurvy in the absence of local irritation.

Granuloma pyogenicum is another type of conditioned gingival enlargement, but the nature of the systemic conditioning factor has not been established. The clinical and microscopic features are similar to those of gingival enlargement seen in pregnancy except that the majority of the cases present surface ulceration and purulent exudation. The lesions tend to become fibroepithelial papillomas or may per-

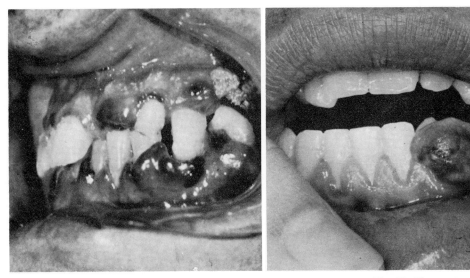

Fig. 20–36   Fig. 20–37

Figure 20–36. *Enlarged gingiva in acute vitamin C deficiency, showing numerous hemorrhagic areas.*
Figure 20–37. *Peripheral giant cell granuloma on the gingiva. Comparison with lesion shown in Figure 20–32. indicates importance of biopsy for definitive diagnosis.*

sist relatively unchanged for years. Treatment consists of removal of the lesion plus the irritating local factors.

The clinical and microscopic features of *leukemic gingival enlargement* were described in a previous section of this chapter.

Epulis. Epulis is the generic term to designate tumors and tumor-like masses located on the gingiva. Neoplasms of the gingiva account for only 8 per cent of all oral tumors and include fibroma, "giant cell epulis," papilloma, hemangioma, carcinoma and, far less frequently, the cellular nevus, myoblastoma, melanoma, fibrosarcoma, lymphosarcoma and reticulum cell sarcoma. Of these, the "giant cell epulis" is the only lesion which occurs only on the gingiva or, in isolated cases, on the mucous membrane covering edentulous ridges.

Giant cell lesions occur on the gingiva as sessile or pedunculated masses protruding from the gingival margin and are referred to as "giant cell epulis" or "peripheral reparative giant cell granuloma." They affect the mandible more than the maxilla, usually appear after age 20 and are often associated with trauma. The lesions are not clinically aggressive or invasive (Bhaskar et al., 1971) and should be distinguished from true neoplastic giant cell tumors.

The lesions vary in appearance from a smooth, spherical mass to an irregularly shaped, multilobulated protuberance with increased firmness (Fig. 20–37). Ulceration of the margin is occasionally seen. The lesions vary in size and, in some instances, may cover several teeth. The consistency may be firm or sponge-like and present gradations in color from pink to deep red or purplish blue, depending upon the degree of vascularity and inflammatory infiltration. Occasionally, the lesions extend into the underlying alveolar bone, resulting in radiographically detectable bone destruction.

With few exceptions, giant cell lesions in the gingiva are giant cell reparative granulomas in response to local injury rather than true neoplasms. The microscopic appearance is essentially the same as that of the giant cell reparative granuloma when it occurs as a central lesion in the jaws (see p. 1444). Surgical removal and curettage of the contiguous structures are followed by uneventful healing.

Benign Oral Mucous Membrane Tumors. *Fibromas* occur usually on the inner surface of the cheeks or lips or on the gingiva or tongue. Unless their size and location are such that they are subjected to trauma, they are covered by intact oral mucous membrane. The lesions usually have the same microscopic appearance

as in their other sites of origin. A variety of other benign neoplasms occur in the oral mucous membrane similar to those arising in other soft tissues.

Uncommon but extremely interesting lesions are the myoblastoma and "congenital epulis." The *myoblastoma* is a benign, slowly growing tumor which occurs at all ages and is seen most often in males. The myoblastoma is not a common oral tumor but is of interest from the standpoint of its histogenesis and morphology discussed in Chapter 31. It occurs most frequently in the tongue and less often in the cheek, lips and alveolar ridge, as a small spherical mass which produces a slightly rounded elevation of the overlying mucosal surface (Fig. 20–38).

The *"congenital epulis"* occurs in the newborn as a soft, spherical, pedunculated mass attached more often to the mucosa of the maxilla than to the mandible.

Microscopically, the tumor resembles the myoblastoma in that it consists of sheets of large polyhedral cells with lightly staining granular cytoplasm and spherical nuclei, which may be eccentrically placed. In addition, it presents groups of cells in apparent transition from a spindle type to the larger polyhedral form. A scattering of discrete masses of epithelium which appear to be odontogenic in origin is also seen.

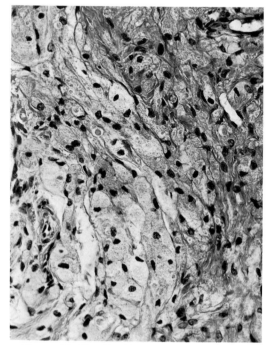

Figure 20–38. *Myoblastoma of the tongue, showing typical nested arrangement of large cells with granular cytoplasm.*

The congenital epulis is a benign but not encapsulated tumor. Opinions differ as to whether it is derived as an embryonic hamartoma of the tooth bud, or from fibroblasts of the oral mucosa or dental follicle, or from peri- and endoneurium and should therefore be considered a granular cell fibroblastoma or neurofibroma (Bauer and Bauer, 1953).

Papillomas appear as hard, wart-like, painless projections from the oral mucosa. *Hemangiomas,* capillary or cavernous, may occur anywhere in the oral cavity, particularly in the tongue, lips and gingiva (Fig. 20–39). A flat, irregularly outlined, congenital form of cavernous hemangioma (vascular nevus) may occur on the oral mucosa with or without contiguous involvement of the face. *Lymphangiomas* occur less frequently than hemangiomas. Common locations are the tongue and lips where they produce macroglossia and macrocheilia. Tumors of salivary gland origin also may occur in the oral mucous membrane. (For a detailed description of these tumors, see p. 895).

Malignant Mucous Membrane Tumors.

Oral malignancies in the U.S. comprise in the neighborhood of 7 per cent of all malignant tumors and annually cause approximately 10,000 deaths (Hinds and Kent, 1971). India leads the world with the highest rate of oral cancer, where it comprises 30 to 50 per cent of all cancers. This remarkable frequency is attributed in some way to the custom of chewing betel nuts. Oral cancer is the leading cause of cancer death in that country (Mehta et al., 1971).

Approximately 90 per cent of the oral malignancies are squamous cell carcinomas. These have many clinical factors common to most malignant tumors but their location in the oral cavity has an important bearing upon the progress and prognosis of individual lesions. Within the oral cavity, about one-half of the lesions occur somewhere in the tongue. The locations of the remaining 50 per cent are roughly equally divided between the palate, floor of the mouth, the gingiva and the buccal mucosa (Bernier, 1972).

Irritation from the jagged edges of carious teeth, ill-fitting prosthetic appliances, chemical and thermal stimulation from tobacco, alcohol and trauma are so common in the oral region that there has been much conjecture regarding their importance in the causation of oral malignancy. Chronic irritation hastens the onset of clinically induced malignancy in experimental animals (Renstrup et al., 1962).

The differential diagnosis of oral lesions must consider the many other conditions that produce lesions which arouse suspicion of malignancy. These include traumatic ulcers, tuberculosis, leukoplakia, syphilis, aphthous stomatitis and many of the benign neoplasms. A simple exfoliative cytology technique is available for preliminary screening of oral lesions (Sandler, 1962), but biopsy is required for definitive diagnosis.

It is important to note that early growth of malignant oral lesions may be entirely symptom-free until secondarily involved by inflammation. Lesions in mobile areas such as the anterior portion of the tongue, the floor of

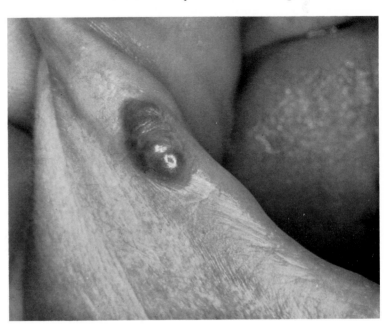

Figure 20–39. *Hemangioma of the lip.*

the mouth or the cheek are more likely to be painful earlier in the disease.

Oral carcinoma follows the same patterns of growth in the mouth as in its other sites of mucosal occurrence. It starts as a small indurated plaque, nodule or ulcer which may become fissured and necrotic on the surface. As it increases in size, it may project as a large cauliflower-like mass into the oral cavity, pushing aside normal structures and interfering with speech and chewing; or it may appear as an extensive ulcerated crater, destroying the soft tissues and bone of the jaws and causing the loss of teeth in the involved areas (Figs. 20-40 and 20-41). In severe cases, the destructive lesion penetrates through to the face, producing disfiguring defects.

As the tumor extends from the oral cavity into the deeper structures, swallowing is difficult and accumulation of saliva results. The lumen of the pharynx may become narrowed, leading to dysphagia. Erosion of blood vessels causes hemorrhage. Pain results when cervical nerve roots are affected; unilateral paralysis of the tongue may result from involvement of the hypoglossal nerve; hoarseness may result from interference with the vagus nerve. Death results from sepsis, malnutrition, dehydration, pain, hemorrhage, respiratory obstruction and metastasis.

In its early stage, oral carcinoma may not metastasize, but regional lymph node involvement invariably occurs as the disease progresses. Metastasis is generally unilateral, except in the case of lesions near the midline which tend to metastasize bilaterally. Ackerman and Regato (1947) present a detailed description of the pathways of lymph node metastasis from carcinomas in different locations in the oral region. Lymph nodes of the submaxillary, submental, cervical, preauricular and postauricular, infraparotid, jugular and subdigastric regions may be affected, depending upon the site of the initial lesion. As a general rule, metastases from oral carcinomas are confined to the region above the clavicle. In uncontrolled carcinoma, cervical metastasis is often followed by metastases to the lungs, liver or bone.

The oral cavity is occasionally the site of multiple primary carcinomas. These occur independently in different locations either simultaneously or at different times. Patients with oral carcinoma may also exhibit a tendency toward multicentric malignancies in the contiguous mucosa of the pharynx, larynx or esophagus.

Carcinoma of the lower lip is the most common site of malignancy in the oral region (including, of course, the oral cavity). These cancers occur predominantly in males (95 per cent) (McCarthy and Shklar, 1964). Females having carcinoma of the lower lip are likely to be predisposed by the

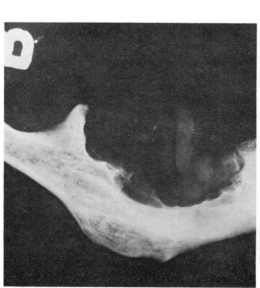

Fig. 20-40

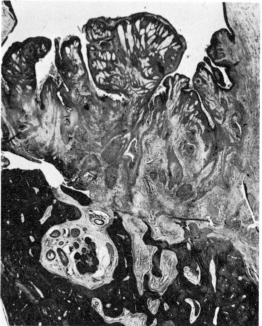

Fig. 20-41

Figure 20-40. Extensive destruction of the mandible resulting from invasion by epidermoid carcinoma from the oral mucosa.

Figure 20-41. Cauliflower-like epidermoid carcinoma of the oral mucosa which has penetrated into the mandible, producing the radiographic appearance shown in Figure 20-40.

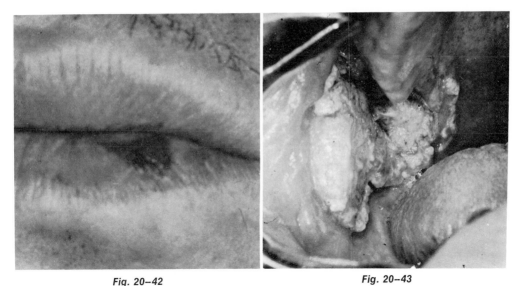

Fig. 20–42   Fig. 20–43

Figure 20–42. Slight persistent encrustation on the lip revealed by microscopic examination to be epidermoid carcinoma.
Figure 20–43. Massive epidermoid carcinoma of the buccal mucosa.

Plummer-Vinson syndrome (p. 000). Blacks are less commonly affected than whites. Leukoplakia is frequently a coexistent finding. It appears in many forms, such as a slight surface encrustation, a papillary mass, an ulcer or a persistent fissure (Fig. 20–42). Any type of lip lesion which persists for two weeks, particularly if it feels firm or button-like when palpated, should be viewed with suspicion. The most frequent site is the exposed vermilion border between the midline and the angle of the lips. Carcinoma of the lower lip shows the least tendency to metastasize of all oral carcinomas and, all other factors being equal, offers the best prognosis. **On the upper lip, malignancy** is comparatively infrequent, but metastasis occurs earlier and is more widespread.

In the **floor of the mouth and the base of the tongue, carcinoma** appears as an elevated indurated ulceration with the major portion of the mass deep in the sublingual and submaxillary areas. Both epidermoid carcinoma and adenocarcinoma occur in this area with otalgia, hypersalivation and speech impairment as common symptoms. In the **buccal mucosa, carcinoma** is frequently preceded by leukoplakia, particularly in the third molar area or intertriginous line. The lesions may appear as cauliflower-like projections from the surface or as ulcerations deep in the cheek (Fig. 20–43). **Carcinoma of the gingiva** occurs on the lower jaw more frequently than on the upper. It extends into the adjacent soft tissues or invades the jaw bone, maxillary sinus or the orbit.

Carcinoma of the tongue occurs most frequently in males in the 50- to 60-year age group. It is second in frequency to carcinoma of the lower lip. Syphilis and leukoplakia are often coexistent findings. The lateral border and ventral surface are more common sites than the tip and dorsal aspects. The lesion usually appears as an indurated mass which infiltrates into the tongue and undergoes surface ulceration. Special mention must be made of localized areas of inflammation on the lateral border of the tongue, apparently from sharp or rough tooth margins, which patients complain of so often. Such areas invariably respond to the elimination of the local irritation. However, the finding of malignancy, often after precious months are lost "waiting for the area to clear up," emphasizes the importance of biopsy whenever the removal of a source of irritation is not followed by prompt return of the tongue to normal. Carcinoma of the tongue tends to metastasize early in its development.

Squamous carcinoma uncommonly occurs on both the **hard and soft palates,** but the glands of the palate are more commonly the site of the malignant salivary gland tumor, the **cylindroma** or **adenocarcinoma.** Malignant tumors on the palate often appear as spherical masses with granular ulcerated surface areas, which distort the contour of the roof of the mouth. Invasive destruction of the palate with involvement of the nasal and paranasal areas is a common feature which complicates the management and darkens the outlook in these cases.

The prognosis of carcinoma in the oral cavity is influenced by the degree of cellular differentiation, the location, the duration and extent of involvement and the presence of metastases. Well differentiated lesions usually grow slowly and are slow to metastasize.

Surgery is the treatment of choice. Anaplastic tumors grow rapidly, metastasize early and are radiosensitive.

Tumors other than the squamous carcinoma account for approximately 10 per cent of the malignancies of the oral mucous membrane. The *adenocarcinoma* may occur anywhere in the oral cavity, but its most frequent locations are the hard and soft palates and the major salivary glands. The *lymphoepithelioma* most often occurs in the nasopharynx but may be found at the base of the tongue. The palate and alveolar mucosa are common locations of the rapidly growing *malignant melanoma* which metastasizes widely through the blood.

Soft tissue fibrosarcoma arises from the periosteum and protrudes into the oral cavity. Invasion of the soft tissues, bone, maxillary sinus and distant metastasis may accompany this tumor. *Neurosarcoma and rhabdomyosarcoma* are extremely rare in the oral cavity. *Lymphosarcoma and reticulum cell sarcoma* are characterized by rapid growth, osteolytic destruction of the adjoining bony structures and widespread metastasis. Although these tumors are uncommon, they do occur in isolated cases in which the initial clinical impression is that of "granulation tissue following extraction" or "Vincent's ulceration" of the palate or nasopharynx.

The *metastasis of tumors* to the oral mucosa is rare.

DISEASES OF THE SALIVARY GLANDS

Congenital anomalies of the salivary glands, such as atresia of the ducts, absence of a gland, aberrant salivary gland tissue or abnormal location of a major salivary gland, are not common. Disturbances in salivary gland function occur more often. Ptyalism or excessive salivary secretion accompanies a variety of conditions, such as metallic poisoning, acute necrotizing gingivitis, various forms of stomatitis, irritation from smoking and psychic stimuli. Decreased salivary secretion or aptyalism is seen in febrile diseases, myxedema, neuropsychiatric disturbances, salivary gland disease, Plummer-Vinson syndrome and pernicious anemia. Xerostomia or "dry mouth" results from decreased salivary secretion and is characterized by a diffuse dryness, erythema and, in extreme cases, fissuring of the oral mucosa, accompanied by a "burning" sensation and glossodynia.

INFLAMMATORY AND OBSTRUCTIVE DISEASE

Inflammatory enlargement of one or more of the salivary glands may occur in a variety of specific and nonspecific infections (Batsakis and McWhirter, 1972). Calculi (sialolithiasis) sometimes form within the ducts of chronically infected salivary glands. Conversely, calculi may form de novo in noninflamed glands and, in turn, predispose to secondary bacterial invasion (Epker, 1972).

The most obvious specific infection of the salivary glands is mumps. No adult needs to be told that painful enlargement, usually affecting the parotid glands, characterizes this viral infection. Occasionally only one side is affected, or the submandibular glands are involved more than the parotids. Infrequently, the salivary glands are infected by the causative agents of actinomycosis, tuberculosis, syphilis, cytomegalic inclusion disease and cat-scratch disease. About 8 per cent of patients with sarcoidosis have involvement of the eye, facial nerve and parotid glands (Heerfordt's syndrome).

Nonspecific bacterial infection and inflammation of the salivary glands (sialadenitis) most often originates in the excretory duct and is caused by invasion of bacteria from the oral cavity or mechanical irritation of the duct followed by infection. It occurs most frequently in the parotid, but other glands may also be affected. Less frequently, inflammation of the salivary gland results from trauma, spread of infection from the oral or tonsillar regions and rarely via the hematogenous route in cases of pyemia and bacteremia.

In acute parotitis there is rapid, painful enlargement of the gland and face, with displacement of the ear lobe and trismus. The ductal orifice is smaller, red and painful, and purulent exudate may be discharged spontaneously or upon digital manipulation. Salivary secretion is interfered with. Locally induced inflammation of the parotid must be differentiated from epidemic parotitis (see p. 436).

Obstruction of the duct by calculi (**sialothiasis**) is a common cause of sialadenitis (Fig. 20–44). The formation of calcified calculi in the salivary gland duct or gland substance occurs in the submaxillary gland far more frequently than the other major glands. In the duct, the calcified calculi assume a cylindrical shape and vary in size. Within the gland substance, the calculi are nodular.

Inflammation of the duct (**sialodochitis**) results in its narrowing and obstruction by exudate, desquamated cells, calculi and mucus. Obstruction,

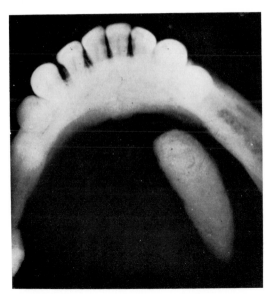

Figure 20–44. *Sialolithiasis. Radiographic appearance of calcified calculus in submaxillary gland duct.*

partial or complete, leads to changes in the glandular tissues and affects their function. The combined inflammatory and functional changes account for the clinical features of sialadenitis. Microscopically there is dilatation of the ducts throughout the gland, associated with retention of saliva. There is infiltration of the connective tissue stroma by leukocytes, which vary according to the acute or chronic nature of the involvement. The acinar appearance varies in different sections of the glands. Some acini are compressed by pressure from the dilated ducts and the inflammation in the connective tissue; others may be dilated and filled with mucus. The secretory cells are distended and may rupture and coalesce. Infiltration by inflammation from the connective stroma often causes necrosis of the glandular epithelium. In chronic involvement, there are areas where only remnants of the glandular epithelium persist in a mass of inflamed fibrotic tissue; and in acute infections, portions of the gland may be destroyed and replaced by focal zones of suppuration.

Chronic infection of the gland generally occurs as a sequel to acute involvement but may also result from persistent low-grade irritation and infection of the duct. With chronic inflammation, the gland is permanently enlarged as a result of the exudate and proliferative changes in the stromal connective tissue. Formation of saliva is interfered with as the result of compression and atrophy of the acini by pressure from the fibrosing stroma. Obstruction of the excretory duct leads to retention of saliva. There may be drainage of purulent or seropurulent exudate from the duct orifice.

SJÖGREN'S SYNDROME

Sjögren's syndrome is a systemic disease of probably autoimmune origin characterized by (1) keratoconjunctivitis sicca (dryness of the eyes with lack of tears), (2) xerostomia (dryness of the mouth), (3) salivary gland enlargement and (4) rheumatoid arthritis. It has been discussed previously in detail on p. 246. Here we should merely note that all of the salivary glands may be enlarged by a diffuse inflammatory reaction marked by dense, lymphocytic and plasma cell infiltration. To a considerable extent, these gland involvements resemble anatomically the changes encountered in the thyroid gland in Hashimoto's thyroiditis. The lymphocytic infiltrate may be accompanied by the formation of lymphoid follicles and may induce partial to complete atrophy of the secretory acini. The replacement of the native architecture may be so complete as to be confused with a leukemic or lymphomatous disorder.

MIKULICZ'S DISEASE (BENIGN LYMPHOEPITHELIAL LESION)

This disorder of unknown etiology causes enlargement of the salivary glands, in particular, the parotids. The glandular enlargement is the result of an extensive replacement of the salivary glands by a dense lymphocytic infiltrate, with atrophy of the acini but preservation of the ducts. Proliferation of the epithelial and myothelial cells of the small ductules creates islands of myoepithelial cells scattered throughout the dense lymphoid background. The anatomic changes are very reminiscent of those in Sjögren's syndrome, suggesting a possible relationship between the two. However, Sjögren's syndrome is systemic in distribution and is accompanied by a variety of immunologic findings and rheumatoid arthritis. None of these findings are present in Mikulicz's disease which is purely a salivary gland disorder.

It is important here to bring up a problem in semantics which has caused considerable confusion in the past. The term Mikulicz's *syndrome* continues to be used to refer to lacrimal and salivary gland enlargement, whatever the cause. Mikulicz s *syndrome*, then, may be encountered in Sjögren's syndrome, sarcoidosis, leukemia and lymphoma, and may also be caused by Mikulicz's *disease* of the salivary glands. For this reason, Mikulicz's *disease* is better referred to as a *benign lymphoepithelial lesion* (Azzopardi and Evans, 1971). From the nature of the morphologic changes, it should be apparent that Mikulicz's disease is easily confused histologically with a malignant lymphoma of the salivary glands. While it is a benign entity, on rare occasion, it has constituted the subsoil for the subsequent development of a malignant lymphoma.

MUCOCELE

Mucocele can best be characterized as a localized collection of extravasated mucus within a minor salivary gland. Its most common location is the lower lip. The cyst appears as a small, bead-like submucosal blister having a bluish tinge. Presumably, they are formed when a duct is ruptured or severed either partially or completely. The mucus extravasates into the surrounding tissue and evokes a scant peripheral inflammatory reaction. Frequently, the mucinous secretion contains distended mucus-laden histiocytes. The ducts distal to the site of injury become distended (Fig. 20–45).

RANULA

Ranula is the term applied to a cyst caused by obstruction of a gland in the floor of the mouth. It presents a smooth rounded prominence with bluish tinge, which elevates the floor of the mouth and pushes the tongue

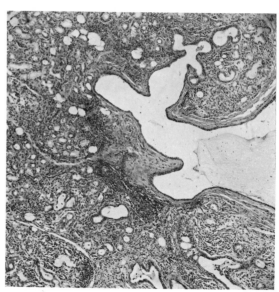

Figure 20–45. *Mucocele with distention of mucus-laden ducts and compression of acini associated with inflammatory infiltration.*

aside (Fig. 20–46). Microscopically, ranula consists of a distended epithelium-lined wall in a thin fibrous capsule with leukocytic infiltration. The contents may be mucous or serous. Surgical treatment is followed by uneventful recovery.

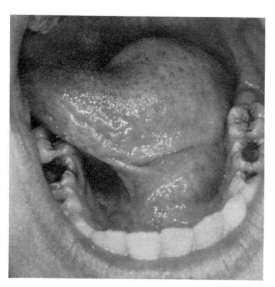

Fig. 20–46

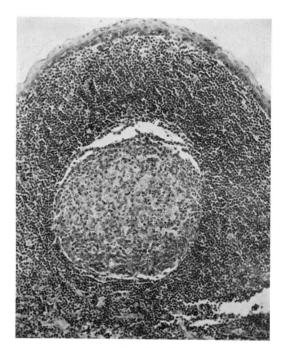

Fig. 20–47

Figure 20–46. *Bulbous elevation of the floor of the mouth and deflection of the tongue caused by ranula.*
Figure 20–47. *Branchial cyst with lymphoid germinal center and surface lining of stratified squamous epithelium.*

DERMOID AND BRANCHIAL CYSTS

Dermoid and branchial cysts are unrelated to the salivary glands but occur in the floor of the mouth and submandibular area and should therefore be presented here. *Dermoid cysts* occur infrequently in the oral region and, when present, are usually situated in the floor of the mouth in the submental region or on either side of the midline more posteriorly. They become apparent later in life between the ages of 15 and 35 but may be seen in young children (see p. 1248 for morphology).

In the embryonic development of the pharyngeal region, the first branchial cleft remains open to the outer surface and the second, third and fourth branchial clefts open into the cervical sinus. The cervical sinus then is closed off from the surface and becomes submerged and the space obliterated. *Branchial cysts* develop from proliferation of the epithelial remnants of the submerged sinus. A *branchial fistula* from the pharynx to the skin develops from the combined circumstances of failure of closure of a branchial cleft which opens into a patent cervical sinus. Branchial fistulas are present at birth and present a draining orifice at the anterior border of the sternomastoid muscle.

Branchial cysts occur as painless swellings in the neck, with the area at the angle of the jaw the favorite location. They appear in all age groups, start as a small spherical mass and extend along the anterior border of the sternomastoid muscle as they enlarge. These cysts are lined with either stratified squamous epithelium or stratified columnar epithelium or a combination of both types (Fig. 20—47). The wall of the cyst is arranged in low papillary projections containing foci of lymphoid tissue with germinal centers in close relation to the epithelial lining. Scattered inflammatory infiltration is a frequent finding in the cyst wall. The cavity is filled with fluid or semifluid material containing cholesterol crystals. Suppuration may be caused by secondary infection of the cyst.

TUMORS OF SALIVARY GLAND ORIGIN

A greater variety of neoplasms arise in the salivary glands than in any other glandular structure of the body. Fortunately, most are quite rare and so our attention can be confined to the more common forms, leaving the rarities to specialized presentations (McFarland, 1936) (Foote and Frazell, 1953) (Bardwil, 1967) (Kauffman and Stout, 1963). The more common lesions and their approximate frequency in the spectrum of salivary gland neoplasms are given in Table 20–1.

Pleomorphic Adenoma (Mixed Tumor). This controversial neoplasm was for many years referred to as a *mixed tumor of salivary gland origin* because it presents a variety of histologic components such as epithelial formations of apparent ectodermal derivation, while other features such as cartilage and myxoid tissue would seem to be derived from mesoderm. Today, the preferred term is *pleomorphic adenoma* since its histogenesis is believed to be from epithelial or myoepithelial cells of ductal origins (Welsh and Meyer, 1968). These cells may differentiate to produce epithelial structures in some areas while, in other areas, they elaborate mucus and islands of pseudocartilage (Eversole, 1971).

The parotid gland is by far the most frequent location of these neoplasms. They occasionally occur in the submaxillary gland and sublingual glands and less frequently in the minor salivary glands in the palate, tongue, lips, cheek, nasopharynx, larynx, trachea, bronchi and jaw. Most frequently, these neoplasms appear in the fourth to sixth decades somewhat more commonly in women.

These tumors are usually slowly growing, painless, ovoid masses which occur anterior to the ear and below it. As they increase in size, they deflect the ear lobe, distend the skin and, in rare instances, may cause pressure necrosis with ulceration. Involvement of the facial nerve results in varying degrees of facial palsy, and involvement of the trigeminal branches gives rise to pain and sometimes the symptomatology of tic douloureux. The tumors vary in size from that of a walnut to that of a large grapefruit; extreme weights of $11\frac{1}{2}$ and 26 pounds have been reported.

Mixed tumors vary widely in microscopic appearance, but each tumor presents some of the structural features which characterize the tumors as a group (Fig. 20—48). Cellular morphology varies in

TABLE 20–1. NEOPLASMS OF MAJOR AND MINOR SALIVARY GLANDS

	Per Cent
Benign	
Pleomorphic adenoma (mixed tumor)	65
Papillary cystadenoma lymphomatosum (Warthin's tumor)	5
Malignant	
Malignant pleomorphic adenoma	5
Cylindroma (adenocystic carcinoma)	5
Mucoepidermoid carcinoma	10 to 15
Acinic cell adenocarcinoma	3

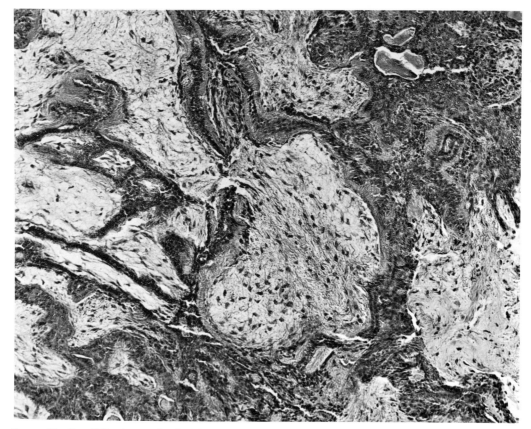

Figure 20–48. *"Mixed tumor" of salivary gland origin showing strand-like and tubular conformations of neoplastic epithelium. Strands of hyaline material bordered by tumor cells are formed in the mucoid connective tissue stroma.*

different areas of the same tumor as well as among different tumors. The neoplastic epithelium may be present in regular or modified ductal or acinar arrangements, in which case the cells tend to be cuboidal or columnar. Amorphous mucinous material is sometimes seen in the ducts and acini. In other areas or other tumors, the epithelium appears as solid sheets or isolated strands and cords. In these tumors, the epithelium tends to take the form of polyhedral cells with ovoid nuclei and eosinophilic cytoplasm. The cells may be well differentiated or anaplastic with occasional mitoses. In many instances, squamous epithelium and patterns resembling the basal cell carcinoma are present as well as areas of transition from cuboidal to squamous epithelium.

The connective tissue stroma which characterizes these lesions understandably suggests a mesodermal origin. It may consist of irregularly distributed fibrous connective tissue with foci of mucinous tissue interspersed with stellate-shaped cells. Interlacing trabeculae or scattered islands of hyaline material bordered by a beard-like layer of large spherical cells, masses of cartilage-like tissue and, less frequently, bone may also be present. The cartilage-like substance is attributed to secretion

from the epithelial tumor cells which becomes modified to form a matrix within which altered epithelial cells become embedded.

Mixed tumors are unencapsulated or poorly encapsulated, and microscopic evidence of penetration into the surrounding parenchyma is a common feature. Occasionally, areas are seen where the tumor blends with the surrounding normal glandular tissue. Recurrences tend to be multicentric, presumably the result of many small peripheral penetrations left behind from the original resection.

Pleomorphic adenomas are usually benign (85 to 95 per cent). The malignant mixed tumors may be obviously more anaplastic than the benign lesions, but some neoplasms may not disclose their biologic aggressiveness by their histologic detail. So some apparently benign-appearing lesions display malignant attributes. Both the benign and malignant forms tend to recur following surgical excision, attributable in all likelihood to incomplete removal. The frequency of such recurrence, as reported in the literature, ranges from 10 to 50 per cent (Molnar et al., 1971). It has been taught in the past that such recurrences tend to acquire more and more malignant attributes. Presently, it is believed that the malignant variants are more difficult to completely excise because of long sinuous projections which extend out into apparent normal glandular substance and are left behind at the time of the original enucleation. Thus, recurrences are more frequent with the infiltrative malignant mixed tumors, but it is doubtful that previously benign lesions undergo transformation to malignant forms. It must be remembered that the facial nerve, which is closely applied to or embedded within the parotid gland, hampers wide excision. Usually, the metastasis of malignant variants is to local nodes, but may be more widespread.

Papillary Cystadenoma Lymphomatosum (Warthin's Tumor). This benign uncommon tumor of salivary glands almost always occurs in the lower portion of the parotid overlying the angle of the mandible. Infrequently, these tumors occur bilaterally or in extraparotid locations. The male preponderance is 5 to 1, usually in the fifth to seventh decades of life (Baum and Perzik, 1964). As will be seen, they present a curious histologic architecture composed essentially of cystic or glandular spaces lined by columnar epithelium embedded within a lymphoid stroma. The histogenesis of such neoplasia has always been an enigma but reasonably has been ascribed to proliferation of heterotopic salivary gland rests, trapped during development, in lymph nodes adjacent to or within the parotid gland (Thompson and Bryant, 1950).

It is a firm, spherical, sometimes coarsely lobulated tumor. It is well differentiated microscopically, with numerous large cystic spaces lined with pseudostratified columnar epithelium resting upon papillary structures projecting into the lumen (Fig. 20–49). The surface cells are cylindrical with pale-staining eosinophilic cytoplasm. The nuclei are aligned near the surface. These cells are sometimes referred to as oncocytes and the lesion, an oncocytoma. The centers of the papillary projections consist of moderately fibrillar connective tissue stroma with closely packed lymphocytes and large germinal centers. The entire mass is encapsulated. The cystic cavity is filled with thick fluid containing lymphocytes, desquamated epithelial cells and fat globules. Almost all of these lesions are benign and are readily excised and cured. Rare malignant variants have been described.

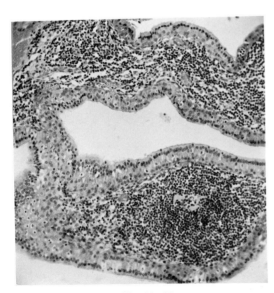

Fig. 20–49

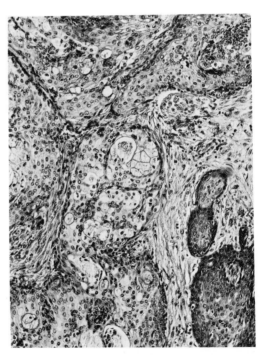

Fig. 20–50

Figure 20–49. *Papillary cystadenoma lymphomatosum showing cystic spaces lined with pseudostratified columnar epithelium. Lymph follicles are contained within the underlying connective tissue.*

Figure 20–50. *Malignant mucoepidermoid tumor showing squamous and mucous neoplastic cells and mucus-filled spaces.*

Cylindroma (Adenocystic Carcinoma).

The cylindroma is a malignant type of mixed salivary gland tumor. Its most frequent location is the mucous glands of the palate. It may occur in the parotid and submaxillary regions and has been reported in the mandible. It is a locally destructive lesion which, in time, almost always metastasizes either to the regional lymph nodes or to distant viscera with a tendency toward pulmonary involvement.

Microscopically, it presents clusters and strands of cuboidal epithelial cells, with large ovoid nuclei and sparse eosinophilic cytoplasm outlining central spherical spaces which may be empty or contain hyaline or mucoid material. Cystic degeneration of the neoplastic cells may be a feature. The fibrous stroma varies in appearance and may present zones of hyalinization or mucoid degeneration.

These tumors are radioresistant and tend to recur after surgery.

Mucoepidermoid Carcinoma.

The *mucoepidermoid tumors* were described as a specific type of salivary gland neoplasm by Stewart et al. (1945). These tumors are derived from mucous and basal cells of the salivary gland ducts.

The basal cells undergo metaplasia and form large polygonal cells which may assume squamous characteristics. The tumors characteristically present a varied structural pattern but may be distinguished by the presence of mucous cells, mucus-filled cystic spaces which often rupture, releasing the contents and eliciting a secondary reaction in the surrounding tissues, squamous differentiation and a diffuse mosaic, sheet-like distribution of the neoplastic cells (Fig. 20–50). Benign or malignant behavior cannot always be predicted from the microscopic appearance. Sparsity of mucous accumulation, predominance of small, round or oval hyperchromic cells or any suggestion of anaplasia favors a diagnosis of malignancy, but all mucoepidermoid tumors should be viewed with suspicion.

Mucoepidermoid tumors constitute about 10 to 15 per cent of all tumors of salivary gland origin. Grossly, they are small, spherical and well circumscribed, but usually not encapsulated, firm masses with numerous small cysts containing mucoid material. Infiltration into the surrounding tissue and relative sparsity of cysts or mucus are likely features of the malignant forms. Metastasis is most often to the cervical lymph nodes, but liver, chest, skin and general metastases have been reported.

Acinic Cell Adenocarcinoma (Clear Cell Carcinoma).

This unusual variant of adeno-carcinoma is characterized by polygonal epithelial cells having a cleared cytoplasm which makes them closely resemble the clear cell patterns of renal cell carcinoma. The neoplastic cells appear to arise from the reserve cells of the intercalated ducts, which differentiate into acinar cells. Although other salivary glands may be affected, most of these tumors arise in the parotid. Histologically, the tumor presents as sheets, cords or masses of cells, some of which are entirely cleared while others have a pink granular cytoplasm. Electron microscopy has highlighted the resemblance of these tumor cells to the serous acinar cells of normal glands (Echevarria, 1967). In general, these neoplasms are well encapsulated and slow-growing, but some are poorly encapsulated and more aggressive. Although most are amenable to complete excision and cure, some lesions are more stubborn, recur locally and eventually metastasize widely to the lungs, bone and brain.

Other Tumors of Salivary Gland Origin.

Other types of tumors are comparatively uncommon in the salivary glands and include lipoma, neurofibroma, fibrosarcoma, melanoma, lymphocytoma, reticulum cell sarcoma and Hodgkin's disease. Under five years of age, salivary gland tumors are rare and are almost exclusively mesenchymal. Hemangiomas, lymphangiomas and xanthomas have been reported (Bhaskar and Lilly, 1963).

TUMORS OF MINOR SALIVARY GLANDS

Only infrequently do tumors arise in the minor salivary glands. The mixed tumor is the most common type, followed in frequency by the cylindromatous adenocarcinoma, mucoepidermoid tumors and adenocarcinoma (Chaudhry et al., 1961). The palate is the favorite site for both benign and malignant minor salivary gland tumors. The second most common site for the mixed tumors is the lip, most often the upper. The tongue and the third molar regions are the second most common sites of the cylindromatous adenocarcinoma and mucoepidermoid tumors.

REFERENCES

Ackerman, L. Y., and Regato, J. A.: Cancer, Diagnosis, Treatment and Prognosis. St. Louis, C. V. Mosby Co., 1947, pp. 217–269.

Afonsky, D.: Saliva and Its Relation to Oral Health. University, Ala., University of Alabama Press, 1961.

Azzopardi, J. G., and Evans, D. J.: Malignant lymphoma of parotid associated with Mikulicz disease (benign lymphoepithelial lesion). J. Clin. Path., 24:744, 1971.

Bardwil, J. M.: Tumors of the parotid gland. Amer. J. Surg., 114:498, 1967.

Batsakis, J. G., and McWhirter, J. D.: Non-neoplastic disease of the salivary glands. Amer. J. Gastroent., 57:226, 1972.

Bauer, W. H., and Bauer, J. D.: The so-called "congenital epulis." Oral Surg., 6:1065, 1953.

Baum, R. K., and Perzik, S. L.: An evaluation of Warthin's tumor: a clinical review of 59 cases. Amer. Surg., 30:420, 1964.

Bernier, J. L.: The effects of atomic radiation on the oral and pharyngeal mucosa. J. Amer. Dent. Ass., 39:647, 1949.

Bernier, J. L.: The prevention of oral cancer. Dent. Clin. N. Amer., 16:747, 1972.

Bernier, J. L.: Tumors of the Odontogenic Apparatus and Jaws. Armed Forces Institute of Pathology. Atlas of Tumor Pathology, Section IV, Fascicle 10a, 1960.

Bernier, J. L., and Bhaskar, S. N.: Lymphoepithelial lesions of the salivary glands. Cancer, 11:1156, 1958.

Bhaskar, S. N., and Lilly, G. E.: Salivary gland tumors of infancy; report of 27 cases. J. Oral Surg., 21:305, 1963.

Bhaskar, S. N., et al.: Giant cell reparative granuloma (peripheral): report of 50 cases. J. Oral Surg., 29:110, 1971.

Burket, L. W.: Recent studies relating to periapical infection including data obtained from human necropsy studies. J. Amer. Dent. Ass., 25:260, 1938.

Cabrini, R. L., et al.: Cysts of the jaws: a statistical analysis. J. Oral Surg., 28:485, 1970.

Cahn, L. R.: Discussion of paper by Blum, T.: Cartilage tumors of the jaws. Report of three cases. Oral Surg., 7:1320, 1954.

Chaudhry, A. P., et al.: Intraoral minor salivary gland tumors. An analysis of 1414 cases. Oral Surg., 14:1194, 1961.

Chauncey, H. H.: Salivary enzymes. J. Amer. Dent. Ass., 63:360, 1961.

Cohen, M. M., and Baty, J. M.: Oral manifestations of erythroblastic anemia. J. Amer. Dent. Ass., 32:1396, 1945.

Christ, T. F.: The globulomaxillary cyst: an embryologic misconception. Oral Surg., 30:515, 1970.

Dean, H. T.: Distribution of mottled enamel in the United States. J. Amer. Dent. Ass., 30:319, 1933.

Dreizen, S.: Oral indications of the deficiency states. Postgrad. Med., 49:102, 1971.

Dreizen, S., and Hampton, J. K., Jr.: Radiosotopic studies of the glandular contribution of selected B vitamins in saliva. J. Dent. Res., 48:579, 1969.

Dummett, C. O., and Barens, G.: Oromucosal pigmentation: an updated literary review. J. Periodont., 42:726, 1971.

Echevarria, R. A.: Ultrastructure of the acinic cell carcinoma and clear cell carcinoma of the parotid gland. Cancer, 20:563, 1967.

Editorial: Tooth discoloration and tetracyclines. Med. J. Aust., 1:954, 1972.

Egelberg, J.: Local effects of diet on plaque formation and development of gingivitis in dogs. Part IV. Odont. Rev., 16:50, 1965.

Eichel, R. A.: A clinical television evaluation of plaque formation in children. I.A.D.R. Abstracts, 1970, No. 491, p. 171.

El-Ashiry, G. M., et al.: Comparative study of the influence of pregnancy and oral contraceptives on the gingivae. Oral Surg., 30:472, 1970.

Epker, B. N.: Obstructive and inflammatory diseases of the major salivary glands. Oral Surg., 33:2, 1972.

Eversole, L. R.: Histogenetic classification of salivary tumors. Arch. Path., 92:433, 1971.

Fitzgerald, R. J., and Keyes, P. H.: Demonstration of the etiologic role of streptococci in experimental caries in the hamster. J. Amer. Dent. Ass., 61:9, 1960.

Foote, F. W., and Frazell, E. L.: Tumors of the major salivary glands. Cancer, 6:1065, 1953.

Frank, R. M., and Brendel, A.: Ultrastructure of the approximal dental plaque and the underlying normal and carious enamel. Arch. Oral Biol., 11:883, 1966.

Gardner, A. F.: Pathology of oral manifestations of systemic diseases. New York, Hafner Publishing Co., 1972, p. 72.

Giansanti, J. S., and Waldron, C. A.: Peripheral giant cell granuloma: review of 720 cases. J. Oral Surg., 27:787, 1969.

Glickman, I.: A basic classification of "gingival enlargement." J. Periodont., 21:131, 1950.

Glickman, I.: Clinical Periodontology. 4th ed. Philadelphia, W. B. Saunders Co., 1972.

Glickman, I.: Fibrous dysplasia in alveolar bone. Oral Surg., 1:895, 1948.

Glickman, I.: Periodontal disease. New Eng. J. Med., 284:1071, 1971.

Glickman, I., and Glidden, H. S.: Paget's disease of the maxilla and mandible, clinical analysis and case reports. J. Amer. Dent. Ass., 29:2144, 1942.

Glickman, I., and Lewitus, M.: Hyperplasia of the gingiva associated with Dilantin (sodium diphenyl hydantoinate) therapy. J. Amer. Dent. Ass., 28:199, 1941.

Glickman, I., and Shklar, G.: The effect of systemic disturbances on the pulp of experimental animals. Oral. Surg., 7:550, 1954.

Glickman, I., and Smulow, J. B.: Histopathology and histochemistry of chronic desquamative gingivitis. Oral Surg., 21:325, 1966.

Glickman, I., et al.: Postsurgical healing in alloxan diabetes. I.A.D.R. Proceedings, 44th General Meeting, 1966, p. 121.

Gold, W.: Dental caries and periodontal disease considered as infectious diseases. Advances Appl. Microbiol., 2:135, 1969.

Gorlin, R. J., et al.: The syndrome of palmar-plantar hyperkeratosis and premature periodontal destruction of the teeth: a clinical and genetic analysis of the Papillon-Lefevre syndrome. J. Pediat., 65:895, 1964.

Guggenheimer, J., et al.: Dental manifestations of the rubella syndrome. Oral Surg., 32:30, 1971.

Hinds, E. C., and Kent, J. N.: Oral lesions. Amer. J. Gastroent., 55:225, 1971.

Hugoson, A.: Gingival inflammation and female sex hormones. J. Periodont. Res., Suppl. 5, 5:7, 1970.

Jaffe, H. L.: Giant cell reparative granuloma, traumatic bone cyst and fibrous (fibro-osseous) dysplasia of the jawbones. Oral Surg., 6:159, 1953.

Jenkins, G. N.: The present status of the fluoridation question. Sci. Basis Med. Ann. Rev., 365:82, 1971.

Kaner, A., et al.: Oral manifestations of congenital heart disease. J. Pediat., 29:269, 1946.

Kaplan, H.: The oral cavity in geriatrics. Geriatrics, 26:96, 1971.

Karmody, C. S., and Gallagher, J. C.: Nasoalveolar cyst. Ann. Otol., 81:278, 1972.

Kauffman, S. L., and Stout, A. P.: Tumors of the major salivary glands in children. Cancer, 16:1317, 1963.

Keene, J. J., Jr.: Observations of small blood vessels in human non-diabetic and diabetic gingiva. J. Dent. Res., 48: Part 2, 967, 1969.

Langeland, K.: Prevention of pulpal damage. Dent. Clin. N. Amer., 16:709, 1972.

Leach, S. A.: Plaque chemistry and caries. Alabama J. Med. Sc., 5:247, 1968.

Leban, S., et al.: The giant cell lesion of jaws: neoplastic or reparative? J. Oral Surg., 29:398, 1971.

Loesche, W. J., and Gibbons, R. J.: Influence of nutrition on the ecology and cariogenicity of the oral microflora. In Nizel, A. E.: The Science of Nutrition and Its Application to Clinical Dentistry. Philadelphia, W. B. Saunders Co., 1966, p. 305.

Lura, H. E.: The caries-pathogenic theories of today. J. Danish Dent. Ass., 73:283, 1969.

Mandel, I. D.: New approaches to plaque prevention. Dent. Clin. N. Amer., 16:668, 1972.

Markowitz, H. A., and Gerry, R. G.: Temporomandibular joint disease (a collective review). Oral Surg., 3:75, 1950.

McCarthy, P. L., and Shklar, G.: Diseases of the oral mucosa. New York, McGraw-Hill Book Co., 1964, p. 313.

McFarland, J.: Three hundred mixed tumors of the salivary glands of which sixty-nine recurred. Surg. Gynec. Obstet., 63:457, 1936.

Mehlisch, D. R., et al.: Ameloblastoma: a clinicopathologic report. J. Oral Surg., 30:9, 1972.

Mehta, F., et al.: Oral cancer and precancerous conditions in India. Bombay, Tata Press Limited, 1971.

Melcher, A. H., and Bowen, W. H.: Biology of the periodontium. London, Academic Press, 1969, p. 485.

Meyer, I.: The value of gingival biopsy in the diagnosis of generalized amyloidosis. J. Oral Surg., 8:314, 1950.

Mittleman, G., et al.: Alveolar bone changes in sickle cell anemia. J. Periodont., 32:74, 1961.

Molnar, L., et al.: Mixed tumors of the parotid gland. Oncology, 25:143, 1971.

Mopsich, E. R., and Gabriel, S. A.: Calcifying epithelial odontogenic tumor (Pindborg tumor). Report of two cases. Oral Surg., 32:15, 1971.

Murray, J. J.: Gingivitis in 15 year old children from high fluoride and low fluoride areas. Arch. Oral Biol., 14:951, 1969.

Oshrain, H. I., et al.: An histologic comparison of supra and subgingival plaque and calculus. J. Periodont., 42:31, 1971.

Pindborg, J. J.: Atlas of Diseases of the Oral Mucosa. Philadelphia, W. B. Saunders Co., 1968, p. 80.

Pruzansky, S.: Description, classification and analysis of un-operated clefts of the lip and palate. Amer. J. Orthodont., 39:590, 1953.

Redman, R.: Prevalence of geographic tongue, fissured tongue, median rhomboid glossitis and hairy tongue among 3,611 Minnesota school children. Oral Surg., 30:390, 1970.

Renstrup, G., et al.: Effect of chronic mechanical irritation on chemically induced carcinogenesis in the hamster cheek pouch. J. Amer. Dent. Ass., 64:770, 1962.

Robinson, I. B., and Sarnat, B. G.: Roentgen studies of the maxillae and mandible in sickle cell anemia. Radiology, 58:517, 1952.

Roper, R. E., et al.: Periodontal disease in aged individuals. J. Periodont., 43:304, 1972.

Rubin, P., and Casarett, G. W.: Clinical Radiation Pathology. Philadelphia, W. B. Saunders Co., 1968, p. 120.

Rud, J.: Cervicofacial actinomycosis. J. Oral Surg., 25:229, 1967.

Rushton, M. A.: Some less common bone lesions affecting the jaws. Oral Surg., 9:284, 1956.

Sandler, H.: Oral Exfoliative Cytology. Washington, D. C., Veterans Administration, Department of Medicine and Surgery, 1962.

Schour, I., and Massler, M.: The effects of dietary deficiencies upon the oral structures. J. Amer. Dent. Ass., 32:714, 871, 1139, 1945.

Selvig, K. A.: The formation of plaque and calculus on recently exposed tooth surfaces. J. Periodont. Res., Suppl. 4, 4:10, 1969.

Sheiham, A.: The prevalence and severity of periodontal disease in Surrey school children. Dent. Pract., 19:232, 1969.

Sheldon, M., et al.: The relationship between microscopic enamel defects and infantile debilities. J. Dent. Res., 24:109, 1945.

Shklar, G.: Oral reflections of infectious diseases II. Postgrad. Med., 49:147, 1971.

Sicher, H., and Bhaskar, S., (eds.): Orban's oral histology and Embryology. 7th ed. Saint Louis, The C. V. Mosby Co., 1972, p. 17.

Small, I. A., and Waldron, C.: Ameloblastomas of the jaws. Oral Surg., 8:281, 1955.

Sognnaes, R. F.: Chemistry and Prevention of Dental Caries. Springfield, Ill., Charles C Thomas, 1962.

Spies, T. D. (ed.): Nutrition and disease. Postgrad. Med., 17:7, 1955.

Stafne, E. C.: Periapical osteofibrosis with formation of cementoma. J. Amer. Dent. Ass., 21:1822, 1934.

Stanley, H.: The effect of systemic diseases on the human pulp. Oral Surg., 33:606, 1972.

Stein, G., and Gold, H.: Correlation between gross appearance and histopathology of the tongue. Oral Surg., 8:1165, 1955.

Stephan, R. M.: Changes in hydrogen-ion concentrations on tooth surfaces and in carious lesions. J. Amer. Dent. Ass., 27:718, 1940.

Stewart, F. W., et al.: Mucoepidermoid tumors of salivary glands. Ann. Surg., 122:820, 1945.

Symposium on solitary bone cysts of the mandible. Oral Surg., 8:899, 1955.

Thoma, K. H.: Oral Pathology. 4th ed. St. Louis, C. V. Mosby Co., 1954, p. 1149.

Thompson, A. S., and Bryant, H. C., Jr.: Histogenesis of papillary cystadenoma lymphomatosum (Warthin's tumor) of the parotid salivary gland. Amer. J. Path., 26:807, 1950.

Trodahl, J. N.: Ameloblastic fibroma. A survey of cases from the Armed Forces Institute of Pathology. Oral Surg., 33:547, 1972.

Turesky, S., et al.: A histochemical study of the keratotic process in oral lesions diagnosed clinically as leukoplakia. Oral Surg., 14:442, 1961.

Van Hassel, H. J.: Physiology of the human dental pulp. Oral Surg., 32:126, 1971.

Waldron, C. A.: Fibro-osseous lesions of the jaws. J. Oral Surg., 28:58, 1970.

Walker, D. G.: Benign nonodontogenic tumors of the jaws. J. Oral Surg., 28:39, 1970.

Weinmann, J. P., and Sicher, H.: Bone and Bones. 2nd ed. St. Louis, C. V. Mosby Co., 1955, p. 253.

Weinstein, L.: Antimicrobial chemoprophylaxis in dentistry. Dent. Clin. N. Amer., 16:760, 1972.

Welsh, R. A., and Meyer, A. T.: Mixed tumors of human salivary gland. Arch. Path., 85:433, 1968.

Wise, J. R., Jr., et al.: Urgent aortic-valve replacement for acute aortic regurgitation due to infective endocarditis. Lancet, II:115, 1971.

Witkop, C. J., Jr., and Wolf, R. O.: Hypoplasia and intrinsic staining of enamel following tetracycline therapy. J.A.M.A., 185:1008, 1963.

World Health Organization: Etiology and prevention of dental caries. Technical Report No. 494, 1972.

21

THE GASTROINTESTINAL TRACT

ESOPHAGUS

NORMAL

Certain features of the normal development and anatomy of the esophagus are helpful in understanding the diseases that affect this structure. The esophagus and the respiratory tract are very closely related developmentally. The respiratory system begins as a ventral groove in the primitive foregut. This groove deepens into a respiratory diverticulum that grows down to form the airways, i.e., trachea and bronchi. The original communication with the gut narrows into a slit that is progressively closed by fusion of its lips. Only the cranial end of this slit normally remains open to become eventually the communication of the larynx with the pharynx.

The esophagus lies throughout most of its course in the posterior mediastinum. It has no serosa and is covered only by the fibrous tissue of the mediastinum, from which it derives numerous small arterial branches. The absence of a serosa and the inadequacy of its own blood supply facilitate the spread of infection and render surgery difficult. The esophagus narrows slightly at three levels: the cricoid cartilage, the bifurcation of the trachea and the diaphragmatic hiatus, creating three areas vulnerable to trauma and perforation by foreign bodies.

There is great controversy and, indeed, confusion over the functional anatomy of the lower third of the esophagus. In question are the sphincteric valve mechanisms that normally block reflux of gastric contents and, when malfunctioning, permit the development of hiatal hernias and erosive inflammations of the lower esophagus. Central to this controversy is the concept of a gastroesophageal vestibule comprising the dilated lowermost end of the esophagus, bounded above by the inferior esophageal sphincter and below by the constrictor mechanism of the gastric cardia. The diaphragm inserts near the midportion of this vestibule, leaving a short segment of intraabdominal esophagus. This vestibule, from the standpoint of its muscular contractions, appears to function independently of the remainder of the esophagus. Presumably, the muscular contractions of the vestibule and the remainder of the esophagus must be coordinated to maintain normal peristalsis.

Venous drainage from the esophagus returns to the heart through both the portal and systemic systems. The coronary vein drains the lower esophagus and empties into the portal vein. It also anastomoses with branches of the esophageal veins which drain upward through the azygos into the superior vena cava. Both physiologically and pathologically, the esophageal venous system can act as a shunt between the portal and systemic systems.

PATHOLOGY

Lesions of the esophagus run the gamut from highly fatal cancers to less life-threatening, but nonetheless disabling, neuromuscular disturbances, inflammations and vascular abnormalities. Because they are lethal, carcinomas of the esophagus are the most important disorders of this level of the gut. These comprise about 5 to 10 per cent of all cancers of the alimentary tract. Second in importance are esophageal varices which, although uncommon in the general population, are dangerous lesions, since their rupture is frequently followed by massive hematemesis (vomiting of blood) and exsanguination. Other lesions, such as cardiospasm, webs, esophagitis and hiatus hernias, are more frequent but less threatening to life. Distressing to the gastroenterologist is the fact that all disorders of the esophagus tend to produce similar symptoms. Dysphagia (subjective difficulty in swallowing) is probably the paramount manifestation of all forms of esophageal pathology. Pain and hematemesis are sometimes evoked, particularly by those lesions associated with ulceroinflammatory changes in the esophageal wall. The clinical differential diagnosis of disorders of the esophagus requires, therefore, intensive investigation including barium swallow, radiography, esophagoscopy, biopsy and other specialized procedures.

CONGENITAL ANOMALIES

Developmental defects in the esophagus are uncommon. Because they cause immediate regurgitation when feeding is attempted, they are usually discovered soon after birth. They must be corrected early as they are incompatible with life.

Agenesis – Atresia. Absence (agenesis) of the esophagus is extremely rare and may affect the entire length or only a portion of it. Much more common are atresia and congenital stenosis. In atresia, a segment of the esophagus is represented by only a thin, noncanalized cord with the resultant formation of an upper blind pouch connecting with the pharynx and a lower pouch leading to the stomach. Most commonly, the atresia is located at or near the tracheal bifurcation. These blind pouches may not be in communication with the respiratory passages, but in about *80 to 90 per cent of the cases, the lower pouch communicates through a fistulous tract with the trachea or main stem bronchi.* The origin of such a maldevelopment is easily understood from the previous discussion of the embryology. The distal slit between the respiratory diverticulum and the primitive foregut fails to close. Much less commonly, a fistulous communication exists between the blind upper esophageal pouch and the respiratory tree.

Excessive salivation, vomiting, coughing from regurgitated aspirated mucus or paroxysmal suffocation from food that passes directly from the upper pouch into the respiratory tree are the prominent clinical manifestations. Even cyanosis and asphyxia may result. When the lower pouch communicates, the stomach tends to fill with air. Reconstructive surgery can effect cures, but if the condition is not recognized promptly, death may occur from asphyxia, aspiration pneumonia, and fluid and electrolyte imbalances. Often associated with such anomalies are congenital heart disease and malformations of the small intestine, rectum and anus.

Stenosis. Abnormal narrowing of the esophagus with the persistence of a constricted lumen may occur as a developmental defect or may be an acquired lesion resulting from inflammation or trauma to the esophagus. As a congenital lesion, agenesis is much less common than stenosis and atresia. The narrowing may be quite limited or may involve up to 10 cm. of the esophagus. When present as a congenital defect, the stenosis is manifested by feeding difficulty from birth.

Acquired stenoses are almost always the late consequence of chronic ulceroinflammatory disease. The initiating disorders are discussed on p. 906. The anatomic changes are nonspecific and consist of fibrous thickening of the esophageal wall associated with atrophy of the muscularis. Chronic inflammatory infiltrates are often present, principally in the submucosa and periesophageal fibrous tissue. The lining epithelium is usually thin and sometimes ulcerated. The extent and location of such changes depend upon the initial disorder giving rise to the fibrotic reaction. In severe acquired stenoses, virtually total obstruction may result.

LESIONS ASSOCIATED WITH NEUROMUSCULAR DYSFUNCTION

Difficulty in swallowing may be caused by one of several closely related entities, i.e., cardiospasm, esophageal ring (web) or hiatal hernia. Although these disorders are fairly well defined clinically and radiographically, the anatomic findings in such patients may be surprisingly scanty. The clinician reminds the pathologist that such disorders are primarily motor functional derangements and hence are difficult to establish in the surgical specimen and postmortem examination. The confusion is rendered more complex because two or more of these disorders, indistinctly separated, are frequently said to coexist in the same patient. It is also known that difficulty in swallowing may be a somatic complaint accompanying an otherwise purely psychologic disturbance—hysteria (globus hystericus) (Kramer, 1965). The line between such a functional disorder and the three previously cited lesions is, at best, poorly defined. We come to further difficulty in the discrepancy between the frequency with which these diagnoses are made clinically and the large number of such patients who have manifested no symptoms of esophageal disease. No less an authority than Palmer (1968) reports that, among 786 patients with clinical diagnoses of hiatus hernia, only 9 per cent had symptoms referable to the lesion. In the vast majority, it was a chance diagnosis made by radiographic studies for other gastrointestinal disorders. The conclusion is inescapable (from the pathologist's vantage) that cardiospasm, esophageal ring and hiatal hernia are abused and overused clinical diagnoses.

Standing apart from these poorly delineated conditions are lacerations of the esophagus also attributed to neuromotor dysfunction. Here the anatomic changes are readily apparent and are usually encountered in a clinical setting quite distinct from those of the other neuromotor dysfunctions.

Cardiospasm (Achalasia). Presumably, cardiospasm is a neuromotor disorder characterized by dysphagia associated with progressive dilatation and irregular tortuosity of the esophagus. It is believed to be the consequence of some functional or structural abnormality in the parasympathetic innervation of Auerbach's myenteric plexus. As mentioned previously, the body of the esophagus and the lowermost portion (called the vestibule) have separate innervations coordinated by the intrinsic plexus of Auerbach. Normally, this intrinsic plexus initiates a wave of muscular relaxation that precedes the peristaltic contraction. In cardiospasm, as a consequence of of neuromuscular incoordination, the vestibule tends to remain closed despite an oncoming wave of peristalsis and thus hampers the passage of food into the stomach. The functional blockage deranges the propulsive waves of peristaltic contraction which become disorganized, purposeless and irregularly segmental.

The underlying cause of such neuromotor disorganization is unknown. A persistent but still not well established theory postulates degeneration or destruction of Auerbach's plexus (Cassella et al., 1964). Both surgical biopsy and necropsy specimens have been reported to demonstrate degeneration or absence of myenteric ganglion cells in approximately 70 per cent of cases. Concomitant

degeneration of the ganglion cells in the vagal nuclei in the brain has been proposed as the primary cause of the myenteric changes. These findings must be accepted cautiously. If impaired vagal function were the basis of achalasia, one would expect interruption of the vagal nerves (vagotomy, a standard method of treating peptic ulcer) to induce the disease, but such patients do not inevitably develop cardiospasm. Moreover, about 30 per cent of cases fail to disclose abnormalities in the myenteric plexus; however, the mere anatomic presence of myenteric ganglion cells does not necessarily imply their normal function. The theory of impaired innervation cannot be lightly dismissed because widespread destruction of intramural ganglion cells in the esophagus sometimes occurs in Chagas' disease and is followed by esophageal dilatation and tortuosity characteristic of cardiospasm (Koberle, 1963).

Other theories propose congenital absence of ganglion cells in the myenteric plexus, deficiency of the B complex of vitamins leading to neural and neuronal degeneration, and psychosomatic causation. It is clear that the genesis of this esophageal dysfunction is still poorly understood.

Classically, the esophagus is dilated, flaccid, elongated and sometimes tortuous (**megaesophagus**). From what has been said above, it is clear that myenteric ganglia may be absent, degenerated or normal anatomically. The vestibule may be contracted and sometimes ulceroinflammatory lesions with fibrotic thickening are seen just above the vestibule. Leukoplakia may appear in the inflammatory regions; rarely these mucosal thickenings progress to cancer.

Cardiospasm affects males and females equally, usually between the ages of 30 and 50 years. The difficulty in swallowing is often paroxysmal and frequently triggered by emotional stress. Some patients complain of a dull ache beneath the lower sternum and of a sensation of food sticking there after swallowing. Indeed, in some severe cases, obstructive vomiting may become so marked as to cause serious debility and weight loss. The majority of patients are satisfactorily treated by muscle-splitting dilatation of the esophagus. Some may require surgical intervention.

Esophageal Rings (Webs). Annular narrowings of the esophagus, sometimes apparent as circumferential mucosal folds (webs), are uncommon lesions encountered in a variety of clinical circumstances. Most patients are over the age of 40. *Webs in the upper esophagus* (above the aortic arch) are generally, although not exclusively, seen in women suffering from severe iron deficiency anemia. The esophageal web is frequently associated with atrophic glossitis. The triad of anemia, atrophic glossitis and dysphagia is known as the *Plummer-Vinson syndrome*. The relationship between the esophageal lesion and the other components of the triad is obscure, but it is interesting that the administration of iron to many patients has ameliorated not only the anemia but also the web defect (Shamma'a and Benedict, 1958).

Lower esophageal rings or webs usually occur close to the squamocolumnar junction and are not associated with iron deficiency anemia or confined to women. The gastroenterologic literature suggests that they are identified at radiologic examination among 0.2 to 14 per cent of patients having routine barium meal examinations (Kramer, 1956) (Keyting et al., 1960). However, in only 0.5 per cent of these patients undergoing study of the upper gastrointestinal tract was the ring responsible for dysphagia. Even if one accepts the one in 200 frequency, these anatomic lesions must be exceedingly subtle, since they are far more rare in routine postmortem series. Undoubtedly, they might be missed by the pathologist, since muscular spasm contributes to their prominence and, once the esophagus is opened, they could virtually disappear (Joyal et al., 1970). About 15 per cent of patients with this anatomic condition have an accompanying hiatus hernia.

Well developed esophageal rings appear as smooth mucosal ledges in the opened esophagus. Virtually all lower rings are found in the caudad 5 cm. and mostly at the squamocolumnar junction. They rarely protrude into the lumen more than 5 mm. and have a thickness in the order of 2 to 4 mm. Histologically, the upper surface is covered by stratified squamous epithelium and the under surface by columnar epithelium. The central core is composed of a vascularized fibrous tissue often containing scattered inflammatory cells (Postlethwait and Musser, 1965).

Symptomatology associated with esophageal webs or rings consists essentially of dysphagia, usually provoked by bolting solid foods. Pain is infrequent. Often the discomfort is episodic with long symptom-free intervals. In some patients, the discomfort progressively worsens with years and is elicited even by soft food; in others, the condition constitutes only a nonprogressive bothersome problem that persists throughout life (Schatzki and Gary, 1956).

Hiatal Hernia. Hiatal hernia is a disorder of the gastroesophageal junction resulting in a sac-like dilatation of the stomach protruding above the diaphragm.

Two anatomic patterns are recognized. In the first, the esophagus ends above the diaphragm, creating a symmetrical bell-like dilatation of that portion of the stomach within the thoracic cavity. The dilatation is bounded below by the diaphragmatic narrowing. This abnormality may result from a congenitally short esophagus or may be an acquired defect secondary to longstanding fibrous scarring of the esophagus. Whatever the basis, traction on the stomach pulls a portion of it into the thorax. Eighty to 90 per cent of all hiatal hernias are of this type (Hagarty, 1960). The supradiaphragmatic herniation of the stomach is accentuated by muscular contraction of the esophagus during the act of swallowing, and so this traction pattern is also called a **sliding hernia**.

The second pattern is designated "paraesophageal hiatal hernia." A portion of the cardiac end of the stomach dissects alongside the esophagus through a defect in the diaphragmatic hiatus to produce an intrathoracic sac. It is usually small and is found alongside the normally positioned lower end of the esophagus. Because the stomach rolls up alongside the esophagus, this form is sometimes called a **rolling hernia**. Less than 10 per cent of hiatal hernias are of this type. More extreme forms of paraesophageal hernia are encountered following traumatic rupture of the diaphragm.

In both forms of hiatal hernia, reflux of gastric contents into the lower esophagus often induces a so-called regurgitative esophagitis (McHardy et al., 1969). In some, as mentioned earlier, an esophageal ring is seen or an apparent upward extension of columnar epithelium (characteristic of the stomach) lines the hernial dilatation.

Enthusiastic roentgenologists report the demonstration of hiatal hernias in 4 to 7 per cent of otherwise normal individuals (Editorial, 1969). However, over half of these patients have no symptoms whatsoever, and only about 9 per cent suffer from such disturbances as retrosternal burning pain ("heart burn") and sometimes regurgitation of gastric juices into the mouth. These manifestations are attributed to incompetence of the esophagogastric sphincter and are accentuated by positions favoring reflux e.g., bending forward or lying supine. Such symptomatic disease is more common in women of advanced age suffering from obesity. It should be cautioned that gastroesophageal reflux and/or heart burn are frequently encountered in the absence of a detectable hiatal hernia (Kramer, 1965). Bleeding is sometimes seen in these patients but very likely is associated with the development of secondary erosive regurgitative esophagitis or gastritis (Palmer, 1963).

Some of the earlier comments about the poor delineation of neuromuscular disorders of the esophagus may be clearer now. Patients with hiatal hernias often have regurgitative esophagitis, and many have esophageal rings. Indeed, these patients also have an increased frequency of peptic ulcers (Montgomery and Wilson, 1963). Which of these many disorders is responsible for the symptomatology and what their interrelationships may be are unclear. Infrequently, such serious complications as stricture formation and the development of carcinoma supervene.

Lacerations (Mallory-Weiss Syndrome). Small tears in the esophagus are fairly uncommon lesions which usually occur as a result of prolonged vomiting. Some are said to occur without antecedent vomiting. These lesions are encountered most commonly, but not exclusively, in chronic alcoholics who usually give a history of massive hematemesis following a bout of excessive vomiting. Normally, a reflex relaxation of the musculature of the gastrointestinal tract precedes the antiperistaltic wave of contraction. One pathogenetic concept speculates that during episodes of prolonged vomiting, this reflex relaxation fails to occur (Weiss and Mallory, 1932). The refluxing gastric contents suddenly overwhelm the contraction of the sphincter of the cardia, and massive dilatation and tearing of

the esophageal wall ensue at the esophagogastric junction. Since these tears also occur in persons who have no history of vomiting, other mechanisms must exist. Recently, several studies have related these tears to underlying inapparent hiatal hernias. It is postulated that the inadequate diaphragmatic support provides an area of weakness that potentiates abnormal dilatation when subjected to increased intragastric pressure. This view contends that lacerations do not occur in the absence of these hiatal defects.

The linear irregular lacerations vary from several millimeters to several centimeters in length. They occur in the long axis of bowel and usually are found in the most distal portion of the esophagus or astride the esophagogastric junction (Fig. 21–1). The tears may involve only the mucosa or they may penetrate deeply enough to perforate the wall.

The histology is not distinctive. The early lesion is a nonspecific traumatic defect accompanied by fresh hemorrhage into the margins of the defect. A nonspecific inflammatory response follows. Infection of the defect may lead to an inflammatory ulcer or to mediastinitis.

Supposedly, healing may occur if the patient survives the initial trauma, but usually these lacerations are followed almost immediately by massive and, not infrequently, fatal bleeding. The importance of these lesions will be discussed later in the differential diagnosis of hematemesis (p. 928).

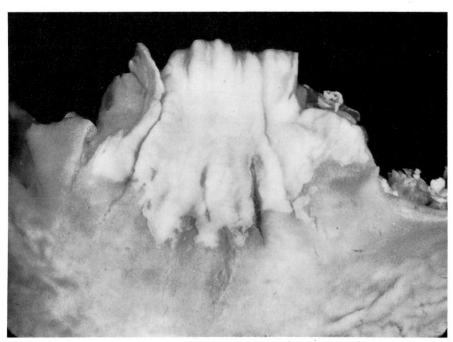

Figure 21–1. Esophageal laceration. A gross view demonstrating a longitudinal laceration extending from esophageal mucosa into stomach mucosa.

INFLAMMATIONS

Inflammatory lesions of the esophagus are relatively common autopsy findings, but only rarely do they cause clinical symptoms. Indeed, in most cases, they represent agonal changes appearing within the last days of life, presumably reflecting profound debility and deranged sphincteric control mechanisms at the cardioesophageal junction. Clinically significant inflammation is encountered in a wide variety of clinical circumstances and may be responsible for disturbing symptoms and even death.

Esophagitis. Only rarely are esophageal inflammations primary disorders. Much more commonly, they are secondary to associated gastric or esophageal lesions or to disease primary elsewhere in the body. The following list indicates the more important associations:

1. Hiatal hernia with reflux of acid gastric juice—regurgitative, reflux or peptic esophagitis.
2. Prolonged gastric intubation.
3. Ingestion (usually suicidal) of corrosive chemicals such as lye, other alkalis or acids.
4. Habitual ingestion of irritant foods such as very hot liquids, exceedingly spicy foods or alcohol.
5. Uremia.
6. Bacteremia with seeding of the esophagus or direct spread of infection in contiguous structures.
7. Fungal infections (moniliasis, mucormycosis, aspergillosis) in debilitated patients, those with an immunologic deficiency, or those receiving immunosuppressive treatment.
8. Plummer-Vinson syndrome.

The anatomic changes depend upon the causative agent, the duration of the process and the severity of the exposure. Simple hyperemia may be the only alteration. More severe degrees of injury result in edema and thickening of the walls, sometimes pseudomembrane formation, or areas of superficial necrosis and ulceration. Typically, moniliasis produces large gray-white inflammatory pseudomembranes teeming with the causative fungus. If the inflammatory process has been severe, fibrosis and stricture formation may follow. Histologically, the reaction pattern depends upon the causative agent, as would be anticipated. One special form merits mention. In esophagitis associated with hiatus hernia and acid reflux, the lower esophagus may become lined by columnar rather than by squamous epithelium, creating what has been referred to as a Barrett esophagus. Very rarely, the chronic irritation and regenerative epithelial efforts lead to superimposed cancer.

The clinical manifestations of esophagitis consist principally of dysphagia, retrosternal pain and sometimes hematemesis or melena.

Esophagitis must be differentiated from agonal or postmortem digestion—*esophagomalacia*. Characteristically, these postmortem lesions produce superficial discolorations or autolysis of the esophageal wall which are brown-black owing to acid digestion of hemoglobin. A spotted or bizarre map-like pattern, often called "leopard spotting," is produced. The ultimate criterion of the nature of such postmortem lesions is the absence of inflammatory response.

Ulcerations. Ulcerations of the esophagus may appear in any of the patterns of esophagitis mentioned earlier. In addition, there are a group of ulcerations often referred to as "peptic ulcerations."

Some so-called "peptic ulcers" occur low in the esophagus within the squamous cell mucosa but are referred to as "peptic" because they are caused by persistent regurgitation of acid peptic chyme. In other instances, the peptic ulceration occurs in gastric mucosa found within the esophagus. Sometimes this mucosa takes the form of ectopic islands. In other instances, the entire lower portion of the esophagus becomes lined by gastric epithelium. Barrett called attention to this aberrant lining, and so the ulceration is designated as a "Barrett ulcer." The origin of this aberrant lining of gastric mucosa is unclear. Either it grows up from the stomach due to some unknown stimulus or it represents a developmental defect. In most of these instances, the ulcer is extremely low within the esophagus and is, in fact, found in the short segment between the diaphragm and the esophagogastric junction.

Esophageal peptic ulcers may occur singly or multiply. They may be superficial or deep and are rarely over 2 cm. in diameter. The inflammatory changes are entirely nonspecific, and when they occur within abnormal gastric epithelium, they resemble quite completely peptic ulceration of the stomach.

In addition to pain, heartburn, dysphagia and vomiting, these lesions are of importance as possible sources of severe bleeding.

MISCELLANEOUS LESIONS

Diverticula. Diverticula of the esophagus may be of two types—pulsion or traction.

Two situations are responsible for producing herniated *pulsion* diverticula. Herniations may result from increased intraluminal pressure, encountered particularly in association with webs, hiatal hernia or cardiospasm (Fig.

21–2). These lesions most often occur in the lower third of the esophagus. Areas of anatomic weakness are the second source of herniation. Such areas occur in the upper third where the esophageal intrinsic musculature is poorly developed and support is partly derived from the constrictor muscles of the pharynx. The spaces between the pharyngeal muscles are foci of maximal weakness.

Traction diverticula result from the pull of inflammatory adhesions of periesophageal or tracheobronchial lymph nodes on the external aspect of the esophageal wall. As these nodes heal and undergo fibrous contraction, they can create a small diverticulum. Such diverticula occur most commonly near the tracheal bifurcation, and tuberculosis is the most common cause of the nodal inflammation.

Traction diverticula rarely cause symptoms because they are small, but pulsion diverticula may produce pain or projectile vomiting. When either become ulcerated as a consequence of the stasis of food, they may lead to hematemesis. Fortunately, only extremely rarely do such ulcerations perforate, leading to fatal mediastinitis.

Systemic Sclerosis (Scleroderma). Involvement of the esophagus in the systemic disease scleroderma is usually accompanied by involvement of other levels of the gut and other internal organs as well. Because these visceral components exist, scleroderma is now more appropriately termed systemic sclerosis. The major consideration of this disease has already been presented (p. 242). The esophageal and lower intestinal lesions consist of submucosal fibrosis, followed by fibrous overgrowth

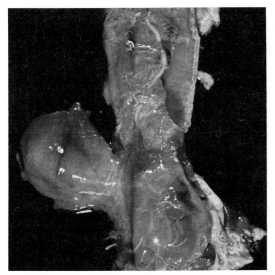

Figure 21–2. *Pulsion diverticulum of the esophagus.*

and atrophy of the smooth musculature. Concomitantly, the overlying mucosa becomes atrophic and sometimes develops large ulcerations. In far advanced cases, extreme rigidity and narrowing of the esophagus develop. Similar narrowing occurs in the affected small and large bowel. When such visceral lesions develop in the course of scleroderma, the prognosis worsens.

VASCULAR

Varices.   Regardless of cause, longstanding obstruction to portal flow through the liver produces portal hypertension and, as a consequence, the normal flow from the coronary veins to the portal vein is reversed. The portal blood is, therefore, shunted via the coronary veins into the esophageal veins and thence into the azygos system. The increase in pressure in the esophageal plexus produces dilated tortuous vessels which are called varices. *Portal hypertension is most commonly caused by cirrhosis,* although rarely it may be produced by portal vein thrombosis, hepatic vein thrombosis (Budd-Chiari syndrome), pylephlebitis, *or tumorous compression or invasion of the major portal radicles.* Varices occur in approximately two-thirds of all cirrhotic patients and are most often associated with alcoholic cirrhosis, sometimes called fatty nutritional cirrhosis. Varices are less commonly found in association with pigment cirrhosis and postnecrotic scarring of the liver and are rarely produced by biliary or cardiac cirrhosis. Contributing to the portal hypertension are abnormal anastomoses that often arise in cirrhotic livers between the finer branches of the hepatic artery and portal vein. Very infrequently, varices are encountered in systemic amyloidosis and sarcoidosis. Furthermore, rare cases have been described without evident cause for the portal hypertension (Palmer and Brick, 1955).

The varices are difficult to visualize in surgical or postmortem material since, in the process of exposing them, veins are transected and drained and the varices collapse. Under optimal conditions, they appear as tortuous dilated veins in the long axis of the bowel, which protrude directly beneath the mucosa or are found in the periesophageal tissue (Figs. 21–3 and 21–4). Varices are most commonly seen in the distal third of the esophagus but are occasionally found in the middle third.

When the varix is unruptured, the overlying mucosa may be normal, but often it is eroded and inflamed because of its exposed position. If rupture has occurred in the past, thrombosis or superimposed inflammation may be seen (Fig. 21–5).

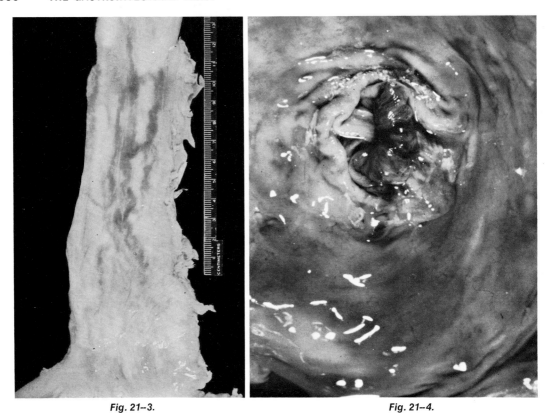

Fig. 21–3.   *Fig. 21–4.*

Figure 21–3. *Esophageal varices. A gross view demonstrating tortuous dilated submucosal varices in the middle and lower thirds of the esophagus.*

Figure 21–4. *Eosphageal varices. A view from below of the unopened cardia showing the remarkable similarity between the varices of the esophagus, as they protrude into the stomach, and their rectal counterparts, hemorrhoids.*

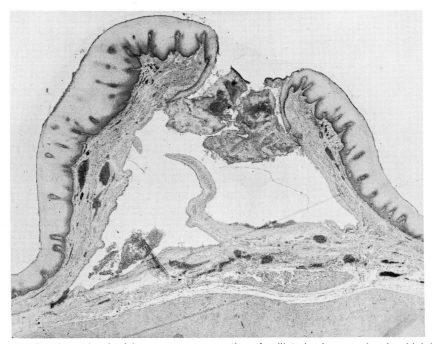

Figure 21–5. *Esophageal varix. A low power cross section of a dilated submucosal varix which has ruptured through the mucosa. A small amount of thrombus is present within the point of rupture.*

Varices produce no symptoms until they rupture, and then calamitous massive hematemesis usually ensues. Among those with well advanced cirrhosis of the liver, over half of the deaths result from rupture of a varix. Some patients die as a direct consequence of the hemorrhage, and others, of hepatic coma triggered by the hemorrhage. Once begun, the hemorrhage rarely spontaneously subsides, and immediate measures are usually required, including multiple transfusions, intraesophageal balloon tamponade and even emergency efforts at surgical varix ligation. Rupture of the varix may occur without an apparent triggering event, usually when there has been silent inflammatory erosion of the overlying thinned mucosa. On the other hand, in many of these patients, vomiting with presumed increase of hydrostatic pressure within the varix is the antecedent to the rupture. In studies of fatal hematemesis from all possible gastric and esophageal causes, rupture of an esophageal varix is responsible for only a small fraction; but when these lesions bleed, death with the first episode occurs in about 70 per cent (Orloff et al., 1967). If the patient survives the first bleed, portacaval shunt may be performed in an attempt to reduce the portal hypertension. The contribution of variceal rupture to hematemesis as a clinical problem is further discussed in the clinical pathologic correlation of causes of hematemesis (p. 928).

TUMORS

BENIGN

A variety of benign tumors occur in the esophagus. These are usually small, rarely over 3 cm. in diameter and occur mostly as intramural, solid, gray, submucosal masses. The most common is the leiomyoma but, in addition, fibromas, lipomas, hemangiomas, neurofibromas and any of the other benign mesenchymal tumors may arise in this location. They usually are chance findings at postmortem and are rarely large enough to cause symptoms.

CARCINOMA

Approximately 4 per cent of all cancer deaths in the United States are caused by carcinoma of the esophagus. These neoplasms occur infrequently relative to those of the stomach and large intestine, but since they remain asymptomatic during much of their development, cure by surgical resection is rare. The striking male preponderance of 5:1 has not been explained but may, in part, be at-tributable to increased exposure to alcohol and smoking. Most patients are over the age of 50.

Pathogenesis. Unlike gastric carcinoma, a genetic predisposition is not substantiated, but a considerable amount of evidence exists that environmental influences and preexisting esophageal dysfunction are important in the causation of esophageal carcinoma (Wynder and Bross, 1961). Among the environmental influences, chronic alcoholism and tobacco smoking contribute most heavily. Esophageal cancer is 25 times more common among heavy drinkers than among controls. Habitual smokers of cigarettes, cigars or pipes have a six- to sevenfold increased frequency of esophageal cancer (United States Department of Health, Education and Welfare, 1968).

Disorders in esophageal structure or function carry an increased risk. Assumed but not established is the concept that prolongation of contact between esophageal mucosa and food and drink is the operative factor in the disorders associated with an increased risk of esophageal carcinoma, e.g., cardiospasm, esophagitis, lye strictures, diverticula, hiatus hernia and the Plummer-Vinson syndrome. It is difficult to express the precise magnitude of the increased risk in each of these settings because of the wide statistical ranges reported in the literature. On the one hand, McConchie (1961) indicates that 8 per cent of his patients with hiatal hernias developed cancers of the esophagus while, on the other hand, Brick (1949) found esophageal and/or gastric malignancy in only 1 per cent of his patients. About 4 per cent of patients with either lye strictures or cardiospasm are said to develop esophageal cancers. The Plummer-Vinson syndrome is said to be associated with esophageal carcinoma proximal to the upper webs in approximately 16 per cent of patients; conversely, about 70 per cent of patients with carcinoma of the *oropharynx* or *upper third* of the esophagus have the Plummer-Vinson syndrome (Calkins, 1964) (Boyd et al., 1964) (Alvarez and Colbert, 1963). Undoubtedly, there is much variation in the criteria used to establish the diagnosis of the preexisting disorder. Despite these uncertainties, it is generally conceded that carcinoma occurs more commonly in the esophagus showing some derangement than in the normal.

Morphology. In the large series of cases collected by Terracol and Sweet (1958), 40 to 50 per cent of these cancers occurred in the lower third of the esophagus, 30 to 40 per cent in the middle third, and the remainder in the upper third. Early lesions are usually discovered incidentally and appear as small, gray-white, plaque-like thickenings or elevations of the mucosa. These extend with time along the long axis of the bowel and, in months to years, encircle the lumen. From this point, three morphologic patterns may evolve. The most common is **a necrotic cancerous ulceration** which excavates deeply into surrounding structures and may erode into the respiratory tree and the aorta or permeate the mediastinum and pericardium (Figs. 21–6 to 21–8).

The second gross pattern is that of **a polypoid fungating lesion** which protrudes into the lumen. The third morphologic variant is **a diffuse infiltrative form** that tends to spread within the wall of the esophagus causing thickening, rigidity and narrowing of the lumen with linear irregular ulcerations of the mucosa. Histologically, 80 to 90 per cent are typical squamous cell carcinomas (Burgess et al., 1951). The remainder are adenocarcinomas which originate either from the esophageal mucous glands or from upward growth of gastric epithelium into the lower esophagus.

These lesions tend to spread by direct continuity, but they also metastasize. Lower third lesions often disseminate not only to mediastinal nodes but also to organs below the diaphragm. Middle and upper third lesions are more often contained within the thorax with spread to the larynx, trachea, thyroid glands and recurrent laryngeal nerves, but

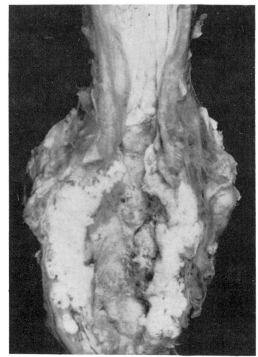

Figure 21–6. *Cancer in the lower third of the esophagus, far advanced with central ulceration and extension into periesophageal tissue.*

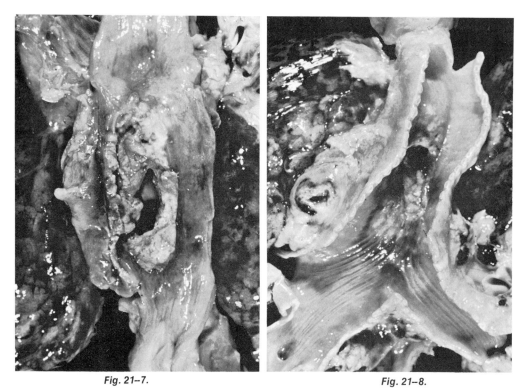

Fig. 21–7.   Fig. 21–8.

Figures 21–7 and 21–8. *Carcinoma of the esophagus. Figure 21–7 viewed from the esophageal aspect showing a large defect in the central necrotic portion. Figure 21–8 viewed from the trachea showing the connecting esophageal-tracheal fistula with extension of tumor along the wall of the trachea.*

even some of these metastasize below the diaphragm.

Clinical Course. Esophageal carcinoma is insidious in onset and produces dysphagia and obstruction gradually and late. The patient subconsciously adjusts to his increasing difficulty in swallowing by progressively altering his diet from solid to liquid foods. Extreme weight loss and debilitation result, both from the impaired nutrition and the effects of the tumor itself. Hemorrhages and sepsis may accompany the ulcerative changes. Occasionally, the first alarming symptom is the aspiration of food which enters the respiratory tree through a cancerous tracheoesophageal fistula. It should be noted that such fistula formation is almost always caused by carcinoma of the esophagus. Bronchogenic carcinoma rarely invades the esophagus and hence rarely produces fistulous tracts. Metastasis occurs as a relatively late phenomenon. In untreated patients with carcinoma of the esophagus, 75 per cent die within one year of the onset of symptoms and, even with surgical resection, five-year survivals are below 10 per cent (Boyd et al., 1958) (Sweet, 1952). The insidious invasive growth of these neoplasms usually leads to large lesions, impossible to resect by the time a diagnosis is established.

SARCOMAS

These are very rare and represent the same types found elsewhere in the intestinal tract. Leiomyosarcoma and fibrosarcoma predominate.

STOMACH

NORMAL

Surprising as it may seem, there is no universally acceptable terminology for the regional divisions of the stomach. Most widely accepted is the following:

1. The *fundus* or cardiac portion is the bulbous upper region of the stomach demarcated by a line drawn directly through the long axis of the esophagus to the greater curvature. The *cardia* includes that region about the esophagogastric junction.

2. The *body* or midregion of the stomach represents that portion lying between the fundus and the incisura angularis.

3. The *antrum* extends from the incisura angularis to the pylorus. Sometimes the narrowed 2.5 cm. segment of the antrum lying just proximal to the pyloric sphincter is designated as the *prepyloric canal*.

4. The *pylorus* is the sphincteric orifice that opens into the duodenum.

Important to understanding the predisposition of regions of the stomach to certain diseases is an appreciation of the mitotic and secretory activity of the gastric mucosa. The surface of the gastric mucosa throughout the stomach is composed of mucus-producing columnar cells. In man, such cells have a life span of approximately 2 to 4 days, and it is estimated that they are shed at the rate of half a million cells *per minute!* (Croft et al., 1966.) These desquamated cells are replaced by proliferation of the cells lining the gastric pits and constant migration of the newly formed cells up the walls of the pits to the surface. The rates of DNA synthesis and mitosis can be imagined. Below the gastric pits, but still within the gastric mucosa, are the glandular or secreting parts, consisting of cells which are quite static and rarely divide. In the body of the stomach, the glands are lined largely by pepsinogen-secreting chief cells and brightly eosinophilic acid-secreting parietal cells. The latter are also thought to be the source of the gastric intrinsic factor. The glands in the pyloric and antral regions, as well as about the cardia, are made entirely of mucus-secreting cells and lack acid-secreting cells. Virtually 95 per cent of peptic ulcers occur in the nonacid-secreting antral and pyloric regions. Presumably, the mucosa here is more vulnerable to the erosive action of the acid-peptic juice. Gastrin, the potent secretagogue, is elaborated principally in the antral region of the stomach.

In clinical and anatomic practice, the stomach is also divided geometrically into anterior and posterior walls with greater and lesser curvatures. In general, infections which result from perforations of the posterior wall and lesser curvature tend to remain localized or to involve only the lesser peritoneal cavity. Perforations of the anterior surface and greater curvature are more likely to produce diffuse peritonitis.

Because the stomach is such a widely expanded segment of the gastrointestinal tract, small lesions may be difficult to detect radiologically. The large mass of barium needed to fill the stomach sometimes obscures lesions lying within the fundus and body. Moreover, lesions in these locations are often clinically asymptomatic because they do not produce obstruction and do not sufficiently impair function to evoke manifestations. For these reasons, the body and fundus of the stomach are sometimes referred to as the "silent area."

PATHOLOGY

From the standpoint of incidence and the seriousness of the resultant clinical disease, the stomach is undoubtedly the most important segment of the entire alimentary tract. Peptic ulcers have become almost a hallmark of so-called "civilized life" and are found in up to 10 per cent of the general population in North America. Gastric carcinoma is one of the leading causes of cancer death in the United States. Gastritis in this day of cigarette smoking, alcohol and pressured existence is one of the everyday causes of "indigestion."

CONGENITAL ANOMALIES

Diaphragmatic Hernias. Weakness or partial to total absence of a region of the diaphragm, usually on the left, may permit the abdominal contents to herniate into the thorax. These hernias differ from hiatal hernias only insofar as the defect in the diaphragm does not involve the hiatal orifice. The hernial wall in these lesions is most often composed only of peritoneum and pleura. Usually, the stomach or a portion of it insinuates into the pouch, but occasionally small bowel and even a portion of the liver accompany it (Fig. 21–9).

Sometimes these hernias are asymptomat-

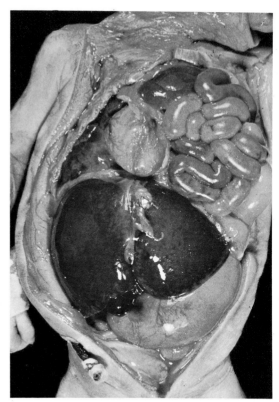

Figure 21–9. Diaphragmatic hernia. An in situ view of the opened trunk of an infant with a diaphragmatic hernia. Numerous loops of small bowel and portions of the colon are evident in the left pleural cavity. The markedly displaced lung can be seen at the very apex of the cavity.

ic and are discovered only by x-ray or by the identification of intestinal sounds within the chest. Large protrusions, however, particularly in infants, may lead to respiratory embarrassment or vomiting.

Pyloric Stenosis. Hypertrophy of the pyloric muscle with narrowing of the lumen is found most often as a congenital defect in the infant. As a rare adult lesion, it may represent either persistence of a childhood defect or an acquired abnormality.

Congenital pyloric stenosis occurs equally in breast-fed and artificially fed infants but is more common in males in the ratio of 4:1. It usually manifests at the third week of life by the development of persistent projectile vomiting following feeding. The pylorus is thick, firm and swollen into a mass about 2 to 3 cm. in length and 1 to 2 cm. in diameter. The enlargement is entirely due to hypertrophy and spasm of the muscular coat. This mass can often be palpated through the thin abdominal wall. The mucosal lining is usually intact, and simple splitting of the hypertrophied muscles without entering the lumen of the pylorus relieves the obstruction. The cause is unknown, but one vague postulation suggests some neuromuscular dysfunction perhaps related to inadequate or incomplete maturation of the pyloric myenteric plexus (Reyes and Friesen, 1967).

Acquired pyloric stenosis is most often encountered in adults secondary to preexisting gastritis, peptic ulceration or prolonged pylorospasm. Occasionally, no antecedent cause is detectable, and it is then considered a persistent infantile lesion. In acquired lesions, there is often extensive intramural fibrosis as well as mucosal changes incident to the underlying cause. Occasionally, considerable hypertrophy of the muscularis is also present.

MECHANICAL LESIONS

Gastric Dilatation. Organic or functional obstruction (pylorospasm) of the pylorus gives rise to retention of gastric contents and progressive gastric dilatation. Occasionally, following surgery or in the presence of peritonitis, atony of the stomach and intestines (paralytic ileus) may allow the accumulation of large amounts of chyme. The stomach may contain as much as 10 to 15 liters of fluid (Fig. 21–10).

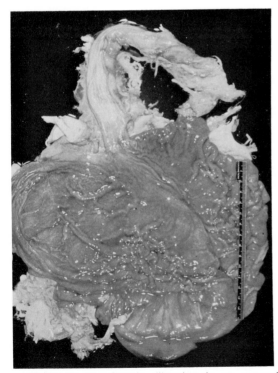

Figure 21–10. *Gastric dilatation in an opened stomach. The extent of the dilatation is apparent by comparison of the stomach with the 15 cm. rule at the right of the picture.*

Grossly, the stomach is not only enormously expanded, but the wall is markedly thinned even to the point of translucency. Usually no intrinsic mucosal involvement is present although occasionally superficial erosions and hyperemia are evident.

Distention of the stomach may be serious, particularly in patients who are already severely ill. The consequent marked elevation of the diaphragm adds sufficient respiratory embarrassment to the underlying disease to prejudice seriously the patient's chances for survival.

INFLAMMATIONS

GASTRITIS

While gastritis is an unquestioned clinical and anatomic disorder, it is a much abused medical term. It is commonly used to explain such transient or seemingly trivial complaints as "sour stomach," "dyspepsia" and "heartburn" without valid substantiating clinical or anatomic evidence. Admittedly, it is extremely difficult to establish the existence of the acute forms since they are generally trivial; and with the remarkable regenerative capacity of the surface lining of the stomach, anatomic evidence of gastritis tends to appear and disappear evanescently.

Innumerable classifications of gastritis have been proposed. Basically, there are two general categories, acute and chronic. However, many subvarieties have been given special designations. All are variations in the pattern of the acute or chronic alterations, e.g., acute hemorrhagic gastritis, acute erosive gastritis, chronic atrophic gastritis and chronic hypertrophic gastritis. Here we shall limit our consideration to acute gastritis, chronic atrophic gastritis and chronic hypertrophic gastritis.

Acute Gastritis. Acute gastritis, as the term implies, is an acute mucosal inflammatory process, usually of transient nature. It tends to recur frequently, and there is much question as to whether repeated episodes of such acute inflammation lead to chronic gastritis (Hurst, 1933) (Joske et al., 1955). This disorder occurs at all ages and in all races.

Pathogenesis. Acute gastritis may best be defined as an inflammation of the gastric mucosa caused by irritants. Increased exfoliation of surface epithelial cells follows. The principal offenders are salicylates (aspirin) and alcohol. Widely unappreciated is the incredible irritant effect of even a few aspirin pills. Markedly increased exfoliation of surface epithelial cells has been shown in the human stomach after 5 to 10 minutes of contact with only 3 aspirin tablets (Croft, 1963). Minor degrees of occult bleeding occur in approximately 70 per cent of patients who take aspirin regularly, as do rheumatoid arthritics (Editorial, 1970b). The irritative effects of this drug depend on both individual susceptibility and dosage. Alcohol as a gastric irritant needs little documentation. Symptoms of alcoholic gastritis may occur within hours but are commonly noted the following morning. Other agents known to produce gastritis include digitalis, iodine, caffeine, cinchophen, phenylbutazone and many of the broad spectrum antibiotics. Obviously, gastritis follows the ingestion of a variety of potent suicidal agents including strong acids, alkalis and mercury salts. Gastric distress is frequently noted by many individuals following dietary excesses of spicy foods, but whether significant histologic changes are associated with such indiscretions remains unproven. The very transient nature of acute gastritis makes it difficult to establish the presence of morphologic changes in these cases.

Special mention should be made of the fulminating forms of gastritis following the ingestion of food contaminated with staphylococcal exotoxin. Little is known of the histologic changes, but the violent vomiting, acute pain and other manifestations referred to the epigastrium strongly suggest some significant form of gastritis.

Depending upon the severity of the insult, the mucosal response may vary from only moderate edema and slight hyperemia to hemorrhagic erosion of the gastric mucosa. In the milder forms, the surface epithelium may be intact and the lamina propria may contain only occasional scattered leukocytes. In the extreme pattern, best referred to as **acute hemorrhagic or erosive gastritis,** there is superficial sloughing of the mucosa, accompanied by hemorrhage into the lamina propria and an acute inflammatory leukocytic infiltrate. Large areas of the gastric mucosa may be denuded, but the involvement is, as stated, superficial and rarely affects the entire depth of the mucosa, sparing the underlying wall. The criteria for differentiating such gastric erosions and acute "stress" ulcers (see below) are exceedingly vague (Ivey, 1971).

Clinical Course. The wide range of morphologic changes embraced by the term "acute gastritis" is paralleled by the range of clinical manifestations. Undoubtedly, minor involvements occur which produce no symptoms. At the other end of the spectrum are the cases with massive hematemesis and acute abdominal pain. In between are those cases manifested by "heartburn," gastric pain, nausea and vomiting. In some instances, the first indica-

tion of the gastritis is the sudden onset of hematemesis or melena. The contribution of acute hemorrhagic gastritis to the clinical pool of massive hematemesis will be discussed on p. 928. It suffices to say here that Valman et al. (1968) have estimated that in Great Britain 25 per cent of all cases of hematemesis and melena arise in severe gastritis related to the widespread use of aspirin.

Chronic (Atrophic) Gastritis. Chronic gastritis is almost always characterized by progressive and irreversible atrophy of the gastric mucosa and hence is often simply designated as atrophic gastritis. It is encountered in two populations of patients, those having pernicious anemia and elderly patients without pernicious anemia. In the first group, there is good evidence that the gastritis is some form of autoimmune disease which selectively destroys parietal cells. These patients cannot elaborate intrinsic factor, so they cannot absorb vitamin B_{12} from the diet and develop a B_{12} deficiency anemia more commonly known as pernicious anemia (p. 715). In elderly patients without pernicious anemia, the mucosal atrophy may be focal or diffuse, mild or severe, and it is not consistently associated with an autoimmune reaction, as will be discussed presently. To this form, the designation *simple* atrophic gastritis is sometimes given. It may well be that we are dealing with a common morphologic end point for more than one pathogenetic pathway.

Pathogenesis. There is a large body of evidence that the atrophic gastritis associated with the adult form of pernicious anemia is caused by an autoimmune reaction (p. 715). It will suffice here to point out that about 90 per cent of these patients have circulating antibodies against parietal cells and about 60 per cent have antibodies against the intrinsic factor itself. The basis for this autoimmune reaction is still uncertain. Some genetic predisposition exists, since it tends to occur in families and, indeed, nonanemic relatives of patients often have chronic gastritis and autoantibodies against parietal cells (Castle, 1970). Further support for a genetic predisposition is found in the higher than chance frequency with which these pernicious anemia patients evidence other forms of autoimmune disease, such as Hashimoto's thyroiditis. Pathologic evidence concurs with the immunologic theory in that significant numbers of lymphocytes and plasma cells are seen in the atrophic gastric mucosa, providing logical sites for the synthesis of autoantibodies.

Simple atrophic gastritis not associated with pernicious anemia is less clearly an autoimmune lesion. Rarely do these patients have antibodies against intrinsic factor. However, about 60 per cent of females and less than 20 per cent of males with simple atrophic gastritis have antiparietal cell autoantibodies. Although these frequencies are significantly above those of the normal population, it is evident that a large number of patients with this form of gastric atrophy have no antibodies. As always, the question arises whether some cause exists for gastric injury which leads secondarily to the elaboration of antibodies. Indeed, habitual smoking, heavy alcohol consumption, hot tea drinking and possibly aspirin abuse may contribute to the development of atrophic gastritis. Croft (1967) makes the statement that an individual over the age of 60 who smokes and drinks heavily has a 60 per cent chance of having simple atrophic gastritis.

Chronic gastritis is also frequently present in patients having a peptic ulcer, gastric carcinoma or iron deficiency anemia.

Morphology. The gross appearance of the stomach varies with the severity of the changes. In the most severe forms associated with pernicious anemia, the stomach wall is thin and the flattened surface red. Rugal folds are flattened or absent, and the velvety appearance of the normal mucosa is replaced by a shiny glazed surface. The redness is the consequence of mucosal thinning to the extent that submucosal blood vessels are visible. Histologically, there are three main alterations in the gastritis related to pernicious anemia: (1) The glandular portion of the mucosa becomes atrophic, ranging from partial loss to almost complete loss. Such glands that persist are shortened and sometimes cystically dilated. There is almost complete absence of parietal cells. Chief cells are replaced by mucus-secreting cells resembling those of the small intestine ("intestinalization"). (2) A marked inflammatory infiltrate is present in the lamina propria of the thinned mucosa. The infiltrate is classically a composite of lymphocytes, occasional plasma cells, neutrophils and eosinophils. (3) The surface epithelial cells undergo megaloid alterations with abnormally large and somewhat atypical nuclei. These nuclear alterations presumably reflect the impact of vitamin B_{12} deficiency on synthesis of DNA and normal replication of cells. The changes may become so severe as to mimic in situ carcinoma and, indeed, they are said to play a causal role in the increased incidence of gastric cancer in pernicious anemia.

Such nuclear and cytoplasmic alterations are not commonly encountered in simple atrophic gastritis. Grossly, the changes are also less impressive; rugal folds are present, though diminished, and mucosal thinning is less. Glands are depleted and distorted, but some parietal cells may persist. The inflammatory infiltrate is less evident.

Clinical Course. The most important clinical association of the atrophic gastritis of pernicious anemia is its predisposition to cancerous transformation. Approximately 10 per cent of patients with this gastric lesion will, over the span of decades, develop cancer of the stomach, a three- to fourfold increase over that expected in normal controls of the same age (Zamchek et al., 1955). There is even some evidence that simple chronic atrophic gastritis has an increased risk of malignant transformation intermediate between pernicious anemia gastritis and normal.

Whatever its clinical setting, the gastric mucosal lesion may be asymptomatic or it may be associated with such vague complaints as upper gastric distress, abdominal pain and, occasionally, nausea and vomiting. Rarely, patients with simple atrophic gastritis have recurrent bleeding, presumably from superficial gastric erosions associated with the mucosal atrophy. In all cases, chronic gastritis produces hypochlorhydria. Those with pernicious anemia have total gastric atrophy, achlorhydria (histamine-fast) and, as mentioned, there is failure to secrete adequate amounts of intrinsic factor, hence the block in absorption of vitamin B_{12}.

Attention should be drawn to the appearance of intercurrent iron deficiency anemia in all patients with atrophic gastritis, whether they have pernicious anemia or not. Chronic bleeding from the gastric mucosa may contribute, but the explanation is more complex. Impaired iron absorption secondary to the hypochlorhydria or achlorhydria, the production by the abnormal gastric mucosa of iron-binding protein, and excessive loss of iron secondary to increased exfoliation of gastric epithelial cells may all participate (Croft, 1963).

Chronic Hypertrophic Gastritis (Menetrier's Disease). This rare entity is better recognized by the designation "giant rugal hypertrophy of the stomach." It is encountered most often in men in their fourth to sixth decades. Most patients have some abdominal distress and pain similar to that caused by a gastric ulcer, but some are asymptomatic. Increased or, in some cases, decreased levels of gastric acid are seen. The gastric rugae are markedly enlarged, and the wall of the stomach is thickened. On gastroscopic or radiographic study, the rugal hypertrophy may simulate a tumorous infiltrate of the stomach. Such changes may be diffuse or may affect only a limited region. Histologically, there is marked cystic dilatation of the glands, along with some evidence of glandular epithelial hyperplasia, which induces tortuosity of the deeper levels of the glands. Biopsy may be necessary to establish the diagnosis and to exclude the possibility of cancer (Butz, 1960).

ACUTE (STRESS) ULCERS

The remarkably labile, fragile gastric mucosa is subject to ulceration in a variety of stressful states:

1. Severe trauma, such as burns, extensive injury and major surgery (Curling's ulcers).
2. Severe infections with or without prior injury.
3. Cerebrovascular accidents, head injury and intracranial surgery (sometimes these are referred to as Cushing's ulcers).
4. Uremia.
5. ACTH or adrenal steroid therapy.
6. In the agonal stages of any fatal illness.
7. Excessive alcohol intake.

From the above listing, it can be deduced that stress ulcers may appear at any age and in either sex.

Pathogenesis. The origins of these acute gastric mucosal erosions are not fully understood, but most of the evidence indicates that they cannot be attributed to a single cause. Those following head injury and intracranial surgery are frequently associated with increased gastric acidity and so are attributed to aggressive acid-peptic digestion. However, in the other clinical settings cited, the lesions are not associated with increased gastric acid levels (Eiseman and Heyman, 1970). Other mechanisms have been invoked. One proposal is that gastric mucous secretion is altered, either quantitatively or qualitatively, such that it less efficiently protects the mucosa (Menguy, 1970). Cortisone and ACTH have been shown to qualitatively alter the gastric mucous secretion. Furthermore, they reduce the rate of shedding of gastric surface epithelial cells, so cell renewal in the gastric mucosa decreases (Max and Menguy, 1970). All forms of stress are known to be associated with increased steroid secretion, presumably acting through the hypothalamus and ACTH. Conceivably, then, many acute gastric erosions result from steroid-mediated mechanisms.

It should be emphasized here that there are no hard lines separating acute stress ulcers from acute erosive or hemorrhagic gastritis. Indeed, the stomach bearing acute ulcers will likely have widespread changes of gastritis. The differentiation that can be made rests largely on the focal erosive nature of the stress ulcer. These ulcers occur as single or multiple discrete lesions in the stomach and rarely in the duodenum. They may be found anywhere in the stomach and do not have the same

predilection for the antral pyloric region and lesser curvature as do chronic peptic ulcers. Stress ulcers tend to be circular and small, usually less than 1 cm. in diameter. They characteristically involve only the mucosa or superficial epithelium and do not penetrate to the muscularis. The ulcer base is frequently stained a dark brown by the acid digestion of the accompanying bleeding (Fig. 21–11). The margins, which rarely show significant hyperemic reaction, are poorly defined because the ulcer is superficial in nature. The rugal pattern is not affected, and the margins and base of the ulcer are not indurated.

Depending upon the duration of the ulceration, there may be some inflammatory infiltration in the margins and base. Red blood cells and fibrin often coat the base. There is usually conspicuous absence of underlying scarring or thickening of blood vessel walls such as is seen in the more chronic forms. Healing with complete reepithelialization occurs as soon as the causative factors are removed. This regrowth of epithelium may be quite active and demonstrate many mitotic figures. It is well known that total replacement of mucosa in animals may occur within 2 days after the formation of the ulcer.

Although these lesions appear and disappear rapidly, potentially they may have great clinical significance, as they can give rise to

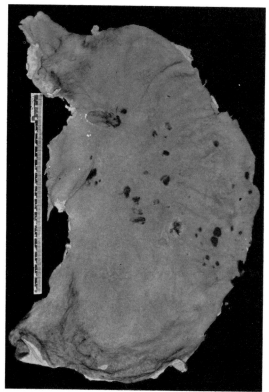

Figure 21–11. *Acute gastric ulcers occurring in a patient dying of severe burns. The dark brown staining is produced by digestion of exuded red cells.*

massive gastrointestinal bleeding. In an analysis of massive hematemesis and melena, acute gastric ulcers were deemed responsible in 3 to 5 per cent of cases (Balasegaram, 1968). Obviously, the severely stressed patient is ill-prepared to cope with the additional complication of gastrointestinal bleeding. If the patient survives, reconstitution of the gastric mucosa can be anticipated in a matter of days. There is no evidence that such acute erosions are antecedents of chronic peptic ulcers.

PEPTIC (CHRONIC) ULCERS

Peptic ulcers are chronic, most often solitary, ulcers occurring in any level of the gastrointestinal tract exposed to the aggressive action of acid-peptic juices. Interestingly, however, the stomach lesions tend to occur in the antral mucosa and only rarely in the acid-secreting parietal cell areas. In economically advanced populations, peptic ulcers are among the commonest clinical problems. They are said to be present in 10 to 15 per cent of the population of the United States. Characteristically, they occur in one of six sites; in descending order of frequency, these are: (1) the duodenum, (2) the stomach, (3) the esophagus, (4) the margins of the stoma of a gastroenterostomy, (5) a Meckel's diverticulum containing heterotopic gastric mucosa and (6) the jejunum in the hypersecretors having the Zollinger-Ellison syndrome. Approximately 98 to 99 per cent of peptic ulcers occur in either the duodenum or the stomach. Most of the following remarks will relate to these lesions.

Wherever they occur, they have a fairly standard, virtually diagnostic gross and microscopic appearance. Despite this uniform morphology, there is much documentation that those ulcers situated in the antral region of the stomach, i.e., gastric ulcers, have a different pathogenesis and represent a "different disease" from the ulcers occurring in the other sites mentioned. Conceivably, as the following discussion will clarify, we may be dealing with a common morphologic expression of more than one pathogenic process.

Incidence. These lesions occur at all ages and in both sexes. Duodenal ulcers have their greatest frequency in middle-aged men (35 to 45 years of age). In contrast, gastric ulcers become progressively more frequent with increasing age. For duodenal ulcer, the ratio of men to women is 7 to 1, but for gastric ulcer, this sex difference is reduced to a ratio of approximately 2 to 1. Indeed, in a recent report from Australia, the incidence of gastric ulcer in women was greater than that in men (Chapman and Duggan, 1969). It is now well documented that among patients with duodenal ulcer, there is a disproportionate number of individuals with blood group O, while those with antral gastric ulcers have blood group A more frequently than chance alone would indicate (Menguy, 1970).

A number of epidemiologic observations are thought-provoking relative to the possible pathogenesis of peptic ulcers. In the United States, for example, duodenal ulcers are much more common than gastric ulcers in a ratio of approximately 7 to 1. In contrast, in Japan gastric ulcers are much more common than duodenal ulcers. During both world wars, the striking increase in the incidence of gastric ulcer in Europe was attributed to psychic stress, dietary restrictions and general deterioration of living conditions. However, in most populations, duodenal ulcer is generally more common in persons working under conditions of tension and high pressure. During the wartime experience, one would have expected the ulcers to be duodenal. Curiously, gastric ulcers tend to occur more often in unskilled workers and in the lower economic classes. It should be evident that there are some striking contrasts in the population distribution of gastric (antral) ulcer and duodenal ulcer.

Pathogenesis. More has been written and less is known about the ultimate genesis of peptic ulcers than perhaps of any other disease in medicine with the possible exception of atherosclerosis. The plethora of writings on this subject are filled with controversy (Kirsner, 1965). In this Augean stable of claim and counterclaim, distinction must be made between observations which are generally accepted and speculations. First, the major well founded observations will be presented, followed by an attempt to integrate them with current proposed mechanisms.

1. Peptic ulcers occur most commonly as single lesions, favoring the duodenum, the nonacid-secreting regions of the stomach and, less often, the other sites listed previously.

2. Peptic ulcers occur only in the presence of acid-peptic digestion. While this statement is made as a flat generalization, some investigators still hold that peptic ulcers may occur in patients with anacidity, but the examples which have been reported as exceptions are open to challenge.

3. On the average, patients with duodenal ulcers have an increased gastric acid-peptic secretion measured both as titrable acidity and maximal histamine response (MHR). Patients with gastric ulcers on the average have a normal to low gastric acidity (both titrable and MHR) but, nonetheless, do have acid-peptic activity in their stomach. There is overlap

between the acid levels encountered in patients with duodenal and those with gastric ulcers as well as overlap between normals and both types of peptic ulcers; the basal level of acid peptic secretion does not differentiate between normals and patients with gastric or duodenal peptic ulcers.

4. The disease appears to be one of civilization and is confined in its spontaneous form to man. In areas where primitive tribes live under identical conditions with more "civilized" populations, ulcers are more frequent in the latter group. Does this association reflect the effects of stressful life?

5. Males are more commonly affected than females.

6. Premenopausal women have a lower incidence of peptic ulcer than postmenopausal women.

7. Gastric ulcer occurs in patients having an active or healed duodenal ulcer with a prevalence variously reported as 10 to 50 per cent (average 25 to 30 per cent). Under these circumstances, the gastric ulcer is referred to as "secondary" to differentiate it from "primary gastric ulcers" that occur in the absence of duodenal ulcers.

8. There is a high level of concurrence (50 to 100 per cent) between chronic gastritis and gastric ulcers (Magnus, 1952).

9. There is a well documented association between the capacity of the gastric mucosa to elaborate acid and its number of parietal cells (Cox, 1963). Patients with duodenal ulcers have a higher parietal cell mass (1.8 billion cells) than normal (1.09 billion cells in the male, and 0.82 in the female). In contrast, patients with gastric ulcers have no elevated parietal cell count and, in fact, tend to have lower than normal values conforming to the observed data on the acid output of these various groups.

10. Multiple and severe peptic ulcerations occur as low in the intestinal tract as the jejunum in the Zollinger-Ellison syndrome with its extreme gastric hypersecretion. These patients usually have a noninsulin-secreting adenoma of the pancreas that produces a gastrin-like substance capable of evoking excessive levels of gastric acidity.

It is impossible to encompass all these observations in any single theory of causation. Indeed, one may ask why the stomach does not normally digest its entire gastric mucosa and why the peptic ulcer occurs most often as a single focus of erosion. Since *acute* gastric ulcers heal rapidly, perhaps we should be asking what factors impede healing and perpetuate the chronic inflammatory erosion. Most theories of causation start with the proposition

that *peptic ulceration reflects an imbalance between the aggressive action of acid-peptic secretions and the defensive forces that protect the normal mucosa. A reasonable argument can be made that gastric (antral) ulcers result from lowered defensive mechanisms, and duodenal ulcers (including those occurring in the esophagus, stomata, Meckel's diverticulum and the Zollinger-Ellison syndrome) are the consequence of the destructive action of increased acid-peptic secretions.*

Turning first to the role of hypersecretion in the causation of the *duodenal ulcer,* it can be said that these lesions never occur unless the gastric mucosa can secrete substantial amounts of acid. Although some patients with duodenal ulcers have normal levels of acid secretion, on the average, they are hyperchlorhydric (Grossman et al., 1963). Consonant with these increased levels of gastric acid are the data on parietal cell mass presented earlier. Most duodenal ulcers heal rapidly when gastric output of hydrochloric acid is reduced by medical or surgical intervention. Duodenal ulcers can be induced in the experimental animal by procedures which increase gastric acid secretion. Perhaps the most convincing evidence of the relationship of hypersecretion of acid-peptic juices and duodenal ulcers is the clinical experiment exemplified by the Zollinger-Ellison syndrome (p. 1074). These patients have pancreatic tumors and multiple peptic ulcers associated with extraordinary gastric acid production (10 to 20 times normal). These ulcers occur in such aberrant locations as the jejunum, third and fourth portions of the duodenum, and esophagus. The isolation of gastrin from some of these tumors has clarified a mechanism of the hypersecretion (Gregory et al., 1960).

If one grants the association between excessive acid-peptic secretion and duodenal ulcers, one must still ask why patients who do not have the Zollinger-Ellison syndrome are hypersecretors. Recall that gastric acid secretion has two phases: (1) a cephalic phase (vagally mediated), in which direct cholinergic stimulation of parietal cells induces gastrin release from the antrum, and (2) a less powerful antral phase when food enters the stomach, causing the liberation of more gastrin from the antral mucosa. Although it is clear that transection of the vagus nerves (vagotomy) substantially reduces the hyperacidity of patients with duodenal ulcers there is no good evidence that abnormal vagal activity is responsible for hypersecretion (Menguy, 1970). Neither is there any substantial evidence that these patients suffer from abnormally high serum gastrin levels. The evidence that patients with duodenal ulcers have an increased parietal cell mass might suggest a genetic predisposition.

However, experimental data indicate that parietal cell hyperplasia can be acquired. It is possible to induce parietal cell hyperplasia in dogs by so-called work-hypertrophy, as when an antral pouch is transplanted to the colon. In short, the basis for the hypersecretion of gastric acid is still unknown.

There are reasons, moreover, for believing that mere levels of acidity are not the whole story. Duodenal ulcer is three times more common in patients with pulmonary emphysema than in control populations. This phenomenon is not related to alterations in the pH of the blood. The basal gastric acidity in these patients does not differ from that of normal subjects (Kramer and Markarian, 1960). Duodenal ulcers are generally thought to be somewhat more common in patients with primary hyperparathyroidism and, conversely, hyperparathyroidism is much more common among patients with duodenal ulcer than in the general population. Here the association is unclear. It may reflect the concurrence of parathyroid and pancreatic adenomas in the condition known as multiple endocrine adenomatosis (p. 1074) with the pancreatic lesion inducing the Zollinger-Ellison syndrome (p. 1074). Alternatively, there may be stimulation of gastric secretion by the increased serum levels of calcium (Black, 1971). Duodenal ulcers are also more common, again for obscure reasons, in patients with alcoholic cirrhosis. There is no clear evidence that such patients have gastric acidity higher than that in cirrhotic patients without an ulcer (Ostrow et al., 1960). There is no simple explanation, then, for the causation of duodenal ulcers.

The pathogenesis of *gastric ulcers* is, if possible, even more mysterious than that of duodenal ulceration. Once more, it should be emphasized that the present usage of the term "gastric ulcer" refers to those peptic ulcers developing in the antral mucosa. Lesions in the pyloric canal are more like duodenal ulcers than gastric ulcers and probably belong to the category "duodenal ulcer disease." Reference has already been made to the many differences relative to age incidence, sex distribution and blood group antigens between persons with gastric antral ulcers and those with duodenal ulcers. An even more important difference is the fact that *patients with gastric ulcer have normal or even abnormally low levels of gastric acid secretion.* Only rarely, if ever, are they achlorhydric. It has been proposed that gastric stasis and prolongation of the gastrin phase of acid secretion lengthen the exposure of the gastric mucosa to acid-peptic aggression (Dragstedt et al., 1954) (Dragstedt, 1954). Delayed gastric emptying cannot always be demonstrated in patients with gastric ulcers. Accordingly, *recourse has been made to the hypothesis that gastric ulceration results largely from lowering of the gastric mucosal resistance.* Principal among the defensive influences is mucus secretion. The increased frequency of gastric ulcers with advancing age might be compatible with progressive inability to secrete a protective layer of mucus. Chronic gastritis is a frequent, if not invariable, concomitant of gastric ulcer, is associated with impaired mucous secretion, and is also age related. It is by no means clear, however, that the gastritis always precedes the ulcer. In experimental animals, it has been demonstrated that protein depletion, avitaminoses and general malnutrition increase the susceptibility to gastric ulceration. Certainly, these influences are more prone to be present in aging patients. Lining epithelial cell renewal might be slowed with advancing age as well. All of these possibilities are purely speculative as, indeed, is the concept of lowered gastric mucosal resistance.

There has never been even a remotely satisfying theory to explain why gastric ulcers most often occur singly in the antral region of the stomach and duodenal ulcers chiefly in the first and second parts of the duodenum. It has been vaguely postulated that the upright position of man allows the drag of the stomach to produce tension on and narrowing of the tortuous left gastric artery, with resultant inadequate blood supply to these regions. Chronic peptic ulcers do not develop spontaneously in quadrupeds. This hypothesis still fails to explain the tendency for ulcers to occur singly. Unfortunately, there are no adequate hemodynamic studies validating relative ischemia to the sites predisposed to ulceration. We can conclude by admitting that the origins of both duodenal and gastric ulcers are the proverbial enigmas wrapped in mystery.

Morphology. The naked-eye appearance of a chronic peptic ulcer is quite characteristic; most can be recognized on sight — a fact of great importance because the differentiation of a benign from a malignant gastric ulcer is an everyday surgical problem. The salient macroscopic features can be considered under the headings of site, size and appearance.

The principal **sites of peptic ulceration** are the stomach and duodenum. Approximately 25 to 30 per cent of gastric ulcers occur in patients who have or have had a duodenal ulcer and, under these circumstances, are termed "secondary gastric ulcers," the remainder being called "primary gastric ulcers." **The favored locations of peptic ulceration are, in order of frequency, the anterior wall of the first portion of the duodenum, the posterior wall of the first portion, the second portion of the**

duodenum, and then the antral region of the stomach along the lesser curvature, most in the immediate prepyloric region (Fig. 21–12).

Gastric ulcers, however, may occur anywhere in the stomach. **In pathologic practice, as many as 14 per cent of benign gastric ulcers occur on or in contact with the greater curvature** (Boudreau et al., 1951). So-called atypical locations, outside of the stomach and duodenum account for not more than 1 or 2 per cent of the total incidence of peptic ulcers.

In terms of **size,** peptic ulcers are usually small; well over 50 per cent are less than 2 cm. in diameter, and 75 per cent are less than 3 cm. However, about 10 per cent of benign ulcers are greater than 4 cm. in diameter. Almost all these larger lesions occur in the stomach. Some carcinomatous ulcers are less than 4 cm. in diameter. **Size, therefore, does not differentiate a benign from a malignant ulcer.**

In **appearance,** the classic peptic ulcer is a round to oval, sharply punched-out defect with relatively straight walls perpendicular to the base. The mucosal margin may overhang the base slightly, particularly on the proximal portion of the circumference. The margins are usually level with the surrounding mucosa or are only slightly elevated (Fig. 21–13). Heaping up or beading of these margins is extremely rare in the benign ulcer but is character-

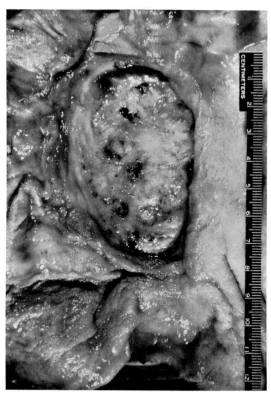

Figure 21–13. A large benign peptic ulcer illustrating the sharply defined margins which overhang on the proximal aspect (right) and shelve on the distal aspect. Note the absence of beading of the margin and apparent absence of necrotic tissue in the clean-appearing base. Despite the 8 cm. diameter, no malignancy is present.

istic of the malignant lesion. The depth of the ulcer varies from superficial lesions involving only the mucosa, down to deeply excavated penetrating ulcers having their base in the muscularis. Penetration of the entire wall may occur and, occasionally, the base of the ulcer may be formed by the adjacent pancreas, omental fat or adherent liver. Characteristically, the base of all peptic ulcers is smooth and clean owing to peptic digestion of any exudate. At times, thrombosed or even patent vessels that provided the site of a fatal hemorrhage project into the base. In most chronic peptic ulcers, underlying scarring causes puckering of the surrounding mucosa so that the mucosal folds radiate out from the crater in spoke-like fashion. Such a mucosal pattern provides a valuable clue to the location of the lesion for surgeon, pathologist and radiologist alike.

The histologic appearance varies with the activity, chronicity and amount of healing. In the stage of active necrosis, four zones are classically demonstrable: (1) the base and margins have a superficial thin layer of necrotic fibrinoid debris not visible to the naked eye; (2) beneath this layer is the

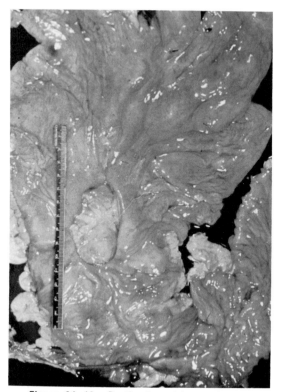

Figure 21–12. Peptic ulcer. A large, deeply excavated peptic ulcer occurring in the prepyloric region of the stomach along the lesser curvature.

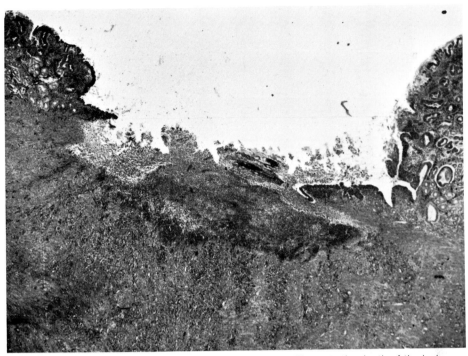

Figure 21–14. A low power view of a peptic ulcer to illustrate the depth of the lesion.

zone of active nonspecific cellular infiltrate with neutrophils predominating; (3) in the deeper layers, especially in the base of the ulcer, there is active granulation tissue infiltrated with mononuclear leukocytes; and (4) the granulation tissue rests on a more solid fibrous or collagenous scar (Fig. 21–14 and 21–15). The scarring characteristically fans out widely and may extend to the serosal surface. To be particularly noted are the mucosal margins which bear the brunt of epithelial regeneration and inflammatory change. Often these glands become totally mucus secreting, a change referred to as "intestinalization." If carcinomatous transformation is imminent, these areas provide the first histologic clue. The vessel walls within the scarred area are characteristically thickened by the surrounding inflammation and occasionally are thrombosed.

Peptic ulcers may heal to varying degrees, depending upon their chronicity and their size. The superficial lesions without significant underlying scarring may completely reepithelialize to leave no residual trace. As the scarring becomes more intense, regeneration of the mucosa is less perfect and healing is retarded presumably because blood supply is impaired.

Clinical Course. The symptoms evoked by peptic ulcers are exceedingly variable; some ulcers are virtually asymptomatic. Nausea and vomiting may be produced by either duodenal or gastric ulcers, but particularly by the latter. The most consistent manifestation, however, is

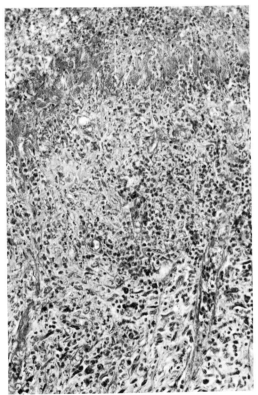

Figure 21–15. A high power detail of the base of an ulcer demonstrating some of the zones that comprise the inflammatory response. The zone of fibrinoid necrosis is above.

epigastric pain described variably as burning, gnawing or boring. Even more important is the episodic nature of the pain, both in the context of a single day and over the span of months. Classically, the duodenal ulcer pain becomes most severe two to three hours after the last meal and persists until it is relieved by food or antacids. For this reason, the pain often recurs in the middle of the night and requires a glass of milk or antacids for its relief. Typically, the patient with a gastric ulcer experiences pain almost immediately after eating and then, after an hour or two, experiences some relief. Such episodic pain may last for a few weeks or months only to abate, usually with a regulated dietary regimen and therapy. For the next few months, the patient may be asymptomatic, only to have a recurrence of symptoms, triggered often by dietary indiscretions or stress.

Under appropriate medical management, i.e., regulated diet and antacids, duodenal ulcers generally respond favorably and, indeed, by radiography, can be seen to "fill in" and apparently heal. Such patients may be free of their disease for the rest of their lives, but most have a recurrence months to years later. Thus, although the lesion is cured, the patient with the duodenal ulcer is never cured. The same may be said of gastric ulcers, but since these respond far less well to conservative medical management, they are more apt to require a vagotomy or a partial gastrectomy, which obviously abort the natural course of this disease.

Although gastric and peptic ulcers produce quite distinctive symptom patterns, the diagnosis and localization of peptic ulcer disease almost invariably requires barium x-ray studies. In general, radiography is about 90 per cent accurate in diagnosing duodenal ulcers and 70 per cent accurate with gastric ulcers. While quantitative studies of gastric acidity, including histamine response, are of some value, as indicated earlier there are overlaps among "normals," gastric ulcer and duodenal ulcer patients.

The complications of peptic ulcer disease are: (1) bleeding, (2) perforation, (3) obstruction from edema or from scarring of the pylorus or duodenum, and (4) malignant transformation. Bleeding, sometimes massive, is the commonest of these complications. It is estimated that one-fourth to one-third of peptic ulcers give rise to significant bleeding and, indeed, massive hematemesis may be the first evidence of the existence of the ulcer in a previously asymptomatic patient (Chandler, 1967). The mortality rate in these bleeding patients ranges from 3 to 10 per cent. Fatal hematemesis is responsible for about one-

fourth of all deaths attributable to peptic ulcer disease. Although perforation of an ulcer is infrequent, occurring in only about 5 per cent of patients, it is a grave complication and accounts for about 65 per cent of all deaths in these patients (Fig. 21–16). Incredibly, perforation may be the first indication of the existence of the ulcer. Obstruction is encountered only in ulcers occurring either within the pyloric canal or duodenum and, while it may produce serious vomiting and fluid-electrolyte disturbances, it rarely is a threat to life. Malignant transformation of an ulcer is unknown with duodenal lesions. The frequency with which gastric ulceration leads to cancer is still a debated issue. Although older reports have cited that 5 to 10 per cent of gastric ulcers may be expected to give rise to a carcinoma, recent studies make it clear that this occurs in 1 per cent or less (Paustian et al., 1960). Much of the controversy stems from the difficulty in distinguishing ulcerative gastric cancers from peptic ulcers which have truly undergone malignant transformation (Mallory, 1940). In the past, many ulcerated gastric cancers have been interpreted as previously benign peptic ulcers with secondary cancerous transformation. Sufficient evidence has now been accumulated to

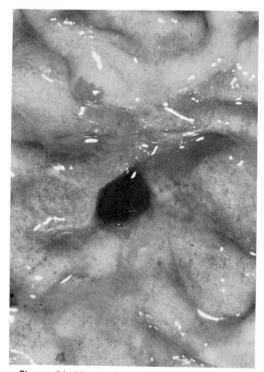

Figure 21–16. *A close-up view of a small, completely penetrating duodenal ulcer. The diameter of the mucosal defect is approximately 1 cm., with the perforation being of almost equal size.*

permit the statement that "cancers commonly ulcerate, but ulcers rarely cancerate."

Despite these complications, most patients with peptic ulcers die with their disease rather than of it. Nonetheless, they bear the burden of an ulcer throughout their life, and many come to surgery because of intractable pain or one of the complications mentioned. In persons with gastric lesions, the inability to rule out the possibility of an ulcerating cancer masquerading as a peptic ulcer often demands surgical intervention.

TUMORS

Of the wide variety of benign and malignant neoplasms that occur in the stomach, the gastric carcinoma is unquestionably the most important. It alone represents about 70 per cent of all stomach neoplasms, including both the benign and malignant. Second in importance in terms of frequency and clinical significance are the gastric adenomas, also known as polyps. All the remainder are encountered infrequently and can be entertained as a clinical diagnosis only when the previously mentioned lesions have first been ruled out.

BENIGN

A review of benign tumors of the stomach listed the following with their relative frequencies (Ochsner and Janitos, 1965):

Name	Per Cent
Adenoma	38
Leiomyoma	26
Lipoma	5
Aberrant pancreas	3
Neurogenic	2
Inflammatory polyp	2
Hemangioma	1
Lymphangioma	1
Carcinoid	1
Fibroma	1

This compilation indicates that adenomas and leiomyomas comprise 64 per cent of all benign neoplasms of the stomach.

Adenomas are important because some tend to become malignant. They may occur singly or multiply and usually are small but sometimes reach diameters of 5 to 10 cm. Some are pedunculated on a slender stalk, while others are sessile and sit upon the gastric mucosa. Virtually identical lesions occur much

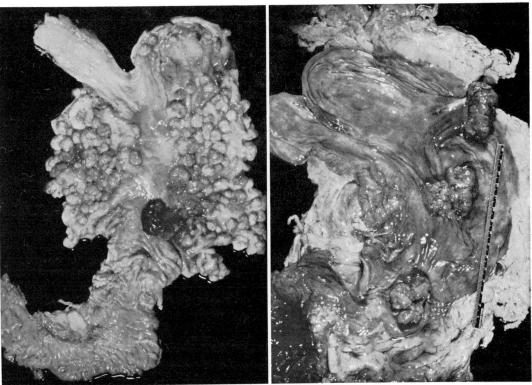

Fig. 21–17.

Fig. 21–18.

Figure 21–17. Gastric polyposis. Innumerable small polyps in a patient with polyposis of the entire gastrointestinal tract (congenital polyposis).

Figure 21–18. Multiple benign pedunculated polyps of the stomach averaging 3 to 4 cm. in diameter.

more frequently in the colon, (p. 962) (Figs. 21–17 and 21–18). Leiomyomas usually appear as small submucosal masses ranging up to 2 to 3 cm. in diameter. Rarely, they exceed this size. They are encapsulated, round to oval gray nodules and are almost invariably overlaid by intact mucosa. They generally do not cause symptoms and are usually discovered incidentally in the course of x-ray examination for other disease of the intestinal tract. The principal importance of these lesions is their differentiation from cancer, since they may appear as small masses that project into the lumen of the stomach.

The aberrant pancreas is included in this listing because it, too, has a radiologic appearance of a neoplasm that must be differentiated from a malignant tumor.

CARCINOMA

Gastric carcinoma is one of the most common and puzzling cancers in man. Only a few decades ago, it was close to the top of the list of lethal cancers in the United States. The incidence of this neoplasm has steadily fallen for the past six decades, and it now rates fifth as a cause of death in this country. The reason for this decline in frequency is totally obscure.

Incidence. Although gastric carcinoma may appear at any age and in either sex, it is rare in the first three decades of life, but thereafter it steadily mounts in frequency throughout life. Males are affected twice as often as females.

Pathogenesis. A number of intriguing hereditary, racial and environmental factors are associated with the appearance of gastric carcinoma. This neoplasm occurs four times more often in families of patients with gastric carcinoma than in the normal population. A disproportionate fraction of those afflicted have group A blood. Gastric carcinoma is far more frequent in Japan, Iceland, Finland, Norway and Chile than it is in the United States. Japanese who have migrated to the United States have an incidence of gastric carcinoma intermediate between those characteristic of their native and adopted countries. Although hereditary influences cannot be excluded, environmental factors are thought to be more important in these national differences (Dawson, 1967). The high incidence in Iceland has been attributed to diets heavy in smoked fish and meat. A polycyclic hydrocarbon (benzpyrene), isolated from these smoked foods, is capable of inducing neoplasms in rats but, strangely, not in their gastrointestinal tracts (Dungal, 1961). Efforts to identify significant dietary differences between groups af-

flicted with gastric carcinoma and control populations in the same country have not been revelatory, however (Acheson and Doll, 1964). Recently, interest has risen in the possible role of food preservatives containing nitrites in the causation of this form of cancer. Recall that nitrosamines are known to be carcinogenic in the experimental animal.

Certain disorders may be considered precancerous insofar as they carry a definitely increased risk of gastric carcinoma. These include the interrelated triad of pernicious anemia, atrophic gastritis and achlorhydria, as well as benign adenomas (polyps) of the stomach. As cited earlier, about 10 per cent of patients with longstanding pernicious anemia and its associated atrophic gastritis may be expected to develop gastric carcinoma (Zamcheck et al., 1955). Patients with simple atrophic gastritis and achlorhydria are also at some increased risk, but not as great as those with pernicious anemia. Conversely, about 75 per cent of patients with gastric cancer have abnormally low levels of gastric acid secretion. In all likelihood, the cancerous transformation relates primarily to the cellular changes encountered in atrophic gastritis rather than to the loss of gastric acid secretion secondary to the atrophic gastritis. The higher risk with pernicious anemia is thought to relate to the impaired DNA synthesis resulting from the deficiency of vitamin B_{12} (p. 715). The evidence supporting the association of gastric polyps with carcinoma is the frequent finding (in approximately 10 to 20 per cent of such lesions) of focal malignant changes.

Studies have also shown that gastric cancers tend to arise over a large area of mucosal surface. They apparently do not arise in a solitary deviant gland or cell. As a consequence, one locus may give origin to one histologic pattern that differs from that of an adjoining area. From this multicentric origin, the separate tumors may eventually coalesce to produce a single cancerous mass (Collins and Gall, 1952). Whatever the nature of the carcinogenic factors, clearly they must be operative over broad areas of mucosa.

Morphology. Over half of gastric cancers originate in the pyloric and prepyloric regions. These have been subdivided on the basis of their gross morphology in various ways, but the simplest and most useful classification recognizes three patterns:

	Per Cent
Ulcerative	28
Fungating or polypoid	23
Spreading or infiltrative	13

The remaining third are so advanced at the time they are seen as to be unclassifiable.

The **ulcerative pattern** differs anatomically in many respects from its benign counterpart. While occurring most often in the prepyloric region, as do benign peptic ulcers, they are more likely to occur on the greater curvature. Nevertheless, as many as 30 per cent arise on or are in contact with the lesser curvature. These malignant ulcers tend to be larger than their benign counterparts, and about half are greater than 4 cm. in diameter. Some become huge excavations, 15 to 20 cm. in diameter. It must not be overlooked that some ulcerating cancers which have caused death are less than 1 cm. in diameter. Classically, the cancerous crater has a very distinctive appearance with heaped-up, beaded, firm overhanging margins and a necrotic shaggy base (Fig. 21–19). In many cases, the ulcer crater sits in the center of an elevated mucosal plaque, suggesting the preexistence of a solid tumor that eventually underwent ischemic necrosis in its center (Fig. 21–20). Mucosal folds do not radiate from the base of malignant ulcers as they do in the benign cases.

The **polypoid cancers** are large fungating cauliflower masses that protrude into the lumen from broad bases. They vary in size from small (3 to 4 cm.) masses to tumors that virtually fill the lumen. It has always been assumed without good proof that most of these cancers arise in preexisting benign adenomas.

The spreading **infiltrative** type may grow superficially along the mucosa or may directly permeate the wall. The superficial spread causes large plaque-like lesions that smooth out the gastric mucosa and flatten the rugal folds. The mucosa loses its normal velvety appearance and becomes opaque, rigid and attached to the deeper layers. More often, the infiltration permeates the entire thickness of the wall to produce the so-called **linitis plastica**. The wall is strikingly thickened up to 2 to 3 cm. and assumes a cartilaginous rigidity. This has been likened to a "leather bottle." On section, such thickening can be seen to be due to a permeation of gritty white tumor, particularly in the submucosal and subserosal regions, spreading the layers of the stomach apart. The mucosa loses its mobility, becomes fused to the underlying wall, and is atrophic and flattened (Fig. 21–21). Shallow ulcerations are often present, and seeding is frequently apparent on the serosal surface.

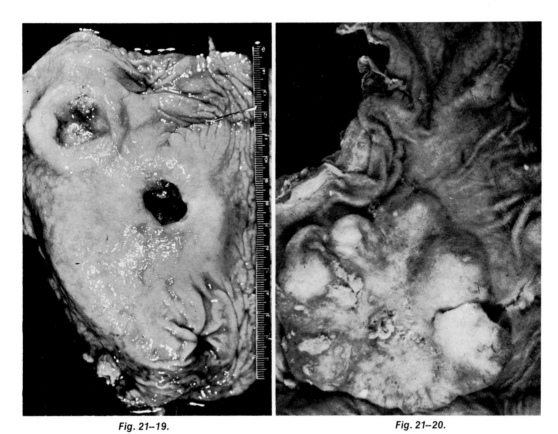

Fig. 21–19. Fig. 21–20.

Figure 21–19. *Ulcerative pattern of gastric carcinoma. A late stage with diffuse infiltration of the wall and two distinct crater formations, one to the left with typical beaded overhanging margins, and one to the right with deep excavation.*

Figure 21–20. *A plaque-like cancer of the stomach showing beginning central necrosis and excavation.*

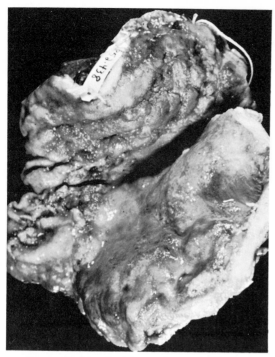

Figure 21-21. *Gastric carcinoma infiltrative pattern (linitis plastica). The anterior wall is diffusely thickened, with flattening of the rugal folds.*

Whatever the gross appearance of the tumor, the histologic pattern is usually that of a well differentiated adenocarcinoma, but one may encounter various stages of differentiation even to a totally undifferentiated growth. There is no correlation between the gross form of tumor and the histologic detail. In the ulcerative pattern, neoplastic tissue is found in the margins and base of the ulcer. The ulcer defect is, as it were, carved out of tumor. The presence of anaplastic glands in the base of the lesion is one of the features that helps to differentiate the ulcerative gastric cancer from the malignant transformation of a benign ulcer. **When a peptic ulcer becomes malignant, the transformation occurs at the mucosal margins and, very often, if the neoplasia is not too far advanced, the base remains free of tumor infiltration. This** criterion is obviously of no value in advanced cases in which spread of tumor obliterates the characteristic inflammatory changes of peptic ulcer and, moreover, totally infiltrates the entire area.

Most polypoid growths produce a glandular, sometimes papillary histologic pattern. Undifferentiated growth generally characterizes the infiltrative tumors. In linitis plastica, the increased thickness of the wall is due not only to the tumor, but also to a massive desmoplastic reaction which accompanies these neoplasms. The thickness of the wall may be due in greatest part to fibrous tissue that contains only scattered isolated or nested tumor

cells. Sometimes it is quite difficult to find the cancer cells.

Mucin secretion is common in any of the histologic types. This secretion may remain within cells to produce "signet ring cells" or be distributed extracellularly as large accumulations of interstitial or intraglandular basophilic mucin. In the light of the multicentric origin of many gastric cancers, it is not surprising that the histologic pattern may vary from one region to another and, for example, be essentially glandular in one area and undifferentiated in another (Stout, 1943).

Mention should be made of in situ carcinoma of the gastric mucosa. It is clear that gastric cancers arise as in situ lesions that remain confined to the glandular epithelium without invading even the lamina propria of the mucosa. Because of the inaccessibility of these lesions, and because these in situ lesions do not evoke symptoms, we have no knowledge as to how long it takes for an in situ lesion to produce an overt cancerous mass. But that such an evolution occurs is well documented by the frequent finding of persistent in situ changes in the margins of frank cancers.

Clinical Course. Little is known of the early manifestations of gastric carcinoma since it so often remains occult for long periods of time. Commonly, when these patients come to medical attention, they have anorexia, epigastric distress, weight loss, melena, anemia and achlorhydria (Lahey and Jordan, 1934). Sometimes an epigastric mass is palpable. By the time symptoms occur, spread to the regional nodes and the liver is common. Widespread metastases to the lungs, brain, bone and, strikingly, the ovaries (so-called Krukenberg tumors) are frequent. Spread to the supraclavicular nodes, sometimes referred to as *Virchow's nodes*, is no longer considered to be pathognomonic of gastric cancer, since it is more commonly a manifestation of lung or esophageal carcinoma or of a primary lymphoma of nodes. However, in many cases of gastric carcinoma, the supraclavicular nodes and particularly, according to recent evidence, the scalene nodes are seeded. It is, therefore, standard practice in many clinics to biopsy the scalene nodes in cases of suspected occult gastric carcinoma, even if the nodes are not palpable. Seeding of the peritoneal cul-de-sac to produce a rectal shelf palpable by digital examination is an additional, peculiarly characteristic form of spread of gastric carcinoma. Direct invasion of adjacent organs sometimes occurs, and necrosis of such tumor tissue may produce fistulas between the stomach and other segments of gut, particularly the colon (gastrocolic fistula).

Most lesions are inoperable at the time of

discovery and permit a survival of 12 to 18 months. Overall, the five-year survival is about 10 per cent. However, it is hoped that this discouraging statistic can be improved with newer and better diagnostic techniques. Examination of properly obtained and prepared smears of the gastric secretions permits a correct cytologic diagnosis of cancer in 70 to 90 per cent of anatomically confirmed lesions. Since even the in situ lesions exfoliate anaplastic cells, they can be diagnosed at a stage when surgical resection may still produce a cure. Periodic cytologic examination has also proved of inestimable value in following pernicious anemia patients with their known vulnerability to gastric cancer.

CARCINOID

While carcinoid lesions of the stomach are rare, they tend, like those in the small and large intestine, to be infiltrative aggressive tumors that metastasize in about a third of the cases. These will be described in greater detail later (p. 942).

SARCOMA

Mesenchymal malignancies are rare in the stomach. When they occur, they produce either large, bulky intramural masses which eventually fungate and ulcerate into the gastric lumen, or otherwise cause marked thickening of the wall with increased prominence of the rugae. A common pattern is that of a large, spherical, intramural mass with a small mucosal ulcer over the prominence of the intraluminal projection. Their large size and gray, soft, yielding substance make them distinctive from carcinoma. Histologically, they may be fibrosarcomas, leiomyosarcomas, endothelial sarcomas or lymphomas.

Lymphomas are of special interest. Anatomically, they resemble their analogues in the small intestines (p. 941). Although they occur as primary neoplasms throughout the gastrointestinal tract, they most often arise in the stomach. Any one of the histologic types discussed earlier (p. 752), including Hodgkin's disease, may arise in the stomach, presumably from lymphoid cells native to the stomach. The gross appearance of these lesions varies. Some grow as bulky, intraluminal masses, often with ulceration of the dome of the mass. Sometimes these masses become polypoid. Others appear as multinodular, multicentric involvements (McNeer and Berg, 1959). Sometimes the lymphoma diffusely permeates the wall, causing massive enlargement of the rugal folds, which simulates giant rugal hypertrophy of the

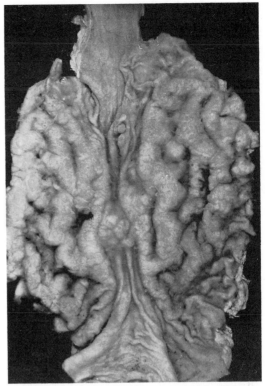

Figure 21–22. A lymphoma of the stomach showing the marked accentuation of the rugal folds produced by the diffuse infiltrative type of growth.

gastric mucosa (p. 915) (Fig. 21–22). All gross patterns are softer, grayer and more rubbery than the usual gastric carcinoma. It is important to caution that chronic gastritis and chronic peptic ulcer may lead to massive inflammatory infiltrates into the stomach wall, creating more than a casual resemblance, both grossly and microscopically, to a true lymphoma. Such inflammatory lesions have been designated *pseudolymphoma*. Gastric lymphomas may arise as isolated lesions without involvement of other sites and thus are amenable to surgical cure.

METASTATIC CARCINOMA

Metastatic involvement of the stomach is a rarity. Although such spread may be produced by carcinomas arising elsewhere, the most common form occurs in generalized lymphomatosis or leukemia (Fig. 21–23). Most lesions are multiple and differ from primary tumors in that they usually affect the submucosa and muscularis primarily and only secondarily invade the mucosa. Central ulceration of these masses may occur.

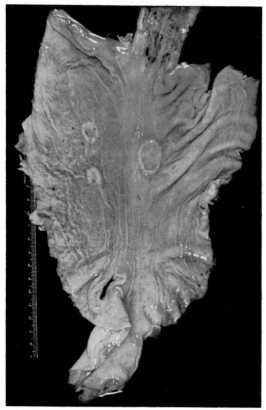

Figure 21–23. *Metastatic foci of Hodgkin's disease in the stomach, showing central ulceration of the implants.*

GASTRIC LESIONS AS CLINICAL PROBLEMS

Differential Diagnosis of Gastric Lesions.
When correlating clinical manifestations with gastric disorders, one must realize that all stomach derangements evoke a fairly limited range of manifestations. Thus, any significant gastric lesion may lead to disturbances of appetite, a sense of fullness, belching, nausea, vomiting, anorexia and/or epigastric pain. Bleeding may result from any disorder that produces a defect in the gastric mucosa. So-called "rhythmic pain," usually associated with peptic ulcer, may be produced by gastric cancer or gastritis. It is, therefore, frequently impossible to arrive at a specific clinical diagnosis without resort to radiography, gastroscopy, gastric chemical analysis and cytologic examination; even then, the issue may remain in doubt.

As with all systems, the probability of a given diagnosis being correct correlates with the epidemiologic frequency of that disease. Gastritis, peptic ulceration and carcinoma together comprise the basis for over 90 per cent of gastric symptomatology. Although we cannot enter here into a definitive differential diagnosis of these three lesions, certain broad generalizations can be made. Gastritis is usually a much more evanescent disease than the other two. The symptoms appear suddenly and disappear equally rapidly. Often the symptoms are related to some dietary indiscretion. Most importantly, simple therapy provides prompt relief. X-ray studies may be necessary to rule out tumors or ulcerations.

The differentiation of a benign peptic ulcer from an ulcerative cancer may be much more difficult. The polypoid and infiltrative tumors are usually readily recognized gastroscopically or radiographically. If the ulcer is found in the duodenum, then it can be safely considered benign. It is the gastric lesion that evokes concern. Cytologic examination is valuable if the smear discloses unmistakably anaplastic cells; however, a negative result does not exclude gastric cancer or make a definite diagnosis of benign peptic ulcer. The radiographic findings are usually fairly definitive in 80 to 90 per cent of cases but, for the remainder, the issue may remain in doubt. As previously mentioned, the size and site of the crater are not very useful in the individual case. The demonstration of increased levels of gastric acidity is also not diagnostic, since patients with gastric cancer may have hypersecretion and patients with gastric peptic ulcers may have abnormally low levels of acid-peptic secretion. The problem must be evaluated from all aspects. Even then, the final diagnosis must often await histologic examination at the time of surgical removal. Some of the more helpful clinical features are included in Table 21–1.

It has been estimated that approximately 10 to 30 per cent of peptic ulcers defy clear-cut clinical appraisal as to whether they are benign or malignant. To quote from the study of Sampson and Sosman (1939): "Proved cases of prepyloric malignant ulcers are herewith reported: (a) in young persons, (b) with high gastric acidity, (c) with clinical improvement under ulcer therapy, (d) with decrease in the size of the ulcer under alkaline therapy, and (e) with roentgen findings simulating benign ulcer."

Hematemesis. The vomiting of blood can be one of the most alarming medical emergencies. The term "massive," as it relates to hematemesis, is here defined as blood loss leading to shock, lowering of the red cell count to 3,000,000 per mm.³ or less and reduction in the hemoglobin level to below 50 per cent. Massive hematemesis of this magnitude produces a mortality rate in the range of 15 per cent (Chandler, 1967). In some series, higher mortality rates have been reported (up to 66 per cent), depending on the patient population

TABLE 21–1. CLINICAL FEATURES OF BENIGN AND MALIGNANT ULCERS

	Benign Ulcer	Malignant Ulcer
Age of patient	Tends to occur in younger individuals	Tends to occur in older individuals
Duration of symptoms	Varies from weeks to many years	Varies from weeks to months, but rarely for years
Sex	Marked male preponderance	Slight male preponderance
Gastric acidity	May be normal or increased—anacidity rare	Usually normal levels, but can be totally absent
Location of lesion	Usually lesser curvature of pyloric or prepyloric region—however, may be on greater curvature or anterior or posterior wall	Greater curvature of pyloric and prepyloric regions—however, may be on lesser curvature or in other sites in stomach
Size of lesion	Usually is less than 2 cm. in diameter and rarely over 4 cm.	Usually greater than 4 cm. in diameter, but may be smaller
Response to medical therapy	Usually shows prompt evidence of healing on adequate treatment	May respond to medical therapy, but usually is refractory
X-ray	Demonstrates a small punched-out niche without involvement of surrounding wall	Demonstrates defect with irregular or heaped-up margins and possible involvement of surrounding wall and mucosa

analyzed. It is difficult to establish generally applicable data on the distribution of upper gastrointestinal lesions responsible for such massive bleeding. The many reported series differ both in the criteria used to define "massive" and in the patient populations analyzed. Most agree, however, that in a large general hospital dealing with a wide variety of clinical problems, peptic ulcers top the list (Weber et al., 1957) (Tanner, 1954). In a recent survey of 326 patients, the following distribution was reported (Balasegaram, 1968).

	Per Cent
Peptic ulceration	63.2
Esophageal varices	12.6
Carcinoma of the stomach	3.4
Drug reaction	1.8
Chronic gastritis	0.9
Miscellaneous causes	6.4
No ascertainable cause	11.7

Notably absent in this analysis is acute hemorrhagic (erosive) gastritis which, in other surveys, is held accountable for 5 to 8 per cent of all massive upper gastrointestinal bleeds. Also missing are such uncommon sources of bleeding as esophageal lacerations and esophagitis which presumably were included under the miscellaneous category. Much depends on the frequency of hepatic cirrhosis (with all of its at-

tendant problems) in the patient population being surveyed. The impact of portal hypertension and alcohol abuse on the previous data is well documented by the analysis of 158 patients with hepatic cirrhosis reported by Merigan et al. (1960). In such patients, the following distribution was encountered:

	Per Cent
Esophageal varices	53
Gastritis	22
Duodenal ulcer	14
Gastric ulcer	6

It should be cautioned that the precise percentages cited are not necessarily applicable to all clinical settings for reasons given earlier. Nonetheless, certain general conclusions can be drawn. In the absence of cirrhosis of the liver, peptic ulceration is unquestionably the commonest cause of massive hematemesis. If the diagnosis of cirrhosis can be established, attention must be shifted to the esophagus, but one should note that even in the presence of hepatic cirrhosis, gastritis and peptic ulcers account for slightly less than half of all upper gastrointestinal bleeds. Obviously, the data just given do not provide a diagnosis for the individual patient. However, this information can aid in establishing priorities for clinical investigation.

SMALL INTESTINE

NORMAL

The term "duodenum" is applied to the first portion of the small intestine because it was originally considered 12 fingers in length. It is the widest and most fixed portion of the small bowel and is shaped like the letter C. Classically, the duodenum is divided into four segments: superior, descending, transverse and ascending. The head of the pancreas nestles in the concavity of the C. The common bile duct, ampulla of Vater and pancreatic ducts make this short segment the most critical area for lesions in the entire small intestine.

The jejunum and ileum together are about 20 feet in length. There is no abrupt anatomic junction of these two levels, but the proximal two-fifths is customarily considered jejunum. The progressive narrowing of the small intestine makes it possible for the examiner to orient proximal and distal ends of a loop. On occasion, it is desirable at the operating table to estimate the location of a lesion in the small intestine. For this purpose, two features are helpful. In the jejunum, the fat in the mesentery usually does not extend out to the mesenteric attachment to the bowel, but leaves cleared windows adjacent to the bowel made only of layers of mesothelium. In the ileum, the mesenteric fat extends directly out to the bowel wall. The second distinction derives from the vascular patterns. In the jejunum, approximately a dozen branches from the superior mesenteric artery fan out radially and terminate in loose wide arcades. From these arcades, small end arteries travel directly to supply the small intestine. In the ileum, there are more tiers of arcades; they are smaller and much more complex, forming loop upon loop producing a lace-like pattern. Here too, small terminal end arteries carry the blood to its ultimate destination in the intestinal wall. These terminal straight portions are shorter than in

the jejunum. In passing, note that this pattern of vascular supply makes it possible for small lesions at the root of the mesentery to produce large areas of damage in the intestine. On the other hand, obstructive lesions of a secondary branch of the superior mesenteric artery will be without effect because of the rich anastomotic supply of the arcades. When vascular lesions occur close to the gut in the small terminal "end arteries," small ischemic lesions will result. Since the lymphatic drainage essentially parallels the vascular supply but does not have the intricate pattern of arcades, involvement of a small focus of lymph nodes or lymphatics produces a rather large segment of intestinal lymphedema.

Normal mucosa of the small bowel appears velvety and gray-pink with characteristic transverse folds known as Kerckring's folds. These are most abundant in the duodenum and become progressively smaller and more widely spaced toward the ileum. They serve as important normal mucosal landmarks in the radiographic barium study of the small bowel.

The histologic identification of the small bowel rests on the recognition of villi. They are most numerous and prominent in the duodenum and become progressively less well defined toward the terminal ileum. Superimposed upon these villi are microvilli seen only by electron microscopy. These are remarkably uniform, tall, straight and regularly spaced over the tips of the villi but become shorter, blunter and more irregular in the crypts of the glands (Fig. 21–24). This detail is important, since alterations in microvilli are used as histologic criteria for certain of the malabsorption syndromes, and it becomes important to know whether the biopsy represents the tip of the villus or the intervening crypt. The lining epithelium of the small bowel is composed of three types of secretory cells. One secretes intestinal enzymes; the second type, the goblet

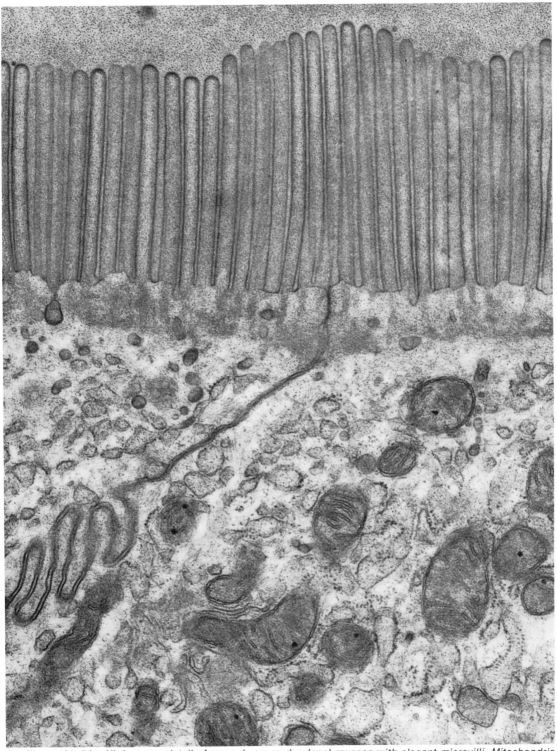

Figure 21–24. *High power detail of normal mouse duodenal mucosa with elegant microvilli. Mitochondria, endoplasmic reticulum and interlocking cell borders are evident. (Courtesy of Dr. L. Gottlieb, Mallory Institute of Pathology.)*

cells, elaborates the mucin; and in the crypts of the glands are found the serotonin-producing argentaffin cells. Covering the mucosal epithelium is a thin coat of mucopolysaccharide that is believed important in the transfer of substance into and out of the cells. Although presumably a secretory product of the columnar cells, it is referred to as "the extraneous coat."

The level of mitotic activity of the intestinal lining epithelial cells is quite remarkable. Cells are continually produced in the crypts of the glands. As new cells are formed, the older ones are pushed outward toward the tip of the villus and are shed. Various studies indicate that the lining epithelium of the small intestine replaces itself virtually every 3 days. Repair of of the mucosa, then, may occur remarkably promptly.

Certain microscopic features aid in the histologic differentiation of the various levels of the small intestine. Brunner's submucosal glands characterize the duodenum. Lymphoid patches begin to appear in the jejunum and become larger and more numerous toward the terminal ileum. In the ileum, they are sufficiently large to produce oval elevated plateaus called Peyer's patches. These become extremely prominent in inflammatory disease and are focal sites of ulceration in many forms of enteritis.

It is important to remember that the major function of the small intestine is absorption of foodstuffs and fluids. Certain lesions and dysfunctions of the small intestine have their most serious significance in that they may give rise to "malabsorption syndromes."

PATHOLOGY

On the whole, lesions of the small intestine are uncommon causes of clinical disease. The principal types of pathology in this segment of the gut are inflammatory disorders and derangements that lead to malabsorption and ulceroinflammatory disease. Because the lumen is narrow, intestinal obstruction is a frequent complication of some of the lesions. In contrast to the stomach and colon, primary tumors are extremely rare.

CONGENITAL ANOMALIES

Numerous developmental defects of rotation, reduplication and atresia occur in the small intestine, but only four congenital anomalies are encountered sufficiently often to merit description.

Duodenal Diverticula. These anomalies are principally of anatomic interest, but rarely they cause clinical manifestations. They are usually discovered incidentally at autopsy or in the course of x-ray studies of the stomach and duodenum. In radiographic studies, they are said to be present in about 1 per cent of all individuals but, in postmortem examinations, their incidence is variously reported as 1 to 10 per cent. Most of these lesions arise in the second, third and fourth portions and project into the concavity of the duodenal loop. They may occur multiply. Although they are designated as congenital, they are infrequent in children. It has been assumed that an area of congenital weakness permits their progressive enlargement. Their chief importance derives from two characteristics: as sites of possible stasis of food, they may become secondarily inflamed; and they sometimes produce inconstant and often puzzling obstructive symptoms as they impinge upon the common bile duct or pancreatic duct.

Multiple Diverticula of the Jejunum and Ileum. In the muscular wall of the small bowel, the points where the mesenteric vessels and nerves enter provide loci of weakness where the mucosa and submucosa may herniate into the mesentery. Such diverticula occur about one-tenth as often as duodenal diverticula and are, therefore, exceedingly rare. They are more frequent in older individuals, perhaps owing to the role continued intraluminal pressure plays in their causation. Because they dissect into the fat of the mesentery, they are easily missed at autopsy. Histologically, the muscular coats of the diverticula are absent or thinned, leaving only the mucosa and submucosa. In rare instances, intestinal stasis within their lumina has led to considerable overgrowth of bacteria which use excessive amounts of vitamin B_{12}, producing a pernicious anemia-like syndrome. Under these circumstances, the diverticula produce an analogue of the blind loop macrocytic anemia of experimental animals. Very rarely, the diverticula are the sites of intestinal bleeding or inflammatory perforation (Thomas et al., 1967).

Meckel's Diverticulum. Persistence of a vestigial remnant of the omphalomesenteric duct may give rise to a solitary diverticulum usually within 12 inches of the ileocecal valve. Rarely, it occurs in more proximal locations, sometimes up to 2 to 3 feet from the ileocecal valve.

These diverticula vary in conformation, from a fibrotic cord to a pouch having a lumen greater than that of the ileum and a length as much as 5 to 6 cm. (Fig. 21–25). The composi-

VASCULAR LESIONS

Mesenteric Thrombosis. Occlusion of either the arterial supply or venous drainage of the small bowel leads, within 18 hours, to infarction of the intestine. *In a series of 100 cases of intestinal infarction, approximately 60 were due to arterial occlusions and were associated with heart disease, embolism or in situ thrombosis precipitated by atherosclerosis.* Because of the rich anastomotic circulation in the mesentery of the small intestine, infarction occurs only when an entire major trunk (or possibly even two) is totally occluded (Rob, 1966). It is obvious from the pathogenesis of the arterial occlusions that this form of mesenteric thrombosis occurs in older individuals, usually in their fifth and sixth decades, when the various types of heart disease and far advanced atherosclerosis are most prevalent. *The remaining 40 per cent were venous in origin and were most often secondary to upper abdominal surgery.* In these cases, venous thrombosis was likely produced in the operative field and extended in the direction of blood flow to involve progressively larger vessels and eventually the main trunks of venous drainage of the bowel (Whittaker and Pemberton, 1938). These venous thromboses may be encountered at any age and tend to occur in somewhat younger individuals than the arterial occlusions. Rarely, liver disease with portal stasis may cause venous thrombosis and mesenteric occlusion. Mesenteric artery thrombosis is more common in males in the ratio of 3 to 2. It is also pointed out that mesenteric thrombosis is especially prone to occur in older diabetics who tend to have severe atherosclerosis. Occasionally, slowly developing or incomplete narrowing of the arterial vessels may occur by *partial* in situ thrombosis or by compression of vessels by adjacent tumor masses, intestinal adhesions or other mechanical pressures.

It is curious that regardless of whether the arterial or venous side is occluded, the infarction always appears grossly hemorrhagic (Kirschner, 1954—55). In the early stages, the segment of bowel appears intensely congested, dusky to purple-red, with small and large foci of subserosal and submucosal ecchymotic discoloration (Fig. 21–26). Later the wall becomes edematous, thickened, rubbery and hemorrhagic. Commonly at this stage, the lumen contains sanguineous mucus or frank blood. In arterial occlusions the demarcation from normal bowel is usually fairly sharply defined; but in venous occlusions, the area of dusky cyanosis fades gradually into the adjacent segments of normal bowel, leaving no clear-cut definition between viable and nonviable bowel. In approximately 24 hours, a fibrinous or fibrinosuppurative exudate appears on

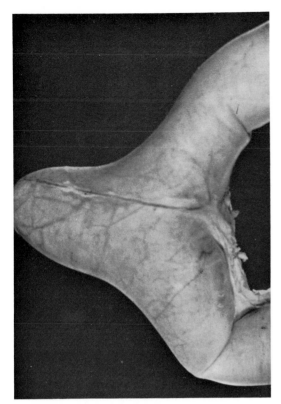

Figure 21–25. *A large Meckel's diverticulum having a diameter equal to that of the small bowel.*

tion of the wall is similar to that of the small bowel, but there are several points of difference. Heterotopic rests of gastric mucosa are found in about one-half of all Meckel's diverticula. Peptic ulceration sometimes occurs in the mucosa of the diverticulum adjacent to the island of gastric mucosa. Mysterious intestinal bleeding or symptoms resembling an acute appendicitis may result. Rarely, perforation occurs or the inflammatory disease causes adhesion to surrounding loops of bowel with resultant intestinal obstruction. Pancreatic rests may occur in Meckel's diverticula and precipitate a Zollinger-Ellison syndrome, but they are infrequent.

Pancreatic Rests. Foci of intramural, essentially normal pancreatic tissue occur anywhere in the small bowel, least often in the jejunum. They are of chief interest to the surgeon since they should not be confused with a primary tumor of the bowel. They are usually not more than 1 or 2 cm. in diameter and present, on cut surface, the typical yellow, lobulated appearance of normal pancreatic tissue. These rests are usually freely movable and are not attached to the underlying muscularis.

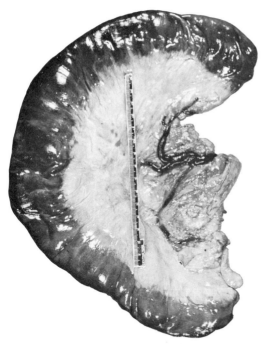

Figure 21–26. *A loop of infarcted small intestine showing the dark hemorrhagic discoloration. A large branching thrombus is evident in the arterial supply.*

the serosa, making it dull or granular. The associated inflammatory reaction depends upon the duration of the disorder. If death occurs within 24 hours, little cellular response may be demonstrable. Later, lesions may show characteristic inflammatory infiltrations and ulcerations. Ulceration of the mucosa, complicated by inevitable secondary bacterial contamination, and perforation of the wall are likely to occur within 3 to 4 days. However, most patients do not live long enough to develop such ulcerations and perforations. Ecchymotic discoloration or extensive hemorrhages in the mesentery accompany the bowel changes. The extent of the lesion depends entirely on the size of the affected vessels. Frequently, the demonstration of the exact point of vascular occlusion is difficult and requires a meticulous dissection of the blood supply. Despite such care, it is often not possible to identify the occlusive lesion, perhaps because the thrombus or embolus shatters and the fragments are sprayed into the distal finer ramifications, where they are impossible to find.

Mesenteric thrombosis is not common. Constant awareness of its possible presence is demanded, however, since it produces signs and symptoms of an acute abdomen that are clinically indistinguishable from all other causes of sudden abdominal pain. Characteristically, these patients have the sudden onset of severe abdominal pain, nausea, vomiting or sometimes diarrhea that may progress rapidly, within 24 to 48 hours, to frank shock. Soon after the onset, peristaltic sounds become diminished or totally absent, and spasm to board-like rigidity of the abdominal wall reflects the development of acute peritonitis. Because these signs are compatible with more common disorders, such as acute appendicitis, perforated peptic ulcer and acute cholecystitis, the diagnosis of mesenteric thrombosis is frequently missed. Since the infarction develops rapidly and is soon followed by permeation of the wall by bacteria, with the subsequent development of suppurative peritonitis, these patients follow an extremely fulminating course. Unless the condition is recognized early and treated within the first 48 hours, too frequently, mortality results from infection, blood loss, perforation of the intestine and shock.

Hyperplasia of Mesenteric Arteries. Attention has recently been drawn to the uncommon finding of infarction of segments of the small and sometimes large intestine by hyperplastic intimal thickening and narrowing of the terminal portions of the mesenteric arteries just before they enter the bowel (Aboumrad et al., 1963). Most of these cases have occurred in older individuals in cardiac failure who were receiving digitalis therapy. There is some question that digitalis toxicity or a sensitivity reaction to digitalis might be the underlying cause.

Acute Hemorrhagic Enteropathy. This intestinal disorder, although observed for many decades by pathologists, only recently has been defined as a distinct entity by Wilson and Qualheim (1954). The anatomic changes have been well described by Freiman (1965): "At autopsy, lesions were found to be widely distributed in segmental fashion through the intestinal tract from stomach to anus. The affected bowel was usually dark red or purple, due in part to accumulated blood in the lumen; the serosa was congested but showed no evidence of peritonitis. The bowel mucosa showed intense hemorrhage ranging from scattered patches in mild cases to involvement of long segments of intestine with shallow mucosal ulcerations in the more severe. Histologic findings range from widely dilated capillaries with a few extravasated red cells to intense hemorrhagic destruction of the mucosa affecting particularly the superficial portion and associated with marked submucosal venous dilatation. Of particular interest was the sparing of the muscular and serosal layers and the scant inflammatory reaction except in ulcerating areas; both of these findings together with the segmental pattern and demonstrated patency of the mesenteric vessels in every case served to distinguish the lesion from intestinal infarction due to vascular occlusion." As mentioned earlier, similar lesions have long been seen in the gut but often have been attributed to postmortem or agonal changes. Many were thought to represent incomplete infarction although the site of vascular occlusion was not found. The anatomic lesions also require differentiation from uremic enterocolitis and pseudomembranous enterocolitis.

The pathogenesis of this disorder appears to be vascular insufficiency to segmental levels of the intestinal tract. Shock with its splanchnic vasoconstriction is the most important underlying cause. Cardiac failure is an undoubted contributor in many cases. Infections play a role, probably by inducing vasomotor changes such as have been described in endotoxic shock (p. 346). Many patients have received digitalis and norepinephrine, raising the possibility that these drugs may have contributed in some way to the pathogenesis of the lesion. In some cases, minute intramural thrombi have been found, possibly representing causative mechanisms. Alternatively, these vascular thromboses may be only secondary to the surrounding inflammatory reaction (Ming, 1965).

Clinically, these patients have the onset of abdominal pain, cramps and bloody diarrhea, often with worsening of the shock state. Although, to this time, most of the diagnoses of this condition have been based on autopsy findings, there are undoubtedly cases of acute hemorrhagic enteropathy that have recovered and, indeed, have complete restoration of the bowel wall as evidenced by failure to find residual changes at a later date.

ULCEROINFLAMMATORY DISEASE

The small intestine is affected in many microbiologic systemic disorders such as the salmonelloses, shigelloses, cholera and staphylococcal bacteremia, as well as in certain of the fungal and parasitic disorders such as actinomycosis and amebiasis. All these have received consideration in Chapter 10. Several inflammations of the small intestine are of sufficient frequency and importance to merit special attention: regional enteritis, acute ileitis, tuberculosis, actinomycosis and potassium chloride enteritis. Only brief mention will be made of some of the others.

CROHN'S DISEASE (REGIONAL ENTERITIS)

Crohn's disease is perhaps best described as a relapsing granulomatous inflammatory disorder which usually affects the terminal ileum or colon but may occur at any site in the gastrointestinal tract. In some patients, the intestinal involvement is associated with inflammatory disorders of the joints, eyes, skin and liver. When first described in 1932 by Crohn and his colleagues, it was thought to affect only the terminal ileum and was thus designated *terminal ileitis*. Later it became apparent that segmental areas of the small bowel might be affected proximal to the terminal ileum—hence the designation *regional enteritis*. Since that time, areas of disease have been identified in the small and large bowel, esophagus, stomach, duodenum, appendix, and there is a single case report of an oral lesion (Thayer, 1970) (Dudeney, 1969).

As will become clear, Crohn's disease bears many similarities to idiopathic ulcerative colitis, not the least of which are that both diseases may produce inflammatory involvement of the colon and both are of unknown etiology. Although ulcerative colitis and Crohn's disease have somewhat distinctive morphologic appearances, they are nonetheless difficult to differentiate in some instances. In fact, for many years, involvement of the colon by Crohn's disease was attributed to ulcerative colitis. It is now appreciated that colonic involvement occurs in at least 25 per cent of all cases and may even precede involvement of the small intestine (Crohn, 1960). These remarks must not be taken to preclude the possibility of the coexistence of ulcerative colitis and Crohn's disease in the individual patient; this does indeed occur.

Incidence. The disease is most prevalent in the Western world and is thought to be rare among blacks. However, the scarcity of case reports from tropical areas may be the spurious consequence of limited case finding and confusion with infective dysentery (Editorial, 1972). The incidence of this disease has increased in the recent past. Regional enteritis has now been identified in Japan and several of the countries in Central and South America. In Norway, new cases of Crohn's disease totaled 2.3 per million per year from 1956–60, rising to 10.5 per million per year in 1964–69 (Myren et al., 1971). In the United States, Crohn's disease is slightly more common in men than in women, and most first attacks occur in the age range of 20 to 30. There is general agreement that Jews are affected more often than non-Jews. About 4 to 6 per cent of cases appear to have a familial distribution, and cases have been reported in each twin of monozygotic pairs. Kirsner and Spencer (1963) report that 11 per cent of their cases disclosed evidence of the familial occurrence of either Crohn's disease, ulcerative colitis or ileocolitis.

Etiology and Pathogenesis. Despite all research efforts and the countless enthusiastic reports, the origins of Crohn's disease remain unknown. The granulomatous inflammatory character of the bowel changes would logically suggest two lines of investigation: (1) search for an infectious agent and (2) interest in a hypersensitivity causation. Virtually every conceivable microbiologic agent, has, at one time, been hailed as the cause and subsequently dismissed. Nonetheless, the belief persists that perhaps organisms difficult to isolate, such as L phase bacteria, anaerobic bacteria or viruses, might be implicated. A recent report under the provocative title, "Agent Transmissible from Crohn's Disease Tissue," indicated that homogenates of tissue from involved gut or lymph nodes inoculated into the footpads of mice induced granulomas closely resembling those encountered in Crohn's disease in man (Mitchell and Rees, 1970). Control studies with normal gut and lymph nodes induced no similar changes. However, no identifiable agent could be isolated, and the interpretation of the experiment remains uncertain, since the granuloma formation might merely indicate an immunologic reaction.

Some abnormal immunologic reaction is the other currently favored view of the causation of Crohn's disease. A number of diverse observations can be offered in support of this theory. Families of patients with Crohn's disease tend to have an increased incidence of eczema, hay fever and arthritis, all probably immunologic in origin. The systemic nature of Crohn's disease, with its often associated arthritis, uveitis and spondylitis, is compatible with systemic immunologic disease. The granulomatous inflammatory reaction is typical of the lesions encountered in tuberculosis and sarcoidosis, in both of which some element of hypersensitivity is thought to be involved. Half of 74 patients with definite or probable Crohn's disease had positive Kveim tests (Mitchell et al., 1970). The Kveim test (p. 469) demonstrates a delayed hypersensitivity skin response to the injection of antigen derived from sarcoid tissue. Since sarcoidosis is thought but not proven to be a hypersensitivity disorder, the positive Kveim reactions in Crohn's disease are held to have some immunologic significance. Elevated serum IgA levels have been reported in persons with extensive or untreated disease (Kraft et al., 1968). Other observations could be cited, but it must suffice for now to conclude that all of these immunologic data comprise hints but no proof.

Repeatedly, allusion is made in the medical writings to the increased frequency of regional enteritis in patients having some form of psychopathology such as depression, dependency conflicts and obsessive-compulsive neuroses. But the consensus would ascribe to these emotional problems importance perhaps in exacerbating existing disease rather than in initiating it.

Morphology. Whatever level of the bowel is affected, Crohn's disease is characterized by **segmental areas of involvement which are abruptly demarcated from contiguous normal gut** (Morson, 1968). In approximately 80 per cent of cases, the terminal ileum is involved, often with additional, more proximal segments of the small intestine as well. Typically, intervening normal bowel separates these involved segments, producing so-called "skip" lesions. Colonic involvement, when present, usually takes the form of perianal lesions, but higher levels of the colon may be affected, closely simulating ulcerative colitis. **In all sites of involvement in the classic disease, the bowel wall is thickened and inflexible and has been likened to a lead pipe or rubber hose** (Fig. 21–27). The serosal surface is granular and dull gray, and often the mesenteric fat "creeps up" over the bowel surface, so that the gut may seem virtually buried. The mesentery of the involved segment is also thickened, edematous and sometimes fibrotic. The striking inflexibility and fibrosis of the bowel wall tend to maintain the cylindrical shape even after opening the bowel, so that it must be propped open for inspection (Fig. 21–28). The lumen is almost always narrowed; this is evidenced on x-ray as the "string-sign," a thin stream of barium. Close examination of the opened bowel reveals separation of the usual anatomic layers by gray, gritty, fibrous tissue, which classically involves mainly the submucosal and subserosal zones. Varying degrees of mucosal edema, ulceration and sloughing are found (Fig. 21–29). Commonly, the ulcers are long and serpentine. On the other hand, they may be extremely narrow and can be virtually hidden between the folds of the mucosa. In chronic cases, the ulcers may penetrate deeply to form fistulous tracts with other loops of bowel. In other instances, penetration of the wall may create abscesses either within the peritoneal cavity or within the mesenteric fat.

The most characteristic histologic features of Crohn's disease are the transmural inflammation (in the form of chronic inflammatory infiltrates and fibrosis) affecting all layers to the serosa and the development of noncaseating granulomas closely resembling those of sarcoidosis. The granulomas are, however, absent or not well developed in approximately 25 to 35 per cent of cases (Williams, 1964). From the inside out, there is variable ulceration and destruction of the mucosa, marked submucosal fibrosis with chronic inflammatory reac-

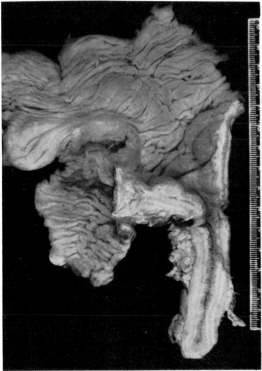

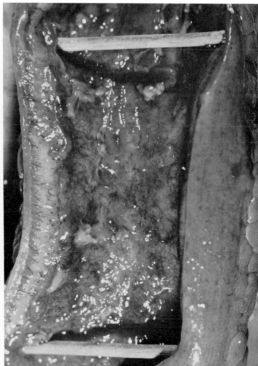

Fig. 21-27.   Fig. 21-28.

Figure 21-27. *Regional enteritis involving the appendix and demonstrating the sharply delineated, marked thickening of the wall characteristic of this lesion in any area.*

Figure 21-28. *Regional ileitis. A close-up of a segment of thickened bowel wall. Note the wooden pegs required to keep the lumen exposed.*

tion, relative preservation of the muscularis and, again, marked subserosal fibrosis with chronic inflammatory changes (Fig. 21-30). The inflammatory response in the mucosal ulcerations is entirely nonspecific and is largely composed of neutrophils, lymphocytes, histiocytes and plasma cells. The preserved mucosa between the ulcers often shows a diffuse nonspecific inflammation, and the glands may be distorted and cystically dilated. Within the submucosal and subserosal zones, the scattered inflammatory foci of mononuclear cells are often aggregated into lymphoid follicles, and some of these contain well formed sarcoid-like granulomas (Fig. 21-31) (Laipply, 1957). The resemblance to sarcoid is complete with the production of multinucleated giant cells, some of which contain Schaumann bodies. However, even when these granulomas are missing from some cases, regional enteritis must still be diagnosed histologically on the basis of the other changes described. Similar chronic inflammatory changes, often replete with granulomas, affect the regional nodes of drainage (Warren and Sommers, 1954).

The histologic changes in the large intestine conform to those cited previously. Fibrosis and thickening tend to be less severe and do not cause the marked stenosis seen in the small intestine. This difference in macroscopic appearance may merely

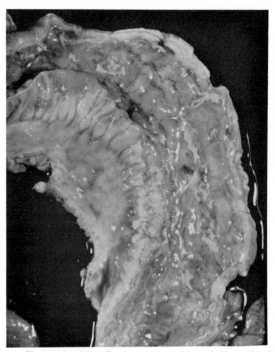

Figure 21-29. *Regional enteritis of the distal ileum demonstrating the fibrosis and thickening of the wall as well as long, serpentine, pale ulcerations of the mucosa.*

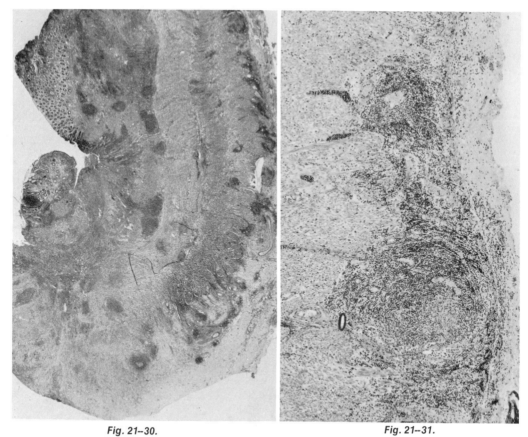

Fig. 21–30.

Fig. 21–31.

Figure 21–30. A low power view of the marked inflammation, thickening and ulceration caused by regional enteritis. Foci of inflammatory cells are evident at points distant from the ulceration. Note the width of the submucosa.

Figure 21–31. Serosal surface of a segment of bowel involved by regional enteritis, illustrating foci of chronic inflammatory cells which sometimes contain central granulomatous responses resembling sarcoid.

reflect differences in the size of the lumina and in the vascular and lymphatic supply of these two levels of the gut. Sarcoid-like granulomas, complete with multinucleated giant cells, are also present in the colon, justifying the sometimes used designation "granulomatous colitis" (Tizes, 1970). Anal lesions are most characteristic in the form of an indolent ulcer or fissure, which sometimes penetrates deeply to produce a fistula. Here again, the histologic changes are those seen in the upper levels of the gut, including granuloma formation and the presence of numerous multinucleated giant cells.

The classic full-blown lesions have just been described. But in many cases seen at what is apparently an earlier stage, there is less prominent fibrosis and more evidence of edema in the submucosal and subserosal regions. These acute stages are not commonly encountered by the pathologist because they are only rarely submitted to surgery.

Clinical Course. These patients have variable abdominal signs and symptoms. Commonly the disease, when localized to the termi-nal ileum, begins with vague right lower quadrant pain associated with cramps, constipation or diarrhea or alternating bouts of both. Exacerbations of symptoms, particularly following emotional upsets, with short or long intervals of remission are quite distinctive of this disorder. As the regional enteritis progresses, the bowel disturbances become more marked and usually then become associated with anorexia, nausea, vomiting and progressive weight loss. Many of the patients have sufficient diarrhea to cause serious disturbances in fluid and electrolyte balance. Melena is present at one time or another in over half the cases. Usually the recurrent abdominal pain brings these patients to medical attention.

Classically, an erratic course is pursued for many years. Some fortunate few have permanent remissions. Usually, however, recrudescences occur, and these patients must be considered as having a potential progressive disease that may recur at any time throughout their lives.

Infrequently, but particularly in young individuals, Crohn's disease manifests with an acute onset, severe right lower quadrant pain and tenderness, vomiting, diarrhea, fever and leukocytosis. Virtually the same syndrome is evoked by acute appendicitis, and laparotomy may be necessary to distinguish these two disorders. With such an acute onset, the prognosis is relatively good, and about half of these patients have no further recurrences once the acute attack has remitted.

The complications of regional enteritis are those that would be anticipated. The impairment of intestinal motility and absorption, plus the accompanying diarrhea and constipation, all lead to severe metabolic disturbances. Hemorrhage, perforation and peritonitis may result from the uclerations. Because the inflammatory response is chronic, adhesion to adjacent segments of bowel frequently develops with occasional penetration and fistula formation.

POTASSIUM CHLORIDE ENTEROPATHY

In 1964, attention was called to small intestinal ulcerations, principally in the jejunum of patients taking thiazide diuretics with potassium chloride supplementation (Baker et al., 1964). It has since become clear that the intestinal lesions are due to the potassium chloride and not the thiazides. The changes in the bowel are unusually distinctive and well defined. They consist basically of focal hemorrhages, congestion and fibrous thickening of the mucosa and occur principally in the jejunum but affect other levels of the small intestine as well. Many of these lesions are sharply segmental and sometimes annular. With progressive fibrosis, they may produce narrowing of the bowel strongly resembling segmental regional enteritis. Unless the possibility of potassium toxicity is borne in mind, the diagnosis may be missed, since the lesions are readily confused with regional enteritis.

ACUTE ILEITIS

Acute inflammatory involvement of the terminal ileum, sometimes of higher levels, is a rare disorder of obscure cause. As would be expected, the intestinal wall is hyperemic, edematous and slightly thickened with minimal to moderate mucosal and submucosal edema. The inflammatory changes are entirely nonspecific. Mucosal ulcerations are infrequent and scarring is generally absent. The mesentery of the affected bowel may be somewhat edematous, but usually its involvement is not as marked as in regional enteritis. That the ana-

tomic changes are all completely reversible corresponds with the transient nature of the clinical disease. There is no evidence that acute ileitis, even when recurrent, progresses to regional enteritis.

TUBERCULOSIS

To the present time, tuberculous involvement of the intestinal tract has always been divided into a primary type, contracted from the ingestion of milk infected with bovine tuberculosis, and a secondary type, which results from swallowing infective material in cases of advanced pulmonary tuberculosis. Primary intestinal tuberculosis has become, in the Western world, virtually nonexistent. Secondary intestinal tuberculosis is found in approximately 80 per cent of cases in which death resulted from far advanced pulmonary tuberculosis (Goldberg, 1947). The organisms are coughed up from "open" lesions in the lung and are then swallowed. Being resistant to acid gastric digestion, they pass into the small intestine and are phagocytized by the lymphatic tissues of the intestine.

The lesions begin in the ileum where the abundant lymphoid tissue traps the M. tuberculosis, providing a nidus of infection. Depending upon whether ulceration or granulomatous hyperplasia dominates, the inflammatory process has been termed "ulcerative" or "hyperplastic." In the more common ulcerative form, many tubercles are formed. Eventually these coalesce, caseate and cause necrosis of the overlying mucosal surface. Sometimes the inflammatory hypertrophy of the lymphoid tissue develops to the point of producing ischemic necrosis of the superficially thinned-out mucosa without the actual development of caseation. Classically, these ulcers extend along the encircling lymphatics of the small bowel (Fig. 21–32). The ulcers may penetrate deeply and may even perforate. In both ulcerative and hyperplastic forms, it is quite typical for small miliary tubercles to extend to the subserosal layer and produce a fine, gray-white seeding apparent on the serosal surface, which may be the most diagnostic feature of the lesion.

In the hyperplastic variety, diffuse granulomatous inflammation causes thickening of the involved bowel wall with ulceration as a less conspicuous feature. The pathognomonic formation of tubercles with caseation is found in both types, either in the margins of the ulcers, in the granulomatous inflammatory tissue or in the muscularis and subserosa. The regional nodes of drainage will disclose tuberculous involvement.

Intestinal tuberculosis may cause signifi-

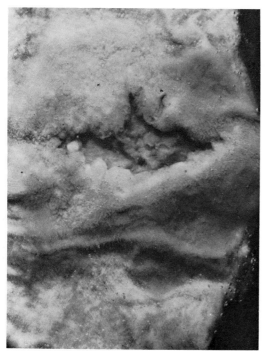

Figure 21–32. *Tuberculous ulcer of ileum transversely oriented with shaggy overhanging margins.*

cant clinical symptomatology such as cramps, diarrhea, pain and disturbances in bowel motility. Ulcerative perforation is rare. As in the lung, the tuberculous inflammatory process tends to produce vascular thrombosis in advance of the caseation necrosis, and bleeding is not a prominent sign. It is to be remembered that in secondary intestinal involvements the clinical picture is dominated by the primary changes within the lung.

ACTINOMYCOSIS

Actinomyces infections uncommonly involve the bowel. They are important, however, because they produce inflammatory suppurative masses that simulate tumors. The fungus gains access to the body through the gastrointestinal tract. In the great preponderance of cases, the infection is confined within the mouth, pharynx or neck region. Occasionally, localization occurs at lower levels in the small intestine, appendix, cecum, colon or rectum. The suppurative inflammation is somewhat distinctive by virtue of its striking tendency to penetrate deeply with the production of large inflammatory masses. These suppurative infections thus tend to burrow into adjacent loops of bowel, into the peritoneal cavity or into the abdominal wall. When the rectum is involved, perianal or ischiorectal abscesses may

develop. The anatomic changes are entirely nonspecific, save for identifiable colony formation of the fungus, producing what has been described macroscopically as "sulfur granules." Positive identification of the agent should be made by cultural methods (p. 442).

TYPHOID AND PARATYPHOID

These systemic bacterial diseases cause prominent ulceroinflammatory lesions in the intestine, described in Chapter 10 (p. 397).

SHIGELLOSES

Although involvement of the small bowel occurs with infections by the Shigella group of organisms, the major lesions occur in the large bowel. The pathologic changes are described in Chapter 10 and also in the consideration of the large bowel (p. 400).

CHOLERA

This fulminating bacterial disease causes extensive damage to the intestines as well as other systemic alterations. It has already been considered in Chapter 10 (p. 402).

TUMORS

BENIGN

Benign tumors of the small intestine rarely evoke clinical symptoms. They are usually discovered as incidental findings at postmortem examination.

Polyps. These small pedunculated lesions occur as solitary or multiple adenomas in the small intestine generally associated with similar involvement in the large intestine. Detailed description of the gross and microscopic features will be given under the discussion of the colon (p. 962). Unlike their analogues in the large bowel, they rarely become malignant.

Miscellaneous. Small, incidental, submucosal, intramural, spherical leiomyomas, fibromas, hemangiomas, lipomas and lymphangiomas occur in the small intestine. Sometimes multiple hemangiomas or vascular hamartomas are present as a part of the systemic disorder, Osler-Weber-Rendu's disease.

MALIGNANT

Cancers occur infrequently in the small intestine but collectively are more common than benign tumors. In an analysis of 132 cases of neoplasms in this level of the bowel, the incidence was as follows (Darling and Welch, 1959):

TABLE 21–2. INCIDENCE OF NEOPLASMS IN THE SMALL INTESTINE

Neoplasms	Duo-denum	Jejunum	Ileum	Per Cent
Benign tumors	14	20	12	35
Argentaffinoma	0	0	15	11
Carcinoma	10	19	4	25
Lymphoma	0	12	17	22
Sarcoma	1	4	4	7
TOTALS	25	55	52	100

Thus, approximately one-third of the neoplasms were benign and two-thirds were malignant. Among the cancers, carcinoma and lymphoma were the two commonest patterns. As a biologic phenomenon worthy of a moment's reflection, why are carcinomas so frequent in the stomach and colon and so rare in the small intestine?

Carcinoma.   In the small bowel, these malignancies grow in a napkin ring, encircling pattern and rarely as polypoid fungating masses (Fig. 21–33). Microscopically, they are almost always adenocarcinomas, some being mucinous. They tend to produce symptoms only when they are well advanced in growth, since early lesions have no obstructive effect on the flow of fluid chyme in this segment of the intestine. In late stages, they spread to regional nodes, liver, lungs and distant organs.

Lymphoma.   This type of neoplasm is one of the more common forms of malignancy to affect the small intestine. These tumors may occur in the lymphoid tissue of the gut as a *primary site of origin*. On the other hand, the lymphomatous lesions may represent *a part of a generalized involvement of the entire body*. In the primary form, the *stomach, followed by the ileum*, is most often affected. As a generalization, *malignant tumors of the upper levels of small bowel are more likely to be carcinomas or argentaffinomas and those of the lower levels, lymphomas.*

Small bowel primary lesions usually become bulky tumors, appearing first as submucosal, irregular, gray, soft masses which apparently arise from the intramural lymphoid patches. As they increase in size, they extend along the long axis of the gut to cause mucosal ulceration, subserosal involvement and finally extension into the mesentery and mesenteric nodes. The tissue has the characteristic soft, gray appearance of sarcomatous growth. The histologic appearance is that of the specific type of lymphoma described under tumors of lymph nodes

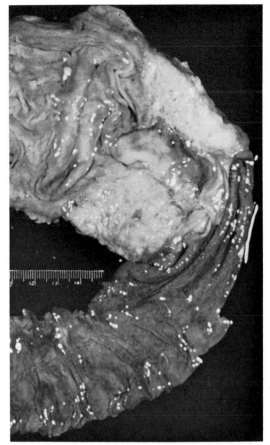

Figure 21–33.   *Carcinoma of small intestine growing in an annular encircling fashion.*

(p. 752). The two most common patterns are lymphocytic lymphoma and histiocytic lymphoma (reticulum cell sarcoma).

In the secondary lymphomatous involvements associated with generalized lymphomatosis, multiple tumor masses may be found along the entire small gut, conforming roughly to the distribution of the lymphoid tissue of the small intestine. Ulceration of the mucosa may be produced. Classically, the ulcers have markedly elevated, heaped-up margins with deeply excavated bases of necrotic tumor. Perforation of these lymphomatous ulcers occurs fairly frequently.

In general, the primary lesions are more common in childhood and show some tendency to a male predilection. As is true for most sarcomas, they grow more rapidly than carcinomas, tend to become more bulky and metastasize more widely and earlier to liver, nodes, bone marrow and lungs. It is important to remember that the primary intestinal lymphoma may be localized to the bowel and, therefore, may be resectable.

Carcinoid (Argentaffinoma). Carcinoids may arise anywhere in the gastrointestinal tract, bronchi, biliary tract, pancreas and wherever enterochromaffin cells are normally found (Wilson et al., 1963). These interesting tumors were called "carcinoids" years ago because it was believed that although they had many of the invasive characteristics of carcinomas, they could not metastasize. The neoplastic cells, like their normal enterochromaffin progenitors, can reduce ammoniacal silver-salts, creating black granules readily visible in formalin-fixed tissues—hence the term argentaffinoma. The preponderance of carcinoids (perhaps 90 per cent) occur in the alimentary tract (in order of decreasing frequency) in the appendix (approximately 60 per cent), the small intestine (approximately 25 per cent), and the rectum and stomach (2 to 5 per cent), conforming to the abundance of enterochromaffin cells in these organs (MacDonald, 1956). *The two most interesting aspects of these neoplasms are: (1) their ability to secrete a variety of catecholamines, particularly serotonin (5-hydroxytryptamine, 5-HT) and (2) the different biologic behavior of appendiceal carcinoids from those in the gut itself.* Although those arising in the gut proper may metastasize, only exceedingly rarely do appendiceal carcinoids metastasize. The reason is unclear. Appendiceal carcinoids may have different natural capabilities, or less metastasis may be seen because these primaries are usually removed easily early in their natural history (Rosenburg, 1966). In contrast, somewhere between 40 and 60 per cent of carcinoids arising in other sites are far more aggressive lesions and metastasize to local nodes and frequently to viscera, particularly the liver and lungs (Pearson and Fitzgerald, 1949).

The elaboration of serotonin results in the *"carcinoid syndrome"* described below.

In the small intestine and other extra-appendiceal sites, argentaffinomas usually occur as small, round to plaque-like, submucosal elevations up to 4 to 5 cm. in diameter (Fig. 21–34). In about 25 per cent of cases, multiple lesions are found. The overlying mucosa is usually intact, and in many instances the lesion is deceptively mobile and unattached to the underlying muscularis. On occasion, they become large, ulcerating or polypoid growths that obviously are bound to the underlying muscularis. Sometimes gross penetration of the bowel wall with

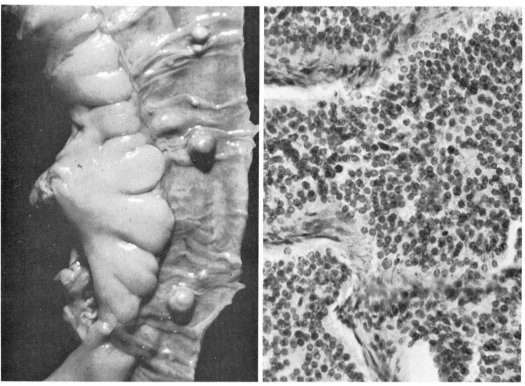

Fig. 21–34.   *Fig. 21–35.*

Figure 21–34. *Multiple small polypoid argentaffinomas involving the small intestine.*
Figure 21–35. *Argentaffinoma. Histologic detail of regularity of cell forms.*

extension into the mesentery of the small intestine or perirectal tissue is evident. On transection, the tissue is classically yellow but is often gray, firm and not distinctive from other types of neoplasms. Argentaffinomas that metastasize generally spread to regional nodes and possibly to the liver, lungs and bones.

Histologically, the lesion is composed of small nests, strands or large masses of regular, polygonal to cuboidal epithelial cells that only occasionally form gland-like patterns. The **individual cells have a striking resemblance to each other with a monotony of cell and nuclear size and shape** (Fig. 21—35). The nuclei are round to oval and deeply chromatic with a fine stippling throughout. Within the cytoplasm, granules of yellow-brown, lipochrome pigment are found which produce the gross coloration. Silver impregnation techniques reveal a fine black granularity throughout the cytoplasm as well. Giant cells, anaplasia and mitoses are virtually absent. Despite the apparently benign appearance, the tumor tends to invade the submucosa and the muscularis and, in the extra-appendiceal sites, frequently penetrates the bowel wall to extend into the adjacent mesentery and fibrofatty tissue. This histologic pattern is faithfully repeated in its metastatic sites.

Carcinoids in the small intestine cause clinical manifestations in one of two ways. As locally invasive lesions, they may cause partial or complete intestinal obstruction. Although they may also metastasize, only rarely is the dissemination of sufficient magnitude to produce the cachectic syndrome so typical of most disseminated cancers. Characteristically, however, they elaborate a variety of catecholamines, which produce the very bizarre and varied symptom complex known as the *carcinoid syndrome* (Baeza, 1969). While the syndrome most often occurs in patients having metastases from their primary lesions, this symptom complex probably reflects only the amount of the tumor; large, nonmetastasizing lesions may also induce the carcinoid syndrome. Colonic and bronchial argentaffinomas may behave similarly. *The clinical features of the syndrome consist of attacks of flushing of the skin, principally the face, that last from minutes to days, cyanosis accompanying these attacks, diarrheal watery stools, bronchoconstrictive attacks, sudden drops in blood pressure during the attacks, edema and ascites. Often there are cardiac murmurs due to development of stenoses of the valves of the right side of the heart, principally of the pulmonary valve.* Serotonin has been isolated from the neoplasm, and increased levels have been demonstrated in the circulating blood. This agent is produced by the tumor from tryptophan, and sometimes this diversion of tryptophan produces a pellagra-like syndrome. However, when administered alone, 5-HT does not reproduce the carcinoid attack, and so it probably is not the sole mediator of the carcinoid syndrome. Recently, kinins as well as other still unidentified products have been isolated from the serum of patients with this disorder. These substances, such as bradykinin, can cause bronchoconstriction, alterations in capillary permeability and, conceivably, by their vasomotor activity, could induce proliferative overgrowth of fibrous tissue leading to the right-sided valvular stenoses. The lungs are rich in monamine oxidases that inactivate these products and thus protect the left side of the heart (Oates et al., 1964). A valuable diagnostic laboratory test of the carcinoid syndrome is the demonstration of increased levels of 5-hydroxyindolacetic acid (5-HIAA) in the urine, the excretory breakdown product of 5-HT.

Sarcoma. As in all levels of the bowel, sarcomas may arise from the various mesenchymal elements of the wall of the small gut. They are all rare, producing the bulky, soft, hemorrhagic necrotic masses typical of sarcomas with their characteristic histologic picture. These lesions apparently grow fast and metastasize widely at an early stage of development.

OBSTRUCTIVE LESIONS

While obstruction to the gastrointestinal tract may be caused by lesions at any level, the narrow lumen of the small intestine makes obstruction most common here. The causes of such obstruction have been well classified by Wangensteen (1937) as follows:

1. *Mechanical obstruction:*
    Strictures, congenital and acquired.
    Atresias.
    Imperforate anus.
    Obstructive gallstones, fecaliths, foreign bodies.
    Adhesive bands or kinks.
    Hernias.
    Volvulus.
    Intussusception.
    Neurogenic paralytic ileus.
2. *Vascular obstruction:*
    Mesenteric thrombosis.

Some idea of the relative frequency of these various causes in clinical practice can be gained from the analysis of 335 cases reported by McIver (1933). Forty-four per cent were caused by hernias; 30 per cent were due to intestinal adhesions and bands (this frequency is somewhat higher than that reported in other series); neoplasm was responsible for 10 per cent; intussusception followed with a frequency of 5 per cent; volvulus, 4 per cent; mesenteric thrombosis, 3 per cent; and all other causes together, the remaining 4 per cent. Tumors and mesenteric thrombosis together accounted for 13 per cent. Four other entities —hernias, intestinal adhesions, intussusception and volvulus—accounted collectively for 80 per cent of obstructions. These four major entities will be considered in detail.

Hernias. A weakness or defect in the wall of the peritoneal cavity may provide an area where persistent intraperitoneal pressure will eventually push out a pouch-like, serosal lined sac called a hernial sac. The usual sites of such weakness in the anterior abdominal wall are the areas of the inguinal and femoral canals, at the umbilicus and in surgical scars. More rarely, similar retroperitoneal defects occur in the posterior wall of the abdominal cavity chiefly about the ligament of Treitz. Hernias are of chief interest because segments of viscera may become trapped in them. This circumstance is more apt to occur in inguinal than in femoral hernias since the former tend to have narrow orifices and large sacs. If the small bowel is involved, partial or complete obstruction to the lumen may follow. Pressure by the neck of the pouch may impair the venous drainage of the trapped viscus. A vicious cycle then develops whereby the edema produced by the venous stasis increases the bulk of the contents of the hernial sac so that the intestinal loops are permanently trapped or *incarcerated*. The increased volume causes further increase of pressure on the collapsible blood vessels and, in time, the venous and possibly the arterial supply may be cut off *(strangulation)*, thus producing infarction of the trapped segment (Fig. 21–36).

If strangulation does occur, the gross and microscopic picture of the affected gut exactly resembles that previously described under mesenteric thrombosis. Not only the small bowel tends to become trapped in these hernial sacs but portions of the omentum and sometimes also segments of the large bowel. When the right side of the colon is loosely attached, or when there are large redundant sigmoid flexures, these segments of bowel may enter a hernial sac. Even ovary, fallopian tube and segments of urinary bladder have been identified in such sacs. All these structures may suffer the same fate described for the small bowel, incarceration or strangulation with infarction. However, involvement of the small bowel is most serious, since it may cause intestinal obstruction or perforation.

Intestinal Adhesions. As peritonitis (an inflammatory reaction of the peritoneal serosa)

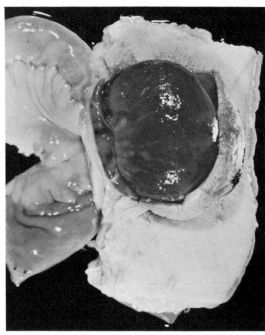

Figure 21–36. A knuckle of small intestine trapped in an inguinal hernial sac is demonstrated en bloc with the encircling skin of the inguinal region in situ. The sac has been opened to demonstrate the hemorrhagic condition of the contents.

heals, adhesions may develop. These fibrous bridges can create closed loops through which other viscera may slide and eventually become trapped, just as in a hernial sac. Intestinal obstruction, partial or complete, ensues and may be complicated by infarction of the trapped segment of bowel (Fig. 21–37). This sequence of events is found most commonly in postoperative patients who develop peritoneal adhesions to the wound in the abdominal wall and within the operative site. Quite rarely, adhesions may occur without prior peritoneal inflammation from fibrous bands arising as congenital defects. Intestinal obstruction and strangulation must be considered, then, even without a history of previous peritonitis or surgery.

Intussusception. This is an uncommon disorder, most often encountered in infants and children, in which one segment of small intestine, constricted by a wave of peristalsis, suddenly becomes telescoped into the immediately distal segment of bowel. Once trapped, the invaginated segment is propelled by peristalsis farther into the distal segment, pulling its mesentery along behind it (Fig. 21–38). The trapped bowel is referred to as the intussusceptum, and the segment which envelops it is known as the intussuscipiens. The pathogenesis of this lesion in children and infants is obscure. There is usually no underlying anatomic lesion or defect in the bowel to explain such an occurrence. However, intussusception also occurs in adults and, in this age group, some intraluminal mass or tumor serves as a point of traction which pulls the base of attachment and segment of gut along with it. In both the spontaneous infantile and the adult cases, not only does intestinal obstruction ensue, but the trapped mesenteric blood supply may eventually become compressed and produce infarction (Fig. 21–39). In the infantile variety, the disorder, if discovered early before infarction has occurred, is readily reduced usually by simply administering a barium enema. In the adult, surgical exploration is necessary not only to determine the cause, but also to deliver the trapped loop.

Volvulus. Complete twisting of a loop of bowel about its mesenteric base of attachment provides another mechanism of producing intestinal obstruction and infarction. This lesion occurs most often in the small bowel; however, large redundant loops of sigmoid are sometimes involved. Recognition of this seldom en-

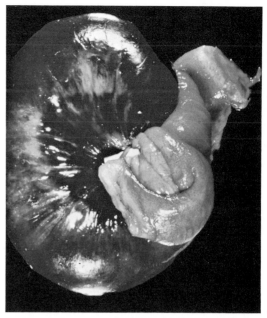

Figure 21–37. *A loop of hemorrhagic infarcted bowel is evident; it has slipped through a peritoneal adhesion visible on top of the central white marker.*

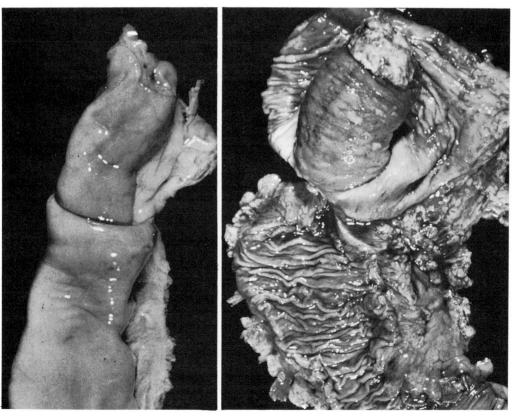

Fig. 21–38.   Fig. 21–39.

Figure 21–38. *Intussusception of the small intestine viewed from the external aspect.*
Figure 21–39. *Intussusception of the small intestine. The bowel has been opened to demonstrate the necrotic tip of the intussusceptum.*

countered lesion demands a constant awareness of its possible occurrence. If the bowel is
not obviously strangulated, a hasty manual exploration at surgery or autopsy may miss the
twisted loop. In most cases, obvious signs of obstruction or infarction develop and require
further therapy.

MALABSORPTION SYNDROMES

Intestinal malabsorption may be defined
as broadly as". . . any state in which there is a
disturbance of the net absorption (insorption-
exsorption) of any constituent across the intestinal mucosa" (Jeffries et al., 1964). In this
sense, diarrhea could be construed as a malabsorption. More often, the term malabsorption
implies largely impaired absorption of fat with
resultant steatorrhea. Many disorders and a
variety of mechanisms may cause steatorrhea,
as is indicated by the classification proposed by
Sleisenger (1967).

Inadequate Digestion:
    Gastric resection.
    Pancreatic insufficiency.
    Biliary obstruction.
    Biliary cirrhosis.
Biochemical Abnormality:
    Celiac disease, adult and childhood.
    Tropical sprue.
    Deficiency of sugar-splitting en-
    zymes.
    Abetalipoproteinemia.
Inadequate Absorptive Surface:
    Jejunal exclusion.
    Gastroileostomy.
    Large fistulas.
    Massive bowel resection.
Disease of the Intestinal Wall:
    Ileojejunitis.
    Amyloidosis.
    Radiation injury.
    Acute bacterial and viral enteritis.
Lymphatic Obstruction:
    Lymphoma.
    Whipple's disease.
    Tuberculosis (tabes mesenterica).
Altered Bacterial Flora:
    Blind loop syndrome.
    Multiple jejunal diverticula.
    Multiple strictures.
    Scleroderma.
    Small fistulas.
    Neomycin therapy.
Miscellaneous:
    Carcinoid syndrome.
    Diabetes mellitus.
    Islet cell tumor of the pancreas.
    Hypoparathyroidism.
    Hypothyroidism.
    Hypogammaglobulinemia.
    Mesenteric artery insufficiency.

From this tabulation, it is apparent that intestinal absorption may be deranged by a
number of dissimilar mechanisms. In biliary
tract disease and pancreatic insufficiency, for
example, there is malabsorption of foodstuffs
within the lumen of the intestine due to deficient enzymic and biliary action. The biochemical abnormalities cited exert their effect
within the epithelial cells lining the intestinal
wall. Lymphatic obstruction acts by blocking
the transport of fats that have already passed
the mucosal barrier. While each of these entities has its own somewhat distinctive characteristics, common to all are diarrhea, steatorrhea,
a variety of malabsorptions, weakness, weight
loss and lassitude. The diarrhea is characterized not only by an increase in the number of
bowel movements but, in addition, the stools
are classically bulky, greasy and have a foul
odor. The impaired absorption of fat leads to
deficient calcium absorption and a resultant
negative calcium balance. The fat-soluble vitamins are absorbed inadequately, and hemorrhagic manifestations may ensue secondary to avitaminosis K. Other hematologic
abnormalities may result from impaired absorption of iron or the B vitamins.

For many years, our understanding of
these malabsorptive disorders was based
largely on such inadequate parameters as measurements of fecal fat and nitrogen and autopsy studies of fatal cases. Newer techniques,
however, have provided an abundance of
knowledge that has helped clarify not only the
anatomic changes but also the underlying abnormalities. Perhaps the most important of
these innovations is the peroral intestinal
biopsy tube described by Shiner (1956). This
technique permits the peroral passage of an intestinal tube carrying at its head a mechanism
by which a small bit of intestinal mucosa may
be sucked into the end of the tube and then
cut off at its base, providing a safe and adequate biopsy of the mucosa in the living patient. The ease with which such bits of intestinal mucosa can be obtained permits serial
studies on the individual patient to evaluate
not only the changing evolution of the disease
but also the effect of various therapeutic measures. When such anatomic data are correlated
with the newer refined methods of bacteriologic study of the intestinal flora derived from
the biopsy specimen and more refined isotopic
measurements of absorption, it is possible
to gain new insights into the effect of structure on function and vice versa. The consider-

ation that follows will be confined to the major causes of malabsorption not already discussed and a few of the newer entities.

CELIAC DISEASE—GLUTEN ENTEROPATHY (NONTROPICAL SPRUE)

Steatorrhea, diarrhea, weight loss and malnutrition may be caused in the adult or child by either a toxic or a hypersensitivity reaction to gluten or one of its fractions found in wheat, oats or rye grains. Although the disease is usually diagnosed in young to middle-aged adults, there is no clear distinction between the disorder in infants and in adults; the differentiation of childhood from adult celiac disease has little meaning. Indeed, over half of affected adults date their initial manifestations back to their childhood.

The characteristic anatomic finding in celiac disease is marked atrophy of the villi and microvilli of the jejunum. These become severely blunted and distorted and may even disappear. There is an accompanying increase in depth of the intervillous crypts and a marked chronic inflammatory reaction in the lamina propria composed of lymphocytes and plasma cells with occasional eosinophils. The surface epithelial cells become cuboidal and stain poorly, and their nuclei assume irregular positions within the cell rather than the regular basal orientation (Samloff et al., 1965). Electron microscopy discloses that the microvilli are markedly distorted and shortened while the mitochondria have abnormal sizes and shapes and show changes in their cristae. The ribonucleoprotein granules are abnormally abundant (Hartman et al., 1960).

The basis for these anatomic changes appears to be some unusual reactivity to the gliadin fraction of gluten. The evidence is mounting that *celiac disease is a form of hypersensitivity response perhaps genetically conditioned*. Family studies indicate that approximately 10 per cent of first-degree relatives are affected (Robinson et al., 1971). Significant increases in the serum level of IgA have been identified in these patients (Asquith et al., 1969). Immunofluorescent studies have also demonstrated localization of IgA in the basement membranes of villous and crypt epithelia in children following challenge diets of gluten (Shiner and Ballard, 1972). Such immunologic reactivity has been linked to some specific genetic predisposition of the immune system in affected individuals. Recalling the close linkage of histocompatibility genes with immune response genes, recent studies indicate that celiac patients tend to have distinctive histocompatibility phenotypes (Stokes et al., 1972).

The clinical expressions of gluten-induced enteropathy are extremely varied and, in one study, were more often "atypical" than "typical." In one series, the classic manifestations of malabsorption, diarrhea, weight loss, steatorrhea and malnutrition were present in only eight of 21 patients (Mann, 1970). The remaining patients presented problems with iron absorption, anemia, osteomalacia and bleeding tendencies secondary to hypoprothrombinemia. Remarkable clinical improvement is achieved within weeks on a gluten-free diet. However, the villous atrophy responds more slowly despite the amelioration of clinical manifestations (Fig. 21–40).

TROPICAL SPRUE

In terms of clinical manifestations, tropical sprue closely resembles its nontropical cousin. In both forms, villous and microvillous atrophy are encountered and, indeed, the two diseases are virtually indistinguishable morphologically (Swanson and Thomassen, 1965). In tropical sprue, the villous atrophy is usually less severe than in the nontropical form of the disease and, indeed, in some patients there may be surprisingly little mucosal change. There are other significant differences. Although tropical sprue is principally encountered in India, the Far East and in Puerto Rico and other Caribbean islands, it is now being seen world-wide in military personnel returning from service in these regions (Sheehy et al., 1965). *Tropical sprue is not related to gluten sensitivity. The evidence points rather to one of two possible mechanisms—dietary deficiency or some microbiologic infection.* Most patients are dramatically improved by the administration of folic acid or vitamin B_{12}. This response is puzzling because, in many cases, the diet does not appear to be deficient. An infectious cause is suggested by several observations. Clinical improvement has been achieved with the use of broad-spectrum antibiotics. In some individuals, the disease is of acute onset, suggesting an infection. Epidemics have been reported, compatible with spread of a transmissible agent. Nonetheless, all efforts to isolate such an agent have been to no avail.

WHIPPLE'S DISEASE

Whipple's disease is an uncommon disorder characterized by steatorrhea, the accumulation of lipids in mesenteric and lymphatic lacteals, and the deposition of carbohydrate-protein complexes, presumably glycoproteins, in histiocytes in the intestinal mucosa as well as elsewhere. For some time, atten-

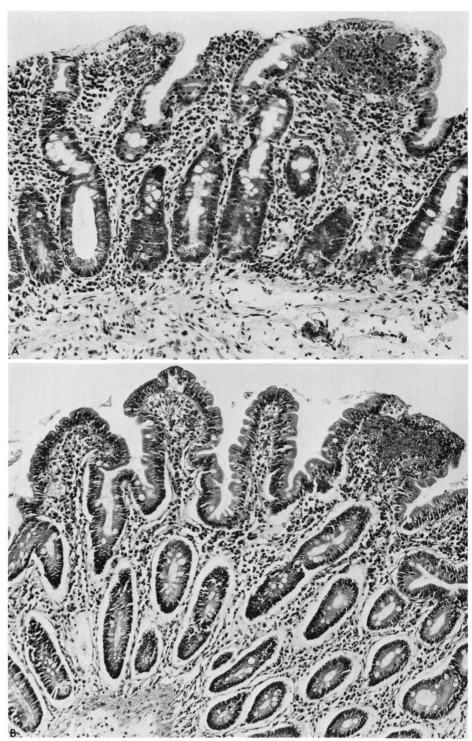

Figure 21–40. A, *Celiac disease — a jejunal peroral biopsy of the gluten enteropathy with atrophy and blunting of villi and an inflammatory infiltrate in lamina propria.* B, *Celiac disease — same patient as in A after 5 days on a gluten-free diet.*

tion was focused on the lipids, and this disease was thought to be caused by obstruction of the mesenteric lymphatics or their lymph nodes of drainage, hence the accumulations of fat. However, it soon became apparent that the accumulation of glycoproteins in the histiocytes was, in fact, universally associated with the disease and was, indeed, more characteristic. Moreover, similar glycoprotein-laden histiocytes were found in many sites throughout the body, indicating the systemic nature of this disorder (Sieracki and Fine, 1959) (Jones et al., 1953). These characteristic cells have been identified in the liver, peripheral lymph nodes, brain and spleen as well as in the small intestine and in virtually every organ where they have been sought.

The disease occurs in the later decades of life with a male predominance in the ratio of 8:1. Because the etiologic considerations are more understandable on the basis of the anatomic changes, the morphology of this condition will be described first.

Morphology. The small intestine is usually totally involved in this disease with thickening of the wall, dulling of the serosa and some thickening and induration of the mesentery. Fine lace-like patterning of the lymphatics can often be seen on the serosal surface. In well advanced cases, **the small intestinal villi are distended and blunted by masses of histiocytes, giving to the intestinal mucosa the appearance of a shaggy bearskin rug** (Fig. 21–41). Histologically, the villi are obviously thickened with bulbous tips. The enlargement of the villi is regarded as being due to masses of foamy histiocytes within the lamina propria. These cells are laden with granular, carbohydrate-protein complexes that are PAS-positive. The mucosal and mesenteric lymphatics are distended with lipids. Some of the lipid material appears within the submucosal fibrous tissue, apparently as a result of rupture of lacteals. Lipogranulomas may form both here and in the mesenteric lymph nodes. Under light microscopic examination, the covering epithelium does not appear to be affected, but the electron microscope discloses some increase in the intercellular spaces.

With the electron microscope, "bacilliform" particles have been identified within the histiocytes, sometimes attached to their outer surface (Cohen, 1964) (Fig. 21–42). These have excited a great deal of attention as possible etiologic agents. Some investigators consider them to be viral inclusions, but most interpret them as some form of bacteria (Chears and Ashworth, 1961). It is of historic interest that these particles were identified by Whipple in his original description of this disorder in 1907, using only the light microscope and the Levaditi stain for bacteria.

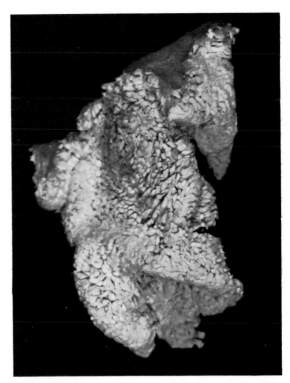

Figure 21–41. Whipple's disease of the small intestine. The hugely distended villi resemble the pile of a shaggy rug.

A second type of inclusion has also been found in the involved histiocytes. These can be resolved as cytoplasmic bodies possibly possessing an internal structure. Fibrils with a regularly repeating periodicity have been identified in these bodies (Cohen et al., 1960). Because these bodies are enclosed within double membranes, they have been thought to represent altered mitochondria or endoplasmic reticulum, but another interpretation is that they are altered lysosomes which contain engulfed bacilliform particles. Many of these bodies are ovoid or sickled in shape and, therefore, have been designated as "sickle-form particles," but these shapes may be merely artefactual.

The extraintestinal histiocytes also contain the granular PAS-positive material as well as the sickle particles and the bacilliform inclusions. The peripheral lymph nodes as well as those draining the small intestine are prominently involved.

Etiology and Pathogenesis. Despite the demonstration of the bacilliform bodies within histiocytes, no microorganisms have yet been isolated from these cases. If these bodies did, indeed, represent some obscure etiologic agent, one would expect them in all instances of Whipple's disease, but occasional reports appear in which they are absent (Adams et al., 1963). It is possible that these patients were in

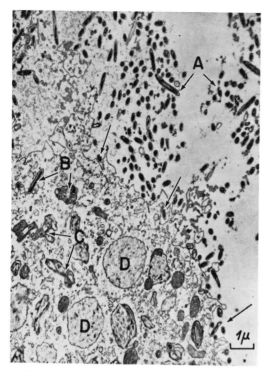

Figure 21–42. *Electron micrograph of an involved histiocyte in Whipple's disease. A indicates bacilliform bodies outside the cell with arrows pointing to loci where they appear to be penetrating cell boundaries. B and C indicate sickle and distorted forms. D indicates uninvolved lysosomes.*

a remission and that the agents had disappeared. However, it is by no means certain that these bodies have anything more than a morphologic resemblance to bacteria. The origins of the glycoprotein and the sickle particle inclusions are equally obscure. It has been postulated that the glycoprotein might represent accumulated bacterial, capsular polysaccharide. On the other hand, Adams proposes the equally plausible explanation that the carbohydrate-protein complexes stored in histiocytes might result from some abnormal function, perhaps genetic in origin, of reticuloendothelial cells. Simple chylous obstruction as the basis of this disorder has been fairly certainly ruled out. At present, therefore, the causation of this disease must be considered unknown.

Clinical Course. These patients are classically emaciated and frequently have gray-brown melanin pigmentations of the skin. The mechanism of this abnormal pigmentation is uncertain. In addition, there are a variety of malabsorptive disturbances along with severe diarrhea and steatorrhea. Many systemic reactions are also present, such as fever, joint pains, cough and weakness. Some of these manifestations may be due to extraintestinal collections of the abnormal histiocytes. The diagnosis can only be suspected in the appropriate adult male on the basis of the symptoms. Sometimes characteristic radiographic findings are present, but final confirmation may require intestinal biopsy disclosing the diagnostic glycoprotein-laden histiocytes in the villi. The wasting is progressive in this disease, and despite present-day efforts to support these patients, most die within two to four years following the diagnosis.

DISACCHARIDE INTOLERANCE

This uncommon entity is mentioned because it is the prototype of heredofamilial malabsorption due to a metabolic defect in the production of an intestinal enzyme. It is now clear that the disaccharides such as lactose and sucrose are hydrolyzed within the intestinal mucosal cell rather than in the lumen of the gut. A deficiency of one or more of the intestinal disaccharidases leads to inadequate breakdown of these sugars and florid proliferation of bacteria in the gut. It is theorized that the diarrhea and steatorrhea reflect the irritating effect of the bacterial overgrowth on the intestinal mucosa.

In closing, it should be stressed that the entities discussed represent only a few of the disorders capable of causing malabsorption. As our knowledge of the ultrastructural and enzymic functions of the small intestine increases, the list of malabsorptive disorders can be expected to grow longer.

COLON

NORMAL

The colon in man is a storage and absorptive organ. It is not essential for life. The subdivisions of the large bowel into the cecum, ascending colon, transverse colon and descending colon are well known. Perhaps somewhat less understood are the exact limits of the sigmoid colon and rectum. The former begins at the pelvic brim, includes the sigmoid flexures and connects below with the rectum at approximately the level of the third sacral vertebra. The rectum is that portion distal to the sigmoid. It is approximately 6 inches long, the proximal portion being within the peritoneal cavity while the distal segment is extraperitoneal. The reflection of the peritoneum from the rectum over the pelvic floor produces a cul-de-sac known as the "pouch of Douglas." This space is a favored site for the implantation of spreading intraabdominal tumors which produce a perirectal mass called a rectal shelf. These masses are within 3 inches of the anus and are, therefore, within reach of the examining finger.

Gross examination of the colon serves to differentiate it readily from the small intestine by three features: (1) the presence of three equally spaced, subserosal bands of muscle known as the taenia coli; (2) the sacculations known as haustrations produced by the shortening of these longitudinal bands; and (3) the abundance of small fatty appendages known as appendices epiploicae which stud the surface of the colon along the margins of the taenia.

The blood supply to the right side of the colon up to the midportion of the transverse colon is derived from the superior mesenteric artery. Occlusion of the superior mesenteric artery, therefore, causes infarction not only of the small bowel, but also of the ascending colon. Almost the entire remainder of the intra-abdominal colon is supplied by the inferior mesenteric artery. The lower rectum receives its supply from the hemorrhoidal branches of the internal iliac or internal pudendal artery, while the upper level is supplied by the superior hemorrhoidal branch of the inferior mesenteric. The venous drainage follows essentially the same distribution. Therefore, within the rectal vasculature there is an anastomotic capillary bed between the superior hemorrhoidal veins draining through the portal system and the inferior hemorrhoidal veins which drain through the inferior vena cava. In portal hypertension, these capillaries can become distended and provide a bypass for portal venous obstruction. Throughout most of its extent, the colon is a fixed retroperitoneal organ. Therefore, it derives considerable accessory blood supply and lymphatic drainage from a wide area of the posterior abdominal wall, making infarction and obstructive lymphedema most uncommon in this level of intestine.

Microscopically, in contrast to the small intestine, the colon has no villi. The normal mucosa contains simple tubular glands rich in mucus-secreting goblet cells. The submucosa, muscularis and subserosa are well defined, resembling the corresponding layers in other levels of the bowel.

While the colon is basically a storage organ, it has important absorptive functions, particularly in conserving water. Because other substances also may be absorbed through the rectal mucosa, certain drugs and anesthetic agents can be administered per rectum. The normal flora (*E. coli*) of the colon is now recognized to be an important protective mechanism in preventing the growth of other, possibly pathogenic, organisms. Antibiotics capable of destroying the normal flora permit the overgrowth of these pathogens and potentiate severe forms of colitis.

PATHOLOGY

Certain lesions that affect the colon comprise some of the most frequently encountered diseases in clinical practice, particularly surgical practice. Cancer of the large bowel is one of the most common tumors in man. It is of the same order of importance as lung, breast and gastric carcinoma. The extremely common hemorrhoid, a comparatively trivial lesion, may produce in the aggregate more clinical discomfort than almost any other lesion to which man is subject. In addition, inflammatory disorders such as ulcerative colitis and functional derangements such as spastic and mucous colitis are by no means uncommon. In terms of clinical and pathologic importance, then, the colon and the stomach are two areas of major importance in the gastrointestinal tract.

CONGENITAL ANOMALIES

Congenital anomalies of the colon are encountered infrequently. *Malrotations* may occur in which the cecum fails to descend to its definitive adult position in the right lower quadrant. Such malpositioning may confuse the diagnosis of acute appendicitis. *Reduplications* of the colon have been described rarely with the occasional formation of entire double large bowels. The most frequently occurring and clinically important anomalies of the colon are megacolon (Hirschsprung's disease) and imperforate anus.

MEGACOLON (HIRSCHSPRUNG'S DISEASE)

Megacolon, marked dilatation and hypertrophy of the colon, occurs as a congenital and as an acquired disorder. The congenital type is encountered more often in infants; the acquired, more often in adults.

Congenital megacolon is also known as *aganglionosis of the colon to indicate the basis of this disorder, namely, an absence of ganglion cells from the myenteric plexus.* Males are affected somewhat more than females and, while the disease is congenital and present from birth, it sometimes does not become manifest until years later. It is now confirmed that ganglion cells are absent from the rectum in 100 per cent of the cases and from the rectosigmoidal region in about 70 per cent (Whitehouse and Kernohan, 1948). Occasional cases are encountered in which the myenteric plexus is absent from the entire colon and even from part of the small intestine. Even more uncommonly, segmental portions of the colon may be involved with normal proximal and distal bowel.

The absence of the myenteric plexus produces a segment of bowel where normal propulsive contraction cannot occur, thus inducing a functional obstruction. Dilatation begins at this point of block

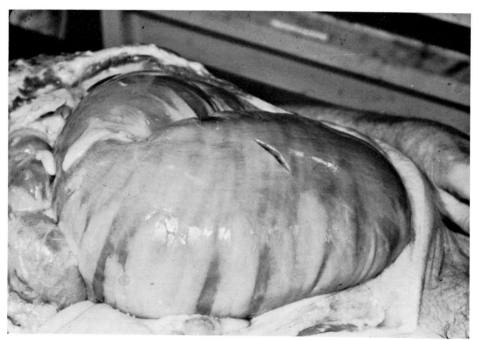

Figure 21–43. *Megacolon. The hugely distended bowel viewed in situ just after the abdomen has been opened in a postmortem examination. The bowel has been accidentally nicked.*

and extends retrogradely with time. Not infrequently, the first portion of the aganglionic bowel undergoes dilatation due to the expansile pressure of the propulsive waves just proximal to it.

In the common pattern in which both the rectum and rectosigmoid are affected, the descending colon undergoes dilatation and hypertrophy first. Eventually, however, the entire colon may become involved back to the ileocecal valve. In far advanced cases, the bowel is distended to a diameter of 15 to 20 cm. and may appear as a huge, elongated balloon (Fig. 21–43). Associated with this dilatation and chronic obstruction, there is usually marked hypertrophy and thickening of the bowel wall. Sometimes, however, the right colon becomes extremely distended with a thinned-out wall. Usually the mucosal lining throughout is intact, but the impacted feces may cause secondary ulcerations. The aganglionic segment of bowel and the normal portions distal to this are not distended because peristalsis does not carry the fecal contents beyond the functional block. When the entire colon is aganglionic, the distention may affect principally the small bowel, but usually in these cases some flow of ileal contents into the cecum produces distention of at least the ascending colon.

The cardinal symptoms of congenital megacolon are constipation, sometimes so severe as to produce obstipation, abdominal distention and vomiting. In the newborn, the vomiting may cause such serious electrolyte imbalance as to produce death within a few days. In less severe instances, the manifestations are principally constipation and abdominal distention. Rarely, diarrhea occurs as a puzzling manifestation. The diagnosis depends on the histologic confirmation of the absence of the myenteric plexus in the rectum. Resection of the aganglionic segment reestablishes effective peristalsis and is curative, although in the newborn with electrolyte imbalances, this procedure may have a high operative mortality (Swenson, 1959).

Acquired megacolon is encountered either in circumstances of chronic organic obstruction such as narrowing of the bowel due to inflammatory disease or neoplasia or as an apparent functional disorder in patients who, for emotional reasons, have chronic constipation. This latter group is composed most often of individuals who have had faulty bowel training during childhood. In acquired cases, the intrinsic innervation of the bowel is normal, and only rarely is the dilatation as massive as that encountered in the congenital form.

IMPERFORATE ANUS

Imperforate anus results when the membrane that separates the entodermal hindgut from the ectodermal anal dimple fails to perforate. An intact membranous septum may completely close the anal canal. This type of anomaly is said to occur in the order of 1 in 5000 births. Many times the occlusion is more serious than a simple membranous covering and takes the form of agenesis, atresia or stenosis of the rectal canal. In a significant number of these developmental failures, fistulous communications occur with the genital tract in the female or with the urinary tract in either sex.

MECHANICAL LESIONS

Because the colon is a relatively fixed retroperitoneal organ, volvulus and herniation involve the large bowel much less commonly than the small intestine. When *herniation* does occur, usually only a small portion of the wall rather than the entire circumference of bowel enters the hernial sac. This so-called Richter's hernia, therefore, does not cause obstruction. The rare cases of *volvulus* of the large bowel have been found almost solely in women during late pregnancy. The reason for this is obscure.

DIVERTICULA (DIVERTICULOSIS, DIVERTICULITIS)

Changing concepts of this disorder would suggest that a better designation might be *diverticular disease* (Painter, 1969). At one time, attention was focused on the numerous small saccular protrusions from the colonic wall along the margins of the taenia coli. These were thought to result from congenital weaknesses in the colonic musculature. The diverticula themselves were considered innocuous, but when fecal impaction led to inflammation (i.e., diverticulitis), clinical manifestations ensued. Within the past decade, several careful studies have indicated that the diverticula may be only secondary changes. Now it is thought that *diverticular disease is primarily characterized by striking hypertrophy of the colonic musculature and that clinical manifestations are produced by abnormal spastic contraction of the colon, as well as by the inflammatory changes of fecal impaction* (Morson, 1963). When diverticulitis does develop, it is an important cause of left lower quadrant pain and fibrotic colonic narrowing (Ming and Fleischner, 1965). Whatever their origins, sacculations of the colonic wall occur in about 10 per cent of Americans over 40 years of age. In most of these individuals, they are either incidental findings at autopsy or are discovered incidentally in the course of barium enema examination. Their prevalence increases with age, and perhaps as many as two-thirds of individuals 85 years or older are affected.

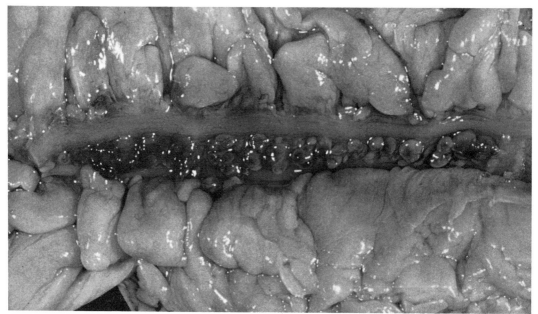

Figure 21–44. *Diverticulosis of the colon viewed from the serosa showing the numerous outpouchings aligned along one margin of the taenia coli.*

Most diverticula are found in the sigmoid (95 per cent), but the descending colon and, indeed, the entire colon may also be affected (Horner, 1958). **Consistently present in all specimens removed for apparent diverticular disease is striking hypertrophy of the musculature of affected segments of colon.** The taenia coli are unusually prominent and have an almost cartilaginous consistency. The circular muscles are also thicker than normal and may impart a corrugated appearance to the gut as viewed from the serosal surface. In addition, in most specimens small flask-like or spherical outpouchings, usually 0.5 to 1 cm. in diameter, can be identified along the margins of the taenia coli (Fig. 21—44 and 21—45). In the absence of secondary inflammation, they are elastic, compressible and easily emptied. Quite characteristically, these sacs dissect into the appendices epiploicae and, therefore, are difficult to identify on casual inspection. They often have small slit-like mouths readily missed on inspection of the mucosal surface. When inflammatory changes supervene, they tend to extend about the diverticula, producing peridiverticulitis, and to dissect into the immediately adjacent pericolic fat. The numerous foci of inflammatory reaction may cause marked diffuse fibrotic thickening in and about the colonic wall. The mucosa may become flattened and bound to the submucosa but, classically, ulceration does not develop. Extension of the infection leads to pericolic abscesses, sinus tracts and sometimes generalized peritonitis.

Histologic examination serves only to confirm the absence or presence of a nonspecific acute or chronic inflammatory reaction, attended in time by considerable fibrosis in and about the bowel wall. Bacterial cultures usually yield a mixed flora, with *E. coli* predominating.

The pathogenesis of diverticula appears to be increased intraluminal pressure with eventual herniation of the mucosa and submucosa through the bowel wall. Whether congenital

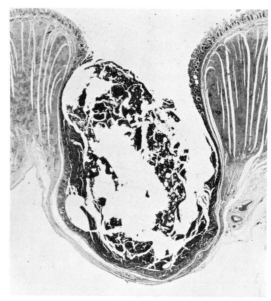

Figure 21–45. *A low power view of a diverticulum of the colon indicating the marked thinning of the wall and absence of muscularis.*

foci of muscular weakness preexist is uncertain, but the extremely high frequency of this condition in the general population argues against any specific congenital defect. The initiating factor appears to be increased muscular tone, leading in time to muscular hypertrophy and eventually to pulsion outpouchings. However, the basis for the muscular hypertrophy is obscure. A host of influences have been questioned. In some individuals, the sigmoid loop is narrow, abnormally redundant and angulated to create possibly a functional obstruction, leading in time to increased muscular contractions and the chain of events described. Chronic constipation and straining, a psychic hazard in some individuals, might contribute. Recent contemporary diets have been incriminated. It is proposed that excessive processing of food products, e.g., white breads, polished rice and dry cereals, has led to diets free of roughage. The fecal stream, thus deprived of its normal bulk, becomes scanty and semifluid. Through some as yet unknown pathways, spastic contraction of the musculature of the sigmoid colon evolves as a compensatory mechanism to slow the fecal stream and prevent overloading of the rectum and the constant urge to defecate (Painter, 1969).

Diverticular disease is unquestionably asymptomatic in most individuals. When manifestations appear, they usually consist of left lower quadrant pain, tenderness, constipation or even acute obstruction in some cases (Editorial, 1970a). Approximately one-third of the specimens surgically resected for such manifestations fail to disclose diverticula; they show only the muscular hypertrophy. When diverticulitis supervenes, the clinical manifestations are accentuated, and pericolic abscesses, fistulous tracts and peritonitis may further modify this symptomatology. But surprisingly, in most cases the manifestations of diverticulitis are not significantly different from those produced by the noninflammatory bowel changes (Parks, 1969). In some patients with diverticulitis, bleeding occurs and may be so severe as to require emergency measures. Worthy of remembering is that longstanding chronic diverticulitis, with its narrowing of the bowel and thickening of the wall, may simulate neoplastic involvement, particularly on barium enema examination.

DEGENERATIVE LESIONS

Melanosis Coli. This curious brown-black discoloration of the mucosa involving either a large segment or the entire large bowel is solely of pathologic interest since it never produces clinical symptoms. It is believed to be due to the deposition of a melanin-like pigment in the phagocytic mononuclear cells of the mucosa. The pigment is probably not melanin but derived from absorbed protein products acted upon by ferments closely related to tyrosinase. It is important to differentiate melanosis coli from hemorrhagic discoloration of the mucosa.

VASCULAR LESIONS

Infarcts. The infrequency of such involvement of the colon is in large measure related to the retroperitoneal location of most of the large bowel. This position allows for the development of a dual blood supply, i.e., the mesenteric vessels as well as the many accessory vessels from the posterior abdominal wall. However, in embolic phenomena, end vessels to a small segment of bowel may be occluded and small foci of hemorrhagic infarction may result. These rarely involve the entire circumference of the colon. Occlusion of the inferior mesenteric artery, especially in the presence of a failing circulation, may give rise to infarction of larger portions of the colon.

Hemorrhoids. Hemorrhoids are variceal dilatations of the anal and perianal venous plexuses. These extremely common lesions affect about 5 per cent of the general population and are rarely encountered under the age of 30 save in pregnant women. They develop secondary to persistently elevated venous pressure within the hemorrhoidal plexus. Although any cause of consistent venous congestion may be responsible, the most important predisposing influences are constipation with straining at stool and venous stasis of pregnancy. The latter state is related to the overall congestion in the pelvis as well as the pressure of the enlarged uterus upon the iliac vessels. More rarely, but much more importantly, hemorrhoids may reflect collateral anastomotic channels that develop as a result of portal hypertension. On this basis, the appearance of hemorrhoids may be a clue to the existence of some diffuse hepatic disease or portal vein occlusion. The varicosities may develop in the inferior hemorrhoidal plexus and be located below the anorectal line (external hemorrhoids), or they may develop from dilatation of the superior hemorrhoidal plexus and produce internal hemorrhoids (Fig. 21–46). Commonly, both plexuses are affected and the varicosities are referred to as combined hemorrhoids.

Histologically, these lesions consist only of thin-walled, dilated, typical varices that protrude beneath the anal or rectal mucosa. In their exposed, traumatized situation, they tend to become thrombosed and, in the course of time, canalized. Occasionally, internal hemor-

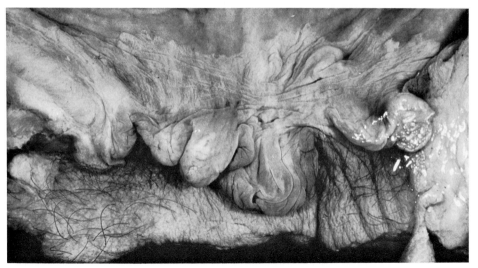

Figure 21–46. *Hemorrhoids. External mucosal protrusions containing markedly dilated veins.*

rhoids may protrude through the anal sphincter and become strangulated by the contraction of the sphincter about their bases. Superficial ulceration, fissure formation and hemorrhagic infarction with strangulation complicate the histologic picture and clinical problem.

INFLAMMATIONS

There are many types of inflammatory disease which affect the colon. All tend to produce anatomic lesions which closely resemble one another. It is often impossible on gross and even microscopic examination to identify the precise etiologic agent. Therefore, an important part of the diagnostic evaluation of inflammation or ulceration of the colon is the bacteriologic and parasitic examination of the lesion and the stools.

IDIOPATHIC ULCERATIVE COLITIS

As the name indicates, this is a mysterious, but common and serious, disorder characterized by extensive ulcerations of the colon. However, although the colon is the primary site of attack, *the disease is systemic in nature and is often associated with arthritis, uveitis, venous thromboses, liver disease and various skin lesions, especially pyoderma gangrenosum. It is also commonly associated with Crohn's disease* and, in a series of 676 cases of Crohn's disease, 60 individuals had concomitant ulcerative colitis (Perlman and Broberger, 1968). Recall that Crohn's disease, too, was associated with extraintestinal manifestations which are virtually identical with those encountered in ulcerative colitis. The intriguing possibility arises that the two disorders

are differing tissue responses to the same insult in anatomically distinct segments of the gut. Indeed, there is overlap in the segments of the bowel affected in the two disorders. Ulcerative colitis classically begins in the rectosigmoid but often extends to affect the entire colon. In 10 to 20 per cent of the cases, the terminal ileum may become involved. Conversely, as was pointed out, the colon may be involved in Crohn's disease; but typically, the inflammatory changes are granulomatous (granulomatous colitis), while in ulcerative colitis the inflammatory changes are nonspecific.

Ulcerative colitis in its typical presentation is a remitting, relapsing disorder marked by attacks of bloody mucoid diarrhea, which may persist for days, weeks or months and then subside only to recur after an asymptomatic interval of months to years or even decades. In the fortunate patient, the first attack is the last. At the other end of the spectrum, the explosive initial attack may lead to such serious bleeding and fluid and electrolyte disturbance as to comprise a medical emergency. Between these extremes are the usually relapsing patterns spanning the life of the patient.

Incidence. A recent review of a large number of patients disclosed a bimodal age distribution for onset of the disease with peaks at 18 and 50 years (DeDombal et al., 1969). In children, the disease tends to be more severe clinically and more extensive anatomically. More than half of the younger patients have involvement of the entire colon, while only 34 per cent of all patients with ulcerative colitis have total colonic disease. The incidence of ulcerative colitis varies widely but, in some respects, it appears to be a disease of civilization. In the United States and Great Britain, approximately 2 to 6 individuals are afflicted per 100,000 population; in Africa, Asia and South America, however, the disease is virtually unknown. In addition to its potentially devastating effects on the health of the individual, of major importance is the high rate at which colonic carcinoma develops in patients with longstanding disease.

Etiology and Pathogenesis. As the term "idiopathic" implies, the causation of this disorder is unknown. Nonetheless, the literature is replete with reports suggesting that the derangement is immunologic and also those contending that all of the immunologic observations represent epiphenomena (secondary phenomena). It is impossible to present more than a survey here. For more details, reference should be made to the excellent recent review by Kraft and Kirsner (1971).

To begin with, it is argued that the large and small intestines are in a sense immunologic organs, in as much as they may be the equivalent of the bursa of Fabricius in fowl. Although such a proposition represents a possibility, it has yet to be established (Watson, 1969a). Anticolon antibodies have been reported in 0 to 50 per cent of these patients, implying that ulcerative colitis is an autoimmune disease (Wright and Truelove, 1966). These autoantibodies cross react with colon tissue extracts, mucopolysaccharide found in intestinal mucin, a membrane-bounded antigen related to human blood group A, "carcinoembryonic antigen" (CEA) (p. 970), and antigens derived from *E. coli* types 0 to 14 polysaccharides (Lagercrantz et al., 1968). Cross reactions between colon tissue antigens and coliform antigens might induce immunologic injury to the colonic mucosa. With respect to these antibodies, it should be pointed out that they have not been identified at all in certain studies, they are not present in more than half of the patients in other studies, they persist after colectomy and they are unrelated to the severity of the colitis. Moreover, when tested against colonic epithelial cells, they are not cytotoxic. Indeed, similar antibodies have been identified in the sera of normal individuals (Kronman, 1971). Therefore, attention has turned to delayed type hypersensitivity. Several reports suggest that lymphocytes from patients with ulcerative colitis are cytotoxic in tissue culture to autologous or allogeneic colon cells (Watson et al., 1966). This cytotoxic effect disappears quickly after colectomy and is undetectable 10 days following surgery, a surprisingly rapid disappearance for cell-mediated immunity. This cytotoxicity does not correlate with the severity of the disease, and the question has been raised as to whether this specific lymphocyte activity is a form of allogeneic inhibition (Watson, 1969b). Many other immunologic observations have been made, but it will suffice to conclude that despite all this evidence, it is not clear that immune mechanisms initiate the ulcerative destruction of the colonic mucosa. An equally plausible explanation would interpret the release of large amounts of antigen as epiphenomena to destruction of colonic cells by other influences. However, this suggestion does not in any way preclude the possibility that immunologic reactions may play a role in perpetuating the disease, whatever its origins.

Brief mention should be made of the persistent theory that ulcerative colitis is a psychosomatic disorder. It is postulated that these patients act out their anxieties, frustrations and hostilities through their gut and, in some way, damage it. It is a well established fact that attacks of ulcerative colitis are often precipitated by emotional stress. However, we do not yet have the tools to measure all variables of homeostasis, so we have little evidence of the mechanisms by which personality structure or emotional problems initiate disease (Hornsby, 1970). Conversely, it is not unreasonable to believe that a disease as severe, disabling and life-threatening as ulcerative colitis may well disrupt a patient's personality structure. One pathogenetic fact is well established—the diagnosis of ulcerative colitis should never be made until all specific known causes of ulcerative lesions of the colon have been excluded.

Morphology. Ulcerative colitis is confined to the colon in about 65 to 75 per cent of all cases, but in 10 to 20 per cent of the cases, it extends to affect the ileum. It should be emphasized that this ileal involvement is quite distinct from regional enteritis and maintains the characteristics of the ulcerative changes in the colon (Warren and Sommers, 1954). The disease usually begins in the rectosigmoid although occasionally it may arise at higher levels, even in the cecum. As the disease progresses, larger areas and sometimes even the entire colon are involved.

At first, pinpoint mucosal hemorrhages appear which in time suppurate to become minute abscesses. Arising in the crypts of the mucosal glands, these abscesses increase in size and undermine the mucosal margins. Superficial sloughing produces small ulcers which may enlarge to involve the submucosa. These defects usually erode only to the muscularis, but deep excavations may penetrate the bowel. In time, the ulcers coalesce to cause large irregular mucosal defects. Sometimes the undermined edges of adjacent ulcers connect to create tunnels covered by tenuous mucosal bridges. In advanced cases, virtually the entire mucosa is destroyed (Figs.

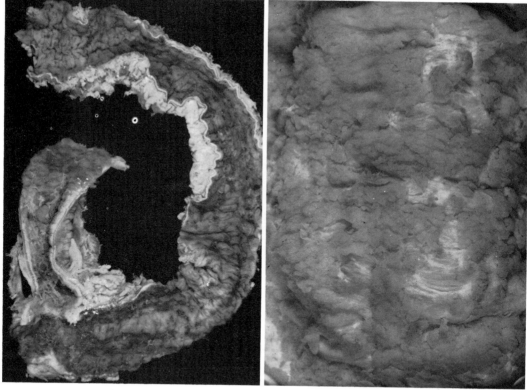

Fig. 21–47.   Fig. 21–48.

Figure 21–47. *Ulcerative colitis. A view of the entire colon showing darker ulcerated areas principally in the cecal region. The pale areas are preserved mucosa. Note the accompanying involvement of the terminal ileum.*

Figure 21–48. *A close-up of the ulcerations in chronic ulcerative colitis. Coalescence of numerous small ulcerations has isolated islands of mucosa which, in the more advanced lesion, would produce the characteristic so-called pseudopolyposis.*

21–47 and 21–48). Residual islands of edematous hyperemic mucosa often persist in such advancing disease. These islands appear elevated above the surrounding ulceration and thus are designated **"pseudopolyps"** (Fig. 21–49). It is important that these pseudopolyps be differentiated from true polyps since the former represent residual foci of preexisting inflammatory epithelium and not neoplasia (Goldgraber et al., 1960).

A number of secondary alterations frequently appear. Active inflammation may penetrate the colonic wall, producing **pericolic abscesses or peritonitis.** In chronic cases, the inflammatory colon may adhere to adjacent viscera, and sometimes **fistulous tracts** result. While edematous thickening is characteristic, late in the disease minimal to moderate fibrous thickening and rigidity of the wall may develop. If the disease can be controlled or remits, reepithelialization of the mucosa may virtually restore the normal architecture if there has not been too much prior damage.

Histologically, **the early acute lesions appear as microabscesses in the depths of the crypts of the mucosal glands** (Fig. 21–50). The ulcerations

which appear later show **nonspecific marked inflammatory bases and margins.** Acute vasculitis is sometimes found in the bases of these ulcers, raising the possibility that immunologic vascular lesions precede and lead to infarction necrosis of the bowel mucosa (Warren and Sommers, 1949). In the acute stages of the disease, the ulcers are usually confined to the mucosa and submucosa. With persistent chronicity the lesions deepen, and the leukocytic infiltrate assumes a more mononuclear pattern. The epithelium of the margins of the ulcers as well as the pseudopolyps consistently have inflammatory metaplasia and dysplasia of the glands, suggesting possible sites of origin of carcinoma. All stages of mucosal regeneration may be seen, often with the production of a more primitive mucosa with cystically dilated and atypical glands. Some fibrosis and inflammatory scarring of the wall are evident in the later stages. The inflammatory reaction and scarring is entirely nonspecific, and bacterial cultures usually reveal a banal flora with *E. coli* predominating. Worth noting as differential features from regional colitis are the absence of granulomas and marked fibrosis.

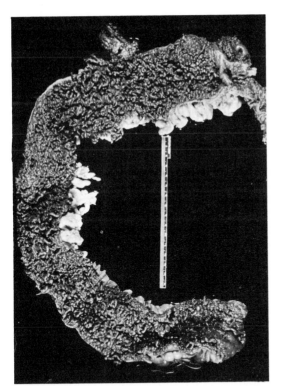

Figure 21–49. Ulcerative colitis with striking pseudopolyposis. The shaggy mucosal surface is produced by myriads of preserved islands of projecting mucosa.

Clinical Course. In most patients, bloody diarrhea containing stringy mucus, lower abdominal pain and cramps, usually relieved by defecation, are the first manifestations of the disease. These appear insidiously but become progressively worse. Often this first attack is preceded by a stressful period in the patient's life. Persistence of the manifestations for even a short time is usually followed by fever and weight loss. Spontaneously, or more often after appropriate therapy, these symptoms abate in the course of days to weeks. An asymptomatic interval of varying length follows, after which typically stress (emotional or physical) may cause a flare-up of the clinical manifestations. In this manner, the disease pursues a relapsing-remitting course, perhaps for decades or for the life of the patient. In the long chronicity of the disease, the bowel may undergo fibrosis with the formation of strictures easily confused with carcinoma, both clinically and radiographically.

With chronic disease, extragastrointestinal manifestations are quite common: ankylosing spondylitis in 17 per cent, arthritis of large joints in another 6 per cent, uveitis in 11 per cent, as well as venous thromboses and skin lesions. Some of these systemic problems may,

indeed, precede the onset of the bowel disease and may persist after colectomy. Hepatic involvement is encountered in about 15 per cent of patients and takes the form of fatty change or pericholangitis. Sudden cessation of bowel function with the production of toxic dilatation of the colon may appear, the so-called "toxic megacolon."

The development of carcinoma is one of the most feared complications. Indeed, multiple carcinomas may appear apparently simultaneously. A range from 0 to 33 per cent has been reported in patients with ulcerative colitis (Felsen and Wolarsky, 1949) (DeDombal, 1968). Important determinants in the development of such cancers are age at initiation of disease, extent of disease and duration of disease. Considering all patients with ulcerative colitis, an average of about 16 years elapses before a tumor develops (Bergen and Cage, 1960). For this reason, the young who develop ulcerative colitis are particularly at risk. In a long-term study of 396 children, a death rate of 20 per cent per decade was found (Devroede, 1971). Most died of cancer at an average of 28 years of age. The risk of cancer in those who first develop their disease in the later decades of life is only slightly greater than that for the general population.

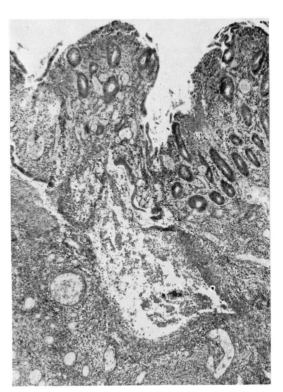

Figure 21–50. A deeply situated mucosal abscess in the early developmental stage of acute ulcerative colitis.

In a minority of patients, the onset of ulcerative colitis is abrupt and fulminant, with uncontrollable diarrhea, bleeding and life-threatening loss of fluids and electrolytes. The mortality rate in this group is extremely high, and often emergency surgical intervention is required.

The diagnosis of ulcerative colitis can often be made on purely clinical grounds, supported by microbiologic studies of stools to rule out specific etiologies. Sigmoidoscopy and biopsy are of great value, since the rectosigmoid is usually involved. Barium enema may offer confirmatory evidence. Few diseases are more debilitating, depressing and threatening. Despite current usage of antibacterial drugs and steroids, the gloomy outlook has not materially improved from previous decades. Because complete control is difficult to effect by conservative therapy, more and more resort to surgery is being made.

TUBERCULOUS COLITIS

This is almost invariably associated with lesions of the small intestine and lung. The ulcerations produced are similar to those found in the small intestine, except that they are not transversely oriented. The microscopic features are identical with those described previously. Uncommonly, anal tuberculous infections may produce chronic perianal fistulous tracts.

AMEBIASIS

In the United States, an estimated 10 per cent of the general population harbor amebas within the large bowel. It was indicated in the general discussion of this disease that few of these infected individuals develop clinical disease (p. 450). Many of these parasites are nonpathogenic *E. hartmanni;* fortunately, the pathogenic *E. histolytica* is much less common. When manifestations are evoked, the condition begins as an amebic colitis.

The lesions affect the entire large bowel in over half the cases but may affect only a small segment of the bowel in the remainder. The parasite penetrates into the depth of a colonic gland. Since it secretes an active proteolytic enzyme, it digests the mucosal surface and penetrates into the lamina propria. As the amebas burrow deeper, they undermine the overlying mucosa. Ischemic necrosis of this overlying mucosa then occurs with the development of ulcers. At first, the ulcers tend to have a narrow neck and a broad base and are appropriately called "**collar button**" **ulcers.** As these ulcers en-

large, they retain their undermined margins so characteristic of amebic colitis. Usually the ulcers are well spaced and do not coalesce to denude the gut.

There is remarkably little cellular exudation and little evidence of exudate in the bases of the ulcerations. However, secondary bacterial invasion soon complicates the picture and chronic suppuration becomes evident. The ulcers may expand to become large defects many centimeters in diameter. The mucosal loss does not, however, approach that seen in nonspecific ulcerative colitis. The ulcers rarely extend below the submucosa and almost never affect the muscularis or serosa or cause penetration. With control of the infection, mucosal regeneration follows.

The diagnosis is made histologically by the demonstration of the vegetative parasites. These are found most abundantly in the base and the advancing undermined margins of the ulcer. The parasites are larger in size than the macrophage (20 to 25 microns in diameter) with which they are often confused. In the **vegetative form,** as contrasted with the encysted parasite, only a **single nucleus** is present and the cytoplasm has a finely granular, pink appearance in the usual tissue stains. These parasites must also be differentiated from their nonpathogenic relatives, the smaller *E. hartmanni* and the *E. coli* normal inhabitants of the colon. *E. coli* never contain phagocytized red cells as do the pathogenic *E. histolytica.* The **encysted form** of *E. histolytica* rarely contains more than **one to four nuclei,** while *E. coli* often have **eight or more nuclei.** The base of the ulcer may show only coagulated amorphous debris beneath which the active parasites are found. Bacterial invasion may totally distort this picture by enhancing the exudation and masking the presence of the parasites.

No adequate explanation exists of why so many individuals harbor the parasites in apparent symbiotic relationship while others develop clinical disease. It is believed that, in many instances, persons harbor the parasite for days, weeks or even years and then, for completely obscure reasons, begin to develop clinical manifestations and anatomic lesions. Usually the disease has an insidious onset with the appearance of diarrhea, abdominal cramps and pain. As it progresses, the diarrhea assumes a bloody mucous quality that may be so severe and so persistent as to cause prostration due to the loss of fluid, electrolytes and blood. Clearly, in any case of persistent diarrhea, it is necessary to examine warm, wet-field fecal smears to rule out the possible presence of amebas.

Amebic colitis is a serious disease, not only because of the bowel disturbances, but also because the organisms erode veins and drain to the liver predisposing to amebic *liver abscesses.* From this site of dissemination, abscesses sometimes burrow through the liver capsule to create *subphrenic abscesses* and then sometimes penetrate the diaphragm to create *empyema, lung abscess* or even pericarditis. In other instances, the amebas may be carried though the blood from the liver to the lungs and thus produce disseminated hematogenous amebic abscesses within the lung. From these pulmonary abscesses, metastatic hematogenous amebic abscesses may occur in other organs, particularly the brain.

BACILLARY DYSENTERY

Ulceroinflammatory disease of the colon and, less frequently, of the small intestine may be caused by a variety of bacteria. The term bacillary dysentery is restricted to those forms of bacterial colitis caused by the Shigella group of organisms. (This disease is discussed in Chapter 10.) The lesions in bacillary dysentery begin in the Peyer's patches as do those of typhoidal enteritis. Progressive inflammatory hyperplasia of these lymphoid masses leads to ulceration of the overlying mucosa and the development of sharp, nonundermined ulcerations with inflammatory hyperemic bases and margins. The ulcers may extend widely and in some instances coalesce, but usually large segments of bowel are not denuded except in the most florid cases. Diffuse edema and hyperemia of the remaining mucosa also may be present. The ulcers rarely extend beyond the submucosa and, only in severe instances, penetrate to produce peritonitis or fistulous communications. Histologically, the ulceroinflammatory disease is entirely nonspecific, manifesting all the characteristic changes of acute suppurative inflammation found anywhere in the body. The identification of bacillary dysentery, then, must rest on bacterial cultures and immunologic procedures that disclose the exact nature of the causative agent.

As in all forms of dysentery, abdominal cramps, pain, diarrhea, mucus, bloody stools, vomiting and variable fluid and electrolyte disturbances characterize the clinical picture. Since the Shigella organisms rarely invade the blood, the bacteremic spread and disseminated lesions characteristic of typhoid fever do not usually occur in bacillary dysentery. However, the dysentery group of organisms elaborate an endotoxin that is released upon the death and proteolytic dissolution of bacterial cells which is capable of producing systemic tissue injury as described on p. 400.

STAPHYLOCOCCIC COLITIS

With the present-day widespread use of antibiotics for all types of infections, the normal flora of the intestinal tract is sometimes eliminated. Freed of their normal bacterial content of *E. coli,* the colon and, less commonly, the small intestine provide an excellent site for the proliferation of antibiotic-resistant organisms, most common of which is *Staphylococcus aureus.* Some patients tolerate this change in bacterial flora well. Others develop a dysentery-like picture and some develop anatomic lesions. Depending on the stage and severity of the disease, the lesions take the form of focal hemorrhages or areas of acute suppurative ulceration. Extensive inflammatory necrosis of the mucosa may produce a pseudomembrane. As in many ulcerative lesions of the gut, no pathognomonic gross or microscopic features are present. Identification of the causative organism by bacteriologic examination is required. Such colonic infections may lead to bacteremias with pyemic abscesses in many other organs and tissues.

PSEUDOMEMBRANOUS COLITIS

Closely allied to staphylococcal enterocolitis is a lesion described only as "pseudomembranous colitis" to designate the characteristic production of a superficial, green-black, necrotic slough on the bowel mucosa. This disease has become more prominent since the widespread use of antibiotics and is generally found in postoperative patients on such therapy (Becker and Brayton, 1958). Presumably the cause is not bacterial, but the etiology remains unknown. Toxicity of antibiotics, interference with the bacterial flora of the gut, ill-defined disturbances in the nutrition of the mucosa, and allergies have been hypothesized as producing the necrotizing pseudomembranous inflammation. At the present time, no one theory has been substantiated. The lesion appears as an ulceroinflammatory disease with characteristic edema and hyperemia, but is specifically designated by the development of a green-brown to black sloughing mucosal surface usually over the regions of the ulcerations. The clinical manifestations are those of the other forms of dysentery. Sometimes the disease is so fulminating and acute as to produce severe fluid and electrolyte loss, vascular collapse and death.

TYPHOID AND PARATYPHOID FEVERS

Typhoid and paratyphoid enterocolitis is a form of ulceroinflammatory intestinal disease that comprises one of the dominant features of these systemic infections. The general discussion of these diseases and intestinal lesions has already been presented (p. 397).

LYMPHOPATHIA VENEREUM

The primary site of origin of this disease in the female is the cervix or vagina (p. 440). Drainage of the infection in this sex occurs to the lymph nodes about the rectum. In the male, with the external genitalia as the primary site, only the inguinal nodes are affected. Therefore, in females, inflammation may extend from the neighboring nodes to involve the rectal wall. While basically a perirectal process, at a far advanced stage it produces sufficient inflammation, fibrosis and scarring of the rectum to cause narrowing of the bowel. Trauma to the wall by the passage of solid feces through the point of narrowing occasionally produces mucosal ulcers. Lymphogranuloma, therefore, must be considered in the differential diagnosis of rectal obstruction in the female.

MISCELLANEOUS COLITIS

Mercury, like many metals, is excreted through the kidneys and large intestine. In cases of mercurial poisoning, toxic damage to the colonic mucosa may occur with the formation of ulcerations. These are invariably secondarily infected and appear, therefore, as nonspecific inflammation. In fatal uremia, changes termed *uremic colitis* are sometimes present. These vary from areas of simple hyperemia to areas of marked ecchymosis which occasionally ulcerate. They are the colonic counterparts of the changes described in the stomach in cases of renal failure. Once again, the gross and microscopic pattern is completely nonspecific, and the diagnosis is made by the presence of other clinical findings of uremia plus exclusion of specific bowel disease.

TUMORS

Cancers and polyps of the colon are two of the most common neoplasms in man. For obscure reasons, gastric carcinoma has declined in frequency and carcinoma of the colon is now the second most common visceral cancer in man. Polyps are not only common (occurring in approximately 10 per cent of the general population), but they also occupy an important albeit controversial role in the development of carcinoma. Both polyps and cancers constitute a great challenge to clinical medicine since they

can be detected by careful clinical and radiographic evaluation at an early stage. Cure is theoretically possible for most patients with these lesions.

BENIGN TUMORS

A polyp may be defined as any outgrowth from a mucosal surface. In the colon, these outgrowths tend to occur in three different but overlapping patterns: (1) the sporadic pedunculated adenoma, (2) the villous or sessile adenoma and (3) heredofamilial patterns in which a profusion of polyps is scattered throughout the colon and sometimes the entire intestinal tract. Each of these patterns has its own distinctive anatomic and clinical features.

Pedunculated Adenoma. *The pedunculated adenoma comprises a small (usually less than 4 cm. in diameter) hemispherical or spherical polypoid head attached to the colon by a stalk.* It is impossible to define in universally acceptable terms what constitutes a stalk, but it has been suggested by Castleman and Krickstein (1962) that if the head of the polyp can be moved freely in all directions through a 90 degree arc, the lesion may be said to be pedunculated. The stalk may be relatively short but at other times may be extraordinarily long, if the head of the polyp is pulled along in the propulsive contractions of the gut.

These lesions are extremely common in both sexes and all age groups with some increased prevalence in the sixth, seventh and eighth decades. The numerous surveys of the frequency of these lesions have yielded results varying from 1 to 50 per cent of the general population. Much of this extraordinary span is due to the techniques used for establishing the diagnosis. Thus, the top level was attained in an autopsy study while the lower levels were generally derived from clinical sigmoidoscopic or radiographic examinations. A reasonable average might be 10 per cent of the general population. Judging from the literature, the distribution of these lesions within the colon is equally controversial. Clinical studies would indicate that over 90 per cent of pedunculated adenomas occur in the rectosigmoid. Autopsy studies indicate that about half occur in the ascending and transverse colon and that only a third are found in the rectum and sigmoid. These differences are readily understood in terms of the limitations of the methods used for identifying these lesions.

Pedunculated adenomas occur throughout the colon as solitary or multiple lesions. In autopsy surveys, about half the patients have an isolated polyp. The remaining half may have two or many more, and about one-sixth of all patients have more than five (Helwig, 1947). All are generally **small, soft, red, raspberry-like masses attached to the colon by a stalk of variable length.** Commonly the heads of these tumors are 1 cm. in diameter or less, but many reach a size of 4 cm. In some, the stalk is quite broad and conical, tapering to the head, while in others it is a long, slender strand. As indicated, to justify the designation "stalk," the head must be movable through a 90 degree arc.

Almost all pedunculated lesions have a central core of fibrovascular tissue which arises in the submucosa and extends in continuity through the center of the stalk and head. The stalk is usually covered by a fairly normal colonic mucosa, but the head may be covered by a wide range of epithelial patterns. At one extreme, the covering glands may be virtually indistinguishable from those of the normal colonic mucosa. At the other extreme, the glands are tall and hyperplastic and sometimes are branching with deep crypts. In this pattern, the epithelial cells are taller, lose their capacity to secrete mucin, and have variably located, somewhat hyperchromatic nuclei. Generally, however, the columnar palisade of the epithelial cells is retained, and some resemblance to colonic mucosa is preserved. These changes are referred to as "polypoid hyperplasia." Mitotic figures give evidence of the proliferative activity of these lesions. In floridly growing lesions, the cells may no longer retain their usual palisade, and some epithelial scrambling and piling up may appear along with the formation of abnormal gland patterns. Sometimes the cytologic abnormality verges on frank anaplasia. Such cellular variation is most frequently found on the surface of the polyp exposed to the irritation of the fecal stream (Fig. 21–51). The benign nature of the lesions is, however, indicated by the absence of invasion of the central fibrous core and by the absence of frank anaplasia of the epithelial cells. However, it must be admitted that the line between polypoid hyperplasia and frank carcinoma is sometimes exceedingly fine and is ultimately drawn on the basis of the pathologist's personal interpretation (Figs. 21–52 and 21–53). Invasion of the underlying fibrous core is usually held to be the most reliable criterion of malignant transformation since cellular changes may not provide a clear basis for distinction between benign and malignant growth.

Clinical Course. Pedunculated adenomas are most often discovered as incidental lesions at autopsy or during sigmoidoscopic or barium enema studies performed for investigation of some other intestinal disease. Occasionally, however, they bleed and are thus discovered. Because cellular atypia is frequently observed in these lesions, described earlier as "polypoid

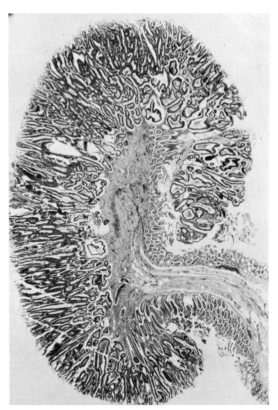

Figure 21–51. *A low power view of a slender-stalked colonic polyp indicating the increased chromaticity and height of the glands covering the head of the lesion.*

hyperplasia," their relationship to colonic cancers was at one time a highly controversial issue. It was felt that these benign lesions were frequent forerunners of carcinoma of the colon. Moreover, because some colonic cancers grow in a polypoid fashion, it was assumed that they had originated from pedunculated adenomas. Virtually all of the recent analyses of large series of patients agree that carcinoma is an extremely rare, but possible, complication of pedunculated adenomas (Enterline et al., 1962) (Spratt and Ackerman, 1960) (Spratt and Watson, 1971). In a recent evaluation of over 1200 adenomatous polyps, there was no instance of malignant transformation (Horn, 1971). Even lesions with frank carcinomatous transformation are probably not "biologic cancer," since in almost all instances there is no recurrence of tumor following removal of the initial lesion. Despite these reassurances, the conservative clinician must take the position that in the individual patient even the remote chance of malignancy demands that these easily resectable lesions be removed. Moreover,

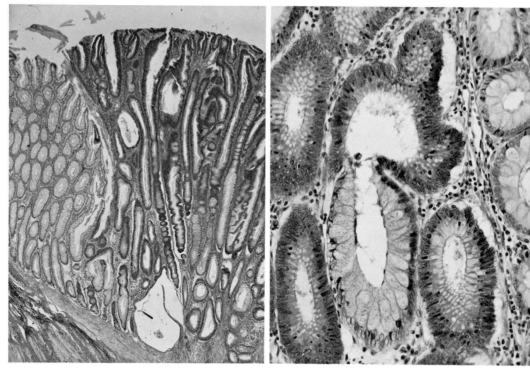

Fig. 21–52.   Fig. 21–53.

Figure 21–52. A low power view of the junction between the normal colonic mucosal covering of the stalk of a polyp and the polypoid change in the adjacent mucosa. Loss of mucus secretion, increase in the height of the glands and variability in the cell size are visible.

Figure 21–53. A high power detail of a junctional group of glands at the point of transition between normal colonic mucosa and polypoid atypicality. A striking comparison is evident between the regular columnar mucus-secreting epithelium and the atypical polypoid epithelium which, however, is not frankly malignant.

the possibility cannot be overlooked that on extremely rare occasions the small polypoid cancer may masquerade as a pedunculated adenoma on clinical and radiologic examination.

Villous or Sessile Adenoma. *The villous or sessile adenoma is a papillary lesion that attaches by a broad base directly to the colonic mucosa.* It is not only distinctive in appearance from the pedunculated lesion but has a totally different clinical significance since it is a known forerunner of colonic carcinoma. At least 30 per cent of these lesions have cancerous areas, and some reports indicate an even higher frequency of malignant transformation (74 per cent) (Swinton et al., 1955) (Wheat and Ackerman, 1958). Some of this reported range is due to variable criteria of malignancy, but more may be attributed to the large size of many villous adenomas requiring innumerable microscopic sections for the total evaluation of the lesion. The more painstaking the search, the higher the likelihood of discovering cancer. In the individual case, it is safest to assume that any villous adenoma is cancerous until exhaustive histologic study rules this out.

Villous adenomas occur six times less frequently than pedunculated adenomas (Horn, 1971). They occur principally in the rectum and sigmoid and are uncommon in the right or transverse colon. Generally they assume a cauliflower, fungating appearance and are frequently over 5 cm. in diameter (Fig. 21–54). Lesions up to 15 to 20 cm. are relatively common. They are pale gray masses that are elevated about 1 to 3 cm. above the surrounding mucosa and often show focal areas of hemorrhage or ulceration on their surface. Although they appear to be superficially attached to the underlying submucosa, in many instances it is apparent that malignant areas have penetrated to deeper levels.

As the term "villous adenoma" implies, these lesions are composed of small, finger-like villi, sometimes branching and complicated, covered by columnar epithelial cells ranging from clearly mature colonic epithelial forms to obviously anaplastic cells. The most valuable histologic criteria of malignancy are (1) piling up of the epithelium to form multilayered masses of cells that have lost their mucinous secretion and have become hyperchromatic, disorderly and anaplastic; (2) formation of small atypical gland patterns within these masses; and (3) invasion of the underlying fibrous core.

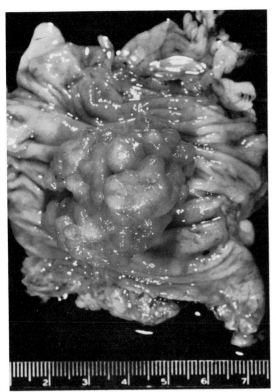

Figure 21-54. *A close-up of a villous sessile polyp of the colon which, on histologic examination, proved to be benign.*

A variant of the villous adenoma is the so-called **hyperplastic polyp.** This lesion appears as a small, broad-based mucosal elevation composed of elongated glands lined by a characteristically scalloped epithelium produced by infoldings of the linings of the glands. Present evidence suggests that hyperplastic polyps are probably antecedents of villous adenomas (Goldman et al., 1970).

Their relationship to colonic cancer clearly gives great importance to villous adenomas. While some of these tumors may be benign, their potential is unmistakable and they should be excised promptly on discovery.

In the recent past, it has also become apparent that these lesions may be hypersecretors of copious amounts of mucoid material and potassium, sometimes causing significant losses of fluid and electrolytes (Davis et al., 1962).

Before closing the discussion of the pedunculated and villous adenomas, it should be noted that many hybrid forms are encountered in which a major portion of the lesion is adenomatous and yet there are focal areas of villous growth. Sometimes the pedunculated lesion has a totally villous glandular pattern

over the head. Therefore, it cannot be assumed because a lesion has a stalk it is a pure pedunculated adenoma and not a villous adenoma. However, as stated previously, in the absence of invasion the stalked lesion will rarely behave as a biologic malignancy.

Heredofamilial Polyposis. In a few instances, the tendency to develop polyps of the colon represents a hereditary trait transmitted as an autosomal dominant (Veale, 1965). In many cases, these polyps are associated with developmental abnormalities outside the intestinal tract. Six distinctive syndromes have been described by McCusick (1962). The four more important of this group are familial multiple polyposis of the colon, Peutz-Jeghers syndrome, Gardner's syndrome and Turcot's syndrome.

Familial multiple polyposis of the colon is made distinctive by the myriads of polyps which may cover virtually the entire mucosa of the colon and sometimes extend into the upper levels of the intestinal tract, including the stomach. Although the disease is hereditary, polyps do not appear before the second and third decades of life. A member of an involved family who has not developed polyps by age 40 is not likely to develop them at a later time.

The individual polyp is usually a small pedunculated adenoma 1 cm. in diameter. When closely packed, the polyps may impart a furry appearance to the mucosal surface (Fig. 21–55). In histologic detail, these adenomas are indistinguishable from the pedunculated lesions already described.

Despite their morphologic resemblance to the benign sporadic pedunculated adenomas, there is a high incidence of malignant transformation of the polyps in this hereditary disorder. It is not uncommon to find certain adenomas larger and presumably more actively growing than the remainder. Such lesions may develop into cancer. Multiple polyps may become cancerous concurrently. Malignancy is more likely if the disease is of long duration, and it is possible that, in time, unless the diseased colon is removed, multiple polyposis inevitably develops into cancer. In the series of heredofamilial polyposis reported by Lockhart-Mummery et al. (1956), there were 154 colonic carcinomas among 218 patients. The average age at death from cancer with this disease is 42 years instead of 67 years for persons in the general population developing a cancer of the colon (Dukes, 1952). It is not clear whether the malignant transformation stems from inherent characteristics of these seemingly benign adenomas or merely reflects the increased probability of malignant change

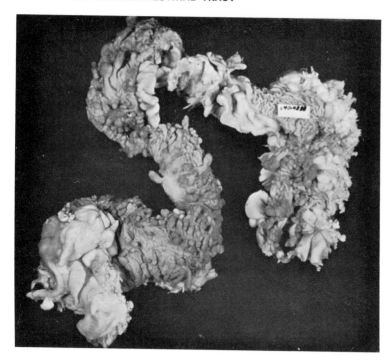

Figure 21–55. Congenital heredofamilial polyposis of the colon. The bowel is studded with numerous small polyps.

among literally hundreds of polyps. The diagnosis can be readily made by either sigmoidoscopic or barium enema study.

The Peutz-Jeghers syndrome is characterized by polyps of the entire gastrointestinal tract, particularly in the small intestine, associated with melanin pigmentation of the buccal mucosa, lips and digits (Dormandy, 1957) (Bartholomew et al., 1957). While the polyps resemble in all anatomic details those of the heredofamilial disorder just described, they rarely give rise to cancer, hence the importance of recognizing this pattern of disease. The reason for this benign behavior is unclear but it is said that the polyps represent hamartomatous overgrowths rather than true neoplasms. All do not take comfort in this reassurance since cases have been reported of apparent Peutz-Jeghers syndrome with carcinomatous transformation (Achord and Proctor, 1963).

The Gardner syndrome refers to the association of polyposis in the colon with neoplasms elsewhere. These extracolonic neoplasms have occurred in the skin, subcutaneous tissue and bone. A systemic derangement in the genetic repressor mechanisms that control cell growth is postulated but not established.

The Turcot syndrome combines polyps of the colon with brain tumors. In contrast to the other entities mentioned, it is transmitted as an autosomal recessive.

Miscellaneous Benign Tumors. The whole gamut of mesenchymal tumors may occur in the colon. These include leiomyomas, fibromas, lipomas, hemangiomas and neurofibromas which are not distinctive from the same lesions occurring elsewhere (Fig. 21–56). Only rarely are these benign lesions of clinical significance. Two other polypoid lesions merit brief mention. Polyps are sporadically found in the colons of children, most frequently in the rectosigmoid; these differ in appearance from the polyps of pedunculated and villous adenoma and are designated *"juvenile polyps."* They tend to be small hemispheric elevations of the mucosa that are rarely pedunculated. Histologically, they are made distinctive by a very abundant loose fibrovascular stroma containing widely spaced glands, some sufficiently dilated to comprise cysts. A scant leukocytic infiltrate is often present in the stroma. Malignant transformation and recurrence are extremely rare if they occur at all.

Lymphoid polyps are an additional rare form of benign tumor consisting of aggregates of lymphoid tissue covered usually by a fairly regular, although sometimes atrophic, colonic mucosa. The lymphoid architecture may be quite regular with prominent lymphoid follicles in a stroma of mature lymphocytes. The pattern resembles that of the nodular lymphoma, and some have considered these to be true lymphomas occurring in the bowel. The preponderant opinion, however, considers these lesions as foci of striking submucosal lymphoid hyperplasia rather than neoplasms (Helwig and Hansen, 1951). In almost all cases, local resection is curative. Occasionally, true neo-

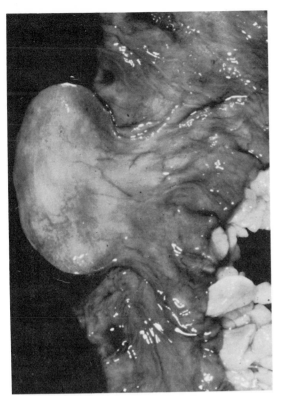

Figure 21–56. *A submucosal lipoma in the colon which has been pedunculated by the traction of the intestinal peristalsis.*

plastic lymphomatous involvement occurs in the rectum as a primary lesion or a systemic dissemination of a lymphoma, and this differential must be borne in mind in the interpretation of these lesions.

MALIGNANT TUMORS

Carcinoma. Virtually 98 per cent of all cancers in the large intestine are carcinomas. They represent one of the prime challenges for the medical profession because they produce symptoms relatively early and are potentially curable by resection. Despite this, colonic carcinoma is the second most common cause of cancer deaths in the United States. In the United States in 1970, bronchogenic carcinoma caused an estimated 62,000 deaths and colonic carcinoma, almost 46,000. Some lesions are virtually silent, but most produce symptoms and signs that should arouse suspicion in the patient and his physician. All too often, these early symptoms are largely ignored by the patient or are not sufficiently investigated by the physician. An interesting study by Bockus et al. (1959) of 418 cases disclosed that a delay of over half a year could be attributed

to the patient in 23 per cent of these cases and to the doctor in 28 per cent. The five-year survival of a group of rectal carcinomas discovered early by careful periodic examination is in the range of 90 per cent. In contrast, the five-year survival for symptomatic cases that have been present for some time is in the order of 40 per cent. The challenge is obvious.

Incidence. The epidemiology of cancer of the colon and rectum has been intensively studied with a number of interesting results. There is a wide range in the prevalence of and mortality from this disease throughout the world. A very high incidence is found in Canada, the United States, the United Kingdom, Australia, New Zealand, France and Denmark. On the other hand, a very low incidence is found in Mexico, Japan and some of the South American countries. The divergence is quite impressive and represents, for example, a six-fold difference between Canada and Japan (Haenszel and Correa, 1971). Immigrants from low incidence countries to high incidence locales acquire the prevalence and mortality rate of their country of adoption, supporting the belief that environmental factors play a major role in the etiology of this form of cancer. Males and females are affected about equally in the high incidence countries. About three-quarters of the cases are discovered in the sixth, seventh and eighth decades of life, with the peak at 67 years of age. However, as will become apparent, certain disorders predispose to cancer in a younger age group. A well defined familial predisposition has been identified. When the family histories of probands are studied, the incidence of cancer of the colon in fathers and mothers is three times greater than would be expected, suggesting genetic susceptibility (Burdette, 1971).

Etiology and Pathogenesis. The geographic and familial data cited above strongly suggest that environmental and genetic factors are operative in the initiation of colonic cancer. However, the precise nature of these influences is still obscure. Single gene mutants for susceptibility to colonic polyps carrying a high risk of cancerous transformation have been identified, e.g., in hereditary familial polyposis. A few pedigrees with high prevalence of carcinoma of the large intestine but without underlying polyps have been reported (Peltokallio and Peltokallio, 1966). Except for these rarities, the nature of the genetic predisposition accounting for the familial data is still obscure. Similarly mysterious are the environmental factors. It has been argued that countries with a high incidence are characterized by low residue diets and those with a low incidence by high residue diets. Speculation arose that low residue diets lead to less regular defecation and prolonged contact between the colonic mucosa and possible carcinogens in the diet such as nitrite food preservatives (Burkitt, 1971). *Better established are certain antecedent disorders of the colon which carry a high risk of the development of carcinoma, e.g., hereditary familial polyposis, villous adenoma and ulcerative colitis.*

Morphology. Colonic carcinoma occurs in a fairly well-defined pattern of distribution: rectum, 50 per cent; sigmoid, 20 per cent; descending colon, 6 per cent; transverse colon and splenic flexure, 8 per cent; cecum and ascending colon, 16 per cent. It is apparent that approximately 70 per cent of colonic carcinomas are within reach of the sigmoidoscope. Infrequently, multiple carcinomas arise concurrently, most often in patients with heredofamilial polyposis (Moertel et al., 1958).

These tumors have been classified descriptively in a number of ways, but it suffices from our standpoint to distinguish two patterns: carcinomas of the left side and those of the right. **Carcinomas of the left side tend to grow in an annular encircling fashion. They produce a so-called "napkin ring" constriction of the bowel with early symptoms of obstruction.** These lesions may begin as sessile masses, but over the span of one to two years, they grow to infiltrate and encircle the circumference. **On the right side, the lesions tend to grow as polypoid fungating masses which extend along one wall of the more capacious cecum and ascending colon. Obstruction is uncommon.** Thus, from the standpoint of morphology and clinical behavior, carcinomas of the left and right colon behave as two distinct tumor types.

The **early lesion on the left side** appears as a small elevated button or as a small polypoid mass. As the tumor grows, it forms a flat plaque which continues to increase in size (Fig. 21–57). It eventually extends circumferentially to encircle the wall (Fig. 21–58). It has been estimated that it takes approximately one to two years for such a lesion to totally encircle the lumen. The deeper layers are invaded slowly and, for a long time, the neoplasm tends to remain superficial. Eventually, ulceration takes place in the middle of the ring as penetration of the bowel wall encroaches on the blood supply. At this time, the annular constriction characteristically shows heaped-up margins with a central ring-like ulceration or excavation. Infrequently, left-sided lesions produce little luminal growth but, instead,

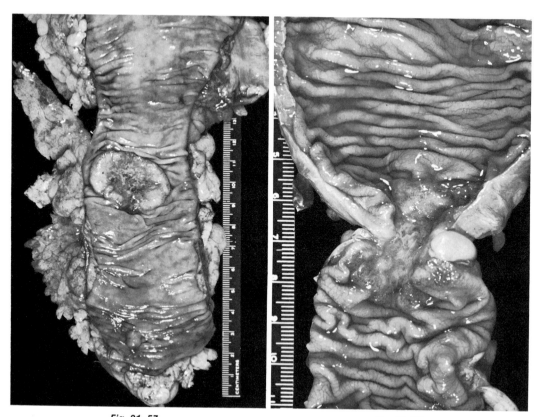

Fig. 21–57.

Fig. 21–58.

Figure 21–57. *An elevated plaque-like adenocarcinoma of the colon.*
Figure 21–58. *Carcinoma of the left colon which has completely encircled the lumen. Dilation of the proximal bowel lumen is evident.*

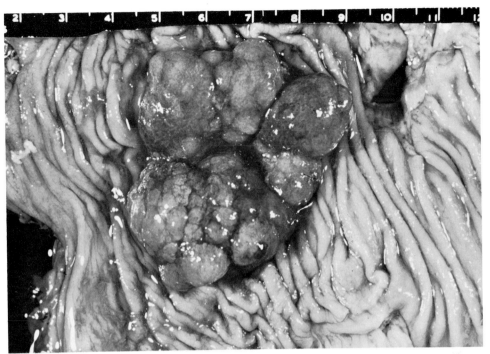

Figure 21–59. *A polypoid fungating carcinoma of the right colon in a male, aged 56 years.*

infiltrate the bowel wall and cause flattening and small ulcerations of the mucosa. Extension of the tumor through the bowel wall into the pericolic fat and regional lymph nodes occurs as these lesions progress. The penetration of bowel wall may, on occasion, produce pericolic abscesses or even peritonitis. Eventually these cancers metastasize to the liver, lungs, bone marrow and other distant organs but not before a considerable period of growth. Rarely, right-sided lesions assume this annular pattern.

The **cancers in the right colon** begin as sessile lesions similar to those of the left but progressively assume a polypoid fungating appearance (Fig. 21–59). They frequently become bulky, cauliflower-like masses or large, irregular spreading papillomatous plaques which protrude into the lumen. Plaque-like or ulcerative lesions of the right side occur but very infrequently. These right-sided lesions eventually penetrate the wall, and extend to the mesentery, regional nodes and more distant sites. Because the lesions occur in the capacious cecum and do not cause obstruction, they may remain clinically silent for long periods of time. Quite uncommonly, colonic carcinomas of the right side grow in an invasive infiltrating fashion with mucosal flattening and ulceration without luminal projections.

Unlike the gross pathology, the microscopic characteristics of right- and left-sided colonic carcinomas are similar. **Ninety-five per cent of all** carcinomas of the colon are adenocarcinomas, many of which produce mucin (Figs. 21–60 and 21–61).

Commonly this mucin is secreted extracellularly either within gland lumina or within the interstitium of the gut wall. Because this secretion dissects the wall, it aids the extension of the malignancy and worsens the prognosis. Occasionally, undifferentiated growth is observed. In the anal region, some of these cancers differentiate as adenoacanthomas.

Clinical Course. It is now appreciated that carcinoma of the colon is present for a considerable time before it produces clinical symptoms. It begins, in all probability, as an "in situ" lesion and then later becomes a small mucosal area of asymptomatic cancerous transformation. In all likelihood, it requires years to become an overt tumor. During this time, the only hope for discovery would be periodic sigmoidoscopic examination coupled with a high index of suspicion. However, even when symptoms are finally produced, the lesion is still small and resectable. In theory, the chance for early discovery and successful removal should be greater with lesions of the left side because these patients usually have prominent disturbances in their bowel function such as melena, diarrhea and constipation. It would be suspected, therefore, that rectosigmoid lesions would yield a better survival rate. However, cancers of the rectum and sigmoid tend to be more infiltrative than those of the proximal levels of colon, and this characteristic is apparently responsible for a somewhat poorer

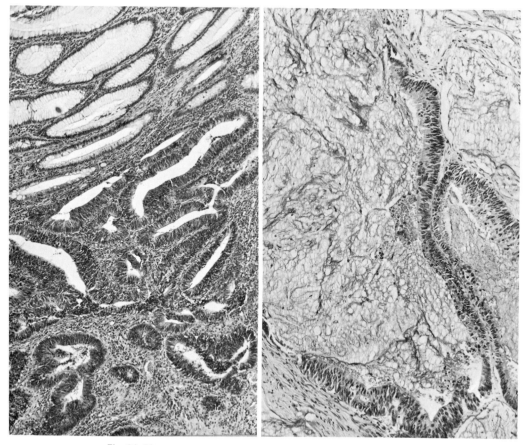

Fig. 21–60.   Fig. 21–61.

Figure 21–60. *The transition zone between the anaplastic glands of an adenocarcinoma of the colon and the normal colonic epithelium.*

Figure 21–61. *A low power field of an invasive cancer of the colon illustrating extensive mucin formation which appears in the figure as stringy coagulated material.*

prognosis for these lesions. Cecal and right colonic cancers are most often called to clinical attention by the appearance of weakness, malaise, weight loss and unexplained anemia. These lesions bleed readily, and the investigation of occult melena sometimes leads to their discovery at an early stage (Gilbertsen, 1960).

All colonic tumors spread by direct extension into adjacent structures and by metastasis through the lymphatics and blood vessels. In order of preference, the favored sites of metastatic spread are the regional lymph nodes, liver, lungs and bones, followed by many other sites including the serosal membrane of the peritoneal cavity, brain and others. In almost half of all cases, spread to regional nodes has occurred by the time of surgery (Grinnell 1950).

Of recent date, a new modality has been added to the standard diagnostic procedures (rectal examination, sigmoidoscopy, biopsy and barium enema) for cancer of the colon. In 1965, Gold and Freedman reported on the demonstration by immunochemical methods of circulating carcinoembryonic antigen (CEA) in patients with proven carcinoma of the colon (Gold and Freedman, 1965*a* and 1965*b*). These antigens are normally present in fetal organs, hence the designation "embryonic." They appear in the circulation in adults having colonic cancer as well as other diseases, as will be detailed. In Gold's original series, he reported a 97 per cent CEA positivity in patients with proven carcinoma of the colon. Since that time, however, the test has proved to be neither so sensitive nor specific. Zamcheck and his colleagues (1972) found a 72 per cent positivity in a large series of cases. The appearance of the circulating antigen appears to be related to the size of the lesion and its spread. In small localized lesions, the approximate positivity is in the order of 20 to 45 per cent, reaching a high of 96 per cent in patients with metastases.

Positive CEA tests may be produced also by cancers of the lung, breast, ovary, urinary bladder and prostate, as well as by alcoholic cirrhosis, pancreatitis, ulcerative colitis and other disorders. When a colonic cancer is found, the test, however, does have value insofar as a negative CEA assay preoperatively suggests a localized tumor and a good prognosis; conversely, a strongly positive CEA bodes ill. Postoperatively, a positive result for serum CEA strongly implies the presence of residual tumor. A negative postoperative test unfortunately does not exclude residual tumor, since a positive assay may be obtained in such patients at a later date, with recurrence of the tumor (Djar et al., 1972).

The prognosis in these cases is dependent upon the extent of bowel involvement and the presence or absence of lymph node metastasis. In the large series of cases analyzed by Dukes and Bussey (1958), the five-year survival of patients without lymphatic metastasis was 83.7 per cent while that of patients with metastasis was 32 per cent. Their study also indicated that the extent of bowel involvement materially modified the outlook for the patient, and they proposed that cancers of the colon be classified into three groups as follows:

1. Growth confined to the rectum, no extrarectal spread, no lymphatic metastasis. Five-year survival rate when corrected for normal attrition, 97.7 per cent.

2. Spread by direct continuity into extrarectal tissues, no lymphatic metastasis; corrected survival rate, 77.6 per cent.

3. Lymphatic metastasis present; corrected survival rate, 32 per cent.

This classification relates to rectal cancer, but relatively similar findings would undoubtedly obtain with lesions at other levels. Generally the site of origin of the cancer, whether left or right, influences the prognosis little. In the report by McSwain et al. (1962), the five-year survival was 40 per cent for all cancers of the right colon, 37.9 per cent for left-sided lesions and 31.3 per cent for those of the rectosigmoid. As mentioned earlier, the probable reason for these small differences is the inherent tendency for rectosigmoidal lesions to infiltrate and spread more rapidly.

It is hardly necessary to point out that five-year survival does not mean cure, and as much as 20 to 40 per cent attrition rate can be anticipated in each successive five-year period. An interesting chart prepared by Welch and Giddings (1951) offers an overview of the results obtained with colonic cancer in a large clinic (Fig. 21–62). While other clinics may report slightly higher levels of survival (average, 50 per cent), this chart is of interest because it highlights the fact that five-year survival rates are generally calculated on the basis of those cases accepted for curative surgery. In the data given in the chart, 30 per cent of the cases were screened out as being too advanced to even attempt curative resections. In the previously cited analysis of Dukes and Bussey (1958), of a total of 3596 rectal cancer patients seen over a 25-year period, only 2447 were treated by a surgical operation which attempted to remove the primary tumor. Thus the outlook for these patients at the present time is still far from favorable, and the goal for the future must be earlier diagnosis.

Squamous Cell Carcinoma. These tumors are largely limited to the anal region. They produce plaque-like thickenings which eventually fungate and ulcerate as do squamous cell carcinomas that occur elsewhere. They tend to be locally invasive and to metastasize eventually to the regional nodes of drainage and then to more distant sites.

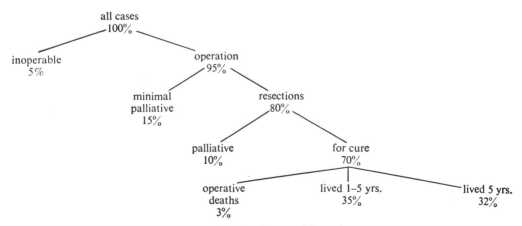

Figure 21–62. Carcinoma of the colon.

Sarcoma. Sarcomas, including lymphomas, occur very rarely in the large bowel. These tumors produce large, fleshy masses which rapidly extend through the bowel wall into adjacent structures. Widespread metastasis to regional nodes is common. Histologically, colonic sarcomas are identical with those at other sites.

Melanocarcinoma. Melanocarcinomas may arise in the pigmented areas of the anus but are extremely uncommon (p. 1401).

Argentaffinoma (Carcinoid). Carcinoid tumors occur preponderantly in the appendix and small intestine. In the series reported by MacDonald (1956), only 3 per cent occurred in the rectum. When they do appear, it is as small nodules covered by an intact mucosa. They are firm and somewhat polypoid. Histologically, they have the same characteristics as those described in the small intestine with the same propensity for metastasis and invasion. The frequency of metastasis is somewhat lower than that of the ileal lesions, and about 15 to 20 per cent spread to regional nodes and the liver. For obscure reasons, even the metastasizing carcinoids that arise in the colon rarely produce the "carcinoid syndrome" (p. 942).

DIFFERENTIAL DIAGNOSIS OF COLONIC MASSES AND ULCERATIONS

Diseases that affect the large bowel are usually made known to the patient in one of three ways: by a change in bowel habit, by abdominal pain or discomfort or by symptomless bleeding evidenced either by tarry stools or the passage of bright red blood. These clinical syndromes are produced most commonly by two types of lesions found in the colon, tumors and ulceroinflammatory disease. It then becomes important to consider the possible types of masses and the various kinds of inflammatory disease that affect this level of bowel.

MASSES IN THE COLON

Left-sided Masses. If the mass is in the left colon, the following lesions must be considered.

1. *Carcinoma of the colon.* From the standpoint of probability, at least 90 per cent of masses in the left colon are carcinoma. If, moreover, the tumor tends to be annular and encircling, the likelihood of such a diagnosis is further enhanced. Sigmoidoscopic biopsy should precede surgery.

2. *Benign polyps of the colon.* These are readily differentiated from carcinoma by barium study. However, many large, apparently benign polyps, especially the villous adenomas, require microscopic examination to differentiate them from polypoid carcinoma.

3. *Diverticulitis.* Longstanding, chronic diverticulitis and peridiverticulitis may produce considerable fibrous narrowing of the colon which may simulate an infiltrative mass or neoplastic constriction. In general, the mucosal involvement is not so prominent, and by x-ray diagnosis one is usually able to exclude true neoplasia. However, biopsy is always necessary for definitive diagnosis.

4. *Lymphopathia venereum in the female.* This lesion may also produce inflammatory narrowing which can closely simulate diverticulitis and, at times, carcinomatous narrowing.

5. *Sarcoma of the large bowel, including lymphoma.* While these lesions tend to be large bulky masses which differ in their growth habits from epithelial malignancy, their final identification can be made only by microscopic examination.

6. *Argentaffinomas* are almost always small lesions but sometimes are difficult to differentiate from carcinomas.

7. *Endometriosis of the pelvic peritoneum* in the female may cause considerable perirectal or sigmoidal fibroses and narrowing, sometimes simulating tumorous involvement.

Right-sided Masses. On the right side as on the left, carcinoma dominates the clinical picture and must be ruled out before any other diagnosis can be reasonably entertained. The only other lesions which occur on this side with sufficient frequency to be considered are sarcoma, lymphoma and argentaffinoma.

ULCEROINFLAMMATORY LESIONS OF THE LARGE BOWEL

In general, such processes rarely simulate masses and hence are readily separable by barium study or sigmoidoscopy from the neoplastic processes previously considered. However, the identification of the precise etiologic agent producing the ulceration may be most difficult. On sigmoidoscopic and direct examination, these ulcers all tend to resemble one another, and often little more can be accomplished by the histologic examination. The only lesions that regularly can be recognized histologically are the tuberculous and amebic ulcers. In general, bacteriology, serologic studies and search for parasites serve best as differential diagnostic procedures. It is impossible to present a list of ulcerative lesions in the precise order of incidence since experience varies in different locales. They may, however, be separated into two groups:

Ulcerative Lesions Which Are Common in the United States:

1. Nonspecific ulcerative colitis.
2. Tuberculous ulcers.
3. Uremic ulcerations.
4. Staphylococcal colitis following antibiotic therapy.
5. Stercoral ulcers.

Ulcerative Lesions Uncommonly Encountered in the United States:

1. Bacillary dysentery.
2. Cholera, producing desquamation of the surface, but no distinct ulceration.
3. Typhoid fever.
4. Mercurial poisoning.

A discussion of clinical disease of the colon would not be complete without mention of perhaps the most common disorder affecting this structure, namely, hemorrhoids. They are particularly important clinically, since all too often rectal bleeding is ascribed to their presence when actually the bleeding comes from a higher level. The possibility that a neoplasm coexists with hemorrhoids is occasionally overlooked, thus delaying the diagnosis of the more important lesion.

APPENDIX

NORMAL
PATHOLOGY
Inflammations
    Acute appendicitis
      Suppurative
      Gangrenous
      In each of these types the
        following qualifying

terms may be added:
With or without
   obstruction
With or without
   perforation
With or without
   periappendicitis

Chronic
Mucocele
Tumors
   Argentaffinoma (carcinoid)
   Carcinoma
   Miscellaneous
Clinicopathologic Correlation

NORMAL

The appendix in man is a mysterious structure with no known function. It varies greatly in size, having an average diameter of 0.5 to 1 cm. It is usually a mobile structure, having a short mesentery called the mesoappendix which carries the blood, nerve and lymphatic supply. It generally lies directly at the extremity of the anterior taenia of the cecum. On occasion, it lies behind the colon in a so-called retrocecal position. It is sometimes enveloped in congenital fibrous bands which may produce torsion, kinking or sharp angulation. These malpositions alone, under certain clinical situations, may cause pain since the angulated lumen may distend with feces or gas and cause colicky pain.

Histologically, the appendix has the same four layers as the remainder of the gut. The distinguishing feature of this organ is the extremely rich lymphoid tissue present in the mucosa and submucosa which, in young individuals, forms an entire layer of germinal follicles and lymphoid pulp. This lymphoid tissue underlying the mucosal epithelium and glands undergoes progressive atrophy during life to the point of complete disappearance in advanced age.

PATHOLOGY

Diseases of the appendix loom large in surgical practice. Appendicitis is the most common acute abdominal condition which the surgeon is called upon to treat. It is, under different conditions, one of the best recognized clinical entities and one of the most difficult diagnostic problems that confront the clinician. A differential diagnosis of this disease must include virtually every acute process that can occur within the abdominal cavity as well as some of the emergencies that affect the organs of the thorax (Thorek, 1952). The more common entities which may produce confusion will be discussed presently.

INFLAMMATIONS

Acute. Acute appendicitis is an extremely common disease that occurs at any age. It occurs relatively less frequently in infancy and in advanced age. It tends to be most prevalent in young adults. Although certain differences in frequency between the two sexes have been described in the various decades, the condition is so common that statistical differences have little clinical significance. The pathogenesis of inflammation of the appendix is poorly understood. While it is well known that the local organisms, such as *E. coli*, enterococci and beta hemolytic streptococci, are most commonly cultured from acute inflammatory lesions of this organ, it is not clear whether these organisms gain access to the wall of the appendix by direct invasion of the mucosa or through lymphatic and vascular spread of bacteria. With little direct proof it has been assumed that intraluminal obstruction is an important underlying factor. The increase in the luminal pressure may collapse the vessels of the wall and thus predispose the appendix to bacterial infection. It is possible that patchy obliteration of vessels may explain the focal character of the inflammation in some cases.

The inflammatory changes seen in developing appendicitis will be presented beginning with the early alterations and then proceeding to the subsequent, more marked reactions as the process progressively worsens. In the earliest recognizable acutely inflamed appendix, there is usually a scant neutrophilic exudation throughout the mucosa, submucosa and muscularis. Occasionally, the mucosal involvement is most prominent. At this phase of the reaction, the subserosal vessels are congested and contain marginated neutrophils, and often there is scant, perivascular, neutrophilic emigration. This serosal reaction transforms the normal glistening serosa to an injected dull, granular, red membrane. This external appearance is that recognized by the surgeon as **early acute appendicitis**. At a later stage, the neutrophilic exudation through the wall is more advanced, with numerous polymorphonuclear leukocytes within the muscularis and a layered fibrinopurulent reaction over the serosa (Fig. 21–63 and 21–64). As the inflammatory process worsens, there are abscess formations within the wall, along with ulcerations and foci of suppurative necrosis in the mucosa. At this stage, the serosa is usually heavily layered with fibrinosuppurative exudate, and the state of the appendix might be termed **acute suppurative appendicitis**. Further worsening of the reaction leads to large areas of hemorrhagic green ulceration of the mucosa, along with similar green-black gangrenous necrosis throughout the wall, extending to the serosa. This level of severity is the immediate antecedent to rupture of **an acute gangrenous appendicitis**. Quite commonly, fecaliths are found in the lumen. When these become impacted, there is distention of the appendix distal to the obstruction with almost invariably enhanced inflammatory reaction in this obstructed segment. The qualifying terms indicated in the outline are used simply to more accurately describe the severity and the extent of the involvement by indicating the presence of abscess formation or gangrene.

The histologic criterion for the diagnosis of acute appendicitis is polymorphonuclear leukocytic

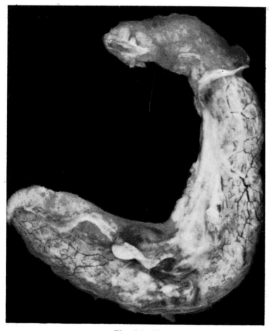

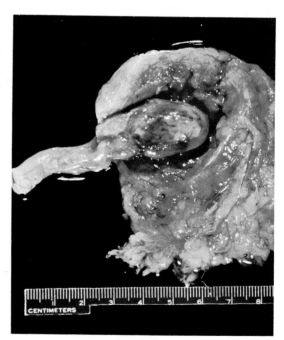

Fig. 21–63.

Fig. 21–64.

Figure 21–63. *A suppurative exudate covering the serosa of the appendix. The uneven dilatation is produced by impacted fecaliths.*

Figure 21–64. *Acute imflammation of the distal third of the appendix together with the segment of the omentum which had become applied to the inflammatory focus.*

infiltration **of the muscularis.** Usually neutrophils and ulcerations are also present within the mucosa. Since drainage of an exudate into the appendix from a focus of infection in a higher level of bowel may also induce some scant neutrophilic infiltrate in the mucosa, it is usually believed that evidence of inflammation within the muscularis is requisite for the diagnosis. The progressively worsening stages of acute appendicitis with suppuration and gangrenous necrosis require no further description since these are entirely nonspecific and follow the pattern of inflammatory reactions in other tissues. The possibility of acute vasculitis or inflammatory thrombosis of the blood vessels in the mesoappendix must always be borne in mind. Such vascular involvement may lead to pylephlebitis or pyemic liver abscesses.

The complications of appendicitis are (1) peritonitis, (2) localized periappendiceal abscess formation, (3) pylephlebitis with thrombosis of the portal venous drainage, (4) liver abscesses and (5) septicemia. Periappendiceal abscesses or peritonitis do not necessarily imply perforation or rupture of the appendix. Organisms can permeate a damaged wall readily without frank rupture of the wall. This method of extension is the more common basis for the development of intraperitoneal infection. Despite the high frequency of acute vasculitis within the inflammatory zone of an acute appendix or its mesoappendix, extension of this intrinsic vascular involvement to the mesenteric and portal veins is rare.

Although the pathologic lesion in acute appendicitis is a simple one, the clinical evaluation of the entity can be extremely difficult. It is frequently said that even the most astute diagnosticians cannot differentiate, in all instances, between acute appendicitis and the following entities which may totally simulate the clinical syndrome of acute appendicitis, i.e., periumbilical or right lower quadrant pain, nausea, vomiting, tenderness and spasm:

1. Mesenteric lymphadenitis, occurring in children in response to a generalized toxic or systemic infection producing enlargement and tenderness of all nodes, particularly the mesenteric.

2. Appendiceal colic secondary to obstruction of the lumen by fecaliths, angulation, fibrous cords or other agents.

3. Intraperitoneal hemorrhage—either from a ruptured ovarian follicle (so-called mittelschmerz) or from a tubal pregnancy.

4. Acute salpingitis.

5. Oxyuriasis vermicularis, infection of the appendix by pinworms, some of which may erode into the mucosa and excite a superficial acute inflammatory reaction.

6. Regional enteritis.

7. Meckel's diverticulitis.

8. Measles appendix in which the lymphoid follicular tissue of the appendix undergoes marked inflammatory hyperplasia coincident with the generalized lymphoid hyperplasia throughout the body (p. 434).

A recent analysis of 5800 cases of appendicitis provides an overview of the clinical problem. The correct diagnosis was made in 82 per cent. The diagnosis was missed (8.3 per cent) most commonly due simply to a lack of sufficient clinical indications to justify surgery. Mesenteric lymphadenitis masqueraded as appendicitis in 4.6 per cent of the cases. The remaining errors were due to the entities mentioned previously that can simulate appendicitis. The mortality rate for surgically treated patients having acute appendicitis without frank gangrene was 0.1 per cent; the mortality rate for patients having a ruptured appendix with an appendiceal abscess not treated immediately by surgery was 13 per cent. It is obvious that the high price of failing to operate justifies operating even under somewhat uncertain clinical indications (Barnes et al., 1962).

Chronic. True chronic inflammation of the appendix is rare. It implies long-continued inflammatory activity. It is characterized grossly by a thickened, fibrotic appendix which shows considerable subserosal fibrosis as well as thickening of the wall and narrowing of the lumen. On microscopic section, the hallmark of chronic appendicitis is the presence of mononuclear white cell infiltration throughout the wall of the appendix, chiefly in the subserosal level, associated with the development of large lymphoid follicles. This type of infiltration indicates a long-continued inflammatory activity.

In some patients, the appendix from birth is a mere fibrous cord. It must not be assumed, therefore, that extensive fibrosis of the appendiceal architecture implies a chronic inflammatory reaction or the end stage of a previous inflammation.

Mucocele. Mucocele of the appendix must be divided into benign and malignant forms. *Benign mucocele* refers to obliteration of the lumen of the appendix usually by inflammatory scarring or fecaliths, with the accumulation of sterile mucus in the isolated segment. Progressive cystic dilatation ensues. In its usual appearance, the distal 3 or 4 cm. of the appendix undergoes spherical or fusiform symmetrical enlargement, commonly reaching diameters of 4 to 6 cm. Rarely, masses up to 15 cm. in diameter have been produced (Fig. 21–65). The wall may be quite thin, and the cyst may appear translucent. Clear glassy mucin is contained. The lining membrane is usually smooth and glistening, produced by marked atrophy

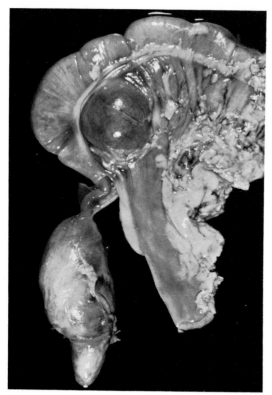

Figure 21–65. *A mucocele of the appendix shown still attached to the terminal ileum and cecum. Narrowing of the proximal one-third is evident and a fusiform dilatation of the distal two-thirds has been produced by stenosis of the lumen.*

of the appendiceal mucosa. Many times the wall is made up only of fibrous tissue and attentuated smooth muscle. Secondary bacterial seeding may introduce an inflammatory component. Exceedingly rarely, these lesions rupture and, if sterile, they cause only a local inflammatory reaction.

Malignant mucocele results from progressive distention of the appendix by proliferating secreting tumor cells. Thus, *the malignant mucocele is a primary mucous cystadenocarcinoma of the appendix.* These are even more rare than the benign form in the ratio of about 1:10. About one-quarter of these cases rupture, seeding the peritoneum with mucus-secreting cancer cells. The peritoneal cavity may thus fill up with mucinous jelly-like secretion, giving rise to the entity termed *pseudomyxoma peritonei* (Shanks, 1961). Buried within this gelatinous secretion are the nests of tumor cells implanted on the peritoneal surfaces. Interestingly, these tumor cells rarely if ever invade the underlying wall, and visceral metastasis is uncommon.

It should be pointed out here that mucinous cystadenocarcinomas of the ovary are more frequent causes of pseudomyxoma peritonei.

TUMORS

Tumors of the appendix are very rare. The most common is the argentaffinoma.

Argentaffinoma (Carcinoid). The most frequent site for carcinoids in the body is the appendix. In the series of cases analyzed by MacDonald (1956), approximately 60 per cent were so located. These appendiceal tumors occur at all ages and are usually discovered as incidental findings at laparotomy or autopsy. The tumor most frequently involves the distal tip of the appendix where it produces a solid bulbous swelling 2 or 3 cm. in diameter which on section is yellow and firm. The lumen and architecture of the wall are obliterated in the area of involvement. Histologically, these tumors have the same appearance as those described in the small intestine (p. 942). The same uniformity of cells and nuclear size and shape is present. Giant cells, anaplasia and mitoses are virtually absent but, despite the benign cytologic appearance, the tumor invades deeply throughout the muscularis and sometimes out to the serosa (Figs. 21–66 and 21–67). Extensions beyond the limits of the appendiceal serosa are extremely rare. These tumors virtually never metastasize and, while regional node involvement may occur, it is very uncommon. These small confined lesions extremely rarely produce the carcinoid syndrome.

Carcinoma. On rare occasions, carcinoma of the appendix may produce a typical neoplastic enlargement of the organ. The mucin-secreting lesions may produce a mucocele (p. 975). Almost all these tumors are shown on histologic examination to be adenocarcinomas. Metastases may follow the pattern of other intestinal carcinomas or may induce pseudomyxoma peritonei.

Miscellaneous Tumors. Benign and malignant mesenchymal growths are reported in this organ as medical curiosities. These neoplasms resemble their counterparts in other areas.

CLINICOPATHOLOGIC CORRELATION

The pathologic evaluation of diseases of the appendix is relatively simple and straightforward. Of the specimens submitted for anatomic diagnosis, 99 per cent concern themselves with the presence or absence of acute

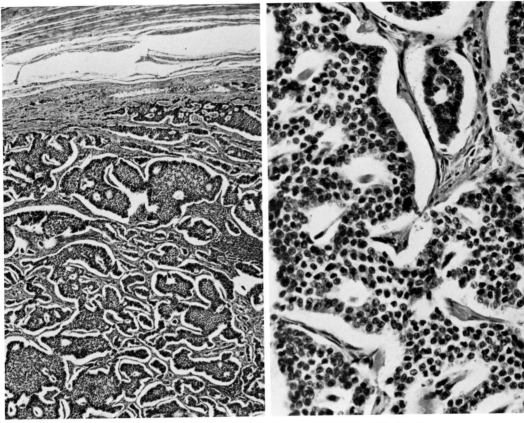

Fig. 21–66.   Fig. 21–67.

Figure 21–66. Argentaffinoma of the appendix. The low power view is taken from one margin of the tumor in contact with the muscularis. The characteristic pattern of growth and invasion of the wall is evident.
Figure 21–67. A close-up of the cellular detail of an argentaffinoma of the appendix. The uniformity of the nuclear size and shape and growth pattern are clearly shown.

inflammation. However, many misunderstandings persist between pathologists and surgeons about the entity of appendicitis. One such misunderstanding arises out of the many clinical syndromes which affect the appendix, simulate appendicitis, and yet are not associated with an acute inflammatory process. Some of these have been listed under the discussion of acute appendicitis, e.g., appendiceal colic produced by fecaliths, minimal focal reactions evoked by pinworms, kinking of the appendix, fibrous constricting bands producing angulation and possibly obstruction of the lumen, and marked hyperplasia of the lymphoid tissue of the appendix or mesenteric nodes. All these disorders may evoke pain virtually indistinguishable from that produced by a true inflammation. For these reasons, it is a well recognized clinical fact that even in the most astute surgical practice, about 15 per cent of appendices removed will not show true acute inflammation. In this connection, it is far

wiser to remove these essentially negative appendices than to be so reluctant to operate upon a possible appendicitis as to miss a true acute process, thus permitting perforation to occur.

Some of this disagreement, in addition, is based upon simple terminology. Chronic appendicitis is a common clinical diagnosis, but is rarely proved anatomically. This is true because the pathologist uses the term only when there is anatomic evidence of true, *persisting*, chronic inflammatory disease, while the clinician is apt to use the term to describe recurrent episodes of right lower quadrant pain over a period of months and perhaps years. Although disease may have been present in this organ for some time, it takes the form of many *recurrent* acute episodes followed by remission or healing and, hence, no true continuing chronic inflammation is ever present. These appendices on microscopic examination disclose either no inflammation or a simple acute suppurative inflammation, depending upon whether the process is interrupted in a stage of remission or relapse. These syndromes are more properly termed "recurrent acute ap-pendicitis," in which case surgeon and pathologist would concur in the diagnosis. The true entity of chronic appendicitis, while it does exist, is a rarity.

PERITONEUM

NORMAL	Pancreatic enzymes	**Mesenteric Cysts**
PATHOLOGY	Surgically introduced	**Tumors**
Inflammation	foreign material	Primary
Sterile peritonitis	Bacterial peritonitis	Secondary
Blood	Sclerosing retroperitonitis	**Causes of "Acute Abdomen"**
Bile		

NORMAL

The abdominal cavity is lined by a glistening membrane called the peritoneum. It is divided into a parietal portion which lines the walls of the cavity and a visceral portion which is reflected over the various organs. In the male, it is a completely closed cavity, but in the female, it communicates with the environment through the hollow viscera of the genital tract. The mesothelial lining of this cavity should always be considered in the same category as the lining of the pleural and pericardial cavities since they all react similarly to inflammation and have a similar type of neoplasia.

The peritoneum is essentially a dialyzing membrane and constantly secretes and absorbs a serous fluid. Accumulation of serous fluid, known as ascites, may be encountered in a variety of conditions, most commonly in cardiac failure and in portal hypertension. Ascites, however, should not be considered a static collection since there is evidence that constant rapid formation and absorption produce a constant turnover. The distinction between a simple collection of ascitic fluid (i.e., transudate) and an exudate is sometimes most important clinically. Commonly, the specific gravity is used as the differential feature, transudates having a specific gravity of approximately 1.010 or lower whereas exudates in general have a specific gravity above 1.020.

The pathologic processes that affect the peritoneum are few in number. The majority of lesions are of an inflammatory type and are called peritonitis. Secondary metastases to the peritoneum are the next most common. Primary tumors are rare.

PATHOLOGY

INFLAMMATION

Peritonitis is an inflammatory process which may be due to either bacterial invasion or chemical irritation. It is, therefore, divided into sterile and bacterial types.

STERILE PERITONITIS

The most common causes of sterile peritonitis in order of frequency are:

Blood. Bleeding into the peritoneal cavity may produce chemical irritation and inflammation. These patients may have signs and symptoms which are indistinguishable from those of acute appendicitis. Some of the more common causes for such bleeding are ruptured ovarian follicles, tubal pregnancy, traumatic or spontaneous rupture of the spleen, perforation of a peptic ulcer, rupture of an intra-abdominal aneurysm, and many other less common involvements of any viscus.

Bile. Perforation or rupture of the biliary system evokes a highly irritating peritonitis. In the early stage, it is usually limited to the right upper quadrant and, in this stage, the peritoneal exudate on examination will be bile-stained. Later the biliary discoloration is masked by the progressive suppuration which ensues concomitantly with superimposed bacterial contamination. Any type of acute inflammatory disease or obstruction within the gallbladder or bile ducts may produce perforation or rupture and spill bile into the peritoneal cavity. Not uncommonly, the bile may gain access to the peritoneal cavity through a perforated peptic ulcer. In almost all these conditions that predispose to the soiling of the peritoneum by bile, bacterial contamination is present and thus places the peritonitis in another category.

Pancreatic Enzymes. Acute hemorrhagic pancreatitis is a calamitous disorder characterized by hemorrhage and necrosis of the pancreas (p. 1061). Concomitantly, pancreatic enzymes leak into the peritoneal cavity. These proteolytic and lipolytic ferments evoke a striking peritoneal reaction and, at the same time, digest lipid tissue. With the release of fatty acids, saponification (formation of soaps) produces chalky white precipitates in focal areas of fat wherever it is exposed to these enzymes. At the same time, globules of free fat may be found floating in the peritoneal fluid which accumulates. Both these features, the formation of soaps and fat globules, are virtually diagnostic of the peritonitis produced by pancreatic necrosis. However, after 24 to 48 hours, bacterial permeation of the bowel wall usually leads to a frank suppurative exudation.

Surgically Introduced Foreign Material, Particularly Talcum Powder. The reaction to such agents is usually localized and minimal. No clinical symptoms may result, and the only significance to such disease is the possibility of the development of chronic inflammatory granulomas, followed by fibrosis and adhesions which may eventually lead to intestinal obstruction or strangulation of the bowel.

BACTERIAL PERITONITIS

This is almost invariably secondary to extension of bacteria through the wall of a hollow viscus or to rupture of a viscus. The common primary disorders leading to such bacterial disseminations are *appendicitis, ruptured peptic ulcer, cholecystitis, diverticulitis, strangulation of bowel and acute salpingitis.* Virtually every bacterial organism has been implicated as a cause of peritonitis, most commonly, *E. coli*, alpha hemolytic and beta hemolytic streptococci, *Staphylococcus aureus*, enterococci, "gram-negative rods" and *Clostridium welchii*. This last organism is a frequent inhabitant of the gut and, therefore, a frequent component of peritonitis. However, it rarely causes true gas gangrene in the abdominal cavity. Seldom encountered today are gonococcal and tuberculous peritonitis, the former arising from an acute salpingitis and the latter secondary to tuberculosis of the intestinal tract or hematogenous dissemination from a primary pulmonary focus. Spontaneous pneumococcal peritonitis is a curiosity occasionally encountered in children with renal disease. Both the source of the organism and mode of spread are obscure.

Depending upon the duration of the peritonitis, the membranes show the following changes. Approximately two to four hours after involvement, the membrane loses its gray, glistening quality and becomes dull and lusterless. There is, at this time, a small accumulation of essentially serous or slightly turbid fluid. Later the exudate becomes creamy and obviously suppurative. In some cases, it may become extremely thick and plastic and even inspissated, especially in dehydrated patients. The volume of such exudate varies enormously. In many cases, it may be **localized** by the omentum and viscera to a small area of the peritoneal cavity, particularly as in an appendiceal abscess, or it may become **generalized** to involve the entire abdominal cavity. In generalized peritonitis, it is important to remember that exudate may accumulate under and above the liver to form **subhepatic and subdiaphragmatic abscesses.** Collections in the lesser omental sac may likewise create residual persistent foci of infection.

The inflammatory process is typical of an acute bacterial infection anywhere and produces the characteristic neutrophilic infiltration with a fibrinopurulent exudate. The reaction usually remains quite superficial and does not penetrate deeply into the visceral structures or abdominal wall. Tuberculous peritonitis tends to produce a plastic exudate studded with minute pale granulomas.

These inflammatory processes can heal either spontaneously or with therapy. In the course of healing, the following results may be obtained: *(1) The exudate may be totally resolved, leaving no residual fibrosis; (2) residual, walled-off abscesses may persist to eventually heal or serve as foci for new infection; or (3) organization of the exudate may occur, with the formation of fibrous adhesive bands termed adhesions.* On occasion, these adhesions may be responsible for later symptoms or pathologic findings, forming potential sources of obstruction to the lumen of the bowel or strangulation of a segment of gut.

SCLEROSING RETROPERITONITIS

Dense fibrotic overgrowth of the retroperitoneal tissues may sometimes develop with no known antecedent infection. This occurrence is designated as sclerosing retroperitonitis. The fibrous overgrowth is entirely nondistinctive and, while infiltrative, does not display frank anaplasia. There is usually an accompanying inflammatory infiltrate of lymphocytes, plasma cells and neutrophils, suggesting inflammatory rather than neoplastic disease. The fibrosis is particularly important because it often encroaches upon the ureters and may produce hydronephrosis. The fibrous tissue insinuates itself into the retroperitoneal fat and about the retroperitoneal organs and, in some ways, is the analogue of the desmoid tumor. Distant metastasis or regional node involvement is not encountered (Hock and Hazard, 1959).

MESENTERIC CYSTS

Large to small cystic masses are sometimes found within the mesenteries in the abdominal cavity or attached to the peritoneal lining of the abdominal wall. These cysts are usually of obscure nature and origin but sometimes offer difficult clinical diagnostic problems because they present on palpation as abdominal masses. Many classifications of these cysts have been proposed which attempt to designate groups according to common pathogenetic origins. On this basis, it has been suggested that mesenteric cysts be divided into (1) those arising from embryonic multipotential cells, (2) those derived from pinched-off enteric diverticula that usually begin during the early development of the fore- and hindgut, (3) those derived from urogenital ridge or its derivatives, i.e., the urinary and male and female genital tracts, (4) those derived from walled-off infections, more properly called pseudocysts, and (5) those of malignant origin.

Usually these cysts are single, but occasionally multiple loculations are found either attached or dispersed throughout the abdominal cavity. They vary from small 1 to 2 cm. nodules to massive structures 15 to 20 cm. in diameter. Commonly, by the time they are discovered, the fluid content is fairly nondescript and may be either serous or mucinous, varying in color from pale yellow to muddy red-brown. Considerable turbidity may be imparted by necrotic tissue or old blood. Histologically, the wall is comprised of fibrous tissue and may have such specialized cytologic detail as permits the identification of the derivation of the cyst. The principal anatomic feature of importance in these cysts is the clear demonstration that they do not arise from any of the definitive organs in the body and therefore merit the designation mesenteric. Since the majority are non-neoplastic and since they are usually fairly mobile or at most are loosely attached structures, surgical resection is the treatment of choice and permits a cure.

TUMORS

Virtually all the tumors of the peritoneum are malignant. These can be divided into primary and secondary.

Primary tumors of the peritoneum are extremely rare and are called mesotheliomas. These exactly duplicate the tumors found in the pleura and the pericardium and grow as spindle cell lesions closely simulating fibrosarcomas. Occasionally they may create a mixed spindle cell and glandular pattern. These gland-like spaces may contain serous secretions similar to those which are normally produced by the mesothelium. Gland-like patterns present in an otherwise spindle cell growth should strongly suggest that the tumor is derived from cells which are both secretory and endothelial in type. They, therefore, closely simulate tumors arising in synovial membranes of joints (synoviomas).

Secondary tumors of the peritoneum are, in contrast, quite common. In any form of advanced cancer, penetration to the serosal membrane or metastatic seeding may occur. The most common tumors which produce a diffuse serosal miliary implantation are ovarian or pancreatic carcinomas. However, it is seen in any type of intra-abdominal malignancy and occasionally represents distant metastases from tumors in other locations within the body. An important procedure aiding the diagnosis of such tumor implants is the aspiration of fluid from the abdominal cavity. Papanicolaou smear of this fluid or microscopic section of the sediment occasionally demonstrates the presence of tumor cells, differentiating the ascites from simple transudation or exudation.

Additional mention is made of the very uncommon tumors that may arise from retroperitoneal tissues, i.e., fat, fibrous tissue, blood vessels, lymphatics, nerves and the lymph nodes alongside the aorta. These native structures may give rise to benign or malignant neoplasms called *retroperitoneal tumors* that resemble their counterparts arising elsewhere in the body.

CLINICOPATHOLOGIC CORRELATION—CAUSES OF "ACUTE ABDOMEN"

Widespread inflammation of the peritoneum, whether caused by bacterial contamination or due simply to the chemical irritation of enzymes or bile, gives rise to common medical emergency known to physician and layman alike as the "acute abdomen." Such peritoneal inflammation is almost invariably caused by some primary disease in the viscera within the abdominal cavity. Only very rarely is it due to bacteremic seeding.

While the list of intra-abdominal diseases that may give rise to such an acute abdomen is long, it is pertinent to consider briefly the most important. In this way, it is possible to appreciate the extent to which a knowledge of intra-abdominal pathology may be extrapolated to arrive at a reasonable differential diagnosis of the acute abdomen.

The principal cause of acute peritonitis is bacterial soiling from an acute appendicitis. Perhaps the second most common cause of an acute abdomen is acute cholecystitis. In both disorders, the bacteria may permeate the unruptured wall of the viscus or may reach the peritoneal cavity in the case of more acute gangrenous infections by rupture of the viscus. Whatever the pathway, the bacteria induce a suppurative inflammation, often with the formation of copious amounts of purulent fluids from which the etiologic agent or agents can be cultured. Under the circumstances mentioned, the common organisms are the coliforms, enterococci and staphylococci.

In the second order of magnitude among the causes of an acute abdomen are the variety of ulcerative lesions of all levels of the gastrointestinal tract. These include peptic ulcer, regional enteritis, ulcerative colitis, diverticulitis of the colon and ulcerating carcinomas wherever they occur. Mesenteric thrombosis and rupture of a loop of gangrenous bowel (trapped in a hernial sac, a volvulus or behind a peritoneal adhesion) are additional causes of peritoneal soiling. Occasionally, an obstructing carcinoma of the left colon may cause sufficient distention of the large bowel to perforate the thinned-out wall of the distensible cecum. In all these instances, there is extensive bacterial contamination of the peritoneal cavity.

As mentioned, not all "acute abdomens" are produced by bacterial infection. Sterile chemical irritation of considerable clinical significance may be caused by the escape of blood, pancreatic enzymes or bile into the abdominal cavity. Hemorrhage into the peritoneal cavity is often due to rupture of a tubal pregnancy and is less often caused by rupture of an intra-abdominal aneurysm. Escape of pancreatic enzymes with its ensuing acute inflammatory reaction is encountered in acute hemorrhagic pancreatic necrosis. This catastrophic disease produces intense pain and is often responsible for vascular collapse and death due to shock. While bile itself is strongly irritant to the peritoneal cavity, bile peritonitis occurs virtually only with rupture of an acute gangrenous gallbladder. Under these circumstances, the bile is not sterile and carries with it a considerable inoculum of bacteria.

The correct evaluation of the cause of an "acute abdomen" is obviously a problem of importance and, at the same time, one that may be extremely difficult. To operate on a case of acute hemorrhagic pancreatic necrosis is, in the opinion of many surgeons, ill advised because there is considerable doubt that operative intervention can shorten or alleviate the natural course of the disease, and the further insult of surgery materially raises the mortality rate. Alternatively, to fail to operate on a blossoming acute appendicitis is to invite rupture. The differential diagnosis of the acute abdomen is one of the major concerns of textbooks of surgery and is beyond our scope. But it is not inappropriate to point out that, before one can achieve a reasonable surgical knowledge of the acute abdomen, it is necessary to have a perspective of the diseases that may potentially be present in the abdominal cavity.

REFERENCES

Aboumrad, M. H., et al.: Intimal hyperplasia of small mesenteric arteries. Occlusive, with infarction of the intestine. Arch. Path., 75:196, 1963.

Acheson, E. D., and Doll, R.: Dietary factors in carcinoma of the stomach. Gut, 5:126, 1964.

Achord, J. L., and Proctor, H. D.: Malignant degeneration and metastasis in Peutz-Jeghers syndrome. Arch. Intern. Med., 111:498, 1963.

Adams, W. R., et al.: Some morphologic characteristics of Whipple's disease. Amer. J. Path., 42:415, 1963.

Alvarez, A. F., and Colbert, J. G.: Lye stricture of the esophagus complicated by carcinoma. Canad. J. Surg., 6:470, 1963.

Asquith, P., et al.: Serum immunoglobulins in adult coeliac disease. Lancet, 2:129, 1969.

Baeza, M.: Carcinoid tumors of the gastrointestinal tract. Dis. Colon Rectum, 12:147, 1969.

Baker, R. D., et al.: Small bowel ulceration apparently associated with thiazides and potassium therapy. J.A.M.A., 190:586, 1964.

Balasegaram, M.: Haematemesis and melaena: a review of 326 cases. Med. J. Aust., 1:485, 1968.

Barnes, B. A., et al.: Treatment of appendicitis at the Massachusetts General Hospital, 1937–1959. J.A.M.A., 180:122, 1962.

Bartholomew, L. G., et al.: Intestinal polyposis: association with muco-cutaneous melanin pigmentation (Peutz-Jeghers syndrome). Gastroenterology, 32:34, 1957.

Becker, I., and Brayton, D.: Acute pseudomembranous enterocolitis. West. J. Surg., 66:1, 1958.

Bergen, J. A., and Cage, R. P.: Carcinoma and ulcerative colitis: prognosis. Gastroenterology, 39:385, 1960.

Black, B. M.: Primary hyperparathyroidism and peptic ulcer. Surg. Clin. N. Amer., 51:955, 1971.

Bockus, H. L., et al.: Early clinical manifestations of cancer of the colon and rectum. Dis. Colon Rectum, 2:58, 1959.

Boudreau, R. P., et al.: Anatomic study of benign and malignant gastric ulcerations. J.A.M.A., 147:374, 1951.

Boyd, D. P., et al.: Carcinoma of the esophagus. New Eng. J. Med., 258:271, 1958.

Boyd, J., et al.: The epidemiology of gastrointestinal cancer with special reference to causation. Gut, 5:196, 1964.

Brick, I. B.: Hiatus hernia and carcinoma of the stomach and esophagus. Gastroenterology, 13:47, 1949.

Burdette, W. J.: Identification of antecedents to colorectal cancer. Cancer, 28:51, 1971.

Burgess, H. M., et al.: Cancer of the esophagus: a clinicopathologic study. Surg. Clin. N. Amer., 31:965, 1951.

Burkitt, D. P.: Epidemiology of cancer of the colon and rectum. Cancer, 28:3, 1971.

Butz, W. C.: Giant hypertrophic gastritis. Gastroenterology, 39:183, 1960.

Calkins, W. G.: Pre-malignant gastrointestinal lesions. Geriatrics, 19:707, 1964.

Cassella, R. R. A. L., et al.: Achalasia of the esophagus: pathologic and etiologic considerations. Ann. Surg., 160:474, 1964.

Castle, W. B.: Current concepts of pernicious anemia. Amer. J. Med., 48:541, 1970.

Castleman, B., and Krickstein, H. I.: Do adenomatous polyps of the colon become malignant? New Eng. J. Med., 267:460, 1962.

Chandler, G. N.: Bleeding from the upper gastrointestinal tract. Brit. Med. J., 4:723, 1967.

Chapman, B. L., and Duggan, J. M.: Aspirin and uncomplicated peptic ulcer. Gut, 10:443, 1969.

Chears, W. C., and Ashworth, E. T.: Electron microscopic study of the intestinal mucosa in Whipple's disease. Demonstration of encapsulated bacilliform bodies in the lesion. Gastroenterology, 1:129, 1961.

Cohen, A. S.: An electron microscopic study of the small intestine in Whipple's disease. J. Ultrastruct. Res., 10:124, 1964.

Cohen, A. S., et al.: Ultrastructural abnormalities in Whipple's disease. Proc. Soc. Exp. Biol. Med., *105*:411, 1960.

Collins, W. T., and Gall, E. A.: Gastric carcinoma: a multicentric lesion. Cancer, *5*:62, 1952.

Cox, J.: Gastric mucosal changes in peptic ulcer. Gastroenterology, *45*:558, 1963.

Croft, D. N.: Aspirin and the exfoliation of gastric epithelial cells. Cytological and biochemical observations. Brit. Med. J., *2*:897, 1963.

Croft, D. N.: Gastritis. Brit. Med. J., *4*:164, 1967.

Croft, D. N., et al.: Cell loss from human gastric mucosa measured by the estimation of deoxyribonucleic acid (DNA). Gut, *7*:333, 1966.

Crohn, B.: Rectal complications of inflammatory disease of the small and large bowel. Dis. Colon Rectum, *3*:99, 1960.

Darling, R. C., and Welch, C. E.: Tumors of the small intestine. New Eng. J. Med., *260*:397, 1959.

Davis, J. E., et al.: Villous adenomas of the rectum and sigmoid colon with severe fluid and electrolyte depletion. Ann. Surg., *155*:806, 1962.

Dawson, J. L.: Carcinoma of the stomach. Brit. Med. J., *4*:533, 1967.

DeDombal, F.: Ulcerative colitis: definition, historical background, etiology, diagnosis, natural history and local complications. Postgrad. Med. J., *45*:684, 1968.

DeDombal, F., et al.: Aetiology of ulcerative colitis. I. A review of past and present hypotheses. Gut, *10*:270, 1969.

Devroede, G. J.: Cancer risk and life expectancy of children with ulcerative colitis. New Eng. J. Med., *285*:17, 1971.

Djar, T., et al.: Carcinoembryonic antigen (CEA) in colonic cancer. J.A.M.A., *221*:31, 1972.

Dormandy, T. L.: Gastro-intestinal polyposis with mucocutaneous pigmentation (Peutz-Jeghers syndrome). New Eng. J. Med., *256*:1093, 1141, 1186, 1957.

Dragstedt, L. R.: The etiology of gastric and duodenal ulcers. Postgrad. Med., *15*:99, 1954.

Dragstedt, L. R., et al.: Antral hyperfunction and gastric ulcer. Ann. Surg., *140*:396, 1954.

Dudeney, T. P.: Crohn's disease of the mouth. Proc. Roy. Soc. Med., *62*:1237, 1969.

Dukes, C. E.: Familial intestinal polyposis. Amer. Eugenics, *17*:1, 1952.

Dukes, C. E., and Bussey, H. J. R.: The spread of rectal cancer and its effect on prognosis. Brit. J. Cancer, *12*:309, 1958.

Dungal, N.: Special problem of stomach cancer in Iceland with particular reference to dietary factors. J.A.M.A., *178*:789, 1961.

Editorial: Asymptomatic hiatus hernia. Lancet, *1*:870, 1969.

Editorial: Diverticular disease. Brit. Med. J., *2*:126, 1970*a*.

Editorial: Epidemiology of Crohn's disease. Lancet, *1*:942, 1972.

Editorial: Susceptibility to aspirin bleeding. Brit. Med. J., *2*:436, 1970*b*.

Eiseman, B., and Heyman, R. L.: Stress ulcers: a continuing challenge. New Eng. J. Med., *282*:372, 1970.

Enterline, H. T., et al.: Malignant potential of adenomas of colon and rectum. J.A.M.A., *179*:322, 1962.

Felsen, J., and Wolarsky, W.: Chronic ulcerative colitis in carcinoma. Arch. Intern. Med., *84*:293, 1949.

Freiman, V. G.: Hemorrhagic necrosis of the gastrointestinal tract. Circulation, *32*:329, 1965.

Gilbertsen, V. A.: Adenocarcinoma of the large bowel. J.A.M.A., *174*:1789, 1960.

Gold, T., and Freedman, S. O.: Demonstration of tumor-specific antigens in human colonic carcinomata by immunological tolerance and absorption techniques. J. Exp. Med., *121*:439, 1965*a*.

Gold, T., and Freedman, S. O.: Specific carcinoembryonic antigens of the human digestive system. J. Exp. Med., *122*:467, 1965*b*.

Goldberg, B.: Clinical Tuberculosis. Philadelphia, F. A. Davis Co., 1947.

Goldgraber, M. B., et al.: The histopathology of chronic ulcerative colitis and its pathogenic implications. Gastroenterology, *38*:596, 1960.

Goldman, H., et al.: Nature and significance of hyperplastic polyps of the human colon. Arch. Path., *89*:349, 1970.

Gregory, R. A., et al.: Extraction of gastrin-like substance from a pancreatic tumor in a case of Zollinger-Ellison syndrome. Lancet, *1*:1045, 1960.

Grinnell, R. S.: Lymphatic metastases of carcinoma of colon and rectum. Ann. Surg., *131*:494, 1950.

Grossman, M. I., et al.: Basal histalog-stimulated gastric secretion in control subjects and in patients with pepetic ulcer or gastric cancer. Gastroenterology, *45*:14, 1963.

Haenszel, W., and Correa, P.: Cancer of the colon and rectum and adenomatous polyps: a review of epidemiologic findings. Cancer, *28*:14, 1971.

Hagarty, G.: A classification of esophageal hiatus hernia with special reference to sliding hernia. Amer. J. Roentgen., *84*:1056, 1960.

Hartman, R. S., et al.: An electron microscopic investigation of the jejunal epithelium in sprue. Gastroenterology, *38*:506, 1960.

Helwig, E. B.: Evolution of adenomas of the large intestine and their relation to carcinoma. Surg. Gynec. Obstet., *84*:36, 1947.

Helwig, E. B., and Hansen, J.: Lymphoid polyps (benign lymphoma) and malignant lymphoma of rectum and anus. Surg. Gynec. Obstet., *92*:233, 1951.

Hock, W. A., and Hazard, J. B.: Sclerosing retroperitonitis and sclerosing mediastinitis. Amer. J. Clin. Path., *32*:321, 1959.

Horn, R. C., Jr.: Malignant potential of polypoid lesions of the colon and rectum. Cancer, *28*:146, 1971.

Horner, J. L.: Natural history of diverticulosis of colon. Amer. J. Dig. Dis., *3*:343, 1958.

Hornsby, L. G.: Ulcerative colitis: a contemporary overview. Dis. Nerv. Syst., *31*:338, 1970.

Hurst, A. F.: The Alvarez lecture on the unity of gastric disorders. Brit. Med. J., *2*:89, 1933.

Ivey, K. J.: Acute haemorrhagic gastritis. Modern concepts based on pathogenesis. Gut, *12*:750, 1971.

Jeffries, G. H., et al.: Malabsorption. Gastroenterology, *46*:434, 1964.

Jones, C. M., et al.: Whipple's disease. New Eng. J. Med., *248*:665, 1953.

Joske, R. A., et al.: Gastric biopsy: a study of 1000 consecutive biopsies. Quart. J. Med., *24*:269, 1955.

Joyal, R. K., et al.: Lower esophageal ring. New Eng. J. Med., *282*:1298, 1355, 1970.

Keyting, W. S., et al.: The lower esophagus. Amer. J. Roentgen., *84*:1070, 1960.

Kirschner, P. A.: Occlusion of the mesenteric arteries and veins with infarction of the bowel. J. Mount Sinai Hosp. N.Y., *21*:307, 1954–55.

Kirsner, J. B.: Peptic ulcer. Review of the literature for 1964. Gastroenterology, *49*:79, 1965.

Kirsner, J., and Spencer, J.: Family occurrences of ulcerative colitis, regional enteritis, and ileocolitis. Ann. Intern. Med., *59*:133, 1963.

Koberle, F.: Enteromegaly and cardiomegaly in Chagas disease. Gut, *4*:399, 1963.

Kraft, S. C., and Kirsner, J. B.: Immunological apparatus of the gut and inflammatory bowel disease. Gastroenterology, *60*:922, 1971.

Kraft, S. C., et al.: Serum immunoglobulin levels in ulcerative colitis and Crohn's disease. Gastroenterology, *54*:1251, 1968.

Kramer, P.: The esophagus. Gastroenterology, *49*:439, 1965.

Kramer, P.: Frequency of the asymptomatic lower esophageal contractile ring. New Eng. J. Med., *254*:692, 1956.

Kramer, P., and Markarian, B.: Gastric acid secretion in chronic obstructive pulmonary emphysema. Gastroenterology, *38*:295, 1960.

Kronman, B. S.: Ulcerative colitis: autoimmune epiphenomena, and colonic cancer. Cancer, *28*:82, 1971.

Lagercrantz, R., et al.: Immunological studies in ulcerative colitis. IV. Origin of autoantibodies. J. Exp. Med., *128*:1339, 1968.

Lahey, F. H., and Jordan, S. M.: Carcinoma of stomach. New Eng. J. Med., *210*:59, 1934.

Laipply, T. C.: Pathologic anatomy of regional enteritis. J.A.M.A., *165*:2052, 1957.

Lockhart-Mummery, H. E., et al.: The surgical treatment of familial polyposis of the colon. Brit. J. Surg., *43*:476, 1956.

MacDonald, R.: A study of 356 carcinoids of the gastrointestinal tract: report of four new cases of the carcinoid syndrome. Amer. J. Med., *21*:867, 1956.

Magnus, H. A.: Gastritis. In Jones, F. A. (ed.): Modern Trends in Gastroenterology. New York, Paul B. Hoeber, Inc., 1952, p. 346.

Mallory, T. B.: Cancer in situ of stomach and its bearing on histogenesis of malignant ulcers. Arch. Path., 30:348, 1940.

Mann, J. G.: The subtle and variable clinical expressions of gluten-induced enteropathy (adult celiac disease, non tropical sprue). Amer. J. Med., 48:357, 1970.

Max, M., and Menguy, R.: Influence of adrenocorticotropin cortisone, aspirin and phenylbutazone and the rate of renewal of gastric mucosal cells. Gastroenterology, 58:329, 1970.

McConchie, I.: Gastro-esophageal carcinoma in hiatal hernia. Aust. New Zeal. J. Surg., 31:6, 1961.

McCusick, V. A.: Genetic factors in intestinal polyposis. J.A.M.A., 182:271, 1962.

McHardy, G. G., et al.: Hiatal hernia and erosive esophagitis. General Practitioner, 40:85, 1969.

McIver, M. A.: Acute intestinal obstruction. Amer. J. Surg., 19:163, 1933.

McNeer, G., and Berg, J. W.: Clinical behavior and management of primary malignant lymphoma of the stomach. Surgery, 46:829, 1959.

McSwain, B., et al.: Carcinoma of the colon, rectum, and anus. Ann. Surg., 155:782, 1962.

Menguy, R.: Pathophysiology of peptic ulcer. Amer. J. Surg., 120:282, 1970.

Merigan, T. C., et al.: Gastrointestinal bleeding with cirrhosis: a study of 172 episodes in 158 patients. New Eng. J. Med., 263:579, 1960.

Ming, S. C.: Hemorrhagic necrosis of the gastrointestinal tract and its relation to cardiovascular status. Circulation, 32:322, 1965.

Ming, S. C., and Fleischner, F. G.: Diverticulitis of the sigmoid colon. Reappraisal of the pathology and pathogenesis. Surgery, 58:627, 1965.

Mitchell, D. N., and Rees, R. J. W.: Agent transmissible from Crohn's disease tissue. Lancet, 2:168, 1970.

Mitchell, D. N., et al.: Further observations on Kveim test in Crohn's disease. Lancet, 2:496, 1970.

Moertel, C. G., et al.: Multiple carcinomas of the large intestine: a review of the literature and a study of 261 cases. Gastroenterology, 34:85, 1958.

Montgomery, D. O., and Wilson, A. C.: Esophageal hiatus hernia and associated intra-abdominal pathology. Amer. Surg., 29:708, 1963.

Morson, B. C.: Histopathology of Crohn's disease. Proc. Roy. Soc. Med., 61:79, 1968.

Morson, B. C.: The muscle abnormality in diverticular disease of the sigmoid colon. Brit. J. Radiol., 36:385, 1963.

Myren, J., et al.: Epidemiology of ulcerative colitis and regional enterocolitis (Crohn's disease) in Norway. Scand. J. Gastroent., 6:511, 1971.

Oates, J. A., et al.: Release of a kinin peptide in the carcinoid syndrome. Lancet, 1:514, 1964.

Ochsner, S. F., and Janitos, G. P.: Benign tumors of the stomach. J.A.M.A., 191:881, 1965.

Orloff, M. J., et al.: The complications of cirrhosis of the liver. Ann. Intern. Med., 66:165, 1967.

Ostrow, J. D., et al.: Gastric secretion in human hepatic cirrhosis. Gastroenterology, 38:303, 1960.

Painter, N. S.: Diverticular disease of the colon. A disease of this century. Lancet, 2:586, 1969.

Palmer, E. D.: Hiatus hernia and hemorrhage. Amer. J. Med. Sci., 246:417, 1963.

Palmer, E. D.: The hiatus hernia—esophagitis—esophageal stricture complex. Amer. J. Med., 44:566, 1968.

Palmer, E. D., and Brick, I. B.: Varices of distal esophagus in apparent absence of portal and superior caval hypertension. Amer. J. Med. Sci., 230:515, 1955.

Parks, T. G.: Natural history of diverticular disease of the colon. A review of 521 cases. Brit. Med. J., 4:639, 1969.

Paustian, F. F., et al.: The importance of the brief trial of rigid medical management in the diagnosis of benign versus malignant gastric ulcer. Gastroenterology, 38:155, 1960.

Pearson, C. M., and Fitzgerald, P. J.: Carcinoid tumors: a reemphasis of their malignant nature. Cancer, 2:1005, 1949.

Peltokallio, P., and Peltokallio, V.: Relationship of familial factors to carcinoma of the colon. Dis. Colon Rectum, 9:367, 1966.

Perlman, N. T., and Broberger, O.: Lower gastrointestinal system. In Miescher, P., and Mueller-Eberhard, H. (eds.): Textbook of Immunopathology. New York, Grune and Stratton, 1968, p. 551.

Postlethwait, R. W., and Musser, A. W.: Pathology of lower esophageal web. Surg. Gynec. Obstet., 120:571, 1965.

Reyes, F. A., Jr., and Friesen, S. R.: Review of the neuromuscular abnormalities in achalasia of the esophagus, congenital pyloric stenosis and congenital aganglionic megacolon. Rev. Surg., 24:153, 1967.

Rob, C.: Surgical diseases of the celiac and mesenteric arteries. Arch. Surg., 93:21, 1966.

Robinson, D. C., et al.: Incidence of small intestinal mucosal abnormalities and of clinical coeliac disease in the relatives of children with coeliac disease. Gut, 12:789, 1971.

Rosenburg, J. C.: Carcinoid and other amine-producing tumors. Progr. Clin. Cancer, 2:297, 1966.

Samloff, I. M., et al.: A clinical and histochemical study of celiac disease before and during a gluten free diet. Gastroenterology, 48:155, 1965.

Sampson, D. A., and Sosman, M. C.: Prepyloric ulcer and carcinoma. Amer J. Roentgen., 42:797, 1939.

Schatzki, R., and Gary, J. E.: The lower esophageal ring. Amer. J. Roentgen., 75:246, 1956.

Shamma'a, M. H., and Benedict, E. B.: Esophageal webs: a report of 58 cases and an attempt at classification. New Eng. J. Med., 259:378, 1958.

Shanks, H. G.: Pseudomyxoma peritonei. J. Obstet Gynec. Brit. Comm., 68:212, 1961.

Sheehy, T. W., et al.: Tropical sprue in North Americans. J.A.M.A., 194:1069, 1965.

Shiner, M.: Jejunal biopsy tube. Lancet, 1:85, 1956.

Shiner, M., and Ballard, J.: Antigen-antibody reactions in jejunal mucosa in childhood coeliac disease after gluten challenge. Lancet, 1:1202, 1972.

Sieracki, J. C., and Fine, G.: Observations of systemic involvement of Whipple's disease. Arch. Path., 67:81, 1959.

Sleisenger, M. H.: Diseases of malabsorption. In Deeson, T. B., and McDermott, W. M. (eds.): Cecil-Loeb Textbooks of Medicine. 12 ed. Philadelphia, W. B. Saunders Co., 1967, p. 883.

Spratt, J. S., Jr., and Ackerman, L. V.: Pathologic significance of polyps of the rectum and colon. Dis. Colon Rectum, 3:330, 1960.

Spratt, J. S., Jr., and Watson, F. R.: The rationale of practice for polypoid lesions of the colon. Cancer, 28:153, 1971.

Stokes, P. L., et al.: Histocompatibility antigens associated with adult coeliac disease. Lancet, 2:162, 1972.

Stout, A. P.: Pathology of carcinoma of stomach. Arch. Surg., 46:807, 1943.

Swanson, V. L., and Thomassen, R. W.: Pathology of the jejunal mucosa in tropical sprue. Amer. J. Path., 46:511, 1965.

Sweet, R. H.: The results of radical surgical extirpation in the treatment of cancer of the esophagus and cardia. Surg. Gynec. Obstet., 94:46, 1952.

Swenson, O.: Hirschsprung's disease (aganglionic megacolon). New Eng. J. Med., 260:972, 1959.

Swinton, N. W., et al.: Papillary adenomas of colon and rectum. Arch. Intern. Med., 96:544, 1955.

Tanner, N. C.: Surgery of peptic ulceration and its complications. Postgrad. Med. J., 30:577, 1954.

Terracol, J., and Sweet, R. H.: Diseases of the Esophagus. Philadelphia, W. B. Saunders Co., 1958.

Thayer, W. R., Jr.: Crohn's disease (regional enteritis). Scand. J. Gastroent., Suppl. 6, 5:165, 1970.

Thomas, C. S., Jr., et al.: Jejunal diverticula as a source of massive gastrointestinal bleeding. Arch. Surg., 95:89, 1967.

Thorek, P. E.: Acute abdominal emergencies. Postgrad. Med., 11:139, 1952.

Tizes, R.: Granulomatous colitis. New Eng. J. Med., 282:1273, 1970.

United States Department of Health, Education and Welfare, Public Health Service Review, 1967: The health consequences of smoking. Public Health Service Publication, No. 1696, 1968, p. 150.

Valman, H. B., et al.: Lesions associated with gastro-duodenal hemorrhage in relation to aspirin intake. Brit. Med. J., 4:661, 1968.

Veale, A. M. O.: Intestinal Polyposis. Cambridge, Cambridge University Press, 1965.

Wangensteen, O. H.: Rationalizing treatment in acute intestinal obstruction. Surg. Gynec. Obstet., *64*:273, 1937.

Warren, S., and Sommers, S. C.: Pathology of regional enteritis and ulcerative colitis. J.A.M.A., *154*:189, 1954.

Warren, S., and Sommer, S. C.: Pathogenesis of ulcerative colitis. Amer. J. Path., *25*:657, 1949.

Watson, D. W.: Immune responses and the gut. Gastroenterology, *56*:944, 1969*a*.

Watson, D. W.: The lymphocyte in ulcerative colitis. Gastroenterology, *56*:385, 1969*b*.

Watson, D. W., et al.: Effect of lymphocytes from patients with ulcerative colitis on human adult colon epithelial cells. Gastroenterology, *51*:985, 1966.

Weber, J. M., et al.: Hemorrhage from the upper gastrointestinal tract. J.A.M.A., *165*:1899, 1957.

Weiss, S., and Mallory, G. K.: Lesions of cardiac orifice of the stomach produced by vomiting. J.A.M.A., *98*:1353, 1932.

Welch, C. E., and Giddings, W. P.: Carcinoma of colon and rectum. New Eng. J. Med., *244*:859, 1951.

Wheat, N. W., Jr., and Ackerman, L. V.: Villous adenomas of large intestine. Clinicopathologic evaluation of 50 cases of villous adenomas with emphasis on treatment. Ann. Surg., *147*:476, 1958.

Whitehouse, F. R., and Kernohan, J. W.: Myenteric plexus in congenital megacolon: study of 11 cases. Arch. Intern. Med., *82*:75, 1948.

Whittaker, L. D., and Pemberton, J. deJ.: Mesenteric vascular occlusion. J.A.M.A., *111*:21, 1938.

Williams, W.: Histology of Crohn's syndrome. Gut, *5*:510, 1964.

Wilson, H. E., et al.: Carcinoid tumors: a study of 78 cases. Amer. J. Surg., *105*:35, 1963.

Wilson, R., and Qualheim, R. E.: A form of acute hemorrhagic enterocolitis afflicting chronically ill individuals. A description of 20 cases. Gastroenterology, *27*:431, 1954.

Wright, P., and Truelove, S. C.: Autoimmune reactions in ulcerative colitis. Gut, *7*:32, 1966.

Wynder, E. L., and Bross, I. J.: A study of etiologic factors in cancer of the esophagus. Cancer, *14*:389, 1961.

Zamcheck, N., et al.: Immunologic diagnosis and prognosis of human digestive tract cancer: carcinoembryonic antigens. New Eng. J. Med., *286*:83, 1972.

Zamcheck, N., et al.: Occurrence of gastric cancer among patients with pernicious anemia at the Boston City Hospital. New Eng. J. Med., *252*:1103, 1955.

22

THE LIVER AND BILIARY TRACT

LIVER

NORMAL
PATHOLOGY
Pathophysiology of Jaundice
  Excess production of
    bilirubin
  Reduced hepatic cell uptake
    of bilirubin
  Impaired conjugation of
    bilirubin
  Impaired excretion of
    conjugated bilirubin
    (cholestasis)
Hepatic Failure
Congenital Defects
  Accessory liver tissue
  Accessory lobes
  Congenital cystic liver disease
  Dubin-Johnson and Rotor
    syndromes
  Crigler-Najjar syndrome
  Gilbert syndrome
Metabolic and Regressive
  Changes
  Brown atrophy
  Hemosiderosis
  Fatty change
  Glycogen accumulation
  Amyloidosis
Circulatory Changes
  Anemia
  Congestion of the liver
  Central hemorrhagic necrosis
    (CHN)
  Cardiac sclerosis
  Infarct

Hepatic vein obstruction
  (Budd-Chiari syndrome)
Portal vein obstruction
Shock
Necroses and Inflammations
Focal and zonal necroses
  Focal random necrosis
  Centrilobular necrosis
  Midzonal necrosis
  Peripheral necrosis
Drug-induced injury and
  cholestasis
Viral hepatitis
Chronic hepatitis
Chronic active (aggressive)
  hepatitis
  Chronic active lupoid
    hepatitis
  Chronic active viral
    hepatitis
Massive hepatic necrosis
Neonatal (giant cell) hepatitis
Other inflammations of the
  liver
  Cholangitis
  Liver abscesses
  Tuberculosis
  Disseminated systemic
    sarcoidosis
  Syphilis
  Weil's disease
  Amebic abscesses
  Actinomycotic infections
  Echinococcus cysts
  Liver flukes

Postmortem Changes
  Postmortem autolysis
  Gas bacillus infection
Tumors
  Benign
    Cavernous hemangioma
    Adenoma
    Regenerative nodules
    Hamartomas
  Primary carcinoma
    Hepatocarcinoma
    Cholangiocarcinoma
    Hepatocholangiocarcinoma
  Metastatic tumors
Cirrhosis
  Portal hypertension –
    pathophysiology
  Associated with alcohol abuse
    (alcoholic, portal,
    Laennec's, nutritional)
  Associated with hemo-
    chromatosis (pigment)
  Postnecrotic scarring
  Posthepatitic (trabecular)
  Biliary
    Secondary obstructive
      and/or infectious
    Primary
  Miscellaneous and
    indeterminate forms
    Cardiac (sclerosis)
    Syphilitic
    Wilson's disease
    Cryptogenic

NORMAL

Beneath the deceptively bland glistening capsule of Glisson that envelops the liver lurks a bewildering host of functional and structural details. Some of the more easily forgotten or less well understood details are selected for presentation. In the adult, the normal liver weighs between 1400 to 1600 gm., varying with the size of the individual. In addition to the right and left lobes the liver normally possesses two additional rudimentary lobes, the quadrate and caudate. The main mass of the liver is made up principally of the right lobe, which is at least six times larger than the left. Clinical estimations of the size of the liver are at best fairly crude approximations. While it is traditionally taught that normally the anterior edge of the liver does not emerge from under the right costal margin, the body build, the level of the right hemidiaphragm and hence the upper margins of the liver, and the configuration of the liver all influence this finding. Mere palpation of the liver beneath the costal margin does not necessarily indicate hepatomegaly. Care must be exercised in delineating both the upper border and the anterior edge to avoid the ptotic organ that may, despite a normal size, hang dependently below the costal margin. Normally the anterior edge is quite sharp. When it becomes rounded or nodular, intrahepatic disorders should be suspected.

According to accepted concepts of the microscopic structure of the liver, it is divided into lobules having in their centers hepatic veins, from which cords of liver cells radiate out to the periphery. The outer boundaries of the lobule are indistinctly demarcated by the portal triads (hepatic artery, portal vein, bile duct). In actual fact, such a conception is highly stylized. In man, no well defined lobules exist. Three-dimensional reconstructions indicate that the liver cells are laid down as bricks in a system of walls or plates. At some points these walls are parallel to each other, while at others they branch or anastomose or double back upon themselves, but they are always separated by intermural spaces called lacunae. These walls are perforated by numerous tunnels which interconnect the lacunae into a vast labyrinth. Through this labyrinth travel the liver sinusoids lined by endothelial cells and specialized reticuloendothelial cells, the Kupffer cells. These sinusoids are not tightly packed into the spaces but are suspended as it were in the overly large lacunae, leaving the space of Disse between sinusoid and surrounding liver substance (Elias, 1949). The surfaces of the liver cells that comprise the outer boundary of the space of Disse are studded by microvilli. Into these vascular sinusoids flow the smallest ramifications of the portal vein and hepatic artery. But before they reach the terminus, there are numerous intercommunications or anastomoses between the radicles of the portal vein and hepatic artery that play important roles in portal vein obstruction and in maintaining the nutrition of the liver cells when either vessel is compromised.

On the other side of the liver cell from the sinusoid, one finds the bile canaliculus. Thus, each liver cell is ingeniously sandwiched between a bile canaliculus and a vascular sinusoid. The bile canaliculus is formed by grooves in the adjoining surfaces of two liver cells so fitted together as to create a tunnel that traverses the entire length of the liver plate along a tier of cells. These canaliculi that extend from the central vein outward to the portal region have no wall of their own and are lined by the plasmal membranes of the liver cells. Numerous microvilli project into the lumina of these canaliculi. In the portal region, many of these canaliculi join to form larger ductules that have been the center of a stormy controversy as to their nature and designation. They have been called intraparenchymal ductules, bile preductules, cholangioles and canals of Hering. These preductules also possess microvilli that become progressively shorter as the larger bile ducts are approached. Once within the portal region, the bile ductules are lined by regularly oriented cuboidal epithelial cells distinctive from hepatic cells.

Turning to the hepatic parenchymal cell itself, one might devote pages to it alone. To quote Bruni and Porter (1965): "The parenchymal liver cell of the rat has been studied more extensively perhaps than any other cell type, not only biochemically but also morphologically." As seen in autopsy sections, the liver cell is polygonal, having a central nucleus with a fairly prominent nucleolus and a homogeneous pink cytoplasm. In freshly fixed biopsy material, the cytoplasm is far more granular and has a reticulated appearance, due perhaps to the preservation of the high content of glycogen. This cell contains the usual organelles with a rich supply of mitochondria as well as endoplasmic reticulum, both smooth and rough, and polyribosomes. The Golgi complex is especially prominent and is often oriented toward the space of Disse. The endoplasmic reticulum often is arrayed in parallel rows with clubbed ends abutting on the Golgi complex (Fig. 22–1).

An elegant level of correlation of ultrastructure with function has been achieved with the liver cell. Both granular and amorphous substances have been identified within the vesicles of the Golgi complex. This material is apparently synthesized by the rough endoplasmic reticulum and is transferred to the Golgi complex where it is separated into the granular substance and the amorphous substance. The granular substance has been identified within the space of Disse, and immunofluorescent and biochemical studies suggest that it represents plasma proteins. Thus, it can be inferred that these proteins are synthesized within the liver cells on the endoplasmic reticulum and are then transferred to the Golgi complex which secretes them into the space of Disse where they will eventually enter the hepatic sinusoids to join the plasma pool. The amorphous substance, in contrast, is transferred from the Golgi complex to lysosomes, suggesting that it represents protein in the form of enzymes. These details are cited only as an example of the depth of penetration of the liver cell.

The intrahepatic circulation is another subject of considerable importance. Well known is the double nutrient supply received through both the portal vein and the hepatic artery. Of the 1.5 liters of blood that the liver

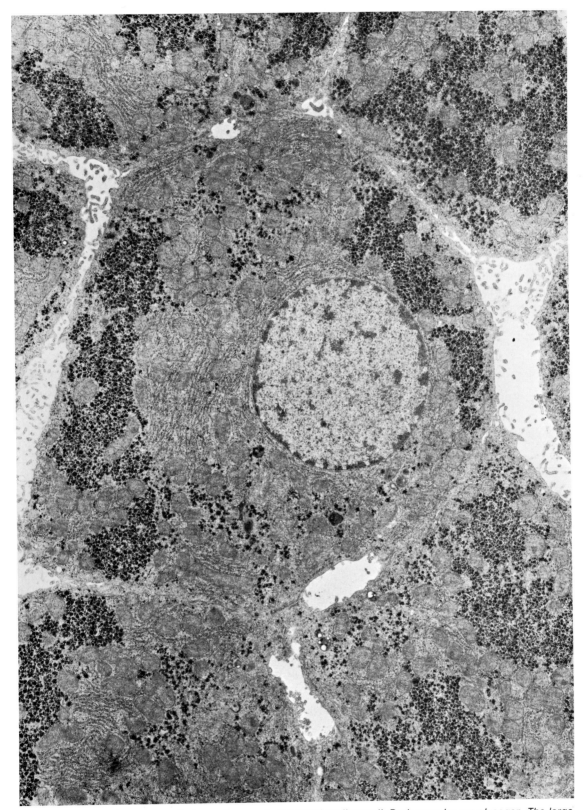

Figure 22–1. Low power electron micrograph of normal rat liver cell. Dark granules are glycogen. The large lateral spaces are vascular sinusoids. Above and below are biliary canaliculi sandwiched between liver cells. Note microvilli in sinusoids and canaliculi. (Courtesy of Dr. Dariush Fahimi, Mallory Institute of Pathology.)

receives per minute, about two-fifths is derived from the hepatic artery and three-fifths from the portal vein. While the arterial blood is the more richly oxygenated, either supply is capable under normal conditions of maintaining the hepatic parenchyma. Hence infarctions in the liver are rare. Previous mention has been made of the anastomoses in the portal areas between radicles of the hepatic artery and the portal vein, providing an additional reinforcement against ischemia of the liver cells. However, because of its high level of metabolism the liver cell is extremely vulnerable to hypoxia, and obviously those cells most removed from the portal region are most precariously situated. Thus, when vascular stasis occurs, as in cardiac failure, the cells about the central part of the lobule are most seriously affected.

It is beyond our limitations of space to discuss the enormously complex physiology of the liver. It has been estimated that over 500 separate metabolic activities occur within a single liver cell. These involve such broad categories as intermediary metabolism of carbohydrates, proteins and lipids; synthesis of proteins such as fibrinogen, albumin, prothrombin and a host of enzymes; conjugation of bilirubin with glucuronide; detoxification and removal of foreign material such as bacteria, drugs and other noxious substances; and the storage of many substances such as proteins, glycogen, vitamins and minerals including iron. One of the most important functions of the liver involves the formation of bile, discussed on p. 989. In the performance of the liver's many roles, literally hundreds of enzymes are involved. Among these, only the transaminases and phosphatases will be discussed here. Later in the chapter, the dehydrogenases and transferases enter into the discussion. All play large roles in the production and detection of hepatic disease. Two parenchymal transaminases, glutamic oxaloacetic (GOT) and glutamic pyruvic (GPT), are most frequently quantitated in the serum as indices of liver cell necrosis. GPT is found virtually only in liver cells, in the cytoplasm, unbound to organelles. It therefore diffuses out of injured hepatocytes and is readily detected in the serum (SGPT). GOT is found in small quantities in tissues other than the liver. Several isoenzymes have been identified; GOT I in the soluble fraction of liver cell homogenates, and GOT II bound to mitochondria. Both isoenzymes are cleared from the blood more rapidly than SGPT. SGPT is then a more specific and sensitive indicator of liver cell damage, and is more useful clinically because the serum levels remain elevated longer.

Alkaline phosphatase is found in many cells (endothelium, epithelial cells of mucosal surfaces, bone, renal tubules), but it is also present in small amounts in liver canaliculi. Its localization within hepatocytes is uncertain. For clinical purposes, serum elevations of alkaline phosphatase are encountered in liver disease, bone disease and pregnancy. Hepatic disorders associated with biliary tract obstruction induce the highest elevations of the serum levels of alkaline phosphatase.

It is not surprising that occasionally deficiencies of an enzyme are encountered as a hereditary defect. An example is the absence of glucuronyl transferase, required for the conjugation of bile, in Crigler-Najjar disease. This particular deficiency was recognized because it involved an easily detectable derangement in the formation and excretion of bile. But there is little question that additional enzyme defects will be uncovered in the future as the level of sophistication of our knowledge rises.

PATHOLOGY

The liver is one of the most frequently damaged organs in the body, and it is indeed fortunate that it has an enormous functional reserve. In the experimental animal, it has been shown that only 10 per cent of hepatic parenchyma is required to maintain normal liver function (Simpson and Finckh, 1963). In man, there is probably an equally large reserve, so that extensive damage may be incurred before it becomes clinically manifested by signs of hepatic insufficiency.

The list of diseases which affect the liver spans a wide range of vascular, metabolic, toxic, obstructive and neoplastic involvements. It is of little use to attempt to ascribe relative frequencies to each, because there is so much geographic variation. In the less well developed countries, where parasitic and fungal infections are common, these might represent the burden of hepatic disease, while in the United States, Great Britain and Europe such disorders are relatively uncommon. In regions of Africa, primary cancer is one of the most common malignancies encountered, but in the United States and Europe these neoplasms are relatively rare. Therefore, only the major hepatic diseases encountered more or less throughout the world will be presented, omitting, for the most part, systemic diseases in which hepatic involvement plays a minor role.

All extensive diseases of the liver which erode the large hepatic functional reserve tend to produce similar clinical signs and symptoms in the patient. *The two most common pathophysiologic syndromes are jaundice and liver failure.* Since both are produced by so many hepatic disorders, they will be considered first before the discussion of the specific diseases of the liver.

PATHOPHYSIOLOGY OF JAUNDICE

Jaundice, or icterus, comprises a yellow-green discoloration of the skin and sclerae produced by accumulations of bilirubin in the tissues and interstitial fluids. It implies hyperbilirubinemia. The normal serum bilirubin levels range from 0.1 mg. per 100 ml. of serum to 1.0 mg. Although an elevation above 1.2 mg. per 100 ml. of serum is abnormal, jaundice only becomes visible when the hyperbilirubinemia exceeds 2 to 3 mg. per 100 ml. of serum (artificial yellow light tends to mask jaundice). Because bilirubin has an affinity for elastic tissue, it is most evident in the sclerae because of their rich content of elastic fibers. The level of hyperbilirubinemia is a determinant of the intensity of the jaundice, but the rate of diffusion of bilirubin from the plasma into the interstitial fluid, and the binding of this pigment in the tissues modify the level of the resultant icterus. In passing, it should be noted that yellowing of the skin may rarely be produced by carotenemia (eating too many carrots), but the sclerae are not particularly affected here.

The consideration of the pathophysiology of jaundice requires an understanding of the formation, transport, metabolism and excretion of bilirubin. Here we can review the subject only briefly, but excellent references are available (Gartner and Arias, 1969) (Robinson, 1968). Approximately 85 per cent of the bilirubin is derived from the breakdown of obsolete red cells in the reticuloendothelial system. The heme pigment is converted by heme oxygenase to biliverdin and thence to bilirubin. The remaining 15 per cent is known as "shunt bilirubin" and is formed, in part, in the bone marrow as a byproduct of hemoglobin synthesis and, in part, in the liver from the rapid turnover of hemoproteins such as the cytochromes and catalases. Whatever its origin, the bilirubin formed outside the liver is promptly bound to albumin and transported through the blood to the liver in this lipid-soluble complex. The bilirubin-albumin complex can be neither excreted in the urine nor taken up by liver cells. In some mysterious fashion, the complex dissociates at the plasma membrane of the hepatocyte, and the bilirubin enters the liver cell where it is accepted by specific binding proteins. In the endoplasmic reticulum, it is conjugated chiefly to glucuronic acid (1 molecule of bilirubin to 2 molecules of glucuronic acid to produce conjugated bilirubin diglucuronide. Involved in such conjugation is the hepatocyte enzyme glucuronyl transferase. *Unconjugated bilirubin is water-insoluble, but the conjugated diglucuronide is water-soluble.* The hepatocyte then secretes the water-soluble diglucuronide into the bile canaliculi. Bilirubin is only the pigment in bile. Also contained are lecithin, bile acids and bile salts mixed with water, trace amounts of calcium and other electrolytes and mucus derived from the epithelial lining of the bile ducts. Bile then passes through the well known biliary apparatus to eventually reach the duodenum. Here the diglucuronide is split, and the released bilirubin is converted by bacterial action in the small intestine to urobilinogen. Thus, in obstructive biliary tract disease, when bile fails to enter the gut, the levels of urobilinogen fall. Normally, some of the urobilinogen is reabsorbed into the portal circulation and passed back to the liver, comprising the so-called enterohepatic circulation, while some is excreted by the kidneys (Poland and Odell, 1971). The fraction remaining in the gut is further transformed to urobilin (stercobilin). Hepatobiliary tract disease may cause elevated serum levels of either the unconjugated or the conjugated forms of bilirubin, and both forms produce jaundice. In most cases of jaundice, there are elevations of both the conjugated and unconjugated pigment.

At the pathophysiologic level, jaundice may be produced by: (1) increased rate of production of bilirubin, (2) decreased uptake in liver cells, (3) derangements in conjugation with glucuronide and (4) impaired secretion (excretion) into the bile canaliculi and biliary tract. The pathophysiology of hyperbilirubinemia can be considered, then, with respect to each of these steps.

Excess Production of Bilirubin. Hemolytic anemias, with the release of increased amounts of heme pigment, cause so-called *hemolytic jaundice.* The hyperbilirubinemia is due to increased levels of unconjugated bilirubin in the serum. Usually, such jaundice is not severe and the serum bilirubin levels rarely exceed 5 mg. per 100 ml. because the normal liver is capable of handling most of the overload. However, damage to the liver, perhaps secondary to the hypoxia attendant on the hemolytic process, or intercurrent hepatic disease, may induce more severe jaundice, sometimes with a conjugated component. Because the bilirubin is bound to albumin, it cannot pass the glomerular filter and so is not excreted in the urine (acholuric jaundice). Neither does the bilirubin-albumin complex pass the blood-brain barrier, and so it has no effect on the central nervous system. In addition to the hemolytic anemias, excess production of bilirubin is encountered in other clinical settings. In pernicious anemia, there is both a small hemolytic component and also an increased synthesis of shunt bilirubin in the bone marrow. A massive pulmonary hemorrhage or infarction, bleeding into the gut or massive hemorrhage in any site in the body may increase the production of bilirubin in the course of resorption of the destroyed red cells.

Reduced Hepatic Cell Uptake of Bilirubin. The precise steps involved in the passage of bilirubin into the liver cell are still poorly understood. All that is clear is that the albumin-bilirubin bond is broken, and the bilirubin is then able to pass the hepatocytic plasma membrane. Once inside the cell, there is evidence that it is immediately picked up by acceptor proteins. Abnormalities of bilirubin uptake are not common but are encountered in the genetic disorder known as Gilbert's disease (p. 995). Inadequate uptake may also occur in certain untoward reactions to drugs. Whatever the cause, there is an unconjugated hyperbilirubinemia which is acholuric because of the binding of the pigment to albumin.

Impaired Conjugation of Bilirubin. Athough glucuronyl transferase is present in other tissues, almost all bilirubin is conjugated in or on the membranes of the smooth endoplasmic reticulum of the hepatocytes. A conjugation defect of genetic origin is encountered in the Crigler-Najjar syndrome characterized by a total or severe lack of glucuronyl transferase. A similar defect has been identified in the inbred Gunn rat, which provides, therefore, an excellent model for study. In some cases of Gilbert's disease, there is a partial deficiency of hepatic glucuronyl transferase. Similarly, jaundice in the newborn may, in some part, be due to immaturity of the hepatic conjugating system. In all of these situations, the jaundice results from unconjugated hyperbilirubinemia. As was pointed out in the earlier discussion of hemolytic disease of the newborn (p. 557), attempts have been made to increase the conjugating capacity of the newborn by inducing increased synthesis of the glucuronyl transferase. It has been found that detoxification of barbiturates involves identical microsomal enzyme systems, and so the administration of barbiturates to the mother late in pregnancy induces synthesis of microsomal enzymes and an increased capacity for conjugation in the newborn.

Impaired Excretion of Conjugated Bilirubin (Cholestasis). The excretion of conjugated bilirubin may be hampered or, indeed, blocked at any level within the hepatobiliary tract from the hepatocyte to the ampulla of Vater. *From the standpoint of clinical management, it is important to distinguish intrahepatic from extrahepatic (posthepatic) obstructive jaundice.* The latter is sometimes amenable to surgical treatment, hence its designation as "surgical" jaundice, while intrahepatic disease is strictly "medical" jaundice.

Intrahepatic causes of hyperbilirubinemia run the gamut of diseases affecting liver cell function. The Dubin-Johnson and Rotor syndromes are hereditary disorders in which there is some defect in the transfer of bilirubin and other organic anions across the hepatocyte membrane. Drugs such as estrogens, certain of the contraceptive agents and anabolic steroids (p. (1002) may, in some patients, hamper the excretion of organic anions from the hepatoctye and thus produce an intrahepatic blockage of bilirubin excretion. Disorganization of the hepatic lobule, as is encountered in many cirrhoses, causes intrahepatic cholestasis. Direct damage to the liver cell which affects the enzyme systems, as for example in viral hepatitis, chemical and drug toxicity and microbiologic infections of the liver, can block conjugation and excretion of bilirubin. Thus, *jaundice is associated with all forms of acute insult to the liver, which seriously damage liver cells.* Intrahepatic causes for cholestasis damage the capacity of the liver cell both to take up bilirubin and to conjugate it. Moreover, in all acute insults to the liver cell, swelling may add an element of intrahepatic obstructive cholestasis with regurgitation of conjugated bilirubin into the blood. Thus, the jaundice is generally a composite of both unconjugated and conjugated hyperbilirubinemia. In general, all these forms of intrahepatic jaundice are associated with elevated levels of SGOT, SGPT and LDH, as well as other evidence of hepatocellular disease such as hypoprothrombinemia.

Extrahepatic cholestasis is seen with significant narrowing or obstruction of the right or left hepatic ducts, common bile duct or ampulla of Vater. Gallstones which become impacted in the common bile duct or carcinomas affecting any one of these ductal structures or the head of the pancreas are the most important causes of posthepatic obstructive jaundice. Much less commonly, acute infections within the biliary tract (cholangitis) may fill the duct with inspissated pus, or congenital anomalies with atresia or agenesis of the extrahepatic ducts may lead to such posthepatic obstruction. Occasionally, diseases arising outside of the ducts impinge on them to produce narrowing, such as subhepatic abscesses, tumorous infiltrates of the portal hepatic nodes or inflammatory swelling of the head of the pancreas. *In all forms of obstructive jaundice, there is a rise in the serum levels of conjugated bilirubin, bile fails to reach the intestines, and the stools lose their normal pigmentation, becoming clay-colored (acholic). Concomitantly, urine urobilinogen levels decline or disappear.* All of these findings are important clinical parameters of extrahepatic obstructive biliary tract disease. Not only is bile pigment impounded, but bile salts also accumulate in the blood, and so an important feature of obstructive jaundice is itching. Moreover, the lack of bile in the gut has serious secondary effects, particularly on the absorption of fats (including fat-soluble vitamins). In this way, a malabsorption syndrome may develop, leading to deficiencies of the fat-soluble vitamins. Avitaminosis K impairs the synthesis of prothrombin. Thus may arise a hemorrhagic diathesis, a serious threat in these patients who may require surgery to alleviate the biliary tract obstruction. Obstructive cholestasis is often associated with elevation of the plasma cholesterol level, and so these patients accumulate lipid-laden histiocytes within the skin, producing xanthomas.

Characteristic of the early state of extrahepatic obstructive jaundice is a conjugated hyperbilirubinemia associated with elevation of the serum alkaline phosphatase level, but no elevation of the SGOT, SGPT or LDH levels. In time, however, extrahepatic obstruction leads to damage of liver cells, and then the element of hepatocellular disease is added to the obstructive disease. Thus, *in well advanced extrahepatic obstructive disease, the hyperbilirubinemia is due to both conjugated and unconjugated bilirubin,* and the profile of serum enzymes reflects the composite effects of both the intra- and extrahepatic disease.

At one time, it was proposed that in all obstructive processes, the conjugated hyperbilirubinemia resulted from regurgitation of bilirubin diglucuronide from the liver cell into the hepatic vascular sinusoids, hence the term *regurgitational jaundice.* More recently, Popper and Schaffner (1970) have suggested a new explanation. They propose that extrahepatic biliary tract obstruction in some way leads to the synthesis, in liver cells, of increased quantities of monohydroxyl bile salts, particularly lithocholate. At body temperature, these salts are abnormally viscous and hamper the conjugating and excretory mechanisms of the liver cell. The intracellular bile stasis further injures the cell and hampers its uptake of bilirubin, adding a component of unconjugated bilirubin to the jaundice. Thus, in extrahepatic obstruction, the jaundice may not be regurgitational but rather may be a reflection of biochemical derangement of the hepatocyte.

There are significant differences in the clinical syndromes produced by unconjugated and conjugated hyperbilirubinemia. As indicated earlier, unconjugated bilirubin is water-insoluble. It, however, is capable of dissolving in the complex lipids encountered in nerve tissues. When high levels of unconjugated bilirubin are present in the blood, particularly in the infant, this pigment may cross the blood-brain barrier to be dissolved in the lipids within the central nervous system, producing the serious disorder known as *kernicterus.* Hyperbilirubinemia is, then, a major clinical problem in hemolytic disease of the newborn. Unconjugated hyperbilirubinemia is acholuric, as well. In contrast, conjugated bilirubin is water-soluble, excreted in the urine and nontoxic to cells. Clinical differentiation of these two forms of jaundice is therefore of major importance. Commonly used to make this distinction is the van den Bergh test, in which the conjugated form gives a prompt, hence a *direct,* reaction, while the unconjugated form gives an *indirect* reaction.

Although virtually any disease of the hepatobiliary system may cause jaundice, in the United States the most frequent causes, in descending order, are: viral hepatitis, cirrhosis, extrahepatic biliary obstruction and drug-induced cholestasis. An overview of the mechanism leading to hyperbilirubinemia and some clinical correlations are offered in Table 22–1.

In summary, then, it is important to recognize that although hemolytic jaundice is rather easily identified, it is frequently extremely difficult to distinguish between hepatocellular and obstructive jaundice. With both of the latter, there is eventually some element of liver cell injury and, therefore, hepatocellular derangement. Moreover, both involve elements of obstruction. With obstructive jaundice, this is primary; with hepatocellular jaundice, the obstruction results from swelling of parenchymal cells and occlusion of bile canaliculi. It requires a careful appraisal of the patient's entire status, in particular, serial studies of the blood, urine and stools and liver function tests, to thoroughly evaluate the underlying disorder. Liver needle biopsy is frequently helpful in making a diagnosis, but in many cases when remediable obstructive disease is suspected, exploratory laparotomy may ultimately be required.

HEPATIC FAILURE

The end result of many of the disorders to be discussed in this chapter is hepatic failure.

TABLE 22–1. CLINICAL CORRELATIONS OF HYPERBILIRUBINEMIA

Postulated Major Mechanism	Clinical Syndrome	Form of Bilirubin*	Bile in Urine	Urobilinogen in Urine
Excessive production: Increased red cell breakdown	Hemolytic disorders	Almost all unconjugated	0	Increased
Direct production in marrow	Shunt bilirubin in hematologic disorders	Almost all unconjugated	0	Increased
Impaired uptake by hepatocyte	Gilbert's syndrome (some cases)	Almost all unconjugated	0	Normal
	?Some forms of drug induced cholestasis	Almost all unconjugated	0	?
Glucuronide conjugation defect	Crigler-Najjar syndrome	Almost all unconjugated	0	Decreased
	Immaturity liver (jaundice of newborn)	Almost all unconjugated	0	Variable
	Gilbert's syndrome (some cases)	Almost all unconjugated	0	Variable
	?Some forms of drug induced cholestasis	Almost all unconjugated	?	?
Impaired secretion or transport into bile sinusoids, or obstructive disease (cholestasis)	?Dubin-Johnson and Rotor syndromes	60 to 80% unconj.; 20 to 40% unconj.	+	Normal
	Some forms of drug induced cholestasis	20 to 40% unconj.	+	Usually decreased
	Hepatitis	20 to 40% unconj.	+	Usually decreased
	Cirrhosis	20 to 40% unconj.	+	Usually decreased
	Posthepatic obstruction	20 to 40% unconj.	+	Low to 0

*Unconjugated forms give indirect van den Bergh test results; conjugated forms give direct van den Bergh test results.

The liver may be likened to the proverbial castle of sand built on the shore. It may be crumbled grain by grain or be lapped away by repeated small waves of erosion. Sometimes it is demolished in one massive wave of destruction. Occasionally, the already tottering castle falls victim to an intercurrent gust of wind, as the patient with marginal liver function is precipitated into hepatic failure by the stress of sudden blood loss or infection. So it is that the enormous functional reserve of the liver may be insidiously depleted, eroded in repeated waves or suddenly overwhelmed. You recall that the experimental animal survives an 80 to 90 per cent hepatectomy and regenerates a normal liver mass. While this extent of hepatic resection has not been approached in man, very large portions of the liver have indeed been resected (for removal of a cancer), and there is no reason to believe that man's reserve liver capacity is less than that of lower animals.

The two major causes of hepatic failure in most industrialized nations are cirrhosis and viral hepatitis. In both of these disorders, the liver is diffusely involved. In general, focal lesions, however numerous, rarely destroy sufficient hepatic parenchyma to wipe out the functional reserve. Widespread cancerous metastases throughout a liver, perhaps producing a two- or even threefold increase in liver weight, are not uncommon in a patient with *no* evidence of hepatic failure.

Disturbance of any one of the hundreds of liver metabolic functions may dominate the expression of hepatic failure. However, certain signs and symptoms are sufficiently common to create a characteristic syndrome. Jaundice is by no means indicative of liver failure, but it is almost invariably present when failure develops. *Personality alterations, confusion and mental obtundation, ranging from mild lethargy to coma, comprise a group of findings often termed metabolic encepha-*

lopathy. Very few anatomic changes have been identified in the brain in this syndrome. The most noticeable is an increase in the number of astrocytes, principally in the cerebral cortex, thalamus, pontine nuclei, ventricular nuclei and substantia nigra. Alterations in the ganglion cells have not been identified, and it can only be assumed that the glial changes reflect some as yet undetected, more significant central nervous system change. A variety of neurologic abnormalities may also appear, most characteristic of which is a flapping tremor of the outstretched hands, usually called a *"liver flap,"* but more scientifically designated asterixis.

Decreased inactivation of steroid hormones, principally estrogens in liver failure, often results in hypogonadism, loss of libido and gynecomastia in the male. Palmar erythema and "spider" angiomas of the skin have been attributed to hyperestrinism but without definite proof. Many patients develop a characteristic pungent sweet-sour odor, known as *fetor hepaticus.* The urine is usually particularly pungent. Renal insufficiency or failure is sometimes present and is designated the *hepatorenal syndrome.* The precise pathophysiology of such renal insufficiency is still obscure and is hotly debated. Indeed, sometimes the hepatorenal syndrome appears in the absence of liver failure following biliary tract surgery or some acute diffuse involvement of the liver. It is by no means correlated with the level of hyperbilirubinemia or the attendant bile pigmentation of renal tubular epithelial cells or bile casts in the tubules. In some cases, there are obvious explanations for the concurrence of hepatic and renal failure, such as can be found in carbon tetrachloride or heavy metal poisonings which damage both organs simultaneously. In those who have had biliary tract surgery, the explanation may be found in an episode of shock related to the surgery. But in the great preponderance of patients, no such obvious mechanisms can be identified. In these mysterious cases, electrolyte imbalances and sequestration of blood in the splanchnic bed with renal vasoconstriction may be causative or at least contributory (Schroeder et al., 1968). Strangely, despite the evidence of functional insufficiency, there may be no renal morphologic changes. Obscure as the mechanism of renal failure may be, it sometimes causes death in these patients.

Any one of a number of additional manifestations may be present. Occasionally, hepatic failure presents simply as extreme hyperpyrexia. Deranged protein synthesis may lead to hypoalbuminemia, hypoglobulinemia and hypoprothrombinemia. The last-mentioned may, in turn, lead to a hemorrhagic diathesis. With such inability to synthesize proteins, increased levels of amino acids may be found in the blood; and the inability to convert ammonia to urea results in increased levels of ammonia and decreased levels of urea in the blood. Many investigators relate the metabolic encephalopathy to the elevated blood levels of ammonia, but here again the issue is controversial, since there is no linear relationship between the severity of the encephalopathy and the blood levels of ammonia. Abnormalities in carbohydrate metabolism may be manifested, such as hypoglycemia resulting from inadequate stores of liver glycogen or, rarely, transient hyperglycemia due to the inability of the damaged liver to absorb and store excesses of blood glucose.

A host of laboratory tests are useful in assaying the extent and probable cause of the liver failure. Primary among them are, of course, the level of hyperbilirubinemia and the nature (conjugated or unconjugated) of the bilirubin. The serum enzyme levels are equally basic to the investigation. The significance of these parameters has been discussed earlier (p. 988). In addition, there are widely used liver function tests which attempt to evaluate some of the metabolic dysfunctions of the damaged liver. Total serum proteins, albumin-globulin ratio and prothrombin level all focus on protein synthetic capacities. The bromsulphthalein (BSP) excretion test evaluates the uptake, conjugation and excretion of the dye by the liver cell through pathways almost identical to those pursued by bilirubin. The serum cholesterol levels are often altered, but in an inconsistent fashion. In some forms of liver disease, the levels are increased and, in others, decreased; but in marked failure, cholesterol esters are usually strikingly reduced. The thymol turbidity and cephalin flocculation tests are often positive in hepatic failure and are thought to be related to imbalances in the synthesis of the various plasma proteins elaborated by the liver. Remarkably, in the individual patient, one parameter of disturbed liver function may be much more abnormal than others, suggesting greater impairment of one metabolic pathway than another. For this reason, it is customary to use many of the tests concomitantly referred to in the jargon as a "liver battery."

Hepatic failure is potentially reversible with the remarkable regenerative capacity of this organ. When the cause is some acute destructive process, the patient's life can sometimes be saved if he can be tided over the immediate stage of severe metabolic and electrolyte imbalance. In the course of days to weeks, regeneration of preserved vital cells may restore at least minimal hepatic function. Quite recently, it has been shown that exchange transfusions may, by presumably lowering blood levels of unknown toxic substances, effect remarkable improvement in patients with hepatic failure and, indeed, start the patient on the road to recovery (Berger et al., 1966).

CONGENITAL DEFECTS

Congenital defects of the liver take one of two forms: those that affect the morphology of the liver, and those that are metabolic in nature. The latter are usually hereditary in origin and do not produce changes to the naked eye but alterations in function and perhaps histologic detail.

Accessory Liver Tissue. Accessory liver tissue is found rarely as small islands in the serosa of the gallbladder at points completely separated from the liver. These islands are of academic interest alone.

Accessory Lobes. Accessory lobes are sometimes produced by capsular furrows that cut the liver substance up into supernumerary lobes. These are of no clinical importance. Sometimes there is marked downward enlargement of the right lobe, creating the erroneous impression of hepatic enlargement. For such an abnormality, the term Riedel's lobe is used. Occasionally, horizontal grooves are encountered on the anterior surface of the liver (Fig. 22–2). Pressure from the lower margin of

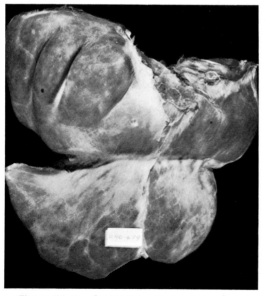

Figure 22–2. Corset liver. Horizontal and vertical furrows due to pressure atrophy from ribs.

the rib cage has been assumed to be the cause and, indeed, in years past such pressure was attributed to tightly laced corsets; hence the designation "corset liver." These grooves are still occasionally encountered in a day when the corset has become more of a medical curiosity than the liver defect. It is more reasonable to classify this unimportant alteration as a congenital abnormality.

Congenital Cystic Liver Disease. Congenital cysts of the liver are found in association with congenital polycystic kidneys. Presumably, these arise from developmental defects in the formation of the bile ducts. These cysts vary in size from a few millimeters up to several centimeters in diameter, tend to be superficial and, when opened, contain clear or slightly bile-tinged fluid. They are lined with cuboidal to columnar epithelium similar to that lining the bile ducts, from which they are presumably derived (Fig. 22–3*A, B*). They do not cause liver enlargement and are rarely palpable clinically. They are chiefly of anatomic interest alone but, when discovered at laparotomy, careful investigation of the kidneys is required.

Dubin-Johnson (Sprinz-Dubin-Johnson) and Rotor Syndromes. These are hereditary disorders having autosomal dominant modes of transmission which often do not become manifest until adulthood. Both are characterized by conjugated and unconjugated hyperbilirubinemia thought to result from some genetic defect in the capacity of the hepatocyte to excrete organic anions, including conjugated bilirubin. The glucuronyl transferase system in liver cells is intact. Conjugated bilirubin builds up in the hepatocyte and blood but, in time, an element of unconjugated hyperbilirubinemia is added as the stasis of bilirubin in liver cells injures them. The basic liver architecture in both syndromes is preserved. In the Dubin-Johnson syndrome, however, the liver is black, because the hepatocytes are diffusely dusted by a pigment (contained within lysosomes) considered by some to be a form of lipofuscin and by others to be melanin-like (Arias et al., 1964) (Fig. 22–4). The origin of the pigment may be related to impaired hepatocyte excretion of metabolites of catecholamines. Interestingly, a similar hepatic disorder is encountered in certain inbred strains of Corriedale sheep. The Rotor syndrome shares the hyperbilirubinemia but does not have the pigment deposits in the liver (Schmid, 1966). In both syndromes, the patients are jaundiced but are rarely very ill, and so they are often described as more yellow than sick (Dubin, 1958) (Dubin and Johnson, 1954).

Crigler-Najjar Syndrome. A hereditary

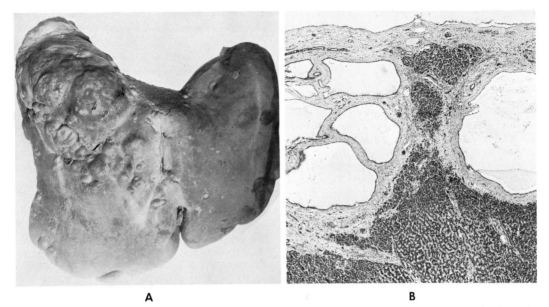

Figure 22–3. A, *Congenital cysts of liver, showing numerous subcapsular cysts.* B, *Microscopically, cysts are surrounded by fibrous tissue and lined by cuboidal epithelium.*

deficiency of hepatic glucuronyl transferase leading to an unconjugated hyperbilirubinemia characterizes the Crigler-Najjar syndrome. It appears in two forms, which appear to have different modes of transmission. The more

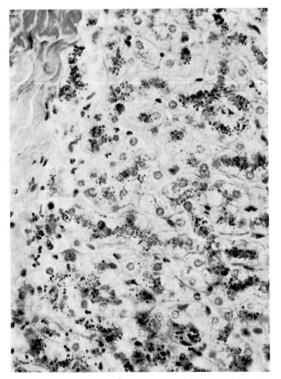

Figure 22–4. *Dubin-Johnson disease, showing fine dust-like pigmentation of the liver cells.*

serious type, characterized by a total lack of transferase, is an autosomal recessive disease most often encountered in infants and children. Because of the complete inability to conjugate bilirubin, there is a rapid buildup of the unconjugated form in the blood, which eventually spills over into the brain and causes serious cerebral damage, previously referred to as kernicterus. Most of those affected die in infancy, but a few have survived into adult life. The second form of the disease is transmitted as an autosomal dominant. These patients have a less severe enzyme lack and so have some glucuronyl transferase in their liver cells and moderate levels of unconjugated hyperbilirubinemia. Jaundice results, but cerebral disease is uncommon, and most patients with this partial lack of transferase survive into adult life. Save for the enzyme defect leading to icteric staining of the liver, there are no other significant morphologic hepatic changes in either genetic pattern of the disease (Fleischner and Arias, 1970). As pointed out earlier, the inbred Gunn rat has a similar enzymatic deficiency (Callahan and Schmid, 1969).

Gilbert Syndrome. This disorder, characterized by unconjugated hyperbilirubinemia, is somewhat poorly defined. It embraces patients who have no apparent hereditary background for hepatic disease and others in which an autosomal dominant mode of transmission is suggested by the family pedigree. In the first category, levels of glucuronyl transferase are normal, and the hyperbilirubinemia is attributed to (1) compensated hemolysis, (2) excessive bilirubin production in the bone marrow, referred to earlier as "shunt bilirubin" or (3) some abnormality of bilirubin uptake into the hepatocytes. In the hereditary form of this syndrome, reduced levels of hepatic transferase have been identified, and it is obvious that such patients with an autosomal dominant genetic defect are very similar to, if not identical with, one of the types of the Crigler-Najjar syndrome (Black and Billing, 1969). The similarities among the various hereditary disorders of bilirubin metabolism make it clear that there is much yet to be learned about the precise metabolic and clinical limits of these diseases.

METABOLIC AND REGRESSIVE CHANGES

Included here are a variety of morphologic alterations in the liver encompassing atrophic changes, abnormal pigmentations, accumulations of metabolites and such abnormal proteins as amyloid.

Brown Atrophy. Brown atrophy of the liver is associated with an overall decrease in the size of the liver reflecting diffuse cellular atrophy. Grossly such a liver is deeper brown, shrunken and has a reduced weight. There is an accompanying deposition of granular yellow brown lipochrome pigment within liver cells. Differentiation of this pigment from hemosiderin requires the use of iron stains. Brown atrophy is seen in chronic wasting disease and old age. Commonly the heart and other organs are affected simultaneously. Almost invariably these alterations are of morphologic interest alone and rarely are associated with hepatic insufficiency.

Hemosiderosis. The liver normally contains small amounts of stored iron in the form of ferritin and trace amounts of hemosiderin. It is not possible with the light microscope to visualize the trace amounts of iron found in the normal. Excesses of iron in the body are almost immediately reflected by the deposit of increased amounts of hemosiderin in the liver. The various circumstances under which such excesses accumulate have already been discussed (p. 273). Suffice it here to recall that hemolytic disorders, multiple transfusions, excess dietary iron, and the systemic disease hemochromatosis are all productive of hemosiderosis of the liver. In hemochromatosis a diffuse fibrous scarring of the liver accompanies the iron deposits producing the entity pigment cirrhosis (p. 277).

Fatty Change. The appearance of visible fat in liver cells implies either significant injury to the liver or some systemic disorder leading either to impaired hepatic metabolism of fat or excessive mobilization of depot fat. Some of the more common systemic disorders associated with fatty change in the liver include: diabetes mellitus, tuberculosis, ulcerative colitis, kwashiorkor, excessive overeating, starvation and the broad category of hyperlipidemic states. Particularly important as a cause of fatty liver in the United States is chronic alcoholism (p. 1025), while in India and Asia, kwashiorkor is a major cause (Fig. 22–5). The metabolic and biochemical derangements and the morphologic changes characteristic of this hepatic lesion were discussed on p. 32 (Fig. 22–6). It is important to recall that the fat may be minimal in amount and grossly undetectable or may accumulate to massive levels, causing hepatomegaly up to 5 to 6 kilos in weight. Fatty change per se is reversible; but, as will be seen in the discussion of the cirrhosis associated with alcohol abuse, it may be followed by severe, irreversible scarring (cirrhosis) of the liver.

Glycogen Accumulation. Glycogen is normally found in the cytoplasm of liver cells in well nourished individuals. This is best seen in promptly fixed biopsy specimens where the glycogen imparts a reticulated appearance to the liver cell. Autopsy sections of liver rarely disclose this pattern since the glycogen is rapidly lysed soon after the patient dies. Excessive

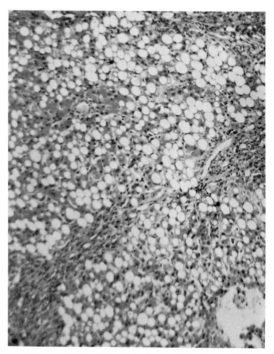

Figure 22–5. Kwashiorkor with fatty changes of the liver. The majority of the liver cells contain single large fat vacuoles.

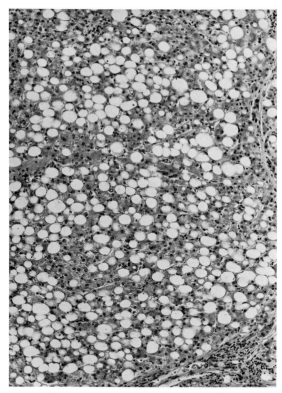

Figure 22–6. Fatty change in the liver.

glycogen accumulation is seen principally in diabetes mellitus (p. 259) and the glycogen storage diseases (p. 296). In diabetes the liver is not altered macroscopically, and the accumulation occurs principally in the hepatic cell nuclei with a lesser increase in the cytoplasm. In the glycogen storage disorders, the accumulation occurs both in the cytoplasm and the nucleus, and the accumulation may be sufficient to produce a pale, enlarged liver.

Except as an indicator of the underlying systemic disorder, the glycogen within the liver cell rarely disturbs its function, is reversible and is not associated with hepatic insufficiency.

Amyloidosis. Deposits of amyloid occur in the liver, principally in the pattern previously described as secondary (p. 281). In the other patterns, the hepatic deposits are usually scant and are restricted to the walls of blood vessels. In secondary amyloidosis, the liver may be markedly enlarged with a pale gray waxy appearance produced by the accumulation of the protein-carbohydrate complex that biochemically characterizes amyloid. For details on the microscopic appearance of this substance and its relationship to the ultra-structure of the liver, reference should be made to the earlier discussion (p. 282). It is important to recall that hepatic insufficiency is one of the mechanisms by which secondary amyloidosis causes death.

CIRCULATORY CHANGES

Circulatory changes merit description because they are so extremely common. These are found in virtually every autopsy because, whatever the underlying cause of death, some element of circulatory failure occurs in the agonal stages of life leading to hepatic alteration. It will be remembered that the liver cells are very sensitive to hypoxia, and therefore vascular stasis is an important cause of hepatocellular injury.

Anemia. In individuals dying of acute exsanguinating hemorrhage, the liver is characterized only by pallor produced by emptying of the sinusoids of their blood. Chronic anemia, however, is an important cause of fatty change in the liver cells. Occasionally, when the anemia is prolonged, particularly in the infant, extramedullary hematopoiesis appears in the liver. Anemia plays an additional important role in rendering the liver more vulnerable to other forms of injury.

Congestion of the Liver. When the right side of the heart fails, as it eventually must in any prolonged cardiac failure, blood backs up through the inferior vena cava and hepatic veins into the liver. The resulting picture is called *chronic passive congestion* (CPC). The nature of the resultant anatomic changes depends upon whether the congestion is of short or long duration. In acute congestion, the liver is swollen and engorged with blood. Much of this escapes when the liver is sectioned. The centers of the lobules stand out as dark, red-purple areas.

When the congestion is prolonged and chronic, the sinusoidal dilatation fans out irregularly toward the periphery and sometimes appears to fuse with dilated sinusoids in adjacent lobules to produce congestive bridges. These appear to the naked eye as red-purple trabeculae surrounded by pale liver substance. Because this picture resembles somewhat the pattern of a nutmeg cut in half, *such chronic passive congestion is spoken of as a "nutmeg liver"* (Fig. 22–7) (p. 322). These chronically congested livers may be slightly enlarged and be tense and tender. Microscopically, the sinusoids are markedly distended and packed with red cells, and there is frequently considerable pressure atrophy of the intervening liver cells (Fig. 22–8). When such congestion is produced by insufficiency of the tricuspid valve, pulsations may be felt in the liver.

Central Hemorrhagic Necrosis (CHN) of the Liver. *Severe chronic passive congestion often leads to rupture of the central portions of the sinusoids and necrosis of the adjacent liver cells designated as central hemorrhagic necrosis. It is very dif-*

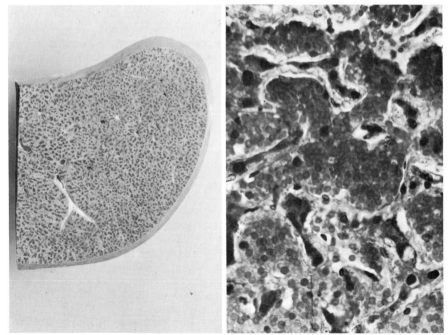

Fig. 22-7.

Fig. 22-8.

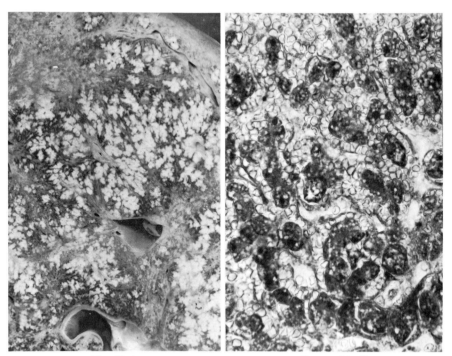

Fig. 22-9.

Figure. 22-10.

Figure 22-7. *Cross section of liver with chronic passive congestion. Congestive bridges give nutmeg pattern.*
Figure 22-8. *Chronic passive congestion. Sinusoids distended with red blood cells. Pressure atrophy of liver cells.*
Figure 22-9. *Cross section of liver. Late central hemorrhagic necrosis with regeneration. Note nutmeg pattern of congestion and pale fern-leaf pattern of regeneration.*
Figure 22-10. *Central hemorrhagic necrosis. Extravasation of red blood cells into subsinusoidal space around necrotic liver cells.*

ficult to differentiate this alteration on macroscopic examination from chronic passive congestion. Sometimes the cut surface of the liver shows slight central depression of the lobules. In late stages, a pale fern leaf pattern of regeneration is seen (Fig. 22–9). *Microscopically, the essential features are rupture of the sinusoids with sinusoidal hemorrhage and necrosis of liver cells.* Usually there is surprisingly scant inflammatory reaction accompanying such necrosis (Fig. 22–10). The necrosis is probably due in part to the increased sinusoidal pressure, but it is unquestionably contributed to by the hypoxia. CHN is seen most often in rapidly progressive cardiac failure, valvular insufficiency of the right side of the heart and obstruction to the venous outflow from the liver such as might be produced by constrictive pericarditis or excessive accumulations of fluid in the pericardial sac.

Cardiac Sclerosis of the Liver. Prolonged severe hepatic CPC or CHN eventually leads to scarring about the central veins of the liver lobules, known as cardiac sclerosis or cardiac cirrhosis.

Central hemorrhagic necrosis probably precedes its development. The necrotic liver cells are removed, but because of the continuing high intrasinusoidal pressure, the cells fail to regenerate and are replaced by fibrous scarring (Fig. 22–11). This scarring is usually quite delicate, fans out from the central veins in irregular strands into the surrounding liver substance but rarely produces interconnecting bridges. Only in the most advanced instances does true bridging of the fibrous trabeculae occur, meriting the term cardiac cirrhosis. Grossly, such livers are slightly shrunken and have a very fine granularity.

All these hepatic congestive changes, i.e., chronic passive congestion (CPC), central hemorrhagic necrosis (CHN) and cardiac sclerosis, reduce liver function to some extent. However, only rarely do they cause hepatic insufficiency because of the large functional reserve. However, when such livers are stressed by other demands, these congestive injuries may contribute to the development of hepatic insufficiency.

Infarct. Infarcts of the liver are very infrequent, probably because of the double blood supply already described. The most common cause of these lesions is polyarteritis nodosa. Embolization from some source within the portal circulation or from a bacterial vegetation on the heart is a rare cause. When infarction occurs, it usually implies an already reduced blood supply to the liver either because of portal vein obstruction or circulatory

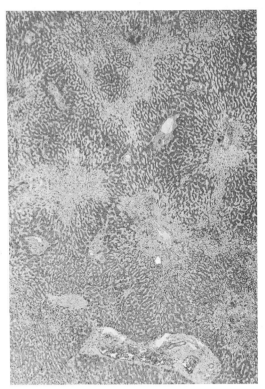

Figure 22–11. *Cardiac sclerosis of liver. Low power. Liver cells in centers of lobules have disappeared and are replaced by fibrous tissue.*

failure. The gross and microscopic picture is similar to that of anemic infarction elsewhere. When the portal branches are involved, the infarct tends to take the form of a small hemorrhagic area sometimes called *Zahn's infarct.*

Hepatic Vein Obstruction (Budd-Chiari Syndrome). Marked narrowing or obstruction of the hepatic vein outflow of the liver by thromboses or tumors produces a symptom complex known as the Budd-Chiari syndrome. Although the venous thrombosis may develop slowly and appear insidiously without apparent predisposing cause, more commonly this syndrome is caused by primary carcinomas of the liver, which grow into the hepatic vein, or by hypercoagulable states such as occur in polycythemia and the use of oral contraceptives. Whatever the cause, the obstruction of the hepatic venous effluent produces marked sinusoidal congestion and, when it occurs acutely, sudden painful enlargement of the liver and intractable severe ascites. In the more slowly developing occlusions, liver enlargement appears more insidiously and is generally less painful, but eventually ascites also develops. In these instances, in addition to having marked central congestion, the liver also exhibits thickening and sclerosis of the central veins, and sometimes atrophy of hepatocytes and delicate fibrosis in the central regions of the liver lobules. Jaundice may or may not be present in both the acute and chronic forms of the disorder. Collateral veins may appear on the lower abdomen when the hepatic vein thrombosis extends into the superior vena cava.

Portal Vein Obstruction. The portal vein may be markedly narrowed or obstructed either in its extrahepatic course or in its intrahepatic distribution. *Extrahepatic obstruction* is most often related to thrombosis, tumorous enlargement of the lymph nodes in the porta hepatis, or direct invasion of the portal vein by cancer possibly arising in the biliary tract or pancreas. In many instances, the portal vein thrombus is initiated by intra-abdominal surgery, which produces a small thrombotic occlusion in one of the tributaries of the portal vein, leading in time to propagation into the main venous channel. In some instances, the portal vein thrombosis is initiated by diffuse acute peritonitis or an abscess cavity lying within the peritoneal sac. If the thrombus itself becomes infected, the extension of the inflammatory thrombotic process into the portal vein creates *pylephlebitis. Intrahepatic obstruction* is most often caused by primary carcinoma of the liver and, less often, by metastases and strategically located liver abscesses. Cirrhosis of the liver induces portal hypertension and some increase in pressure within the radicles of the portal vein. However, these hemodynamic changes probably reflect enlargement of preexisting normal anastomoses between hepatic artery and portal vein and the formation of abnormal arteriovenous anastomoses within the microcirculation of the liver rather than true obstruction of the portal vein or its ramifications. Unlike hepatic vein obstruction, the liver is not acutely enlarged or tender in portal vein obstruction and, surprisingly, there may be little or no ascites and no jaundice. Congestive splenomegaly is, however, usual in any form of portal hypertension (p. 771).

Shock. The peripheral circulatory insufficiency of shock, when sufficiently prolonged and intense, produces hepatic changes. These vary from subtle centrilobular fatty change in liver cells to hypoxic necrosis. In most cases of shock, liver functional impairment is trivial, if present at all. The morphologic hepatic changes are reversible; regeneration replaces lost cells and, at a subsequent date, no residual evidence of damage is present (p. 351).

NECROSES AND INFLAMMATIONS

The liver, with its myriad enzymes and metabolic functions, is particularly vulnerable to all manner of toxic, metabolic and microbiologic attacks. The most important causes of liver necrosis are viral hepatitis and chemical and drug toxicity. The same agent may cause death of individual cells or small clusters of cells but, at higher dosage-intensity levels, destroy massive areas. Here our attention is directed to the unicellular or focal necroses; massive necrosis will be considered later.

FOCAL AND ZONAL NECROSES

Unicellular to small necroses may occur randomly without relationship to any particular region of the lobule and are referred to as focal; but at other times the necroses have a zonal distribution, i.e., centrilobular, midzonal or peripheral.

The ultimate cause of all liver cell necroses must be damage to enzyme systems within the hepatocyte. Why certain agents induce random lesions and others localize their effect to zonal regions is a mystery. In the case of centrilobular necrosis, it can be argued that this region of the lobule is most hypoxic and therefore most vulnerable to superimposed stress. However, we have no rationale for those occurring in the midzonal or peripheral regions.

It is impossible to present a comprehensive list of all of the causes of focal and zonal

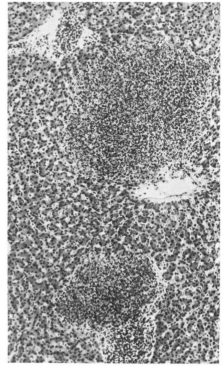

Figure 22–12. *Liver. Focal necrosis. Areas of necrosis with no definite relationship to lobular architecture.*

necroses in the liver because so many agents have been indicted. Many microbiologic agents and chemicals (including drugs) are hepatotoxic, some in all patients, and others only in some patients. Here we are concerned with those whose effect is dose-related and extends to all individuals exposed. These are so-called direct hepatotoxins. Later, in the consideration of drug-induced cholestasis, the inconstant indirect hepatotoxins are presented.

Focal random necroses are most characteristic of microbiologic infections with bacteremic or viremic involvement of the liver. Typhoid fever and viral infections, including viral hepatitis, may induce destruction of single cells or small clumps of cells without specific localization. In most instances, the regressive changes in the liver cells are nonspecific and, depending on the extent of the lesion, are accompanied by little or no inflammatory reaction. Occasionally, the site of cell death accu-

mulates neutrophils, macrophages and swollen Kupffer cells (Fig. 22–12). In the case of typhoid fever, often there is a predominant mononuclear infiltrate with striking hypertrophy of Kupffer cells in the lesions. Tuberculosis, sarcoidosis, syphilis, tularemia and brucellosis also produce focal liver lesions. In these instances, the pattern of histologic reaction to each specific etiologic agent provides a strong clue to the nature of the injurious agent, for example, noncaseating granulomas in sarcoidosis.

Centrilobular necrosis is most often the result of ischemia and is usually associated with cardiac failure and congestion. The hepatic changes were described as central hemorrhagic necrosis (p. 999). Centrilobular necrosis without significant congestion is typical of carbon tetrachloride and chloroform poisoning (Fig. 22–13). Often, as has been indicated earlier, the necrosis is preceded by fatty change

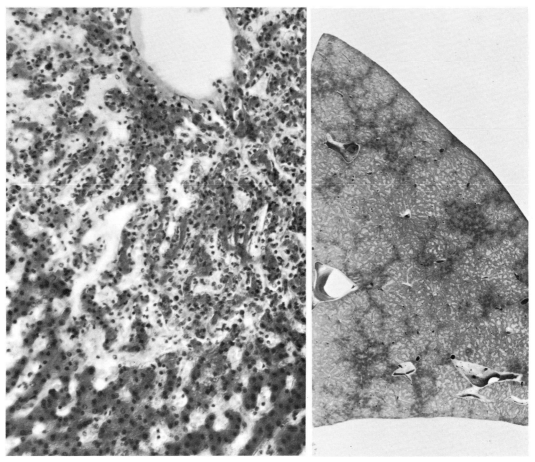

Fig. 22–13.   **Fig. 22–14.**

Figure 22–13.   *Central necrosis. Liver cells adjacent to central vein are necrotic and surrounded by polymorphonuclear infiltrate.*
Figure 22–14.   *Liver. Fatty change and central necrosis. Centers of lobules are pale and somewhat depressed.*

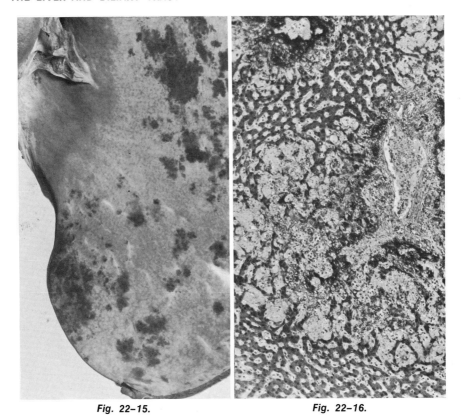

Fig. 22–15.   **Fig. 22–16.**

Figure 22–15. *Eclampsia. Numerous areas of subcapsular hemorrhage.*
Figure 22–16. *Eclampsia. Periportal areas of necrosis.*

(Fig. 22–14). The specific etiology of the lesion cannot be determined from the morphologic changes.

Midzonal necrosis is a distinctive feature of yellow fever. The hepatocytes undergo a peculiar coagulative necrosis, converting the dead cells into acidophilic, rounded masses known as "Councilman bodies." Often, infected liver cells develop nuclear inclusions.

Peripheral necrosis occurs in phosphorous poisoning and eclampsia. In the latter, the necrotic foci may also be hemorrhagic and sometimes have sinusoidal thromboses (Figs. 22–15 and 22–16).

DRUG-INDUCED INJURY AND CHOLESTASIS

Cholestasis implies obstruction, partial or total, of bile flow. While in theory the obstruction might be anywhere from the hepatocyte to the outflow into the duodenum, as generally used, the term cholestasis applies to obstructive processes at the level of liver cells and bile canaliculi. Here, our main concern is with those disorders resulting from the use of ther-

apeutic drugs, rather than the hepatic problems encountered in drug addicts. The latter are often complicated by the introduction of bacteria and contaminants into the blood (p. 529). Undesirable side-effects from therapeutic drugs have become a problem of significant proportions for contemporary man with his indiscriminate affection for pills. A great many of these drugs have been associated with cholestasis and, indeed, necroses within the liver. Many efforts have been made to classify the drugs into (1) those causing injury in most individuals *(direct hepatotoxins)*, (2) those causing injury in only occasional individuals *(indirect hepatotoxins)* and (3) those having little direct toxicity but which cause injury by hypersensitivity or idiosyncratic reactions *(hepatic allergens)*. Regrettably, the drugs do not always run true to form in every patient, and it is better to divide them into morphologic groups: (1) those causing only cholestasis, (2) those causing cholestasis and necrosis and (3) those causing principally necrosis. Obviously, the first category is least threatening and, while it may be associated with jaundice, it is usually mild. Recovery is prompt when the use of the inciting agent is discontinued. The last category is far more ominous and may, indeed, be sufficiently extreme to cause massive liver necrosis and death.

The *major drugs producing only cholestasis* include: anabolic steroids, methyltestosterone, chlorpromazine and some of the oral contraceptives. Only rarely do they cause death of liver cells. It should be pointed out here that occasionally pregnant women become jaundiced (called *benign jaundice of pregnancy*), presumably related to high levels of estrogens. The jaundice promptly clears after delivery. Similarly, contraceptive pills having a high content of estrogen, particularly the 17-alpha-alkyl-19-norsteroids, are often implicated in cholestasis (Schaffner, 1966). The mode of action of these cholestatic agents is poorly understood. One theory suggests that they interfere with hepatocytic mechanisms involved in the excretion of bilirubin and other organic anions (Popper and Schaffner, 1970). Morphologically, all that can be seen are bile pigment within swollen hepatocytes and Kupffer cells, as well as small bile plugs within canaliculi, particularly in the centers of the lobules (Fig. 22–17). Electron microscopy will almost always reveal blunting or disappearance of the microvilli of the hepatocyte. When exposure

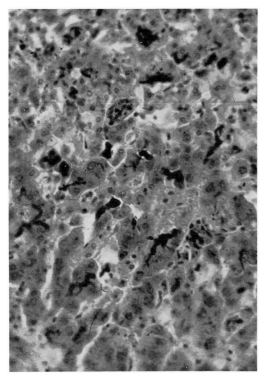

Figure 22–17. *Liver—bile stasis. Bile canaliculi distended with inspissated bile. Kupffer cells contain phagocytized bile.*

to the causative agent is stopped, the cholestasis and morphologic changes promptly disappear.

The drugs which cause both *cholestasis and variable amounts of necrosis* include: sulfonamides, some antibiotics (particularly tetracycline), thiouracil, cinchophen, tolbutamide, mercaptopurine and occasionally phenothiazine deriviatives such as chlorpromazine. There is a wide range of susceptibility to these agents and, in most instances, no untoward effects are encountered; but for mysterious reasons, some individuals become jaundiced because of cholestasis and focal necroses within the liver. It has been speculated, but without proof, that a specific idiosyncrasy or sensitivity lies behind the hepatic changes caused by many of these agents. The histologic findings are variable and include evidence of cholestasis (as described above) and focal swelling or coagulative necrosis of cells, accompanied by only a scant infiltrate of macrophages locally. The adjacent portal triads often have a lymphocytic infiltrate admixed with eosinophils where sensitivity is involved. Rarely, granulomas appear in the portal areas, further suggesting a hypersensitivity response. The changes induced by tetracycline are somewhat distinctive. This agent blocks RNA synthesis of protein; hence, lipoproteins cannot be synthesized, and fine droplets of fat accumulate within liver cells, accompanied by focal death of cells. The hepatic changes are rarely serious in all of these forms of liver injury and promptly remit when further drug therapy is stopped.

A third category of drugs is far more dangerous and may produce either *zonal or massive necrosis.* Included here are halothane, isoniazid, iproniazid, para-amino-salicylic acid, phenylbutazone, urethane and 6-mercaptopurine. Special attention should be given to the anesthetic agent halothane. A number of cases of focal to massive necrosis of the liver have been described following its use. In an analysis of 150 cases of fulminant hepatic necrosis, 80 patients had a form of viral hepatitis, and 35 patients developed the hepatic necrosis less than three weeks after halothane anesthesia (Trey et al., 1968). In three-fourths of these halothane cases, the liver injury only appeared after the second or third exposure to the anesthetic. Fulminant hepatic necrosis is the extreme, untoward effect of this agent. Many more patients have transient episodes of jaundice, which disappear in the course of a few days or weeks. There is a suspicion that the halothane-induced necrosis is more related to some sensitivity reaction than to direct toxicity. Recall that most patients only developed untoward reactions on second or third exposure. Lymphocyte transformation, presumed to be an indicator of immunologic stimulation, has been described in some of these patients with posthalothane hepatitis (Paronetto and Popper, 1970). Despite such evidence, some patients develop liver injury following a first exposure, and so both individual idiosyncrasy and sensitization may be operative. The morphologic changes encountered in these chemical and drug reactions extend from focal necroses (resembling the lesions described above) to confluent areas of necrosis and even massive destruction of the liver (massive hepatic necrosis).

The clinical manifestations associated with these undesirable effects of drugs vary with the severity of the morphologic change. Agents causing only cholestasis induce only a mild benign jaundice, which promptly remits as soon as the use of the drug is stopped. Elevations of alkaline phosphatase levels may be present, but there are no biochemical indications of liver cell death. Those drugs inducing necrosis of liver cells cause not only jaundice and elevated alkaline phosphatase levels but also elevated transaminase levels and other positive liver function tests. As will be seen later, when the necrosis becomes massive, as may occur with drug-induced injury, hepatic failure and death may result.

VIRAL HEPATITIS

The subject of viral hepatitis is one of the most exciting and rapidly unfolding areas in medicine. New observations are accumulating at an ever-faster pace; only a reasonable overview of this rapidly evolving subject can be given now, with the recognition that new information will inevitably require revision of present concepts. Although there is a substantial body of evidence that at least one virus or possibly two viral agents cause two somewhat distinctive forms of viral hepatitis, many problems persist (Prince et al., 1970). The exact nature of the relationship of the two forms of hepatitis, their causative agents and the meaning of a specific hepatitis-associated antigen (HAA) identified in the sera of many of these patients remain to be discovered. This much now seems clear: exposure to the viral agent(s) may occur with no resultant liver injury; the hepatic involvement may be subclinical and only detectable by biochemical tests of liver function; an acute, febrile, usually reversible, benign viral hepatitis may result; but in some individuals, a chronic liver disease or massive liver necrosis may develop. *The term viral hepa-*

titis is usually limited to the acute form of the disease, characterized by moderate liver injury and symptoms such as malaise, fever and jaundice, which generally clear over the span of weeks to a few months and rarely cause death. The other presentations will be considered later under the headings of "chronic hepatitis" and "massive necrosis of the liver." The two patterns of viral hepatitis are now referred to by a variety of names and, indeed, our concepts of their relationship to each other have undergone considerable change. It is desirable, therefore, to retrace the evolution of our understanding of viral hepatitis (Krugman and Giles, 1970).

In the classic historic view, *the two patterns of viral hepatitis were known as: (1) infectious hepatitis (IH) and (2) serum hepatitis (SH). Infectious hepatitis* was characterized as follows: it was orally acquired, had an incubation period of 15 to 50 days, tended to occur in children and young adults sporadically and occasionally in epidemics, was of acute onset and usually mild and, after an illness of six to eight weeks, cleared and left no residuals. In contrast, *serum hepatitis* was held to have the following features: it was parenterally transmitted, had an incubation period of 50 to 160 days, occurred sporadically at any age but more often in the elderly, often developed insidiously, but produced a severe illness which sometimes persisted for months (Havens, 1970). While most patients recovered, some developed protracted disease and eventually died of the late sequelae of chronic liver injury. While the mortality from classic infectious hepatitis was not more than a fraction of 1 per cent, up to 10 to 15 per cent of those with serum hepatitis died of their disease (Sherlock, 1972). Subsequent studies identified an agent, then called MS-1, in the pooled sera of hepatitis patients which, when given by the oral route, induced a short-incubation type of hepatitis (30 to 38 days) (Krugman et al., 1967). This same agent could also be extracted from the stools. A second agent, known as MS-2, was also isolated. It was most infective when administered parenterally but had a low infectivity by the oral route. The incubation period for MS-2 was between 41 and 108 days. The two agents were immunologically distinctive. It thus appeared that agent MS-1 caused infectious hepatitis and MS-2 produced serum hepatitis. At about this time, to provide uniform terminology, infectious hepatitis was designated "hepatitis A" and its causative agent, "virus A," and serum hepatitis was designated "hepatitis B" and its causative agent, "virus B."

Concomitantly, in the course of studies of population genetics using serum marker proteins to identify population cohorts, Blumberg et al. (1965) made the epochal observation that serum from two hemophiliac patients formed a precipitin line when tested against serum from an Australian aborigine. Further studies revealed that the aboriginal serum contained a protein-antigen, tentatively called "Australia antigen," which was cross reactive with antibodies in the hemophiliac sera. Thereafter, a spate of studies associated this antigen and its related antibodies to viral hepatitis which, presumably, the two hemophiliacs had contracted in the course of receiving numerous transfusions (Blumberg et al., 1967). Now the Australia antigen (Au) is generally referred to as the hepatitis-associated antigen (HAA), or sometimes as hepatitis B surface antigen (HBs) for reasons which will become clear. More about the interrelationship of these two forms of hepatitis will follow later, but first we should consider the nature of HAA and its relationship to the specific causative agents of the two forms of viral hepatitis.

Nature of HAA. It is now quite clear that HAA is a specific marker for hepatitis B. Apparent complete virions, having icosahedral symmetry and an inner core or nucleoid surrounded by a protein envelope, have been visualized in the serum and liver cells of patients with hepatitis B (Dane et al., 1970). These have an outer diameter of about 42 nm and are called Dane particles. In addition, small spherical particles approximately 20 nm in diameter as well as tubular particles have also been seen in these patients. These are thought to represent viral envelope protein without the RNA containing nucleoid. The tubular particles may comprise aggregates of the small spherical 20 nm particles. The core nucleoid is antigenically dissimilar from the small spherical particles and the tubular aggregates. The core antigen is referred to as HBc (hepatitis B core antigen), while the outer envelope, including the small spherical and tubular particles, is now referred to as HBs antigen (hepatitis B surface antigen). Thus, according to our present understanding, HAA in the serum comprises the small spherical or tubular particles (HBs antigen) made up of envelope proteins of the complete virus. In other words, the Australia antigen, the hepatitis B associated antigen (HAA) and the HBs antigen are different designations of the same envelope proteins but are not complete virions of virus B (Skikne and Talbot, 1974).

Types of Viral Hepatitis. The evidence is now near-incontrovertible that hepatitis B, so-called serum hepatitis, and hepatitis A, previously called infectious hepatitis, are separate and distinct entities. This view has long been championed by Prince (1968). The evidence is both clinical and immunologic. As pointed out earlier, hepatitis A has a much shorter incubation period than hepatitis B, tends to have an acute onset and in almost all cases follows a brief, benign course terminating within six to eight weeks in complete recovery (Blumberg, 1970a). In contrast, hepatitis B has a much longer incubation period, a more insidious onset and in a significant fraction of patients does not entirely clear but instead gives rise to chronic hepatitis and sometimes massive necrosis of the liver, both of which may be fatal. Immunologically the two diseases are distinct (Shulman, 1970; London et al., 1972). Recovery from hepatitis A does not confer immunity against hepatitis B and vice versa. Moreover, in the recent past a virus-like particle has been identified in the liver cells and in the stools of patients with hepatitis A. This particle has an inner core and an outer envelope, and is 27 nm in diameter. These particles specifically interact with the antibodies from patients with hepatitis A but not those from patients with hepatitis B (Dienstag et al., 1975).

Much of the confusion in the past about the separate identities of hepatitis A and hepatitis B was occasioned by our poor understanding of the mode of transmission of these two forms of the disease. The classic concept that serum, or long incubation, hepatitis B is acquired by parenteral inoculation and short incubation, infectious, hepatitis A is contracted by fecal-oral transmission is no longer tenable (Mosley, 1972). We now understand that hepatitis B virus can be found in the saliva, urine and semen, and in virtually almost every other body fluid. Thus, hepatitis B can be transmitted orally, by fecal-oral contamination and even by sexual intercourse. On this basis sporadic hepatitis occurring in a patient having no apparent parenteral exposure may well be hepatitis B. In contrast, hepatitis A, while usually transmitted by fecal-oral contamination, may also be transmitted parenterally. Fecal-oral pathways of transmission are particularly common in closed population groups such as summer camps, school dormitories and groups of individuals living together. It seems likely, therefore, that *the long-incubation HAA-positive disease can be spread by nonparenteral routes. It is now proposed that the classic serum hepatitis and sporadic infectious hepatitis may both be caused by virus B and so may be associated with HAA. In contrast, the virus A infectious hepatitis may largely be limited only to epidemic spread of the disease and, under these circumstances, yields an HAA-negative syndrome.* Admittedly, virus A may cause sporadic disease, but probably far less often than virus B. Evidence in support of this view is the inability to detect HAA in epidemic outbreaks of infectious hepatitis (Mosley et al., 1970). In essence, then, lack of a history of parenteral exposure may not be sufficient grounds for calling a case hepatitis A or infectious hepatitis. Classification as short-incubation or long-incubation disease is not satisfactory because of uncertainty as to when the individual acquired his infection. It seems preferable, therefore, at the present time and until further data clarify the issue, to consider the two patterns of viral hepatitis to represent, on the one hand, epidemic hepatitis, which we shall continue to refer to as hepatitis A and, on the other hand, serum and sporadic hepatitis, here referred to as hepatitis B.

Incidence. Hepatitis A, here equated with epidemic hepatitis, occurs in young individuals in closed population groups such as schools, institutions and military barracks. The outbreak of this form of the disease among many members of a football team in the United States exemplifies the spread and occurrence of epidemic hepatitis. However, because the agent can clearly be transmitted by fecal-oral contamination, isolated cases or sporadic patterns of spread may occur. Both sexes are affected equally. Most of the population is presumed to have been exposed and to have acquired a protective immunity by the age of 30, and so the disease is uncommon to rare in middle and later life.

Hepatitis B, here called sporadic and/or serum hepatitis, used to be considered principally a disease of middle to later life, a distribution reflecting the more common use of parenteral medications and blood transfusions in this older, more ailing population. Using HAA as a tracer, it is apparent that this pattern of disease is far more widespread. About 0.1 per cent of the general population of the United States and Northern Europe are HAA-positive; 1 to 4 per cent, in Japan and the Mediterranean countries; and up to 20 per cent in the tropics (Blumberg et al., 1970b). The great preponderance of these cases are asymptomatic carriers. High prevalence groups for HAA in all countries are patients with Down's syndrome, lymphocytic leukemia, those with chronic renal disease receiving renal dialysis and multiply transfused patients (Sutnick et al., 1972). The reasons for this high incidence in these groups are apparent, comprising closed populations, immunologic incompetence and repeated parenteral exposure. Another high incidence group comprises drug addicts, with their sharing of "needles," in whom it is found in about 4 per cent. As is well known, viral hepatitis is a major threat to life in these individuals (Sutnick et al., 1971). The contribution of drug abuse to the incidence of this disease can be appreciated from the following data derived from the California State Department of Public Health. The rate per 100,000 population for viral hepatitis in 1954 was approximately 21; in 1961, approximately 78; and in 1968, approximately 218 (Brewin, 1972). In a study of so-called serum hepatitis from 1967 through 1969, 90 per cent of the cases occurred in young adults, in contrast to past experience where 90 per cent of cases occurred in those over the age of 40 (Tartakow, 1971). So drug addiction has made hepatitis B, or serum hepatitis, a disease preponderantly of the young.

Recently, hepatitis virus has been identified in mollusks such as clams and oysters, gathered from polluted sea regions. They have been shown to concentrate the virus and, when ingested raw or partially cooked, transmit the disease (Dougherty and Altman, 1962). Obviously, the extent of the hazard is related to the level of fecal contamination of the local seawater. It has been calculated that habitual consumers of raw mollusks have approximately a 1 in 10,000 chance of contracting hepatitis; one wag admonishes that one should never consume more than 9999 of these delicacies.

Morphology. The morphologic changes encountered in hepatitis A and B are indistinguishable. They range from very subtle alterations in those with mild disease to extensive hepatic necrosis in those with the more severe expressions of this viral infection. During the incubation and prodromal period, liver biopsies reveal only slight, widespread hepatocellular swelling, along with some swelling and hyperplasia of Kupffer cells. A sparse lymphocytic infiltrate, admixed with a few macrophages, can be seen in the portal areas. Sometimes lymphocytes are unusually abundant in the sinusoids. Isolated liver cell necrosis with disappearance of the necrotic cells, sometimes called "cell dropout," may be present but is not prominent and is difficult to detect. At this stage of the disease, the liver would be of normal color and perhaps slightly swollen, hence increased in weight.

With the onset of symptoms, the classic features of viral hepatitis appear. Three major features are evident: (1) liver cell injury and necrosis, (2) evidence of regeneration of liver cells and (3) a reticuloendothelial reaction accompanied by portal infiltration of macrophages and lymphocytes (Popper, 1972). The liver cell reaction is usually diffuse and ranges from marked swelling of cells to frank necrosis. As the parenchymal cells swell, the cytoplasm appears watery and vacuolated, classically referred to as "ballooning degeneration" (Fig. 22–18). These changes are most evident in the centrilobular regions. Isolated liver cell dropout or small focal areas of necrosis now become more prominent, particularly in the centrilobular regions. Some of the necrotic cells literally disappear, leaving no trace, hence the name "dropout." Others undergo a peculiar coagulation and appear as round, anuclear, eosinophilic inclusions—"Councilman bodies." The acidophilic inclusion bodies have been resolved to contain shadowy remains of many cell organelles, confirming that they are derived from dead, shrunken hepatocytes (Klion and Schaffner, 1966). The combination of cellular swelling and liver cell necrosis disrupts the normal liver cords and produces a disarray of the lobule under low power examination (Fig. 22–19). Electron microscopy has disclosed virus-like particles in the cy-

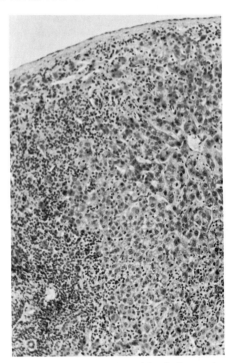

Figure 22–19. Viral hepatitis. Subcapsular area showing lobular disarray and periportal and intralobular inflammatory infiltration.

toplasm and intranuclear inclusions, though whether these represent the causative agent, HAA, or intracellular products secondary to the viral infection remains uncertain (Caramia et al., 1972) (Scotto and Caroli, 1972) (Yasuzumi et al., 1968). Intrahepatic cholestasis is seen in some cases in the form of small droplets of bile pigment in liver and Kupffer cells, along with inspissated bile within the canaliculi. For unknown reasons, some livers have no evidence of bile stasis.

Concurrent with the hepatocellular damage, evidence of regeneration may be found in the form of occasional mitotic figures and nests of crowded, helter-skelter cells, suggesting proliferative foci.

The reticuloendothelial reaction is quite prominent and takes the form of swelling and reduplication of Kupffer cells. Within the focal areas of liver cell necrosis, nests of lymphocytes and macrophages are present, the latter sometimes containing obvious cellular debris. Similar aggregations of cells are found in the portal triads, occasionally accompanied by a sparse infiltrate of eosinophils and, rarely, neutrophils. The eosinophilic component raises the issue of the possible emergence of an immunologic reaction to either the causative agent (conceivably HAA) or the necrotic products of destroyed hepatocytes.

At this stage of the disease, the liver is classically heavy, swollen and tense and, depending on the amount of bile stasis, more or less jaundiced.

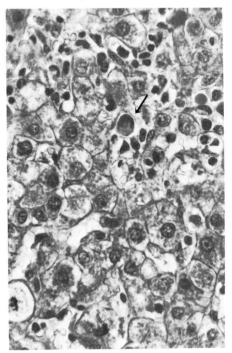

Figure 22–18. Viral hepatitis. Lobular disarray with swelling (ballooning) of liver cells and an isolated hyaline body (arrow).

Although the previous description pertains to the usual changes encountered in both forms of viral hepatitis, a great many variations on this theme are encountered. The hepatocellular necrosis may be more extensive and extend from one lobule to another, so-called bridging necrosis (Boyer and Klatskin, 1970). The hepatitis may be quite severe and may induce massive necrosis, as will be described in later sections of this chapter. In still other patients, the hepatitis may not resolve in the anticipated time and may become persistent or chronic. At the present time, it is believed that epidemic hepatitis does not contribute to this chronic pool and invariably resolves. On the other hand, hepatitis B, referred to as sporadic and serum hepatitis, carries a much greater risk of chronicity and sometimes leads to postnecrotic scarring of the liver and/or hepatic failure.

Clinical Course. Many of the clinical features of the two forms of viral hepatitis have already been cited. After the incubation period, which is short in hepatitis A and long in hepatitis B, malaise, fever, jaundice, elevated levels of SGOT, SGPT and LDH appear in both patterns of the disease. The hyperbilirubinemia is caused by both conjugated and unconjugated bilirubin. With these manifestations common to both forms, there are significant differences. The onset of hepatitis A tends to be more acute and is marked by nausea, vomiting, anorexia and frequently a distaste for cigarettes. In contrast, the onset of viral hepatitis B is more insidious, and there is a two to three-week period when the patient has a poorly defined illness, often described as flu-like or serum sickness-like. Many of these patients have arthritis involving the distal joints and an erythematous or urticarial rash, representing manifestations of allergy to some antigenic trigger, as yet poorly understood. Following this nonspecific prodrome with hepatitis B, the classic manifestations of hepatic involvement appear.

Epidemic hepatitis A usually runs a course of four to six weeks and is almost always followed by return of hepatic functions to normal, disappearance of the jaundice and steady improvement. In this pattern, fatalities are rare. In contrast, the course of hepatitis B is far more unpredictable. The illness is more prolonged, tends to be more severe and more often fails to completely clear. About 10 to 15 per cent of these patients suffer protracted or chronic illness, as will be described later. In these patients, progressive liver damage may ultimately lead to either hepatic failure or cirrhosis. In general, the prognosis with hepatitis B is related to the age of the patient and to his immunologic status. Younger, previously healthy individuals tend to have complete recovery, while the elderly and those unusually vulnerable by virtue of underlying debilitating illness or immunodeficiency have a much worse prognosis. In this long-incubation disease, the mortality can be as high as 1 in 8 in the predisposed, but, overall, is in the range of 2 to 4 per cent.

It should be pointed out that some patients are converted to carriers of HAA. Moreover, it is likely that many patients have subclinical disease, leaving only an HAA antigenemia as a residual. Obviously, carriers provide a hazardous reservoir of infection, particularly when they serve as donors for transfusions. It has been estimated that the risk of acquiring the disease from blood transfusions is as high as 20 per 1000 units of blood (Taswell et al., 1970).

CHRONIC HEPATITIS

Almost all patients who have had an acute attack of hepatitis A and approximately 80 per cent of those with hepatitis B recover completely from their acute viral hepatitis. But some, mostly those with hepatitis B, continue to exhibit persistently elevated SGOT or SGPT levels in their sera for years. This "biochemical lesion" has been called "transaminitis" or unresolved viral hepatitis. Some of these individuals are HAA-positive. Many of these patients with "transaminitis" and persistent HAA in their sera are predisposed to chronic viral infection by immunosuppressive therapy, lymphomatous disease, chronic renal failure or other debilitating chronic illnesses. Sherlock and her colleagues have, indeed, raised the possibility that chronic antigenemia reflects, in all patients, some impaired T-lymphocyte function (Giustino et al., 1972). Whether this mild disorder reflects incomplete eradication of the viral infection, the emergence of some postviral immunologic reaction or, instead, some other form of chronic hepatic involvement, conceivably an autoimmune reaction, has not been resolved. It is clear that HAA evokes antibodies. Conceivably, a persistent HAA antigenemia and the resultant immune complexes might bind complement in the liver cells and cause hepatocellular necrosis (Fox et al., 1971).

Another more serious pattern of chronic disease is represented by the group of patients who have overt clinical evidence of chronic hepatitis for months or even years. It is known that approximately 10 per cent of patients who develop viral hepatitis have clinically evident hepatic disease for months and years. About 25 per cent of these cases have persistent HAA in their sera (Fox et al., 1969a). Those who are

HAA-negative raise the same question of a secondary immune reaction as was mentioned above. This pattern of disease has been called variously *chronic hepatitis, protracted hepatitis and persistent hepatitis.* Ultimately, however, in most patients it is a reversible condition. Hepatic biopsies in such patients reveal a prominent portal mononuclear infiltration, varying degrees of fibrosis and focal hepatocellular necrosis. Some of these patients do not recover and eventually die of liver failure. In general, younger patients recover, but the elderly have a much higher mortality.

There are, however, less fortunate individuals who develop a progressively destructive form of chronic hepatitis, leading, in the great majority of cases, to either liver failure or massive scarring of the liver known as postnecrotic cirrhosis. This group has been segregated under the designation of *chronic active (aggressive) hepatitis* (discussed in the following section). So it becomes clear that viral infection of the liver, or possibly an immunologic reaction following such an infection, may pursue a myriad of courses ranging from a benign "biochemical disorder" to fatal massive necrosis. Intermediate between these extremes are the instances of protracted or persistent hepatitis, which usually eventually resolve, and the destructive, chronic active (aggressive) hepatitis which generally leads eventually to liver failure with or without cirrhosis.

CHRONIC ACTIVE (AGGRESSIVE) HEPATITIS

The term "chronic active or aggressive hepatitis" implies persistent, smoldering, progressive damage to the liver, punctuated sometimes by recurrent episodes of acute viral hepatitis. Most patients in the course of time suffer massive scarring of the liver, known as postnecrotic cirrhosis, and hepatic failure (Mistilus and Blackburn, 1970). It is highly likely that several etiologies are involved, which produce similar clinical changes and the same endpoint, i.e., an extensively damaged liver.

The etiology and pathogenesis of chronic active hepatitis is still poorly understood. As will be seen, there is evidence that in some patients it represents persistence or recurrence of viral infection. In others, it may be an immune reaction. The mere presence of immunologic findings does not, of course, exclude an initial injury (viral infection or a toxic chemical or drug reaction) as the trigger for the immunologic response. Autoimmunity has also been proposed. In still other patients, there are no clues, and the disease is sometimes called "cryptogenic chronic active hepatitis."

Whatever the presumed etiology, the morphologic changes are quite similar in all cases (Sherlock, 1972). In general, these can be categorized as acute liver cell necrosis admixed with evidence of liver cell regeneration and other areas of scarring. The acute cellular changes are remarkably similar to those of viral hepatitis (p. 1006). A chronic inflammatory infiltrate of lymphocytes and plasma cells in the portal areas, accompanied by focal but widely scattered areas of hepatocellular necrosis, comprise the most prominent findings. The foci of liver cell necrosis may be large enough to bridge adjacent liver lobules (Boyer and Klatskin, 1970). Generally, there is no fatty change in the liver cells. Usually, liver cell regeneration is scant but, sometimes, disorganized masses of cells, termed regenerative nodules, are seen. In most instances, scarring which is quite irregular in distribution eventually appears. Typically, the scarring is in the form of broad, varying-sized bands of fibrous tissue, which crisscross the entire liver, isolating islands of liver substance of markedly differing size. In some instances, many distorted lobules are found within such an island; in other instances, only a small nest of cells is isolated by the scar. Most typical of such scarring is its irregularity and the variable width of the bands of fibrous tissue, with consequent variation in the size of the isolated hepatic islands. In effect, the pattern is that found in postnecrotic cirrhosis.

Acknowledging that the causation of these disorders is uncertain, two clinical variants are sufficiently distinctive to merit individual consideration: (1) chronic active lupoid hepatitis and (2) chronic active viral hepatitis.

Chronic Active Lupoid Hepatitis. This entity is poorly named because of an earlier belief that it was a manifestation of systemic lupus erythematosus. In these early reports, much significance was attached to the positive LE cell tests found in such patients, as well as to other manifestations suggesting lupus erythematosus, such as arthralgia, hyperglobulinemia and fever (Bearn et al., 1956). Moreover, at first it was also thought that the disease occurred preponderantly in women. Since then, it has become apparent that both sexes and all ages may be affected, although most patients are women at the beginning and end of their reproductive lives. Few patients are HAA-positive and their disorders may not be correctly categorized as lupoid hepatitis. The sequence of events is now thought to be some form of injury to the liver, whatever its origin, followed by a host of immunologic reactions. Over three-fourths of these patients have antinuclear antibodies, positive LE tests and, mysteriously, antibodies against smooth muscle and mitochondria (Maclachlan et al., 1965) (Whittingham et al., 1966). Of interest in relation to the following discussion of chronic active *viral* hepatitis, preliminary data suggest that HAA and smooth muscle antibodies do not occur in the same patient (Vischer, 1970). Possibly, then, lupoid hepatitis is immunologically induced, and there is another form of chronic active hepatitis that is viral in origin. Other immunologic findings are: 50 per cent of the patients have a positive latex fixation test for rheumatoid arthritis; most have marked hyperglobulinemia, occasionally over 8 gm. per 100 ml. of serum; most have elevations of IgG and IgM; and some have increased levels of IgA (Feizi, 1968).

Recently, it has been found that 60 to 68 per cent of patients with active chronic hepatitis possess specific genetic histocompatibility genes (HL-A1 and HL-A8) in contrast to about 25 to 30 per cent of patients with other forms of liver disease, and 18 to 30 per cent of normal individuals. The known link in animals between the genetic control of immune responses and the major histocompatibility gene system raises the possibility that individuals with this disease are genetically predisposed to this immune disorder (MacKay and Morris, 1972). The evidence thus supports the proposition that lupoid hepatitis is, in some way, an immunologic disorder, perhaps triggered by an initial viral or toxic liver injury. Perhaps antibodies to HAA play a major role not only in eradicating the antigen but also in evoking the cellular damage. Of considerable interest is the fact that antibodies to liver antigens have not been identified.

Chronic Active Viral Hepatitis. This pattern of persistent liver disease is probably distinct from lupoid hepatitis discussed above. The discovery of HAA has made it possible to identify apparent protracted viral infection. In these patients, persistent antigenemia has been reported in 10 to 25 per cent (Simon, 1971) (Gitnick et al., 1969). Smooth muscle antibodies do not occur in this form of hepatitis, and surprisingly HAA antibodies are inconstantly demonstrated. Recrudescence of acute hepatitis is rare.

It must be emphasized that the mere demonstration of HAA in the blood does not necessarily prove a viral causation for this form of chronic active hepatitis, since there are carriers of this antigen who might well develop hepatic disease of unrelated causation. Indeed, most patients with this chronic disease are HAA-negative, there is *no* history of an antecedent acute attack and the manifestations appear insidiously. Males and females are affected with equal frequency (in contrast to the female preponderance in lupoid hepatitis), and these patients show few of the systemic symptoms such as involvement of the skin and joints, and the immunologic findings so typical of the lupoid form of the disease. Nonetheless, the belief persists that, in some way, the development of an immunologic reaction to damaged liver tissue perpetuates this apparent viral infection (Dudley et al., 1971). It must be cautioned that it may be exceedingly difficult to differentiate clinically between chronic active viral hepatitis and a primary cirrhosis from other causes such as chronic alcoholism, with persistence only of an HAA antigenemia.

Other forms of chronic active hepatitis have been described in addition to the two better-defined entities discussed above. These even more mysterious patterns are less clearly characterized and include: persistent hepatic disease related to drug ingestion, toxic exposure to chemical agents or spread of infections up the biliary tree to eventually involve the hepatic substance. In still other cases, when there are no hints as to the pathogenetic pathway, the disorder is termed "cryptogenic." Whatever the pathogenesis, it is clear that there exists a form of aggressive chronic inflammatory hepatic disease, fortunately uncommon, which pursues a relentless course to advanced scarring and liver failure in almost all patients.

MASSIVE HEPATIC NECROSIS

Necrosis of large areas, whole lobes or even the entire liver may be caused by fulminant viral infections, as well as by hepatotoxic chemicals and drugs. In years past, this form of necrosis was referred to as "acute yellow atrophy of the liver," a complete misnomer, since the liver is neither yellow nor atrophic but rather red and necrotic. The liver damage may slowly develop in the form of chronic active (aggressive) hepatitis, or it may take the form of an acute, overwhelming attack leading to death within 24 hours. The causative agent may be viral or hepatotoxic chemicals and drugs, i.e., those already mentioned in the causation of focal and zonal necroses (p. 1000) and drug-induced injury (p. 521 and p. 1003). Among these latter agents, some are particularly dangerous, including carbon tetrachloride, chloroform, cinchophen, mushroom poisoning, arsenicals, iproniazid, para-aminosalicylic acid, tetracyclines, gold compounds, phosphorus and halothane. As mentioned earlier, among 150 cases of fulminant hepatic failure, 80 patients were presumed to have a form of viral hepatitis, and an additional 35 patients, halothane toxicity (Trey et al., 1968).

The factors that determine the amount of necrosis that will be caused by the various etiologies are poorly understood. Alcohol abuse, malnutrition and systemic diseases known to injure the liver and produce fatty change may all be potentiating influences. Could, for example, prior malnutrition influence the severity of a viral infection? With some of the hepatotoxic chemicals, including drugs, there is a definite dose relationship, but with others, the amount of liver necrosis appears to be far more quixotic. Sensitization and idiosyncrasy have been postulated without proof. It is, however, known that most cases of halothane-induced massive necrosis occur on the second or third exposure to the anesthetic. The issue of sensitization to this agent was raised on p. 1003. Answers are not yet available to the many questions, and the knowledge must suffice that certain agents are potentially destructive to the liver and may, without warning, induce massive necrosis.

Morphology. The morphologic changes depend upon the length of survival of the patient. During the first days of massive necrosis, the liver is slightly enlarged, tense and dusky red, reflecting vascular congestion and edema. Patchy areas of hemorrhage may appear. Over the ensuing few days, the necrotic areas become yellow to red to green, depending upon the amount of fat, hemorrhage and bile leakage that appears. In the course of the next few weeks, the involved areas begin to collapse as the necrotic cells are removed. Thus, the necrotic area sinks below the surrounding uninvolved liver. An entire liver or a lobe may shrink to become a soft, flabby mass covered by a wrinkled, too large capsule (Fig. 22—20). Subtotal involvement may be referred to as submassive necrosis. Sometimes the liver weight is reduced to 600 gm. These livers are virtually mushy and can easily be folded back upon themselves without fracture. In two to three weeks, regeneration becomes apparent in the form of irregular, yellow-brown to green firm nodules that bulge above the surface. Sometimes these nodules are surrounded by still soft areas of necrosis. The pattern of regeneration is totally haphazard and reflects the areas of liver substance that were spared and thus remained capable of growth and mitotic division. Where all liver substance is destroyed, regeneration is impossible and these areas remain as bands of traversing fibrous tissue which create the pattern that will be described as postnecrotic scarring (p. 1031).

Histologically, the patterns of drug- or chemical-induced necrosis and fulminant viral hepatitis are similar. Presumably, the necrosis begins in the center of the lobules and then rapidly extends to destroy the entire lobule. In this fashion, large areas of liver substance are literally erased, leaving only islands of preserved portal triads separated by amorphous cellular debris (Fig. 22 -21). These portal areas converge on each other as the intervening substance collapses. Hemorrhages and bile pigment can sometimes be identified in these necrotic zones. During this early stage, there is very

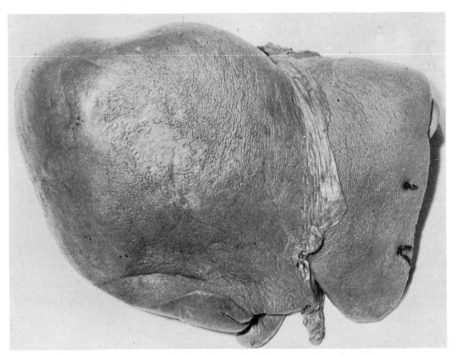

Figure 22–20. Massive necrosis. Liver is small (700 gm.), pale and soft in consistency.

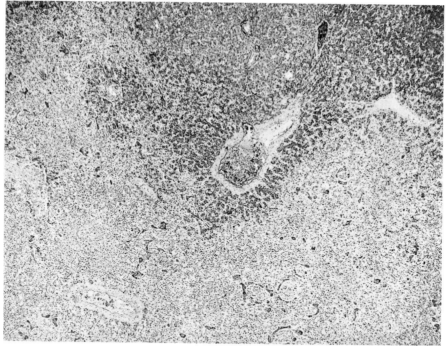

Figure 22–21. *Massive necrosis. In lower portion of field, complete necrosis is apparent with removal of all liver cells in many adjacent liver lobules.*

little inflammatory reaction in the liver substance. Marginal cells in spared areas may show the histologic details described under viral hepatitis.

In the course of the first week, the mononuclear inflammatory infiltrate previously described in viral hepatitis appears in the portal regions. There may be surprisingly few neutrophils in this leukocytic infiltrate. By this time, much of the necrotic debris has undergone proteolysis and has been removed, and the bands of collapsed reticular framework and beginning fibrosis become evident. Often, the Kupffer cells attached to the reticular framework are preserved. Fatty change and regenerative activity can be identified in the cells in the margins of the necrotic areas, presumably because they were spared the full brunt of the attack. There is congestion of the sinusoids imparting the red color seen in the gross. Inconspicuous bile duct reduplication may also be present. Over the next weeks, if the patient survives, the proliferative activity in the spared areas produces the regenerative nodules described, and the areas of necrosis are progressively replaced by the ingrowth of fibroblasts to produce the massive scarring characteristic of postnecrotic cirrhosis (Lucke, 1944).

It must be remembered from animal experimentation and clinical observation that large areas of the liver may be destroyed without causing death. Thus, livers with only a small fraction of preserved substance are capable of extraordinary regeneration. However, when an entire lobule is destroyed and the framework collapses, the regeneration cannot reconstitute the lobule and so normal liver function is not restored in these areas. Haphazard masses of regenerative cells do not have normal orientation to sinusoids and canaliculi, and hence such foci often have intense bile stasis and appear deep green.

Changes in other organs are found in fatal massive hepatic necrosis. There is often fatty change in the renal tubular epithelium as well as bile pigmentation of the collecting tubules (cholemic nephrosis). Acute splenitis and degenerative changes in the ganglion cells of the central nervous system also sometimes occur. A hemorrhagic diathesis may be encountered, presumably due to depletion of both prothrombin and fibrinogen.

Clinical Course. The course of fulminant hepatic necrosis is obviously extremely variable and depends on the amount of liver substance destroyed. Some patients collapse and die within 24 hours, before manifestations of liver failure can appear. In others, hepatic failure appears within days, and death follows soon thereafter. In still others with less extensive damage, the course of the disease may be more prolonged. In these individuals, the major manifestations include: malaise, fever and jaundice, leading eventually to the other features of hepatic failure discussed earlier (p. 991). In general, the issue is decided within the first two weeks, because if the patient can be kept alive this long, regeneration can be expected to bring about improvement. Obviously, all of the liver functions are deranged, and hypoprothrombinemia, with its hemorrhagic diathesis, constitutes a serious problem. As might be expected, elevated serum levels of GOT, GPT and LDH are always present, but it should be noted that they do not necessarily parallel the severity of the liver damage.

While once a rare disease of middle to later life, fulminant viral necrosis of the liver is now seen with greatly increased frequency in many younger patients because of the large pool of drug-associated hepatitis B. In municipal general hospitals across the United States, about 90 per cent of patients are under 30 years of age, and the number of deaths from this disease has increased two- to threefold over the past 10 years (p. 1006). Possibly, massive hepatic necrosis is fulminating in drug addicts because of associated malnutrition or intercurrent infections. Younger patients (first three decades of life) enjoy a better prognosis than the elderly, perhaps because of limitations of hepatic regeneration in advanced life. Nonetheless, because of the epidemic nature of this disease among drug addicts, 60 to 70 per cent of all deaths occur in the group of patients under 30 in contrast to former years when 60 to 70 per cent of the fatalities occurred in those over 30 years of age. There is no effective treatment for this disorder other than supportive, but exchange transfusions have been beneficial in some patients even though we do not really understand why (Berger et al., 1966).

NEONATAL (GIANT CELL) HEPATITIS

Neonatal hepatitis is not merely hepatitis occurring in the newborn and infant. It is specifically characterized by the transformation of liver cells into large multinucleate syncytium-like cells. While a number of known etiologies (mentioned later) may all induce these hepatocellular alterations, in the majority of instances, no specific causation can be identified, and it is to this idiopathic disorder that our attention is presently directed.

Macroscopically, the liver is usually enlarged, sometimes slightly granular and intensely bile stained. The extrahepatic biliary ducts as well as the major intrahepatic ducts are patent. Histologically, the normal liver cells are replaced throughout by large giant cells having an abundant, often swollen cytoplasm with many small nuclei, sometimes up to 100. These cells resemble, to a considerable degree, foreign body type giant cells. Some normal liver cells may be interspersed but, in the

well advanced case, the giant liver cells occupy the entire lobule from central vein to portal area (Fig. 22–22). The normal lobular architecture is obliterated by the disarray of these cells. Bile stasis is prominent, and bile can be seen within the cytoplasm of these altered hepatic cells. The bile canaliculi are lost in the lobular disarray, but the small bile ducts in the portal region are usually unaffected and do not contain inspissated bile. This detail helps to differentiate these livers from extrahepatic obstruction of the bile ducts. Usually, the central veins and portal areas are unaffected, save for a periportal mononuclear exudation. It is obvious that this pattern differs from the usual viral hepatitis.

The relationship of this form of obscure liver disease in infants to viral hepatitis remains obscure. Placental transmission of HAA does not usually occur; but conceivably, in rare instances, the *virus* may be passed from mother to infant at the time of delivery (Schweitzer and Spears, 1970). However, there is a considerable amount of evidence that hepatitis virus is not responsible for this neonatal disease. Infants in general and even infants born of mothers with viral hepatitis rarely develop intrauterine or postnatal infections, presum-

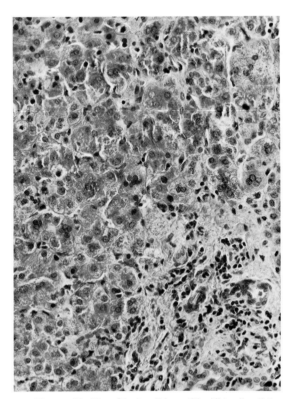

Figure 22–22. *Giant cell hepatitis. Virtually all the parenchyma is replaced by enlarged, often multinucleate cells with total disarray of the architecture.*

ably due to some placental transfer of gamma globulins from the mother (Mansell, 1955). When viral hepatitis occurs in older infants after the third month of life, the histologic changes are indistinguishable from those of the adult disease and are not associated with the formation of the large multinucleate giant cells. The morphologic changes, then, in neonatal hepatitis differ significantly from those of infantile viral hepatitis.

Craig and Landing (1952) have commented on the similarity of the histologic changes in giant cell hepatitis to those in biliary atresia. Smetana (1963) concurs by pointing out that biliary stasis in the infant will itself induce the formation of giant cells in the liver. He further points out that, in the livers with neonatal hepatitis, bile canaliculi cannot be demonstrated, implying that their loss or destruction represents a reasonable basis for the biliary stasis.

Much of the confusion about the nature and etiology of giant cell hepatitis stems from the fact that, in the newborn, the liver reacts to a variety of injuries by the formation of giant cells. Thus, giant cell transformation is encountered in hemolytic disease of the newborn, excessive iron overload, cytomegalic inclusion disease, congenital syphilis and other conditions. In these disorders, only some of the hepatocytes are transformed to giant cells. The presence of occasional giant cells scattered among otherwise usual liver cells does not constitute giant cell hepatitis.

The clinical course is one of prolonged persistent jaundice, sometimes intermittent, rarely progressive, leading to cirrhosis of the liver. The jaundice may appear to be obstructive with acholic stools, bile in the urine and depressed levels of urinary urobilinogen. Some patients recover. The differentiation of this disorder from extrahepatic biliary tract obstruction is difficult and sometimes requires surgical exploration to rule out congenital atresia or other extrahepatic obstructive disease.

OTHER INFLAMMATIONS OF THE LIVER

Cholangitis is a term that should be restricted to those inflammations of the liver characterized by bacterial purulent infection in the intrahepatic bile ducts. Grossly, pus can be expressed from the bile ducts and, histologically, they contain numerous polymorphonuclear leukocytes (Fig. 22–23). Almost invariably, there is an accompanying inflammatory infiltrate in the surrounding portal fibrous tissue. Cholangitis is only rarely seen in the ab-

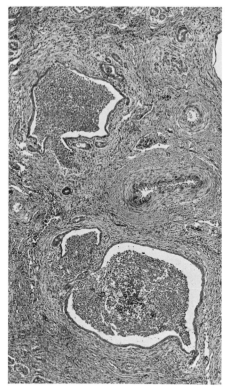

Figure 22–23. *Acute cholangitis. Bile ducts dilated and filled with exudate. Fibrosis of surrounding tissue.*

sence of either extra- or intrahepatic obstruction of the major ducts and so is encountered as a complication of obstruction of the common duct by gallstones, carcinomas of the head of the pancreas, papilla of Vater or bile ducts and occasionally in malformations of the extrahepatic ducts. Usually, cholangitis is accompanied by a similar inflammatory process in the gallbladder.

The method by which the infection reaches the intrahepatic bile ducts is not completely understood. It is most commonly postulated that the ascending infection traverses the peribiliary tract lymphatics, although bloodborne and direct intraductal spread has not been ruled out.

Clinically, cholangitis causes a large tender liver and a septic febrile course. Frequently, mild degrees of jaundice are present. The signs and symptoms are often confused with those of acute cholecystitis. Severe cholangitis may lead to the formation of abscesses in the liver.

Liver abscesses result whenever pyogenic bacteria seed the liver in sufficient numbers to create a focus of suppuration. Such seeding may reach the liver through the bile ducts, portal vein, hepatic artery and lymphatics and by direct spread of contiguous infections. As previously mentioned, when cholangitis destroys the wall of the bile ducts, the spread of the infection to the adjacent liver parenchyma produces a liver abscess. These are referred to as *cholangitic abscesses.* The most common causative agent is *E. coli,* but any of the enterobacteria may also be involved.

Suppuration within the abdominal cavity may give rise to a pylephlebitis that may seed the liver *(pylephlebitic abscesses)* (Bakst and Jeghers, 1937). Usually in these cases, suppurative thrombi in the intrahepatic radicles of the portal vein can be demonstrated (Fig. 22–24).

Septic emboli or bacteria may seed the liver through the branches of the hepatic artery in bacterial endocarditis or other bacteremias. In this mode of spread, the abscesses are usually small and widely distributed *(hematogenous abscesses).* It is also believed but less well documented that organisms may reach the liver through the lymphatics by direct spread from infections in the peritoneal cavity.

Much less commonly, perforations of the gastrointestinal tract or other intraperitoneal infections give rise to either *subdiaphragmatic or subhepatic abscesses* which burrow into the liver. These often produce obscure and confusing clinical pictures that can only be resolved by a high index of suspicion.

Tuberculosis of the liver almost always takes the form of miliary seeding and is therefore accompanied by the manifestations of miliary tuberculosis throughout the body. Occasionally, the tubercle bacilli can be seen within the Kupffer cells (Fig. 22–25). Eventually, characteristic tuberculous miliary granulomas are produced. Needle biopsy of the liver provides, at times, one of the better diagnostic methods of establishing the diagnosis of miliary tuberculosis.

Disseminated systemic sarcoidosis may involve the liver, providing sometimes a site from which diagnostic tissue can be obtained in difficult diagnostic problems.

Syphilis of the liver takes one of two forms, an interstitial hepatitis or multiple gummas. The interstitial form is seen usually in congenital syphilis, while the gummas represent a tertiary manifestation of the disease. In the course of the fibrous healing of the gummas, large scars result that create a form of cirrhosis known as hepar lobatum (p. 1036).

Weil's disease prominently affects the liver. These patients are characteristically jaundiced during the height of their leptospirosis, owing to a diffuse interstitial hepatic inflammatory process. Histologically, there is swelling and prominence of Kupffer cells, swelling of the liver cells, some unicellular necrosis and widespread mitotic, proliferative and regenerative activity. Sometimes with very industrious

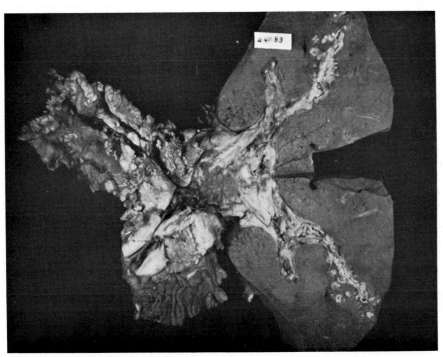

Figure 22–24. *Liver with portal vein. Pylephlebitic abscesses with suppurative phlebitis of branches of the portal vein, found as complication of acute appendicitis.*

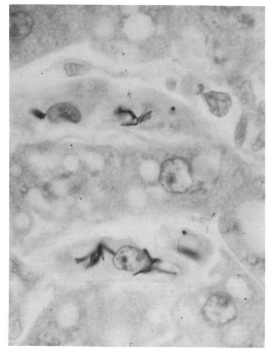

Figure 22–25. *Tuberculosis of liver. Tubercle bacilli in Kupffer cells in early miliary tuberculosis.*

search, spirochetes can be found in the interstitial tissue and sinusoids. As previously described in the consideration of Weil's disease, changes are also commonly present in other organs in these patients (p. 388).

Amebic hepatic abscesses are one of the feared complications of amebic dysentery. The parasites presumably reach the liver through the portal vein. The abscess characteristically contains a brown paste exudate rather than pus, but the diagnosis depends upon the histologic identification of the parasites in the wall of the abscess (p. 450). From the liver, these abscesses may burrow through the subdiaphragmatic space to enter the lungs and occasionally may embolize from there to the brain.

Actinomycotic infections may also be carried by the portal blood to the liver and give rise to multiple suppurative abscesses. These have quite a characteristic gross appearance in that the center of the abscess does not break down completely but is somewhat sponge-like, with purulent material in the interstices of the framework. Microscopically, the colonies of the fungus with their characteristic radical mycelia can be demonstrated (p. 442). Sometimes these colonies produce the so-called "sulfur granules" distinctive of actinomycosis.

Echinococcus cysts are extremely common in the liver in the regions of the world where this parasite is endemic (p. 464). When severely involved, the liver may contain one to many cysts virtually replacing whole lobes. These large cysts are referred to as mother cysts. They contain bile-stained fluid in which can be found multiple, small, thin-walled daughter cysts (Fig. 22–26). Histologic examination of the mother cyst discloses its wall to be composed of

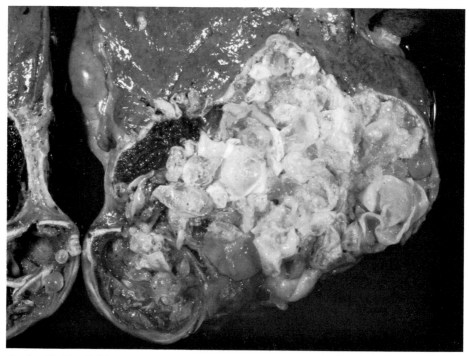

Figure 22–26. *Echinococcus cyst of liver. Mother cyst containing numerous daughter cysts.*

laminated layers of chitinous material, and prolonged and careful search may reveal the scolices or hooklets of the echinococcus.

Liver flukes are common infections of the biliary tree in the Orient. *Fasciola hepatica*, by selective predilection, localizes in the lumina of the larger bile ducts where it may cause obstruction. The parasite is readily identified on histologic examination and is surounded by a prominent inflammatory reaction. This hepatic infection is believed to be related to the increase in frequency of bile duct carcinoma in these regions (p. 466).

POSTMORTEM CHANGES

When the peritoneal cavity is opened during a postmortem examination, it is fairly common to find those portions of the liver which are in contact with the large bowel to be black-brown in color. This change is most frequently found when the lower edge of the right lobe is in contact with the hepatic flexure of the colon. Incision of such a discolored area shows the change to be quite superficial, extending only 1 or 2 mm. into the liver substance. This is a postmortem change, the result of substances passing from the bowel to the liver and depositing sulfides in the adjacent liver tissue. Often when there is an increased deposit of iron salts in the liver, as in systemic hemosiderosis or hemochromatosis, this black discoloration is accentuated.

Postmortem Autolysis. Postmortem autolysis of the liver usually starts about 24 hours after death. The consistency of the liver becomes considerably softer. Softening of the liver may also occur as an antemortem change as the result of toxic damage. It is important to differentiate between the ante- and postmortem causes of this change. This can be done by histologic examination of the liver. Microscopically, in autolysis the changes are similar to autolysis in other tissues, and are devoid of inflammatory response.

Gas Bacillus Infection. Agonally, *Clostridium welchii* may be carried by the portal vein from the gastrointestinal tract into the liver. After death, particularly if high fever existed prior to death and the body is not promptly refrigerated, these organisms proliferate, form gas and produce many gas blebs throughout the liver substance. When this is extreme, the liver substance is, to a large extent, replaced by these bubbles. The name *foamy liver* is sometimes applied to this change. Histologically, examination of such a bleb will show masses of large gram-positive bacilli in the center of the bleb and compression of the surrounding liver cells as a result of the pressure of the gas produced by the bacilli. No inflammatory response is found to this bacterial invasion.

TUMORS

Tumorous involvement of the liver ranks as one of its commonest disorders. The great preponderance of these tumors are metastatic, particularly from cancers arising in the abdomen. But the liver is also seeded by cancers arising outside the abdominal cavity, for example, carcinoma of the breast or lung and melanocarcinoma of the skin. Hepatic metastases are found in over half of all postmortems on patients whose death was caused by neoplasia.

Primary tumors in the liver are much less common, the most important being the carcinomas. These may have origin in the hepatic parenchymal cell (hepatocarcinoma) or the bile duct epithelium (cholangiocarcinoma), while some are mixed. Benign tumors are not only infrequent but are also usually small and of no clinical significance save for their differentiation from cancers.

BENIGN

The histogenesis of benign tumors reflects all the cell types found in the liver and, therefore, runs the gamut from hepatic cell adenomas and bile duct adenomas to the variety of mesenchymal tumors that include hemangiomas, fibromas, leiomyomas (presumably from blood vessel walls) and the like. The most common pattern is the hemangioma, followed in order by the adenomas (Henson et al., 1956) (Henson, 1956).

Cavernous hemangiomas are the most common type of benign tumor in the liver, but they are still infrequent incidental findings at autopsy. There is some question as to whether they should be considered neoplasms or hamartomatous malformations. They are generally 1 to 3 cm. nodules embedded in liver substance, red, blue or gray, depending on the amount of sclerosis. Histologically, they are composed of large, vascular, endothelium-lined spaces filled with red cells. Some become sclerosed and are replaced by fibrous tissue. They are almost invariably of no clinical importance. In one rare pattern known as *peliosis hepatis*, diffuse angiomatoid lesions are found throughout the liver.

Two types of *benign adenoma* occur in the liver: the bile duct adenoma and the liver cell adenoma. Bile duct adenomas are usually small, spherical, encapsulated, yellow-white nodules rarely over a few centimeters in diameter. Histologically, they are composed of multiple small acini lined by epithelium similar to that present in the small bile ducts. These epithelial channels are surrounded by a variable amount of fibrous tissue stroma. Liver cell adenomas, on the other hand, may not be so easily recognized grossly. Some tend to be larger, less sharply demarcated from the surrounding liver tissue and of usual liver color. Others are green and easily spotted. Histologically, they are composed of well differentiated liver cells forming cords and sinusoids. They are not, however, broken up into normal lobules. In those that have not made connection with the biliary system, bile stasis is present, and these are readily recognized by their green pigmentation.

Regenerative nodules are mentioned here because there may be considerable difficulty in distinguishing them from a liver cell adenoma. Well known is the liver's remarkable capacity to regenerate following injury. Such regeneration presumably occurs from preserved hepatic cells, but there is some controversy regarding the possibility that the bile duct epithelium at the level of the preductules may have the capacity to differentiate into liver cells. Whatever the histogenetic origin of these regenerative cells, they are capable of reconstituting the liver lobule to an almost perfect degree, when the necrosis has not been too massive, the underlying reticular framework has not been destroyed, and when at least some of the cells within the lobule are still vital. According to our present concepts, when the total lobule and its framework are destroyed in the human it cannot be reconstituted. However, adjacent liver cells may proliferate to produce nodules of hepatic cells that obviously do not have the normal canalicular-sinusoidal relationships. These cells may function in many of the metabolic activities of the liver but cannot function normally in secretion and excretion of bile. Hence these nodules are bile-stained if the cells are sufficiently differentiated to elaborate this product. Such a regenerative nodule may be quite difficult to distinguish from a liver cell adenoma.

Hamartomas are solitary, usually small, masses occurring in the liver, occupying an intermediate biologic position between true benign neoplasms and regenerative nodules. For uncertain reasons, they often occur on the liver surface and project as hemispheric masses sometimes up to 5 to 7 cm. in diameter. Discrete and encapsulated, they may have the same appearance as the surrounding hepatic substance, may be slightly darker in hue, or may appear trabeculated by traversing fibrous bands. As with all hamartomas, they are composed of mature cell types indigenous to the liver, principally fibrous tissue, blood vessels and usually well organized bile ducts. These masses rarely contain well differentiated hepatocytes. It is probable that they arise in hepatogenesis and, on this account, are sometimes encountered in infants and children (Stephens and Jenevein, 1965).

PRIMARY CARCINOMA

Primary malignant hepatic tumors are practically always epithelial in origin and are known as primary carcinomas of the liver. Sarcomas having origin in blood vessels or the fibrous stroma are rarities. The epithelial cancers can be divided histologically into three types: (1) the primary liver cell carcinoma or *hepatocarcinoma*, (2) the primary bile duct carcinoma, or *cholangiocarcinoma* and (3) the mixed pattern, the *hepatocholangiocarcinoma*. The hepatocarcinoma comprises approximately 80 per cent of these three. By long, but regrettable, precedent, the hepatocarcinoma and the cholangiocarcinoma have been known as hepatoma and cholangioma, terms that unfortunately carry a benign implication.

The hepatocarcinoma is a particularly interesting form of cancer on three counts: (1) the many influences now thought to be implicated in its causation, (2) its association with cirrhosis of the liver and (3) the incredible number of paraneoplastic syndromes and unusual products produced by these neoplasms. These issues are dealt with in the discussion which follows.

Pathogenesis. Among the influences thought to contribute to the development of hepatocarcinoma, the most important are: (1) hepatocarcinogens in food, (2) cirrhosis of the liver, (3) persistent viral infection and (4) parasitic infections of the liver. Other less important influences would include: ionizing radiation, particularly that derived from compounds such as thorotrast, used in past years for radiographic visualization of the biliary tract; and possible food additives, such as "butter yellow" (N-methyl-4-aminoazobenzene), known to be capable of inducing hepatic cancers in laboratory animals.

Several naturally occurring potent hepatocarcinogens for animals have been identified. All exist in nature in possible foodstuffs for man and so may have relevance to the production of hepatocarcinoma in man. Aflatoxin B_1, mycotoxin of the fungus *Aspergillus flavus*, is a well documented carcinogen in rats, fowl and fish. Microgram amounts will induce cancer in these animals. The Aspergillus grows readily on improperly stored corn, grains and ground nuts (peanuts). Could the growth of this mold be relevant to the extraordinary incidence of primary carcinoma of the liver in African native populations consuming large amounts of inadequately stored moldy corn and ground nuts? Epidemiologic studies have shown a correlation between the incidence of hepatocarcinoma in specific locales and the apparent content of aflatoxin in the diet (Alpert and Davidson, 1969) (Alpert et al., 1968). Cycasin, found in cycad nuts, is another naturally occurring carcinogen which may have neoplastic potential. A variety of plants in Africa, South America and Asia have been found to produce alkaloids which may be carcinogenic for man (Schoental, 1968). The question is obvious: could diet account for the remarkable differences in the incidence of hepatocarcinoma around the world?

Eighty per cent of hepatocarcinomas and 30 per cent of cholangiocarcinomas develop in already cirrhotic livers. Certain types of cirrhosis have a higher level of association than others. Thus, in the series reported by MacDonald (1957), primary hepatic cancer was found in 13.1 per cent of the cases that would now be called postnecrotic scarring (healed acute yellow atrophy), 7.7 per cent of the pigment cirrhoses, 2.4 per cent of the cirrhoses associated with alcohol abuse and 2.1 per cent of the biliary cirrhoses. It should be pointed out that there is some disagreement over the frequency of liver cancer in the cirrhosis of alcohol abuse, and many investigators would disagree with a rate of 2.4 per cent, contending that it is a rarity. While, then, the precise percentages vary among clinics, there is good agreement that postnecrotic scarring is the most common subsoil for primary hepatic cancers (Gall, 1960*b*). In the United States, about 5 per cent of all patients with cirrhosis may be expected to develop a primary carcinoma. In Africa, in contrast, over half of all males with cirrhosis of the liver develop carcinoma, and carcinoma of the liver represents 50 per cent of all cancers encountered in men and 20 per cent of those in women. The occurrence of cancer in cirrhotic livers could be simplistically interpreted as an extension of active regeneration beyond the bounds of control into neoplasia. The variability in cell size and morphology seen in regenerative nodules is reminiscent of the anaplasia of tumor cells, making such an explanation seductive, but still unestablished.

Of recent date, a significant proportion of patients with hepatocarcinomas in high incidence regions of the world have been shown to have HAA antigenemia. In Greece and Uganda, 30 to 40 per cent and, in Taiwan, 80 per cent of patients with this form of neoplasm are HAA-positive (Vogel et al., 1970). In these same locales, a high percentage (3 to 15 per cent) of the general population is HAA-positive, but this frequency does not begin to approximate that found in the liver cancer subset. In Great Britain, 10 of 46 patients with liver cell cancer were HAA-positive (Sherlock, 1972). In contrast, in the United States, where liver cell carcinoma is not common and where less than 1 per cent of the general population has HAA, little or no correlation has been reported between the hepatitis antigen and hepatocarcinoma (Moertel et al., 1970). Perhaps the correlation between HAA and liver cancer stems from the development of postnecrotic scarring as a consequence of a severe or persistent viral infection of the liver. However, the geographic differences suggest that other influences must also be operative in certain nations to explain the high incidence of antigenemia in general and its association with liver cell cancer.

Liver flukes (*Clonorchis sinensis*) cause primary liver cell carcinoma in the Orient, and Schistosoma in Africa causes cirrhosis and frequently hepatocarcinoma. There are many hints, therefore, that cancer of the liver is, to some extent, an environmental disease.

Incidence. Striking differences in the world-wide incidence of hepatic cancers have already been mentioned, possibly related to the predisposing influences discussed above. In the United States and Europe, cancers of the liver are encountered in about 0.2 to 0.7 per cent of all autopsies. In certain African and Asian countries, the incidence rises to 5.5 per cent (Lin, 1970). Indeed, there are local regions in Africa where the frequency reaches 10 to 20 per cent of all autopsies and where it is the most common form of cancer found in men. In these regions, the peak incidence is encountered in the third and fourth decades of life. In the low incidence countries such as the United States, hepatic cancers are most often encountered in the sixth and seventh decades of life. Among these adults, there is a male-female ratio of 3 to 1. A second smaller peak *not* associated with cirrhosis is encountered in the first decade (Patton and Horn, 1964).

Morphology. Both the hepatocarcinoma and the cholangiocarcinoma, as well as the occasional mixed pattern, assume one of the following three macroscopic appearances in the liver: (1) a solitary massive tumor, sometimes described as monolobular, that may virtually replace one lobe or sometimes over half the liver; (2) multiple nodules scattered throughout the liver, virtually indistinguishable from metastatic implantation within the liver; and (3) a diffuse infiltrative type which is sometimes extremely difficult to differentiate from the underlying cirrhosis. It is not clear whether the multiple nodules represent dissemination of a single primary focus or multicentric origins of the neoplasm. Rarely, the diffuse infiltrative pattern may induce a stromal fibroblastic reaction to create a so-called "carcinomatous cirrhosis." In all three patterns, the tumor may be yellow-white or varying shades of green. Bile pigmentation is generally associated with the hepatoma since the bile duct epithelium of the cholangioma cannot elaborate bile. However, the cholangioma destroys ducts and may thus cause bile stasis, but usually the pigmentation is spotty or peripheral and is not as marked as in the hepatocarcinoma. All these tumors usually cause hepatic enlargement, particularly the monolobular variety where the enlargement is typically asymmetrical (Fig. 22–27). The multinodular pattern tends to produce scattered nodules up to 5 cm. in diameter. The enlargement may be only

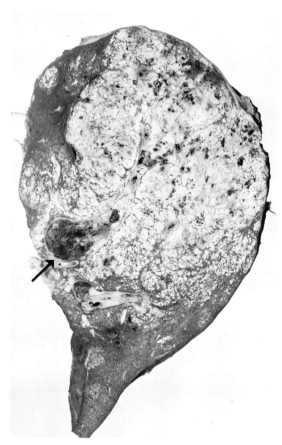

Figure 22–27. *Primary liver cell carcinoma complicating pigment cirrhosis. Tumor thrombus in branch of portal vein* (arrow).

slight in the diffuse infiltrative pattern. Hemorrhages and necroses are particularly prominent in the monolobular pattern, but are also encountered in the multinodular form. All these tumors, particularly those arising in hepatocytes, have a propensity for invading the hepatic veins and are one of the causes of the Budd-Chiari syndrome. Sometimes they extend in direct continuity from the hepatic vein up into the vena cava and even into the right side of the heart.

Histologically, the cells in the hepatoma more or less resemble hepatocytes. When the tumors are sufficiently well differentiated, the cells have a tendency to form cords which sometimes are separated by sinusoids. In the better differentiated lesions, the tumor cells elaborate bile, comprising when present a reliable diagnostic feature (Fig. 22–28). The less well differentiated tumors are usually composed of large anaplastic giant cells with abundant cytoplasm and multiple nuclei that are often seen in mitotic division (Fig. 22–29). Rarely, the cells take a spindle form. There is surprisingly scant fibrous stroma in the usual hepatocarcinoma.

The cholangiocarcinoma arising from bile ducts usually is an adenocarcinoma, but sometimes it is less well differentiated. Characteristically, this tumor evokes an abundant fibroblastic stroma. Mucin production may be present. No bile is found within the tumor cells, as previously mentioned, but bile pigment may be trapped within the tumor mass. The differentiation of a multicentric cholangiocarcinoma from metastatic adenocarcinoma may be most difficult and often rests with the exclusion of other primary sites of origin for the cancer. An infrequent primary hepatic cancer partakes of the characteristics of both the hepato- and cholangiocarcinoma.

Primary hepatic tumors in about half the cases metastasize to extrahepatic sites, particularly the regional nodes, lungs, bones, adrenal gland and elsewhere. They often, as previously mentioned, invade smaller veins as well as the larger radicles including the hepatic veins. Portal vein involvement is also encountered, but less frequently (Patton and Horn, 1964).

Clinical Course. The most common clinical features of these neoplasms are a palpable mass in the liver, rapid liver enlargement, an unexplained fever of mild degree and the chain of symptoms and signs associated with the underlying cirrhosis. The frequently associated ascites is often bloody. Weight loss, gastrointestinal disturbances and extreme weakness are additional nonspecific features. Rarely, spontaneous hypoglycemia may occur, attributed to replacement of liver substance by tumor and hence low reserves of hepatic glycogen. Involvement of the hepatic vein may produce the Budd-Chiari syndrome. Pain and

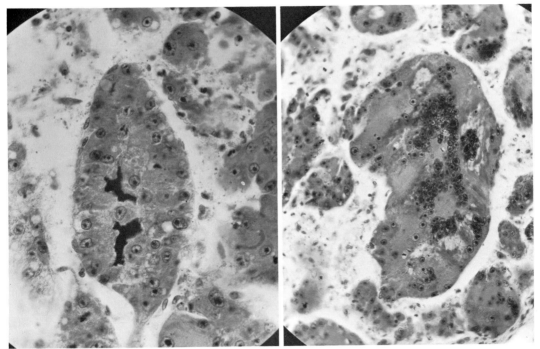

Fig. 22–28.   Fig. 22–29.

Figure 22–28. *Primary liver cell carcinoma. Bile stasis in tumor cells.*
Figure 22–29. *Primary liver cell carcinoma. Large tumor giant cells.*

tenderness over the liver region may be a consequence of necrosis or hemorrhage into the tumor. The diagnosis of primary liver carcinoma should be suspected when a patient with cirrhosis shows sudden worsening of his condition or has sudden progressive enlargement of the liver and bloody ascites.

Recently, a new laboratory diagnostic test has become available. Approximately 50 to 75 per cent of patients with primary hepatocarcinoma (but not cholangiocarcinoma) have an alpha feto-globulin in their serum (Smith, 1970) (Abelev, 1968). This serum globulin is normally present in the fetus, but disappears soon after birth. Presumably, its synthesis is repressed in postnatal life. Its production by hepatocarcinomas may reflect genetic mutations in cancer cells, permitting expression of codons normally repressed. It is important to emphasize that liver function studies may show surprisingly little abnormality since there appears to be remarkable tolerance on the part of the liver to growth of tumor. Only when a large part of the hepatic substance is destroyed do the laboratory tests become abnormal. Unless some of the larger bile ducts are blocked, jaundice may be absent. The clinical problem is further complicated by the fact that cirrhosis is such a frequent concomitant that it alone may be an adequate explanation for the

clinical signs and symptoms. Once the diagnosis becomes apparent, the average duration of survival is less than six months, although patients with well differentiated solitary nodules survive longer.

METASTATIC TUMORS

The majority arise in the gastrointestinal tract, particularly in the colon, and spread through the portal system to the liver. Typically, metastatic tumors will form many scattered nodules of tumor tending to be very uniform in size. Metastatic tumors can cause livers to weigh from 5000 to 8000 gm. Nonetheless, interference with the function of the liver by metastatic tumors is the exception rather than the rule (Figs. 22–30 and 22–31).

CIRRHOSIS

There is no universally accepted definition of cirrhosis. At first approximation, it can be characterized as widely distributed scarring of the liver which follows death of islands or small aggregates of cells throughout the liver. This oversimplified definition has been variously qualified by adding that (1) the fibrosis must represent an actual or relative

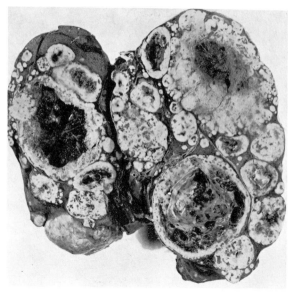

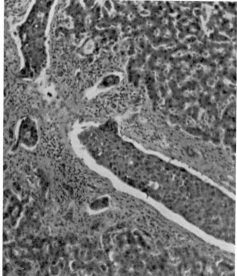

Fig. 22–30.   **Fig. 22–31.**

Figure 22–30. *Liver. Metastatic malignant tumor from stomach. Replacement of majority of liver by tumor. Ischemic necrosis of central portions of large nodules.*

Figure 22–31. *Metastatic carcinoma from colon in branches of portal vein and invading periportal portions of lobule.*

increase in connective tissue and (2) the necrosis must be associated with nodular regeneration of liver cells. According to this definition, focal scarring, such as follows the healing of an abscess, an infarct, or loss of hepatic cells with condensation of preexisting fibrous framework, is not a form of cirrhosis. *The cirrhotic liver then is characterized by widely distributed scars and more or less widely distributed regeneration of hepatocytes.*

The difficulties in arriving at a universally accepted definition of cirrhosis are somewhat amusing when viewed within the limited strict meaning of the term "cirrhosis" itself. Derived from the Greek word *kirrhos*, it means tawny. The term was originally applied to one form of cirrhosis now associated with alcohol abuse which is, indeed, tawny in color. But all the other forms of cirrhosis are not tawny.

Many influences may induce widespread injury to the liver, resulting in many morphologic patterns of scarring. To some extent, the size and distribution of the scars is conditioned by the specific agent causing the injury. However, the resultant morphologic patterns are not sharply delimited from each other and, in many instances, the end-stages of scarring tend to overlap. For these reasons, it has been exceedingly difficult to establish a classification of cirrhosis on morphologic grounds. Clinical differentiation is equally difficult because, with all forms of injury, scar tissue results, hyperplastic regenerative nodules appear, jaundice is com-

mon and liver function is impaired. Moreover, a pathogenetic classification is made difficult because the precise sequence of events at the biomolecular level leading to the ultimate cirrhotic process is still poorly understood. It is no surprise, then, that there is no single universally accepted classification. Acknowledging all of these difficulties and imperfections, here we shall offer a classification based on presumed pathogenesis. It has the virtue of simplicity and focuses attention on the need to further explore the causation of these important disorders. An approximate relative distribution among the forms of cirrhosis is given as a percentage range after each type.

Type		Per Cent
1.	Cirrhosis associated with alcohol abuse (Laennec's, portal, nutritional, alcoholic)	30–60
2.	Cirrhosis associated with hemochromatosis (pigment cirrhosis)	2–5
3.	Postnecrotic scarring	10–30
4.	Posthepatitic cirrhosis	(rare)
5.	Biliary cirrhosis (primary and secondary)	10–20
6.	Indeterminate and miscellaneous types	15–25

The distribution offered above will, of course, vary with the population surveyed. Indeed, the frequency of the various forms of cirrhosis may differ from one hospital to another, perhaps reflecting varying exposure of the patient population to the many influences inducing cirrhosis. At the Boston City Hospital, cirrhosis is encountered in 10 to 15 per cent of all autopsies. The form associated with alcohol abuse alone accounts for the preponderance of these cases (MacDonald, 1957). In the Los Angeles County Hospital, the incidence of cirrhosis in the Mexican population was reported as 22 per cent, three times that found in the remainder of the hospital population (Hall et al., 1953). Among other hospitals in the United States, the incidence ranges from 3 to 6 per cent. In Africa, Chile and parts of Asia, a frequency of up to 8 per cent is reported. Whatever the precise figure, it is clear that cirrhosis of the liver is a common disorder and, in 1964, represented the fifth most common cause of death in men 25 to 64 years of age (Terris, 1967).

The prevalence of cirrhosis has increased in the United States during the recent past. At the Boston City Hospital, there has been a twofold increase over the past 45 years. To some extent, this increase in frequency reflects better medical care, permitting patients to survive liver injury and to develop the diffuse fibrosis characteristic of cirrhosis. Whether other factors are also involved is less clear. Is alcoholism becoming more common? Is there greater exposure to hepatotoxic drugs and chemicals? Have viral infections become more frequent, or has there been some change in the virulence of the agent? Conversely, is there some basis for increased susceptibility in those exposed? Whatever the reasons, cirrhosis is world-wide in distribution and is on the increase.

Both its prevalence and its impact on liver structure and function make cirrhosis of the liver one of the most important forms of clinical disease. Before presenting the many types of cirrhosis, it is desirable to consider one of its most important pathophysiologic consequences, the production of portal hypertension.

PORTAL HYPERTENSION—PATHOPHYSIOLOGY

Portal hypertension is almost always (in more than 90 per cent of cases) due to cirrhosis. Rarely, it may be caused by disorders that obstruct the portal vein before it enters the liver, so-called *prehepatic* portal hypertension, or by lesions that hamper the venous outflow from the liver, so-called *posthepatic* portal hypertension. Prehepatic hypertension may be produced by neoplastic obstruction or thrombosis of the extrahepatic portal vein. Causes of posthepatic hypertension include: neoplastic obstruction or thrombosis of the hepatic vein

or inferior vena cava, and prolonged congestive heart failure.

Our major interest here is in the *intrahepatic* form of portal hypertension associated with cirrhosis of the liver. Surprisingly, its genesis is not entirely clear. Obstruction of the intrahepatic radicles of the portal vein, caused either by the fibrous scarring or expansion of regenerative nodules within the liver, undoubtedly contributes. But other mechanisms must also be operative for the following reasons. The hepatic sinusoidal pressures are elevated to levels higher than those in the extrahepatic portal vein. When a clamp is placed on the extrahepatic portal vein, the pressure on the hepatic side of the clamp is higher than it is on the splanchnic side (Reynolds et al., 1969) (Mikkelsen et al., 1962). Moreover, in the cirrhotic liver, the normal anastomoses between portal vein and hepatic artery are enlarged, and abnormal shunts develop as a consequence of the inflammatory and reparative process occurring in the genesis of the scarring. So it seems reasonable to conclude that a major contribution to the portal hypertension is made by shunting of arterial blood (at arterial pressure) into the portal vein. In cirrhosis, the pressure in the portal vein often rises to 20 or 30 mm. Hg, in contrast to normal pressures in the range of 5 to 10 mm. Hg.

When portal hypertension develops, it is followed by a host of changes, among which three are predominant: (1) ascites, (2) the formation of collateral venous channels and (3) splenomegaly. In a series of patients with cirrhosis, 46 per cent presented with ascites, 23 per cent with gastrointestinal bleeding as a consequence of the abnormal venous collaterals, 18 per cent with signs and symptoms of hepatic failure and 9 per cent with jaundice (Blaisdell and Cohen, 1961). Among the various cirrhoses to be described, portal hypertension is most often encountered in that associated with alcohol abuse and is less frequently encountered in pigment cirrhosis, postnecrotic scarring and posthepatitic cirrhosis. Only very rarely do biliary cirrhosis, cardiac sclerosis and the other forms of diffuse hepatic scarring induce portal hypertension.

Ascites is an intraperitoneal accumulation of watery fluid containing proteins (largely albumin) in the range of 1 to 2 gm. per 100 cc., which impart a specific gravity of 1.008 to 1.012. Solutes such as glucose, sodium and potassium have essentially the same concentration in the ascitic fluid as in the blood. Many liters of such fluid may collect to produce massive abdominal distention. In some patients, because of the discomfort produced by the fluid, large volumes are drained by abdominal tapping. It is evident that in this process a considerable amount of proteins and electrolytes are lost, which may have serious consequences on the fluid and electrolyte metabolism. Ascitic fluid may also contain mesothelial cells and lymphocytes but, in uncomplicated cases, red cells and neutrophils are absent. This point is worthy of note, since the appearance of red cells in ascitic fluid may well indicate cancerous seeding of the peritoneal surfaces, and any significant number of neutrophils indicates peritoneal irritation, most commonly by bacterial infection. Ascitic fluid does not constitute a stagnant pool. It is in dynamic equilibrium with the blood plasma. The rate of exchange is fantastic and has been estimated to be as high as 80 per cent per hour. It is no surprise, then, that after tapping it has the distressing potential of rapidly reaccumulating.

It would be natural to assume that the ascitic fluid is a transudate resulting from the increased pressures within the portal venous system. While this mechanism undoubtedly contributes, the genesis of ascites is much more complex. Impaired synthesis of albumin due to the liver disease induces hypoalbuminemia. The increase in sinusoidal pressure described earlier results in increased transudation and formation of lymph within the liver, and the liver surface literally "weeps" volumes of fluid. Similar weeping may occur throughout the splanchnic bed. With portal hypertension and sequestration of considerable volumes of blood in the splanchnic bed, there is reduced renal blood flow and reduced glomerular filtration with consequent sodium retention. It has also been suggested that, in some unexplained fashion, liver disease impairs the kidney's ability to excrete sodium (Lieberman et al., 1969). Increased levels of aldosterone are also commonly encountered in the plasma and urine, elaborated in response to the secretion of renin in the juxtaglomerular apparatus as the renal blood flow drops (Davis, 1964). The aldosterone further induces sodium retention (Liebowitz, 1969). With the sodium retention the blood volume increases, compounding the portal hypertension. Increased levels of ADH may appear, either because of the liver's inability to metabolize it or in response to reduction in effective circulating blood volume, as much of it is sequestered in the splanchnic bed. Thus, the ascites is the result of a constellation of influences. In about 20 per cent of patients, the ascitic fluid passes through transdiaphragmatic lymphatics into the pleural cavities, particularly on the right, to cause *hydrothorax.*

Whatever its genesis, ascites, when present, implies cirrhosis of the liver until proved otherwise. The fluid accumulations

may cause massive distention of the abdomen, accentuated by the concomitant muscle wasting and the scrawny extremities, which take on the appearance of appendages of the enormously rounded, protuberant abdomen.

Collateral venous channels develop as portal vein bypasses. These appear wherever the systemic and portal circulations share common capillary beds. The most important are found in the lower esophageal plexus and have already been described in the production of esophageal varices (p. 907). Varices occur in about 67 per cent of patients with advanced cirrhosis (Palmer and Brick, 1953), cause hematemesis in about 25 per cent and, indeed, when ruptured, are the principal cause of death in almost this same number. Once varices rupture, the hematemesis is massive and is usually fatal. Portal vein bypasses also develop in the anorectal region, where the superior mesenteric vein of the portal system communicates, via the inferior mesenteric system, with the hemorrhoidal plexus of the caval system. About 30 to 50 per cent of patients with cirrhosis of the liver develop hemorrhoids. While serious hemorrhage rarely arises from such sources, hemorrhoids constitute a significant source of discomfort. In some patients, when the fetal umbilical vein has not become totally obliterated, it may communicate with dilated venous channels about the umbilicus to produce a *caput medusae.*

The *splenomegaly* associated with cirrhosis has already been described as congestive splenomegaly (p. 771). Weights of up to 1000 gm. may be encountered. As was indicated in the previous discussion, the hypersplenic syndrome may then appear and produce a variety of hematologic abnormalities, including anemia, leukopenia and thrombocytopenia. The last-mentioned, in turn, may induce a hemorrhagic diathesis in concert with the hypoprothrombinemia of cirrhosis.

A host of other manifestations may be encountered in the cirrhotic patient. Peptic ulceration is more frequent in these patients than in the normal population. Renal disturbances, both morphologic and functional, occur in a small percentage of patients with cirrhosis. Tubular and glomerular changes of obscure etiology are encountered in 5 to 10 per cent of cirrhotics (Baxter and Ashworth, 1946). The glomerular abnormalities have been characterized as proliferative and membranous glomerulonephritis and as cirrhotic glomerulosclerosis (Jones et al., 1961) (Fisher and Hellstrom, 1959).

Still other clinical findings are attributable to hepatic failure; these were discussed earlier (p. 991). However, the consequences of hepatic failure may also be induced by any destructive process. Thus, the most diagnostic signs and symptoms of an underlying cirrhosis comprise those findings attributable solely to portal hypertension, remembering that pre- and posthepatic disorders are rare causes of this same syndrome.

CIRRHOSIS ASSOCIATED WITH ALCOHOL ABUSE (ALCOHOLIC, PORTAL, LAENNEC'S, NUTRITIONAL)

On a global basis, the cirrhosis associated with alcohol abuse is not only the most common type but is also referred to by a greater variety of names. It has variously been called Laennec's, portal, nutritional and alcoholic cirrhosis. It is apparent from the many designations that there is still disagreement as to whether the liver injury is primarily nutritional in origin or related to direct hepatotoxicity of alcohol. In either event, there is a clear association between chronic alcoholism and this form of cirrhosis of the liver. For this reason, the more noncommittal term is used here — "cirrhosis associated with alcohol abuse."

In the United States and in other affluent societies, the growing problem of chronic alcoholism undoubtedly underlies the increasing incidence of this form of cirrhosis (Popper et al., 1969). It is impossible to scientifically define chronic alcoholism. Facetiously, it has been said that "a chronic alcoholic is anyone who drinks whom you don't like." More rigorously, it represents a form of addiction which interferes with one's life. So defined, this form of addiction occurs in all levels of society and in both sexes at all ages of adult life. Once predominantly a male disease, it is now encountered with increasing frequency in both sexes, with a peak incidence in the fourth and fifth decades of life. The view that this disorder occurs mainly among the derelicts of life is grossly erroneous, as all hospital files would confirm.

Pathogenesis. Few subjects have evoked more heated controversy than the role of alcohol in the production of this form of cirrhosis. Central to this debate is the issue of whether the alcohol itself is a direct hepatotoxin or merely a calorie-substitute predisposing to malnutrition in those who preferentially "drink their calories." *Two observations are noncontroversial: (1) there is a well established association between alcohol consumption and the appearance of this form of cirrhosis and (2) the fibrous scarring is almost invariably preceded by fatty change throughout the liver.* Epidemiologic data indicate that, around the world, mortality rates from cirrhosis are directly related to per capita consumption of alcoholic beverages (Terris, 1967). A history of chronic alcoholism can be obtained in up to 90 per cent of these patients.

The general consideration of fatty change in the liver was presented on p. 32. It was indicated that, in general, the mechanisms implicated in the accumulation of fat in the liver include: (1) increased transport of fat from the periphery to the liver, (2) reduced fatty acid oxidation in the liver, (3) increased synthesis of triglycerides and, possibly, (4) impaired mobilization of lipids as lipoproteins (Lieber, 1969). Abundant evidence has been marshalled that alcohol can induce fatty change in the liver. But it has not been established beyond doubt that chronic alcohol abuse with its fatty change inevitably leads to fibrous scarring and cirrhosis. Elevated blood alcohol levels increase the transport of fat from the periphery to the liver. Simultaneously, the ethanol is transported to the liver where it is metabolized, as discussed on p. 517. The hepatic metabolism of alcohol has a profound effect on the oxidative capacity of liver cells (Rubin and Lieber, 1968). The effect of ethanol on the liver is to produce increased amounts of $NADH_2$ and thus increase the $NADH_2/NAD$ ratio. As a consequence, oxidative pathways in the liver cell are hampered, and there is a marked decrease in hepatic lipid oxidation and in the oxidation of chylomicrons (Lieber, 1968). Since alcohol mobilizes depot fat, increases its transport to the liver, and simultaneously blocks hepatic utilization of lipids, it accumulates within hepatocytes. This effect of alcohol is remarkably quick.

Young, nonalcoholic volunteers developed fatty change in the liver within 2 days when they consumed 18 to 24 ounces of alcohol per day, despite a concomitant substantial caloric intake high in protein and low in fat (Rubin and Lieber, 1968). In these volunteers, the livers were presumably normal at the outset and, indeed, the subjects continued to consume a better-than-average diet. Smaller amounts of alcohol over a longer time span had the same effect. Popper and Orr (1970) believe that a long-term intake below 80 ml. of ethanol per day rarely leads to significant liver injury, while levels above 160 ml. often lead to hepatic damage and cirrhosis. Whether chronic consumption of alcohol and persistent fatty change will inevitably lead to cirrhosis has, however, not been established. It has been impossible in experimental animals to produce a reasonable facsimile of the cirrhosis of alcohol abuse by feeding of alcohol along with an adequate diet for long periods of time.

A second school of thought maintains that nutritional imbalances play a large role in the genesis of the cirrhosis in chronic alcoholics

(Porta et al., 1970). Proponents of this view suggest that, along with the chronic alcoholism, the diet is deficient in protein and, consequently, in lipotropes. The lipotropes, choline and methionine, are requisite for the synthesis of phospholipids and lipoproteins, in which form fat is mobilized from the liver (Porta and Gomez-Dumm, 1968). A protein-deficient diet alone will induce fatty change in the liver. Fatty change and diffuse fibrosis can be induced by a diet containing alcohol but deficient in lipotropes and, indeed, by a choline deficiency alone, but these models are not generally accepted as faithful replicas of the human disease. Moreover, there is considerable doubt that man can survive on a diet sufficiently inadequate in proteins to produce a lipotrope deficiency.

Can these differing viewpoints be reconciled? At the present writing, it seems well established that ethanol alone can induce fatty change (Lieber and Rubin, 1969). Whether it alone induces the cirrhosis associated with alcohol abuse in the patient remains controversial because of the likelihood that many or most of these individuals also suffer from nutritional deficits. It should be noted that profound fatty change in the liver is encountered in infants suffering from the protein deficiency state known as kwashiorkor (Cook and Hutt, 1967). Cirrhosis almost never develops in these infants. Malnutrition alone, then, does not cause cirrhosis of the liver in this setting. On the other hand, sufficient levels of alcohol will induce not only fatty change but also liver cell injury (Rubin et al., 1971). In the experimental animal and in man, the administration of alcohol causes mitochondrial swelling, megamitochondria, swelling of endoplasmic reticulum and often disruption of organelles (Figs. 22–32 and 22–33). Simultaneously, a pink hyaline deposit with a fibrillar substructure, known as "alcoholic hyalin," appears within the cytoplasm of these damaged liver cells. This hyalin will be described subsequently, but it should be noted here that some investigators have interpreted it as aggregates of destroyed organelles, while others believe that it is an abnormal synthetic product secondary to serious injury to the hepatocyte (Iseri and Gottlieb, 1971). Whatever its interpretation, it reflects liver cell injury and, in some instances, is associated with liver cell death and localized polymorphonuclear infiltrations. Here, then, could be a mechanism for cell injury, cell death and consequent scarring. On balance, then, *the weight of evidence is on the side of alcohol's being a direct hepatotoxin, but it must be admitted that in chronic alcoholics it may well be abetted by nutritional deficits.*

Whatever the precise pathways, it is clear that the chronic alcoholic almost always first develops a massively fatty liver and, over the span of years, scarring slowly appears, accompanied by progressive shrinkage of the liver. In some individuals, symptoms of liver disease first become manifest after a spree of excessive drinking and grossly inadequate food intake. In most individuals, the disease becomes manifest far more insidiously. While many are obviously heavy drinkers with a record of habitual drunkenness, some, it should be noted, lead stable, productive lives, living with their families, and eating, as best as can be determined, an adequate diet.

Morphology. The evolution of the cirrhosis associated with alcohol abuse follows a fairly predictable course, unless the process is arrested by abstinence from alcohol and an appropriate diet. The early stage is a large, smooth, yellow, obviously fatty liver, weighing perhaps up to 6 kilos. At body temperature, such a liver is soft and greasy when cut. Histologically, the alterations resemble those already described as fatty change (p. 32). In this early stage, the liver cells may be so swollen as to produce some bile stasis within canaliculi and hepatocytes. In some patients, usually those who have been on a spree, alcoholic hyalin can be found within the cytoplasm of scattered liver cells. This takes the form of numerous coarse hyaline granules or irregular skeins or networks, usually disposed about the nucleus (Fig. 22–34). The material is acidophilic and stains intensely with phloxine, but can also be seen in ordinary hematoxylin and eosin preparations. Often, cells containing such hyalin are seriously damaged; some are necrotic and have provoked a local infiltration of a few neutrophils. During this early stage of fatty liver, there is little or no evidence of increased fibrous tissue or scarring.

Figure 22–32. *Liver cell in male rats maintained for 7 days on nutritionally adequate diet in which ethanol isocalorically replaces sucrose up to 36 per cent of the total calories. The early changes comprise the appearance of fat vacuoles (dark inclusions), slight vesiculation of the endoplasmic reticulum and slight swelling of the mitochondria. (Compare with Figure 22–1).*

Figure 22–33. *The same experimental model at 27 days. Note greater vesiculation of endoplasmic reticulum and swelling of mitochondria. Inset (lower right) shows detail of mitochondrion with loss of cristae and disruption of outer layer of mitochondrial membrane. (Figures 22–32 and 22–33 courtesy of Dr. O. Iseri, Mallory Institute of Pathology.)*

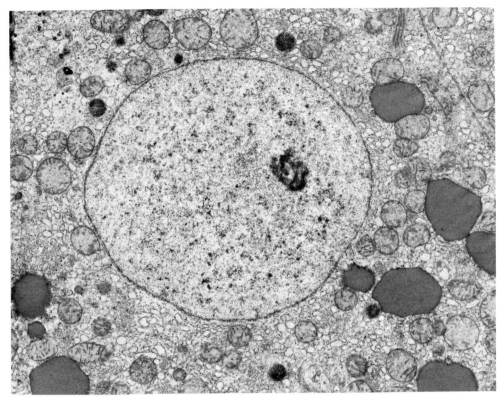

Fig. 22-32.

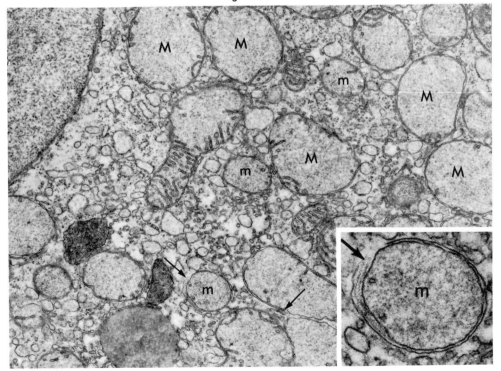

Fig. 22-33.

(See opposite page for legend)

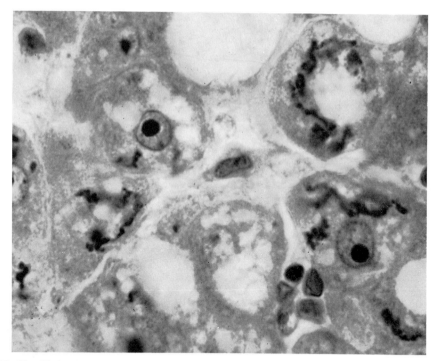

Figure 22–34.   *Cirrhosis of alcohol abuse. Alcoholic hyalin stands out as skeins of dark-staining material with a tendency to surround nuclei. Numerous fat vacuoles are also present.*

As the lesion evolves, the liver decreases in size and gradually but progessively becomes finely nodular to produce a so-called classic hobnail pattern (Figs. 22–35 and 22–36). Now the liver is yellow-orange and diffusely scarred, and this stage of the disease probably accounts for the original use of the term cirrhosis. The nodules vary in size from 0.1 to 1 cm. in diameter, with the larger nodules presumably resulting from regeneration. They are produced by the progressive development of fibrous scarring which begins about the portal areas and extends eventually to interconnect adjacent portal triads. The scarring simultaneously invades individual lobules and, in this manner, the nodules apparent on macroscopic examination represent at times individual lobules, perhaps several lobules, or small islands of cells representing only a portion of a lobule. It should be emphasized that the fibrous tissue derives from active fibroblastic proliferation and not merely condensation of collapsed stromal framework (Popper and Hutterer, in press). The remaining hepatocytes still often contain fat and, in many, alcoholic hyalin is visible. With active disease, unicellular necroses are evident, eliciting a local neutrophilic infiltrate. Bile stasis may be present in individual cells or canaliculi and often the bile ducts trapped within scarred portal areas show some reduplication and regeneration.

With the advance of the disease, the liver progressively shrinks to a small, fibrotic, indurated organ, frequently weighing less than 1200 gm. As the fibrous tissue accumulates, the fat disappears, and so the liver becomes progressively more brown. Alcoholic hyalin and cell necrosis now are generally absent (Figs. 22–37, 22–38 and 22–39). However, the regenerative activity may have produced greater variation in the prominence of nodules. In the far advanced cirrhosis associated with alcohol abuse, the scarring may become quite heavy and produce broad bands which simulate those encountered in postnecrotic cirrhosis. So it is that end-stage cirrhoses come to resemble each other.

Clinical Course.   The course of this form of cirrhosis is usually the slow evolution of scarring over the span of decades. In many patients, the disease is entirely asymptomatic and, in one series, a clinical diagnosis had only been made in 33 per cent of the cases (Stone et al., 1968). Symptoms, when they occur, may take such nonspecific forms as weight loss, loss of appetite, nausea, vomiting and ill-defined digestive disturbances. In time, more specific signs and symptoms become manifest, pointing toward the existence of portal hypertension caused by the cirrhosis. These include ascites, splenomegaly and gastrointestinal bleeding arising in esophageal varices or acute gastritis, as well as other findings discussed on p. 1023. In some cases, the first manifestation of the liver disease is jaundice. The hyperbilirubinemia is made up of both conjugated and unconjugated bilirubin, reflecting both

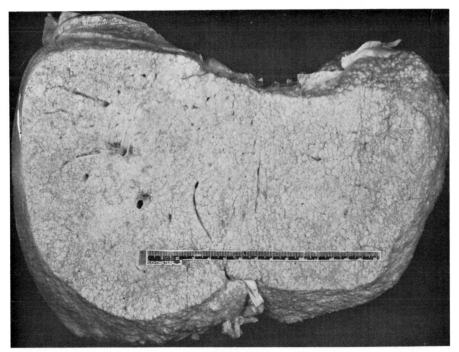

Fig. 22–35.

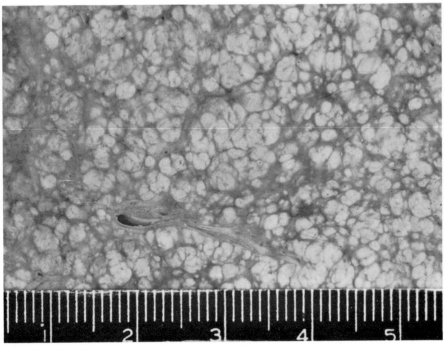

Fig. 22–36.

Figure 22–35. *Cirrhosis of alcohol abuse. Fine nodularity of capsular and cut surface. Liver is somewhat contracted.*

Figure 22–36. *Cirrhosis of alcohol abuse. Somewhat enlarged gross photograph to show variation in size of nodules and large amounts of intervening connective tissue.*

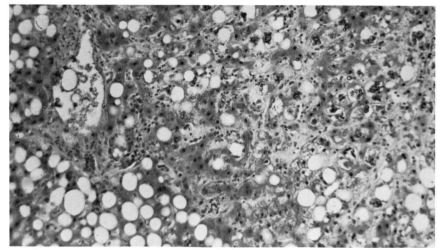

Fig. 22–37.

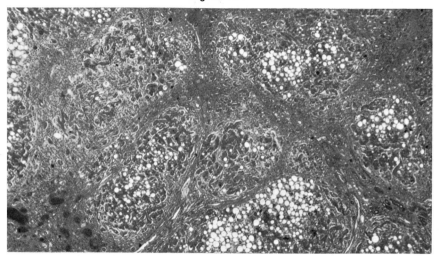

Fig. 22–38.

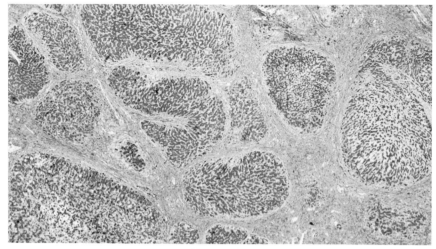

Fig. 22–39.

Figure 22–37. *Cirrhosis of alcohol abuse. Early stage with much fat and alcoholic hyalin but little, if any, fibrosis.*

Figure 22–38. *Center. Cirrhosis of alcohol abuse. Intermediate stage with considerable fat but also large amounts of fibrous tissue.*

Figure 22–39. *Cirrhosis of alcohol abuse. Late stage with no fat and large amounts of fibrosis.*

cholestasis and direct liver cell injury. Not infrequently, the cirrhosis becomes manifest after some unusual stress. The patient may have been on an alcoholic spree for a period of time, presumably eroding the last remnants of hepatic reserve. At other times, a massive hemorrhage from esophageal varices may be the initial manifestation of the disease or the hemorrhage may superimpose sufficient hypoxic injury to tip the liver into insufficiency. Intercurrent infections and surgical emergencies can also trigger hepatic decompensation.

It deserves emphasis that hepatic failure may appear long before the scarring becomes marked. The liver may still be extremely fatty and may have sufficient liver cell injury to produce hepatic insufficiency. When ascites and the other manifestations of portal hypertension are present, it can be assumed that fibrous scarring has already occurred and usually such livers are not massively enlarged and may, indeed, be shrunken and nonpalpable on abdominal examination. Obviously, those with active liver cell disease almost invariably have elevated levels of SGOT, SGPT and LDH.

The outlook for these patients is unpredictable and is dependent on the stage of advancement of the scarring and the patient's ability to abstain from further use of alcohol. At the fatty stage before fibrous scarring has occurred, the fat can be mobilized, with reversion of the liver to a remarkably normal state (Powell and Klatskin, 1968). When the scarring has become well advanced and portal hypertension has developed, it is doubtful that more than arrest of the disease can be achieved. Although there is a belief that some resorption of fibrous tissue may occur, accounting for some clinical improvement, it is more likely that under an appropriate regimen the liver regenerates enough to improve hepatic function. Such patients may have a long survival if they escape the serious effects of portal hypertension, such as intractable ascites or hemorrhage from a ruptured esophageal varix. However, the psychodynamics of chronic alcoholism are such that very few patients totally restructure their lives, and about 80 to 90 per cent of those with the cirrhosis of alcohol abuse die within five years of diagnosis. The causes of death are predominantly liver failure, intercurrent infections, gastrointestinal hemorrhages and, rarely, the development of a hepatocarcinoma.

Remember, that alcoholic injury to the liver predisposes it to intercurrent viral hepatitis, as well as drug and chemical injury. Thus at death, mixed or, more likely, indeterminate patterns of scarring may be found which account for the miscellaneous category of cirrhosis mentioned at the outset.

CIRRHOSIS ASSOCIATED WITH HEMOCHROMATOSIS (PIGMENT CIRRHOSIS)

Hemochromatosis has been discussed previously, and reference should be made to this earlier consideration (p. 277). It was indicated then that pigment cirrhosis is associated with a pattern of fibrous scarring quite similar to that encountered in the moderately advanced stages of alcohol abuse. However, the chocolate-brown color of the liver makes this form of cirrhosis quite distinctive. Special stains for iron will be of further diagnostic aid, highlighting the increased amounts of hemosiderin found in these livers. The pigment is found not only within the cytoplasm of liver cells but also within Kupffer cells, bile duct epithelium and in the scars. The clinical manifestations in these patients stem not only from the cirrhosis of the liver but also from the diabetes so often present in hemochromatosis. In most patients, however, hepatic failure or evidence of portal hypertension dominates. Pigment cirrhosis and postnecrotic scarring comprise the two most common antecedents of hepatocarcinoma in the United States.

POSTNECROTIC SCARRING (CIRRHOSIS)

Massive liver necrosis, whether it be due to viral hepatitis (p. 1010) or to drug or chemical toxicity (p. 1002), will in the course of time lead to irregular massive scarring of the liver if, of course, the patient survives the initial assault. However, the antecedents of this form of scarring may not be obvious. In less than half, there is a history of an episode of acute viral hepatitis or acute toxic damage to the liver. In most, the postnecrotic scarring develops insidiously and may be the end-stage of some form of chronic hepatitis, viral or immunologic (p. 1009). Possibly, the liver damage occurred at a subclinical level here. However, it is perhaps more accurate to say that some cases are cryptogenic.

The pattern of the scarring is entirely dependent, of course, on the distribution of the necrosis. Occasionally, a single large area or one lobe may be affected, producing a massive area of fibrosis, leaving the remainder of the liver unaffected. For this reason, there is some objection to designating such postnecrotic scarring as cirrhosis. However, more often the necrosis is widely distributed and patchy, and the scarring is sufficiently diffuse and acccompanied by regeneration to create a nodular, distorted liver, satisfying the more stringent criteria of cirrhosis. In the past, this form of cirrhosis has been called healed acute yellow atrophy, but the inappropriateness of such a designation has been alluded to earlier (p. 1010).

Morphology. Postnecrotic scarring, as the name implies, is a completely random haphazard process that often produces a grotesquely misshapen, usually small or somewhat contracted liver. The weight may be reduced to 1000 gm. or less. Large regenerative nodular areas with a smooth capsule are alternated with depressed scars of variable size. These scars are characteristically broad with fine wrinkling. One entire lobe may be reduced to a shriveled fibrotic appendage (Fig. 22–40). At other times, the scarring is more diffuse and creates nodules 3 to 4 cm. in diameter. The liver is basically brown with areas of green or red due to bile stasis or hemorrhage. The nodules result from regeneration and hence are composed of yielding liver substance in contrast to the gritty resistance of the gray-brown intervening scarred areas. It is not the pattern of nodularity that is distinctive in this form of cirrhosis but rather the broad scarring.

Histologically, the dominant feature is the irregular coarse nature of the scarring. In the large scars, only scattered bile ducts and blood vessels can be seen (Fig. 22–41). There is some proliferative reaction within these ducts but usually no striking reduplication such as that seen in biliary cirrhosis. Occasionally, islands of preserved liver cells are trapped in these scars. In other areas, the fibrosis may be more delicate, but characteristic of postnecrotic scarring is the total destruction of entire

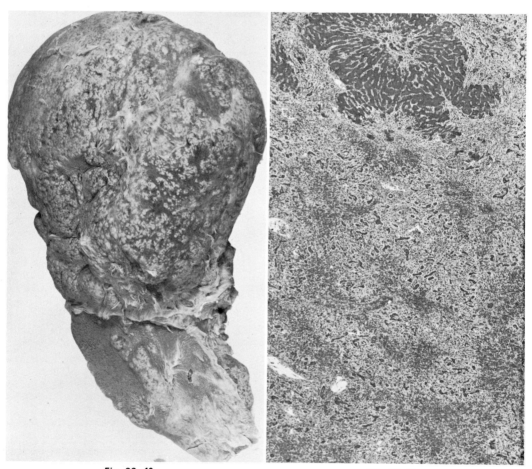

Fig. 22–40.

Fig. 22–41.

Figure 22–40. Postnecrotic cirrhosis. A small cirrhotic liver with marked atrophy of left lobe (below). Coarse nodules of regeneration in all lobules.

Figure 22–41. Postnecrotic cirrhosis. Low power photomicrograph. Small nodule of regenerated liver cells (above). Elsewhere, in many adjacent liver lobules, all liver cells have disappeared, leaving collapsed lobules with thickening of connective tissue and proliferation of bile ducts.

lobules and the agglomeration of the more resistant portal triads. An inflammatory infiltrate of mononuclear leukocytes is present in these scars. This pattern represents the late, well healed stages, but earlier one may see more active granulation tissue with still remaining necrotic liver cells. Between the scars, the persistent parenchyma may be completely normal but, in other areas, regeneration of injured liver cells may produce large disorganized masses of liver cells (Gall, 1960a). Such regenerative nodules often have prominent bile stasis.

Distinguishing the postnecrotic scarring from the cirrhosis of alcohol abuse are the size of the scars, total destruction of entire lobules, agglomeration of portal triads and the absence of fat. However, in some instances, it may be very difficult to differentiate between the late advanced stages of these two forms of liver disease.

Clinical Course. In many patients, the liver disease is entirely asymptomatic and is only discovered at postmortem. Manifestations, when they do appear, are those of liver failure or those related to the development of portal hypertension. On occasion, the irregularity of the scarring may produce a lobularity that can be appreciated on abdominal palpation.

One would assume that once the liver had become scarred, hepatic function would stabilize. However, because some of these patients may be suffering from continuing liver destruction, as in chronic active hepatitis, or because the scarring may progressively encroach on the blood supply, causing marginal zones of liver cells to die, the functional reserve ebbs and a progressive downhill course is followed. Over 50 per cent of all patients die within the first year of the appearance of major manifestations, most of liver failure or intercurrent infections. An additional 25 per cent die within the next three to five years usually because of portal hypertension and its sequelae. As indicated previously, this form of liver disease represents one of the important subsoils for the development of primary liver cell cancers, representing yet another fatal pathway.

POSTHEPATITIC (TRABECULAR) CIRRHOSIS

Posthepatitic or trabecular cirrhosis is a poorly defined lesion of somewhat obscure origin. Despite the designation posthepatitic, it does not necessarily imply a prior viral infection. Indeed, most of the evidence indicates that hepatitis A (infectious hepatitis) rarely, if ever, leads to scarring. On the other hand, it is generally believed that hepatitis B (serum hepatitis) may lead to scarring and this may be

one of the origins of this pattern of cirrhosis. As described by Gall (1960a, 1966), posthepatitic cirrhosis is characterized by a fine trabecular scarring, enclosing single or multiple liver lobules with relative preservation of the intralobular architecture. How such scarring comes about is still pure conjecture. Necrosis bridging several adjacent lobules has, indeed, been seen in classic cases of viral hepatitis, and this type of liver injury could lead to the pattern of scarring seen in this form of cirrhosis (Boyer and Klatskin, 1970). Chronic active hepatitis, whether of viral or immunologic origin, could be another pathway for the induction of trabecular scarring. We may be dealing, then, with a morphologic lesion having many origins, the common denominator being widespread submassive injury to the liver and consequent widely distributed but delicate scarring.

Morphology. The liver is usually of normal weight and color. The delicate scarring creates nodules ranging from 0.5 to 1.5 cm. in diameter. No fat is evident grossly or microscopically nor is cholestasis usually present. The fibrous trabeculae are narrow and tend to stretch from one portal tract to another, sometimes isolating individual lobules, and at other times several lobules. Only rarely does the fibrous tissue bridge an individual lobule, as is so characteristic of the cirrhosis associated with alcohol abuse. Thus, the basic architecture of the lobule is relatively well preserved. Within the fibrous septa there is a variable chronic inflammatory reaction, in some cases a scant infiltrate of lymphocytes, and in other cases an abundance of lymphocytes admixed with histiocytes and plasma cells. The portal tracts are not destroyed entirely, and bile ducts are readily evident.

Clinical Course. Most likely, this pattern of cirrhosis results from chronic hepatitis. Accordingly, as was pointed out earlier, the disease in many of these patients is totally submerged, and so this form of cirrhosis is often encountered unexpectedly at autopsy. Uncommonly, the fibrous scarring becomes manifest by the development of portal hypertension and its attendant disruptions.

BILIARY CIRRHOSIS

The term biliary cirrhosis embraces two quite distinctive patterns: (1) *secondary* obstructive and/or infectious biliary cirrhosis and (2) *primary* biliary cirrhosis. Both types are characterized by widespread but delicate and orderly scarring of the liver arising about the bile ducts in the portal triads and extending to eventually interconnect adjacent triads. Thus, the individual lobules are enclosed by fibrous bands. The *secondary obstructive/infectious biliary cirrhosis* is caused by: (1) prolonged, usually extrahepatic, bile duct obstruction or (2) upward spread of infection through the biliary tree into the bile ducts within the portal tracts. The common causes of biliary obstruction are gallstones, neoplasms (usually in the head of the pancreas, ampulla of Vater or extrahepatic bile ducts), biliary atresia or stricture of the extrahepatic bile ducts. Eventually, such obstruction of the outflow of bile produces intrahepatic cholestasis with damage to the intralobular bile ducts, cholangioles and canaliculi. Often, in these cases, ascending secondary infection by gram-negative bacilli and enterococci adds to the damage induced by the inspissated bile. Rarely, in the absence of biliary obstruction, bacterial infections may ascend the biliary tree to initiate this form of cirrhosis sometimes designated as *infectious biliary cirrhosis.* The inflammatory exudate may so plug the bile ducts as to add an element of biliary obstruction to the infectious process.

Primary biliary cirrhosis is a less well understood entity. It has been attributed to viral infection with involvement principally of the intrahepatic bile ducts, so-called *cholangiolitic viral hepatitis.* The validity of such an entity is challenged, and HAA cannot be identified in most of these patients. Alternatively, an immunologic causation has been proposed. Immune complexes, containing principally IgM, transformed lymphocytes and plasma cells, have been identified in the portal areas in some cases of primary biliary cirrhosis (Fox et al., 1969*b*). *Antimitochondrial* antibodies have been identified in the sera of some of these patients (Doniach et al., 1966). Why such antibodies should only damage the liver remains mysterious. Despite the presence of humoral antibodies, it is believed that most of the immunologic damage is due to a cell-mediated immune response, and it has therefore been proposed that this form of biliary cirrhosis is an autoimmune disorder (Doniach et al., 1970). It must be admitted, however, that the immunologic evidence is still scanty and its interpretation still debatable. Still a third possible pathway has been proposed, namely, drug-induced cholestasis. Here again, the evidence is insubstantial and, in most well studied cases of drug cholestasis, periportal damage and cirrhosis do not develop. So we deal with an entity of obscure nature.

Morphology. Common to all forms of biliary cirrhosis is a diffuse, regular, delicate scarring which imparts a pigskin or fine sandpaper texture to the serosal surface. No irregular nodularity is evident (Fig. 22—42). In the secondary form of obstructive biliary cirrhosis, the liver is intensely green. In the rare case of secondary biliary cirrhosis, where ascending infection without significant biliary tract obstruction causes the damage, the liver is unchanged in color, as it is in most cases of the primary form of biliary cirrhosis. Neither are these livers significantly reduced in size.

Histologically, the distinctive features are: (1)

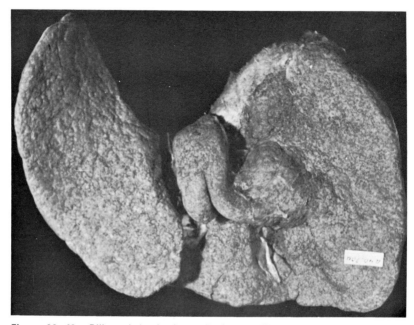

Figure 22–42. Biliary cirrhosis. A very finely and diffusely nodular cirrhotic liver.

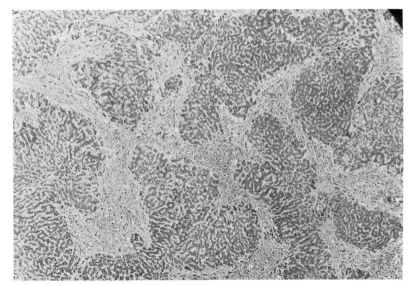

Figure 22–43. Biliary cirrhosis. Low power photomicrograph showing zone of proliferated bile ducts and connective tissue tending to surround each lobule.

regularity of the delicate periportal scars extending out to interconnect adjacent portal triads, (2) bile duct and ductular injury, proliferation and regeneration within the scars and (3) a heavy, leukocytic infiltration in the scars (Fig. 22–43). Additional changes may be present, depending on the particular pathogenetic mechanism involved.

In the obstructive form, inspissated bile is obviously prominent. Bile can be found within liver cells, canaliculi, ductules and ducts. In many areas, canaliculi appear to have ruptured to produce large accumulations of bile pigment, referred to as "bile lakes," causing necrosis of surrounding hepatocytes. About these foci, there may be a neutrophilic exudation or sometimes a granulomatous reaction. In the purely obstructive form of this cirrhosis, the periportal scarring is heavily infiltrated with lymphocytes. Where infection plays a more prominent role, neutrophilic exudation is not only readily evident within bile ducts and ductules but may also extend out into the pericholangitic regions.

The primary form of biliary cirrhosis is made distinctive by the prominence of plasma cells within the periportal scarring and the occasional formation of large lymphoid aggregates and even follicles in these regions. In some cases, lipid-filled macrophages (lipophages) crowd into the periductal portal regions and are sometimes associated with sarcoid-like granulomas. This granulomatous reaction may be a sequel to the death of the lipophages, but it has also been offered as proof of a possible immunologic mechanism. As mentioned in the discussion of causation, immunofluorescent techniques disclose immune complexes within macrophages in the periportal regions in some cases of primary biliary cirrhosis (Paronetto et al., 1967). The lipophages are particularly abundant in those

cases with marked hypercholesterolemia, and this form of biliary cirrhosis is sometimes designated **xanthomatous biliary cirrhosis.**

Clinical Course. The clinical findings in the secondary obstructive biliary cirrhosis differ significantly from those in the primary form of the disease. When there is posthepatic obstruction, jaundice and itching are the most characteristic findings. The itching is related to retention of bile salts. Where there is a significant element of infection, fever, right upper quadrant pain and marked leukocytosis are evidenced.

In those with the primary form of the disease, hypercholesterolemia is sometimes seen, although for reasons that are still obscure. Such patients have a predilection for xanthomas of the skin, florid atherosclerosis and myocardial infarction.

In all forms of biliary cirrhosis, the liver is rarely palpable, no nodularity is evident and these patients almost never develop portal hypertension. However, the deficient flow of bile into the duodenum impairs lipid absorption and sometimes leads to a hemorrhagic diathesis related to inadequate absorption of vitamin K. Although extensive destruction of liver substances is not common in biliary cirrhosis, in some patients hepatic failure may eventually ensue.

MISCELLANEOUS AND INDETERMINATE FORMS OF CIRRHOSIS

There are several varieties of well defined cirrhosis which are so uncommon today as to not merit separate description. In longstanding severe cardiac decompensation, centrilobular hemorrhagic necrosis of the liver may lead to centrilobular scarring, known as *cardiac cirrhosis* or *cardiac sclerosis*. Such scarring is rarely of sufficient magnitude to cause more than a slight pigskin graining of the liver. There is rarely significant reduction in liver size and, on macroscopic cut section, the changes are virtually indistinguishable from the nutmeg pattern of chronic congestion. Some increase in liver consistency may suggest the existence of the central fibrosis. The scarring does not often interconnect with the adjacent centrilobular regions, and neither is regeneration a common feature of this form of liver disease. Thus, although this entity has been referred to as cardiac cirrhosis, most investigators prefer to call it cardiac sclerosis. These patients virtually never have evidence of portal hypertension or hepatic failure.

In both congenital and tertiary acquired syphilis, cirrhosis of the liver with many of the signs and symptoms characteristic of the whole group of cirrhoses may be found. In areas where syphilis is well controlled and treated, this is becoming a very rare type of cirrhosis. In the Boston City Hospital series, it comprised only 1.5 per cent of the group.

Syphilitic cirrhosis must be divided into the forms seen in congenital syphilis and those found in acquired syphilis. In *congenital syphilis*, if the liver is severely involved, it is *enlarged, firm and somewhat pale unless bile stasis has occurred.* Histologically, there is a very diffuse proliferation of fibroblasts in the subsinusoidal spaces throughout the lobules. As a result, the cells lining the sinusoids are separated from the liver cells by a layer of fibroblasts (Fig. 22–44). The sinusoids are somewhat compressed. With the Levaditi stain, numerous treponema can be demonstrated between the fibroblasts, and the fibroblastic proliferation is evidently a reaction to their presence. Occasionally, miliary gummas may be scattered throughout these livers.

The syphilitic cirrhosis of acquired syphilis is known as *hepar lobatum*. It is a tertiary manifestation and results from the development and healing of multiple large gummas in the liver substance (Symmers and Spain, 1946). Grossly, such livers are broken up into many coarse lobules, varying from 3 to 5 cm. in diameter, by deep, depressed scars extending into the liver substance (Fig. 22–45). The cut surface may reveal active or healing gummas in the scars. Histologically, sections taken through the centers of the lobules show essentially normal-appearing liver tissue with normal lobular architecture. Sections through the

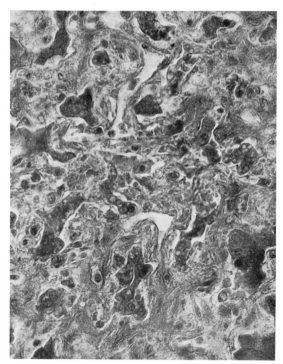

Figure 22–44. *Liver in congenital syphilis. Diffuse proliferation of fibroblasts around liver cells in subsinusoidal space.*

scar show fibrous scar tissue and sometimes evidence of active or healing gummas.

There are no specific findings indicating a diagnosis of hepar lobatum, which happily has become a rare entity. A positive serologic test for syphilis in a patient with a palpably lobular liver would point toward this diagnosis but, of

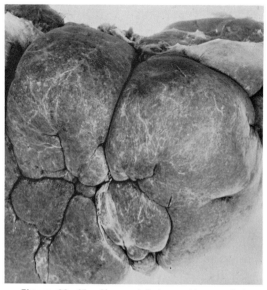

Figure 22–45. *Hepar lobatum. Liver substance cut up into coarse lobes by deep furrows.*

course, a positive serology might well be found in a patient with one of the more common forms of cirrhosis.

Wilson's disease, an inborn error of copper metabolism, is characterized by cirrhosis of the liver and brain damage and so is also referred to as *hepatolenticular* degeneration. The disorder is inherited as an autosomal recessive trait manifested in the homozygote, usually in the second or third decade of life. The fundamental defect appears to be inadequate synthesis of the plasma copper-binding ceruloplasmin. Copper, after absorption from the diet, is normally transported complexed to this copper-binding protein. It is believed that in those patients with Wilson's disease, the inadequate levels of ceruloplasmin permit copper to be transported loosely complexed with albumin. In this state, it is readily dissociated and so is deposited in the liver, basal ganglia, cerebral cortex, kidney and cornea, causing damage to all of these structures. The copper deposits in the eye are found in Descemet's membrane at the limbus of the cornea, producing the *Kayser-Fleischer* ring pathognomonic of Wilson's disease. The deposits in the brain are described on p. 1539.

Early in the course of Wilson's disease, hepatocellular necrosis has been observed, often accompanied by the formation of hyaline acidophilic inclusions extremely reminiscent of those seen in the liver of alcohol abuse (Levi et al., 1967). Scarring follows the stage of necrosis. The scarring may produce delicate trabeculae, somewhat similar to those in posthepatitic cirrhosis, or broad, massive areas of collapse, suggesting postnecrotic cirrhosis (Fig. 22–46). Electron microscopic studies have revealed accumulations of copper in the hepatocytic lysosomes as well as mitochondrial abnormalities (Goldfischer and Sternlieb, 1968).

The diagnosis of Wilson's disease can often be made by the pathognomonic Kayser-Fleischer ring in the cornea. Strongly confirmatory evidence includes: a low serum copper, low serum ceruloplasmin and increased excretion of copper in the urine. Spectrographic analysis of a needle biopsy of the liver will disclose abnormal deposits of copper here. In this particular disease, an early diagnosis before damage has already developed in the liver

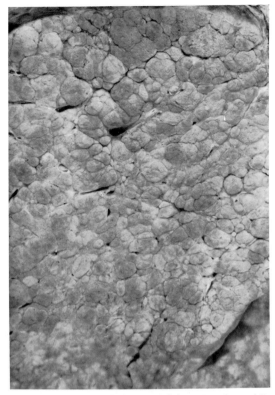

Figure 22–46. *A close-up of the cut surface of the nodular cirrhotic liver of Wilson's disease.*

and brain can be lifesaving, since it has been shown that treatment with chelating agents and penicillamine will control the accumulation of excess amounts of copper and protect these patients from subsequent damage.

In any collection of cirrhoses of the liver, as many as 20 to 25 per cent will conform to none of the previously described morphologic or pathogenetic categories. The temptation is to discern suggestive findings and thus to assign these cases to one or another of the better characterized entities. However, it may be wiser to retain a wastebasket designation of *indeterminate or cryptogenic cirrhosis* as a reminder of the mysteries shrouding the genesis of scarring of the liver. It is entirely possible that these indeterminate cases reflect multiple causes of liver injury, for example, the concurrence of alcohol abuse and chronic viral hepatitis or other such combinations.

THE BILIARY SYSTEM

NORMAL

The extrahepatic biliary system—the gall-bladder and the extrahepatic bile ducts—maintains a direct connection between the liver and the gastrointestinal tract and thus serves as an essential link in the enterohepatic circulation. The ducts passively transfer bile from the liver to the duodenum directly or via the gallbladder. The gallbladder is not vital for life and, in its absence, man thrives and usually suffers no physiologic disturbance.

In the adult, the gallbladder is a conical, musculomembranous sac lying in a fossa in the under surface of the right lobe of the liver. It is divided into three regions: (1) the fundus, the hemispheric blind end which is most inferior; (2) the body, the portion between the fundus and the neck; and (3) the neck, a narrow tube-like structure which tapers into the cystic duct. The relaxed gallbladder measures 7 to 10 cm. in length and 2 to 3 cm. in width, and has a capacity of 30 to 50 cc. From each lobe of the liver, a hepatic duct emerges. These soon unite to form the common hepatic duct which passes between the two layers of the lesser omentum for about 4 cm. It is joined at an acute angle by the cystic duct to create the common bile duct, having an approximate diameter of 0.5 to 0.7 cm. This normal value is of some importance because the question of dilatation of this duct often arises in certain disease states. The common bile duct empties into the second portion of the duodenum through a small dilatation (the ampulla of Vater). In approximately 60 to 70 per cent of persons, the pancreatic duct joins with the common bile duct to drain through a common orifice in the ampulla of Vater. In the remainder of individuals, the ducts enter separately. These anatomic details are of some interest in the pathogenesis of acute cholecystitis and pancreatic necrosis (p. 1061). The ampullary orifice in the duodenum is marked by a 0.7 to 1 cm. hemispheric protrusion of the duodenal mucosa known as the papilla of Vater.

Histologically, the gallbladder wall has four distinct layers: (1) The mucosa of the gallbladder is formed of a single layer of tall columnar cells that are thrown up into nu-merous, interlacing, tiny folds creating a honeycombed surface to the mucosa. Simple tubuloalveolar, mucus-secreting glands are present only in the neck while the body and fundus have none. Similar lining epithelium and glands are found throughout the major extrahepatic biliary ducts. The mucosa of the gallbladder neck is thrown into a varying number of crescentic folds forming the spiral valves of Heister. The mucosal columnar epithelium of the gallbladder and ducts is based upon a delicate connective tissue stroma, but there is no well developed submucosa in the gallbladder, a feature differentiating the gallbladder from the intestines histologically. (2) Beneath the mucosa is a fibromuscular layer composed of smooth muscle cells and elastic fibrils. This layer provides contractility to the gallbladder. (3) A perimuscular layer of connective tissue and elastic fibers, often sparsely infiltrated with lymphocytes, is interposed between the muscular wall and the outer wall of the gallbladder. (4) A serous peritoneal layer covers all but the bare area of the hepatic bed.

Two common histologic variants merit mention here. These variants are so common as to virtually constitute normal details. Small duct-like structures (ducts of Luschka), lined by typical epithelial cells, are often found in the perimuscular connective tissue layer (Fig. 22-47). These do not communicate with the lumen, but are occasionally connected with the bile ducts and are assumed to represent aberrant supernumerary ducts. As sites for the inspissation of bile and stasis of bacteria and debris, they may contribute to the genesis of inflammatory disease. *Rokitansky-Aschoff sinuses* are small outpouchings of the mucosa of the gallbladder that extend into the underlying connective tissue and sometimes into the muscular layer. These obviously communicate directly with the lumen of the gallbladder. They are lined by typical columnar epithelium and are occasionally found in normal and often in diseased gallbladders (Fig. 22-48). Their higher incidence in inflamed gallbladders raises the possibility that preexisting injury to the wall may predispose to their development. However, their infrequent occurrence in com-

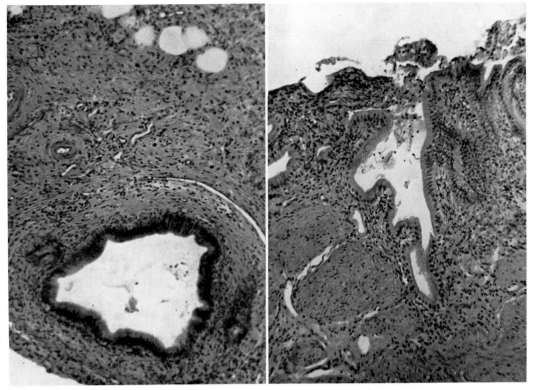

Fig. 22–47.   Fig. 22–48.

Figure 22–47. *Duct of Luschka deep within wall close to serosa.*
Figure 22–48. *Rokitansky-Aschoff sinus in an inflamed gallbladder.*

pletely normal gallbladders suggests that they may also represent a minor deviation from the norm—possibly attributable to the herniation of the mucosa through minute points of muscular weakness.

The blood supply to the extrahepatic biliary system is derived from the hepatic artery, the arterial branch to the gallbladder being known as a cystic artery. Many variable patterns of arterial supply are encountered that are of principal interest to the surgeon.

The extrahepatic biliary system has two principal functions: storage and concentration of bile and the delivery of bile to the duodenum. Bile, as it is secreted by the liver, contains water, cholesterol, bile salts, bile acids, bilirubin, lecithin in micellar complexes, inorganic ions and mucoproteins secreted by the epithelium of the biliary tract. The bile salts (sodium salts of taurocholic and glycocholic acids) aid in maintaining cholesterol in solution. As secreted by the liver, bile is composed of about 3 per cent solids, the remainder being water. One of the principal functions of the gallbladder is the concentration of this bile by selective absorption of water, inorganic ions,

and small amounts of bile salts to a volume possibly five to 10 times smaller than the original hepatic secretion. Cholesterol is not significantly reabsorbed in the gallbladder.

The delivery of bile to the duodenum involves mechanisms that are still somewhat controversial. The sphincter of Oddi or some sphincteric mechanism (since there is doubt about the existence of an anatomic sphincter) is usually closed except when fatty food enters the duodenum and bile is thus diverted into the gallbladder. Contraction and partial emptying of the gallbladder occurs when foods, especially fatty ones, or other stimulants enter the duodenum. This gallbladder activity is probably mediated through a hormone, cholecystokinin, which is released from the duodenum into the blood. At the same time, the sphincter of Oddi is relaxed, thereby facilitating the passage of concentrated bile into the duodenum. There is persistent question as to whether the gallbladder actually contracts or merely selectively resorbs. It is possible that the diminution in size that can be visualized radiographically may, in fact, be due to rapid reabsorption, but most evidence favors a definite motor contraction. It is estimated that the gallbladder is capable of resorbing half its volume within one hour.

The remarkable resorptive capacity of the gallbladder provides the basis for the radiographic diagnostic technique of cholecystography, the so-called *Graham-Cole test*. A variety of radiopaque substances, when taken by mouth or administered intravenously, are taken up by the liver and excreted in the bile and so reach the gallbladder. Since they are not resorbed by the gallbladder, they become concentrated as the water in the bile is resorbed. Thus, levels are achieved which are readily visualized roentgenographically. In this way, the outline of the gallbladder can be seen on x-ray, and the normal contractile response of the gallbladder to a fatty meal can be visualized. This diagnostic procedure sometimes also discloses the presence of radiolucent gallstones, seen as "holes" in the radiopaque shadow representing the gallbladder lumen.

PATHOLOGY

Diseases of the gallbladder loom large in clinical practice and in pathologic specimens. Inflammations of the gallbladder comprise the second most common cause (next to appendicitis) of abdominal pain and abdominal surgery. Frequently, the formation of stones within the gallbladder (cholelithiasis) accompanies this gallbladder inflammation and, at times, may be responsible for obstruction of the common duct, leading to such serious sequelae as obstructive jaundice and biliary cirrhosis. Neoplasms in the gallbladder and extrahepatic biliary ducts are relatively common and are invariably extremely serious, because most are malignant and are often totally asymptomatic until they have either extended into the liver or caused serious ductal obstruction. Congenital anomalies also merit consideration because of their importance in surgery on the biliary tract.

CONGENITAL ANOMALIES

Developmental anomalies of the gallbladder and bile ducts take many forms and are of varied clinical significance. Most are chiefly of interest to the surgeon and embryologist and do not affect the patient's health. A few, to be mentioned below, have clinical importance. With respect to the gallbladder, there may be complete *agenesis, hypoplasia, hyperplasia, total reduplication* to form a double gallbladder, or

subtotal division of the fundus and body to create a *bilobed* structure. The gallbladder may be abnormally located within the left lobe, is sometimes totally embedded within the liver substance *(intrahepatic)* or, at other times, is described as a *floating gallbladder,* having a long pendulous mesentery. Angulation, kinking or a circumferential constriction of the body of the gallbladder gives rise to an apparently expanded bulbous end to the fundus, known as a *phrygian cap.* The bile ducts frequently do not conform to the classic anatomic form and have a variety of anomalous connections and patterns, the most important of which are total *agenesis of all or any portion of the hepatic or common bile ducts,* or *atresic narrowing* of these channels. Agenesis, or severe stenosis, is incompatible with life and is usually discovered shortly after birth by the progressive development of jaundice. Unless it is surgically corrected, death ensues within months to years.

CHOLELITHIASIS

The development of calculi or gallstones in the biliary tract is called cholelithiasis. Almost all form in the gallbladder, but occasionally stone formation may occur within the major bile ducts or liver. They are composed of three constituents of the bile: cholesterol (cholesterol stones), calcium bilirubinate (pigment stones) and calcium carbonate (calcium carbonate stones). Most stones contain either bilirubin or cholesterol. The former are usually pure concretions of bile pigment, the latter are most often mixtures of cholesterol with pigment and carbonates, although sometimes pure cholesterol stones are found. Pure calcium carbonate stones are very rare. Gallstones, whatever their composition, are commonly found in chronically inflamed gallbladders. Which comes first, the stones or the inflammation, is a time-hallowed problem. As will soon be discussed, the evidence now favors the view that gallstones may be formed in the absence of inflammation of the gallbladder and, indeed, the same influences leading to their formation may also contribute to the inflammatory changes in the gallbladder wall.

Incidence. In the United States, about 10 to 20 per cent of the adult population harbors gallstones. They are rare in the first two decades of life, but the prevalence progressively increases to reach a peak in the sixth and seventh decades. Women are affected far more often than men in a ratio of 4 to 1, reflecting, in some part, the predisposition to stone formation during pregnancy. The population with the highest incidence of gallstones can be characterized by the four "F's": female, fat, fertile (multiparous) and forty. For obscure reasons, blacks are less frequently affected than whites. There is a predisposition to cholelithiasis in diabetes mellitus and in anemias characterized by abnormal hemolysis and increased production of bilirubin pigment, i.e., the hemolytic anemias and pernicious anemia.

Pathogenesis and Types of Stones. Here we enter an arena of controversy. The pathogenesis of the stones varies with their composition. Nonetheless, *for all forms, three factors are important: (1) abnormalities in the composition of the bile, (2) stasis and (3) infection.* It has been exceedingly difficult to segregate the contribution of each of these factors because one, in time, introduces the others.

Currently, it is believed that *abnormalities of the bile — either an absolute or relative increase in one of the constitutents —* is the most important factor in stone formation (Small, 1968, 1970). Pigment stones are usually encountered in patients with hemolytic anemia or some other cause of destruction of red blood cells. In these disorders, there is increased breakdown of hemoblogin, and the excess of bile pigment excreted in the bile precipitates to form pigment stones. For stones containing cholesterol, whether pure or mixed, there is now substantial evidence that in most patients the *bile becomes supersaturated with cholesterol because of the elaboration of an abnormal bile by the liver.* The levels of bile salts and lecithin relative to the cholesterol content are extremely critical (Carey and Small, 1972). Cholesterol is, of course, water-insoluble. It is maintained in solution by the creation of micelles having a central core of cholesterol surrounded by a hydrophilic shell made up of bile salts and lecithin. Theoretically, then, in this system an increase in cholesterol concentration or a decrease in bile salts or lecithin could lead to instability of micelles and to precipitation of cholesterol (Juniper, 1965). Although Small (1972) has described a number of pathways by which cholesterol may accumulate in the bile, the most important involve the elaboration of an abnormal bile by the liver (Small, in press). Thus, for cholesterol-containing stones, the liver, not the gallbladder, appears to be responsible in most instances for producing a bile having too high a content of cholesterol to be maintained in micellar solution by the bile salts and lecithin. Stones are formed, therefore, by the precipitation of crystals out of an unstable solution, followed by progressive accretion of more stone-forming substances or by the sticking together of individual crystals.

The *roles of inflammation and infection* are probably not as important as abnormalities in the composition of the bile. Certainly, cholelithiasis occurs in the absence of bacterial infection. However, in most of these gallbladders, some element of inflammation can be found. It is doubtful that such cholecystitis is always bacterial in origin. Rather, the evidence points to chemical irritation secondary to the alteration in the composition of the bile, such as high levels of bile salts or bile acids. Secondary invasion by bacteria may then ensue. However, in some patients, it is entirely possible that a primary infection alters the normal resorptive function of the gallbladder wall and thereby leads to instability of the bile. The pathologic gallbladder may resorb excessive amounts of bile salts, leaving the cholesterol in excess. This pathogenetic mechanism probably accounts for only a small fraction of cholesterol stone formation. Bacteria might also serve as a nidus for the precipitation or accretion of bile constituents. Similarly, inflammatory necrosis of the gallbladder lining could provide additional foreign bodies. If necrotic debris, bacteria and nidus formation were important, however, it would hardly explain the frequent finding of families of stones within a gallbladder, all having virtually identical size and composition, strongly suggesting some episode of supersaturation rather than random seeding.

Stasis, such as might result from obstruction of the outflow tract at any level within the cystic or common duct, could have several effects. It would predispose to bacterial infection and favor increased resorption of water. Concentration of the bile might then permit the accumulation of mucoproteins from the bile duct epithelium. Any one of these events might alter the stability of the bile. Stasis might also favor selective resorption of one or the other constituents of bile thus leading to the imbalance mentioned earlier. An earlier comment might now be clearer; it is impossible to determine whether abnormalities in the compostion of the bile, inflammation or stasis is most fundamental to stone formation because all three influences so frequently coexist.

PURE STONES

Cholesterol Stones. Approximately 10 per cent of all gallstones are pure composition, cholesterol being the commonest type. Cholesterol stones usually occur singly, varying in size up to egg-shaped structures 5 to 6 cm. in greatest dimension. Smaller stones are more often spherical. They have a gray-yellow translucency and, when small, have an obvious crystalline external appearance. As they get larger, and perhaps polished in the gallbladder, they develop a smooth, egg-shell surface. However, when transected, a glistening, crystalline, radiating palisade becomes evident (Fig. 22–49). In some instances, gallbladders containing such stones develop cholesterolosis (p. 1047). As will be evident later, the pure cholesterol stone may become overlaid by other constituents of the bile, principally calcium carbonate. Patients developing cholesterol stones do not usually have hypercholesterolemia. Instead, the formation of these stones appears to result from local influences, i.e., the elaboration of an abnormal bile by the liver, leading to an imbalance between the levels of cholesterol and those constituents important in maintaining it in solution, i.e., bile salts and lecithin.

Calcium Bilirubinate Stones. These are less common than the pure cholesterol stones and are principally encountered in diseases characterized by excessive production of bilirubin, principally the hemolytic anemias and pernicious anemia. Other causes of hemolysis, such as infections (malaria) or chemical toxicity, may also lead to the formation of these stones. They almost invariably take the form of multiple jet black jackstones, ranging from 0.5 to 1 cm. in greatest diameter. Classically, all stones within a gallbaldder will be very similar in size, suggesting a similar age and a single event which initiated the formation of all of them. They almost never occur singly. Their genesis appears to reside entirely

in increased levels of bilirubin to the point of supersaturation of the bile.

Calcium Carbonate Stones. This is the rarest type encountered. These appear gray-white with smooth, usually articulated surfaces, as adjacent stones wear off abutting surfaces. Calcium is not a major constituent of the bile, and the source of the mineral salts making up these calculi is poorly understood. Conceivably, some cause for increased alkalinity of the bile might favor the precipitation of calcium carbonate, with the slow build-up of stones over the course of years. They generally vary in size from sand-like grains to faceted polyhedral shapes up to 2 cm. in diameter.

MIXED AND COMBINED GALLSTONES

These gallstones account for approximately 90 per cent of all biliary calculi in surgically removed gallbladders. The term *mixed gallstones* refers to those having varying proportions of all three of the stone-forming constituents of the bile. In contrast, *combined gallstones* refers to those in which either the central core or external layers are pure, and the remainder of the stone is a mixture of constituents. One could deduce that combined stones would result from intervals in the life of

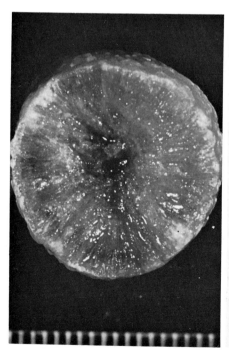

Fig. 22–49.

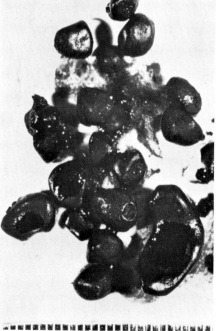

Fig. 22–50.

Figure 22–49. *Cholesterol stone transected, showing translucence and radial crystalline pattern.*
Figure 22–50. *Mixed pigment stones.*

the patient which favor the formation of pure gallstones, with other intervals creating opportunities for mixed gallstone formation. Mixed gallstones almost invariably occur in great profusion within the individual gallbladder. In contrast, combined stones are sometimes solitary. When one encounters a gallbladder literally stuffed with hundreds of stones, it is almost certain that they are of the mixed variety. They vary in size up to 2 cm. in diameter, and there is usually great variation in the size of the stones. Their appearance and structure depend, of course, on which of the stone-forming constituents predominates. As might be anticipated, bilirubinate is black, cholesterol is yellow and calcium carbonate is gray-white (Fig. 22–50). While frequently articulated, some have a mulberry external contour and others are totally grotesque. It is the mixed stones which are so frequently associated with cholecystitis. The view is favored that imbalances in the composition of the bile lead not only to the formation of stones but also to the inflammation of the gallbladder. In about half of the cases, however, bacteria can be cultured from these gallbladders. Presumably, the chemical inflammatory changes prepare the soil for bacterial invasion.

Clinical Implications. In perhaps 80 per cent of the cases, gallstones remain within the gallbladder and evoke no clinical manifestations if they are not associated with active cholecystitis. They may, however, be much more invidious and produce a variety of clinical problems. Paradoxically, larger calculi, too big to enter the cystic duct, are more harmless than their smaller counterparts. The most serious consequence of calculous disease of the gallbladder is obstruction of the cystic duct or, worse, of the common bile duct. Once within the ductal system, or even in the neck of the gallbladder, they may give rise to severe biliary colic, resulting apparently from spastic, episodic contraction of the musculature. Complete blockage of the cystic duct leads, in time, to so-called *hydrops of the gallbladder* (p. 1048). Common duct stones may, of course, cause obstructive jaundice. One of the most difficult and serious clinical dilemmas is the differentiation of jaundice due to obstructive disease, i.e., gallstones or cancer (in the head of the pancreas, bile ducts, ampulla of Vater) from that caused by hepatocellular disease. Obviously, to permit a stone to cause fatal obstructive jaundice would be a dire tragedy. On the other hand, to perform a surgical laparotomy in an extremely ill, jaundiced, hypoprothrombinemic patient having acute liver disease is no step to be taken lightly. Perhaps no less critical is the differentiation of calculous biliary tract obstruc-

tion from neoplastic obstruction. In this situation, *"Courvoisier's law"* (unfortunately marked by many exceptions) may be of some help. In calculous obstruction, the gallbladder is often not distended and may even be smaller than normal, presumably because such gallbladders frequently are fibrotic from concurrent chronic cholecystitis. In contrast, neoplastic obstruction of the common duct is more likely to be unassociated with chronic cholecystitis, and so the continued formation of bile within the liver leads to distention of the gallbladder. Satisfying as this postulate may sound, its unreliability generally dictates the need to explore such patients surgically, in the hope of finding a readily curable cause for the biliary obstruction, namely, an impacted gallstone.

Calculous obstruction of the cystic or common bile ducts predisposes to bacterial infection, either in the gallbladder or in the ductal system (cholangitis). Presumably stasis, distention of the biliary system, impaired lymphatic drainage and vascular supply, and chemical irritation are all operative factors here. The cholangitis or cholecystitis may spread upward (ascending cholangitis and cholangiolitis) to produce widespread involvement of the intrahepatic bile ducts and portal traids. Thus, calculous disease may lead to either a purely obstructive or infectious biliary cirrhosis or one in which both influences contribute.

Rarely, when gallstones are present along with acute inflammatory disease of the gallbladder, the stone may erode through the gallbladder wall and adherent intestinal loops to create cholecystointestinal fistulas. Most such stones pass unnoticed through the alimentary tract. But under extraordinary circumstances, exceedingly large ones may impact at points of narrowing, usually at the ileocecal valve, to produce intestinal obstruction—so-called *gallstone ileus*.

Whether gallstones play a causal role in the development of carcinoma of the gallbladder is one of the oldest controversies in medicine. Autopsy studies indicate that there is a high incidence of stones (65 to 95 per cent) in cancerous gallbladders. The association, however, between these two diseases does not indicate which is primary and which is secondary, and it would seem equally plausible that abnormal cancerous gallbladders might favor stone formation. Nonetheless, surgeons are wont to recall a patient with known asymptomatic cholelithiasis for many years, who later developed a carcinoma of the gallbladder. Even more controversial is the role of gallstones in the production of cholecystitis, an issue which has been discussed in the preceding paragraphs. It suffices to say that current opinion favors the view that it is not the stones which induce the inflammation but, rather, the abnormalities in the constitution of the bile which excite not only stone formation but also a chemical cholecystitis, providing a fertile soil for bacterial seeding. Because of these controversies, there is still no agreement on the treatment of patients with "silent gallstones." All would agree that symptomatic stones are a justifiable indication for cholecystectomy but, when the patient is asymptomatic and the stones are discovered incidentally, surgeons are wont to operate, while many internists prefer a "wait and see" policy. Before concluding the controversial issues relating to calculous disease, mention should be made of the possible role of stones within the common duct in the production of pancreatitis, as discussed on p. 1061.

CHOLECYSTITIS

Inflammation of the gallbladder, cholecystitis, may be acute or chronic. Often the acute response is subdivided on the basis of the severity of the inflammatory response into acute, suppurative and gangrenous cholecystitis. Sometimes the acute cholecystitis is superimposed on a preexisting chronic cholecystitis. These inflammations, which are essentially varying stages of a single inflammatory disease, are extremely common and, as mentioned, are second only to appendicitis as causes for abdominal laparotomies.

Incidence. The prevalence of cholecystitis as reported in the literature is extremely variable because of the differing criteria used in establishing this diagnosis. In some reported series, gallstones alone are interpreted as evidence of cholecystitis. Other investigators demand evidence of inflammatory exudation or chronic fibrosis in the wall to establish the diagnosis. Thus, the condition is cited as occurring in 70 per cent of all adults or, when more rigid criteria are used, in less than half of all adults. These data are, however, derived from autopsy studies, and many of these lesions are incidental findings without clinical significance. Though found in all age groups, cholecystitis does not occur in significant numbers until the mid-thirties, and reaches a peak in the fifth and sixth decades of life. Females are affected about three times as often as males. Because obesity is a common accompaniment of cholecystitis, the classic clinical pattern is well characterized by the adage, "female, fat, forty and fertile."

Etiology and Pathogenesis. Not long ago, acute cholecystitis was regarded by most investigators as a primary bacterial infection of the gallbladder. Considerable recent evidence, however, casts some doubt on this simplified version (Womack and Bricker, 1942). *Three factors are probably important: chemical irritation by concentrated bile, bacterial infection and pancreatic reflux,* given in the order of importance. The theory of *primary chemical inflammation* is supported by the fact that the morphologic changes in early acute cholecystitis are not those of a classic infection and, moreover, cultures are negative in approximately 25 per cent of cases. It is fairly widely accepted that obstruction, partial or complete, of the outflow of bile creates the appropriate conditions for progressive concentration of bile and chemical irritation of the gallbladder wall. Stones obstructing the cystic duct can be implicated in up to 80 per cent of the cases of acute cholecystitis. Even in the absence of stones at surgery or autopsy, their obstructive role cannot be excluded, since they may have passed into the gastrointestinal tract and, moreover, kinking of the gallbladder or ducts and pressure from anomalous vessels and from adjacent structures may serve to explain noncalculous obstruction. Experimental reproduction of acute cholecystitis has been effected by injecting concentrated bile into the obstructed gallbladder.

Venous or lymphatic stasis may play a contributory role in these chemical irritations, since it is entirely possible that impaction of a stone or extrinsic pressures may interfere with the blood supply of the gallbladder and predispose to the acute inflammatory reaction. Once chemically injured, however, these gallbladders are prone to develop secondary bacterial infections, and bacteria are present in up to 75 per cent of the cases of acute cholecystitis and in 30 per cent of cases of chronic cholecystitis.

In the minority of cases (5 to 10 per cent) in which evidence for *bacterial infection* as the initiating etiologic agent is strong, there is usually some concomitant severe infection elsewhere or septicemia. Bacteria may reach the gallbladder via the blood, lymphatics (particularly from the liver) or bile ducts, or by direct extension from neighboring organs. The most common offending microorganisms are the staphylococci, enterococci and the gram-negative rods.

The role of *pancreatic reflux* as a possible etiologic mechanism has been well established, but the frequency with which this reflux assumes importance in the clinical problem is not certain. Experimentally, the injection of pancreatic enzymes excites a definite inflammatory response. Moreover, active lipases, amylases and proteases can be identified in the bile of a few cases of acute cholecystitis in man.

The evolution of *chronic cholecystitis* is very obscure, but only rarely is it preceded by a well defined bout of acute cholecystitis. Much of the difficulty stems from the lack of criteria for distinguishing between a true chronic inflammatory disease of the gallbladder and the vague, atrophic, fibrotic changes—so-called wear and tear—which are inevitable accompaniments of aging. All too often, slight fibrosis of the gallbladder wall, especially when accompanied by cholelithiasis, is automatically interpreted as chronic cholecystitis. While true chronic inflammatory reactions undoubtedly occur and may be related to the same factors which cause acute cholecystitis, in only 30 per cent of the cases can bacterial infection be identified in such surgically removed gallbladders. Although gallstones are encountered in perhaps 90 per cent of these cases, it is doubtful that the gallstones play a direct role in inducing the alterations in the gallbladder wall. If there is any relationship between the stones and the inflammatory disease, it more likely lies in abnormalities in bile predisposing to both.

In **acute cholecystitis**, the gallbladder is usually enlarged (two- to threefold) and tense, and often assumes a bright red or a blotchy, violaceous to green-black discoloration, imparted by subserosal hemorrhages. The serosal covering is frequently layered by fibrin and, in the very intense reaction, by a definite suppurative, coagulated exudate. On being opened, the lumen is tensely filled with a cloudy or turbid bile that may contain large amounts of fibrin and frank pus, as well as hemorrhage. When the contained exudate is virtually pure pus, the condition is referred to as **empyema of the gallbladder.** Gallstones are present in up to 80 per cent of these cases, and often a fine, sandy gravel is mixed in with the contained biliary contents. The gallbladder wall is thickened up to 10 times the normal and has a rubbery, yielding consistency. Edema fluid, exudate and hemorrhage flow out from the cut surface. The mucosa may be merely patchily or totally hyperemic in the milder cases, transformed to a green-black necrotic surface in the more severe cases (**gangrenous cholecystitis**), or may have small to large ulcerations which may penetrate the wall to give rise to pericholecystic abscesses or generalized peritonitis (Hallendorf et al., 1948).

Histologically, the inflammatory reactions are not distinctive and consist of the usual patterns of acute inflammation, i.e., edema, leukocytic infiltration, vascular congestion, frank abscess formation or gangrenous necrosis, when vascular stasis complicates the edematous inflammatory response. As mentioned earlier, based upon the severity of the inflammatory reaction and the possible presence of vascular stasis, these acute reactions are divided into acute cholecystitis, suppurative cholecystitis and acute gangrenous cholecystitis (Fig. 22–51).

The inflammatory reaction may subside and the neutrophils then are replaced by eosinophils to comprise the diagnostic features of subacute cholecystitis. Alternatively, in other cases, the deposition of calcium within the gallbladder wall gives rise to the so-called calcified gallbladder or **porcelain gallbladder**. In an unknown number of instances, the subsidence of the acute response leads to chronic cholecystitis.

The morphologic features of **chronic cholecystitis** are quite variable. The gallbladder may be contracted, normal in size or enlarged. The size of the organ depends upon the balance between the development of fibrosis in the wall and the element of obstruction in the genesis of the inflammation. The serosa is usually smooth and glistening, but oftentimes it is dulled by subserosal fibrosis. In other instances, dense fibrous adhesions may remain as sequelae of preexistent acute inflammation. On section, the wall is variably thickened, rarely to more than five times normal. It has an opaque gray-white cut section and may be less flexible and translucent than normal. In the uncomplicated case of cholecystitis, the lumen usually contains fairly clear, green-yellow, mucoid bile. Stones are present in up to 90 per cent, depending upon the criteria used in establishing the diagnosis of chronic cholecystitis (Fig.

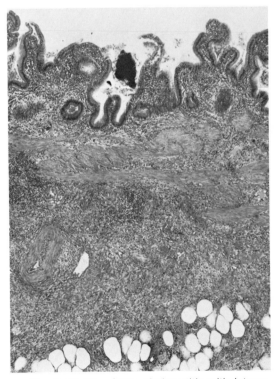

Figure 22–51. *Acute cholecystitis with intense leukocytic infiltration of wall throughout all layers.*

22–52). The mucosa itself is usually preserved and has no loss of the usual mucosal folds that create the normal honeycombed pattern. In other instances, when the lumen of the gallbladder is partially or totally obstructed, the gallbladder contents may be under sufficient pressure to cause flattening of the mucosal folds and thinning and atrophy of the mucosa.

Histologically, the degree of inflammatory reaction is quite variable. In the mildest cases, only scattered lymphocytes, plasma cells and macrophages are found beneath the columnar lining epithelium and in the subserosal fibrous tissue. In the better developed cases, there is some increase of fibrous tissue subepithelially and subserosally, accompanied by a mononuclear cell infiltration (Fig. 22–53). In the more extreme instances, the wall may be permeated by fibrous scar, with considerable obliteration of the smooth musculature. Rokitansky-Aschoff sinuses are found in up to 90 per cent of these chronically inflamed gallbladders, presumably because the inflammatory damage to the wall predisposes to the herniation of the lining epithelium. Inflammatory proliferation of the mucosa and fusion of the mucosal folds may give rise to buried crypts of epithelium within the gallbladder wall, designated as **cholecystitis glandularis.**

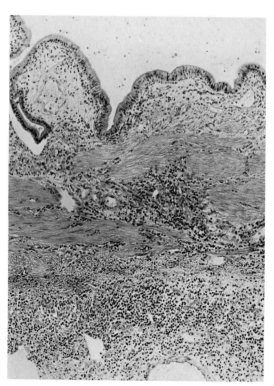

Figure 22–53. Chronic cholecystitis with increased subepithelial fibrosis and marked leukocytic infiltration. The mucosal folds are somewhat flattened.

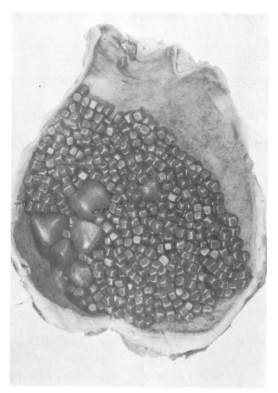

Figure 22–52. Chronic cholecystitis with cholelithiasis. The gallbladder wall is thickened, but the mucosa is intact.

Not infrequently, the anatomic changes of acute cholecystitis are superimposed upon the chronic changes just described, implying acute exacerbation of a previously chronically injured gallbladder.

Clinical Course. Acute cholecystitis usually presents as an acute abdominal emergency, with right upper quadrant pain that is often referred to the right shoulder, when the inflammatory exudate treks up beneath the diaphragm to cause irritation of the phrenic nerve. Fever, nausea, vomiting, leukocytosis, rigidity of the abdominal wall, especially in the right upper quadrant, and palpable gallbladder are the outstanding features. Jaundice is found in up to 25 per cent of the cases, but is usually not severe. The management of these acute cases is a controversial surgical problem in which the decision whether to operate upon the patient during the height of the attack hangs upon the question of whether the acute reaction will promptly begin to subside, permitting surgery to be carried on at a later date under more appropriate conditions, or whether the increasing exudation within the gallbladder lumen and destruction of the gallbladder wall will lead to perforation. The complications of the acute attack, i.e., pericholecystic abscesses due to permeation of the infection or perforation of the gallbladder, generalized peritonitis, ascending cholangitis, liver abscesses, subdiaphragmatic abscesses and septicemia, are more hazardous than the disease itself.

Chronic cholecystitis is a vague, insidious disorder. It usually manifests itself by intolerance to fatty foods, belching, postcibal epigastric distress, nausea or vomiting. Many times it is called to attention by biliary colic due to the gallstones which so frequently accompany this inflammatory state. The differential diagnosis of chronic cholecystitis must include peptic ulcer, esophageal hiatal hernia, appendicitis, myocardial infarction, pleuritis and renal stones. The diagnosis is usually only established by cholecystography that discloses either a malfunctioning gallbladder or the presence of stones. Two of the most feared but infrequent complications of chronic cholecystitis and cholelithiasis are the development of car-

cinoma of the gallbladder, previously discussed, or the passage of an associated gallstone into the common duct, with resultant biliary tract obstruction.

CHOLESTEROLOSIS

Cholesterolosis is also commonly designated as a "strawberry" gallbladder, because the focal deposits of lipid in the epithelium and subepithelial region of the gallbladder evoke a similarity to the pale yellow-gray seeds that punctuate the surface of a strawberry (Feldman and Feldman, 1954). Although this condition afflicts approximately 10 per cent of the general autopsy population, cholesterolosis rarely causes clinical symptoms and, therefore, is not of great clinical significance. It does not, as far as we know, predispose to cholecystitis.

This condition apparently represents a local disturbance in cholesterol metabolism and is not associated with any derangement in

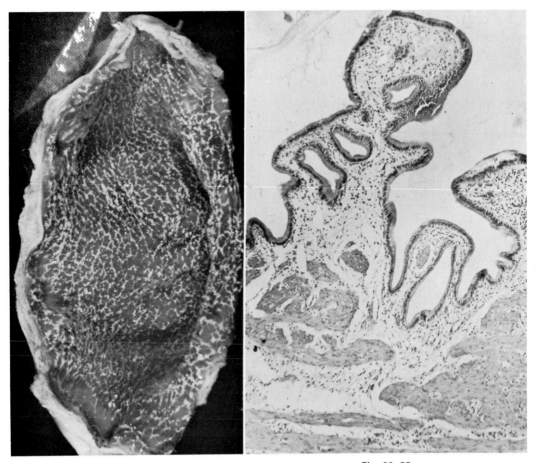

Fig. 22–54.   Fig. 22–55.

Figure 22–54. *Cholesterolosis. The typical flecking of a "strawberry" gallbladder.*
Figure 22–55. *Cholesterolosis. The mucosal folds are expanded at their tips by aggregates of lipid-laden histiocytes.*

the blood levels of cholesterol. There is wide disagreement as to the mechanisms by which the cholesterol becomes deposited in the gall-bladder wall. Some investigators propose that it is essentially due to an excessive abnormal absorption of cholesterol from the bile by the epithelial cells of the gallbladder wall. Alternatively, it is proposed that local lymphatic and venous stasis predisposes to the accumulation of cholesterol absorbed from the bile contents. Others maintain that there is failure of the mucosa to secrete cholesterol, resulting in abnormal accumulation within the mucosa and submucosa. Whatever the mechanism, the *mucosa of the gallbladder is studded with minute yellow flecks,* imparting the strawberry appearance (Fig. 22–54). Usually, the intervening mucosa is yellow-green and intact but, occasionally, accompanying cholecystitis modifies the macroscopic appearance.

Histologically, the diagnostic features are *enlargement and distention of the mucosal folds into club shapes with aggregations of round to polyhedral*

histiocytes within these clubbed ends (Fig. 22–55). These cells have a foamy, reticulated, fat-laden cytoplasm and small, round, darkly prominent nuclei. When the deposit becomes more massive, these cells may die, and the release of lipids gives rise to the precipitation of cholesterol crystals in the subepithelial region and a subsequent inflammatory reaction of white cells, giant cells and fibroblasts. This inflammatory pattern is, however, quite uncommon. It is not known whether the process is reversible, since it is asymptomatic and is only discovered incidentally at surgery or postmortem. When symptoms are present, they are usually due to accompanying cholecystitis.

HYDROPS OF THE GALLBLADDER

Hydrops of the gallbladder is also known as *mucocele* of the gallbladder, referring to *distention of the gallbladder by a clear, watery, mucinous secretion.* This condition may occur in a

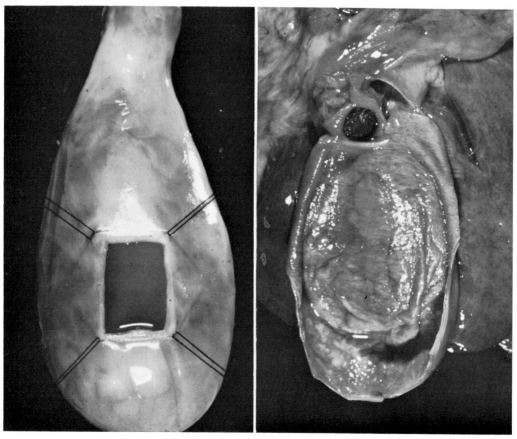

Fig. 22–56.

Fig. 22–57.

Figure 22–56. *Hydrops of the gallbladder. A window has been cut out to reveal the clear, translucent, mucoid contents.*

Figure 22–57. *Hydrops of the gallbladder caused by a stone impacted in the cystic neck. The mucosa is atrophic and replaced by a glazed, shiny surface.*

normal or previously inflamed gallbladder and is invariably due to total obstruction of the cystic duct. Presumably, the trapped bile is resorbed and the gallbladder becomes filled with a clear, mucinous secretion derived from the gallbladder wall. Anatomically, the gallbladder is usually tense and enlarged, and has a translucent appearance before being opened. The serosa is usually not involved; the wall is not thickened and, in fact, is often quite thin. On opening the gallbladder, the clear mucinous contents disclose the nature of the condition (Fig. 22–56). Stones may, of course, be present but are not intrinsic to the hydrops. When the condition is longstanding, the mucosa of the wall becomes atrophic or thinned out and the lining may have a pale gray-red, smooth, glazed surface.

Histologically, depending upon the severity of the condition, there is more or less atrophy of the epithelium so that, in far advanced cases, no columnar or flattened cuboidal epithelial cells are present, and the wall of the gallbladder is composed only of an inner layer of connective tissue surrounded by the usual muscularis and other layers. As mentioned earlier, a prominent anatomic feature is the demonstration of the underlying cause for the cystic obstruction, most often a stone, but less frequently neoplasia within the cystic duct or kinking of the duct (Fig. 22–57). The condition is usually asymptomatic, but occasionally there are manifestations of epigastric pain, discomfort, nausea, vomiting and other features suggestive of nonspecific cholecystitis. No serious clinical sequelae attend this lesion and, following operative removal, the condition is cured.

TUMORS

Tumors of the biliary system range from benign to malignant and occur in all possible sites within the ducts and gallbladder (Babcock and Eyerly, 1957). Although fibromas, myomas, neuromas, hemangiomas and the malignant counterparts of these lesions as well as carcinoids have been described in these organs, the only neoplasms of sufficient frequency and clinical importance to merit description are the papilloma, adenoma and adenomyoma of the gallbladder, carcinoma of the gallbladder and carcinoma of the bile ducts (including carcinoma of the papilla of Vater).

PAPILLOMA, ADENOMA AND ADENOMYOMA OF THE GALLBLADDER

Papillomas and adenomas of the gallbladder are very infrequent, benign epithelial tumors (Shepard et al., 1942). They both represent localized overgrowths of the lining epithelium, the papilloma growing as a pedunculated, complex, branching structure and the adenoma as a flat, sessile thickening. While these lesions are small and easily missed unless careful inspection is carried out, there is a greater tendency to overdiagnose these conditions, since inflammatory hyperplasia or edema of the wall may create local projections that are often interpreted as benign neoplasms. The papilloma may occur singly or multiply as small, branching, pedunculated masses less than 1 cm. in diameter, that project into the lumen of the gallbladder. They are usually connected to the underlying wall by a slender stalk. In contrast, the adenoma is a broad-based, hemispheric elevation, again less than 1 cm. in diameter, that is firmly attached to the underlying wall.

Both are composed histologically of a vascularized connective tissue stroma covered by a single layer of well oriented, well differentiated columnar lining epithelial cells. The adenoma also has contained glands in the stroma. Rarely, there is concomitant proliferation of the smooth muscle cells to create a leiomyomatous tumor enclosing cystic gland spaces lined by columnar epithelial cells — the so-called *adenomyoma*. In all macroscopic patterns, the cellular proliferation is regular, does not invade the underlying wall and is entirely well differentiated. These lesions are only of clinical significance insofar as they may be detected on cholecystography and then require differentiation from more ominous malignancies. Papillomas, by fragmentation, may further provide a nidus for the formation of a gallstone. None of these benign lesions is believed to predispose to the development of a cancer.

CARCINOMA OF THE GALLBLADDER

While other forms of malignancy may arise in the gallbladder, carcinoma is much more frequent than the aggregate of all other types of malignancy and is a much more common lesion than the benign adenomas and papillomas described (Illingworth, 1936). Carcinoma of the gallbladder ranks fifth in frequency among gastrointestinal malignancies and comprises about 1 to 3 per cent of all malignancies. It is more common in advanced ages, particularly in the sixth and seventh decades of life, although significant numbers of these tumors are found in the forties and in the very elderly. These tumors are more common in whites than in blacks, and there is a female preponderance in the ratio of approximately 4 to 1. Considerable interest centers about the role of gallstones and cholecystitis in the genesis of these tumors. Gallstones are found in from 65 to 95 per cent of carcinomatous gallbladders, strongly suggesting an etiologic role. Inflammation is another common accompaniment. For these reasons, it is postulated that chronic irritation is an important factor in the origin of these malignancies, and stones, even when asymptomatic, are prophylactically removed upon discovery by some surgeons. In this connection, it is interesting to remember that derivatives of cholic acid, a bile component, are some of the most powerful carcinogenic agents known.

Morphologically, carcinomas of the gallbladder are usually divided into two gross patterns, infiltrating and fungating. The most common sites of involvement are the fundus and the neck, while about 20 per cent involve the lateral walls. The **infiltrating type** is more common and usually appears as a poorly defined area of diffuse thickening and induration of the gallbladder wall that, when discovered, may cover several square centimeters or may involve large portions or the entire gallbladder (Fig. 22–58). The tumors are scirrhous and,

therefore, have an extremely firm consistency. The luminal surface may be ulcerated, and often the tumor extends beneath the serosa in small, irregular, nodular projections or may directly penetrate the gallbladder wall to invade the liver bed. On cross section of these masses, the architecture of the wall is entirely obscured and replaced by a gritty, hard, white, solid tissue. Deep ulceration of the center of the mass may cause direct penetration of the gallbladder wall or fistula formation to adjacent viscera into which the neoplasm has grown.

The **fungating pattern** grows into the lumen as an irregular, small cauliflower mass but, at the same time, invades the underlying wall. The luminal portion may be necrotic, hemorrhagic and ulcerated. By the time that these neoplasms are discovered, **most have invaded the liver centrifugally** and many have extended to the cystic duct and adjacent bile ducts and portahepatic lymph nodes (Fig. 22–59). This state of advancement is made possible by the fact that these neoplasms, in their developmental stages, are entirely asymptomatic and can thus grow for a long time until they are discovered by their extension into surrounding structures. If the cystic duct is occluded, the trapped bile is resorbed

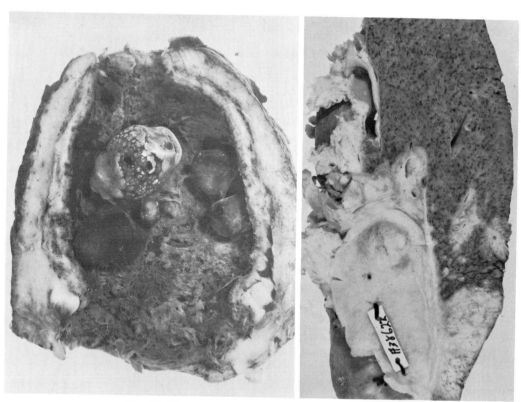

Fig. 22–58.

Fig. 22–59.

Figure 22–58. Carcinoma of gallbladder. Infiltrating pattern with diffuse, irregular thickening of the gallbladder wall.

Figure 22–59. The gallbladder and its liver bed have been transected longitudinally to disclose the direct permeation by carcinoma of the contiguous liver substance.

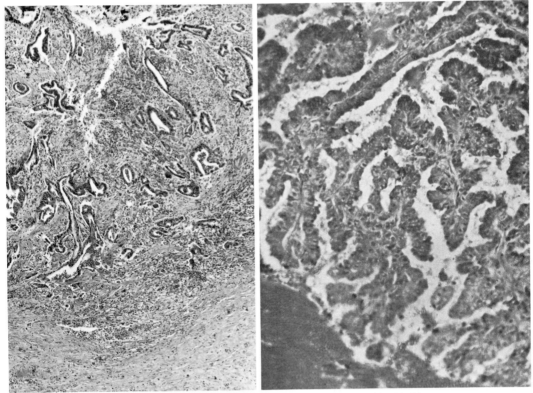

Fig. 22-60.   Fig. 22-61.

Figure 22-60. *Adenocarcinoma of gallbladder with typical abundant fibrous stroma.*
Figure 22-61. *Papillary carcinoma of gallbladder.*

and replaced by mucinous secretion (white bile), creating hydrops of the gallbladder.

Histologically, over 90 per cent of these growths are adenocarcinomas. The infiltrating variety usually has an extensive fibrous tissue stroma that accompanies the irregular gland patterns of columnar epithelium (Fig. 22-60). Most neoplasms are well differentiated, but occasionally anaplastic growths are encountered that do not form well developed glands. The fungating variety also grows in an adenomatous pattern, but often assumes papillary qualities (Fig. 22-61). Mucinous secretion is often present in all these histologic variants. Uncommonly, in 5 to 10 per cent of the cases, the infiltrating patterns may take squamous cell forms. Presumably, this squamous cell epithelium originates as a metaplastic differentiation of the columnar lining epithelium of the gallbladder. And still less frequently, mixtures of squamous and adenomatous growth are encountered, meriting the designation of adenoacanthoma.

The clinical course of these carcinomas is extremely insidious and frequently asymptomatic over long periods of time. Symptoms, when present, take the form of loss of appetite, nausea, vomiting, intolerance to fatty foods and belching, all suggesting some form of gallbladder involvement, usually inflammatory in nature. Jaundice does not appear until the tumor has infiltrated major biliary ducts or extended into the liver bed to obstruct an intrahepatic bile duct, or until metastasis has occurred to portahepatic nodes which then cause extrinsic pressure on the bile duct. A palpable mass is present in about one-half of the cases, and right upper quadrant pain or colic is experienced in somewhat over half of the cases. As the tumor advances in size, weakness, weight loss and other signs of advanced malignancy become apparent. The average duration of life, after establishment of the diagnosis, is in the order of one to one and a half years and only rare five-year survivals have been reported. At autopsy, direct penetration of the liver, metastasis to the regional nodes about the porta hepatis and pancreas, and disseminated metastases to the liver, lungs and other viscera are found in these far advanced malignancies.

CARCINOMA OF THE BILE DUCTS AND AMPULLA OF VATER

The designation, carcinoma of the bile ducts, is meant to include involvement of all the extrahepatic bile ducts as well as the intraduodenal segment. The latter form is usually distinguished as *carcinoma of the ampulla of Vater.* Carcinomatous involvement of these ducts in the aggregate occurs somewhat less frequently than carcinoma of the gallbladder (Kirshbaum and Kozoll, 1941). However, these malignancies far outnumber in frequency all the other rather uncommon benign neoplastic (papilloma and adenoma) involvements of these structures (Chu, 1950). The same age range is affected as in carcinoma of the gallbladder but, in contrast to this last-mentioned neoplasm, males are said to be affected more often than females. The predisposing influences of inflammation and gallstones are less well established for carcinoma of the ducts than for carcinoma of the gallbladder. Accompanying stones are found in only about one-third of the cases.

The sites of location of these tumors in descending order of frequency are the common bile duct, especially the lower end; the junction of the cystic, hepatic and common ducts; the hepatic ducts; the cystic duct; and last, in order of frequency, the duodenal portion of the common bile duct that includes lesions arising from the periampullary region. **These tumors are almost always extremely small when found** and usually have few metastases, presumably because, in their strategic location, they give rise to prominent obstructive symptoms early in their course and, therefore, do not pass through a long developmental evolution. The tumors appear as gray-white, scirrhous thickenings of the duct wall with narrowing of the lumen of the duct. Rarely, nodular excrescences project into the lumen and appear on the external aspect. At other times, fungating growths are present within the lumina of these channels. In the region of the papilla, small, hemispheric, intraduodenal masses may develop that rarely exceed 2 to 3 cm. in diameter and 1 cm. in height (Fig. 22–62). In most instances, the overlying duodenal mucosa is intact but, occasionally, permeation of the duodenal wall may cause ulceration of the mucosa and small excavated defects on the surface. It is for this reason that periampullary carcinomas are associated with bleeding into the bowel.

Histologically, these lesions are almost invariably adenocarcinomas composed of gland formations lined by cuboidal to columnar epithelial cells that may or may not be mucin-secreting. Infrequently, papillary growth is produced and, quite rarely, squamous metaplastic differentiation occurs.

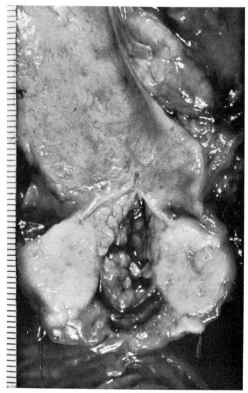

Figure 22–62. *Carcinoma of papilla of Vater. The widened common bile duct comes down from above. The neoplasm has been split open to demonstrate the 1.5 cm. size of the mass.*

For the most part, an abundant fibrous stroma accompanies the epithelial proliferation. As mentioned earlier, metastases to regional nodes may occur but, in general, **these lesions cause such early clinical disturbances that extensive dissemination is uncommon.** Significant, clinically detectable hydrops of the gallbladder is a frequent sequel to those lesions originating in the cystic duct.

Despite their insidious development, most of these tumors present themselves with the symptoms of an acute onset of right upper quadrant pain, biliary colic, jaundice, loss of weight and nonspecific digestive disturbances. It should be stressed at this point that despite the progressive growth of these tumors, the jaundice may temporarily remit if necrosis reestablishes a passage for the bile. It is also to be stressed that while, classically, obstructive jaundice associated with pain is considered to be due to gallstones impacted within the common duct, carcinomas of the bile duct also cause pain in about half the cases. Ultimately, when untreated, obstructive jaundice with its associated pruritus, decolorized (acholic) stools, bile-stained urine and frequent accompaniments of cholangitis and biliary cirrhosis dominate the clinical symtpom complexes. Thus, in any diagnostic problem involving obstructive jaundice, the three major differential diagnoses are common duct stone, carcinoma of the head of the pancreas and carcinoma of the extrahepatic bile ducts (including those of the papilla of Vater). This is a most difficult differential diagnosis to establish on clinical grounds.

While classically it is taught, according to Courvoisier's law, that obstruction due to stones is associated with a small gallbladder, in only approximately one-half of the cases of obstruction due to neoplasia is the gallbladder enlarged; in the remainder, it is not palpable. Because the lesions are small, even though they produce symptoms, a palpable mass due to the neoplasm is extremely rare. Although their strategic location precludes sufficient time for widespread dissemination, metastases to the regional lymph nodes, the liver and other sites do occur in a number of instances. Despite early manifestations, the overall outlook in these tumors is poor, and most patients have a survival of three to six months after diagnosis. Adequate surgical resection and reconstruction of the resected ducts, although not simple, can now be accomplished, and successful surgery in cases of carcinoma of the ampulla of Vater is becoming moderately common.

REFERENCES

Abelev, G. I.: Production of embryonal serum alpha-globulin by hepatomas: review of experimental and clinical data. Cancer Res., 28:1344, 1968.

Alpert, M. E., and Davidson, C. S.: Mycotoxins, a possible cause of primary carcinoma of the liver. Amer. J. Med., 46:325, 1969.

Alpert, M. E., et al.: Hepatomas in Uganda: a study in geographic pathology. Lancet, 1:1265, 1968.

Arias, I. M., et al.: Black liver disease in Corriedale sheep: a new mutation affecting hepatic excretory function. J. Clin. Invest., 43:1249, 1964.

Babcock, J. R., and Eyerly, R. C.: A 5 year survey of 1055 consecutive patients with extrahepatic biliary tract disease. Surg. Gynec. Obstet., 105:711, 1957.

Bakst, H. J., and Jeghers, H.: Pylephlebitis of extraportal origin: report of a case with review of the literature. Amer. J. Med. Sci., 193:690, 1937.

Baxter, J. H., and Ashworth, C. T.: Renal lesions in portal cirrhosis. Arch. Path., 41:476, 1946.

Bearn, A. G., et al.: The problem of chronic liver disease in young women. Amer. J. Med., 21:3, 1956.

Berger, R., et al.: Transfusions in the treatment of fulminating hepatitis. New Eng. J. Med., 274:497, 1966.

Black, M., and Billing, B. H.: Hepatic bilirubin. U.D.P.-glucuronyl transferase activity in liver disease and Gilbert's syndrome. New Eng. J. Med., 280:1266, 1969.

Blaisdell, F. W., and Cohen, R.: Cirrhosis of the liver. Clinical course in 2,377 patients at the San Francisco General Hospital. Calif. Med., 94:353, 1961.

Blumberg, B. S., et al.: A new "antigen" in leukemia serum. J.A.M.A., 191:541, 1965.

Blumberg, B. S., et al.: A serum antigen (Australia antigen) in Down's syndrome, leukemia, and hepatitis. Ann. Intern. Med., 66:924, 1967.

Blumberg, B. S., et al.: Australia antigen and hepatitis. New Eng. J. Med., 283:349, 1970a.

Blumberg, B. S., et al.: Australia antigen as a hepatitis virus. Variation in host response. Amer. J. Med., 48:1, 1970b.

Boyer, J. L., and Klatskin, G.: Pattern of necrosis in acute viral hepatitis. Prognostic value of bridging (subacute hepatic necrosis). New Eng. J. Med., 283:1063, 1970.

Brewin, A. W.: Current concepts of viral hepatitis. J. Amer. Coll. Health Ass., 20:328, 1972.

Bruni, C., and Porter, K. R.: The fine structure of the parenchymal cell of the normal rat liver. I. General observations. Amer. J. Path., 46:691, 1965.

Callahan, E. W., Jr., and Schmid, R.: Excretion of unconjugated bilirubin in the bile of Gunn rats. Gastroenterology, 57:134, 1969.

Carey, C. M., and Small, D. M.: Micelle formation by bile salts. Arch. Intern. Med., 130:506, 1972.

Chu, P. T.: Benign neoplasms of the extrahepatic bile ducts. Arch. Path., 50:84, 1950.

Cook, G. C., and Hutt, M. S. R.: The liver after kwashiorkor. Brit. Med. J., 3:454, 1967.

Craig, J. M., and Landing, B. A.: A form of hepatitis in the newborn suggesting biliary atresia. Arch. Path., 54:321, 1952.

Dane, D. S., et al.: Virus-like particles in serum of patients with Australia-antigen-associated hepatitis. Lancet, 1:695, 1970.

Davis, J. O.: Aldosterone and angiotensin. J.A.M.A., 188:1062, 1964.

Dienstag, J. L., et al.: Faecal shedding of hepatitis-A antigen. Lancet, 1:765, 1975.

Doniach, D., et al.: Current concepts: "autoallergic" hepatitis. New Eng. J. Med., 282:86, 1970.

Doniach, D., et al.: Tissue antibodies in primary biliary cirrhosis, chronic-active hepatitis, cryptogenic cirrhosis and other liver diseases and their clinical implications. Clin. Exp. Immunol., 1:237, 1966.

Dougherty, W. J., and Altman, R.: Viral hepatitis in New Jersey 1960–1961. Amer. J. Med., 32:704, 1962.

Dubin, I. N.: Chronic idiopathic jaundice: a review of 50 cases. Amer. J. Med., 24:268, 1958.

Dubin, I. N., and Johnson, F. B.: Chronic idiopathic jaundice with unidentified pigment in liver cells. A new clinicopathologic entity with a report of 12 cases. Medicine, 33:155, 1954.

Dudley, F. J., et al.: Relationship of hepatitis-associated antigen (HAA) to acute and chronic liver injury. Lancet, 2:2, 1971.

Elias, H.: A re-examination of the structure of the mammalian liver. Amer. J. Anat., 84:311, 1949.

Feizi, T.: Immunoglobulins in chronic liver disease. Gut, 9:193, 1968.

Feldman, M., and Feldman, M., Jr.: Cholesterolosis of the gallbladder. Gastroenterology, 27:641, 1954.

Fisher, E. R., and Hellstrom, H. R.: The membranous and proliferative glomerulonephritis of hepatic cirrhosis. Amer. J. Clin. Path., 32:48, 1959.

Fleischner, G., and Arias, I. M.: Recent advances in bilirubin formation, transport, metabolism and excretion. Amer. J. Med., 49:576, 1970.

Fox, R. A., et al.: Hepatitis-associated antigen in chronic liver disease. Lancet, 2:609, 1969a.

Fox, R. A., et al.: Impaired delayed hypersensitivity in primary biliary cirrhosis. Lancet, 1:959, 1969b.

Fox, R. A., et al.: The serum concentration of the third component of complement β1C/β1A in liver disease. Gut, 12:574, 1971.

Gall, E. A.: Posthepatic, postnecrotic and nutritional cirrhosis. A pathologic analysis. Amer. J. Path., 36:241, 1960a.

Gall, E. A.: Posthepatitic cirrhosis: fact and fancy. In Ingelfinger, F., Relman, A. S., and Finland, M. (eds.): Controversies in Internal Medicine. Philadelphia, W. B. Saunders Co., 1966, p. 244.

Gall, E. A.: Primary and metastatic carcinoma of the liver: relationship to hepatic cirrhosis. Arch. Path., 70:226, 1960b.

Gartner, L. M., and Arias, I. M.: Formation, transport, metabolism and excretion of bilirubin. New Eng. J. Med., 280:1339, 1969.

Gitnick, G. L., et al.: Australia antigen in chronic liver disease with cirrhosis. Lancet, 2:285, 1969.

Giustino, V., et al.: Thymus-dependent lymphocyte function in patients with hepatitis-associated antigen. Lancet, 2:850, 1972.

Goldfischer, S., and Sternlieb, I.: Changes in the distribution of hepatic copper in relation to the progression of Wilson's disease (hepatolenticular degeneration). Amer. J. Path., 53:883, 1968.

Hall, E. M., et al.: Portal cirrhosis: clinical and pathologic review of 782 cases from 16,600 necropsies. Amer. J. Path., 29:993, 1953.

Hallendorf, L. C., et al.: Gangrenous cholecystitis: a clinical and pathologic study of 100 cases. Surg. Clin. No. Amer., 28:979, 1948.

Havens, W. P.: Viral hepatitis. Med. Clin. N. Amer., 54:455, 1970.

Henson, S. W., Jr.: Benign tumors of the liver. 2. Hemangiomas. Surg. Gynec. Obstet., 103:237, 1956.

Henson, S. W., Jr., et al.: Benign tumors of the liver. 1. Adenomas. Surg. Gynec. Obstet., 103:23, 1956.

Illingworth, C. F. W.: Carcinoma of the gallbladder. Brit. J. Surg., 23:4, 1936.

Iseri, O., and Gottlieb, L. S.: Alcoholic hyalin and megamitochondria as separate and distinct entities in liver alcoholism. Gastroenterology, 60:1027, 1971.

Jones, W. R., et al.: The renal glomerulus in cirrhosis of the liver. Amer. J. Path., 39:393, 1961.

Juniper, K., Jr.: Physiochemical characteristics of bile and their relation to gallstone formation. Amer. J. Med., 39:98. 1965.

Kirshbaum, J. D., and Kozoll, D. D.: Carcinoma of the gallbladder and extrahepatic bile ducts. Surg. Gynec. Obstet., 73:740, 1941.

Klion, F. M., and Schaffner, F.: The ultrastructure of acidophilic "councilman-like" bodies in the liver. Amer. J. Path., 48:755, 1966.

Krugman, S., and Giles, J. P.: Viral hepatitis: new light on an old disease. J.A.M.A., 212:1019, 1970.

Krugman, S., et al.: Infectious hepatitis: evidence for two distinctive clinical, epidemiological and immunological types of infection. J.A.M.A., 200:365, 1967.

Levi, A. J., et al.: Presymptomatic Wilson's disease. Lancet, 2:575, 1967.

Lieber, C. S.: Metabolic derangement induced by alcohol. Ann. Rev. Med., 18:35, 1969.

Lieber, C. S.: Metabolic effects produced by alcohol in the liver and other tissues. Advances Intern. Med., 14:151, 1968.

Lieber, C. S., and Rubin, E.: Current concepts: alcoholic fatty liver. New Eng. J. Med., 280:705, 1969.

Lieberman, F. L., et al.: Effective plasma volume in cirrhosis with ascites. Evidence that a decreased value does not account for renal sodium retention, a spontaneous reduction in glomerular filtration rate (GFR), and a fall in GFR during drug-induced diuresis. J. Clin. Invest., 48:975, 1969.

Liebowitz, H. R.: Pathogenesis of ascites in cirrhosis of the liver. II. New York J. Med., 69:2012, 1969.

Lin, T. Y.: Primary cancer of the liver. Scand. J. Gastroent. Suppl., 6:223, 1970.

London, W. T., et al.: Current status of Australian antigen. In Ioachim, H. L. (ed.): Pathology Annual, 1972. New York, Appleton-Century-Crofts, 1972, p. 207.

Lucke, B.: The pathology of fatal epidemic hepatitis. Amer. J. Path., 20:471, 1944.

MacDonald, R. A.: Primary carcinoma of the liver: a clinicopathologic study of 108 cases. Arch. Intern. Med., 99:266, 1957.

MacKay, I. R., and Morris, P. J.: Association of autoimmune active chronic hepatitis with HL-A$_{1, 8}$. Lancet, 2:793, 1972.

Maclachlan, M. J., et al.: Chronic active ("lupoid") hepatitis: a clinical, serological, and pathological study of 20 patients. Ann. Intern. Med., 62:425, 1965.

Mansell, R. V.: Infectious hepatitis in the first trimester of pregnancy and its effect on the fetus. Amer. J. Obstet. Gynec., 69:1136, 1955.

Mikkelsen, W. P., et al.: Portacaval shunt in cirrhosis of the liver. Clinical and hemodynamic aspects. Amer. J. Surg., 104:204, 1962.

Mistilus, S. P., and Blackburn, R. B.: Active hepatitis. Amer. J. Med., 48:484, 1970.

Moertel, C. G., et al.: Australia antigen and primary liver cancer. Amer. J. Dig. Dis., 15:983, 1970.

Mosley, J. W.: Viral hepatitis: a group of epidemiologic entities. Canad. Med. Ass. J., Suppl., 106:427, 1972.

Mosley, J. W., et al.: Failure to detect an antigen associated with hepatitis in a community epidemic. Nature, 225:953, 1970.

Palmer, E. D., and Brick, I. D.: Sources of upper gastrointestinal bleeding in cirrhotic patients with esophageal varices. New Eng. J. Med., 248:1057, 1953.

Paronetto, F., and Popper, H.: Lymphocyte stimulation induced by halothane in patients with post halothane hepatitis. New Eng. J. Med., 282:277, 1970.

Paronetto, F., et al.: Antibodies to cytoplasmic antigens in primary biliary cirrhosis and chronic active hepatitis. J. Lab. Clin. Med., 69:979, 1967.

Patton, R. B., and Horn, R. C., Jr.: Primary liver carcinoma: autopsy study of 60 cases. Cancer, 17:757, 1964.

Poland, R. L., and Odell, G. B.: Physiologic jaundice: the enterohepatic circulation of bilirubin. New Eng. J. Med., 284:1, 1971.

Popper, H.: The pathology of viral hepatitis. Canad. Med. Ass. J., Suppl., 106:447, 1972.

Popper, H., and Hutterer, F.: Hepatic fibrogenesis and disturbance of hepatic circulation. Ann. N.Y. Acad. Sci., in press.

Popper, H., and Orr, W.: Current concepts of cirrhosis. Scand. J. Gastroent., Suppl., 6:203, 1970.

Popper, H., and Schaffner, F.: Pathophysiology of cholestasis. Hum. Path., 1:1, 1970.

Popper, H., et al.: The social impact of liver disease. New Eng. J. Med., 281:1455, 1969.

Porta, E. A., and Gomez-Dumm, C. L. A.: New experimental approach in the study of chronic alcoholism. Lab. Invest., 18:352, 365, 379, 1968.

Porta, E. A., et al.: Recent advances in molecular pathology: a review of the effects of alcohol on the liver. Exp. Molec. Path., 12:104, 1970.

Powell, W. J., and Klatskin, G.: Duration of survival in patients with Laennec's cirrhosis. Influence of alcohol withdrawal and possible effects of recent changes in general management of the disease. Amer. J. Med., 44:406, 1968.

Prince, A. M.: An antigen detected in the blood during the incubation period of serum hepatitis. Proc. Nat. Acad. Sci., 60:814, 1968.

Prince, A. M., et al.: Immunologic distinction between infectious and serum hepatitis. New Eng. J. Med., 282:988, 1970.

Reynolds, T. B., et al.: Portal hypertension without cirrhosis in alcoholic liver disease. Ann. Intern. Med., 70:497, 1969.

Robinson, S. H.: The origins of bilirubin. New Eng. J. Med., 279:146, 1968.

Rubin, E., and Lieber, C. S.: Alcohol-induced hepatic injury in nonalcoholic volunteers. New Eng. J. Med., 278:869, 1968.

Rubin, E., et al.: Ethanol and the liver: an example of injury and adaptation. Hum. Path., 2:343, 1971.

Schaffner, F.: The effect of oral contraceptives on the liver. J.A.M.A., 198:1019, 1966.

Schmid, R.: Hyperbilirubinemia. In Stanbury, J. B., Wyngaarden, J. B., and Fredrickson, D. S. (eds.): The Metabolic Basis of Inherited Disease. 2nd ed. New York, McGraw-Hill Book Co., 1966, p. 871.

Schoental, R.: Toxicology and carcinogenic action of pyrrolizidine alkaloids. Cancer Res., 28:2237, 1968.

Schroeder, E. T., et al.: Renal failure in patients with cirrhosis of the liver. III. Evaluation of internal blood flow by para-amino hippurate extraction and response to angiotensin. Amer. J. Med., 43:887, 1968.

Schweitzer, I. L., and Spears, R. L.: Hepatitis-associated antigen (Australia antigen) in mother and infant. New Eng. J. Med., 283:570, 1970.

Shepard, D. V., et al.: Benign neoplasms of the gallbladder. Arch. Surg., 45:118, 1942.

Sherlock, S.: Long incubation (virus B, HAA-associated) hepatitis. Gut, 13:297, 1972.

Shulman, N. R.: Hepatitis-associated antigen. Amer. J. Med., 49:669, 1970.

Simpson, G. E. C., and Finckh, E. S.: The pattern of regeneration of rat liver after repeated partial hepatectomies. J. Path. Bact., 86:361, 1963.

Skikne, M. I., and Talbot, J. H.: The identification and structural analysis of viral particles in serum hepatitis. Lab. Invest., 31:246, 1974.

Small, D. M.: The formation of gallstones. Advances Intern. Med., *16*:243, 1970.

Small, D. M.: Gallstones. New Eng. J. Med., *279*:588, 1968.

Small, D. M.: Personal communication, 1972.

Small, D. M.: The treatment of gallstone disease. In Ingelfinger, F., Relman, A., and Friedman, M. (eds.): Controversies in Medicine. 2nd ed. Philadelphia, W. B. Saunders Co., in press.

Smetana, H.: In Schiff, L. (ed.): Diseases of the Liver. 2nd ed. Philadelphia, J. B. Lippincott Co., 1963, p. 401.

Smith, J. B.: Alpha-fetoprotein: occurrence in certain malignant diseases and review of clinical application. Med. Clin. N. Amer., *54*:797, 1970.

Stephens, C. L., and Jenevein, E. P., Jr.: Mesenchymal hamartoma of liver. Arch. Path., *80*:413, 1965.

Stone, W. D., et al.: The natural history of cirrhosis. Experience with an unselected group of patients. Quart. J. Med., *37*:119, 1968.

Sutnick, A. I., et al.: Australia antigen posttransfusion hepatitis and the chronic carrier state. Amer. J. Dis. Child., *123*:392, 1972.

Symmers, D., and Spain, D. M.: Hepar lobatum. Arch. Path., *42*:64, 1946.

Tartakow, I. J.: Narcotic-induced hepatitis. Amer. J. Med., *50*:313, 1971.

Taswell, H. F., et al.: Hepatitis-associated antigen in blood donor populations. Relationship to posttransfusion hepatitis. J.A.M.A., *214*:142, 1970.

Terris, M.: Epidemiology of cirrhosis of the liver: national mortality data. Amer. J. Public Health, *57*:2076, 1967.

Trey, C., et al.: Fulminant hepatic failure. New Eng. J. Med., *279*:798, 1968.

Vischer, T. L.: Australia antigen and autoantibodies in chronic hepatitis. Brit. Med. J., *2*:695, 1970.

Vogel, C. L., et al.: Hepatitis-associated antigen in Ugandan patients with hepatocellular carcinomas. Lancet, *2*:621, 1970.

Whittingham, S., el al.: Smooth muscle autoantibody in "autoimmune" hepatitis. Gastroenterology, *51*:499, 1966.

Womack, A., and Bricker, E. M.: Pathogenesis of cholecystitis. Arch. Surg., *44*:658, 1942.

Yasuzumi, G., et al.: The fine structure of nuclei revealed by electron microscopy. V. Intranuclear inclusion bodies in hepatic parenchymal cells in cases of serum hepatitis. J. Ultrastruct. Res., *23*:321, 1968.

23

THE PANCREAS

NORMAL

In its posterior location in the upper abdomen, the pancreas is one of the "hidden" organs in the body. It is virtually impossible to palpate clinically. Diseases that impair its function only evoke signs or symptoms when far advanced, because there is such a large reserve of both endocrine and exocrine function. Lesions in this organ are, therefore, frequently only manifested by impingement or encroachment on neighboring structures. For example, carcinoma of the pancreas may be discovered only when it invades the vertebral column, occludes the biliary system or causes disturbances in the stomach or colon.

The pancreas arises from two duodenal buds that are referred to, respectively, as the dorsal and ventral pancreas. The ventral bud grows more slowly and eventually swings around the gut to fuse with the larger dorsal mass. Fusion of the two creates the adult organ, after which the two contributions can no longer be distinguished. In general, the entire body and tail of the pancreas are derived from the dorsal anlage, and the remainder, from the ventral bud. The ductal drainage systems anastomose, and the major excretory duct of the dorsal pancreas, draining into the duodenum, persists as the duct of Wirsung. Usually, the duct of the ventral pancreas disappears but, if it persists, it creates the accessory duct of Santorini. However, there is much variability in this ductal system. In somewhat more than 60 per cent of adults, the major pancreatic duct does not empty directly into the duodenum but into the common bile duct just proximal to the ampulla of Vater, thus providing a common channel to the pancreatic and biliary drainage.

In the adult, the pancreas averages about 15 cm. in length, 3 to 5 cm. in width and 2 to 3 cm. in maximal thickness. Its gross anatomic relationships are well known and include immediate proximity to the duodenum, ampulla of Vater, common bile duct, superior mesenteric artery, portal vein, spleen and its vascular supply, stomach, transverse colon, left lobe of the liver and lower recesses of the lesser omental cavity. Inflammatory and neoplastic processes within the pancreas, therefore, may cause secondary involvement of many adjacent structures. It is, in fact, these secondary involvements that produce, in many cases, the so-called characteristic signs and symptoms of pancreatic disease.

Mention should be made of the extremely firm consistency of this organ. Frequently at laparotomy, the problem arises of identification of a possible malignancy in the pancreas. Unless the observer is familiar with the normal firm consistency of the pancreas, it is all too easy to confuse its normal substance with a malignant tumor.

Histologically, the pancreas has two separate components, exocrine and endocrine glands. The islets of Langerhans have already been considered with diabetes mellitus (p. 262) and will be further described in the section on islet cell lesions (p. 1072). The exocrine portion is made up of numerous small glands aggregated into the lobules seen in the gross. These glands are separated by a scant connective tissue stroma. The cells that comprise these glands are columnar to truncated pyramids radially oriented about the gland circumference. The central lumen of the gland is extremely small in the normal state and may not even be visible. Small microvilli project from the apical surfaces of the secretory cells into the gland lumen. The exocrine secretory cells are deeply basophilic in routine tissue stains because of their abundance of granular endoplasmic reticulum with its attached RNA-containing ribosomes. The Golgi complex is well developed in these cells and, along with the endoplasmic reticulum, appears to be oriented toward the basal region. The apical regions of the cells contain abundant membrane-bounded sacs enclosing zymogen granules.

The ductal system of the pancreas is produced by progressive anastomosis of the extremely fine radicles which begin within the secretory glands. These small ducts eventually drain into the main excretory ducts of Wirsung and Santorini. At first cuboidal, their lining epithelium becomes progressively higher to produce tall, columnar, regularly aligned cells. This ductal epithelium is mucus-secreting. About the larger ducts, there are numerous accessory branching ducts and mucous glands which may be sufficiently agglomerated in the region of the duodenum to create the false impression of an invasive, well differentiated glandular carcinoma.

It is hardly necessary here to reiterate the secretory functions of the pancreas and the regulatory mechanisms that control such activity. Several points, however, are directly pertinent to disease processes and merit reemphasis. The secretory activity of the pancreas is well adjusted to the workload that it is called upon to perform. In the intact animal, the quantity and distribution of the various pancreatic enzymes are nicely adjusted to the volume and character of the intestinal contents. The regulation of this secretion is a complex problem that involves humoral, vagal and local neurogenic reflexes. Perhaps the most important of these regulators is the humoral agent, secretin, produced in the duodenum. Fats and alcohol are particularly active stimulators of secretin production and, therefore, indirectly of the pancreas. On this basis, pancreatic secretory activity is directly correlated with the ingestion of food, and it is thought that sometimes the ingestion of large meals or alcohol may initiate pancreatic disease when the volume of secretion exceeds the drainage capacity of the ducts.

A second point of interest relates to the elaboration of the proteolytic enzymes. Trypsin and chymotrypsin secreted as inactive precursors are the most important of the protein-digesting ferments. In addition to the proteases, the pancreas secretes amylases, lipases, phospholipases and elastases. All of these enzymes are elaborated as inactive precursors and are activated in the duodenum on contact with the succus entericus. One of the most important pancreatic diseases, acute hemorrhagic pancreatic necrosis, may be initiated by activation of these enzymes within the pancreatic ducts.

An elegant level of correlation of structure with function has been achieved with the pancreas (Palade et al., 1961) (Sjostrand, 1961). It has been possible to identify synthesis of the pancreatic enzymes within the endoplasmic reticulum where apparently the RNA granules elaborate these protein complexes. These proteins are then apparently transmitted to the region of the Golgi complex where membrane-bounded granules are formed. When the pancreas is stimulated to secretory activity, these zymogen granules, apparently enclosed within membranous sacs, migrate to the apical region of the cell. Here the sac becomes attached to the plasma membrane, and rupture at the point of attachment releases the enzyme-rich zymogen granules into the acinus of the gland. The secretory cycle of insulin has been equally well elucidated, as was discussed on p. 262.

PATHOLOGY

The most significant disorders of the pancreas consist of diabetes mellitus (p. 259), fibrocystic disease of the pancreas (p. 560), inflammations and tumors, benign and malignant. It should be emphasized that, from the standpoints of both morbidity and mortality, diabetes mellitus alone overshadows all the other pancreatic disorders now to be considered. However, a knowledgeable alertness to all pancreatic disease is most necessary, since almost all these disorders are difficult to diagnose because of the hidden position and large reserve function of this organ and because they appear under such diverse guises as a catastrophic "acute abdomen" or the silent growth of a carcinoma.

CONGENITAL ANOMALIES

The pancreas is subject to a variety of congenital anomalies, most of which are either quite uncommon or of little clinical significance. The gland may be totally absent (agenesis). Complete agenesis is quite regularly associated with widespread severe malformations that are incompatible with life. The endocrine and exocrine elements may be *hypoplastic*. The gland may exist as two separate structures representing the persistence of the dorsal and ventral pancreas. The head of the pancreas may encircle the duodenum as a collar *(annular pancreas)* and sometimes may cause subtotal duodenal obstruction and consequent clinical symptoms. Two additional anomalies occur with sufficient frequency or have sufficient clinical significance to merit separate consideration.

Aberrant Pancreas. Aberrant, or ectopic, displaced pancreatic tissue is found in about 2 per cent of all routine postmortems. These aberrant rests are usually chiefly of anatomic interest, but occasionally they arouse clinical concern. The most favored sites for such ectopia follow the order of the descent of the intestinal tract; that is, they are most common in the stomach and duodenum, with about equal frequency, next in the jejunum, then in Meckel's diverticulum, and then in the ileum. Ectopic pancreatic tissue also occurs in other viscera, but only with great rarity. Usually, the masses vary from a few millimeters up to 3 to 4 cm. in diameter. They appear as single or multiple, firm, yellow-gray nests within the wall of the gut subjacent to the mucosa, lying usually within the submucosa or mucosa (Fig. 23–1). Occasionally, they are found in the muscularis or subserosa. They are composed histologically of glands that appear completely normal and, not infrequently, islets of Langerhans are also present.

In such locations, they may be discovered accidentally in the course of a laparotomy or be visualized radiographically as sessile lesions that project slightly into the lumen of the bowel. Sometimes, therefore, they are confused with considerably more serious tumors. On transection, however, the usual racemose, yellow-white pattern of the pancreas should reveal their identity and establish their innocence. Ectopic pancreatic rests have caused clinical symptoms in the form of pain due to inflammatory involvement of the aberrant tissue, intestinal obstruction and other disturbances in intestinal motility, although such cases are quite infrequent. They are rare sites of tumorigenesis.

Anomalies of the Ducts. Anomalies of the pancreatic duct comprise a second type of congenital defect that is sometimes of clinical importance. The duct of Wirsung and the duct of Santorini may both persist as totally separate structures. The major excretory pancreatic duct, the duct of Wirsung, may drain into the common bile duct or may drain through an abnormally high orifice in the duodenum. These variations would seem to be of little importance except that this particular region is the focal point of a considerable amount of surgery, for example, on duodenal ulcers. These aberrations, unless recognized, may potentiate ligation or severance of the ducts and serious sequelae.

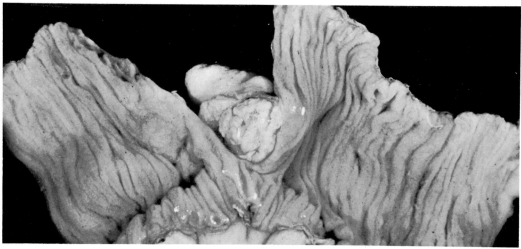

Figure 23–1. Aberrant pancreas. The mucosa of the jejunum has been incised to disclose the rest of pale, yellow-white, submucosal, lobulated pancreatic tissue.

REGRESSIVE CHANGES

The pancreas is an extremely labile organ susceptible to a great variety of adverse influences. Following death, it undergoes postmortem autolysis almost as rapidly as the brain. It is likewise affected by any severe febrile or systemic toxic disorder and reacts by cell swelling and hydropic degeneration. For the most part, these cytologic alterations are of little clinical import. Certain retrogressive changes, however, are of some significance. Most have already been discussed in the earlier sections of the book, but are briefly reiterated for emphasis.

Pigmentation. Pigmentation of the pancreas occurs in hemochromatosis (p. 280). This deposit, principally of hemosiderin, in the acinar and islet cells accounts for the distinct brown discoloration of the pancreas which comprises one of the most readily detectable anatomic changes in this systemic disorder.

Stromal Fatty Infiltration or Fatty Ingrowth. These alterations enlarge the apparent size of the pancreas by spreading apart the lobular structure (p. 38). The dispersion of the parenchyma may create the impression that the pancreas has been totally replaced by a mass of adipose tissue. However, the fat is confined to the interstitial stroma and does not disturb the parenchymal elements and, if the fat is dissolved out, a normal amount of pancreatic substance can be recovered. It was pointed out that the genesis of this condition is entirely obscure. Fatty ingrowth of the pancreas is unrelated to any apparent pancreatic dysfunction.

Islet Changes in Diabetes Mellitus. It will suffice to recall that the islets in the diabetic may appear normal with light microscopy or may disclose a variety of alterations. Even the apparently normal islets under closer scrutiny such as with electron microscopy or biochemical analysis almost invariably reveal beta cell degranulation and depleted stores of insulin. Juvenile diabetics sometimes have evidence of active beta cell necrosis provoking an eosinophilic or lymphocytic infiltration. In the adult, the most common alteration is hyaline deposits, encountered in approximately 40 per cent of maturity-onset diabetics (Fig. 23–2). According to present evidence, these deposits represent a form of amyloid. Fibrosis of the islets is encountered in approximately 25 per cent, and vacuolation of beta cells due to glycogen accumulation, in about 4 per cent. The infant born of a diabetic mother may also have evidence of active beta cell necrosis accompanied by an eosinophilic infiltration or enlargement of the islets. More details on these lesions are given on p. 265.

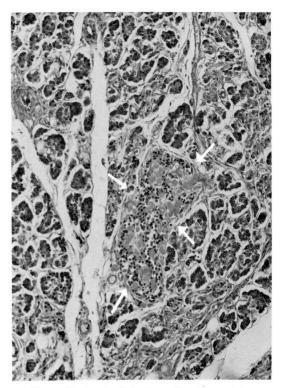

Figure 23–2. Hyalinization of the islets of the pancreas in a 45-year-old diabetic (arrows).

Pancreatic Atrophy. The usual cause of atrophy is *ischemia* due to atherosclerosis of the pancreatic arteries. Under these circumstances, the parenchymal atrophy affects both the endocrine and exocrine elements but is usually minimal and of little functional significance. Most often, there is only an increase of stromal connective tissue without obvious loss of pancreatic substance. More important, atrophy may be caused by *obstruction of the pancreatic ducts*. In this form, the islets of Langerhans are totally spared, but the exocrine glands undergo progressive disuse or pressure atrophy to the point of total disappearance (Fig. 23–3). The discovery that such exocrine atrophy could be induced by ligature of the pancreatic ducts paved the way for the pioneer experiments on the extraction and identification of insulin. In these early experiments, it was known that the pancreas contained some factor responsible for the prevention of the metabolic abnormalities recognized as diabetes mellitus, but it was impossible to isolate this principle because of the presence of the proteolytic enzymes of the exocrine glands. Ligature of the pancreatic duct induced total atrophy of the enzymatically active exocrine component, and permitted the extraction of the active insulin.

In man, such exocrine atrophy may be caused by congenital stenosis or atresia of ducts, inflammatory stenoses of the ducts, surgical ligature of ducts, obstructive pancreatic calculi, squamous metaplasia of the lining epithelium with piling up of epithelial debris, or neoplastic obstruction. Whatever the cause, the pancreas becomes reduced to a small, irregular, nodular, fibrous mass that may be one-quarter to one-sixth of its normal volume. On section, only fibrous tissue can be identified, usually traversed by dilated ducts that are sometimes ballooned out into cystic enlargements. When the obstruction affects only tributaries of the main pancreatic duct, the atrophy involves only regional portions of the pancreas. The histologic identification of such atrophy is readily made by the preservation of islets, with total disappearance and fibrofatty replacement of the acinar glands. Such atrophy only very infrequently leads to digestive disturbances but, as might be anticipated, there is no disturbance of insulin secretion or carbohydrate metabolism.

Uremic Alterations. These changes in the pancreas are only detectable microscopically. Careful study of the pancreas in patients who have died of renal failure discloses, in approximately 40 to 50 per cent, histologic alterations that, to the present time, are of only aca-

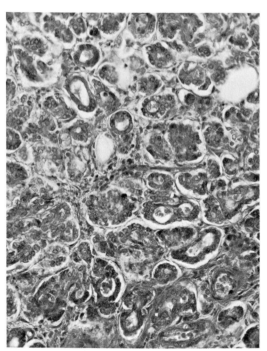

Figure 23–4. Uremic alterations in the pancreas. The acinar glands are dilated and filled with a mucinous secretion.

demic interest (Baggenstoss, 1948). These changes consist essentially of dilatation of the acinar glands to create small central lumina, dilatation of the pancreatic ducts, inspissation of pancreatic secretion within dilated acinar glands and ducts, and a scant increase of interstitial stroma accompanied by a minimal scattering of lymphocytes within the stroma (Fig. 23–4). The genesis of these alterations is unknown. Similar changes are encountered in certain nonuremic states, such as fibrocystic disease of the pancreas, and as incidental findings in some routine autopsies (20 per cent). However, the so-called uremic changes are found in a sufficient number of cases of renal failure to make them helpful, along with uremic pericarditis, gastritis and colitis, in anatomically establishing the diagnosis of uremia.

VASCULAR CHANGES

Cardiac failure or diseases in the liver with attendant portal hypertension may cause intense congestion and edema in the pancreas. Such changes are of little more than passing interest.

Not uncommonly, at postmortem examination, extensive areas of hemorrhage are found in the pancreas (*pancreatic apoplexy*), principally localized to the interstitium. When

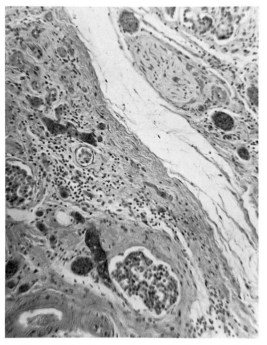

Figure 23–3. Pancreatic atrophy due to ductal obstruction. The acinar glands are totally replaced by fibrous tissue, but the islets are preserved.

these hemorrhages are widespread, they may convert the organ into a red-blue mass. These hemorrhages are unassociated with either macroscopic or microscopic evidence of inflammatory reaction or tissue necrosis. The absence of inflammatory reaction clearly indicates that such bleeding must have occurred in the agonal stages of life and that, therefore, the lesion is without clinical significance. Its major importance lies in differentiating such hemorrhage from the more significant hemorrhages found in certain acute necroses of this organ.

INFLAMMATIONS

ACUTE HEMORRHAGIC PANCREATIC NECROSIS (ACUTE HEMORRHAGIC PANCREATITIS)

Acute pancreatic necrosis refers to a sudden, more or less diffuse, enzymic destruction of pancreatic substance, caused presumably by the sudden escape of active lytic pancreatic enzymes into the glandular parenchyma. These enzymes characteristically cause focal areas of fat necrosis in and about the pancreas and in other fatty depots in the abdominal cavity. They also lead to rupture of pancreatic vessels and relatively insignificant or massive hemorrhages into the parenchyma of this organ. This sudden necrotizing destruction of the pancreas often follows an alcoholic debauch or an excessively large meal, suggesting some pathogenetic relationship. The designation acute hemorrhagic pancreatic necrosis is preferred to acute hemorrhagic pancreatitis, since it is more descriptive of the basic enzymic necrotizing character of the tissue destruction. Because the fate of the patient depends, to a considerable extent, upon the recognition and appropriate treatment of this condition, familiarity with its anatomic and clinical characteristics is mandatory.

Incidence. This condition occurs about once in every 500 to 600 medical and surgical admissions to a general hospital and, although it is by no means common, it can be expected that one such case might be admitted weekly to any large hospital. Acute pancreatic necrosis occurs most often in middle life in patients who are obese, and slightly more commonly in females than in males. It is particularly frequent among alcoholics, for reasons that will soon become clear. Recently, a hereditary predisposition to pancreatitis has been identified, transmitted apparently as an autosomal dominant trait (Logan et al., 1968). While such familial disease may be very severe in the individual patient, this hereditary form of pancreatitis makes an insignificant contribution to the total pool of this disease.

Etiology and Pathogenesis. The anatomic changes in this disease strongly suggest that acute pancreatic necrosis is caused by the destructive lytic effects of pancreatic enzymes. Why they run amok is still uncertain. Equally uncertain is which enzymes are of major importance. These issues have been intensively studied and, indeed, reasonable facsimiles of the clinical disease can be produced by a wide variety of interventions. However, the pertinence of these experimental observations to the patient is still unestablished (Banks, 1971) (Barraclough et al., 1972).

Turning to the issue of which enzymes are the principal culprits, it is evident from the morphology that proteolysis, lipolysis and hemorrhage are the three major morphologic features of this disorder. It would be natural to assume that trypsin, chymotrypsin and the lipases were the keys to such pancreatic destruction. Indeed, reflux of proteases into the pancreatic ducts initiates pancreatic inflammation in the experimental animal (Anderson et al., 1969). However, in the disease in man, activated trypsin or chymotrypsin is not found in large amounts in the damaged pancreas. Conceivably, small amounts of these proteases play a role in the initiation of a chain reaction, as will become clear. The contribution of lipase is equally unsettled. Clearly, it has great potential for causing enzymic necrosis of fat and, with ductal reflux of activated lipase in the experimental animal, a severe form of pancreatitis results. Whether lipase plays a significant role in the initiation of the disease in man is uncertain. On balance, the evidence indicates that it assumes principal importance after a chain reaction has already begun. Currently, there is greatest interest in elastase and phospholipase A. Elastase has been identified in high concentrations in the zymogen granules of acinous cells. It is present in pancreatic secretion as an inactive precursor. It can be activated by trypsin and, in the active form, causes dissolution of elastic fibers of blood vessels and ducts (Trowbridge and Moon, 1969) (Geokas et al., 1968). Tissues taken from patients who have died of this form of pancreatic disease disclose histologic features strongly suggestive of elastase activity. Similarly, phospholipase A may be important. When activated, it has two effects: destruction of cell membranes and the conversion of lecithin in bile to lysolecithin. This last-mentioned compound is believed to be highly toxic and capable of damaging the ductal system of the pancreas (Schmidt and Creutzfeldt, 1969).

It is difficult at the present time to single out one or even two enzymes that are most important in the causation of this disease in man. In fact, the only major enzymes which can be excluded are the amylases. *At the present time, we can only speculate that elastase and phospholipase A are probably key factors.* Trypsin may be implicated in their activation, but it is entirely possible that the formation of lysolecithin from lecithin initiates ductal injury and paves the way for the chain reaction.

It is not enough to identify the implicated enzymes. One must also ask how they are activated. Here the trail is even fainter. Theories abound, largely based on animal models, but facts are scanty. The possibility must be entertained that many pathways may all lead to activation of enzymes. The proposals can be categorized as follows:

1. Bile reflux
2. Hypersecretion-obstruction
3. Alcohol-induced changes
4. Duodenal reflux

Biliary reflux has long been considered an important mechanism of activation of pancreatic enzymes. Opie (1901) directed attention and perhaps overemphasized the role of a "common channel" in the production of pancreatitis. He noted, at autopsy of a patient who died of this disease, a gallstone impacted in the ampulla of Vater, which thereby blocked the outflow of both the pancreatic and common bile ducts. In effect, the two ductal systems were joined. As was pointed out earlier, in the majority of adults, the pancreatic duct and common bile duct join together before emptying into the duodenum. However, impaction of a gallstone in the ampulla of Vater is rarely seen in acute pancreatitis. Nonetheless, there is a substantial amount of evidence that biliary tract disease and bile reflux, even in the absence of a stone, contribute to the causation of this disorder. Pancreatitis is much more common among those with prior biliary tract disease than among those without it (Coghill and Song, 1970). In the experimental animal, when bile is instilled into the pancreatic ducts at high pressures, it induces a significant inflammatory reaction, but at low physiologic pressures it is without effect (Sum et al., 1970). Moreover, reflux of bile apparently occurs frequently in normal individuals without inducing any untoward effect. If bile, then, is to play an important role, the secretory pressures in the gallbladder must be increased, and perhaps this is a role for biliary tract disease. Alternatively, the bile might be rendered more toxic. Two constituents of bile have been found to be potentially injurious to ductal epithelium in the pancreas: unconjugated bile salts and lecithin. As pointed out earlier, the lecithin may be converted to the highly toxic lysolecithin by the action of phospholipase A, derived from pancreatic secretions. Unconjugated bile salts are formed from normal conjugated bile salts by bacterial action. Adding these observations together, one could propose increased biliary secretory pressures, perhaps due to prior biliary tract disease; reflux of bile into the pancreatic ducts at higher than normal pressures; and injury to pancreatic ducts, with leakage and activation of trypsin which, in turn, activates elastase and phospholipase A, the latter possibly producing lysolecithin. Interesting as such a proposal might be, it is still unsubstantiated.

The *hypersecretion-obstruction theory* proposes that rupture of ducts by pancreatic hypersecretion is the initial event possibly potentiated by partial ductal obstruction. Partial ductal obstruction is more dangerous than total obstruction, since pancreatic duct ligation in experimental animals does not evoke acute pancreatitis and, indeed, leads rapidly to suppression of pancreatic secretory function. On the other hand, partial obstructions, such as might be produced by small pancreatic stones or ductal metaplasia, might provide the appropriate setting for rupture (Fig. 23–5). With rupture of ducts, activated enzymes and lysolecithin are provided access to the interstitial tissue to there initiate the characteristic inflammatory changes. The hypersecretion pathway well fits the common story of the gargantuan meal just prior to an acute attack.

The *role of alcohol* is considered to be so important in the production of this disease that it has been dignified by the term "alcoholic pancreatitis." Alcohol is a potent stimulator of pancreatic secretions and, at the same time, it may lead to partial obstruction to pancreatic ducts (Kalant, 1969). Its secretory effect is mediated by increased acid secretion in the stomach and augmented release of secretin from the duodenal mucosa secondary to the high levels of gastric acidity. The mechanism by which alcohol induces partial ductal obstruction is less clear. In the dog, it has been reported that alcohol increases pancreatic sphincteric tone (Schapiro et al., 1970). Alcohol may also induce edema of the duodenal mucosa. It has also been considered to render pancreatic tissue vulnerable to injury by impairing the metabolism and enzymic activity of acinar cells (Darle et al., 1970). With these potential effects, alcohol could induce hypersecretion, rupture of ducts and further poten-

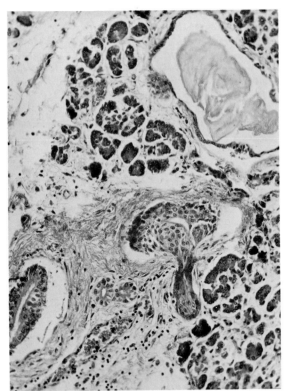

Figure 23-5. *Pancreas with squamous metaplasia of one of the small ducts virtually obliterating its lumen. Note the dilated duct above filled with inspissated secretion.*

tiate these damaging actions by direct injury to the homeostasis of the acinar cells.

Duodenal reflux would offer another possible means by which pancreatic enzymes could be activated within ducts. In this situation, bacteria might contribute to intraductal activation of enzymes. Indeed, suppression of the bacterial flora of the gut in the experimental animal reduces the incidence of pancreatitis induced by other interventions (Williams and Byrne, 1968). If for any reason the hypothetic sphincteric mechanism of the pancreatic duct is deranged, perhaps by alcohol-induced injury or inflammatory disease within the duodenum, reflux of duodenal juice might occur and initiate the disease.

Before closing this discussion, note should be made of the increased frequency of acute pancreatitis in patients having hyperparathyroidism and hypercalcemia (Banks and Janowitz, 1969). Approximately 7 to 19 per cent of patients having either a parathyroid adenoma or a parathyroid carcinoma develop acute pancreatitis (Banks, 1971). The basis for this association is not clear, but two possibilities exist: Increased levels of calcium in the blood and increased concentrations of calcium in pancreatic juice may induce an increase in the trypsin level of the pancreatic secretion. This has been documented in animals but not in man (Kelly, 1968). Hypercalcemia might also lead to intraductal stones and, thus, partial ductal obstruction. However, the great majority of patients with hyperparathyroidism and pancreatitis do not have pancreatic stones, and hypercalcemia has been shown to produce pancreatitis without the prior development of ductal stones. More often, when stones are present, the pancreatic changes take the form of chronic inflammatory fibrosis and atrophy, i.e., chronic pancreatitis (p. 1065).

Morphology. The histologic changes are presented first because they can be predicted, to a considerable extent, from the presumed pathogenesis of this disease. The basic alterations are four in number: **proteolytic destruction of pancreatic substance, necroses of blood vessels with subsequent hemorrhage, necrosis of fat by lipolytic enzymes, and an accompanying inflammatory reaction** (Roberts et al., 1950). The extent and predominance of each of these alterations depend upon the duration and severity of the process and vary from one case to the other. In the very early stages, a phase that has usually passed by the time the patient comes to postmortem examination, only interstitial edema is present. Soon after, focal and confluent areas of frank necrosis of endocrine and exocrine cells are found, but usually the resistant stroma remains fairly well preserved. The affected cells assume a glassy clouded appearance and then progressively undergo granular coagulative necrosis. The accompanying neutrophilic inflammatory reaction is usually confined to the margins of the necrotic foci. These lesions represent the proteolytic destruction. Hemorrhagic extravasation may be minimal to extreme. In the milder cases, the interstitium is suffused with red blood cells and fibrin clots; in severe instances, large areas of the pancreatic substance are virtually converted to a mass of blood clot.

Perhaps the most characteristic histologic alteration of acute pancreatic necrosis is the focal areas of fat necrosis that occur in the stromal, peripancreatic fat and fat depots throughout the abdominal cavity. These lesions consist of enzymic destruction of fat cells, in which **the vacuolated fat cells are transformed to shadowy outlines of cell membranes filled with pink, granular, opaque precipitate.** Presumably, this contained granular material is derived from the hydrolysis of fat. The liberated glycerol is reabsorbed, and the released fatty acids combine with calcium (a process referred to as saponification, or the formation of soaps) to form insoluble salts that are precipitated in situ.

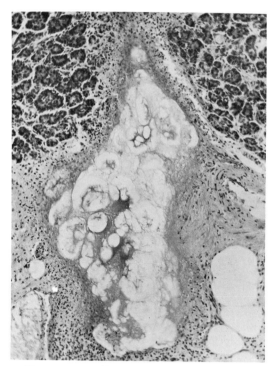

Figure 23–6. *Acute pancreatic necrosis. The central focus of necrotic fat is surrounded by a rim of leukocytic infiltration.*

Depending on the amount of calcium deposition, amorphous basophilic precipitates may be visible within the necrotic focus. It is to be particularly noted that the leukocytic exudate is confined to the periphery of these areas and there is no white cell infiltration in the central areas of the fat necrosis (Fig. 23–6). Moreover, the shadowy outlines of the cell membranes are readily visible.

The leukocytic reaction is also present between the areas of hemorrhage and necrosis of both fat and protein elements, but usually the white cell response is less marked in intensity than would be anticipated from the amount of tissue damage, highlighting the essential enzymic character of the destruction. In extreme cases, almost the entire pancreas may be wiped out but, at the other end of the spectrum, the damage may involve focal scattered areas and spare most of the gland. Secondary bacterial invasion, a common occurrence after the passage of 3 to 4 days, may modify this picture by converting many areas into foci of characteristic suppurative necrosis or frank abscess formation. If the patient survives, the acute necrotizing damage may slowly resolve and be replaced by diffuse or focal parenchymal or stromal fibrosis, calcifications and irregular ductal dilatations. Occasionally, liquefied areas are walled off by fibrous tissue to form small or large cystic spaces, known as **pseudocysts.**

Macroscopically, the dominant characteristics of acute pancreatic necrosis are **areas of gray-white proteolytic destruction of parenchymal substance, hemorrhage and chalky white areas of fat necrosis.** In the early stages, the edema may cause an increase in the size and consistency of the gland. However, soon thereafter, the classic features mentioned appear and produce in the typical case a very variegated map-like patterning in the pancreas, with areas of blue-black hemorrhage, other areas of gray-white necrotic softening, alternating with sprinkled foci of yellow-white chalky fat necrosis (Fig. 23–7). In individual cases, any one of these three components may dominate. Thus, occasionally the pancreas appears to be transformed to a solid mass of red-blue to black coagulated blood while, in other cases, it appears to have been converted into a soft, opaque, necrotic mass and, in still other instances, the hemorrhage may be largely absent and only foci of parenchymal and fatty necrosis are present.

Characteristically, there are accompanying changes in the remainder of the abdominal cavity.

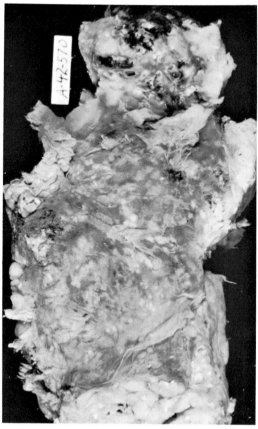

Figure 23–7. *Acute hemorrhagic pancreatic necrosis. The destruction here is moderate in severity and consists principally of scattered foci of white necrotic fat with several darker areas of hemorrhage above.*

In the majority of instances, the peritoneal cavity contains a serous, slightly turbid, brown-tinged fluid in which globules of oil can be identified (so-called "chicken broth" fluid). The liquid fat globules are quite characteristic of the lipolytic action of enzymes on the adult fat cells. In late cases, this fluid may become bacterially infected to produce suppurative peritonitis. Additionally, foci of fat necrosis may be found in any of the fat depots, such as in the omentum, mesentery of the bowel and properitoneal deposits. Occasionally, fat necrosis has been described in fat depots outside the abdominal cavity. This clearly indicates that the released enzymes cause their damage not only by direct escape into the peritoneal cavity, but also, in all probability, by absorption into the blood and lymphatic systems with transport throughout the body. It should be emphasized that the characteristic chalky white foci of fat necrosis and the peritoneal fluid are important findings in establishing the diagnosis of pancreatic necrosis on laparotomy. Associated biliary tract disease, cholecystitis and cholelithiasis, has been reported in as many as 80 to 90 per cent of cases of acute pancreatic necrosis. The relationship between this biliary tract disease and pancreatitis has already been noted, but obstructing stones are not found in the majority of such instances.

Clinical Course. Full-blown, acute pancreatic necrosis is a medical emergency of the first magnitude. These patients usually have the sudden calamitous onset of an "acute abdomen" that must be differentiated from such other causes as acute appendicitis, perforated peptic ulcer, acute cholecystitis with rupture, and occlusion of mesenteric vessels with infarction of the bowel, to mention a few. Characteristically, the pain appears without prodromal symptoms, usually soon after a large meal or an alcoholic debauch. The pain is constant and intense, and is often referred to the upper back. It appears to be aggravated by motion, probably due to peritoneal irritation. In many cases, soon thereafter, the agonizing pain leads to peripheral vascular collapse, and is sometimes followed by a profound shock-like state. Many explanations have been offered for this rapid development of shock. Absorption of necrotic proteinous debris, involvement of the celiac plexus, electrolyte disturbances such as the rapid withdrawal of calcium from the circulation, and bacterial toxicity have all been proposed.

On physical examination, when some time has elapsed between the onset and the examination, a fluid wave may be demonstrable. Jaundice sometimes appears after the first day and is presumed to be due to edematous narrowing of the common bile duct. The laboratory may provide direct support for the diagnosis. Characteristically, there is an elevation of the serum amylase level within the first 24 hours and the serum lipase level somewhat later (72 to 94 hours). Both remain elevated during the height of the active destructive disease in the pancreas and fall to basal levels 2 to 5 days after the acute phase passes. Elevated enzyme levels may also be produced by acute cholecystitis, perforated peptic ulcer and other inflammatory conditions in the upper abdomen that impinge on the pancreas.

Glycosuria develops in about 5 to 10 per cent of cases, apparently as an expression of acute disturbance in islet cell function. Classically, such glycosuria appears only during the acute phases and is transient, disappearing with the improvement of the condition. However, in a few cases the destruction of the islets may be so widespread as to cause permanent diabetes, a very uncommon occurrence. The presumptive diagnosis of acute necrosis of the pancreas can sometimes be established by aspiration of the characteristic "chicken broth" fluid from the abdomen. This diagnostic technique can be attempted only when there is a demonstrable accumulation of fluid in the abdomen. Recently, it has been reported that patients with this disease may have a positive test for carcinoembryonic antigen (CEA) (Delwiche et al., 1973). The CEA test was originally thought to be specific for cancer of the colon, but, since then, it has been found to be positive with many other diseases, as is pointed out on p. 970.

About 20 to 50 per cent of these patients die during the acute stages of peripheral vascular collapse and shock during the first week of the clinical course. If the patients survive this period, a variety of complications may follow: abscess, pseudocyst (p. 1067), paralytic ileus and hematemesis (Editorial, 1972).

CHRONIC INTERSTITIAL PANCREATITIS

This entity might more appropriately be termed recurrent acute pancreatitis or relapsing pancreatitis, because it undoubtedly represents progressive destruction of the pancreas by repeated acute flare-ups of inflammation. In former years, it was the custom to refer to acute interstitial pancreatitis and to a separate entity, chronic pancreatitis. However, follow-up of these cases over a long period of time indicated that these two entities merely represented two phases of the same disorder. If the organ was examined early in the course of events during an acute episode, it would disclose acute interstitial pancreatitis. With the repeated waves of destruction, a later phase would reveal the changes of chronic pancreatitis.

The condition is more common in males than females and is particularly common in alcoholics. The association between this pattern of pancreatic injury and alcoholism is paid eloquent tribute by the intern's designation, "rum belly" (Howat, 1963).

Its cause is as obscure as is the genesis of acute pancreatitis. Generally, it is believed that each wave of acute inflammation encountered in this entity is merely an attack of acute pancreatic necrosis in miniature. Perhaps some of the many factors that synergize each other to cause massive necrosis are absent from these less severe attacks of acute destruction encountered in relapsing pancreatitis. There is a high incidence of biliary tract disease among cases of relapsing pancreatitis, but some cases of this chronic pancreatic disease are encountered in the complete absence of biliary tract disorders. Moreover, it should be noted that biliary tract disease is more common in women than in men, quite the converse of relapsing pancreatitis. A few cases of chronic pancreatic disease have been reported in patients with hyperlipemia and in patients who have a strong hereditary background of similar disease in members of the family. However, these interesting syndromes represent a minority of the cases of chronic pancreatitis, and these observations are of principal importance because of their possible but as yet not understood pathogenetic significance.

Thal et al. (1959) have called attention to isoantibody formation in cases of chronic pancreatitis. But these antibodies were also found in patients with carcinoma of the pancreas and in a rare case of some presumed nonpancreatic disorder. It seems more reasonable to assume that these antibodies merely reflect injury to the pancreas, with the release of pancreatic proteins causing a secondary antibody reaction, rather than to ascribe any causal role to this immunologic observation.

Morphologically, there is a wide spectrum of changes. In the earlier stages of this disorder during the height of an acute attack, the gland may be slightly enlarged because of edema but is otherwise not grossly abnormal. Microscopically, acute interstitial edema with a minimal leukocytic infiltrate (neutrophils, lymphocytes and histiocytes) may be the only changes found. In the more severe attacks, there are foci of necrosis and, indeed, abscess formation. Sometimes the lesion takes the form of a subsiding acute inflammatory reaction denoted by large numbers of eosinophils and by areas of shadowy outlines of fat cells surrounded by a fibroblastic inflammatory zone containing foreign body type giant cells. In the long chronicity of this disorder, there is progressive destruction of pancreatic substance with shrinkage in the size of the gland and progressive accumulation of fibrous scarring with replacement of both acinar and islet cell elements (Fig. 23–8). Such glands are nodular and firm to hard with areas of calcification and possible pseudocyst formation. These pseudocysts may be small collections of essentially clear to slightly turbid fluid not more than 1 cm. in diameter, or they may be many centimeters in diameter and contain fluid of varying degrees of turbidity often with flecks of blood pigment, cholesterol clefts and gritty fragments of calcium. Analysis of such cystic contents often discloses high levels of pancreatic enzymes. Squamous metaplasia of ducts, deposits of interstitial amorphous calcium or laminated pancreatic ductal stones are additional common features (Edmondson et al., 1949).

During the early phases of the disease, the reserve capacity of the pancreas is sufficient to block the development of metabolic disturbances, and these disorders may present themselves as recurrent attacks of abdominal discomfort that are extremely difficult diagnostic problems. Elevations of the serum amylase and lipase levels are very helpful findings but raise the serious differential diagnosis of acute

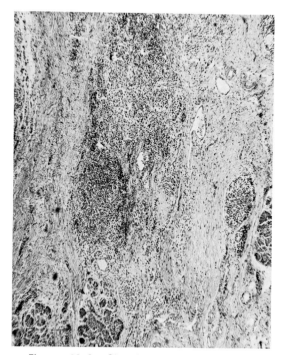

Figure 23–8. Chronic pancreatitis. The large fibrous scar with lymphocytic infiltration occupies the center of the field.

hemorrhagic pancreatic necrosis. Between attacks, during the early stages of the disease, the patient may be entirely asymptomatic. Later, as more and more pancreatic substance is wiped out, manifestations of functional insufficiency may appear, such as steatorrhea, glycosuria and the appearance of calcifications on abdominal x-ray. Because of the wide spectrum of clinical manifestations, the recurrent nature of this condition and the variable severity of the attacks, chronic relapsing pancreatitis is a difficult clinical diagnosis (Gross and Comfort, 1956).

TUMORS

The heading "tumors of the pancreas" is used to include a variety of non-neoplastic and neoplastic masses that involve this organ. The non-neoplastic masses almost invariably take the form of cysts, while the neoplasms are of both benign and malignant, and primary and secondary types. The most important primary neoplasms are carcinomas and islet cell tumors.

CYSTS

Cysts are infrequent findings in the pancreas, but are of considerable clinical significance since they may present as abdominal masses that are suspected of being malignant. They vary from minute lesions found only on serial section of the gland to large masses up to 30 to 40 cm. in diameter that are readily palpable through the abdominal wall. They may be found in any location within the pancreas, but are somewhat more common in the body and tail regions. They arise from a variety of causes (Abeshouse, 1953).

Congenital Cysts of the Pancreas. Congenital cysts are believed to result from anomalous development of the pancreatic ducts. In the genesis of the pancreas, it is postulated, a succession of duct systems develop and degenerate until the adult definitive pattern is created. Persistence and segmentation of some of the primitive ducts may give rise to small sequestered nests of ductal secretory cells that fill up with fluid to create cysts. This pathogenetic mechanism is analogous to the one proposed as the origin of congenital cysts in the kidney and liver and, in fact, congenital cystic disease of the pancreas, liver and kidney coexists not infrequently. Usually these cysts are multiple, but occasionally they occur singly. They range in size from microscopic lesions to larger spaces up to 3 to 5 cm. in diameter. They are lined by a smooth, glistening membrane that may, on histologic section, have total atrophy of the lining epithelial cells, or may show preservation of flattened pavement or low cuboidal epithelial cells. They are usually enclosed in a thin fibrous capsule and are filled with a clear to turbid, mucoid or serous fluid. Occasionally, hemorrhage or infection modifies the appearance of the lining epithelium and the cystic contents.

In one rare entity, *Lindau-von Hippel disease*, angiomas are found in the retina and cerebellum or brain stem in association with such cysts in the pancreas, as well as in the liver and kidney.

Retention Cysts. Retention cysts have already been referred to under the discussion of obstruction of pancreatic ducts. These cysts are usually considerably smaller than the congenital cysts, and many have a communication with adjacent ducts. They are usually multiple, rarely exceed several centimeters in diameter and are of little clinical significance.

Pseudocysts of the Pancreas. This term is applied to a collection of fluid that arises from loculation of inflammatory processes, necroses or hemorrhages (Waugh and Lynn, 1958). The accumulation of fluid may follow traumatic injury to the abdomen with direct damage and hemorrhage in the pancreas. These cysts are usually solitary and are frequently quite massive, with isolated cases having recorded diameters in the range of 20 to 40 cm. Such cysts may be situated within the pancreatic substance but, *more often, they are found adjacent to the pancreas, particularly in the region of the tail.* Sometimes these pseudocysts are formed by the accumulation of fluid in the lesser omental sac adjacent to the tail of the pancreas. Depending upon the genesis of the collection of fluid, the wall may be moderately thin, but is usually quite thick and fibrous (Fig. 23–9). The contents vary from turbid, serous fluid to purulent exudate, modified sometimes by fresh or changed blood. Characteristically, they do not have an epithelial lining and have no connection or communication with surrounding ductal systems. There is usually a marked inflammatory reaction in the fibrous capsule and often organizing blood clot, old blood pigment, precipitates of calcium and cholesterol clefts. Many cysts are lined by organizing granulation tissue. Usually, by the time the lesion is removed, the fluid contents have been transformed to a turbid serous fluid and, even though the initial lesion may have been bacterially infected, the bacterial contamination may have long since died out and the exudate been digested to a thin watery fluid.

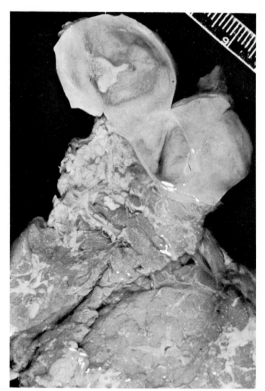

Figure 23–9. Pseudocyst of pancreas. The cyst has been opened and contents drained. A small plaque of white calcium is visible in the wall.

Their major clinical significance lies in their being discovered as an abdominal mass in a location that strongly suggests a primary intra-abdominal malignancy. Occasionally, such cysts rupture and cause generalized peritonitis. They are treated by drainage, marsupialization or resection but are often difficult to manage.

Neoplastic Cysts. These lesions are cystadenomas or cystadenocarcinomas. They are very uncommon tumors of the pancreas, and are presumed to arise as cystic neoplasms from the ducts. These neoplasms are usually solitary, and generally vary in diameter from 5 to 15 cm. Histologically, they have a well defined lining epithelium characteristically thrown up into numerous papillary projections that form branching villous processes. Frequently, these cysts are multilocular and resemble, to a considerable degree, the cystadenomas of the ovary (p. 1242). In the benign form, the columnar epithelial lining cells are well oriented to their basement membrane, are regularly aligned and have no evidence of anaplasia, piling up or invasiveness. However, in the cystadenocarcinomatous varieties, the epithelium assumes the anaplasia of all malignancy, becomes piled up into irregular proliferative masses and invades the underlying wall and adjacent structures.

CARCINOMA OF THE PANCREAS

The term carcinoma of the pancreas is meant to imply carcinoma arising in the exocrine portion of the gland. For unknown reasons, virtually all these cancers begin in the ductal epithelium; the glands themselves virtually never give origin to a malignant tumor. Tumors that arise from the islets of Langerhans are specifically designated as islet cell lesions and will be considered later (p. 1072). Pancreatic cancers, while not common, are highly fatal. Thus, they cause about 6 per cent of all neoplastic deaths in the United States and rank high among fatal cancers. The relative frequency of these lesions appears to be on the increase perhaps because cancer of the digestive system as a whole is on the decrease (Glenn and Thorbjarnarson, 1964). These malignancies are of great importance because of their silent growth habits already mentioned. Cures by surgical resection are extremely rare. These tumors occur most often in the sixth, seventh and eighth decades of life, although about 10 per cent of the patients are much younger. There is a male preponderance in the ratio of about 2:1 (Bell, 1957).

While these lesions may arise anywhere in the pancreas, all studies show a fairly standard distribution: head of the pancreas, 60 to 70 per cent; body of pancreas, 20 to 30 per cent; and tail of pancreas, 5 to 10 per cent (Goswitz, 1961). In some cases, the tumor has spread so widely by the time of discovery as to preclude localization of its precise site of origin. From the standpoints of their clinical significance, usual life history and manner of spread, carcinomas of the head of the pancreas differ strikingly from those of the body and tail. Tumors of the head of the pancreas are in a strategic location to impinge upon the ampulla of Vater, common bile duct and duodenum and thus cause obstructive biliary symptoms relatively early in their life history. These lesions, therefore, tend to be discovered while still small and before widespread metastasis has occurred. In contrast, cancers in the body and tail may grow silently for longer periods of time and become manifest only by extension to adjacent structures and by metastatic dissemination. Both forms, however, are intrinsically similar anatomic lesions that differ only in their location and hence in their resultant clinical manifestations (Leach, 1950).

Carcinoma of the Head of the Pancreas. Grossly, tumors in this region of the pancreas are fairly small lesions that frequently cause little or only moderate expansion of the head of the pancreas. Sometimes they are totally inapparent on external examination of the organ and only create the impression of some increased consistency and irregular nodularity in the glandular substance. Other lesions create masses up to 8 to 10 cm. in diameter. They are most readily visualized by transection of the gland. The gray-white scirrhous, homogeneous tumor infiltrates and replaces the usual yellow lobular architecture. Characteristically, such lesions have poorly defined, obviously infiltrative margins with few, if any, foci of hemorrhage (Fig. 23—10). Occasionally, small areas of yellow-white opaque infarct necrosis are present. The tumor frequently narrows the common bile duct and pancreatic duct and may cause atrophy of the distal pancreas. It extends usually to the margin of the duodenum and frequently invades the wall as well as the common bile duct. In a small percentage of cases, it extends directly through the wall either to produce a small fungating lesion within the duodenal lumen or, more often, to cause a shallow, irregular, obviously malignant ulceration (Fig. 23—11). In this infiltrative growth, it frequently surrounds and compresses, and less commonly directly invades, the common bile duct or ampulla of Vater. Invasion of the portal vein, hepatic flexure of the colon and the stomach is uncommon. This local spread of cancer of the pancreas usually is blocked by the confinement of the surrounding organs.

As a consequence of the involvement of the common bile duct, there is marked distention of the gallbladder in about 50 per cent of the patients. You recall that, according to Courvoisier's law (p. 1043), neoplastic obstruction of the biliary outflow tract induces gallbladder distention, while calculous obstruction implies chronic cholecystitis, and such fibrotic changes prevent gallbladder enlargement. This so-called "law," however, has repeatedly been proved to be unreliable. Cholecystitis is a not infrequent accompaniment of pancreatic disease and may, therefore, prevent distention of the gallbladder. On the other hand, the inflammatory fibrosis of cholecystitis and cholelithiasis may not be of sufficient magnitude to prevent distention of this organ when the common duct is blocked.

As a consequence of the biliary tract obstruction, patients who die of carcinoma of the pancreas almost invariably have intense bile stasis in the liver and other tissues and often have well developed biliary cirrhosis (p. 1033).

Most of the carcinomas of the pancreas grow in more or less well differentiated glandular patterns and are thus adenocarcinomas (Fig. 23—12). The tumors may be either mucinous or nonmucin secreting. The gland patterns, however, may be atypical, irregular, small and bizarre, and lined by anaplastic cuboidal to columnar epithelial cells. Other variants grow in an undifferentiated pattern. Rarely, some assume an adenoacanthomatous pattern or the uncommon pattern of extreme anaplasia with giant cell formation, numerous mitoses and bizarre pleomorphism.

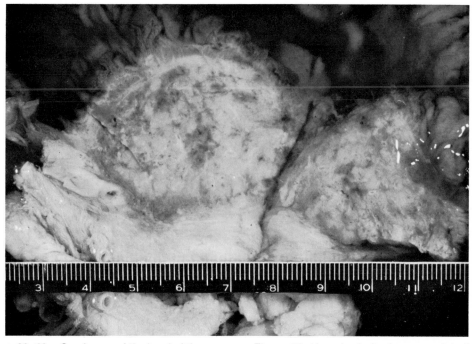

Figure 23—10. Carcinoma of the head of the pancreas. The mottled invasive lesion has grown into the wall of the duodenum which appears at the upper extent of the tumor.

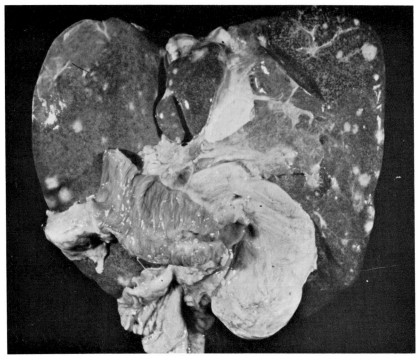

Figure 23–11. Carcinoma of the head of the pancreas with bile stasis and metastases in liver. The primary lesion has caused a small ulceration in the exposed wall of the duodenum.

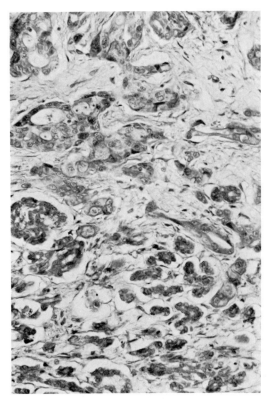

Figure 23–12. Adenocarcinoma of the pancreas. The atypical glands are invading the pancreatic substance seen at the bottom of the photograph.

Invasion of ducts, obliteration of ducts, destruction of islets, invasion of lymphatics and vessels can often be identified. Notwithstanding this gross and microscopic evidence of invasiveness, carcinoma of the head of the pancreas is usually not a widely disseminated lesion when found at autopsy. Extension to peripancreatic and portohepatic nodes with isolated, small metastases in the liver is not uncommon. But because these tumors produce biliary tract obstruction and jaundice at an early date, they usually have not had a long life history before discovery, and patients die of their hepatobiliary dysfunction before the tumor has become widely disseminated. However, in many cases, metastases involve the lungs, bone marrow, peritoneum, pleura and other organs.

Carcinoma of the Body and Tail of the Pancreas. These tumors are usually large, hard, irregular masses that may sometimes wipe out virtually the entire tail and body of the pancreas. Rarely, they reach a diameter of 10 to 15 cm. and are readily palpable, particularly in the thin patient. On cross section, the tumors exactly resemble those of the head of the gland and, microscopically, the same cytologic and architectural patterns are repeated. In this location, **these carcinomas frequently extend more widely than those of the head.** They impinge upon the adjacent vertebral column, extend through the retroperitoneal spaces inferiorly and superiorly and occasionally invade the adjacent spleen or adrenal. They may extend into the transverse colon or stomach (Fig. 23–13). Peripancreatic, gastric, mesenteric, omental and portohepatic nodes are frequently involved, and the liver is often strikingly seeded with tumor nodules to produce hepatic enlargement two to three times the normal size. Such massive hepatic metastases are quite characteristic of carcinoma of the tail and body of the pancreas, and are attributed to invasion of the splenic vein that courses directly along the margins of this organ. Penetration into the retroperitoneal lymphatics and vessels as well as into the peritoneal cavity leads to distant metastases in the lungs, bone and other organs, and to peritoneal carcinomatosis (Duff, 1939). On the other hand, extension to the head of the pancreas, with involvement of the duodenum and biliary tract, is infrequent.

Clinical Course. Carcinomas of the pancreas, even those of the head of the pancreas, are insidious lesions that undoubtedly are present for months and possibly years before they produce symptoms referable to their expansile growth. The major symptoms include weight loss (approximately 70 per cent), abdominal pain (approximately 50 per cent), back pain (approximately 25 per cent), anorexia, nausea, vomiting and generalized malaise, and weakness. Carcinoma of the pancreas was often considered a painless disease until far advanced. It is classically held out as a cause of painless jaundice. It should, therefore, be specifically noted that the majority of the patients have pain. Jaundice is present in about 50 per cent

of patients with carcinomas of the head of the pancreas but is a rare finding in those lesions that arise in the tail and body. The gallbladder is enlarged and palpable in about half of the patients with tumors in the head of the pancreas. There is an additional widely prevalent misconception that jaundice, when it appears, is progressive and unremitting due to the continued expansile growth of these tumors. However, necrosis of the tumor sometimes permits transient flow of the bile, and so there may well be fluctuations in the mounting serum bilirubin levels.

Because these tumors are so insidious, many efforts have been made to establish laboratory procedures, such as enzyme determinations, which might provide a clue to the existence of these cancers. However, none of these procedures, such as the leucine aminopeptidase levels, has withstood the test of time.

Within the very recent past, it has been shown that 80 to 90 per cent of patients with cancer of the pancreas have positive diagnostic tests for carcinoembryonic antigen (CEA) (Zamcheck et al., 1972). Formerly thought to be quite specific for cancer of the colon, it is now clear that the CEA assay is positive in a number of other conditions such as pancreatitis, liver disease, cancer of the lung, cancer of the breast and ulcerative colitis. At the present time, therefore, the interpretation of a positive CEA test must be done with great caution. It has become apparent that only the standard techniques that indicate biliary tract obstruc-

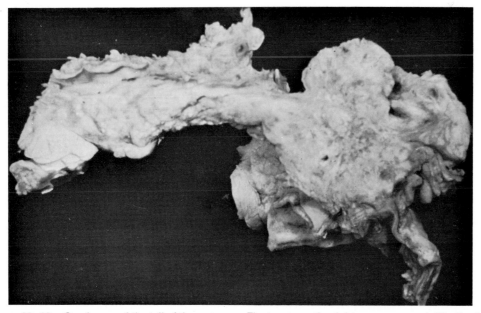

Figure 23–13. *Carcinoma of the tail of the pancreas. The tumor on the right appears as an infiltrative irregular mass.*

tion are of help in this diagnostic quandary. As would be expected, in any form of obstructive jaundice, there are elevations of the serum bilirubin levels, principally of the conjugated form. The increased levels of conjugated bilirubin are excreted through the kidneys to produce bile in the urine. With the decreased excretion of bile into the intestinal tract, the stools become clay-colored and the urobilinogen levels of the urine fall. The alkaline phosphatase levels, as a sensitive indicator of biliary tract obstruction, are almost always elevated.

Spontaneous venous thrombosis, also referred to as migratory thrombophlebitis and clinically known as Trousseau's sign, is sometimes encountered in patients with pancreatic carcinoma. Ironically, Trousseau diagnosed his own fatal disease as cancer of the pancreas when he developed migratory thrombophlebitis. These spontaneously appearing and disappearing thromboses are also encountered in other forms of cancer, but the two highest levels of correlation are with pancreatic and pulmonary neoplasms (Fusco and Rosen, 1966). The pathogenesis of the thromboses probably involves a number of factors, including confinement to bed and surgical interventions but, in addition, it has been suggested that the necrotic products of the tumor may induce a hypercoagulable state (Sise et al., 1962).

While surgical resection is attempted in the appropriate cases, five-year survivals are exceedingly rare. Ninety per cent of patients with this disease die within six to 12 months of the appearance of clinically recognizable signs and symptoms. Death is usually occasioned by obstructive biliary disease, hepatorenal failure or progressive spread of the tumor and its associated malignant cachexia. At the time of autopsy, metastases are found in the liver in three-quarters of the cases and, in descending order of frequency, in the peripancreatic lymph nodes, peritoneal cavity, lung, pleura and skeletal system.

ISLET CELL LESIONS

Three distinctive cells have been identified in the islets of Langerhans in man: the beta, alpha and delta cells, and some investigators would add a gamma cell (Arky and Knopp, 1971). The beta cell has been most intensively studied because it produces insulin. Lacy (1967) has been able to demonstrate, by some elegant electron microscopic and functional studies, the cycle of elaboration and secretion of insulin. He followed the synthesis of the insulin-containing beta granules within the endoplasmic reticulum, their transfer to the region of the Golgi complex, where the granules are apparently enclosed within a smooth membranous sac, and the subsequent migration of this sac to the periphery of the cell, where it fuses with the cell membrane and later opens to eject its insulin content into the intercellular pericapillary space. Hyperplasia and neoplasia of these cells are responsible for the important clinical syndrome of hyperinsulinism to be described. The alpha cells of the islets secrete glucagon. This substance induces hyperglycemia by its glycogenolytic activity in the liver. Tumors of alpha cells are exceedingly rare and are sometimes called glucagonomas. The role of delta cells is still somewhat uncertain, but recent studies utilizing the fluorescent antibody technique suggest that these cells may secrete gastrin (Lomsky et al., 1969) and/or secretin. This observation may help to explain islet cell lesions with the Zollinger-Ellison syndrome.

Three distinctive clinical syndromes are associated with hyperfunction of the islets of Langerhans: hyperinsulinism, multiple endocrine adenomatosis and the Zollinger-Ellison syndrome. Each of these three clinical entities may be caused by (1) diffuse hyperplasia of the islets of Langerhans, (2) benign adenomas that occur singly or multiply and (3) malignant tumors. It should be emphasized that nonfunctioning adenomas and carcinomas also arise in the islets, albeit quite rarely.

Hyperinsulinism—Beta Cell Lesions. Hyperplasia or neoplasia of the beta cells may be responsible for the elaboration of sufficient insulin to induce clinically significant hypoglycemia. The characteristic clinical manifestations that result from these pancreatic lesions were well detailed by Whipple in his classic triad: (1) attacks of hypoglycemia occur with blood sugar levels below 50 mg. per 100 ml. of serum; (2) the attacks consist principally of such central nervous system manifestations as confusion, stupor and loss of consciousness and are clearly related to fasting or exercise; (3) the attacks are promptly relieved by the feeding or parenteral administration of glucose. While there are other causes for hypoglycemia when a patient manifests Whipple's triad, the cause should first be sought in the pancreas.

Analysis of pancreatic islet lesions inducing hyperinsulinism indicates that about 70 per cent are solitary adenomas, approximately 10 per cent are multiple adenomas, 10 per cent are metastasizing tumors that must be interpreted as carcinomas and the remainder are a mixed group of diffuse hyper-

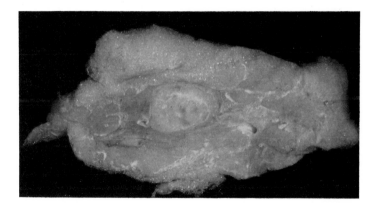

Figure 23–14. *Islet cell adenoma of the pancreas. The small, pale tumor is seen on transection of the pancreas.*

plasia of the islets and adenomas occurring in ectopic pancreatic tissue. The insulin-producing adenomas, often called insulinomas, vary in size from minute lesions difficult to find even on the dissecting table to huge masses of over 1500 gm. (Fig. 23—14). While most occur singly as indicated earlier, in about one case in seven, multiple adenomas are found scattered throughout the pancreatic substance. They are usually encapsulated, firm, yellow-brown nodules that, by expansile growth, compress the surrounding pancreatic substance. Histologically, they are composed of cords and nests of well differentiated beta cells that do not differ from those of the normal islet (Fig. 23—15). Not even the malignant lesions display much evidence of anaplasia and, in fact, it may be impossible from the histologic evaluation of the tumor to determine its biologic behavior. Rupture of the capsule and extension into the surrounding pancreatic substance are not reliable criteria of malignancy, and the diagnosis of carcinoma of the islets should not be made in the absence of unmistakable evidence of metastasis or local invasion beyond the substance of the pancreas. In a study of approximately 400 cases of islet cell tumors, Howard et al. (1950) reported that 313 were morphologically and clinically benign, 48 were morphologically malignant but clinically benign and 37 were both clinically and morphologically malignant. Not cited in this analysis are the other cases that appear morphologically benign but are clinically malignant.

Hyperinsulinism may be caused also by diffuse hyperplasia of the islets. This change is found occasionally in adults but is rather characteristic of infants born of diabetic mothers. Long exposed to the hyperglycemia of the maternal blood, the infant responds by an increase in the size and number of its islets. In the postnatal period, these hyperactive islets may be responsible for serious episodes of hypoglycemia.

The differential diagnosis of hypoglycemia must also include a consideration of a variety of functional and organic disorders in addition to the beta cell lesions already discussed. Functional hypoglycemia is sometimes encountered quite mysteriously in patients without apparent underlying cause and may here be referred to as idiopathic hypoglycemia. It is also encountered in so-called insulin sensitivity states, early diabetes mellitus, after partial gastrectomy, in starvation and in certain leucine-sensitive states. The organic causes for hypoglycemia

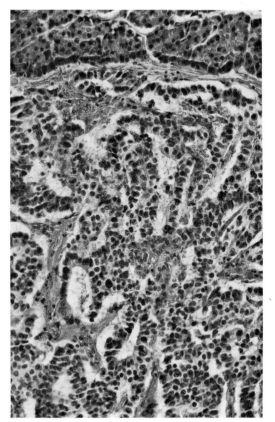

Figure 23–15. *Islet adenoma of pancreas. The well defined margin of an islet cell tumor. Note the resemblance of the tumor cells to normal islet cells.*

include, in addition to the beta cell lesions already described, diffuse liver disease, the glycogenoses, hypofunction of the anterior pituitary and adrenal cortex, and a variety of extrapancreatic neoplasms. The association of hypoglycemia with these extrapancreatic neoplasms has excited considerable interest in the effort to elucidate the underlying mechanisms. Fibromas and fibrosarcomas located in the retroperitoneal space adjacent to the diaphragm or in the thorax predominate among these interesting problems. Also responsible, although less commonly, are such varied tumors as hepatic, adrenal, gastric and bile duct carcinomas. All these tumors generally are of large size and, while many have metastasized, there is no linear correlation between the production of hypoglycemia and the total mass of tumor. Several studies have identified elevations of a circulating insulin-like substance in patients with these tumors, but its precise nature has not been further characterized (Field et al., 1963).

Zollinger-Ellison Syndrome. Reference has been previously made, in the consideration of peptic ulcer, to the syndrome described by Zollinger and Ellison (1955), comprising *the association of pancreatic islet cell lesions with gastric hypersecretion and peptic ulceration.* When first described in 1955, attention was focused on the occurrence of these ulcers in the jejunum. Since that time, however, it has become clear that the ulcers occur most often in the usual sites within the stomach and duodenum, and only 25 per cent occur in atypical locations such as the jejunum. As indicated earlier, most investigators suggest that the islet cell adenomas are derived from delta cells capable of elaborating gastrin (Grossman et al., 1961). However, several recent studies indicate that gastrin cannot be isolated from all neoplasms associated with the Zollinger-Ellison syndrome, and raise the question of whether certain neoplasms elaborate a secretin-like hormone. If, indeed, this observation is validated, it poses the intriguing question of whether delta cells elaborate both gastrin and secretin or, alternatively, if there is a fourth secretin-producing cell in the islets (Zollinger et al., 1968).

The pancreatic lesions that underlie the Zollinger-Ellison syndrome are non-beta cell neoplasias and hyperplasias. The cell of origin now appears to be the delta cell, but further questions remain, as was pointed out earlier. In an extensive review of these lesions in 1964, approximately 60 per cent were malignant, two-thirds having metastasized at the time of discovery, and 40 per cent

were benign. Among the benign lesions, 30 per cent were adenomas and 10 per cent showed hyperplasia of the islets alone. Some of the benign adenomas occurred multiply and in association with endocrine adenomas elsewhere, justifying their being classified as examples of multiple endocrine adenomatosis (Ellison and Wilson, 1964). As with the insulin-secreting lesion of the pancreas, the cytologic evaluation of the tumor is not a reliable criterion of its biologic behavior. Evidence of invasion and spread to lymph nodes or extrapancreatic sites is required for the unmistakable diagnosis of malignancy. The regional lymph nodes about the pancreas are the most commonly affected extrapancreatic sites, followed in order of frequency by local invasion into peripancreatic tissues and metastasis to the liver. Infrequently, the metastases spread to the lung.

As mentioned, these patients have a fulminant, intractable, ulcerogenic diathesis. Seventy-five per cent of the ulcers occur in the usual sites within the stomach or, more often, in the first and second portions of the duodenum. Abnormally located peptic ulcers in the distal portions of the duodenum and jejunum occur in 25 per cent of the cases. In one of ten patients, there are multiple ulcerations.

Patients with the Zollinger-Ellison syndrome constitute formidable problems in clinical management. They have striking gastric hypersecretion which presumably produces the intractable ulcers. In addition, diarrhea is often sufficiently extreme to cause serious problems in fluid and electrolyte control, and many patients develop malabsorption syndromes (Rawson et al., 1960) (Summerskill, 1959). Moreover, the lesions in the pancreas may not only be malignant but, even when benign, may be very small or multiple and difficult to discover at surgical exploration. It is not uncommon, therefore, for symptoms to be recurrent following removal of an apparent solitary lesion, with later discovery of additional lesions within the pancreas (Smith, 1965).

Multiple Endocrine Adenomatosis. This fascinating syndrome, as first described, comprised the common association of "multiple endocrine adenomas" of the pituitary, pancreas and parathyroid glands. Wermer (1963) expanded this entity when he noted the frequent occurrence of peptic ulcers in these patients. He further postutated a familial distribution, now defined as an autosomal dominant mode of transmission with incomplete penetrance. Virtually contemporaneously, the Zollinger-Ellison syndrome was described, associating some noninsulin-producing islet cell tumors of the pancreas with peptic ulcers. Since these original descriptions, the Zollinger-

Ellison syndrome has been noted in individuals with multiple endocrine tumors, and families have been identified in which one member had the Zollinger-Ellison syndrome while others had multiple adenomas (Way et al., 1968). Currently, it is believed that multiple endocrine adenomatosis and the Zollinger-Ellison syndromes are phenotypic variants of the same mutant gene.

In addition to the pituitary, pancreas and parathyroids, it is recognized that the adrenals may also be involved and, in all of these sites, although adenomas are usual, occasionally the lesions take the form of hyperplasia or even carcinoma. The concurrence of such pluriglandular involvement and peptic ulcers has now been designated multiple endocrine adenomatosis I to contrast it with yet another variant. Multiple endocrine adenomatosis II comprises concurrent pheochromocytomas and medullary carcinoma of the thyroid, sometimes associated with endocrine gland adenomas, cutaneous and mucosal neurofibromatosis and sometimes increased levels of circulating calcitonin. Table 23–1 indicates the areas of overlap of MEA I and MEA II. It is evident that MEA I comprises, in essence, polyendocrine involvement associated with peptic ulcers. In contrast, MEA II is better remembered as the medullary carcinoma-pheochromocytoma syndrome not associated with peptic ulcers. Both patterns of MEA are familial and may be phenotypic variants of the same mutant gene. Not all the multiple components are necessarily encountered in the same patient in either MEA I or MEA II, but families appear to run true to form (Croughs et al., 1972) (Baum, 1971). Other variants have been segregated, strongly suggesting a spectrum of familial disorders arising out of specific gene mutations or variable expressions of a common mutant gene.

Classically, the pathogenesis of MEA I is

thought to be a genetic defect leading directly to cellular proliferation in affected endocrine glands (Weichert, 1970). According to this hypothesis, the polyglandular syndrome represents a systemic disease of the neuroectoderm. However, since adrenal adenomas figure prominently in these patients and the adrenal cortex is of mesodermal origin, there are obvious deficiencies in such a proposition. Alternatively, attention is focused on a single glandular lesion as the primary disorder in MEA I, and all of the other wide-ranging findings are interpreted as changes secondary to the secretory products of the primary lesion. The primary culprit might be the pancreatic islets. Thus, it is proposed that pancreatic islet hyperplasia or a pancreatic adenoma secretes a variety of hormones including insulin, glucagon and gastrin, as well as inappropriate ACTH, MSH and serotonin. Gastrin secretion would, of course, lead to peptic ulcer formation. Glucagon has a hypocalcemic effect, due either to promotion of bone uptake of calcium or to the release of calcitonin from the thyroid gland (Avioli et al., 1969). The hypocalcemia would, in turn, lead to parathyroid hyperplasia and conceivably, in time, to adenoma formation. Supporting such a proposition is the recent review of 15 such patients with hyperparathyroidism, in 12 of whom islet cell hyperplasia could be demonstrated (Paloyan et al., 1967). In another study, six members of a family with this syndrome were shown to have evidence of islet cell hyperactivity with increased insulin, glucagon and gastrin secretion. In these patients, the increased levels of glucagon could induce the hypocalcemia. The chronic hyperinsulinism could lead directly or indirectly to the secretion of growth hormone, ACTH, glucocorticoids and epinephrine, thus conceivably stimulating the formation of functioning tumors of the pituitary gland, adrenal cortex and adrenal medulla (Vance et al., 1969). Speculation is rife in the attempt to reconcile the multiplicity of endocrine derangements in these enigmatic disorders.

It is impossible to even summarize the range of clinical presentations which may be encountered in MEA I and MEA II. In the individual patient, one or two of the functioning lesions usually overshadow the others. Among the more frequent presentations are: (1) intractable peptic ulcer disease, (2) evidence of hyperparathyroidism, (3) manifestations arising in the pancreatic islet lesions such as hyperinsulinism, (4) Cushing's syndrome and (5) hypertension related to the pheochromocytomas.

TABLE 23–1. MULTIPLE ENDOCRINE ADENOMATOSIS SYNDROMES

Lesions	MEA I	MEA II
Pituitary	++++	0
Medullary carcinoma of thyroid	++	++++
Parathyroid	++++	++
Adrenal cortex	++++	+
Pheochromocytoma	0	++++
Pancreas	++++	0
Peptic ulcer	++++	0
Neuromas	0	++++

MISCELLANEOUS TUMORS

While lipomas, myxomas, fibromas, perineural fibromas, angiomas, lymphangiomas and their malignant counterparts have been described in the pancreas, they are all exactly comparable to such lesions found elsewhere, and are, moreover, of such rare occurrence as to merit no further discussion.

SECONDARY MALIGNANCY OF THE PANCREAS

In general, the pancreas is infrequently involved by the dissemination of other primary malignancies. When it is secondarily involved, it is most often due to the direct contiguous growth of a cancer arising in an anatomically closely situated organ such as the stomach, colon and biliary tract. Metastases from distant sites affect the pancreas itself quite uncommonly but, on the other hand, are by no means unusual in the peripancreatic nodes. When such surrounding nodes are involved, the tumor may extend through the capsule of these structures to invade the pancreatic substance. It is often difficult to differentiate true involvement of the pancreatic substance from metastasis to adjacent nodes with secondary extension to the pancreas. The differentiation is of little more than academic interest, but it is nonetheless of some significance to note the infrequency with which the true pancreatic parenchyma is the initial site of hematogenous dissemination.

REFERENCES

Abeshouse, B. S.: Differential diagnosis of pancreatic and renal disease with particular emphasis on differentiating pancreatic cysts from renal cysts. Int. Abstr. Surg., 96:1, 1953.

Anderson, M. C., et al.: Further inquiry into the pathogenesis of acute pancreatitis. Arch. Surg., 99:185, 1969.

Arky, R. A., and Knopp, R. H.: Evaluation of islet-cell function in man. New Eng. J. Med., 285:1130, 1971.

Avioli, L. V., et al.: Role of the thyroid gland during glucagon-induced hypocalcaemia in the dog. Amer. J. Physiol., 216:939, 1969.

Baggenstoss, A. H.: The pancreas in uremia. Amer. J. Path., 24:1003, 1948.

Ballard, H. S., et al.: Familial multiple endocrine adenoma-peptic ulcer complex. Medicine, 43:481, 1964.

Banks, P. A.: Acute pancreatitis. Gastroenterology, 61:382, 1971.

Banks, P. A., and Janowitz, H. D.: Some metabolic aspects of exocrine pancreatic disease. Gastroenterology, 56:601, 1969.

Barraclough, B. H., et al.: Acute pancreatitis: a review. Aust. New Zeal. J. Surg., 41:211, 1972.

Baum, J. L.: Abnormal intradermal histamine reaction in the syndrome of pheochromocytoma, medullary carcinoma of the thyroid gland and multiple mucosal neuromas. New Eng. J. Med., 284:963, 1971.

Bell, E. T.: Carcinoma of the pancreas. I. A clinical and pathologic study of 609 necropsied cases. II. The relation of carcinoma of the pancreas to diabetes mellitus. Amer. J. Path., 33:499, 1957.

Coghill, C. L., and Song, K. T.: Acute pancreatitis. Arch. Surg., 100:673, 1970.

Croughs, R. J. M., et al.: Glucagonoma as part of the polyglandular adenoma syndrome. Amer. J. Med., 52:690, 1972.

Darle, N., et al.: Ultrastructure of the rat exocrine pancreas after long-term intake of ethanol. Gastroenterology, 58:62, 1970.

Delwiche, R., et al.: Carcinoembryonic antigen in pancreatitis. Cancer, 31:328, 1973.

Duff, G. L.: The clinical and pathological features of carcinoma of the body and tail of the pancreas. Bull. Johns Hopkins Hosp., 65:69, 1939.

Editorial: Acute pancreatitis. Lancet, 1:416, 1972.

Edmondson, H. A., et al.: Chronic pancreatitis and lithiasis. A clinicopathologic study of 62 cases of chronic pancreatitis. Amer. J. Path., 25:1227, 1949.

Ellison, E. H., and Wilson, S. D.: The Zollinger-Ellison syndrome: reappraisal and evaluation of 260 registered cases. Ann. Surg., 160:512, 1964.

Field, J. B., et al.: Insulin-like activity of nonpancreatic tumors associated with hypoglycemia. J. Clin. Endoc., 23:1229, 1963.

Fusco, F. D., and Rosen, S. W.: Gonadotropin-producing anaplastic large-cell carcinomas of the lung. New Eng. J. Med., 275:507, 1966.

Geokas, M. C., et al.: The role of elastase in acute hemorrhagic pancreatitis in man. Lab Invest., 19:235, 1968.

Glenn, F., and Thorbjarnarson, B.: Carcinoma of the pancreas. Ann. Surg., 159:945, 1964.

Goswitz, J. T.: Carcinoma of the pancreas. A comprehensive review of 173 cases emphasizing inadequacy of our diagnostic techniques. Ohio State Med. J., 57:1255, 1961.

Gross, J. B., and Comfort, M. W.: Chronic pancreatitis. Amer. J. Med., 21:596, 1956.

Grossman, M. I., et al.: Zollinger-Ellison syndrome in a Bantu woman, with isolation of a gastrin-like activity from the primary and secondary tumors. Gastroenterology, 41:87, 1961.

Howard, J. M., et al.: Hyperinsulinism in islet cell tumors of the pancreas (with 398 recorded tumors). Int. Abstr. Surg., 90:417, 1950.

Howat, H. T.: Chronic pancreatitis. Practitioner, 191:42, 1963.

Kalant, H.: Alcohol: pancreatic secretion and pancreatitis. Gastroenterology, 56:380, 1969.

Kelly, T. R.: Relationship of hyperparathyroidism to pancreatitis. Arch. Surg., 97:267, 1968.

Lacy, P. E.: The pancreatic beta cell. Structure and function. New Eng. J. Med., 276:187, 1967.

Leach, W. B.: Carcinoma of the pancreas (a clinical and pathologic analysis of 39 autopsy cases). Amer. J. Path., 26:333, 1950.

Logan, A., Jr., et al.: Familial pancreatitis. Amer. J. Surg., 115:112, 1968.

Lomsky, R., et al.: Immunohistochemical demonstration of gastrin in mammalian islets of Langerhans. Nature, 223:618, 1969.

Opie, E. L.: The relation of cholelithiasis to disease of pancreas and to fat necrosis. Amer. J. Med. Sci., 121:27, 1901.

Palade, G. E., et al.: Structure, chemistry and function of the pancreatic exocrine cell. In Ciba Foundation Symposia: The Exocrine Pancreas. Boston, Little, Brown & Co., 1961.

Paloyan, E., et al.: Alpha cell hyperplasia in calcific pancreatitis with hyperparathyroidism. J.A.M.A., 200:97, 1967.

Rawson, A. B., et al.: Zollinger-Ellison syndrome with diarrhea and malabsorption: observations on a patient before and after pancreatic islet cell tumor removal without resort to gastric surgery. Lancet, 2:131, 1960.

Roberts, N. J., et al.: Acute pancreatic necrosis. A clinicopathologic study. Amer. J. Clin. Path., 20:742, 1950.

Schapiro, H., et al.: The effect of chemical and mechanical stimulation on canine pancreatic sphincter pressure. Amer. Surg., 36:365, 1970.

Schmidt, H., and Creutzfeldt, W.: The possible role of phospholipase A in the pathogenesis of acute pancreatitis. Scand. J. Gastroent., 4:39, 1969.

Sise, H. S., et al.: On the nature of hypercoagulability. Amer. J. Med., 33:667, 1962.

Sjostrand, F. S.: The fine structure of the exocrine pancreas cells. In Ciba Foundation Symposia: The Exocrine Pancreas. Boston, Little, Brown & Co., 1961.

Smith, R.: The Zollinger-Ellison syndrome. Ann. Roy. Coll. Surg. Eng., 37:160, 1965.

Sum, P. T., et al.: Pathogenesis of bile-induced acute pancreatitis in the dog. Amer. J. Dig. Dis., *15*:637, 1970.

Summerskill, W. H. J.: Malabsorption and jejunal ulceration due to gastric hypersecretion with pancreatic islet cell hyperplasia. Lancet, *1*:120, 1959.

Thal, M. B., et al.: Isoantibody formation in pancreatic disease. Lancet, *1*:1128, 1959.

Trowbridge, J. O., and Moon, H. D.: Elastase in human pancreas. Immunologic and fluorescent antibody studies. Lab. Invest., *21*:288, 1969.

Vance, J. E., et al.: Nesidioblastosis in familial endocrine adenomatosis. J.A.M.A., *207*:1979, 1969.

Waugh, J. M., and Lynn, T. E.: Clinical and surgical aspects of pseudocyst: analysis of 58 cases. Arch. Surg., *77*:47, 1958.

Way, L., et al.: Zollinger-Ellison syndrome. An analysis of 25 cases. Amer. J. Surg., *116*:293, 1968.

Weichert, R. F.: The neuroectodermal origin of the peptide-secreting endocrine glands. A unifying concept for the etiology of multiple endocrine adenomatosis and the inappropriate secretion of peptide hormones by non-endocrine tumors. Amer. J. Med., *49*:232, 1970.

Wermer, P.: Endocrine adenomatosis and peptic ulcer in a large kindred: inherited multiple tumors and mosaic pleiotropism in man. Amer. J. Med., *35*:205, 1963.

Williams, L. F., Jr., and Byrne, J. J.: The role of bacteria in hemorrhagic pancreatitis. Surgery, *64*:967, 1968.

Zamcheck, N., et al.: Immunologic diagnosis and prognosis of human digestive-tract cancer: carcinoembryonic antigens. New Eng. J. Med., *286*:83, 1972.

Zollinger, R. M., and Ellison, E. H.: Primary peptic ulcerations of the jejunum associated with islet cell tumors of the pancreas. Ann. Surg., *142*:709, 1955.

Zollinger, R. M., et al.: Identification of the diarrheogenic hormone associated with nonbeta islet cell tumors of the pancreas. Ann. Surg., *168*:502, 1968.

24

THE KIDNEY

NORMAL

Few organs of the body are as clever and can simultaneously carry out as many complex and diverse functions as the kidney. Involved as it is in filtration, concentration and secretion, it is not surprising that it has a complex structure. An understanding of diseases of the kidney requires a thorough knowledge of its structure and the intimate interrelationships and interdependence of its various components. An effort will be made to select those features and details of special importance to the following consideration of renal pathology.

The adult kidney, the metanephros, is formed only after two primitive attempts have developed and regressed. The collecting system of the definitive kidney is derived from the main excretory duct of the earlier pronephros, now termed the wolffian duct. This duct branches forming the renal calyces and the collecting tubules. The functioning nephrons, derived from the metanephric anlage, become attached to the growing ends of the collecting system. Thus it is possible to have developmental failure of the metanephric anlage in the presence of a well developed collecting system.

Each adult kidney weighs approximately 150 gm. On section, the red-brown cortex is normally well defined from the medulla and is approximately 1.2 to 1.5 cm. in thickness. Within the medulla the pale gray, readily apparent pyramids are separated by broad bands of renal substance, the columns of Bertin. The pyramids end in blunt tips, referred to as papillae, which protrude into the open ends of the funnel-shaped calyces.

From the standpoint of its diseases, the kidney can be divided into four components: glomeruli, tubules, interstitium and blood vessels. Each kidney contains approximately one to two million nephrons. The *vascular supply to the glomeruli* represents a marvelous adaptation of structure to function. The short renal arteries, once within the renal parenchyma, branch into interlobar arteries which course between the pyramids. In the peripheral medulla, these interlobar arteries give off right angle branches, an arcuate arterial system possessing numerous anastomoses. From the arcuate arteries, the *interlobular* arteries course through the intervening medulla and renal cortex, virtually to the cortical periphery, giving off in their passage a succession of afferent arterioles, each of which terminates in an individual glomerular vascular tuft, better known as the glomerulus. Once the afferent arteriole enters the glomerular tuft, it divides into about eight branches, each of which supplies one of the glomerular lobules. These branches again di-

vide into anastomosing capillary networks, one for each lobule. Collectively, these lobules comprise the glomerular vascular tuft (Fig. 24–1). The capillaries eventually rejoin to leave the glomerulus as a second arteriole, the efferent arteriole, from which is derived a second capillary network, the peritubular capillary system. It is this peritubular capillary network which supplies the cortical tubules and eventually dips into the medulla to form the vasa recta which supply the medullary tubules. Long redundant loops of the vasa recta course down into and out of the pyramids to drain eventually into the interlobular veins. Anastomoses permit blood to leave the cortical peritubular system and drain directly into the interlobular veins, short-circuiting much of the medullary blood supply.

These anatomic details are important in understanding both normal renal function and diseases of the kidneys. Slightly more than 20 per cent of the cardiac output passes through the kidneys under basal conditions. Over 90 per cent of this volume-flow goes to the cortex. The unique location of the glomerular capil-

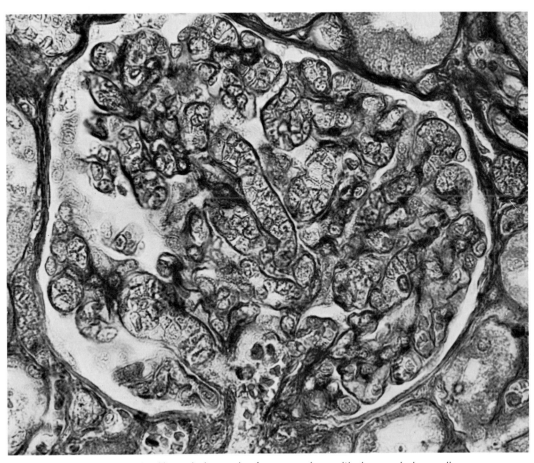

Figure 24–1. Normal glomerulus for comparison with damaged glomeruli.

laries, interposed as they are between two sets of arterioles, coupled with the short length of the renal, arcuate and interlobular arteries, provides a filtration blood pressure in the glomerular capillaries about threefold that found in other capillary beds. The hematocrit in the cortical capillaries, normally about 30 per cent, is similar to that found in other tissue capillaries. However, shunting of red cells directly into interlobular veins through anastomoses produces a hematocrit in the vasa recta on the order of 10 per cent. Plasma proteins are thus concentrated in the vasa recta and so the viscosity of the blood is increased, slowing the blood flow. With such slow blood flow, there is opportunity for sodium chloride to diffuse into the blood in the descending limb of the vasa recta and to escape into the ascending limb before the blood once again returns to the interlobular veins. Thus, there is ample time for the enormous exchange of salt between the loop of Henle, the interstitium and the vasa recta fundamental to the countercurrent mechanism in the medulla. The medullary interstitium becomes very hypertonic as a consequence of the salt exchange between tubules and blood vessels. Such hypertonicity impairs leukocyte phagocytic function, rendering the medulla vulnerable to bacterial invasion.

The anatomy of the renal vasculature has many other implications. It is evident that glomerular disease which interferes with blood flow through the glomerular capillaries must have profound effects on the tubules, within both the cortex and the medulla, since all tubular capillary beds are derived from the efferent arterioles. The peculiarities of the blood supply to the renal pyramids render them especially vulnerable to ischemia. The remarkably low hematocrit in the capillary loops descending into the pyramids is one predisposing factor. Moreover, the entire blood flow into and out of the pyramids is easily impaired by otherwise inconsequential lesions which happen to be located at the critical corticomedullary junction. Thus, acute infections in the kidney involving the base of the pyramids may so reduce the blood supply that renal papillary ischemic necrosis develops. The renal cortex, on the other hand, is peculiarly vulnerable to hypertensive changes. As pointed out earlier, even normal pressure in the glomerular capillaries is higher than in other capillary beds, and any elevation of blood pressure in the aorta is readily transmitted to the afferent arterioles. An earlier remark may now be more clear, namely, that an understanding of the normal is requisite for understanding the abnormal.

A brief review of the *fine structure of the glomerulus* will be helpful in understanding glomerular diseases. The capillaries here are lined by a unique fenestrated endothelium perforated by pores about 1000 Å in diameter. These endothelial cells rest on a basement membrane which comprises a continuous sheet laid over the entire glomerular vascular tuft. The sheet is tucked in snugly, but does not completely encircle each capillary since it is reflected onto the adjacent capillary. There is, therefore, a narrow zone of the capillary wall that is devoid of basement membrane. The defect is filled either by the endothelial cells themselves or by deeper, underlying cells, the mesangial cells (Fig. 24–2).

The basement membrane itself can be resolved into three layers, a central electron-dense layer (lamina densa) sandwiched between two layers of lesser density (lamina rara interna and externa). On cross section, the basement membrane is of uniform thickness, averaging about 0.3 microns. It is composed of glycoprotein but, while the protein moiety is rich in hydroxylysine, implying the presence of collagen, fibrils have not been visualized by electron microscopy. As will become clear, the basement membrane represents the ultimate filter in the glomerulus. Thus, the questions of its porosity and its response to disease are matters of great interest. Unfortunately, they are also matters of some obscurity. All that can be

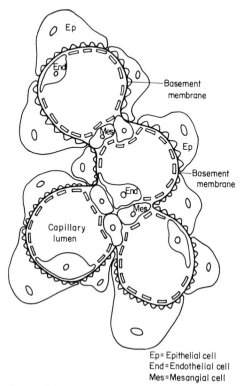

Ep= Epithelial cell
End=Endothelial cell
Mes=Mesangial cell

Figure 24–2. *Schematic representation of ultrastructure of glomerular lobule.*

said with certainty is that no anatomically demonstrable true pores have been visualized, even with the highest resolution electron microscope. Pores can be seen neither in the normal basement membrane nor in diseased kidneys which leak large quantities of plasma proteins. External to the basement membrane are the glomerular visceral epithelial cells, or podocytes. These cells may be likened to an octopus with only the extended tentacles (foot processes) reaching out to contact the basement membrane. In any cross section, the foot processes are separated by filtration slits on the order of 200 to 500 Å in width. Some investigators have proposed that a thin membrane interconnects the foot processes, but this has not been clearly demonstrated and its existence is in doubt. It is evident, then, that in places where an endothelial cell pore is directly apposed to an epithelial cell filtration slit, the only filtration barrier is the glomerular basement membrane. These morphologic details are vital to an understanding of glomerular diseases.

The entire glomerular tuft is supported by mesangial cells lying between the capillaries. Basement membrane-like mesangial matrix comprises a meshwork through which the mesangial cells are scattered. These cells are presumably of mesenchymal origin and are closely related to pericytes. However, the mesangial cell has been shown to be phagocytic and to be capable of laying down both matrix and collagen fibers. Mesangial cells, you recall, may fill the gaps left open by the reflected basement membrane. Sometimes such cells have a slightly distinctive morphology and are called deep endothelial cells. Mesangial matrix and glomerular basement membrane yield a positive tinctorial reaction with the periodic acid-Schiff (PAS) stain. This fact is of great value in visualizing these structures under the light microscope. In the ordinary H & E stain, it is almost impossible to discern the glomerular basement membrane, sandwiched as it is between endothelial cells and podocytes (Fig. 24–3).

A remarkable structure, the *juxtaglomeru-*

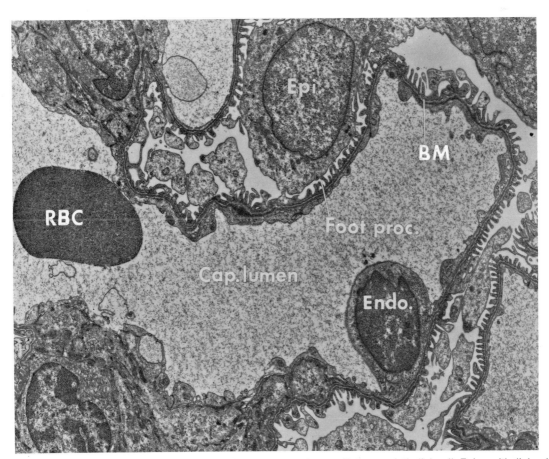

Figure 24–3. *Normal rabbit kidney.* BM, *basement membrane.* Endo., *endothelial cell.* Epi., *epithelial cell.* Cap. lumen, *capillary lumen.* RBC, *red blood cell.* Foot proc., *foot processes.* × *12,200. (Electron micrograph courtesy of Alan S. Cohen, M.D., Department of Medicine, Boston University School of Medicine.)*

lar *(JG) apparatus,* snuggles closely against the glomerulus where the afferent arteriole enters. The JG apparatus of a single glomerulus is composed of: modified granular cells in the media of its afferent arteriole, closely massed epithelial cells of the adjacent distal convoluted tubule of the same nephron known as the macula densa and, between arteriole and tubule, a few closely packed lacis cells. The granulated cells in the media of the afferent arteriole are thought to be the site of renin production in the kidney, and the intensity of the granulation is related to the level of renin output. Renin itself is not a pressor substance. It is an enzyme which acts on a plasma alpha-2-globulin to produce a decapeptide known as angiotensin I. This, in turn, is converted by a plasma-converting enzyme to angiotensin II, which is a potent vasoconstrictor acting on renal and extra-renal arterioles. Renin also stimulates aldosterone secretion in the adrenal cortex. It will come as no surprise that excessive elaboration of renin is thought to be one possible cause of hypertension. *The secretory activity of the JG apparatus is responsive to arteriolar pressure, the sodium content of the arteriolar blood and the sodium content of the filtrate passing through the distal convoluted tubules.* If, for example, the sodium content in the arteriolar blood rises, the renin-angiotensin system is depressed and the afferent arteriole dilates to increase the glomerular filtration rate, thus tending to lower the plasma level of sodium. As another example, the renin-angiotensin system is activated to constrict afferent arterioles and to reduce GFR as a compensatory mechanism to conserve plasma and blood volume when there is a reduction in cardiac output or blood volume.

With these details on a few of the specialized features of the kidney, we can turn to a consideration of its diseases.

PATHOLOGY

Disorders primary in the kidneys are responsible for a great deal of morbidity, but fortunately are not major causes of mortality. To place the problem in some perspective, in the United States in 1967, approximately 29,000 deaths were attributed to renal disease. In contrast, approximately 700,000 deaths were attributable to heart disease, 300,000 to cancer and 200,000 to "stroke." But the mortality data do not give a true picture of the clinical importance of renal disease because, although the total number of deaths is fortunately not great, the morbidity is by no means insignificant. To cite only a few examples, urinary tract infections are exceedingly common and disabling,

but only rarely cause death. Similarly, dialysis and transplantation programs keep many patients alive who would formerly have died and so added to the pool of renal morbidity. Renal disease also has special importance to the clinician because so many of the deaths occur in young people.

The correct clinical and anatomic diagnosis of the various disorders of the kidney may be simple or very difficult. The functional reserve of the kidneys is large (approximately 90 per cent) and much damage may occur before there is evident functional impairment. Moreover, many forms of renal disease tend to produce similar signs and symptoms as well as remarkably similar anatomic changes. The anatomic interdependence of the component parts of the kidney implies that damage to one will secondarily affect the others. Disease primary in the blood vessels, for example, must inevitably affect all of the structures dependent on this blood supply. Severe glomerular damage, as mentioned earlier will impair the flow through the entire peritubular vascular system. Thus, there is a tendency for all forms of renal disease ultimately to destroy all four components of the kidney, culminating in what has been called *"end-stage contracted kidneys."* Because of the large functional reserve, manifestations of renal disease may not become evident until there is extensive damage and, at this stage, it may be extremely difficult to differentiate, both clinically and morphologically, one disease entity from another. For these reasons, the early signs and symptoms are particularly important to the clinician. The major early clinical presentations are: (1) hematuria, (2) generalized edema and other manifestations of the nephrotic syndrome (described later), (3) pain and (4) palpably enlarged kidneys. Infrequently, there is acute renal failure.

Some suggestions for a reasonable approach to the histologic diagnosis of renal disease may be worth detailing. In the gross inspection of the kidney, attention must be directed to its *size, shape, color and conformation.* It is apparent that *kidneys which are larger than normal must contain some added substances or structures* to account for the greater volume, such as excessive amounts of blood or fluid, accumulation of fat or hypertrophied nephrons. It can also be generalized that *kidneys larger than normal cannot reasonably be the seat of pure chronic inflammatory processes,* which inevitably produce scarring, atrophy and loss of substance. The shape and conformation of the kidney may give important clues to congenital anomalies and tumors, and particularly to focal lesions which cause irregular distortions. The distribution of the scarring, whether diffuse or focal, symmetrical or asymmetrical, unilateral or bilateral, suggests, for example, whether the process is a generalized derangement which affects both kidneys symmetrically or is a disease characterized by haphazard involvement. It would be unreasonable, as will be seen later, to entertain the single diagnosis of glomerulonephritis with asymmetrical renal involvement.

The cut section of the kidney should be closely scrutinized to detect the apparent gross localization of the pathologic change. The color of the kidney is of significance, since it may be hyperemic, suggesting increased amounts of blood, or it may be pale, which would imply rather ischemia, the deposition of fat, the collection of edema fluid or some other abnormal accumulation.

In the histologic examination of the kidney, it is well to bear in mind that each of the four basic morphologic components—glomeruli, tubules, blood vessels and interstitium—requires individual attention. By this approach, it is usually possible to distinguish the principal point of attack from the secondary concomitant alterations. It is implied, then, that in the study of histologic sections, each of these four basic components should be thoroughly and systematically surveyed serially, rather than randomly scanning the kidney for general impressions.

The kidney reacts to tissue injuries as do all the other tissues of the body. Acute inflammation evokes the same pattern of exudation, white cell accumulation and tissue damage when it occurs in the kidney as it does elsewhere. By the same token, chronic longstanding inflammation produces scarring and permanent destruction of elements. So it is that in acute glomerulonephritis, the glomeruli have the hallmarks of acute inflammatory changes, i.e., edema and polymorphonuclear infiltration, while in chronic glomerulonephritis, permanent fibrous scarring of the glomeruli results. However, the problem of the morphologic diagnosis of disease in an organ as complex as the kidney frequently requires special techniques to highlight specific morphologic and functional details. Some of these aids are listed with their specific indications:

Schiff-McManus periodic acid stain. This stain offers two special features:
1. the demonstration of glycogen within tubular epithelium, and
2. delicate rose-violet outlining of the basement membranes of the glomeruli.

Sudan stains. These demonstrate fat within tubular epithelium.

Silver impregnation stains. These outline glomerular and tubular basement membranes.

Immunofluorescent stains. These identify and localize antigen, antibody or antigen-antibody complexes.

Many other techniques are of specialized value, such as alkaline phosphatase stains to detect early lesions that injure tubular enzymes without causing morphologic damage. Occasionally, stains for fibrin and pigments are of value for specific problems. With glomerular disease in particular, electron microscopy is of inestimable value in resolving the finer details of lesions and is often necessary to identify subtle lesions inapparent with light microscopy.

Because all forms of serious renal disease may ultimately lead to renal failure, it is appropriate first to present this pathophysiologic entity before the consideration of the individual diseases of the kidney.

RENAL FAILURE

Although the term renal failure would appear to be quite explicit—implying renal function which is inadequate to maintain an internal milieu normal in both volume and composition—it has come to have a variety of interpretations. Some terminology must therefore be clarified. *Azotemia* is, strictly speaking, a biochemical abnormality and refers to an elevation in the blood urea nitrogen (BUN) and creatinine levels. It implies a decrease in renal function resulting in the retention of nitrogenous wastes. Azotemia may, of course, be produced by many renal disorders but it may also arise from extrarenal disorders. *Prerenal azotemia* is encountered whenever there is hypoperfusion of the kidneys, such as occurs in congestive heart failure, shock, volume depletion and hemorrhage, all of which impair renal function without parenchymal damage. If this hypoperfusion becomes sufficiently severe, it can, of course, lead to morphologic damage. But, in most instances, correction of the extrarenal problem returns the kidney function to normal and the azotemia clears. Similarly, *postrenal azotemia* is seen whenever there is obstruction to urinary flow below the level of the kidney. If the obstruction is severe and protracted, it will inevitably produce renal lesions. But until such time, relief of the obstruction will be followed by prompt correction of the azotemia.

When azotemia becomes associated with a constellation of clinical signs and symptoms and biochemical abnormalities, it is termed uremia. Thus, uremia is a clinical syndrome and not merely a biochemical abnormality. It is characterized by two types of manifestations: those directly referable to deranged renal excretory function, and those related to secondary gastrointestinal, neuromuscular and cardiovascular involvement. The second group of clinical changes is necessary for the diagnosis of uremia. Before delving into the individual characteristics of the uremic syndrome, the terms *renal insufficiency* and *renal failure* should be clarified. Many nephrologists reserve the term uremia for the terminal stage of renal failure. They would, therefore, apply the terms renal insufficiency and renal failure to the preuremic patient who has mild to moderate azotemia, acidosis, hyponatremia, hypocalcemia, hyperphosphatemia and sometimes mild hyperkalemia. At this stage of renal functional impairment, anemia, nocturia (urinating in the night) and polyuria (increased frequency of urination) are often present. It is clear, then, that renal insufficiency and renal failure are characterized largely by renal excretory and regulatory dysfunction and are not necessarily associated with all of the extrarenal manifestations characteristic of uremia. Renal failure may develop relatively suddenly or slowly. *Acute renal failure is encountered principally in acute tubular necrosis, acute glomerulonephritis and acute pyelonephritis, especially with papillary necrosis.* The importance of recognizing acute renal failure lies in the fact that it is usually reversible. Careful medical management of fluid balance and the biochemical milieu will generally permit the renal lesion to subside. This, indeed, occurs with acute tubular necrosis and in some cases of glomerulonephritis and acute pyelonephritis. On the other hand, *chronic renal failure is usually caused by slowly progressive, irreversible disorders* (chronic glomerulonephritis and chronic pyelonephritis) and, almost inevitably, these patients develop uremia unless they are maintained on dialysis or receive a renal transplant.

To return to the uremic syndrome, the manifestations directly referable to deranged renal function will first be considered. These are best understood in terms of the principal functions of the kidneys: (1) volume regulation, (2) acid-base balance, (3) electrolyte balance and (4) excretion of waste products.

Deranged volume regulation may lead either to dehydration or to retention of salt and water, with resultant edema. Dehydration tends to appear early in the course of some forms of renal disease in which there is impairment of concentrating ability and consequent excretion of large volumes of water. With progression of most significant forms of renal disease, glomerular filtration is ultimately impaired, with retention of both salt and water. Moreover, in most forms of chronic renal disease, an activated renin-angiotensin system

leads to hyperaldosteronism which further compounds the retention of salt and water. Renal edema is systemic in distribution. When severe, it is termed anasarca. In these cases, the edema is usually compounded by hypoproteinemia caused by the excessive loss of serum proteins through the damaged glomeruli. Because the tissue about the eyelids is loosely attached to deep structures, periorbital edema is often the first manifestation. The volume overload may also lead to congestive heart failure and pulmonary congestion as will be discussed later.

Severely damaged kidneys lose their capacity to regulate *acid-base balance,* leading to metabolic acidosis. The details of the deranged physiology producing such acidosis are beyond our scope but have been well reviewed by Relman (1968). It suffices to say that the major defect may be a reduced capacity to produce ammonium. As a consequence of severe renal failure, there is commonly a decreased serum bicarbonate level, a lowered blood pH and variable degrees of compensatory hyperventilation. Occasionally, the sighing respiration through somewhat pursed lips comprises the classic Kussmaul breathing. The acidosis has far-reaching implications for intracellular metabolism throughout the body and undoubtedly contributes to the secondary derangements in carbohydrate and protein metabolism, as well as the electrolyte imbalances encountered in renal failure.

Electrolyte imbalances, the most important of which are hyperkalemia and hypocalcemia, are among the most threatening aspects of uremia. Both hyperkalemia and hypocalcemia may initiate potentially fatal cardiac arrythmias as well as alterations in myocardial contractility. They also lead to generalized muscle weakness and an increase in neuromuscular excitability. The muscle twitching, "restless leg syndrome," and muscular cramps are related to both the hypocalcemia and the generalized metabolic disturbance of the central nervous system (Merrill and Hampers, 1970). The hypocalcemia also has secondary effects on calcium and bone metabolism as will be indicated.

Nitrogenous wastes are retained, producing elevations of the BUN and the blood levels of creatinine, which are invariably encountered in renal failure and, indeed, are usually considered clinical indices of the severity of the problem. As will become clear, however, there is no proof that the nitrogenous wastes account for the extrarenal manifestations of the uremic syndrome.

In addition to the evidence of impaired renal regulatory and excretory function, uremia is characterized by:

1. Neurologic changes.
2. Gastrointestinal signs and symptoms.
3. Cardiovascular abnormalities.
4. Hematologic disorders.
5. Derangements in calcium and bone metabolism.
6. Dermatologic changes.

The *neurologic alterations* take many forms including disorientation, delusions, frank psychoses and obtunded mentation to the level of frank coma. In addition, peripheral neuropathy may be encountered as an early sign of the metabolic derangement. In turn, the neuropathy may lead to paresthesias as well as motor and sensory defects. Although, as we shall see, the precise basis for these neurologic manifestations is not clear, they are reversible with adequate dialysis or transplantation.

Gastrointestinal signs and symptoms of uremia may consist of only nausea and vomiting. In some patients, however, gastrointestinal bleeding occurs. The hemorrhage arises in diffuse or patchy ulcerations which may affect virtually any level of the gut, from the oral cavity to the anus. Uremic esophagitis, gastritis and colitis are the more common localizations of the gastrointestinal lesions.

The *cardiovascular abnormalities* are varied. Congestive heart failure, probably in part secondary to salt retention and increased blood volume, is one of the most common manifestations. However, it is by no means certain that hypervolemia is the only influence. Abnormalities in the myocardium have been identified, suggesting that some of the metabolic derangements may have a direct effect on the myocardial cells. Hypertension is often present. To some extent, the elevated blood pressure may be caused by the hypervolemia but there is also evidence that, even with advanced renal failure, sufficient functioning renal tissue remains to elaborate increased amounts of renin (Merrill and Hampers, 1970). Uremic pericarditis is a frequent complication of chronic uremia (Bailey et al., 1968). Characteristically, it takes the form of a marked fibrinous exudate and is sometimes accompanied by a fibrinous pleuritis. To the clinician, these are manifested as pericardial and pleural friction rubs. Both have been shown to clear with adequate dialysis and only rarely do they give rise to significant fibrous adhesions. Pulmonary edema is yet another cardiovascular abnormality in uremia. It may, of course, be secondary to congestive heart failure. In addition, it has been attributed to overhydration and to increased capillary permeability (Gibson, 1966).

The most prominent *hematopoietic manifestation* of uremia is anemia. Its severity does not necessarily correlate with the severity of the renal disease as measured by the BUN. Generally, it is normochromic and normocytic but sometimes it is hypochromic. The basis for the anemia is still unclear. While a shortened red cell survival has been identified, a normally responsive bone marrow could compensate for this. Hence, there is a suspicion that some extracorpuscular factor may be involved which depresses the bone marrow or, alternatively, that there is inadequate production of erythropoietin (Eschbach et al., 1967) (Henkin et al., 1964). Some uremic patients develop a bleeding diathesis with or without depressed platelet counts. This is, at least in part, related to a qualitative defect in the remaining platelets (Eknoyan et al., 1969).

Abnormalities in *calcium and bone metabolism* are important aspects of chronic uremia. Classically, the patient with chronic renal failure will exhibit a decrease in serum calcium levels and a corresponding increase in serum phosphate levels. In turn, the hypocalcemia leads to compensatory activity in the parathyroid glands, with increased levels of parathyroid hormone in the serum and progressive hypertrophy and hyperplasia of the parathyroid glands (Berson and Yallow, 1966). Thus, in longstanding uremia, skeletal abnormalities characteristic of hyperparathyroidism may appear, sometimes referred to as *renal osteodystrophy*. Morphologically, these changes resemble those seen in osteomalacia and/or osteitis fibrosa cystica (Kleeman et al., 1967) (p. 1444). The basis for the hypocalcemia eludes us, but a host of influences have been implicated. Defective absorption of calcium from the gut may be one of the prime factors. Resistance to the effects of vitamin D has been well established (p. 483). Increased fecal calcium excretion may contribute when calcium phosphate insoluble complexes are formed in the gastrointestinal tract. But, in addition, there are reasons for believing that other as yet unidentified mechanisms contribute to the calcium imbalance of uremia.

The *dermatologic changes* comprise principally a peculiar sallow coloration to the skin and itching. The skin color is, in part, the consequence of anemia but may also result from the accumulation, in the skin, of urinary pigment, principally urochrome (which normally gives urine its characteristic color). Much has been made, in the past, of a uremic frost caused by the precipitation of crystals of urea on the skin, but it is rarely seen in the well cared for patient. The origin of uremic itching remains unexplained, but it can be very distressing to the patient.

Having discussed all the manifestations of uremia, we should ask what produces them.

The innumerable studies to identify the causative factor or factors "have much in common with the attempts to identify the Yeti or Abominable Snowman. Evidence of its presence is clearly visible, but attempts to identify and isolate the factor have yet to be successful" (Merrill and Hampers, 1970). One observation appears to be well established. While the severity of uremic signs and symptoms correlates roughly with the blood concentration of urea, this nitrogenous waste is not their prime cause. When uremic patients are dialyzed with fluid containing sufficient urea to prevent a fall in the concentration of urea in blood, the manifestations of uremia nevertheless clear (Merrill et al., 1953). Without going into all of the leads which have been followed, the two most enticing observations relate to guanidines and to some ill-defined factor which is known to be humoral. Chronic intoxication with methylguanidine in dogs has been shown to produce anemia, anorexia, vomiting, ulcerative lesions in the stomach and duodenum, central and peripheral nervous system changes and many (but it should be noted, not all) of the manifestations of the uremic syndrome in man (Giovannetti et al., 1969). With respect to the humoral factor, it has been shown that uremic serum impairs the growth of white cells in tissue culture and inhibits cellular metabolism presumably by altering cell membrane permeability (Welt, 1969). Interesting as these leads may be, the precise biochemical culprit which is responsible for all the far-ranging manifestations of the uremic syndrome has not been identified. Against this background of the clinical syndrome of renal failure, we can turn to the consideration of the renal diseases which may cause it.

CONGENITAL ANOMALIES

AGENESIS OF THE KIDNEY

Total bilateral agenesis of the kidneys is obviously incompatible with life, and is only encountered in stillborn infants. *Unilateral renal agenesis* is an infrequent anomaly compatible with adequate renal function. It is presumed to be due to the unilateral absence of a nephrogenic primordium or to a failure of the wolffian duct to make contact with the mesodermal mass out of which the functioning nephrons develop. Occasionally, a small undifferentiated mass of connective tissue, 2 to 3 cm. in size, may mark the site of the developmental failure. The renal artery and vein may be absent or rudimentary. Sometimes a recognizable ureteral remnant may be defined. With unilateral agenesis, the opposite kidney is usually enlarged (compensatory hypertrophy). Since it has been established experimentally that one-fourth of the normal renal substance is sufficient to maintain function, the development of "compensatory" hypertrophy by the normal kidney is somewhat mysterious.

HYPOPLASIA

Renal hypoplasia refers to failure of the kidneys to develop to *normal size*. In the adult, hypoplastic kidneys vary in weight from a few grams up to approximately 80 to 100 gm. This anomaly may occur bilaterally, but is more commonly encountered as a unilateral defect (Fig. 24–4). Such small kidneys usually have corresponding hypoplasia of the renal vessels, but the pelves and ureters may be of normal size and thus not in proportion to the renal parenchyma. However, superimposed renal disease (infection, stone formation) is a common complication of malformed kidneys. It may, therefore, be very difficult to determine whether a small kidney is the result of an underlying developmental failure or is entirely due to marked scarring and contraction of a previously normal organ.

Although such a differentiation may be

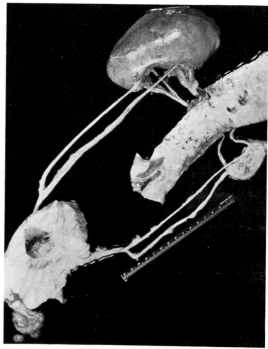

Figure 24–4. *Multiple congenital anomalies of the urinary tract. The right kidney is hypoplastic. The ureters bilaterally are bifid (divided in their upper regions) and there are accessory anomalous renal arteries.*

impossible, the following features are helpful: The presence of a kidney on the opposite side which is not larger than normal suggests that scarring had occurred after the uninvolved kidney became permanently fixed in size. Compensatory hypertrophy would be anticipated in a congenitally hypoplastic kidney. A normal renal artery suggests, but does not confirm, that the organ may, at one time, have been normal in size. And finally, a renal weight below 50 gm. is rarely encountered in contraction due to chronic renal disease. Scattered clinical reports have suggested hypoplasia of the kidneys as the basis of renal ischemia and consequent hypertension, but the evidence for this is not well established.

DISPLACEMENT OF THE KIDNEYS

The development of the definitive metanephros may occur in ectopic foci, usually at abnormally low levels. Commonly, these kidneys lie either just above the pelvic brim or sometimes even within the pelvis. They are usually normal or slightly smaller in size, but are otherwise not remarkable. Because of their abnormal position, kinking or tortuosity of the ureters may cause some obstruction to urinary flow which predisposes to bacterial infections. This anomaly may produce a palpable pelvic mass which has, at times, been confused with a pelvic tumor.

HORSESHOE KIDNEY

Fusion of the upper or lower poles of the kidneys produces a horseshoe-shaped structure continuous across the midline anterior to the great vessels. This anomaly is quite common and is found in about 1 in 500 to 1000 autopsies. The majority of such kidneys are fused at the lower pole, although approximately 10 per cent are fused at the upper pole. In those which have a bridge at the lower pole, the ureters usually pass anterior to the renal parenchyma. These malformed kidneys are capable of normal function and are not more predisposed to renal disease than the normal. Renal calculi are said to be slightly more common, perhaps owing to angulation of the ureters with stasis of urinary flow through the ureters.

CYSTS OF THE KIDNEY

Cysts of the kidney are sometimes of anomalous developmental origin. They may occur singly or multiply, or be so numerous as to transform the kidney into a multicystic mass, creating *polycystic kidneys.* Sometimes inflammatory scarring and pinching off of tubules create cystic dilatations in the proximal nephrons. These cysts are usually less than 1 cm. in diameter and multiple, and are found in kidneys which are obviously the seat of marked renal disease. The single or multiple congenital cysts which dot an otherwise adequate renal parenchyma are known as *simple cysts.* The polycystic variant is a heredofamilial disorder of far greater clinical significance (Spence et al., 1957). This division of cystic involvements finds its exact counterpart in isolated polyps of the colon and the heredofamilial congenital polyposis.

Simple Cysts. These occur as multiple or single cystic spaces which vary in diameter over wide limits. Commonly, they are 1 to 5 cm. in size, translucent, lined by a gray, glistening, smooth membrane, and filled with clear fluid. Microscopically, these membranes are composed of a single layer of cuboidal or flattened cuboidal epithelium which, in many instances, may be completely atrophic. These cells rest on an outer enclosing thin fibrous capsule. While these cysts are usually confined to the cortex, they may sometimes occur in the medullary portion of the kidney, where they must be differentiated from hydronephrotic dilatation of the collecting system. It is apparent that, in the latter disease, connections with the pelvis and the ureter can be demonstrated, while in the true cysts no such connection exists. Rarely, large massive cysts are encountered up to 10 cm. in diameter. These massive cysts are sometimes the cause of great clinical concern as palpable masses.

Simple cysts are extremely common postmortem findings which have no clinical significance. On occasion, hemorrhage into them may cause sudden distention and pain. Calcification of the hemorrhage sometimes gives rise to bizarre x-ray shadows.

Polycystic Kidney Disease. This designation should be limited to those kidneys which are so completely cystic that the *intervening renal parenchyma appears to be virtually completely obliterated.* Since multiple simple cysts may occur and may indeed be numerous, it is sometimes difficult to clearly define the limits of true polycystic disease, and the definition just given has proved to have the greatest meaning. Polycystic kidney disease occurs in approximately 1 in 400 to 500 autopsies.

Within the recent past, our understanding of polycystic kidneys has been immeasurably clarified by the definitive study of Osathanondh and Potter (1964). By beautiful microdissections, they demonstrated that all polycystic kidneys arise from abnormalities in the formation of the fetal kidneys. Some are incompatible with survival and, therefore, are only found in the newborn. Others are sufficiently mild to permit life to continue for decades. These workers demonstrated quite clearly that polycystic kidney disease is *not* caused by (1) failure of branches of the ureteral bud to unite with distal tubules arising from the metanephric blastema, (2) cystic enlargement of persisting vestigial generations of nephrons, (3) cystic dilatation of nephrons which detach and fail to reattach to collecting tubules, (4) failure of canalization of tubules or (5) neoplastic adenomatous proliferation.

Three patterns of polycystic disease were delineated. **Type I, due to dilatation and hyperplasia of collecting tubules,** is characterized by saccular or cylindrical dilatations in all collecting tubules. The disease is, therefore, bilaterally symmetrical and produces a uniform sponge-like appearance of the kidneys. With the hand lens, it is possible to visualize the dilated elongated channels at right angles to the cortical surface. These channels completely replace the medulla and cortex and have a uniform lining of cuboidal epithelial cells, reflecting their origin from collecting tubules. Osathanondh and Potter (1963) postulate that hyperplasia of portions of the collecting tubules is responsible for the cystic dilatations and point out that **these kidneys are incompatible with extended life and are, therefore, found only in infants.** In these cases, the bile ducts are also invariably cystic and siblings may be affected, suggesting a heredofamilial trait.

Type II, due to inhibition of ureteral ampullary activity, is characterized by asymmetrical involvement which may affect both kidneys, one kidney or only a portion of a kidney. Involved regions are converted into masses of large, grossly visible, thick-walled cysts, up to many centimeters in diameter, enclosed within dense fibrous tissue. Between the cysts, there is dense fibrous tissue with occasional normal nephrons. In addition, irregularly distributed abnormal blood vessels, abnormally large nerve trunks and occasional islands of cartilage may be present. It is postulated that the cysts develop because of failure of the ureteral ampullary regions to branch. This results not only in absence of the collecting tubules, but also in failure of the nephron to develop, since ampullary branching is a necessary stimulus to nephron formation. **If the disease is bilateral, it is totally incompatible with life, and it is found therefore only in stillborn infants and in those who die soon after birth.** If the disease is unilateral or segmental, the unaffected regions of the kidney may be adequate to sustain life.

Type III, due to multiple abnormalities of development, is characterized by an admixture of normal and abnormal nephrons. **This variant is the most frequent type of polycystic disease encountered in adults.** If the number of normal nephrons is sufficiently large, life can be sustained for decades. Many of these patients die in the fifth and sixth decades, when bacterial infection and vascular complications compromise the residual renal function. If the involvement is more severe, the renal function may be insufficient to sustain life and cause death at any time after birth. This pattern is usually, but not always, bilateral, and the kidneys are most often larger than normal, even in the newborn. In the adult they may achieve enormous sizes, and weights up to 4 kg. for each kidney have been recorded. These very large kidneys are readily palpable abdominally as masses extending into the pelvis (Fig 24–5). On gross examination, this type of polycystic kidney seems to be composed solely of a mass of cysts (up to 3 to 4 cm. in diameter) with no intervening parenchyma. However, microscopic examination reveals functioning nephrons dispersed between the cysts. The cysts themselves may be filled with a clear serous fluid or, more usually, with turbid red to brown, sometimes hemorrhagic fluid. As these cysts enlarge, they may encroach upon the calyces and pelves to produce pressure defects.

The cysts arise either from tubules or from portions of the nephron, and they therefore have a variable lining. Occasionally, Bowman's capsules are involved in the cyst formation and, in these cases, glomerular tufts may be seen within the cystic

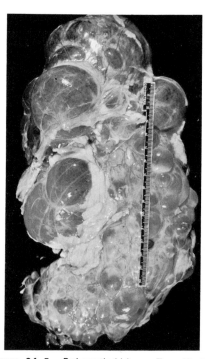

Figure 24–5. Polycystic kidney—Type III. Note its length of over 20 cm.

space. Since the pressure of the expanding cysts leads to ischemia of the intervening renal substance, progressive atrophy narrows the functional reserve. Superimposed bacterial infection and vascular disease due to concomitant hypertension are common accompaniments which further encroach upon the already precarious renal reserve.

Clinical Course. As has been indicated, polycystic kidney disease may lead to renal failure during infancy. In its more benign forms, it is compatible with life into later decades (Bell, 1935). Many of these patients may be entirely asymptomatic until indications of renal insufficiency announce the presence of an underlying kidney disease. In others, hemorrhage or progressive dilatation of cysts may produce pain. The large masses of type III, which are usually apparent on abdominal palpation, sometimes even on pelvic examination, may produce a dragging sensation. Occasionally, the disease begins with the insidious onset of hematuria, followed by other features of progressive, chronic renal disease, such as albuminuria, polyuria and, commonly, hypertension. Elevation of blood pressure occurs in over 50 per cent of the patients. This form of chronic renal failure is quite remarkable in that patients may survive for many years with azotemia slowly progressing to uremia. Ultimately, about one-third of the adult patients die of renal failure; in another third, the hypertension is responsible for death through the development of cardiac disease; the remaining third die of unrelated causes. Often, superimposed renal infection precipitates the renal failure.

In many patients with polycystic disease, other forms of congenital anomalies are also present, such as polycystic liver disease, polycystic pancreatic disease, hemangiomas of the pancreas and brain and congenital berry aneurysms of the circle of Willis.

MISCELLANEOUS ANOMALIES

There is a heterogeneous group of developmental anomalies that affect the kidney, most of which are of no clinical significance. A double or an extrarenal pelvis may occur with otherwise normal kidneys. These are of interest only insofar as they may produce modifications in the patterns of the pyelogram. Anomalous renal arteries may arise either directly from the aorta or as branches from the renal artery. Sometimes such vessels are of benefit, since they maintain the blood supply to a portion of the kidney if the main renal artery is occluded. However, some of these anomalous vessels to the lower pole have been repeatedly described as causes of ureteral obstruction when they cross anterior to the ureter and compress it.

DISEASES OF GLOMERULI

The glomerulus is the prima ballerina of the kidney. All else pivots on its structure and function. Damage it and you impair renal function and injure or destroy renal structure. It is no surprise, then, that severe damage to the glomerulus has far-ranging implications. Indeed, in glomerular disease, the commonly measured indices of renal function correlate better with the secondary tubular changes than with the glomerular involvement (Schainuck et al., 1970). Anatomically, then, the late stages of glomerular disease are associated with widespread alterations in the other three major components of the kidney, i.e., the tubules, interstitium and blood vessels. For this reason, identification of disorders primary to the glomeruli is best made early because later it becomes difficult to determine whether the primary attack was on the tubules, blood vessels, interstitium or glomeruli.

The response of the glomerulus to all forms of injury is remarkably limited. In essence, it takes one of four forms:

1. Cellular Proliferation. Many inflammatory involvements of the glomerulus are reflected by an increase in the number of endothelial, mesangial and epithelial cells. In certain disorders, the proliferation is limited largely to endothelial and mesangial cells while, in others, the epithelial cell proliferation is more prominent.

2. Leukocytic Infiltration. Surprisingly, leukocytic infiltration is not prominent in most inflammatory involvements of the glomeruli. However, in a few where there is an acute, intense reaction, neutrophils and sometimes monocytes are found within the glomerular capillary lumina, in Bowman's space and sometimes in the periglomerular interstitial tissue.

3. Glomerular Basement Membrane (GBM) Thickening. By light microscopy, this change appears as thickening of the capillary walls, best seen in the outer capillary loops of the individual glomerular lobules. Special stains, such as the PAS, which selectively stain the GBM, are helpful if not necessary. Under the electron microscope, however, thickening of the basement membrane is readily resolved as being due either to increased deposition of basement membrane substance itself and/or to the deposition of foreign materials such as immunoglobulins, immune complexes or fibrin on either the endothelial or epithelial side of the membrane.

4. Hyalinization. This commonly used term, as applied to the glomerulus, connotes the accumulation within the glomerular-vascular tuft of material which is homogeneous and eosinophilic by light microscopy and which resembles increased amounts of basement membrane or mesangial matrix by electron microscopy. In some cases, the hyalinization is the consequence of extreme GBM thickening, with collapse of glomerular capillary lumina. In the course of hyalinization of glomeruli, the glomerular capillaries are narrowed or obliterated, and the structural detail of the vascular tuft is lost, becoming a blur of eosinophilic substance. Hyalinization implies irreversible injury to glomerular structure and function.

The nature of the glomerular injury can, to an extent, be deduced by determining which of these reactions to injury is prominent. Glomerulonephritis (GN), an inflammatory disorder, is characterized principally by cellular proliferation and leukocytic infiltration. Sometimes basement membrane thickening is also present. In most of these conditions, more or less all glomeruli are equally affected in both kidneys. In one disease, the glomeruli are affected patchily, hence its designation, focal glomerulonephritis. That is, one glomerulus among many might be involved and, at the same time, the change might be segmental within the glomerular tuft, sparing some lobules and affecting others. In contrast to the inflammatory disorders are the diseases characterized primarily by degenerative glomerular changes, i.e., basement membrane thickening and hyalinization, as is seen in diabetic glomerulosclerosis.

Regrettably, the terminology of glomerular disease is plagued by a multiplicity of synonyms and individual preferences, but Table 24–1 offers a listing of the common forms, employing the most widely used designations.

In the section on glomerular diseases which follows, all seven forms of primary glomerular involvement will be considered in some detail. Only a brief review of the secondary involvements is provided since the systemic diseases associated with glomerular damage have been considered already.

Any one of these diseases, primary or secondary, may eventually cause uremia but, before reaching this late stage, they tend to segregate into those characterized principally by a nephritic syndrome and those evoking a nephrotic syndrome (although, as will be seen, there is overlap). The nephritic patient classically has azotemia, hematuria, mild to moderate edema and hypertension. The nephrotic syndrome will be described in detail later but,

TABLE 24–1. GLOMERULAR DISEASE

I. Primary Glomerular Disease
  A. Poststreptococcal (proliferative) glomerulonephritis (PGN)
  B. Rapidly progressive glomerulonephritis (RPGN)
  C. Lipoid nephrosis (LN), minimal change glomerulonephritis (MCGN)
  D. Membranous glomerulonephritis (MGN), membranous nephropathy
  E. Membranoproliferative nephritis
  F. Chronic glomerulonephritis (CGN)
  G. Focal glomerulonephritis (FGN)
II. Secondary Glomerular Disease
  A. Lupus nephritis, lupus glomerulonephritis
  B. Glomerulitis secondary to other "autoimmune" disease, e.g., scleroderma, polyarteritis
  C. Goodpasture's syndrome
  D. Diabetic glomerulopathy (including diffuse and nodular glomerulosclerosis)
  E. Amyloidosis

briefly, it is characterized by heavy proteinuria, hypoalbuminemia and severe edema. In these patients, at least at first, there may be little or no azotemia, hematuria or hypertension. It is important to emphasize that the nephritic may become nephrotic and, conversely, the nephrotic may, with the advance of his disease, develop manifestations of nephritis.

Several forms of primary glomerular involvement (poststreptococcal GN, rapidly progressive GN) and the secondary glomerular involvements encountered in systemic lupus erythematosus and the other "autoimmune diseases" are believed to result from immunologic injuries to the glomeruli. For this reason, a general discussion of immune mechanisms of glomerular disease will precede separate discussion of the different diseases.

IMMUNE MECHANISMS OF GLOMERULAR DISEASE

A wealth of clinical and experimental evidence indicates that many forms of glomerulonephritis are caused by immunologic mechanisms (Lewis and Couser, 1971) (McCluskey, 1970) (Seymour et al., 1971). Basically, two patterns of immunologic injury are involved: (1) deposition of circulating immune complexes (*immune complex disease*) and (2) fixation of antiglomerular basement membrane antibody to the GBM (*anti-GBM disease*). First, these two patterns of immune disease will be briefly characterized before discussing them in greater detail.

Immune Complex Disease. Here the glomerular injury is caused by the trapping of circulating antigen-antibody complexes within glomeruli. The antigens are nonglomerular and thus the glo-

merulus is, in a sense, an innocent victim of its own filtration function. The antibodies have no specificity for glomerular constituents, and the complexes localize within the glomeruli probably because of their physical properties or other influences discussed later. The immune complexes can be visualized by electron microscopy or by immunofluorescent techniques as characteristic granular lumps adjacent to the GBM. The evocative antigens are of two origins:

1. Exogenous, as in human serum sickness nephritis, poststreptococcal PGN, and experimental foreign protein nephritis.

2. Endogenous, as in systemic lupus erythematosus where circulating DNA and its antibodies form complexes which are trapped in the glomeruli.

Anti-GBM Disease. In this immunologic pattern, antibodies directed against antigens in the GBM localize in the glomerulus and cause injury. Examples of such disease are nephrotoxic nephritis in animals and Goodpasture's syndrome in man. In the former, kidney extract from one species of animal (e.g., the rat) is injected into another species (e.g., the rabbit). When the antirat kidney serum derived from the rabbit is administered to a rat, anti-GBM glomerulonephritis results. The relevance of this experimental model to man is evident with Goodpasture's syndrome where anti-GBM antibodies evoke the glomerulonephritis.

Immune Complex Nephritis. A host of studies have all documented that trapping of immune complexes against the GBM will induce glomerular injury (Benacerraf et al., 1947) (McCluskey et al., 1962) (Dixon et al., 1961). GN can be induced in animals by the infusion of preformed immune complexes or by the induction of serum sickness with heterologous protein. Serum sickness nephritis is the classic prototype of immune complex disease. Dixon and his collaborators (1961) demonstrated that when serum sickness is induced in rabbits by the injection of some foreign protein, such as bovine serum albumin, the amount of antibody formed in response to the antigenic challenge is critical in the development of nephritis. Animals producing large amounts of antibody developed transient acute serum sickness and nephritis. The large insoluble antigen-antibody aggregates formed in these animals were cleared by the reticuloendothelial system, and the glomerular injury was fleeting. At the other end of the spectrum were those animals with no immune response. In the absence of immune complexes, glomerulonephritis did not develop. Only in those animals with a weak antibody response, such that small soluble immune complexes formed in the presence of antigen excess, did a significant GN develop. So it is clear that *requisite for immune complex glomerulonephritis is the development of soluble an-tigen-antibody complexes formed in antigen excess,* which tend to persist in the circulation and are trapped against the GBM as the plasma is filtered.

In addition to the quantity of antibody, a host of other factors may be important in the production of immune complex glomerulonephritis. The quality of the antibody may play an important role. Pincus et al. (1968) have shown that nonprecipitating antibodies are more likely to induce this form of glomerular injury than antibodies which induce immune precipitation. To help explain the localization in glomeruli, increased vascular permeability in glomerular capillaries is postulated. The development of immune complex glomerulitis can be prevented by pretreatment of rabbits with antihistamines, antiplatelet antiserum or other antivasoactive agents (Cochrane, 1963). The size of the complexes may be significant. Those with sedimentation rates greater than 19S tend to become trapped, while smaller complexes may filter through. But of greatest importance in the production of immune complex nephritis is the role of complement. The antigen-antibody complexes must bind complement, principally C3 but possibly other components as well (Ward and Cochrane, 1965). Activation of complement is probably necessary for the induction of glomerular injury. *The chemotactic factors of activated complement attract leukocytes, and the destructive proteolytic lysosomal enzymes of the white cells constitute the ultimate mediator of the injury.* Questions persist as to whether the lytic action of activated C8–9 (Bokisch et al., 1969) (Cochrane et al., 1965) or activated chemical mediators of the inflammatory response alone may injure the glomerulus. More about the role of complement and leukocytes will follow later. *In this immunogenetic pattern of nephritis, the immune complexes appear, by electron microscopy and immunofluorescent methods, as granular deposits (humps) usually trapped between the GBM and the epithelial cells* (Fig. 24–6). In one particular instance, namely, lupus nephritis, the immune complexes localize preferentially on the endothelial side of the GBM but, as the disease advances, they are also found on the epithelial side. The factors significant to the development of immune complex glomerulonephritis can be recapitulated as follows:

1. Formation of antigen-antibody complexes in antigen excess.

2. Qualitative nature of antibody—nonprecipitating.

3. Some influence by vasoactive amines in localization of immune complexes.

4. Trapping of immune complexes against the GBM.

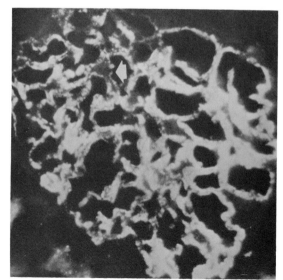

Figure 24-6. *Immune complex glomerulo-nephritis with granular ("humps") immunofluorescent deposits* (arrow) *along glomerular basement membrane. Compare with Figure 24-7.*

5. Complement binding by immune complexes.

6. Production of leukocyte chemotactic factors from complement.

7. Basement membrane damage resulting most likely from the release of neutrophilic lysosomal enzymes.

Anti-GBM Nephritis. As induced in experimental animals, this entity provided one of the first insights into immune mechanisms in nephritis. In 1934, Masugi showed that glomerulonephritis similar to human disease could be produced in rats by antirat kidney antibodies prepared by immunizing rabbits and ducks with rat kidney tissue. This experimental disease is known as nephrotoxic or Masugi nephritis (Masugi, 1934). The circulating antibodies bind along the entire length of the glomerular basement membrane which comprises their specific antigen, resulting in a so-called linear pattern as visualized by immunofluorescent techniques (Hammer and Dixon, 1963). *It should be particularly noted that anti-GBM reactions create linear patterns of immunofluorescence as contrasted with the granular humps of immune complex disease* (Fig. 24-7). Complement is fixed in this union. As an immune complex disease, attracted leukocytes probably mediate the injury in anti-GBM disease but, as will become clear, other mechanisms may also be involved.

This form of nephrotoxic nephritis may have considerable relevance to disease in man. In Goodpasture's syndrome, it is well established that antibodies to glomerular basement membrane and to lung basement membrane (which presumably have antigenic similarities) induce lesions in both organs. Steblay's (1962) observations lend further importance to anti-GBM mediated nephritis as a possible mechanism of disease in man. He showed that sheep could be induced to make autologous anti-GBM antibody when immunized with glomeruli from another species. Presumably, there are antigenic similarities in the glomerular basement membrane among several species. It is, therefore, possible that in man the release of glomerular basement membrane or other antigens into the circulation could induce glomerulonephritis, if the antigens induce antibodies cross reactive with the GBM. Antiserum to the placenta, aorta or lung can induce nephrotoxic nephritis in animals (Baxter and Goodman, 1956). Alternatively, glomerular antigens might be slightly modified by a biologic agent such as a virus which renders them foreign to the immune system and thus provokes an immune response reactive against the GBM.

It is necessary to appreciate that, in both immune complex and anti-GBM nephritis, the ultimate mechanisms of glomerular injury involve complement and leukocytes. Glomerular damage is significantly diminished by depletion of either serum complement or polymorphonuclear leukocytes (Hammer and Dixon, 1963). However, the glomerular damage is not

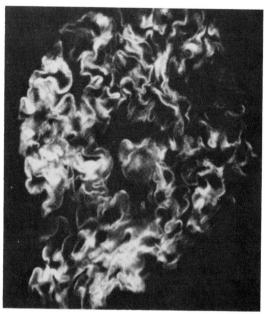

Figure 24-7. *Antiglomerular basement membrane disease with its linear pattern of immunofluorescence. Compare with Figure 24-6.*

totally blocked and other mechanisms may be operative. Antigen-antibody complexes may directly activate the kinin-forming system, which could result in increased glomerular and vascular permeability, emigration and destruction of neutrophils and release of damaging lysosomal enzymes (Cochrane, 1969). The coagulation system may also be a mediator of glomerular damage (McCluskey et al., 1966) (McIntosh et al., 1971). In nephrotoxic nephritis fibrin thrombi appear in glomerular capillaries and fibrinogen may leak into Bowman's space. The fibrin precipitated in Bowman's space may serve as a stimulus to epithelial cell proliferation (Vassalli and McCluskey, 1964). It is this proliferation which induces masses of epithelial cells in Bowman's space, called "crescents." Similar deposits of fibrin or fibrinogen derivatives have been demonstrated in several forms of glomerular disease in man (McCluskey et al., 1966).

In the following sections, the glomerular diseases are divided into the two principal clinical categories: nephritic and nephrotic syndromes.

NEPHRITIC SYNDROME

Certain forms of glomerular disease are characterized anatomically by inflammatory alterations in the glomeruli and clinically by a complex of findings classically referred to as *the syndrome of acute nephritis*. For example, the nephritic patient with widespread glomerular involvement usually presents with hematuria, azotemia, hypertension and red cell casts in the urine. While the patient also commonly has proteinuria and edema, these are not as severe as when encountered in the nephrotic syndrome, discussed later. Although certain forms of nephritis are reversible in a high percentage of cases, all of these inflammatory diseases have the potential of progressing to widespread destruction of the kidney and loss of renal function, leading to uremia. Focal glomerulonephritis, as will be seen, is an exception and is almost always a benign condition.

Poststreptococcal (Proliferative) Glomerulonephritis. This glomerular disease is basically a form of immune complex nephritis which develops in the course of the immune response to a streptococcal infection anywhere in the body. The majority of cases occur 5 to 30 days after a streptococcal throat infection and classically present with hematuria, proteinuria, oliguria, edema and hypertension. Most of those afflicted are children, but no age is immune. For unknown reasons, males are affected about twice as often as females.

Etiology and Pathogenesis. *Only certain strains of group A beta hemolytic streptococci are nephritogenic.* Over 90 per cent of cases of poststreptococcal glomerulonephritis can be traced to three types of streptococci—types 12, 4 and 1. Rarely, epidemics of this renal disease have been traced to other uncommon types, for example, Red Lake. It should be noted, however, that other etiologic agents have been implicated, but only rarely, in the causation of an apparently similar disease. A morphologically indistinguishable form of glomerulonephritis has been seen in acute staphylococcal endocarditis (Tu et al., 1969) and in a variety of viral infections including mumps, measles and chickenpox. Recent reports describe glomerulonephritis following viral hepatitis and HAA antigenemia (Combes et al., 1971). Collectively, however, the nonstreptococcal etiologies are very uncommon.

The evidence that poststreptococcal glomerulonephritis is, indeed, of immunologic origin is quite convincing. The kidneys, blood and urine are sterile. The latent period between the streptococcal infection and the onset of nephritis is very similar to that in serum sickness and is compatible with the time required for the buildup of antibodies. Elevated titers of antistreptolysin O (ASO) are present in the great majority of patients. The serum complement levels are usually low, compatible with involvement of the complement system as a mediator of the immune reaction (Lewis et al., 1971b). The similarity of the granular immune deposits along the GBM in serum sickness and poststreptococcal nephritis lends considerable support to the immune complex concept. Immunofluorescent stains reveal deposits of IgG, C3 and fibrin in the diseased glomeruli. However, it should be noted that, despite numerous efforts, it has not been convincingly demonstrated that the immune complexes contain identifiable antigenic components of streptococci even in those cases indisputably following streptococcal infections. Perhaps the closest approach has been that of Treser et al. (1970). They demonstrated that fluorescein-labeled IgG fractions of serum from patients with acute poststreptococcal glomerulonephritis would react with the damaged glomeruli obtained from renal biopsies of the same patients during the early phase of the disease. Preabsorption of such serum with the plasma membrane fraction of certain group A streptococci abolished the staining reaction. From this indirect evidence, they concluded that antigenic streptococcal plasma membrane components must be present in the immune complexes in the diseased glomeruli.

To date, it has not been possible to produce an acceptable facsimile of poststreptococcal disease in experimental animals by the injection of either live streptococci or streptococcal products (Lewis and Couser, 1971). Many still believe that poststreptococcal nephritis is the consequence of antigenic similarities between components of streptococci and GBM (Markowitz, 1969). If previous concepts of immune mechanisms are correct, such anti-GBM antibodies should induce a linear pattern of immunofluorescent staining in the disease of man but, with rare exception, the deposits are in the form of "humps" (Lewis et al., 1971a). It must suffice to say here that questions remain relative to the pathogenesis of this disease, but the evidence is substantial that it is a form of immune complex nephritis, triggered, in the great majority of cases, by an antecedent streptococcal infection.

Morphology. In the very early phase of the disease, the kidneys may appear normal, but soon they become moderately enlarged, perhaps up to 180 gm. each. The cortical surface is red-brown and smooth but is often dotted by fine punctate petechiae produced by the acute inflammatory rupture of glomerular capillaries (Fig. 24—8). On

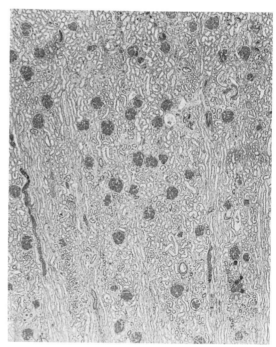

Figure 24–9. Poststreptococcal glomerulonephritis. A low power view to show the prominence of the acutely congested glomeruli.

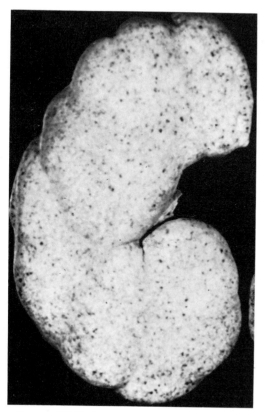

Figure 24–8. Poststreptococcal glomerulonephritis with pallor of the parenchyma and prominent petechial hemorrhages. The fetal lobulations are incidental.

sectioning, the cortex is widened by inflammatory edema and is usually clearly differentiated from the medulla. Early in the disease, close inspection with a hand lens may reveal enlarged congested glomeruli (Fig. 24—9). As the disease reaches its fully developed phase, the glomeruli become bloodless and their capillaries are compressed by swelling and proliferation of cells.

Microscopically, the stage of glomerular congestion passes rapidly and is replaced by **the classic diagnostic picture of enlarged, hypercellular, relatively bloodless glomeruli.** The hypercellularity is caused by the proliferation of both endothelial and mesangial cells which compress the lumina of capillaries and distort the native architecture of the glomerular vascular tuft. An exudation of leukocytes, principally neutrophils, in the glomeruli may be quite prominent particularly in children, but may be very scant in adults (Fig. 24—10). Small deposits of fibrin within capillary lumina and within the mesangium can sometimes be demonstrated by special stains for this plasma protein. In addition to the glomerular lesions, there may be interstitial edema and inflammation and the epithelial cells of the proximal convoluted tubules may show hyaline droplets, presumably reflecting reabsorption of protein from the glomerular filtrate. Frequently, the tubules contain red cell casts which, for the clinician, comprise the most diagnostic urinary finding of acute nephritis.

The more specific morphologic features of post-

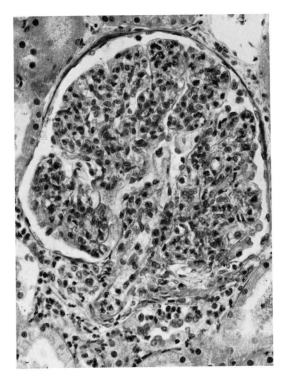

weeks after the onset of the disease. However, in some cases they persist for years and are accompanied by the deposition of excessive mesangial matrix. The persistence of glomerular abnormalities beyond a year is generally interpreted to mean latent disease which may progress to chronic GN either insidiously or following repeated exacerbations.

Clinical Course. The clinical course of poststreptococcal nephritis varies with the age of the patient. In the classic case, a young child abruptly develops malaise, fever, nausea, oliguria and hematuria some 5 to 30 days after apparent recovery from a streptococcal infection. Characteristically, the urine is smoky brown as its content of red cells is hemolyzed, with transformation of the hemoglobin to hem-

Figure 24–10. *Poststreptococcal glomerulonephritis. The glomerular hypercellularity is due to an immigrant leukocytic infiltrate and an edematous enlargement of the native cells. There is also an infiltrate of white cells in the renal interstitium about the glomerulus.*

streptococcal glomerulonephritis become evident only under the electron microscope and with immunofluorescent stains. With higher resolution, the endothelial and mesangial cell swelling and proliferation are clearly evident. Leukocytes can be seen eroding the endothelium, with baring of the basement membrane. Electron dense granules can now be visualized along the GBM as subepithelial "humps." Immunofluorescence confirms the fact that these humps contain both IgG, C3 and possibly other components of complement (Fig. 24–11). In most cases, the epithelial cells have not lost their foot processes nor is the basement membrane thickened. Occasionally, particularly in those having severe proteinuria, foot processes are lost and the epithelial cells become directly applied to the external aspect of the GBM. As will be seen later, loss of foot processes generally implies that the patient has developed the so-called nephrotic syndrome (p. 1102). Rarely, epithelial cells from both the parietal and visceral layer of Bowman's capsule proliferate to fill Bowman's space and create so-called crescents. Proliferation of epithelial cells occurs only in severe involvements and indicates a poor prognosis for the return of normal renal function.

In the great majority of cases, the glomerular changes begin to subside approximately four to six

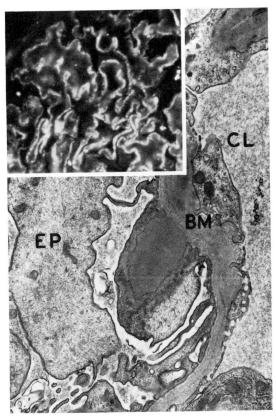

Figure 24–11. *An electron micrographic detail of the basement membrane (BM) of the glomerulus in the "immune complex" form of diffuse PGN. A lumpy immune complex deposit is attached to the epithelial surface of the basement membrane (BM) just to the left of the symbol BM. It is enclosed within a cytoplasmic process of the epithelial cell (EP). The inset at upper left is a detail of an immunofluorescent stain of the glomerulus in this disease. Seen are the irregular, luminescent, lumpy deposits arrayed about the margins of the glomerular capillaries. (CL, capillary lumen.)*

atin in the relatively acid urine. Red cell casts in the urine are one of the most diagnostic findings. Proteinuria is generally mild but may be massive, resulting in the nephrotic syndrome, as was mentioned earlier. In the typical child, there is little or no edema, azotemia or hypertension.

In adults, the onset is more apt to be atypical, with back pain and fever suggesting pyelonephritis, or the disease may become manifest by the sudden appearance of hypertension or pulmonary edema. The urinary findings are identical to those in the child, but the BUN is more likely to be elevated. *Characteristic of the acute phase of the disease in both children and adults are depressed levels of serum complement and elevated ASO titers.* Indeed, the activity of the disease can be monitored by the extent of lowering of the serum complement level; when it begins to rise to normal levels, the active phase of the disease is over.

The course and prognosis of the disease are very different in children from those in adults. *Over 95 per cent of children with poststreptococcal glomerulonephritis totally recover following progressive amelioration of the renal involvement over the course of four to six weeks.* Less than 1 per cent die in the acute phase in uremia or acute congestive heart failure. Another 1 per cent pursue a rapidly downhill course and die in uremia in a few months. The disease is then termed *rapidly progressive glomerulonephritis* and will be discussed below. Additional rare patients (approximately 1 per cent) show slow progression to chronic glomerulonephritis, with or without recurrent bouts of active nephritis. Generally, the exacerbations are triggered by recurrent infections. The most detailed study of this course has been that of Dodge et al. (1968, 1972) who biopsied all children with acute glomerulonephritis at onset and at specified intervals for five years after the acute attack. They found that persistent glomerular hypercellularity, deposition of mesangial matrix and failure of the glomeruli to promptly return to normal after the acute disease were all indices of a poor prognosis.

In adults, this renal disease is probably far more sinister. Only about 60 per cent promptly recover. In as many as 40 per cent of patients, the glomerular lesions may fail to resolve completely. Adults have a higher mortality during the acute phase of the disease and a much greater incidence of progression, either rapidly or slowly, to renal failure. Some of those with persistent proteinuria, hypertension, azotemia and hematuria may show eventual resolution, but no precise data are available on their number. Similarly, the rare patient with acute glomerulonephritis following some other type of infection has a somewhat less favorable prognosis than those with poststreptococcal nephritis.

Goodpasture's Syndrome. Goodpasture's syndrome is an acute, often fulminating disorder characterized by the sudden onset of *pulmonary hemorrhages and acute glomerulonephritis typical of anti-GBM disease* (Proskey et al., 1970). It is seen mostly in young adults, principally in men. The pulmonary involvement usually precedes the onset of the nephritis and is, in fact, the dominant cause of morbidity and mortality as is discussed on p. 828. Here our interest is in the glomerulonephritis.

The pathogenesis of the pulmonary and renal lesions resides in the appearance of circulating antibodies directed against antigens common to both the pulmonary and glomerular basement membranes (Koffler et al., 1969). Experimentally, it is possible to induce the nephritis readily with antiserum directed against pulmonary basement membrane. The trigger which provokes the production of these antibodies in man is still uncertain. In the original description of this syndrome, the pulmonary lesions were thought to be influenzal and, conceivably, the virus could have altered the pulmonary basement membranes, antigenically rendering them "foreign" (Goodpasture, 1919). Alternatively, could this disorder be an autoimmune disease?

Morphology. The macroscopic appearance of the kidneys in Goodpasture's syndrome may be indistinguishable from those of acute poststreptococcal glomerulonephritis. On renal biopsy, the early changes comprise mild segmental proliferative changes, usually involving all glomeruli. Small foci of glomerular capillary necrosis and deposits of fibrinoid may then develop. In time, the classic enlarged hypercellular, bloodless glomeruli become apparent. These are identical with those in poststreptococcal glomerulonephritis, as far as can be determined by light microscopy. However, at this phase of the renal involvement, electron microscopy fails to disclose the hump-like deposits characteristic of immune complex disease. Instead, **immunofluorescent stains for both immunoglobulins and complement reveal the uniform linear pattern outlining the entire glomerular basement membrane characteristic of anti-GBM disease** (see Fig. 24–7 on p. 1092). Deposits of fibrin have been demonstrated between the capillary endothelium and the GBM by electron microscopy.

As the renal involvement progresses in Goodpasture's syndrome, the proliferative changes in the glomeruli, at first largely endothelial and mesangial, soon are dominated by striking **epithelial cell proliferation with the formation of crescents.**

Crescents comprise masses of epithelial cells (parietal and visceral layers of Bowman's epithelium) which fill the uriniferous space of the glomerulus. Thus emerges, in almost all of these patients, the form of renal involvement mentioned earlier called rapidly progressive glomerulonephritis.

Clinical Course. The clinical course of this disease has been discussed on p. 829. It suffices here to indicate that the fatality rate is very high, death usually being caused either by massive pulmonary involvement or by renal failure. Steroids and other immunosuppressive therapeutic agents have been used, and some patients have recovered, but too few have been so treated to express a precise prognosis with this therapy. Of great theoretical interest, reversal of the pulmonary lesions has been reported after bilateral nephrectomy, followed by long-term dialysis or renal transplantation (Siegel, 1970). Why should removal of the kidneys and the GBM antigens permit the pulmonary disease to resolve if the lung basement membranes are also antigenic triggers? This remarkable finding, if confirmed, indicates that much is yet to be learned about this disease. It should be emphasized here that, early in its course, the histologic pattern of glomerulonephritis in this anti-GBM disease is indistinguishable by light microscopy from that of immune complex nephritis as seen in poststreptococcal glomerulonephritis. However, in Goodpasture's syndrome, there is a far greater tendency toward the glomerular crescent formation typical of rapidly progressive glomerulonephritis.

Rapidly Progressive Glomerulonephritis (RPGN).

This form of proliferative glomerulonephritis is much less common than acute poststreptococcal GN but much more serious. *It is characterized anatomically by widespread crescent formations throughout all glomeruli in both kidneys and, clinically, by rapidly worsening renal failure, leading to death in uremia within weeks or months unless dialysis or transplantation is instituted.* For these reasons, this entity is also called "malignant glomerulonephritis" or "glomerulonephritis with extensive epithelial crescents" (Cameron, 1970). It is not a distinctive immunologic entity but, instead, is best viewed as an ominous pathway which may be followed by any form of acute glomerulonephritis. Some cases of RPGN arise as immune complex disease while others originate as anti-GBM disease. Thus, RPGN may occur in poststreptococcal glomerulonephritis, Goodpasture's syndrome, lupus glomerulonephritis or the Henoch-Schönlein syndrome. However, most cases are idiopathic and arise without apparent antecedent infections or history of acute nephritis. It has, therefore, been suggested that rapidly progressive glomerulonephritis be divided into three categories—immune complex type (e.g., poststreptococcal), anti-GBM type (e.g., Goodpasture's) and nonstreptococcal (idiopathic) (Richardson et al., 1970).

The majority of cases examined by immunofluorescence and electron microscopy have linear fluorescence of immunoglobulins and complement along the GBM typical of anti-GBM nephritis. Also, circulating antikidney antibodies are sometimes found in the serum of these patients. What triggers such an immune response is unknown (? autoimmunity). Lewis et al. (1970) have raised the question of whether immune responses eliciting selective subclasses of IgG may be responsible for producing such progressive renal disease.

Morphology. The kidneys are always bilaterally and symmetrically involved and are enlarged and pale. Petechial hemorrhages are frequently evident on the cortical surface but may be absent. By light microscopy, the glomeruli are hypercellular with some proliferation of the endothelial and mesangial cells, but characteristic is the **striking proliferation of the epithelial cells to form crescents throughout most glomeruli** (Fig. 24–12). Renal biopsies have indicated that these crescents form extremely rapidly and may be fully developed within a few days of onset of the nephritis. Indeed, these crescents may compress and distort the vascular glomerular tuft. Small or large portions of the glomerular tuft may become necrotic. Electron microscopy and immunofluorescence may disclose changes typical of immune complex disease, particularly in those cases of streptococcal origin, or these techniques may, instead, reveal linear deposits conforming to anti-GBM disease. Electron microscopy will also disclose fibrin strands between the proliferating epithelial cells forming the crescents. Indeed, it is currently believed that it is the fibrin which is the stimulus to epithelial proliferation. A very recent ultrastructural study indicates that some of the cells comprising these crescents are monocytic epithelioid cells which have emigrated from the blood in response to the immunologic injury (Kondo et al., 1972). There is usually concomitant marked interstitial edema and infiltration by inflammatory cells, and the tubules may show degenerative changes (Seymour et al., 1971). In most cases, with the advance of the disease, there is organization of the crescents to form collagen with eventual total hyalinization of the glomeruli. In rare fortunate cases, it has been reported that the crescents apparently disappear, but such evidence is derived from renal biopsies which may not have adequately sampled the total kidney (McCluskey and Baldwin, 1963).

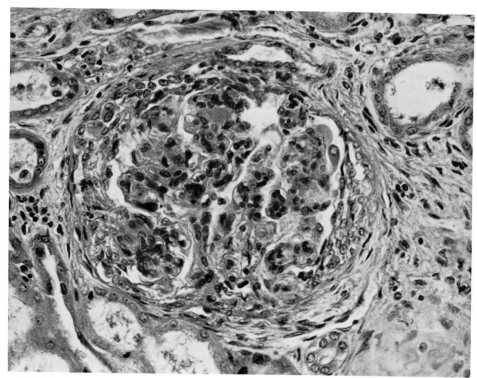

Figure 24–12. *Rapidly progressive glomerulonephritis, with characteristic proliferation of the visceral epithelial cells producing crescents.*

Clinical Course. Generally, when renal biopsy discloses widespread crescent formation characteristic of RPGN, the prognosis is bleak. Some patients begin with a classic history of poststreptococcal glomerulonephritis which fails to resolve in the usual four to six weeks and progressively worsens over the following weeks to months. Urinary findings are similar to those in acute glomerulonephritis, i.e., hematuria, proteinuria, oliguria and red cell casts. But in RPGN, the oliguria may worsen and lead to virtually complete anuria. The BUN and creatinine levels progressively mount and hypertension is very pronounced. Obviously, when the patient is rendered virtually anephric, fluid and electrolyte problems become severe. Most patients die in uremia unless they are dialyzed or receive a renal transplant. However, as indicated in the discussion of morphology, in a few cases the crescents may resolve and the patient may eventually recover although this favorable outcome has not yet been definitely proved for this disorder. Leonard et al. (1970) propose a better prognosis in patients with good evidence of a poststreptococcal etiology. As mentioned earlier in the discussion of Goodpasture's syndrome, steroids or immunosuppressive therapy and bilateral nephrectomy followed by transplantation have led to recovery in a few cases of Goodpasture's syndrome with RPGN.

Chronic Glomerulonephritis. Chronic GN is the final common outcome of many forms of longstanding glomerular disease. *It is best considered as an end-stage pool of glomerular disease fed by a number of streams of glomerulonephritis, some of known and others of unknown origin.* Perhaps 10 to 20 per cent of these cases result from the slow progression of poststreptococcal GN. Most of these instances represent adults, who in general fare less well than children with this disease. The chronic glomerular destruction takes place over the span of years during which time the patient may suffer repeated exacerbations of acute nephritis or the disease may smolder and progress without acute crises. An additional 30 to 50 per cent of chronic GN is derived from the stream of unresolved membranous glomerulonephritis, soon to be discussed (p. 1103). *The remainder of the cases, perhaps representing 40 to 50 per cent, arise mysteriously with no clear antecedent history of renal disease.* These patients first come to attention with well advanced chronic glomerulonephritis and, often, all of the features of chronic renal failure discussed earlier (p. 1083).

Whatever its origin, chronic glomerulonephritis is one of the two most frequent causes of death from uremia. The other, chronic pyelonephritis, is probably the more common clinical condition, but is less lethal than chronic GN, and studies vary as to whether chronic GN or chronic pyelonephritis is the most frequent cause of uremia. Any age may be affected, but because many of the streams feeding this pool arise at an early age, most fatalities occur in the first five decades of life. Males are affected somewhat more often than females.

Pathogenesis. The pathogenesis of chronic GN relates to the origins of poststreptococcal glomerulonephritis, membranous glomerulonephritis and the large fraction of cases of idiopathic nature. As is evident from the designation, little is known about the latter. One might speculate that they represent subclinical forms of one of the better defined entities, but there is no evidence to either support or contradict such a proposition. As would be anticipated from the several etiologies of chronic GN, immunofluorescent studies have shown, in some cases, the immune complex and, in others, the anti-GBM patterns of fluorescence (Dixon, 1968). But, in many cases, there are no immunologic findings, and the question arises whether they were once present and disappeared or were never present.

Morphology. The kidneys are symmetrically contracted and have red-brown, diffusely granular, cortical surfaces (Fig. 24–13). Each generally weighs in the range of 100 gm. Such symmetrical contraction must be differentiated from that caused by benign nephrosclerosis, characterized usually by more pallor and less marked diminution in size and weight, and the rare case of bilateral symmetrical diffuse chronic pyelonephritis which generally shows more profound contraction and weights of less than 100 gm. On sectioning, the cortex of the kidney in chronic GN is markedly thinned, to 1.5 cm. or less, and the demarcation between cortex and medulla is often obscured. The glomerular histology depends on the stage of the disease and, to some extent, on whether the lesion follows proliferative or membranous glomerulonephritis. Some vestiges of glomerular hypercellularity and crescent formations may be evident, or membranous thickening of the capillary walls may be apparent (Fig. 24–14). However, in either case, there eventually ensues eosinophilic hyaline obliteration of total glomeruli, transforming them into acellular, collagenous masses (Fig. 24–15). Generally some glomeruli are less affected, even in advanced disease, or the patient would have died sooner (unless, of course, he had been maintained on dialysis for a long time). Cases seen in the end-stage of uniformly advanced glomerular hyalinization provide no clues as to their origin. The obstruction of blood flow between the afferent and efferent arterioles has secondary effects upon the other components of the kidney. Thus, there is secondary atrophy of tubules, increased interstitial fibrosis and occasionally a scant, scattered interstitial lymphocytic infiltrate. The small arteries and arterioles are frequently thick-walled with narrowed lumina, perhaps secondary to the commonly associated hypertension, as well as to atrophic alterations. Although immunofluorescence may reveal immunoglobulins and complement in either of the distinctive patterns mentioned earlier, in the great preponderance of

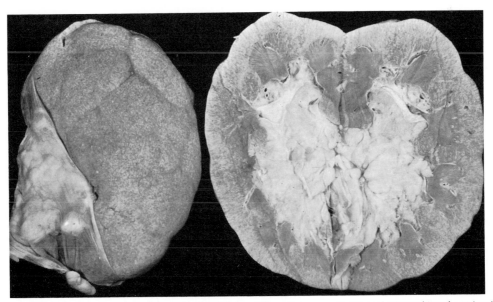

Figure 24–13. Chronic glomerulonephritis with its diffuse fine granularity and parenchymal contraction as evidenced by narrowing of the cortex and increase of peripelvic fat.

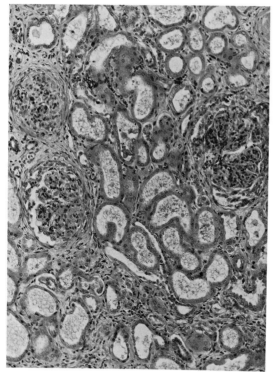

Figure 24–14. Three glomeruli in a kidney with chronic glomerulonephritis. The glomerulus at the lower left is least involved; the one on the right has complete obliteration of the Bowman space; the one on the upper left is almost totally destroyed.

cases, by the time the changes have reached the chronic stage, there is no immunologic evidence to suggest the nature of the antecedent disease.

Clinical Course. In most patients, chronic GN develops insidiously and slowly progresses to death in uremia over a span of years or possibly decades. Not infrequently, patients present with such nonspecific complaints as loss of appetite, nausea, vomiting or weakness. In some, the renal disease is first suspected with the discovery of proteinuria, hypertension or azotemia on routine medical examination. In others, the underlying renal disorder is discovered in the course of investigation of edema. *Most patients are hypertensive, and sometimes the dominant clinical manifestations are cerebral or cardiovascular.* In all, the disease is relentlessly progressive, although at widely varying rates, and 10 or more years may elapse between onset of symptoms and death unless the patients are treated by dialysis or transplantation. In about 20 per cent of these cases, the slow progression is punctuated by bouts of active nephritis with its attendant hematuria, red cell casts and oliguria. In other instances, episodes of marked proteinuria may evoke the nephrotic syndrome but, in general, as the

disease advances and the glomeruli become progressively obliterated, the protein loss in the urine diminishes and so does the likelihood of nephrotic episodes. Save for those patients maintained on continued dialysis or receiving renal transplants, the outcome is invariably death.

Focal Glomerulonephritis (FGN), Focal Nephritis. Focal glomerulonephritis is a pathologic entity characterized anatomically by irregular random involvement of glomeruli and segments of individual glomeruli throughout the kidney. Clinically, it is principally associated with transient episodes of hematuria and proteinuria without azotemia. *The phase of active disease is usually self-limited and resolves within days to weeks* only possibly to recur months or years later. Focal glomerulonephritis is associated with a host of systemic diseases, including bacterial endocarditis, lupus erythematosus, polyarteritis nodosa, Henoch-Schönlein purpura, Goodpasture's syndrome, Wegener's granulomatosis and hypersensitivity drug reactions. Irregular resolution of poststreptococcal glomerulonephritis can sometimes leave an apparent focal pattern. But, in addition, FGN may appear in the absence of an underlying systemic or renal dis-

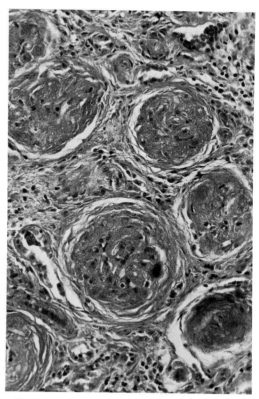

Figure 24–15. Chronic glomerulonephritis. The glomeruli are totally replaced by hyaline connective tissue.

ease, usually 1 to 3 days after an acute febrile illness. It is not particularly related to streptococcal infection and sometimes follows respiratory disorders. It may occur at any age and in both sexes, but mainly affects children and young adults.

Etiology and Pathogenesis. Present evidence favors the view that FGN is an immunologic disease. Widespread deposits of immunoglobulins, complement and fibrinogen within the mesangium and along the glomerular basement membrane can be seen in many but not all cases. Interestingly, the distribution of these immune deposits may be far more generalized than the focal nature of the lesions suggests. These immunologic findings are present in FGN associated with SLE, Goodpasture's syndrome, Wegener's granulomatosis and hypersensitivity drug reactions (Hayslett et al., 1968), and are also found in patients with Henoch-Schönlein purpura. In this condition they are also found in the small vessels of the skin, intestine, joints and afferent arterioles of the kidney, a distribution which suggests the development of a systemic hypersensitivity vasculitis (Heptinstall, 1966). One form of FGN, Berger's disease, is characterized by the deposit of principally IgA in the mesangium of glomeruli (Berger, 1969). This disorder, principally of young males, is not associated with any underlying disease. FGN occurring in patients with infective endocarditis was once called focal embolic glomerulonephritis. However, bacteria-laden emboli are almost never visualized, and this lesion also is likely to have immunologic origins. Thus it is suspected that immune mechanisms underlie all forms of FGN, but the evidence is still fragmentary. It should be noted that serum complement levels are almost never depressed in this disease.

Morphology. Grossly, the kidneys are usually of normal size and color but often have irregularly scattered petechial hemorrhages, whence arises the designation **"the flea-bitten kidney"** (Fig. 24–16). On sectioning the kidney, the gross architecture is normal, save for the petechial hemorrhages in the cortex. Microscopically, randomly scattered glomeruli (usually only one or two segments of each) are involved. In the acute stage, there is proliferation of endothelial and mesangial cells usually adjacent to a focus of necrosis in the vascular tuft (Fig. 24–17). In the areas

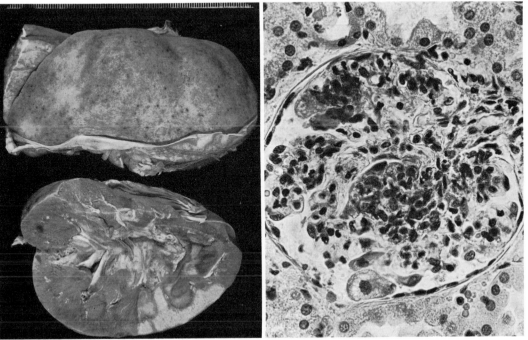

Fig. 24–16   Fig. 24–17

Figure 24–16. The kidneys in bacterial endocarditis. The cortical surface of the upper kidney has the "flea-bitten" petechiae. The cut surface of the lower kidney demonstrates a large pale infarct.

Figure 24–17. Focal glomerulonephritis with several focal acute necroses within the glomerular tuft.

of involvement, fibrin deposition and capillary thromboses are common. Minimal lesions may demonstrate only platelet aggregates and fibrin thrombi within glomerular capillary lumina, while more severe involvement may be accompanied by epithelial cell proliferation with crescent formation. Later, the involved areas undergo fibrosis with obliteration of a segment of the glomerulus. Adhesions may form between the affected segment and the visceral layer of Bowman's capsule. The severity of the disease clinically correlates well with the number of glomerular lesions in the kidney and, in cases with an abundance of glomerular lesions, the anatomic and, indeed, the clinical findings may resemble diffuse proliferative glomerulonephritis.

Clinical Course. As indicated earlier, FGN manifests itself as transient episodes of hematuria and proteinuria, rarely associated with azotemia or hypertension. In some instances, the hematuria may be quite massive and may be accompanied by red cell casts. In others, the urinary abnormalities are transient and minimal. Serum complement levels are normal, as are the ASO titers, and rarely is the glomerular filtration rate affected. Since FGN is frequently encountered in systemic diseases, the renal manifestations may be overshadowed or may comprise only a trivial part of the underlying disorder. Severe FGN is most likely to be encountered in bacterial endocarditis and, in a few such cases, may cause sufficient glomerular damage to produce renal failure and death in uremia.

NEPHROTIC SYNDROME

Certain glomerular diseases (membranous GN, lipoid nephrosis), to be presented, virtually always produce the nephrotic syndrome. In addition, many of the forms of glomerulonephritis already discussed may evoke it. It is convenient, therefore, before presenting its two major causes, to discuss this clinical complex. *The nephrotic syndrome comprises the following findings:*

1. Massive proteinuria with the daily loss, in the urine, of 4 gm. or more of protein.

2. Hypoalbuminemia with plasma albumin levels less than 3 gm. per 100 ml.

3. Generalized edema.

4. Hyperlipidemia.

Whenever glomerular diseases alter the GBM and make it abnormally permeable, large molecules (such as albumin and sometimes even the larger plasma proteins) freely escape into the glomerular filtrate, producing massive proteinuria. It will be remembered from the earlier discussions that the GBM comprises the filtration barrier in the glomerulus. Despite the unmistakable pathophysiologic evidence of increased permeability, e.g., massive proteinuria, it has been impossible to identify, with the highest resolution electron micrography, actual defects in the membrane. As will be seen, in membranous GN, the membrane is unmistakably altered and paradoxically thickened, but no structural pores are visible. The heavy proteinuria leads to depletion of serum albumin levels below the compensatory synthetic abilities of the liver, with consequent hypoalbuminemia and a reversed albumin-globulin ratio. The generalized edema is, in turn, the consequence of the loss of colloid osmotic pressure of the blood. With the accumulation of fluid in the interstitial tissues, the hypovolemia diminishes the glomerular blood flow and filtration rate. Compensatory secretion of aldosterone, mediated by the JG apparatus, follows, further promoting retention of salt and water and further aggravating the edema. The edema may be quite massive, termed anasarca. Characteristically, it is soft and pitting, most marked in the periorbital regions and dependent portions of the body. In some patients, pleural effusions and ascites appear as manifestations of the retention of salt and water. The genesis of the hyperlipidemia is less clear. It is proposed that the serum concentration of lipoproteins becomes elevated as the albumin falls. Presumably, the low albumin level stimulates increased synthesis, in the liver, of all forms of plasma proteins including lipoproteins, particularly the beta and pre-beta classes. Hence, these patients have hyperlipidemia and hypercholesterolemia corresponding to the Frederickson types II, III and IV. Lipiduria follows the hyperlipidemia, since not only albumin molecules but also lipoproteins are able to pass the glomerular basement membrane. The fat may appear in the urine sediment as oval fat bodies representing lipoprotein resorbed into tubular epithelial cells and then shed along with the cells.

There are additional extrarenal consequences of the nephrotic syndrome. The associated hyperlipidemia and hypercholesterolemia evoke an increased tendency toward atherosclerosis in general and atherosclerotic coronary heart disease in particular. In addition, the patients are particularly vulnerable to infection, especially with staphylococci and pneumococci. The basis for this vulnerability is not clear but could be related to loss of immunoglobulins through the leaky glomeruli.

As mentioned above, the nephrotic syndrome may be caused by a variety of glomerular involvements. In some patients, the renal disease is primary; in others, the renal involvement is part of a systemic disorder. Both children and adults may be affected. A recent compilation from the University of Chicago of the forms of renal involvement that give rise to the nephrotic syndrome is presented in Table 24–2 (Seymour et al., 1971). Several features are noteworthy in this table. Among children, the great preponderance of cases of the nephrotic syndrome are the consequence of primary renal disease. The outstanding cause is lipoid nephrosis (65 per cent), but membranous glomerulonephritis accounts for 7 per cent, and proliferative (immune complex or anti-GBM disease) glomerulonephritis, for 24 per cent. In adults, primary renal disease is less predominant. Most important is membranous glomerulonephritis (29 per cent). However, it should be noted that adults also suffer from lipoid nephrosis. Diabetic glomerulosclerosis, amyloidosis and lupus nephritis make a substantial contribution to the spectrum of the nephrotic syndrome in adults.

It is important to note that, at the outset, the pure nephrotic with MGN or lipoid nephrosis has little or no azotemia, hematuria or hypertension. However, as these diseases advance, the patient with MGN frequently develops sufficient glomerular damage to eventually suffer renal failure. While this same course is sometimes followed by those with lipoid nephrosis, fortunately it is uncommon. In the other less common causes of this syndrome, such as proliferative GN, manifestations of nephritis and nephrosis are both present, and the patient is sometimes called a nephritic nephrotic.

Membranous Glomerulonephritis (MGN).

Membranous glomerulonephritis, a major cause of the nephrotic syndrome, is characterized anatomically by subepithelial electron-dense immune deposits often associated with thickening of the GBM. Some investigators prefer the terms *epimembranous* or *membranous nephropathy* since, as will be clear, there is little evidence of inflammatory change within the glomeruli. Although the previous analysis of causes of the nephrotic syndrome indicates that children may suffer from this disease, it is most common in young adults and in middle life. As will be discussed later in the consideration of lipoid nephrosis, there was for some long time controversy as to whether MGN and lipoid nephrosis were separate and distinct entities or merely two stages of the same disease. Current evidence favors the view that they are not related.

Etiology and Pathogenesis. MGN is probably an immune disorder but of uncertain etiology. It is occasionally encountered in secondary syphilis and following hypersensitivity reactions to drugs, particularly gold therapy, compatible with immune reactions. Furthermore, *the anatomic changes, as visualized by the electron microscope and immunofluorescence, reveal irregular lumpy deposits which contain immunoglobulins and complement between the GBM and the epithelial cells.* While all of these observations

TABLE 24–2. CAUSES OF THE NEPHROTIC SYNDROME

Lesion	Adult		Less Than 15 Yrs.		Total Series	
	No.	Per Cent	No.	Per Cent	No.	Per Cent
Primary Renal Disease						
Lipoid nephrosis	20	18	43	65	63	35.5
Membranous glomerulonephritis (MGN)						
Idiopathic	30	27	5	7	35	20
Gold therapy	1	1	—	—	1	0.5
Secondary syphilis	1	1	—	—	1	0.5
Renal vein occlusion	1	1	—	—	1	0.5
Proliferative glomerulonephritis	18	16	16	24	34	19
SUBTOTALS		64		96		76
Systemic Disease						
SLE	15	13	1	2	16	9
Diabetes mellitus	14	12	—	—	14	8
Amyloidosis	9	8	—	—	9	5
Other	3	3	1	2	4	2
SUBTOTALS		36		4		24
TOTALS	112	100	66	100	178	100

Modified from Seymour, A. E., et al.: Contributions of renal biopsy studies to the understanding of disease. Amer. J. Path., 65:550, 1971.

suggest an immune causative mechanism, the nature of the antigenic trigger is completely obscure. The disease is not related to streptococcal infection, and it has not been associated with any other known infectious agent. Thus, although the anatomic evidence points to some form of "immune-complex disease," its origin is still mysterious.

In addition to the immune deposits, the GBM undergoes striking changes, leading eventually to its irregular thickening. Why such thickening should increase its permeability is unknown, except that we must postulate that ultrastructural or biochemical alterations increase its porosity. The proteinuria is heavy and nonselective. *The epithelial podocytes lose their foot processes, which is generally believed to be an adaptive response to the leakage of proteins.* Thus, the epithelial cells appear as cytoplasmic smears applied to the GBM. In experimentally induced aminonucleoside nephrosis, scanning electron microscope studies have shown that disappearance of foot processes results from cell swelling and compression of the filtration slits, rather than fusion of the foot processes (Arakawa, 1970).

Morphology. Just as the patient is large, swollen and pale due to systemic edema, the kidneys are large, swollen and pale. On sectioning, the cortex is widened but the medulla and other gross features are undisturbed. By light microscopy in the fully developed case, there is marked, uniform, diffuse thickening of glomerular capillary walls which, as will be seen, results from GBM and epithelial cell changes. There may be some swelling of mesangial, endothelial and epithelial cells, but there is no significant evidence of cellular proliferation in the pure form of idiopathic MGN. The diagnostic features of MGN become evident only under the electron microscope. **Irregular, lumpy, dense deposits can be seen between the basement membrane and the overlying smeared epithelial cells.** Basement membrane material is laid down between these deposits, appearing as irregular spikes protruding from the GBM. In time, these spikes thicken to produce dome-like protrusions and, with progression of the disease, these eventually close over the immune deposits, burying them within a markedly thickened, irregular membrane (Ehrenreich and Churg, 1968). In this fashion, the membrane assumes a "moth-eaten" appearance, but eventually the holes fill in. Visualization of these membranous details requires either electron microscopy or, with light microscopy, silver impregnation stains (Jones, 1957) (Fig. 24–18). Immunofluorescence, as has been indicated, demonstrates that the immune deposits contain both immunoglobulins and complement (McCluskey et al., 1966). As

the disease advances, the membranous thickening progressively encroaches upon the capillary lumina and some proliferation of endothelial and mesangial cells occurs. Thus, the glomeruli become relatively sclerosed and, in the course of time, may eventually become totally hyalinized (Fig. 24–19). The epithelial cells of the proximal tubules contain hyaline droplets, reflecting reabsorption of protein from the urinary filtrate and lipid vacuolation as a consequence of lipoprotein reabsorption. In the advanced stage of the disease, tubular atrophy and interstitial fibrosis occur and, indeed, the kidneys may become contracted, finely granular and scarred, closely resembling, or identical to, those of chronic GN.

Clinical Course. In a previously healthy individual, this disorder usually begins with the insidious onset of the nephrotic syndrome (discussed earlier on p. 1102). In the majority of patients (70 to 90 per cent), the disease is irreversible and progresses slowly to renal failure over the span of five to 10 years. The fatal uremia results from the slow sclerosis and eventual destruction of the glomeruli—referred to earlier as the development of chronic GN. Perhaps 10 to 30 per cent of patients have regression of their anatomic changes and recover (Rosen, 1971). The course of the disease is notoriously irregular, with exacerbations of the nephrotic syndrome, followed by remissions for months or even years. For this reason, it has been difficult to evaluate the validity of the reports contending that steroids are effective in controlling the disease (Rastogi et al., 1969). Indeed, some investigators believe that steroids may be harmful in this condition (Black et al., 1970).

Lipoid Nephrosis (Minimal Change Glomerulonephritis, Foot Process Disease). The various designations of this condition indicate its essential features, namely, accumulation of lipids in renal tubular epithelial cells accompanied by virtually no change in glomeruli other than loss of the foot processes of the epithelial cells. This entity is the most common cause of the nephrotic syndrome in children, accounting for two-thirds of all cases in children under 15 years of age. Adults may also be affected but, among them, lipoid nephrosis accounts for only about one-fifth of the total incidence of this syndrome. *While MGN is usually irreversible and unresponsive to steroid therapy, lipoid nephrosis is reversible and responsive to such treatment* (White et al., 1970). It is evident, then, that it is critically important to differentiate, in the patient, between these two causes of the nephrotic syndrome, and the patient's age alone is not sufficient. While it is true that adult

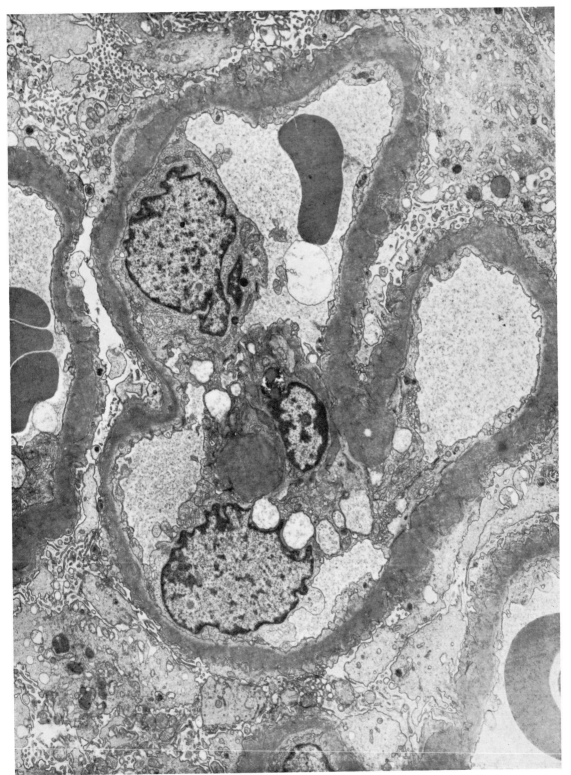

Figure 24–18. A low power (× 7200) electron micrograph of a capillary loop in a glomerulus from a patient with membranous glomerulonephritis. Note the irregularly thickened basement membrane with direct application of the podocytes to the outer surfaces. The foot processes have largely disappeared. (Courtesy of Dr. Paul Kimmelstiel, Professor of Pathology, University of Oklahoma Medical Center.)

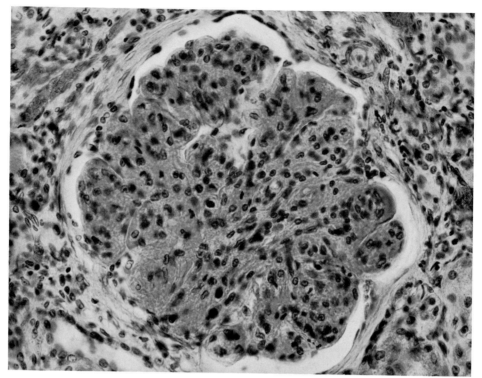

Figure 24–19. *Advanced membranous glomerulonephritis. The glomerular tuft is dense and compact, but the Bowman's space is relatively clear.*

nephrotics are more likely to have MGN, and childhood nephrotics, lipoid nephrosis, the reverse may obtain.

Controversy has long existed as to whether lipoid nephrosis may eventually evolve into MGN. As will be seen, in longstanding lipoid nephrosis, focal glomerular changes may appear which would cause morphologic diagnostic confusion but, at the present time, it is believed that the two entities are distinct.

Etiology and Pathogenesis. While there are indications that immune mechanisms are operative in MGN, there is *no* evidence of an immune pathogenesis for lipoid nephrosis. Immunofluorescent studies are characteristically negative for immunoglobulins, complement and fibrin (Drummond et al., 1966). Rarely, lipoid nephrosis erupts in a child following exposure to some allergen, such as a bee sting. There are rare reports of depressed serum complement levels in this disease but, on the whole, the evidence for an immuno-pathogenetic basis is virtually nonexistent (Ellis and Walton, 1958). The genesis of this disorder is therefore totally unknown.

Morphology. The kidneys tend to be slightly larger and heavier than normal. They are often pale or even yellowed by the combination of edema and the accumulation of lipid in tubular epithelial cells (Fig. 24 -20). With the light micro-scope, the only anatomic alteration is striking lipid vacuolation of the epithelial cells in the proximal tubules. The glomeruli appear normal. The diagnosis, therefore, rests upon negative criteria. However, with the electron microscope, **the epithelial cells show a uniform and diffuse loss of foot processes** (Churg et al., 1970). This abnormality of the epithelial cells is present only in active disease, that is, while there is heavy proteinuria. With improvement clinically, there is restoration of the normal architecture of the podocytes. In a small number of cases, perhaps more frequently in adults, focal areas of capillary collapse and sclerosis appear. Such foci may be visible with the light microscope and have been referred to as **focal glomeru-losclerosis**. Some investigators, therefore, divide lipoid nephrosis into two patterns — "minimal lesions" and "focal glomerulosclerosis" (Habib and Kleinknecht, 1971). The latter lesion is mentioned because it undoubtedly provides the basis for the former erroneous concern that lipoid nephrosis might, over the span of years, progress to MGN. Very rarely, the focal glomerulosclerosis progresses and involves sufficient glomeruli to cause renal failure (Hoyer et al., 1972). Only rarely does such an unhappy outcome occur in children (Hayslett et al., 1969).

Clinical Course. This disease manifests itself by the insidious development of the nephrotic syndrome. Despite massive protein-

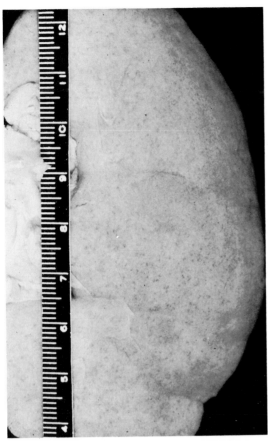

Figure 24–20. *Lipoid nephrosis to illustrate the pallor of the cortex. The color approaches that of the white markings on the millimeter rule.*

uria, renal function remains good and there is usually no hypertension. It may be impossible, short of renal biopsy, to differentiate lipoid nephrosis from MGN in the early stages of both diseases. With lipoid nephrosis, the manifestations of the nephrotic syndrome may persist for weeks to months, but usually they remit spontaneously or with steroid therapy. In a few patients, the nephrotic phase may recur and remit. The prognosis is, on the whole, very good, particularly when steroid therapy is instituted within six months of the onset of the disease. Approximately 95 per cent of children recover entirely. With adults, the prognosis is somewhat less favorable, and some go on to progressive glomerulosclerosis. One study indicates that about one-quarter of adult patients fail to respond to steroid therapy, and some follow a long remitting-relapsing course, ending ultimately in uremia (Hopper et al., 1970).

Renal Vein Thromboses. Venous thromboses are sometimes encountered with the nephrotic syndrome. The association of thromboses and the nephrotic syndrome is of particular interest when the renal veins are involved. It has long been a clinical puzzle as to which event occurs first. For many years, it was postulated that the *renal vein thromboses* induced membrane thickening in the glomeruli, loss of foot processes and the nephrotic syndrome, but the question has been raised recently as to whether the venous thromboses are not merely a manifestation of the generalized predisposition to thrombosis rather than the cause.

In contrast to the pure idiopathic form of MGN, the nephrotic syndrome associated with renal vein thrombosis may be reversible. The relationship between the venous thrombi and the glomerular lesions is completely enigmatic, and it should be noted that attempts to reproduce the combination experimentally have been unsuccessful (Fisher et al., 1968).

Other Causes of the Nephrotic Syndrome. Among adults, glomerular involvement in lupus erythematosus, diabetes mellitus or amyloidosis accounts for approximately 40 per cent of instances of the nephrotic syndrome. These are rare causes of the nephrotic syndrome in childhood.

Lupus nephritis or lupus nephropathy was described in the general consideration of this disease (p. 233). Only a few details will be given here to facilitate recall. In SLE, the kidney is involved in approximately 50 to 70 per cent of cases (Pollak and Pirani, 1969). The glomerular lesions can be roughly divided into four categories:

1. Focal basement membrane thickening, not associated with immune complex deposits.

2. Diffuse basement membrane thickening with irregular subepithelial immune deposits, reproducing the pattern of membranous glomerulonephritis.

3. Granular *subendothelial* immune deposits accompanied by proliferation of mesangial and endothelial cells. The glomerular hypercellularity is identical to that seen in poststreptococcal glomerulonephritis (Comerford and Cohen, 1967).

4. Focal glomerulonephritis indistinguishable from that encountered in other diseases.

Both the focal and diffuse forms of membrane involvement create eosinophilic thickening of the walls of capillaries, giving rise to the "wire loop" lesions said to be classic of SLE but found in all forms of membranous glomerulopathy (Fig. 24–21). In the pattern likened to membranous glomerulonephritis, there is loss of foot processes in the podocytes, and such patients almost always manifest the nephrotic syndrome. The proliferative pattern is indis-

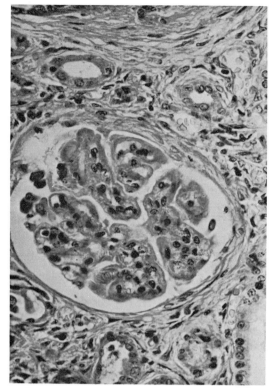

Figure 24–21. *Marked basement membrane thickening in the membranous glomerulonephritis of lupus erythematosus now sufficiently advanced to be visible with the light microscope. There is some increased cellularity with obliteration of lobules.*

tinguishable, with the light microscope, from poststreptococcal nephritis. However, with electron microscopy and immunofluorescence, it is evident that the immune complexes (presumably DNA–anti-DNA antibodies) localize first between the *endothelial* cells and the GBM. In later stages, the immune complexes may be found both subendothelially and subepithelially. The subendothelial location is virtually diagnostic of SLE, but why it occurs remains a mystery.

In longstanding diabetes mellitus, the kidney rarely escapes damage. Acute and chronic pyelonephritis, necrotizing papillitis, glycogen and fat deposits in the tubular epithelial cells, hyaline arteriolosclerosis of both the afferent and efferent arterioles and glomerulopathy are the principal forms of the diabetic nephropathy (p. 268). The glomerular involvement takes the form of diffuse or nodular glomerulosclerosis (Kimmelstiel-Wilson's disease) or, more often, the concurrence of both patterns (Figs. 24–22 and 24–23). It will be recalled that these glomerulopathies are related to the dura-

tion of the disease rather than to its severity, and one or both almost inevitably appear within 15 to 20 years. Both the diffuse and nodular forms of glomerulosclerosis may evoke the nephrotic syndrome but, whenever there is nodular glomerulosclerosis, there is almost inevitably concomitant diffuse involvement of the GBM and so, in all probability, it is this overall basement membrane change which leads to the nephrotic syndrome. In such patients, loss of the podocytic foot processes is usually, but not invariably, present.

Disseminated amyloidosis, whether it conforms to the so-called primary or secondary pattern of distribution, may be associated with deposits of amyloid within the glomeruli. Beginning in the mesangium, the fibrillar deposits of amyloid reach out to affect the basement membranes of the capillary loops, eventually to obliterate the glomerulus (p. 284) (Fig. 24–24). Before the stage of total obliteration is reached, the amyloid deposits are first seen along the subendothelial side of the GBM, but then flood through the basement membrane and appear subepithelially as well. In this fashion, the basement membrane is markedly thickened. There is also loss of podocytic foot processes. You recall that deposits of amyloid also appear in blood vessel walls and in the renal interstitium (Fig. 24–25). Thus, the patient with glomerular amyloidosis may present with the nephrotic syndrome and later, with destruction of the glomeruli, may die in uremia.

The nephrotic syndrome may be encountered in patients with poststreptococcal proliferative glomerulonephritis and, in rare instances, is produced by chronic glomerulonephritis, by rapidly progressive glomerulonephritis and by membranoproliferative glomerulonephritis (p. 1110). Whenever these inflammatory involvements of the glomeruli cause massive proteinuria, it is almost always associated with podocytic changes.

Although a compilation of major causes of the nephrotic syndrome was given on p. 1103, there are in addition a host of exotic causes. For example, it is sometimes encountered in unexpected settings such as transplant rejection, malaria, congestive heart failure and, indeed, as a congenital, apparently hereditary, disorder in infants. Patently, in the differential diagnosis of a patient with this syndrome (frequently requiring renal biopsy), the major causes must be exluded first, but it is important to realize that the appearance of massive proteinuria, followed by generalized edema in a patient with, for instance, congestive heart failure, does not necessarily imply the development of a primary glomerular disease.

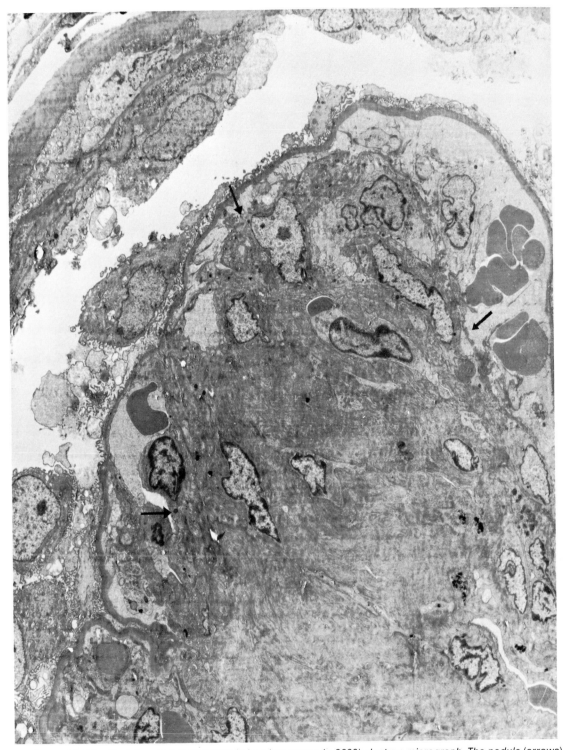

Figure 24–22. *Nodular glomerulosclerosis in a low power (× 3600) electron micrograph. The nodule (arrows) represents the irregularly deposited basement membrane-like material that has trapped so-called mesangial cells and has compressed portions of the peripheral capillaries. (Courtesy of Dr. Paul Kimmelstiel, Professor of Pathology, University of Oklahoma Medical Center.)*

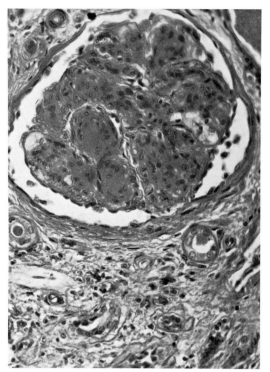

Figure 24–23. Nodular glomerulosclerosis in high power detail. The lesion is far advanced and there is beginning obliteration of the glomerular vascular tuft, but the globular masses are still evident.

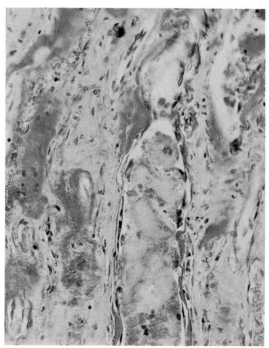

Figure 24–25. Amyloidosis of the interstitial tissue and basement membranes of the renal tubules. A large proteinous cast is present in one tubule.

RARE GLOMERULAR DISEASES

A few words are in order about some seldom encountered forms of glomerulopathy, if only to indicate the wide range of involvements that must be considered in any patient with clinical or physiologic evidence of glomerular dysfunction.

Membranoproliferative Glomerulonephritis (Chronic Hypocomplementemic Glomerulonephritis). A syndrome of chronic proliferative glomerulonephritis is encountered in children, sometimes accompanied by low serum levels of complement, particularly the C3 component. Many features of this disorder warrant its separation from the other glomerulopathies already described. It has been variously called mixed membranous and proliferative glomerulonephritis (Burkholder et al., 1970), membranoproliferative glomerulonephritis (Cameron et al., 1970) and chronic hypocomplementemic glomerulonephritis (West et al., 1965). The glomerular changes comprise essentially enlarged, hypercellular glomerular tufts, with exaggeration of the lobular architecture. The increased cellularity is produced by mesangial and endothelial proliferation and, in some cases, by polymorphonuclear exudation. Silver impregnation techniques reveal either splitting of the basement

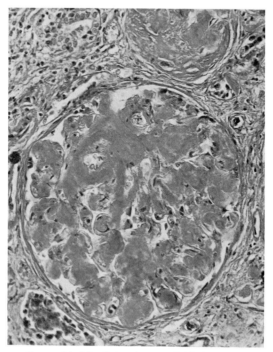

Figure 24–24. Extensive amyloid deposit within the glomeruli.

membrane, giving the capillary wall a "tram track" appearance, or sometimes merely thickening of the GBM. The splitting and thickening of the glomerular capillary walls is continuous with an increase in mesangial matrix. Immunofluorescence sometimes discloses granular staining for beta-1-complement, but generally immunoglobulins are absent (Burkholder et al., 1970). In time, this proliferative phase is passed and there is hyalinization of the individual lobes, producing a pattern closely resembling nodular diabetic glomerulosclerosis. The meaning of low serum complement levels and complement deposits in the glomeruli not associated with immunoglobulins is still obscure. Although some investigators hold that this is a variant of progressive poststreptococcal glomerulonephritis, most believe it is a distinctive entity, albeit of unknown origin. Despite the usually depressed serum complement levels, there is no good evidence for an immune causation and, indeed, the serum complement levels do not correlate with the course of the disease (West and McAdams, 1970).

Hereditary Nephritis (Familial Nephritis, Diffuse Familial Nephropathy). A form of familial nephritis has been described in several families, which is associated with hearing loss (nerve deafness) and ocular disturbances, in a more than chance frequency (Kaufman et al., 1970). While both males and females are affected, curiously the renal lesion tends to be progressive only in males and may, indeed, lead to renal failure in this sex. Females, in contrast, remain well throughout their lives and few die of their kidney disease. The nephropathy appears usually in the first two decades of life, and most males die before the age of 40. The syndrome appears to be transmitted as an autosomal dominant with greater penetrance in the male, although other modes of inheritance such as partial sex-linkage have been proposed (Perkoff et al., 1958).

The morphologic renal changes are neither distinctive nor pathognomonic. Moreover, the histologic features vary among patients but tend to be similar within families. In some instances, changes reminiscent of proliferative GN are seen. In others, only glomerular basement membrane thickening is present while, in still others, podocytic proliferation, thickening of Bowman's capsule or periglomerular fibrosis is present. Often the glomerular changes are accompanied by interstitial fibrosis and tubular atrophy. A somewhat distinctive finding, seen only in a small percentage of cases, is the appearance of foam cells either within the proliferated glomerular cells or within the interstitium. It is to be emphasized

that the foam cells are not a common finding, nor are they limited to hereditary nephritis. Immunofluorescent studies are almost always negative.

The pathogenesis of this disorder is unknown. Some hereditary predisposition to viral infections, such as a slow-virus has been suspected, but is unproven. A genetic metabolic or enzymic defect leading to the formation of a toxic metabolite injuring the kidneys, auditory nerves and eyes is also postulated, but without proof. Some aberration in lipid metabolism would fit the appearance of the foam cells in the kidneys, but no distinctive abnormalities in plasma lipids have been documented in all cases. In summary, the disorder is still idiopathic in origin but, whatever its genesis, it requires recall whenever nephritis appears in a member of a family having other affected members.

Hemolytic-Uremic Syndrome (Microangiopathic Hemolytic Anemia). A uremic syndrome associated with hemolytic anemia has been observed in children and adults. In this entity, the glomerular anatomic changes reported in the literature vary widely, but common to all are platelet aggregations and fibrin thrombi within the glomerular capillary lumina. In addition, swelling of endothelial and mesangial cells, as well as proliferation of these cells, is seen, affecting in some instances only segments of the individual glomerulus or, in other instances, the entire glomerulus. Subendothelial deposits of variable electron density (perhaps fibrin) have also been described (Gianantonia et al., 1964, 1968). Thus, the glomerular lesions sometimes resemble those encountered in focal glomerulonephritis or, in other cases, those of diffuse proliferative glomerulonephritis. In time, total glomerulosclerosis may eventuate.

The etiology of this disorder is unknown, but many consider it to be one component of disseminated intravascular coagulation in which the thrombotic process is not sufficiently widespread in the kidneys to cause ischemic necrosis but is, nonetheless, sufficiently severe to induce a microangiopathic hemolytic anemia (Franklin et al., 1972). The trigger initiating the vascular coagulation is still obscure. Immunologic and microbiologic mechanisms have been proposed, but not substantiated.

DISEASES OF THE TUBULES

Nephrosis is the morphologic term used for all types of renal disease which primarily attack the tubules, differentiating these disorders from those primary to the glomeruli, interstitial tissue or blood vessels. The anatomic term nephrosis is *not* synonymous with the clinical symptom complex known as the nephrotic syndrome. Paradoxically, diseases primary to the tubules virtually never produce the nephrotic syndrome.

ACUTE TUBULAR NECROSIS (ATN)

Acute tubular necrosis is the generic designation for all forms of acute renal failure resulting from widespread destruction of tubular epithelial cells. Two distinctive patterns were defined by Oliver in his classic studies (Oliver et al., 1951). The toxic form, also called *nephrotoxic nephrosis,* results from the ingestion or inhalation of some toxic agent which kills tubular cells, principally those in the proximal convoluted segments of the nephron. The other form of ATN is the *ischemic or tubulorrhectic pattern.* Here, both distal convoluted tubules and the loops of Henle are affected, giving rise to the older designation of "lower nephron nephrosis." Together *these two patterns of ATN are the major cause of acute renal failure.* Their clinical recognition is of particular importance because they represent reversible disorders, compatible with complete recovery of the renal lesions and the patient. The renal failure may, however, be quite severe. In patients having some underlying serious disorder contributing to the ATN, the mortality rate is on the order of 50 per cent (Balsløv and Jørgensen, 1963). As will be apparent from the following discussion, any age and both sexes may be affected.

Nephrotoxic ATN is caused by a wide variety of renal poisons including: heavy metals (mercury, lead, gold, arsenic, bismuth, chromium, uranium); organic solvents (carbon tetrachloride, chloroform, methyl alcohol); phenol; antibacterials (polymyxin, neomycin, sulfonamides, methicillin); mushroom poisoning; ethylene glycol; and pesticides. Recently, it has been observed that methoxyflurane (penthrane), commonly used as an anesthetic, may cause nephrotoxic acute renal failure (Hollenberg et al., 1972).

Characteristic of all these nephroses is acute necrosis, usually most prominent in the proximal convoluted tubules. The kidneys, when examined during the acute phase of the poisoning, are swollen and pale. Histologically, the tubular necrosis may be entirely nonspecific but is somewhat distinctive in poisonings with certain agents. With mercury (mercury nephrosis, p. 522), severely injured cells not yet dead may contain large acidophilic inclusions—"hyaline droplets"—representing reabsorption of protein (Fig. 24–26). Later, these cells become totally necrotic, are desquamated into the

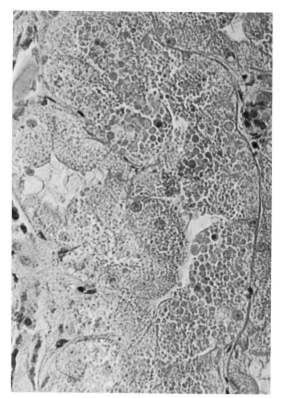

Figure 24–26. *Mercurial nephrosis. High power detail to demonstrate the "hyaline droplets" alteration in the tubular epithelial cells.*

lumen and may undergo striking calcification. Carbon tetrachloride poisoning, in contrast, is characterized by the accumulation of large amounts of neutral lipids in injured cells but, again, such fatty change is followed by necrosis. Ethylene glycol produces marked ballooning and hydropic or vacuolar degeneration of proximal convoluted tubules. Calcium oxalate crystals are often found in the tubular lumina in such poisonings. Whatever the etiology, if the patient survives, toward the end of the first week and extending into the second and third weeks, epithelial regeneration occurs, lining the tubular basement membranes with elongated, flattened cells containing mitotic figures. In the course of time, this regeneration repopulates the tubules so that, at some later date, no residual evidence of damage can be seen. Two features differentiate nephrotoxic ATN from the ischemic pattern: (1) the tubular basement membranes are preserved and (2) generally the distal tubular segments of the nephron are spared.

The ischemic tubulorrhectic pattern of ATN appears most often after an episode of shock. It has, therefore, been described earlier in the general consideration of the subject (p. 349), and remarks here can be confined to a brief summary. ATN is most common in those shock states produced by severe bacterial infections, large cutaneous burns, massive crushing injuries and any medical, surgical or obstetric event complicated by an episode of peripheral circulatory insufficiency. ATN is surprisingly uncommon when the shock is due to massive hemorrhage alone, e.g., following rupture of an aneurysm or laceration of a large artery. Mismatched blood transfusions or massive hemolysis from any cause may lead to this form of renal tubular lesion. Hence the ischemic pattern of ATN has also been called *"shock kidneys," "hemoglobinuric nephrosis"* and *"lower nephron nephrosis."*

Morphologically, there is patchy segmental necrosis of tubular cells, often accompanied by rupture of the tubular basement membrane — tubulorrhexis. These changes affect all levels of the nephron segmentally but are most prominent in the distal convoluted tubules. Tubular casts most often seen in the collecting tubules and loops of Henle accompany the cell death. These may be proteinaceous and made up of cell debris, but most characteristically take the form of pigment casts containing either hemoglobin or myoglobin. As indicated in the earlier discussion, toward the end of the first week, mitotic regenerative activity can be seen in vital cells adjacent to the areas of tubular necrosis and, over the course of the next week or two, the tubules are remarkably reconstituted.

Clinical Course. The nephrotoxic and ischemic forms of ATN are the important causes of acute and reversible renal failure. Evidence of renal insufficiency usually begins abruptly within the first 24 hours of the insult—toxic exposure or an ischemic episode. Characteristic are oliguria, proteinuria and a progressive rise in BUN and creatinine. Casts identical to those in the renal tubules may be seen in the urine. The total urine output may be reduced to a few milliliters per day and, at this time, water and salt overload and hyperkalemia become life-threatening problems requiring scrupulous clinical management. With appropriate attention to water balance and blood electrolytes, the patient can be tided over this oliguric crisis. Toward the end of the second week, a massive diuresis often follows, but the BUN and creatinine usually remain elevated. Classically, the specific gravity of the urine is at first very low but, nonetheless, large amounts of electrolytes are lost in the urinary flood. The low urinary specific gravity has been attributed to failure of the countercurrent mechanism. Some time in the third week, renal tubular function is restored, with improvement in the concentrating ability. At the same time, the BUN and creatinine levels begin to return to normal. For a consideration of the mechanisms leading to such acute anuric insufficiency, reference should be made to the earlier discussion (p. 352).

The prognosis of ATN depends, to a considerable extent, on the clinical setting surrounding its development. In general, it is much better in the nephrotoxic form of the disease when the poison has not caused serious damage to other organs such as the liver or heart. With tubulorrhectic ATN due to pure hemorrhagic shock, the mortality rate may be as low as 3 per cent. In shock related to overwhelming sepsis or extensive burns or caused by some other serious underlying disorder (such as an obstetric, surgical or medical emergency), the mortality rate rises to 80 per cent. In some large part, this extensive mortality is attributable to inability to control the underlying disease producing the shock state—for example, massive myocardial infarct and cardiogenic shock. Overall, in a study of 499 patients with this form of acute renal insufficiency, the mortality rate averaged approximately 50 per cent (Balsløv and Jørgensen, 1963). However, it is obvious that most of these deaths are not attributable to uremia.

VACUOLAR (OSMOTIC) NEPHROSIS

This nonspecific term is applied to a tubular injury characterized by the formation of small to large, clear vacuoles filled apparently with simple tissue fluids. These tubular lesions may be encountered in a wide variety of clinical situations. The most important cause is hypokalemia *(hypokalemic nephrosis)*. This electrolyte abnormality is encountered in any setting associated with marked alteration in fluid balance, particularly gastrointestinal and renal disorders producing severe vomiting, diarrhea or disturbances in fluid or electrolyte balance. Patients who have been administered hypertonic solutions, particularly mannitol, sucrose and rarely glucose, may also show these renal changes. The morphologic lesions are principally localized to the proximal convoluted tubules but sometimes affect the loops of Henle and the collecting tubules (Oliver et al., 1957). The vacuoles do not contain fat, glycogen, mucus or other foreign substances. These abnormal collections of fluid are presumed to be due to disturbances in the normal osmotic relationships within the cells, and thus the lesions are sometimes referred to as *osmotic nephrosis.*

The manner in which potassium deficiency causes injury to the renal tubular cells is still unclear. It is known that potassium is an essential activator of some of the enzymic reactions within tubular cells. Presumably, derangements in biochemical reactions might deplete energy reserves within the cell, and slowing of the sodium pump could lead to marked cellular hypertonicity, followed in time by the accumulation of water.

No gross alterations are evident. Microscopically, there are a great variety of tubular changes localized principally to the proximal convoluted tubules, but the loops of Henle and collecting tubules may also be affected. Granularity of the cytoplasm, coagulation necrosis, sloughing of the cells and even calcification of the tubular cells have been described, but the most prominent and distinctive feature is the appearance of small to large, clear vacuolar spaces having sharply defined margins that virtually fill the entire cell. Often the luminal border of the cell bulges into the tubular space, and the nucleus is displaced basally (Fig. 24–27).

The impact of these lesions on renal function is still not clear. In animals, potassium depletion leads to loss of renal concentrating power, and this has also been described in some patients. However, blood nitrogen levels have as a rule not been elevated, and there is good evidence that restoration of normal potassium stores is followed by a prompt recovery, in both structure and function, of the kidney (Relman and Schwartz, 1958).

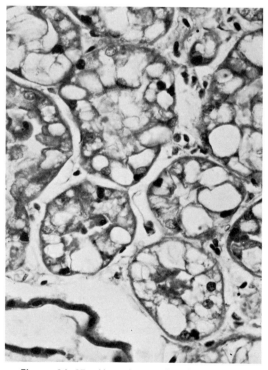

Figure 24–27. Vacuolar nephrosis. High power detail of the large clear intracytoplasmic vacuoles within the tubular cells.

GLYCOGEN (NEPHROSIS) ACCUMULATION

Glycogen vacuolation within the proximal convoluted tubules and the loops of Henle occurs, to all intents and purposes, in two clinical conditions: *diabetes mellitus* and the *glycogenoses*. These tubular changes have been described earlier, and it is only to be emphasized at this point that, in the diabetic, these tubular changes are reversible as far as is known and are rarely the cause of clinical dysfunction (p. 270).

CHOLEMIC NEPHROSIS

This type of tubular damage is encountered in many types of hepatic or biliary dysfunction, particularly those associated with obstructive jaundice. Rarely, cases have been described in the apparent absence of jaundice although, in these cases, minimal amounts of jaundice may have been present which were not clinically detected.

The exact manner in which these kidneys are injured is not clear. Bilirubin glucuronide is not toxic to cells. It may be that the elevated levels of unconjugated bile, such as are found in severe hepatocellular disease, are injurious to tissues. Alternatively, perhaps the bile salts in biliary obstruction are toxic to cells. There is, however, a growing suspicion that cholemic nephrosis may be caused by the excretion of abnormal amounts of amino acids in severe liver disease. Indeed, in the experimental animal, renal tubular damage can be caused by the urinary excretion of such amino acids as cystine, arginine, histidine and tryptophan.

Grossly, the kidneys may appear quite unremarkable. In more marked cases, the kidneys are slightly enlarged and may have a diffuse icteric cast to the cortex and medulla. Sometimes the bile staining is more evident in the renal pyramids. This pigmentation is sharply accentuated by previous formalin fixation which transforms the pigment to biliverdin and produces a distinct green hue to the affected areas.

Microscopically, deposits of granular or amorphous, yellow-green to brown bile may be found in the tubular epithelium of the proximal nephron as well as in the loop of Henle. Bile pigments may also be found in the epithelium of the collecting tubules, but more often these tubules only contain irregular, amorphous or granular, yellow-brown casts which are sometimes quite difficult to distinguish from hemoglobinuric precipitates. Degenerative changes and necrosis of the proximal tubular epithelial cells with associated interstitial, lymphocytic and plasma cell infiltration are present only in the most severe instances. Usually, however, the bile pigmentation of the tubular cells is not associated with cell necrosis. In certain instances, crystalline or spherical starch-like bodies are found in the tubular lumina, particularly in cases of severe hepatocellular damage with the excretion of large amounts of amino acids. The exact nature of these concrements is, however, still unknown.

The cholemic nephrosis encountered in the usual case of obstructive jaundice, in contrast to the hepatorenal syndrome, is not productive of significant renal dysfunction, although it occasionally leads to some elevation in the blood urea nitrogen.

MYELOMA KIDNEY (MYELOMA NEPHROSIS)

All plasma cell neoplasias, particularly those involving osseous lesions, produce a variety of abnormal serum and urinary proteins and proteoses (p. 248). Most of these abnormal proteins are globulins, which move with the gamma fraction; others are found in the beta and alpha fractions, and still others produce abnormal peaks, known as "M" or myeloma proteins. These are of particular interest since they are virtually limited to the myeloma diseases and are, therefore, of great diagnostic significance. In addition, there occur smaller abnormal proteins termed Bence Jones proteoses (p. 249). It has been shown that they have a small molecular size, in the range of 40,000, and are readily filtered through the glomerular capillary endothelium apparently without injuring the glomeruli, and thus appear promptly in the urine (Osserman, 1959). However, the passage of Bence Jones proteoses injures the tubular epithelial cells, which become swollen and develop hyaline droplets considered to be aggregates of the Bence Jones proteoses possibly complexed with cellular proteins. In some cases, crystals are formed within the epithelial cells. As the cells accumulate these products, they become progressively more swollen and eventually rupture. Large, characteristic casts are found in the myeloma kidney, presumably derived from both necrotic tubular epithelial cells and the abnormal proteins of the urine (Lichtenstein and Jaffe, 1947).

Grossly, the kidneys are usually normal but sometimes are shrunken and pale because of extensive interstitial scarring. The most prominent changes are histologic. The tubular casts appear as pink to blue amorphous masses, sometimes concentrically laminated, filling and distending the tubular lumina. Many of the casts are partially or com-

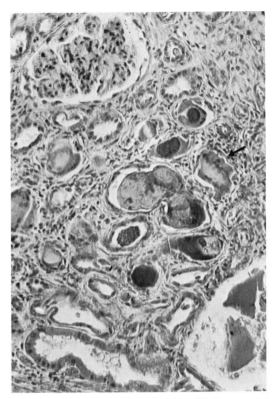

Figure 24–28. Myeloma kidney with large protein casts in the tubules and several multinucleate giant cells (arrow) visible in the microscopic field.

pletely surrounded by multinucleate giant cells derived from reactive tubular epithelium. The epithelium surrounding the cast is often necrotic, and the adjacent interstitial tissue usually shows a nonspecific inflammatory response (Fig. 24–28) (Oliver, 1944–45). Occasionally, the casts erode their way from the tubules into the interstitium and here evoke a granulomatous inflammatory reaction. At a later stage, such areas become fibrotic, producing the contracted kidney already mentioned. Sometimes metastatic calcification occurs in these kidneys due to the hypercalcemia commonly associated with disseminated multiple myeloma.

FANCONI SYNDROME

The *Fanconi syndrome* is an uncommon but interesting disorder of infants or adults, characterized by multiple defects in renal tubular function. The major manifestation is the excessive excretion in the urine of phosphate, amino acids and glucose due to failure of tubular reabsorption. As a consequence, severe skeletal disturbances ensue, such as rickets resistant to vitamin D in children and osteomalacia in adults, as well as acidosis, dehydration and other fluid derangements. These patients usually present with signs and symptoms of rickets or osteomalacia involving disturbances in gait and predisposition to multiple fractures. The disease is believed to be a metabolic defect of hereditary origin. However, in adults there is also an acquired form, presumably due to tubular lesions caused by exposure to such heavy metals as lead, cadmium and uranium. Microdissections have shown, in the hereditary disease, an anomaly of the neckpiece of the proximal convuluted tubule, i.e., a narrowed "swan's neck" (Clay et al., 1953). The cells are flattened and often deficient in phosphatase. It is not clear whether the tubular lesions are the primary inherited defects or merely acquired morphologic reflections of a systemic metabolic defect. In line with the latter possibility, it has been postulated that the continued excretion of cystine produces tubular injury leading to the changes described.

URATE DEPOSITS IN THE KIDNEY

Yellow-white streaks are occasionally observed in the tips of the kidney pyramids in newborn infants and rarely in leukemic or polycythemic adults. The lesions have erroneously been called uric acid infarcts. Since there is no evidence of tissue necrosis or infarction, there appears to be no justification for the perpetuation of the term infarct. The lesions consist of deposits of amorphous or crystalline urates in the collecting tubules of the kidneys (Fig. 24–29). With progressive deposition, the lining epithelial cells and the peritubular connective tissue may be affected. The urates are derived from the excessive breakdown of nucleoprotein, pre-

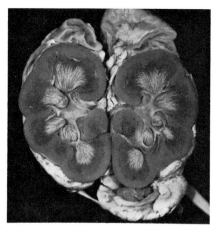

Figure 24–29. *Urate deposits in the kidney. The crystalline deposits in the tubules and peritubular connective tissue form linear white streaks in the renal pyramids.*

sumably from the destruction of red cells in infants, and from the destruction of white and red cells in affected adults.

There is no associated clinical evidence of renal damage. These lesions are anatomic changes which have importance only insofar as they must be differentiated grossly from deposits of calcium in the interstitial tissue of the pyramids of the kidneys.

DISEASES OF THE INTERSTITIUM

Interstitial disease is the generic designation for three important entities: acute pyelonephritis, chronic pyelonephritis and chronic interstitial nephritis. Although the disease, in all three entities, starts in the interstitium, it invariably spreads to the tubules where the most prominent changes appear. It may also extend to damage the glomeruli. Hence "diseases of the interstitium" are clearly not forever confined to the interstitium. On the other hand, it is important to recognize that some interstitial changes are seen in all renal diseases. It is evident from earlier discussions that interstitial fibrosis occurs in many forms of glomerular and vascular disease and, indeed, is a universal reaction to all forms of injury to the parenchymal elements of the kidney. However, these *secondary* interstitial changes are not the subject of our concern here.

A more confusing issue lies in the varying usages of the terms chronic interstitial nephritis and chronic pyelonephritis. At heart is the continuing debate over the etiology of chronic pyelonephritis. Traditionally, it was thought to represent continuing or recurrent bacterial infection of the kidneys. Clearly, acute pyelonephritis is a bacterial infection. Similarly, many cases of chronic pyelonephritis are bacterial in origin. However, in some instances, renal morphologic changes indistinguishable from those of chronic bacterial pyelonephritis are found in patients in whom there is no clinical, pathologic or bacteriologic evidence of infection. As we shall see, plausible abacterial etiologies may exist for such changes. Customarily, such definite abacterial disease has been termed chronic interstitial nephritis rather than chronic pyelonephritis. Whether this distinction is still tenable, in view of the many instances of this disease that may or may not be bacterial, is questionable. Certainly, the distinction has become blurred. *In my view, it is preferable to speak of this distinctive anatomic form of chronic renal disease as chronic pyelonephritis, and to recognize that this entity may have both bacterial and nonbacterial causations* (Kimmelstiel, 1964). Examples abound where one morphologic lesion may have many causes, e.g., the numerous causes of gastric erosions and the many pathways involved in the production of chronic glomerulonephritis.

ACUTE PYELONEPHRITIS (PN)

Acute PN is an acute suppurative bacterial infection of the kidney and renal pelvis, which is usually benign and controllable by appropriate treatment. As a form of clinically significant infection, it probably ranks second only to respiratory infections (Kleeman et al., 1960). The term urinary tract infection (UTI) implies involvement either of the kidneys and their collecting systems (pyelonephritis) or of only the bladder (cystitis). While cystitis may occur as the sole localization of UTI, it does not exist for long without retrograde spread of the infection to the kidneys. Conversely, acute pyelonephritis continually seeds the bladder with organisms to perpetuate the cystitis. Thus, infection in the urinary tract is rarely localized to either the bladder or the kidneys alone, and all UTI carries the potential of damage to the kidneys and, indeed, death from overwhelming sepsis or renal failure. Both cystitis and acute pyelonephritis are valid entities, but it is preferable, from the standpoint of their significance, to consider them as expressions of UTI.

The existence of a urinary tract infection is readily established by a few simple laboratory tests, urine culture and direct microscopy of the urine for the detection of bacteria. Kass (1956), employing gram-stained uncentrifuged urine, and Kunin (1961), using centrifuged unstained sediments, both documented that microscopic visualization of bacteria correlated well with colony counts of 10^5 or more organisms per ml. of urine. Bacteriuria of this magnitude generally, but not always, implies UTI. In other words, lower bacterial counts may be due only to bacterial contamination and postvoiding multiplication of organisms. However, it must be recognized that even counts below 10,000 organisms per ml. may be significant in the individual patient and, indeed, it has been estimated that between 5 and 10 per cent of patients with true UTI have counts between 10^4 and 10^5 organisms per ml. In any event, so-called "significant bacteriuria" is a sine qua non of acute pyelonephritis. While it is frequently accompanied by pyuria, the absence of pus cells in the urine does not exclude the diagnosis, nor is pyuria alone diagnostic of acute pyelonephritis.

Incidence and Pathogenesis. The genesis of acute pyelonephritis has an important bearing on its distribution among individuals,

so both incidence and causation can be discussed here. The organisms infecting the kidneys fall into three categories of importance. The dominant etiologic agent, accounting for at least 80 per cent of cases (when there is no urinary tract obstruction, previous antimicrobial treatment or urologic manipulation) is *E. coli.* Of second order importance are: Proteus, Psuedomonas, Klebsiella, Aerobacter, Enterococci and Staphylococci. Rare etiologies extend to virtually every other bacterial and fungal agent. In general, the agents of second and third order importance are more apt to be encountered in special circumstances: e.g., infections acquired in hospitals, following antimicrobial therapy or instrumentation of the urinary tract (Kessner and Lepper, 1967).

Granted that acute pyelonephritis is a bacterial infection, how do the organisms reach the kidney? *Three pathways are theoretically possible: hematogenous, lymphatic and urinary.* While hematogenous seeding of the kidney undoubtedly occurs under certain circumstances, the evidence is strongly against its being the major pathway of causation of this disease (Beeson, 1955). In the experimental animal, it has been shown that on the average only one in 10,000 microorganisms inoculated into the blood stream will lodge in the kidneys (Guze and Beeson, 1956). The coliform bacilli, the most common pathogens in man, are unable to establish infection in normal animal kidneys when introduced hematogenously. The few bacteria that lodge in the kidneys rapidly disappear without causing injury. However, *if urinary tract obstruction is produced, as by ligation of a ureter, blood-borne organisms will localize in the obstructed kidney to produce a unilateral acute pyelonephritis* without affecting the unobstructed kidney (Mallory et al., 1940). In man, then, urinary tract obstruction, e.g., by a stone in the ureter or by prostatic enlargement, may lead to hematogenous seeding of the kidney(s). Virtually no evidence exists for the lymphatic route.

An abundance of clinical and experimental evidence indicates that *the most common pathway of infection of the kidneys is passage of bacteria up the urinary stream from the bladder cavity* (Vivaldi et al., 1959) (Andersen and Jackson, 1961). Retrograde ascending infection of the kidney begins with bacterial contamination of the bladder urine or bacterial infection of the bladder. Bladder urine is normally sterile. In man, bacteria are normally present in the lower urethra, but their numbers progressively dwindle toward the bladder. *Indeed, in both the experimental animal and man, it is exceedingly difficult to colonize bladder urine or induce an infection in the normal bladder,* for many reasons. First, bacteria are continually flushed out by voiding. In addition, the urethral and bladder mucosa have been shown to have a number of antibacterial protective mechanisms, although their precise nature is somewhat uncertain. Phagocytosis and killing of bacteria by neutrophils may be one of the bladder antibacterial mechanisms (Cobbs and Kay, 1967). Clumping of bacteria in the secretions of the bladder and urethral mucosa would favor their being washed out. Recently, much attention has been directed to the local synthesis of antibody by immunologically competent cells in the mucosal surfaces (Hand et al., 1971). Immunofluorescent studies have identified IgG and IgA in the bladder mucosa (Feldman, 1971). While the IgG does not appear to be particularly effective in killing bacteria, the IgA may be more potent. Other more mysterious antibacterial secretions have been proposed. Whatever their nature, it is clear that the normal bladder urine is usually sterile. In this context, it must be remembered that urine is an excellent medium for bacteria. Were it not for these antibacterial defense mechanisms, organisms might proliferate in urine as freely as they do in culture media. Surprisingly, urine from women, particularly from pregnant women, seems to support bacterial growth better than that from men (Asscher et al., 1966).

The factors which play a role in bacterial infection of the urinary tract can be listed as:

1. Instrumentation of the urinary tract.
2. Obstruction.
3. Vesicoureteral reflux.
4. Age and sex of the patient.
5. Pregnancy.
6. Vulnerability of the renal medulla to infection.
7. ? Diabetes mellitus.

Catheterization of the bladder or any type of urethral instrumentation, even under the best circumstances, almost inevitably carries organisms into the bladder. Indwelling catheters are especially dangerous. Unquestionably, in all of these circumstances, trauma as well as the introduction of organisms are operative. Patients at particular risk are those with neurologic diseases, who have difficulty in bladder control. The necessity for constant bladder drainage imposes a high risk of acute pyelonephritis.

Urinary tract obstruction makes a major contribution to the pathogenesis of pyelonephritis. Strictures, congenital valves, stones, tumors, prostatic enlargement, prolapse of the uterus and neurogenic disorders all predispose to renal infection. It should be noted that obstruction above the level of the bladder is prob-

ably less important than urethral obstruction, since it is the urinary tract stasis within the bladder which is of chief pathogenic significance. The mechanisms by which interference with urine flow increases the susceptibility of the kidney to infection are still poorly understood. Stasis and incomplete emptying of the bladder would obviously favor bacterial multiplication. In addition, distention of the bladder compresses its blood supply, and the slowed vascular flow probably impedes the delivery of leukocytes as well as other possible antibacterial factors. The flushing action of normal voiding is also lost with urethral obstruction or narrowing. All of these influences favor bacterial colonization of the bladder urine, and the stage is set for retrograde extension to the kidneys.

Vesicoureteral reflux has been widely emphasized as facilitating the passage of bacteria from the bladder to the kidneys. It has been clearly documented that, when the vesicoureteral sphincteric mechansim is grossly incompetent, bladder contraction yields a retrograde urinary gush which flows directly into the collecting system of the kidneys (Rosenheim, 1963). Milder forms of incompetence are also thought to play an important role in the upward spread of bacterial contamination. It is difficult to be certain how many cases of acute pyelonephritis involve vesicoureteral reflux. It is said to be present in 30 to 40 per cent of children having acute pyelonephritis. Hodson (1969) contends that it is present in every case of bacterial chronic pyelonephritis in children. Recently, it has been noted that vesicoureteric reflux may have a familial distribution, suggesting that, at least in some instances, it represents a genetic trait. However, it should be emphasized that one does not need to postulate abnormal reflux to provide a pathway of ascending spread of bacterial contamination. Many studies have documented that, with each normal ureteral contraction propelling the urine toward the bladder, there is backward turbulence and, indeed, dye introduced into the bladder will, in this manner, reach the renal collecting system.

Age and sex contribute significantly to the predisposition to this disease. Most of the epidemiologic data are based on studies of the prevalence of bacteriuria (Kunin, 1970). The frequency of bacteriuria increases with age in both sexes but, at all ages, females far outnumber males (Mond et al., 1970). In a large-scale survey of bacteriuria among healthy schoolchildren between the ages of five and nine, the overall prevalence was 0.03 per cent in boys and 1.2 per cent in girls; in girls 12 to 16 years of age, the prevalence rose to 3 per cent (Kunin, 1969). In the overall adult female population, the prevalence ranges between 3 and 6 per cent. In males, the comparable rate is approximately 0.5 per cent. However, males over the age of 70 have a 3.5 per cent rate, undoubtedly related to prostatism and instrumentation of the urinary tract. Except, then, for the advanced years of life, UTI is rare among males. These sex differences have been attributed to the shorter female urethra with greater likelihood of contamination of the bladder. Intercourse, with its attendant urethral trauma in the female, may favor the extension of organisms from the lower urethra into the bladder, accounting for the well recognized entity "honeymoon cystitis." However, there is also evidence that prostatic fluid may have some antibacterial properties and, as mentioned earlier, for unknown reasons the urine in women constitutes a better medium for bacterial growth than that in men.

In *pregnancy*, the prevalence of UTI increases, and bacteriuria has been detected in up to 13 per cent of pregnant women, the rate increasing with age, parity and lower socioeconomic status (Norden and Kass, 1968). This prevalence has been attributed to urinary stasis resulting from the pressure of the enlarging uterus on the ureters and the normal physiologic dilation of the ureters as well.

The *vulnerability of the renal medulla* to bacterial infection has received intensive study. Less than 10 coliform bacilli injected into the medulla are necessary to instigate an infection, whereas approximately 100,000 are required to infect the cortex. A number of factors may be involved in this phenomenon, including poorer vascular supply and consequent delay in inflammatory response, production of ammonia in the renal medulla which has been shown to inactivate the fourth component of complement (Beeson and Rowley, 1959), conversion of bacteria to cell-wall deficient forms (protoplasts, L-forms) which can survive in the hyperosmolality and are antibiotic resistant (Alderman and Freedman, 1963), and interference with leukocyte function because of the high osmolality (Lancaster and Allison, 1966). Thus, once bacteria reach the renal collecting system, they find a favorable environment for their growth in the medulla and may then extend to infect the cortex.

Before concluding the discussion of the genesis of acute PN, two common controversial issues should be brought up, i.e., the importance of diabetes mellitus as a predisposing influence, and the impact of UTI on neonatal mortality. Many studies have shown a significantly higher prevalence of bacteriuria among adult female diabetics than among nondiabetic controls, comparable rates being, 18.8 per cent and 7.9 per cent respectively (Vejlsgaard, 1965). On the other hand, no increase in the prevalence of asymptomatic bacteriuria could be identified among diabetic schoolgirls as compared with nondiabetic controls (Pometta et al., 1967). It thus appears that diabetics acquire higher rates later in life probably because of more frequent instrumentation and their generalized vulnerability to infection. Bacteriuria in the diabetic pregnant woman is a serious hazard since the rate of perinatal infant mortality is 50 per cent as compared to only 15 per cent among similar nonbacteriuric diabetic women (Pometta et al., 1967). The issue of urinary infections and perinatal mortality in general is still unsettled, but Norden and Kass (1968) have suggested that bacteriuric women have an increased frequency of premature birth and a higher rate of perinatal mortality. The reasons for these findings are complex and probably involve many of the socioeconomic factors known to contribute to the prevalence of bacteriuria during pregnancy.

Morphology. Suppuration necrosis is the characteristic hallmark of acute pyelonephritis. The suppuration may occur as discrete focal abscesses involving one or both kidneys, or as large areas of coalescent suppuration which destroy large segments or even the entire kidney (Fig. 24–30). The distribution of these lesions is totally unpredic-

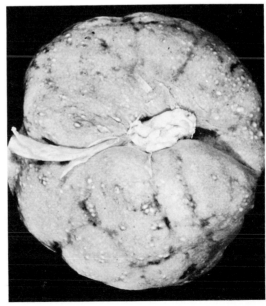

Figure 24–30. Acute pyelonephritis. The cortical surface is dotted with small abscesses.

table and haphazard. Sometimes the infection manifests itself as a very few widely scattered abscesses; in other instances, one or both kidneys are dotted with these lesions, or perhaps the infection is limited to one pole of the kidney, while in other patients massive areas of one or both kidneys are affected.

Externally, the lesions consist of small, yellow to white, softened, raised abscesses on the cortical surface, usually rimmed by narrow zones of hyperemia or large, confluent yellow to red areas of suppuration necrosis. The capsule strips readily from these surfaces and may, at times, rupture the abscesses or tear the softened areas of suppuration. On section, the necrotic foci are usually distributed throughout the kidney and, although the medulla is usually involved, paradoxically the suppuration is often most evident in the cortex. Presumably, once the bacteria have proliferated in the medulla, they then invade the cortex and here stimulate a more pronounced inflammatory response. The greater blood supply of the cortex allows more inflammatory cells to reach the area, and the lower levels of interstitial pressure enable easier movement from the vessels to the inflammatory area. Depending on the severity of the involvement, the kidney may or may not be enlarged. In the typical cases, pelvic changes are not marked. However, hyperemia, granularity of the pelvic mucosa or even suppuration is occasionally present. If the renal infection is severe and confluent, producing massive abscess formation which virtually wipes out the entire kidney, it is referred to as a **carbuncle of the kidney.** Extension through the capsule into the perirenal tissues may produce a **perinephric abscess.**

The pathognomonic histologic feature of acute pyelonephritis is suppurative necrosis or abscess formation within the renal substance. In the very early stages, the suppurative infiltrate is limited to the interstitial tissue. However, by the time most kidneys are examined, the reaction has ruptured into tubules and produced a characteristic abscess with destruction of the engulfed tubules (Fig. 24–31). Since the tubular lumina present a ready pathway for the extension of the infection, large masses of polys frequently extend along the involved nephron into the collecting tubules. Characteristically, the glomeruli appear to be rather resistant to the infection, and often abscess formations surround glomeruli without actually invading them. Large areas of severe necrosis, however, eventually destroy the glomeruli. Necrosis of exudate within the tubular lumina gives rise to granular or white cell casts. In the more severe cases, bacteria may be seen within the focal areas of suppuration.

Two variants are encountered in special circumstances. One is known as **necrotizing papillitis or renal papillary necrosis.** This special form of acute pyelonephritis is seen in diabetes and in those with urinary tract obstruction, for example, elderly males with prostatism. Necrotizing papillitis is

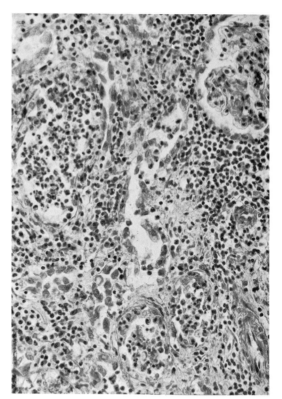

Figure 24–31. Acute pyelonephritis marked by an acute neutrophilic exudate within the tubules and renal substance.

usually bilateral, but may be unilateral. One or all of the pyramids of the affected kidney may be involved. These papillary necroses may or may not be associated with the usual types of cortical or medullary abscesses. The pathognomonic gross feature of this condition is evident only on cut section. The tips or distal two-thirds of the pyramids have gray-white to yellow necrosis which resembles infarction. The junction of the necrotic papillae with the preserved proximal portion of the pyramid is usually sharply defined and outlined by a narrow zone of hyperemia (Fig. 24–32).

Microscopically, the ischemic character of the process is readily evident. The necrotic tissue shows characteristic coagulative infarct necrosis, with preservation of outlines of tubules. There is no inflammatory infiltrate within the necrotic tips, and the leukocytic response is limited to the junctions between preserved and destroyed tissue (Fig. 24–33). Large masses of proliferating bacteria are sometimes found within the acellular necrotic foci and, strikingly, there is often little or no white cell response about these bacterial growths, confirming the absence of blood supply in these regions. In the better defined cases, acute vasculitis and thrombosis of the vascular supply may be evident in the peripheral zone of inflammation, but such changes are often difficult to visualize.

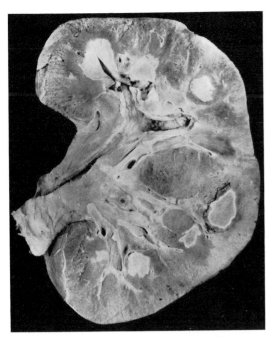

Figure 24–32. *Necrotizing papillitis. The areas of pale gray necrosis are limited to the papillae.*

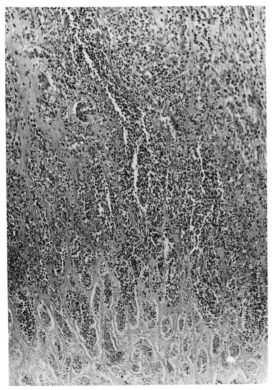

Figure 24–33. *Necrotizing papillitis. The inflammatory junction of the necrotic papilla (below) with the preserved renal parenchyma (above).*

The second special variant of acute pyelonephritis is seen when there is total or almost complete urinary tract obstruction, particularly when it is high in the urinary tract. The suppurative exudate is unable to drain and thus fills the renal pelvis, calyces and ureter, producing **pyonephrosis**. The kidney may be converted virtually to a sac of pus, as the renal damage characteristic of hydronephrosis (p. 1136) is added to that caused by the bacterial infection.

Clinical Course. Although acute pyelonephritis is often a benign, self-limiting disease, the possibility that it may develop into serious chronic pyelonephritis demands that each case be treated with vigorous antibiotic therapy and removal of predisposing influences, if any. When acute pyelonephritis is clinically apparent, the onset is usually sudden, with pain at the costovertebral angle and systemic evidence of infection, such as fever and malaise. Urinary findings include pyuria and bacteriuria. In addition, there are usually indications of bladder and urethral irritation, i.e., dysuria, frequency and urgency. Renal functional abnormalities are typically absent, save in those cases with widespread involvement. The symptomatic phase of the disease usually lasts no longer than a week, although bacteriuria may persist much longer and should be treated.

If necrotizing papillitis develops, the prognosis is markedly worsened. Patients having this specialized form of pyelonephritis usually present one of two clinical syndromes: signs and symptoms of an overwhelming septic infection or the sudden onset of acute urinary insufficiency. Death may, therefore, eventuate from generalized sepsis or from uremia. This form of nephropathy is usually, but not invariably, fatal. In patients with unilateral papillitis, surgical removal of the kidney or prompt antibacterial therapy may abort the disease and produce a cure. Quite rarely at postmortem examination, kidneys are observed in which autoamputation of the pyramids has occurred. These cases suggest that the necrotic papillae have sloughed, and thus relieved the urinary blockage imposed by these selective sites of tubular destruction.

The genesis of necrotizing papillitis is still obscure (Robbins et al., 1946). This pattern of necrosis may be an expression of the vulnerability of the medulla to infection and of the peculiar pattern of blood supply to the pyramids. It is to be remembered that the papillary blood supply comprises vasa recta which descend from the corticomedullary junction and then return to drain into efferent veins. Chance localization of organisms in the bases of pyramids and rapid spread of the infection in the diabetic could embarrass the blood supply to the tip of the pyramid. Remember also that leukocytic function is depressed in the medulla, further favoring rapid spread of infection (Bryant et al., 1972). In the nondiabetic patient with urinary tract obstruction, it is assumed that increased urinary pressure may produce sufficient compression and ischemia of the pyramids to predispose to the same sequence of events. It should, however, be noted that papillary necrosis is also seen with analgesic abuse (p. 1125) in the absence of bacterial infection.

CHRONIC PYELONEPHRITIS (CHRONIC PN)

The two most important forms of fatal renal disease are chronic glomerulonephritis and chronic pyelonephritis. Both cause progressive scarring and contraction of the kidneys but, whereas chronic glomerulonephritis is invariably bilateral and symmetrical, chronic pyelonephritis generally produces asymmetrical irregular destruction of the renal parenchyma. It will be remembered from an earlier discussion that, as employed here, the term chronic pyelonephritis embraces both bacterial and nonbacterial etiologies. Furthermore, *there are two well-recognized clinical patterns of this disease: chronic obstructive PN and chronic nonobstructive PN. There is complete agreement that, in the presence of obstruction, bacterial infection is the usual cause of the chronic renal damage.* Here, persistence of an acute infection or recurrence of acute infections as a result of urinary tract obstruction provides readily accepted pathogenic mechanisms for the renal damage. The nonobstructive form of the disease is less well understood. *In a significant number of cases of chronic nonobstructive PN, there is no clear history of an antecedent UTI, nor can organisms be cultured in the urine over the span of years and repeated examinations.* Moreover, organisms cannot be isolated at postmortem culture of the kidneys (Angell et al., 1968). Some investigators prefer to call such cases chronic interstitial nephritis but, as pointed out earlier, the morphologic changes are indistinguishable from those encountered in documented chronic bacterial infections. It will become clear in the following discussion that many, perhaps all, cases of chronic nonobstructive PN are indirectly related to renal infection possibly in the remote past. Unless otherwise specified, the use of the term chronic PN will include both the obstructive and the nonobstructive forms of the disease.

Incidence. Chronic PN, particularly the nonobstructive form, has been grossly over-diagnosed in the past, both clinically and morphologically (Freedman, 1967). Chronic PN was said to be present in 3 to 7 per cent of all autopsies. It soon became apparent that there was a tendency to interpret all focal renal scars as chronic PN unless there was clear evidence of some other cause. Thus, old infarcts and focal obstructive atrophy were sometimes mistaken for chronic PN. At that time, it was not appreciated that *pelvic and calyceal deformities resulting from papillary and medullary scarring were requisite morphologic features of chronic PN*, and so the diagnosis was made merely on the basis of chronic cortical scarring (Hodson, 1959) (Heptinstall, 1967). With more strict anatomic criteria, the incidence of chronic PN at autopsy falls to about 2 per cent or less, and approximately 85 per cent of such cases are chronic obstructive PN (Heptinstall and Farmer, 1970). Unlike acute PN in which there is a large female preponderance, chronic PN occurs equally frequently in both sexes and at all ages and, as would be expected, is much more common in the advanced years of life because of the major role of urinary tract obstruction in its genesis.

Etiology and Pathogenesis. Nothing further needs to be said about chronic obstructive PN except to reiterate that it is clearly a bacterial infection whose chronicity or recurrence is often related to urinary tract obstruction as was discussed on p. 1118. It is generally, but not universally, believed that chronic nonobstructive PN results from bacterial infection perhaps in the remote past. In many instances, there is clinical evidence of some bacterial infection of the urinary tract in the past, but not sufficient to explain the severe loss of renal tissue (Kleeman et al., 1960). Vesicoureteral reflux is present in almost all such cases. Reasons exist for suspecting that some renal infection, perhaps even subclinical, might initiate mechanisms which could perpetuate a chronic inflammatory state and, in time, produce extensive renal damage. Fluorescent antibody techniques have demonstrated bacterial antigens in the scarred areas of the kidney in models of this disease induced in rats (Cotran, 1963). However, it must be admitted that, in this experimental model, the disease was not progressive as it often is in man. Recently, there was a report of the demonstration of bacterial antigens in the pyelonephritis scars of man (Aoki et al., 1969). However, this report has not been confirmed and the findings have, indeed, been challenged (Cotran, 1972). An additional hint of a bacterial mechanism is the finding of macrophages containing PAS-positive granules thought to represent bacterial debris in experimental models of chronic PN (Cotran, 1969). Similar cells are encountered, albeit infrequently, in the disease of man. One peculiar form of disease, known as xanthogranulomatous pyelonephritis caused by Proteus organisms, is characterized by masses of these distinctive cells (Hooper et al., 1962). The evidence, then, for persistent bacterial antigens as a mechanism for the progressive disease in man is still fragmentary.

Could there be other etiologies for chronic PN besides persistent bacterial antigens? Mention has already been made of the ability of protoplasts (L-forms) to survive in the hyperosmolar environment of the renal medulla. Such forms cannot be identified by the usual cultural methods and so urine and/or kidneys would be interpreted as sterile. The additional possibility must be raised that there are entirely abacterial causes for the scars characteristic of chronic nonobstructive pyelonephritis. Reverting to the almost invariable association of vesicoureteral reflux with chronic PN, Hodson (1969) raises the question of whether prolonged severe reflux may itself eventually induce medullary atrophy followed, in time, by damage to the cortex, leading to changes indistinguishable from those of bacterial causation. Furthermore, as will be seen, analgesic abuse produces renal damage indistinguishable from documented chronic bacterial PN (p. 1125). If infections indeed lie behind all forms of chronic PN, it is surprising to note that males and females are affected equally, since urinary tract infections are much more common in females.

Morphology. At the outset, it should be emphasized that cortical scars indistinguishable from chronic pyelonephritis may be caused by primary vascular disease or by localized obstruction in the absence of infection. **The diagnosis of chronic pyelonephritis thus requires not only cortical scarring but also evidence of involvement of the collecting system in the form of calyceal scarring, pyramidal blunting or, in other words, deformity of the normal pelvic-calyceal system.** Weiss and Parker (1939), in their classic description of these kidneys, provided the following major anatomic characteristics: (1) The kidneys are usually grossly scarred and contracted; (2) in the scarred areas, the tubules are atrophic and contain colloid casts; (3) the areas of involvement contain an interstitial infiltrate of lymphocytes, plasma cells and occasional polys; (4) glomerular changes are largely confined to concentric fibrosis about the parietal layer of Bowman's capsule, termed periglomerular fibrosis; and (5) vascular changes similar to those of either benign or malignant arteriolosclerosis are often present. The cortical scarring may be either diffuse or patchy. When diffuse, an irregular or sometimes a fairly uniform contraction results (Fig. 24–34). This may be quite extreme and may reduce kidney weights to less than 50 gm. each (renal weights that are rarely encountered in any other form of chronic renal disease). Patchy or asymmetrical contraction is more

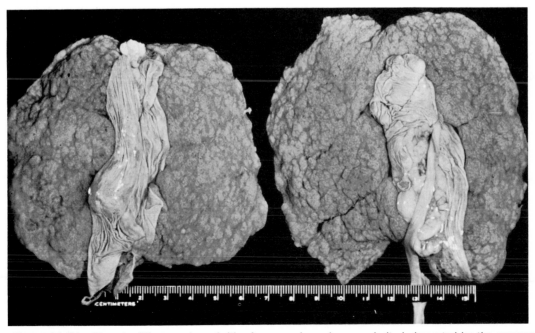

Figure 24–34. Chronic diffuse pyelonephritis. A coarse, irregular granularity is imparted by the numerous focal areas of scarring.

usual, and so one kidney may be virtually normal and the other, severely involved. The characteristic scar of focal chronic pyelonephritis is flat, broad-based, U-shaped and has a red-brown granular base (Fig. 24–35).

The microscopic changes can be further characterized as disproportionate damage to tubules as compared with glomeruli. Indeed, the glomeruli may be remarkably preserved, but those trapped in scars often show shrinkage of the capillary tuft and not only periglomerular fibrosis but also the deposition of collagen within Bowman's space. The collagen may literally fill this space and, at times, fuse with the atrophic glomerular vascular tuft to produce totally hyalinized spheres. The most prominent change, however, is found in the tubular regions of both the cortex and the medulla. There is a marked increase in the fibrous interstitium, with concomitant atrophy of the tubules. Tubules may be lost completely or, in other places may be filled with neutrophils or amorphous colloid casts (Fig. 24–36). Indeed, collections of tubules with colloid casts create a classic pattern referred to as **thyroidization** (Fig. 24–37). The medulla shows similar interstitial fibrosis, atrophy of tubules and, indeed, in some cases, the papillae may have undergone total fibrosis and blunting. In some cases, there is thickening of the epithelial lining of the calyces, while in others, it is destroyed as a consequence of the protracted chronic inflammation. The calyceal changes also include a marked chronic inflammatory infiltrate. Lymphoid follicles may appear in this inflammatory infiltrate in the calyceal wall.

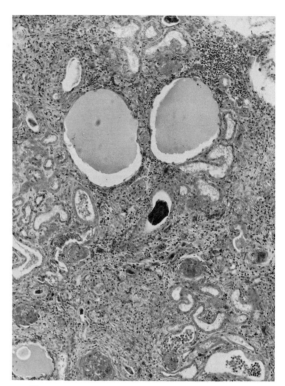

Figure 24–36. A focus of chronic active pyelonephritis with interstitial scarring, tubular atrophy, mononuclear infiltration (lymphocytes and plasma cells), colloid casts and a neutrophilic exudate in tubules in lower right. Several trapped glomeruli are destroyed.

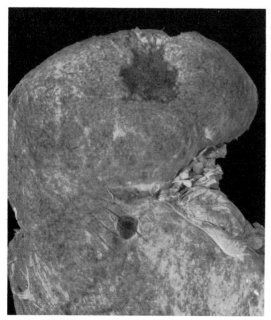

Figure 24–35. Focal chronic pyelonephritis. A small scar with a dark inflammatory base.

Clinical Course. Chronic bacterial obstructive pyelonephritis may be insidious in onset or may present many of the clinical manifestations of acute pyelonephritis, i.e., back pain, fever, frequency and pyuria. Chronic nonobstructive pyelonephritis is almost always insidious. With this form of disease, only a minority of patients show a definite history of symptomatic urinary tract infection. The remainder come to medical attention relatively late in the course of their disease, because of the gradual onset of renal insufficiency and hypertension, or because of the discovery of pyuria or proteinuria on routine examination. Since glomerular damage occurs relatively late in the course of chronic PN, renal functional impairment is first referable to the tubules. Loss of tubular function, in particular of concentrating ability, gives rise to polyuria and nocturia. Mild proteinuria is typical, but proteinuria sufficient to cause the nephrotic syndrome is rare. *Pyelography is virtually requisite for the clinical diagnosis. Pyelograms will show the affected kidney or kidneys to be smaller than normal, often asymmetrically contracted, with blunting and deformity of the calyceal system.* The

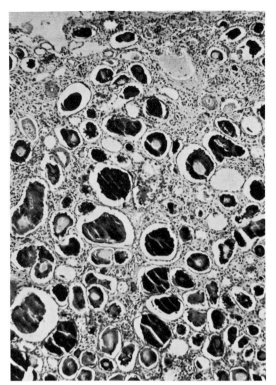

Figure 24–37. *A large area of scarring to illustrate a "thyroid-like" area.*

diagnosis of chronic pyelonephritis is strongly supported if examination of the urine sediment discloses leukocyte casts and numbers of leukocytes. In contrast to glomerulonephritis, chronic PN is not usually associated with red cell or hemoglobin casts. Significant bacteriuria, when found in cases with pyelographic abnormalities and urinary tract obstruction, is virtually diagnostic; but its absence does not rule out chronic PN. In the case of unilateral chronic pyelonephritis, nephrectomy may be the treatment of choice, primarily to protect against the development of renal hypertension, as will be explained later. If the disease is bilateral and progressive, glomerular damage eventually occurs, with consequent azotemia as well as acidosis leading, in time, to death in uremia.

Before closing the discussion of chronic PN, its relationship to hypertension should be brought up. Between 50 to 75 per cent of patients with this form of renal disease are hypertensive. The question is which comes first. Unravelling this issue is made difficult by the fact that hypertension causes severe renal vascular disease which, in turn, induces renal atrophy and scarring. Could such scarring predispose to secondary bacterial infection? Contrariwise, the progressive scarring of chronic PN is a perfectly reasonable basis for secondary renal hypertension. On balance, the weight of evidence favors the view that chronic pyelonephritis with its marked fibrosis, atrophy of renal substance and vascular narrowing are plausible causes for renal ischemia, which might then activate the renin-angiotensin system (Weiss and Parker, 1939). While it is difficult to sort out which comes first in adults, the frequent appearance of hypertension in children with chronic PN lends considerable support to the view that the renal disease is primary. Moreover, with unilateral chronic PN, hypertension is sometimes cured by nephrectomy.

CHRONIC INTERSTITIAL NEPHRITIS

The designation interstitial nephritis, as used here, is reserved for an anatomic picture often indistinguishable from chronic PN, but which is definitely *not* caused by direct suppurative bacterial infections of the kidneys. Thus, the distinction between chronic PN and chronic interstitial nephritis is an etiologic one. Morphologic changes of this nature are encountered in certain systemic nonsuppurative microbic infections, i.e., those producing powerful exotoxins and those characterized by dissemination of spirilla throughout the body. Thus, renal interstitial infiltrates of lymphocytes, plasma cells and neutrophils are sometimes encountered in patients having beta hemolytic streptococcal infections, diphtheria or clostridial infections somewhere in the body (Fig. 24–38). Syphilis and Weil's disease, with their widely disseminated microorganisms, may produce similar renal changes, in this instance, accompanied by seeding of the renal interstitium with spirochetes. Acute to chronic interstitial nephritis is sometimes encountered as a manifestation of a hypersensitivity reaction to drugs—penicillin, sulfonamide, diphenylhydantoin, as well as others. In these instances, the inflammatory infiltrate may contain an admixture of eosinophils. In addition to these fairly well defined etiologies, there are two important forms of chronic interstitial nephritis of more mysterious origin—the nephropathy of analgesic abuse and Balkan nephritis.

The *nephropathy of analgesic abuse* is the term used for a form of chronic interstitial nephritis and renal papillary necrosis related to the intensive intake of analgesics. The entity was first called to attention in 1953 by Spuhler and Zollinger. In these early reports, most of the patients, over long periods of time, had taken large quantities of analgesic mixtures

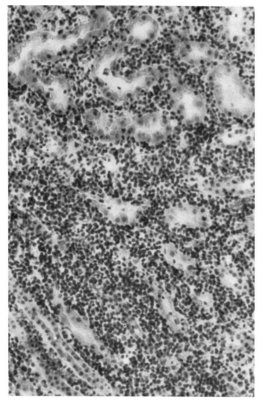

Figure 24–38. Interstitial nephritis with an intense mononuclear leukocytic infiltrate between the tubules.

(containing aspirin, phenacetin, caffeine and sometimes codeine). Subsequent studies have confirmed an unmistakable association between the analgesic abuse and the renal disease which has all the earmarks of the usual chronic bacterial pyelonephritis accompanied by papillary necrosis (Gault et al., 1968).

In Europe where the first cases were identified, proprietary preparations containing mixtures of analgesics were extremely popular as cures for headaches, depression and, indeed, all manner of ailment. Without definite proof, phenacetin was singled out as the toxic agent in the mixtures (Burry et al., 1966). This implication was drawn largely because it appeared to be the common denominator in the wide variety of proprietary preparations associated with this renal disease. However, the administration of phenacetin to experimental animals failed to induce the disease. Accordingly, intensive investigations were undertaken in the hope of finding a metabolite in man that might be incriminated. Phenacetin is rapidly and almost completely metabolized by the microsomal enzymes in the liver. It is largely broken

down to paracetamol, but other metabolites have been identified as well (Prescott, 1970). Without going into all of the details, it will suffice to state that *there is no substantial evidence that phenacetin or any of its metabolites has high nephrotoxicity,* although relatively massive doses will induce renal damage in rats.

Recently, Kincaid-Smith and her collaborators (1970) suggest that it is aspirin which is the cause of nephropathy (Nanra et al., 1970). This group points out that, for years, salicylates have been known to be capable of causing renal damage. Renal papillary necrosis has been produced in animals with aspirin alone, and cases of analgesic nephropathy have been reported in man following excessive intake of aspirin alone. In their studies in rats, they found that aspirin would induce papillary necrosis at a dosage level six times lower than that of phenacetin. The controversy over which particular drug is implicated continues.

The renal damage in analgesic abuse may be as severe as that encountered in advanced cases of chronic bacterial obstructive PN and need not be further detailed here. It is, however, important to point out that *bilateral papillary renal necrosis is almost invariably present in analgesic nephropathy.* It is heartening to report that in a follow-up of 52 patients with this disease, after complete abstinence from drugs, renal function improved in 25, deteriorated in 8 and remained unchanged in 19 (Kincaid-Smith et al., 1970).

Closely related to the nephropathy of analgesic abuse is so-called *Balkan nephropathy.* It too manifests itself as a chronic interstitial nephritis accompanied by papillary necrosis. It is a most mysterious entity occurring in a limited zone, about 40 km. wide and 200 km. long, which includes adjacent regions of Rumania, Bulgaria and Yugoslavia. Affected families live in the valleys and are mostly agricultural workers. The nature of this disease has been vigorously pursued but remains mysterious. Toxic fungi, water pollutants, industrial wastes, metal residues, microbiologic agents, dietary influences and genetic predisposition have all been, at one time or another, suspected but not established. Further details on this mystery disease are available in a recent publication (Wolstenholme and Knight, 1967).

RENAL TUBERCULOSIS

Tuberculosis of the kidneys arises almost always from a blood-borne spread of pulmonary tuberculosis. Occasionally, the primary infection may be in the intestines, tonsils or even the skin. The renal involvement takes one of several forms: (1) isolated, small tubercles which occur as one part of systemic hematogenous spread *(miliary tuberculosis)*; (2) large, caseating, necrotic areas *(nodular tuberculosis)*; or (3) cavitation of the tuberculous necrosis with sloughing of the pyramids *(cavitating renal tuberculosis)*. All patterns are believed to be hematogenous in origin. Occasionally, the primary focus of infection may heal or disappear, and thus the renal disorder remains as the dominant site of tuberculous involvement in the body, in which form it is referred to as an *isolated organ-renal tuberculosis*. It is thus the renal counterpart of isolated tuberculosis of bone and isolated tuberculous salpingitis.

Miliary tuberculosis of the kidneys requires no detailed description, resembling miliary tuberculosis in any organ. The tubercles tend to be somewhat more concentrated in the cortex, principally in the interstitium. In the nodular form, the tubercles coalesce to produce large conglomerate areas of caseous necrosis. Sometimes these masses achieve sufficient size to be dignified by the term **tuberculoma** (Fig. 24–39). In the progression of the nodular pattern, the involvement may extend into the pyramids and be followed by sloughing of the tips of the pyramids. Thus, the papillae are excavated and converted into cup-shaped cavitations lined by shaggy, yellow-white, caseous debris. The caseation necrosis may progressively extend to-ward the cortex to virtually wipe out the pyramids. At the same time, the infection spreads into the calyces and pelves which become filled with caseous debris and lined by granular inflammatory surfaces. Such renal tuberculous involvement may be unilateral or bilateral, and may be limited to one or several pyramids in a kidney or may involve all of them. More commonly, it begins in one pole of one side and eventually spreads to affect the major portions of both kidneys.

In far advanced renal tuberculosis, the kidney is converted into a hollowed, cavitated, sac-like structure. Occasionally in these cases, the ureter becomes plugged by the inflammatory tissue and debris and the kidney is transformed into a closed cystic mass. Under these circumstances, spontaneous sterilization of the infection may occur and, in the course of time, the cyst wall becomes fibrotic and calcified. This process is referred to as **autonephrectomy**. In all forms of renal tuberculosis, **there is almost always an associated tuberculous infection of the bladder, which is clinically significant because the cystitis is often responsible for more prominent symptoms than the renal tuberculosis.**

Miliary renal tuberculosis is completely overshadowed by the systemic infection. The isolated organ form is usually dominated, from the standpoint of clinical signs and symptoms, by the concomitant tuberculous cystitis. Patients, therefore, most often complain of frequency, dysuria and nocturia. Hematuria may be quite prominent. The findings of such a sediment in the absence of culturally demonstrable organisms should raise the question of a tuberculous etiology. The diagnosis is confirmed by the demonstration of tubercle bacilli either on smear of the urine sediment or on special culture. Renal tuberculosis may lead to death from either uremia or the chronic wasting resulting from an uncontrolled tuberculous infection.

DISEASES OF BLOOD VESSELS

The blood vessels are affected in virtually all forms of renal disease. Here we are concerned with those disorders in which vascular lesions are the primary cause of the renal disease, i.e., benign nephrosclerosis, malignant nephrosclerosis, senile arteriosclerotic kidney, renal infarct and acute cortical necrosis. Within this group, benign and malignant nephrosclerosis are of preeminent importance. Both are almost always associated with hypertension and may well be caused by it. Because the kidney and its diseases are intimately related to hypertension, it is necessary to review this subject briefly.

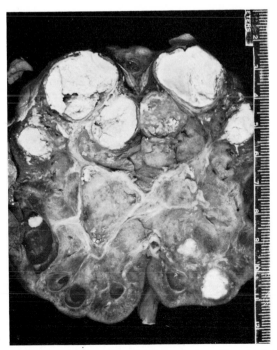

Figure 24–39. *Renal tuberculosis with massive areas of conglomerate caseous necrosis.*

PATHOPHYSIOLOGY OF HYPERTENSION

Elevated levels of blood pressure cause vascular changes throughout the body, particularly in the kidneys; conversely, kidney disease plays an important role in the causation of certain forms of hypertension. Ironically, there is no universally accepted definition of hypertension. Probably, it should be defined as any level of blood pressure deleterious to the patient, but such vagueness is of little use. Most investigators would agree that a sustained diastolic pressure above 90 mm. Hg is an essential feature. A sustained systolic pressure above 140 mm. Hg may also constitute hypertension, but systolic elevations are generally thought to be less significant than elevation of the diastolic pressure.

Approximately 90 to 95 per cent of hypertension is of uncertain origin and is called primary or essential hypertension. The remaining 5 to 10 per cent would obviously be called secondary hypertension, for reasons which will become clear later. Essential hypertension might equally well be called idiopathic hypertension. It is estimated to be present in about 5 per cent of the adult population of the United States, and it generally arises mysteriously in previously healthy individuals. Females are affected more often than males, usually beginning in the fourth to fifth decades of life. The incidence of this disease rises with age, and as many as 25 per cent of the population of the United States over the age of 50 may have essential hypertension. In most instances, even if not treated, it is characterized by extremely slow, progressive elevation of the blood pressure over the span of decades. It may eventually lead to cardiovascular and cerebrovascular disorders, but the rate of development of these complications is a function of the severity of the blood pressure elevations. In many of the milder expressions, the hypertension exerts little untoward effect. Moreover, in general, it is readily controlled by antihypertensive therapy. In other words, the disorder is relatively benign and so is sometimes referred to as *benign hypertension.* In time, benign essential hypertension does cause thickening of the walls of small arteries and arterioles in the kidney, but the renal ischemia rarely causes significant damage or renal failure. Even in former years before the advent of effective antihypertensive therapy, *only about 5 per cent of patients with benign essential hypertension died of uremia; the remainder died largely of coronary or hypertensive heart disease, of cerebrovascular accidents, and of unrelated causes.*

Some cases of idiopathic hypertension pursue an accelerated course characterized by rapidly mounting blood pressure usually to diastolic levels over 110 mm. Hg. The systolic pressure is often well over 200 mm. Hg. This more serious form is called *accelerated or malignant hypertension,* the latter term denoting its ominous prognosis unless controlled by therapy. Although malignant hypertension is considered in more detail later, here it should be pointed out that although it may arise de novo in previously normotensive individuals, more often, it develops in those already having preexisting essential or secondary hypertension.

The search for the origins of essential hypertension has been most frustrating. Clearly, the increased diastolic pressure implies increased peripheral resistance in the vascular, probably arteriolar, tree. Hyaline arteriolar thickening, so-called hyaline arteriolosclerosis, is a common postmortem finding in patients with essential benign hypertension, particularly in the kidneys. However, biopsy of the kidneys in patients with essential hypertension has shown that as many as 25 to 30 per cent have little or no vascular change, and so the evidence suggests that the arteriolar narrowing is a consequence of the hypertension rather than a primary event explaining increased peripheral resistance. It has also not been possible to document increased levels of angiotensin in this form of hypertension.

Recourse has, therefore, been made to a theory of vasomotor lability. Presumably in affected individuals, transient episodes of blood pressure elevation, in time, induce the anatomic vascular changes described. Such vasomotor constriction could be mediated through the autonomic nervous system, perhaps in response to mental and physical stress. The predisposition to such functional vasomotor hypertension may involve both environmental and hereditary influences. Chinese people, for example, living in their native country have a much lower incidence of hypertension than do the Chinese living in the United States. Another environmental influence, obesity, is correlated with hypertension. Evidence of genetic predisposition comes from several sources. Black Americans have a higher incidence of hypertension and more severe forms than white Americans in the same geographic locale. Elevated blood pressure is more often encountered in those with short, heavy body builds than in those who are tall and slender. When both parents are hypertensive, approximately 50 per cent of the offspring will develop the same disorder, compared with only 3 per cent of the children of normotensive parents. A host of other pathogenetic mechanisms have been postulated, including defective catecholamine metabolism, deranged function of the autonomic nervous system and others; but it is clear that the origins of essential hypertension are as yet not elucidated.

In contrast to essential or primary hypertension, *secondary hypertension* is uncommon and accounts for only 5 to 10 per cent of the general spectrum of hypertension in the general population. *In most instances, it is secondary to renal disease, but it may also occur with narrowing of a renal artery (renovascular hypertension), adrenal lesions including primary aldosteronism, Cushing's disease, pheochromocytoma, and central nervous system disorders associated with increased intracranial pressure or brain stem lesions.* Coarctation of the aorta also causes hypertension in the portion of the arterial tree deriving its blood supply from the segment of the aorta proximal to the narrowing. Secondary hypertension, then, occurs with disorders which are thought to be the cause of the elevation of the blood pressure.

Much is known about the pathogenesis of secondary hypertension. Pheochromocytomas elaborate catecholamines, particularly norepinephrine. The adrenal disorders are all characterized by excess secretion of aldosterone, which induces salt and water retention leading to hypervolemia. The secondary renal hypertension is more complex. It has long been known that most patients with chronic renal disease, most importantly, chronic glomerulonephritis and chronic pyelonephritis, have hypertension. Other renal disorders implicated are polycystic kidneys, hydronephrosis and involvement of the kidneys in "connective tissue diseases."

The significance of these observations was considerably clarified when Goldblatt, in his epochal experiments in 1934, demonstrated that hypertension could be produced consistently in animals by partially constricting a renal artery (Goldblatt et al., 1934) (Goldblatt, 1948). He proposed, and it is now abundantly confirmed, that *renal ischemia leads to hypertension through the mediation of the renin-angiotensin-aldosterone system* (Vander, 1967). Renal ischemia reduces blood flow through the renal arterioles and activates the J-G apparatus to elaborate renin which, as was explained earlier, is converted to angiotensin II. Not only does the angiotensin have direct vasomotor pressor effect, but it also stimulates the adrenal glands in man to produce aldosterone, leading to salt and water retention and hypervolemia, aggravating the pressure elevation (Carpenter et al., 1961). Despite establishment of the fact that renin is released in increased amounts from the ischemic kidney, the extent of its participation in the sustained hypertension of man is still somewhat controversial. To date, consist-

ently elevated levels of renin or angiotensin in the chronic sustained form of renal hypertension have not been documented. This may merely reflect technical difficulties in identifying small amounts of renin and angiotensin. Improved laboratory methods for renin assay and radioimmunoassay for angiotensin may shed light on this problem.

In support of the proposition that renal ischemia leads to hypertension are the numerous clinical reports of unilateral renal or renovascular disease inducing hypertension which remitted following nephrectomy. For example, reconstruction of a renal artery to relieve a narrowing, or nephrectomy, in the case of unilateral chronic pyelonephritis, has been followed by remarkable lowering of the blood pressure. However, such improvement occurs only in about 50 to 70 per cent of these cases. In those in which no relief is achieved, it is postulated that the longstanding hypertension eventually caused arteriolar disease in the healthy kidney, rendering it ischemic and a continuing source of renin.

The relationship between hypertension and the kidney may be more complex than the production of renin alone. In the experimental animal, when hypertension is produced by narrowing of one renal artery, the elevation of blood pressure becomes much more severe when the healthy kidney is removed (Goldblatt, 1937). Similarly, bilateral nephrectomy, followed by dialysis, induces hypertension. These observations have been interpreted by some investigators to mean that the kidneys normally exert some protective effect, possibly the elaboration of some *hypotensive* agent. Conceivably, then, renal disease might interfere with the production of this agent, producing hypertension by default or "renoprival" hypertension (Grollman et al., 1949). Others, however, have interpreted these same experiments to mean that removal of the normal kidney(s) induces hypertension merely from loss of excretory capacity for water and electrolytes. The validity of "renoprival" hypertension remains very uncertain, but recently several factors have been extracted from the normal kidney—vasodepressor renomedullary prostaglandins and vasodepressor renomedullary lipid—which once again light the fire of some renoprival mechanism (Hickler et al., 1964) (Muirhead et al., 1968). In addition, a phospholipid has been found in the normal kidney which has the capability of inhibiting renin (Smeby et al., 1967). It is possible, therefore, that the kidney may elaborate both hypertensive and hypotensive factors involved in some delicately balanced feedback system controlling blood pressure.

Malignant hypertension may appear de novo in previously normotensive individuals, or it may be superimposed upon preexisting mild hypertension, primary or secondary. In this accelerated form of hypertension, the pressure elevation rapidly mounts over the span of weeks to months, reaching, as mentioned, diastolic pressures of over 100 mm. Hg and systolic pressures frequently over 200 mm. Hg. But pressure levels alone do not characterize this form of hypertension, and most investigators would agree that *this diagnosis should not be made unless the patient also has bilateral retinal hemorrhages and exudates, with or without papilledema.* In its pure form, malignant hypertension is encountered usually in the fourth and fifth decades of life. In those with preexisting mild hypertension, it may appear later in life. Fortunately, the accelerated pattern is encountered in only about 5 per cent of all patients with elevated blood pressure. As the name implies, it is a malignant disease and, unless controlled by therapy, causes death in over half of the patients within two years. Ninety-five per cent of these deaths are due to uremia; the remainder are due to cardiac disease and cerebrovascular accidents.

Significant elevations of blood pressure, whether relatively mild or accelerated, will, in time, produce generalized narrowing of the arterioles and small arteries throughout the body. The more severe the hypertension, the more marked the vascular changes. In general, *benign hypertension, whether primary or secondary, induces, as was mentioned earlier, a hyaline arteriolosclerosis, most prominently in the kidneys.* But all other arterioles of the body are affected to a greater or lesser extent. *Malignant hypertension causes necrotizing and hyperplastic changes in arterioles and small arteries.* When a patient has had benign hypertension before developing the accelerated phase, the vascular changes comprise a composite of hyaline and malignant arteriolosclerosis. In the patient, the arteriolar thickening and narrowing are most easily identified in the fundi and, as mentioned, malignant hypertension may be associated with retinal hemorrhages and patches of exudates representing ischemia and edema of the choroid (hypertensive retinopathy).

Hypertension has many other side effects. Hypertensive or coronary heart disease is the most frequent cause of death in the overall spectrum of all forms of hypertension. As was indicated in an earlier discussion, hypertension accelerates the progression of atherosclerosis. In those with accelerated hypertension, headaches, confusion and transient episodes of loss of consciousness or convulsions are encountered. These episodes are known as *hypertensive crises,* probably reflecting bouts of cerebral edema. Intracerebral hemorrhages or subarachnoid hemorrhages may occur in both the benign and accelerated forms of hypertension but are, of course, more frequent with marked elevations of pressure. Subarachnoid hemorrhages are related to rupture of thin-walled congenital berry aneurysms at the base of the brain. So it is evident that hypertension has far-reaching clinical implications to many organs throughout the body, including the kidneys, and conversely, the kidneys are deeply involved in the genesis of some and perhaps most forms of hypertension.

BENIGN NEPHROSCLEROSIS (HYALINE ARTERIOLAR NEPHROSCLEROSIS)

Benign nephrosclerosis is the form of renal disease that is associated with benign hypertension and hyaline arteriolosclerosis. It is the most frequent form of anatomic nephropathy and is found in over three-fourths of postmortems on individuals over the age of 60. However, benign nephrosclerosis may also be encountered in younger individuals, for example, in diabetics who have a predisposition to arteriosclerosis and in those circumstances involving a known underlying cause for hypertension, such as pheochromocytoma. Benign nephrosclerosis is somewhat more frequent in males than females, probably because women appear to tolerate elevated blood pressure with greater impunity. Rarely, these vascular changes are found in the apparent absence of clinical hypertension, and the issue arises: Did these patients at some time in their lives have a period of hypertension, or are there as yet undiscovered causes of hyaline arteriolosclerosis?

Pathogenesis. As mentioned in the discussion of hypertension, the thickening of the small arteries and hyaline arteriolosclerosis are thought to be secondary to prolonged benign hypertension. As was pointed out earlier, patients with benign hypertension may have, at postmortem examination, essentially normal kidneys with normal vasculature. It is assumed that the hypertension was of too short duration to have induced morphologic changes. Still unexplained is the problem of how the elevated blood pressure leads to the anatomic vascular changes. Electron microscopic study offers two not mutually incompatible alternatives: (1) the hyaline thickening of the arterioles may be the consequence of reduplication or thickening of the intimal basement membrane or (2) vascular injury may lead to increased permeability of small vessel walls, with mural accumulation of water and plasma proteins (Weiner et al., 1965). Whatever the pathway, in time, these small vessels undergo collagenous fibrosis with marked narrowing of their lumina. Although the small arteries and arterioles throughout the body are affected, those in the kidney, spleen, pancreas, adrenal glands and brain bear the brunt of the hypertensive changes. As a consequence, the kidneys are rendered ischemic and undergo slow, progressive atrophy and fibrosis.

Morphology. From the preceding outline of the pathogenesis, it can be anticipated that **the kidney changes take the form of slowly developing, symmetrical, diffuse, ischemic atrophy and scarring** (Kimmelstiel and Wilson, 1936). In the advanced case, which may require many years and decades for its development, decrease in kidney size occurs to average levels of approximately 110 to 130 gm. The cortical surfaces have a fine, even granularity which resembles grain leather. Because the process is primarily an ischemic one, the kidneys

are usually more pale and gray than normal (Fig. 24—40). On section, the loss of mass is mainly due to cortical narrowing, but inevitably medullary atrophy ensues and is accompanied by an increase in peripelvic fat. The corticomedullary demarcation is usually not markedly disturbed. On close inspection, thickening of the walls of the small arteries may be apparent, producing the so-called "pipe-stem" appearance. In the process of fibrous atrophy, nephrons may be pinched off, giving rise to small cysts under 2 mm. in diameter, usually in the cortex.

The primary characteristic of benign nephrosclerosis is marked narrowing of the lumina of arterioles and small arteries caused by thickening and hyalinization of their walls (Fig. 24—41). Unlike the situation with the diabetic, in which both afferent and efferent arterioles are affected, in benign nephrosclerosis only the afferent arterioles are involved. The nature of this hyaline material has been discussed above. The hyalinization often obliterates the underlying native cellular detail.

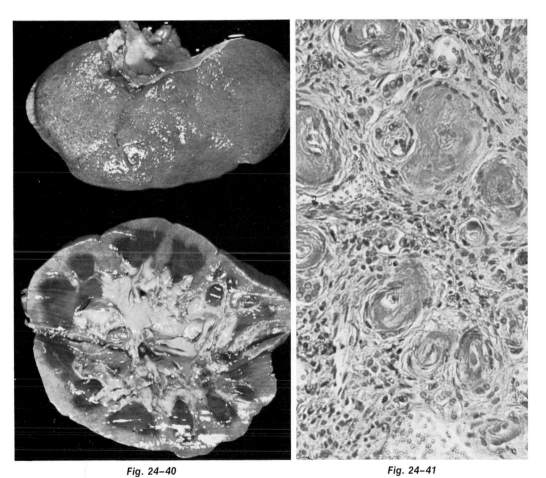

Fig. 24—40   Fig. 24—41

Figure 24—40. Benign nephrosclerosis illustrating the fine granularity of the cortical surface and narrowing of the cortex.

Figure 24—41. Benign nephrosclerosis. The hyaline arteriolosclerosis is presumed to reflect prolonged moderate hypertension.

Consequent to the diffuse vascular narrowing, there is widespread ischemic atrophy of all structures in the kidney. Thus, the glomeruli show thickening of the periglomerular interstitial tissue, together with collagenous fibrosis of the uriniferous space and thickening of the entire axial framework of the glomerular tufts. The latter thickening is, in large part, due to basement membrane thickening and is designated **diffuse intercapillary glomerulosclerosis**. This diffuse pattern should not be confused with the nodular glomerulosclerosis of the diabetic, previously discussed (p. 268). In far advanced cases of benign nephrosclerosis, the diffuse glomerulosclerosis may obliterate the glomerular tuft. Tubular atrophy is diffuse and accompanied by a progressive increase in the interstitial fibrous tissue. A scant interstitial lymphocytic infiltrate commonly accompanies the renal atrophy.

The anatomic changes are frequently superimposed on other forms of renal disease which initially produced the hypertension. Thus, the patient with pyelonephritis or polycystic kidney disease may, because of his secondary renal hypertension, develop hyaline arteriolosclerosis and the anatomic changes of benign nephrosclerosis.

Clinical Course.

Benign nephrosclerosis alone rarely causes severe renal insufficiency or uremia. Not more than 5 per cent of the patients with well developed benign nephrosclerosis die of renal failure. The clinical signs and symptoms of these patients relate to other manifestations of prolonged hypertension, such as heart disease or cerebral accidents. However, most patients with benign hypertension die of diseases not directly related to their hypertension.

MALIGNANT NEPHROSCLEROSIS (HYPERPLASTIC ARTERIOLAR NEPHROSCLEROSIS)

Malignant nephrosclerosis is the form of renal disease associated with malignant hypertension. This pattern of hypertension may develop in previously normotensive individuals or may be superimposed upon preexisting benign hypertension, whether primary or secondary. Malignant nephrosclerosis may therefore appear as a pure form of nephropathy, or it may be superimposed upon an underlying chronic renal disease, particularly benign nephrosclerosis, glomerulonephritis and pyelonephritis.

Incidence.

Malignant hypertension is uncommon, occurring in less than 5 per cent of all patients with elevated blood pressure. In its pure form, it usually affects younger individuals, under the age of 45. As a complication of preexisting hypertension, it is found at any age.

Pathogenesis.

The basis for the development of malignant hypertension is obscured in the darkness of the cause of essential hypertension. The rapidly mounting levels of arterial pressure often appear without antecedent signs or symptoms or apparent cause. Elevated levels of renin and aldosterone have been found in many patients, but why the kidney should suddenly hypersecrete renin is not understood. Whatever its basis, malignant hypertension profoundly affects all vessels of the body, particularly the small arteries and arterioles of the kidney. The small arteries tend to develop hyperplastic thickening of their walls, creating an appearance referred to as "onion-skinning" (Fig. 24–42). This has been attributed to proliferation of both muscular cells within the media and fibroblasts within the intima (Spiro et al., 1965). The arterioles may also show hyperplastic thickening, but more often develop a lesion known as "fibrinoid necrosis." This takes the form of thickening of the arteriolar wall by an amorphous, proteinous precipitate smudging and obliterating the underlying details (Fig. 24–43). Frequently, a neutrophilic infiltrate is found within this deposit. The "onion-skin" thickening can be interpreted as a hyperplastic cellular reaction to stress, but the nature of the proteinous deposit is still uncertain.

Linton et al. (1969) have recently postulated that the vascular stress causes increased permeability of the arteriolar wall, with seepage and intramural deposition of plasma proteins, including fibrinogen. He further postulates that the arteriolar narrowing induces mechanical trauma to red cells, resulting in hemolysis and anemia known as microangiopathic hemolytic anemia. The lysed red blood cells activate the clotting mechanism, favoring the deposition of fibrinogen not only within the lumen but also within the vessel walls. Thus is the appearance of "fibrinoid necrosis" achieved. Interesting as such a proposition is, it is still speculative. For the present, the mechanism by which the malignant hypertension induces the vascular changes must still be considered unsettled.

Morphology.

Renal parenchymal changes develop as a consequence of the vascular lesions described above. The macroscopic appearance of the kidney is dependent upon the preexisting state of the kidneys before the development of the malignant hypertension and on the duration and severity of the hypertensive disease. In pure malignant nephrosclerosis, the gross alterations may be quite minimal. Commonly, vascular congestion produces some slight increase in size. A frequent pattern is that of irregular congestive mottling. Because of

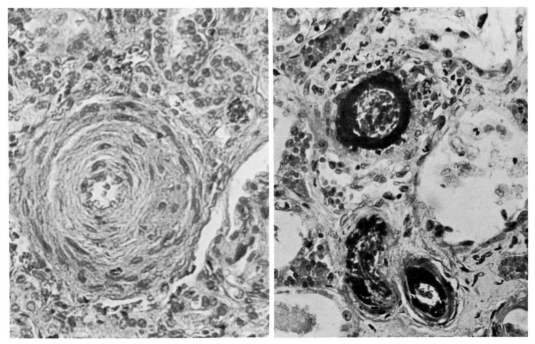

Fig. 24-42   Fig. 24-43

Figure 24-42. The hyperplastic arteriolosclerosis of malignant hypertension.
Figure 24-43. Necrotizing arteriolitis of malignant nephrosclerosis with fibrinoid degeneration of the walls of the arterioles and small arteries.

the extremely rapid course of the disease, ending in death, there is not sufficient time for scarring and contraction to develop. **Small, pinpoint petechial hemorrhages** may appear on the cortical surface from rupture of arterioles or glomerular capillaries. Often, however, petechiae are absent. On cut section, the kidneys may be quite normal in appearance, save for the possible presence of petechiae within the cortex. When the malignant nephrosclerosis is superimposed upon preexisting renal disease, its presence may be completely undetectable grossly. Sometimes it is suspected only by the appearance of small petechial hemorrhages in a nephropathy in which petechiae are not anticipated.

In its pure expression, malignant nephrosclerosis is characterized by proliferative or hyperplastic "onionskinning" of the small arteries and afferent arterioles and by fibrinoid necrosis of arterioles (described in the consideration of the pathogenesis). The narrowed lumina induce marked renal ischemia and further parenchymal alterations. The proximal convoluted tubules which are particularly sensitive to ischemia may undergo regressive changes manifested by granularity of the cytoplasm or fatty change. If the arteriolar lumina are obstructed, the involved glomeruli may become necrotic, and infiltrated with neutrophils, and the glomerular capillaries may thrombose (necrotizing glomerulitis). Rupture of these necrosed capillaries

gives rise to hemorrhages into the glomerular spaces and draining tubules, providing the microscopic basis for the petechiae seen grossly.

Pure malignant nephrosclerosis is encountered much less often than malignant nephrosclerosis superimposed on an underlying chronic renal disease such as benign nephrosclerosis, chronic glomerulonephritis, or chronic pyelonephritis. When superimposed on benign nephrosclerosis, the arterioles and small arteries show changes characteristic of both disorders, referred to facetiously as "benignant" nephrosclerosis.

Clinical Course. Usually the clinical manifestations of malignant hypertension appear abruptly, and initially are referable to the cardiovascular or central nervous systems. Cardiac decompensation, manifested principally as left ventricular failure, may be the first manifestation. Rarely, patients with malignant hypertension present in oliguric acute renal failure (Mattern, 1972). More often, the early symptoms are related to increased intracranial pressure and include headaches, nausea, vomiting and visual impairments, particularly the development of scotomas or spots before the eyes. "Hypertensive crises" are sometimes encountered, characterized by episodes of loss of consciousness or even convulsions. At the onset of the rapidly mounting blood pressure, there is marked proteinuria and microscopic or sometimes macroscopic hematuria but no significant alteration in renal function. So the BUN may be normal or minimally elevated. However, in time, the renal damage leads to progressive renal failure. In the untreated patient, once signs of renal decompensation set in, the course lasts for only a few months, and 95 per cent of these patients die in uremia. The remaining 5 per cent of deaths are about evenly divided between cerebrovascular accidents, usually cerebral hemorrhages, and cardiac failure. Effective therapy has improved the outlook and, with treatment, the five-year survival is in the range of 50 per cent. There is every reason to believe that, with early diagnosis and improved forms of antihypertensive therapy, still more progress will be made in the control of this disorder.

SENILE ARTERIOSCLEROTIC KIDNEY

Arteriosclerotic narrowing of the main renal arteries or their major branches may give rise to ischemic atrophy of the affected renal parenchyma. The resultant alterations thus involve the entire kidney or sharply demarcated segmental areas supplied by branches. With narrowing of the main renal artery, diffuse, symmetrical contraction of the entire kidney produces a pale, granular, small kidney resembling that described in benign nephrosclerosis. When the renal branches are affected, the lesions are patchy and asymmetrical so that contracted, depressed focal scars are produced on the renal surface, resembling focal areas of benign nephrosclerosis or healed pyelonephritis or infarctions. These are characteristically pale, granular, depressed areas which, on section, appear as wedge-shaped areas of fibrosis extending into the medulla. In these focal involvements, the renal size may or may not be affected.

Microscopically, if the vascular occlusion is marked, the scarred areas show fibrous obliteration of glomeruli with atrophy and fibrous replacement of the tubules by dense, collagenous scar tissue. A lymphocytic infiltrate is usually also present within the scar. The vessels within the scarred area have thickened walls and narrowed lumina, so-called *vascular atrophy*. The adjacent preserved parenchyma may show some tubular dilatation and some cast formation, probably due to the fact that the distal portions of these preserved nephrons have been blocked by scar at some lower level. The margins of the scar extend into the interstitium in the form of an increase in the intertubular connective tissue. This histologic appearance of these focal areas of ischemia may be extremely difficult to differentiate from infarcts described below. The precise diagnosis rests upon the identification of the arteriosclerotic involvement of the affected vessels.

RENAL INFARCTS

The kidneys are favored sites for the development of infarcts, presumably because approximately one-fourth of the entire cardiac output passes through these organs. The infarcts are almost entirely arterial, although very rarely venous thrombosis has been described as the basis for infarction. Although thrombosis in advanced atherosclerosis and the acute vasculitis of polyarteritis nodosa may occlude arteries, almost all arterial infarcts are due to embolism. The major source of such emboli are the heart, more specifically mural thrombosis in the left auricle and mural thrombosis in the ventricle on the basis of myocardial infarction. Vegetative endocarditis and thromboses in aortic aneurysms and aortic atherosclerosis are less frequent sites for the origin of emboli. Paradoxical embolism in congenital heart disease is a very rare source of renal infarction. The uncommon venous infarcts are usually caused by infections within the abdominal cavity or by a perinephric abscess that excites a renal thrombophlebitis. Infarcts are therefore encountered in any age group, under the great variety of clinical circumstances just mentioned.

Because the arterial supply to the kidney is essentially of the "end-organ" type, most infarcts are of the anemic type. They may occur as solitary lesions or be multiple and bilateral. When the main renal artery is affected, the entire kidney may be involved. In the very early stages, anemic infarcts appear externally as slightly elevated map-like areas which may show only slight congestive discoloration due to initial capillary hemorrhage. Within 24 hours, infarcts become sharply demarcated, pale, yellow-white areas which may contain small irregular foci of hemorrhagic discoloration. They are usually ringed by a zone of intense hyperemia.

On section, they characteristically assume a wedge shape, with the base against the cortical surface and the apex pointing toward the medulla. Close inspection may disclose a very narrow rim of preserved subcortical tissue which has been spared by the collateral capsular circulation. In time, these acute areas of ischemic necrosis undergo progressive fibrous scarring, giving rise to depressed, **pale, gray-white scars** which characteristically assume a V shape on section and are associated with wedge-shaped strands of fibrous tissue extending into the underlying kidney substance. These areas of scarring may be indistinguishable from the more slowly developing ischemic atrophy due to arteriosclerotic narrowing of major vessels. They may also at times be difficult to differentiate from focal, healed pyelonephritis. Not infrequently, infarcts of varying ages are encountered in the same kidney, denoting recurrent embolic episodes (Fig. 24–44). The histologic changes in renal infarction have already been covered in Chapter 9 (p. 341). It suffices for now to recall that, in common with all infarctions, there is at first progressive coagulative necrosis of cells, with preservation of shadowy cell outlines (Fig. 24–45) (Sheehan and Davis, 1958, 1959b).

The signs and symptoms of renal infarction are acute in onset, with pain and tenderness localized to the costovertebral angle. These two features associated with the showers of red cells in the urine are almost diagnostic. When the infarction is more massive and bilateral, signs of renal dysfunction and even insufficiency may arise. Occasionally, massive unilateral infarction may produce sudden oliguria or anuria, presumably due to "sympathetic" suppression of the unaffected side. Massive infarction of one kidney is a well known basis for a "Goldblatt kidney."

DIFFUSE CORTICAL NECROSIS

Bilateral, symmetrical, renal cortical necrosis is an extremely rare entity of sudden onset, causing acute renal failure. The cortical

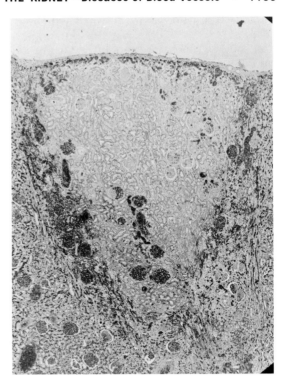

Figure 24–45. Renal infarction at low power, illustrating the wedge shape, the shadowy outlines of necrotic renal substances and the darker peripheral zone of leukocytic infiltration.

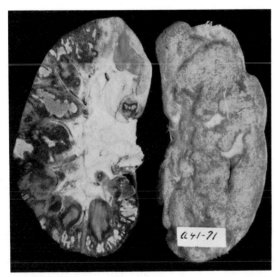

Figure 24–44. Renal infarcts recent and old. The cross section of the left kidney has fresh pale infarcts involving almost the entire renal parenchyma surrounded by wide zones of hemorrhage. The right kidney presents focal depressed pale scars of healed infarcts.

destruction has all of the earmarks of ischemic necrosis. This renal disorder is encountered in a very wide variety of clinical settings: shock, accidents of childbirth (toxemia, premature separation of placenta), burns, chemical poisonings, gram-negative and gram-positive septicemias and thrombotic thrombocytopenic purpura. In all likelihood, the common denominator among all these clinical conditions is the development of disseminated intravascular coagulation (DIC) (p. 744). In support of this view, cases have been reported with bilateral renal cortical necrosis and pituitary insufficiency strongly suggestive of intravascular coagulation affecting both the kidneys and pituitary (Chervony et al., 1965) (McKay, 1965). Indeed, as will be seen, thromboses within small vessels in the cortex and the glomerular capillaries characterize cortical necrosis. And so the best evidence suggests that this form of renal necrosis is one manifestation of DIC. However, another pathogenic mechanism has been proposed for some or possibly all cases. Studies by Trueta et al. (1947) on the war-wounded suggest the existence of juxtamedullary shunts by which most of the cortical blood flow is shunted through the medulla, bypassing the cortex. Conceivably, in any form of severe stress, bypassing of the cortex might occur. The two possible mechanisms, i.e., DIC and shunting, are not mutually exclusive and may act in concert or individually in specific cases.

The gross alterations of the massive ischemic necrosis of the parenchyma are sharply limited to the cortex. On external examination, the kidney is usually enlarged and the surface has a variegated color of marked congestion and hemorrhage, interspersed with pale, yellow-white, irregular, geographic areas of massive infarction. On section, these changes are limited to the cortex and more or less completely spare the medulla. The histologic appearance is that of acute ischemic infarction. Later stages are not observed because this lesion is incompatible with long survival. Rarely, there may be areas of apparently better preserved cortex. The mechanism for such uneven involvement is completely obscure. At the deeper levels, in contact with the preserved medulla, there is usually a massive leukocytic infiltration. Intravascular thromboses may be prominent, and occasionally acute necroses of small arterioles and capillaries may be present. Hemorrhages occur into the glomeruli, together with the precipitation of fibrin in the glomerular capillaries.

This form of acute renal necrosis is of grave significance since it is almost invariably bilateral and gives rise to sudden anuria terminating rapidly in uremic death. Rare instances of unilateral involvement have been described and are compatible with survival. The recent beneficial use of anticoagulants in some of these patients lends clinical support to the thrombotic concept of pathogenesis.

OBSTRUCTIVE AND CALCULOUS NEPHROPATHY

HYDRONEPHROSIS

Hydronephrosis is the term used to describe dilatation of the renal pelvis and calyces associated with progressive atrophy and cystic enlargement of the kidney due to obstruction to the outflow of urine. The urinary obstruction may exist at any level, from the urethra up to the renal pelvis, and may be partial or complete, intermittent or total. Complete, sudden obstruction usually evokes only little hydronephrosis because of abrupt suppression of renal glomerular filtration. However, it has been shown that sudden, total obstruction may still lead to significant dilatation of the collecting system and parenchymal atrophy, since there is continued glomerular filtration as pyelovenous com-

munications permit resorption of the urine (Sheehan and Davis, 1959a). The genesis of the dilatation of the collecting system involves more than mere obstruction, since much evidence points to concomitant circulatory disturbances as important in the development of this lesion. Presumably, as the pelvis and calyces expand, they compress the renal vessels and thus add elements of venous stasis and arterial insufficiency to the damaging influences (Hinman and Morison, 1926).

In addition, it is proposed that the anatomic configuration of the pelvis may be important in the development of hydronephrosis (Hanley, 1960). The normal ureteropelvic junction in 90 per cent of individuals is funnel-shaped and, in these individuals, hydronephrosis almost never develops despite angulation, kinking or external pressures. On the other hand, about 10 per cent of renal pelves are rounded, ball-shaped structures in which the ureter arises rather abruptly and at a slight angle. There is often a high degree of ureteropelvic tone in these latter anatomic arrangements, adding to the tendency for these collecting systems always to remain filled or even distended with urine. It may take very little inflammatory edema or congestion or extrinsic pressure to further aggravate this tendency for distention and thus lead to hydronephrosis.

The common causes for urinary retention can be conveniently grouped into two categories: congenital and acquired. The *congenital* causes include atresia of the urethra, congenital valve formations in either the ureters or the urethra, aberrant renal arteries and torsion or kinking of the ureter due to displacement of the kidney. The *acquired* causes are most commonly prostatic hypertrophy, carcinoma of the prostate, uterine procidentia producing angulation of the urethra, calculi, spinal cord damage with neurogenic paralysis of the bladder and neoplastic invasion of the ureters or bladder such as occurs in carcinomas of the bladder, cervix and uterus. The mild hydronephrosis of pregnancy is an apparently reversible physiologic change. It is not certain whether it is due to direct pressure on the ureters by the uterine enlargement or to endocrinologic relaxation of all smooth muscle of the body. However, there is a slight tendency for the hydronephrosis to be more marked on the right where the pressure of the enlarged fundus is somewhat greater. In most instances, the hydronephrosis disappears promptly after delivery.

Hydronephrosis may be unilateral or bilateral. When the obstruction is sudden and complete, the suppression of glomerular filtration usually leads to mild dilatation of the pelvis and calyces but sometimes to atrophy of the renal parenchyma. When the obstruction is subtotal or intermittent, glomerular filtration is not suppressed and progressive dilatation ensues. Depending upon the level of the urinary block, the dilatation may affect first the bladder or ureter and then the kidney. Usually in low obstruction in which both kidneys are affected, uremia cuts short the development of far advanced hydronephrotic changes. The unilateral involvements display the full range of changes.

Grossly, the kidney may have slight to massive enlargement. The earlier features are those of **simple dilatation of the pelvis and calyces.** Progressive blunting of the apices of the pyramids occurs, and eventually these become cupped to form small, multilocular cavities which communicate through broad openings with the calyces and pelves. In far advanced cases, the kidney may become transformed into a thin-walled cystic structure having a diameter of up to 15 to 20 cm. (Fig. 24–46) with striking parenchymal atrophy, total obliteration of the pyramids and thinning of the cortex. The kidney is thus converted to a thin-walled, fibrous, hugely dilated sac.

The characteristic microscopic feature of hydronephrosis in cases which are not too extreme is **tubular atrophy and fibrosis with sparing of the glomeruli.** The lesion begins with tubular dilatation, but it eventually leads to obliteration of the tubules, leaving only compressed atrophic glomeruli separated by dense fibrous tissue (Fig. 24–47). Only in the more advanced stages do the glomeruli become atrophic and eventually disappear. There may be little inflammatory infiltrate in the pure form. However, it has already been indicated that, in the presence of urinary tract obstruction, pyelonephritis is a common complication, and it is not unusual therefore for pyelonephritis to develop in hydronephrotic kidneys thus to produce **pyonephrosis** and **pyoureter.**

Clinically, hydronephrosis may remain completely silent for long periods of time. This is particularly true when the disease is unilateral and the unaffected kidney is capable of adequate function. The early symptoms, if any,

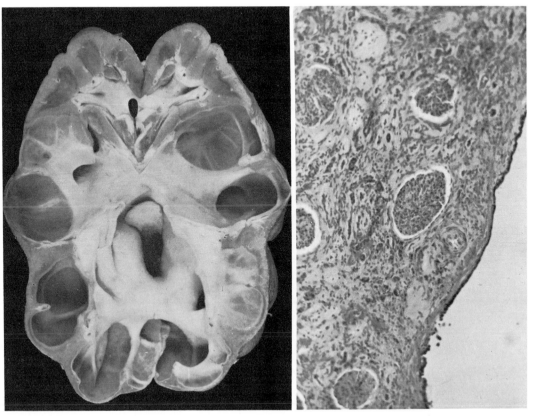

Fig. 24–46   **Fig. 24–47**

Figure 24–46. *Hydronephrosis of the kidney with marked dilatation of the pelvis and calyces and thinning of the renal parenchyma.*

Figure 24–47. *Hydronephrosis, illustrating the atrophy and fibrosis of the tubules with relative sparing of the glomeruli.*

are usually produced by the basic cause of the hydronephrosis. Thus, calculi lodged in the ureters may give rise to renal colic, and prostatic enlargements give rise to bladder symptoms. Unilateral hydronephrosis is frequently discovered on routine physical examination as a mass in the costovertebral angle. Sometimes its existence first becomes apparent in the course of pyelography. It is regrettable that this disease tends to remain asymptomatic, since it has been shown that in its very early stages, perhaps the first few weeks, relief of such obstruction is compatible with a reversion to normal of renal structure and function. However, after this period of time, despite the fact that much preserved renal parenchyma may be left, relief of the obstruction does not appear to prevent the progressive atrophy of the affected kidney. Apparently, even with minimal hydronephrotic damage on one side, total urinary formation is taken over by the unaffected kidney, and disuse atrophy causes progressive destruction of the affected kidney. If, however, the process is bilateral, as may be caused by prostatic enlargement, and not too far advanced, removal of the obstructing prostate is compatible with preservation of the remaining renal function and considerable reconstitution of the kidney.

UROLITHIASIS

Stones may form at any level in the urinary tract but most arise in the kidney. Urolithiasis is a frequent clinical problem. In a large series, kidney stones were found in 1.12 per cent of autopsies (Bell, 1950). From the clinical standpoint, it is said that one in every 1000 individuals in the United States needs hospitalization each year because of kidney stones. Males are affected somewhat more often than females and most patients are over the age of 30. A familial and hereditary predisposition to stone formation has long been known. Many of the inborn errors of metabolism, such as gout, cystinuria and primary hyperoxaluria, provide good examples of hereditary disease characterized by the excessive production and excretion of stone-forming substances. In addition, a genetic predisposition to calcium oxalate urolithiasis has been identified, presumably inherited as a polygenic trait (Resnick et al., 1968).

Pathogenesis. The composition of stones varies with the underlying disorder responsible for their production, but all contain crystalloids as well as complex mucoproteins called matrix. In one of the largest studies of the problem, it was found that approximately 90 per cent of stones contain calcium; about 70

per cent, oxalate; 5 to 10 per cent, urates; and 2 to 3 per cent, cystine (Prien and Prien, 1968). The great majority of stones contain varying mixtures of these crystalloids although some are relatively pure, for example, the uric acid stones of gout.

In some instances, the formation of stones appears to reflect increased urinary concentrations of the crystalloids. But in other instances, there are normal concentrations of crystalloid, and physicochemical changes favoring stone formation are postulated. These concepts can be summarized as follows:

A. Mechanisms leading to increased concentration of crystalloids.
 1. Reduction in urine volume—dehydration.
 2. Excessive excretion of crystalloid constituents.
B. Mechanisms favoring stone formation at normal concentrations of crystalloids.
 1. Alterations in pH of the urine.
 2. Alterations in the stone matrix.
 3. Stasis.
 4. Foreign bodies.
 5. ? Deficiency of stabilizing factors.

The influence of *reduction in urine volume* on stone formation is attested to by the nearly epidemic proportions of renal stones in troops sent to tropical climates.

The circumstances favoring *excessive excretion* of crystalloid varies with the particular constituents involved. Hypercalciuria is encountered in any disorder causing resorption of bone (metastatic cancer, multiple myeloma, hyperparathyroidism, osteoporosis, Cushing's syndrome, steroid therapy, immobilization, Fanconi's syndrome), or in situations favoring excessive absorption of calcium (milk-alkali syndrome, vitamin D intoxication, sarcoidosis). Hypercalciuria is also encountered in both adults and infants without apparent cause. High concentrations of other stone-forming crystalloids are excreted in specific metabolic disorders, gout and cystinuria being prime examples. Infections in the urinary tract by urea-splitting organisms may lead to increased levels of ammonia and the formation of magnesium-ammonium phosphate stones.

As mentioned, *physicochemical changes in the urine* favor stone formation despite normal concentrations of crystalloids. Most important in this respect are extremes of urinary pH. An alkaline pH favors the formation of calcium and magnesium-ammonium phosphate stones, while an acid pH is associated with both uric acid and cystine stones.

The *role of the mucoprotein matrix* is not well understood. Perhaps the mucoprotein matrix provides the skeletal structure on which the crystalloids precipitate (Boyce, 1968).

It is clear from clinical observations that *stasis* predisposes to stone formation, but how is still not readily evident. It may favor reabsorption of water and concentration of crystalloids, provide time for crystallization to occur and predispose to infection. Conceivably, with stasis and infection, bacteria serve as foreign bodies to which crystalloids may adhere.

Foreign bodies such as desquamated epithelial cells encountered in the squamous metaplasia of vitamin A deficiency provide appropriate niduses for the precipitation of stone-forming constituents.

Factors must exist to stabilize the solution of urinary crystalloids, since equimolar concentrations in water promptly crystallize out. The precise nature of these protective substances is still obscure.

This consideration of the pathogenesis of urinary tract stones indicates that when there is no overt basis for the excretion of excessive amounts of stone-forming constituents, attention should be directed to possible influences favoring solution instability of the urinary crystalloids.

Morphology. Stones are unilateral in about 80 per cent of patients. The favored sites for their formation are within the renal calyces and pelves and in the bladder. If formed in the renal pelvis, they tend to remain small, having an average diameter of 2 to 3 mm. These may have smooth contours or may take the form of an irregular, jagged mass of spicules. Often, many stones are found within one kidney (Fig. 24–48). Occasionally, progressive accretion of salts leads to the development of branching structures known as "staghorn" stones, which create a cast of the pelvic and calyceal system (Fig. 24–49).

Stones are of importance only when they obstruct urinary flow or produce sufficient trauma to cause ulceration and bleeding. Stones may be present without producing any symptoms or significant renal damage. In general, smaller stones are most hazardous, since they may pass into the ureters, producing pain referred to as renal colic (one of the most intense forms of pain) as well as ureteral obstruction. Larger stones cannot enter the ureters and are more likely to remain silent within the renal pelvis. Commonly, these larger stones first manifest themselves by hematuria. Stones also predispose to superimposed infection, both by their obstructive nature and by the trauma they produce.

TUMORS OF THE KIDNEY

Many types of benign and malignant tumors occur in the kidney. In general, the be-

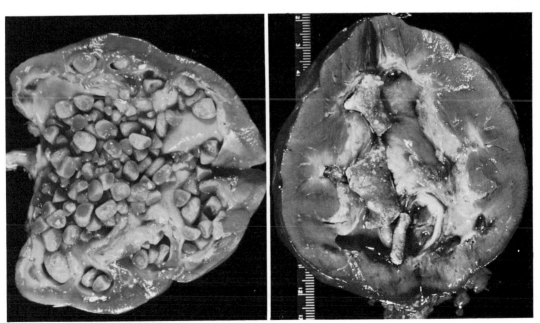

Fig. 24–48   **Fig. 24–49**

Figure 24–48.   Nephrolithiasis. Multiple, somewhat rounded stones are present in the expanded pelvis and calyces.

Figure 24–49.   Nephrolithiasis. A fractured stag-horn calculus is present in the somewhat dilated pelvis.

nign tumors are usually of anatomic interest only, and rarely have clinical significance. Malignant tumors, on the other hand, are of great importance clinically and deserve considerable emphasis. The majority of these malignant tumors are primary renal cell carcinomas (Riches et al., 1951) (Solway, 1938). Perhaps the second most common malignancy is Wilms' tumor found in children. Primary tumors of the calyces and pelves, while relatively infrequent, represent the third most important tumor of the kidney.

BENIGN

Cortical Adenoma. Small, discrete adenomas having origin in the renal tubules are found rather commonly at autopsy.

These are usually under 2 cm. in diameter. They are present invariably within the cortex and appear grossly as pale yellow-gray, discrete, seemingly encapsulated nodules. Rarely, these may achieve a diameter of 5 cm. or more. Microscopically, several variants are recognizable. Some tumors are composed of complex, branching, papillomatous structures with numerous complex fronds which project into a cystic space. Sometimes these papillomatous growths are sufficiently complicated and branching to produce apparent solidification of the cyst. The nodule may then appear as a solid tumor composed of double cords of cells. Solid variants are found in which the cells grow in tubules, glands, cords and totally undifferentiated masses of cells.

The cell type for all these growth patterns is quite regular and free of anaplasia. They are cuboidal to polygonal in shape with distinct cell membranes, round, regular small central nuclei and a highly granular cytoplasm which may be partially or totally vacuolated. The vacuoles contain neutral fats and, in addition, anisotropic lipids, presumably cholesterol. Despite the apparent discrete margin on gross inspection, it is common to find no well defined capsule histologically. At times, small extensions of cells project between the renal tubules, giving the apparent impression of invasiveness. This characteristic may make it difficult to differentiate large adenomas from small, well differentiated renal cell carcinomas. In this differential, it has been suggested that the size of the tumor can be used as a diagnostic feature. All tumors over 3 cm. in diameter are considered by some investigators as malignant. This postulate is obviously useful as a rule of thumb only.

Cortical adenomas are most often confused histologically with *adrenal rests,* which sometimes are sequestered under the capsule of the kidney. Most of these rests are located in the upper pole. They appear as 0.5 to 2.0 cm., flat, yellow plaques either incorporated into the capsule or located directly beneath it. Usually, however, there is some resemblance between the architectural pattern of the adrenal rest and that of the normal adrenal, aiding in the differentiation of these rests from cortical adenomas. At one time, these ectopic cells were proposed as the site of origin of carcinomas of the kidney. This view, however, first propounded by Grawitz, is no longer held tenable.

Fibroma. Occasionally at autopsy, small foci of gray-white firm tissue, usually under 1 cm. in diameter, are found within the pyramids of the kidneys. Characteristically, they tend to occur at the junction of the distal and middle thirds of the pyramids. Microscopic examination of these almost invariably discloses mature, well differentiated fibroblasts. While they are not encapsulated and are poorly defined from the surrounding interstitial tissue, they have no malignant propensities. Rarely, one finds small gray hamartomatous nodules within the renal substance, composed of abundant amounts of fibrous tissue, small cords of tubular cells and prominent vessels.

Miscellaneous. As might be anticipated, any other form of mesenchymal benign tumor may occur in the kidney, such as angiomas, lipomas, lymphangiomas and the entire category of tumors derived from mesenchyme. These are all rare and of no clinical significance.

MALIGNANT

Renal Cell Carcinoma (Grawitz Tumor; Hypernephroma, Hypernephroid Carcinoma). Renal cell or hypernephroid carcinomas (to indicate their resemblance to adrenal tissue) are interesting clinical and pathologic problems. Clinically, they are among the most unpredictable tumors of man (Grabstald, 1964). In one patient, the primary site of origin may remain totally silent and the neoplasm is first suspected when it metastasizes. These metastases have masqueraded as primary brain, primary bone and primary lung tumors. In another patient, the tumor may silently achieve massive size without metastasizing, and in yet others, the growth and spread may be virtually explosive.

Incidence. These tumors represent about 3 per cent of all visceral cancers, and account for over 75 per cent of all renal cancers. They occur most often in older individuals, usually in the fifth, sixth and seventh decades of life, showing a definite male preponderance in the ratio of 2 to 1.

Pathogenesis. The relationship of these

malignancies to cortical adenomas is most interesting. On purely morphologic grounds, there is evidence to suggest that renal cell carcinomas may arise from previously benign cortical adenomas based on the fact that large cortical adenomas may be histologically indistinguishable from small carcinomas. Such evidence suggests a possible transition of a benign to a malignant growth. Renal cell carcinomas are characterized by the presence of large amounts of lipid within the tumor cells. For this reason, they were at one time considered to arise from displaced lipid-laden adrenal cells, hence the designation hypernephroma. This origin is now considered as untenable. There is ample evidence to indicate that renal tubular epithelium can elaborate lipids and cholesterol just as do the adrenal cells. Moreover, the total spectrum of renal tumors, varying from minute, clearly defined tubular adenomas to large, obviously malignant carcinomas, offers further circumstantial evidence of their renal cell origin. For this reason, these tumors should be referred to as *renal cell carcinomas or hypernephroid carcinomas* rather than hypernephromas.

Morphology. In its macroscopic appearance, the tumor is quite characteristic. It may arise in any portion of the kidney, but more commonly affects the poles, particularly the upper one. Usually these neoplasms occur as solitary unilateral lesions, but occasionally bilateral neoplasms have been said to have arisen simultaneously. **They are spherical masses, 3 to 15 cm. in diameter, composed of bright yellow-gray-white tissue,** which distort the renal outline. Commonly there are large areas of ischemic, opaque, gray-white necrosis, foci of hemorrhagic discoloration and areas of softening. The margins of these tumors are usually sharply defined, confined within the renal capsule and deceptively give the appearance of encapsulation (Fig. 24–50). This characteristic is due to the expansile growth, which pushes the renal parenchyma ahead of it, rather than insidiously infiltrating. However, at times small processes project into the surrounding parenchyma, and small satellite nodules are found in the surrounding substance, providing clear evidence of the aggressiveness of these lesions. As the tumor enlarges, it may bulge into the calyces and pelves, and eventually may fungate through the walls of the collecting system even to extend into the ureter. One of the striking characteristics of this tumor is its tendency (over one-half) to **invade the renal vein and grow as a solid column of cells within this vessel.** Further extension of this growth may produce a continuous cord of tumor in the inferior vena cava and even into the right side of the heart. Yet despite this intravascular growth, discrete metastases may not be evident. Occasionally, the

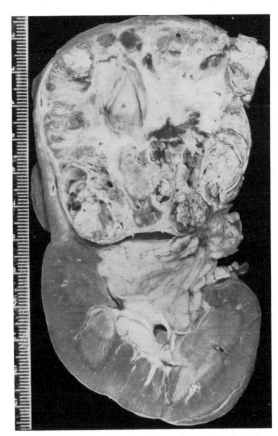

Figure 24–50. Renal cell carcinoma. Typical cross section of spherical neoplasm in one pole of kidney. Note necroses and hemorrhages in the tumor.

tumor grows through the capsule to invade the adrenal and perinephric fat.

Formerly, it was the practice to divide renal cell carcinomas into a variety of histologic types based upon the degree of vacuolation of the cells and their patterns of arrangement, i.e., papillary, glandular, tubular and undifferentiated. **In any single tumor, all variations in cytologic patterns of growth may be present.** The subdivision of these neoplasms, then, into histologic patterns is at best arbitrary, and all have equal clinical significance. On the one extreme, the cells may resemble cuboidal tubular epithelium having round, small regular nuclei with granular pink cytoplasm and great regularity and constancy of the cytologic detail. Such so-called **solid cell tumors** may at times have more anaplasia with variation in cell size, the formation of giant tumor cells with irregular, multilobate or multiple nuclei, numerous mitotic figures, both typical and atypical, and an undifferentiated growth pattern (Fig. 24–51).

On the other extreme from the solid cells are the so-called **clear cells** with complete vacuolation of the cytoplasm so that only distinct cell membranes

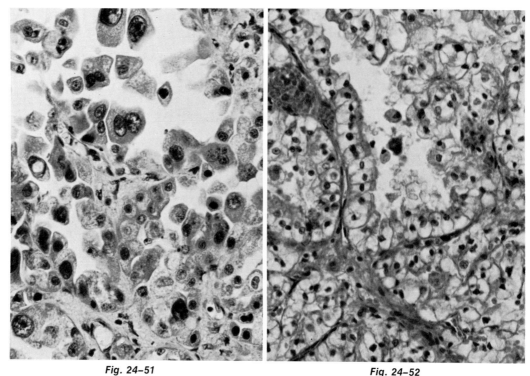

Fig. 24–51.   *Fig. 24–52.*

Figure 24–51.   *Renal cell carcinoma. Solid cell anaplastic variant.*
Figure 24–52.   *Renal cell carcinoma. The pathognomonic clear cell type.*

are preserved which demarcate the outer limits of the cell. The nuclei are usually pushed basally and are small and somewhat pyknotic. These cells are heavily laden with lipids. **This form of cytology is quite distinctive of renal cell carcinomas and virtually permits the identification of a metastasis wherever it is located** (Fig. 24–52). Between the extremes of solid cells and cleared cell forms, all intergradations may be found. Most tumors demonstrate many of these variants, but almost invariably in some foci the clear cell growth can be identified. As was mentioned, these cells are arranged in masses, cords, glands, papillae and, occasionally, as a lining to small cystic spaces. The stroma is usually scanty, but highly vascularized. Hemorrhages, scars, blood pigment and calcification are common additional histologic features.

Clinical Course. The three classic diagnostic features of *hypernephroid carcinoma are costovertebral pain, palpable mass* and *hematuria* (Creevy, 1935). However, in any single case, any or all of these features may be absent. Perhaps the most reliable of the three is hematuria, present eventually in about 90 per cent of the cases. In certain cases, the tumor may remain silent locally and only give rise to generalized constitutional symptoms, such as fever, malaise, weakness and weight loss. This

pattern of silent, asymptomatic growth occurs in many patients so that, at the time of discovery, the tumor may have reached a diameter of over 10 cm.

One of the common characteristics of this tumor is its *tendency to metastasize widely before giving rise to any local symptoms or signs.* It is not uncommon for metastases to be discovered before the primary is detected. The histologic pattern of the excised lesion may disclose that it is, in reality, a metastatic site of latent renal carcinoma. The most common locations of metastasis are the lungs (over 50 per cent) and bones (33 per cent), followed in order by the regional lymph nodes, liver and adrenals and brain. In approximately 10 to 15 per cent of the cases, the primary tumor metastasizes across the midline to the opposite kidney. In addition to these favored sites, renal cell carcinoma has been described as having metastasized to virtually every organ and every site in the body, sometimes to such uncommon locations as the eye and vagina.

These tumors pursue some of the most bizarre growth behaviors in the realm of neoplasia. Sudden explosive growth with widespread metastasis is matched by slow, silent, asymptomatic growth for years. In a number of cases, solitary metastases have occurred so that removal of the metastasis and the primary tumor has produced a cure. In still other instances, the metastases have mysteriously appeared in patients who have had nephrectomies 10 to 20 years prior to the discovery of the metastatic focus. For these reasons, *renal cell carcinoma is classified as one of the great mimics in medicine, having been confused at one time or another with almost every disease.*

The average five-year survival rate following surgery is not more than 35 per cent. When the tumor is confined to the kidney, the five-year survival is about 50 per cent. With renal vein invasion or extension into the perinephric fat, this figure is reduced to approximately 5 to 10 per cent. Better results have been reported by Robson et al. (1968) with radical surgery.

Wilms' Tumor (Embryoma, Embryonal Mixed Tumor, Carcinosarcoma). These tumors, while somewhat uncommon in adults, are the second most common visceral tumor in children under the age of 10, preceded in importance in this age group only by neuroblastomas (Klapproth, 1959). These tumors make up about one-fourth of malignant neoplasms in children, and about 65 per cent occur in those under three years of age. Because they contain a variety of cell and tissue components, they are closely allied to the teratomas. However, all the various elements are derived from one single germ layer—the mesoderm—rather than from the three primitive germ layers. This heterogeneous growth pattern has produced much speculation as to the possible origin of such growths. The present consensus maintains that the various elements all arise from the primitive renal blastema, which differentiates into all possible lines of mesenchymal development.

Grossly, these tumors are generally large, expansile, spherical masses which totally dwarf the kidney. In certain cases, **they may grow so large as to produce distention of the abdomen and a readily observable mass on casual inspection.** In a child, one is reported to have achieved the weight of 30 pounds! They are usually unilateral but, in 7 to 10 per cent of the cases, bilateral tumors are encountered. On section, these tumors have a very variegated surface dependent upon the tissue types produced. Myxomatous, soft, fish-flesh areas, solid gray, hyaline cartilaginous tissue and areas of hemorrhagic necrosis are the common components. The aggressive nature of these neoplasms is manifested by their propensity to rupture through the renal capsule and extend locally into the perirenal tissues. Sometimes they invade the mesentery of the bowel. Although they may invade the adrenal, more

often they tend to push it ahead of the advancing neoplasm. Involvement of the other kidney occurs in about 20 per cent of the cases.

Histologically, the characteristic features are primitive or abortive glomeruli with apparent or poorly formed Bowman spaces, and abortive tubules enclosed within a spindle cell stroma (Fig. 24–53). This combination of mesenchymal spindle cells and tubules has led to these tumors being called adenosarcomas and carcinosarcomas. In addition, **striated muscle,** smooth muscle, collagenous fibrous tissue, cartilage, bone, fat cells and areas of necrotic tissue containing cholesterol crystals and lipid macrophages may all be seen. The most consistent of these various elements are the striated muscle cells. The ultimate histologic diagnosis rests upon the identification of the primitive organoid structures of the glomeruli and tubules as well as the strongly supportive evidence of striated muscle fibers.

Most children with these neoplasms present with a large abdominal mass which may be unilateral or, when very large, may extend across the midline and down into the pelvis. Hematuria, pain in the abdomen following some hemorrhagic incident, intestinal obstruction and the appearance of hypertension are other patterns of presentation. In a considerable number of these patients, pulmo-

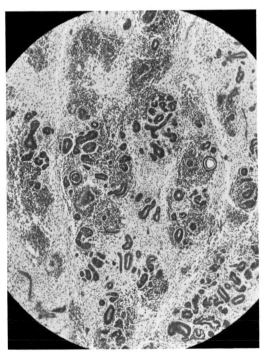

Figure 24–53. Wilms' tumor, illustrating tubule formation and abortive glomeruli in a loose fibrous stroma.

nary metastases are present at the time of the primary diagnosis.

Up to the recent past, the five-year survival of these patients was tragically low (10 to 40 per cent), a tragedy rendered the more poignant because of the age of the patients. However, it has recently been discovered that the combined use of chemotherapy, radiotherapy and surgery may produce remarkable results. At the Children's Hospital in Boston, if these tumors are available for primary treatment with the three modalities mentioned, there is over a 90 per cent two-year survival (unpublished communication). These results are all the more remarkable since in many of these patients pulmonary metastases, unquestionably present by x-ray, miraculously melted away under the therapeutic regimen. When metastases occur in other sites, such as the brain, bone and liver, the results of treatment are far less successful and only about one-third of the patients survive two years. In some instances, after primary treatment had apparently eradicated all existing neoplasia including pulmonary metastases, recurrence of the neoplasm as long as five to eight years later was still successfully controlled by chemotherapy and radiotherapy. The lesson to be learned from these cases is that an aggressive therapeutic attitude must be maintained despite recurrences, because long survivals can be effected with present-day methods of treatment.

Tumors of the Renal Pelvis. Approximately 5 to 10 per cent of primary renal tumors occur in the renal pelvis. These tumors span the range from apparently benign papillomas to frank papillary carcinomas but, as with bladder papillomas, these lesions tend to recur and all these tumors are best considered as low-grade cancers.

Renal pelvic tumors usually become clinically apparent within a relatively short time because they lie within the pelvis and, by fragmentation, produce noticeable hematuria (Higgins, 1939). They are almost invariably small when discovered (Fig. 24–54). These tumors are almost never palpable clinically; however, they may block the urinary outflow and lead to palpable hydronephrosis. Pain is rarely present. Pelvic tumors are the exact counterpart of those found in the urinary bladder and, for further detail, reference should be made to this section (p. 1160).

Infiltration of the wall of the pelvis and calyces is common, and renal vein involvement likewise occurs. For this reason, despite their apparent small, deceptively benign appearance, the prognosis of these tumors is not

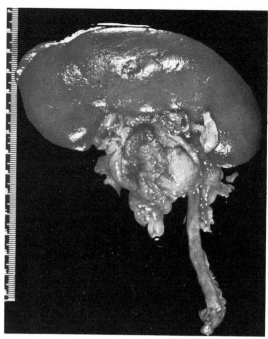

Figure 24–54. *Squamous cell carcinoma of the renal pelvis. The pelvis has been opened to expose the nodular irregular neoplasm.*

good. Less than 10 per cent of the patients survive five years, despite what appears to be adequate surgical removal, which usually implies nephrectomy. Again their similarity to bladder tumors is emphasized by the fact that apparently histologically benign tumors may recur.

Miscellaneous. A variety of sarcomas may arise in the kidney from the various connective tissue elements found in this organ. These are all extraordinarily rare and resemble their prototypes in all other organs.

Metastatic Tumors. The kidney, because of its large volume of blood flow, is frequently the site of metastatic tumor growth of both carcinomas and sarcomas arising in other organs of the body. The only specific malignancy which tends to selectively metastasize to the kidney is a primary neoplasm in the other kidney. The mechanism for such across-the-midline spread is still obscure, but it may occur by way of the lymphatic drainage to the para-aortic nodes and thence retrogradely across to the opposite kidney.

REFERENCES

Alderman, M. H., and Freedman, L. R.: Experimental pyelonephritis. X. The direct injection of E. coli protoplasts into the medulla of the rabbit kidney. Yale J. Biol. Med., 36:157, 1963.
Andersen, B. R., and Jackson, G. G.; Pyelitis: an important factor in the pathogenesis of retrograde pyelonephritis. J. Exp. Med., 114:375, 1961.

Angell, M. E., et al.: "Active" chronic pyelonephritis without evidence of bacterial infection. New Eng. J. Med., *278*:1303, 1968.

Aoki, S., et al.: "Abacterial" and bacterial nephritis. Immunofluorescent localization of bacterial antigen. New Eng. J. Med., *281*:1375, 1969.

Arakawa, M.: A scanning electron microscopy of the glomerulus of normal and nephrotic rats. Lab. Invest., *23*:489, 1970.

Asscher, A. W., et al.: Urine as medium for bacterial growth. Lancet, *2*:1037, 1966.

Bailey, G. L., et al.: Uremic pericarditis: clinical features and management. Circulation, *38*:582, 1968.

Balsløv, J. T., and Jørgensen, H. E.: A survey of 499 patients with acute anuric renal insufficiency. Causes, treatment, complications and mortality. Amer. J. Med., *34*:753, 1963.

Baxter, J. H., and Goodman, H. C.: Nephrotoxic serum nephritis in rats. I. Distribution and specificity of the antigen responsible for the production of nephrotoxic antibodies. J. Exp. Med., *104*:467, 1956.

Beeson, P. B.: Factors in the pathogenesis of pyelonephritis. Yale J. Biol. Med., *28*:81, 1955.

Beeson, P. B., and Rowley, D.: The anticomplementary effect of kidney tissue: its association with ammonia production. J. Exp. Med., *110*:685, 1959.

Bell, E. T.: Cystic disease of the kidneys. Amer. J. Path., *11*:373, 1935.

Bell, E. T.: Renal calculi. In Bell, E. T. (ed.): Renal Diseases. Philadelphia, Lea & Febiger, 1950, p. 414.

Benacerraf, B., et al.: The pathologic effects of intravenously administered soluble antigen-antibody complexes. II. Acute glomerulonephritis in rats. J. Exp. Med., *85*:571, 1947.

Berger, J.: IgA deposits in renal disease. Transplant. Proc., *1*:939, 1969.

Berson, S. A., and Yalow, R. S.: Parathyroid hormone in plasma in adenomatous hyperparathyroidism, uremia and bronchogenic carcinoma. Science, *154*:907, 1966.

Black, D. A. K., et al.: Controlled trial of prednisone in adult patients with the nephrotic syndrome. Brit. Med. J., *3*:421, 1970.

Bokisch, V. A., et al.: Isolation of a fragment (C3a) of the third component of human complement containing anaphylotoxin and chemotactic activity and description of an anaphylotoxin inactivator of human serum. J. Exp. Med., *129*:1109, 1969.

Boyce, W. H.: Organic matrix of human urinary concretions. Amer. J. Med., *45*:673, 1968.

Bryant, R. E., et al.: Effect of osmolalities comparable to those of the renal medulla on function of human polymorphonuclear leukocytes. J. Infect. Dis., *126*:1, 1972.

Burkholder, P. M., et al.: Mixed membranous and proliferative glomerulonephritis: a collative light, immunofluorescence and electron microscopic study. Lab. Invest., *23*:459, 1970.

Burry, A. F., et al.: Phanacetin and renal papillary necrosis: results of a prospective autopsy investigation. Med. J. Aust., *1*:817, 1966.

Cameron, J. S.: Glomerulonephritis. Brit. Med. J., *4*:285, 1970.

Cameron, J. S., et al.: Membrane proliferative glomerulonephritis and persistent hypocomplementaemia. Brit. Med. J., *4*:7, 1970.

Carpenter, C. C. J., et al.: Relation of renin, angiotensin II, and experimental renal hypertension to aldosterone secretion. J. Clin. Invest., *40*:2026, 1961.

Chervony, A. M., et al.: Bilateral renal cortical necrosis, malignant hypertension, probable pituitary insufficiency with survival. Amer. J. Med., *39*:147, 1965.

Churg, J., et al.: Pathology of the nephrotic syndrome in children: a report for the International Study of Kidney Disease in Children. Lancet, *1*:1299, 1970.

Clay, R. D., et al.: The nature of the renal lesion in the Fanconi syndrome. J. Path. Bact., *65*:551, 1953.

Cobbs, C. G., and Kay, E. D.: Antibacterial mechanisms in the urinary bladder. Yale J. Biol. Med., *40*:93, 1967.

Cochrane, C. G.: Mediation of immunologic glomerular injury. Transplant. Proc., *1*:949, 1969.

Cochrane, C. G.: Studies on the localization of circulating antigen-antibody complexes and other macromolecules in vessels. II. Pathogenetic and pharmacodynamic studies. J. Exp. Med., *118*:503, 1963.

Cochrane, C. G., et al.: A role of polymorphonuclear leukocytes and complement in nephrotoxic nephritis. J. Exp. Med., *122*:99, 1965.

Combes, B., et al.: Glomerular nephritis with deposition of Australia antigen-antibody complexes in glomerular basement membrane. Lancet, *2*:234, 1971.

Comerford, F. R., and Cohen, A. S.: The nephropathy of systemic lupus erythematosus: an assessment by clinical, light and electron microscopic criteria. Medicine, *46*:425, 1967.

Cotran, R. S.: Personal communication, 1972.

Cotran, R. S.: The renal lesion in chronic pyelonephritis: immunofluorescent and ultrastructural studies. J. Infect. Dis., *120*:109, 1969.

Cotran, R. S.: Retrograde proteus pyelonephritis in rats: localization of antigen and antibody in treated sterile pyelonephritic kidneys. J. Exp. Med., *117*:813, 1963.

Creevy, C.: Confusing clinical manifestations of malignant renal neoplasms. Arch. Intern. Med., *55*:894, 1935.

Dixon, F. J.: The pathogenesis of glomerulonephritis. Amer. J. Med., *44*:493, 1968.

Dixon, F. J., et al.: Experimental glomerulonephritis: the pathogenesis of a laboratory model resembling the spectrum of human glomerulonephritis. J. Exp. Med., *113*:899, 1961.

Dodge, W. F., et al.: Poststreptococcal glomerulonephritis. A prospective study in children. New Eng. J. Med., *286*:273, 1972.

Dodge, W. F., et al.: The relationship between the clinical and pathological features of poststreptococcal glomerulonephritis: a study of the early natural history. Medicine, *47*:227, 1968.

Drummond, K. N., et al.: The nephrotic syndrome of childhood. Immunologic, clinical and pathologic correlations. J. Clin. Invest., *45*:620, 1966.

Ehrenreich, T., and Churg, J.: Pathology of membranous nephropathy. In Sommers, S. C. (ed.): Pathology Annual. New York, Appleton-Century-Crofts, 1968, p. 145.

Eknoyan, G., et al.: Platelet function in renal failure. New Eng. J. Med., *280*:677, 1969.

Ellis, H. A., and Walton, K. W.: Variations in the serum complement in the nephrotic syndrome and other forms of renal disease. Immunology, *1*:234, 1958.

Eschbach, J. W.: Erythropoiesis in patients with renal failure undergoing chronic dialysis. New Eng. J. Med., *276*:653, 1967.

Feldman, B. H.: Local immunomechanism of the urinary tract. Invest. Urol., *8*:575, 1971.

Fisher, E. R., et al.: Experimental renal vein constriction. Its relation to renal lesions observed in human renal vein thrombosis and nephrotic syndrome. Lab. Invest., *18*:689, 1968.

Franklin, W. A., et al.: The hemolytic-uremic syndrome. Arch. Path., *94*:230, 1972.

Freedman, L. R.: Chronic pyelonephritis at autopsy. Ann. Intern. Med., *66*:697, 1967.

Gault, M. H., et al.: Syndrome associated with the abuse of analgesics. Ann. Intern. Med., *68*:906, 1968.

Gianantonia, C. A., et al.: The hemolytic uremic syndrome. J. Pediat., *64*:478, 1964.

Gianantonia, C. A., et al.: The hemolytic uremic syndrome. J. Pediat., *72*:757, 1968.

Gibson, D. G.: Hemodynamic factors in the development of acute pulmonary oedema in renal failure. Lancet, *2*:1217, 1966.

Giovannetti, S., et al.: Uraemic symptoms in dogs chronically intoxicated with methylguanidine. Presented at the 4th International Congress of Nephrology, Stockholm, June 22, 1969, p. 43.

Goldblatt, H.: The Renal Origin of Hypertension. Springfield, Ill., Charles C Thomas, 1948.

Goldblatt, H.: Studies on experimental hypertension. V. The pathogenesis of experimental hypertension due to renal ischemia. Ann. Intern. Med., *11*:69, 1937.

Goldblatt, H., et al.: Studies in experimental hypertension. I. The production of persistent elevation of systolic blood pressure by means of renal ischemia. J. Exp. Med., *59*:347, 1934.

Goodpasture, E. W.: The significance of certain pulmonary lesions in relation to the etiology of influenza. Amer. J. Med. Sci., *158*:863, 1919.

Grabstald, H.: Renal cell cancer. I. Incidence, etiology, natural history and prognosis. II. Diagnostic findings. III. Types of treatment. New York J. Med., *64*:2539, 2658, 2771, 1964.

Grollman, A., et al.: Role of the kidney in pathogenesis of hypertension as determined by a study of the effects of bilateral nephrectomy and other experimental procedures on the blood pressure of the dog. Amer. J. Physiol., *157*:21, 1949.

Guze, L. B., and Beeson, P. B.: Experimental pyelonephritis. I. Effect of ureteral ligation on the course of bacterial infection in the kidney of the rat. J. Exp. Med., *104*:803, 1956.

Habib, R., and Kleinknecht, C.: The primary nephrotic syndrome of childhood. Classification and clinical pathologic study of 406 cases. Sommers, S. C. (ed.): Pathology Annual. New York, Appleton-Century-Crofts, 1971, p. 414.

Hammer, D. K., and Dixon, F. J.: Experimental glomerulonephritis. II. Immunologic events in the pathogenesis of nephrotoxic serum nephritis in rats. J. Exp. Med., *117*:19, 1963.

Hand, W. L., et al.: The antibacterial effect of normal and infected urinary bladder. J. Lab. Clin. Med., *77*:605, 1971.

Hanley, H. G.: Hydronephrosis. Lancet, *2*:664, 1960.

Hayslett, J. P., et al.: Focal glomerulitis due to penicillamine. Lab. Invest., *19*:376, 1968.

Hayslett, J. P., et al.: Progression of "lipoid nephrosis" to renal insufficiency. New Eng. J. Med., *281*:181, 1969.

Henkin, R. I., et al.: Evidence for the presence of substances toxic for HeLa cells in the serum and in the dialysis fluid of patients with glomerulonephritis. J. Lab. Clin. Med., *64*:79, 1964.

Heptinstall, R. H.: Focal glomerulonephritis. Pathology of the Kidney. Boston, Little, Brown & Co., 1966, p. 315.

Heptinstall, R. H.: The limitations of the pathological diagnosis of chronic pyelonephritis. In Black, D. A. K. (ed.): Renal Disease. 2nd ed. New York, Blackwell Scientific Publications, Oxford Press, 1967, p. 350.

Heptinstall, R. H., and Farmer, E. R.: Chronic-nonobstructive pyelonephritis: a reappraisal. In Kincaid-Smith, P., and Fairley, K. F. (eds.): Renal Infection and Renal Scarring. Proceedings of an International Symposium on Pyelonephritis, Vesico-ureteric Reflux, and Renal Papillary Necrosis. Melbourne, Australia, Mercedes Pub. Serv., 1970, p. 233.

Hickler, R. B., et al.: Vasodepressor lipid from the renal medulla. Canad. Med. Ass. J., *90*:280, 1964.

Higgins, C. C.: Squamous cell carcinoma of the pelvis. Arch. Surg., *38*:224, 1939.

Hinman, F., and Morison, D. M.: Experimental hydronephrosis. Surg. Gynec. Obstet., *42*:209, 1926.

Hodson, C. J.: The effects of disturbance of flow in the kidney. J. Infect. Dis., *120*:54, 1969.

Hodson, C. J.: The radiological diagnosis of pyelonephritis. Proc. Roy. Soc. Med., *52*:669, 1959.

Hollenberg, N. K., et al.: Irreversible acute oliguric renal failure. A complication of methoxyflurane anesthesia. New Eng. J. Med., *286*:877, 1972.

Hooper, R. G., et al.: Xanthogranulomatous pyelonephritis. J. Urol., *88*:585, 1962.

Hopper, J., et al.: Lipoid nephrosis in 31 adult patients. Renal biopsy study by light, electron and fluorescent microscopy with experience in treatment. Medicine, *49*:321, 1970.

Hoyer, J. R., et al.: Recurrence of idiopathic nephrotic syndrome after renal transplantation. Lancet, *2*:773, 1972.

Jones, D. B.: Nephrotic glomerulonephritis. Amer. J. Path., *33*:313, 1957.

Kass, E. H.: Asymptomatic infections of the urinary tract. Trans. Ass. Amer. Physicians, *69*:56, 1956.

Kaufman, D. B., et al.: Diffuse familial nephropathy. J. Pediat., *77*:37, 1970.

Kessner, D. M., and Lepper, M. H.: Epidemiologic studies of gram-negative bacilli in the hospital and community. Amer. J. Epidem., *85*:45, 1967.

Kimmelstiel, P.: The nature of chronic pyelonephritis. Geriatrics, *19*:145, 1964.

Kimmelstiel, P., and Wilson, C.: Benign and malignant hypertension and nephrosclerosis. Amer. J. Path., *12*:45, 1936.

Kincaid-Smith, P., et al.: Analgesic nephropathy: a recoverable form of chronic renal failure. In Kincaid-Smith, P., and Fairley, K. F. (eds.): Renal Infection and Renal Scarring. Proceedings of an International Symposium on Pyelonephritis, Vesico-ureteric Reflux and Renal Papillary Necrosis. Melbourne, Australia, Mercedes Pub. Serv., 1970, p. 385.

Klapproth, H. H.: Wilms' tumor: a report of 45 cases and an analysis of 1,351. J. Urol., *98*:566, 1959.

Kleeman, C. R., et al.: Divalent ion metabolism and osteodystrophy in chronic renal failure. Yale J. Biol. Med., *40*:1, 1967.

Kleeman, C. R., et al.: Pyelonephritis. Medicine, *39*:3, 1960.

Koffler, D., et al.: Immunologic studies concerning the pulmonary lesions in Goodpasture's syndrome. Amer. J. Path., *54*:293, 1969.

Kondo, Y., et al.: Cellular aspects of rabbit Masugi nephritis. II. Progressive glomerular injuries with crescent formation. Lab. Invest., *27*:620, 1972.

Kunin, C. M.: Epidemiology of bacteriuria and its relation to pyelonephritis. J. Infect. Dis., *120*:1, 1969.

Kunin, C. M.: The natural history of recurrent bacteriuria in schoolgirls. In Kincaid-Smith, P., and Fairley, K. F. (eds.): Renal Infection and Renal Scarring. Proceedings of an International Symposium on Pyelonephritis, Vesico-Ureteric Reflux and Renal Papillary Necrosis. Melbourne, Australia, Mercedes Pub. Serv., 1970, p. 3.

Kunin, C. M.: The quantitative significance of bacteria visualized in the unstained urinary sediment. New Eng. J. Med., *265*:589, 1961.

Lancaster, M. G., and Allison, F., Jr.: Studies on the pathogenesis of acute inflammation. VII. The influence of osmolality upon the phagocytic and clumping activity of human leukocytes. Amer. J. Path., *49*:1185, 1966.

Leonard, C. D., et al.: Acute glomerulonephritis with prolonged oliguria. Ann. Intern. Med., *73*:703, 1970.

Lewis, E. J., and Couser, W. G.: The immunologic basis of human renal disease. Ped. Clin. N. Amer., *18*:467, 1971.

Lewis, E. J., et al.: Gamma G globulin subgroup composition of the glomerular deposits in human renal diseases. J. Clin. Invest., *49*:1103, 1970.

Lewis, E. J., et al.: Immunopathologic study of rapidly progressive glomerulonephritis. Hum. Path., *2*:185, 1971*a*.

Lewis, E. J., et al.: Serum component levels in human glomerulonephritis. Ann. Intern. Med., *75*:555, 1971*b*.

Lichtenstein, L., and Jaffe, H. L.: Multiple myeloma: a survey based on 35 cases, 18 of which came to autopsy. Arch. Path., *44*:207, 1947.

Linton, A. L., et al.: Microangiopathic hemolytic anemia and the pathogenesis of malignant hypertension. Lancet, *1*:1277, 1969.

Mallory, G. K., et al.: Pathology of acute and healed pyelonephritis. Arch. Path., *30*:330, 1940.

Markowitz, A. S.: Streptococcal-related glomerulonephritis in the rhesus monkey. Transplant. Proc., *1*:985, 1969.

Masugi, M.: Über die experimentelle Glomerulonephritis durch das spezifische Antinierenserum. Bietr. Path. Anat., *92*:429, 1934.

Mattern, W. D.: Oliguric acute renal failure in malignant hypertension. Amer. J. Med., *52*:187, 1972.

McCluskey, R. T.: Evidence for immunologic mechanisms in several forms of human renal disease. Bull. N.Y. Acad. Med., *46*:769, 1970.

McCluskey, R. T., and Baldwin, D. S.: Natural history of acute glomerulonephritis. Amer. J. Med., *35*:213, 1963.

McCluskey, R. T., et al.: An immunofluorescent study of the pathogenic mechanisms in glomerular diseases. New Eng. J. Med., *274*:695, 1966.

McCluskey, R. T., et al.: Passive acute glomerulonephritis induced by antigen-antibody complexes solubilized in excess. Proc. Soc. Exp. Biol. Med., *111*:764, 1962.

McIntosh, R. M., et al.: Glomerular localization of fibrinogen: clinical, pathologic, prognostic and therapeutic considerations. J. Chron. Dis., *24*:787, 1971.

McKay, D. G.: Disseminated Intravascular Coagulation: An Intermediary Mechanism of Disease. New York, Harper & Row, 1965, p. 175.

Merrill, J. T., et al.: Observations on the role of urea in uremia. Amer. J. Med., *14*:519, 1953.

Merrill, J. T., and Hampers, C. L.: Uremia. New Eng. J. Med., *282*:953, 1014, 1970.

Mond, N. C., et al.: Study of childhood urinary tract infection in general practice. Brit. Med. J., *1*:602, 1970.

Muirhead, E. E., et al.: Lapine renomedullary lipid in murine hypertension. Arch. Path., *85*:72, 1968.

Nanra, R. S., et al.: Renal papillary necrosis in rats produced by aspirin, A.P.C. and other analgesics. In Kincaid-Smith, P., and Fairley, K. F. (eds.): Renal Infection and Renal Scarring. Proceedings of an International Symposium on Pyelonephritis, Vesico-ureteric Reflux and Renal Papillary Necrosis. Melbourne, Australia, Mercedes Pub. Serv., 1970, p. 347.

Norden, C. W., and Kass, E. H.: Bacteriuria of pregnancy: a critical appraisal. Ann. Rev. Med., 19:431, 1968.

Oliver, J.: New direction in renal morphology: method, its result and its future. Harvey Lect., 40:102, 1944–45.

Oliver, J., et al.: The pathogenesis of acute renal failure associated with traumatic and toxic injury, renal ischemia, nephrotoxic damage and the ischemuric episode. J. Clin. Invest., 30:1307, 1951.

Oliver, J., et al.: The renal lesions of electrolyte imbalance. J. Exp. Med., 106:563, 1957.

Osathanondh, V., and Potter, E. L.: Development of human kidney as shown by microdissection. I. Preparation of tissue with reasons for possible misinterpretation of observations. II. Renal pelvis calyces and papillae. III. Formation and interrelationship of collecting tubules and nephrons. Arch. Path., 76:271, 277, 290, 1963.

Osathanondh, V., and Potter, E. L.: Pathogenesis of polycystic kidneys. Type I due to hyperplasia of interstitial portions and collecting tubules. Type II due to inhibition of ampullary activity. Type III due to multiple abnormalities of development. Arch. Path., 77:466, 474, 485, 1964.

Osserman, E. F.: Plasma cell myeloma. II. Clinical aspects. New Eng. J. Med., 261:1006, 1959.

Perkoff, G. T., et al.: A follow-up study of hereditary chronic nephritis. Arch. Intern. Med., 102:733, 1958.

Pincus, T., et al.: Experimental chronic glomerulitis. J. Exp. Med., 127:819, 1968.

Pollak, V. E., and Pirani, C. L.: Renal histologic findings in systemic lupus erythematosus. Mayo Clin. Proc., 44:630, 1969.

Pometta, D., et al.: Asymptomatic bacteriuria in diabetes mellitus. New Eng. J. Med., 276:1118, 1967.

Prescott, L. F.: The absorption, metabolism, excretion and CNS effects of phenacetin. In Kincaid-Smith, P., and Fairley, K. S. (eds.): Renal Infection and Renal Scarring. Proceedings of an International Symposium on Pyelonephritis, Vesico-ureteric Reflux, and Renal Papillary Necrosis. Melbourne, Australia, Mercedes Pub. Serv., 1970, p. 359.

Prien, E. L., and Prien, E. L., Jr.: Composition and structure of urinary stones. Amer. J. Med., 45:654, 1968.

Proskey, A. J., et al.: Goodpasture's syndrome (a report of 5 cases and review of the literature). Amer. J. Med., 48:162, 1970.

Rastogi, S. P., et al.: Idiopathic membranous glomerulonephritis in adults. Remission following steroid therapy. Quart. J. Med., 38:335, 1969.

Relman, A. S.: The acidosis of renal disease. Amer. J. Med., 44:706, 1968.

Relman, A. S., and Schwartz, W. B.: The kidney in potassium depletion. Amer. J. Med., 24:764, 1958.

Report of "The Committee on Chronic Dialysis" ("Gottschalk" Report), September 1967.

Resnick, M., et al.: Genetic predisposition to formation of calcium oxalate renal calculi. New Eng. J. Med., 278:1313, 1968.

Richardson, J. A., et al.: Kidney transplantation for rapidly progressive glomerulonephritis. Lancet, 2:180, 1970.

Riches, E. W., et al.: New growths of kidney and ureter. Brit. J. Urol., 23:297, 1951.

Robbins, S. L., et al.: Necrotizing renal papillitis: a form of acute pyelonephritis. New Eng. J. Med., 235:885, 1946.

Robson, C. J., et al.: The results of radical nephrectomy for renal carcinoma. Trans. Amer. Ass. Genitourin. Surg., 60:122, 1968.

Rosen, S.: Membranous glomerulonephritis. Current status. Hum. Path., 2:209, 1971.

Rosenheim, M. L.: Problems of chronic pyelonephritis. Brit. Med. J., 1:1433, 1963.

Schainuck, L. I., et al.: Structural-functional correlations in renal disease. II. The correlations. Hum. Path., 1:631, 1970.

Seymour, A. E., et al.: Contributions of renal biopsy studies to the understanding of disease. Amer. J. Path., 65:550, 1971.

Sheehan, H. L., and Davis, J. C.: Complete renal ischemia. J. Path. Bact., 76:569, 1958.

Sheehan, H. L., and Davis, J. C.: Experimental hydronephrosis. Arch. Path., 68:185, 1959a.

Sheehan, H. L., and Davis, J. C.: Patchy permanent renal ischemia. J. Path. Bact., 77:33, 1959b.

Siegel, R. R.: The basis of pulmonary disease resolution after nephrectomy in Goodpasture's syndrome. Amer. J. Med. Sci., 259:201, 1970.

Smeby, R. R., et al.: A naturally occurring renin inhibitor. Circ. Res., Suppl. II, 21:129, 1967.

Solway, H. M.: Renal tumors: review of 130 cases. J. Urol., 40:477, 1938.

Spence, H. M., et al.: Cystic diseases of the kidney: classification, diagnosis and treatment. J.A.M.A., 163:1466, 1957.

Spiro, D., et al.: The cellular pathology of experimental hypertension. I. Hyperplastic arteriolar sclerosis. Amer. J. Path., 47:19, 1965.

Spuhler, O., and Zollinger, H. V.: Die chronisch-interstitielle nephritis. Z. Klin. Med., 151:1, 1953.

Steblay, R. W.: Glomerulonephritis induced in sheep by injections of heterologous glomerular basement membrane and Freund's complete adjuvant. J. Exp. Med., 116:253, 1962.

Treser, G., et al.: Partial characterization of antigenic streptococcal plasma membrane components in acute glomerulonephritis. J. Clin. Invest., 49:762, 1970.

Trueta, J., et al.: Studies of the Renal Circulation. Springfield, Ill., Charles C Thomas, 1947.

Tu, W. H., et al.: Acute diffuse glomerulonephritis in acute streptococcal endocarditis. Ann. Intern. Med., 71:335, 1969.

Vander, A. J.: Control of renin release. Physiol. Rev., 47:359, 1967.

Vassalli, P., and McCluskey, R. T.: The pathogenic role of fibrin deposition in immunologically induced glomerulonephritis. Ann. N.Y. Acad. Sci., 116:1052, 1964.

Vejlsgaard, R.: Bacteriuria in patients with diabetes mellitus (a controlled study). In Kass, E. H. (ed.): Progress in Pyelonephritis. Philadelphia, F. A. Davis Co., 1965, p. 478.

Vivaldi, E., et al.: Ascending infection as a mechanism in the pathogenesis of experimental non-obstructive pyelonephritis. Proc. Soc. Exp. Biol. Med., 102:242, 1959.

Ward, P. A., and Cochrane, C. G.: Bound complement and immunologic injury of blood vessels. J. Exp. Med., 121:215, 1965.

Weiner, J., et al.: The cellular pathology of experimental hypertension. II. Arteriolar hyalinosis and fibrinoid change. Amer. J. Path., 47:457, 1965.

Weiss, S., and Parker, F., Jr.: Pyelonephritis: its relation to vascular lesions and to arteriolar hypertension. Medicine, 18:221, 1939.

Welt, G.: Red cell sodium and uremia. Presented at the 4th International Congress of Nephrology, Stockholm, June 22, 1969, p. 46.

West, C. D., and McAdams, A. J.: Serum beta-1-C globulin levels in persistent glomerulonephritis with low serum complement. Variability unrelated to clinical course. Nephron, 7:193, 1970.

West, C. D., et al.: Hypocomplementemic and normocomplementemic persistent (chronic) glomerulonephritis. Clinical and pathologic characteristics. J. Pediat., 67:1089, 1965.

White, R. H. R., et al.: Clinical pathological study of nephrotic syndrome in children. Lancet, 1:1353, 1970.

Wolstenholme, G. E. W., and Knight, J. (eds.): The Balkan Nephropathy. Ciba Foundation Study Group No. 30. Boston, Little, Brown & Co., 1967.

25

THE LOWER
URINARY TRACT

URETER

NORMAL

The ureters arise as bud-like outgrowths from the mesonephric or wolffian ducts. These buds elongate to produce the long, definitive tubular structures found in the adult. They grow into the metanephric anlage which covers them in the form of a cap. Tubular projections from the blind end give rise to the collecting tubules. These eventually anastomose with the distal convoluted tubule of the renal nephron, and thus provide drainage for the functioning nephron. The genesis of the important renal disorder, polycystic kidney disease, is probably not due to failure of union of the collecting tubules of ureteric origin with the nephrons of metanephric origin.

In the normal adult of average size, the ureters are approximately 30 cm. in length and about 5 mm. in diameter. They lie throughout their course in a retroperitoneal position. As they enter the pelvis, they pass anterior to either the common iliac or external iliac artery. In the female pelvis, they lie close to the uterine arteries and are, therefore, vulnerable to injury in operations upon the female genital tract. There are three points of slight narrowing: at the ureteropelvic junction, where they enter the bladder and where they cross the iliac vessels.

On histologic section, they are composed of three distinct coats: an outer fibrous invest-ment; a thick muscular coat with the fibers traveling, for the most part, in a circular fashion but with, however, a less well developed longitudinal layer of muscle; and a lining mucosa of transitional epithelium (urothelium) resembling that which is found in the renal pelvis and bladder. This epithelium rests upon a well developed basement membrane. Active peristaltic waves propel urine through the ureters into the bladder. As the ureters enter the bladder, they pursue an oblique course, terminating in a slit-like orifice. This orifice is marked by a slight papilliform elevation in the floor of the bladder. The obliquity of this ureteral orifice permits the enclosing bladder musculature to act as a sphincteric valve, blocking the regurgitation of urine even in the presence of marked distention of the urinary bladder.

PATHOLOGY

As a generalization, the ureters are remarkably seldom affected by disease. The processes in which they become involved are most commonly primary in either the kidney or the bladder. Ureteral involvement, then, is usually overshadowed clinically and anatomically by the accompanying underlying disorders. The most important category of lesions to affect them falls under the heading of obstructive disease.

CONGENITAL ANOMALIES

Congenital anomalies of the ureters occur in about 2 or 3 per cent of all autopsies. They are, for the most part, of only incidental interest and have little clinical significance. Rarely, certain anomalies may contribute to obstruction to the flow of urine and thus cause clinical disease.

Double and Bifid Ureters. Double ureters (derived from a double or split ureteral bud) are almost invariably associated either with totally distinct double renal pelves or with the anomalous development of a very large kidney, having a partially bifid pelvis terminating in separate ureters. Double ureters may pursue separate courses to the bladder, but commonly are joined within the bladder wall and drain through a single ureteral orifice. Separate ureteral orifices into the bladder are extremely unusual. More commonly with a double origin, they unite at some midway point to create a Y-shaped structure. Division of a proximally single ureter in the pelvis into two ureters, forming essentially an inverted Y, is a very infrequent occurrence. These anomalies are completely consistent with adequate function, and have little clinical significance.

Aberrant Renal Vessels. Occasionally an aberrant vein, but more usually an artery, is found supplying the lower pole of the kidney. These aberrant vessels are derived from the major renal vessels or even from the aorta. When they cross anterior to the ureter, these vessels, particularly arteries, may compress the ureter usually at the ureteropelvic junction, causing obstruction and marked narrowing. *While these anomalies are not common, they nonetheless account for a large percentage of urinary tract obstructions at the ureteropelvic junction.* While similar aberrant vessels may sometimes traverse to the upper pole of the kidney, in these locations they do not affect the ureter.

Miscellaneous Congenital Anomalies. Congenital valves, narrowing or strictures, kinks and torsions of the ureters usually occur at the level of the ureteropelvic junction. Although infrequent, they may be important as causes of obstruction. *Diverticula,* saccular outpouchings of the ureteral wall are uncommon lesions. They appear as congenital or acquired defects and are of importance as pockets of stasis and secondary infection, Dilatation, elongation and tortuosity of the ureters *(hydroureter)* may occur as congenital anomalies or as acquired defects. Congenital hydroureter is thought to reflect some neurogenic defect in the innervation of the ureteral musculature. The acquired form is encountered when there is some low ureteral obstruction or in pregnancy. In the latter circumstance, pressure of the enlarged uterus and relaxation of the smooth muscle both contribute. Massive enlargement of the ureter is known as *megaloureter.* These anomalies are usually associated with some congenital defect of the kidney, particularly polycystic disease. While they are more frequently encountered in patients who die early in life from this associated renal disorder, they are sometimes found in adults with congenital polycystic kidney disease. Megaloureter may cause some functional impairment of urinary flow and thus may secondarily lead to dilatation of the renal collecting system.

INFLAMMATION

Ureteritis almost invariably develops secondary to infection elsewhere in the body, particularly in the kidneys or bladder. Only infrequently does such ureteritis make a significant contribution to the clinical problem and, therefore, these lesions are usually only of academic interest.

ACUTE NONSPECIFIC URETERITIS

Acute inflammatory involvement of the ureters occurs as a secondary complication of bacterial infection within the kidney or bladder. It occurs most often with pyelonephritis and acute or chronic cystitis. In both of these circumstances, it is assumed that the infection spreads through the urine; however, lymphatic or blood transmission cannot be ruled out. The causative organisms are those commonly associated with pyelonephritis and cystitis: i.e., coliform bacilli, staphylococci, enterococci and the gram-negative rods. Quite rarely, acute ureteritis may occur in the course of the systemic spread of infection from a focus elsewhere in the body.

The morphologic changes are usually quite minimal and consist of hyperplasia and granularity of the ureteral mucosa with a histologic reaction characteristic of acute inflammation. Most of the inflammatory changes are confined to the submucosal connective tissue. The overlying epithelium is only sometimes ulcerated in these acute conditions.

CHRONIC NONSPECIFIC URETERITIS

Persistence of infection or repeated acute exacerbations may give rise to chronic inflammatory changes within the ureters. The pathogenesis of this type of reaction is identical with that described under acute ureteritis, and the causative organisms are the same.

In the more usual form, the chronic inflammatory changes comprise reddening and granularity of the ureteral mucosa, both of which are more marked than those found in acute inflammation. Superficial ulcerations or areas of sloughing necrosis may be present in the more virulent infections and merit the designation of **ulcerative gangrenous ureteritis**. Noteworthy is the possible causation of gangrenous ureteritis by roentgen radiation of the abdomen and pelvis for the treatment of a malignancy.

Histologically, the reaction follows the pattern of all chronic inflammations, and consists of vascular congestion, fibroblastic activity and neutrophilic, lymphocytic, plasma cell and histiocytic infiltration chiefly in the submucosal tissues. The epithelium overlying these sites may have inflammatory metaplasia. Necrosis and sloughing of the mucosa are the cause of the grossly demonstrable ulcers. The chronic fibroblastic proliferations may at times produce some narrowing of the ureteral lumen and thickening of the wall, but rarely of sufficient magnitude to cause obstruction.

In certain cases of longstanding chronic ureteritis, specialized reaction patterns are sometimes observed. The accumulation or aggregation of lymphocytes in the subepithelial region may cause slight elevations of the mucosa and produce a fine granular mucosal surface **(ureteritis folicularis)**. At other times, the mucosa may become sprinkled with fine cysts varying in diameter from 1 to 5 mm. **(ureteritis cystica)**. Chronic pyelonephritis is the most common antecedent of this interesting lesion. Nests of epithelium become pinched off and buried in inflammatory reaction. These sequestered epithelial nests give rise to small submucosal cysts. These may increase in size slowly over the course of months or years. The process usually affects only the upper third of the ureter but, in more severe cases, may involve the lower regions. The cysts appear on the surface of the mucosa as small (0.1 to 0.5 cm.), clear, thin-walled (hemispheric) vesicles (Fig. 25–1). They may aggregate to form small grape-like clusters. When they are opened, clear serous or slightly viscid fluid escapes. Histologic sections through such cysts demonstrate a lining of modified transitional epithelium with some flattening of the superficial, tall, pyramidal cells. The epithelium undergoes progressive flattening as the cysts enlarge and, in very large cysts, the epithelium may consist of only a single layer of pavement cells, or the cells may become completely atrophic. The usual chronic inflammatory response surrounds the cystic areas.

Both follicular and cystic ureteritis are variants of nonspecific chronic ureteritis; these variants frequently coexist. Rarely, large cysts may obstruct the ureter.

TUBERCULOSIS

Tuberculous involvement of the ureters occurs commonly in cases of renal tuberculosis or tuberculosis of the urinary bladder. It usually takes the form of minute submucosal miliary lesions but, on occasion, these may coalesce to form larger caseous masses. In far advanced cases, tuberculous ulcers may develop. The tuberculous reaction is usually entirely overshadowed by the primary focus of infection, and does not contribute materially to the underlying disease.

TUMORS

Primary neoplasia of the ureter is very rare; the most common forms are malignant. Metastatic seeding from other primary lesions occurs much more often than primary growths.

BENIGN TUMORS

Small benign tumors of the ureter are very uncommon, but are generally of mesenchymal

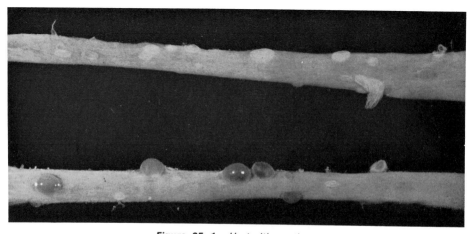

Figure 25–1. Ureteritis cystica.

origin. They include the usual variety of neoplasms derived from fibrous tissue, blood vessels, lymphatics and smooth muscle. These are almost invariably well encapsulated, submucosal nodules less than 1 cm. in diameter, which are rarely of sufficient size to cause obstruction of the ureteral lumen.

MALIGNANT TUMORS

The primary malignant tumors of the ureter follow the identical patterns described in the renal pelves and calyces. They are found most frequently during the fifth and sixth decades of life.

They are usually unilateral and single, and vary from **slender-stalked, delicately branched, friable papillomas to sessile ulcerative lesions**. They occur most often in the lower third of the ureter. The more malignant forms are the broad, sessile growths. Sometimes plaque-like, ulcerating, fungating lesions develop. The pedunculated papillomas are ordinarily less than 1 cm. in diameter. Frequently, numerous foci of hemorrhage are evident where small fragments have broken off. The larger sessile or ulcerating lesions cover a surface area 1 to 2 cm. in longest diameter, but occasionally they may cover greater lengths of the ureter.

The histology of these tumors follows a fairly regular pattern. The more benign forms are composed of well differentiated, easily recognizable transitional epithelium covering the slender connective tissue stalks of the papilloma (Riches et al., 1951). In fact, the covering of the papillary fronds in the very well differentiated tumors almost completely resembles the normal ureteral mucosa. However, from clinical experience, it has been amply demonstrated that even benign-appearing lesions have a great tendency to recur and become locally invasive and, therefore, all are considered in the category of cancers. With progression toward the malignant forms, the transitional epithelium becomes more anaplastic with loss of the usual stratified architecture. The cells vary in size and shape and have atypical nuclei and mitotic figures. Invasion of the stalk and piling up of cells are evident. In more malignant growths, there is usually a change in the transitional growth pattern to a stratified squamous type or epidermoid carcinoma. This is the histologic pattern most often found in the frankly ulcerating, fungating lesions. Invasion into the underlying ureteral wall and extension into the periureteral tissues occur in far advanced lesions. Metastases may occur in the regional nodes, liver, lungs, bone marrow or any other organ.

Ureteral tumors rarely grow to large size because they become clinically evident at a very early stage. By the papillary, fungating character of their growth, they are subject to constant trauma, fragmentation and hemorrhage. *Hematuria is an almost invariable clinical finding from the onset of the neoplastic growth*. If this presenting feature is ignored by the patient, the tumor may increase to sufficient size to produce urinary tract obstruction or to metastasize. Another sequel, i.e., obstruction, will be cited in the next section. However, death from dissemination of the tumor is a very rare phenomenon.

OBSTRUCTIVE LESIONS

A great variety of pathologic lesions may obstruct the ureters and give rise to hydroureter, hydronephrosis and sometimes pyelonephritis. Obviously, it is not the ureteral dilatation that is of significance in these cases, but the consequent involvement of the kidneys. These various causes may be conveniently separated into intrinsic ureteral disease and extrinsic lesions which compress the ureters.

INTRINSIC OBSTRUCTIVE DISEASES

These will be mentioned in the order of their clinical importance.

Calculi. Calculous obstruction of the ureters not only is the most frequent cause of obstruction but, at the same time, is the cause of one of the most intense forms of pain encountered in clinical practice—renal colic. Ureteral calculi almost invariably arise within the kidney and are more fully considered on p. 1138. They vary from small, round to ovoid formations to irregular crystalline deposits, usually less than 0.5 cm. in diameter. Stones larger than this do not enter the ureteropelvic junction and, therefore, remain within the pelvis. Intrapelvic calculi are usually quite innocuous, save for the possible production of traumatic injury to the pelvic mucosa. Stones rarely arise within the ureters, but it is quite impossible to determine from simple morphologic observation whether or not the primary site of origin was the renal pelvis or the ureter.

Strictures. Narrowing by strictures may occur from either congenital anomalous development or acquired deformities. Acquired strictures may be caused by operative trauma. Because of the close anatomic relationship of the ureter to the uterine arteries, ureteral damage occasionally occurs in pelvic surgery. Inclusion of the ureter into a surgical ligature or even transection of a ureter is encountered, fortunately rarely. The early recognition of this accident permits reconstructive procedures and restoration of normal urinary flow. Intrinsic inflammation or periureteral inflammatory reactions, occurring, for example, in chronic salpingitis, chronic diverticulitis with peridiverticulitis and adhesions following peritonitis, may also lead to narrowing or obstruction. Congenital strictures usually occur at the sites of physiologic narrowing, particularly the ureteropelvic junction and the entrance of the ureter into the urinary bladder. Other common causes of such narrowing are aberrant renal vessels, congenital valves or stenosis.

Tumors. Malignant tumors and, quite rarely, benign tumors may give rise to obstruction. The manner in which they produce impairment of urinary flow is twofold: first, by formation of an intraluminal mass and, second, by invasion and thickening of the underlying wall with consequent narrowing of the lumen.

Blood Clot. Hematuria arising in the kidney or in a ureteral lesion may be sufficiently massive to permit the formation of clots which may lodge and cause obstruction. This magnitude of bleeding is most often associated with calculi and tumors. The hematuria associated with various forms of inflammatory and degenerative disease of the kidneys is usually sufficiently diluted by urine to prevent the formation of clots. Organization of the blood clot at its site of lodgment may anchor the obstruction and produce progressive narrowing of the constriction by the fibroblastic response.

EXTRINSIC OBSTRUCTIVE DISEASES

Pregnancy. Ureteral dilatation is a frequent accompaniment of pregnancy. It is still not known whether the dilatation results from endocrine causes, physiologic relaxation of smooth muscle or pressure upon the ureters at the pelvic brim. The greater tendency for the right than for the left ureter to be dilated suggests that the latter explanation is more likely, since the uterine fundus twists slightly to the right with increase in size.

Tumors. Malignant tumors of the rectum, prostate, bladder and female pelvic organs, particularly endometrial and cervical carcinoma, are major causes of narrowing of the ureters, either by external pressure or by direct invasion of the ureteral wall. This sequence of events comprises one of the major complications of advanced carcinoma of the cervix. Retroperitoneal sarcomas, including lymphomas, and metastatic involvement of periureteral lymph nodes all behave in a similar fashion.

Inflammation. It has already been indicated that periureteral inflammations may involve the ureters secondarily or, in the course of healing, cause scarring which may give rise to significant narrowing. The dilated ureter loses its peristaltic efficiency and thus causes urinary stasis. Sclerosing retroperitonitis, while not a true inflammation, may compress and obstruct the ureters.

Ureteral narrowing and urinary stasis from any cause is a serious clinical problem, since it leads to hydroureter and hydronephrosis. The resultant renal destruction, if bilateral, may lead to renal failure. Stasis of urine always carries with it the potentiality of infection of the kidney. It is for this reason that pyelonephritis is so commonly associated with the pregnant state. In most of the cases just mentioned, the obstruction develops slowly and, by the time it becomes manifest, severe renal damage may have occurred. However, calculous obstruction, surgical trauma and impacted blood clots may produce immediate symptoms which, by bringing the patient to early clinical attention, allow for removal of the obstruction before renal damage has occurred.

BLADDER

NORMAL

The terminal segment of the endodermal tube, which comprises the hind gut, gives rise to a common intestinal and urinary channel known as the cloaca. In early fetal development, the allantois is connected with this common excretory passage through an elongated tapering urachus. A septum then divides the cloaca into an anterior urogenital sinus and bladder, and a posteriorly situated rectum. The ureters connect with this anterior segment, which gives rise to the bladder. Later, a constriction in this anterior portion separates it into a distal urethra and proximal bladder. Differentiation of this endodermal anlage gives rise to the mucosal lining of the bladder, and a downgrowth of mesoderm invests it with a musculature, creating the thick-walled, muscular, urinary bladder. Throughout fetal development, the connection with the allantois persists but, at birth, the urachus separates from the umbilicus and becomes obliterated down to the level of the apex of the bladder.

Only those anatomic features which have pertinence to pathology will be mentioned at this time. The bladder exists almost entirely as an extraperitoneal structure situated deeply within the pelvis. It is in contact with the peritoneal cavity only in its most superior anterior aspect, where the peritoneum reflects from the anterior abdominal wall over the dome of the bladder. In the female, this peritonealized area is somewhat smaller than in the male, owing to the posteriorly situated uterus. The close relationship of the female genital tract to the bladder is of considerable significance. It makes possible the spread of disease from one tract to the other and, in middle-aged and elderly females, relaxation of pelvic support leads to prolapse (descent) of the uterus, pulling with it the floor of the bladder. In this fashion, the bladder is protruded into the vagina, creating a pouch—*cystocele*—which fails to empty readily with micturition. Frequency, loss of sphincteric control, with dribbling and predisposition to urinary tract infections, may follow. In the male, the seminal vesicles and prostate have similar close relationships, being situated just posterior and inferior to the neck of the bladder. Thus, enlargements of the prostate (prostatism), so very common in middle to later life, constitute an important cause of urinary tract obstruction.

The act of micturition involves a complex coordination of many reflexes, i.e., relaxation of the internal urethral sphincters and the external sphincter (existing only in the male), accompanied by constriction of the ureteral sphincters and contraction of the detrusor muscles in the wall of the bladder. In the normal state, this sequence of events is entirely under voluntary control and can be initiated or inhibited by will. In pathologic states, when the nervous impulses to the brain are interrupted, spinal reflex pathways take over control of urination, producing automatic emptying of the bladder whenever the retained volume reaches a critical level. Under these circumstances, the bladder functions as a *"cord bladder."*

PATHOLOGY

Diseases of the bladder, particularly inflammation (cystitis), comprise an important source of clinical signs and symptoms. Usually, however, these disorders are more disabling than lethal. Cystitis is particularly common in the older age group and is, therefore, commonly found at autopsy. Tumors of the bladder constitute an important source of both morbidity and mortality. In the overall perspective, however, the bladder is not often the source of lethal disease.

CONGENITAL ANOMALIES

The bladder is involved in a great variety of anomalous developmental defects. They are often associated with malformations of other levels of the urinary and sometimes genital tracts. Most of these are of rare occurrence and require brief citation. Diverticula, exstrophy of the bladder and persistent urachus will be accorded some detailed consideration.

DIVERTICULA

A bladder or vesical diverticulum consists of a pouch-like eversion or evagination of the bladder wall. Diverticula may arise as congenital defects or as acquired lesions from persistent urethral obstruction. The acquired forms are more frequent. Because they resemble each other in their morphologic features and clinical significance, they will be considered together. Diverticula, both of congenital and of acquired origin, are frequently encountered in approximately 5 to 10 per cent of the routine autopsy population of older individuals. They are extremely uncommon under the age of 50, and are more prevalent in males, presumably because of the causal role of enlargement of the prostate.

The *congenital form* may be due to a focal failure of development of the normal musculature, with resultant herniation of the mucosa at this point, or to some urinary tract obstruction during fetal development that creates increased intravesical pressure and consequent weakening of the wall at one point. Alternatively, diverticula may develop from bud-like outgrowths of the fetal bladder. In any event, *some musculature is retained within the wall* of such diverticula, although it may be thinner than normal. These may occur as single defects or, at most, are few in number (Fig. 25–2).

The *acquired variety* presumably implies the presence of a normal bladder at the time of birth, with consequent urinary tract obstruction causing pouch-like eversions at points of decreased resistance to pressure. Usually, these occur between the large interlacing bundles of muscles that create the bladder wall. The sequence of events can be set forth as follows: (1) urinary tract obstruction, (2) hypertrophy of the bladder muscle with trabeculation of the wall, (3) formation of small primitive sacculations (cellules) between the muscle trabeculae and (4) creation of large, sac-like pouches which expand between muscle groups. The diverticula have markedly thinned musculature and, in the more advanced lesions, may have virtually *no intrinsic musculature* but only a mucosa with tunica propria. This form occurs as multiple lesions throughout the bladder (Fig. 25–3). In both forms, the diverticulum usually consists of a round to ovoid sac-like pouch which varies from less than 1 cm. to 5 to 10 cm. in diameter. The mucosal lining of the bladder is continu-

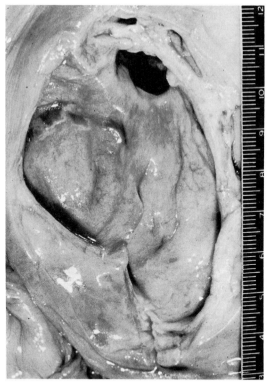

Figure 25–2. *The mouth of a bladder diverticulum of congenital origin, situated high in the dome of the bladder.*

ous into it and throughout the diverticulum and resembles that of the bladder. There may be some thinning and flattening of the normal transitional mucosa. In very extreme instances, the wall may appear to consist of a few layers of transitional cells, based upon an extremely thinned-out tunica propria.

Diverticula are of clinical significance because they constitute sites of urinary stasis that tend to become infected. The thinness of the wall predisposes to bacterial penetration or perforation and the possible development of perivesical infections or spread of infection into the peritoneal cavity. Urinary stasis in these structures also predisposes to the precipitation of urinary salts and the formation of bladder calculi. Perhaps it is the chronic irritation that further predisposes these lesions to the development of carcinomas.

EXSTROPHY OF THE BLADDER

Exstrophy of the bladder, according to the derivation of the term, refers to a turning out of the bladder. More specifically, it implies the presence of a developmental failure in the anterior wall of the abdomen and the bladder so that the bladder either communicates directly

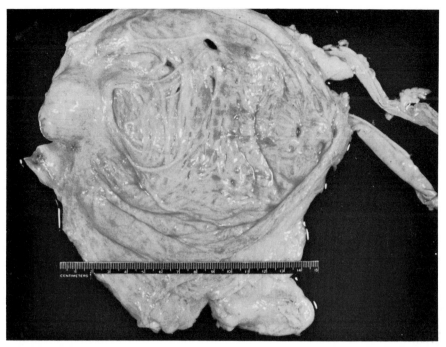

Figure 25–3. *Acquired diverticula of the bladder. Note the bladder distention as indicated by the 15 cm. rule and the trabeculation of the wall.*

through a large defect with the surface of the body in the suprapubic region, or lies as an opened sac. It is believed to have its origin in the failure of downgrowth of the mesoderm over the anterior aspect of the bladder. The anterior musculature of the bladder and adjacent abdominal wall never develops, and the bladder ruptures anteriorly to communicate with the skin surface (Gross and Cresson, 1952). Exstrophy of the bladder is associated not only with developmental defects in the musculature of the abdominal wall, but also with defective closure or formation of the symphysis pubis. This pattern of anomaly is extremely rare. The exposed bladder mucosa is subject to the development of infections that often spread to upper levels of the urinary system. In the course of the persistent chronic infections, the mucosa often becomes converted into an ulcerated surface of granulation tissue, and the preserved marginal epithelium becomes transformed into a stratified squamous type. There is an increased tendency toward the development of carcinoma. Death from pyelonephritis or urinary failure is common. Children with such anomalies have a markedly shortened life expectancy. This lesion, however, is not incompatible with life, and cases are on record of survival into adult life. Moreover, in less extreme instances, surgical correction is possible.

PERSISTENT URACHUS

In the discussion of the embryogenesis of the bladder, it was indicated that the urachus connects the apex of the bladder, known as the dome, with the allantois through the umbilical stalk. In the normal course of events, this connection atrophies and fibroses at birth and the dome of the bladder completely closes. Sometimes a narrow vestigial cord can be found below the umbilicus lying beneath the peritoneal covering of the anterior abdominal wall, marking the course of the fibrotic remnant. Rarely, the urachus may remain patent in part or in whole. When it is totally persistent, a fistulous urinary tract is created which connects the bladder with the umbilicus. At other times, the umbilical end or the bladder end remains patent, while the central region is obliterated. No direct communication exists under these circumstances, but a sequestered umbilical epithelial rest or bladder diverticulum is formed that may provide a site for the development of an infection or the origin of an epithelial cyst or malignancy.

MISCELLANEOUS ANOMALIES

Absence of the bladder and hypoplasia are very uncommon congenital defects. Occasionally, an incomplete transverse septum may create a so-called hourglass deformity. Abnormal connections between the bladder and the vagina, rectum or uterus may create congenital vesicovaginal, vesicorectal and vesicouterine fistulas. All these conditions are rare and will not be further described.

INFLAMMATIONS OF THE BLADDER

Cystitis is the most common form of lesion encountered in the bladder. This disorder is encountered in a wide variety of circumstances but, in almost every instance, there is some underlying derangement that predisposes to infection and inflammation. The urinary bladder is normally extremely resistant because of its many antibacterial protective mechanisms (discussed on p. 1117). Thus, infection of the urinary bladder virtually always implies some predisposing cause, e.g.:

1. Exstrophy.
2. Urethral obstruction.
3. Fistulous communications (congenital or acquired) to rectum or vagina.
4. Catheterization or instrumentation of the lower urinary tract.
5. Cystocele.
6. Bladder calculi.
7. Bladder neoplasms.
8. Trauma (frequent coitus in the female).
9. Debilitating illnesses, particularly diabetes mellitus.
10. Pyelonephritis.
11. Pregnancy.
12. Derangements in the bladder innervation (cord bladder).

Up to the middle years of life, cystitis is much more prevalent in females, presumably because the shorter female urethra, pregnancy and the trauma of coitus all render the young woman more vulnerable than the male to spread of bacteria into the bladder. In later years, males are affected as often as females, because of the high incidence of prostatism in those over the age of 50.

While many bacterial and mycotic agents have been identified as the underlying cause of such inflammation, in many instances the etiology remains obscure (Mathe, 1949). An etiologic classification is, therefore, long and complex, and it is necessary to resort to a descriptive morphologic classification. Cystitis is thus divided into categories based upon the dominant anatomic alteration in the bladder structure. In many instances, the lines of division remain indistinct, and the entities, therefore, overlap to some extent. The following presentation will only consider the better defined, most frequently encountered variants.

ACUTE AND CHRONIC CYSTITIS

The great majority of cases of cystitis take the form of nonspecific acute or chronic inflammation of the bladder.

The pathogenesis of cystitis and the common bacterial and mycotic etiologic agents were already discussed in some detail in the consideration of urinary tract infections (UTI) on p. 1117. For recall, the common etiologic agents are the coliforms (*E. coli*, Proteus, Pseudomonas). As with acute pyelonephritis, less common offenders are *A. aerogenes*, enterococci, Klebsiella, staphylococci, streptococci and *N. gonorrheae*. Tuberculous cystitis is an almost inevitable sequel to renal tuberculosis. Infrequently, cystitis is due to monilial or torula agents, particularly in patients on long-term antibiotics. More rarely seen are the trichomonas and schistosome parasites. As was emphasized earlier, in most instances, bacterial pyelonephritis (acute or chronic) is preceded by infection of the urinary bladder, with retrograde spread of microorganisms into the kidneys and their collecting systems. Once active bacterial pyelonephritis has become established, the constant seeding of the bladder perpetuates cystitis. Any of the other influences cited on p. 1118 may also be involved. Less frequently, cystitis may result from blood-borne seeding of the bladder; and equally unusual are vaguely defined, suspected allergic mechanisms (to drugs, chemicals or foods).

Morphology. The bladder size depends entirely upon the volume of contained urine at the time of death. In patients who have been catheterized just prior to death, or in whom an indwelling catheter has been used, the bladder may be quite contracted. Usually, however, the predisposing causes of urinary retention create dilatation and thinning of the wall so that, in extreme instances, the dome of the bladder is at the level of the umbilicus. Preexisting obstruction may have caused hypertrophy and trabeculation of the wall.

The first alteration, in the acute stages, is hyperemia of the mucosa. At this stage, the normal velvety character of the mucosa is preserved. In the more advanced cases, hyperemia may become transformed to focal or diffuse hemorrhagic discolorations associated with the precipitation of gray-white to yellow suppurative exudate. As the inflammatory reaction progresses in severity, the normal velvety mucosa is replaced by a friable, hemorrhagic, granular surface with many shallow, focal ulcers filled with exudate. When the hemorrhagic component is a dominant feature, it is designated as **hemorrhagic cystitis.** The accumulation of large amounts of suppurative exudate may merit the designation of **suppurative cystitis** (Fig. 25–4). Progression of the infection may give rise to sloughing

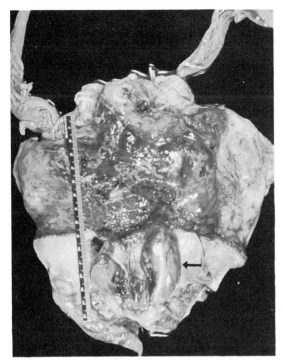

Figure 25–4. Suppurative cystitis. The mucosa is darkened by hemorrhage and congestion and is also layered by patches of pale exudate. Note the enlarged prostate predisposing to stasis (arrow).

and ulceration of large areas of the mucosa or, sometimes, the entire bladder mucosa, known as **ulcerative cystitis.** Coagulation of the exudate and necrotic mucosa may produce an inflammatory reaction similar to that evoked by diphtheria, referred to as **diphtheritic or membranous cystitis.** The infection may extend into the underlying wall to cause deeply excavated ulcerations and intramural abscesses. Inflammatory edema may cause sufficient ischemia to produce **gangrenous cystitis.** Under these circumstances, the surface mucosa may appear green-black and totally necrotic. In the far advanced cases, when the organisms are particularly virulent, the infection may extend through the bladder to cause perivesical abscesses, perforation, sinus tracts to neighboring structures and pelvic peritonitis. However, in most cases, the inflammatory reaction is not intense and the infection appears to be limited to the mucosa and tunica propria.

Persistence of the infection leads to chronic cystitis, which differs from the acute form only in the character of the inflammatory infiltrate. The mucosa is more edematous, and the inflammatory reaction tends to cause more extreme heaping up of the epithelium with the formation of a red, friable, granular, sometimes ulcerated, surface. Chronicity of the infection gives rise to fibrous thickening in the

tunica propria and consequent thickening and inelasticity of the bladder wall.

The histologic findings of most of these variants of acute and chronic nonspecific cystitis are exactly those that can be anticipated in any such nonspecific inflammation. Mention might be made of a special form of chronic inflammatory reaction, the accumulation of lymphocytes into lymph follicles within the bladder mucosa and underlying wall, creating a variant of chronic cystitis known as **cystitis follicularis.**

It is important to mention the extreme susceptibility of the bladder mucosa to postmortem artefactual shedding or sloughing. Under ordinary laboratory conditions, the bladder epithelium desquamates within a few hours after death. Unless fixation of the bladder is accomplished before this, considerable loss of the mucosa may occur, which may be confused with antemortem ulceration. Absence of inflammatory reaction, however, distinguishes this form of shedding from true inflammatory sloughing.

All forms of cystitis are characterized by a triad of symptoms: (1) frequency, which in acute cases may necessitate urination every 15 to 20 minutes; (2) lower abdominal pain localized over the bladder region, or in the suprapubic region; and (3) dysuria—pain or burning on urination. Associated with these localized changes, there may be systemic signs of inflammation, such as elevation of temperature, chills and general malaise. In the usual case, the bladder infection does not give rise to such a constitutional reaction.

The major clinical significance of cystitis is its predisposition to pyelonephritis. The local symptoms may be disturbing but, in general, these infections are more uncomfortable than serious. For the most part, cystitis is usually a secondary complication of some underlying disorder, such as prostatic enlargement, cystocele of the bladder or kidney infections. These primary diseases must be corrected before the cystitis can be relieved. The threat of retrograde extension of bladder infections to the kidneys is ample justification for their prompt and effective treatment (Kretschmer, 1945).

SPECIAL FORMS OF CYSTITIS

There is a multiplicity of so-called special variants of cystitis that are distinctive by either their morphologic appearance or their causation.

Encrusted Cystitis. This term is applied to those instances of nonspecific cystitis characterized by the precipitation of urinary salts, particularly phosphates, upon the bladder surface. The crystalline, gray-white, granular precipitate creates a focal or diffuse encrustation on the bladder mucosa. Chronic cystitis with its attendant changes invariably underlies this condition. Usually urea-splitting bacteria are found in such infections. These produce alkalinity of the bladder urine, and favor precipitation of chemical salts.

Bullous Cystitis. This refers to the formation of large vesicles in the bladder mucosa from the collection of large amounts of submucosal edema fluid. These vesicles appear as grape-like masses directly beneath the mucosal surface. With some loss of fluid, the bullae appear as loose, flaccid, wrinkled, low elevations. This variant may occur in the acute stages of cystitis when the organism produces a high degree of toxicity and an intensive serofibrinous exudate.

Interstitial Cystitis. This condition is characterized by chronic edematous thickening, with ulceration of the mucosa and tunica propria of the bladder. It was first described by Hunner in cases which showed accompanying ulceration of the mucosa of the dome of the bladder. Hence, interstitial cystitis is sometimes known as *Hunner's ulcers.* The etiology of this interstitial inflammation is best explained by the lymphogenous spread of infection to the bladder, with simultaneous obstruction of the lymph nodes of drainage. Lymphedema and interstitial inflammatory reaction cause thickening of the bladder wall and, in the more severe cases, sloughing and ulceration of the mucosa which, peculiarly, *spares the trigonal area.* It occurs almost entirely in menopausal females, frequently after pelvic surgery. Endocrine imbalance has been postulated as important in its production.

Irradiation Cystitis. Roentgen or radium irradiation to the bladder may result in inflammatory changes known as "irradiation cystitis." Usually such radiation is used in therapy of tumors in the uterus or bladder. Congestive hyperemia, followed by hemorrhagic cystitis, is the first change noted. In more severe cases, the bladder mucosa may ulcerate and slough extensively. Accompanying these changes, there is widespread edema and interstitial leukocytic infiltration of the bladder wall, associated with radiation injury to the blood vessels. Vascular thromboses may lead to deeply penetrating ulcerations and sometimes to perforation of the bladder and formation of fistulous tracts with the vagina, uterus, rectum or the skin surface. Secondary infections frequently complicate the clinical and anatomic picture.

Malakoplakia. Malakoplakia (soft plaque) is a term applied to a distinctive form of cys-

titis, characterized by the development of soft, broad, sessile, polypoid plaques in the bladder mucosa (Fig. 25–5). These occur under totally obscure circumstances although, in all instances, the entire organ is the site of a marked, chronic inflammatory reaction. A variety of etiologic agents has been indicted, such as the colon bacilli, parasites, tubercle bacilli and systemic sarcoidosis, but none has been well established. The lesion is identified morphologically by yellow-gray to brown, circumscribed, slightly elevated, soft plaques which vary from a few millimeters up to several centimeters in diameter. The edges are slightly overhanging, but sharply defined, and are separated by intervening zones of relatively normal but inflamed mucosa. Histologically, the plaques are composed of massive submucosal aggregates of large macrophages, interspersed with numerous lymphocytes, plasma cells and foreign body giant cells. Inclusions may be present in these giant cells or in the large macrophages. These intracellular structures appear as laminated, deeply basophilic, round to irregular, clearly demarcated microspherules (Michaelis-Gutmann bodies), which vary in size from one to many microns. Their similarity to the Schaumann inclusions in Boeck's sarcoid has suggested the possible relationship of this form of cystitis to systemic sarcoidosis. They contain calcium and iron and probably represent encrusted debris.

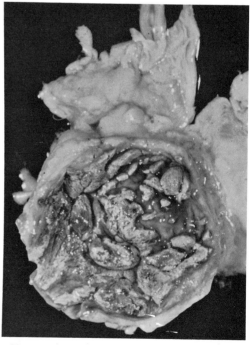

Figure 25–5. *Malakoplakia of the bladder showing the classic, broad, flat inflammatory plaques.*

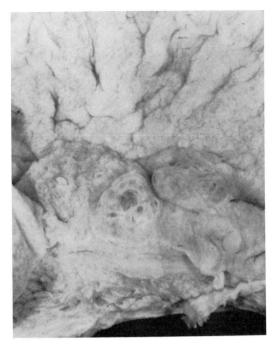

Figure 25-6. Cystitis cystica. A close-up of the bladder mucosa with heaped-up cystic formations in the trigonal region.

Cystitis Cystica. Cystitis cystica represents the vesical analogue of pyelitis and ureteritis cystica. In longstanding chronic inflammation, nests of bladder mucosa may become buried and give rise to small, cystic, mucosal inclusions. The gross and microscopic histologic features are identical with those already described in the renal pelvis and ureter (Fig. 25–6). Occasionally, by metaplasia the epithelium becomes columnar mucus-secreting to produce cystitis glandularis.

Tuberculous Cystitis. This is almost invariably an accompaniment of renal tuberculosis. *Secondary vesical involvement occurs in over two-thirds of the cases of renal tuberculosis* and is responsible for some of the major clinical features of the tuberculous nephropathy. Frequency, pain, dysuria and pyuria, all referable to the bladder, are often the first overt manifestations of tuberculous infection in the kidneys.

The morphologic alterations in the bladder vary with the duration of the infection. The trigonal area is usually the first affected but, in advanced cases, the entire bladder is involved. In early cases, minute tubercle formations may be identified in the bladder as small, 1 to 2 mm., yellow-white, submucosal elevations. With progression of the lesion, these tubercles may coalesce to form large caseous nodules which, in the course of time, ulcerate and produce characteristic, irregular, slightly under-mined ulcers having necrotic, ragged bases. Deep ulcerations may give rise to fistulas into adjacent structures. If secondary infection has not modified the inflammatory reaction, the typical caseous character of the inflammatory debris suggests the appropriate diagnosis. Histologically, the characteristic inflammatory tuberculous response permits a ready diagnosis.

The clinical diagnosis is usually made by the failure to isolate a usual bacterial agent in a patient having an apparent cystitis. Only then are acid-fast smears and special techniques performed to identify the appropriate causal agent.

The chief clinical significance of tuberculous cystitis is the implication of associated renal involvement. Although the vesical lesion is the dominant source of clinical symptoms, the renal involvement constitutes the major threat to life.

Miscellaneous Forms of Cystitis. *Monilia albicans* infection of the bladder may occur, as in any other mucosal surface of the body. The characteristic opaque white growth of this fungus is readily identified on histologic section, as well as on examination of the urine sediment, and constitutes the diagnostic feature of this lesion. Syphilis, systemic trichinosis and schistosomiasis are infrequent causes of specific forms of cystitis in the U.S.

TUMORS OF THE BLADDER

Over 95 per cent of bladder (vesical) tumors are cancers. The infrequent benign neoplasms have importance only insofar as they must be distinguished, clinically, from the far more serious malignant lesions. Cancers arising in the bladder are the most frequent tumors of the entire urinary tract, including the kidney. Approximately 95 per cent arise from the epithelial lining of the bladder and are known as urothelial tumors. These epithelial neoplasms constitute a spectrum from innocuous, benign-appearing lesions to those that are obviously malignant. While the benign lesions have traditionally been called papillomas to differentiate them from the malignant papillary carcinomas, clinical experience indicates that many papillomas tend to recur when excised and tend to become progressively more anaplastic with each recurrence so that their innocent histologic appearance belies their biologic aggressiveness (Dean et al., 1954). Moreover, on anatomic grounds alone, there is no sharp line of distinction between the benign-appearing papillomas and the better differentiated papillary carcinomas. For these reasons, all the urothelial tumors are considered clinically to be malignant or potentially malignant and will be considered together (Ash, 1940) (Kerr and Colby, 1951).

MALIGNANT TUMORS

Papilloma-Carcinoma. With rare exception, bladder cancers are of epithelial (urothelial) origin. They account for about 3 per cent of cancer deaths in the United States annually. The anatomic classification and the biologic behavior of the urothelial tumors of the bladder are two of the most nebulous areas in oncology. It is clear that these tumors grow in three distinctive cytologic patterns, i.e., transitional cell carcinoma, squamous cell carcinoma and adenocarcinoma. Pure adenocarcinomas are relatively noncontroversial since they present distinctive histologic patterns, having clearly delimited biologic significance. Foci of adenocarcinoma may be found in a predominantly transitional cell carcinoma, in rare instances. The major area of confusion involves the transitional cell and squamous cell patterns. While pure forms of each of these histologic patterns are encountered, some neoplasms are mixed. In an analysis of a large series of epithelial cancers, about 90 per cent were basically transitional cell carcinomas; 7 per cent, squamous cell carcinomas; and 1 to 2 per cent, adenocarcinomas (Pugh, 1959). About 20 per cent of the invasive transitional cell carcinomas contained areas of squamous differentiation. The prevailing practice is to call such neoplasms transitional cell carcinoma with areas of squamous change. Some pathologists would call all neoplasms with any squamous transformation simply squamous cell carcinomas. The problem is not merely academic, since long-term follow-up indicates that well differentiated, pure, squamous cell carcinomas have a better prognosis than transitional cell neoplasms with foci of squamous change (Pugh, 1959).

An additional area of confusion has already been alluded to. It stems from the dichotomy between the histologic appearance of the transitional cell tumor and its biologic behavior. Some pathologists define well differentiated lesions that are histologically quite benign in appearance as benign papillomas, and the more anaplastic tumors are then segregated into Grades I to III carcinoma. Others classify the papilloma as transitional cell carcinoma Grade I because of its known tendency to recur and to become progressively more anaplastic with each recurrence. Thus, Grade I lesions have different levels of anaplasia in the two systems, a difference which, as will be seen, may have clinical significance in terms of prognosis.

Incidence. Cancer of the bladder causes about 10,000 deaths annually in the United States. Whatever the histologic type, it is rarely encountered under the age of 40. The peak incidence is in the sixth decade. Males are affected three or four times more often than females. In populations where parasitic infections of the bladder by *Schistosoma haematobium* are common, there is a marked increase in the incidence of bladder cancer, which occurs at a younger age. In Egypt, for example, where over 90 per cent of the population harbor Schistosomes in their bladders, the incidence of squamous cell carcinoma of the bladder is almost 10 times that in the United States, and young adults in the third or fourth decades of life are affected.

Pathogenesis. No genetic or familial predisposition to bladder cancer has been identified, but there is a large body of evidence suggesting that the following environmental factors are important: exposure to (1) industrial carcinogens; (2) metabolites of tryptophan; (3) tobacco tars; and (4) mechanical irritation (including parasites).

Occupational exposure to certain dye intermediates is associated with a high incidence of transitional cell bladder cancer. The most potent of these carcinogens is beta-naphthylamine encountered in industries concerned with the manufacture of rubber products, aniline dyes and electric cables. Bladder cancers occur after a mean exposure time of approximately 23 years; a fifty-fold increased incidence is observed among workers (Kleinfeld et al., 1966). Additional occupational hazards include parabiphenylamine, benzidine, alpha-naphthylamine and auramine (McDonald, 1968). The common denominator among these agents appears to be the excretion and concentration, in the urine, of orthohydroxylated metabolites complexed to sulfates or glucuronic acid. The pH of urine is closer to optimal for the enzyme beta glucuronidase than is the pH of tissue or blood. Thus, the glucuronides are split in the urine, exposing the bladder epithelium to higher levels of the hydroxylated carcinogens than any other tissue of the body. Herein may lie the explanation of the carcinogenic effect of naphthylamine being limited to the bladder.

Metabolites of tryptophan have been shown to induce bladder tumors in mice (Bryan et al., 1964). Excessive quantities of tryptophan metabolites have been identified in patients with bladder tumors, and administration of tryptophan to such patients leads to the excretion of greater than normal quantities of carcinogenic metabolites. The carcinogenic metabolites are normally excreted in conjugated form, and there is speculation that urinary enzymes may split these conjugates to liberate the proximate (immediate) carcinogen. However, in clinical trials, efforts to block urinary glucuronidase have not proved efficacious in correcting the excretion of metabolites proved to be carcinogenic in animals.

Heavy cigarette smoking has been implicated, on epidemiologic grounds, in the production of cancer of the bladder (Cobb and Ansell, 1965). The evidence is somewhat circumstantial, but recently it has been suggested that smokers excrete increased amounts of tryptophan metabolites, providing a possible causative mechanism (Kerr et al., 1965).

Mechanical irritation may account for the increased incidence of vesical carcinoma in patients with Schistosomiasis of the bladder and in those having the congenital anomaly, exstrophy of the bladder. Implantation of parasitic eggs in the bladder wall induces a chronic inflammatory response with epithelial hyperplasia and regeneration, presumably leading in time to neoplasia. Similarly, protracted nonspecific chronic infections induce a variety of mucosal changes including inflammatory hyperplastic polyps and leukoplakia, considered to be important soils for the development of malignant tumors.

Morphology. The three major forms of bladder cancer—(1) transitional cell, (2) squamous cell and (3) adenocarcinoma—will be discussed separately. It is important to emphasize at the outset that, for all histologic patterns, the clinical behavior, optimal method of treatment (radiation, fulguration, local or radical resection) and the prognosis for the patient depend heavily on the degree of anaplasia of the neoplastic cells and the extent of infiltration of the tumor. There have been developed, therefore, elaborate systems both for grading the degree of anaplasia and for staging the extent of the cancer. As will become clear, there is a high level of correlation between the degree of anaplasia and the invasiveness of the lesion (approximately 80 per cent). But for the sake of clarity, it should be emphasized that anaplasia is judged entirely by cytologic characteristics, while staging of the extent of the cancer depends upon clinical and pathologic estimates of its depth of penetration and spread.

Transitional cell tumors range from well differentiated, usually benign lesions to highly anaplastic, aggressive cancers. Although many have been devised, two systems to express the degree of anaplasia are in current usage. The first is based on Broder's classification recognizing Grades I to IV. In this classification, Grade I (transitional cell carcinoma) represents a lesion which others call benign papilloma. The American Registry of Bladder Tumors and the World Health Organization, in con-

trast, recommend retention of the benign papilloma designation, with further subdivision of the carcinomas into Grades I to III. In this classification, the benign papilloma therefore conforms to the Grade I transitional cell carcinoma in the Broder's classification. Recognizing this area of ambiguity, the benign papilloma can be characterized as a papillary neoplasm having a complicated fern-like structure composed of a delicate connective tissue stalk covered by transitional epithelium that is as regular as the normal lining of the urinary bladder (Figs. 25–7 and 25–8). Such tumors appear as small, red, elevated excrescences varying in size from less than 1 cm. in diameter to large masses up to 5 cm. in diameter. They occur more often about the trigone. Multicentric origins may produce separate tumors (Fig. 25–9). The long slender fronds often create a velvety consistency and, when viewed within the urinary bladder through the cystoscope, resemble aquatic grasses waving in water currents. Fragmentation of the tips of the papillae, ulceration, necrosis and hemorrhage may complicate the basic macroscopic appearance.

In the American Registry classification, which recognizes the existence of benign papillomas, Grade I transitional cell carcinoma may be charac-

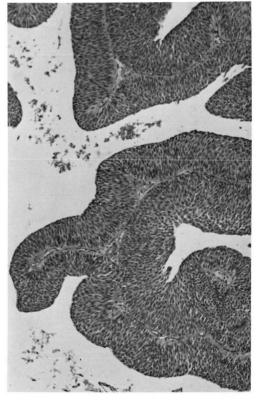

Figure 25–7. *Low power view of typical papillomatous growth of the bladder. Note the delicate axial stromal framework.*

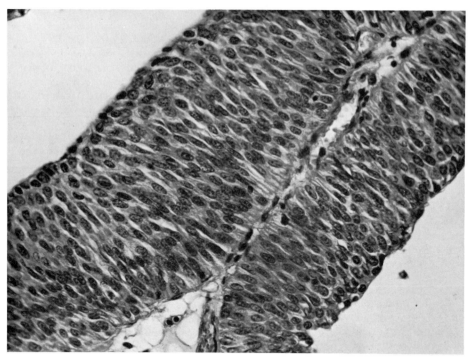

Figure 25–8. *Papilloma of the bladder. Compare the well differentiated transitional epithelium with the lesion in Figure 25–10.*

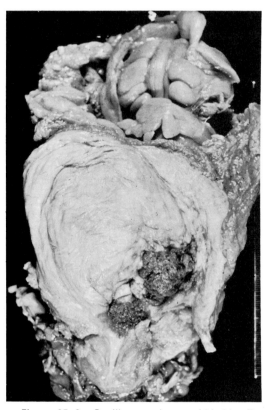

Figure 25–9. *Papillary carcinoma of bladder. Two discrete lesions in the trigonal area.*

terized as a tumor, having the gross morphology of a benign papilloma but differing insofar as the transitional epithelium is thickened, with some slight variation in nuclear and cell size, and some increased chromaticity of the nuclei. Mitotic figures are rare. In other words, the tumorous transitional epithelium presents minor variation from the normal bladder lining. The Grade III transitional cell carcinomas represent the other end of the spectrum of anaplasia and contain large numbers of tumor giant cells, abundant atypical mitotic figures and most of the standard features recognized as marked anaplasia (Fig. 25–10). Between these two extremes are the Grade II transitional cell carcinomas having intermediate degrees of cytologic anaplasia.

The depth of infiltration and the extent of spread are the parameters used in the clinical staging of tumors. The clinician arrives at his judgement by bimanual examination of the patient and cystoscopic study. The pathologist can make his judgement only postoperatively from morphologic examination of the specimen. In general, papillomas and Grade I carcinomas appear as exophytic papillomatous lesions. The papilloma is superficially attached to the bladder mucosa, and the neoplastic epithelial cells do not invade either the stalk of the neoplasm or the underlying wall of the bladder itself. The Grade I carcinomas often progressively enlarge to cauliflower-like masses, but these too are somewhat superficially attached to the underlying bladder wall. As the scale of anaplasia is

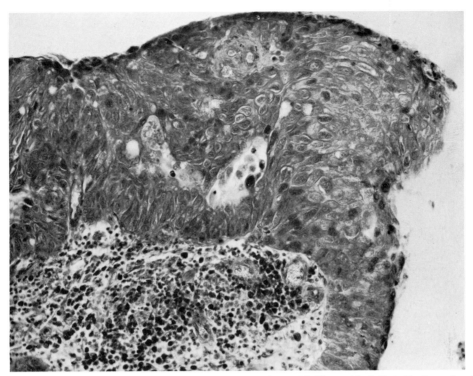

Figure 25–10. *Papillary carcinoma of bladder for comparison with Figure 25–8. Note the loss of orderly normal transitional growth.*

ascended, the neoplasms tend to produce larger cauliflower masses or broad-based plaques until one reaches the Grade III cancers which are usually infiltrative, ulcerative lesions that invade, penetrate and spread beyond the bladder (Figs. 25–11 and 25–12). Some tumors progressively spread into the adjacent prostate, seminal vesicles and retroperitoneum. About 40 per cent of deeply invasive tumors metastasize to regional lymph nodes. Hematogenous dissemination generally occurs late and only with highly anaplastic tumors. About one-third of fatal bladder cancers metastasize widely, principally to the liver, lung and bone marrow. Infrequently, ulcerative lesions produce fistulous communications to the vagina or rectum.

All transitional cell neoplasms, including the papillomas, have a tendency to recur following excision, and usually the recurrence exhibits greater anaplasia. In some instances, the recurrence occurs at a different site and the question of a new primary tumor must be entertained. Transitional cell tumors seem to be prime examples of neoplasia arising in a "restless epithelium." As mentioned earlier, in almost one-fourth of these transitional cell tumors, foci of squamous change are encountered, almost always in the more anaplastic transitional cell tumors. Thus, tumors exhibiting such squamous metaplasia tend to be more aggressive cancers.

The two most widely used classifications of the

stages of bladder cancer are those of Jewett and Strong (1946) and Union Internationale Contre le Cancrum (1967). The international classification essentially uses the TNM system presented on p. 156. A somewhat simplified correlation of the two methods of classification is given in Table 25–1.

The cytologic grade of anaplasia and the stage of the cancer are closely interrelated, and both heavily influence the prognosis for the patient. While there is a high level of correlation (at the 80 per cent level) between the degree of anaplasia and the invasiveness of a lesion, i.e., the more anaplastic the more invasive, the correlation is not always perfect. About 7 to 10 per cent of Grade I carcinomas invade lymphatics and these patients have a poor prognosis. Conversely, the Grade III carcinoma may not have extended beyond the bladder wall and, therefore, may be curable by total cystectomy.

The **squamous cell carcinoma** in pure form accounts for about 7 per cent of all bladder carcinomas. Transitional cell carcinomas with areas of squamous metaplasia are much more frequent. This pattern of neoplasia was discussed above. Squamous cell carcinomas may be fungating tumors projecting into the bladder lumen, but more often are infiltrative and ulcerative. The level of cytologic differentiation varies widely from the highly differentiated lesions producing abundant keratohyaline pearls to very anaplastic giant cell tumors

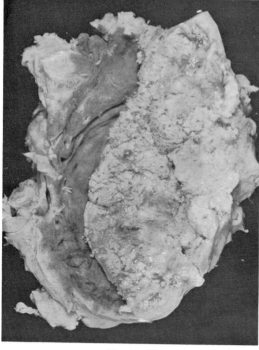

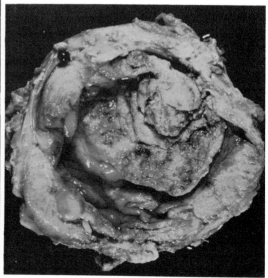

Fig. 25–11

Fig. 25–12

Figure 25–11. Transitional cell carcinoma Grade II. The entire right side of the bladder is overgrown by the spreading lesion.

Figure 25–12. Infiltrative transitional carcinoma Grade III of the bladder seen as a fungating ulcerative mass occupying almost the entire floor.

showing no evidence of squamous differentiation. No system of classification has been provided for these lesions but, in general, the same principles apply. Namely, the prognosis depends on the grade of anaplasia and the extent of infiltration and spread. It is believed that some of these squamous cancers arise from preexisting leukoplakia, but others appear to represent metaplastic differentiation of neoplastic transitional cells.

Adenocarcinoma of the bladder is rare. These tumors may arise from urachal remnants, from periurethral and periprostatic glands, from cystitis cystica or from metaplasia of transitional epithelium. The glandular neoplastic components may secrete mucin, making it impossible to unmistakably differentiate such primary bladder neoplasms from those arising in adjacent structures such as the prostate or seminal vesicles, with secondary extension into the bladder.

Clinical Course. All bladder tumors classically produce painless hematuria. This is their dominant and sometimes only clinical manifestation. Occasionally, frequency, urgency and dysuria accompany the hematuria. The use of cytologic examination of urinary sediment for the desquamated tumor cells deserves special mention in the clinical in-

TABLE 25–1. CLASSIFICATIONS OF BLADDER CANCER

Classification of Jewitt and Strong	Classification of International Union Against Cancer	Description of Tumor
Stage 0	T1S	Carcinoma in situ
Stage A	T1	Tumor with infiltration into subepithelial tissue
Stage B1	T2	Tumor with infiltration into superficial muscle
Stage B2 or C	T3	Tumor with infiltration into deep muscle
Stage D	T4	Tumor with infiltration into adjacent organs
Stage D1	N+ (regional)	Tumor with lymph node invasion below bifurcation of iliac arteries
Stage D2	M+ (distant)	Tumor with lymph node invasion in periaortic region

vestigation of these patients. While a negative result does not exclude the presence of a tumor, the identification of anaplastic cells dictates the need for cystoscopic or radiographic studies.

The prognosis depends on the histologic pattern of the neoplasm, the grade of anaplasia and the clinical stage when first diagnosed. For the benign papilloma, there is good agreement that the five-year survival is over 90 per cent, with simple local resection or fulguration. For the frankly malignant lesions, the five-year survival data not only vary among reports but also are complicated by the choice of treatment—supervoltage irradiation or total cystectomy (Caldwell, 1970). The following five-year survival figures represent ranges for both forms of therapy. For Stages 0, A and B1, 25 to 80 per cent; for B2 or C, 8 to 30 per cent; and for D, 0 to 10 per cent. Death is usually due either to progressive infiltration of the ureters leading to bacterial and obstructive renal disease or to dissemination of the cancer.

Other Primary Malignancies. A great variety of sarcomatous growths may involve the bladder, paralleling the benign mesodermal tumors described below. As a group, they tend to produce large masses (varying up to 10 to 15 cm. in diameter) which protrude into the vesical lumen. Their soft, fleshy, gray-white gross appearance suggests their sarcomatous nature. Identification of the precise neoplastic cell type depends upon histologic study.

One form, rhabdomyosarcoma, deserves special mention. It tends to grow in large, polypoid projections into the bladder lumen, producing grape-like clusters of soft, fleshy tissue. These malignancies, called *sarcoma botryoides*, are identical with those that occur in the female genital tract (p. 1213).

BENIGN TUMORS

Since the epithelial tumors of the bladder have all been considered in the preceding discussion, attention here can be focused on the great variety of benign mesodermal tumors. These include fibromas, fibromyxomas, myxomas, leiomyomas, neurofibromas, xanthomas, angiomas, granular cell myoblastomas, dermoids and osteomas. They all tend to grow as isolated intramural, encapsulated, oval to spherical masses, varying in diameter up to several centimeters. Occasionally, they assume submucosal pedunculated positions. They have the histologic features of their counterparts elsewhere. As a group they are somewhat more common in adults, but certain lesions such as the myxomas and angiomas tend to occur in children. The clinical significance of these benign tumors is usually minimal, except insofar as they may cause ulceration of the thinned-out overlying mucosa and so produce hematuria or obstruct one of the ureteral orifices. While malignant sarcomatous transformation of such benign lesions remains a possibility, it is from clinical experience an extremely infrequent occurence.

SECONDARY TUMORS

Secondary malignant involvement of the bladder may reach it by one of three pathways: by direct extension from primary lesions in nearby organs, by implantation from primary lesions within the upper urinary tract or by spread through lymphatics and blood from such primaries as the stomach, lungs, breast and elsewhere. Direct extension is the most common form of secondary involvement, from carcinomas of the cervix, uterus, prostate and rectum, in the order given. Carcinoma of the cervix, in the advanced stages, is particularly prone to extend into the bladder wall and, since it is in contact with the floor of the bladder, is in a position to invade the wall in the region of the orifice of the ureters as well as the urethra. Since most of these carcinomas are squamous cell lesions, they may, on casual inspection of the bladder, appear as primary squamous cell carcinomas of this organ. Hemorrhage, ureteral obstruction and vesicovaginal fistulas are the common sequelae.

Endometrial carcinomas less commonly affect the bladder, but may produce essentially the same sequence of events. In the male, far advanced prostatic carcinoma may extend into the bladder wall, but more usually affects the seminal vesicles and the perivesical connective tissue. In the bladder, it may occlude the urethral orifice and cause obstruction at this level, but extension within the bladder wall may likewise cause compression of the ureteral orifices.

MECHANICAL LESIONS

OBSTRUCTION TO THE BLADDER NECK

Obstruction to the bladder neck is of major clinical importance, not only for the changes induced in the bladder, but also because of its eventual effect on the kidney. A great variety of intrinsic and extrinsic diseases of the bladder may narrow the urethral orifice and cause partial or complete vesical obstruction. In the male, the most important lesion is enlargement of the prostate gland due either to nodular hyperplasia or to carcinoma (Fig. 25–13). Vesical obstruction is somewhat less common in the female, and is most often caused by cystocele of the bladder. The more infrequent causes can be listed as (1) congenital narrowings or strictures of the urethra; (2) inflammatory strictures of the urethra; (3) inflammatory fibrosis and contraction of the bladder following varying types of cystitis; (4) bladder tumors—either benign or malignant—when strategically located; (5) secondary invasion of the bladder neck by growths arising in perivesical structures, such as the cervix, vagina, prostate and rectum; (6) mechanical obstructions caused by foreign bodies and calculi; and (7) injury to the innervation of the bladder causing cord bladder.

The morphologic alterations in the bladder are the same, irrespective of the underlying cause. In the early stages, there is only some thickening of the bladder wall, presumably due to hypertrophy of the smooth muscle. The mucosal surface at this time may be entirely normal. With progressive hypertrophy of the muscular coat, the individual muscle bundles greatly enlarge and produce trabeculation of the bladder wall. These submucosal cord-like thickenings run in all directions and produce a crisscross pattern of mucosal ridging. The overlying mucosa may be entirely normal but, more commonly, the urinary stasis leads to bladder infection, and changes of cystitis are present. Persistent obstruction leads to more marked trabeculation, and the prominent ridging produces crypt-like depressions between the interlacing bands which resemble small diverticula. In the course of time, these crypts may become converted into true acquired diverticula. The histologic alterations may be very slight. The mucosal surface may be entirely normal or may show some thinning of the normal multilayered transitional epithelium. Slight inflammatory changes may be present, representing the development of a superimposed cystitis. The hypertrophy of smooth muscle is difficult to evaluate histologically, and can only be surmised by an increase in the total thickness of the muscular layer of the bladder wall.

In some cases of acute obstruction or in terminal disease when the patient's normal reflex mechanisms are depressed, the bladder may become extremely dilated. The enlarged bladder may reach the brim of the pelvis or even the level of the umbilicus. In these cases, the bladder wall is markedly thinned and the trabeculation becomes totally inapparent. Catheterization and too rapid decompression of such hugely dilated bladders may cause massive hemorrhage into the mucosa and bladder lumen. The mechanism for this decompression hemorrhage is not completely clear, but it is assumed to be based upon sudden release of urinary pressure, permitting massive dilatation of the submucosal vessels and their consequent rupture.

MISCELLANEOUS LESIONS

FOREIGN BODIES

Foreign bodies may be encountered within the bladder. These are usually present under one of two circumstances; physicians' accidents or self-induced manipulations. The list of such foreign bodies ranges from such objects as fragments of catheter or total intact coiled rubber catheters to such nonmedical objects as hairpins and nails. Rarely, these objects migrate into the abdomen by the formation of inflammatory fistulous tracts through the bladder wall. The chief significance of these bodies is their causation of urethral obstruction, chronic cystitis and potentiation of the formation of vesical calculi by the superimposed precipitation of urinary salts (Fig. 25–14).

CALCULI

Bladder calculi may either be of primary origin within the bladder or pass into the bladder from a renal or ureteral focus of origin

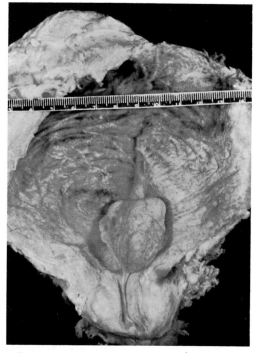

Figure 25–13. *Hypertrophy and trabeculation of the bladder wall secondary to polypoid nodular hyperplasia of the prostate.*

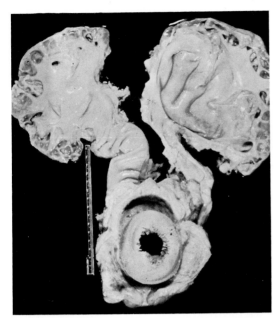

Figure 25–14. A huge doughnut-shaped bladder calculus with secondary urinary tract obstruction and resultant marked hydronephrosis and hydroureter. The barely visible coils of a catheter can be made out within the calculus.

(McKay et al., 1948). The latter types are referred to as secondary bladder calculi. Most occur in adults over the age of 40, although younger persons may also be affected. The factors favoring the formation of bladder calculi are the same as those involved in the formation of renal calculi (p. 1138).

The stones contain calcium, ammonium and magnesium salts, such as phosphates, carbonates, oxalates, urates and occasionally other compounds. They are commonly of mixed composition, although other forms are encountered. Phosphate and carbonate calculi tend to have a rounded appearance with a chalky gray-white consistency. These are most common in the presence of infection. Noninflammatory calculi may be composed largely of urates, producing yellow-brown, small stones under 1 cm. in diameter. Oxalates produce brown-colored stones (Fig. 25–15). Most often, on fracture of the stones, multiple lamellations are encountered, suggesting their mixed composition. A single calculus is most characteristic, but occasionally multiple stones are present. These commonly achieve a diameter of 2 to 3 cm., although sometimes massive concretions are formed which virtually fill the bladder lumen. Occasionally, fracture of a large, apparently homogeneous calculus discloses the unanticipated presence of a centrally placed foreign body.

Vesical calculi usually merely reside within the capacious bladder lumen and remain entirely asymptomatic, since they are too large to enter the urethral orifice. They may cause symptoms by producing chronic irritation and inflammation of the bladder wall, or by becoming lodged in the neck of the bladder and producing urinary tract obstruction. Under these circumstances, frequency and urgency may be evoked by the partial obstruction, and dysuria, pyuria and hematuria may be caused by the inflammatory changes in the mucosa. The diagnosis can only be suspected clinically and must be confirmed by cystoscopic or radiographic examination.

NEUROGENIC OR CORD BLADDER

A cord bladder may be defined as one in which normal vesical function is disturbed by interruption of the neural pathways of the bladder. Depending upon the level of cord injury, various types result. The understanding of this impaired function requires a knowledge of the normal neural connections which control bladder function. Two totally separate sets of pathways exist. *Voluntary micturition is under the control of the brain,* acting by way of somatic nerves which control the internal sphincter of the bladder. In addition to this volitional mechanism, there is an *automatic conditioned emptying reflex, actuated by autonomic nerve im-*

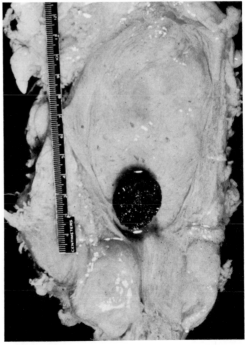

Figure 25–15. A relatively pure brown oxalate bladder calculus.

pulses which pass through a spinal reflex arc. When the *connections with the brain* are severed, volitional control of the bladder function is lost, and totally automatic function ensues. Consequently, any form of injury to the spinal cord *above* the level of the spinal reflex arc causes an automatic cord bladder. Trauma, tumors, inflammations and central nervous system degenerations may all cause such interruption of the pathways between the brain and the bladder. *Lower cord injuries to the corda equina and sacral plexus may destroy the automatic mechanism* so that reflex activity is abolished and *evacuation of the bladder occurs only by overflow (autonomic neurogenic bladder).* Peripheral nerve lesions may also sever these pathways and produce total interruption of nervous control of vesical function. Depending upon the level of the nerve lesion, the bladder may be either atonic or hypertonic and, consequently, may show either contraction and thickening of the wall or marked dilatation and thinning of the wall.

Neurogenic dysfunction is an important disorder because of the vulnerability of such bladders to infection. Urinary stasis and the necessity for catheterization provide the appropriate circumstances for the introduction of bacterial contamination. Only meticulous attention to asepsis, irrigation of the bladder and appropriate techniques of catheterization (tidal drainage) can stave off these serious sometimes fatal, complications.

FISTULAS

Abnormal fistulous tracts may occur between the bladder and the vagina, uterus, rectum, small intestines or the skin. The most common form is the *vesicovaginal fistula*, in which a communication between the bladder and vagina develops secondary to a carcinoma of the cervix or some severe cystitis. Inevitably, superimposed infection complicates the morphologic changes, causing inflammatory necrosis of the margins of the fistulous tract and severe acute to chronic cystitis. Less commonly, connections may exist to the uterus, known as *vesicouterine fistulas*. Neoplastic disease and postirradiation necrosis are the common antecedents. Superimposed infection is slightly less prone to occur. In both instances, the major presenting clinical finding is the escape of urine from the vaginal orifice. Those uncommon cases which are due to inflammatory disease permit successful reconstructive surgery. Abnormal communication may occur between the bladder and the rectum (*vesicorectal fistula*) and between the bladder and loops of small intestine (*vesicoenteric fistula*). These are most commonly caused by infections, tumors and irradiation necrosis. It is obvious that infection immediately complicates the presence of such fistulous tracts, and severe acute and chronic cystitis invariably results. Gross intestinal and fecal contamination may cause the accumulation of large amounts of foreign material within the bladder and may give rise to urethral obstruction. The most striking clinical finding is the passage of grossly contaminated, turbid urine, containing recognizable fecal contents. In addition, the entrance of gas and air from the intestinal tract into the bladder produces the passage of bubbles of gas in the urine referred to as *pneumaturia*.

URETHRA

It is hardly necessary to devote a special section to the sole consideration of diseases of the urethra. These are in the first place uncommon, and second, they rarely consist of disorders which affect the urethra alone. Much more often, urethral involvements arise in diseases of the male and female genital tract or urinary tract which, in turn, involve the urethra as one part of the genitourinary system. Such disorders will be taken up more appropriately in later sections. Only the tumors, perhaps, merit the designation of primary urethral lesions.

TUMORS

CARUNCLE

Urethral caruncle is the designation applied to small, red, painful masses that occur about the external urethral meatus in the female. They may be found at any age, but are more common in later life. The lesion usually consists of a hemispherical, friable, 1 to 2 cm. nodule that usually occurs singly, either just outside or just within the external urethral meatus. It may be covered by an intact mucosa, but is extremely friable and the slightest trauma may cause ulceration of the surface and bleeding. Histologically, it is composed of a *highly vascularized, young, fibroblastic connective tissue, more or less heavily infiltrated with leukocytes.* The overlying epithelium, where present, is either transitional or squamous cell in type. When there is no ulceration, the white cell infiltration is considerably less prominent. The question of whether the urethral caruncle represents merely a mass of inflammatory granulation tissue or a capillary hemangioma has been disputed for years. The consistent failure of this lesion ever to grow beyond 1 to 2 cm. in size argues strongly against a neoplastic origin. Surgical excision affords prompt relief and complete cure.

PAPILLOMA

Papillomas of the urethra occur usually just within or on the external meatus. In this location, they also fall within the scope of papillomas of the external genitalia, and are discussed there.

CARCINOMA

Carcinoma of the urethra is an uncommon lesion. It tends to occur in advanced age and, in the majority of instances, begins about the external meatus or on the immediately surrounding structures, such as the glans penis, or the introitus in the female. Some apparently begin just inside the external meatus or even at a higher level within the urethra. Those which occur at and protrude from the external meatus appear as warty, papillary growths that at first resemble the sessile papillary carcinomas described in the bladder. As they progress, they tend to become ulcerated on their surfaces and to assume the characteristics of a fungating, ulcerating lesion (Fig. 25–16). Tumors that arise higher in the urethral canal are more apt to have an invasive, ulcerative character from the onset. It is not known whether this represents a difference in biologic growth patterns or merely the difference imposed by the confinement of the higher positioned growths.

Most of these malignancies assume a squamous cell pattern of growth and resemble other squamous cell carcinomas in all histologic details. The papillary lesions that protrude from the external meatus are apt to show a transitional cell growth that further heightens their similarity to bladder carcinoma. Uncommonly, an adenocarcinomatous growth pattern is found and presumably suggests origin in the periurethral glands. These tumors invade locally, ulcerate and destroy, then eventually metastasize to the regional nodes and thence to the distant organs. In the male, lymph node spread tends to involve first the external inguinal nodes, thus permitting a good chance for radical excision of the primary tumor and the nodes of drainage. In the female, the drainage sites include the internal nodes about the iliac and hypogastric vessels, thus hampering the possibility of successful surgical excision.

SECONDARY TUMORS

More common than primary neoplasia of the urethra is secondary involvement of this

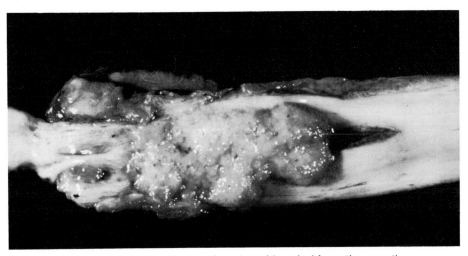

Figure 25–16. *Carcinoma of urethra with typical fungating growth.*

structure by extension of malignancies from the penis, prostate, bladder, vulva, vagina, cervix and uterus. In such involvements, fistulous communications may be produced which are similar to those described in the bladder.

REFERENCES

Ash, J. E.: Epithelial tumors of the bladder. J. Urol., *44*:135, 1940.

Bryan, G. T., et al.: Incidence of mouse bladder tumors following implantation of paraffin pellets containing certain tryptophan metabolites. Cancer Res., *24*:582, 1964.

Caldwell, W. L.: Cancer of the Urinary Bladder. St. Louis, Green Publishing, 1970.

Cobb, B. G., and Ansell, J. S.: Cigarette smoking and cancer of the bladder. J.A.M.A., *193*:329, 1965.

Dean, A. L., et al.: A restudy of the first 1400 tumors in the Bladder Tumor Registry, Armed Forces Institute of Pathology. J. Urol., *71*:571, 1954.

Gross, R. E., and Cresson, S. L.: Exstrophy of bladder: observations from eighty cases. J.A.M.A., *149*:1640, 1952.

Jewett, J. H., and Strong, G. H.: Infiltrating carcinoma of the bladder. Relation of depth penetration of the bladder wall to incidence, local extension and metastases. J. Urol., *55*:366, 1946.

Kerr, W. K., et al.: Effect of cigarette smoking on bladder carcinogenesis in man. Canad. Med. Ass. J., *93*:1, 1965.

Kerr, W. S., Jr., and Colby, F. H.: Carcinoma of the bladder: a correlation of pathology with treatment and prognosis. J. Urol., *65*:841, 1951.

Kleinfeld, M., et al.: Bladder tumors in a coal tar dye plant. Industr. Med. Surg., *35*:570, 1966.

Kretschmer, H. L.: The diagnosis and treatment of cystitis in women and children. New Eng. J. Med., *233;* 339, 1945.

Mathe, C. P.: Cystitis: classification and treatment. Discussion of type occurring after transurethral resection. J. Urol., *62*:308, 1949.

McDonald, B. F.: Carcinogens and chemical causes. (Symposium on bladder tumors.) J.A.M.A., *206*:1774, 1968.

McKay, H. W., et al.: Analysis of 200 cases of urinary calculi with particular reference to methods of management of ureteral stones. J.A.M.A., *137*:225, 1948.

Pugh, R. C. B.: The pathology of bladder tumors. In Wallace, D. M. (ed.): Neoplastic Disease at Various Sites: Tumors of the Bladder. Vol. 2. Edinburgh, Livingston Ltd., 1959, p. 116.

Riches, E. W., et al.: New growths of the kidney and ureter. Brit. J. Urol., *23*:297, 1951.

Union Internationale Contre le Cancrum: Malignant tumors of the urinary bladder. Clinical stage, classification and applied statistics. Geneva, 1967, p. 3.

26

MALE
GENITAL SYSTEM

EMBRYOGENESIS

The male genital tract is derived from the urogenital ridge. It begins to differentiate at about the sixth week of fetal life. The medial portion of the urogenital ridge proliferates to form a specialized genital ridge which parallels the mesonephric urinary ridge. During the second month of fetal development, the genital ridge of mesenchyme differentiates into an outer, germinal epithelium and an inner, loosely arranged epithelial mass. To this point, there is no sex differentiation and the primitive gonad is intersexual. By differential rates of growth, and by more marked proliferation of the caudal end of this ridge, a recognizable intracelomic testis is produced. It comes to lie just above the pelvis by about the third month of fetal development, a process termed the *internal descent*.

The further passage of the testis into its definitive adult position in the scrotum occurs in the eighth to ninth months of fetal development and is designated as the *external descent*. The internal structure of the testis develops during the third month of gestation. The external germinal epithelium differentiates into the tunica coverings of the testis. The inner epithelial mass or included totipotential cells give rise to the tubular structures of the testis including the rete testis. At the time of birth, a well developed branching system of seminiferous tubules is present. These still lack a lumen and continue as solid cords until puberty. At puberty, the testis cords acquire lumina and mature. Differentiation of secondary spermatocytes into spermatids and spermatozoa, which begins at this age, characterizes the adult form of spermatogenesis, which continues throughout life into extreme old age.

It is during the early ambisexual period that aberrations of development may give rise to both male and female sex organs in the same individual, producing a true hermaphrodite, or to various intergrades of sexual differentiation that create pseudohermaphrodites.

The external genitals begin to appear at about the sixth week of fetal life in the form of a conical protuberance in the midline of the body about midway between the umbilical cord and tail. This protuberance is designated as the genital tubercle. In the course of time, it will develop a shallow ventral groove with lateral ridges that fuse to create a urethral canal. Progressive growth of this tubercle creates a cylindrical phallus that gives rise to either the penis in the male or the clitoris in the female. Later swellings are the first indication of the developing scrotum or the labia in the female. As with the primitive gonad, the genital tubercle is a sexually undifferentiated structure that may give rise to either male or female external genitals. Aberration in its early development, therefore, accounts for the occurrence of intergrades between the definitive patterns of adult genital structure found in each sex.

PENIS

NORMAL

The body of the penis is made up of three intimately attached erectile structures, two lateral penile corpora cavernosa and the medial corpus cavernosum urethrae, containing the penile urethra. The glans penis is molded over the distal extremities of these three longitudinal corpora. The penis is covered with pigmented skin which is folded over at the distal extremity to form the prepuce. The prepuce is attached about the coronal sulcus. In the normal state it is readily retracted. When this epithelial sheath is abnormally small it sometimes cannot be retracted. When forcibly retracted, it may be caught about the glans and impinge upon the urethra or even the blood supply to the tip of the penis.

The arterial supply to the penis is derived from the internal pubic arteries, which are branches of the hypogastrics. These vessels enter the erectile corpora at the penile base. Traumatic injuries and lesions in the pubic region may thus impair this arterial supply. The venous drainage of the penis joins the prostatic plexus. Conceivably, therefore, disease in the prostate may embarrass such venous drainage but, for obscure reasons, this rarely occurs. Moreover, it is quite uncommon for disease processes to extend through these common vascular channels from one organ to the other. The lymphatic drainage of the penis and scrotum passes through the superficial inguinal and subinguinal lymph nodes. These nodes are often involved in inflammatory and neoplastic processes arising in the penis.

PATHOLOGY

The most important diseases of the penis comprise inflammations and tumors. The venereal infections syphilis and gonorrhea are, in their early stages, limited to the penis and the penile urethra. Carcinoma of the penis, while not one of the more common neoplasms in the male, still accounts for about 1 to 3 per cent of cancers in this sex. Despite the fact that this malignancy is readily apparent in its earliest stages, these cancers are often not brought to medical attention until they are well advanced and beyond cure. Penile cancer, therefore, is a significant cause of mortality.

CONGENITAL ANOMALIES

The penis is the site of many varied forms of congenital anomalies, most of which are of little clinical significance. These range from congenital absence and hypoplasia to hyperplasia, duplication and other aberrations in size and form. For the most part, these deviations in size and form are extremely uncommon and readily apparent on inspection. Certain other anomalies are more frequent and, therefore, have greater clinical significance.

Hypospadias and Epispadias. Malformation of the urethral groove and urethral canal may create abnormal openings either in the *ventral surface of the penis (hypospadias)* or in the *dorsal surface (epispadias)*. Such anomalies are commonly associated with failure of normal descent of the testes and with malformations of the urinary bladder. Frequently, the penile anomalies are accompanied by other severe congenital defects which are incompatible with life. Even the isolated urethral defects may have clinical significance, because frequently the abnormal opening is constricted and produces partial urinary obstruction and an attendant hazard of spread of bacterial contamination from the obstructed penile urethra into the bladder and remainder of the urinary tract. Moreover, these anomalies may have more serious consequences. When the orifices are situated near the base of the penis, normal ejaculation and insemination are hampered or totally blocked. These lesions are, therefore, possible causes of sterility in the male.

Phimosis. When the orifice of the prepuce is too small to permit its normal retraction, the condition is designated as phimosis. Such an abnormally small orifice may result from anomalous development, but may also be produced by inflammatory scarring of the prepuce. Phimosis is important since it interferes with cleanliness and permits the accumulation of secretions and detritus under the prepuce, favoring the development of secondary bacterial infections. When a phimotic prepuce is forcibly retracted over the glans penis, marked constriction and subsequent swelling may block the replacement of the prepuce creating the condition known as *paraphimosis*. This condition is not only extremely painful, but may also be a potential cause of urethral constriction and serious acute urinary retention.

INFLAMMATIONS

Inflammations of the penis almost invariably involve the glans and prepuce and include a wide variety of specific and nonspecific infections. For the most part, these inflammatory disorders are of little clinical significance, except for certain specific diseases to be mentioned.

Balanoposthitis. Balanoposthitis is a nonspecific infection of the glans and prepuce caused by a wide variety of organisms, i.e., staphylococci, streptococci, coliform bacilli, and less often by the gonococci. It is usually encountered in patients having phimosis or a large, redundant prepuce which interferes with cleanliness and predisposes to bacterial growth within the accumulated secretions and smegma. Such nonspecific inflammations may, if neglected, lead to frank ulcerations of the mucosal covering of the glans (Fig. 26–1). If they persist and become chronic, they lead to further inflammatory scarring of the phimosis, with aggravation of the underlying condition. The inflammatory reaction in the urethral and periurethral glands in gonorrheal balanoposthitis is indistinguishable morphologically from the nonspecific forms of balanoposthitis, and correct identification of the specific agent requires bacterial smears and cultures.

Syphilis. The primary hard chancre in the male usually occurs on the glans or on the inner surface of the prepuce. It may less commonly be situated on the shaft of the penis. The morphologic characteristics and clinical significance of this lesion have already been discussed in Chapter 10 (p. 378).

Chancroid. Chancroid, otherwise known as soft chancre, is a local bacterial infection of the penis, caused by the short, thick, gram-negative bacillus, *Hemophilus ducreyi*. While the infection usually arises as a local ulceration on the glans or prepuce of the penis, the disease is characterized by the extension of the infection to the inguinal nodes as described in Chapter 10 (p. 377).

Granuloma Inguinale. Granuloma inguinale is a chronic, specific, granulomatous infection that most commonly occurs in the genital regions of the male and female, characterized by a spreading, suppurating, ulcerating infection of the skin and mucous membranes. It has already been described (p. 389).

Lymphogranuloma Inguinale. Lympho-

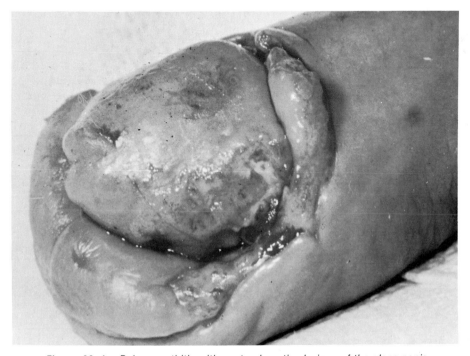

Figure 26–1. *Balanoposthitis with acute ulcerative lesions of the glans penis.*

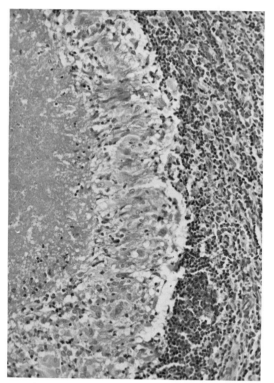

Figure 26–2. *Lymphogranuloma inguinale. The margin of a characteristic "stellate" abscess rimmed by a granulomatous reaction.*

granuloma inguinale, also known as *lymphogranuloma venereum* and *lymphopathia venereum,* is a venereal disease caused by Chlamydiae, minute organisms intermediate in size between bacteria and viruses. The disease is characterized by local lesions, usually about the external genitals of the male and female, followed in a period of weeks by marked inflammatory enlargement and suppuration within the inguinal nodes to constitute buboes (Fig. 26–2). (For further details, refer to p. 440.)

Other Infections. Many other miscellaneous infections may occur on and about the male genitals, such as herpes progenitalis, tuberculosis, diphtheria, fusospirochetal infections and a variety of others. Individually, and as a group, they are so uncommon as not to merit further consideration in a general survey of this type.

TUMORS

Tumors of the penis are, on the whole, uncommon. The most frequent neoplasms of the penis are carcinomas arising in the covering epithelium. Benign tumors are exceedingly rare. However, in addition to the clearly defined benign and malignant categories, there are several conditions that fall into an intermediate zone commonly designated as precancerous lesions.

BENIGN TUMORS

While lipomas, neuromas, fibromas and angiomas occur in the penis, they are so rare as to be medical curiosities.

Papilloma and Condyloma Acuminatum. The only benign tumor of any significant frequency is the epithelial papilloma. Commonly, these are divided into the condyloma acuminatum and the simple papilloma. Considerable importance was attached to the differentiation between these two lesions because the former was considered to be the result of a viral infection transmitted sexually, while the latter was considered as a sporadic new growth. However, it has become clear that the distinction between these two lesions is not always well defined. Some papillomas may indeed be new growths, but others may be of viral origin. Trauma and irritation may act as inciting or aggravating factors rather than initiating causes.

On the penis, these lesions occur most often about the coronal sulcus and inner surface of the prepuce. They consist of sessile or pedunculated, red papillary excrescences that vary from minute lesions 1 to several millimeters in diameter up to large, raspberry-like masses several centimeters in diameter. Histologically, a branching, villous, papillary connective tissue stroma is covered by a thickened hyperplastic epithelium that may have considerable superficial hyperkeratosis and thickening of the underlying epidermis (acanthosis) (Fig. 26–3). The normal orderly maturation of the epithelial cells is preserved, but may be slightly modified by increased mitotic activity in the basal layers and by some widening of the prickle cell layers. The basement membrane is usually intact, and there is no evidence of invasion of the underlying stroma. As far as is presently known, these lesions remain benign throughout their course and only rarely undergo cancerous transformation.

MALIGNANT TUMORS

With very rare exceptions, malignancy of the penis is virtually synonymous with squamous cell carcinoma. The rare exceptions, so infrequent as to barely merit citation, include melanocarcinomas, endotheliosarcomas and fibrosarcomas.

Carcinoma of the Penis. Squamous cell carcinoma of the penis represents about 1 to 3 per cent of cancer in the male in the United States. Since protection against this malignancy

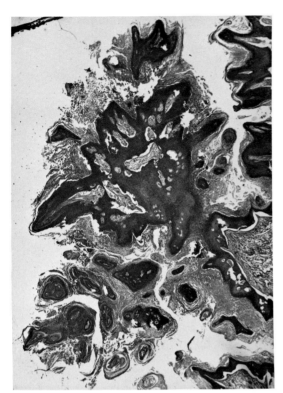

Figure 26–3. *Condyloma of penis. A low power view to illustrate the papillary excrescences covered by epithelium.*

carcinoma of the penis is virtually unknown. It is extremely rare among Mohammedans, in whom circumcision is performed before the tenth year of life. However, it is of interest that there is a somewhat higher incidence among Mohammedans than among those of the Hebrew faith. In other regions of the world where circumcision is not routinely practiced, carcinoma of the penis is correspondingly more common, so that it is reported to represent about 18 per cent of all malignant tumors in the Orient. Carcinomas are usually found in patients between the ages of 40 and 70. Phimosis, balanoposthitis, syphilis and chronic irritation are thought to play important predisposing roles. Presumably, circumcision protects against tumorigenesis by preventing the accumulation of smegma (carcinogenic in animals) and minimizing the tendency to irritation and infections.

The lesion usually begins on the glans or prepuce near the coronal sulcus. The first observable changes are a small area of epithelial thickening accompanied by graying and fissuring of the mucosal surface. With progression, an elevated leukoplakic papule is produced that often ulcerates when a diameter of approximately 1 cm. is reached. Despite the obviousness of such lesions, by the time most patients seek medical attention, large characteristic malignant ulcers are present, having necrotic, secondarily infected bases with ragged, irregular, heaped-up margins (Fig. 26–4). In far advanced lesions, the ulceroinvasive disease may have destroyed virtually the entire tip of the penis or large areas of the shaft.

is apparently conferred by circumcision, the incidence among different population groups varies widely throughout the world. In the Hebrew religion in which circumcision is performed ritually within the first two weeks of life,

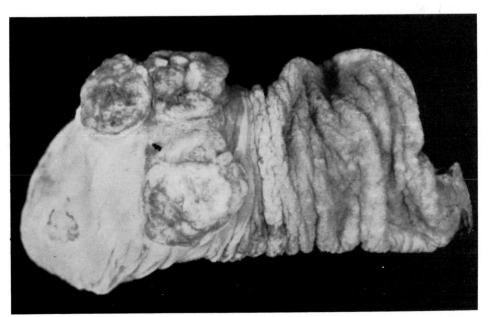

Figure 26–4. *Squamous cell carcinoma of penis with typical shaggy, fungating ulcerations.*

A second pattern of macroscopic tumor growth is the papillary tumor that simulates the condyloma and progressively enlarges to form a cauliflower-like, fungating mass. As this tumor enlarges, it undergoes central ulceration and may become transformed to a pattern that resembles the ulcerative lesion just described.

Histologically, both the papillary and ulceroinvasive lesions are squamous cell carcinomas exactly resembling those that occur elsewhere on the skin surface.

Clinical Course. Carcinoma of the penis is a slowly growing, locally metastasizing lesion that usually has run a clinical course of one or two years by the time the patient seeks treatment (Lenowitz and Graham, 1946) (Sauer and Leighton, 1944). Occasionally, such delay is occasioned by the existence of a phimosis that completely hides the developing lesion, but more often an unawareness of the significance of the developing papule underlies this regrettable delay. The lesions are nonpainful until they undergo secondary ulceration and infection. Frequently they bleed. At the time when most patients are first diagnosed, about one-third have inguinal node metastases. Metastasis to local nodes characterizes the early stage, and widespread dissemination is ex-

tremely uncommon until the lesion is far advanced. Surgical amputation and regional node dissection produce about 50 per cent three- to five-year survivals. It is of interest that the papillary lesions metastasize much less frequently.

PREMALIGNANT LESIONS

There is a group of dysplastic epithelial changes which may occur anywhere in the body, but tend to occur somewhat more frequently in the penis, that have been related to the genesis of frank malignancy. These entities are *leukoplakia, erythroplasia of Queyrat and Bowen's disease.* Only the erythroplasia is limited to the penis. The exact cause of these epithelial dysplasias and their precise relationship to the development of carcinoma are still obscure. However, in repeated clinical studies, such lesions have been identified months to years before the development of frankly invasive carcinoma (Melicow and Ganem, 1946). Only the leukoplakia is considered to be due to persistent, chronic irritation. The genesis of Bowen's disease and erythroplasia is unknown.

Leukoplakia is recognized as a pearly white

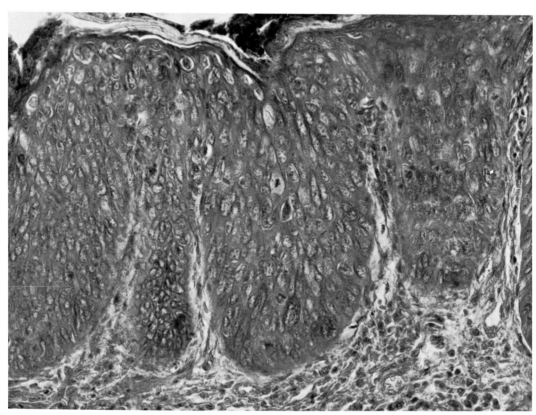

Figure 26–5. *Bowen's disease illustrating the dysplasia and anaplasia of the epithelial cells.*

thickening of the mucosa, characterized microscopically by a variety of changes, including hyperkeratosis, epithelial thickening, acanthosis, epithelial dysplasia and chronic inflammation of the submucosal connective tissue. The *erythroplasia of Queyrat* produces similar hyperkeratosis, but there is a more marked hyperplasia and dysplasia of the epithelium, with considerably greater thickening of the epidermis and more striking loss of orientation and variability in the size and shape of the epithelial cells (Payne, 1957). Frequently, it is extremely difficult to distinguish lesions which are considered to be erythroplasia from carcinoma in situ. Approximately 5 to 10 per cent of individuals with this condition eventually

develop a squamous cell carcinoma. *Bowen's disease* is even more similar to overt malignancy and is considered by many authors to be identical to carcinoma in situ (Fig. 26–5). All these lesions are given more complete consideration under the discussion of the vulva, but it merits reemphasis, at this time, that these dysplastic epithelial changes may be importantly related to the genesis of cancer. It should also be pointed out here that leukoplakia is a clinical term used to describe an area of mucosal thickening that may be caused by hyperkeratosis or unusual hyperplasia within the deeper layers. Therefore, all leukoplakias do not have the same pattern of epithelial changes or clinical significance, as will be brought out later.

TESTIS AND EPIDIDYMIS

NORMAL

In the adult, the testis weighs approximately 12 gm. and measures about $5 \times 3 \times 3$ cm. It is covered by a serosal membrane, the visceral layer of the tunica vaginalis, which is reflected off the hilus of the testis to form an inner lining of the scrotal sac, the parietal tunica vaginalis. Thus, in the normal adult, there is a completely closed serosa-lined potential space folded about the testes, much as Bowman's capsule envelops the glomerular tuft. The lining of this space is derived from the processus vaginalis of the peritoneum. Beneath the visceral tunica vaginalis there is the dense, white, fibrous tunica albuginea and deep to it a so-called tunica vasculosa which is, in reality, merely a condensation of fibrous tissue and blood vessels on the inner surface of the tunica albuginea. All the arteries, veins, lymphatics and nerves enter through the hilus. The epididymis is a crescentic tubular organ lying along the posterolateral border of the testis. The rete tubules of the testis drain into the collecting tubules of the head of the epididymis, while the tail of the epididymis communicates with the vas deferens.

Histologically, the testis consists of branching tubular glands separated from adjacent glands by a scant, loose, connective tissue stroma. These glands have distinct basement membranes that increase in thickness with age. The testis is divided into many lobules by condensed fibrous septa which all radiate from the hilus of the testis. Within the testicular tubules are found the sustentacular supporting cells and the maturing germinal epithelium that has already been mentioned in the embryology of this organ. Within the stroma, there are scattered groups and nests of round to polygonal, epithelial-like Leydig cells having abundant acidophilic cytoplasm and large nuclei that contain coarse chromatin granules and a prominent nucleolus. In the cytoplasm of these cells are found lipofuscin, lipid granules and long, slender, crystalline structures, the crystalloids of Reinke. These interstitial cells are presumed to be a site of formation of androgens. The number of these Leydig cells bears an inverse ratio to the preservation and activity of the tubular germinal epithelium. In advanced age or acquired disease, with atrophy of the germinal epithelium, there is an accompanying proliferation of the Leydig cells.

The histology of the epididymis is composed essentially of a coiled, twisted, single duct which is formed by the agglomeration of the vasa efferentia. This duct is lined by extremely tall, pseudostratified, columnar, ciliated epithelium, having nuclei for the most part disposed basally, and luminal portions of the cells composed only of cytoplasm containing fat droplets, pigments and fat vacuoles.

PATHOLOGY

The major pathologic involvements of the testis and epididymis are quite distinct. In the case of the epididymis, the most important and frequent involvements are inflammatory diseases while, in the testis, the major lesions consist of tumors. However, their close anatomic relationship permits the extension of any of these processes from one organ to the other.

CONGENITAL ANOMALIES

With the exception of incomplete descent of the testes, congenital anomalies are extremely rare and include: absence of one or both testes, fusion of the testes (so called *synorchism*), the formation of relatively insignificant cysts within the testis and the formation of the testis in an aberrant location (ectopic testis).

CRYPTORCHIDISM

Cryptorchidism is synonymous with undescended testes. It is found in about 4 per cent of prepubertal boys. This anomaly represents a complete or incomplete failure of the intra-abdominal testes to descend into the scrotal sac. From the preceding embryogenesis of the male genital tract, it will be recalled that in the fetus the testis arises within the celomic cavity and then, by differential growth of the body, as well as more rapid proliferation of the caudal end of the urogenital ridge, the testis comes to lie within the lower abdomen or brim of the pelvis, a process referred to as the internal descent. Following this, it descends through the inguinal canal into the scrotal sac, the external descent. On this basis, *malpositioned testes may be found at any point in this pathway of descent.* The precise cause of cryptorchidism is still poorly understood. In a small percentage of cases, it is believed to be a congenital, hereditary disturbance. In another small group, it is related to some hormonal imbalance with incomplete sexual development. But in the majority of cases it will represent an isolated, random, congenital anomaly or some mechanical obstruction to the complete external descent. A short spermatic cord, a narrow inguinal canal, inadequate development of the gubernaculum testis and fibrous adhesions in the pathway of descent are all attributed causal significance. The condition is completely asymptomatic, and is found only by the patient or the examining physician when the scrotal sac is discovered not to contain the testis.

Cryptorchidism may be unilateral or bilateral. When unilateral, it is somewhat more common on the right side. When discovered before the age of puberty, the organ is essentially normal in size, shape and consistency, and is only malpositioned. However, at about the time of puberty, progressive atrophy ensues and the organ shows progressive decrease in size and progressive increase in consistency and, on cut surface, discloses an increased amount of fibrous tissue, replacing, apparently, the testicular substance (Fig. 26–6A). At this stage, the testicular tubules fail to string out as do the normal.

Histologically, the gross atrophy is accompanied by progressive hyaline thickening of the basement membranes of the tubules, with progressive increase of the interstitial connective stroma. Concomitantly, spermatogenic activity is diminished and then totally ceases. The germinal epithelium then undergoes progressive atrophy until only a few primitive spermatogonia and Sertoli cells persist (Cohen, 1967). During this time, the basement membranes show increasing hyalinization and thickening, so that eventually the tubules become replaced by dense cords of hyaline connective tissue outlined by the prominent thickened basement membranes (Fig. 26–6B). There is a concomitant increase of interstitial stroma and usually some hyperplasia of the interstitial cells of Leydig. However, in certain cases, these cells may appear to remain normal or even be decreased in number when pituitary insufficiency underlies the condition.

Cryptorchidism is of more than academic interest since, from the morphologic changes, it is apparent that it may result in sterility when the process is bilateral. The atrophy pubertally is attributed to the higher temperature in the environment of the nonscrotal testis (Newman and Wilhelm, 1950). When it lies in the inguinal canal, it is particularly exposed to trauma and crushing against the ligaments and bones. A concomitant inguinal hernia frequently accompanies such malposition of the testis.

One of the most controversial questions is whether cryptorchidism is related to a higher than usual incidence of the development of testicular cancer. There is wide disagreement on this subject, and regrettably there has been

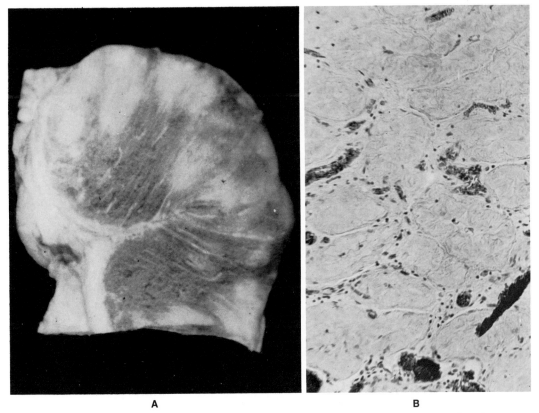

Figure 26–6. A, *Fibrosis of testis viewed on cut section. The pale white fibrous scars replace large areas of the darker testicular tubules.* B, *Atrophy of testis. The tubules are visible as shadowy structures totally replaced by collagenous fibrous tissue.*

repetitious quotation of a very few articles with little new definitive work. On the one hand, Gross and Jewett (1956) take the view that there is no solid evidence that the likelihood of cancer is much higher in the cryptorchid than in the normally positioned testis. To quote from their article, "Unfortunately in some quarters there is the feeling that all undescended testes should be excised as a measure to prevent neoplastic disease. We feel very strongly that in the light of present knowledge such a step is completely unwarranted." They concede that there might possibly be an increased chance of tumor formation but doubt that it is clinically significant.

From this extreme, there are reports indicating an eleven-fold, and even one with a 48-fold, increased incidence of malignancy. Sovhal (1956) states that the incidence of cancer in the undescended testis is 11 per cent, whereas the incidence in the normally located testis is only 0.0013 per cent. He goes further to point out that testicular tumors that occur in normally positioned testes may, indeed, arise in foci of tubules of the prepubertal type, suggesting that tumors do not arise in completely normal testes. Campbell (1942) states unequivocally that there is statistical validity to the differing incidence of malignant change in the undescended and normally descended testes. Be it noted, however, that all agree that placement of the testis within the scrotum does not preclude the possibility of a cancer developing at a later date.

The opinions are so varied that the subject can only be summarized by stating from personal experience that, in all probability, the undescended testis is more vulnerable to neoplasia than the scrotal testis, but the magnitude of this danger is probably small. Moreover, when the malposition is corrected before six years of age, the hazard is further reduced to virtually control levels.

REGRESSIVE CHANGES

Atrophy. Atrophy is the only important regressive change that affects the scrotal testis. Atrophy may occur from a number of causes. These can be listed as (1) progressive atherosclerotic narrowing of the blood supply in old age, (2) the end-stage of an inflammatory orchitis, whatever the etiologic agent, (3) generalized avitaminosis, (4) hypopituitarism, (5) generalized malnutrition or cachexia, (6) obstruction to the outflow of semen and (7) irradiation. (8) Prolonged administration of female sex hormones, such as is used in treatment of patients with carcinoma of the prostate, may lead to atrophy. (9) Exhaustion atrophy may follow the persistent stimulation produced by high levels of follicle-stimulating pituitary hormone. The gross and microscopic alterations follow the pattern already described in cryptorchidism. When the process is bilateral, as it frequently is, sterility results. Atrophy or sometimes improper development of the testes occasionally occurs as a primary failure of genetic origin. It may produce an interesting endocrine derangement (Klinefelter's syndrome) to be described next.

Klinefelter's Syndrome. This uncommon cause of testicular atrophy and primary hypogonadism represents a sex chromosomal disorder discussed in detail on p. 181. The karyotype is usually XXY but may be XXXY, XXYY or XXXXY. Any one of these karyotypes which have in common extra X chromosomes in the male leads to aberrations in testicular development, resulting in small testes, alterations in somatic development, reduced fertility to complete sterility and sometimes reduced intelligence. The more X chromosomes, the greater the reduction in intelligence. Thus, in the investigation of infertility in the male, Klinefelter's syndrome must be considered and can be diagnosed by the demonstration of Barr bodies (sex chromatin) in smears of somatic cells such as buccal epithelial cells. You recall that all but one X chromosome is inactivated, and so all additional X chromosomes are transformed to Barr Bodies (sex chromatin). According to Grumbach et al. (1957), Klinefelter's syndrome accounts for about 3 per cent of all cases of subfertility in males.

INFLAMMATIONS

Inflammations are distinctly more common in the epididymis than in the testis. It is classically taught that, of the three major specific inflammatory states, *gonorrhea and tuberculosis almost invariably arise in the epididymis, while syphilis affects first the testis.*

NONSPECIFIC EPIDIDYMITIS AND ORCHITIS

Nonspecific epididymitis and possible subsequent orchitis are commonly related to infec-

tions in the urinary tract (cystitis, urethritis, genitoprostatitis), which presumably reach the epididymis and the testis through either the vas deferens or the lymphatics of the spermatic cord. On this account, *epididymitis is a common complication of operations on the prostatic gland unless the vasa deferentia have been previously ligated.* Rarely, the testis or epididymis is seeded hematogenously from some other focus of infection. The common organisms involved are the coliform bacilli and the pyogenic staphylococci and streptococci.

The bacterial invasion sets up a nonspecific acute inflammation characterized by congestion, edema and a white cell infiltration chiefly by neutrophils, macrophages and lymphocytes. While the infection, in the early stage, is more or less limited to the interstitial connective tissue, it rapidly extends to involve the tubules and may progress to frank abscess formation or complete suppurative necrosis of the entire epididymis (Fig. 26-7). Usually, having involved the epididymis, the infection extends either by direct continuity or through tubular channels or lymphatics into the testis to evoke a similar inflammatory reaction within the testis. Such inflammatory involvement of the epididymis and testis is often followed by fibrous scarring which, in many cases, leads to permanent sterility. Sterility may result from inflammatory obstruction of the excretory pathways or may be due to the intense pressure

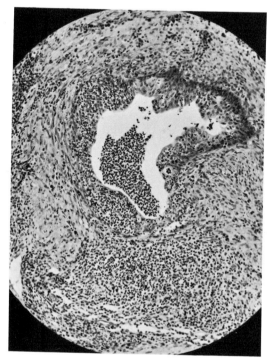

Figure 26-7. *Nonspecific acute epididymitis. The inflammation has partially destroyed the tubule and has caused inflammatory metaplasia of the lining epithelium.*

placed upon the blood supply of the testis by the development of edema within a tight, fibrous, enclosing tunica albuginea. Thus, even when suppurative necrosis has not occurred, extensive inflammations may be followed by considerable atrophy of spermatic tubules and loss of spermatogenesis. Usually the interstitial cells of Leydig are not totally destroyed and are believed to be capable of regeneration when partially injured so that sexual activity is, therefore, not disturbed. Any such nonspecific infection may become chronic.

GRANULOMATOUS ORCHITIS

Among middle-aged men, a rare cause of unilateral testicular enlargement is nontuberculous, granulomatous orchitis. Often, the testicular swelling develops after an interval of a week to months after some trauma to the testis. Histologically, the orchitis is distinguished by granulomas which are seen both within spermatic tubules and in the intertubular connective tissue. The lesions closely resemble tubercles but differ somewhat in having plasma cells and occasional neutrophils interspersed within the enclosing rim of fibroblasts and lymphocytes. The causation of these lesions remains unknown, but traumatic destruction of spermatocytes within tubules or rupture of tubules with extravasation of sperm is postulated. It has been shown in hamsters that lipid extracts of human spermatozoa will induce granulomas (Berg, 1954). Granulomatous orchitis may be a form, then, of autoimmune disease to sequestered antigens in the individual's own spermatozoa. Death of spermatozoa or rupture of tubules may be the trigger which releases these antigens and initiates the inflammatory response.

SPECIFIC INFLAMMATIONS

Gonorrhea. Extension of infection from the posterior urethra to the prostate, seminal vesicles, and thence to the epididymis is the usual course of a neglected gonococcal infection. Inflammatory changes similar to those described in the nonspecific infections occur, with the development of frank abscesses in the epididymis, resulting in extensive destruction of this organ. In the more neglected cases, the infection may thence spread to the testis and produce a suppurative orchitis.

Mumps. In about one-quarter to one-third of cases of parotitis in adults, an acute interstitial orchitis develops about one week following the onset of the swelling of the salivary glands. Rarely, cases of mumps orchitis have been described without apparent or significant

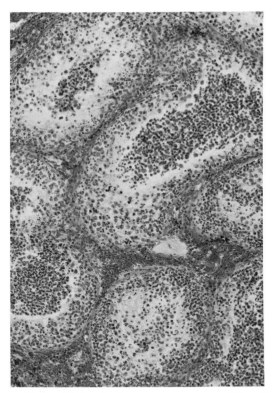

Figure 26–8. Acute severe mumps orchitis with extensive interstitial and intratubular exudation.

involvement of the salivary glands. In the acute stage, the inflammatory reaction is characterized by intense interstitial edema and mononuclear infiltration, consisting chiefly of lymphocytes, plasma cells and macrophages. Neutrophils are usually not prominent but, in the more intense inflammatory responses, frank suppuration may develop and the tubular lumina may become filled with purulent exudate (Fig. 26–8). Since the process usually remains largely interstitial and is, characteristically, patchy and haphazard, healing of the inflammatory reaction may not be followed by any late residuals. However, when the edema has been intense, atrophy of the germinal epithelium may remain and give rise to sterility.

Tuberculosis. *Tuberculosis almost invariably begins in the epididymis and may spread to the testis.* In all but rare exceptions, such lesions reflect a tuberculous infection elsewhere in the body, almost invariably in the lungs. Rarely, tuberculous epididymitis has followed apparently isolated renal tuberculosis. In many of these cases, there is associated tuberculous prostatitis and seminal vesiculitis, and it is believed by some that epididymitis usually represents a secondary spread from these other involvements of the genital tract. However, the epididymal involvement as a metastatic dissemination through the blood cannot be excluded, even in those cases with involvement of the organs in the urogenital system. The infection invokes the classic morphologic reactions of tuberculosis. Numerous tubercles become confluent to produce large caseous masses that, in the course of time, may obliterate the entire epididymal structure. By continuity or lymphogenous spread, such infections may extend into the testis but, for long periods of time, this organ is spared in most cases (Figs. 26–9 and 26–10). Tuberculous orchitis usually remains confined to the regions proximal to the epididymis. The inflammatory involvement is followed, in the course of weeks or months, by progressive fibrous scarring and sometimes calcification. Infrequently, exudate accumulates within the tunica vaginalis and, equally

rarely, tuberculous scrotal skin sinuses develop.

Syphilis. The testis and epididymis are affected in both acquired and congenital syphilis, but *almost invariably the testis is involved first by the infection.* In many cases, the orchitis is not accompanied by epididymitis. The morphologic pattern of the reaction takes two forms: the production of gummas, or a diffuse interstitial inflammation characterized by edema and lymphocytic and plasma cell infiltration with the characteristic hallmark of all syphilitic infections, i.e., obliterative endarteritis with perivascular cuffing of lymphocytes and plasma cells. In the early case, the gummas cause a nodular enlargement and the characteristic yellow-white foci of necrosis. The diffuse reaction causes swelling and induration. In the course of time, whether or not the

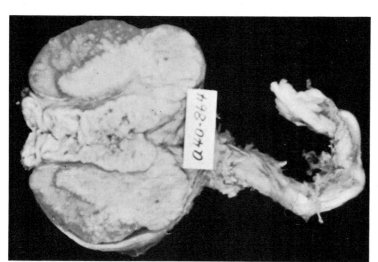

Figure 26–9. *Tuberculous epididymo-orchitis with extensive confluent caseous necrosis.*

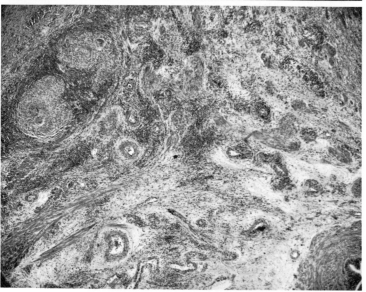

Figure 26–10. *Tuberculous epididymitis with two characteristic tubercles in the upper left corner and an epididymal tubule in the lower right corner.*

morphologic reaction is that of the already described gumma formation or diffuse inflammation, progressive fibrous scarring follows, which in turn leads to considerable tubular atrophy and, sometimes, sterility. Usually the testes shrink and become pale and fibrotic. The interstitial cells of Leydig are spared, and sexual potency is not impaired. However, when the process is extremely advanced, the Leydig cells may be destroyed, resulting in loss of libido. Sterility occurs less often with the gumma than with the diffuse inflammation.

Miscellaneous Infections.   The testis and epididymis are involved by hematogenous metastatic dissemination of organisms in a wide variety of infectious diseases, such as leprosy, typhoid fever, brucellosis and meningococcal and rickettsial infections, and in some fungus diseases such as blastomycosis and actinomycosis. In all these instances, the testicular and epididymal involvement is only one small component of the systemic disorder, and the local inflammatory changes resemble those found in the systemic disease.

VASCULAR DISTURBANCES

Torsion.   Twisting of the spermatic cord may cut off the venous drainage and the arterial supply to the testis. Usually, however, the thick-walled arteries remain patent so that intense vascular engorgement and venous infarction follow. The usual precipitating cause for such torsion is some violent movement or physical trauma. In the majority of instances, however, predisposing causes, such as incomplete descent, absence of the scrotal ligaments or the gubernaculum testis, atrophy of the testis so that it is abnormally mobile within the tunica vaginalis, abnormal attachment of the testis to the epididymis and other abnormalities, predispose to such twisting. Depending upon the duration and severity of the process, the morphologic changes may be those of merely intense congestion to widespread extravasation of blood into the interstitial tissue of the testis and epididymis. In the more extreme instances, hemorrhagic or even ischemic infarction of the entire testis may occur (Fig. 26–11). In these late stages, the testis is markedly enlarged and is converted virtually into a sac of soft, necrotic, hemorrhagic tissue. The leukocytic reaction is very variable and depends upon the free access of blood via the arterial system. Usually the blood flow is so impaired that leukocytic infiltration is not a prominent feature and the process essentially resembles one of pure coagulative infarction necrosis without considerable inflammatory reaction.

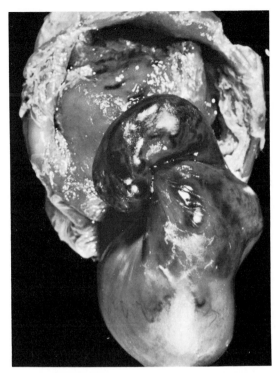

Figure 26–11.   *Torsion of the testis.*

TESTICULAR TUMORS

No other organ of the body is victim to such a wide variety of neoplasms as the testis. Approximately 97 per cent arise from germ cells. Most of the remainder, the nongerminal tumors, originate from the interstitial cells of Leydig or the Sertoli cells, and most of these neoplasms produce steroids and consequent systemic endocrinopathies. The nongerminal tumors tend to be small, rarely cause testicular enlargement and are generally benign. Those arising in germ cells often cause testicular enlargement, and almost all are highly malignant cancers capable of widespread metastasis. In addition to these neoplasms are the extremely rare, nondistinctive tumors arising from connective tissue and blood vessels, producing fibromas, leiomyomas and angiomas entirely like their counterparts elsewhere.

GERM CELL TUMORS

Tumors arising in germ cells may occur at any age, with a large peak incidence between the ages of 25 and 35 and a much smaller peak in the advanced years of life. Indeed, germinal neoplasms comprise the most common form of cancer in males between the ages of 25 and 35. Overall, they have an incidence of 3 per

100,000 male population, and represent about 5 per cent of all genitourinary tract neoplasms.

Pathogenesis. As with all neoplasms, little is known about the ultimate causes of germinal tumors. However, several predisposing factors may be important. As indicated earlier (p. 1178), cryptorchid testes have an increased vulnerability, but the precise magnitude of the risk is still highly controversial. Genetic factors may contribute but the evidence is still fragmentary. The occurrence of testicular tumors in siblings, identical twins and related members of a family suggests hereditary influences. Infrequently, bilateral tumors are encountered in the same individual. In a survey in New York, an ethnic differential was found among young men, with Jews being affected twice as often as non-Jews, and Protestants twice as often as Catholics (Editorial, 1968). Could these ethnic differences reflect genetic factors? In support of the role of hereditary predisposition, it has been possible to develop inbred strains of laboratory animals bearing an exceedingly high incidence of testicular tumors. Yet another influence has been suspected, namely, trauma to the testis. But here, as in other settings, it is uncertain whether the trauma played a causative role or merely called attention to a preexisting neoplasm.

Classification. Over the years, there has been continued difficulty in establishing a universally acceptable classification of testicular, germinal tumors. Fundamental to the argument has been the issue of whether all testicular tumors arise from primordial germ cells or, instead, from spermatic epithelium of the seminiferous tubule. In the United States, most experts hold to the germ cell concept as proposed by Friedman, Dixon and Moore (Friedman and Moore, 1946) (Dixon and Moore, 1953). The Testicular Tumor Panel and Registry of the Pathological Society of Great Britain and Ireland (1964) favor the spermatic epithelial origin. We need not enter this arena of controversy and will follow the most widely used classification proposed by Friedman and Moore, in which five distinctive histologic and clinical patterns are recognized:

1. Seminoma.
2. Embryonal carcinoma.
3. Choriocarcinoma.
4. Teratoma.
5. Teratocarcinoma.

Despite the identification of five distinctive types, in approximately 40 per cent of cases, mixed patterns are encountered and, indeed, Dixon and Moore (1952) have identified as many as 15 combinations.

Morphology. Seminoma. The seminoma is the most common testicular tumor and accounts for about 40 per cent of all germ cell neoplasms. Compared with the teratoid tumors, it tends to occur in slightly older individuals and, while it frequently metastasizes to pelvic and para-aortic lymph nodes, its susceptibility to radiation therapy permits cures in many cases even when spread has already occurred. Three somewhat distinctive histologic variants are recognized: (1) the classic pattern accounting for 90 per cent of these neoplasms, (2) an anaplastic variant and (3) the rare spermatocytic seminoma. They all produce grey to yellow-white nodules or masses in the testis that, on cut section, often have a lobulated, soft, fleshy encephaloid appearance. Centrifugal growth eventually replaces all of the native architecture and causes symmetrical testicular enlargement. However, even in bulky lesions which double or triple the size of the testis, growth is for a long time confined within the tunica albuginea, and only in far advanced cases does the tumor penetrate into adjacent structures (Fig. 26–12).

Microscopically, the classic seminoma presents sheets of uniform so-called "seminoma cells" divided into lobules by delicate septa of fibrous tissue. The "seminoma cell" is highly distinctive and can be recognized even in disseminated metastases. It comprises a large, round to polygonal cell having a cleared or watery-appearing abundant cytoplasm in the center of which is found a round, moderately large nucleus having clumped chroma-

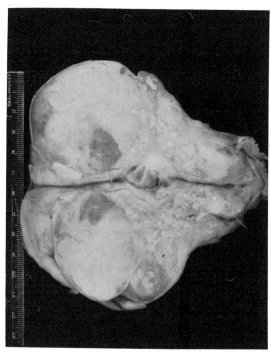

Figure 26–12. *Seminoma of the testis with virtual obliteration of the testis and invasion beyond the tunica albuginea.*

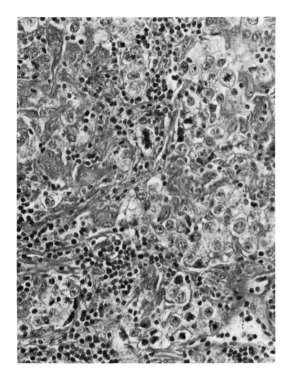

Figure 26–13. Seminoma of the testis demonstrating the large "cleared" seminoma cells and lymphocytic stroma.

tin and one or two prominent nucleoli (Fig. 26—13). In the classic neoplasm, mitoses are infrequent as are giant cells, hemorrhages or areas of necrosis. The fibrous septa are also made distinctive by virtue of a sparse to abundant infiltrate of mature lymphocytes and, less often, foci of granulomatous inflammation. The granulomatous lesions may have necrotic caseous-like centers and contain Langhans' type giant cells producing more than a passing similarity to tubercles. It is believed that the lymphocytic infiltrate and granulomatous reaction are both manifestations of an immunologic defensive reaction of the host against the neoplasm.

A few seminomas (less than 10 per cent) are much more anaplastic, have greater variability in cell and nuclear size and contain numerous mitotic figures. Foci of hemorrhage and necrosis are frequently present, suggesting rapidity of growth which outpaces the available blood supply.

As would be anticipated, anaplastic seminomas tend to be larger than the classic variant, have a poorer prognosis, macroscopically are softer, and have more variegated cut surfaces because of the areas of cystic softening and red-brown hemorrhagic discoloration. The rarest pattern—the spermatocytic seminoma—also exhibits, on gross inspection, areas of cystic softening and, under the microscope, tumor cells which grow in cords or columns, mimicking testicular tubules. In this pattern, the neoplastic cells do not have the cleared cyto-

plasm seen in the classic variant. Instead, the tumor cells resemble the spermatic epithelium of the normal testicular tubules.

Although all variants of the seminoma tend to remain confined within the testis for a long time, they eventually extend into the epididymis and spermatic cord and metastasize to inguinal, para-iliac, para-aortic and even mediastinal and cervical nodes. Visceral metastasis may occur, but is uncommon. With orchiectomy followed by radiation of the possible pelvic and abdominal sites of involvement, the five-year survival rate is approximately 98 per cent in cases with no nodal metastasis, 90 per cent in those with nodal spread but no visceral metastasis, but only 20 per cent when visceral metastases are present.

Foci of embryonal carcinoma or choriocarcinoma may be encountered in seminomas, and the prognosis then becomes that of these more aggressive neoplasms. Indeed, the primary tumor within the testis may appear to be a pure seminoma, but foci of choriocarcinoma or embryonal carcinoma may appear in the metastases. It is reasonable to assume that the primary neoplasm had similar foci which were not detected, but conceivably the multipotentiality of the germinal epithelium makes possible several lines of differentiation in the metastatic sites.

Embryonal Carcinoma. These tumors are much more aggressive and lethal than the seminomas and represent about 15 to 20 per cent of testicular neoplasms. They tend to be smaller, producing asymmetrical nodular distortion of the testis in contrast to the bulkier seminoma which often produces symmetrical enlargement. On cross section, the nodules are basically gray-white, but foci of hemorrhage and necrosis create a heterogeneous surface (Fig. 26—14). Far more infiltrative than seminomas, these cancers penetrate the tunica albuginea, epididymis and spermatic cord. As the term embryonal implies, the neoplastic cells have the potential of growing in a wide variety of patterns, including glandular, papillary, tubular or microcystic arrangements and, rarely, even solid sheets of highly anaplastic cells (Fig. 26—15). In the glandular, papillary and microcystic variants, the cells are cuboidal to columnar, but in the tubular and sheet-like array, there is great cytologic variability ranging from polyhedral to spindle shapes. Tumors composed of spindled cells have a remarkable resemblance to sarcomas. Tumor giant cells, mitoses, foci of ischemic necrosis and hemorrhages are common. The stroma is generally scant and is distributed about and between the glandular, cystic and tubular structures when formed. Lymphoid infiltrate and granulomatous reactions are not present in the stroma of embryonal carcinomas.

Even when the primary nodule is small, the embryonal carcinoma tends to locally invade and then spread to lymph nodes and internal viscera.

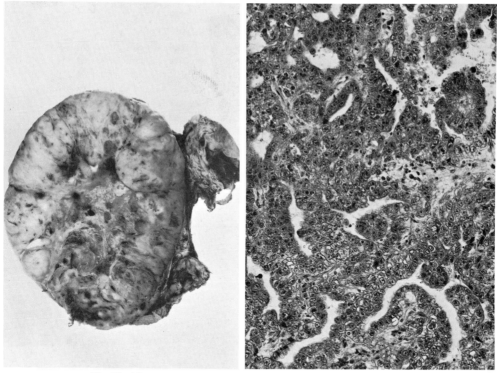

Fig. 26-14   Fig. 26-15

Figure 26-14. *Embryonal carcinoma with extensive mottled necrosis and hemorrhage.*
Figure 26-15. *Embryonal carcinoma growing in glandular and papillary fashion.*

Widespread visceral metastasis is not uncommon with these tumors and, since they are less radiosensitive than seminomas, the five-year survival rate following orchiectomy, regional node dissection, radiation and chemotherapy is on the order of 25 to 35 per cent. As with other testicular tumors, foci of aberrant differentiation may be encountered, particularly in the form of choriocarcinoma.

Choriocarcinoma. The choriocarcinoma is a highly malignant, rapidly metastasizing tumor that is characterized by three features. There must be (1) recognizable syncytiotrophoblast and (2) cytotrophoblast, and (3) the cells must be arranged in definite papillae or villi. While these highly malignant tumors may arise in the testis, ovary or primitive rests, they comprise only 1 per cent of so-called germinal tumors of the testis. Most often, the choriocarcinoma develops in the placenta itself.

These tumors are frequently very small in their primary sites, and many would have escaped clinical and anatomic recognition were it not for their metastases. Metastases from a choriocarcinoma have been identified at postmortem examination in patients with no apparent primary lesion. Only when serial sections of the testis were made could minute microscopic foci of primary neoplasm be identified. In other instances, the tumor may occupy the entire testicular structure and may produce nod-

ular enlargement. On cut section, the tumor is characteristically variegated, having small foci of pale gray-white, apparently well preserved tissue, interspersed with areas of yellow-white infarction necrosis and other areas of red to black hemorrhage. These tumors are usually quite soft and necrotic, with the best preserved areas to be found in the margins of the specimen.

Histologically, the characteristic cytologic detail of the choriocarcinoma is the biphasic cellular growth — the cytotrophoblast composed of masses, sheets or cords of cuboidal cells with round, central, darkly pigmented nuclei, and the syncytiotrophoblast represented by irregular masses or sheets of syncytial epithelium with an abundant pink vacuolated cytoplasm and very pleomorphic nuclei, many of which are giant sized and contain large clumps of chromatin and dark-staining nucleoli. In certain cases, these two elements align themselves about fibrovascular stalks, reduplicating quite faithfully the architecture of the mature placenta. In some of these malignancies, foci of the other types of germinal cancer are also found; nonetheless, in all instances, the tumor remains as a choriocarcinoma because of the dominating behavior of this pattern of growth. Conversely, as has already been mentioned, foci of choriocarcinoma may be found in any of the other germinal tumors. Unlike its counterpart arising in the placenta, the choriocarcinoma in the male is relatively unaffected by radiation or by methotrexate which is so effective in the treatment of these tumors arising in the placenta (p. 1261).

Teratoma and Teratocarcinoma. The designation teratoma according to Dixon and Moore (1953) refers to tumors that demonstrate areas of cellular differentiation which resemble normal adult tissues. Such structures as muscle bundles, cartilage or clusters of squamous epithelium are most often found. Sometimes these tissues have differentiated to the point of producing organoid structures such as thyroid gland complete with acini containing colloid, recognizable lining of bronchiolar epithelium or bits of intestinal wall or brain substance. These well differentiated tumors in which no histologically malignant elements are observable are designated **teratoma** or **teratoma differentiated.** These tumors occur with relatively greater frequency in children. These differentiated neoplasms often are multicystic on cross section. Microscopic examination discloses that the cysts are lined by variable epithelial patterns separated by a variety of connective tissue elements. In some instances, the tumors differentiate along epidermal lines and create one large solitary cyst lined by skin replete with hair, sebaceous glands and other usual adnexal structures. Such specialized differentiation is designated a **cystic dermoid teratoma** and is much more frequent and characteristic of ovarian teratomas. In the **teratocarcinomas** or malignant teratomas, one of the epithelial components shows all the features of anaplasia, and frequently the carcinomatous area resembles the pattern of a seminoma or embryonal carcinoma. Occasionally, sarcomatous transformation is encountered. However, even when no histologic areas of malignancy are observed in solid teratomas, experience demonstrates that metastasis may occur. Malignant behavior is even more likely when these tumors occur in young adults.

As a group, the teratomas and teratocarcinomas comprise about 30 per cent of testicular tumors. They produce moderate enlargement of the testis, but they are usually contained within the tunica albuginea. In about 10 per cent of those in which malignant elements are observed, extension beyond the testicular capsule is also found. They have a fairly characteristic cut surface distinctive in the incorporation of numerous cystic spaces within the tumor. Sometimes a honeycombed effect is produced. Often there are focal areas of definite cartilaginous translucent tissue. Occasionally, spicules of hard calcification can be found that can later be identified as bone. Necrosis and hemorrhage may occur, but are not usually prominent.

The distinctive feature of these tumors is the multiplicity of tissue and organoid structures present (Fig. 26—16). Occasionally, the tumor may differentiate completely along a single line, for ex-

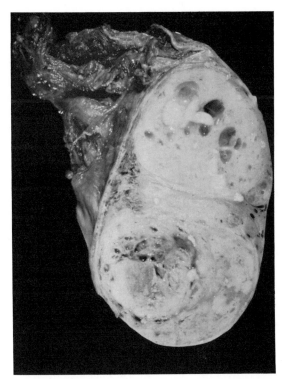

Figure 26–16. *Teratoma of the testis. The variegated cut surface reflects the multiplicity of tissue types found histologically.*

ample, thyroid gland acini (struma ovarii). According to some experts, all cases of malignant teratoma ought to be classified on the basis of the best differentiated areas present. On this basis, a tumor with only one-tenth of its area occupied by a malignant, moderately well differentiated teratoma and nine-tenths occupied by an anaplastic, poorly differentiated teratoma would still be classified as a moderately well differentiated lesion. The exception to this rule occurs when areas of malignant (trophoblastic) teratoma are present. Here the controlling character of this element in the clinical behavior is recognized, and classification of the entire tumor as malignant teratoma trophoblastic is made. But again it should be emphasized that **the anatomic distinction between teratoma and teratocarcinoma (teratoma differentiated and malignant teratoma) is not always of value clinically in predicting metastasis.** The overall five-year survival for teratomas and teratocarcinomas is approximately 70 per cent. Only one distinctive pattern, the cystic dermoid tumor (p. 1248), has a distinctly better prognosis because, as mentioned above, even the apparently well differentiated solid teratomas may behave as cancers.

Clinical Course. The clinical course of all testicular tumors discussed above is similar in many respects. The neoplasms are usually manifested by enlargement or palpable hardness of the affected testis, a feeling of heaviness and, less frequently, pain. Often these lesions induce serous secretion within the tunica vaginalis to produce a persistent hydrocele. These findings alone should suggest to the examiner the possible presence of testicular tumor. Sometimes symptoms which result from metastasis are the presenting complaints.

It has already been pointed out that testicular tumors may arise in scrotal testes, but undescended and ectopic testes are more vulnerable (Campbell, 1942) (Gross and Jewett, 1956). The predisposition to neoplasia is greater in abdominal testes than in those confined within the inguinal canal. Approximately half of the germ cell tumors arising in abnormally situated testes are seminomas.

In many of these patients, particularly those with choriocarcinomas, there is a high secretion of gonadotropic hormone which can be readily detected in the urine. The origin of this hormone may be the tumor but might be destruction of the testis with elaboration of the hormone by the unopposed pituitary. Comparison of the preoperative and postoperative levels in patients who initially showed elevated amounts of this hormone can give some information on the prospects for the patient and can provide a means for detecting clinical recurrence or metastatic dissemination at a later date. High levels of estrogen secretion are also sometimes observed in these patients, but only when metastases are present.

TUMORS ARISING IN GONADAL STROMA

The stroma of the testis bears many similarities to the ovarian stroma. It has the capacity to differentiate along a variety of lines and to elaborate both androgens and estrogens, predominantly the former. The varying patterns of specialization of the stroma may give rise to a variety of distinctive cytologic variants including interstitial cell tumors (Leydig cell tumors), granulosal and thecal cell tumors, as well as more exotic variants designated by Mostofi et al. (1959) as androblastomas and gynandroblastomas (indicative of the major hormonal output of the neoplasms). Only the interstitial cell tumors occur with sufficient frequency to merit inclusion here.

INTERSTITIAL CELL TUMORS

The interstitial cell tumor derived from the cells of Leydig is an uncommon and generally benign growth which constitutes about 1 per cent of all testicular tumors. Hyperplasia of the Leydig cells may result from atrophy of the seminiferous epithelium due to age, injury or developmental failure, and the distinction between hyperplasia and neoplasia of these cells is often a difficult one. Some of the factors related to hyperplasia may also play a role in the development of neoplasms, but this is not known for certain. Most interstitial cell tumors occur between the ages of 40 and 60, but the literature contains many cases above and below this range.

The testicular tumor in these cases is often asymptomatic. In other cases, testicular swelling, heaviness or pain is the initial symptom. However, the principal significance of this tumor is related to its ability to produce hormones having largely androgenic effects. Sexual precocity may result when these tumors develop in male children. In male adults, the relative increment of androgens is not sufficient to produce symptoms. Feminization associated with some of these tumors reflects, in all likelihood, the elaboration of estrogens together with androgens. Certainly, gynecomastia is a common finding. Rarely, corticosteroids are also produced.

Most interstitial cell tumors are small, 1 to 2 cm. nodules of firm, essentially spherical, yellow-brown tissue within the testicular substance. Occasionally, the neoplasms are larger and cause an increase in testicular size.

Microscopically, these tumors are composed of nests or sheets of mature Leydig cells traversed by fibrous septa. Usually there is very little anaplasia, and the cells are readily recognizable as the interstitial cells found within the normal testicular stroma. Some tumors, however, manifest considerable variation in cell or nuclear size though, in other respects, the cells appear normal. Eosinophilic granular cytoplasm, lipid vacuoles, cytoplasmic brown pigment granules and the occasional slender, rod-shaped crystalloids of Reinke within the cytoplasm further identify the nature of the cells. The only constant criterion for malignant behavior seems to be the actual occurrence of metastases or invasion. The proportion of these tumors having malignant behavior is probably less than 10 per cent.

ADENOMATOID TUMORS

These are benign, slow-growing nodules that arise in the epididymis or in sequestered remnants of the müllerian ducts. They usually have an encapsulated, firm, gray-white macroscopic appearance and are rarely larger than a few centimeters in size. On microscopic examination, they contain variable amounts of stroma and an admixture of cells which would seem to have an epithelial origin. In some instances, these apparent epithelial cuboidal cells line cystic spaces. At other times, they form small apparent glandular patterns and, at still other times, they are disposed in cords and nests. Occasionally, these cells contain vacuoles that do not react with the usual fat or glycogen stains. Tumors of identical gross and histologic appearance also occur in the female genital tract. The origin of this uncommon tumor is uncertain, and its histogenesis has been ascribed to such varied sources as müllerian duct vestiges, mesothelium, endothelium and mesonephric tissue.

MISCELLANEOUS LESIONS OF THE TUNICA VAGINALIS

Brief mention should be made of the tunica vaginalis. As a serosa-lined sac immediately proximal to the testis and epididymis, it may become involved by any lesion arising in these two structures. Clear serous fluid may accumulate from neighboring infections or tumors (*hydrocele*). Usually about 100 cc. of fluid is found, but amounts of up to 300 cc., rarely larger, have been described. The tunica may fill up with fluids when there is systemic edema, as in cardiac failure or renal disease; at other times, when the processus vaginalis has failed to close completely, peritoneal fluid may seep in and accumulate. Considerable enlargement of the scrotal sac is produced which can be readily mistaken for testicular enlargement. However, by transillumination it is usually possible to define the clear, translucent character of the contained substance and, many times, the opaque testis can be outlined within this fluid-filled space. When infected, as in the course of a tap or by the extension of organisms directly from infections within the testis or epididymis or through the lymphohematogenous route, the serosa-lined membrane may be converted to a shaggy, thickened, fibrous wall and the serous fluid may be transformed to frank pus (Fig. 26–17). In the course of time, overgrowth of the organisms may halt their multiplication, and the process may undergo autosterilization with organiza-

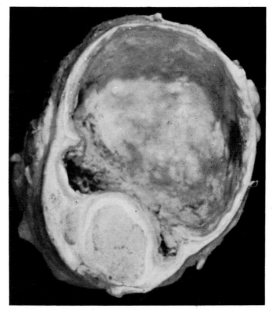

Figure 26–17. *An infected hydrocele sac. The wall is thick and fibrous and has a shaggy lining.*

tion of the exudate and destruction of the original serosa-lined space.

Hematocele indicates the presence of blood in the tunica vaginalis. It is an uncommon condition which usually is only encountered when there has been either direct trauma to the testis or torsion of the testis with hemorrhagic suffusion into the surrounding vaginalis, or in hemorrhagic diseases associated with widespread bleeding diatheses. Tumorous invasion may evoke a hydrohematocele.

Chylocele refers to the accumulation of lymphatic fluid in the tunica and is virtually only found in patients with elephantiasis who have widespread, severe, lymphatic obstruction. For clarity's sake, mention should be made, at this point, of the *spermatocele* and *varicocele*, which refer respectively to small cystic accumulations of either semen or blood in the spermatic cord. In the spermatocele, the cyst usually represents a dilatation of one of the ducts in the head of the epididymis and, in the case of the varicocele, it might be more properly described as a cystic varix of one of the veins of the spermatic cord.

PROSTATE

NORMAL

In the normal adult, the prostate weighs approximately 20 gm. It is a retroperitoneal organ encircling the neck of the bladder and urethra and is devoid of a distinct capsule. Classically, the prostate has been divided into five lobes to which are attributed distinctive significance in the development of tumors and benign enlargements. These five lobes include a posterior, middle, anterior and two lateral lobes. However, other investigators deny the clear definition of these five lobes and suggest that, in the course of development, the five lobes become fused into only three distinct lobes—two major lateral lobes and a small median lobe, which presumably includes the classic posterior lobe. Cross section of the gland, however, fails to disclose well defined lobes and only two lateral masses can be found on either side of the urethra, as well as a much thinner median lobe, which forms the floor of the urethra. In the normal adult, the prostate has a homogeneous, pale gray, cut surface in which it is possible, with a low power lens, to identify small, discrete, yellow-white, minute cystic areas representing prostatic glands from which may be extruded, by slight pressure, a milky fluid.

Histologically, the prostate is a compound tubuloalveolar gland which, in one plane of section, presents small to fairly large glandular spaces lined by tall to low columnar epithelium. Characteristically, this epithelial layer is usually one cell thick but, occasionally, small, basal, cuboidal cells may be found distributed along the basement membrane, which create the appearance of stratification. In many areas, there are small villous projections or papillary inbuddings of the epithelium. These glands all have a distinct basement membrane and are separated by an abundant fibromuscular stroma. Franks (1954a) has called attention to two apparent distinct glandular divisions within the prostate. On cross section, the outer regions of the prostate are composed of long "external" glands which curve toward the base of the prostate eventually to drain into the posterolateral grooves of the urethra, and an inner mass made up of branching, as well as extremely short, glands that drain much more

directly into the urethra. This distinction into an outer and inner mass of prostatic tissue may have some significance in the etiology of the common nodular hypertrophy to be described shortly.

The prostate is an endocrine-dependent organ and, in one sense, is the counterpart of the breast in the female. However, our knowledge of its endocrine relationships is still somewhat confused. It is clear that castration produces atrophy of the prostate and that administration of androgens delays the development of such atrophy. But estrogen also is capable of delaying the atrophy of castration. Numerous attempts have been made, none of them entirely satisfactory, to explain the paradox of apparently opposing hormonal influences exerting a similar effect on the prostate. Perhaps the most ingenious explanation suggests that the outer glandular zone comprises the so-called "male prostate" responsive to androgens, while the inner prostatic mass represents a so-called "female prostate" responsive to estrogens. While this postulate is not clearly established, it would help to explain the development of abnormal enlargement of the prostate in older males. The increase in prostate size usually arises in the inner mass which presumably responds to the decrease in androgen secretion and the relative or absolute increase in estrogen levels.

PATHOLOGY

The only three pathologic processes that affect the prostate gland with sufficient frequency to merit discussion are inflammation, benign nodular enlargement and tumors. Of these three, the benign nodular enlargements are by far the most common and occur so often in advanced age that they can almost be construed to be a "normal" aging process. Prostatic carcinoma is also an extremely common lesion in the male and one, therefore, that merits careful consideration. The inflammatory processes are, for the most part, of much less clinical significance, and can be treated briefly.

INFLAMMATIONS

Prostatitis may be divided into nonspecific acute and chronic, and granulomatous prostatitis.

NONSPECIFIC ACUTE AND CHRONIC PROSTATITIS

Acute prostatitis consists of an acute focal or diffuse suppurative inflammation in the prostatic substance, caused by the usual pyogenic organisms, i.e., staphylococci, streptococci, gonococci and coliform bacilli. These organisms become implanted in the prostate usually by direct extension from the posterior urethra or from the urinary bladder, but occasionally seed the prostate by the lymphohematogenous routes from distant foci of infection. One of the most common clinical sequences encountered is prostatitis following some surgical manipulation on the urethra or prostate gland itself, such as catheterization, cystoscopy, urethral dilatation or resection procedures on the prostate (Ghormley and Needham, 1953).

Acute prostatitis may appear as minute, disseminated abscesses, as large, coalescent focal areas of necrosis, or as a diffuse edema, congestion and boggy suppuration of the entire gland (Fig. 26—18). When these reactions are fairly diffuse, they cause an overall, soft, spongy enlargement of the gland.

Histologically, depending upon the duration and severity of the inflammation, there may be minimal stromal leukocytic infiltrate accompanied by increased elaboration of prostatic secretion or leukocytic infiltration within gland spaces (Fig. 26—19). When abscess formation has occurred, focal or large areas of the prostatic substance may become necrotic. Such inflammatory reactions may totally subside and leave behind only some fibrous scarring. These acute reactions may become chronic, particularly when the excretory ducts are plugged and the infection continues to smolder within walled-off minute abscesses in the prostatic substance.

Chronic prostatitis, when correctly diagnosed, should be restricted to those cases of inflammatory reaction in the prostate characterized by the aggregation of numerous lymphocytes, plasma cells, macrophages, as well as neutrophils, within the prostatic substance. It should be pointed out that in the normal senile changes, aggregations of lymphocytes are prone to appear in the fibromuscular stroma of this gland. All too often, such nonspecific aggregates are diagnosed as chronic prostatitis,

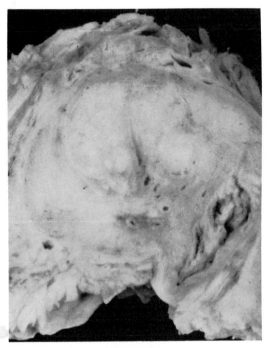

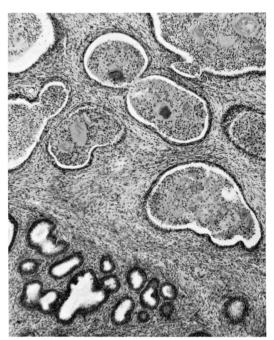

Fig. 26–18   *Fig. 26–19*

Figure 26–18. *A cross section through the prostate to demonstrate the cavitated abscesses in the posterior-lateral aspect of the right lobe.*

Figure 26–19. *Acute prostatitis. The gland lumina are filled with neutrophils and the stroma contains a sprinkling of similar leukocytes.*

even though the pathognomonic inflammatory cells, i.e., the macrophages and neutrophils, are not present.

On the basis of such erroneous criteria, chronic prostatitis is frequently said to be an extremely common disorder, and much stress has been laid upon its clinical significance as a source of chronic infection in the body, predisposing to arthritis, iritis, myositis and neuritis. No sound evidence for such a causal role has yet been established, and the disease is probably much more uncommon than generally considered. The term "chronic prostatitis," then, should be restricted to those cases in which there is clear-cut evidence of persistent smoldering infection in the form of neutrophilic infiltration, along with the other mononuclear cells described, as well as evidence of destruction and fibroblastic proliferation.

GRANULOMATOUS PROSTATITIS

Two forms of granulomas are found in the prostate. Nonspecific granulomas may occur secondary to acute or chronic prostatitis. In these conditions, there may be inspissation of secretions, followed by surrounding focal aggregations of neutrophils, lymphocytes and plasma cells, enclosed within a fibroblastic proliferative response. The granuloma production is further augmented by the appearance of foreign body giant cells. These granulomas do not have caseous centers, nor do they contain acid-fast bacilli. They are nonspecific inflammatory reactions to the accumulation of inspissated secretion or necrotic tissue. An autoimmune causation has also been postulated.

The other pattern of granulomatous prostatitis consists of tuberculosis of the prostate that almost invariably follows tuberculosis of some other region of the genitourinary tract, such as renal or urinary bladder tuberculosis. Less commonly, miliary spread to the prostate may occur from distant pulmonary tuberculosis. Under these circumstances, the prostate may be the first or the only organ affected in the genitourinary system. In the miliary disseminated type, the lesions may be entirely microscopic in character and not evident grossly. However, in the course of time, many tubercles may become confluent to produce frank foci of caseous necrosis. In far advanced cases, the process may destroy large areas of the prostate and extend into the neighboring seminal vesicles. Considerable enlargement may attend such tuberculous prostatitis.

BENIGN ENLARGEMENT

NODULAR HYPERPLASIA (BENIGN PROSTATIC HYPERTROPHY OR HYPERPLASIA)

Benign prostatic hypertrophy or, more properly, nodular hyperplasia, is an extremely common disorder of men over the age of 50. It is characterized by the production of large, fairly discrete nodules that involve the middle and lateral lobes of the prostate and progressively encroach upon the urethra to cause partial to sometimes virtually complete obstruction of urinary flow. Although the designation, benign hypertrophy of the prostate, is firmly fixed in medical writing, it is obviously an inappropriate term, since hypertrophy is by definition a benign process and, moreover, there is abundant histologic evidence that proliferation of cells occurs, which more properly should be designated as hyperplasia. However, benign hyperplasia is equally redundant and therefore, most authors favor the use of nodular hyperplasia, although the usage of benign prostatic hypertrophy is difficult to dislodge.

Incidence. Beginning at approximately the age of 45, there is a progressive increase in incidence with each decade of life, until about 80 per cent of men beyond the age of 80 are affected. With this prevalence, it may be truly questioned whether this condition should be considered as a disease or as a normal aging process. Despite this frequency, not more than 5 to 10 per cent of affected men require surgical treatment for relief of the urethral obstruction and, in the remainder, the lesion is of little clinical significance.

Etiology. The cause of nodular hyperplasia is still unknown, but the accumulating evidence fairly well invalidates the older concepts that the disorder is essentially neoplastic, a response to chronic inflammation, or irregular hyperplasia following atherosclerotic involution. Current opinion strongly favors some endocrine imbalance as its basis. Both clinical and experimental evidence indicate that maintenance of the normal prostate is dependent on a constant level of androgen secretion. The progressive increase in the incidence of this disease with age strongly suggests that decreased testicular function underlies nodular hyperplasia. With age, it is known that there is a progressive drop in androgen secretion and hence a relative hyperestrinism (largely contributed by adrenal secretion). Nodular hyperplasia may then be due to an absolute or relative hyperestrinism. In support of this view, it is postulated that the inner so-called female prostate is estrogen-dependent and the hyperestrinism may induce its major changes here (Franks, 1954a). Indeed, most of the enlargement encountered in nodular hyperplasia involves the periurethral portion of the gland. A number of alternative proposals have been made. Perhaps with aging there is some chemical alteration in the nature of the androgens, or the gonadal stroma may produce increased amounts of estrogens. Possibly, the absolute or relative hyperestrinism exerts its principal effect upon the stroma of the prostate, and the glandular changes are secondary to the stromal alterations. Conceivably, with aging, the testicular Sertoli cells become more active in the production of estrogens at the same time that androgen production by the Leydig cells lags. It is evident from all of these speculations that the etiology of nodular hyperplasia remains a mystery.

Morphology. In the usual case of nodular enlargement, the **prostatic nodules** weigh between 60 and 100 gm. However, not uncommonly, aggregate weights of up to 200 gm. are encountered, and even larger masses have been recorded. **These nodules usually occur in the lateral and middle or median lobes and do not involve the posterior portion of the median lobe, the so-called posterior lobe,** which is the usual site of the development of carcinoma (Moore, 1943). These nodular enlargements

may encroach upon the lateral walls of the urethra to compress it to a slit-like orifice while, at the same time, nodular enlargement of the median or middle lobe may project up into the floor of the urethra as a hemispheric mass directly beneath the mucosa of the urethra (Figs. 26–20 and 26–21). At other times, the middle lobe enlargement may assume even a long, slender, delicate, polypoid appearance attached by a narrow neck; and in many of these instances, it appears to act as a ball-valve obstruction to the mouth of the urethra.

On cross section of the affected prostate, the nodules are usually fairly readily identified because of the compression of the remainder of the prostatic tissue about the nodule. They usually arise from the inner prostatic mass, and only rarely do they extend to the outer perimeter of the gland (Fig. 26–22). The nodule itself varies in color and consistency, depending, as will be shown, upon whether it is primarily due to fibromuscular stromal hypertrophy and hyperplasia or to glandular proliferation. In those which are primarily glandular, the tissue has a yellow-pink, soft consistency, which is fairly discretely demarcated from the more gray, glistening, firm, compressed prostatic capsule. Usually a milky-white prostatic fluid oozes out of these areas. In those due primarily to fibromuscular involvement, the nodule itself is also pale gray, tough and fibrous, does not exude fluid, and is less clearly demarcated from the surrounding prostatic capsule.

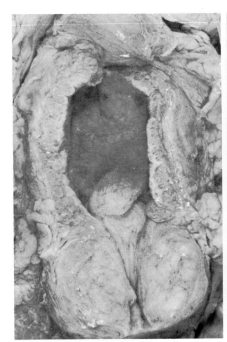

Fig. 26–20

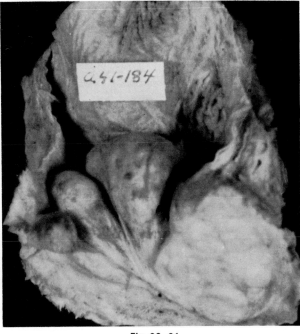

Fig. 26–21

Figure 26–20. *Nodular prostatic hyperplasia. The prostatic enlargement has caused marked thickening of the bladder wall.*
Figure 26–21. *An irregular nodularity of the so-called median lobe.*

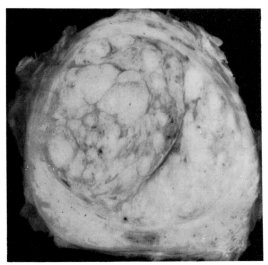

Figure 26–22. *A cross section of nodular hyperplasia of the prostate with compression of the urethra into a slit-like cleft.*

While the nodules do not have true capsules in the sense that benign neoplasms are encapsulated, the compressed surrounding prostatic tissue creates a plane of cleavage about them, utilized by the surgeon in the enucleation of prostatic masses in so-called suprapubic prostatectomies. A considerable amount of prostatic tissue remains behind so

that, at a later date, it is entirely possible for recurrent nodules to develop or for the patient to develop a carcinoma.

Microscopically, **there are many patterns of nodular hyperplasia.** Ultimately, all are differentiated on the basis of whether the enlargement is due mainly to glandular proliferation, or dilatation, or to fibrous or muscular proliferation of the stroma. All three elements are involved in almost every case although, in individual instances, one may predominate over the others. Usually the epithelial element predominates in the form of aggregations of small to large to cystically dilated glands, lined by a single regular layer of tall columnar or flattened cuboidal epithelium, based upon an intact basement membrane. The epithelium is characteristically thrown up into numerous papillary buds and infoldings, which are more prominent than in the normal prostate (Fig. 26–23).

In certain cases, many small glands are formed which may simulate the pattern of adenocarcinoma. Usually the glandular size is sufficiently large to be visible on hand lens inspection of the tissue section. Frequently these glands contain inspissated secretion, granular, desquamated epithelial cells and numerous corpora amylacea. When the fibromuscular hypertrophy or hyperplasia predominates, it may produce nodules of almost solid spindle cells, free of glands, that have sometimes been designated as **fibromatous hyperplasia, or leiomyoma-**

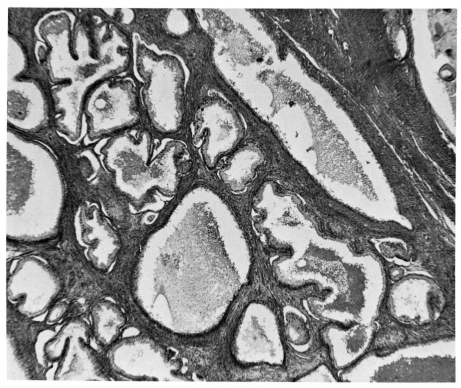

Figure 26–23. *Nodular hyperplasia of the prostate. The field contains glands of large and small size. Small papillary buds are evident in the linings of the glands.*

tous hyperplasia of the prostate. However, such differentiation is probably not clinically useful. Not infrequently, aggregates of lymphocytes are found within the stroma that are frequently construed as implying inflammation, but are more likely due to the senile changes already described. Nonspecific infections may produce secondary alterations in the gross and microscopic appearances just described.

Clinical Course. Although nodular enlargement is an extremely common condition, it has been pointed out already that in only a small percentage of those affected does the lesion produce clinical symptoms. Symptoms, when produced, relate to two secondary effects: compression of the urethra with difficulty in urination; and retention of urine in the bladder with subsequent distention and hypertrophy of the bladder, infection of the urine and the development of cystitis and renal infections.

These patients have frequency, nocturia, difficulty in starting and stopping the stream of urine, overflow dribbling and dysuria (painful micturition). In many cases, sudden, acute urinary retention appears for unknown reasons, and persists up until the time that the patient receives emergency catheterization. In addition to these difficulties in urination, prostatic enlargement results in the inability to completely empty the bladder. Presumably this is due to the raised level of the urethral floor so that, at the conclusion of micturition, a considerable amount of residual urine is left. This residual urine provides a static fluid that is vulnerable to infection. On this basis, catheterization or surgical manipulation provides a real danger of introducing organisms and leading to pyelonephritis.

Many secondary changes occur in the bladder which have already been described, such as hypertrophy, trabeculation and pseudodiverticulum formation (p. 1165). Hydronephrosis or acute retention with secondary urinary tract infections, and even azotemia or uremia, may develop.

SECONDARY CHANGES IN NODULAR HYPERPLASIA

Two related morphologic changes are so frequently encountered in nodular hyperplasia as to almost represent intrinsic features of this disease. The first is squamous metaplasia and hyperplasia of the periurethral glands. These glands become transformed to masses or nests of small, regular, polygonal to spindle cells which resemble squamous epithelial cells. But the basement membranes remain intact even though the glandular lumina become filled. The cells are fairly uniform in size and shape, and have no evidence of anaplasia. The major significance of these changes is that they are frequently mistaken for carcinoma.

The second alteration that accompanies nodular hyperplasia relates to the occurrence of small areas of infarction necrosis within the nodules or in the surrounding prostatic tissue. These foci are usually extremely small, less than 1 cm. in diameter, but may be microscopic in size. Histologically, they present the characteristic shadowy outlines of infarcted, necrotic tissue. Inflammatory reaction about the margins may be slight to moderate. However, most noteworthy is the tendency for squamous metaplasia to occur in the preserved margins of the focus of infarction.

TUMORS

CARCINOMA

Carcinoma of the prostate is the most common malignancy in the adult male, and is found at autopsy in 14 to 46 per cent of men over the age of 50 years. However, in the majority of cases, it is discovered as an incidental finding either at postmortem examination or in a surgical specimen removed for other reasons. In almost all these instances, the lesion is small, totally latent and without clinical significance. On the other hand, it may come to attention as a clinically aggressive, spreading neoplasm that kills. Prostatic cancer, then, exists in two biologic forms: a common, small, incidental lesion sometimes referred to in the literature as a "localized form," and the much less frequent, clinically significant disease that may metastasize and kill, termed an "advanced form." It has always been assumed, without proof, that the small localized lesion would, in time, become a clinically significant lesion, but with the known variation in the inherent growth potential of tumors, many of the small lesions may have persisted and continue to persist as such for years.

Incidence. Cancer of the prostate is a disease of men over 50 years of age. It is rarely seen in younger individuals. The median age for clinically overt disease is 70 years. Despite the fact that histologic evidence of carcinoma of the prostate is found at autopsy in approximately 14 to 46 per cent of men, the age-adjusted incidence of the *clinical disease* in the United States in 1950 was 36 per 100,000 male population. Moreover, carcinoma of the prostate was a cause of death in only 1.38 per cent of men over the age of 50 in Britain in 1952 (Franks, 1954*b*). There is obviously a wide discrepancy between the frequency of carcinoma of the prostate as a cause of clinical disease and death and its prevalence as an anatomic lesion. Nonetheless, the clinically significant form of cancer is sufficiently common to account for its being the third most common cause of cancer deaths in the male preceded only by bronchogenic and colorectal carcinomas.

There are some striking racial and national differences in the prevalence of this disease. Blacks in the United States are affected significantly more often than whites, in a ratio of 3:2. In Japanese men, the disease is far more rare than in American men and, in a study quoted by Strahan (1963), autopsy examination of 12,127 Japanese men disclosed only 15 cases of prostatic carcinoma. The basis of these racial and national differences is obscure.

Etiology. Little is known about the etiology of carcinoma of the prostate, particularly considering its extremely high incidence. Inflammation has been shown to have no significant role as a precursor. Some studies suggest that prostatic carcinoma may be related to elevations in the circulating levels of androgens or lowering of the estrogen levels, both changes resulting in relative excesses of androgens. However, there are reasons to doubt this hypothesis. Prostatic cancer is a disease of advanced life when the androgen levels normally diminish. Patients administered androgens for long periods of time have no apparent increased attack rate of carcinoma of the prostate. Alternatively, alterations in the sensitivity of prostate cells to these steroids may be the key to the induction of neoplasia. Prostatic cancers are endocrine dependent and can be inhibited in their growth, though probably not destroyed by orchiectomy or estrogen therapy. It may be that steroid hormonal imbalances are important coupled with some increased pituitary gonadotropin activity. Alterations in the distribution of cells in the pituitary glands as well as modifications in the testis and other endocrines consistent with pituitary hyperactivity have been identified in some of these cases. The significance of preexistent hyperplasia of the prostate is highly controversial. Some investigators contend that 15 to 20 per cent of hyperplastic glands harbor cancer but, since hyperplasia also occurs in the later decades and since prostatic cancer has been found in up to 46 per cent of all prostatic glands in American men, the finding of coexistent cancer and hyperplasia may be merely coincidental. In my experience, hyperplasia does not constitute a precancerous lesion.

Morphology. Carcinoma of the prostate arises in the posterior lobe in about 75 per cent of

the cases and, in all but rare instances, it arises in subcapsular locations within this lobe. In contrast, benign nodular hyperplasias are confined to the inner prostatic mass. In its early developmental stages, the carcinoma is extremely difficult to identify macroscopically. Characteristically, the neoplastic tissue is gritty and firm but, when embedded within the prostatic substance, it may be extremely difficult to visualize and be more readily apparent on palpation. At times the tumor tissue is somewhat yellower than the surrounding tissues and is therefore distinctive but, at other times, it is gray-white and therefore blends imperceptibly into the background of the prostate gland. Only when the tumor has extended beyond the confines of the prostate to invade the seminal vesicles or the adjacent rectum or bladder can it be clearly identified (Fig. 26–24). Such extraprostatic extension will ultimately occur in almost all advanced, biologically aggressive lesions.

Histologically, most cases are adenocarcinomas with varying degrees of differentiation (Kahler, 1939). Morphologic studies have failed to disclose any anatomic differences between the la-

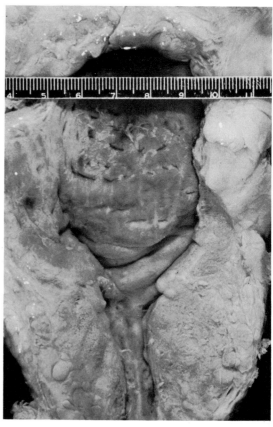

Figure 26–24. Carcinoma of the prostate. The carcinomatous tissue cannot be distinguished within the prostate itself, but has invaded the floor of the urethra and infiltrated into the vesicle neck.

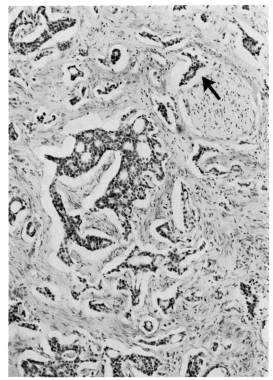

Figure 26-25. *Carcinoma of the prostate. The cords of tumor cells permeate the stroma. Perineurial invasion is present* (arrow).

of the prostate itself. The exceptional cases that do not fall into the category of adenocarcinoma are squamous cell carcinomas that presumably arise from metaplastic glands.

In an effort to provide more homogeneous groups of patients for comparison of the results of various forms of therapy, **carcinomas of the prostate are graded on the basis of cytologic levels of differentiation of the neoplasm and staged on the basis of the extent of the spread.** Histologically, they are divided into Grades I, II and III; well differentiated adenocarcinomas are classified as Grade I while those neoplasms growing in undifferentiated cords or sheets of cells are classified as Grade III. With this approach, Jewett et al. (1968) have shown that Grades I and II permit a 30 to 35 per cent 15-year survival after radical prostatectomy, while virtually no patients with Grade III carcinoma are alive at 15 years following similar therapy. Numerous systems have been devised for the staging of the extent of these cancers, regrettably using different terminology (Commission on Clinical Oncology, 1968) (Flocks, 1965) (Rubin, 1969). The two most widely used systems divide these neoplasms into four categories called Stages A to D in one system and Stages 0 to III in the other. While the four categories do not completely correspond in the two systems, it will suffice to cite the divisions into Stages A to D:

Stage A: Occult cancer.

Stage B: Cancer nodule confined within the prostatic capsule.

Stage C: Cancer with extracapsular extension into surrounding structures or confined within the capsule, with elevation of serum acid phosphatase. Pelvic nodes may be involved.

Stage D: Demonstrated bone or extrapelvic involvement.

Based on this staging, it has been shown that, at the time of the initial diagnosis of carcinoma of the prostate, only 5 to 20 per cent of patients are in Stages A or B and, even with such local lesions, 10 per cent of these patients with presumably "early disease" later develop lymph node or bone marrow metastases (Flocks, 1969).

Clinical Course. As the term implies, occult or "localized" carcinomas are asymptomatic and may only represent microscopic foci of cancer identified either at postmortem examination in patients dying of other causes or merely chance findings in surgical specimens removed for nodular hyperplasia. The clinically significant form of this disease comes to attention either by the finding, on rectal examination, of stony hard nodules in the prostate or because of the development of symptoms reflecting encroachment on the urethra. Only when the patency of the urethral lumen or the

tent and clinically overt forms of carcinoma. Most tumors produce well defined, readily demonstrated gland patterns but, in other instances, the gland patterns may be scant in number, and the tumor may grow in cords, nests or sheets of cells (Fig. 26-25). The epithelial cells themselves, whether in glands or in undifferentiated masses, are surprisingly uniform in size and shape. They tend to be cuboidal or polygonal with small, round, central, deeply pigmented nuclei and scant cytoplasm surrounded by clearly defined cell borders. Mitotic figures are uncommon and tumor giant cells are rare. Stromal production may be scant or quite extensive in certain lesions, to produce a scirrhous-like consistency to the neoplasm.

Uniformity of the cells and the lack of anaplasia contribute to the histologic difficulties of diagnosing carcinoma of the prostate. It is, moreover, sometimes difficult to distinguish between nodular hyperplasia, with small gland formation, and well differentiated adenocarcinoma. It is necessary to resort to clear evidence of invasion, the best defined indicators being invasion of blood vessels, invasion of capsule and invasion of perineurial and perivascular spaces. Only by the demonstration of such invasiveness can carcinoma of the prostate be diagnosed with complete certainty in tissue sections

action of the internal sphincter is disturbed do manifestations such as difficulty in starting or stopping the urinary stream, dysuria and frequency appear. Hematuria is found in a small percentage of cases but only when the tumor has invaded the mucosa of the bladder or the urethra. Pain is a late finding reflecting invasion of perineurial spaces. The first manifestation of a prostatic malignancy is often the development of symptoms incident to widespread metastases. Characteristically, spread occurs principally to the skeletal system; usually the vertebral column is first affected, producing back pain (Fig. 26–26). In 90 per cent of cases, the metastases are *osteoblastic* as the neoplasm stimulates bone formation. Spread to the regional lymph nodes occurs regularly, but involvement of internal organs is less common.

Rectal palpation of the gland is an important part of the clinical examination for suspected prostatic carcinoma. Since the tumor arises in the posterior lobe, which is closely applied to the rectum, it is frequently possible to feel the hard irregularity through the rectal wall. Moreover, the tumor tends to spread to the seminal vesicles and rectal wall, thus further providing opportunity for its detection.

Acid phosphatase is elaborated by the normal prostate but ordinarily it is only present in the blood in small quantities. However, in cases of metastatic prostatic carcinoma, the acid phosphatase produced by the neoplasm leads to elevated blood levels which usually imply skeletal metastases. However, not all metastatic cancers produce elevated levels of acid phosphatase. In Mellinger's (1965) words: "When levels are normal, metastases may be present or may not." Elevated levels above the upper limits of normal (1.5 to 4.0 Bodansky units) are readily detectable in the serum in about 40 per cent of cases. There is still no agreement as to whether the increased acid phosphatase is due to the greater amount of neoplastic prostatic tissue producing enzyme or to the more ready absorption of this enzyme into the blood from the bony metastatic sites. Few locally invasive lesions produce elevated levels of enzyme. It may be noted in passing that, with widespread osteoblastic metastases, elevated levels of alkaline phosphatase may be encountered also.

The survival rates in prostatic carcinoma depend on many factors: the histologic grade, clinical stage and the form of therapy employed. Stage A cancer is occult and represents

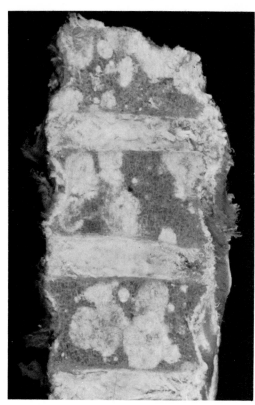

Figure 26–26. *Metastatic prostatic carcinoma within vertebral bodies.*

only a histologic diagnosis. In general, radical prostatectomy is the treatment of choice for patients with Stage B disease. With this favorable group and this form of therapy, about a 33 per cent five-year survival is achieved. When patients do not qualify for surgery, estrogen therapy and/or orchiectomy are used. When these forms of therapy fail to control the disease or provide relief from symptoms, resort is then made to radiation or chemotherapy. The great majority of patients with prostate carcinoma respond favorably, at least for some time, to estrogens or orchiectomy and have a reduction in prostatic size, relief of urinary symptoms and seeming disappearance of bony metastases. However, in the course of time (years), the tumor usually once again escapes control. Some experts are currently enthusiastic about supervoltage radiation or radiogold insertion directly into the prostate in Stage B disease and claim almost a 50 per cent five-year survival with these modalities (Flocks, 1969).

INTERPRETATION OF TESTICULAR MASSES

The most important clinical problem related to the subject matter of this chapter is the differential diagnosis of enlargement of the testis. More properly, this problem should be expressed as the consideration of diseases that cause enlargement of the scrotum. Often, it is extremely difficult to differentiate between those enlargements that are of testicular origin and those that are due to diseases within the tunica vaginalis or scrotal tissues. The list of possible diagnoses is quite long and would, of necessity, include many extemely uncommon disorders. In usual clinical practice, the following conditions would include at least 98 per cent of cases encountered:

1. Hydrocele. While of little clinical significance, abnormal accumulations of fluid in the tunica vaginalis are undoubtedly the most common cause of scrotal enlargement. The differentiation of this condition from true testicular masses has already been presented. It should be reemphasized that rarely, but significantly, the development of hydrocele may reflect an underlying tumor of the testis with invasion of the scrotal sac.

2. Scrotal Hernia. Scrotal enlargement is often caused by descent of loops of intestine into the tunica vaginalis in an indirect inguinal hernia. This type of scrotal enlargement may be quite massive, but usually can be differentiated from other conditions by exerting gentle pressure on the scrotal contents and thus replacing the intestinal loops into the abdominal cavity. When such a hernia has existed for a long time, fibrous adhesions may bind the loops into the scrotal sac and prevent such reduction. Usually, however, marked relaxation or widening of the external inguinal ring permits the ready identification of the nature of the condition.

3. Neoplasms of the Testis. All enlargements of the scrotum should be considered as neoplastic until proved otherwise. While these cancers are uncommon in terms of all forms of malignancy in the male, they are of great importance because they disseminate at early stages in their development. Every effort, therefore, should be directed toward their early detection when, perhaps, only slight nodularity or thickening of the testis is present without much overall enlargement of the organ. Regrettably, careful palpation of the testes is all too frequently not performed in routine physical examination.

4. Nonspecific Epididymitis or Orchitis. Such inflammatory involvements are usually secondary complications of prostatic surgery or infections elsewhere. These conditions are usually bilateral and are attended by the classic manifestations of acute inflammation, i.e., pain, heat and edema.

5. Specific Inflammations of the Epididymis and Testis. Tuberculosis and syphilis are infrequent, but possible, causes of scrotal enlargement. As has been pointed out, tuberculosis almost invariably affects first the epididymis, while syphilis is primarily a testicular infection.

6. Torsion of the Testis. Torsion of the testis causes considerable hemorrhagic and edematous enlargement of this organ, but usually the differential diagnosis is readily apparent from the acute onset, exquisite pain and rapid appearance of swelling. Usually, the patient seeks medical advice before the seepage of blood has caused discoloration of the scrotum.

7. Spermatocele and Varicocele. These conditions are uncommon and rarely cause scrotal enlargement. However, they may produce nodular swellings that require differentiation from neoplasm.

8. Scrotal Edema. Scrotal edema is a not infrequent accompaniment of generalized systemic edema, and is particularly prominent in those conditions that produce severe anasarca, such as kidney disease and cardiac failure. Usually the soft, doughy thickening of the scrotum can be readily differentiated from intrascrotal lesions. Lymphatic obstruction is a rare cause of scrotal edema.

9. Scrotal Inflammatory Disease. Here, again, the inflammatory reaction is usually readily distinguished from intrascrotal disease and is usually accompanied by inflammatory changes in the genital tract and regional nodes, which represent the probable primary source of the scrotal infection.

The two most common causes of scrotal enlargement in this list are hydrocele and scrotal inguinal hernia. While it is not germane in such a discussion as this to present all the clinical features that distinguish these conditions from other causes of enlargement, the major problem centers about the detection of malignancies. It is a clinical maxim that, when in doubt, surgical exploration is indicated to establish the nature of the scrotal enlargement.

When, at exploration, the problem still cannot be resolved by palpation of the testis, orchiectomy may be justified to exclude the possibility of an occult tumor. Moreover, infarction necrosis and hemorrhage into the tumor may have produced sufficient softening so that no palpable nodularity can be identified to explain the apparent enlargement. Such a radical approach is reasonable because of the aggressive nature of testicular tumors, with their tendency to metastasize at an early stage, often when the primary lesion is still very small. Only in this way can the mortality figures on malignancies of the testis be improved.

REFERENCES

Berg, J. W.: An acid-fast lipid from spermatozoa. Arch. Path., 57:115, 1954.

Campbell, H. R.: Incidence of malignant growth of the undescended testicle. Arch. Surg., 44:353, 1942.

Cohen, D. B.: Histology of the cryptorchid testis. Surgery, 62:536, 1967.

Commission on Clinical Oncology of the Union Internationale Contre Cancrum: TNM Classification of Malignant Tumors. Geneva, International Union Against Cancer, 1968.

Dixon, F. J., and Moore, R. A.: Testicular tumors: clinicopathological study. Cancer, 6:427, 1953.

Dixon, F. J., and Moore, R. A.: Tumors of the male sex organs. In Atlas of Tumor Pathology, Section VIII, fascicles 31B and 32. Armed Forces Institute of Pathology, 1952.

Editorial: An epidemic of testicular cancer? Lancet, 2:164, 1968.

Flocks, R. H.: Carcinoma of the prostate. J. Urol., 101:741, 1969.

Flocks, R. H.: Clinical cancer of the prostate. A study of 4,000 cases. J.A.M.A., 193:89, 1965.

Franks, L. M.: Benign nodular hyperplasia of the prostate: a review. Ann. Roy. Coll. Surg. Eng., 14:92, 1954a.

Franks, L. M.: Latent carcinoma of the prostate. J. Path. Bact., 68:603, 1954b.

Friedman, N. B., and Moore, R. A.: Tumors of the testis. Military Surgeon, 99:573, 1946.

Ghormley, K. O., and Needham, G. M.: Chronic prostatitis: a urologic quandary, J.A.M.A., 153:915, 1953.

Gross, R. E., and Jewett, T. C., Jr.: Surgical experience from 1222 operations for undescended testis. J.A.M.A., 160:634, 1956.

Grumbach, M. M., et al.: Sex chromatin pattern in seminiferous tubule dysgenesis and other testicular disorders: relationship to true hermaphroditism and to Klinefelter's syndrome with a review of gonadal ontogenesis. J. Clin. Endocr., 17:703, 1957.

Jewett, H. J., et al.: The palpable nodule of prostatic cancer. J.A.M.A., 203:115, 1968.

Kahler, J. E.: Carcinoma of prostate gland: a pathologic study. J. Urol., 41:557, 1939.

Lenowitz, H., and Graham, A. P.: Carcinoma of the penis. J. Urol., 56:458, 1946.

Melicow, M. M., and Ganem, E. J.: Cancerous and precancerous lesions of the penis: a clinical and pathological study based on 23 cases. J. Urol., 55:486, 1946.

Mellinger, G. T.: Carcinoma of the prostate. Surg. Clin. N. Amer., 45:1413, 1965.

Moore, R. A.: Benign hypertrophy of the prostate: a morphological study. J. Urol., 50:680, 1943.

Mostofi, F. K., et al.: Tumors of specialized gonadal stroma in human male patients: androblastoma, Sertoli cell tumor, granulosa-theca cell tumor of the testis, and gonadal stroma tumor. Cancer, 12:944, 1959.

Newman, H. F., and Wilhelm, S. F.: Testicular temperature in man. J. Urol., 99:288, 1950.

Payne, R. A.: Erythroplasia of Queyrat. Brit. J. Urol., 29:163, 1957.

Rubin, P.: Cancer of the urogenital tract: prostatic cancer. Current Concepts in Cancer. J.A.M.A., 210:320, 1072, 1969.

Sauer, D., and Leighton, W. E.: Carcinoma of the penis. Surg. Clin. N. Amer., 24:1211, 1944.

Sovhal, A. R.: Testicular dysgenesis in relation to neoplasm of the testicle. J. Urol., 75:285, 1956.

Strahan, R. W.: Carcinoma of the prostate: incidence, origin, pathology. J. Urol., 89:875, 1963.

Testicular Tumor Panel and Registry of the Pathological Society of Great Britain and Ireland in association with the British Empire Cancer Campaign for Research: The pathology of testicular tumors. Brit. J. Urol., Suppl., 36: 1964.

27

FEMALE GENITAL TRACT

NORMAL

Embryology. The many congenital anomalies of the female genital tract can only be understood from the standpoint of the embryology of this system. At about the sixth week of fetal development, invagination of the celomic lining epithelium to form a furrow creates a groove whose lips later fuse to form the lateral müllerian (paramesonephric) ducts. These arise parallel to the paired wolffian (mesonephric) ducts that are destined, in the male, to form the epididymis and vas deferens. The müllerian ducts first become apparent high on the dorsal wall of the celomic cavity and then progressively grow caudally to enter the pelvis where they swing medially to fuse. Further caudal growth brings these fused ducts into contact with the urogenital sinus. With relatively uncomplicated transformations, the unfused portions mature into the fallopian tubes and the fused caudal portion, into the uterus and the vagina. The upper portion of the vagina is generally held to be of müllerian origin, and the lower portion is probably derived from the urogenital sinus. It is apparent that the entire lining of the uterus and tubes is derived from celomic epithelium. The embryogenesis here serves to explain the origin of such congenital anomalies as a bicornuate or totally septate uterus and a septate or double vagina. The primitive celomatous origin of the endometrium of the uterus serves also to explain the possible differentiation of foci of peritoneum in the adult into endometrial tissue, one of the presumed origins of the common disease endometriosis.

Normally, the mesonephric duct regresses in the female. Remnants, however, may persist into adult life as epithelial inclusions about the hilus of the ovary and mesosalpinx, designated respectively as the epoophoron and paroophoron. If the caudal portions of this meso-

nephric anlage persist, they may appear as epithelial inclusions within the wall of the lower uterine segment and cervix and as epithelial rests in the lateral walls of the vagina. Sometimes in the vagina these rests produce cysts that are designated as Gartner's duct cysts. These inclusions may also be the origin of rare tumors in the femal genital tract designated as mesonephromas.

The ovary, like the testis, arises from a medial proliferation of the urogenital ridge specified as the genital ridge. At six weeks of fetal development, this sexless gonad has three components: a covering of differentiated celomic lining epithelium, now designated as germinal epithelium; an underlying undifferentiated fibroblastic stroma, the mesenchyme; and primitive germ cells. The germinal epithelium grows into the inner mesenchyme to provide the progenitors of the granulosa cells of the graafian follicles, although it is possible that differentiation of the mesenchyme also provides an origin for these granulosa cells. The inner mesenchyme gives origin to the theca cells of the follicle. It is generally believed that the germ cells are set aside as totipotential gametes in the earliest stage of formation of the embryonic disk. As the embryo develops, they migrate or are carried into the primitive mesenchyme destined to become the ovary. It is of interest that these divide during the first half of fetal development to reach a maximum number of 6 to 7,000,000, but subsequently some regress so that at birth approximately 1 to 2,000,000 oocytes remain. None are formed after the fifth month of fetal development and, indeed, there is a progressive loss so that at puberty the number has dwindled into the hundreds of thousands, still more than needed to provide 12 per year during the woman's active reproductive life.

Certain details of the embryogenesis of the ovary assume importance in the histogenesis of ovarian tumors. The germinal epithelium included within the inner mesenchyme may be the cytologic origin of some of the epithelial cysts, cystadenomas and carcinomas of the ovary. The concept that the mesenchyme may differentiate into both granulosal and thecal elements provides a reasonable origin for neoplasms such as the granulosa cell tumors and arrhenoblastomas which synthesize estrogens, androgens or both, and which span a morphologic range from epithelial to stromal patterns.

Measurements. Certain normal dimensions of the female genital tract are of value, since so much importance attaches to various diseases that cause enlargement of the ovaries and uterus. During active reproductive life, the ovaries measure about 4 cm. in length, 2.5 to 3 cm. in width and 1 to 1.5 cm. in thickness. It should be emphasized that in the majority of ovaries removed in the course of surgical procedures on the pelvic organs, small follicle cysts, to be described presently, are found so commonly as to represent virtually normal anatomic features. Postmenopausally, as is well known, the ovaries atrophy to wrinkled "encephaloid" nodules 2.0 ×1.0 × 0.5 cm. or smaller.

The uterus varies in size, depending upon the age and parity of the individual. During active reproductive life, it weighs about 50 gm. and measures 8 cm. in length, 5 to 6.5 cm. in breadth in the fundic region and 3 cm. in thickness. Pregnancies may leave small residual increases in these dimensions (up to 70 gm. in weight) since the uterus rarely involutes to its original size completely. Postmenopausally, the atrophic changes may cause diminution to 5 to 6 cm. in length, 3 cm. in width, and 1.5 to 2 cm. in thickness. In the menstruating female, the myometrium of the body and fundus of the uterus averages 1.2 to 1.5 cm. in thickness. Certainly an upper limit of 2 cm. can be placed, beyond which myometrial thickening must be postulated. Considerable clinical importance attaches to all these measurements since, in certain obscure conditions such as uterine fibrosis (myometrial hypertrophy), the major basis for diagnosis lies in precise measurements of the uterus that indicate an abnormal increase over usual measurements.

Histology. Several histologic details that are apt to be forgotten are of some pathologic importance. In the ovary, the covering germinal epithelium becomes flattened to assume the characteristics of the peritoneum. In histologic sections, these cells are so thinned out that they cannot be identified. When portions of this covering epithelium are incorporated into fibrous scars, the cells may revert into readily visible cuboidal cells to create small gland lumina (germinal inclusions) that are sometimes confused with neoplastic infiltrations.

The ovarian substance is divided into a cortex and medulla. Ordinarily, the cortex comprises a layer of closely packed spindle cells that resemble plump fibroblasts separated by only a scant intercellular ground substance. The very outermost portion directly beneath the covering serosa is compacted into a thin layer of relatively acellular collagenous connective tissue. Thickening of this layer may give rise to ovarian dysfunction, since it may prevent follicular rupture and ovulation. By puberty, ova in varying stages of maturation are found within the outer cortex. Corpora lutea of varying ages as well as nodules of collagenous connective tissue, the corpora albicantia, are also present in the cortex.

The medulla of the ovary is made up of a more loosely arranged mesenchymal tissue. Occasionally, large, round to polygonal, epithelial-appearing cells are buried within the medulla in the so-called hilar region. These cells are presumed to be vestigial remains of the gonad from its primitive "ambisexual" phase. The large epithelial-appearing cells are thought to derive from the sequestered remnants of the wolffian duct. The "hilus" cells thus resemble the interstitial cells of the testis, and sometimes contain identical crystalloids of Reinke. Rarely, these cells give rise to masculinizing tumors.

In the tube, the mucosa is thrown up into numerous high, delicate folds that, on cross section, produce a papillary or frond-like appearance. In the normal, these mucosal folds are not interadherent and hence the folds form deep crypts. In the absence of fusion of these folds, no sequestered, buried, cystic or follicle-like spaces are found. When gland-like or cystic patterns are produced, it can be assumed that inflammatory fusion of adjacent folds has occurred. It will be remembered that the lining epithelium of the tube is made up of three cell types: ciliated, columnar cells; nonciliated, columnar, secretory, mucous cells; and so-called intercalated cells that may simply be progenitors of these secretory cells.

The uterus has three distinctive anatomic and functional regions: the cervix, the lower uterine segment and the corpus. The cervix is further divided into the vaginal or anatomic portio and the endocervix. The anatomic portio is that portion of the cervix visible to the eye on vaginal examination. It is covered by a stratified squamous nonkeratinizing epithelium reflected off the vaginal vaults onto the cervix. This squamous epithelium covers the entire anatomic portio and extends more or less up to the central dimple that comprises the external os. In the nulliparous normal cervix, this os is virtually closed. The endocervix is normally not exposed and is lined by columnar mucus-secreting epithelium that dips down into the underlying stroma to produce crypts sometimes designated as endocervical glands. This narrow endocervical channel ends at the so-called internal os, a poorly defined region where the central lumen of the uterus begins to open up into the more capacious lower uterine segment. Congenital malformation, inflammation or childbirth injuries may cause small bits of the endocervical columnar lining epithelium to become everted and, therefore, to become apparent externally. Such eversion is particularly susceptible to inflammation and trauma and is, therefore, often the site of erosion.

The lower uterine segment has no clear delimitation. It is lined by columnar mucus-secreting epithelium that progressively becomes transformed to nonmucus-secreting epithelium resembling the basal resting glands of the endometrium. This epithelium is frequently removed in curettage and can be recognized by virtue of its nonendometrial fibromuscular stroma. Since it does not participate in the cyclic changes of the functional endometrium, failure to identify this lower uterine segment mucosa in curettings leads to the erroneous impression that the endometrium is nonfunctional. Care must also be taken not to confuse endocervical mucus-secreting glands with secretory endometrium.

Menstrual Cycle. A review of the menstrual cycle follows. The anterior lobe of the pituitary under the neuroendocrine control of the hypothalamus cyclically produces follicle-stimulating hormone (FSH) and luteinizing hormone (LH). Under the influence of FSH, usually several ovarian follicles, each containing an ovum, begin to develop, but eventually one becomes ascendent and the others regress. This selected follicle continues to evolve until it reaches the stage where a small antral cavity is formed within the follicle. Further development requires the addition of LH. Under the combined influence of FSH and LH, ripening continues and ovulation occurs at about the midpoint in the classic 28 day menstrual cycle but, in longer or shorter cycles, ovulation may in retrospect be timed at about 14 days prior to the onset of the next menstrual period. Once ovulation has taken place, the follicle is transformed, under the influence of FSH and LH, to the corpus luteum, but luteotropic hormone (LTH) is needed, it is currently believed, for the complete functional activity of the corpus luteum and its production of progesterone.

Under the influence of the gonadotropic hormones, estrogen production by the follicle progressively rises during the first two weeks. It reaches a peak, presumably just prior to ovulation, and then falls. The precise events that trigger ovulation are still poorly understood, but one of the contributing factors may be this sudden drop in estrogen level. Alternatively, ovulation may antedate the drop in estrogen levels and, indeed, be responsible for this drop. It is of interest that, at this time in the midphase of the 28 day cycle, some women have minimal amounts of vaginal bleeding, referred to as "ovulatory bleeding." Following ovulation, the estrogen levels again begin to rise to a plateau at about the end of the third week, but these levels are never as high as the preovulatory peak. The level of this hormone then progressively falls, beginning 3 to 4 days before the onset of the menstruation. Progesterone of uncertain origin makes its appearance even before ovulation and progressively rises throughout the last half of the menstrual cycle to fall to basal levels just prior to the onset of menstrual bleeding.

The cyclic endometrial changes are keyed to this rise and fall of the ovarian steroids. We can begin the review of these changes with the shedding of the upper one-half to two-thirds of the endometrium during the menstrual period. The basal third does not respond to the ovarian steroids and is retained at the conclusion of the menstrual flow. From this basal third, during the first half of the menstrual cycle the surface epithelium is regenerated and, during the preovulatory proliferative phase of the cycle, there is extremely rapid growth of both glands and stroma. The glands are straight, tubular structures lined by quite regular, tall, columnar cells. During the proliferative phase, the columnar cells are rich in ribonuclease and alkaline phosphatase, but contain little acid phosphatase or glycogen (McKay et al., 1956). The nuclei in these cells are not aligned, mitotic figures are numerous and there is no evidence of mucus secretion or vacuolation. The gland lumina are relatively tubular and devoid of secretion (Fig. 27–1). The endometrial stroma is composed of thickly compacted spindle cells that have very scant cytoplasm but abundant mitotic activity. Although one can readily identify a proliferative endometrium, *there are no characteristic cell or architectural changes that permit precise dating of this phase of the menstrual cycle.* The height of glands is an unreliable criterion.

At the time of ovulation, under the combined influence of estrogen and progesterone, the endometrium slows in its growth and ceases apparent mitotic activity within days immediately following ovulation. The postovula-

Fig. 27–1

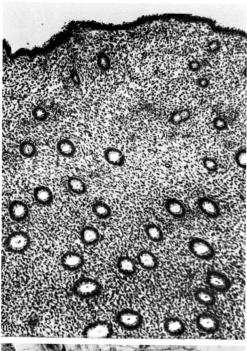

Figure 27–1. *Normal proliferative endometrium, illustrating the tube-like pattern of the glands.*

Figure 27–2. *Postovulatory endometrium with prominent subnuclear vacuoles and alignment of the nuclei.*

Figure 27–3. *Late secretory endometrium with tortuosity of the glands, producing the serrate margins.*

(All three figures through the courtesy of Dr. Arthur Hertig, from Fertility and Sterility, Vol. 1, 1950.)

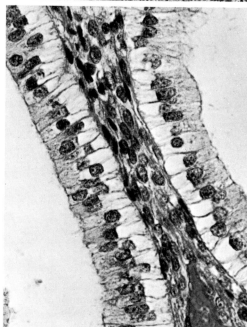

Fig. 27–2

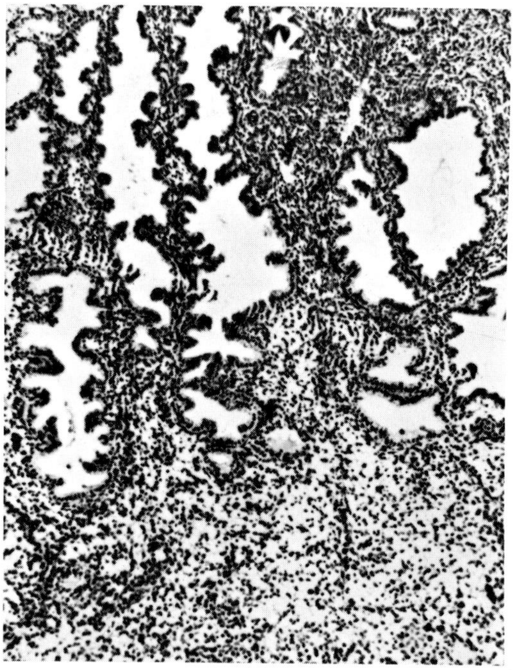

Fig. 27–3

tory endometrium is marked by basal secretory vacuoles beneath the nuclei in the glandular epithelium (Fig. 27–2). The secretory activity becomes more prominent during the third week of the menstrual cycle, and the basal vacuoles appear to push past the nuclei of the columnar lining epithelial cells to now appear above and below the nuclei. The nuclei are thus aligned at midpoint in the cell. Although glandular proliferation ceases during the secretory phase, there is marked secretory activity. Tortuosity of the glands appears and is well developed by the fourth week. This tortuosity produces a serrate margin to the glands when cut in their long axis (Fig. 27–3). During the last week of the cycle, rupture of some of the columnar epithelial cells releases mucus secretion into the gland lumina. The cells thus are emptied to produce so-called secretory exhaustion, and the glands become progressively dilated, with mucus secretion enhancing their tortuosity. The stroma between the glands becomes edematous, and the spiral arterioles become more prominent. There is now a considerable increase in ground substance and edema between the stromal cells. In the nonpregnant state just prior to the menstrual flow, the somewhat edematous stromal cells become hypertrophied and accumulate a considerable amount of pink cytoplasm to produce so-called predecidual changes.

The escape of blood into the stroma marks the beginning of menstrual shedding. This stromal bleeding is apparently initiated by necrosis and rupture of the walls of the spiral arterioles. The imminence of such necrosis is usually marked by hyaline pink smudging of the walls of these vessels. In the premenstrual and menstrual phases, the endometrial stroma contains scattered neutrophils and occasional lymphocytes. The normal presence of such leukocytes is to be particularly noted since these white cells are ordinarily considered to be indicators of an inflammatory reaction.

In summary, the proliferative phase should therefore be readily differentiated from the secretory phase. Ovulation should be fairly well denoted by the basal vacuolation of the columnar epithelial cells of the glands. When ovulation fails to occur and progesterone is not produced, the entire secretory phase drops out and, even though menstrual bleeding may occur, there is no secretory vacuolation in the endometrial glands and the characteristic stromal edema and later decidual transformation are absent. For these reasons, endometrial biopsy to determine ovulation should not be performed before the twentieth day and preferably on or about the twenty-fifth day, at which time it can be assumed that the secretory changes in glands and stroma are well developed.

Some fascinating insights have been gained into the mode of action of steroid hormones on the endometrium, insights which may have great relevance to the treatment of hormone-dependent endometrial carcinomas. We glibly say that estrogen promotes endometrial regrowth, but how does it work at the cell level? What signal initiates cellular proliferation? Currently, it is believed that steroid molecules (estradiol or metabolites of progesterone) bind to receptor cytoplasmic proteins in the endometrial epithelial cells. The steroid-receptor complex enters the nucleus where it links up to an acceptor protein attached to DNA and, in so doing, derepresses or "turns on" codes within the cell's genome (O'Malley, 1971). Fundamental to this concept is the identification of specific binding proteins in target cells. Thus, endometrial cancers, if they possess binding proteins, are estrogen-dependent and so may be suppressed by high levels of progesterone (Richardson, 1972).

Functional Abnormalities in the Ovary and Endometrium. In the active cyclic ebb and flow of the ovary and endometrium, minor abnormalities may produce a wide variety of changes that, while deviations from the normal, are hardly of sufficient significance to be designated pathologic. First, with respect to the ovary, when ovulation fails to occur, the follicles may persist and become increasingly enlarged to produce *solitary or multiple follicle cysts*. These may be sufficiently large (up to 3 to 4 cm. in diameter) or numerous to increase the size of the ovary. The aggregate estrogenic production of these follicles may induce hyperplasia in the endometrium. Obviously, such failure of ovulation implies sterility.

When ovulation occurs normally, there is scant escape of blood into the peritoneal cavity. Sometimes more profuse hemorrhage from the follicle causes sufficient intraperitoneal bleeding to evoke the classic midcycle pain known as "*mittelschmerz*." While this hemorrhage is usually minimal, it sometimes can be quite marked and be responsible for significant loss of blood and manifestations of an "acute abdomen."

Cysts may form within corpora lutea "luteal cysts" to produce increased levels of progesterone; in turn, these may give rise to hyperplastic secretory endometrium.

With respect to the endometrium, many patients show curious focal unresponsiveness of portions of the endometrium to the ovarian steroids. In these cases, certain areas may show proliferative changes, while others are in the appropriate secretory phase. Such endometria do not go through regular menstrual cycles and are susceptible to persistent bleeding or "*irregular shedding.*"

PATHOLOGY

Diseases of the female genital tract are numerous and extremely common in clinical and pathologic practice, to the point at which they have been segregated into specialities unto themselves in gynecology and gynecologic pathology. The following discussion attempts to present the major entities that comprise the bulk of the clinical problem.

VULVA

Diseases of the vulva in the aggregate comprise only a small fraction of gynecologic practice. The great variety of inflammations that occur here are usually amenable to therapy and do not constitute significant threats to the patient. Only malignant neoplasms can be considered as diseases of major clinical significance.

CONGENITAL ANOMALIES

Of the various malformations of the vulva, only hypoplasia, duplication and imperforate hymen merit mention. The *imperforate hymen* sometimes escapes recognition in the infant and remains uncorrected until the onset of menstruation. At this time, the absence of menstrual bleeding and clinical manifestations of pelvic pain and discomfort reflect the progressive accumulation of menstrual blood in the vagina *(hematocolpos)*, in the uterus *(hematometria)* and in the tubes *(hematosalpinx)*. If the condition persists long enough, the overflow of blood may spill into the pelvic cavity and produce signs of pelvic peritonitis. The accumulated blood may organize within the tubes, with resultant permanent sterility.

Duplication of the vulva is quite rare and is almost invariably accompanied by a septate double vagina and double uterus.

Hypoplasia of the vulva or external female genitals may arise as a congenital developmental defect. More often, it implies a failure of normal growth response. The hypodevelopment may be due to an ovarian or pituitary insufficiency, or may reflect an end organ unresponsiveness to normal levels of hormone. Such infantilism is usually accompanied by hypodevelopment of the remainder of the genital tract and by inadequate development of the secondary sex characteristics.

INFLAMMATIONS

The inflammatory lesions that affect the vulva parallel, in general, those that involve the penis. Since the histologic features of these inflammatory conditions are essentially identical, whether they occur in the male or female, it is necessary here to cite only the differences that occur when these diseases arise in the female.

PELVIC INFLAMMATORY DISEASE (PID)

Pelvic inflammatory disease (PID) is considered here because it begins in the vulva or its accessory glands, but usually the infection spreads upward through the entire genital tract involving more or less all the structures in the female genital system. While at one time the gonococcus was the most common causative agent, the prophylaxis of gonorrhea and the effective treatment of early gonococcal infection by antibiotics have markedly reduced not only the incidence of gonorrhea but also such serious complications as PID. Puerperal infections by a variety of organisms including the staphylococci, streptococci, coliforms and *Clostridium welchii* have assumed increased importance in the production of PID.

Whatever the etiologic agent, the anatomic changes that result are virtually the same. The mechanism of spread of these various organisms may, however, differ. Gonococcal inflammation usually begins in Bartholin's glands, Skene's ducts, the minor perivulvar or periurethral glands or sometimes the endocervical glands. From any of these loci, the organisms spread upward over the mucosal surfaces to eventually involve the tubes and tubo-ovarian region. In such spread, the vagina in the adult is remarkably resistant. In the child, presumably because of a more delicate lining mucosa, vulvovaginitis may develop. The nongonococcal infections that follow induced abortion, dilatation and curettage of the uterus and other surgical procedures on the female genital tract are thought to spread upward through the lymphatics or venous channels rather than on the mucosal surfaces. These infections therefore tend to produce less mucosal involvement but more reaction within the deeper layers.

With the gonococcus, approximately 4 to 6 days after inoculation of the organism, nonspecific inflammatory changes appear in the affected glands. Wherever it occurs, gonococcal disease is characterized by an acute suppurative reaction accompanied by the copious outpouring of yellow pus. The involved structures become hyperemic, edematous and tense. The infection usually but not invariably affects both sides. Histologically, there is little to indicate the nature of the organism since the reaction is entirely nonspecific. In gonococcal infections, the inflammatory changes are largely confined to the superficial mucosa and underlying submucosa. Only rarely do microabscesses develop in the deeper layers. Smear of the exudate should disclose the intracellular gram-negative diplococcus, but absolute confirmation requires cultural identification. In most acute cases, with therapy, the infection promptly subsides and does not involve the upper levels of the genital tract. If spread occurs, a gonorrheal endometritis may develop, but more often the endometrium is remarkably spared for obscure reasons. Once within the tubes, an **acute suppurative salpingitis** ensues. The tubal serosa becomes hyperemic and layered with fibrin, the tubal fimbriae are similarly involved and the lumen fills with purulent exudate which may leak out of the fimbriae. In the course of days or weeks, the tubal fimbriae may seal or become plastered against the ovary to create a **salpingo-oophoritis**. Pus may collect in these sealed tubes to cause distention, sometimes to diameters of 10 cm. or more. Characteristically, the distention is most marked at the fimbriated end and gradually subsides toward the uterine portions, creating the pattern referred to as "**retort tubes**." So enclosed, the infection tends to smolder and become chronic for months and even years. In the course of time the limiting factors of inadequate nutrition, progressive anaerobiosis and increasing acidity all bring about death of the organisms and eventual sterilization of the infection. The pus then undergoes slow proteolysis and the contents of the tube are transformed to a thin, serous fluid **(hydrosalpinx)**. Sometimes these large cystic masses imbibe additional water because of their hyperosmolarity and thus achieve massive size. **Tubo-ovarian abscesses** may result from collections of exudate where the tube is sealed against the ovary. This inflammatory process is not truly an ovarian abscess since the underlying ovarian substance is remarkably spared save for the most superficial layers.

PID caused by the staphylococci, streptococci and the other puerperal invaders tends to have less exudation within the lumina of the tube and less involvement of the mucosa, with correspondingly greater inflammatory response within the deeper layers. The infection tends to spread throughout the wall to involve the serosa and may often trek into the broad ligaments, pelvic structures and peritoneum. Bacteremia is a more frequent complication of streptococcal or staphylococcal pelvic inflammatory disease than of gonococcal infections.

PID causes pelvic pain, dysmenorrhea, disturbance in intestinal function, menstrual abnormalities and sometimes manifestations of an acute abdomen. In the chronic disorders, adhesions between the small bowel and the genital system may produce intestinal obstruc-

tion. In addition to these local significances, the bacteremias have the potential of inducing meningitis, endocarditis and suppurative arthritis. Sterility is one of the feared complications of longstanding pelvic inflammatory disease. In the early stages, gonococcal infections are readily controlled with antibiotics. However, when the infection becomes walled off in suppurative tubes or tubo-ovarian abscesses, it is difficult to achieve a sufficient level of antibiotic within the centers of such suppuration to effectively control these infections. The cases of pelvic inflammatory disease caused by other organisms are also amenable to antibiotics but are far more difficult to control than the gonococcal infections.

SYPHILIS

As in the male, the primary lesion of syphilis is the chancre, which may occur anywhere on the vulva or sometimes is located on the cervix. Its gross and microscopic characteristics are identical with those in the male, and its clinical significance and sequelae have already been generally considered on p. 378.

MISCELLANEOUS INFECTIONS

Chancroid, granuloma inguinale and lymphogranuloma inguinale all pursue virtually parallel courses in the male and the female, and have already been adequately considered (Chapter 10). It is only necessary here to point out that, in the female, lymphogranuloma of the vulva tends to drain not only to the inguinal nodes but also to the deep nodes about the rectum. Intense scarring may follow and produce rectal strictures in the female. Such drainage does not occur in the male.

Tuberculosis of the vulva is extremely uncommon and is almost invariably secondary to a primary infection at some higher level in the genital tract or in the urinary tract. Mycotic and yeast infections on the vulva have also been described. Of these latter forms, monilial vulvitis is the most common.

Any of the dermatologic conditions that affect hair-bearing skin elsewhere in the body may also occur on the vulva so that nonspecific vulvitis may be encountered in erysipelas, eczema and allergic dermatitis. The vulva is particularly prone to such infections, since it is constantly exposed to secretions and moisture. Nonspecific vulvitis is particularly likely to occur in the blood dyscrasias involving both the red and white cells, uremia, diabetes mellitus, malnutrition and the avitaminoses. Because itching is the most prominent feature of these conditions, secondary trauma from scratching complicates the clinical and histologic picture.

KRAUROSIS VULVAE

This designation refers to an obscure progressive atrophy and fibrosis of the vulva that occurs in advanced age. Since the external genitals physiologically atrophy in postmenopausal life, kraurosis may represent simply an accentuation or exaggeration of this physiologic atrophy.

The skin becomes pale gray, thin and parchment-like, the labia atrophy and the introitus narrows. The entire vulvar area smooths out with loss of the usual skin folds and, many times, the skin assumes a glazed red appearance as the subcutaneous vessels become more apparent. Histologically, there is atrophy and thinning of the epidermis, with disappearance of the rete pegs and replacement of the underlying dermis by dense collagenous fibrous tissue (Fig. 27–4). A nonspecific mononuclear cell infiltrate about blood vessels may also occur. The avascular skin and mucosa are particularly susceptible to trauma and infections, and kraurosis is therefore frequently complicated by chronic inflammatory changes, fissuring, ulceration and even frank abscess formations.

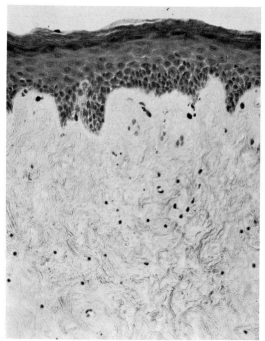

Figure 27–4. Kraurosis vulvae, illustrating atrophy of epidermis and dense sclerosis of dermis with total atrophy of dermal adnexal structures. (Courtesy of Dr. Arthur Hertig.)

Clinically, this disease occurs in the advanced years of life and, on this basis, it has been postulated that it is caused by estrogen deficiency. However, occasionally kraurosis is encountered in women in active reproductive life, invalidating such a hormonal basis. At all ages, it tends to be a slowly developing, insidious, progressive disorder which, while producing considerable discomfort and predisposing to acute infection, is usually of little systemic significance. The superimposed development of malignancy has been described, but it is doubtful whether the incidence of cancer in these women is significantly higher than in the normal population.

Lichen sclerosus et atrophicus must be considered in the differential diagnosis of kraurosis. It is essentially a dermatologic disorder which induces identical histologic findings including sclerosis and atrophy of the vulva indistinguishable from kraurosis. However, the lichenification tends to extend beyond the vulvar mucosa onto the adjacent skin (Janovski and Ames, 1963). It may well be that the two conditions are identical and, when the vulva alone is affected, it is designated kraurosis.

TUMORS OF THE VULVA

Tumors of the vulva are the most important lesions to affect this region. Many types have been recorded, both benign and malignant, including fibromas, neurofibromas, angiomas, sebaceous cysts, sweat gland tumors, melanocarcinomas and various types of mesenchymal sarcoma. But all these forms are extremely uncommon and, moreover, are exactly analogous to similar tumors occurring elsewhere in the body. Therefore, attention is focused on the more frequent tumors and other proliferative lesions distinctive of the vulva.

LEUKOPLAKIA

Leukoplakia is a rather poorly defined morphologic entity, but is a useful clinical term to refer to an opaque, white, plaque-like mucosal thickening—in this instance, the mucosa of the vulva. It is included under the heading of tumors because it is believed to be an important predisposition to the development of carcinoma.

Leukoplakia is an insidious lesion that affects the vulva patchily or totally. The epithelium progressively hypertrophies and thickens due to either an increase in surface keratinization or hyperplasia of the underlying cells, principally the prickle cell layer. In the hyperplastic form there is increased mitotic activity in both the basal and prickle cell layers (Fig. 27-5). Usually the orderly transition from basal to surface cell is preserved but, in some cases, dysplasia is evidenced by variability in nuclear and cell size. The epithelial changes may begin to approximate frank anaplasia and thus merit the designation of carcinoma in situ (Bowen's disease). At times, therefore, it is quite difficult to differentiate markedly dysplastic leukoplakia from frank malignancy. In most instances, there is a marked dermal leukocytic infiltrate composed chiefly of lymphocytes, plasma cells and histiocytes. These histologic changes are recognized grossly as patchy or diffuse, gray-white thickenings of the vulvar skin and mucosa. Commonly, the surface is scaly and wrinkled, and may even be fissured. The margins are usually fairly sharply demarcated with a map-like perimeter.

According to some authors, this hyperplastic pattern may enter a phase of marked atrophy of the epithelium, with fibrosis of the dermis that resembles kraurosis vulvae. On this basis, leukoplakia is sometimes referred to as hypertrophic kraurosis vulvae, but this designation is only confusing, since the term "kraurosis" specifically means shrinkage (Montgomery et al., 1934). Alternatively, the dermal infiltrate has led to another erroneous term, "leukoplakic vulvitis," implying an inflammatory state.

As mentioned, leukoplakia may consist only of innocuous hyperkeratosis or, in other instances, may have an important relationship to the development of carcinoma. It has been shown that over one-half of the patients who develop cancer of the vulva have some leukoplakic patches elsewhere on the vulva and, conversely, about 10 per cent of the patients with leukoplakia develop a carcinoma. However, these data must be interpreted against the background of the known difficulty in drawing a line between the marked cellular atypicality of the leukoplakia and frank carcinoma, and the understandable tendency to examine the patient with vulvar carcinoma more meticulously for possible leukoplakia (Langley et al., 1951).

BARTHOLIN'S CYST

Obstruction of the excretory duct of Bartholin's glands by inflammatory scarring, epithelial metaplasia or the accumulation of inspissated secretion may give rise to cystic dilatation of the ducts or the racemose glands, designated as a Bartholin's cyst. This lesion is quite common and occurs at all ages. It is readily recognized grossly by the hemispheric enlargement and discrete tumor mass produced in the labia minora. These cysts are usually unilateral, vary up to 3 to 5 cm. in diameter and, when uncomplicated by infection, are filled with a clear, mucous secretion. Infection is prone to occur in these cysts. The suppurative exudation creates a *Bartholin's abscess*. Beyond the pain and local discomfort produced by these conditions and the required differentiation from gonorrheal infection, these lesions are usually of no systemic significance.

PAPILLOMA

There is considerable disagreement whether the simple papilloma is different from the so-called condyloma acuminatum. The *papilloma* usually occurs singly and microscopically is composed of many finger-like fibrous cores covered by thickened, sometimes hyperkeratotic layers of stratified squamous epithelium. Sometimes the epithelial coverings have sufficient hyperplasia and dysplasia to make them difficult to differentiate from malignancy and, in fact, these lesions are believed to be the forerunners of carcinomas in a small but definite percentage of cases. In contrast, the *condyloma acuminatum* plays no role in the development of cancers, is frequently multiple, is believed to be of viral origin and is often transmitted from husband to wife or vice versa.

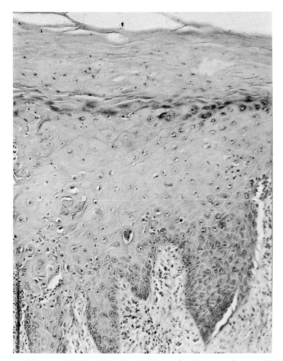

Figure 27-5. Leukoplakia of the vulva with marked epithelial thickening and hyperkeratosis. (Courtesy of Dr. Arthur Hertig.)

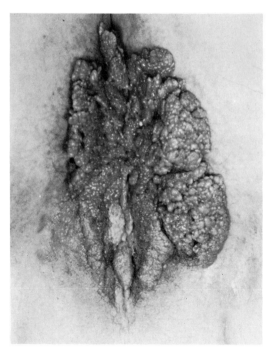

Figure 27–6. *Numerous condylomas of the vulva, almost obscuring the labia minora. (Courtesy of Dr. Arthur Hertig.)*

They usually occur as large, fungating, cauliflower-like masses that are superficially ulcerated and infected (Fig. 27–6). These are sometimes referred to as *venereal warts*, a misleading term since there is no relationship to other venereal infections. More aptly, these lesions should be construed as the mucosal counterparts of the common viral warts of the fingers and hands.

CARCINOMA

Carcinoma of the vulva is an uncommon malignancy that represents about 3 per cent of all cancers in the female. It is rarely seen under the age of 60. In a considerable number of instances, these malignancies are preceded by leukoplakia and, in a small percentage of cases, by benign papillomas.

Any region of the vulva may be affected and, in fact, a small percentage arise from the perineal skin about the rectum as well. These tumors begin as small areas of epithelial thickening that resemble leukoplakia but, in the course of time, progress to create firm indurated, elevated, map-like areas that become fissured and frequently secondarily infected. In the course of time, the central regions may ulcerate to produce the characteristic malignant ulceration with heaped-up, firm margins and a dirty, necrotic, irregular, indurated base. Destruc-

tive ulceration wipes out all structures in its path (Fig. 27–7). Histologically, these tumors are almost invariably squamous cell carcinomas, showing good differentiation with the formation of keratohyalin pearls and prickle cells (Fig. 27–8). (Collins et al., 1963).

The tumors grow by local invasion for a period of weeks to months and tend to metastasize at a relatively early stage to the regional nodes (Palmer et al., 1949). In about 65 per cent of cases, vulvar carcinoma has metastasized to the regional nodes at the time of discovery. The nodes affected are the inguinal nodes and the nodes within the pelvis, about the rectum and about the iliac vessels and bifurcation of the aorta. Such nodal metastasis is correlated more with the size and duration of the lesion than with the degree of differentiation of the squamous cell growth. Ultimately, lymphohematogenous dissemination involves the lungs, liver and other internal organs.

Although these lesions are superficial tumors that are obviously apparent to the patient and to the clinician, many are misinterpreted as dermatitis, eczema or leukoplakia for long periods of time.

The clinical manifestations which they evoke are chiefly those of pain, local discomfort, itching and exudation, since superficial secondary infection is common. If biopsies were performed on all questionable alterations on the vulva, many of these tumors would be discovered at an earlier date. Early lesions, defined as those less than 3 cm. in diameter, have a 60 to 80 per cent five-year survival rate, while larger lesions yield less than a 10 per cent five-year survival (Merrill and Ross, 1961).

Basal cell carcinomas, adenocarcinomas and sweat gland tumors have also been reported in the vulva, but are extremely uncommon.

EXTRAMAMMARY PAGET'S DISEASE

This rare lesion of the vulva, and sometimes the perianal region, comprises a form of submucosal glandular or ductal carcinoma that invades the perineal mucosa. It is the counterpart of the Paget's disease of the breast (p. 1283). This vulvar neoplasm manifests itself as a red, crusted, sharply demarcated, map-like area occurring usually on the labia majora. It is often accompanied by a palpable submucosal thickening or a discrete tumor mass. In most instances, *the neoplasm arises in a carcinoma of one of the mucous or sebaceous glands of the perineum and then grows along the excretory ducts of these glands to invade the mucosa.* The diagnostic microscopic feature of this lesion is the presence of large anaplastic tumor cells lying singly or in

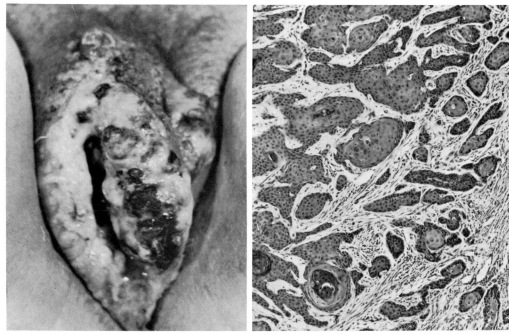

Fig. 27-7   **Fig. 27-8**

Figure 27-7. Carcinoma of the vulva, far advanced, with total destruction and erosion of the external genitals. (Courtesy of Dr. Arthur Hertig.)

Figure 27-8. Carcinoma of the vulva at medium power, illustrating the invasive cords of cells.

small clusters *within the epidermis.* These cells are rendered distinctive by a clear halo that sets them off from the surrounding epithelial cells. In many of these cases, the underlying ductal or glandular involvement is also readily identified. However, in some reports, the intraepidermal cancerous cells have been found in the apparent absence of an underlying glandular or ductal malignancy. In these particular instances, it is postulated either that the small primary site of the malignancy was missed or that the intraepithelial cells represent a form of melanocarcinoma that is easily confused with Paget's disease.

MELANOCARCINOMA

Melanocarcinomas of the vulva are uncommon, representing 2 to 3 per cent of all vulvar cancers. Many times, they are preceded by nevi, although by no means do all melano-carcinomas arise in such previously benign lesions; in fact, there is much controversy about the role of benign nevi in the origin of melanocarcinomas. Some investigators maintain that nevi on the vulva tend to be of the junctional variety (p. 1400), and that these junctional nevi are more likely to undergo malignant transformation than the same lesions occurring elsewhere. The melanocarcinomas of the vulva have the same biologic characteristics of those that occur elsewhere and are capable of widespread metastatic dissemination.

Early in the evolution of the melanocarcinoma, it is sometimes confined to the skin, where it may produce pagetoid cellular changes within the epidermis. As already indicated, the differentiation of Paget's disease of the vulva from an intraepithelial superficial melanocarcinoma may be extremely difficult if not impossible.

VAGINA

The vagina is a portion of the female genital tract that is remarkably free from primary disease. In the adult, inflammations often affect the vulva and perivulval structures and spread through the vagina to the cervix without intrinsic involvement of the vagina. The only significant primary lesion of this structure is the seldom found primary carcinoma. The remaining entities can then be cited quite briefly.

CONGENITAL ANOMALIES

Atresia and total absence of the vagina are both extremely uncommon. The latter virtually occurs only when there are severe malformations of the entire genital tract. Septate, or double, vagina is also a very uncommon anomaly that arises from failure of total fusion of the müllerian ducts. Congenital cysts, however, are relatively common defects that are fairly innocuous. These arise usually from *Gartner's ducts*, vestigial remnants of the wolffian ducts. Occasionally, these cysts arise from persistent inclusions of müllerian ductal epithelium. Most of these lesions are found along the lateral walls of the vagina, and commonly they are 1 to 2 cm. fluid-filled cysts that occur submucosally. Rarely, they may enlarge up to 5 to 6 cm. The lining epithelium is at times cuboidal, at times columnar or may even be transitional in form. Mixtures of these epithelial types are frequent. The cysts are of no consequence, save for their differentiation from more ominous tumor masses.

INFLAMMATIONS

While any vulvar inflammation may extend through the introitus and thus affect the vagina, the only types of intrinsic vaginal inflammation that are of any consequence are gonorrheal vulvovaginitis in the child, already cited (p. 1206), trichomonal and monilial vaginitis that occur at any age and senile vaginitis in the postmenopausal woman.

Trichomonal Vaginitis. Acute or chronic vaginal infections may be caused by *Trichomonas vaginalis*, a large, flagellated, ovoid protozoan measuring up to 30 microns in length and 10 to 15 microns in diameter. It is readily recognized by several tufted, elongated flagella at one end, matched usually by a solitary flagellum at the opposite pole. Infections with this organism may occur at any age, but are somewhat more common in postmenopausal women.

When the inflammation is well developed, the underlying vaginal and cervical mucosa has a characteristic brilliant fiery red, sometimes called "strawberry," appearance. Histologically, there is a suppurative inflammatory reaction, but it is usually quite superficial and involves only the vaginal mucosa and immediate subjacent tissues. This reaction may extend over the vulva and perineum, into the urethra and even the urinary bladder.

Monilial Vaginitis. As presented in Chapter 10 (p. 448), *Candida albicans* may implant on the mucosa of the vagina and produce its characteristic anatomic changes.

Senile Vaginitis. Senile vaginitis is something of a misnomer that is applied to the atrophic changes found in the vaginal epithelium postmenopausally. With this physiologic atrophy, the epithelium becomes thin and keratinization less well developed, and the mucosa is rendered more susceptible to nonspecific inflammations and other irritations. Accordingly, some mononuclear cell infiltration may be found submucosally, hence the designation as a vaginitis.

TUMORS

The only tumors of the vagina of clinical significance in terms of frequency and biologic behavior are the carcinoma and sarcoma botryoides. However, other forms of benign neoplasms and non-neoplastic lesions that simulate tumors also arise in the vagina. Epithelial papillomas, fibromas, leiomyomas and hemangiomas are uncommon and resemble their counterparts in other sites. Small red nodules of granulation tissue may simulate tumors in the vagina. These usually follow hysterectomy or the longstanding chronic inflammation induced by pessaries. Because these nodules bleed freely, they are often mistaken for hemangiomas. Foci of endometriosis may arise in the vagina and masquerade as a neoplasm (p. 1225). Cystic dilatation of remnants of the mesonephric duct may produce laterally situated Gartner's cysts.

PRIMARY CARCINOMA

Primary carcinoma of the vagina is an extremely uncommon cancer accounting for about 1 per cent of malignant neoplasms in the female genital tract. Its peak incidence is in the fifth and sixth decades of life but, rarely, it occurs in younger women (Whelton and Kottmeier, 1962).

Most often, it affects the upper regions of the vagina, particularly along the posterior wall at the junction with the exocervix. It follows the characteristic course of malignancies in such mucosal surfaces, beginning as a focus of epithelial thickening and progressing to a plaque-like mass that extends centrifugally and invades, by direct continuity, the cervix and perivaginal structures such as the urethra, urinary bladder and rectum. The lesions in the lower two-thirds metastasize to the inguinal nodes, while upper lesions tend to involve the regional iliac nodes and, in late, advanced stages, distant organs via the blood. As ulcerating, invasive lesions, they may produce malignant urethrovaginal, vesicovaginal or rectovaginal fistulas. Almost all are squamous cell lesions. Rarely (5 per cent), an adenocarcinoma arises, presumably in the associated mucous glands or in an endometrial inclusion.

These lesions first come to the patient's attention by the appearance of irregular spotting or the development of a frank vaginal discharge (leukorrhea). At other times, they remain totally silent and only become clinically manifest by pain on coitus or, late in their life history, by the onset of urinary or rectal fistulas. Recently, it was observed that the administration *of diethylstilbestrol to pregnant women induced an increased frequency of vaginal adenocarcinoma in the exposed offspring* (Herbst et al., 1971). Most of the exposed offspring were 15 to 20 years old when they developed cancer. A subsequent report has confirmed these findings (Greenwald et al., 1971). Because of their insidious, invasive growth, all forms of vaginal cancer (squamous and adenocarcinoma) are difficult to cure. With radiotherapy or radical surgery, the 5-year survival rate is on the order of 20 to 30 per cent; the ten-year survival rate, about 15 per cent. Extension of cervical carcinoma to the vagina is much more common than primary malignancies of the vagina. Accordingly, before a diagnosis of primary vaginal carcinoma can be made, it is requisite that a preexisting cervical lesion be ruled out.

SARCOMA BOTRYOIDES (MIXED MESODERMAL TUMOR)

Sarcoma botryoides is an extremely interesting anatomic, but very uncommon, clinical lesion. *The tumor is distinctive since it is composed of all the various mesodermal histogenetic cell types,* i.e., fibrous tissue, myxomatous tissue, striated or smooth muscle cells, cartilage, bone and, less commonly, epithelial or glandular structures similar to those found in the mucosal lining of the female genital tract. These tumors are found at all ages. Some occur in children under the age of three years. From the very pleomorphic character of the cell types found within the neoplasm, it is assumed that they arise from primitive pluripotential mesodermal cells. Some tumors arise in the vagina, but others have uterine origins.

Grossly, these tumors tend to grow as large, rounded, bulbous, multilobate, bulky masses that sometimes fill and project out of the vagina (Fig. 27–9). Because of the resemblance of these masses, on external examination, to grape-like clusters, they are designated sarcoma botryoides (grape-like). They have a soft gray to yellow, almost gelatinous consistency, are extremely friable, and frequently break off in the course of their growth, with subsequent bleeding and secondary infection. Histologically, the characteristic features consist of the clear demonstration of many mesodermal cell types. In most tumors, loose fibromyxomatous stroma and well defined striated muscle cells predominate. However, in many instances, well differentiated epithelial masses or gland formations are present,

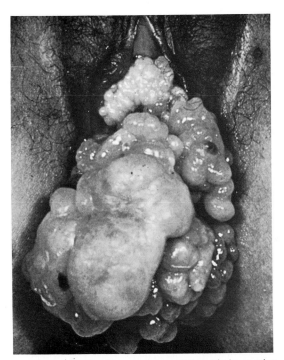

Figure 27–9. *Sarcoma botryoides of the vagina appearing as a polypoid mass protruding from the vagina. (Courtesy of Dr. Arthur Hertig.)*

as well as cartilage and bone, reflecting the multipotentiality of the mesoderm.

Those tumors that arise in children tend only to invade locally and cause death by penetration into the peritoneal cavity or by obstruction of the urinary tract. In adults, the local spread is often accompanied by metastases, not only to the regional nodes but also to distant organs. The prognosis in the adult is extremely poor, and death usually occurs within one to two years of the diagnosis (Wurtz, 1949).

CERVIX

Congenital Anomalies	Tumors	Polyps
Inflammations	Carcinoma	Papilloma
Cervicitis (acute and chronic)		

Lesions of the cervix are extremely common if one includes the great abundance of minor inflammatory changes designated as nonspecific cervicitis. In fact, excessive inflammatory vaginal discharge, referred to clinically as leukorrhea, constitutes one of the most common clinical complaints of gynecologic practice. However, in addition to these for the most part innocuous inflammatory lesions, the cervix is extremely vulnerable to the development of cancer. As will be reemphasized presently, cervical carcinoma alone is responsible for about one-tenth of all cancer deaths in women.

CONGENITAL ANOMALIES

Hypoplasia of the cervix usually accompanies infantile development of the uterus and is frequently only one feature of general underdevelopment of the female genital tract. Duplication of the cervix almost invariably implies a septate, totally bifid uterus. Stenosis and atresia of the cervical os may occur as congenital developmental defects. In this condition, the narrowing may be so extreme as to represent a complete absence of the cervical canal. In most instances, the developmental narrowing is at least probe-patent. Stenosis of the cervix is more commonly an acquired defect from chronic cervicitis, with subsequent fibrosis and scarring. Both the developmental and acquired stenoses may result in sterility and retention of menstrual blood and secretions.

INFLAMMATIONS

Inflammations of the cervix are extremely common and are present, to some extent, in virtually every multipara. However, the preponderance of these infections are relatively insignificant. They are caused by a variety of bacteria, many of which comprise the normal flora of the vagina. This form of banal inflammation is referred to as nonspecific cervicitis. However, it should not be inferred that all nonspecific cervicitis is without serious significance because, as will be pointed out, in a small percentage of cases it may predispose to serious complications. In addition to this commonplace type of cervicitis, there are many types of specific cervical inflammations, i.e., gonorrhea, syphilis, chancroid and tuberculosis, that have been adequately described in other sections.

ACUTE AND CHRONIC CERVICITIS

Depending upon the histologic criteria that are selected for the establishment of this diagnosis, some degree of cervical inflammation may be found in virtually all multiparous and in many nulliparous adult women. It is extremely doubtful that the minor involvements are of any clinical consequence.

Etiology and Pathogenesis. Despite its commonplace occurrence, few data have been accumulated on the precise causes of this disorder. It is clear that bacteria can be isolated from the cervical secretions in all instances. The most commonly identified organisms are *E. coli*, alpha and, less commonly, beta hemolytic streptococci and a variety of staphylococci. However, the vagina and the cervix normally contain a mixed flora that includes similar organisms. Predisposing causes to infection must then be sought. Trauma of childbirth, instrumentation in the course of gynecologic treatment, hyperestrinism, hypoestrinism, intercourse, excessive secretion of the cervical glands, high alkalinity of the cervical mucus and congenital eversion of the endocervical mucosa have all been cited as predisposing influences.

Morphology. Cervicitis may be divided into an acute and a chronic phase.

Excluding gonococcal infections, **acute cervicitis** is most commonly encountered postpartally and is usually caused by either staphylococci or streptococci. The inflammatory changes are similar to those already described under nonspecific pelvic inflammatory disease (p. 1206). However, in the lesion referred to as cervicitis, the process is largely limited to the tissues in and about the exocervical os (**exocervicitis**). In the more marked cases, the inflammatory infiltration extends to involve the superficial endocervical mucosa and endocervical glands (**endocervicitis**). In general, the acute changes are quite rare and, more often, the condition is of fairly long duration and merits the designation chronic cervicitis.

Chronic nonspecific cervicitis is far more common than acute cervicitis. It begins or is most marked within the endocervix, in and about the external cervical os. In its simplest form, chronic cervicitis appears as a slight reddening, swelling and granularity limited to the margins of the external cervical os. With progression, the reddening and granularity extend out to produce a progressively widening ring of inflamed mucosa (Fig. 27–10). The changes are not necessarily uniformly distributed about the circumference of the os. With persistence of the inflammation, superficial irregular cervical ulcerations or erosions develop, particularly about the external os. In far advanced, neglected cases, the continual inflammatory-reparative process creates granulation tissue that causes irregular, friable nodularity and distortion of the exocervix to the point at which it can be readily confused with a neoplasm. Inflammatory stenosis of the cervical glands may yield cystic dilatations designated as **nabothian cysts.** Chronic inflammatory changes

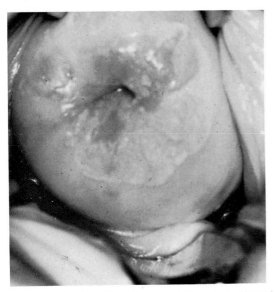

Figure 27–10. *Chronic cervicitis as viewed through a speculum. The inflammatory area rims the external os. (Courtesy of Dr. Arthur Hertig.)*

and scarring may cause deformity of the cervix with protrusion of the endocervical mucosa, designated by the terms **ectropion** and **eversion.** The chronic inflammatory cells may accumulate into lymphoid follicles, **follicular cervicitis.** All these anatomic lesions are merely variations on the basic theme of nonspecific cervicitis.

Histologically, the inflammatory infiltrate is usually found subjacent to the endocervical mucosa in close proximity to the squamocolumnar junction of the exocervical os. The leukocytic population is preponderantly mononuclear, but many "polys" are present as well. The infiltrate is usually limited to the superficial regions and extends about the endocervical mucus-secreting glands as well as into the gland lumina. The ulcerations are usually quite shallow but, in neglected cases, may destroy a considerable portion of the endocervical glands (Fig. 27–11).

The cervical and endocervical mucosa is an additional site of significant changes. Commonly, the epithelium has minimal inflammatory dysplastic changes. In the more marked cases with erosions and eversion, these inflammatory epithelial alterations may produce considerable dysplasia with downgrowth of epithelial pegs into the inflammatory granulation tissue (Fig. 27–12). In the course of these inflammatory changes, the epithelial cells are depleted of their normal content of glycogen (Fig. 27–13). This loss of glycogen is an important biochemical alteration, since it accounts for the failure of these areas to stain brown with Schiller's solution (an iodine preparation), thus suggesting a neoplasm (p. 1219). Hence, cervicitis may produce confusion in the interpretation of this valuable diagnostic clinical procedure.

In certain cases, in the region of the external os, tongues of stratified squamous epithelium may extend down from the surface mucosa immediately subjacent to the columnar mucus-secreting lining cells of the endocervical glands. In some instances, this apparent downgrowth may completely encircle glands and sometimes narrow or totally compress the gland lumina (Fig. 27–14). These changes are designated as **epidermidization.** This form of epithelial alteration merits careful anatomic attention because it can be mistaken, on casual inspection, for the infiltrative growth of a squamous cell carcinoma.

In addition to these characteristics of nonspecific cervicitis, dilatation of endocervical glands to comprise the nabothian cyst described, the formation of lymphoid aggregates or even true lymphoid follicles replete with germinal centers, and hyperplasia of the cervical mucus-secreting glands may all be encountered in this condition. Inflammatory proliferative thickening of squamous epithelial cells of the exocervix may create white plaques of **leukoplakia.** These too may create areas depleted of glycogen, which fail to stain with the Schiller test.

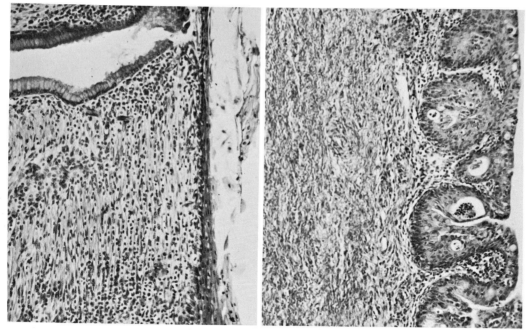

Fig. 27–11

Fig. 27–12

Figure 27–11. *Chronic ulcerative cervicitis with previous loss and partial regrowth of the surface epithelium. An inflammatory infiltrate is present in the subjacent tissue.*

Figure 27–12. *Chronic cervicitis with inflammatory metaplasia and dysplasia of the exocervical epithelium. (Both figures by courtesy of Dr. Arthur Hertig. Figure 27–12 from Amer. J. Obstet. Gynec., Vol. 8, 1949.)*

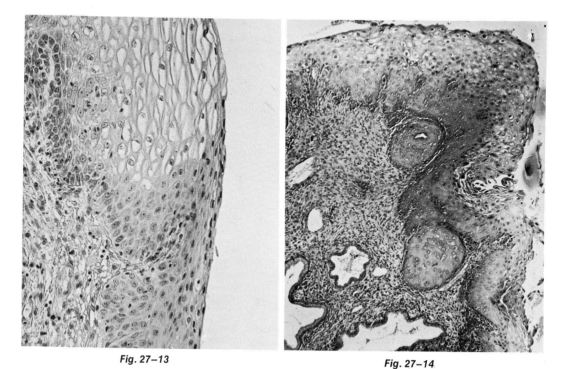

Fig. 27–13

Fig. 27–14

Figure 27–13. *The junction between normal glycogen-laden vacuolated epithelium (above) and inflammatory glycogen-depleted cells (below).*

Figure 27–14. *Chronic cervicitis with marked epithelial thickening and downgrowth of epithelium (epidermidization) that has totally obliterated the endocervical glands. (Both figures by courtesy of Dr. Arthur Hertig.)*

Clinical Course. It has already been indicated that nonspecific cervicitis may be a completely banal, asymptomatic lesion that is discovered only when the cervix is removed for other causes. However, most cases are discovered either in the course of routine gynecologic examination or because of leukorrhea. The diagnosis may be made by simple visual examination of the cervix when the changes are well defined or, at times, may be extremely difficult to differentiate from the much more serious condition of cancer of the cervix. The cervical distortion, destruction of cervical epithelium and overgrowth of inflammatory tissue may sometimes make this lesion resemble a granular, necrotic, ulcerated neoplasm. The ultimate differentiation rests on histologic examination of biopsy specimens.

While generally of little systemic consequence, cervicitis may be responsible for sterility and, more importantly, is believed to predispose to the development of carcinoma.

TUMORS

While the cervix may develop a wide variety of both benign and malignant tumors that include such rare entities as hemangiomas, adenomas, fibromas, fibrosarcomas and leiomyosarcomas, at least 95 per cent of cervical tumors are represented by the three lesions, carcinomas, polyps and papillomas. On this basis, further discussion is limited principally to these entities.

CARCINOMA OF THE CERVIX

No form of clinical cancer better documents the remarkable effects of early diagnosis and curative therapy on the mortality rate than cancer of the cervix. The United States Bureau of the Census does not codify cancer of the cervix but only cancer of the uterus which predominantly represents carcinoma of the cervix and carcinoma of the endometrium. The mortality rate from cancer of the endometrium has not altered significantly over the decades, but the net result of the better cure of cervical cancer has reduced the death rate from uterine cancer from 27 per 100,000 female population in 1930 to 12 per 100,000 in 1967 (National Vital Statistics Division, Bureau of the Census, United States). This most heartening trend has occurred despite the fact that the incidence of cervical cancer has remained constant for the past 40 years, averaging about 30 cases per 100,000 females. The lowered mortality rate reflects the earlier discovery of curable lesions. Today about 50 per cent of cervical cancers are detected when they are small localized lesions (Stage 0 and 1) while only a decade ago, only 20 per cent were discovered in these curable stages. Thanks for these impressive improvements are largely owed to the Papanicolaou cytologic test for detection of cancer. However, the disease has not been conquered and it still accounts for approximately 13,000 deaths per year. It is still the third or fourth most important cause of cancer deaths in females in the United States (Lund, 1961).

More is known about the life history of this form of cancer than of any other. Cervical cytology and the accessibility of the cervix to biopsy provide the opportunity for the early discovery and close follow-up of these lesions. The entire concept of "in situ" cancer originated with studies of this neoplasm and it is, therefore, appropriate to consider here in some detail the relationship of carcinoma in situ to overt clinical malignancy.

Incidence. Carcinoma of the cervix may occur at any age from the second decade of life to senility. The peak incidence of clinically obvious lesions occurs around 50 years of age, but in situ lesions have their peak 10 to 15 years earlier. The frequency of this form of cancer in young women in the second and third decades of life appears to have significantly risen in the recent past, suggesting increasingly earlier exposure of women to carcinogenic influences. As will become apparent in the discussion of etiology and pathogenesis, many social and personal factors may be implicated in this trend.

Etiology and Pathogenesis. A high incidence of carcinoma of the cervix has been correlated with each of the following:

1. It is more common among low income classes.

2. Blacks have a higher incidence than whites in the United States, but this is probably related to socioeconomic influences rather than to racial predisposition.

3. Early marriage and increasing parity is correlated with an increased frequency.

4. There is a correlation between the incidence of this disease and age at onset of sexual relations and frequency of coitus (Malhotra, 1971).

5. The incidence of this disease rises with the number of consorts (Elliot, 1964).

6. There is a high incidence in prostitutes and a low incidence in nuns. Gagnon (1950) found no case of cervical carcinoma in 13,000 nuns over a 20-year period.

7. Chronic cervicitis is believed to predispose to this form of cancer.

8. The incidence of cervical carcinoma has been shown to be markedly lower in Jews and Indian Muslims and Parsees, correlated with early circumcision of males in these groups.

Many of these observations have raised the issue of whether personal hygiene in the male and penile smegma may be important considerations in the development of cervical carcinoma in females. Trace amounts of chemical carcinogens have been isolated from human smegma. When placed into the mouse vagina, human smegma can induce cervical cancer. A transmissible, possibly oncogenic, virus is also currently under suspicion. A number of studies point toward herpes simplex virus (type 2) infections as possibly playing a role in the induction of cancer of the cervix. Neutralizing antibodies to this serotype have been reported in 80 to 90 per cent of women with carcinoma of the cervix as compared with a frequency of 20 to 55 per cent in controls (Rawls et al., 1969) (Plummer and Masterson, 1971). Viral antigens have been detected by immunofluorescent techniques in cervical cancer cells in vivo and also in those grown in tissue culture. However, attempts to isolate the virus from cervical lesions have been largely unsuccessful. The high incidence of neutralizing antibodies in cancer subjects must be interpreted in the light of the extraordinarily high incidence in controls, ranging up to 55 per cent. The viral infection and cervical cancer might be independently related to promiscuity or, alternatively, the virus might preferentially grow in preneoplastic or neoplastic cervical tissue (Editorial, 1972). There is much uncertainty, but the possibility that the virus plays a causative role is attractive, since it would explain many of the previously mentioned correlations relating the incidence of cancer of the cervix to early intercourse, frequency of intercourse, multiple consorts and penile hygiene, all of which could relate to the possible spread of an infectious agent.

Relationship of Carcinoma In Situ to Overt Carcinoma. There is substantial evidence that all overt carcinomas of the cervix begin as in situ lesions. The focal point of the controversy involves the frequency with which in situ lesions progress into invasive cancer. Stated in another way, when a diagnosis of in situ carcinoma is made, will it invariably later become an invasive tumor? Or is it possible that in situ lesions may remain as such without progression or, even more important, may they regress and disappear? Studies of serial biopsies of patients have clearly shown that in situ lesions arise through sequential epithelial alterations that might be designated as basal cell hyperplasia, atypical basal cell hyperplasia, dysplasia or metaplasia, and atypical dysplasia or metaplasia ultimately becoming unmistakable anaplasia (Johnson et al., 1964). These changes usually begin at the squamocolumnar junction and often arise in the presence of surrounding chronic cervicitis and endocervicitis. The cytologic alterations represent a continuum of progressively severe cellular deviations from the normal.

Much of the dispute about the progression and regression of in situ carcinoma involves the problem of clearly identifying the degree of cytologic abnormality requisite for the diagnosis of in situ carcinoma. Where is the line between inflammatory atypia and tumorous anaplasia? It is well known that the cytologic abnormalities which attend chronic inflammation are reversible when the underlying inciting stimulus is removed. It is, therefore, not surprising that, were such lesions to be termed in situ carcinoma, progression into invasive cancer would not be inevitable and regression might well occur. Much of this controversy then arises from the lack of clearly defined limits for the diagnosis of in situ carcinoma. In recognition of this problem, Nieburgs (1963) proposes that atypical cellular changes in the cervix be divided into three classes: benign dysplasia, atypical dysplasia and incipient carcinoma. With this approach, he was able to demonstrate that no invasive carcinoma occurred over an eight-year period in 12 patients having benign dysplasia. Of the group of 12 patients with atypical dysplasia, four developed carcinoma on an average of four and a half years later, while eight of nine patients with incipient carcinoma progressed to invasive carcinoma in three and a half years. He summarizes this clinical course by stating: "It is suggested that benign dysplasia is a reversible lesion with uncertain preneoplastic significance. Atypical dysplasia reflects a potentially malignant alteration while incipient carcinoma may be regarded as an irreversible malignant alteration."

In contrast to these findings, in which all but one of the incipient carcinomas progressed, we can turn to a somewhat different study done of 23 patients who were found, in retrospect, to have had unrecognized in situ carcinoma in a biopsy six to 10 years prior to the time of the report (Old and Jones, 1965). Of these 23 patients, 78 per cent had no detectable residual neoplasia some six to 10 years later *as judged by pelvic examination and Papanicolaou smear.* Biopsy material was not available on all these patients. Persistent carcinoma in situ as proved by biopsy was present in three of the 23 patients eight to 10 years later. Only one of the 23 patients had developed invasive carcinoma. This study implies that carcinoma in situ is frequently reversible and, in some patients, may persist without progression. However, the study suffers from the lack of adequate histologic evaluation of all patients at the end of the time span and from the usual hazards of the criteria used to establish the diagnosis of in situ carcinoma; for example, the original biopsy required to establish the diagnosis might conceivably have totally removed a small lesion. Moreover, most patients with these borderline lesions have many forms of treatment for the concomitant inflammation and erosion that are so often present. Thus, in a large series of 93 cases of in situ carcinoma studied at the New York Memorial Hospital, there were 27 cases of disappearing lesions but, among these 27, only three regressed spontaneously (Koss et al., 1963). The remaining patients all had a variety of forms of treatment, such as douches, antibiotics and other anti-inflammatory measures that might have influenced the lesion. Nonetheless, three untreated cases had regressed, in which the diagnosis had been established by cytologic examination, no biopsy had been performed, and no medical therapy had been administered. So, at least in these instances, carcinoma in situ represented a reversible lesion.

The present consensus is best summarized by the following quotation: "Carcinoma in situ is a lesion of the cervical epithelium that beyond a doubt is a precursor of invasive cervix cancer. Carcinoma in situ is very fragile and poorly established and may be readily eradicated by a variety of minor procedures. Its natural course may be profoundly modified by even small biopsies, drugs and possibly physiological trauma such as delivery. Spontaneous disappearance of carcinomas in situ apparently does occur but it is an extraordinarily rare event" (Koss et al., 1963). To this statement, it should be added that carcinoma in situ may also persist without progression for many years.

Morphology. Carcinoma of the cervix begins at or close to the squamocolumnar junction of the exocervical os. This junction may not coincide with the anatomic os when there has been previous eversion or ectropion (Wheeler and Hertig, 1955). Carcinomas rarely if ever arise from the more lateral regions of the exocervix. In its in situ stage, carcinoma of the cervix produces no recognizable alteration to the naked eye. The diagnosis can only be suspected by either the Schiller test or the Papanicolaou smear. The Schiller test involves painting the cervix with a solution of iodine and po-

tassium iodide. The normal cervical epithelium is rich in glycogen and stains a mahogany brown. The cancerous focus, because it is depleted of glycogen, fails to stain. It should be cautioned that both methods may yield false-positive results since areas of inflammation may also fail to stain with the Schiller solution and sometimes these dysplastic foci shed inflammatory atypical cells that are confused with cancer. At this in situ stage, one sees characteristic cellular anaplastic changes within the cervical mucosa without invasion of the stroma. Sometimes the anaplastic changes extend along the surface into the underlying endocervical glands, but such superficial spread should not be construed as invasion since the basement membranes of these glands are not penetrated. As previously emphasized, **rarely these in situ lesions undoubtedly regress but most develop into clinically overt invasive cancers.**

Overt cervical carcinoma presents in three somewhat distinctive macroscopic patterns: fungating, ulcerating and infiltrative cancer. The most common variant is the fungating tumor which produces an obviously neoplastic cauliflower mass which projects above the surrounding normal mucosa. Such a lesion appears by progressive thickening of the epithelium followed by slight nodularity which, in the course of time, eventuates in the irregular papillary nodular appearance of the fungating tumor (Fig. 27–15). The ulcerating pattern is a modification of the fungating tumor. Here the progressive epithelial thickening leads to sloughing

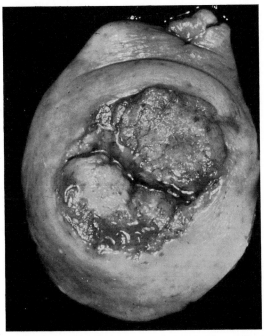

Figure 27–15. Carcinoma of the cervix, well advanced.

necrosis of the surface of the tumor with the production of a necrotic neoplastic ulceration. The infiltrative pattern is the most uncommon variant in which the tumor grows downward into the underlying stroma of the cervix, causing only irregular thickening of the mucosal surface without ulceration or fungation. This infiltrative pattern may also represent a precursor to the more obvious variants already described. In the course of time, all cervical carcinomas infiltrate the underlying cervix, obliterate the external os, grow up into the endocervical canal and lower uterine segment and eventually extend into the wall of the fundus. Advanced lesions infiltrate surrounding organs, as is indicated in Table 27–1.

It is obvious that cervical carcinoma extends by direct continuity to involve every contiguous structure. At the same time, local and distant lymph nodes are involved. The paracervical, hypogastric, obturator and external iliac nodes are affected in about half the cases and more distant periaortic nodes in about the same number. Distant metastasis occurs, in the late stages, to the liver, lungs, bone marrow and other structures.

The histology of 95 per cent of carcinomas of the cervix is that of a typical squamous cell carcinoma of varying differentiation and growth rate. Some of the tumors are extremely well differentiated, producing keratohyalin, epithelial pearls and prickle cells, while others are composed of more undifferentiated squamous cells. It is usually possible to identify in situ carcinoma in the margins of overt invasive lesions. This finding is a vital key that quite assuredly links the in situ lesions to the later developing overt neoplasms.

Many systems of classifying these carcinomas have been devised, but all comprise essentially either **grading** the degree of differentiation of the neoplasm or expressing its extent in **stages.** As would be suspected, the better differentiated tumors generally yield a better survival rate than the anaplastic undifferentiated lesions. With comparable radiation therapy, differentiated lesions yielded a 51 per cent five-year survival rate as compared with 28 per cent for anaplastic tumors

TABLE 27–1. PELVIC ORGAN INVOLVEMENT FOUND IN 356 AUTOPSIES PERFORMED ON WOMEN WITH CERVICAL CARCINOMA

Pelvic Organ Involvement	Nontreated Patients (%)	Treated Patients (%)
Uterus	39	17
Bladder wall	30	20
Bladder	19	21
Vagina	32	20
Rectum	24	18

From Henriksen, E.: The dispersion of the cancer of cervix. Radiology; 54:812, 1950.

(Glucksman, 1965). The most widely accepted classification of staging was proposed by the General Assembly of Nations of the International Federation of Gynecology and Obstetrics in 1961 (McGarrity, 1963).

Preinvasive Carcinoma of the Cervix

Stage 0—Carcinoma in situ or intraepithelial carcinoma.

Invasive Carcinoma of the Cervix

Stage 1—Includes carcinoma which is strictly confined to the cervix. It may be subdivided into:

Stage I-A (cases of early stromal invasion) and Stage I-B (all other cases of Stage I).

Stage II—The carcinoma extends beyond the cervix but has not extended onto the pelvic wall. The carcinoma involves the vagina, but not the lower third.

Stage III—The carcinoma has extended onto the pelvic wall. On rectal examination, there is no cancer-free space between the tumor and the pelvic wall. The tumor involves the lower third of the vagina.

Stage IV—The carcinoma has extended beyond the true pelvis or has involved the mucosa of the bladder or rectum. This stage obviously includes those with metastatic dissemination.

The remaining 5 per cent of cervical carcinomas constitute either adenocarcinomas or adenoacanthomas. The adenocarcinomas presumably arise in the endocervical glands. Rarely, such adenocarcinomas may arise in remnants of the mesonephric ducts. These look and behave as do the squamous cell lesions. They arise, however, in a slightly older age level. **The mixed squamous and adeno-patterns comprise the adenoacanthomas.** These are thought generally to arise from the squamocolumnar junction. According to some reports, these lesions are prone to develop during pregnancy and account for a disproportionate percentage of the cervical cancers in this group of women. Anatomically, they are distinguishable from the more common squamous cell lesions only by histologic examination.

Clinical Course. It is apparent from the preceding discussion that cancer of the cervix evolves slowly over the course of many years. In situ lesions have their peak incidence in the mid-thirties and early forties, but invasive carcinoma does not achieve its maximum prevalence until 10 years later. Long before the in situ lesion appears, variable cellular changes begin that themselves require many years to achieve the level of in situ carcinoma. During this long evolution, the cytologic abnormalities produce no clinical manifestations. Such symptoms as increased vaginal discharge may be present, but this is related more to accompanying chronic cervicitis than to the incipient neoplasm. For these reasons, it is generally acknowledged that periodic Papanicolaou smears should be performed on all women over the age of 20. This low age limit is suggested because, as has been indicated, cervical cancer sometimes appears in the second and third decades of life, particularly in those who have borne many children and have been sexually active. The excellent opportunity is afforded by such periodic examinations to detect these incipient cancers when they can be eradicated with almost complete certainty. *The remarkable effectiveness of cervical cytology in detecting early lesions has been documented by a number of studies.* With mass screening of population groups, invasive carcinoma has virtually disappeared from individuals screened regularly each year (Dunn, 1958). Presumably, those with carcinoma in situ were discovered, treated and thus spared the development of invasive cancer. Screening clinics report a 30 per cent decrease in clinically invasive carcinoma over the past five years (Boyes et al., 1962). It must be emphasized, however, that the cytologic examination merely detects the possible presence of a cervical cancer; it does not make an absolute diagnosis. The latter requires histologic evaluation of appropriate biopsy specimens. Ultimately, when these cancers become clinically overt, they usually produce irregular vaginal bleeding, leukorrhea, pain on coitus and dysuria as the dominant clinical manifestations.

The treatment of carcinoma of the cervix depends on the stage of the neoplasm. Virtually all clinicians advocate surgery for Stage 0, but controversy arises over the preferred mode of treatment for the various stages of invasive cancer. Among three therapeutic modalities—surgical excision, radiation alone or combined surgery and radiation—all are equally ardently sponsored. Most of these carcinomas are radiosensitive, and many clinicians advocate radiation for all stages. Graham (1947) has proposed that the degree of radiosensitivity (RR) can be evaluated from the appearance of the *benign* desquamated vaginal cells, after a test dose of radiation therapy has been administered. Others, however, prefer surgical excision for Stage I on the grounds that these lesions can be readily excised and the patient is spared the potential hazards of radiation therapy. Recent reports of end results clearly indicate that, for Stages I and II, there is little difference in five-year survival rates with all three forms of therapy (Rutledge, 1965).

All writings now stress that there is no need for hasty possibly injudicious treatment of the early incipient stages of this neoplasm. Years will elapse before *in situ lesions become invasive.* Many so-called in situ lesions may, indeed, represent atypical dysplasia that will disappear under simple forms of medical therapy. As long as the patient can be kept under observation, much can be gained from intelligent delay without jeopardizing the patient's life.

The prognosis and survival of these patients depends largely upon the stage at which the disease is first discovered. If these lesions are discovered at Stage 0, 100 per cent cure should be effected. With current methods of treatment, there is a five-year survival rate of about 80 to 90 per cent with Stage I, 75 per cent with Stage II, 55 per cent with Stage III and 10 to 15 per cent with Stage IV disease. Most patients with Stage IV cancer die as a consequence of local extension of the tumor for example, into and about the urinary bladder and ureters, leading to fatal renal infections rather than of metastatic disease (DeAlvarez, 1947).

A word is necessary about the occurrence of cervical cancer during pregnancy. The diagnosis of these lesions is extremely difficult at this time because pregnancy itself induces a certain amount of variability in the morphology of the stratified squamous cells of the cervical mucosa. However, these "pregnancy changes" should theoretically be distinguishable from true carcinoma. Nonetheless, many clinicians prefer, with in situ lesions during pregnancy, to reevaluate the patient after delivery at a time when the changes of pregnancy may be assumed to have disappeared. Since there is no real hazard to the patient's life in delaying therapy for this period of time, such a conservative approach seems justifiable. Obviously, invasive carcinomas would cause no difficulty in diagnosis and should be treated as soon as possible compatible with the stage of pregnancy and the clinical circumstances.

No better conclusion to this discussion of cancer of the cervix can be given than to quote Lund (1961): "The epitaph for cervical cancer has been inscribed. The methods, skills and techniques are available to destroy it. The date of death remains unwritten in the hands of the practising physicians and their patients."

POLYPS

Cervical polyps are extremely common, relatively innocuous tumors that occur in 2 to 5 per cent of adult women, usually in the fourth and fifth decades of life. They are frequently associated with chronic cervicitis, although it is doubtful that the two conditions have a causal relationship (Aaro et al., 1963). Perhaps the major significance of polyps lies in their production of irregular vaginal "spotting" or bleeding that arouses suspicion of some more ominous lesion.

Polyps may occur singly (approximately 90 per cent) or multiply. They are extremely variable in size and shape. Most arise within the endocervical canal and are barely, if at all, apparent on external examination of the cervix. They vary from small, hemispheric, sessile projections several millimeters in diameter to large, bulbous masses that are pedunculated and may protrude or hang out through the cervical os, having external diameters of up to 2 to 3 cm. and lengths of up to 4 to 5 cm. (Fig. 27–16). Many times these lesions cause dilatation of the endocervical canal and exocervical os. All characteristically are soft, almost mucoid, and contain hypertrophied or cystically dilated mucous glands. When they protrude through the cervix, they frequently develop superficial erosions and interstitial hemorrhage, transforming their usual pale gray color to a red-blue cyanosis. Almost all can be demonstrated to have a very superficial attachment to the endocervical mucosa.

Histologically, polyps are composed of a loose fibromyxomatous stroma harboring hypertrophied or cystically dilated mucus-secreting endocervical glands. The covering epithelium is usually columnar-mucous in type, resembling that of the endocervix. Ulceration and chronic inflammation may lead to squamous metaplasia or considerable inflammatory epithelial alterations. Occasionally, polyps may originate low within the cervical canal at the junction of the squamous and columnar epithelium. Such polyps may be covered by stratified squamous epithelium.

In almost all instances, simple currettage or surgical excision effects a cure, although reformation of an additional polyp may occur. Although cancer arising in a polyp has been seen, it is rare indeed.

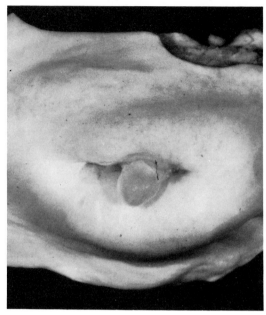

Figure 27–16. *Endocervical polyp, protruding through the external os.*

PAPILLOMA

Several types of papilloma arise on the cervix. They take one of three forms: (1) The cockscomb papilloma or polyp almost invariably occurs during pregnancy and regresses following delivery. It is a small, red lesion that projects above the surrounding mucosa and has a resemblance to a cockscomb. (2) The condyloma accuminatum is similar to those lesions occurring in the vulva (p. 1209). As pointed out, these are probably of viral etiology. (3) The solitary, true neoplastic papillomas range up to 1 cm. in diameter and are broad-based papillary proliferations of the cervical mucosa usually arising from the squamocolumnar junction. As proliferative lesions, this form of papilloma may, on occasion, convert to a squamous cell cervical cancer.

BODY OF THE UTERUS AND ENDOMETRIUM

The uterus, stimulated daily by hormones, denuded monthly of its endometrial mucosa and invaded spasmodically by fetuses, is subject to a variety of disorders, the most common of which result from endocrine imbalances, complications of pregnancy and neoplastic proliferation. Together with the lesions that affect the cervix, the lesions of the corpus of the uterus and the endometrium account for the great preponderance of gynecologic practice. Excluding the disorders relating to pregnancy, to be considered subsequently, the major conditions that merit consideration are endometriosis, abnormalities of the endometrium and neoplasms of both the endometrium and myometrium.

CONGENITAL ANOMALIES

Hypoplasia of the uterus is encountered in a variety of endocrine disorders. Such small uteri are referred to clinically as infantile. Most are due to ovarian or pituitary hypofunction. Strictly speaking, such failure of growth is not a congenital anomaly, but rather is an acquired defect.

Various anomalies may derive from the imperfect fusion of the primitive müllerian ducts. These consist of many patterns that vary from simple notching of the fundus to a partial septum that divides the fundus but not the cervix, to total division of the uterus by a septum into two endometrial cavities, a *septate uterus.* The most extreme anomaly is a completely *double uterus with double cervix,* each organ receiving only one tube. Such anomalies are perfectly compatible with normal fertility and normal menstrual cycles, but sometimes result in interesting and confusing clinical problems. Pregnancy in one half of a septate uterus may be accompanied by bleeding from the unaffected half of the uterus or by a second conception. Pregnancy may occur in one half of the uterus after the other half has already developed a pregnancy, so-called superfetation.

INFLAMMATIONS

The endometrium and myometrium are remarkably resistant to infections. Endometritis and myometritis are, therefore, uncommon clinical problems. Acute reactions are virtually limited to bacterial infections that arise following delivery or miscarriage. Retained products of conception are the usual predisposing influence. The most common causative agents are the group A hemolytic streptococci, although the staphylococci and other bacteria are sometimes involved. The inflammatory response is chiefly limited to the interstitium and is entirely nonspecific in nature. Removal of the retained gestational fragments by curettage is promptly followed by remission of the infection.

Chronic Endometritis. Chronic inflammation of the endometrium is encountered in patients suffering from pelvic inflammatory disease, in the miliary spread of extragenital tuberculosis or the drainage of a tuberculous salpingitis producing a tuberculous endometritis, and in postpartal, bacterially contaminated uterine cavities (Fig. 27–17). The chronic endometritis in these cases represents a secondary disease and, under these circumstances, there is a plausible cause for the endometrial infection.

Occasionally, no such primary infection in the tubes or previous pregnancy is present and yet plasma cells are found in the endometrium. It will be remembered that, in the normal menstrual cycle, the endometrial mucosa is suffused with neutrophils, lymphocytes and histiocytes during the late premenstrual phase. Therefore, only one type of white cell, the plasma cell, is not a normal inhabitant of the endometrium. Some of these women have such gynecologic complaints as abnormal bleeding, pain, discharge or infertility that appear to be based upon the diagnosis of primary chronic endometritis. Moreover, increased numbers of plasma cells accompanied

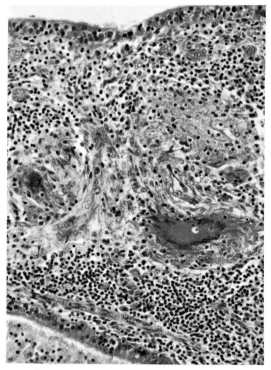

Figure 27–17. Tuberculous endometritis.

by irregularities of the endometrial glands are consistently present in patients with the secondary forms of chronic endometritis. On this account, it would appear to be justified to accept the entity of primary chronic endometritis when plasma cells alone are present, even though we fail to understand the cause for the changes.

Pyometria. Pyometria designates the accumulation of suppurative or necrotic exudate within the uterine cavity. It implies stenosis of the cervical canal, the most common cause being a cervical carcinoma. In less than one-half of the cases, the stenosis is inflammatory or is due to irradiation for a previous carcinoma. Very infrequently, marked retroversion of the uterus may angulate the canal sufficiently to cause obstruction. The causative organisms are usually the common pyogens, but frequently the infection is a mixed one, with relatively nonpathogenic saprophytes and anaerobes. Remarkably, the low-grade inflammatory reaction is usually confined to the endometrium and immediately adjacent myometrium and rarely represents a spreading infection or one that gives rise to periuterine or tubal secondary involvement.

ENDOMETRIOSIS

Endometriosis is the term used to describe the presence of endometrial glands or stroma, or both, in abnormal locations. It is divided into two types that have quite different clinical significance. *Internal* or *direct endometriosis*, also known as *adenomyosis*, refers to abnormal nests of endometrium within the myometrium of the uterine wall. *External* or *indirect endometriosis* is the much more important condition that is referred to when the unqualified term "endometriosis" is used clinically. It designates abnormal foci of endometrium in the tubes, ovaries or peritoneum, for example, or in any other site in the body outside the uterus. The two forms may occur separately or may coexist and, while they have a close kinship, are believed to arise through different pathogenetic mechanisms and certainly have differing importance to the patient.

ENDOMETRIOSIS INTERNA (ADENOMYOSIS)

Internal endometriosis, better referred to as adenomyosis, is currently believed to represent an abnormal growth activity of the endometrium. It is found at postmortem examination in 10 to 50 per cent of uteri, depending upon the criteria used for the diagnosis and the zeal with which it is sought. The glands and stroma penetrate between the muscle bundles of the myometrium to produce a diffuse, apparent invasion of the myometrium. In one plane of section, these nests may appear to be entirely sequestered and not in contact with overlying endometrium. However, serial section studies have demonstrated, in most cases, direct continuity between the mucosa of the uterine cavity and the apparent, buried nests of endometrial stroma or glands. A minority proposes that the appearance of endometrium within the myometrium arises from metaplasia of myometrial mesenchymal connective tissue stroma or from included rests of either wolffian or müllerian duct origin. The pathogenesis, as it is currently accepted, is well summarized by Novak, who likens the endometrial downgrowth to the proliferation of an inverted endometrial polyp.

Because the penetrations are derived from the nonfunctional stratum basalis of the endometrium, these abnormal foci rarely bleed at the time of the period.

Adenomyosis usually causes slight uterine enlargement although, in many cases, the uterus is normal in size. Usually the contour and the serosal surface of the uterus are unaffected although, as will be mentioned, in certain cases the endometrium penetrates the serosa. The uterine wall is often thickened to 2 to 2.5 cm., sometimes irregularly. The endomyometrial junction may be less sharply defined than usual. The myometrium itself appears en-

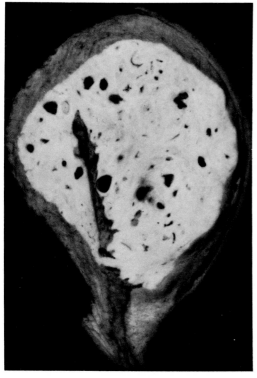

Fig. 27–18

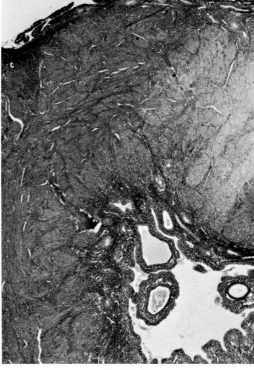

Fig. 27–19

Figure 27–18. *Internal endometriosis (adenomyosis). An unusual variant with function of the endometrial nests producing foci of hemorrhage within the uterine wall.*

Figure 27–19. *Internal endometriosis. A nest of typical endometrium within the uterine wall, well down below the endometrial surface* (at top).

tirely unremarkable in the majority of cases. In very florid instances, small nests of somewhat yellow-white soft tissue may be seen with the naked eye or by hand lens inspection. In less than 10 per cent of the cases, the included endometrium is functional, menstruates and, therefore, produces small nests or masses of red-brown blood pigmentation within the myometrium (Fig. 27–18).

The histologic diagnosis of adenomyosis rests upon the identification of buried endometrial stroma or glands, or both, between the muscle bundles of the myometrium. In most instances, the nests are composed of typical glands enclosed within a spindle cell stroma (Fig. 27–19). Occasionally, the nests are composed only of stroma, sometimes designated as **stromal endometriosis.** For a justifiable diagnosis of adenomyosis, the endometrial nests should be more than one high power field away from the overlying endometrial layer. In those few instances in which the glands function, blood accumulates within the ectopic foci to cause considerable hemosiderosis of the endometrial stroma and surrounding connective tissue stroma of the myometrium. If there are penetrations to the serosa and these bleed with each period, periuterine adhesions to surrounding viscera and structures, such as the tubes, small intestine and rectum, may develop.

Patients with internal endometriosis frequently have menorrhagia, colicky dysmenorrhea, dyspareunia and drawing pelvic pain, particularly during the premenstrual period. While the colicky menstrual pain and pelvic pain can be attributed to premenstrual edema and tension within the uterus, the exact basis for the excessive vaginal bleeding at the time of the menstrual period is still obscure. It has been superficially attributed to hyperestrinism but without valid evidence.

ENDOMETRIOSIS EXTERNA

This form of endometriosis is also referred to as pelvic endometriosis, since it is prone to occur in the following sites in descending order of frequency: (1) ovaries, (2) uterine ligaments, (3) rectovaginal septum, (4) pelvic peritoneum, (5) umbilicus, (6) laparotomy scars, and in other rare sites such as the vagina, vulva, nasal mucosa and appendix (Groseclose, 1954).

Incidence. This disorder is principally a disease of women in active reproductive life, most often in the third and fourth decades. There is a higher incidence of this condition in women in the higher economic groups, who tend to marry later in life, have fewer children and have a lower fertility rate than lower income groups. Pregnancy is a period of high progesterone levels. Moreover, the relative infertility of the endometriosis group suggests ovulatory difficulties and the failure of formation of corpora lutea. It has, therefore, been proposed that endometriosis results from prolonged relative hyperestrinism. However, there has been no direct experimental or clinical evidence of hyperestrinism, relative or absolute, in these women.

Pathogenesis. The derivation of the nests of aberrant endometrium has long been argued. Of the two principal schools of thought, one proposes that endometrium is regurgitated through the fallopian tubes at the time of the normal menstrual period and spills out through the fimbriated ends to become implanted in various sites. This concept is known as the *implantation theory.* Regurgitation can indeed be demonstrated during menstruation, particularly when the cervix is stenotic or narrowed. Moreover, the tendency for endometriosis to be localized within the pelvis further fits the implantation theory. However, obviously it does not suffice to explain the development of endometriosis in the umbilicus or in sites removed from the pelvis.

The metaplastic theory favors the abnormal differentiation of celomic epithelium. The endometrium of the uterus is derived from the lining of the müllerian duct, itself a derivative of the lining of the celomic cavity in the fetus. The lining of the müllerian duct is then identical in origin with the peritoneum and the serosal coverings of the ovaries, tubes and intra-abdominal viscera. Thus, the peritoneum and serosa are potentially capable of abnormal differentiation into endometrial glands and stroma. The two theories are not mutually incompatible, and external endometriosis may encompass both pathways described.

Morphology. External endometriosis may present in many varied patterns. The foci of endometrium, unlike adenomyosis, are almost invariably under the influence of the ovarian hormones and, therefore, undergo the cyclic menstrual changes with periodic bleeding. As a result, these foci appear as red-blue to yellow-brown nodules implanted on the serosal surfaces or apparently lying beneath the serosa in the sites mentioned. They vary from microscopic lesions to 1 to 2 cm. in diameter. Individual lesions may enlarge and coalesce. In the course of time, these nodules may evoke a marked fibroblastic proliferation as the result of the irritative effect of the blood to produce dense fibrous nodules. When the accumulation of blood is extensive, its organization causes interadherence of structures, obliteration of the pouch of Douglas, distortion and total fibrosis in and about the tubes and ovaries and sometimes virtually a frozen pelvis. The ovaries may become markedly distorted by large cystic spaces (3 to 5 cm. in diameter) filled with brown blood debris to form so-called **chocolate cysts** (Fig. 27–20). When these cysts achieve a diameter of 8 to 10 cm., they are sometimes dignified by the term **endometriomas.** As the blood undergoes organization, these areas are converted into dense fibrous scars that characteristically contain large amounts of hemosiderin pigment and lipid debris.

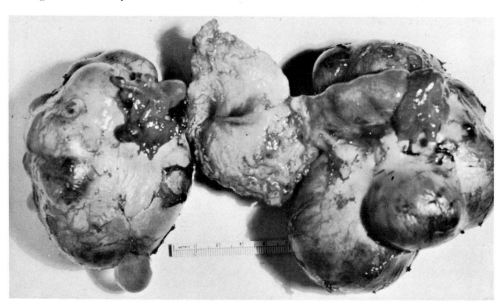

Figure 27–20. *External endometriosis. The ovaries are converted into enlarged irregular masses by large "chocolate cysts." (Courtesy of Dr. Arthur Hertig.)*

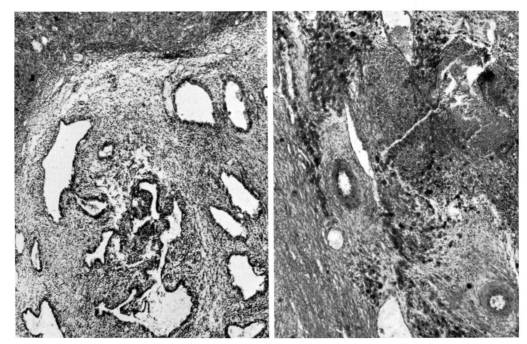

Fig. 27–21   Fig. 27–22

Figure 27–21. Classic diagnostic endometriosis of the ovary with readily recognized, well formed endometrium within the ovarian stroma.

Figure 27–22. An area of "burned out," fibrosed, pigmented scarring in a focus of old endometriosis within the ovary.

The histologic diagnosis of endometriosis is sometimes readily made but, at other times, it may be most obscure (Fig. 27—21). Paradoxically, **the diagnosis is most difficult in the advanced, florid, longstanding cases** because, as the disease progresses, the fibroproliferative response to the retained blood progressively obliterates recognizable features. In late cases, then, it may only be possible to identify hemosiderin pigment and nests of macrophages containing green-brown granular debris within areas of dense fibrosis (Fig. 27–22). A definite histologic diagnosis requires two of the three following features: glands, stroma or hemosiderin pigment.

Clinical Course. The clinical manifestations of endometriosis are entirely dependent upon the distribution of the endometrial lesions and on their functional activity. It may, therefore, be present as an asymptomatic lesion. When clinical signs and symptoms become manifest, they usually consist of severe dysmenorrhea and pelvic pain due to the intrapelvic bleeding and periuterine adhesions (Meigs, 1942). Dyspareunia may be present on the same basis. As the disease advances and affects neighboring structures, pain may result from tension on the suspensory ligaments of the uterus. Pain on defecation reflects rectal wall involvement, and dysuria reflects the involvement of the serosa of the bladder. Intesti-

nal disturbances may appear when the small intestine is affected. Menstrual irregularities are common for obscure reasons. As the tubes become embedded in fibrous tissue and the ovaries are deformed by the bleeding process, sterility is a late serious complication. These clinical manifestations, it will be appreciated, are almost identical with those that accompany chronic salpingitis and, accordingly, the diagnosis of pelvic endometriosis should always be entertained when the physical findings suggest inflammatory involvement of pelvic viscera or thickenings or masses in the cul-de-sac or tubo-ovarian regions.

MYOMETRIAL HYPERTROPHY

Myometrial hypertrophy, also known as *fibrosis uteri* and *subinvolution of the uterus,* is an obscure condition characterized by diffuse symmetrical enlargement of the uterus.

The enlargement is caused by moderate to marked, usually symmetrical thickening of the myometrium of the uterine corpus. In the fundic region, the myometrial wall may measure up to 3 to 4 cm., but usually it averages about 2 to 2.5 cm. (normal thickness, approximately 1.5 cm.). The endometrium and serosa of the uterus are usually normal, but occasionally there is some endometrial hyperplasia or polypoid hypertrophy. Histologically, the myometrial muscle bundles and individual cells appear entirely normal on routine microscopic section. There may be a slight increase in the interstitial connective tissue, hence the designation fibrosis uteri. This alteration is not sufficiently marked to account for the increased thickness of the myometrium. On this basis, the thickening has been attributed to hypertrophy of individual muscle cells, demonstrable only by careful micrometric studies (Williams and Kinney, 1944).

Since the uterus undergoes some cyclic alterations in size with the menstrual cycle and since it undergoes enormous alterations in size with pregnancy, it is argued that such enlargement represents merely subinvolution of the uterus following pregnancy. However, myometrial hypertrophy occurs in women who have never borne children and, at least in these instances, some other mechanism must be operative. The possibility has also been raised that so-called hypertrophy may merely represent an unusually large but normal variant of uterine size. Many of these patients develop abnormal uterine bleeding, particularly menorrhagia, as well as pain and excessive vaginal discharge. The status of this entity remains unsettled and, while the term myometrial hypertrophy may be used to designate this condition, it should be understood that further studies may indicate the need for a revision of our concepts of this entity.

ENDOMETRIAL HYPERPLASIA

During active reproductive life, the normal monthly cyclic shedding and regrowth of the endometrium is a finely balanced mechanism. It is controlled by the rise and ebb of pituitary and ovarian hormones not only in regulated, absolute amounts, but also in carefully integrated, relative levels. Normal endometrial function not only requires certain levels of estrogen and progesterone, but also is dependent upon the levels of one hormone relative to the other. Failure of production of progesterone results in a relative excess of even normal amounts of estrogen, and normal levels of progesterone may be overbalanced by excessive estrogenic formation. This finely adjusted proliferation of a new endometrial mucosa each month is subject to many aberrations that cause either abnormal hyperplasia or atrophy of the endometrium. These endometrial abnormalities account for 15 to 20 per cent of all gynecologic problems and, next to leiomyomas of the uterus, are the most common causes of abnormal uterine bleeding.

The many variable patterns are embraced by four entities—polyps and polypoid hyperplasia, cystic hyperplasia, adenomatous hyperplasia and atypical hyperplasia of the endometrium. Endometrial hyperplasia is important because of its relationship to endometrial carcinoma. Almost 30 years ago, Hertig and Sommers (1949) proposed, and many others have since confirmed, a progression of endometrial changes from polyp formation to cystic hyperplasia to adenomatous hyperplasia to atypical hyperplasia, leading eventually to endometrial carcinoma (Foster and Montgomery, 1965). *Every carcinoma does not necessarily evolve through such an orderly sequence. Implied, instead, is the concept that all of these lesions carry an increasing risk of cancerous transformation as one advances along the progression cited.* Thus, the most dangerous lesions are adenomatous and atypical hyperplasia.

ENDOMETRIAL POLYPS AND POLYPOID HYPERPLASIA

Endometrial polyps are small, sessile, projecting masses that tend to arise multiply. They may occur at any age, but are somewhat more common at or near the menopause. These lesions are best construed as focal areas of cystic hyperplasia, described below. Indeed, in some instances, the polyps are so numerous that they create an overall *polypoid hyperplasia* which is almost indistinguishable from cystic hyperplasia. The individual polyps ordinarily vary from 0.5 to 3 cm. in diameter and are usually hemispheric in contour. Sometimes they are poorly defined from the surrounding endometrial mucosa. Others are larger and pedunculated (Fig. 27–23). They are soft, pale gray and fleshy and have the same consistency as the surrounding mucosa. On histologic examination, they have an edematous stroma and cystically dilated glands that resemble those described in cystic hyperplasia (Fig. 27–24). Glandular atypicalities may appear in these polyps, including foci of adenocarcinoma (Peterson and Novak, 1956).

CYSTIC HYPERPLASIA (SWISS CHEESE ENDOMETRIUM)

Cystic hyperplasia designates an abnormal growth and thickness of the endometrium caused by an absolute or relative excess of estrogen. This condition is most often found just before or at the menopause, when ovulatory and progestational activity slows and relative hyperestrinism is present. It is also encountered in states with absolute increases in estrogen production, i.e., in persistence of follicle cysts in the ovary, such as may occur in the

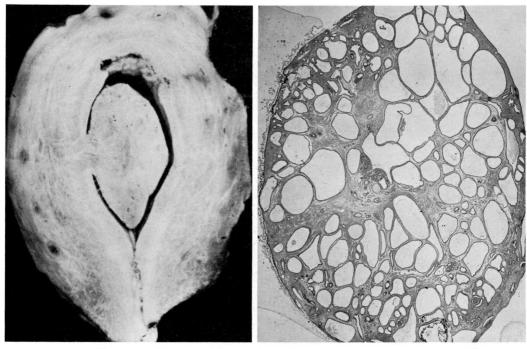

Fig. 27–23   Fig. 27–24

Figure 27–23. *A large pedunuclated polyp within the endometrial cavity, viewed on cross section.*
Figure 27–24. *Endometrial polyp at low power, illustrating the cystic dilatation of the glands. (Courtesy of Dr. Arthur Hertig.)*

Stein-Leventhal syndrome, in the hyperestrinism of functioning granulosa and theca cell tumors of the ovary, in excessive adrenocortical function and in the prolonged therapeutic administration of estrogenic substances.

The endometrium grossly is thick, velvety, lush and pale gray. Its surface is often slightly granular due to the cystic dilatation of the endometrial glands. Histologically, the dominant characteristic of this lesion is cystically dilated glands that are visible in the tissue section on naked eye inspection (Fig. 27–25). The cribriform lacunar appearance of the tissue section accounts for the colloquial designation, **Swiss cheese hyperplasia.** In addition to the cystically dilated glands, other small glands may be present and, in fact, are usually more abundant in amount than normal. The glands are lined by regular, well oriented, tall, columnar epithelial cells that are **nonsecretory.** Uncommonly, the cells may pile up to produce small, abortive, papillary excrescences with some loss of the alignment of the cells. It is particularly to be noted that secretory changes are rarely present in the epithelial cells. Very rarely, some secretory activity is found in undisputed cystic hyperplasias so that this criterion cannot be considered as an absolute. The intervening stroma often contains large, dilated, thin-

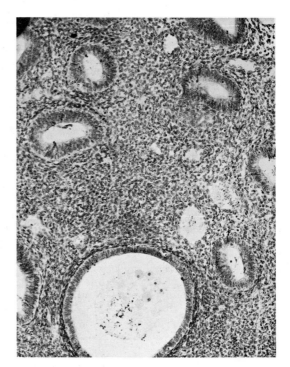

Figure 27–25. *Cystic hyperplasia of the endometrium with marked dilatation of only one gland. (Courtesy of Dr. Arthur Hertig.)*

walled vascular sinusoids, the source of the associated abnormal bleeding.

Cystic hyperplasia results usually in excessive uterine bleeding, most often at the time of the period (menorrhagia), but occasionally also causes irregular, spotty bleeding between periods (metrorrhagia). The condition is of further significance as an indicator of hyperestrinism. It should, therefore, be thoroughly investigated to discover the possible coexistence of a functioning ovarian tumor or other basis for the endocrinopathy. The relationship of this form of hyperplasia to carcinomatous change is a very moot point. In a certain number of patients who later develop endometrial carcinoma, cystic hyperplasia has been present in earlier curettage specimens. There is fairly general agreement that the hazard of malignancy is probably in the order of 1 to 2 per cent. Certainly, cystic hyperplasia has not been accorded the serious import of the adenomatous and atypical hyperplasia to be described.

ADENOMATOUS HYPERPLASIA AND ATYPICAL HYPERPLASIA

Adenomatous and atypical hyperplasia are varying shades of the same color. *Both are characterized by abnormal endometrial proliferation which results in both an increase in the number of glands and atypical patterns of gland growth.* There is no sharp line of demarcation between these hyperplasias, and differentiation is based on the orderliness of the epithelium lining the glands. Both conditions occur in women during active reproductive life and are frequently observed in patients who subsequently develop endometrial carcinoma.

The genesis of these conditions is uncertain. While they are ascribed to hyperestrinism, there is substantial evidence that these changes, as well as endometrial carcinoma, may begin, rather, in prolonged hyperpituitary stimulation of the ovaries which, in turn, affects the endometrium.

Adenomatous hyperplasia results in a markedly thickened, lush, gray, velvety endometrial mucosa that macroscopically resembles cystic hyperplasia. The mucosal surface may be somewhat more irregular and nodular and may even have small, abortive, polypoid projections. Histologically, too, many and atypically formed glands are present within an otherwise unremarkable endometrial stroma. Usually the change is diffuse, but sometimes it may be patchy (Fig. 27–26). The glands are unevenly distributed so that focal aggregates are found closely packed together with scant intervening endometrial stroma. Many times, the glands are backed up to each other and are in apparent contact. Papillary inbuddings into the glands are formed, as well as finger-like outpouchings into the adjacent endometrial stroma. The lining epithelial cells vary from cuboidal to columnar and are usually slightly hyperchromatic. Secretory activity may be evident, but is more often absent.

Atypical hyperplasia is indistinguishable grossly from adenomatous hyperplasia. Here, too, there are too many glands, too tightly packed. In contrast to adenomatous hyperplasia, the epithelial cells lining the glands are often no longer neatly palisaded, but piled up and atypical. There is a tendency toward variability in nuclear size and shape, and mitotic figures are usually readily evident, although atypical mitoses are not found. It is apparent that the cellular and glandular abnormalities approach those that might be interpreted as anaplastic changes (Fig. 27–27).

Both adenomatous and atypical hyperplasia produce abnormal bleeding in the form of either spotting between the periods or excessive menstrual flow. Distressing as these manifestations may be, their role in the genesis of endometrial cancer is far more important. It is apparent from their morphology that adenomatous hyperplasia and atypical hyperplasia (even more so) approach the glandular alterations characteristic of endometrial carcinoma. Indeed, an additional subgroup has been segregated by Hertig and his colleagues (1949), showing further cellular and glandular atypicality, to which the term endometrial anaplasia or endometrial carcinoma in situ has been applied. We see, then, a continuum of atypicality ranging from adenomatous hyperplasia through atypical hyperplasia to endometrial anaplasia. Because of this sequence of morphologic changes and the frequency of these changes in patients who later develop carcinoma, adenomatous and atypical hyperplasia are accorded serious significance. *Retrospective studies of patients with endometrial carcinoma who have had prior endometrial biopsies have disclosed these patterns of hyperplasia in 3 to 25 per cent* (Hertig and Sommers, 1949) (Foster and Montgomery, 1965). Among 774 patients with endometrial atypias, 92 women had repeated curettages with the following findings (Wentz, 1964). Three patients with a prior diagnosis of in situ carcinoma had progressed to invasive cancer. Among the remaining 89 patients, 12 with prior adenomatous or atypical hyperplasia had developed carcinoma. From studies such as this, we learn that carcinoma in situ is the infant which will almost always evolve into a full-grown cancer. We also learn that these forms of hyperplasia must be consid-

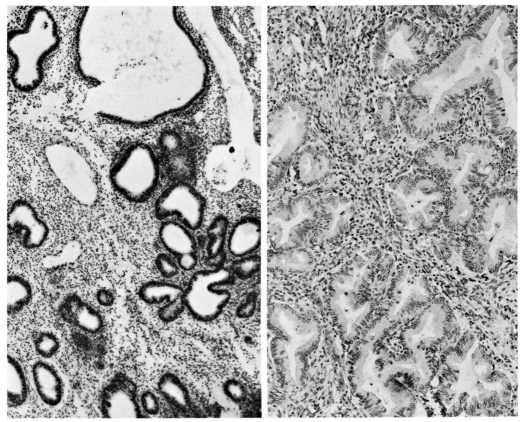

Fig. 27-26   Fig. 27-27

Figure 27-26. *Focal adenomatous hyperplasia of a nest of closely packed glands in the right side of the field.*
Figure 27-27. *Atypical hyperplasia merging into frank anaplastic carcinoma. (Both figures by courtesy of Dr. Arthur Hertig from Cancer, Vol. 2, 1949.)*

ered as fertile soils for cancer although predictions cannot be made in the individual patient.

MISCELLANEOUS ENDOMETRIAL CHANGES

This unsatisfactory designation is applied to: (1) senile cystic endometrial atrophy, (2) irregular menstrual shedding and (3) endometrial changes induced by oral contraceptives.

SENILE CYSTIC ENDOMETRIAL ATROPHY

In the postmenopausal woman, the endometrium normally atrophies and becomes a rudimentary, thin layer composed only of the stratum basalis glands. For obscure reasons, in some women the glands, instead of atrophying, become cystically dilated.

Grossly, the atrophic endometrium has a flat, thin, glazed gray-red appearance, and histologically consists of compact endometrial stroma containing simple tubular, nonproliferative, nonsecretory resting glands. Against this background are scattered, large, cystically dilated glands lined by flattened or totally atrophic epithelial cells. Such cystic change should not be confused with cystic "Swiss cheese" hyperplasia in which the cystic glands are lined by lush, active, tall columnar cells.

Senile cystic atrophy is virtually a physiologic phenomenon in the postmenopausal woman. For obscure reasons, it sometimes gives rise to postmenopausal vaginal bleeding. Occasionally, similar endometrial atrophy is seen in the premenopausal woman when it usually implies a pituitary or ovarian deficiency.

IRREGULAR MENSTRUAL SHEDDING

For completely obscure reasons, the endometrium may respond irregularly to normal ovarian hormonal influences. Thus, focal areas of proliferative endometrium are interspersed with areas of secretory change. This phenomenon is somewhat vaguely ascribed to irregular unresponsiveness of endometrial loci to progesterone. As a result, there is continual and irregular focal menstrual shedding and, consequently, vaginal bleeding intermittently throughout the cycle. The curettage specimen discloses fragments of endometrium in the proliferative phase and other fragments in all stages of the postovulatory, secretory phase. This form of *"chronic menstrual shedding"* is an obvious cause for considerable distress and excessive blood loss to the patient but otherwise is not threatening. Following curettage, when the patient's ovarian hormones are supported by administration of estrogen and progesterone timed to the normal rise and fall of these steroids, the patient's normal cyclic endometrial growth and shedding are frequently resumed.

ORAL CONTRACEPTIVES AND THE ENDOMETRIUM

As might be suspected, the use of oral contraceptives containing synthetic or derivative ovarian steroids induces a wide variety of endometrial changes. The precise pattern of morphologic change varies with the specific compound (its content, both absolute and relative, of estrogenic and progestational agents), the dosage and the schedule of administration. A common reaction pattern can be best characterized as a discordance between glandular and stromal activity. Implied here is the presence of inactive, virtually atrophic glands lined by extremely low, nonproliferative, nonsecretory cells surrounded by a very lush stroma showing large cells with abundant cytoplasm and considerable mitotic activity. This morphologic pattern is reminiscent of the decidua of pregnancy. Indeed, when encountered in a curettage, it is easy to confuse such endometrial changes with those of early pregnancy. The inactive glands, however, are inconsistent with such a diagnosis. In other instances, with other contraceptives, employed on a different schedule, the glandular epithelial cells are sometimes vacuolated and embedded within a less reactive stroma, once again readily confused with pregnancy changes. When such therapy is discontinued, the endometrium eventually reverts to its normal pattern. As far as is now known, the changes have no untoward implications and there is no evidence that they predispose to cancer. However, the cautious clinician points out that oral contraceptives have not been in use long enough to pass final judgement.

The cervical epithelium also undergoes modifications with the use of oral contraceptives. Striking glandular proliferation is frequently seen in the region of the squamocolumnar junction (Candy and Abell, 1968) (Gall et al., 1969). The glandular proliferation may be so exuberant as to produce small polypoid projections along the endocervical canal or, in other circumstances, to raise the suspicion of a neoplasm. When the oral contraceptive therapy is stopped, the changes apparently revert to normal but, during the height of the reaction, they can be quite confusing to the unwary pathologist.

TUMORS

The uterine corpus and endometrium are frequently affected by a great variety of neoplastic growths. Virtually every form of benign and malignant mesenchymally derived tumor, such as fibromas, lipomas, hemangiomas and their malignant counterparts, has been described in the uterus. The most common lesions, however, are leiomyomas, endometrial adenocarcinomas and adenoacanthomas.

LEIOMYOMA (FIBROMYOMA)

Leiomyomas are benign tumors of smooth muscle origin. They are the most common tumors in women. They are also referred to as myomas and, in colloquial clinical usage, as "fibroids."

Incidence. These tumors are responsible for at least one-third of all gynecologic admissions to hospitals and are found in the general population in about one in four women in active reproductive life. While they are most common in the third and fourth decades, they are not infrequent in girls in the second decade of life and, of course, may persist and be discovered in advanced age.

Pathogenesis. There is much controversy over the role of hyperestrinism in the production of these tumors. It is known that they shrink and become fibrosed and even calcified postmenopausally. They rarely arise following the menopause. Castration makes them atrophy premenopausally. Perhaps most importantly, during pregnancy there is a rapid increase in their size, accompanied by striking cellular proliferation. On all these bases, these tumors are thought to be caused by excessive estrogenic stimulation. However, experimental proof in animals is still lacking, and there is no evidence that estrogen initiates their formation or does more than maintain their size. It is perhaps more accurate, then, to consider leiomyomas as endocrine-dependent lesions whose growth or size is dependent upon estrogens.

Morphology. Leiomyomas, wherever they occur, are sharply circumscribed, unencapsulated but discrete, usually round, firm, gray-white masses that have a characteristic whorled cut surface. Except in rare instances, they are found within the myometrium of the corpus. Only infrequently do they involve the uterine ligaments, lower uterine segment or cervix. Descriptive terms have been applied to their various situations within the myometrial wall. Those embedded within the myometrium are referred to as **intramural.** When they occur beneath the covering serosa of the uterine corpus, they are called **subserosal.** Some occur in immediate proximity to the endometrium and are designated as **submucous.** Frequently, the submucosal and subserosal masses protrude either from the outer contour of the uterus or into the endometrial cavity (Fig. 27—28). These may become **pedunculated.** The pedunculated subendometrial lesions may appear as bulbous polyps totally covered by endometrium, but having a firm, round head (Fig. 27—29).

It is worthy of note that despite their projection into the uterine cavity, **these masses rarely, if ever, cause ulceration or sloughing of the overlying endometrial mucosa.** Uncommonly, the pedunculated subserosal lesion may develop an extremely long, tenuous stalk and is sometimes designated as a **wandering or migratory leiomyoma.** Occasionally, such bizarre tumors become adherent to sur-

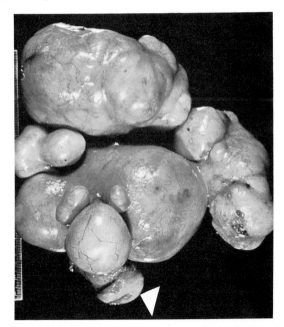

Figure 27—28. Multiple subserosal leiomyomas of the uterus. The uterine body is "lost" in the irregular mass, but the cervix is visible as the most dependent portion of the specimen (arrow).

rounding structures or omentum, develop an auxiliary blood supply, and lose their original attachment to the uterus and are then termed **parasitic** leiomyomas. In other cases, the subserosal mass may protrude into the broad ligament to create the **intraligamentous** leiomyoma.

Only infrequently do these tumors occur singly.

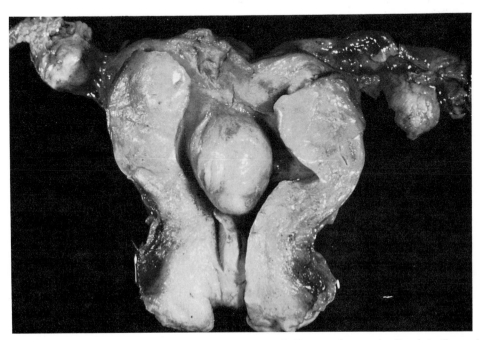

Figure 27—29. A submucosal leiomyoma appearing as a bulbous polyp, protruding into the endometrial cavity.

They vary in size from barely visible, pale gray seedlings to massive tumors that may simulate a pregnant uterus. While not encapsulated, they are sufficiently discrete so that they can be readily shelled out. Whatever their size, the characteristic whorled pattern of smooth muscle bundles on cut section, likened to watered silk, usually makes these lesions readily identifiable on gross inspection. Several modifications in this fairly uniform pattern may be encountered. Large tumors may develop areas of yellow-brown to red softening, referred to as **necrobiosis** or **red carnaceous degeneration** (Fig. 27–30). Occasionally, the necrotic areas undergo proteolytic liquefaction to produce cystic degeneration. In advanced ages, particularly postmenopausally, as the masses atrophy they tend to become distinctly more collagenous and firm and sometimes partially or completely **calcified.**

Histologically, the leiomyoma is composed of whorling bundles of smooth muscle cells that more or less exactly resemble the architecture of the uninvolved myometrium (Fig. 27–31). The similarity of the cytology may be such that it is difficult to recognize the existence of a neoplasm unless low power examination discloses the contour of the margin of the tumor and the surrounding compressed myometrium. Usually the individual muscle cells are completely uniform in size and shape, and have the characteristic oval nucleus and long, slender, bipolar cytoplasmic processes. Mitotic figures are scarce and giant cells and anaplasia are not present. Tumors that occur in advanced age groups, as well as occasionally in younger individuals, may have an increase of the connective tissue with dense hyalinization of this stroma. When degenerative or cystic changes occur, the foci appear as areas of ischemic necrosis with hemorrhages and more or less complete proteolytic digestion of dead cells. In older individuals, the smooth muscle cells progressively atrophy so that the tumor is converted into a collagenous mass composed principally of fibrous tis-

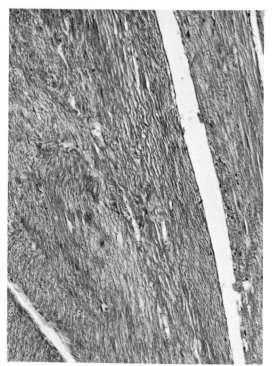

Figure 27–31. *Leiomyoma. Low power view showing similarity of structure between myometrium to the right of the cleft-like space and leiomyoma to the left.*

sue. Basophilic precipitates of calcium are found in many of these atrophic lesions.

Clinical Course. Leiomyomas of the uterus may be entirely asymptomatic and are frequently only discovered in routine physical examinations. However, they may cause a variety of symptoms, the most important of which is profuse bleeding at the time of the menstrual period. Abnormal, irregular vaginal bleeding may also occur. The exact mechanism by which these tumors produce abnormal bleeding is still unknown. It may indeed be related to an accompanying hyperestrinism, although the endometrium infrequently has hyperplastic changes consistent with such hyperestrinism. Some investigators state that, by pressure on the endometrium, these tumors cause bleeding. However, histologic examination of such lesions fails to disclose ulceration of the overlying mucosa, even in those that are submucosal. While, then, there is a relationship between abnormal bleeding and these tumors, the exact basis for it remains unknown.

Leiomyomas frequently undergo rapid increase in size during pregnancy and, at this time, these tumors may have considerable hypertrophy of individual cells with some variabi-

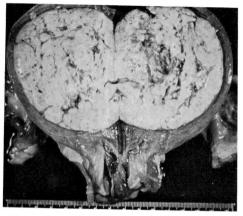

Figure 27–30. *A leiomyoma on cut section, illustrating the whorling bands of tissue and several areas of "red" degeneration.*

lity in nuclear and cell size, as well as frequent mitotic figures. Such changes are sometimes alarming as histologic observations, since they can be confused with malignant transformation. Malignant transformation is said to occur; it will be discussed in the consideration of leiomyosarcomas (p. 1237).

CARCINOMA OF THE ENDOMETRIUM

Carcinoma of the endometrium is ever increasingly becoming a common disease. At one time, it was far more infrequent than cancer of the cervix, in a ratio of 1 to 4. Earlier detection and eradication of in situ cervical cancer has lowered its prevalence as a form of life-threatening cancer. In addition, the longer life expectancy has led to a real increase in the number of endometrial carcinomas so that the ratio of clinically overt endometrial to cervical cancer is now 1 to 2. Carcinoma of the endometrium is fast becoming the third most frequent form of fatal cancer in the female, ranking below cancers of the breast and colon.

Incidence. These neoplasms tend to occur in a slightly older age group than cervical carcinoma. They have, on rare occasion, been reported in the second decade of life, but the incidence steadily rises with each passing decade to reach a high plateau in the sixth decade. The disease is more frequent among spinsters and childless married women. To quote or paraphrase a remark attributed to Meigs (1942): "By marrying a woman may look forward to carcinoma of the cervix. If she prefers to stay single she may look forward to carcinoma of the endometrium." Other significant correlations have been made. Carcinoma of the endometrium appears to be more frequent in patients with obesity, diabetes mellitus, hypertension, thyroid disease and breast carcinoma. As will become apparent, endocrine imbalances may predispose simultaneously to both breast and endometrial carcinoma.

Pathogenesis. Currently, it is believed that carcinoma of the endometrium results from prolonged, unbalanced (by progesterone) estrogen stimulation (Speert, 1948). Evidence in support of this belief is as follows. Endometrial cancer is exceedingly rare in women with ovarian agenesis or in those castrated early in life. Cortical stromal hyperplasia of the ovaries is found in a significant percentage of patients with endometrial cancer. These ovarian changes are associated with increased steroid secretion but, in all probability, they have their origin in primary pituitary hyperfunction. Patients with estrogen-secreting granulosa-theca cell tumors of the ovaries (p. 1251) have a much higher incidence of this form of cancer than age-matched controls. Scattered reports have attributed the induction of this form of carcinoma to prolonged therapy with estrogens (Bromberg et al., 1959), but most experts attribute the concurrence to coincidence.

It will be recalled that this form of neoplasia is sometimes preceded by endometrial hyperplasia, also related to hyperestrinism (Gore and Hertig, 1962) (p. 1230). The more aytpical the hyperplasia, the greater the likelihood of subsequent cancer (Campbell and Barter, 1961). The incidence of cancer in postmenopausal women rises from about 2 to 3 per cent with cystic hyperplasia to as high as 10 to 25 per cent with adenomatous and atypical hyperplasia. Supporting this general proposition is the work of Wagner and his colleagues (1967) who observed progressive increments of DNA in the glandular epithelial cells of the various forms of hyperplasia which correlated with the advance from the less risky cystic forms to the more atypical patterns. Thus, they sometimes observed tetraploidy in adenomatous hyperplasia and completely aberrant quantities of DNA consistent with aneuploidy in the cells of a few cases of atypical hyperplasia (possibly representing carcinoma in situ).

There is a strong suggestion that endometrial carcinoma has a life history resembling that of cervical carcinoma (Gusberg et al., 1954). The retrospective studies on the development of carcinoma following endometrial hyperplasia indicate a progressive series of glandular atypicalities that precede, for many years, the development of carcinoma in situ and eventually invasive cancer. The time interval between the atypical hyperplasia or carcinoma in situ may vary from a few years to well over a decade (Chamlian and Taylor, 1970).

Morphology. Carcinoma of the endometrium tends to assume one reasonably constant macroscopic growth pattern, but nonetheless consists of two distinctive histologic types. About 85 per cent are adenocarcinomas and virtually all the remainder are adenoacanthomas (tumors that produce both glandular and squamous cell patterns). These tumors arise first as in situ lesions that later become isolated foci of endometrial thickening in any part of the uterine cavity or lower uterine segment. Some tumors develop into firm, nodular, polypoid masses; others grow down into the wall in an infiltrative fashion. Both forms, in time, fungate into the endometrial cavity at the same time that they invade (Fig. 27–32). The uterine cavity thus becomes filled with a nodular, firm to soft, partially necrotic neoplasm. With this accumulation of tissue, the uterus becomes enlarged, often asymmetrically, rarely more than twofold.

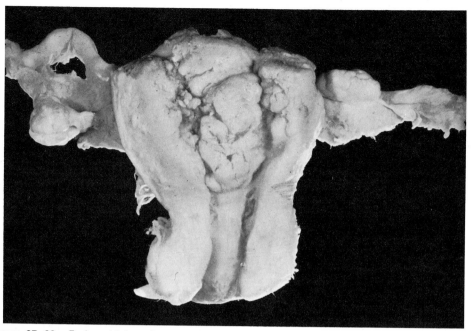

Figure 27–32. Endometrial carcinoma, presenting as a fungating mass in the fundus of the uterus.

As these tumors infiltrate and slough, deep irregular ulcerations or cavities are produced. In the course of time, the tumor extends through the myometrial wall to produce subserosal and serosal nodules, and eventually the tumor spreads to periuterine structures by direct continuity. The broad ligaments and lateral pelvic vaults may thus become filled with neoplasm to create clinically palpable masses. Eventual dissemination to the regional iliac, aortic, inguinal and hypogastric lymph nodes occurs and, in the late stages, the tumor may be hematogenously borne to the lungs, liver, bones and other organs. In a few cases (approximately 5 per cent), the tumor spreads to the tubes or to the ovaries.

Occasionally, this cancer grows as a huge polyp attached by a slender or broad base. Such cancerous polyps always have a markedly increased firmness that differentiates them from benign endometrial polyps and are usually much larger in size than the benign forms.

Histologically, the adenocarcinoma is characterized by more or less well defined gland patterns lined by obviously anaplastic cuboidal to columnar epithelial cells (Fig. 27–33). Not infrequently, papillary formations are produced. Rarely, these cells have mucinous secretory activity giving rise to the unusual "secretory carcinoma." Endometrial carcinoma may grow as an adenoacanthoma, composed of both glands and foci of squamous cells (Fig. 27–34). More accurately, these two cytologic patterns are encountered within individual glands so that, along one arc of the circumference, the epithelial lining is columnar in type and, by gradual metaplasia, the cells are transformed to squamous cells. It is generally believed that such squamous transformation represents a metaplasia of the neoplastic columnar lining epithelial cells.

As for all neoplasms, several systems for classifying endometrial carcinomas have been proposed. On the basis of the cytologic differentiation of the cancer, they are divided into Grades I to III. In most large analyses of these cancers, approximately 60 per cent conform to Grade I; 25 per cent, to Grade II; and 15 per cent, to Grade III. The extent of the cancer permits the establishing of clinical stages. The American Joint Committee for Cancer Staging and End Result Reporting has adopted the designations of Stage 0 to IV-B. These can be correlated with the TNM classification as follows:

Stage 0: (T0, N0, M0)—Preinvasive carcinoma; carcinoma in situ.

Stage I: (T1, N0, M0)—Carcinoma strictly confined to the corpus uteri.

Stage II: (T2, N0, M0)—Carcinoma involves corpus uteri and the cervix.

Stage III: (T3, N0, M0)—Carcinoma has extended outside the uterus but not outside the true pelvis.

Stage IV-A: (T4, N0, M0)—Carcinoma has extended beyond the true pelvis to perhaps involve the bladder and rectum.

Stage IV-B: (T1–4, N+, M+)—Any of the above stages associated with nodal spread and metastasis outside the pelvis.

Clinical Course.   Carcinoma of the endo-

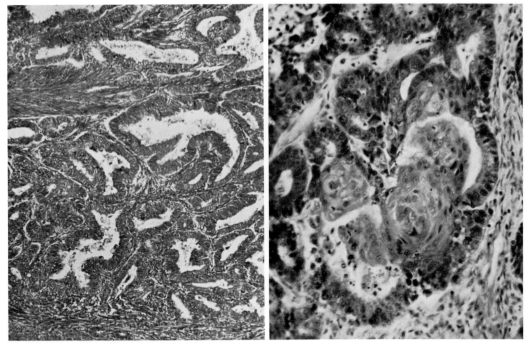

Fig. 27–33   **Fig. 27–34**

Figure 27–33. *Endometrial carcinoma in the classic "adeno" pattern.*
Figure 27–34. *Endometrial adenoacanthoma showing the transition between glandular and squamous growth.*

metrium may be asymptomatic for a long time. It produces symptoms only when the tumor erodes the endometrial surface or penetrates beyond the uterine body. The most common manifestation is irregular vaginal bleeding accompanied by excessive leukorrhea. While this tumor may extend down through the endocervical canal and appear at the external os, most often these patients have a completely negative-appearing cervix. Uterine enlargement may, in the early stages, be deceptively absent. Cytologic examination of vaginal smears by competent observers is highly accurate, but ultimately the diagnosis must be established by curettage and histologic examination of the tissue.

As would be anticipated, the prognosis is heavily dependent on the clinical stage of the disease when discovered and somewhat less dependent on the histologic grade. Stage 0 endometrial carcinoma is entirely curable by hysterectomy. Surgery alone, or in combination with irradiation, yields a 70 to 75 per cent five-year survival in Stage I disease. This rate drops to 50 per cent in Stage II and to less than 10 per cent with any of the other more advanced stages of the disease (Thiede and Lund, 1962).

SARCOMA

Virtually all forms of mesenchymal malignancies may arise in the uterine wall, including fibrosarcomas, but only three occur with significant frequency to merit further mention. Collectively, all comprise 3 per cent or less of uterine tumors (Ober, 1959). Leiomyosarcoma is the most common and represents about 75 per cent of all uterine sarcomas. The second most common variant is endometrial stromal sarcoma. The third, the sarcoma botryoides, has already been described (p. 1213).

Leiomyosarcoma. These infrequent malignancies almost always arise directly from the myometrium. Their origin from a preexisting leiomyoma is a highly controversial issue although, in one recent series, slightly less than half of the leiomyosarcomas of the uterus arose in previous benign leiomyomas (Spiro and Koss, 1965). Another recent study presents the view that they virtually never arise in a benign leiomyoma. It was pointed out in this study that proof of the previous existence of a benign lesion is almost impossible to achieve and that most reports of malignant transformation of a leiomyoma are lacking in undisputed proof (Taylor and Norris, 1966). While there is no answer to this controversy, the consensus would hold that these cancers are extremely rare complications of the very common benign leiomyoma.

Leiomyosarcomas grow within the uterus in two somewhat distinctive patterns: bulky, fleshy masses that invade the uterine wall, or polypoid masses that project into the uterine lumen. Histologically, they show a wide range of anaplasia, from those that are extremely well differentiated and have sometimes been referred to as benign metastasizing leiomyomas to very anaplastic lesions that have all the cytologic abnormalities of wildly growing sarcomas (Wheelock and Warren, 1942). Many of the borderline, well differentiated sarcomas are difficult to delineate from cellular leiomyomas and, in the report by Taylor and Norris (1966), much importance is attributed to the frequency of mitotic figures. They offer as a guideline that, when a tumor has more than ten mitoses in ten high power fields, it represents a sarcoma. It follows from this that the benign leiomyoma may have mitoses, but fewer than the number just cited.

Leiomyosarcomas have a striking tendency to recur after removal, and over half the cases eventually metastasize to distant organs such as the lungs, bone and brain. Dissemination throughout the abdominal cavity is also encountered. The five-year survival averages about 20 to 40 per cent. The better differentiated lesions have a better prognosis than the anaplastic lesions, which have a very low five-year survival in the range of 10 to 15 per cent.

Endometrial Stromal Sarcoma. Strands and nests of more or less well differentiated endometrial stroma are sometimes encountered in the myometrium. The cytologic differentiation of the stromal cells ranges from patterns virtually indistinguishable from the normal endometrial stroma to obviously sarcomatous anaplasia. Although there is uncertainty as to the interpretation of the benign-appearing patterns, these involvements have been divided into three large categories: (1) stromal endo-

metriosis (discussed on p. 1224), (2) endolymphatic stromal myosis and (3) endometrial stromal sarcoma. It should be emphasized that these lesions represent a spectrum, and many bridging patterns defy clear-cut categorization.

Endolymphatic stromal myosis refers to the appearance of masses of well differentiated endometrial stroma lying between muscle bundles of the myometrium, which can only be differentiated from stromal endometriosis by the tendency of the stromal nests to penetrate lymphatic channels (hence the term endolymphatic stromal myosis). Occasionally, blood vessels are also invaded. Despite such permeation, spread to regional nodes is exceedingly rare, but has been reported as has distant metastasis. The cases found in the literature citing aggressive behavior for this lesion probably represent true endometrial stromal sarcoma. It would seem preferable to restrict the term endolymphatic stromal myosis to the well differentiated lesion which is a low-grade stromal sarcoma incapable of spread beyond the uterus.

Endometrial stromal sarcoma is the overtly cancerous counterpart of endolymphatic stromal myosis. Here the neoplasm arising in the stromal cells forms large fleshy tumor masses which project into the endometrial cavity and penetrate the underlying myometrium. Commonly, these cancers arise high in the fundus. The cells display a wide range of anaplasia from fairly well differentiated stromal cells, which nonetheless present variability in size and shape and frequent mitoses, to highly undifferentiated lesions with wild pleomorphic tumor giant cells. As with all sarcomas, these cancers invade blood vessels and are capable of widespread metastasis.

FALLOPIAN TUBES

Inflammations	matory disease)	Physiologic
Suppurative (pelvic inflam-	Tuberculous	**Tumors**

The most common disorders in these structures are inflammations. Next in frequency is ectopic (tubal) pregnancy, to be discussed presently.

INFLAMMATIONS

Suppurative Salpingitis (Pelvic Inflammatory Disease). Salpingitis may be caused by

any of the pyogenic organisms, i.e., streptococci, staphylococci, coliforms and gonococci. In years past, the gonococcus accounted for at least half the cases of suppurative salpingitis. However, undoubtedly this distribution has changed in recent years with the fall in the incidence of untreated gonorrhea. In almost all instances, these tubal infections are a part of the pelvic inflammatory disease (PID) previously described (p. 1206) (Fig. 27–35).

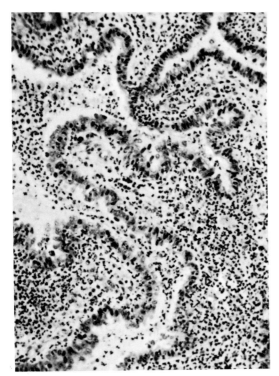

Figure 27–35. *Acute salpingitis with a diffuse neutrophilic exudate within both the mucosal folds and the lumen.*

TUMORS

Only rarely do tumors arise within the tubes. The most common forms of tumor, which hardly merit such a designation, are minute, 0.1 to 2 cm., translucent cysts filled with clear serous fluid, found near the fimbriated end of the tube or in the broad ligaments, referred to as *parovarian cysts or hydatids of Morgagni.* These cysts are presumed to arise in remnants of wolffian duct and are of little more than academic significance. Carcinoma of the fallopian tubes is exceedingly rare, to the point of being a medical curiosity. These tumors arise from the mucosal lining of the tube, usually near the distal ends, grow as adenocarcinomas, spread by continuity to adjacent structures and, in the isolated case reports of the literature, metastasize in the late stages to distant organs, such as the lungs and bones. The condition is so uncommon that the diagnosis can only be made at exploration when an intrapelvic mass of obscure nature is found clinically. Equally rarely, adenomatoid tumors occur subserosally on the tubes or sometimes in the mesosalpinx. These small nodules are the exact counterparts of those already described in relation to the testes or epididymides (p. 1188).

Tuberculous Salpingitis. The only other type of salpingitis encountered with sufficient frequency to merit mention is tuberculous salpingitis. It is almost invariably a secondary complication of a focus of tuberculosis elsewhere in the body. Presumably, the tubes are seeded hematogenously and then the process spreads to other organs in the genital tract, such as the endometrium, and to the peritoneal cavity (Fig. 27–36). Tuberculous salpingitis is, however, extremely uncommon at present and accounts for probably not more than 1 to 2 per cent of all forms of salpingitis.

Physiologic Salpingitis. It should be pointed out that acute inflammatory changes may be encountered in the tubes at the time of the menstrual cycle. These changes are generally of little significance but, at times, may cause pelvic pain. In a study of a series of pelvic viscera removed at the time of the menstrual period, minimal inflammatory changes and edema were observed in the tubes in about 60 per cent. This type of physiologic salpingitis is mentioned to indicate the caution that must be observed in making the diagnosis of a clinically significant form of salpingitis, especially when the specimens are removed at the time of the menstrual period.

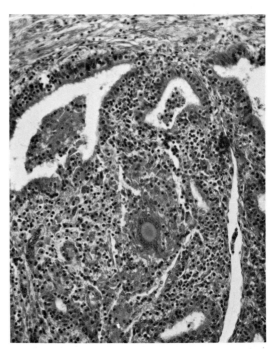

Figure 27–36. *Tuberculous salpingitis with a typical tubercle in the mid-field. Note the fusion of mucosal folds that has produced buried epithelial crypts (gland-like spaces).*

OVARIES

Tumors are the most common type of lesion encountered in the ovary. With the exception of these neoplasms, the ovary appears remarkably resistant to disease. Intrinsic inflammations of the ovary are extremely uncommon, and usually periovarian inflammations are secondary to involvement of the adjacent tube. Endometriosis does affect the ovary, but usually in conjunction with the pelvic endometriosis described. Save for the important subject of tumors, only two entities merit separate treatment.

MISCELLANEOUS LESIONS

Walthard Rests. Walthard rests are small inclusions of glands found either in contact with the serosal covering of the ovary or immediately beneath it. These glandular inclusions are microscopic in size and are lined by regular cuboidal to transitional epithelium. They are presumed to arise from pinched off nests of the surface epithelium that embryologically represent the germinal epithelium of the ovary. These rests are important for two reasons: they must not be confused with endometriosis or with metastases of glandular carcinomas, and they provide considerable support to the concept that the covering celomic or germinal epithelium may, indeed, be the site of origin of primary epithelial tumors of the ovary. In fact, it is possible that such tumors may arise within Walthard rests.

Cortical Stromal Hyperplasia. Careful study of the ovaries in patients with endometrial hyperplasia and endometrial carcinoma has revealed that, in a significant percentage of instances, there is marked thickening and cellularity of the ovarian stroma. These cortical stromal cells are somewhat plumper than the usual cells of the ovarian stroma, and histochemical studies indicate that such cells contain a scant amount of lipid material that may rep-

resent functionally active steroids. Occasionally, these cells form small subserosal, almost granulomatous, nodules. Because of these unusual changes in the ovarian cortex and the higher than chance relationship between this lesion and endometrial hyperplasia and carcinoma, there is reason to suspect that cortical stromal hyperplasia may represent an increase of steroid secreting stroma that plays a causal role in the development of the endometrial lesions.

PRIMARY TUMORS AND CYSTS

Tumors of the ovary are a common form of neoplasia in women. Among cancers of the female genital tract, the incidence of ovarian cancer ranks below only carcinoma of the cervix and endometrium (Allan and Hertig, 1949) (Dockerty, 1945). However, because many of these ovarian neoplasms are highly aggressive and lethal, they account for a disproportionate number of fatal cancers among the female genital tract malignancies (Anderson, 1962).

The ovary is covered by celomic epithelium that embryologically has the potential of differentiating into ciliated, serous, columnar cells, such as are found in the tube, and nonciliated, mucous, columnar cells, such as occur in the endometrium. The stroma of the ovary is made up of connective tissue that is capable of differentiation into granulosal, thecal and luteal cells and further harbors ova that are totipotential. It can be anticipated, therefore, that ovarian tumors run a wide gamut of anatomic types. The classification of these lesions presents a problem on which there is no unanimity of opinion. The classifications differ, depending upon whether the criteria employed are based upon the macroscopic appearance of the tumors, their microscopic architecture, their clinical behavior or their histogenesis.

An excellent and detailed classification of

TABLE 27-2. OVARIAN NEOPLASMS

I. Tumors of Surface Epithelial and Ovarian Stromal
   Origin
   Serous
   Mucinous
   Endometrioid   Benign
   Cystadenofibroma   Borderline
   Clear cell (mesonephric)   Malignant
   Brenner

II. Germ Cell Tumors
    Dysgerminoma
    Cystic (dermoid) teratoma
    Solid teratoma (well differentiated and embryonal)
    Choriocarcinoma

III. Sex Cord—Mesenchymal Tumors
     Granulosa cell-theca-luteal tumors
     Arrhenoblastoma (Sertoli-Leydig cell tumors)

IV. Tumors Derived from Connective Tissue
    Fibroma and fibrosarcoma

V. Secondary Tumors
   Krukenberg

Adapted from Scully, R. E.: Recent progress in ovarian cancer. Hum. Path., *1*:73, 1970.

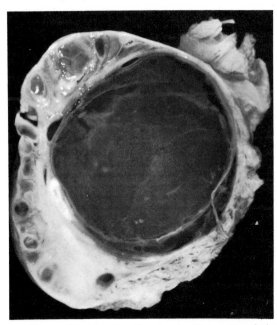

Figure 27-37. *Functional retention cysts of the ovary, one large one and multiple subcortical smaller cavities.*

these neoplasms, including more than 30 forms, has been provided by Scully (1970). Only the more frequent and clinically significant lesions are presented in the preceding modified classification (Table 27–2). Before discussing these neoplasms, it may be well to call attention to some common non-neoplastic causes of ovarian enlargement readily mistaken clinically for true neoplasms.

NON-NEOPLASTIC FUNCTIONAL CYSTS OF THE FOLLICLE AND CORPUS LUTEUM

Follicle cysts in the ovary are so commonplace as to be virtually physiologic variants. They originate in unruptured graafian follicles or in follicles that have ruptured and immediately sealed. These cysts may be single, but are usually multiple. They rarely exceed 1 to 1.5 cm. in diameter, are filled with a clear serous fluid and are lined by a gray, glistening membrane. They are usually found within the cortex of the ovary immediately subjacent to the serosal covering. Histologically, granulosal lining cells can be identified when the intraluminal pressure has not been too great. But as the cysts increase in size, the lining cells atrophy under the pressure of contained fluid (Fig. 27–37). When the lining becomes totally atrophic, further secretion ceases and the cyst no longer enlarges. On this basis, these cysts

always remain small and are of little clinical significance. Rarely, the increased production of estrogen stimulates endometrial hyperplasia.

Luteal cysts may be formed in much the same way, usually by the immediate sealing of a corpus hemorrhagicum. The liquid contents of the follicle are retained, and the corpus luteum cannot fill with hemorrhage and hence cannot become fibrosed. Clear serous fluid may accumulate to produce small cystic spaces up to 2 to 3 cm. in diameter. These cysts are characteristically lined by a rim of bright yellow luteal tissue. Luteal cysts are much less common than follicle cysts, but are of the same innocuous significance as the latter. When numerous, the aggregate production of hormone may induce endometrial hyperplasia.

The *Stein-Leventhal syndrome* is another disorder characterized by the accumulation of many follicle cysts within the ovary. It occurs in girls in their late teens or early twenties and is characterized by obesity, hirsutism, menstrual irregularity, often amenorrhea, and reduced fertility or even sterility. The ovaries are usually but not invariably enlarged, contain multiple follicle cysts and sometimes have a thickened outer tunica recognized by the terms *large white ovary* and *cortical stromal fibrosis*. It is tempting to attribute the accumulation of the follicle cysts to collagenous fibrosis of the outer tunica but, since this latter alteration is sometimes absent, it is probably not fundamental to the syndrome. In about one-third of the cases, some evidence of ovulation is present in the form of corpora lutea (Chamberlain and Wood, 1964) (Goldzieher and Green, 1962). However, in the classic case, the patients do not ovulate and are sterile.

To explain the masculinization in these patients and other endocrinologic abnormalities, an enzymic block in the production of estrogen has been postulated, yielding increased levels of androgens. More specifically, a deficiency of a dehydrogenase necessary for the hydroxylation of estrogen precursors has been reported, but the evidence is still contradictory and confusing (Richardson, 1966). A recent report describes the identification of a chromosomal defect in some of these patients, suggesting that the abnormality in steroid synthesis is hereditary in origin (Netter, 1961).

TUMORS OF SURFACE EPITHELIAL AND OVARIAN STROMAL ORIGIN

The great preponderance of primary neoplasms in the ovary fall within this category. These tumors may be composed largely of epithelial cells with a scant connective tissue framework or, alternatively, may be predominantly made up of stroma with a scant epithelial component. The epithelium may be serous, mucinous or endometrioid, recapitulating the tubal epithelium or the mucinous epithelium lining the endocervix or the epithelium of the endometrium. In some tumors, the epithelium is so anaplastic it is unclassifiable. Neoplasms composed of the three better differentiated cell types range from those which are clearly benign to frank cancers. Between these extremes falls a group of intermediate tumors which are best considered as low-grade cancers called borderline carcinomas. *The classification of a tumor into benign, borderline or malignant depends, in general, upon two microscopic features: (1) the amount of nuclear atypicality and mitotic activity and (2) the presence or absence of stromal invasion by the neoplastic epithelial cells.* Obviously, benign neoplasms have regularity of cells and no evidence of stromal invasion, while the cancers are characterized by cellular anaplasia, stromal invasion, permeation of the tumor capsule and spread beyond the primary site. Identification of the borderline lesions offers the greatest difficulty. In general, they are distinguished either by having some degree of anaplasia but no evidence of stromal invasion or, conversely, by having some stromal invasion despite the virtual absence of anaplasia. In other words, they ambiguously present features of both benign and malignant tumors. Rarely, tumors considered to be borderline implant on the peritoneum or metastasize via the lymphohematogenous routes. With such dissemination, the justification for the borderline classification rests entirely with the degree of differentiation and regularity of the epithelial component. As will become apparent, the borderline carcinomas, despite such aggressive behavior, have a distinctly better prognosis than the overt cancers.

Epithelial neoplasms run the gamut from small to massive tumors that sometimes fill the pelvis and even the abdominal cavity. Although most are cystic, some are solid. The cysts may be quite massive. Some have only a single cavity (cystoma), but more often they are multilocular (cystadenoma or cystadenocarcinoma). As one ascends the scale of aggressiveness, papillary projections into the cystic lumina become more prominent, multiloculation more complex and solidification of the cystic spaces more complete. In general, unilocular cysts with little papillation tend to be benign, while multiloculated, highly papillated cysts or solid epithelial neoplasms are likely to be malignant.

Serous Cystadenoma and Cystadenocarcinoma. These common *cystic neoplasms are lined by tall, columnar, ciliated epithelial cells and are filled with serous fluid,* the two distinctive features of these tumors. Together the benign, borderline and malignant types account for about 30 per cent of all ovarian tumors. In the overall spectrum of serous tumors, about 10 per cent are benign, 30 per cent borderline and 60 per cent malignant. Thus, the ratio of benign to malignant serous tumors is 1 to 9. The cystadenocarcinomas account for approximately 60 per cent of all cancers of the ovary. As with all ovarian tumors, these serous tumors occur at any age, but are most common between 20 and 50 years of age. They are quite uncommon prior to puberty.

The benign, borderline and malignant variants are usually large, spherical or ovoid cysts that vary up to 30 to 40 cm. in diameter. The smaller masses usually have only a single cystic cavity but, as they enlarge, they are more often multilocular and then lose their symmetrical external aspect (Fig. 27–38). In the benign form, the serosal covering is smooth and glistening. The cystadenocarcinomas often have small, solid nodularities or irregular thickenings either directly beneath the serosa or protruding through it. These serosal irregularities are important indicators of penetration of the capsule by invasive tumor. On being opened, both the benign and malignant forms are filled with a clear serous fluid in most instances, but occasionally there is mucinous content to the fluid because some tumors are mixed serous and mucin-secreting. In many cases, intracystic hemorrhage or necrosis of tumor

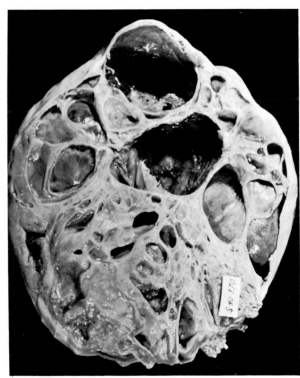
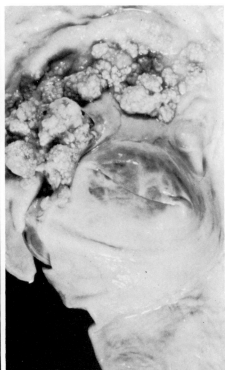

Fig. 27–38   Fig. 27–39

Figure 27–38. *Multilocular serous cystadenoma of the ovary on cross section.*
Figure 27–39. *Multilocular serous cystadenocarcinoma of the ovary. A close-up of the papillary excrescences that have penetrated the covering serosa.*

creates a turbidity and discoloration to the fluid. The character of the lining varies. The usual small (up to 10 cm.), unilocular cyst has a smooth, glistening lining. Only infrequently are papillary formations or projecting intracystic masses identified in these small tumors.

As the tumors enlarge, they tend to develop multiloculation and papillary projections or large masses or thickenings of the wall that jut into the cystic cavities. All these features are correlated with malignant potentiality. Occasionally, some of the smaller locules in these multicystic lesions are filled with solid, obvious tumor tissue. As a whole, **most serous cystic tumors are multilocular and have a greater tendency to become papillomatous than mucinous lesions to be described.** It should be emphasized that the papillary tendency, the solid projecting masses, the presence of totally solid locules and penetration or nodularity of the capsule are all important indicators of probable malignancy (Fig. 27–39). However, the exception should be noted that, occasionally, papillary ingrowths of benign cystomas grow into the wall to appear on the serosa. These are, however, small and widely scattered, and are not readily confused with the malignant form.

Histologically, the lining epithelium in the

smooth areas of the cysts is composed of a single layer of tall columnar epithelium. The cells are, in part, ciliated and, in part, dome-shaped and serous-secreting (Fig. 27–40). Microscopic papillae may be found, but are more characteristic of those neoplasms that have gross papillary structures or the projecting masses described. These papillae in the benign variants have a delicate fibrous core covered by a single layer of well oriented columnar cells (Fig. 27–41). Typical psammoma bodies are often found in the stroma of these tumors, their exact significance being totally unknown.

There is no sharp line of demarcation between this histologic pattern in the cystadenoma and the progressive anaplastic changes that denote borderline or frank malignancy in the tumors designated as cystadenocarcinomas. The histologic features that denote malignancy consist of piling up of the epithelial lining into more than one layer, invasion of the underlying stroma or capsule of the cyst, the formation of large, solid, epithelial masses that usually represent the jutting areas described in the gross, and frank penetration or invasion of the cyst wall (Fig. 27–42). In the more solid cellular areas, papillary growth can still be made out and usually gland lumina are produced. The individual tumor cells in the carcinomatous lesions display the usual

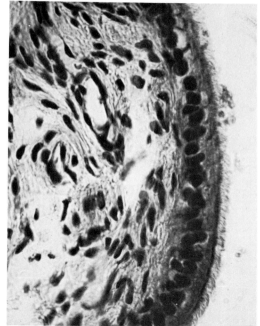

Fig. 27–40

Fig. 27–41

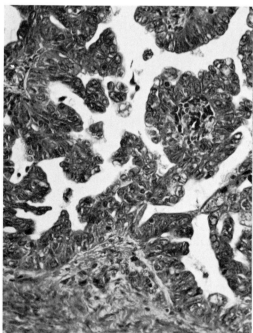

Fig. 27–42

Figure 27–40. *Histologic detail of the classic ciliated columnar lining epithelial cells of a serous cystadenoma.*

Figure 27–41. *Papillary serous cystadenoma of the ovary, illustrating the uniform layer of the epithelium covering the papillae in the benign neoplasms.*

Figure 27–42. *Papillary serous cystadenocarcinoma of the ovary with loss of orientation and piling up of the anaplastic epithelium.*

anaplastic features of all malignancy and, with the more extreme degrees of anaplasia, the cells may become quite undifferentiated. To express this range of differentiation, the malignant tumors may be classified as Grades I to III. While only 20 to 30 per cent of the benign tumors occur bilaterally, approximately two-thirds of the borderline and malignant forms affect both ovaries. It should be noted that half of these bilateral borderline and malignant lesions remain confined to the female genital tract and are, therefore, amenable to surgical extirpation.

All ovarian neoplasms derived from surface epithelium and/or ovarian stroma tend to produce similar clinical manifestations which will be discussed later. Here it is important to cite some of the prognostic data for the borderline and cancerous lesions. The 10-year survival rate for the overt cancers is on the order of 10 to 13 per cent but, for the borderline serous neoplasms, it is approximately 75 per cent (Santesson and Kottmeier, 1968). Even when borderline tumors give rise to extraovarian implants, surgery and radiation have yielded a 10-year survival rate of over 70 per cent. Such borderline neoplasms pursue a leisurely course and, indeed, rare spontaneous regression has been reported (Taylor, 1959).

Mucinous Cystadenoma and Cystadenocarcinoma. These tumors closely resemble their serous counterparts. They are somewhat less common than the serous forms and account for about 20 per cent of all ovarian neoplasms. They occur principally in middle adult life and are rare before puberty and after menopause. The benign variants are much more common than the malignant in the ratio of approximately 7 to 1. Indeed, mucinous cystadenocarcinomas are rare and account for only 3 per cent of all ovarian cancers. You recall that, for serous neoplasms, the ratio of benign to malignant is 1 to 9. The mucinous neoplasm differs from the serous in the character of the lining epithelium. It is composed of nonciliated, tall, columnar, mucus-secreting cells. The nuclei are disposed basally and the mucoid secretion is found in the luminal portion of the cell. The cystic spaces are filled with this sticky, slightly gelatinous fluid rich in glycoproteins.

Grossly, the mucinous tumors closely resemble the serous cystadenomas and cystadenocarcinomas. However, in contrast to the serous tumors, the mucinous tumors are more apt to be unilateral. Approximately 5 per cent of the benign forms and only 20 per cent of the carcinomas are bilateral. In general, mucinous tumors tend to produce larger cystic masses and some have been recorded with weights of over 60 pounds! They tend to be more strikingly multiloculated and, on cross section, often present a honey-combed appearance. Despite these features, it is not possible on gross inspection to unmistakably distinguish between the serous and mucinous forms of cystadenomas except by the nature of the cystic content (Fig. 27–43).

One gross feature of these mucinous tumors unmistakably distinguishes them from serous lesions. Metastases from these cystadenocarcinomas or rupture of a malignant tumor may give rise to a clinical condition designated as **pseudomyxoma peritonei.** The peritoneal cavity becomes filled with a glairy mucinous material resembling the cystic contents. Multiple tumor implants are found on all the serosal surfaces, and extensive interadherence and adhesion of the viscera produces a complete matting together of all the abdominal contents (Fig. 27–44). This form of pseudomyxoma peritonei is clearly a manifestation of malignant dissemination and, therefore, is similar in significance to the pseudomyxoma peritonei encountered in rupture of a carcinomatous mucocele of the appendix (p. 976).

Histologically, these mucinous tumors are identified by the apical mucinous vacuolation of the tall columnar lining epithelial cells and the absence of cilia (Fig. 27–45). However, it should be emphasized that, not uncommonly, mixtures of epithelium may be encountered that make it impossible to distinguish clearly serous from mucinous tumors. The same characteristics that applied to the serous cystadenocarcinomas, i.e., piling up of epithelium, formation of papillae, anaplasia of epithelial cells, invasion of the capsule and formation of solid masses of tumor, also apply to the segregation of the mucinous variants into benign, borderline and malignant tumors.

Because of the complexity of the loculation in mucinous tumors, it may be exceedingly difficult to differentiate histologically between benign, borderline and malignant lesions. Often, minute locules filled with epithelial cells present as invasive nests of tumor. Hence, greater reliance must be placed on the level of differentiation of the epithelial components and, where the cells are quite regular, displaying only slight anaplasia, the borderline classification may be applied. **Infrequently, in these mucinous tumors, nodules of a dermoid cyst or a Brenner tumor are found in the wall of a cystic space.**

The importance of differentiating between borderline and malignant mucinous tumors is made clear by the reported 68 per cent 10-year survival in patients with borderline lesions in contrast to a 34 per cent rate for the overt carcinomas (Santesson and Kottmeier, 1968).

Endometrioid Tumors. These neoplasms account for approximately 15 per cent of all ovarian cancers. *While benign and borderline forms may occur, most are true carcinomas* (Gray and Barnes, 1967). They are distinguished from serous and mucinous tumors by the presence of tubular glands bearing a close resemblance to benign or malignant endometrium. *Approximately one-third of endometrioid carcinomas are accompanied by a carcinoma of the endometrium* (Scully et al., 1966). Is one tumor primary and the other a metastasis? Pertinent to this question is the observation that the five-year survival rate of endometrioid carcinoma confined to the ovary is 55 per cent, while the comparable figure in cases of endometrioid carcinoma accompanied by carcinoma of the uterus is 44 per cent (Scully, 1970). The small difference

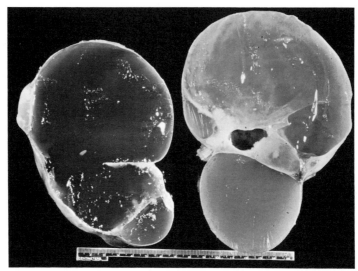

Fig. 27--43

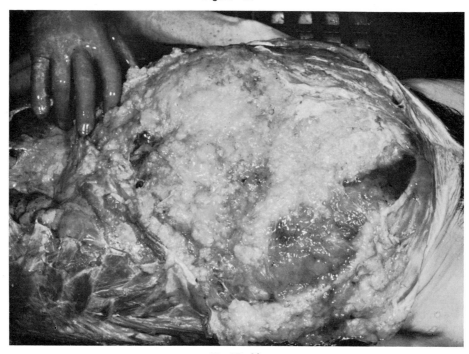

Fig. 27--44

Figure 27--43. Bilateral mucinous cystadenomas of the ovary. The tumors were fixed previous to sectioning to demonstrate the gelatinous nature of the cystic contents. Note 15 cm. rule.

Figure 27--44. Pseudomyxoma peritonei (ovarian), viewed at autopsy with the abdominal wall laid back to expose the massive overgrowth of gelatinous metastatic tumor.

between these two rates (having questionable statistical validity) argues against the concept of metastasis from one site to the other. If this phenomenon represented metastatic disease, one might reasonably expect more widespread dissemination and a significantly worse prognosis.

Grossly, endometrioid carcinomas present either in the form of a cyst or a solid mass. These tumors do not achieve the monstrous proportions of their mucinous cousins. The cysts are lined by a velvety surface from which may protrude polypoid masses or papillae. Multiloculation and papillation such as is seen in the mucinous or serous tumors are uncommon. About one-third of patients with endometrioid carcinoma have involvement of both ovaries. When such bilaterality is found, it usually, but not always, implies extension of the neoplasm beyond the female genital tract. Histologically,

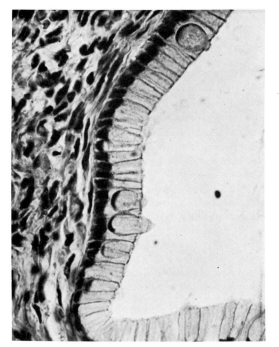

Figure 27–45. Histologic detail of the classic non-ciliated, mucin-secreting, columnar lining epithelium of a mucinous cystadenoma of the ovary. (Courtesy of Dr. Arthur Hertig.)

glandular patterns are seen bearing a strong resemblance to those of endometrial origin. On occasion, there are foci of squamous differentiation, recapitulating the pattern of adenoacanthomas of the endometrium. Similarly, some tumors have foci resembling serous or mucinous carcinomas. The survival data cited earlier are modified by the level of differentiation of the epithelial component.

Cystadenofibroma. The cystadenofibroma is essentially a variant of the serous cystadenoma in which there is more pronounced proliferation of the fibrous stroma that underlies the columnar lining epithelium. These tumors are usually small and multilocular and have rather simple papillary processes that do not become so complicated and branching as those found in the ordinary cystadenoma. The epithelial lining is usually quite regular and does not have the tendency to develop anaplastic changes. These cystadenofibromas are of interest because the stromal e ement behaves as thecal cells that sometimes give rise to hyperestrinism. Carcinomatous transformation is rare.

Clear Cell Tumors. This uncommon pattern of surface epithelial tumor of the ovary is characterized by large epithelial cells with abundant clear cytoplasm reminiscent of those encountered in the clear cell hypernephroid carcinoma of the kidney. Thus, these ovarian clear cell tumors were years ago designated as a form of "mesonephroma" on the presumption that they arose from renal anlagen. Morphologically identical tumors are occasionally encountered in the broad ligament, cervix and vagina, presumably arising in mesonephric remnants.

The clear cell tumors of the ovary can be dominantly solid or cystic. In the solid neoplasm, the clear cells are arranged in sheets or tubules. In the cystic variety, the neoplastic cells line the spaces. Occasionally, the cystic spaces are filled with hemorrhagic, chocolate-colored fluid. These neoplasms range in cellular differentiation from benign to borderline to malignant. They are occasionally bilateral.

The five-year survival rate is in the range of 40 per cent when the tumors are confined to the ovary(s). With spread beyond the ovary, five-year survival is exceptional.

Brenner Tumor. This usually solid ovarian neoplasm is characterized by a dense fibrous stroma punctuated by nests of transitional cells resembling those lining the urinary bladder. Less frequently, the nests comprise microcysts or glandular spaces lined by columnar mucin-secreting cells. Brenner tumors are uncommon and account for no more than 2 per cent of ovarian neoplasms. They are encountered at all ages, from childhood to the advanced years of life, with a peak incidence between the ages of 40 and 70. As cited earlier, Brenner tumors are occasionally encountered in mucinous cystadenomas.

These neoplasms are usually unilateral (approximately 90 per cent) and vary in size from small lesions less than a centimeter in diameter to massive tumors up to 20 to 30 cm. in diameter. Although generally solid, occasionally they are cystic. The fibrous stroma, resembling that of the normal ovary, is marked by sharply demarcated nests of epithelial cells. The epithelial cells are generally regular and uniform, with little evidence of anaplasia or mitotic activity. Those nests resembling the epithelium of the urinary tract tend to be solid masses of cells, while the mucinous variety often comprise microscopic cysts or glands. Infrequently, the stroma is composed of somewhat plump fibroblasts resembling theca cells. Such neoplasms may have hormonal activity and in support of such a notion are the reported instances of the concurrence of Brenner tumors and endometrial carcinoma (Tighe, 1961). With rare exception, Brenner tumors are benign.

Clinical Course of Surface Epithelial and Stromal Tumors. All these tumors of the ovary tend to produce the same clinical manifestations. The two most prominent complaints found in these cases are low abdominal pain and abdominal enlargement. The extraordinary size of some of these masses frequently causes marked distention of the abdomen, and sometimes it is impossible to identify clearly the upper border of the neoplasm, especially when it is under the edge of the costal margin or liver. Under these circumstances, gastrointestinal complaints, frequency, dysuria, pelvic pressure and many other symptoms may appear. When benign, the lesions are easily resected with cure. However, the malignant forms tend to cause the progressive weakness, weight loss and cachexia characteristic of all malignancies.

The carcinomas extend through the capsule of the tumor to seed the pleural and peritoneal cavities. Massive ascites is common with such dissemination to the abdominal cavity. Characteristically, this fluid is filled with diagnostic exfoliated tumor cells. The peritoneal seeding which these malignancies produce is quite distinctive. They tend to seed all serosal surfaces diffusely with 0.1 to 0.5 cm. nodules of tumor. These surface implants rarely invade the underlying parenchyma of the organ. In addition to this form of spread, these malignancies may metastasize through lymphatics and blood vessels. The regional nodes are often involved and intraparenchymal visceral metastases may be found in the liver, bones, lungs and elsewhere. Metastasis across the midline to the opposite ovary is discovered in about half the cases by the time of surgical laparotomy and, from this point, the patients usually run a progressive downhill course to death within one to two years.

Several complications may punctuate the course of these neoplasms. *The large, bulky ovarian masses may become twisted on their pedicles (torsion) and undergo hemorrhagic infarction and thus evoke symptoms of an acute abdomen.* The cystic lesions may rupture spontaneously, or during palpation, to produce acute abdominal symptoms.

GERM CELL TUMORS

Dysgerminoma. The dysgerminoma is best remembered as the ovarian counterpart of the seminoma of the testis. It is composed of large vesicular cells having a cleared cytoplasm, well defined cell boundaries and centrally placed regular nuclei. These cells are thought to be derived from primordial germ cells of the sexually undifferentiated embryonic gonad. Relatively uncommon tumors, the dysgerminomas account for about 1 per cent of all ovarian neoplasms. They are encoun-

tered at all ages from infancy to late life, with a peak incidence in the second and third decades.

Usually unilateral (80 to 90 per cent) for obscure reasons, they occur more frequently in the left ovary (50 per cent) than in the right (35 per cent). Generally, they are solid tumors which range in size from barely visible nodules to masses that virtually fill the entire abdomen. On cut surface, they have a yellow-white to gray-pink appearance and are often soft and fleshy. Histologically, the dysgerminoma cells are dispersed in sheets or cords separated by scant fibrous stroma. As in the seminoma, the fibrous stroma is infiltrated with mature lymphocytes and, occasionally, has focal granulomatous lesions strongly reminiscent of tuberculosis or sarcoidosis. Occasionally, small nodules of dysgerminoma are encountered in the wall of an otherwise benign cystic teratoma or, conversely, a predominantly dysgerminomatous tumor may contain a small cystic teratoma.

All dysgerminomas must be considered to be malignant although cures can be effected, in many instances, by salpingo-oophorectomy. It is impossible, from histologic examination, to distinguish those lesions amenable to curative surgery from those destined to behave more aggressively. These neoplasms are radiosensitive, and even those which have extended beyond the ovary can generally be controlled or eradicated by such therapy, yielding overall a five-year survival rate between 70 and 90 per cent (Asadourian and Taylor, 1969).

Cystic Teratoma (Dermoid). Cystic teratomas are better known in clinical parlance as *dermoid cysts.* This designation alludes to the fact that they are lined by apparent skin with all of its associated adnexal structures and are typically filled with a sebaceous cheesy secretion in which is found matted hair. These neoplasms are almost invariably benign and are presumably derived from the ectodermal differentiation of totipotential cells, although frequently, within the wall of the cyst, mesodermal and endodermal elements are encountered (Marcial-Rojas and Medina, 1958).

Cystic teratomas are relatively common and account for about 25 per cent of all ovarian neoplasms. They are found usually in young women during the active reproductive years.

The tumors are unilateral in about 80 per cent of the cases and are characteristically relatively small compared to other ovarian neoplasms. Three-quarters are less than 10 cm. in diameter and only rarely do they exceed 15 cm. Characteristically, they are unilocular cysts enclosed within a smooth, glistening serosa, which have a doughy, yielding consistency. On section, they have a thin wall lined by an opaque gray-white, wrinkled, apparent epidermis. From this epidermis, hair shafts and tooth structures frequently protrude (Fig. 27–46). Within the wall, it is common to find areas of calcification that prove to be bony spicules. The lumen of the cyst is filled with a thick, yellow-white, sebaceous secretion that is more or less heavily admixed with matted strands of hair.

Histologically, the dominant characteristic is the mature development of stratified squamous epithelium with underlying sebaceous glands, hair shafts and other skin adnexal structures (Fig. 27–47). However, in the majority of cases, structures from other germ layers can be identified, such as cartilage, bone, thyroid tissue or other organoid formations (Fig. 27–48). On this basis, it is better to refer to these lesions as cystic teratomas (Marcial-Rojas and Medina, 1958). Tumors such as these are sometimes incorporated within the wall of a pseudomucinous cystadenoma. In about 1 per cent of the dermoids, malignant transformation of the epithelium is found. Malignancy developing from other contained structures is a rare occurrence.

The clinical symptoms are those of all ovarian neoplasms, i.e., abdominal pain, mass and, occasionally, gastrointestinal complaints or disturbances in the menstrual cycle. There is apparently some unknown influence of these tumors upon the uterus and contralateral ovary, since these patients have a higher than usual rate of sterility. Torsion of a dermoid tumor on its pedicle is a not uncommon complication and produces signs and symptoms of an acute abdominal emergency. Dermoids appear to twist more often than other types of ovarian neoplasms for completely obscure reasons. Occasionally, the diagnosis of a dermoid can be made radiographically by the shadows caused by teeth, bones, areas of calcification or even the markedly thickened epidermal lining of the cyst. Except in the rare instance of malignant transformation (1 to 2 per cent), these tumors are resectable and curable. The malignant component may take the form of a squamous cell carcinoma, a thyroid carcinoma, melanocarcinoma or sarcoma.

An extremely rare variant of the cystic teratoma is entirely composed of mature thyroid tissue and is designated a *struma ovarii*. Interestingly, these thyroidal neoplasms may hyperfunction, producing hyperthyroidism.

Solid Teratoma (Well Differentiated and Embryonal). The solid teratoma differs from the dermoid in that it has a more heterogeneous collection of tissues and organoid structures derived from all three germ layers. Although these tumors presumably have the

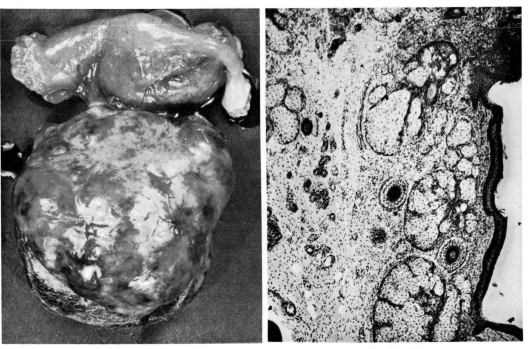

Fig. 27–46   Fig. 27–47

Figure 27–46. Dermoid teratoma of the ovary. The cut margin (below) shows protruding hair shafts.
Figure 27–47. Dermoid teratoma. Low power view of the lining epithelium, illustrating the almost complete resemblance to skin. (Both figures courtesy of Dr. Arthur Hertig.)

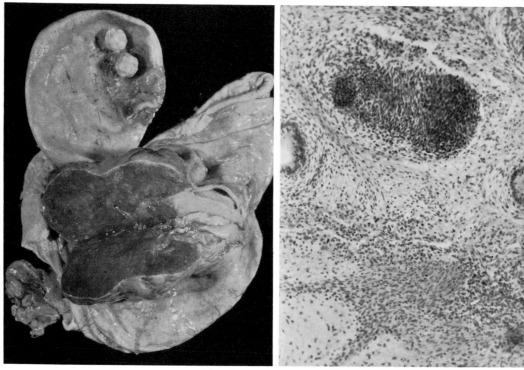

Fig. 27–48   Fig. 27–49

Figure 27–48. *Dermoid cyst of the ovary, opened to illustrate several abortive tooth structures (above) and a darker area of thyroid substance (below).*

Figure 27–49. *Embryonal teratoma of the ovary, illustrating the heterogeneity of the organoid structures.*

same histogenetic origin as dermoids, there is no preponderant differentiation into ectodermal derivatives. *They tend to occur in a younger age group and are sometimes found in the prepubertal years.* In some tumors, all of the germ layer derivatives are well differentiated, and such tumors may well be benign (Thurlbeck and Scully, 1960). In contrast to such well differentiated solid teratomas are those which contain more embryonal and anaplastic components including foci of choriocarcinoma.

Externally, they may resemble the dermoids described, but often are larger, bulkier masses. On section, they have a solid or preponderantly solid structure containing small locules or cystic spaces. The transection usually discloses an essentially yellow-white to brown tissue that is of varying consistency and, in many areas, may contain recognizable islands of gelatinous hyaline cartilage and focal areas of red-brown meaty tissue that may prove to be muscle or thyroid. The well differentiated tumors are characterized histologically by a complete heterogeneity of more or less adult structures, sprinkled through a loose connective tissue stroma. Thus, one may recognize masses of bronchial epithelium, islands of well formed salivary

glands and brain tissue; indeed, scanning these lesions takes on the aspect of a treasure hunt.

Embryonal solid teratomas present a wide variation of elements in varying stages of differentiation. Frequently, there are nests of highly embryonic stellate cells with other sarcomatous areas reminiscent of fibrosarcoma or rhabdomyosarcoma and, in yet other areas, foci of primitive neural tissue (Fig. 27–49). Islands of cartilage, bone, glandular structures and lymphoid tissue may also be present but are usually more difficult to identify than in the well differentiated lesions. Although embryonal teratomas are usually unilateral, in about 10 per cent of cases, they arise in both ovaries simultaneously (Woodruff et al., 1968).

It is probable that the well differentiated solid teratomas and the embryonal forms represent expressions of a range of biologic behavior extending from benign lesions at one end to highly malignant tumors at the other extreme. The degree of differentiation of the various components heavily influences whether a cure can be effected by salpingo-oophorectomy or whether, instead, the five-year survival will be below 10 per cent (Breen and Neubecker, 1963).

Choriocarcinoma. More commonly of

placental origin, the choriocarcinoma may arise in the ovary from the teratogenous development of germ cells. It is generally held that such an origin can only be certified in the prepubertal girl since, after this age, the neoplasm may well have arisen in an ovarian ectopic pregnancy.

These neoplasms may exist in pure form or in dysgerminomas (Neigus, 1955). The pure choriocarcinomas may be minute or range up to 10 to 15 cm. in diameter. They may be entirely encapsulated or have ruptured through the capsule. Cut section usually discloses a hemorrhagic, often necrotic mass which resembles old blood clot more than tumor. Areas of yellow-white preserved tumor tissue may be evident. Histologically, they are identical with the more common placental lesions (p. 1261). These ovarian primaries are ugly tumors which generally have metastasized widely through the blood stream to the lungs, liver, bone and other viscera by the time they have been diagnosed.

As with all choriocarcinomas, they elaborate high levels of chorionic gonadotropins which are sometimes helpful in establishing the diagnosis or in highlighting recurrences. In contrast to its effectiveness in choriocarcinomas arising in the placenta, methotrexate therapy is of no avail in these highly fatal cancers.

SEX CORD—MESENCHYME TUMORS

Included within this category are all ovarian neoplasms originating either from the sex cords of the embryonic gonad or from the mesenchyme of the ovary. As is well known, granulosal cells, theca cells and luteal cells are derived from such sex cords or from the ovarian mesenchyme, and so neoplasms having such histogenetic origins fall within this category. Moreover, since theca cells are the source of ovarian steroids, many of these neoplasms are functional and have feminizing effects. The embryonic sex cords may differentiate along masculine lines to give rise to Sertoli-Leydig cell tumors, better known as arrhenoblastomas. However, some of these Sertoli-Leydig cell tumors either have no function or have estrogenic effects.

Granulosa-Theca-Luteal Cell Tumors.

This designation embraces ovarian neoplasms composed of varying proportions of granulosal cells, theca cells and luteinized cells. At one end of the spectrum are those tumors composed almost entirely of granulosal cells and at the other are the pure thecomas sometimes showing sufficient luteinization to merit the designation luteoma. Collectively, these neo-

plasms account for about 5 to 10 per cent of all ovarian tumors. Although they may be discovered at any age, approximately two-thirds occur in the postmenopausal woman.

These tumors are usually unilateral and vary from microscopic foci to large, solid, discretely encapsulated masses up to 20 to 30 cm. in diameter. Generally, they range from about 5 to 10 cm. in diameter when discovered. On external inspection, they have a smooth encapsulated surface which may be somewhat lobulated. Tumors that are endocrinologically active have a yellow coloration to their cut surfaces, produced by contained lipids, and in the most active tumors, such as the relatively pure thecomas or the less common luteomas, the coloration may be a bright orange-yellow.

The granulosa cell component of these tumors takes one of many histologic patterns. The small, cuboidal to polygonal, epithelial-appearing follicle cells may grow in anastomosing cords, sheets or strands. In occasional cases, small gland-like patterns or abortive follicles are produced that are filled with an acidophilic secretion resembling an ovum (Call-Exner bodies) (Fig. 27–50). When these folliculoid structures are evident, the diagnosis is rendered considerably more simple. In still other variants, well developed gland patterns are formed that make the tumor resemble an adenoma. In the theca luteoma, the cells may be disposed in large sheets of cuboidal to polygonal cells that gradually

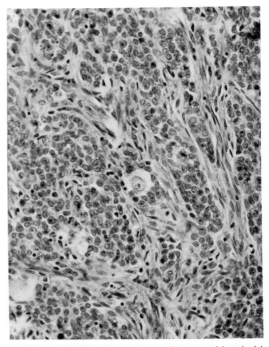

Figure 27–50. *Granulosa cell tumor with cuboidal epithelial cells, forming in the center field an abortive follicle.*

change into plump spindle cells resembling the theca lutein cells. The theca cells, in turn, blend rather deceptively with the surrounding stroma of the ovary.

The variation in the architectural pattern of these tumors makes it quite difficult, in certain instances, to determine whether the cells are granulosal in nature or are more like theca cells. Pure theca luteomas are composed of large sheets or poorly defined areas of plump spindle cells that closely resemble those of the fibroma (Fig. 27–51). The distinction between the theca cell and the fibrocyte can be made with certainty only by histochemical techniques. Characteristically, theca cells contain sudanophilic droplets, many of which can be proved by special procedures to give the staining reaction of steroids. The pure luteoma is composed largely of epithelium-like, acidophilic, granular, apparent luteal cells. These cells are extremely rich in the lipids mentioned.

In the study by Mansell and Hertig (1955), the granulosa cell type predominated in about 17 per cent, mixtures of granulosa cell and theca cell were found in 15 per cent, and relatively pure theca cell types in 67 per cent. The pure luteoma is rare. Most of the predominantly granulosa cell patterns contained only a scant amount of lipid substance, and most of these tumors were relatively inactive endocrinologically. This finding is consonant with the well established belief that the granulosa cell of the ovarian follicle does not produce the estrogens, but rather that the endocrinologic activity of the follicle resides in the theca cells. The functional activity of the theca and luteal cell variants is, to a considerable extent, correlated with their lipid content.

This group of mesenchymal tumors have clinical importance for two reasons: (1) their potential elaboration of large amounts of estrogen and (2) the hazard of malignancy in the granulosal cell forms. Functionally active tumors (usually those having a large thecal component) may produce precocious sexual development in the prepubertal girl. In the adult woman, the elaboration of estrogens leads to a variety of important consequences, including endometrial hyperplasia, cystic disease of the breast, breast carcinoma and endometrial carcinoma. About 10 to 15 per cent of patients with steroid-producing tumors eventually develop an endometrial carcinoma. In the postmenopausal woman with a functionally active tumor, the incidence of endometrial carcinoma may be as high as 25 per cent (Mansell and Hertig, 1955).

The additional clinical significance of these tumors is the possibility that the granulosal cell lesion may be malignant. It is not implied that a benign tumor becomes malignant but, rather, that granulosal cell neoplasms range de novo from those clearly benign to those overtly cancerous. It is extremely difficult, from the histologic evaluation of granulosa cell tumors, to predict their biologic behavior (Norris and Taylor, 1968). Some are anaplastic and present variation in cell and nuclear size and very likely exhibit aggressive behavior. However, other apparently innocent-appearing lesions have been known to recur following removal. Overall, such recurrence is seen in 25 per cent of tumors composed almost entirely of granulosa cells. Such cancers show the same metastatic potential as all other forms of ovarian carcinoma and spread to the regional lymph nodes, peritoneum and eventually to visceral organs. The five-year survival rate is approximately 85 per cent (Sjostedt and Wahlen, 1961). In contrast, tumors composed predominantly of theca and luteal cells are almost never malignant.

Arrhenoblastoma (Sertoli-Leydig Cell Tumor). Some authors object to the designation arrhenoblastoma because it connotes masculinization. While these neoplasms do, indeed, commonly produce masculinization, or at least defeminization, a few have estrogenic effects (Scully, 1970). They occur in women of all ages and have been recorded as early as the first decade of life although the

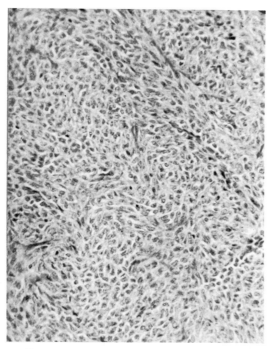

Figure 27–51. *Theca luteoma composed of plump differentiated stromal cells. Note the resemblance to a fibroma. (Courtesy of Dr. Arthur Hertig and Armed Forces Institute of Pathology.)*

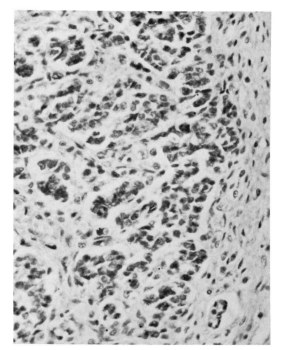

peak incidence is in the second and third. When masculinizing, they inhibit ovulation and are responsible for sterility. Virilization is usually associated with increased urinary excretion of 17-ketosteroids but, in some patients, the levels are not unusually high or may even be normal, and the elaboration of small amounts of more potent testosterone is postulated. The embryogenesis of such male-directed stromal cells remains a puzzle, and it can only be theorized that it represents masculine differentiation of the mesenchyme derived from the embryonic "ambisextrous" primitive gonads.

Macroscopically, these tumors are usually unilateral (95 per cent) and exactly resemble the granulosa-theca cell neoplasms. The cut surface is usually gray-white and solid. Larger tumors may have areas of hemorrhage and necrosis and sometimes small cysts.

Histologically, they present a great variation in cytologic detail, so much so that it is difficult at times to establish the identity of this neoplasm unless clear clinical evidence of masculinization is present. Abortive testicular tubules, cords or masses of epithelial cells, which closely resemble those in the granulosa cell tumor, and undifferentiated spindle cell sarcomatous patterns encompass the variability of these tumors (Fig. 27—52).

These Sertoli-Leydig cell tumors are more often malignant than the granulosa cell lesions. In the literature, the mortality rates range from 10 to 30 per cent (O'Hern and Neubecker, 1962). In addition to malignant potential, these neoplasms may cause defeminization of adult females manifested by atrophy of the breast, amenorrhea and loss of hair. This syndrome may progress to striking virilization, i.e., hirsutism, male distribution of hair, hypertrophy of the clitoris and lowering of the voice. In the prepubertal child, they of course block normal female sexual development and eventually lead to virilization.

TUMORS DERIVED FROM CONNECTIVE TISSUE

Fibroma and Fibrosarcoma. Fibromas arising in the ovarian stroma are a relatively common form of ovarian neoplasm and account for about 10 per cent of all types.

The fibromas of the ovary do not have any distinctive gross or anatomic features that differentiate them from fibromas elsewhere. They are unilateral in about 90 per cent of the cases and usually are solid, spherical or slightly lobulated, encapsulated, hard, gray-white masses covered by glistening, intact ovarian serosa (Fig. 27-53). Commonly, they have a diameter of 5 to 10 cm. when excised, but larger masses have been described. Histologically,

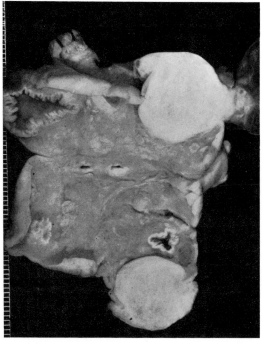

Figure 27-53. A small fibroma of ovary apparent as a discrete, small, pale mass.

they are composed of well differentiated fibrocytes and fibroblasts having a more or less scant collagenous connective tissue interspersed between the cells. The cells are uniform and mature, and mitotic figures are, on the whole, uncommon. Rare mitoses may be found in completely benign lesions. Probably less than 1 per cent of these fibrous lesions are malignant, i.e., a fibrosarcoma.

Clinically, these tumors are of considerable interest. In addition to the characteristic nonspecific findings of pain, pelvic mass and possibly intestinal disturbances due to pressure, ascites is found in about 40 per cent of the cases in which the tumors measure more than 6 cm. in diameter. The genesis of the ascites in these cases is somewhat obscure. It is usually ascribed either to marked venous stasis within these tumors, perhaps due to twisting of the pedicle of the ovary, or to increased transudation through markedly dilated lymphatics. Uncommonly, these patients with ascites also have hydrothorax, usually only of the right side. This combination of findings, i.e., *ovarian tumor, hydrothorax and ascites, is designated as the "Meigs syndrome."* The passage of fluid into the pleural cavities is presumed to occur through transdiaphragmatic lymphatics. It should be emphasized that this curious association of ovarian neoplasm with abdominal and pleural fluid is not restricted to fibromas. It has been reported in other forms of ovarian neoplasm, perhaps in not the same high incidence as with fibromas. An awareness of the Meigs syndrome is of considerable clinical importance, because all too frequently the findings of ovarian tumor, ascites and pleural fluid are interpreted as indicative of a malignancy with peritoneal and pleural metastases.

SECONDARY TUMORS OF THE OVARY

The ovary is more often involved by metastatic processes than any of the other pelvic genital organs. Two groups of malignancies contribute to this incidence: carcinomas arising within the other pelvic organs and carcinomas arising within the upper gastrointestinal tract, i.e., stomach, biliary tract and pancreas. In the first group, the spread to the ovary occurs ei-

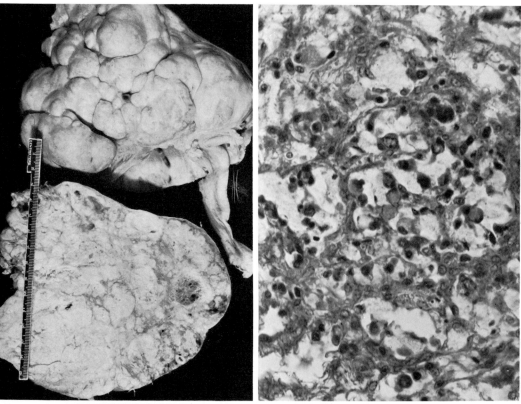

Fig. 27–54

Fig. 27–55

Figure 27–54. Bilateral Krukenberg tumors of the ovary metastatic from the stomach.
Figure 27–55. Krukenberg tumor of the ovary, illustrating the signet ring forms dispersed through the fibrous stroma.

ther via the lymphatics or by direct continuity, and the ovarian involvement tends to duplicate, in histologic detail, the primary neoplasm. The second group of primary cancers that often metastasize to the ovary raises many issues that have not been resolved and that bear on the question—what is a *Krukenberg tumor?* Krukenberg originally described bilateral ovarian neoplasms appearing as large, solid, gray-white tumors composed of a fibromyxomatous stroma through which were scattered mucin-secreting "signet ring" cells. To these tumors, he applied the name *"fibrosarcoma ovarii mucocellulare carcinomotodes"* (Figs. 27–54 and 27–55). He conceived of these tumors as primary ovarian neoplasms. Subsequent to this original description, it was demonstrated that the Krukenberg tumors were actually metastatic from other primary malignancies, principally in the stomach, and that the signet rings were, indeed, metastatic

mucus-secreting epithelial cells. It was then accepted that Krukenberg tumors were metastases of gastric carcinoma to the ovary. Since that time, there has been a growing tendency to expand the concept of a Krukenberg tumor to include all ovarian metastases from gastrointestinal primary carcinomas, as well as those from the pancreas and biliary tract.

The problem of how the metastases spread from the gastrointestinal tract to the ovary has not been solved. Peritoneal sedimentation and lymphatic and hematogenous spread have all been cited as the pathways. While most investigators favor peritoneal sedimentation, there are equally strong proponents of the other routes. However, the major clinical significance of this discussion lies in the fact that when bilateral, or even unilateral, solid ovarian tumors are found, careful investigation for a primary site elsewhere is definitely in order.

PLACENTAL DISEASES

Toxemia of Pregnancy— Eclampsia Inflammations of the Placenta Syphilis Tuberculosis	Spontaneous Abortion Ectopic Pregnancy Tumors Hydatidiform mole Choriocarcinoma	(chorionepithelioma) Syncytial endometritis Chorioadenoma destruens Choriocarcinoma

The present discussion concerns itself only with those disorders of the placenta in which a knowledge of the morphologic lesion contributes to the understanding of the clinical problem.

TOXEMIA OF PREGNANCY— ECLAMPSIA

Toxemia of pregnancy refers to a symptom complex characterized by elevations of blood pressure, proteinuria and edema, often accompanied by variable gastrointestinal and central nervous system symptoms. Certain of these patients become more seriously ill to develop frank coma, and some have episodes of severe convulsions. To this more severe form, the term *eclampsia* is applied. Many of these eclamptic patients develop lesions in the liver, kidneys, heart, placenta and sometimes the brain. This is not true of all cases. Moreover, there is no absolute correlation between the severity of eclampsia and the magnitude of the anatomic changes.

The nature of toxemia of pregnancy is still

unclear. Recent studies suggest that it may be one of the many presentations of disseminated intravascular coagulation (p. 744) (McKay, 1964) (Merskey et al., 1967). Conceivably, maternal sensitization to placental antigens, followed by a sudden release of a challenge dose of antigens, might induce an immunologic reaction triggering widespread intravascular microcirculatory coagulation. Alternatively, placental thromboplastin might be the mediator of widespread clotting. Whatever the mechanism, widespread thromboses in arterioles and capillaries throughout the body are seen, particularly in the liver, kidneys, brain, pituitary and placenta.

The *liver* lesions, when present, take the form of irregular, focal, subcapsular and intraparenchymal hemorrhages. On histologic examination, there are fibrin thrombi in the portal capillaries with foci of necrosis in the hepatic parenchyma subcentrally or in the periportal regions. These foci of necrosis are accompanied by an inflammatory reaction.

The *kidney* lesions are quite variable, both in severity and in type. Swelling of the endothelial cells of the glomeruli may be the only

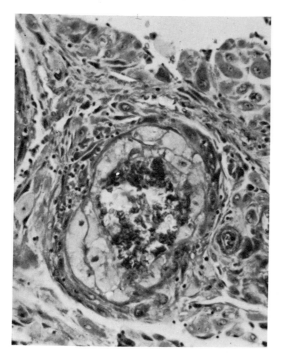

Figure 27–56. Acute atherosclerosis of vessels in an eclamptic placenta. Note the foamy subendothelial macrophages.

manifestation. More often, these changes are accompanied by marked swelling and fatty changes and, in a rare instance, by complete necrosis of the cells of the proximal convoluted tubules. In the more well defined cases, there are membrane changes (p. 1103) and fibrin thrombi present in the glomeruli and capillaries of the cortex. These lead to focal areas of glomerulitis as well as microinfarcts throughout the cortex. When the lesion is far advanced, it may produce complete destruction of the cortex in the pattern already referred to as bilateral renal cortical necrosis (p. 1135).

The *brain* may have gross or microscopic foci of hemorrhage along with small vessel thromboses. Similar changes are often found in the *heart* and in the anterior pituitary. It is entirely possible that this type of vascular lesion may account for significant degrees of *pituitary* infarction to reproduce the entity known as Sheehan's postpartum pituitary necrosis (p. 1358).

The *placenta* is the site of variable changes. The principal alterations may be interpreted as *premature aging.* Occasionally, this overall pattern is accompanied by large, pale, retracted areas of infarction that affect whole cotyledons or only a part of one. The aging changes consist principally of an accentuated atrophy of the syncytial trophoblast during the last trimester. Normally in the first two trimesters of

pregnancy, the villi are covered by fairly evenly distributed cytotrophoblast and syncytiotrophoblast. In the last trimester, the syncytiotrophoblast undergoes atrophy so that it is disposed unevenly above the villi to create areas devoid of syncytium punctuated by small, piled-up masses of trophoblast—the so-called syncytial knots. Such villi are characteristically referred to as "naked villi." In the normal process of maturation and aging of the placenta during the last trimester, about one-third of the villi pass through this phase of epithelial atrophy. However, in eclampsia, this alteration may affect as many as 90 to 100 per cent of the villi. These alterations are often accompanied by capillary thromboses and, once in a while, by florid, degenerative alterations in the walls of the small vessels (Fig. 27–56).

INFLAMMATIONS OF THE PLACENTA

Bacterial infections may occur in the placenta *(placentitis)* and in the fetal membranes *(chorioamnionitis).* In the majority of instances, these bacterial invasions arise as ascending infections through the birth canal and, in almost all such instances, premature rupture of the membranes provides the portal of entry for the organisms. The hazard of infection is much increased by prolapse of the umbilical cord or one of the extremities. However, bacterial infections may also be introduced in the course of an induced abortion. Very uncommonly, bacterial infections of the placenta and fetal membranes may arise by the hematogenous spread of bacteria and, under these circumstances, the fetal membranes may be intact. The amniotic fluid is cloudy and contains purulent exudate. The chorioamnion, when involved, is thickened and opalescent, and histologically is the site of a leukocytic polymorphonuclear infiltration with accompanying edema and congestion of the vessels. When the infection extends beyond the membranes, it may involve the placental villi with similar inflammatory changes. The vessels often have acute vasculitis. In general, in the usual form of chorioamnionitis encountered in induced abortions, the infection is limited to the fetal membranes.

Syphilis. Syphilis was, at one time, a not uncommon infection in the placenta. It is, at the present time, very rare. It is characterized by enlargement of the placenta caused by bulbous swelling and fibrosis of the villi. The characteristic histologic alterations of syphilis, i.e., obliterative endarteritis and perivascular plasma cell and lymphocytic infiltrations, are sometimes evident. Subsequent atrophy and fibrosis of the more severely ischemic areas may develop.

Tuberculosis. Tuberculous infections of the placenta are almost invariably initiated by hematogenous miliary tuberculosis. While such placental seeding is an infrequent localization of miliary tuberculosis, it provides the possible genesis for the development of congenital tuberculosis in the offspring.

SPONTANEOUS ABORTION

Approximately 15 to 20 per cent of pregnancies terminate in spontaneous abortion, most often in the 10th to 13th week of gestation. The term abortion implies miscarriage of a medically nonviable pregnancy of less than six months' gestation. As was discussed in an earlier section (p. 551), spontaneous abortion represents the natural processes of selection whereby defective ova and fetuses which are either nonviable or have reduced viability are shed. Thus, fetuses which are less defective may survive longer, only to die in the last trimester of pregnancy or immediately following delivery.

The causes of spontaneous abortion are both fetal and maternal. Defective implantation, inadequate to support fetal development, or death of the ovum or fetus in utero because of some genetic or acquired abnormality comprise the major origins of spontaneous abortion. Numerous studies have indicated bizarre chromosomal abnormalities in over half of spontaneous abortuses (Singh and Carr, 1967) (World Health Organization, 1970). Induced abortions are now commonplace; in most of these instances, the abortus is normal.

Maternal influences are less well understood and include vaguely postulated inflammatory diseases, both localized to the placenta and systemic, uterine abnormalities and possibly trauma. The role of trauma is generally overemphasized and it must be considered a rare to exceptional cause of spontaneous abortion.

The morphologic changes depend, of course, on the time interval between fetal death and passage of the products of conception. Generally, there are focal areas of decidual necrosis with intense neutrophilic infiltrations, thromboses within decidual blood vessels and considerable amounts of hemorrhage, both recent and old, within the necrotic decidua. The changes encountered in the ovum or fetus are highly variable. In many spontaneous abortions, no fetal products can be identified. In others, the fetus has undergone almost total autolysis. Placental villi may be markedly distended with fluid and devoid of blood vessels (hydropic degeneration of placenta). Such changes are interpreted as a *blighted ovum*, with failure of development of the fetal circulation within the villus leading to the progressive accumulation of hydropic fluid.

As indicated earlier, special studies often yield striking karyotypic abnormalities in many of the defective fetuses.

ECTOPIC PREGNANCY

Ectopic pregnancy is the nonspecific term applied to implantation of the fetus in any site other than the normal uterine location. The most common abnormal location is within the tubes (approximately 85 per cent). The other, far less frequently involved sites are the ovary, abdominal cavity and the intrauterine portion of the fallopian tube (interstitial pregnancy). Ectopic pregnancies are by no means uncommon and occur about once in every 100 to 150 pregnancies. It will be remembered that, according to our present knowledge, the ovum is fertilized within the tube. Any delay or obstruction to the passage of the ovum into the uterus may result in ectopic implantation. The most important pathologic condition that retards the passage of the ovum is preexisting chronic inflammatory disease within the tubes. Intrauterine tumors and previous intratubal hemorrhage are far less common causes for delayed migration of the ovum.

Ovarian pregnancy is presumed to result from the rare fertilization and trapping of the ovum within the follicle just at the time of its rupture (Fig. 27–57). Abdominal pregnancies may develop when the fertilized ovum drops out of the fimbriated end of the tube, or may occur when an implantation in the fimbriated end does not become firmly attached and either drops out and becomes reimplanted or becomes attached to adjacent organs and then predominantly develops in these extratubal sites. In all these abnormal locations, the fertilized ovum undergoes its usual development with the formation of placental tissue, amniotic sac and fetus, and the host implantation site develops decidual changes.

Anatomically, tubal pregnancy causes localized dilatation of the tube by hemorrhage (Fig. 27–58). Tubal pregnancy is the most common cause of hematosalpinx and, when such intratubal hemorrhage is found, this underlying cause should always be suspected. Histologically, the characteristic immature products of conception are present, usually fairly well preserved because the acute symptoms cause immediate surgical exploration. However, with delay, the fetal and placental tissues undergo

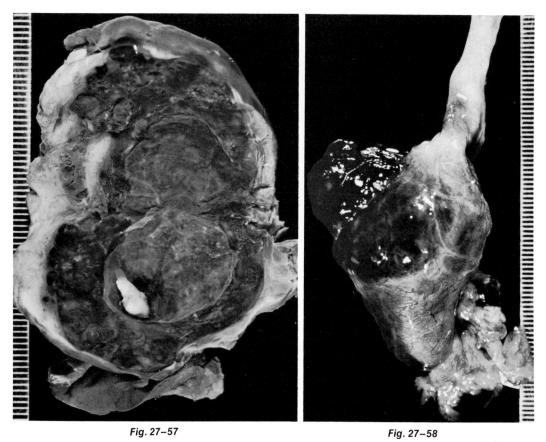

Fig. 27–57   **Fig. 27–58**

Figure 27–57. *Ovarian pregnancy. The transected ovary reveals an amniotic sac containing a deformed, pale, blighted ovum.*

Figure 27–58. *Tubal pregnancy with marked dilatation and rupture of the distal end of the tube by the contained pregnancy and subsequent hemorrhage.*

progressive necrosis, accompanied by an acute neutrophilic inflammatory infiltration. Characteristically, the implantation site within the tube is modified by the development of large, plump, decidual cells. This form of decidual reaction may also be present on the serosal covering of the tube.

The placenta is poorly attached to the wall of the tube in most instances. Intratubal hemorrhages may thus occur from partial placental separation without tubal rupture. More often the burrowing, invasive placental tissue invades the wall, sometimes penetrates the serosa and thus weakens the tubal wall. Tubal rupture and intraperitoneal hemorrhage follow. This is the usual fate of tubal pregnancies that commonly ensues two to six weeks after the onset of pregnancy. In other instances, but less commonly, the tubal pregnancy may undergo spontaneous regression due to the poor placental attachment, leading to necrosis of the products of conception, followed by proteolytic digestion and resorption of the entire gesta-

tion. If fetal death occurs within the tube at a later stage, the fetus may be retained and eventually may become calcified or mummified, sometimes to form a *lithopedion*.

Still less commonly, the tubal pregnancy is extruded through the fimbriated end into the abdominal cavity *(tubal abortion).* Under these circumstances, the placenta may retain its original site of attachment within the tube. More often, the placenta follows the fetus and becomes implanted on adjacent intrapelvic or intra-abdominal structures. The capacious abdominal cavity may then permit the full-term development of the fetus.

The clinical course of the usual form of ectopic pregnancy is punctuated by the onset of severe abdominal pain when rupture of the tube leads to a pelvic hemorrhage. In an analysis of almost 2000 ectopic pregnancies, approximately 75 per cent had ruptured, 12 per cent had been aborted into the abdomen and 14 per cent were still in situ within the tube (Beacham et al., 1956). Very often with tubal rupture, the patients rapidly pass into a shock-like state, accompanied by all the classic signs of an acute abdomen. Physical examination may disclose the tenderness in the tubal regions as well as an apparent tubal mass. In about one-third to one-half of the cases, if the patient is studied soon after the onset of symptoms, the blood serum or urine will give a positive pregnancy test. However, in the remainder of the cases, the poor implantation and vascularization, followed by the partial separation, necrosis and death of placental tissue, all militate toward low serum and urinary levels of placental hormones so that they cannot be detected by the pregnancy tests. A negative pregnancy test, then, does not rule out a tubal pregnancy. The diagnosis can sometimes also be supported by the aspiration of fresh blood from the pouch of Douglas through the posterior vaginal fornix. Endometrial biopsy may be helpful. Decidual changes develop here in less than half the cases. It must be remembered that rupture of a tubal pregnancy constitutes a major medical emergency, since about 1 in 400 of these patients dies before the hemorrhage can be controlled.

TUMORS

The two highly important tumors of the placenta are the hydatidiform mole and choriocarcinoma (chorionepithelioma). These two growths are grouped together because, in at least half the instances, choriocarcinoma is preceded by a hydatidiform mole. However, these tumors should be considered separately because, in the majority of patients, the mole is a benign lesion and many such patients subsequently have normal pregnancies, while the choriocarcinoma, contrariwise, is fatal in some instances.

HYDATIDIFORM MOLE

Hydatidiform mole is a cystic, hydropic swelling of the chorionic villi, accompanied by variable hyperplastic and anaplastic changes in the chorionic epithelium. No fetus develops. Because similar hydropic swellings of the villi occur in certain instances of fetal death, the mole is sometimes referred to as a "*hydatid degeneration,*" implying that the lesion is not a true neoplasm. Many moles are indeed completely innocuous and have little evidence of anaplasia or even hyperplasia. Such cases might be construed as degenerations. However, there is a continuum of morphologic variants from these banal forms to those that have unmistakable abnormal anaplastic proliferation of the chorionic epithelium to the ex-

treme of transformation to invasive choriocarcinomas. It is, therefore, best to consider all moles as tumors.

Incidence. They can occur at any age during active reproductive life. About one in every 2000 pregnancies results in hydatidiform mole.

Pathogenesis. Approximately one in five pregnancies terminates in spontaneous abortion and, in about half of these, the development of the ovum or fetus is pathologic or blighted. In the majority of these blighted ova, the placental tissue has variable degrees of hydatid swelling and, on microscopic examination of the affected villi, the fetal circulation is usually totally absent or, at best, is imperfectly developed. It is believed that this edema of the villi is related to the absence of an adequate functioning fetal circulation. Fluid elaborated cannot be reabsorbed and so accumulates to produce the progressive swelling. Parenthetically, it might be noted that *hydropic swelling of villi in chorionic tissue derived from abortions is a valuable morphologic criterion of a blighted ovum.* A hydatidiform mole is presumed, then, to represent an accentuation or continuance of the hydropic swelling encountered in the blighted ovum. Possibly, the development of a full-blown mole simply reflects the fact that moles are usually not delivered until the fourth to fifth months of gestation, while blighted ovum abortions almost invariably occur within the first two months. Over this longer time span, the cystic swelling of the villi becomes more accentuated, to produce the classic mole.

Morphology. In the majority of instances, hydatid moles develop within the uterus, but they may occur in any ectopic site of pregnancy. When discovered, usually in the fourth or fifth month of gestation, the uterus is usually larger (but may be normal, or even smaller) than is anticipated for the duration of the pregnancy. The uterine cavity is filled with a delicate, friable mass of thin-walled, translucent, cystic, grape-like structures that rupture easily and collapse with release of clear fluid (Fig. 27–59). These grape-like clusters are held together by delicate, filamentous fibrous strands. This "cluster of grapes" architecture is best demonstrated by floating the mole in isotonic saline solution. Careful dissection may disclose a small, usually collapsed, amniotic sac. Even when the sac is intact and filled with fluid, no ovum or, at best, only a small blighted nubbin representing the ovum, can be demonstrated. The individual cysts vary from microscopic size to locules up to 2 to 3 cm. in diameter. Theca lutein cysts are found in the ovaries bilaterally in about one-fifth of these cases. These cysts regress upon removal of the source of the chorionic gonadotropic hormone, namely, the mole.

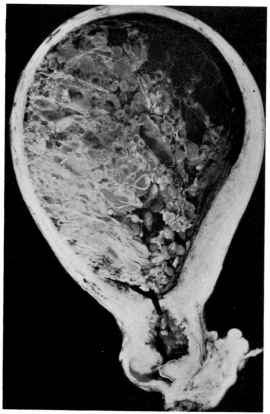

Figure 27–59. Hydatidiform mole, The uterus is filled with the classic mass of grape-like clusters. (Courtesy of Dr. Arthur Hertig from Anderson: Textbook of Pathology, C. V. Mosby Co., 1971.)

Microscopically, the principal characteristics of the mole consist of: **hydropic swelling of chorionic villi, virtual absence or inadequate development of vascularization of villi and variable degrees of hyperplasia and anaplasia of the chorionic epithelium.** In the morphologically and clinically benign forms, the villi have only small capillary channels and not the well formed vessels of the normal placenta. The central substance of the villi is a loose, myxomatous, edematous stroma, and they are covered by a thin layer of chorionic epithelium, both cytotrophoblast and syncytial trophoblast (Fig. 27–60). The epithelium is usually not multilayered and more or less resembles that found in the normal placenta.

At the opposite end of the spectrum are found moles having similar cystic dilatation of villi, accompanied, however, by striking proliferation of the chorionic epithelium to produce sheets and masses of both cuboidal and syncytial cells. Many of these epithelial masses have no clear attachment to villi in the plane of the histologic section. Anaplasia is present in this placental epithelium. However, it is extremely difficult to identify. Even in the normal

state, this epithelium is characterized by marked variability in cell morphology. Supporting this view, Park and Lees (1950) state, "Morphologically a trophoblast with a benign future is exactly like a trophoblast with a cancerous future."

For these reasons, the curettings obtained after the molar tissue has been evacuated have greatest importance as diagnostic material. These fragments will provide the more significant evidence of the extent to which the chorionic epithelium has invaded the uterine wall and blood vessels, and will thus indicate the destructiveness and probable clinical potential of the mole. By morphologic study of the curettings, moles have been divided into various grades of anatomic and probable clinical malignancy. The many groups run the gamut from the superficial noninvasive lesions that are clearly benign to the infiltrative lesions that are frankly cancerous and have become transformed into obvious choriocarcinoma. Between these extremes are found many intergrades that are designated as possibly benign, probably benign, possibly malignant and probably malignant (Hertig and Sheldon, 1947). Within these intergrades are found special types of growths that have been designated as invasive moles or chorioadenomas destruens, morphologic lesions that are characterized by abnormal inva-

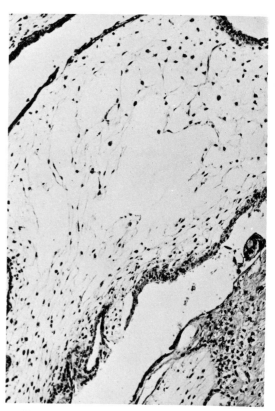

Figure 27–60. Hydatidiform mole. Histologic appearance of cystically edematous villi.

sion of the uterine wall and penetration and perforation of the uterine wall (described below). However, even these invasive moles lack the striking cancerous and metastatic potential of the aggressive choriocarcinoma to be described.

Clinical Course. From the morphologic description of the very variable nature of hydatidiform moles, it is apparent that the resultant clinical syndrome will be equally variable. In general, these patients have abnormal uterine bleeding that usually begins early in the course of the pregnancy and is frequently accompanied by the passage of a thin, watery fluid and bits of tissue that the observant patient may describe as small, grape-like masses. The uterine enlargement is more rapid then anticipated, and may even cause tension on supporting structures and lower abdominal pain. No fetus can be palpated or visualized radiographically.

Quantitative analysis of the chorionic gonadotropin may also provide valuable support. In the classic case, there are abnormally high levels of hormone in both the blood and urine. These levels greatly exceed those produced by a normal pregnancy of similar age. However, no absolute level can be cited as diagnostic. The magnitude of the abnormal elevation of the hormones can be best expressed thus: Whereas pregnancy produces titers of gonadotropic units in terms of thousands, moles elaborate titers in the tens and even hundreds of thousands. However, the hormone level may be very variable in individual cases and may, therefore, not be diagnostic. Some moles elaborate little hormone. Others may be partially necrotic or have a poor communication with the maternal circulation, with little absorption of the hormone into the maternal blood. Frequently, serial hormone determinations will indicate a rapidly mounting level that climbs faster than the usual normal single or even multiple pregnancies.

Once the diagnosis is made, the mole must be removed and the uterus curetted either through the cervix or by abdominal hysterotomy. The future clinical course of the patient depends entirely upon the malignant potential of the removed uterine contents. From many studies, it is clear that at least 80 per cent of these moles remain benign and give no further difficulty. The remaining 20 per cent, including those that fall into the categories of chorioadenoma destruens and choriocarcinoma, may cause further complications. The incidence of the development of choriocarcinoma in hydatidiform moles is probably not greater than 2 to 3 per cent.

CHORIOCARCINOMA (CHORIONEPITHELIOMA)

Choriocarcinoma is an epithelial malignancy of trophoblastic cells derived from any form of previous normal or abnormal pregnancy or from a teratogenous origin. While the majority of cases arise in the uterus, ectopic pregnancies and teratomas provide extrauterine and even extragenital sites of origin. *Choriocarcinoma should be differentiated from the locally invasive, but nonmetastasizing, forms of malignancy described as syncytial endometritis and chorioadenoma destruens.* In this strict usage, the choriocarcinoma is one of the most rapidly invasive, widely metastasizing malignancies.

Incidence. It is, fortunately, an uncommon condition that arises in probably not more than one in 20,000 to 30,000 pregnancies. It is preceded by the following conditions: 50 per cent arise in hydatidiform moles, 25 per cent in previous abortions, approximately 22 per cent in normal pregnancies, the others in ectopic pregnancies and genital and extragenital teratomas. It should be realized that, *in such teratogenous origin, choriocarcinomas may occur in males.* It can be further computed that about one in 40 hydatidiform moles may be expected to give rise to a choriocarcinoma, in contrast to one in approximately 15,000 abortions and one in approximately 150,000 normal pregnancies. It is evident, then, that the more abnormal the pregnancy, the greater the hazard of the development of this tumor.

Considerable variation in these data is encountered in the literature. Much of this variation is based upon the fact that the nonmetastasizing, clinically more benign conditions, i.e., syncytial endometritis and chorioadenoma destruens, are included in the compilation of choriocarcinomas. Obviously, such an all-inclusive use of the term provides a higher frequency of so-called choriocarcinomas or, as they are more apt to be called in such usage, chorionepitheliomas. Moreover, the clinical patterns ascribed to this broader group are much more variable and are, in many instances, nonmetastasizing and not usually fatal. It is desirable, then, to describe these variants as well as the pure form of choriocarcinoma.

Syncytial Endometritis. Syncytial endometritis is a somewhat controversial lesion characterized by the appearance of plump, syncytium-like cells in the deeper levels of the myometrium. It usually follows a hydatidiform mole. It may simply represent an exaggeration of the normal tendency for syncytial or decidua-like cells to appear within the intermuscular septa of the myometrium in any placental implantation site. Alternatively, the syncytium-like cells might actually be derived from chorionic epithelium that has invaded the myometrium. In any event, a sufficient number of cases have been treated by simple curettage to indicate that the condition is benign, probably not a true neoplasm and, undoubtedly, not even a remote relative to the true choriocarcinoma.

Chorioadenoma Destruens. Chorioadenoma destruens is defined as a cellular, invasive mole that penetrates or even perforates the uterine wall. It differs from syncytial endometritis in that there is clear invasion of the myometrium by **well developed chorionic villi, accompanied by proliferation of both cuboidal and syncytial chorionic epithelial components.** This tumor is more cellular and more invasive than the syncytial endometritis, but is only locally destructive and does not metastasize. By penetration of the uterine serosa, it may locally invade adjacent structures and, therefore, give rise to considerable difficulty in its excision.

Choriocarcinoma. Choriocarcinoma is a purely epithelial cellular malignancy that does **not** produce chorionic villi and grows, as do other cancers, by the abnormal proliferation of both the cuboidal and syncytial cells of the placental epithelium. It is sometimes possible to identify anaplasia within such abnormal proliferation replete with abnormal mitoses. The tumor invades the underlying myometrium, frequently penetrates blood vessels and lymphatics and extends out, in some cases, onto the uterine serosa and adjacent structures (Figs. 27–61 and 27–62). In its rapid growth, it is subject to hemorrhage, ischemic necrosis and secondary inflammatory infiltration. From this histologic pattern, the characteristic macroscopic features can be deduced.

Classically, the choriocarcinoma is a soft, fleshy, yellow-white tumor with a marked tendency to form large pale areas of ischemic necrosis, foci of cystic softening and extensive hemorrhage. This pattern of friable hemorrhagic tissue may be encountered as a small area within a previous mole, as a small mural mass recurring after previous evacuation of the uterus or as a large, bulky tumor that fills and expands the uterine cavity. However, attention should be called to one bizarre macroscopic pattern. Because of its predisposition to undergo infarction necrosis, not uncommonly metastatic, unmistakable choriocarcinoma is found in the lungs, bone marrow, liver and other favored sites of spread in the complete absence of a primary lesion in the uterus or in any extrauterine site. This paradoxical situation is encountered not only in the female but also in the male when the tumor may be primary in the testis or some teratoid tumor. Under such circumstances, it is postulated that the primary focus underwent total necrosis and resorption after it had metastasized.

Clinical Course. Classically, the uterine choriocarcinoma does not produce a large, bulky mass. It becomes manifest only by irregular spotting of a bloody, brown, sometimes foul-smelling fluid. This discharge may appear

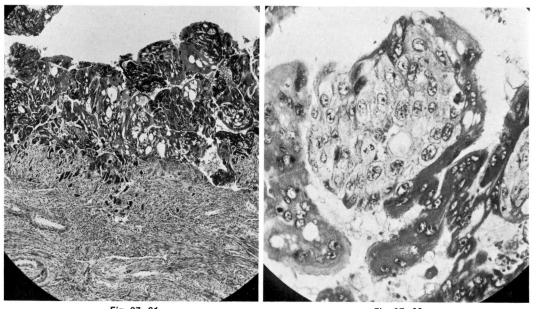

Fig. 27–61

Fig. 27–62

Figure 27–61. *Low power view of choriocarcinoma of uterine wall showing invasion of underlying myometrium.*

Figure 27–62. *High power detail of choriocarcinoma illustrating the two types of epithelial cells—cytotrophoblast and syncytiotrophoblast.*

in the course of an apparently normal pregnancy, may begin after a miscarriage or may become manifest following a curettage for retained products of conception. Sometimes the tumor does not appear until months later. Usually, by the time the tumor is discovered locally, x-ray films of the chest and bones already disclose the presence of metastatic lesions. The hormone titers are markedly elevated by choriocarcinoma to levels above those encountered in hydatidiform moles. Hormone titers of hundreds of thousands to millions of gonadotropic units are not uncommon. When such extreme elevations are found, the diagnosis of choriocarcinoma is virtually established. However, occasional tumors have been recorded as not having produced any hormone, and many tumors have become so necrotic as to become functionally inactive. Therefore, low levels of gonadotropins that fall within the range of normal pregnancy are sometimes encountered. But the final diagnosis must rest upon the histologic demonstration of unmistakable cancerous invasiveness in the curettings or other tissue biopsies. In the male, the demonstration of gonadotropin in the urine or blood provides a very valuable indicator of this form of malignancy. Rarely, in the unusual cases mentioned, the primary site may fail to disclose tumor tissue.

Widespread metastases are characteristic of these tumors. Favored sites of involvement are the lungs (50 per cent) and vagina (30 to 40 per cent), followed in descending order of frequency by the brain, liver and kidney. However, in the dissemination of this tumor through the vascular system, any organ or tissue may be involved.

It may be recalled from an earlier discussion (p. 147) that the therapy of choriocarcinomas arising in the placenta represents a triumph for both chemotherapy and probably the immune response of the host. Chemotherapy (principally methotrexate) has achieved over an 80 per cent cure rate with these placental cancers which were once almost universally fatal (Hertz et al., 1961) (Bagshawe, 1969). As was pointed out, no such control can be achieved with choriocarcinomas of teratogenous origin in either the male or the female. It is postulated that the therapy reduces the viability of the cancer, permitting the immune response to histocompatibility antigens of paternal origin in the placental neoplastic cells to effect the ultimate control.

REFERENCES

Aaro, L. A., et al.: Endocervical polyps. Obstet. Gynec., 21:659, 1963.

Allan, M. S., and Hertig, A. T.: Carcinoma of the ovary. Amer. J. Obstet. Gynec., 58:640, 1949.

Anderson, M. D.: Carcinoma of the Uterine Cervix and Ovary. Hospital and Tumor Institute, Houston, Texas, Year Book Medical Publishers, 1962.

Asadourian, L. A., and Taylor, H. B.: Dysgerminoma. An analysis of 105 cases. Obstet. Gynec., 33:370, 1969.

Bagshawe, K. D.: Choriocarcinoma. In The Clinical Biology of the Trophoblast and its Tumours. Baltimore, Williams and Wilkins Co., 1969.

Beacham, W. D., et al.: Ectopic pregnancy at New Orleans Charity Hospital. Amer. J. Obstet. Gynec., 72:830, 1956.

Boyes, D. A., et al.: Significance of in situ carcinoma of the uterine cervix. Brit. Med. J., 1:203, 1962.

Breen, J. L., and Neubecker, R. D.: Malignant teratoma of the ovary. An analysis of 17 cases. Obstet. Gynec., 21:669, 1963.

Bromberg, Y. M., et al.: Early endometrial carcinoma following prolonged estrogen administration in an ovariectomized woman. Obstet. Gynec., 14:221, 1959.

Campbell, P. E., and Barter, R. A.: The significance of atypical endometrial hyperplasia. J. Obstet. Gynaec. Brit. Comm., 68:668, 1961.

Candy, J., and Abell, M. R.: Progestogen-induced adenomatous hyperplasia of the uterine cervix. J.A.M.A., 203:323, 1968.

Chamberlain, G., and Wood, C.: Stein-Leventhal syndrome. Brit. Med. J., 1:96, 1964.

Chamlian, D. L., and Taylor, H. B.: Endometrial hyperplasia in young women. Obstet. Gynec., 36:659, 1970.

Collins, C. G., et al.: Cancer involving the vulva. A report on 109 consecutive cases. Amer. J. Obstet. Gynec., 87:762, 1963.

DeAlvarez, R. R.: Causes of death in cancer of cervix uteri. Amer. J. Obstet. Gynec., 54:91, 1947.

Dockerty, M. B.: Ovarian neoplasms: a collective review of the recent literature. Int. Abstr. Surg., 81:179, 1945.

Dunn, J. E., Jr.: Preliminary findings of the Memphis-Shelby County uterine cancer study and their interpretation. Amer. J. Public Health, 48:861, 1958.

Editorial: Carcinoma of the cervix and herpesvirus. Brit. Med. J., 2:548, 1972.

Elliot, R. I. K.: On the prevention of carcinoma of the cervix. Lancet, 1:231, 1964.

Foster, L. N., and Montgomery, R.: Endometrial carcinoma: a review of prior biopsies. Amer. J. Clin. Path., 43:26, 1965.

Gagnon, F.: Contribution to the study of the etiology and prevention of cancer of the cervix of the uterus. Amer. J. Obstet. Gynec., 60:516, 1950.

Gall, S. A., et al.: The morphologic effects of oral contraceptive agents on the cervix. J.A.M.A., 207:2243, 1969.

Glucksman, A.: Can radiosensitivity and histopathology of cervical cancer be correlated? J.A.M.A., 193:823, 1965.

Goldzieher, J. W., and Green, J. A.: The polycystic ovary. I. Clinical and histological features. J. Clin. Endocr., 22:325, 1962.

Gore, H., and Hertig, A.: Premalignant lesions of the endometrium. Clin. Obstet. Gynec., 5:1448, 1962.

Graham, R.: The effect of radiation on vaginal cells in cervical carcinoma. Surg., Gynec. Obstet., 84:166, 1947.

Gray, L. A., and Barnes, N. L.: Endometrioid carcinoma of the ovary. Obstet. Gynec., 29:694, 1967.

Greenwald, P., et al.: Vaginal cancer after maternal treatment with synthetic estrogens. New Eng. J. Med., 285:390, 1971.

Groseclose, E. S.: Clinical significance of endometriosis. Virginia Med. Monthly, 81:253, 1954.

Gusberg, S. B., et al.: Precursors of corpus cancer. II. A clinical and pathological study of adenomatous hyperplasia. Amer. J. Obstet. Gynec., 68:1472, 1954.

Herbst, A. L., et al.: Adenocarcinoma of the vagina. Association of maternal stilbestrol therapy with tumor appearance in young women. New Eng. J. Med., 284:878, 1971.

Hertig, A. T., and Sheldon, W. H.: Hydatidiform mole: a pathologicoclinical correlation of 200 cases. Amer. J. Obstet. Gynec., 43:1, 1947.

Hertig, A. T., and Sommers, S. C.: Genesis of endometrial carcinoma. I. Study of prior biopsies. Cancer, 2:946, 1949.

Hertig, A. T., et al.: Genesis of endometrial carcinoma. III. Carcinoma in situ. Cancer, 2:964, 1949.

Hertz, R., et al.: Five years' experience with the chemotherapy of metastatic choriocarcinoma and related trophoblastic tumors in women. Amer. J. Obstet. Gynec., 82:631, 1961.

Janovski, N. A., and Ames, S.: Lichen sclerosus et atrophicus of the vulva: a poorly understood disease entity. Obstet. Gynec., 22:697, 1963.

Johnson, L. D., et al.: The histogenesis of carcinoma in situ of the uterine cervix. Cancer, 17:213, 1964.

Koss, L. G., et al.: Some histological aspects of behavior of epidermoid carcinoma in situ and related lesions of the uterine cervix. A long-term prospective study. Cancer, 16:1160, 1963.

Langley, I. I., et al.: Relation of leukoplakic vulvitis to squamous carcinoma of the vulva. Amer. J. Obstet. Gynec., 62:167, 1951.

Lund, C. J.: Epitaph for cervical carcinoma. J.A.M.A., 175:98, 1961.

Malhotra, S. L.: A study of carcinoma of uterine cervix with special reference to its causation and prevention. Brit. J. Cancer, 25:62, 1971.

Mansell, H., and Hertig, A. T.: Granulosa theca cell tumors and endometrial carcinoma: a study of their relationship in a survey of 80 cases. Obstet. Gynec., 6:385, 1955.

Marcial-Rojas, R. A., and Medina, R.: Cystic teratomas of the ovary: a clinical and pathologic analysis of 268 tumors. Arch. Path., 66:577, 1958.

McGarrity, K. A.: Recent modifications to the international clinical staging of cancer of the cervix and the corpus uteri and a new staging of vaginal carcinoma. Med. J. Aust., 1:92, 1963.

McKay, D. G.: Clinical significance of the pathology of toxemia of pregnancy. Circulation, Supp. II, 30:66, 1964.

McKay, D. G., et al.: Histochemical observations on the endometrium. Obstet. Gynec., 8:22, 1956.

Meigs, J. V.: Endometriosis. New Eng. J. Med., 226:147, 1942.

Merrill, J. A., and Ross, N. L.: Cancer of the vulva. Cancer, 14:13, 1961.

Merskey, C., et al.: The defibrination syndrome. Clinical features and laboratory diagnosis. Brit. J. Haemat., 13:528, 1967.

Montgomery, H., et al.: Kraurosis, leukoplakia and pruritus vulvae: correlation of clinical and pathologic observations with further studies regarding resection of the sensory nerves of perineum. Arch. Derm. Syph., 30:80, 1934.

Neigus, I.: Ovarian dysgerminoma with chorionepithelioma: report of a case. Amer. J. Obstet. Gynec., 69:838, 1955.

Netter, A. P.: The Stein-Leventhal syndrome. Proc. Roy. Soc. Med., 54:1006, 1961.

Nieburgs, H. E.: The significance of tissue cell changes preceding uterine cervix carcinoma. Cancer, 16:141, 1963.

Norris, H. J., and Taylor, H. B.: Prognosis of granulosa-theca cell tumors of the ovary. Cancer, 21:255, 1968.

Ober, W. B.: Uterine sarcomas: histogenesis and taxonomy. Ann. N.Y. Acad. Sci., 75:568, 1959.

O'Hern, T. M., and Neubecker, R. D.: Arrhenoblastoma. Obstet. Gynec., 19:758, 1962.

O'Malley, B. W.: Mechanisms of action of steroid hormones. New Eng. J. Med., 284:370, 1971.

Old, J. W., and Jones, D. G.: Squamous carcinoma in situ of the uterine cervix. III. A long term follow-up of 23 unsuspected cases of 6 to 10 year duration without interim treatment. Cancer, 18:1622, 1965.

Palmer, J. P., et al.: Carcinoma of the vulva: report of 313 cases. Surg. Gynec. Obstet., 88:435, 1949.

Park, W. W., and Lees, J. C.: Choriocarcinoma: a general review with an analysis of 516 cases. Arch. Path., 49:73, 205, 1950.

Peterson, W. F., and Novak, E. R.: Endometrial polyps. Obstet. Gynec., 8:40, 1956.

Plummer, G., and Masterson, J. G.: Herpes simplex virus and cancer of the cervix. Amer. J. Obstet. Gynec., 111:81, 1971.

Rawls, W. E., et al.: The association of herpesvirus type 2 and carcinoma of the uterine cervix. Amer. J. Epidem., 89:547, 1969.

Richardson, G. S.: Endometrial cancer as an estrogen-progesterone target. New Eng. J. Med., 286:645, 1972.

Richardson, G. S.: Ovarian physiology. New Eng. J. Med., 274:1064, 1183, 1966.

Rutledge, F.: Can irradiation destroy metastatic pelvic lymph nodes? J.A.M.A., 193:1102, 1965.

Santesson, L., and Kottmeier, H. L.: General classification of ovarian tumors. In Gentil, F., and Junqueira, A. C. (eds.): Ovarian Cancer. U.I.C.C. Monograph Series, Vol. 3. New York, Springer-Verlage, 1968, p. 1.

Scully, R. E.: Recent progress in ovarian cancer. Hum. Path., 1:73, 1970.

Scully, R. E., et al.: The development of malignancy and endometriosis. Clin. Obstet. Gynec., 9:384, 1966.

Singh, R. P., and Carr, D. H.: Anatomic findings in human abortions of known chromosome constitution. Obstet. Gynec., 29:806, 1967.

Sjostedt, S., and Wahlen, T.: Prognosis of granulosa cell tumors. Acta Obstet. Gynec. Scand., Suppl. 6, 40:1, 1961.

Speert, H.: Corpus cancer. Clinical, pathological, and etiological aspects. Cancer, 1:584, 1948.

Spiro, R. H., and Koss, L. G.: Myosarcoma of the uterus: a clinico-pathologic study. Cancer, 18:571, 1965.

Taylor, H. B., and Norris, H. J.: Mesenchymal tumors of the uterus. IV. Diagnosis and prognosis of leiomyosarcomas. Arch. Path., 82:40, 1966.

Taylor, H. C., Jr.: Studies on the clinical and biological evolution of adenocarcinoma of the ovary. J. Obstet. Gynaec., Brit. Comm., 66:827, 1959.

Thiede, H. A., and Lund, C. J.: Prognostic factors in endometrial carcinoma. Obstet. Gynec., 20:149, 1962.

Thurlbeck, W. M., and Scully, R. E.: Solid teratoma of the ovary. A clinicopathologic analysis of 9 cases. Cancer, 13:804, 1960.

Tighe, J. R.: Brenner tumors of the ovary: a clinico-pathological study. J. Obstet. Gynaec. Brit. Comm., 68:292, 1961.

Wagner, D., et al.: Deoxyribonucleic acid content of presumed precursors of endometrial carcinoma. Cancer, 20:2067, 1967.

Wentz, W. B.: Effect of a progestational agent on endometrial hyperplasia and endometrial cancer. Obstet. Gynec., 24:370, 1964.

Wheeler, J. D., and Hertig, A. T.: The pathologic anatomy of carcinoma of the uterus. I. Squamous carcinoma of the cervix. Amer. J. Clin. Path., 25:345, 1955.

Wheelock, M. C., and Warren, S.: Leiomyosarcoma of the uterus. Ann. Surg., 116:882, 1942.

Whelton, J., and Kottmeier, H. L.: Primary carcinoma of the vagina: a study of a Radiumhemmet series of 146 cases. Acta. Gynec. Scand., 41:22, 1962.

Williams, J. T., and Kinney, T. D.: Myometrial hypertrophy (so-called fibrosis uteri). Amer. J. Obstet. Gynec., 47:380, 1944.

Woodruff, J. D., et al.: Ovarian teratomas. Relationships of histologic and ontogenic factors to prognosis. Amer. J. Obstet. Gynec., 102:702, 1968.

World Health Organization: Five years of research on human genetics. W.H.O. Chron., 24:248, 1970.

Wurtz, K. G.: Mixed mesodermal tumors of the female genital tract. Illinois Med. J., 96:264, 1949.

28

THE BREAST

NORMAL

Embryogenesis and Development. The breast is a modified skin sweat gland that develops into a complex functional structure in the female, but remains as a rudimentary organ in the male. It arises from an epidermal thickening on the ventral surface of the body at approximately the sixth week of fetal development. Bilateral ridges (the milk line) develop between the upper and lower limb buds. These ridges totally atrophy save for several persistent cephalad thickenings which later give rise to the nipples. During the second trimester of fetal life, cords of cells grow downward from the basal layer of the epidermis, and later give rise to the primary mammary ducts. At first solid, the cords eventually develop lumina so that, at the time of birth, rudimentary branching ducts are present, which fan out in a small area about the region of the nipple and the areola. Development of the breast is by no means complete at the time of birth. Progressive growth and branching of the mammary ducts occur at a very slow pace during prepubertal life. Mammary development ceases at about this stage in the male. In the female, prior to the onset of menstruation, the growth rate increases with branching of ducts and proliferation of the interductal stroma. During adolescence, stromal growth is responsible for most of the increases in the mass of the breast but, at the same time, the terminal small ducts give rise to many small, blind, saccular outpouchings—rudimentary gland buds. Under the influence of the ovarian hormones and the hormones of pregnancy, further changes occur which will be described.

Anatomy. Only a few features of the gross anatomy, of special interest to the pathologist, bear repetition at this time. While it is common to consider each breast as a large, single, secretory gland, in reality each is comprised of 15 to 20 separate branching glands, each of which is totally autonomous and has no anastomotic communications with its neighbors. These individual glands are wedge-shaped segments. Each drains through a separate main excretory or lactiferous duct into the nipple. The orifices of these mammary ducts are readily identified about the outer margin of the nipple. These anatomic details aid in the understanding of pathologic processes which arise from obstruction of a single major duct.

Commonly a long tongue-like process of breast tissue, the axillary appendage, extends from the main mass up into the anterior axillary line toward and even into the axilla. This minor deviation is sometimes of considerable significance, since it is, on occasion, mistaken for a tumor mass arising in the breast and, at other times, it may give rise to tumors or other abnormalities which are mistaken for involvements of the axillary lymph nodes.

It is the condensations of the fibrous stroma that create the suspensory ligaments which anchor the breast to the deep fascia of the thoracic wall. The stroma is largely dense collagenous connective tissue heavily admixed with fat. It is this stromal element which gives the breast its characteristic yielding consistency. The epithelial component, comprising approximately 10 to 15 per cent of the bulk of the virginal breast, is virtually inapparent on palpation and on gross inspection.

Histology. The histology of the female breast is constantly changing under the influence of the ovarian hormones and is markedly modified by the hormones of pregnancy. At the time of puberty, the breast consists only of a complex system of branching ducts that drain into the nipple; each duct terminates at the other end in a number of small saccular gland buds that comprise an individual duct lobule. These terminal buddings are enclosed in a loose, delicate, myxomatous stroma that contains a scattering of lymphocytes, and the individual lobules are enclosed within a more dense, collagenous, fibrous, interlobular stroma.

Just as the endometrium rises and ebbs with each menstrual cycle, so does the breast. Following the menstrual period, with the progressive rise in estrogen, the ductal epithelium and the epithelium of the gland buds proliferate and continue to develop throughout the menstrual cycle. During this time, the ducts and gland buds become slightly dilated and hypertrophied. It is believed that during the last half of the menstrual cycle, under the influence of progesterone, stromal growth and edema begin. This combined stimulatory effect of estrogen and progesterone upon the intralobular loose connective tissue accounts for the sense of fullness commonly experienced by women during the premenstrual phase of the cycle. At this same time in the cycle, abortive secretory activity appears in the gland buds and further accentuates the ductal dilatation. At the time of the menstrual period, the fall in estrogen and progesterone levels is followed by desquamation of epithelial cells, atrophy of the intralobular connective tissue, disappearance of the increased interstitial edema fluid, and overall shrinkage in the size of the ducts and gland buds. In the nonpregnant female, then, the size of the ducts and gland buds and the prominence of the epithe-

lial linings and periductal and intraductal stroma vary according to the phase of the menstrual cycle.

Understanding these cyclic changes, we can now present the basic histology of the breast. The stratified squamous epithelium that covers the areola and nipple extends only superficially into the mouths of the main lactiferous ducts. It soon becomes transformed into a pseudostratified columnar and double-layered cuboidal epithelium that lines the major breast ducts. As the ducts branch and become smaller, the epithelium tends to become a single layer of cells but, in the smaller ducts and sometimes even in the gland buds, a low flattened layer of cells (reserve and myoepithelial cells) can be identified beneath the more prominent lining epithelium. The intralobular and periductal connective tissue has a loose, myxomatous appearance, and is, therefore, readily distinguished from the surrounding interlobular denser stroma. During the late phases of each menstrual cycle, considerable numbers of lymphocytes accumulate in the periductal tissue. The interpretation of these cells as indicators of inflammatory disease, particularly when found in pathologic breasts, has led to the erroneous concept that cystic disease of the breast is an inflammatory condition, thus, the designation chronic mastitis. In the sections to follow, it will be indicated that deviations from the normal cycle of proliferation and regression underlie the development of this important entity, better known as cystic hyperplasia of the breast.

It is only with the onset of pregnancy that the breast assumes its complete morphologic maturation and functional activity. From each gland bud, numerous true secretory glands pouch out to form grape-like clusters. As a consequence, the breast is converted into an almost solid glandular structure that, indeed, comes to resemble the pancreas. As a consequence, there is a reversal of the usual stromal-glandular relationship so that, by the end of pregnancy, the breast is composed almost entirely of glands separated by a relatively scant amount of stroma. The secretory glands are lined by a single layer of cuboidal cells which, in the third trimester, begin to assume secretory activity. Vacuoles of lipid material are found within the cells, and immediately following birth, the secretion of milk begins. The lipid material formed prior to birth accounts for the secretion of colostrum.

Following lactation, the glands once again regress and atrophy, the ducts shrink, and the total breast size diminishes remarkably. However, complete regression to the stage of the normal virginal breast usually does not occur, and some increase of glandular parenchyma remains as a permanent residual. With this postlactation atrophy, the stromal connective tissue once again proliferates to reconstitute, to a greater or lesser extent, the former volume of the breast. Inadequate stromal growth accounts for the loss in consistency and volume of the involutional breast.

With the menopause, the ducts and gland buds further atrophy with more shrinkage of the intra- and interlobular stroma. The gland buds may almost totally disappear in the very aged, and leave only ducts to create a morphologic pattern that comes close to that of the male. However, in most women, there is sufficient persistent estrogenic stimulation, possibly of adrenal origin, to maintain vestigial remnants of gland buds that differentiate even the very aged female breast from the male breast.

Before closing the consideration of the normal breast, mention should be made of the influence of maternal hormones on the neonatal breast. These may cause considerable proliferation of the ductal epithelium and periductal connective tissue in the newborn. Accordingly, it is not uncommon to find hypertrophy and swelling of the breasts in the postnatal infant. Sometimes the maternal hormones of pregnancy cause abortive secretory activity with the actual appearance of secretion at the nipple. These changes are entirely normal and should not be confused with inflammation or tumor formation. As the levels of the maternal hormones fall in the infant after birth, these breast changes promptly regress and are usually gone by the second week of infant life.

PATHOLOGY

FEMALE BREAST

Lesions of the breast are preponderantly confined to the female. In the male, the breast is a rudimentary structure relatively insensitive to endocrine influences and apparently resistive to neoplastic growth. In the female, on the other hand, the more complex breast structure, the greater breast volume and the extreme sensitivity to endocrine influences all predispose this organ to a number of pathologic conditions.

The breast is the most common site of development of cancer in the female and alone accounts for about one-fifth of all malignancies in this sex. Notwithstanding this high incidence, benign tumors and tumor-like conditions are more frequent than these malignant neoplasms.

It is obvious, then, that diseases of the female breast have great importance in clinical medicine. Therefore, the major portion of this chapter is devoted to exclusive consideration of the female breast. Only at the conclusion will brief reference be made to disorders of the male breast. The two disorders of the female breast that assume preponderant importance are cystic hyperplasia and carcinoma. Since both these entities give rise to masses or lumps in the breast, the entire consideration of the pathology of this organ should be oriented within the framework of: What lesions produce masses? What is the significance of the mass? May it be confused clinically with a carcinoma? Does the lesion have a tendency to become malignant?

CONGENITAL ANOMALIES

These anomalies run the gamut from congenital absence of the breasts to abnormal numbers of breasts, but as a group these entities are rare and of limited clinical significance.

Supernumerary Nipples or Breasts. These result from the persistence of epidermal thickenings along the line of the ventral ridges, referred to in the embryogenesis of this organ as the milk line. Development of these aberrant foci gives rise to the formation of nipples, or even rudimentary breast structures, along the milk line, both below the adult breast and above it in the anterior axillary fold. They are usually readily identified on clinical examination, and only rarely produce confusion with a skin or subcutaneous tumor. Rarely the disorders that affect the normally situated breast may arise in these heterotopic foci, and occasionally the cyclic changes of the menstrual cycle cause painful premenstrual enlargements of these supernumerary structures.

Accessory Breast Tissue. Extension of breast tissue into the anterior axillary fold or axilla has already been described as being so common that it hardly merits designation as an anomaly. However, these minor aberrations may be the site for the development of tumors or abnormal proliferative or cystic changes. The chief importance of such lesions lies in the fact that they may create masses which appear to be outside the breast and are, therefore, commonly misidentified as lesions of the axillary lymph nodes or even as metastases from an occult breast cancer.

Congenital Inversion of the Nipples. This occurs in many women, particularly those who have large or pendulous breasts. The cause of this abnormality is obscure. It may be related to failure of normal elongation of the ducts and tension upon the nipple, made more apparent by the accumulation of large amounts of subcutaneous fat and enlargement of the breast. Commonly, this inversion is corrected during the growth activity of pregnancy, or it may sometimes be corrected by simple traction upon the nipples. Nipple inversion is of clinical significance, since it may frustrate attempts at nursing, and may also be confused with acquired retraction of the nipple, sometimes observed in mammary cancer and in inflammations of the breast.

INFLAMMATIONS

Inflammations of the breast are, on the whole, uncommon and consist of only a relatively few forms of acute and chronic disease. Of these, the most important is nonspecific acute mastitis, virtually confined to the lactating period. Breast abscesses are included under the heading of acute mastitis. The other forms of mastitis consist of tuberculosis, usually a complication of tuberculous mediastinal lymphadenitis; syphilis in the form of a chancre on the nipple or areola, or possibly a skin syphilid; and mammary duct ectasia or plasma cell mastitis, an entity of obscure etiology.

ACUTE MASTITIS AND BREAST ABSCESS

During the early weeks of nursing, the breast is rendered vulnerable to bacterial infection by the development of cracks and fissures in the nipples. The disease is not confined, however, to the postpartum state and may be predisposed to by eczema and other dermatologic conditions of the nipples. From this portal of entry, *Staphylococcus aureus* usually, or streptococci less commonly, invade the breast substance.

Usually the disease is unilateral. The staphylococcus tends to produce a focalized area of inflammation that may progress to the formation of single or multiple abscesses. The streptococcus tends to cause, as it does in all tissue, a diffuse spreading infection that eventually involves the entire organ. Both agents produce characteristic reddening, swelling, pain and increased consistency in the affected breast substance, commonly with considerable edema and thickening of the overlying skin. During this early stage, the inflammatory changes may consist largely of the collection of pus within the affected ducts accompanied by periductal neutrophilic infiltration with involvement of the gland buds and surrounding stroma. However, in the course of time, the suppurative necrosis may destroy large, but usually only focal, areas of breast substance. Surgical drainage may limit the spread of the infection, but whatever its extent, the destroyed breast substance is replaced by fibrous scar as a permanent residual of the inflammatory process. Such scarring creates a localized area of increased consistency often accompanied by retraction of the skin or the nipple, changes that may later be mistaken for a neoplasm. The similarity to a breast tumor is further heightened by the inflammatory enlargement of the axillary nodes that drain the infection. The skin and nipple retraction usually regresses in time as the fibrous scar stretches. Only rarely are sufficient breast substance or main excretory ducts involved to seriously impair future secretory activity of the breast.

MAMMARY DUCT ECTASIA (COMEDOMASTITIS)

Mammary duct ectasia is the designation of choice given to the entity that is also called *plasma cell mastitis. It is an obscure entity characterized chiefly by dilatation of ducts, inspissation of breast secretion, and marked periductal and interstitial chronic inflammatory reaction in which lymphocytes and plasma cells are prominent.* This disorder tends to occur in the fifth decade of life and is somewhat more common in women who have borne children. Its genesis is obscure and, as can be appreciated from the various designations applied to this condition, it is thought to be due possibly to inspissation of lipid debris, bacterial infection or virus infections. The inspissation of secretion within the ducts is the favored view.

Supporting this theory, about half the patients have some difficulty such as inverted nipples, difficulties in nursing their young and cracked nipples. The accumulated debris excites a sterile ductal inflammation followed by escape of the lipid material into the surrounding stroma with resultant, more widespread, chronic inflammatory reaction to the necrotic lipid material. According to this concept, then, the terms mammary duct ectasia and comedomastitis are applicable (Haagensen, 1951) (Tice et al., 1948). On the other hand, it is considered by others as an inflammatory reaction to some bacterial, viral or other obscure agent and is thus designated as plasma cell mastitis.

But it should be pointed out that there is disagreement as to whether mammary duct ectasia and plasma cell mastitis are, indeed, identical entities. The majority hold the view that these lesions reflect one and the same entity and create varying tissue patterns only by virtue of the differing stages of chronicity at which the lesions are examined.

Anatomically, the condition usually affects a single area of breast substance drained through one of the major excretory ducts. A poorly defined area of induration, thickening or ropiness results. Rarely, however, the entire breast is affected when all the ducts are involved, or the disease may even be bilateral. Dilated, firm, ropy ducts are frequently palpable through the skin, and become more readily apparent on section. Thick, cheesy material can be extruded from these cut ducts by slight pressure. The interductal connective tissue is of increased consistency and sometimes contains, on section, foci of yellow necrosis. Retraction of the nipple by the inflammatory scarring may heighten the similarity to malignancy.

On histologic examination, **the dominant features are (1) duct dilatation, (2) occlusion of ducts by inspissated secretion and white cells, (3) periductal inflammation and (4) foci of lipid granulomatous inflammation.** The affected ducts are filled by granular, necrotic, acidophilic debris (secretion), which sometimes contains mixed white cells, principally lipid-laden macrophages (Fig. 28–1). The lining epithelial cells of the ducts may persist in small foci but, for the most part, they are necrotic and atrophic. The periductal and interductal inflammation in the full-blown disease, caused by inflammatory erosion of the duct walls, is manifested by heavy infiltrates of inflammatory cells, i.e., neutrophils, lymphocytes and histiocytes, with a striking predominance of plasma cells. Occasionally, foci of inflammation about lipid debris create small, granulomatous, inflammatory reactions (pseudotubercles or pseudosarcoid lesions), composed of central masses of foamy macrophages and precipitated spicules of cholesterol and fatty acids, surrounded by a fibroblastic proliferation and scattered foreign body giant cells. The axillary lymph nodes that drain the focus may also be the site of chronic lymphadenitis and secondary enlargement.

This lesion is of clinical significance because it produces a focal or ill-defined diffuse area of pain, tenderness, induration and ropiness in the peri- or subareolar region. Fixation to the skin, with retraction of the skin or nipple, may easily cause the lesion to be mistaken for a neoplasm. The concurrence of axillary node enlargement further heightens the similarity by raising the possibility of metastatic spread. Although neoplasia may occur in these breasts, it is highly doubtful that the two are causally related.

FAT NECROSIS

Focal necrosis of fat tissues in the breast, followed by an inflammatory reaction, is an uncommon lesion that tends to occur as an isolated, sharply localized process in one breast. *The subsequent inflammatory scarring may give rise to a focus of increased consistency* that is potentially capable of confusion with a new growth, hence the clinical importance of this otherwise innocuous condition. This entity has been known as *traumatic fat necrosis*, since in about one-half of the cases a history of trauma can be obtained. However, in its exposed position, the breast is subject to almost daily trauma of varying severity, yet fat necrosis is an uncommon lesion. Moreover, in about one-half of the cases, there is no history of trauma, although here it might be argued that the daily exposure to trauma lowers the threshold of awareness so that the actual initiating injury may pass unnoticed. However, fat necrosis occurs in other fat depots outside the breast, sometimes in areas that are considerably more protected from trauma. The causal role of physical injury should, therefore, not be too quickly accepted.

The morphologic changes depend upon the duration of the lesion and the stage of the inflamma-

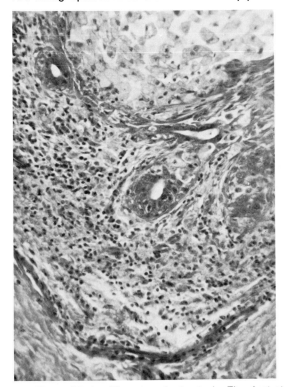

Figure 28–1. *Mammary duct ectasia. The duct at the top is partially filled with lipid-laden macrophages. The ductal epithelium is destroyed and the periductal tissues infiltrated with leukocytes.*

tory reaction. In the early stages, the focus may consist of hemorrhage and, later, central liquefactive necrosis of fat surrounded by a zone of increased consistency. Still later, it may be a more or less well defined nodule of gray-white, increased consistency, containing possibly small **foci of chalky white or hemorrhagic debris.** In the course of time, the area is converted to a dense fibrous scar, or the central focus of necrosis may become encysted, pigmented and sometimes calcified. Usually such focal areas are extremely small and are rarely over 2 cm. in diameter (Adair and Munzer, 1947).

Histologically, the central focus of necrotic fat cells is surrounded by lipid-filled macrophages and an intense neutrophilic infiltration. Then, over the next few days, progressive fibroblastic proliferation, increased vascularization and lymphocytic and histiocytic infiltration wall off the focus. By this time, the central necrotic fat cells have disappeared and may be represented only by foamy, lipid-laden macrophages and spicules of crystalline lipids (Fig. 28–2). Still later, foreign body giant cells, calcium salts and blood pigments make their appearance, and eventually the focus is replaced by scar tissue or is encysted and walled off by collagenous tissue.

This condition is without clinical significance save for its possible confusion with a tumor, when fibrosis has created a clinically palpable mass. The tendency for the focus of fibrosis to be attached to the skin, sometimes causing dimpling or retraction, and the focal calcifications seen on mammography further heighten the resemblance to cancer.

GALACTOCELE

A galactocele represents a cystic dilatation of a duct occurring during lactation. It implies some cause for ductal obstruction, such as inflammation, fibrocystic disease or neoplasia. Occasionally, a single duct is affected to produce an isolated cyst, but more often multiple ducts are involved. During the acute phase, the palpable nodules are tender and, when exposed, contain a milky fluid enclosed within thin, dilated ductal walls. In the course of time, the tenderness abates and the cystic dilatations become more firm. At this time, transection may disclose an inspissated cheesy content. Secondary infection may convert these areas to foci of acute mastitis or abscess formation. Occasionally, even in the absence of bacterial contamination, rupture of ducts produces a change similar to that described as mammary duct ectasia.

ENDOCRINE IMBALANCES

CYSTIC HYPERPLASIA (MAMMARY DYSPLASIA, FIBROCYSTIC DISEASE)

This most common involvement of the female breast is included under the heading of endocrine imbalance because it is now almost universally accepted that it results from *an exaggeration and distortion of the cyclic breast changes that normally occur in the menstrual cycle.* Notice should be taken, however, that there are still dissenters to this etiologic concept. The terminology of this condition is unfortunately one of its most confusing aspects, and a complete citation of all the terms that have been used in the past would require the completely nonproductive use of a full text page. The most persistent, most widely used and, paradoxically, most inappropriate term is chronic cystic mastitis. The disease is not invariably chronic, not always cystic, and certainly it is not an inflammation. Cystic hyperplasia is considerably more appropriate, since it at least denotes two of the principal characteristics of this condition. Alternatively, the term fibrocystic disease is currently in vogue as an equally explanatory designation. Mammary dysplasia has the advantage of being noncommittal but has not received wide usage.

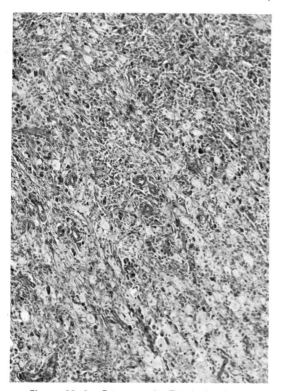

Figure 28–2. Fat necrosis. The lesion is well advanced and now represents a focus of lipophages interspersed with fibroblasts and leukocytes.

Cystic hyperplasia or fibrocystic disease encompasses a wide variety of morphologic changes and resultant clinical manifestations that run the gamut from lesions that consist principally of an overgrowth of the fibrous stroma, to lesions in which both stromal and epithelial proliferation participate, to the other types in which epithelial proliferation predominates (Foote and Stewart, 1945) (Warren, 1946). It is a notoriously pleomorphic disorder in which variable morphologic patterns are encountered in different patients, in different areas of the same lesion or even in different microscopic fields of one slide. Despite this variable behavior, it is possible to distinguish three dominant patterns of morphologic change. Since these patterns conform fairly well to specific age distributions, have somewhat distinctive clinical manifestations and are of different significance with respect to malignant transformation, it seems desirable to present each separately. It should be emphasized, however, that there is much overlap and considerable concurrence in these patterns. It is difficult, therefore, to categorize every case. Nonetheless, by the separate consideration of these three subdivisions, the full spectrum of cystic hyperplasia can be presented. The three basic patterns are here referred to as fibrosis of the breast, cystic disease and adenosis.

Incidence. Together these three variants comprise the single most common disorder of the breast and account for over one-half of all surgical operations on the female breast. It is difficult to express an incidence of this condition in the general adult female population because of the variable criteria used for its diagnosis and because of the selective nature of the material studied. In a study of the so-called "normal breast," i.e., unselected postmortem cases, significant disease was found in 28 per cent by Frantz et al. (1951). Minimal disease was found in 24 per cent additionally, giving a total incidence, then, of 52 per cent. These cases, however, were weighted with older age groups and, therefore, do not represent a true sample of the general population. It is clear, however, that fibrocystic disease is a commonplace autopsy finding (Sandison, 1962) and clinical problem. It does not occur before adolescence and rarely, if ever, develops after the menopause. However, premenopausal lesions may persist into more advanced life.

Pathogenesis. Hyperestrinism is considered to be basic to the development of this multipatterned disorder. The excess of estrogens may represent an absolute increase, as in the rarely associated functioning ovarian tumors, or the excess of estrogen may be relative to a deficiency of progesterone as is seen in the anovulatory woman. Accordingly, the morphologic changes in the breast are considered to reflect overstimulation of ductal epithelial and stromal growth, resulting in the changes to be described.

Fibrosis of the Breast. Also known as *mastodynia*, this variant is characterized principally by *stromal fibrous tissue overgrowth unaccompanied by prominent epithelial hyperplasia*. It is usually not associated with the formation of grossly demonstrable cysts. This pattern tends to occur in young women from *30 to 35 years of age*, and is more usually unilateral, but may affect both breasts.

Classically, the upper outer quadrant is most often involved and the increase in fibrous tissue results in a **poorly defined area of rubbery consistency** which commonly varies from 2 to 10 cm. in diameter. The line of demarcation from the surrounding normal breast is poorly defined. There is no fixation to the skin or underlying structures. Sometimes, by insertion of the palpatory hand between the breast and pectoral muscles in the anterior axillary fold, a plate-like thickening is demonstrable. On section, the affected area has a dense, rubbery consistency that yields readily to pressure, but resists cutting. The overall appearance is that of a homogeneous, white-pink, collagenous connective tissue devoid of fat, within which minute yellow-pink areas of glandular parenchyma may be barely visible. Cysts are usually microscopic in size when present, but are more often absent.

In milder cases, the increase in stromal connective tissue may be so minimal that it may appear inadequate as an explanation for the formation of a clinical mass. However, in the more classic examples, **the overgrowth of collagenous stroma engulfs the epithelial structures and obliterates the loose periductal and lobular myxomatous stroma.** Sometimes it compresses the ducts and buds to the point at which they become markedly flattened or even atrophic (Fig. 28-3). Occasionally, small cysts and other epithelial changes to be described are also present. However, in the better defined examples, the lesion is principally one of fibrosis, and epithelial changes are insignificant.

Clinical Course. The clinical features of this variant can be surmised from the morphologic description. It most commonly affects the upper outer quadrant, but other regions may be affected and the condition may be bilateral. The lesion is usually palpable as a reasonably well delimited, but not sharply circumscribed, area of induration. Sometimes the focus has a sufficiently sharp lateral margin to be described as "saucer-like." It is frequently painful and tender to palpation, particularly in the days preceding menstruation. In the classic

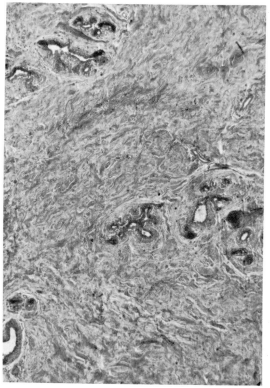

Figure 28–3. *Fibrosis of the breast. The entire interductal breast substance is replaced by hyaline connective tissue. The ducts and glands are compressed and atrophic.*

of the cyclic changes rather than as a consequence of obstruction to the ducts.

Rarely, an isolated cyst may be formed within one breast, but usually the disorder is multifocal and often is bilateral (Fig. 28–4). As a result of the stromal overgrowth and cystic dilatation of the ducts, the involved areas have an **ill-defined diffuse increase in consistency and discrete nodularities.** Closely aggregated, small cysts produce a shotty texture. Larger, particularly solitary, cysts evoke the greatest alarm as isolated firm masses that are deceptively unyielding. Occasionally, multiple cysts aggregate to produce a large, irregular, multilobular mass. On section, the cysts vary up to 4 or 5 cm. in diameter (some are larger). Unopened, these cysts are brown to blue owing to the contained semitranslucent, turbid fluid (Fig. 28–5). Usually the cysts are filled with serous, turbid fluid that flows out readily to disclose a smooth, glistening, membranous lining devoid of areas of thickening or papillary projection. However, intracystic hemorrhage, inspissation of secretions or inflammation may modify the contents. Sometimes the cystic walls are thickened or calcified by complicating hemorrhages and infections.

The histologic hallmark of this variant is **cystic dilatation of ducts.** In larger cysts, the lining

case, the tenderness may regress following the menstrual period, with recurrence of pain and tenderness with the next cycle. The significance of this variant and its management will be considered later, along with the other patterns.

Cystic Disease. This variant, also designated as *Bloodgood's disease, Schimmelbusch's disease* and *blue dome cyst*, is the form of mammary dysplasia characterized by both *stromal and epithelial hyperplasia with the formation of cysts.* Haagensen (1971a) pleads for restricting the term cystic disease to those cases having macroscopically palpable cysts, *i.e.,* over 2 to 3 mm. in diameter. He points out that microcysts are found so commonly in all women in the middle years of life that they cannot be construed as disease nor as justification for surgery. True cystic disease usually occurs in women near or at the age of menopause, that is, *between the ages of 45 and 55.* It is considered to be due to abnormal hyperplasia of the ductal epithelium and dilatation of the ducts with each menstrual cycle, not balanced by the sequential regressive changes of atrophy, desquamation of cells and shrinkage of the ducts. Accordingly, the cystic dilatation arises within the ducts as a distortion

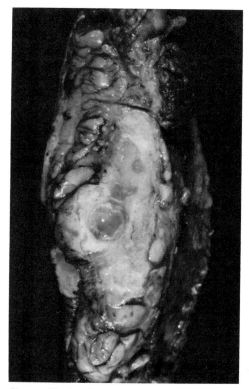

Figure 28–4. *Cystic disease of the breast. The cross section reveals an area of diffuse fibrosis containing a solitary cyst in the plane of section.*

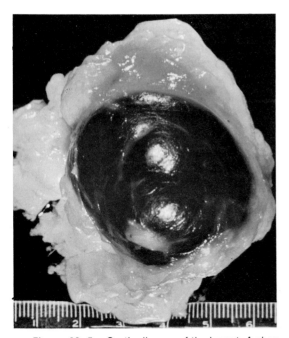

Figure 28–5. *Cystic disease of the breast. A characteristic excised, unopened, blue dome cyst.*

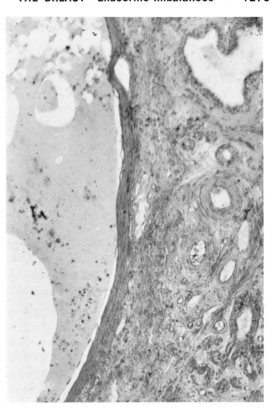

Figure 28–7. *Cystic disease of the breast. A detail of the wall of a large cystic space with complete atrophy of the lining epithelium.*

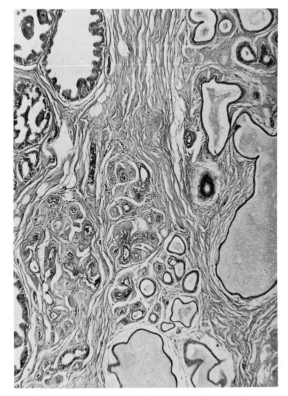

Figure 28–6. *Cystic disease of the breast. Multiple cystic spaces—some are filled with precipitated fluid. Others have a somewhat high epithelium, thrown up into papillary projections.*

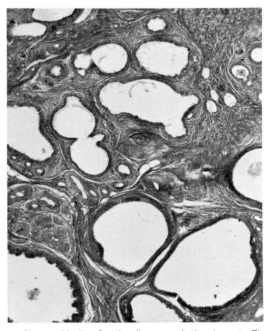

Figure 28–8. *Cystic disease of the breast. The smaller cysts have preserved cuboidal to columnar cell lining epithelium.*

epithelium may be flattened, or may even be totally atrophic, so that the surface is composed only of compressed collagenous fibrous tissue. In smaller cysts, the epithelium is more cuboidal to columnar and is frequently multilayered in focal areas (Figs. 28–6, 28–7, and 28–8). Occasionally, epithelial proliferation leads to piled-up masses or small papillary excrescences. In most instances, a clearly defined, intact basal membrane is present, and only rarely are epithelial extensions found outside the basement membrane, changes interpreted as "spillage" of the epithelium rather than true invasion. Occasionally, cysts are lined by large polygonal cells having an abundant granular, eosinophilic cytoplasm, with small, round, deeply chromatic nuclei, **so-called apocrine epithelium.** Such apocrine epithelium is found not uncommonly in the normal breast, and is presumed to represent a specialized differentiation of breast parenchyma along the line of sebaceous gland cells. Epithelial overgrowth and papillary projections are common in cysts lined by apocrine epithelium (Fig. 28–9).

The stroma about all forms of cysts is usually compressed fibrous tissue, having lost its normal, delicate, myxomatous appearance. Occasionally, the interlobular stroma is of the dense fibrous collagenous type previously described and, in other cases, overgrowth of epithelium in the form of small

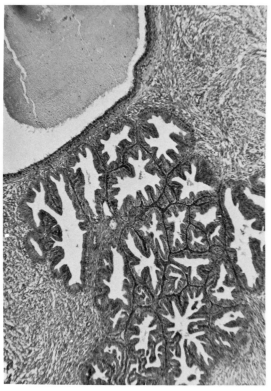

Figure 28–9. *Cystic disease of the breast. The apocrine epithelium is hyperplastic and thrown up into papillary processes.*

glands, strands or cords of cells embedded within the fibrous tissue creates changes that conform to those to be described under adenosis.

Clinical Course. The clinical characteristics of this variant of fibrocystic disease have virtually been presented in the morphologic description. When cysts are macroscopic in size, they are readily palpable as discrete nodules, and since they usually occur multiply and are commonly bilateral, the existence of this diffuse, irregular nodularity is readily distinguished from the characteristic discrete, solitary focus of carcinoma. However, solitary cysts may be difficult to distinguish from a cancer on gross palpation. Commonly, the cysts produce pain, are tender to palpation and are more distressing during the period of premenstrual tension.

Benign Epithelial Hyperplasia (Adenosis). This variant is also known by a variety of names and includes many special patterns encompassed by these terms: *ductal hyperplasia, ductal papillomatosis, sclerosing adenosis, sclerosing and fibrosing benign epithelial hyperplasia, blunt duct adenosis and adenomatosis.* All are characterized by *dominance of the proliferation of the epithelial parenchyma,* but may also be accompanied by fibrosis and cystic disease. These lesions are most commonly found *between the ages of 35 and 45.*

Adenosis is more apt to be unilateral than is cystic disease, and is often focal, affecting the upper outer quadrant of the breast. However, other localizations and bilateral involvement are by no means uncommon.

Depending upon the extensiveness of the morphologic changes, the area may have a **hard cartilaginous consistency that begins to approximate that found in breast cancer, or may be only an illdefined area of firmness.** Cystic nodules are more commonly present in this variant than in the pattern described as fibrosis. On section, the involved area is not well localized, is gray-pink and firm and, on close inspection, has small, elevated, pink-gray foci that can be later identified as glandular epithelial structures. Minute and large cysts are commonly present. Characteristically, however, the chalky yellow-white foci and streaks of necrosis that identify breast carcinoma are absent, an important gross differential feature. Many times, the ducts have an increased ropy consistency and, on pressure, exude a pulpy yellow-white debris.

The histologic pattern of epithelial hyperplasia is extremely varied and consists principally of the following features: **(1) intraductal hyperplasia, (2) intraductal papillomatosis, (3) glandular reduplication and proliferation, and (4) increase of stroma compressing and distorting the epithe-**

lial overgrowth (Foote and Stewart, 1946). The ductal proliferation causes multilayering of epithelium and the formation of small, abortive papillary projections **(intraductal papillomatosis).** The larger ducts may be partially or completely plugged with cuboidal cells which, although somewhat disoriented, are nonetheless regular in size and do not have variations in nuclear size or shape, nor are they hyperchromatic. Characteristically, the ductal overgrowth preserves some tendency toward gland formation. Such mitotic figures as are present are invariably normal in type. The basal membranes of the ducts are intact, and there is usually no extension of the intraductular epithelium into the surrounding stroma.

Proliferation of small ducts, canaliculi and gland buds may yield masses of small gland patterns, or nests and cords of cells embedded within a fibrous stroma. Usually in such an area, many or at least some well defined glands can be identified, but frequently they are closely aggregated so that glands lined by single or multiple layers of cells are backed up to each other **(adenosis).** At other times, the stromal overgrowth distorts and compresses the glands; however, usually the cell aggregates preserve some vestige of a central lumen and some resemblance, therefore, to normal gland patterns. However, occasionally the fibrous growth may totally compress the lumina to create the appearance of solid cords or strands of cells lying within the dense stroma, a histologic pattern **(sclerosing adenosis)** that, at times, verges on the appearance of infiltrative carcinoma (Urban and Adair, 1949).

To the inexperienced, the histologic differentiation of a florid case of sclerosing adenosis from frank cancer is most difficult (Figs. 28–10 and 28–11). When clearly defined cysts and apocrine elements are present, or when the epithelial structures preserve their glandular regularity, the distinction is made more readily.

Clinical Course. Just as the morphologic differentiation of adenosis from cancer may be difficult, the clinical distinction is equally vague. This lesion characteristically produces a hard localized mass on palpation, reasonably well delimited, but not sharply defined from

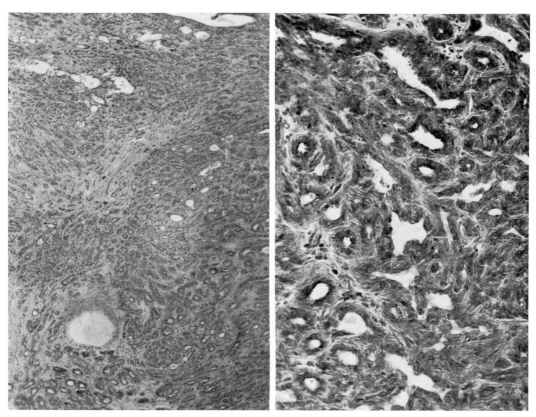

Fig. 28–10   Fig. 28–11

Figure 28–10. *Adenosis. A low power view of a florid case of benign epithelial proliferation, readily mistaken on casual inspection for carcinoma.*
Figure 28–11. *Adenosis. A high power view of same lesion as in Figure 28–10. The epithelial overgrowth forms many gland patterns that are lined by somewhat distorted but not anaplastic cells.*

the surrounding breast substance. It has, therefore, many of the clinical characteristics of malignancy. When the disorder is bilateral, or when cysts are present, the clinical diagnosis is more apparent, but unfortunately such accompanying changes are not invariably present. The pain and tenderness of florid adenosis may also serve to differentiate this lesion from neoplasia.

Clinical Significance of Fibrocystic Disease. The many patterns of breast pathology included under the designation fibrocystic disease have great clinical importance for two reasons: (1) they produce masses in the breast that require differentiation from carcinoma, and (2) they may predispose to the subsequent development of carcinoma.

Any mass or lump in the breast must be viewed as a possible carcinoma. While certain clinical features of fibrocystic disease tend to differentiate it from cancer, the only certain way of making this distinction is biopsy and pathologic examination. However, the following features favor the diagnosis of fibrocystic disease. Bilateral involvement and multiple nodules are more characteristic of fibrocystic disease than carcinoma. Fibrocystic disease tends to be painful prior to the menstrual period as breast engorgement occurs. These benign lesions occur in a somewhat younger age group but, unless the patient is in the first two decades of life, when carcinoma of the breast is rarely encountered, the age of the patient is a slender thread. Frequently, fibrocystic disease regresses and even disappears during pregnancy. Despite these clinical features, it is an unwise clinician who relies solely on clinical examination of the breast to rule out carcinoma, the more so because, as will be pointed out, carcinoma may supervene on preexisting mammary dysplasia.

What is the relationship between fibrocystic disease and carcinoma? This question has been hotly argued from time immemorial. Two diametrically opposite viewpoints have long been held equally vehemently: that fibrocystic disease predisposes to cancer, and that there is no causal relationship between the two disorders. *The evidence is becoming more substantial that patients with fibrocystic disease have a higher than expected attack rate of cancer of the breast.* Warren (1946), in a five-year follow-up of 1200 cases of this disease, cites a cancer rate 4.5 times greater than that in patients with normal breasts. In the patterns that have florid epithelial overgrowth within the ducts, he cites a twelve-fold increased attack rate. Haagensen (1971*b*), in an authoritative study of 1693 patients, points out that on the basis of age-adjusted risk-years and expected incidence of cancer, women with this disease have a greater

than fourfold increased attack rate of cancer. It should be noted, however, that in about half of the instances, the cancer occurred in the contralateral breast, not in the one with cystic hyperplasia. Evidently, the influences predisposing to cystic disease also favor the development of cancer. Despite all of this evidence, doubt persists about the association between cystic hyperplasia and cancer of the breast. As recently as 1972, an editorial appeared still urging caution in accepting "benign disease" as an important subsoil for breast cancer (Editorial, 1972*a*).

The temptation is often great to treat patients with fibrocystic disease by "watchful waiting." It is chastening to realize that at the New York Memorial Hospital, one of the worldwide centers for the treatment of neoplasia, in a series of 329 breast cancers the clinical impression as to the nature of the lesion was equivocal or erroneous in about 20 per cent. In other words, the cancer had been clinically diagnosed as some form of benign disease. The clinical differentiation of these diseases is then, at the least, imperfect.

HYPERTROPHY OF THE BREAST

Abnormal hypertrophy of one or both breasts may occur at any age, presumably when the breast tissue either is excessively sensitive to normal amounts of hormone or is abnormally stimulated by high levels of ovarian hormones. When hypertrophy is unilateral, it is postulated that there is a differential sensitivity of the breasts. Neonatal hypertrophy has already been described (p. 1267). Prepubertal hypertrophy is commonly bilateral and almost invariably suggests abnormal levels of ovarian hormone. This condition is, therefore, encountered in functioning ovarian tumors, choriocarcinomas, adrenal cortical tumors and pituitary tumors. Control or lowering of hormone production permits regression of the breast size. However, in other instances, the condition is more obscure and arises without known cause. Sometimes, in the adolescent or preadolescent girl, the hypertrophy of one or both breasts is irreversible. The increase in size may be quite exaggerated, and one or both breasts may assume a bulk three or four times normal. This form of overgrowth is sometimes referred to as virginal hypertrophy. Histologically, there are no distinguishing features, and sections disclose only an abnormal increase of fibrous stroma, accompanied by some proliferation of the ducts and canaliculi.

TUMORS

Neoplasms constitute the most important, albeit not the most common, lesions of the female breast. A great variety of tumors may occur in the female breast, made up as it is of a covering integument, adult fat, mesenchymal connective tissue and epithelial structures. These tumors run the gamut of virtually all the neoplasms that may arise from stratified squamous epithelium, glandular structures and mesenchymal connective tissue. Some of these neoplasms may be listed as skin papillomas, squamous cell carcinomas of the skin, adenomas, papillomas of ducts, carcinomas of glandular or duct origin, and virtually every variety of benign and malignant mesodermal tumor, such as fibroma and fibrosarcoma, granular cell myoblastoma, chondroma and chondrosarcoma, lipoma and liposarcoma, osteoma and osteogenic sarcoma and angioma and angiosarcoma. Only the more common tumors specialized to the breast, however, will be discussed. The majority of those just listed exactly resemble the analogous neoplasms which occur elsewhere in the body and do not have any special properties when they occur in the breast.

The unqualified term breast cancer implies a carcinoma arising in the glandular and ductal structures of the breast. Breast carcinoma is the number one cause of cancer deaths among females. This form of cancer has been called "the foremost cancer" in women. An eloquent justification of this designation was given in 1971 by H. Marvin Pollard, President of the American Cancer Society (Pollard, 1971): "It is the most feared of cancers, the most frequently self discovered and the most controversially treated of all cancers. It ranks first among cancers in number of surgical procedures, in radiation therapy treatments, in the number of hormone and chemotherapy administrations. In cancer diagnosis it is first in the number of biopsies. It is the foremost of all cancers, too, from the standpoint of cost in physicians' fees and hospital bills. One cannot compute its ranking to heartache and suffering."

Understandably, then, breast cancer has been the focus of intensive study relative to its origins, diagnostic methods and therapy. Despite all the efforts, little ground has been gained and the age adjusted death rate from breast cancer in the female in the United States has virtually remained stable over the past 30 years at about 25 to 26 per 100,000. In highly personal terms, it has been calculated that slightly more than 5 women per 100 will develop cancer of the breast during their lives (Randall et al., 1954). It is a disease, then, of preeminent importance.

CARCINOMA OF THE BREAST

This foremost cause of cancer death in the female accounts for approximately 30,000 deaths annually in the United States. While the mortality rates for most of the other major cancers in women have shown a steady decline over the past few decades, the death rate from breast cancer continues to climb slowly (see p. 151). The small gains that have been made in the early diagnosis and treatment of this disease cannot keep pace with its rising incidence in the female. In contrast, cancer of the breast is quite rare in males, the ratio being 100 to 1. It is both ironic and tragic that a neoplasm, arising in an exposed organ, readily accessible to self-examination and clinical diagnosis, continues to exact such a heavy toll.

Incidence. Cancer of the female breast is rarely found under the age of 25. It may occur at any age thereafter, with a peak incidence shortly before, during or after the menopause. Data derived from the State of Connecticut indicate that the age-adjusted incidence of cancer of the breast in the female has slowly but steadily increased from 55 per 100,000 in 1940–44, to 72 in 1965–68 (Cutler et al., 1971). Virtually identical trends have been reported in other North American studies. This increase has occurred among all ages including young, premenopausal women (Feinleib and Garrison, 1969). The explanation for this upward trend still eludes us.

Few cancers have been subjected to more intensive epidemiologic study. A host of observations has emerged. For example, there are striking geographic differences in its prevalence. The incidence and death rate of breast cancer in Japan and Taiwan is approximately one-sixth that of the United States (MacMahon et al., 1970). Observations bearing on the incidence of this disease can be summarized as follows.

Breast cancer is more common:
1. In Jews than in gentiles.
2. In higher socioeconomic classes.
3. In those with a family history of breast cancer.
4. In those with previous breast disease.
5. In single women than in married women.
6. In nonparous than in parous married women.
7. In those whose menarche was early (before the age of 12).

From these epidemiologic observations, it is possible to identify groups at high risk (Zippin and Petrakis, 1971). Some order of magnitude of the increased risk is cited in Table 28–1 (modified from Shapiro et al., 1968).

Most of the influences productive of a higher attack rate appear to reflect increased exposure to steroid (estrogen) hormones, and to familial and genetic influences (MacMahon and Cole, 1969) (Mirra et al., 1971).

TABLE 28–1. RELATIVE RISK OF BREAST CANCER IN DIFFERENT GROUPS

Conditions	Relative Risk of Breast Cancer
Breast conditions (1 or more vs. none)	3.1
Never married vs. married	2.3
Nonparous vs. parous	2.0
1–2 Pregnancies vs. 3 or more	2.0
Sisters (1 or more with breast cancer vs. none)	1.9
Age at menarche (under 12 vs. 15 or over)	1.7
30 Years or more aggregate menstrual activity vs. less than 30 years	1.4

Modified from Shapiro, S., et al.: The search for risk factors in breast cancer. Amer. J. Public Health, 58:820, 1968.

In previous years, it was believed that lactation in some way had a prophylactic effect against the development of breast cancer. It was held that the risk of this disease was inversely related to total nursing time. Recent studies suggest, however, that although pregnancy itself confers some protection, there is no consistent difference in duration of lactation between breast cancer patients and controls, once the factor of fewer pregnancies among the breast cancer patients has been allowed (MacMahon et al., 1970) (Yuasa and MacMahon, 1970).

Etiology and Pathogenesis. The search for the origins of breast cancer has been greatly aided by animal studies. Mouse mammary cancer is an excellent model of the human disease. In these animals, it is well documented that four sets of influences are important: (1) genetic factors, (2) hormones, (3) a virus or viruses and (4) environmental factors (Dmochowski, 1971). All of these are not directly applicable to women, since it is impossible in humans to establish the rigorous controlled studies of environmental factors achieved with mice. Therefore, the following consideration will deal with three major concerns: genetic factors, hormones and viruses.

The *role of genetic factors* in the development of cancer, although poorly understood, is unmistakably evident. The risk of breast cancer in women with a familial history of similar disease is approximately two to three times greater than that in control groups. The mode of transmission of the genetic predisposition is unknown, but is believed to be multifactorial.

The *role of hormones* can be summarized in the statement that *unopposed estrogen activity over a long reproductive life span is considered to be highly significant in the genesis of breast cancer.* Estrogens are known to induce proliferative changes in the ducts during the normal ebb and flow of hormones in the menstrual cycle.

Most breast carcinomas arise in ducts, and it would be reasonable to expect that excessive estrogenic effects might lead to accentuated hyperplasia. Such cellular proliferation is probably a requisite for cancerous transformation.

We are just beginning to understand how steroid hormones exert their proliferative effect. It is now clear that steroids regulate gene activity (Editorial, 1972b). Target cells possess binding proteins, and it has been shown that normal cells, in such target organs as the breast and endometrium, selectively bind steroids such as 17-beta-estradiol (Korenman and Dukes, 1970). Similar binding proteins have been identified in breast cancer cells and, moreover, these cells may possess enzyme systems not present in normal mammary tissue, rendering them capable of converting androgens to estrogens (Jones et al., 1970). As discussed on p. 1205, the steroid hormone-binding protein complex may serve as a key which, in some way, turns on DNA synthesis and replicative activity in target cells. In this sense, it is perhaps more proper to speak of hormones as promoters in the carcinogenic process rather than as initiators.

Much of the epidemiologic data cited earlier supports a role for hyperestrinism in the genesis of breast cancer. The prototype of the unmarried female with no pregnancies and early menarche exemplifies a long reproductive life span, with unremitting exposure to the estrogen peaks of every menstrual cycle. Pregnancies, and a late menarche, shorten such exposure to estrogens. In this context, it is of interest that in dairy cows, which are bred virtually yearly, mammary carcinoma is almost nonexistent. Functioning ovarian tumors and ovarian cortical hyperplasia which elaborate estrogens are associated with breast cancer in postmenopausal women. This neoplasm rarely occurs in the prepubertally castrated. These same hormonal influences are thought to be operative in the genesis of fibrocystic disease of the breast and probably account for the increased incidence of breast cancer in women having preexisting fibrocystic disease. As pointed out earlier, the carcinoma often arises in the opposite breast, which did not have clinically apparent cystic disease, consonant with the systemic effect of the hormonal influence.

Remarkably, in the light of all this evidence, studies have failed to disclose an increased incidence of breast cancer in women taking oral contraceptives or in those receiving estrogen therapy (Arthes, 1971) (Vessey et al., 1971). It should be pointed out, however, that the use of oral contraceptives dates back only a short span of years, and it is necessary to maintain close scrutiny of this problem before final judgement is made.

A *viral etiology* of mouse mammary tumor has long been established, dating back to the pioneer observations of Bittner (1936). The agent is an RNA virus identifiable as cytoplasmic, so-called B-type, particles in mammary tumor cells. It is transmitted vertically in the mother's milk to the suckling newborn. It has been shown to contain RNA-dependent DNA polymerase. A similar viral agent has been identified in a spontaneous breast tumor in a subhuman primate (Chopra et al., 1971). The simian agent has also been shown to possess RNA-dependent DNA polymerase (Schlom and Spiegelman, 1971).

A number of observations lead us close to establishing a human mammary tumor virus. Virus-like (type B) particles similar to, or identical with, those found in mammary tumors in mice have been identified in milk samples from women in an inbred Parsi community. These women have an unusually high incidence of breast cancer (Moore et al., 1971). Thirty-nine per cent of milk samples obtained from these Parsi women contained these particles, as did 31 per cent of milk samples from women of high-risk American families. Only 12 per cent of samples from 181 controls revealed the same. Spiegelman and his colleagues have recently identified an RNA-dependent DNA polymerase in the particle-containing milk. You recall that this so-called reverse transcriptase is peculiar to tumor viruses (Schlom et al., 1971). Hybridization experiments have shown similarities between the murine and monkey viruses, indicating a close nucleic acid relationship which suggests that the same agent may be responsible for mammary tumors in more than one species and, conceivably, in man. Sera from women who have had a breast cancer are capable of significantly neutralizing the mouse virus. In summary, there is a considerable body of evidence suggesting, but certainly not proving, a viral etiology for breast cancer in women (Seman et al., 1971) (Feller and Chopra, 1971). To date, it has not been possible to isolate the human virus-like particles and, of course, it is not possible to fulfill Koch's postulate for obvious reasons.

In the final analysis, *while the etiology of human breast cancer is still unknown, the accumulated evidence points strongly towards an RNA oncogenic viral initiator and hormonal promotion acting on a genetically predisposed or vulnerable soil.* It might be well, at this point, to mention that trauma is a nonetiologic influence. There has been no documented association between a blow to the breast and the subsequent development of cancer.

Morphology. Curiously, carcinoma is more common in the left breast than in the right, in a ratio of 110:100. The cancers are bilateral or sequential in the same breast in 4 per cent or more of cases. They may be either infiltrating or noninfiltrating and have a great deal of fibrous stroma or very little. Some of these neoplasms secrete mucin and some occasionally extend up into the skin to produce Paget's disease (p. 1283). Over 90 per cent of breast cancers arise in the ductal epithelium. The mammary lobules are rare sites of origin. An overview of the range in tumor types is provided by the following simplified classification.

Breast cancer arising in mammary lobules:
  A. Noninfiltrating—in situ lobular carcinoma.
  B. Infiltrating—lobular carcinoma.
Breast cancer arising in mammary ducts:
  A. Noninfiltrating—intraductal carcinoma.
  B. Infiltrating:
    1. Fibroplastic-scirrhous carcinoma
    2. Medullary carcinoma.
    3. Colloid or mucinous carcinoma.
    4. Paget's disease (ductal carcinoma with extension to skin).

The rare special forms such as sweat gland carcinoma and squamous cell carcinoma arising within the breast will be omitted from this consideration.

Among breast carcinomas small enough that their general areas of origin can be identified, approximately 50 per cent arise in the upper, outer quadrant; 10 per cent in each of the remaining quadrants; and about 20 per cent in the central or subareolar region. As will be seen, the site of origin influences the pattern of nodal metastasis to a considerable degree.

Lobular Carcinoma. Lobular carcinoma may be either noninfiltrating—**in situ**—or infiltrating. The noninfiltrating lesions produce no gross morphologic changes. Only when such a tumor becomes infiltrative is it palpable as a mass. These cancers are of particular interest for a number of reasons. As was mentioned, only about 10 per cent of breast carcinomas arise in these structures, but lobular carcinomas tend to be bilateral far more frequently than those arising in ducts (Robbins and Berg, 1964). It is standard clinical practice now to do large and possibly multiple biopsies on the contralateral breast when a lobular carcinoma is found in one. The likelihood of cancer in the contralateral breast is on the order of 20 per cent (Urban, 1967). Moreover, these cancers tend to be multicentric in origin within the same breast. With such diffuse involvement, the **in situ** lobular carcinoma is exceedingly difficult to differentiate histologically from the wide variety of proliferative atypicalities encountered in fibrocystic disease, especially the adenosis variant.

Ductal Carcinoma. The noninfiltrating intraductal carcinoma will be discussed first, followed by a presentation of the four major variants of infiltrating tumors arising within the ducts: the scirrhous, medullary and colloid types, and Paget's disease.

Intraductal Carcinoma (Noninfiltrating). As previously stated, over 90 per cent of breast carcinomas arise within the ducts. As long as the tumor remains within the confines of the ductal basement membranes, it comprises a noninfiltrating intraductal carcinoma. These begin as **anaplastic proliferations of ductal epithelium which eventually completely fill and plug the ducts with neoplastic cells.** The tumor exists as a poorly defined focus of slightly increased consistency caused by the marked dilatation and solidification of the ducts. Occasionally, ductal carcinomas create no change in the consistency of the breast substance. It is only when the breast is sectioned that cord-like ducts are found filled often with necrotic and cheesy tumorous tissue. This substance can be readily extruded upon slight pressure, hence the designation **comedocarcinoma.** Histologically, the ducts are dilated and filled with neoplastic epithelial cells which completely plug the lumina. At times, some small glandular pattern or papillary growth may be distinguished, but eventually the compressive proliferation obliterates all architectural detail and only solid cords of anaplastic disoriented cells are visible. As the lesion advances, the intraductal neoplasia eventually extends through the basement membrane, and the tumor becomes an infiltrative ductal carcinoma, to be described (Fig. 28—12).

Scirrhous Carcinoma. The scirrhous carcinoma is the most common of the infiltrating ductal tumors, and accounts for about three-fourths of all mammary carcinomas. These growths occur as fairly sharply delimited nodules of **stony hard** consistency that average 2 cm. in diameter and rarely exceed 4 to 5 cm. On palpation, they may appear deceptively discrete, but in many cases the focus of malignancy is ill-defined and obviously has an infiltrative attachment to the surrounding structures with fixation to the underlying chest wall, dimpling of the skin and retraction of the nipple (Fig. 28—13). Only rarely is there ulceration through the skin. The mass is quite characteristic on cut section. **It is retracted below the cut surface, has a hard, cartilaginous consistency and produces a grating sound when scraped.** Within the central focus, there are small pinpoint foci or streaks of chalky white, necrotic tumor (Fig. 28—14). Sometimes obvious long prolongations of fibrous tissue or tumor extend into the surrounding fibrofatty stroma of the breast, with no sharply defined outer limit or encapsulation.

Histologically, **the tumor is composed principally of dense, collagenous, hyaline, fibrous stroma, in which are found scattered, isolated small nests or long, filamentous, irregularly disposed strands of "Indian-file" epithelial cells** (Fig. 28—15). Small sheets or masses may create gland patterns. The individual cells are round to poly-

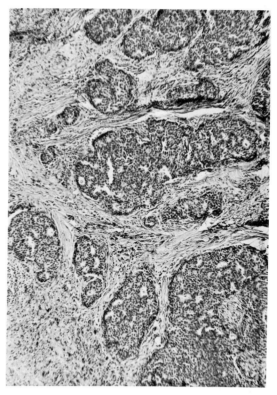

Figure 28–12. *Ductal carcinoma. The tumor cells fill the ducts and have invaded the stroma.*

gonal or compressed, and contain small, deeply chromatic nuclei that are surprisingly uniform in size and shape, and usually display remarkably few mitotic figures. At the margins of the main tumor mass, the neoplastic cells infiltrate into the surrounding fibrofatty tissue, and frequently invasion of perivascular and perineural spaces, as well as of blood vessels, is readily evident (Fig. 28—16).

Medullary Carcinoma. This is a distinctly uncommon variant (5 to 10 per cent of all mammary carcinomas) that tends to produce **large, fleshy tumor masses up to 5 to 10 cm. in diameter.** These tumors do not have the striking desmoplasia (formation of fibrous tissue) of the scirrhous carcinoma and, therefore, are distinctly more yielding on external palpation as well as on cut section. The tumor does not retract when cut, but rather bulges above the level of the native tissue about it and has a soft, fleshy, almost brain-like consistency. These masses grow centrifugally along a broad front and are often deceptively sharply delimited from the surrounding substance (Fig. 28—17).

Histologically, **the dominant features are a scant stroma and the large, irregular masses, sheets and cords of cells that usually form no well identified gland or papillary structures** (Fig. 28—18). Occasionally, well differentiated gland formations are present and, in these cases, the tumor is

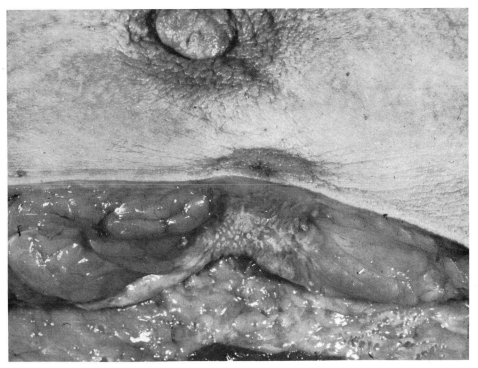

Fig. 28-13

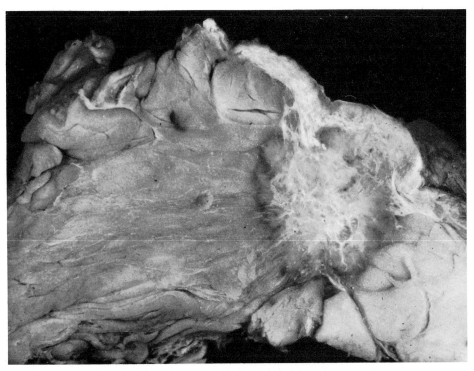

Fig. 28-14

Figure 28-13. *Carcinoma of breast, scirrhous type. The tumor is transected through the middle, and the breast is viewed obliquely to illustrate the retracted mass and the fixation to and dimpling of the attached skin.*

Figure 28-14. *Carcinoma of breast, scirrhous type. The cut surface illustrates the lack of demarcation, the fixation to the skin and the chalky foci of necrosis within the mass.*

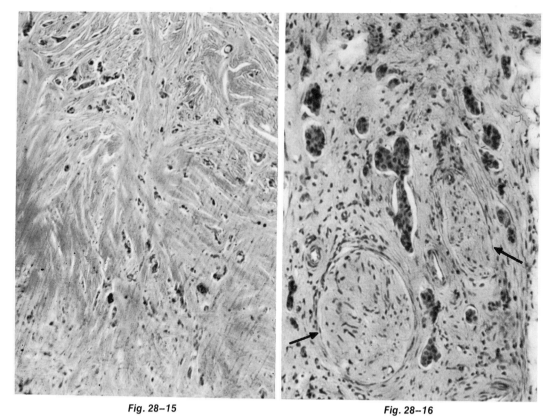

Fig. 28–15   Fig. 28–16

Figure 28–15. *Carcinoma of breast, scirrhous type. The small nests of tumor cells are embedded within a dense fibrous stoma.*

Figure 28–16. *Carcinoma of breast, scirrhous type. The tumor has surrounded nerve fibers (arrows) and is lying within a lymphatic space.*

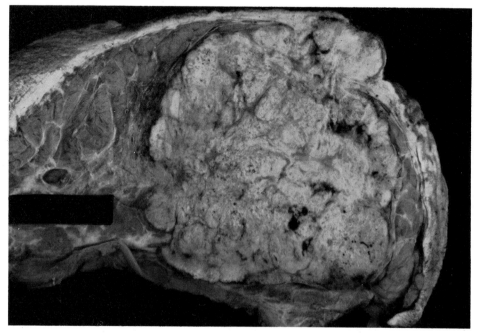

Figure 28–17. *Carcinoma of breast, medullary type. The large bulky mass appears deceptively discrete.*

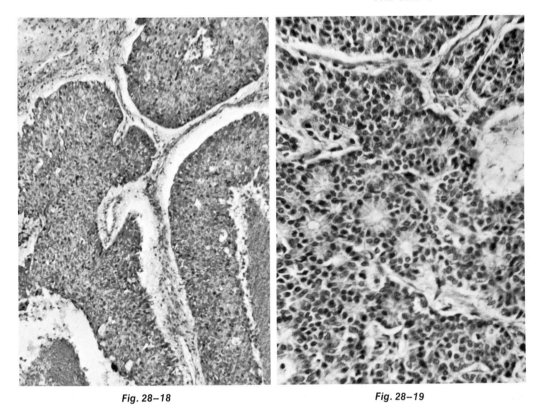

Fig. 28–18   Fig. 28–19

Figure 28–18. Carcinoma of breast. The tumor cells grow in large undifferentiated masses.
Figure 28–19. Carcinoma of breast. The medullary tumor has reproduced well formed glands meriting the designation of medullary adenocarcinoma.

designated a medullary adenocarcinoma (Fig. 28–19). There may be a striking lymphocytic infiltration in the scant connective tissue stroma within these tumors.

Colloid or Mucinous Carcinoma. This is another unusual variant, which tends to grow slowly over the course of many years, and may produce bulky, gelatinous masses which appear to be circumscribed on palpation but, on cut section, are found to blend imperceptibly into the surrounding tissue zones. The tumor is extremely soft and has the consistency and appearance of pale gray-blue gelatin. Commonly, the tumor undergoes central cystic softening and hemorrhage.

Histologically, this tumor usually takes on one of three patterns of growth, but all three may coexist in a single lesion. There may be **large lakes and masses of basophilic, amorphous mucin that dissect and extend into contiguous tissue spaces and planes of cleavage. Floating within this mucin are small islands and isolated neoplastic cells sometimes forming glands** (Fig. 28–20). Vacuolation of at least some of the cells is characteristic. In other colloid tumors, the histologic appearance may be essentially that of an **adenocarcinoma, with well defined glands, the lumina of which contain mucinous secretions.** Some mucin may also be found in the interglandular spaces and in the surrounding fibrous stroma. The cells lining the glands usually contain obvious vacuoles of similar substance. Alternatively, the tumor may grow as an **undifferentiated mass of cells, many or most of which are distended with large vacuoles of mucin to produce the characteristic signet ring pattern** so frequently encountered in the undifferentiated tumors of the stomach and gastrointestinal tract.

Basic to all three of these variants is the production of mucin, either intra- or extracellularly. The neoplastic cells show the usual anaplasia and invasive characteristics.

Paget's Disease. Paget's disease of the breast is a **specialized form of intraductal carcinoma that arises in the main excretory ducts of the breast, and extends to involve the skin of the nipple and areola.** As a consequence of this malignant invasion of the skin, eczematoid changes occur in the nipple and areola, so that for many years Paget's disease was considered to be only an inflammatory involvement of the skin of the breast. Careful morphologic study of these lesions has demonstrated beyond doubt that intraductal carcinoma invariably antedates the skin change. This disease tends to occur in an age group slightly older than

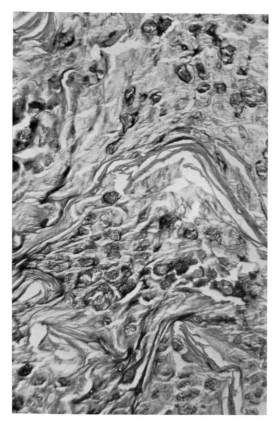

Figure 28-20. Carcinoma of breast—mucinous undifferentiated pattern. The neoplastic cells are dispersed throughout the collection of stringy mucin.

that with the common forms of breast carcinoma. Since Paget's disease of the nipple implies extension to the skin, the prognosis is somewhat less favorable than in the simple noninvasive ductal carcinoma. About 30 to 40 per cent of these women have metastases at the time of surgery.

The most striking gross characteristics of this lesion involve the skin. The skin of the nipple and areola is frequently fissured, ulcerated and oozing. There is surrounding inflammatory hyperemia and edema. In the far advanced cases, total ulceration of the nipple and areola may occur (Fig. 28-21). Superimposed bacterial infection may cause a localized suppurative necrosis, which masks the eczemalike changes. An underlying lump or mass is only rarely present.

Section through the lesion invariably reveals marked proliferation within ducts similar to the other forms of ductal carcinoma. In the far advanced lesion, the tumor extends through the duct basement membrane, at which time the other characteristics of the scirrhous carcinoma may be present.

The histologic hallmark of this entity is the invasion of the epidermis by malignant cells, referred to as **Paget cells.** These cells are large, anaplastic and hyperchromatic, and are usually surrounded by a clear zone or halo. This zone of clearing has been referred to as "ballooning degeneration" (Fig. 28-22). The use of the term degeneration presumably refers to the hypothesis that such cells result from alterations in the epidermal cells produced by the ductal carcinoma. Majority opinion, however, favors the view that these intraepidermal cells are neoplastic cells of the ductal carcinoma that have invaded the epidermis. In addition to the pathognomonic Paget cells, the other histologic criteria of ductal carcinoma are also present.

There are **additional morphologic features common to all infiltrative breast carcinomas,** whatever the histologic type. As focal lesions, they extend progressively in all directions. In the course of time, they may become adherent to the deep fascia of the chest wall and thus become **fixed in position.** Extension to the skin may cause not only fixation but **retraction and dimpling of the skin,** an important characteristic of malignant growth. At the same time, the lymphatics may become so involved as to block the local area of skin drainage, and cause lymphedema and thickening of the skin, a change that has for years been referred to as **"orange peeling."** When the tumor involves the main excretory ducts, particularly in the intraduct variety, **retraction of the nipple** may develop. Certain carcinomas, particularly during pregnancy, tend to infiltrate widely through the breast substance, involve the majority of the lymphatics and produce acute swelling, redness and tenderness of the breast, a picture referred to clinically as **"inflammatory carcinoma."** This is not a special morphologic pattern of carcinoma but merely a clinical variant that implies widespread dissemination. Very late lesions may cause ulceration of the skin or extension within the skin to produce the form that was, at one time, illustrated in medical texts as **"carcinoma en cuirasse"** (Fig. 28-23).

Spread of the tumor eventually occurs through the lymphohematogenous routes. The pathways of lymphatic dissemination are in all possible directions: **lateral** to the axilla, **superior** to the nodes above the clavicle and the neck, **medial** to the other breast, **inferior** to the abdominal viscera and lymph nodes and **deep** to the nodes within the chest, particularly along the internal mammary arteries. The two most favored directions of drainage are the axillary nodes and the nodes along the internal mammary artery.

Overall, about two-thirds of all patients have metastases to lymph nodes at the time of the initial diagnosis of the breast cancer. **The pattern of nodal spread is heavily influenced by the location of the cancer in the breast.** Tumors arising in the outer quadrants involve the axillary nodes alone in about 50 per cent of cases, and have both

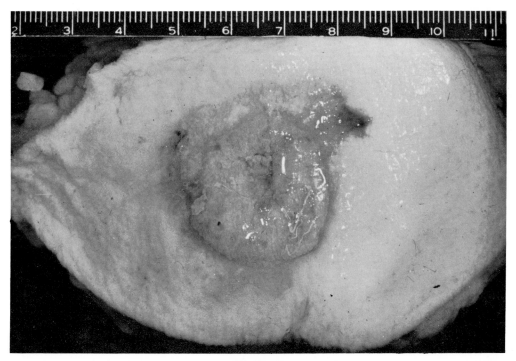

Fig. 28–21

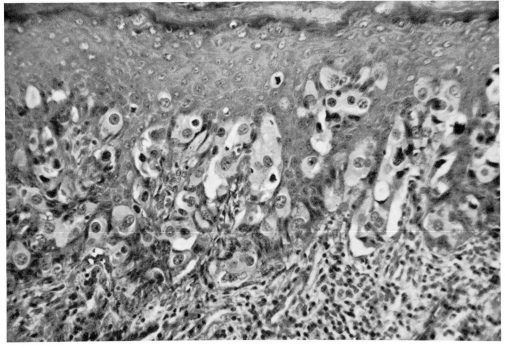

Fig. 28–22.

Figure 28–21. Paget's disease of breast. The lesion is far advanced and has destroyed the nipple.
Figure 28–22. Paget's disease of breast. The classic Paget cells dot the epithelium.

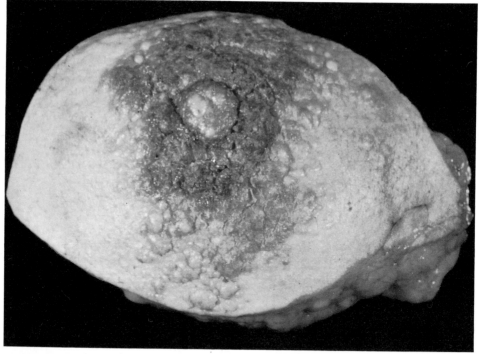

Figure 28–23. Carcinoma of breast. The tumor has extensively invaded the skin in the pattern referred to as "carcinoma en cuirasse."

internal mammary and axillary involvement in an additional 15 per cent of cases. In contrast, cancers arising in the inner quadrants and center of the breast affect the axilla alone in about 25 per cent of cases. In an additional 40 per cent, internal mammary nodes are affected, often with axillary involvement (Haagensen et al., 1969). The supraclavicular nodes are the third most favored site of nodal spread. As will be seen, nodal involvement seriously prejudices the prognosis. Distant metastases via the blood stream may affect virtually any organ of the body and, on occasion, extremely widespread dissemination is encountered. Favored sites for metastases are the lungs, bones, liver and adrenals. Some of the most bizarre metastatic involvements, such as spread to the pituitary gland, eyes and skin, are seen in this form of cancer.

Classification of Breast Cancer. The many histologic grades and stages of breast cancer have been subdivided into smaller homogeneous groups to standardize comparisons of results of various therapeutic modalities among clinics. A plethora of classifications has led to mass confusion but, at the present time, three are widely used, one based on histologic details and the other two on the extent of spread of the cancer.

The histologic classification of cancers arising in ducts is as follows:

Type 1. Nonmetastasizing: intraductal or comedocarcinoma without stromal invasion.

Type 2. Rarely metastasizing: pure extracellular mucinous or colloid cancer, medullary cancer with lymphocytic infiltration, well differentiated adenocarcinoma.

Type 3. Moderately metastasizing: scirrhous carcinoma, intraductal carcinoma with stromal invasion.

Type 4. Highly metastasizing: undifferentiated carcinoma.

The classification of the extent of spread of the neoplasm promoted by the Union Internationale Contre le Cancrum (UICC) employs the TNM terminology (p. 156) (Commission on Clinical Oncology, 1968), as shown below:

T1 < 2 cm. in diameter—no skin fixation.

T2 2 to 5 cm. in diameter—skin infiltration or ulcerative—no pectoral fixation.

T3 5 to 10 cm. in diameter—infiltrative or ulcerative—pectoral fixation.

T4 > 10 cm. in diameter—skin involvement but not beyond the breast—chest wall fixation.

N0 No nodes.

N1 Axillary nodes, present but movable.

N2 Axillary nodes, fixed.

N3 Supraclavicular nodes, edema of arm.

M0 No metastases.

M1 Metastases, including skin involvement beyond breast and contralateral nodes.

The American Joint Committee on Cancer Staging more or less follows the recommendations of the UICC and divides the clinical stages as follows (Copeland, 1962):

Stage 1. A tumor less than 5 cm. in diameter without nodal involvement and no metastases.

Stage 2. A tumor less than 5 cm. in diameter with movable axillary nodes, but no metastases.

Stage 3. All breast cancers of any size with possible skin involvement, pectoral and chest wall fixation, nodal involvement including axillary nodes, fixed, but without disseminated metastases.

Stage 4. Any form of breast cancer with or without nodal involvement, pectoral fixation, skin ulceration or chest wall fixation, but having disseminated metastases.

Clinical Course. Cancers of the breast are usually first discovered by the patient or physician as a solitary, painless mass in the breast. The older the patient with a single breast mass, the more likely is it cancer. When first discovered, these cancers are deceptively freely movable and delimited. Accordingly, the differential diagnosis extends to virtually every disorder in this chapter, including the variants of fibrocystic disease, fat necrosis, scarring of an abscess, and benign tumors. Most cancers are first detected by the patient during self-examination. On the average, these lesions are 4 cm. in diameter when first found, and approximately two-thirds have already spread to axillary or other nodes. Intraductal cancers, which rarely produce palpable masses, more often come to attention by the appearance of a discharge (sometimes hemorrhagic) from the nipple.

Because mastectomy or radiation is still the most reliable means of cure of localized disease, an enormous effort has been made to identify breast cancers while they are still in Stage 1. For some time, the hope was held that health education and frequent self-examination would accomplish this goal, but recent studies challenge this optimism (Thiessen, 1971). A number of factors influence the validity of the self-examination technique, principally the size of the breast. Currently, emphasis is being placed on more frequent, regular medical examinations and mammography as a screening technique. The latter method discloses the increased density and spotty calcifications characteristic of breast cancer. It is capable of detecting lesions smaller than can be identified by palpation and, in several surveys, provided the only evidence for the existence of as many as one-third of the cancers discovered (Strax, 1971). However, mammography yields a false-negative diagnosis in about 15 per cent of proven breast carcinomas. In addition to clinical examination and mammography, newer approaches such as thermography, ultrasonic studies and xerography are being employed to provide more meticulous evaluation of women known to be at high risk.

At the present time, it is impossible to present a concise consensus of the most effective methods of treating the varying stages of breast cancer. Contention continues about the effectiveness of the following approaches:

1. Radical mastectomy (which includes removal of axillary nodes and pectoral muscles).

2. Superradical mastectomy (usually following biopsy of the supraclavicular and internal mammary nodes) which includes, in addition to the radical mastectomy, removal of internal mammary nodes and supraclavicular nodes on the same side.

3. Simple mastectomy or local excision of the lesion along with intensive irradiation (McWhirter technique).

4. Radical mastectomy with prophylactic, postoperative irradiation.

5. Radiation alone.

The prognosis in breast cancer is obviously modified by the histologic grade of the lesion, the clinical stage at time of discovery and such other variables as concomitant pregnancy (the disease appears to be more virulent during pregnancy) and the adequacy of primary treatment. Bad prognostic signs include:

1. Extensive edema of the skin over the breast.

2. Edema of the arm.

3. Satellite nodules in the skin over the breast.

4. Extensive skin ulcerations.

5. Fixation to the chest wall.

6. Fixation of axillary nodes.

7. Spread to internal mammary nodes.

8. Supraclavicular metastases.

9. Inflammatory carcinoma (redness, swelling, and increased heat in the affected breast due to diffuse permeation of the cancer into the regional lymphatics and blood vessels.

10. Distant metastases.

In the overall view of breast cancers, the five-year survival is about 35 to 40 per cent. This rate is heavily weighted by the fact that approximately 25 per cent of breast cancers are found to be inoperable at the time of discovery. The five-year survival rate for all patients treated by radical mastectomy is on the order of 50 to 55 per cent. Surprisingly, this survival rate has not changed significantly in the past decade. Indeed, at one time there was a prevailing view that therapy did little to alter the natural course of this disease, accounting for the unchanging survival rate despite modifications in therapy. Recent studies have dispelled this notion and document that untreated cases yield a five-year survival rate of approximately 20 per cent (Bloom et al., 1962). Stage 1 cancers with adequate therapy yield an 80 per cent five-year survival rate and a 62 per cent 10-year survival, without evidence of residual disease. It should be noted that recurrence may appear late, even after 10 years but, with each passing year free of disease, the prognosis improves. Thus, less than 20 per cent of patients free of disease after five years died during the next five years. Stage 2 cancer, with nodal involvement, yields only a 36 per cent five-year survival and a 22 per cent 10-year survival without evidence of residual disease. The McWhirter technique of local excision and radiation therapy has yielded approximately the same survival rates for Stage 1 disease and slightly better survival rates (50 to 55 per cent) for Stage 2 (Guttman, 1968). Despite these small differences, there is still much uncertainty as to which is the best method of treatment of breast cancer, and more data must be gathered on carefully controlled and matched series.

In addition to surgery and radiation, which are generally utilized as primary forms of treatment, a host of other interventions are employed either to support the primary treatment or as secondary measures in those who fail to respond or suffer recurrences. Ovariectomy may be performed in premenopausal women in an effort to reduce levels of circulating estrogens. Sex steroids, adrenalectomy, hypophysectomy and chemotherapy are additional measures employed in patients with progressive disease and pain (usually arising in bone metastases), in the hope of prolonging life.

Efforts are currently being made to explore immunologic methods for control of this cancer. There are many suggestions that specific antigens are present in the cancer cells. Antibodies against such antigens can be identified in the sera of these patients (Priori et al., 1971). It has not, however, been possible to document that these antibodies favorably alter the course of the disease. The lymphocytic infiltrate of the medullary carcinoma is generally interpreted as a response of the host to the neoplasm. Sinus histiocytosis in the regional lymph nodes is also interpreted as a defensive reaction. Many studies have attempted to correlate improved prognosis with such lymphoidal reactions with equivocal results (Berg, 1971). Nonetheless, Crile (1965) argues against

removal of axillary lymph nodes (i.e., radical mastectomy) in patients not having solid evidence for nodal metastases. He suggests that the nodes serve as defense barriers and their removal favors more distant spread. Immunotherapy remains, for the present, only a fond hope.

Thus, this discussion of breast cancer ends virtually where it began. The clinical problem is monumental; despite great efforts to solve it, there is much yet to be learned.

PAPILLOMA AND PAPILLARY CARCINOMA

Neoplastic and papillary growths may develop within ducts or cysts (*intraductal and intracystic papillomas or papillary carcinomas*). These lesions are *rarely* palpable and are usually called to the patient's attention by a bloody, serous or turbid discharge from the nipple (Haagensen et al., 1951). They run a wide gamut of morphologic patterns from the benign to the malignant forms, and from those that occur as an isolated solitary excrescence within a duct or cyst to diffuse papillary growths, sometimes designated as *papillomatosis*. The diffuse papillomatous variant is encountered most often in breasts involved with cystic hyperplasia, while the isolated lesion is more apt to occur in an otherwise normal breast. These patterns of neoplastic growth occur most often in women just prior to or during the menopause. The solitary lesion is best considered as a random new growth and, in common with all neoplasms, its precise etiology is unknown. In the diffuse papillomatosis, it is assumed that the genesis of the epithelial hyperplasia is that of mammary dysplasia.

Anatomically, these lesions may be confined to a single focus within one duct, or may involve a large segment of a single duct or many ducts. Commonly, the duct is dilated and contains fresh or changed blood, along with a serous or turbid secretion produced by the obstruction and the necrosis and desquamation of the surface epithelium of the papilloma. **The isolated solitary papilloma is usually an extremely minute lesion, rarely more than 1 cm. in diameter, and is extremely difficult to locate both clinically and anatomically.** It is a small, friable, delicate, villous, branching growth within a dilated duct or cyst. It may be sessile or delicately pedunculated.

On histologic examination, these lesions vary from delicate, branching papillary patterns with slender to broad stalks, to papillary heaping up of epithelial cells without well defined stalks of fibrous stroma. **The isolated papilloma tends to have the**

central connective tissue framework covered by
one to two layers of small, regular, cuboidal
epithelial cells. In the benign papilloma, these
cells are of uniform size and shape and are well
oriented to their basement membrane. The innocent
forms do not produce piled-up masses of cells, nor
do the cells invade the stalks or base of attachment
to the ducts (Fig. 28–24). However, all gradations
of atypicality are encountered, to the frank papillary carcinoma in which the epithelium is more apt
to be piled up in irregular knots and masses on the
fibrous core (Fig. 28–25). This increased cellular
proliferation in the malignant variants is frequently
accompanied by considerable anaplasia of the
epithelium, as well as by invasion of the underlying
stroma, stalk and even the base of the duct.

In the diffuse papillomatosis, no well developed stromal stalk or framework is present, and
the small papillary masses of cells protrude from
the base of the duct or cyst into the lumen as irregular, heaped-up masses of cells that sometimes produce abortive, villous, branching patterns. Usually
these papillomatous projections do not have the
branching complexity of the isolated lesion just
described. There is frequently considerably more
distortion of the cells in the diffuse papillomatosis,
and cell orientation appears to be lost. The individual cells, however, are not anaplastic in the benign
forms. However, malignant characteristics occur in
some cases and are usually accompanied by frank
evidence of invasion of the surrounding ducts.

There is, then, on histologic examination,
a complete spectrum of lesions from those that
are clearly benign with regular, small, uniform

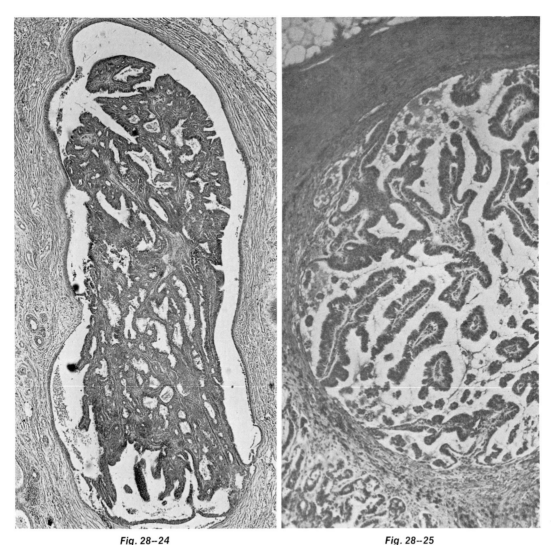

Fig. 28–24

Fig. 28–25

Figure 28–24. Intraductal papilloma.
Figure 28–25. Intraductal papillary carcinoma. The covering epithelium is disorderly and piled up in small
masses on the fibrous stalks. Anaplastic invasive glands are apparent in left lower field.

epithelial cells and no evidence of significant piling up or atypicality of the cells, to those that are frankly anaplastic and give evidence of invasive tendencies. Between these two extremes there are, however, many borderline lesions that produce considerable difficulty in anatomic diagnosis. Fortunately, experience teaches in these borderline cases that most of these lesions behave in a benign fashion and are effectively cured by local excision. In other words, when the biologic behavior of the new growth is that of frank cancer, there is usually little doubt about the anaplastic characteristics of the histologic detail.

It is in relation to this type of borderline new growth that many simple mastectomies are performed, because the lesion is neither frankly malignant nor frankly benign. To escape the responsibility of missing a diagnosis of carcinoma, the entire breast is removed (simple mastectomy), but radical mastectomy with its excision of the pectoral muscles and axillary lymph nodes is not performed. While this course of action may be necessary in some instances, fear dictates its use perhaps too often. Simple mastectomy is generally considered to be, except in rare instances, an unwarranted type of surgery, since in the words of Halsted, "It is too radical for benign disease, and inadequate for malignant disease."

MISCELLANEOUS MALIGNANCIES

Malignant neoplasia may arise from the skin of the breast, from the sweat glands, sebaceous glands and hair shafts, or from the connective tissues and fatty stroma. These tumors are identical with their counterparts found in other sites of the body. Those arising from the skin grow as epidermoid or squamous cell carcinoma. Cancers arising in the skin adnexa grow as carcinomas of sweat glands or sebaceous gland origin (p. 1406). Malignancies of the stroma are, of course, sarcomas. The most common of these types is the fibrosarcoma. Many fibrosarcomas have areas of myxomatous tissue, justifying the designation fibromyxosarcoma. Liposarcomas are quite infrequent. Equally rare are malignancies, such as chondrosarcomas and osteogenic sarcomas, derived from metaplastic differentitaion of the fibroblasts. Of the same origin are the extremely rare reticulum cell sarcomas and other varieties of lymphosarcoma. As a general rule, the sarcomas occur in the same age range as carcinomas, and differ chiefly in their rate of growth. They tend to produce large, bulky, fleshy masses which cause rapid increase in the size of the breast with considerable distortion of the breast contour. Attachment to the skin surface and ulceration are, perhaps, more common with this rapid growth than with carcinomas. Sarcomas as a group spread via the lymphatics to the axillary nodes, but also frequently metastasize via the blood to distant organs, particularly the lungs. The clinical outlook in these cases is poor, and successful removal is rarer than with carcinomas.

FIBROADENOMA AND GIANT FIBROADENOMA (CYSTOSARCOMA PHYLLODES)

The most common benign tumor of the female breast is the fibroadenoma. As the name implies, it is *a new growth composed of both fibrous and glandular tissue*. Occurring at any age within the reproductive period of life, it is somewhat more common before 30. This tumor is said to develop as the result of increased sensitivity of a focal area of the breast to estrogen. On this basis, it may not in reality warrant the designation of new growth, but possibly might be included as a variant of mammary dysplasia. Supporting this dysplastic concept, areas closely resembling a fibroadenoma are found in many cases of mammary dysplasia. Sometimes these areas are poorly defined and merge with the cystic hyperplasia so that the designation *fibroadenomatosis* has been applied to these diffuse lesions to distinguish them from the more common, more typical, focal, discrete nodules called fibroadenomas.

The fibroadenoma usually grows as **a centrifugal, small nodule that is usually sharply circumscribed and freely movable from the surrounding breast substance.** These tumors usually occur in the upper outer quadrant of the breast, but rarely multiple nodules or other locations are encountered. They vary in size up to giant forms 6 to 10 cm. in diameter, but most are removed when 2 to 4 cm. in diameter (Figs. 28–26 and 28–27). As benign lesions, they are encapsulated and tend to be spherical but, on occasion, they may be multilobular and somewhat irregular. Expanding pressures give a firm to hard consistency to the mass. On section, it is composed of uniform, gray-white, apparent fibrous tissue, punctuated by elevated, minute, yellow to pink, softer areas (the glandular structures), which protrude slightly above the level of the surface and impart a granularity or shagginess to the cut section. Occasionally, soft somewhat gelatinous areas are present which have a slightly more opalescent gray appearance or more pink, hemorrhagic coloration. Foci of gritty calcification or opaque hemorrhagic infarction are only rarely encountered.

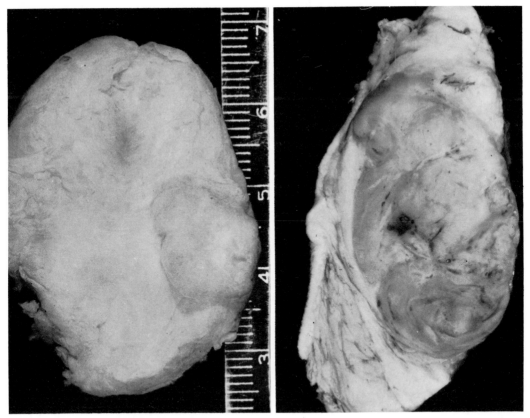

Fig. 28–26   Fig. 28–27

Figure 28–26. Fibroadenoma. The mass is enucleated and has a broad elevated lobule toward the right side.
Figure 28–27. Fibroadenoma. A cross section of breast through the nipple at left of illustration. The large discrete mass occupies a large part of the breast substance.

The histologic pattern is essentially one of **delicate, cellular, fibroblastic stroma enclosing glandular and cystic spaces lined by epithelium.** The connective tissue tends to have a loose, reticulated appearance, and is sometimes myxomatous in nature. The glands show considerable variation in form in different tumors, and in different areas within the same tumor. **Intact, round to oval gland spaces may be present, lined by single or multiple layers of cells (pericanalicular fibroadenoma).** The cells are regular, cuboidal to polygonal in shape. The basement membranes of these glands are intact and usually well defined. The connective tissue immediately surrounding these gland spaces tends to be somewhat compressed and denser than the intervening stroma. In other areas, the connective tissue stroma appears to have undergone more active proliferation with compression of the gland spaces. In consequence, **glandular lumina are collapsed or compressed in slit-like, irregular clefts, and the epithelial elements then appear as narrow strands or cords of epithelium lying within the fibrous stroma (intracanalicular fibroadenoma).**

Quite rarely, **the connective tissue element is scant in amount, and the entire tumor may be composed of fairly densely packed glandular or acinar spaces lined by a single or double layer of cells.** These glands may be separated only by a scant, delicate, fibrous stroma. Cellular regularity is, however, preserved and the encapsulation is unimpaired. This pattern is most often encountered in the lactating breast and frequently the tumor epithelium shows secretory activity similar to that in the surrounding breast substance **(lactating adenoma).**

There does not appear to be valid justification for the sharp differentiation of the pericanalicular pattern from the intracanalicular, since there is so much overlap between the two, and both patterns are so common within a single nodule (Figs. 28–28 and 28–29). Only rarely does one growth pattern exist in pure form, most commonly in the type designated as the adenoma, almost invariably related to the abnormal stimulation of pregnancy and lactation.

The clinical characteristics of the fibroadenoma are apparent from the description given. It usually appears as a solitary, discrete,

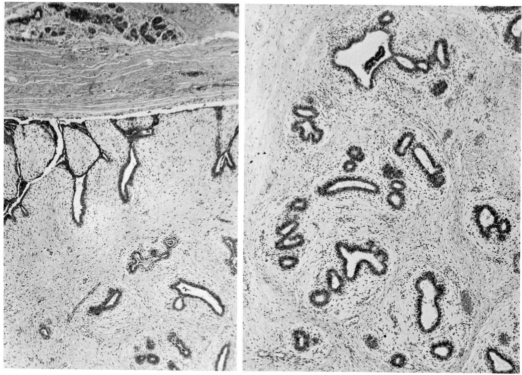

Fig. 28–28   *Fig. 28–29*

Figure 28–28. *Fibroadenoma. The margin of the nodule, showing distinct separation from compressed breast substance above. The growth is in part intracanalicular, particularly near the capsule, with compression of gland spaces. Toward the bottom the pattern is pericanalicular.*

Figure 28–29. *Fibroadenoma. The center of nodule with little compression of glands—the morphology referred to as the pericanalicular variant.*

freely movable nodule within the breast. Quite rarely, several such nodules may be present within a single breast or may involve both breasts. There is no attachment to the overlying skin or underlying fascia. Rounded, fairly smooth margins can usually be made out. Differentiation from a solitary cyst may, at times, be difficult. Slight increase in size may occur during the late phases of each menstrual cycle, and pregnancy may stimulate the growth. Postmenopausally, regression may occur and total calcification may eventuate. Although this lesion presents fairly distinctive clinical characteristics, it nonetheless requires surgical enucleation for absolute verification of its benign nature, a diagnostic procedure that, at the same time, effects a cure.

Infrequently, fibroadenomas may grow to very massive proportions, reaching diameters of 10 to 15 cm., the so-called *giant fibroadenomas.* These large, bulky tumors are also called *cystosarcoma phyllodes,* an unfortunate designation for a lesion which is often benign. They may distort the breast, produce bulges in the contour of the skin and even cause pressure necrosis of the overlying skin. In these ul-

cerated lesions, the capsule of the tumor may rupture, and the growth may fungate through the skin to appear as an irregular malignancy. However, even this bizarre clinical behavior does not of necessity imply malignancy. Histologically, these lesions tend to have a more cellular myxoid stroma than do the fibroadenomas. Lymphomatous, chondromatous or osteoid foci may appear in the stroma (Smith and Taylor, 1969); but the most ominous change is the appearance of increased cellularity with frank anaplasisa of the stroma denoting cancerous transformation. In one large series of 77 cases of these giant tumors, 41 were benign, 18 malignant, and 18 borderline (Treves and Sunderland, 1951). In another study of 94 cystosarcomas, 17 per cent of the patients developed metastases (Norris and Taylor, 1967). Malignant transformation is invariably accompanied by rapid increase in size. Despite malignant transformation, these tumors tend to remain as localized lesions for some time. However, in time, metastases to axillary lymph nodes and distant sites may result. These tumors, even those that are malignant, can be successfully excised to produce a cure in the majority of cases. Most writers caution that, in many instances, anaplastic changes may be found in masses that nonetheless are innocent clinically, and therefore overdiagnosis and overtreatment must be guarded against.

MALE BREAST

The rudimentary male breast is relatively free from pathologic involvement. Only two processes occur with sufficient frequency to merit consideration.

GYNECOMASTIA

The embryogenesis and development of the male breast parallel those of the female breast up to the age of puberty. At this point, only the major breast ducts are formed, with a scant amount of secondary duct branching. *Gland lobules are not found in the normal male breast.* As in the female, the male breast is subject to hormonal influences, but is considerably less sensitive than the female. Nonetheless, enlargement of the male breast (gynecomastia) may occur in response to excesses of estrogen. It is encountered under a variety of normal and abnormal circumstances. It may be found at the time of puberty or in the very aged, in the latter presumably due to a relative increase in the adrenal estrogens as the androgenic function of the testis fails. It is one of the manifestations of Klinefelter's syndrome (p. 181) and may occur in those with functioning testicular neoplasms. It may occur at any time during adult life when there is cause for hyperestrinism. The most important cause for hyperestrinism in the male is cirrhosis of the liver, since the liver is responsible for metabolizing estrogen. *Gynecomastia, then, is the male analogue of cystic hyperplasia in the female.*

Grossly, the lesion may be unilateral or bilateral. Unilateral disease is explained as an increased sensitivity of the tissues in one breast. A button-like, subareolar enlargement develops. In the farther advanced cases, the swelling may simulate the adolescent female breast. On section, the breast tissue is white and rubbery and has minute, elevated, pinkish spots dispersed throughout it. This architectural pattern is reminiscent of that found in certain forms of cystic hyperplasia.

Microscopically, there is proliferation of a dense, periductal hyaline, collagenous connective tissue, but more striking are the changes in the epithelium of the ducts. There is marked hyperplasia of the ductal linings with the piling up of multilayered epithelium (Fig. 28–30). The individ-

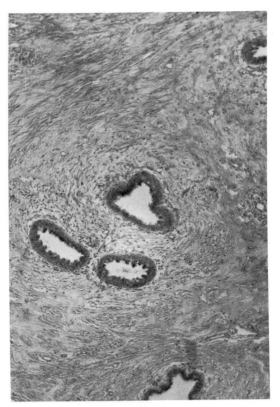

Figure 28–30. *Gynecomastia. There is diffuse interductal fibrosis and hyperplasia of the lining epithelium.*

ual cells are fairly regular, columnar to cuboidal, with regular nuclei. Occasionally there may be some variation in cell size and considerable disorientation of the heaped-up lining cells. Anaplasia is absent. The basal membranes are intact and the lumina of the ducts are rarely filled. There is minimal periductal lymphocytic and plasma cell infiltration. The microscopic changes are, then, similar to the ductal hyperplasia found in cystic hyperplasia in the female.

The lesion is readily apparent on clinical examination, and must only be differentiated from the seldom-occurring carcinoma of the male breast. Gynecomastia is chiefly of importance as an indicator of hyperestrinism, suggesting the possible existence of a functioning testicular tumor (choriocarcinoma), or the possible presence of cirrhosis of the liver. According to Karsner (1946), gynecomastia is *not* related to the development of carcinoma.

CARCINOMA OF THE MALE BREAST

Carcinoma arising in the male breast is a very rare occurrence with a frequency ratio to breast cancer in the female of 1 : 100. It occurs in advanced age. Because of the scant amount of breast substance in the male, the malignancy rapidly infiltrates to become attached to the overlying skin and underlying thoracic wall. Ulceration through the skin is perhaps more common than in the female. These tumors behave exactly as do the invasive scirrhous carcinomas in the female but, on the whole, tend to have less striking desmoplasia and, hence, less of the hard, scirrhous quality. Dissemination follows the same pattern as in women, and axillary lymph node involvement is present in about one-half of the cases at the time of discovery of the lesion. Distant metastases to the lungs, brain, bone and liver are common (Treves and Holles, 1955).

INTERPRETATION OF BREAST MASSES

The differential diagnosis of a mass in the breast is obviously the most important clinical problem that arises in relation to this organ. It is a common clinical problem and is all too often incorrectly handled. The general principle to which most adhere is that *all suspicious areas in the breast must be considered as possible cancer until proved otherwise.* On this basis, the consensus would favor immediate biopsy investigation of all such lesions. While this alarmist attitude may result in a certain number of "unnecessary" surgical procedures, in the long run the greatest good will be done for most patients. Admitting the difficulties in clinical differential diagnosis of breast masses, it is, nonetheless, desirable to consider the various lesions that may be present according to the age group of the patient. Such a consideration provides a foundation for the clinical approach to the problem and aids in arriving at a correct *preoperative* diagnosis.

MASSES IN THE BREAST IN WOMEN UNDER THIRTY-FIVE

Cystic Hyperplasia. Cystic hyperplasia or fibrocystic disease is, without question, the most important cause of abnormalities in the breast in this age group. The most common variant is simple fibrosis. However, cystic disease and epithelial hyperplasia may also occur. These lesions occasionally produce single, unilateral masses but, as has been indicated, many cause multifocal and bilateral involvement that aids in the appropriate diagnosis.

Fibroadenoma. This solitary, circumscribed, well delimited benign tumor is the most common neoplasm in this age group.

Mastitis. These focal or diffuse infections develop particularly during pregnancy and nursing. They are usually accompanied by local and systemic signs of inflammation, rendering the diagnosis reasonably apparent. In the presence of these inflammatory reactions, it may be justified to observe the process for a reasonable period of time to determine whether or not it may totally disappear. Persistence of the mass, however, requires biopsy.

Traumatic Fat Necrosis. This is a rare disorder, which can be diagnosed only in the presence of a well defined clinical history of injury. In the absence of such a history, a characteristic of at least one-half of the cases, this diagnosis can be established only by histologic examination.

Carcinoma of the Breast. Although malignancy is uncommon in this age group, it cannot be excluded on this basis. In clinical practice, it is distinctly more common than traumatic fat necrosis.

MASSES IN THE BREAST BETWEEN THE AGES OF THIRTY-FIVE AND FIFTY

This age range is most subject to the development of breast masses.

Cystic Hyperplasia. This is the most common cause of abnormal lesions in the breast in this age group also. All three variants of this disorder may be encountered, but the variants which show epithelial hyperplasia are, perhaps, more frequent. Since this lesion is associated with a higher than usual attack rate of cancer, surgical exploration is strongly indicated. The presence of a diffuse or bilateral involvement cannot be accepted as an indication for nonoperative observation.

Carcinoma. Mammary cancer is frequent in this age range, and ranks second only to cystic hyperplasia as a cause of masses. Any one of the many forms of carcinoma may be present, but the invasive, scirrhous variety is unquestionably the most prevalent.

Fibroadenoma. This benign tumor is distinctly less common in this age group than in younger women.

Traumatic Fat Necrosis. Since no age is immune to this lesion, it also occurs in this group.

Mastitis. Acute inflammations are less common in this somewhat older age group, presumably because of the lower pregnancy rate.

Papilloma. Papillomas of the breast must be included in the differential diagnosis of lumps, although it is recognized that these lesions are frequently so small as to be entirely occult. The abnormal discharge from the nipple is the most common presenting feature, but occasionally this secretion may be accompanied by alterations in the consistency of the breast.

MASSES IN THE BREAST IN THE AGE GROUP OVER FIFTY

Carcinoma. This is the most common cause for abnormal masses in this age group.

Cystic Hyperplasia. Cystic disease occurs at or just after the menopause and, therefore, must also be considered as an important cause of breast pathology in this group.

Fat Necrosis. In the postmenopausal group, the atrophy of the breast parenchyma causes a relative increase in the amount of fat in the stroma. Accordingly, the breast in this age group is perhaps more subject to injury than in younger women.

Paget's Disease of the Breast. This is given a separate heading, because clinically it is often confused with dermatitis. In this age group, involutional atrophy of the skin predisposes to inflammatory conditions, and hence the eczematoid nature of the nipple lesion may deceive the patient into considering the process as a simple dermatitis.

Acute Mastitis. Inflammations in this age group are quite rare.

Papilloma. These benign tumors may occur, producing abnormal discharge.

The chief value of any such differential diagnosis, it should be pointed out, lies merely in the collection of a list of entities that require consideration in attempting to establish a correct preoperative diagnosis. Under no circumstances is it to be implied that the differential features permit a definite diagnosis without further investigative procedures.

REFERENCES

Adair, F. E., and Munzer, J. T.: Fat necrosis of the female breast: a report of 110 cases. Amer. J. Surg., 74:117, 1947.

Arthes, F. G.: The pill, estrogens and the breast. Epidemiologic aspects. Cancer, 28:1391, 1971.

Berg, J. W.: Morphological evidence for immune response to breast cancer. An historical review. Cancer, 28:1453, 1971.

Bittner, J. J.: Some possible effects of nursing on mammary gland tumor incidence in mice. Science, 84:162, 1936.

Bloom, H. J. G., et al.: Natural history of untreated and treated cases according to histological grade of malignancy. Brit. Med. J., 2:213, 1962.

Chopra, H. C., et al.: Studies on virus particles resembling oncogenic RNA virus in monkey breast carcinoma. Cancer, 28:1406, 1971.

Commission on Clinical Oncology of the Union Internationale Contre le Cancrum (International Union Against Cancer—UICC): TNM classification of malignant tumors. Geneva, International Union Against Cancer, 1968.

Copeland, M. (ed.): Clinical Staging System for Carcinoma of the Breast. American Joint Committee for Cancer Staging. An End Result Reporting. June, 1962.

Crile, G., Jr.: Rationale for clinical stage 1 cancer of breast. Surg. Gynec. Obstet., 120:975, 1965.

Cutler, S. J., et al.: Increasing incidence and decreasing mortality rates for breast cancer. Cancer, 28:1376, 1971.

Dmochowski, L.: Viruses and breast cancer. Cancer, 28:1404, 1971.

Editorial: Benign and malignant breasts. Lancet, 2:218, 1972a.

Editorial: Steroid hormones and breast cancer. Lancet, 2:521, 1972b.

Feinleib, M., and Garrison, R. J.: Interpretation of the vital statistics of breast cancer. Cancer, 24:1109, 1969.

Feller, W. F., and Chopra, H. C.: Virus-like particles in human milk. Cancer, 28:1425, 1971.

Foote, F. W., and Stewart, H. E.: Comparative study of cancerous vs. noncancerous breasts. Ann. Surg., 121:6, 197, 1945.

Foote, F. W., and Stewart, H. E.: A histologic classification of carcinoma of the breast. Surgery, 19:74, 1946.

Frantz, V. K., et al.: Incidence of chronic cystic disease in so-called "normal breasts." A study based on 225 postmortem examinations. Cancer, 4:762, 1951.

Guttman, R.: Trends in radiotherapy for breast cancer. In Cancer Management. Philadelphia, J. B. Lippincott Co., 1968, p. 131.

Haagensen, C. D.: Diseases of the Breast. Philadelphia, W. B. Saunders Co., 1971, p. 155a.

Haagensen, C. D.: Diseases of the Breast. Philadelphia, W. B. Saunders Co., 1971, p. 169b.

Haagensen, C. D.: Mammary duct ectasia. A disease that may simulate carcinoma. Cancer, 4:740, 1951.

Haagensen, C. D., et al.: Metastasis of carcinoma of the breast to the periphery of the regional lymph node filter. Ann. Surg., 169:174, 1969.

Haagensen, C. D., et al.: Papillary neoplasms. Ann. Surg., 113:18, 1951.

Jones, D., et al.: Steroid metabolism by human breast tumours. Biochem. J., 116:919, 1970.

Karsner, H. T.: Gynecomastia. Amer. J. Path., 22:235, 1946.

Korenman, S. G., and Dukes, B. A.: Specific estrogen binding by the cytoplasm of human breast carcinoma. J. Clin. Endocr. Metab., 30:639, 1970.

MacMahon, B., and Cole, P.: Endocrinology and epidemiology of breast cancer. Cancer, 24:1146, 1969.

MacMahon, B., et al.: Lactation and cancer of the breast: a summary of an international study. Bull. W.H.O., 42:185, 1970.

Mirra, A. P., et al.: Breast cancer in an area of high parity, Sao Paulo, Brazil. Cancer Res., 31:77, 1971.

Moore, B. H., et al.: Some aspects of a search for human mammary tumor virus. Cancer, 28:1415, 1971.

Norris, H. J., and Taylor, H. B.: Relationship of the histologic features to behavior of cytosarcoma phyllodes. Cancer, 20:2090, 1967.

Pollard, H. M.: Welcoming remarks in a breast cancer symposium. Cancer, 28:1368, 1971.

Priori, E. S., et al.: Immunofluorescence studies on sera of patients with breast carcinoma. Cancer, 28:1462, 1971.

Randall, C. L., et al.: The probability of the occurrence of the more common types of gynecologic malignancy. Amer. J. Obstet. Gynec., 68:1378, 1954.

Robbins, G. F., and Berg, J. W.: Bilateral primary breast cancer: a prospective clinicopathological study. Cancer, 17:1501, 1964.

Sandison, A. T.: An autopsy study of the adult human breast, National Cancer Institute, Monograph No. 8, U.S. Department of Health, Education and Welfare, 1962.

Schlom, J., and Spiegelman, S.: DNA polymerase activities and nucleic acid components of virions isolated from a spontaneous mammary carcinoma from a rhesus monkey. Proc. Nat. Acad. Sci., 68:1613, 1971.

Schlom, J., et al.: RNA dependent DNA polymerase activity in virus-like particles isolated from human milk. Nature, 231:97, 1971.

Seman, G., et al.: Studies on the presence of particles resembling RNA virus particles in human breast tumors, pleural effusions, their tissue cultures, and milk. Cancer, 28:1431, 1971.

Shapiro, S., et al.: The search for risk factors in breast cancer. Amer. J. Public Health, 58:820, 1968.

Smith, B. H., and Taylor, H. B.: The occurrence of bone and cartilage in mammary tumors. Amer. J. Clin. Path., 51:610, 1969.

Strax, T.: New techniques in mass screening for breast cancer. Cancer, 28:1563, 1971.

Thiessen, E. U.: Breast self examination in proper perspective. Cancer, 28:1537, 1971.

Tice, G. I., et al.: Comedomastitis. A clinical and pathologic study of data in 172 cases. Surg. Gynec. Obstet., 87:525, 1948.

Treves, N., and Holles, A. I.: Cancer of the male breast. Cancer, 8:1239, 1955.

Treves, N., and Sunderland, D. A.: Cystosarcoma phyllodes of the breast. A malignant and benign tumor. A clinicopathologic study of 77 cases. Cancer, 4:1286, 1951.

Urban, J. A.: Bilaterality of cancer of the breast. Cancer, 20:1867, 1967.

Urban, J. A., and Adair, F. E.: Sclerosing adenosis. Cancer, 2:625, 1949.

Vessey, M. P., et al.: Investigations of the possible relationship between oral contraceptives and benign and malignant breast disease. Cancer, 28:1395, 1971.

Warren, S.: The prognosis of benign lesions of the female breast. Surgery, 19:32, 1946.

Yuasa, S., and MacMahon, B.: Lactation and reproductive histories of breast cancer. Bull. W.H.O., 42:195, 1970.

Zippin, C., and Petrakis, N. L.: Identification of high risk groups in breast cancer. Cancer, 28:1381, 1971.

29

THE ENDOCRINE SYSTEM

ADRENAL CORTEX

NORMAL

The adrenals, although small and tucked incongruously away as seeming appendages to the kidneys, are remarkably crucial to homeostasis and adaptation to stress. We do not know why the cortex and medulla are in such close relationship, for they have little in common. The medulla is of neural crest ectodermal origin and thus is essentially a part of the nervous system. The cortex is mesodermal in origin, derived from the urogenital ridge. In its development, the human adrenal passes through three stages: (1) fetal, (2) childhood and (3) adult. Prior to birth, the adrenal cortex is largely composed of a wide juxtamedullary fetal zone. Precisely at the time of birth, irrespective of whether the infant is full term, premature or postmature, the fetal zone begins to atrophy. In a few months, the three definitive cortical zones appear: the subcapsular zona glomerulosa, the zona fasciculata and the zona reticularis (adjacent to the medulla).

The precise weight of the adrenal glands is a detail of considerable importance. Many striking adrenal endocrinopathies (for example, adrenal cortical hyperplasia) are associated with nothing more than a subtle increase in adrenal weight. The gland weights vary with age. At birth, the adrenals are large and heavy, relative to body weight, and weigh in the aggregate 4 to 8 gm. Over the age of 10 to 15 years, when the periadrenal fat is carefully stripped, they should normally weigh, in the aggregate, 7 to 8 gm. in the female and 8 to 9 gm. in the male (Symington, 1962). Normally, the adrenal cortex is yellow to yellow-brown. Often, the lipid and steroid content of the adrenal cortex is judged by its yellowness. Thus, it is sometimes said that a brown hue implies lipid and steroid depletion. In point of fact, the lipids of the adrenal cortex consist principally of free cholesterol and its esters, triglycerides and phospholipids, all of which are essentially colorless. There is very little preformed steroid in the normal adrenal cortex since, as steroid is synthesized, it is rapidly released into the circulation. The yellow cortical coloration is due to lipochrome pigments which bear no relationship to the steroid secretory activity of the cortex.

Of the three distinct zones in the human adrenal cortex, the outer or *zona glomerulosa* is poorly formed and consists of small cells with dark nuclei and scanty cytoplasm, arranged in small groups that lie parallel to the fibrous capsule of the gland. Not infrequently, this zone is present in some areas and absent in others. The *zona fasciculata*, constitutes fully 80 per cent of the normal gland. The cells are stocked with lipid, most of which is cholesterol, cholesterol esters and unsaturated lipids, which appear as vacuolated spaces in the usual paraffin sections. This cell of the zona fasciculata is referred to appropriately as the *clear cell*. It is poor in stainable enzymes, such as alkaline and acid phosphatase, as well as the dehydrogenase enzymes of the Krebs cycle, and few mitochondria are seen. Little stainable ribonucleic acid is found. The zona fasciculata ends abruptly in the narrow *zona reticularis*, which abuts on the adrenal medulla. The cells of the zona reticularis are arranged in small alveoli, which are widely separated by thin-walled, blood-filled channels. The cells of this zone are poor in lipid, have an eosinophilic cytoplasm but differ from the clear cells of the zona fasciculata in that they are rich in alkaline and acid phosphatase, ribonucleic acid, as well as the Krebs cycle dehydrogenases. Abundant mitochondria are present in the cytoplasm. These cells of the zona reticularis are referred to as *compact cells*.

The compact cell of the zona reticularis is the normal, functionally active cell of the cortex, supplying the daily usual needs of steroids (Symington, 1959). The zona fasciculata with its clear cells represents a storage zone of precursor lipid, available on stimulation of the gland for synthesis of increased amounts of steroid. Thus, *in prolonged or chronic stress or after exogenous ACTH (corticotropin) stimulation, the clear cells of the fasciculata are converted into compact cells as the clear cell becomes activated* and the stored lipid is converted to steroid hormones (Fig. 29–1). Concomitantly, this transformed cell becomes rich in phosphatases, dehydrogenase enzymes and ribonucleic acid, all attributes of cellular activity. The zona fasciculata thus comes into full activity in response to unusual demands on the cortex for increased amounts of steroid, and so the zona reticularis and zona fasciculata must be regarded as variants of the same zone (Braunstein and Yamaguchi, 1964). This same transformation of clear cells to compact cells is also found in the hyperfunctioning, hyperplastic or neoplastic gland, as will be seen later.

As would be anticipated with active steroid synthesis, cortical cells abound with smooth endoplasmic reticulum. The mitochondria are somewhat distinctive in each of the three cortical zones. In the glomerulosa they are round or elongated, with lamellar cristae. In the fasciculata, they tend to be round and have tubular cristae, while those in the reticularis are long or round but have tubular cristae (Long and Jones, 1967).

Steroid Biosynthesis. All steroid hormones are of basically similar structure with relatively minor chemical differences which,

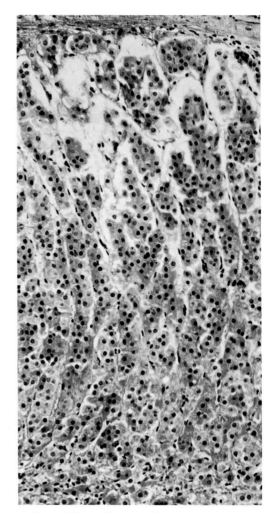

Figure 29–1. Human adrenal cortex in stress— complete lipid depletion. The cells of the cortex are exclusively compact in type.

however, lead to striking specificities in biologic activity. All have a basic skeleton of 17-carbon atoms labeled in a definite order, and to this common denominator are added 1-, 2- or 4-carbon atoms. As is well known, the steroids fall into three major groups: glucocorticoids, synthesized largely in the zona reticularis and fasciculata; mineralocorticoids, formed in the zona glomerulosa; and sex steroids, also formed in the reticularis and fasciculata. The most important are the glucocorticoids (C_{21} steroids), among which cortisol (hydrocortisone) is the most active. Glucocorticoids exert their major effect upon intermediary metabolism by converting endogenous protein to carbohydrate. The glucocorticoids appear to block hepatic cell repressors or, in some way, to turn on DNA sequences required for the translation of an mRNA coded for the synthesis of enzymes involved in gluconeogenesis (Catt, 1970).

The major mineralocorticoid is aldosterone (a C_{21} steroid), produced in the zona glomerulosa. Aldosterone, as is well known, is involved in the maintenance of sodium homeostasis. The major triggers of aldosterone secretion are sodium deficiency, potassium excess, angiotensin II and, to a lesser extent, ACTH. The renin-angiotensin system is itself responsive to plasma sodium levels and volume changes.

The adrenal secretes small quantities of testosterone and estradiol. Testosterone is a C_{19} and estradiol a C_{18} steroid. The amounts are not of great biologic significance compared with those produced in the gonads.

A simplified concept of the complex biosynthesis of these steroids is shown in Figure 29-2. Cholesterol, and possibly acetate, in the adrenal cortex under the stimulus of pituitary ACTH is converted via Δ^5-pregnenolone to progesterone under the action of the Δ^5-3β-hydroxysteroid dehydrogenase (Δ^5-3β-HSD). Subsequent conversion of progesterone to the important hormone, cortisol, requires the presence of three enzymes, 17-alpha, 21-alpha and 11-beta hydroxylase. The function of these enzymes is to insert hydroxyl groups at carbon atoms 17, 21 and 11. The 17 and 21 hydroxylases are present in the microsomal fraction of the cell and insert the -OH groups in the alpha (α) position; the 11-hydroxylase is in the mitochondria and puts the -OH group in the beta (β) position. The importance of these enzymes will be seen in the discussion of the etiology of the adrenogenital syndrome. The pathway of synthesis of aldosterone is believed to be via corticosterone, and the biosynthesis of the C_{19} (androgens) and C_{18} (estrogens) steroids arises via 17-alpha hydroxypregnenolone or 17-alpha hydroxyprogesterone.

Many metabolites occur in the urine from C_{18}, C_{19} and C_{21} steroids, and there are three stages in the degradation of the C_{21} hormones (Fig. 29-2). The first results in saturation of ring A with the formation of tetrahydro compounds. This is followed by saturation at C-20 with the formation of the cortols. These substances are estimated in urine as ketogenic steroids. The third stage is removal of the C-20 and C-21 side chains and the formation of the 17-oxosteroids or 17-ketosteroids. Estimation of the different groups has proved valuable in differentiation of the syndromes that result

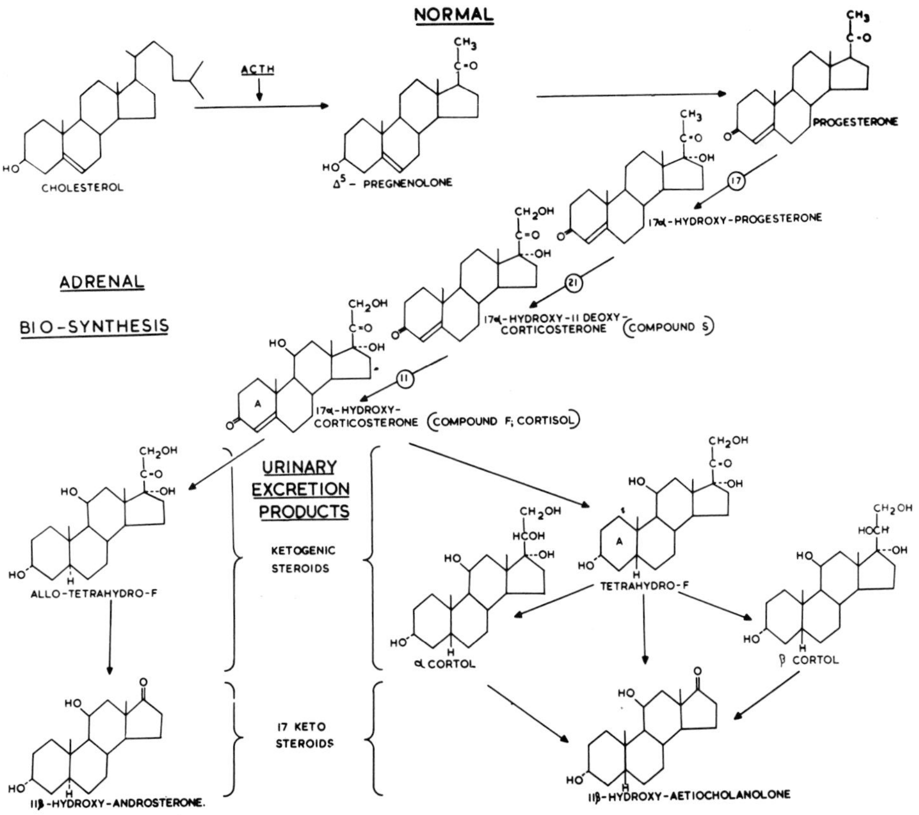

Figure 29-2.

from hypercorticalism. (For further details of steroid assay methods, reference may be made to the work of Loraine, [1958]).

Regulation of Adrenocortical Secretion.

Adrenocorticotropin (ACTH) maintains and regulates cortical structure and function, stimulating predominantly glucocorticoid secretion and exerting a permissive or supportive action on aldosterone secretion. It is secreted by basophils and sparsely granulated chromophobes in the anterior pituitary in response to corticotropin-releasing factor (CRF), formed in the hypothalamus. CRF maintains a circadian rhythm in the adrenal steroid secretion. In those having usual working and sleeping schedules, plasma cortisol levels are low during the night and peak in the morning. There is, in addition, a reciprocal inhibition feedback system between the plasma cortisol levels and ACTH release. The feedback mechanism makes it possible to use suppression tests which employ the administration of glucocorticoids or cortisol-like steroids to inhibit ACTH release. With this procedure, it is sometimes possible to distinguish between hypersecretion of corticosteroids by hyperplastic processes which are pituitary dependent and autonomous neoplastic adrenal sources of steroid hypersecretion. A further independent system, which apparently overrides the basal homeostatic control, is capable of inducing elevations of plasma cortisol during acute stress, such as trauma, infection, emotional tension and delivery.

ACTH appears to act on membrane receptor sites on cells in the zona glomerulosa and fasciculata, stimulating adenyl cyclase and the formation of cyclic AMP. In turn, this nucleotide is believed to act upon messenger RNA involved in the synthesis of a specific regulator protein which modulates steroid synthesis (Catt, 1970). The steroids produced in response to ACTH are predominantly cortisol, corticosterone, ketosteroids and small amounts of androgens and estrogens.

As mentioned above, ACTH is not a major regulator of aldosterone secretion but possibly plays a supportive or permissive role in maintaining the zona glomerulosa. Hypophysectomy induces a fall in aldosterone secretion and causes some slight atrophy of the zona glomerulosa. However, patients with adrenal hyperplasia and increased levels of ACTH do not show elevated levels of aldosterone. ACTH also has a weak melanocyte-stimulating hormone activity. The major control of melanin synthesis in man is still somewhat controversial but is thought to reside in a melanocyte-stimulating hormone (MSH) also known as intermedin. As is discussed later (p. 1355), amino acid sequences in ACTH are identical to porcine MSH, and ACTH also may have an MSH-like activity. In any event, both ACTH and MSH are secreted in high concentrations simultaneously. Thus, in disorders which damage the adrenal and reduce the circulating levels of plasma corticoids, the loss of feedback inhibition leads to increased levels of both ACTH and MSH, resulting in the skin and mucosal hyperpigmentation of adrenal insufficiency (Addison's disease).

The regulation of aldosterone secretion is still under intensive study. As mentioned, salt depletion and increased levels of potassium and angiotensin II all stimulate aldosterone secretion. The main influence of salt depletion, however, is not hyponatremia, but rather hypovolemia. In hypovolemic states, the renin-angiotensin system is called into play, and so the precise ultimate signal for aldosterone secretion is still somewhat uncertain (Bransome, 1968).

Reaction of the Adrenal to Stress.

The role of the adrenal gland in the response to stress is a most controversial one. Selye is the leading proponent of the view that this organ regulates and determines the body's capacity to respond to unusual demands. There is, in fact, no question that the adrenal reacts to stress. However, does the adrenal initiate the adaptive responses to stress, or is its role simply a permissive one allowing these responses to occur? According to Selye, stress acts upon the hypothalamus and, through the hypophyseo-thalamic axis, acts indirectly on the pituitary. There is increased elaboration of ACTH, which acts upon the adrenal to stimulate the production of increased amounts of steroids. These steroids are then responsible for a number of metabolic changes that have the general purpose of preparing the body for an emergency "fight or flight" or for a long-term adaptation to chronic stress.

This entire concept is encompassed within the term *general adaptation syndrome* (Selye, 1946). This syndrome is classically divided into three phases; the alarm reaction, the stage of resistance and the stage of exhaustion. During the alarm reaction, the pulse and blood pressure rise; there is sweating and all the changes we associate with fright. In the stage of resistance, the alterations include the breakdown of protein. Moore and Ball (1955) noted that following an operation there is a negative nitrogen and potassium balance, a positive sodium and water balance and an undue loss of weight. These changes are associated with hyperglycemia and increased levels of urinary 17-ketosteroids and ketogenic steroids. All these alterations are considered by Selye

(1948) to represent various adaptive responses mediated by the adrenal. In the stage of exhaustion, the stored lipid precursor in the adrenal may be depleted, *but there is no valid evidence that there is an insufficiency of circulating adrenal steroids.* Rather, it appears that in the stage of exhaustion there may be failure on the part of the body to utilize the available steroids. It is to be noted, therefore, that even in patients dying of prolonged stressful disease, there is no substantial evidence of adrenal failure or insufficiency.

Ingle and his colleagues doubt that the adrenal is the pivotal organ in this reaction to stress (Crane et al., 1960). They have shown that the whole process can occur in adrenalectomized animals maintained on small constant doses of adrenocortical hormones. These workers therefore propose that the adrenal plays a permissive role in maintaining homeostasis, thus permitting the metabolic alterations to occur in the stressed animal. This conflict of views has, at times, achieved rather epic proportions.

PATHOLOGY

The pathology of the adrenal cortex is of particular clinical significance by virtue of the capacity of diseases to affect the types and amounts of hormones secreted by this organ. Inflammatory and regressive processes and, rarely, some tumors may destroy sufficient functioning cortical tissue to lead to hypoadrenalism or hypocorticalism (Addison's disease). The adrenal cortex has an enormous reserve of functional activity. The destructive processes, then, must wipe out probably over 90 per cent of the functioning cortical tissue before insufficiency develops.

On the other hand, hyperplastic or neoplastic processes may, by the production of increased amounts of steroids, lead to hyperadrenalism, also called hypercorticalism. To understand these syndromes, the biosynthesis of the steroids and the enzyme systems that play a role in this synthetic process must be known. In this area of pathology, as in so many others, function cannot be separated from structure. In the sections which follow, the major disorders of the adrenal will be discussed under the headings of hyper- and hypoadrenalism. Developmental anomalies and nonfunctioning tumors are dealt with separately.

DEVELOPMENTAL ANOMALIES

Adrenocortical hyperplasias are the most important of the congenital anomalies. Since all cause striking alterations and increases in steroid synthesis resulting in adrenogenital syndromes. They will be discussed in the section on hyperadrenalism. Several fairly rare anomalies remain to be considered here.

CONGENITAL ADRENAL HYPOPLASIA

Two distinct adrenal lesions occur in the newborn or young child. In one, the small adrenals are seen in the anencephalic usually stillborn fetus, and the term *anencephalic type* is applied. The gland consists only of a provisional or adult cortex and no fetal zone. The cause is either cerebral, hypothalamic or pituitary in origin.

In the second, the *cytomegalic type*, an equally small adrenal (combined weight less than 1 gm.) and a distinctive histologic pattern are found. The cortex consists uniformly of large compact eosinophilic cells several times the size of normal adrenal cells, referred to as cytomegaly. They extend in irregular columns up to the capsule of the gland. They resemble the large cells seen occasionally in the fetal zone. This cytomegalic type of adrenal hypoplasia should not be confused with cytomegalic inclusion disease, which is a very different condition. The cause of cytomegalic adrenal hypoplasia is still unknown, but is possibly familial. When recognized promptly and replacement steroid therapy is instituted, long survival is possible (Lindgren, 1967).

ECTOPIC ADRENALS

Accessory adrenal tissue may be found retroperitoneally anywhere from the diaphragm to the pelvis. Surprisingly, some of these aberrant adrenals contain both cortex and medulla. Rests of adrenal tissue are also found in the subcapsular regions of the kidney, testis and ovarian cortex. These curious ectopias may assume importance, as in the patient with advanced breast cancer who is ovariectomized and adrenalectomized to ablate all sources of estrogen secretion.

HYPERADRENALISM OR HYPERCORTICALISM

There are three major clinical forms of hyperadrenalism: (1) the adrenogenital (A/G) syndrome, (2) Cushing's syndrome and (3) Conn's syndrome. Common to all is increased biosynthesis of one or more of the adrenocortical steroids. Such cortical hyperfunction may be associated with diffuse or nodular hyperplasia, an adenoma or a carcinoma of the cortex.

Rarely, apparently normal glands are found, but such instances may merely represent the early phase of adrenal hyperplasia. Each of the three clinical forms of hyperadrenalism, then, may be associated with a variety of adrenal lesions. The morphology of the hyperplasia seen in each of these three syndromes is quite distinctive and should, in fact, permit a shrewd guess as to the nature of the clinical syndrome. The neoplasms associated with these three syndromes are, however, not significantly different morphologically from nonfunctioning tumors. Conn's syndrome is usually caused by an adenoma of the adrenal gland, which cannot, on anatomic grounds, be differentiated from an incidental nonfunctioning adenoma. In the A/G and Cushing's syndrome, the neoplasia is very similar and, again, on purely morphologic grounds, resembles nonsteroid-producing tumors.

ADRENOGENITAL (A/G) SYNDROME

The term adrenogenital syndrome encompasses a variety of specific entities. Each is associated with an adrenal enzyme deficiency blocking normal steroid production. Thus, the biosynthesis is shunted into androgenic and other pathways, which, in part, produce virilism. Both infants and adults may be affected. *In the infant or child, the usual cause is some inborn error leading to a lack of a specific adrenal enzyme which blocks the normal biosynthesis of cortisol.* As a consequence of the loss of feedback inhibition, ACTH is elaborated in excess, inducing the congenital adrenal hyperplasia. Similar mechanisms may be operative in the older child or adult, or more precisely, the congenital enzyme defect may not be so severe and thus may not be recognized until later in life. *More often, an autonomous hyperfunctioning adenoma or carcinoma is the cause of the A/G syndrome in adults.*

Among the many patterns of congenital adrenal hyperplasia described by Bongiovanni et al. (1967), only the three most common will be described here: (1) simple virilism, (2) virilism with salt-losing crises and (3) virilism with hypertension. Common to all three is virilism. Both sexes may be affected. The newborn or young female child may present as a pseudohermaphrodite with a phalloid organ but with a uterus and ovaries. In the male child, there may be slight enlargement of the penis, but frequently it is the vomiting and dehydration of the salt-losing crises which direct attention to the possibility of the A/G syndrome. Often, such children die of what is considered to be gastroenteritis or pyloric stenosis. Isosexual precocity develops in the older male child, and signs of hirsutism and enlarged clitoris draw attention to the condition in the older female child. Occasionally, this condition occurs in females in a latent form that only becomes manifest at puberty. The young girls menstruate normally and then, as a result of some emotional stress, develop amenorrhea and hirsutism as manifestations of this condition. In both male and female children, there is a considerable increase in bone age with premature closure of the epiphyses. Virilism characterizes this condition in adult females, manifested by hirsutism, enlarged clitoris, male distribution of hair, baldness of the scalp and male musculature. The breasts are often small. As might be anticipated, virilism alone is virtually impossible to detect in the adult male without laboratory evidence of deranged steroid production or evidence of additional manifestations such as hypertension or derangements in salt metabolism.

Etiology. The etiology of these syndromes lies in the excess of specific steroids. In infants and children with congenital adrenal hyperplasia, the lack of a specific enzyme is inherited as a genetic defect transmitted by an autosomal recessive mutant gene. *A 21-hydroxylase deficiency accounts for about 90 per cent of all congenital adrenal hyperplasias. A partial deficiency of this enzyme produces almost pure virilism.* The dominant steroids elaborated are 17-hydroxyprogesterone and androsterone. Testosterone is also synthesized. C_{21}-hydroxysteroids are inadequately synthesized, and there are reduced levels of cortisol in the blood. As a result, the pituitary gland overproduces ACTH, which appears in increased amounts in the blood. Concomitantly, there is increased urinary excretion of 17-ketosteroids (Fig. 29–3). Pregnanetriol and 11-ketopregnanetriol are also increased. Urinary estimation of these latter two compounds forms an important part of the diagnosis of this condition.

A complete lack of 21-hydroxylase results in inadequate production of both aldosterone and cortisol. Hence the patient manifests virilism with salt-losing crises.

An 11-hydroxylase deficiency is the major cause of virilism with hypertension. In this syndrome, there is increased production of deoxycorticosterone and other mineralocorticoids, and the hypertension may be attributable to sodium retention and hypervolemia.

Adenomas and carcinomas of the adrenal gland may also cause the adrenogenital syndrome, although less is known about the precise biosynthetic pathways in these neoplasms. It can only be assumed that enzymic defects must exist in these tumors. Rapaport et al.

STEROID   BIOSYNTHESIS

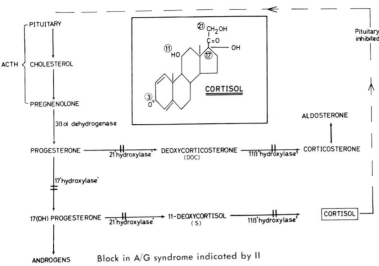

Block in A/G syndrome indicated by ‖

Figure 29--3.

(1952) and Heinbecker et al. (1957) found in the literature, during the years 1930 to 1955, only 113 tumors causing the adrenogenital syndrome. About 50 per cent of these tumors occurred before the age of 12.

Morphology. The adrenal hyperplasia of the A/G syndrome may be either diffuse or nodular. The gland may vary in weight from 2 to 12 gm. in the newborn and up to 30 gm. in the adult female. It has a typical brown color and is depleted of lipid. Microscopically, the histologic appearance closely resembles that found in the normal adrenal after repeated corticotropin stimulation. The zona reticularis and zona fasciculata form a unified zone of compact cells, which extends up to an extremely broad zona glomerulosa (Fig. 29–4). Sometimes a thin layer of clear cells appears in the outer zona fasciculata under the zona glomerulosa.

The adenomas associated with this condition vary from small nodules weighing as little as 10 gm., up to rather massive tumors weighing 200 gm. (Patients with these somewhat bulky but benign tumors have been alive and well 10 years after the surgical removal.) These adenomas are usually well encapsulated and are soft and fleshy (Figs. 29–5 and 29–6). On section, they are red-brown, resembling the zona reticularis of the normal adrenal. Occasionally, the adenomas contain pale yellow streaks of apparent lipid deposit. In the larger adenomas, the tissue is more lobulated and friable and is punctuated by areas of hemorrhage, necrosis or even calcification.

The cells of these benign tumors resemble the compact cells described in the normal adrenal under conditions of stress or corticotropin stimulation. In the small lesions, the cells are almost

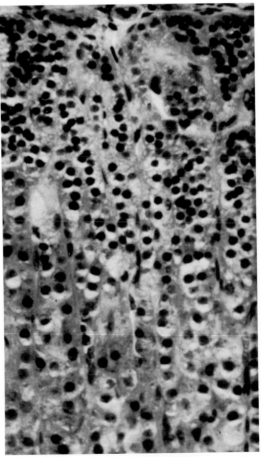

Figure 29--4. Adrenogenital syndrome—adrenal hyperplasia. There is a very broad zona glomerulosa on the surface of the gland. The rest of the cortex consists of compact cells, only a few of which contain lipid globules.

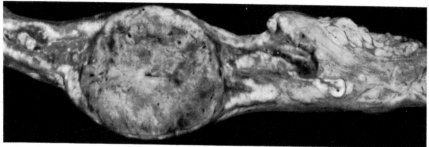

Figure 29–5. A cross section of the adrenal gland illustrating a sharply defined benign adrenal adenoma which appears to occupy a central position.

exclusively of the compact variety, and are often arranged in small distinct alveoli. Occasionally there are focal areas of clear cells (Fig. 29–7). In the larger benign adenomas, the alveolar arrangement is less obvious. The cells are usually compact, but often the cytoplasm loses its granularity and takes on a hyaline appearance. In these larger adenomas, some nuclear and cytoplasmic degeneration may be found progressing to focal areas of necrosis. Occasionally, lesions are encountered with some nuclear enlargement, slight pleomorphism and increased chromatin content. Sometimes these tumors behave clinically as adenomas, and occasionally some behave as carcinomas. The histologic assessment of these borderline lesions is difficult if not, at times, impossible.

In the well established cases of adrenal carcinoma causing the adrenogenital syndrome, the tumors are large, usually weighing over 100 gm., and frequently weighing as much as 4 kg. (Fig. 29–

8). These may be lobulated masses that on section consist of brown, friable tissue with large intervening areas of necrosis and hemorrhage.

Microscopically, the viable cells are usually compact in type and have an ovoid vesicular nucleus. The cells are arrayed in solid sheets around dilated vascular spaces, which are lined by flattened epithelium. Cellular pleomorphism and mitotic figures may or may not be prominent. Some of these carcinomas are composed almost entirely of giant cells with extreme anaplasia and invasion of capsule and blood vessels (Fig. 29–9). It is obvious

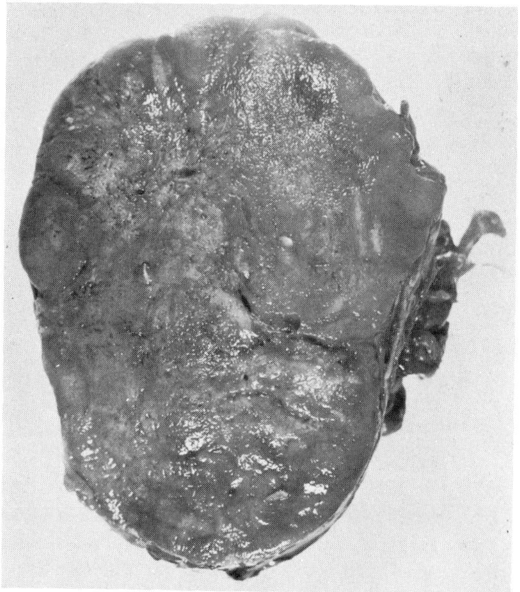

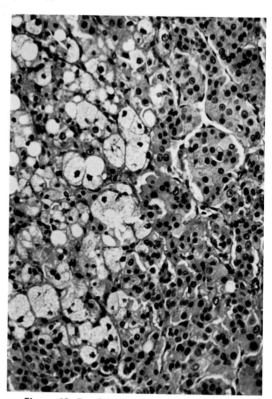

Figure 29–7. Adrenogenital syndrome—adenoma. Most of the tumor consists of compact cells arranged in alveoli of different sizes. There is little or no nuclear or cellular pleomorphism. Some collections of large clear cells are shown.

Figure 29–6. Adrenal adenoma weighing 130 gm. from a patient suffering from adrenogenital syndrome.

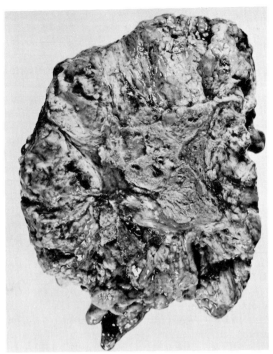

Figure 29–8. *Adrenal carcinoma. The tumor is large, hemorrhagic and necrotic. Very little viable tissue is present.*

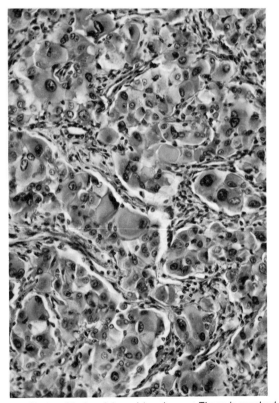

Figure 29–9. *Adrenal carcinoma. There is marked anaplasia and pleomorphism of the neoplastic cells.*

that the cellular morphology of these tumors spans a complete spectrum from innocent regular adenomas to wildly growing carcinomas.

Whatever the symptom complex produced by these carcinomas, all have the potential of metastasizing, commonly to the para-aortic lymph nodes, liver, lungs or brain.

Clinical Course. The clinical manifestations of this condition have already been presented. Cortisol therapy has produced gratifying control of the adrenogenital syndrome associated with hyperplasia of the adrenal (Jailer et al., 1952). Presumably, the administered cortisol suppresses ACTH function and thus diminishes the stimulation of the adrenal cortex that leads to the overproduction of androgenic steroids.

Mention should here be made of the uncommon feminizing pattern of the adrenogenital syndrome, manifested by isosexual precocity in the female before the age of puberty. In the male, feminization occurs with gynecomastia, loss of libido and, in some instances, diminution in the size of the penis. About 52 cases have been reported in the literature (Gabrilove et al., 1965). All are due to tumors (10 to 2800 gm.) that are macroscopically and microscopically identical to those described in the adrenogenital syndrome. A whole range of cellular pleomorphism and mitotic activity has been recorded, and some of these lesions have therefore been diagnosed as adenomas and some as carcinomas. It is interesting that the cellular pleomorphism in some of these cases recorded as adenomas appears to be no less than in others, recorded as carcinomas. Long periods of reappraisal are required before the diagnosis of a benign tumor can be accepted, since metastases may develop as long as seven years later.

CUSHING'S SYNDROME

Only now, after 30 years of study, is the fascinating disorder Cushing's syndrome reasonably well understood. It is characterized biochemically by excess production of glucocorticoids and clinically by central obesity, moon face, buffalo hump, diabetes mellitus, osteoporosis, hypertension, plethora, hirsutism, amenorrhea, acne, weakness and emotional lability. In the original description of this entity in 1932, Harvey Cushing drew attention to the presence of basophil adenomas in the pituitary glands of several of these patients (Cushing, 1932). For a long time, this syndrome was thus thought to be a primary pituitary disorder having secondary effects on the adrenals. Since then, it has become apparent that *there are three general categories of Cushing's syndrome. One is the autonomous production of cortisol by a primary neoplasm (benign or malignant) of the adrenal cortex. The second is excessive secretion of ACTH by the pituitary, stimulating hypersecretion of cortisol. The source of the increased ACTH may be either a pituitary tumor (usually an adenoma, sometimes basophilic hyperplasia) or some functional derangement at the hypothalamic-pituitary level. The third category is the ectopic production of ACTH by nonpituitary neoplasms.*

At this point, the distinction should be made between the terms Cushing's *syndrome* and Cushing's *disease*. The term Cushing's *disease* is reserved for cases identical to those first described by Cushing himself, in which a basophilic adenoma is the primary cause of the hypercorticalism. Cushing's *syndrome* is the more generic term applied to the clinical and metabolic disorder, whatever its cause. It should be noted that *the therapeutic administration of large doses of cortisol, or cortisol-like synthetic steroids, for sufficiently long periods of time will induce an iatrogenic disorder indistinguishable from the natural disease.*

Cushing's syndrome may occur in a "pure" form, when most of the signs and symptoms are attributable to the overproduction of C_{21} steroids, or in a "mixed" form, when features relating to the C_{21} steroids are associated with those relating to excess production of androgens. Adult females are most frequently affected, but this disorder may occur in male or female children, as well as in adult males.

Etiology. Analyses of patients with Cushing's syndrome disclose the following clinicopathologic types (Freeark and Waldstein, 1969).

	Per Cent
Pituitary "tumor" (includes focal hyperplasia)	20
Hypothalamic-pituitary hyperfunction	40
Adrenal adenoma	10
Adrenal carcinoma	15
Nonendocrine ACTH-producing tumor	15

The simplest type of Cushing's syndrome to comprehend is that resulting from the autonomous secretion of cortisol by an adrenocortical neoplasm. As would be expected, the increased levels of cortisol suppress ACTH production (Liddle and Shute, 1969). Since ACTH is not involved in the autonomous hyperfunction of the neoplasm, the excessive steroid synthesis is not affected by suppressing the function of the pituitary, as can be done by the administration of large doses of steroids, such as dexamethasone.

Next simplest to understand is Cushing's

syndrome resulting from ectopic ACTH secretion by nonendocrine tumors (Liddle et al., 1965). A variety of cancers have been implicated, the most common being oat cell carcinoma of the lung, thymomas, thyroid medullary carcinoma and pancreatic islet cell tumors. ACTH can be extracted from these neoplasms. Most patients are cured by surgical removal of the tumor; when the tumor tissue is cultured in vitro, it continues to elaborate ACTH (Liddle et al., 1969). As a consequence of this ACTH excess, either nodular or diffuse hyperplasia occurs in the adrenal gland. Obviously, suppression of the pituitary gland by dexamethasone has no effect on the ectopic elaboration of ACTH. It should be noted that in patients with cortisol-secreting neoplasms primary in the adrenal, the circulating plasma ACTH level is low, while in those with ectopic production of ACTH, it is high.

A third major form of Cushing's syndrome originating in increased secretion of ACTH by a hyperfunctioning pituitary or a pituitary adenoma is less easy to understand. Most of these adenomas are composed of basophils. There is convincing evidence that, in all of these cases, there is inappropriate hypersecretion of ACTH (Ney et al., 1967). As a consequence of the increased levels of ACTH, the adrenals undergo hyperplasia and elaborate excessive amounts of cortisol and other steroids. The adenomas may represent a form of excessive hyperplasia rather than true autonomous neoplasia, since some lesions are exceedingly small and poorly defined. Why the increased levels of steroids do not suppress ACTH production by the pituitary remains a mystery. It has been suggested that the primary defect is hypothalamic with increased production of corticotropin-releasing factor. However, the administration of very large doses of steroids, such as the potent dexamethasone, will, in most instances, suppress the excess pituitary function.

Morphology. In most cases of Cushing's syndrome, changes can be found in the pituitary gland in the form of **Crooke's hyaline degeneration of the basophils** (p. 1363). The cells first lose their specific granulations, and this is followed by progressive hyalinization of the cytoplasm. Electron microscopy indicates that the hyaline deposit has a fibrillar substructure in which the granules of the basophils are scattered (Decicco et al., 1972). Approximately 20 per cent of all patients have a pituitary tumor but, in many, the lesion is small, produces no enlargement of the sella turcica and, more accurately, might be described as a focus of hyperplasia. In most of the instances, the focus of hyperplasia or the adenoma is basophilic in nature, but occasionally the cells appear on light microscopy to be chromophobes, presumably the type now referred to as the sparsely granulated basophil. Because of this variation in precise cytology and in the extent of the proliferative lesion in the pituitary—whether nodular hyperplasia or adenoma—many have resorted to the relatively nonspecific term Cushing's basophilism.

Hyperplasia of the adrenal gland, either diffuse or nodular, is found in 75 per cent of the cases. About half of these hyperplastic adrenals weigh, in the aggregate, 10 to 12 gm. and are sometimes called normal. However, careful analysis of the weights of normal adrenals removed at operation from patients with breast cancer and those found post mortem in healthy young males who have died suddenly from trauma disclosed that the true, normal, single right or left adrenal weighs only 4 gm. Accordingly, the Cushing's adrenals removed at operation that weigh 10 to 12 gm. are not truly normal. It is, however, useful to retain the term normal adrenal, since it depicts the small-sized gland that can occur in Cushing's syndrome as distinct from the much larger hyperplasia encountered in the adrenogenital syndrome. In these cases of Cushing's syndrome, the hyperplastic adrenal retains its normal shape and color, but the edges are slightly rounded in contrast to the sharp margins of the normal gland. In some cases, both adrenals together weigh up to 25 gm., and in these there may be an increase in the width of the cortex.

Histologically, in both the so-called normal and the more frankly hyperplastic glands, there is a prominent zona reticularis, which occupies the inner half of the cortex, and an equally prominent zona fasciculata (Fig. 29—10). The clear cells of the zona fasciculata may be unusually large in the hyperplastic gland but are of usual size in the so-called normal gland. The clearing of the cytoplasm can be resolved under the electron microscope to be due to dilatation and hyperplasia of the smooth ER (Hashida et al., 1970). The hyperplasia is nodular in approximately 15 per cent of patients with Cushing's syndrome (Fig. 29—11).

In about 25 per cent of the cases of Cushing's syndrome, an adenoma or carcinoma is found. Rapaport et al. (1952) and Heinbecker et al. (1957) collected 172 such tumors over a period of 25 years (1930 to 1955).

These tumors are in no way distinctive from those described in the adrenogenital syndrome except in certain minor respects. The adenomas in Cushing's syndrome are more apt to be yellow in color due to enlarged lipid-laden cells scattered throughout the background of the more common compact cells. The same range in cellular pleomorphism is encountered in the cancers of Cushing's syndrome as in those described in the adrenogenital syndrome, as well as the same bizarre patterns of metastatic dissemination (Fig. 29—12).

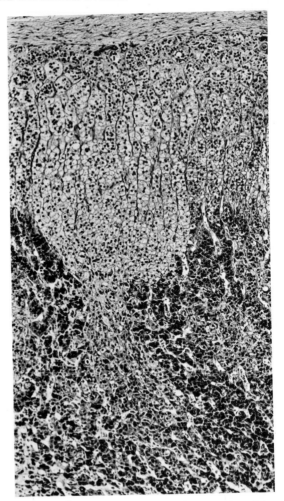

Figure 29–10. Cushing's syndrome—adrenal hyperplasia. A broad zona reticularis, shown below, projects irregularly into the zona fasciculata, shown above. The zona glomerulosa is seen lying under the capsule.

Clinical Course. The full-blown symptom complex of Cushing's syndrome with its rather characteristic facies, obesity, hypertension and osteoporosis, and occasionally derangements in glucose metabolism and menstruation, constitutes a not easily missed clinical syndrome (Sprague et al., 1956).

Cushing's syndrome in childhood differs in several respects from that seen in later life. In adults, ectopic ACTH secretion by nonendocrine tumors and pituitary hyperfunction are the most common causes of Cushing's syndrome. Adrenocortical tumors are less frequent in this age group. In contrast, adrenal tumors are the most common origin of Cushing's syndrome in children during the first two years of life. Such tumors often produce some concurrent virilization (Editorial, 1972).

The differential diagnosis of the major ca-

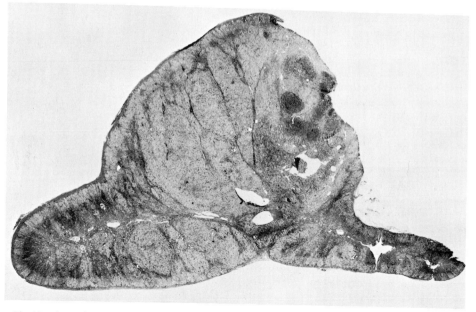

Figure 29–11. Irregular, nodular adenomatous hyperplasia of the adrenal in a case of Cushing's syndrome.

tegories of Cushing's syndrome, with respect to dexamethasone suppression tests and plasma ACTH levels, has already been presented in the consideration of the etiology of this disorder. We need only emphasize here that, although the full-blown syndrome is striking and the moon face can be recognized on entering the patient's room, many times the manifestations are far more subtle and the diagnosis more difficult. In young infants, for example, the major clue may be obesity, not considered at first glance to be significantly abnormal. In older children, retarded growth may be the only manifestation. Frequently, we must rely upon the laboratory to provide definitive evidence. When encountering a case, the vital question must not be forgotten, "Have you been receiving medications from any physician?"

PRIMARY HYPERALDOSTERONISM—CONN'S SYNDROME

This now well recognized syndrome first described by Conn (1955) is characterized by periodic muscle weakness, hypertension, polydipsia and polyuria. When these manifestations are accompanied by an alkaline urine with an elevated serum sodium, hypokalemic alkalosis and renal potassium loss, the diagnosis of primary hyperaldosteronism is almost certain. The diagnosis can be confirmed by the demonstration of an elevated serum level of aldosterone. Renin is characteristically sup-

pressed in Conn's syndrome, the primary form of hyperaldosteronism. In contrast, secondary hyperaldosteronism (as is seen in chronic renal disease, renal artery stenosis and renin-secreting renal tumors) is characterized by increased circulating levels of renin (Brown et al., 1972).

At first, Conn's syndrome was thought to be produced only by cortical adenomas, which secreted an excess of mineralocorticoids. *Indeed, a solitary adenoma is responsible for about 90 per cent of cases.* However, rare instances are associated with multiple adenomas, carcinoma and cortical hyperplasia (Robertson, 1972). Indeed, in those under 20 years of age, bilateral diffuse or nodular cortical hyperplasia is more frequent than an adenoma (Conn et al., 1964) (Omae et al., 1971).

Solitary adenomas are the usual cause of Conn's syndrome in adults. They vary from 1 to 4 cm. in size and appear as encapsulated yellow nodules. Microscopically, the cells are mostly large, lipid-laden clear cells similar to those seen in the zona fasciculata (Fig. 29–13). Recent studies have shown that the histologic pattern in these tumors can be variable (Fig. 29–14) and, despite their zona fasciculata-like appearance, these lipid-laden cells can form aldosterone and corticosterone, as well as cortisol. Sometimes the tumor is composed exclusively of cells of the zona glomerulosa (Fig. 29–15), but more often they are mixed with other cell patterns. Electron microscopic studies have confirmed that either the cells in these adenomas possess lamellar cristae identical to those in the normal glomerulosa cells, or the cells constitute hy-

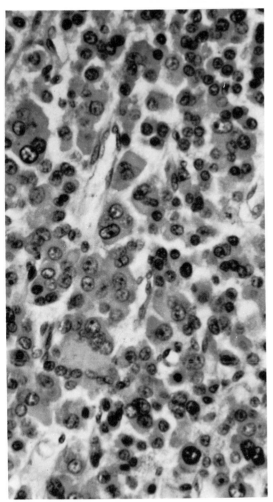

Figure 29–12. *Cushing's syndrome—carcinoma. The tumor in this case weighed 1100 gm. The cells are almost exclusively compact, but show some nuclear and cellular pleomorphism. Mitotic figures are not prominent. A similar histologic appearance occurs in adrenogenital syndrome, feminization and malignant aldosteronism.*

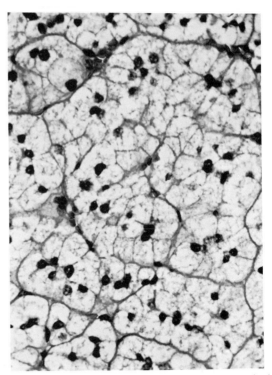

Figure 29–13. *Conn's syndrome—the typical clear zona fasciculata-like cells.*

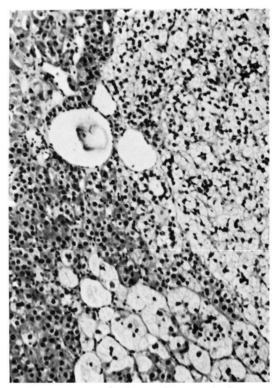

Figure 29–14. *Conn's syndrome—mixed pattern; compact cells to the left, hybrid cells to the right, and a tongue of zona glomerulosa cells in between, with an area of large zona fasciculata-like cells at the bottom.*

brids which possess mixtures of lamellar and tubulovesicular cristae, intermediate between those found in the zona glomerulosa and zona fasciculata.

The most characteristic adrenal alteration in adolescents with this syndrome is diffuse or nodular cortical hyperplasia resulting from widening of the zona glomerulosa. Infrequently, a carcinoma of the adrenal produces hyperaldosteronism in adults.

As mentioned, renin is suppressed in these patients, and the renal juxtaglomerular cells are classically atrophic.

While the diagnosis of Conn's syndrome can often be made readily, it is sometimes extremely difficult to determine the location of the adrenal adenoma before surgery (right or left side). As indicated, the adenomas are

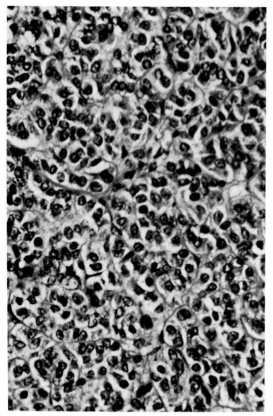

Figure 29–15. A Conn's tumor consisting exclusively of zona glomerulosa-like cells.

usually extremely small and are not clinically palpable. Pyelograms, perirenal air insufflation, radiographic studies and catheterization of the adrenal vein effluent to identify elevated levels of aldosterone must often be employed. Removal of the hyperfunctioning adenoma is curative. If adrenal hyperplasia is found, bilateral subtotal adrenalectomy is performed.

It may be well to mention *Bartter's syndrome* in the differential diagnosis of hyperaldosteronism. This syndrome occurs in infants and is characterized by increased plasma renin, juxtaglomerular cell hyperplasia, hyperaldosteronism and hypokalemia (Wald, 1971). It therefore differs from Conn's syndrome by having increased levels of plasma renin. It has been suggested, but not established, that the hyperaldosteronism is related to the overproduction of renin.

RÉSUMÉ OF ADRENOCORTICAL LESIONS CAUSING HYPERADRENOCORTICALISM

When corticotropin is injected into a normal individual, it exerts its effect on the clear cells of the zona fasciculata nearest the zona re-

ticularis and converts them into compact cells (Symington, 1959). This results in an apparent widening of the zona reticularis and, if sufficient corticotropin is injected, this morphologic transformation will involve the whole of the zona fasciculata and the change may extend out to the capsule. A similar histologic appearance is found in congenital adrenal hyperplasia causing the adrenogenital syndrome, and this is quite expected since there is a marked increase in circulating corticotropin in this condition. However, since the normal biosynthetic process in the adrenal is interfered with in congenital adrenal hyperplasia as a result of a defect in one or more of the hydroxylating enzymes, cortisol formation is defective, androgens are formed in abundance and virilism develops. The increased levels of circulating corticotropin in Cushing's syndrome are lower than those seen in the adrenogenital syndrome and cause less broadening of the zona reticularis. Since there is no defect in the hydroxylating enzyme systems in Cushing's syndrome, the effect of the moderately increased blood corticotropin results in an increase in cortisol production.

In the hyperplastic gland in both syndromes, the effect of corticotropin is to convert the clear fasciculata cell to a compact cell but to a different extent, depending on the amount of circulating corticotropin. The resultant steroids formed depend on the presence or absence of intact hydroxylating enzyme systems. It now becomes clear why the reticularis-fasciculata cell can form C_{21} steroids, such as cortisol and C_{19} androgens, and why, in Cushing's syndrome due to adrenal hyperplasia, the formation of cortisol predominates while, in the adrenogenital syndrome, androgens are formed to a greater extent.

An understanding of this principle makes it clear why tumors causing Cushing's and the adrenogenital syndromes have a similar histologic appearance of compact cells with varying mixtures of clear cells. Again, since there will be a relative lack of many of the enzyme systems, it becomes easier to understand why carcinomas can produce corticosteroids, androgens or estrogens which give rise to a mixed Cushing or adrenogenital syndrome. Likewise, one can understand why it is impossible from simple histologic examination of an adrenal tumor to predict what hormones it is producing or, in fact, if it is producing any hormones at all. It is only by cooperation among the clinician, pathologist and biochemist that a true assessment of adrenocortical lesions will be achieved.

It is now fully established that aldosterone is formed by the cells of the zona glomerulosa and that, in Conn's syndrome not due to a tumor, there is bilateral hyperplasia of the zona glomerulosa. Although the clear, lipid-laden zona fasciculata-like cell is the most common pattern found in recorded adenomas, such cells can produce and secrete aldosterone and its precursors as well as cortisol. This is the basis for referring to such cells as "hybrids."

HYPOADRENALISM OR HYPOCORTICALISM

Adrenal insufficiency may manifest itself as an adrenal crisis or may develop insidiously in a chronic form on which acute insufficiency may be superimposed at any time. Chronic hypoadrenalism is far more common and is better known as *Addison's disease*.

The effects of chronic adrenal steroid deficiency (Addison's disease) include sodium loss; potassium retention; decreases in blood volume, blood lipids and blood sugar; and impairment of renal function with reduced excretion of water, ammonium and urea. More nonspecific manifestations comprise fatigue, muscle weakness, weight loss, anorexia or gastrointestinal symptoms. Hypotension and increased melanin pigmentation of the skin and mucous membranes are often present. Many of the above manifestations become accentuated when sudden loss of cortical function occurs in the course of the chronic illness or in a previously healthy individual.

Acute adrenal insufficiency may constitute a crisis with low blood pressure, rapid pulse and sometimes even circulatory collapse. Patients with such crises often have vomiting, diarrhea and sometimes abdominal pain, and at times these fulminating syndromes are so atypical that adrenal insufficiency is not considered. If the diagnosis is not made promptly and therapy instituted at once, death may occur virtually within hours. Replacement steroid therapy has completely altered the prognosis in patients with both acute and chronic adrenocortical insufficiency.

Adrenocortical insufficiency may result from: (1) disorders primary in the adrenal cortex, (2) diminished ACTH production as a consequence of hypothalamic or pituitary disease or (3) suppression of the hypothalamic pituitary axis by treatment with corticosteroids. When the adrenal insufficiency is secondary to hypothalamic or pituitary disease, such as in Simmonds' disease or Sheehan's syndrome, varying levels of hypofunction of the other pituitary-dependent endocrine glands are seen.

The anatomic lesions of the adrenal cortex responsible for significant depression of cortical function are all characterized by loss, acute or chronic, of cortical cells. Acute insufficiency is most often caused by necrotizing hemorrhagic inflammations of the adrenals, although it may sometimes be induced iatrogenically. Chronic insufficiency (Addison's disease) is usually related to (in decreasing order of importance): (1) atrophy of the adrenals, (2) tuberculosis, (3) amyloidosis, (4) carcinomatosis and (5) fungal infections. Tuberculosis (p. 411), amyloidosis (p. 281) and carcinomatosis have already been the subjects of earlier discussions. It might be pointed out here that bilateral adrenal tuberculosis still accounts for 5 to 10 per cent of cases of Addison's disease. At one time, it was the predominant cause of this syndrome, but better control of the infection has reduced the frequency and severity of adrenal tuberculosis. Metastases to the adrenal rarely cause Addison's disease, even though the cancerous involvement of the adrenals is massive, as it so frequently is with bronchogenic carcinomas. Conceivably, the adrenocortical insufficiency is overlooked because its manifestations are so similar to those of malignant cachexia (Eisenstein, 1968). In the sections that follow, the remaining causes of acute and chronic insufficiency are considered under the broad headings of: (1) hemorrhage, inflammation and necrosis and (2) atrophy.

HEMORRHAGE, INFLAMMATION AND NECROSIS

Hemorrhage, acute and chronic inflammation, and cortical cell necrosis may follow a wide variety of infectious and stressful disorders. The cortical damage may be focal and widely scattered or confluent and quite extensive.

Hemorrhages may be seen in the adrenals in the neonate, usually following prolonged and difficult delivery associated with considerable trauma and asphyxia. Whether such hemorrhages are a reflection of infantile stress or are anoxic in origin is unclear. They are particularly common in breech deliveries, and so hypoxia is thought to be the more important cause. The neonatal adrenal is particularly predisposed to hemorrhage, since it is relatively large for the body size, has little periadrenal fat and its large medullary venous sinuses are fragile and have poorly developed, unequally distributed supporting muscular walls. In addition, newborn infants are often deficient in prothrombin for at least several days after birth.

The appearance of the hemorrhagic adrenal is very variable, and the characteristic patterns en-

HEMORRHAGIC ADRENAL

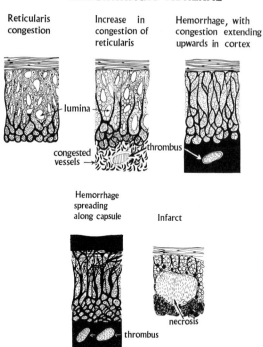

Reticularis congestion — lumina — congested vessels → — thrombus → Increase in congestion of reticularis — Hemorrhage, with congestion extending upwards in cortex — Hemorrhage spreading along capsule — Infarct — thrombus → — necrosis →

Figure 29–16. Diagrammatic representation of the patterns of congestion, hemorrhage and ischemic necrosis in the adrenal.

countered are shown in Figure 29–16. Sometimes all that occurs is marked congestion of the zona reticularis accompanied by lumen formation. This appearance may be associated with a thrombus in the central vein or its muscular branches. In those with more marked hemorrhage, rupture of the vessels of the zona reticularis compresses the medulla and presents as if the hemorrhage had arisen in the medulla. Often, the hemorrhages extend to the capsule of the gland and compress the cords of cells in the zona fasciculata. Other appearances consist of periadrenal hemorrhage or hemorrhagic infarcts. In some patients, the adrenal hemorrhage is accompanied by widespread ecchymoses and petechiae throughout other viscera and surfaces.

Whether such adrenal hemorrhage pro duces much steroid insufficiency is uncertain. More likely, the primary cause of death is fetal trauma and asphyxia.

Inflammation, necrosis and hemorrhages in the cortex may occur in severe diphtheria and systemic streptococcal, pneumococcal and meningococcal infections. The most severe expression of such acute necrotizing destruction is seen in overwhelming meningococcal infections associated with bacteremia, known as the *Waterhouse-Friderichsen syndrome.* Here the abrupt onset of the infection, usually in infants, children and young adults, is followed in a matter of hours by the appearance of cutaneous petechiae and later a purpuric eruption. The patient may go into circulatory collapse and die within 24 hours. Blood cultures will invariably disclose a meningococcal bacteremia, and the organisms can also be cultured from the purpuric hemorrhages which may become focally necrotic if the patient survives long enough. This syndrome may also be encountered with overwhelming nonmeningococcal bacteremias.

Anatomically, widespread petechiae, purpura and hemorrhages are found throughout the body, particularly in the skin, mucous membranes and serosal surfaces. The adrenals are likewise hemorrhagic and partially necrotic. In some children, the adrenals appear as virtual sacs of clotted blood. The bleeding begins in the zona reticularis or the medulla and may be confined to these regions. More often, it extends throughout the medulla and cortex, at first penetrating between the cords of cortical cells toward the capsule and eventually engulfing these cells. Classically, even in those cases where the entire adrenal appears to be replaced by blood clot, microscopic examination discloses nests and strands of preserved cortical cells. In essence, the morphologic changes are those of a bleeding diathesis, and there is a suspicion that the bacterial infection triggers a form of disseminated intravascular coagulation leading to the hemorrhagic state (p. 744).

The cause of the circulatory collapse appears to be predominantly the overwhelming bacteremia and toxemia; however, the acute adrenocortical insufficiency may play a significant contributory role. When this condition is recognized promptly (within hours) and appropriately treated with massive doses of antibiotics and steroids, survival and complete recovery are possible.

Focal necroses may occur with any form of acute stress, such as severe burns, shock, postoperative complications and longstanding debilitating illnesses. The precise pathophysiology of such lesions is poorly understood. It has been vaguely attributed to exhaustion and death of individual cortical cells as a consequence of overwork. In support of such a theory, the zona fasciculata is often converted into maximally functioning compact cells.

Histologically, there is death and dropping out of individual cells in the outer border of the zona fasciculata, creating a small pseudotubule with a lumen, sometimes referred to as **tubular degeneration of Rich.** The lumina may contain a granular coagulum of fibrin or histiocytes. It is assumed that the peripheral collar of epithelial cells reflects, in some part, a regenerative response of the viable surrounding fasciculata cells.

ATROPHY

Atrophy of the adrenal glands now accounts for about 60 per cent of all cases of Addison's disease. Atrophy is a poorly defined condition which represents the end-point of a variety of inhibitory and destructive processes, some understood and others quite mysterious. One well defined mechanism is chronic administration of glucocorticoids, which suppress the adenohypophyseal axis. In addition to such iatrogenic disease, there are instances of adrenal atrophy for which there is no clear-cut explanation. Such cases are called idiopathic atrophy although, as will be seen, autoimmune mechanisms are suspected in some.

Suppression of the adenohypophysis by corticosteroids (iatrogenic atrophy) may lead to adrenocortical deficiency in patients whose corticosteroid therapy is omitted for some reason, or when the dose is not sufficiently increased during an acute intercurrent illness. The steroid deficiency may also become manifest during periods of too rapid withdrawal of therapy. In most patients, the hypothalamic-pituitary-adrenal axis recovers spontaneously with time but, in a few, collapse and sudden death may occur, particularly if the patients are subjected to surgery or any other form of acute stress. The extent of the suppression is related to the dose, duration and nature of the therapy. Hartog (1972) indicates that doses of 30 mg. of cortisol daily or its equivalent (approximately 5 mg. of prednisone, 0.75 mg. of dexamethasone) will produce this effect if given for prolonged periods. Smaller doses may also be suppressive if the duration of therapy is more extended.

Iatrogenic adrenal atrophy is best documented by the appearance of the adrenal glands removed at operation from patients on steroid therapy for breast cancer. In one group, corticosteroids had been administered for periods between seven and 16 weeks prior to operation and for a period of up to 2 days after operation. Each gland weighed between 1.8 and 4.8 gm. (mean, 3.4 gm.), a significant decrease from the normal mean operation weight of 4 gm. The adrenals were leaf-like in appearance, yellow in color and, on histologic examination, had an extremely thick fibrous capsule. The cortex consisted almost exclusively of a thin, clear cell zona fasciculata and a thin or absent zona reticularis. The weight of the single glands removed at postmortem from patients who were on steroids up to the time of death varied between 2 and 7 gm. (mean, 4.1 gm.), some showing a marked decrease in weight when compared with the normal gland usually found at autopsy.

These atrophic changes are quite similar to those in patients with Cushing's syndrome (a form of hyperadrenalism) due to a benign or malignant tumor. Atrophy of the adjacent cortex and contralateral gland is found. Accordingly, such patients must have steroid cover during and for a long time after operation. When adenomatous hyperplasia causes Cushing's syndrome, the process is bilateral and so the contralateral adrenal will be hyperplastic, not atrophic, and steroid therapy is required only after the second adrenal has been removed.

Idiopathic atrophy is currently thought to be an autoimmune disorder. Evidence in support of such a proposition is as follows. Approximately 50 to 70 per cent of these patients have circulating autoantibodies against adrenocortical antigens (mitochondrial and microsomal) (Wuepper et al., 1969). Other antibodies against thyroid gland and gastric mucosa are often present in these patients and, indeed, concurrent Addison's disease and Hashimoto's thyroiditis is now recognized as a specific entity—*Schmidt's syndrome*. The gland has histologic changes reminiscent of those encountered in Hashimoto's thyroiditis, such as a lymphocytic infiltration accompanied by an interstitial fibrosis and atrophy. Similar lesions can be produced in the experimental animal by the injection of autologous adrenal tissue admixed with Freund's adjuvant.

Morphologically, idiopathic atrophy appears as small, irregularly contracted adrenal glands with a combined weight reduced to as little as 2 to 3 gm. Indeed, it may be difficult to identify such glands in the periadrenal fat. The medulla is unaltered, but the cortex appears to have collapsed about it. There is focal absence of cortical epithelium, and such intervening cells as are present may be large, with an abundant eosinophilic cytoplasm, and possess somewhat atypical nuclei. A loose fibrous tissue, infiltrated with lymphocytes and plasma cells, occupies the spaces between the islands of residual epithelial cells. Because of this mononuclear infiltrate, this condition has also been called **primary atrophic adrenalitis.**

Additional cases of adrenal cortical atrophy are encountered, in which there is no history of suppressive therapy or evidence for an immunologic reaction. These instances are truly idiopathic, and it can only be speculated that they represent the end-stage of one of the more acute inflammatory necrotizing disorders discussed previously.

NONSTEROID-PRODUCING TUMORS OF THE CORTEX

It is evident from preceding sections that the proliferative lesions of the adrenal cortex range from diffuse hyperplasia to nodular hyperplasia to benign and malignant tumors, and that all of these proliferative processes may be associated with steroidogenesis. Nonfunctioning tumors may also occur and are briefly reviewed here.

Adrenal adenomas are found in about 2 per cent of adult autopsies, and most are nonsteroid-producing. For years, however, the controversy has persisted as to whether some apparently nonfunctional adenomas may produce hypertension in the nature of a "forme fruste" of Conn's syndrome (Russell et al., 1972). It is also important to remember that adrenal adenomas may be one part of the multiple endocrine adenomatosis syndrome (p. 1074). Usually adenomas are poorly encapsulated masses of yellow-orange adrenal cortical tissue ranging from 1 to 5 cm. in diameter. They may achieve much larger size and exhibit areas of hemorrhage, cystic degeneration and calcification. The encapsulation may be poorly defined and appear at places to be deficient. The nonsteroid-producing adenomas differ from their functioning relatives principally because they are composed of lipid-filled cells that reflect their secretory inactivity. **The cells may show some variation in size and nuclear characteristics which, indeed, verges on anaplasia.** Thus, many lesions fall into an intermediate category and are neither clearly benign nor clearly malignant.

Even more difficult is the differentiation of a true adenoma from a focus of nodular hyperplasia. Adenomas, as you recall, are not necessarily well encapsulated and so may be easily mistaken for a focus of hyperplasia. In general nodules which are larger than 1 cm. in diameter are likely to be adenomas. If nodules are multiple, bilateral or located in the capsule or outside of it, they are more likely to be expressions of nodular hyperplasia.

Cortical carcinomas usually produce steroids (90 per cent) and are associated with one of the hyperadrenal syndromes; however, some cannot. They are exceedingly rare, and most are highly malignant. Usually large when discovered, many exceed 20 cm. in diameter. On cut surface, they are predominantly yellow but frequently have hemorrhagic, cystic and necrotic areas. Many appear to be more or less encapsulated. Histologically, they range from lesions showing mild degrees of atypia, not dissimilar from that seen in some large adenomas, to wildly anaplastic neoplasms composed of monstrous giant cells. Between these extremes are found cancers with moderate degrees of anaplasia, some predominantly composed of spindle cells.

Adrenal cancers have a strong tendency to invade the adrenal vein, vena cava and lymphatics. Metastases to regional and periaortic nodes are common, as well as distant hematogenous spread to the lungs and other viscera. Bone metastases are unusual (Hutter and Kayhoe, 1966).

Carcinomas which have no steroid functional capability are often silent and are called to attention by their metastases. Because of their silent growth, these tumors generally remain undiscovered until inoperable, and the mean survival time for patients after diagnosis is in the range of three to four months (Macfarlane, 1958). In a series of cases reported by Lipsett et al. (1963), less than half produced local manifestations in the form of displacement or obstruction of the kidney, pain secondary to sudden hemorrhages within the tumor, abdominal distention or a large abdominal mass. Infrequently, these nonsteroid-producing tumors elaborate inappropriate hormones, such as gonadotropins, insulin-like products and catecholamines.

Miscellaneous Primary Tumors. As might be expected in an organ having abundant fibrous stroma, blood vessels, neural connections and periadrenal fat, a wide variety of benign and malignant mesodermal tumors have been recorded in the adrenal. These are uncommon to the point of extinction. One bizarre lesion merits mention. Infrequently, a mass of bone marrow and fat is found in the adrenal. This curious combination is designated as a *myelolipoma* or *myeloid metaplasia*. It is not known whether it is a true neoplasm or an aberration of mesodermal differentiation. Alternatively, it has been attributed to marrow embolism or extramedullary hematopoiesis, even though no anemia was present. The lesion is only of academic interest and is without clinical significance.

Secondary Tumors Although it is not certain whether metastatic tumors are more prone to affect the cortex or the medulla, metastasis to the adrenal is common in disseminated malignancy of all types. For obscure reasons, bronchogenic carcinoma sometimes singles out the adrenals as sites of spread. Approximately 60 per cent of all lung cancers affect these organs.

ADRENAL MEDULLA

NORMAL
PATHOLOGY
Pheochromocytoma

Neuroblastoma and
Ganglioneuroma

Tumors of the Chemoreceptor
System

NORMAL

The adrenal medulla is derived from the primitive cells of the neural crest, which migrate into the center of the fetal adrenal cortex and form the medulla with its complement of mature cells—pheochromocytes. In the fetus, similar collections of cells are found along the abdominal aorta, mainly in relation to the origin of the inferior mesenteric artery, and constitute the organs of Zuckerkandl. Other groups are scattered throughout the sympathetic nervous system in relation to the cervical and thoracic ganglia, the gastrointestinal system, the bladder, the heart and the gonads. These islands are usually replaced by lymphatic tissue shortly after birth, but may persist and lead to extra-adrenal pheochromocytomas in later life.

The cells of the neural crest are also capable of forming the ganglion cells of the sympathetic nervous system, which are produced by way of the intermediate cell—the neuroblast.

The pheochromocytes in the adrenal medulla are responsible for producing the catecholamines epinephrine and norepinephrine, and their formation from the amino acids phenylalanine and tyrosine is illustrated in Figure 29–17. Epinephrine is the major product; together with norepinephrine, it is stored in the adrenal medulla in a ratio of 9:1. Both catecholamines are bound to adenosine triphosphate (ATP) in pheochromocytes and form granules which are responsible for the positive chromaffin reaction obtained following fixation of the gland in a suitable solution of chromium salts. On release, the catecholamines are metabolized as shown in Figure 29–17, the enzymes catechol-O-methyl transferase and monoamine oxidase occupying key roles in this process. The principal end products are metanephrine, normetanephrine and 3-methoxy-4-hydroxymandelic acid (VMA:MHMA). Only a small amount of unchanged catecholamine is excreted free in the urine.

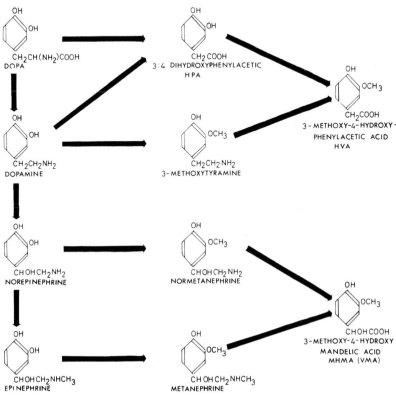

Figure 29-17. Pathways of catecholamine biosynthesis and metabolism.

PATHOLOGY

The only significant pathologic lesions which affect the medulla are tumor formations such as pheochromocytoma, neuroblastoma and ganglioneuroma.

PHEOCHROMOCYTOMA

Pheochromocytoma is a tumor which arises from pheochromocytes. These cells have an affinity for chrome salts and secrete norepinephrine or epinephrine. The majority of these tumors are found in the adrenal medulla and almost all are benign. They are important because they cause a rare but curable form of hypertension.

Over 1000 cases of pheochromocytoma have been reported since Fränkel recorded the first tumor in 1886. The tumor is found in both adults and children and affects the right gland more often than the left (48:33 per cent). Bilateral lesions are found in about 9 per cent of cases and occur more frequently in patients with a familial multiple endocrine adenomatosis syndrome.

Extra-adrenal tumors can develop and have been noted in about 7 per cent of patients. Most of them occur in the organs of Zuckerkandl, but some have been discovered in other sites where chromaffin tissue develops in the embryo. Multiple pheochromocytomas (3 per cent) have been described. They may involve one or both adrenal glands and an ectopic site, or they may occur exclusively in extra-adrenal situations.

The tumor in adults is found between 30 and 50 years of age and occurs equally in males and females, but in children it occurs more often in males. The clinical features are due to the release of catecholamines, chiefly norepinephrine, which, in contrast to the normal gland, is usually the major product elaborated by the tumor. Hypertension, either paroxysmal or sustained, is the most frequent presenting feature, and differentiation from essential hypertension may be difficult if the hypertension is sustained. However, other symptoms occur which are rare in essential hypertension. They include headache, sweating, pallor, tachycardia, postural hypotension and a raised basal metabolism. Many patients have glycosuria and even frank diabetes mellitus. Nervousness is a frequent complaint and, along with the raised basal metabolism, tends to suggest the possibility of thyrotoxicosis. Rare instances of Cushing's syndrome have been attributed to cortisol-secreting pheochromocytomas.

No single investigation is satisfactory for the accurate diagnosis of this condition. The diagnostic aids in current use are both pharmacologic and chemical, the latter being the more accurate.

Two types of pharmacologic tests are available, the histamine vasopressor or provocative test, and the Regitine vasodepressor test. Histamine is suited for patients who are normotensive at the time of the examination, but it carries a high morbidity, and even death has been reported with its use. Age, coronary artery insufficiency and allergic diseases are absolute contraindications to its use. Regitine is of more value for patients who have sustained hypertension, but equivocal results have often been observed.

Chemical methods are less liable to produce misleading results, and the measurement of free catecholamines in the urine, although not infallible, is the best single test available at present. If performed along with an estimation of the urinary metabolites of the catecholamines, the diagnosis will be established in almost every case.

When the tumor is situated in the adrenal medulla, it usually produces both norepinephrine and epinephrine. If an extra-adrenal pheochromocytoma is present, norepinephrine alone is formed in excess. By estimating the concentration of the free catecholamines in the urine, some indication of the site of the tumor can be obtained.

Aortography, especially when combined with presacral air insufflation, is also an excellent method for localizing the larger tumors.

The average weight of a pheochromocytoma is 100 gm., but variations from just over 1 gm. to almost 4000 gm. have been recorded. The tumors are well encapsulated by either connective tissue or compressed adrenocortical tissue. Fibrous trabeculae pass into the tumor and produce a lobular pattern. In many tumors, remnants of the adrenal gland can be seen, stretched over the surface or attached at one pole. On section, the cut surface has a pale gray or light brown color and areas of hemorrhage or necrosis can be observed, particularly in the larger lesions (Fig. 29–18). When fixed in formalin, the fixative turns yellow; when a suitable chrome-dichrome fixative is employed, the tumor becomes black.

The histologic diagnosis of pheochromocytoma is never complete or even established unless the presence of catecholamines is ascertained by both biochemical and histochemical methods. A known weight of the tumor, approximately 10 gm., is minced and placed in 3 ml. of 0.01 N HCl. This can be conveniently stored in the refrigerator until the catecholamine content of the growth can be esti-

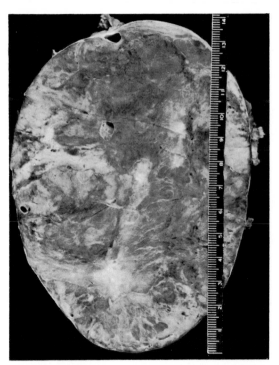

Figure 29–18. An adrenal pheochromocytoma of unusually large size. The variegated coloration is due to necrosis and hemorrhage.

which subsequently behave in a benign fashion. Occasionally, tumor cells can be found lying in the capillaries or sinusoids. This is not indicative of malignancy, as it has been observed in tumors which are benign in their behavior.

Chromaffin granules can be demonstrated in paraffin sections from chrome-fixed material by the Schmorl or Sevki Giemsa techniques, or simply by staining with 1 per cent methylene blue. The granules are stained olive green in color (Fig. 29–21).

Since malignant and benign pheochromocytomas may have a similar histologic appearance, the diagnosis of malignancy cannot be made by histologic examination of the tumor alone. The accepted histologic criteria of malignancy generally applicable to nonendocrine growth, if used, only lead to misdiagnosis, and the only absolute criterion upon which a diagnosis of malignancy can be made is the presence of distant metastases. The exact incidence of malignancy is difficult to gauge, but recent reports cite a frequency as high as 10 per cent (Raker, 1971). Metastases may be functional or nonfunctional. They occur most frequently in the related lymph nodes, the liver, lungs and bones, and survival after diagnosis rarely exceeds three years. Urinary dopamine levels are stated to be elevated in cases which behave in a malignant manner, and this may prove to be an index of considerable importance in the future assessment of these patients.

mated by a chemical method. The chromaffin reaction, which is used to demonstrate the presence of catecholamines in the tumor cells, is best performed by using a solution containing 100 parts of 5 per cent potassium dichromate and seven parts of 5 per cent potassium chromate. This yields a pH of about 5.8. It is important to fix the tumor in such a solution; if the pH exceeds 6 or is less than 4, false-negative results will be obtained. The chromaffin test is positive even in autopsy material and, when a negative reaction is elicited, the pH of the fixative should be checked. In these circumstances, it is even more important to establish the presence of catecholamines by chemical means.

The cytologic patterns in pheochromocytomas are quite variable (Symington and Goodall, 1953). The tumors are composed of mature pheochromocytes, which possess a faint granular basophilic cytoplasm in which granules can be demonstrated by the use of chrome salts. The cells are arranged in either large trabeculae, punctuated by thin-walled sinusoids often lined by the tumor cells themselves (Fig. 29–19), or in small alveoli, each surrounded by a fibrovascular trabecula derived from the tumor capsule (Fig. 29–20). Various patterns may be found in any one tumor. Cellular and nuclear pleomorphism are often noted, especially in the alveolar group of lesions, and giant and bizarre cells are commonly seen. Mitotic figures are usually not present in these lesions, but they can occur in tumors

Pheochromocytoma can occur as a familial disease, inherited as a dominant gene with a high degree of penetrance. The incidence of bilateral tumors in such familial cases (approximately 50 per cent) is a fact of considerable surgical and therapeutic interest.

The association of pheochromocytoma and the heredofamilial disorder neurofibromatosis is now a well recognized entity. Both diseases are derived embryologically from neuroectoderm. In recent years, a number of reports on the concurrence of pheochromocytoma and another member of the neurocutaneous disorders, von Hippel-Lindau disease, have appeared. It is important to realize that these defects may not manifest themselves in full and may only be represented as a "forme fruste," e.g., café au lait spots in neurofibromatosis. The left gland is involved more often than the right in this group of disorders. Between 5 and 10 per cent of patients with pheochromocytomas will also suffer from one of the neurocutaneous disorders.

There is an increased frequency of thyroid carcinomas and parathyroid adenomas in patients who also have a chromaffin tumor. The thyroid lesion may develop before or after the appearance of the pheochromocytoma. The most common type of thyroid tumor is the

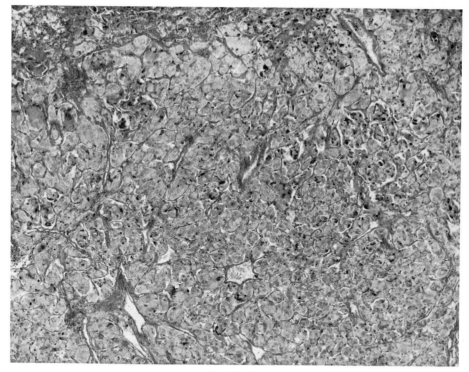

Fig. 29–19

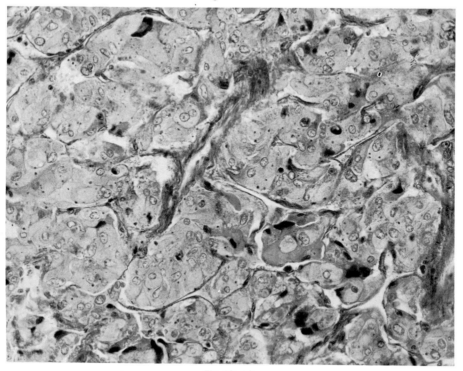

Fig. 29–20

Figure 29–19. *A low power microscopic view of a pheochromocytoma showing nests of cells resembling those normally found in the medulla.*

Figure 29–20. *A high power detail of a field from Figure 29–19 illustrating cellular detail consisting of fairly regular nuclei and abundant granular cytoplasm. The chromaffin pigment is not visible in the photograph.*

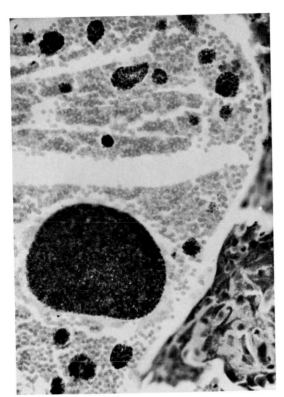

Figure 29-21. *Pheochromocytoma. A large sinusoid is shown at high power. It contains granular pheochromocytes specially stained by Sevki's method to show the positive chrome reaction.*

medullary carcinoma, although other cellular patterns have also been found. It has been suggested that this particular type of tumor of the thyroid is genetically determined and that this, rather than any humoral cause, is the relationship between the two tumors. The association of tumors of the adrenal medulla, thyroid and parathyroid probably represents, then, a manifestation of one of the *familial multiple endocrine adenomatosis syndromes* (p. 1074).

NEUROBLASTOMA AND GANGLIONEUROMA

Neuroblastoma is a highly malignant tumor which occurs most frequently in children and young adolescents. Approximately 80 per cent are found in children under the age of five, and only infequently are they encountered in those over the age of 15 years. Rarely, these neoplasms are encountered at birth. The neuroblastoma is one of the most common tumors in childhood and ranks along with Wilms' tumor, glioma and leukemia as a principal form of cancer in childhood (Willis, 1962). Males are affected more frequently than females.

Between 40 and 50 per cent of all neuroblastomas are found in the adrenal gland; the remainder are located in the region of the cervical, thoracic and lower abdominal sympathetic chain. They can occur in other sites, such as the jaw, bladder, lip, nose and other abdominal viscera, and this is understandable on the basis of the embryologic development of their component cells. Primary involvement of the central nervous system by neuroblastoma is very rare. *A closely related tumor in the retina is called a retinoblastoma.*

Macroscopically, the growths are lobular, soft in consistency and weigh between 80 and 150 gm. The cut surface is gray in color, and areas of hemorrhage and necrosis may be obvious as the tumor increases in size. Calcification is not infrequent, and this can help in their radiologic localization.

Histologically, the cells are small and dark like lymphocytes and frequently are arranged in masses without any true pattern. In characteristic lesions, rosettes are formed when the tumor cells occupy the periphery and young nerve fibrils grow into the center of each rosette. Careful search of any tumor will almost always reveal this type of structure.

Metastases develop rapidly and widely. In addition to local infiltration and lymph node metastases, there is a pronounced tendency to spread by the blood to liver, lungs and bones. Profuse bony metastases, particularly to the skull and orbit, with exophthalmos is referred to clinically as Hutchinson-type neuroblastoma. Massive metastasis to the liver is designated the Pepper-type syndrome. Many cases of assumed Ewing's tumor of bone represent metastases from a primary neuroblastoma, which may remain undiscovered unless a thorough search is made.

In the developing embryo, neuroblasts undergo maturation to form ganglion cells. Similarly, *some neuroblastomas may undergo spontaneous maturation to form the benign tumor called a ganglioneuroma.* During the transition, both elements are present and the growth is referred to as a ganglioneuroblastoma. The basis for such transformation of a highly lethal neuroblastoma to a much less aggressive, potentially resectable, benign ganglioneuroma is still mysterious. There are many hints that it is related to the emergence, in the host, of an effective immunologic reaction against the tumor antigens (Bill, 1969). Indeed, complete regression of neuroblastomas has been reported, possibly in the fortunate patient with a potent immunologic response.

There is a better prognosis if the tumor is situated outside the adrenal gland or if the lesion is detected before the age of two years.

The prognosis is also improved if ganglion cells are present. Radiotherapy and/or chemotherapy has yielded improved survival rates but, in general, few children with metastatic pure neuroblastomas live longer than a year (Report of the Subcommittee on Childhood Solid Tumor Task Force, National Cancer Institute, 1970). When resection is possible, coupled with radiation and chemotherapy, children who are tumor-free 14 months from the last evidence of tumor are likely to be cured. Such cures are achieved largely in those under one year of age.

In recent years, some neuroblastomas and ganglioneuromas have been associated with endocrine function. Such cases show a wider diversity of catecholamine metabolites in the urine than occurs in cases of pheochromocytoma. Not only norepinephrine and epinephrine and their metabolites are found in elevated amounts in the urine, but also their precursors, dopamine and even dopa and the related metabolites.

TUMORS OF THE CHEMORECEPTOR SYSTEM

The chemoreceptor system is represented principally by the carotid body, the aortic pulmonary bodies and the glomus jugulare, although similar collections of tissue have been demonstrated in other sites. These structures respond to variations in the blood oxygen and carbon dioxide tensions and may be concerned with the regulation of respiration. Tumors which arise from them are called chemodectomas or nonchromaffin paragangliomas. They resemble carotid body tumors described in greater detail on p. 632.

Such tumors are rare, occur in both males and females and are found mostly between the ages of 30 and 60 years. They tend to be small and to weigh between 15 and 60 gm. Almost all are single, but bilateral or multiple tumors involving more than one structure have been recorded. Like pheochromocytomas, they can occur in families.

Typical tumors are composed of polyhedral cells, which are epithelioid in appearance and grouped in small nests, each surrounded by vascular connective tissue trabeculae. There is thus a remarkable similarity to the appearance of the normal glands.

Most of these lesions are benign indolent growths, and they are more likely to cause difficulty at the time of removal than to become malignant.

Functional chemodectomas are known to occur, and catecholamines have been extracted from some of these lesions. If these organs are formed in part from neuroectoderm, there is no reason why pheochromocytomas cannot arise in these structures. Thus, it is false to refer to them as functional chemodectomas or chemodectoma-like tumors when they would be called pheochromocytomas in any other site in the body. A true chemodectoma will be chrome negative. Greater care in classification is required in all future examinations of tumors of this type or in those tumors which arise near the chemoreceptor bodies.

THYROID GLAND

NORMAL
PATHOLOGY
Hyperthyroidism
Hypothyroidism
  Cretinism
  Myxedema
Congenital Anomalies
  Thyroglossal duct or cyst
  Hypoplasia or aplasia
Regressive Changes
  Atrophy
  Amyloidosis
  Pigmentation
Thyroiditis
  Infectious (acute or chronic)

Secondary to trauma or radiation
Subacute (de Quervain's, granulomatous)
Invasive fibrous (Riedel's struma)
Hashimoto's disease (struma lymphomatosa)
Lymphocytic
Goiter Arising in Functional Derangements
Colloid (simple) goiter
Nodular or multiple colloid adenomatous goiter
Familial
Iatrogenic

Graves' disease (primary hyperthyroidism, diffuse primary thyroid hyperplasia)
Tumors
  Benign
    Follicular adenoma
    Teratoma
  Malignant
    Papillary carcinoma
    Follicular carcinoma
    Medullary carcinoma with amyloid stroma
    Anaplastic carcinoma
  Miscellaneous
    Sarcomas

NORMAL

The thyroid gland develops as a tubular invagination from the root of the tongue called the foramen cecum. It grows downward in front of the trachea and thyroid cartilage to reach the position it will occupy as the adult gland. The distal end of this structure proliferates to form the adult gland, while the remainder degenerates and disappears, usually by the fifth to sixth week of fetal development.

A large number of developmental anomalies (some discussed in greater detail later) may have clinical importance. Thyroid aplasia leads to serious physical and mental underdevelopment, known as athyrotic cretinism. Less complete failure of organogenesis may substitute an imperfectly formed mass of connective tissue, ducts, lymphatic nodules and scattered thyroid follicles for the normal mature thyroid architecture. Persistence of the vestigial tubular structure, which grows down from the root of the tongue, provides a source for the later development of thyroglossal cysts or ducts. Incomplete descent may lead to the formation of the thyroid at loci abnormally high in the neck, producing, for example, a lingual thyroid or aberrant subhyoid or paratracheal thyroid tissue. Excessive descent leads to substernal thyroid glands. Infrequently, lateral aberrant thyroid nodules develop, but it should be noted that these developmental anomalies are largely confined to locations medial to the sternocleidomastoid muscle. It scarcely needs mention that any of these aberrantly located thyroid glands or thyroid nodules may be the site of origin of disease, such as tumors, identical with those arising in the definitive thyroid. Malformations of branchial pouch differentiation may result in intrathyroidal portions of the thymus or parathyroid glands. The implication of these deviations from the norm may become all too evident in the patient who has a total thyroidectomy and subsequently develops hypoparathyroidism.

In the adult, the thyroid gland weighs between 20 and 30 gm. Two large lateral lobes are connected in the midline by a broad isthmus from which, on occasion, a pyramidal lobe may protrude superiorly. Occasionally, in a very thin person, this normal pyramidal structure may be mistaken for a thyroid nodule. The close relationship of the recurrent laryngeal nerve and the parathyroid glands makes them extremely vulnerable to injury during thyroid surgery as well as to involvement by spreading malignancy or inflammation.

Histologically, the thyroid is composed of acini or follicles of variable size that, in three dimensions, comprise spheroidal sacs. These are lined by regular cuboidal cells having a height of 14 to 15 microns. In the normal thyroid, the follicles are separated by a delicate fibrous tissue stroma which is compacted in some places into fibrous septa that traverse the gland. Small collections of lymphocytes are occasionally found in the stroma. Dispersed within the follicles are the parafollicular or so-called C cells. These cells are not identifiable by light microscopy except with special stains. They elaborate calcitonin, a polypeptide hormone having a hypocalcemic effect (Englund, 1972). The C cells are thought to be the site of origin of one form of thyroid tumor, the medullary carcinoma.

In the normal state of functional activity, the follicles are filled with the glycoprotein—thyroglobulin—synthesized by thyroid epithelial cells. In the usual tissue stain, it has a pink, refractile appearance and is termed colloid. Release of active thyroid hormones, as will be discussed, involves proteolysis of the colloid (thyroglobulin). The electron microscope discloses numerous tentacles or pseudopods projecting from the luminal surfaces of the epithelial cells into the colloid (Herman, 1960). The processes enormously expand the cell-colloid interface.

The active, circulating hormones of the thyroid are triiodothyronine (T_3) and thyroxine (T_4), both being derived from thyroglobulin. The synthesis of these hormones has been delineated in elegant detail (Rapoport and DeGroot, 1971) (Davies, 1972). The following steps are involved:

1. Iodide trapping, an active process requiring energy. Normally in man the thyroid-serum iodide ratio is about 50 to 1.

2. Oxidation of iodide to iodine within the thyroid cell which covalently attaches to tyrosine residues in thyroglobulin to form mono- and diiodotyrosine (MIT and DIT).

3. Iodination, occurring at the microvillous interface between colloid and thyroid cell.

4. While still incorporated in the thyroglobulin molecule, coupling of MIT and DIT to form T_3 or coupling of two DIT's to form T_4.

5. Both the oxidation of iodide to nascent iodine and the coupling of MIT and DIT involve peroxidases in the particulate fraction of the thyroid epithelial cell.

The release of T_3 and T_4 from thyroglobulin involves two sequences, the phagocytosis of thyroglobulin and the proteolysis of the thyroglobulin. The first step in thyroid hormone release involves endocytosis (phagocytosis) of thyroglobulin. The pseudopods apparently reach out and close over small fragments of the colloid and, in this manner, membrane-bounded vesicles containing colloid material are incorporated within the thyroid epithelial cells (Stein and Gross, 1964). Lysosomes migrate apically to meet the incoming membrane-bounded vesicles containing the thyroglobulin-colloid, and fusion of the lysosome with the colloid-bearing vesicles produces a phagolysosome (Seljelid, 1968). The phagolysosome migrates to the basal portion of the epithelial cell and, during this passage, lysosomal proteinases and peptidases split off T_3 and T_4, which are discharged at the base of the cell into perifollicular capillaries. Over 99 per cent of T_3 and T_4 in the blood is bound to protein, mainly to thyroxine-binding globulin. The serum protein-bound iodine (PBI) level is thus a measure of this fraction and a valuable index of thyroid function.

The PBI value does not measure physiologically active, unbound hormones which ultimately are the mediators of thyroid function. T_4 can be assayed directly. The concentration of free T_4 in the circulation is about three times greater than that of T_3, but the potency of T_3 is three times greater than that of T_4, so, in physiologic terms, both hormones contribute equally to the metabolic function of the thyroid. Recent evidence suggests that T_3 may be formed from T_4 by extrathyroidal conversion (Sterling, 1970). In passing, it should be noted that alterations in the levels of thyroid-binding globulin can depress or elevate the PBI value. In hypoproteinemia, for example, the binding proteins are reduced, and so the PBI level may be low and give a spurious index of thyroid function. Conversely, estrogens and contraceptive pills elevate the PBI level by increasing the synthesis of binding protein.

Thyroid functional activity is controlled by thyroid-stimulating hormone (TSH) of pituitary origin and, in turn, TSH secretion is regulated through feedback inhibition by the circulating levels of thyroid hormone. TSH is elaborated by basophils (and possibly other cells) of the anterior pituitary in response to thyrotropin-releasing factor (TRF) produced in the adenohypophysis. TRF passes through the adenohypophyseal axis into the anterior pituitary and stimulates both the synthesis and release of TSH. It is not clear whether the thyroid hormones exert their feedback inhibition by direct action on the anterior pituitary or, instead, indirectly by suppressing hypophyseal function.

It has been shown that TSH, when released, is carried through the blood to bind to thyroid epithelial cell membranes. Here it activates adenyl cyclase, thus catalysing the formation of cyclic AMP within the cell. Ultimately, it is cyclic AMP which stimulates iodide trapping, iodination of tyrosine, synthesis of thyroid hormones and release of these hormones (Schell-Frederick and Dumont, 1970). The maintenance of normal thyroid function and the thyroid gland is thus dependent on the pituitary. Total loss of TSH, as may occur in hypopituitarism, results in depressed thyroid function and, in time, in atrophy of the thyroid gland. Conversely, depressed levels of thyroid hormones lead to increased levels of TSH. Failure, therefore, of the synthesis of normal amounts of thyroid hormones may result in enlargement of the gland due to TSH-induced hyperplasia.

From the physiologic standpoint, the thyroid gland is one of the most sensitive organs in the body. It responds to many stimuli and is in a constant state of adaptation. During puberty, pregnancy and physiologic stress from any source, the gland increases in size and becomes more active functionally. Changes in activity and size may even be noted during a normal menstrual period. This extreme functional lability is reflected in transient hyperplasia of the thyroidal epithelium. At this time, thyroglobulin is resorbed and the follicular cells become tall and columnar, sometimes forming small infolded buds. When the stress abates, involution occurs, i.e., the height of the epithelium falls, colloid accumulates and the acinar cells resume their normal size and architecture. Failure of this normal balance between hyperplasia and involution may produce major or minor deviations from the usual histologic pattern.

Drugs commonly used in the therapy of hyperthyroidism significantly modify the histology of the gland. The thioureas inhibit oxidation of iodide to iodine by competing with iodide as a substrate for peroxidase (Randall, 1946). Thus, thyroid hormones cannot be produced; there is diminished negative feedback on the adenohypophysis, and the result is increased levels of TSH and proliferation within the thyroid gland. Pharmacologic doses of iodide are likewise used in the treatment of hyperthyroidism. Iodide inhibits the proteolytic enzyme systems involved in the release of hormone. Hence, proteolysis of thyroglobulin is blocked and colloid accumulates, distending the follicles and flattening the follicular epithelium. Although thiourea and iodide both effectively suppress excess thyroid function, one drug leads to an extremely cellular, seemingly hyperactive gland, and the other leads to a seemingly inactive gland with too much colloid.

PATHOLOGY

Diseases of the thyroid, while not common in clinical practice, are nonetheless of great importance because most are amenable to medical or surgical management. They present principally as hyperthyroidism, hypothyroidism or enlargement of the thyroid gland known as *goiter*. The enlargement may be diffuse and symmetrical or irregular and focal (nodular). Some concept of the relative frequency of the more common lesions can be gained from the following experience in an institution dealing principally with the thyroid (Hurxthal and Heineman, 1958). Roughly one-third of the cases presented with hyperthyroidism, 85 per cent of these having diffuse thyroid hyperplasia (Graves' disease), and the remaining 15 per cent being toxic nodular goiters (toxic colloid adenomatous goiter). Two-thirds of the patients presented with nontoxic nodular goiters, 80 per cent representing nontoxic colloid adenomatous goiters; 10 per cent, solitary adenomas; and 4 per cent, carcinomas. The small residual comprised a miscellaneous category of thyroidal cysts and thyroiditis.

Before presenting the various disorders of the thyroid gland, the clinical syndromes of hyperthyroidism and hypothyroidism will be discussed to provide more effective clinical correlation.

HYPERTHYROIDISM

Hyperthyroidism is caused by an overproduction of thyroid hormone. It is manifested clinically by a state of hypermetabolism associated with cardiovascular and neuromuscular alterations. It is most commonly caused by diffuse primary hyperplasia of the thyroid (Graves' disease). Less frequently, hyperthyroidism is caused by: (1) a hyperfunctioning focus within a colloid adenomatous goiter, (2) a tumor, benign or malignant, possessing the capacity to elaborate thyroid hormone and (3) rarely by Hashimoto's thyroiditis.

The clinical manifestations of hyperthyroidism are varied and include: warm, moist skin; sweating; increased sensitivity to heat; nervousness; a fine tremor of the hands, particularly when outstretched; weight loss; increased appetite; fatigability; muscular weakness; tachycardia; elevation of systolic blood pressure and sometimes, in older patients, cardiac arrhythmias. Eye changes, particularly exophthalmos, are encountered in Graves' disease but only rarely with other forms of hyperthyroidism (Hall, 1970). Graves' disease is, therefore, sometimes called *exophthalmic goiter* (Fig. 29–22). The protrusion of the eyes is probably not directly related to the thyroid hyperfunction, and so Graves' disease is best considered as having two components: (1) hyperthyroidism and (2) eye changes. Similarly, the cardiovascular alterations in the hyperthyroid patient, such as tachycardia and cardiac arrhythmias, may not

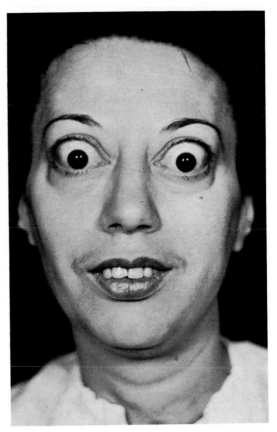

Figure 29–22. *Exophthalmic goiter in a young woman 27 years of age.*

be directly related to the increased elaboration of thyroid hormone but, instead, may be the consequence of thyroid hormone-induced increased sensitivity of the cardiovascular and nervous systems to catecholamines. Present evidence, however, is against such an indirect mechanism (Levey and Epstein, 1969).

A variety of clinical laboratory procedures are available both to measure the extent of increased thyroid activity and to help determine its cause. Measures of thyroid function include: the basal metabolic rate (BMR), the levels of protein-bound iodine (PBI) in the serum, the uptake of radioiodine (RaI), and direct quantitation of circulating T_4 in the serum. The causes of abnormal thyroid function can be investigated by tests in which thyroid function is stimulated (by TSH) or suppressed (by T_3) and by the search for autoantibodies.

In most patients with hyperthyroidism, the clinical manifestations just mentioned begin insidiously and are present for some time before the clinical diagnosis is made. In clinical parlance, such patients are said to be toxic, and hence an often-used designation for this condition is toxic hyperthyroidism. Physical or emotional stress frequently exacerbates the manifestations and may, indeed, precipitate an acute crisis, termed thyroid storm. The latter is characterized by extreme hyperpyrexia, delirium, dehydration, gastrointestinal disturbances, marked elevation of the blood pressure, extreme tachycardia, serious cardiac arrhythmias, and ultimately, in many patients, vasomotor collapse. This clinical crisis is believed to result from sudden excesses of thyroid hormone, and unless the thyroid hyperfunction is promptly controlled, thyroid storms often terminate in death.

The anatomic alterations in the patient with hyperthyroidism are inconstant and frequently minimal, save for the underlying lesion within the thyroid gland. Lymphoid hyperplasia throughout the body is common and appears to be due to depression of the pituitary by the increased amounts of circulating thyroid hormone. As a consequence, there is decreased formation of ACTH, depressed levels of adrenal steroids and resultant overgrowth of the lymphoid tissues. Skeletal decalcification and degenerative changes in the voluntary muscles have been described. Focal necrosis in the heart muscle along with focal aggregations of lymphocytes occur in some cases. Focal necroses, cell swelling and fatty degeneration have been noted in the liver.

It can be said of these anatomic changes that none of them is pathognomonic of hyperthyroidism. Even the evaluation of the thyroid gland does not permit a correct estimate of its functional activity. It is to be remembered that the patient receiving thiourea or its derivatives will possibly be euthyroid, but because thyroid hormone output is blocked, hyperactivity of the pituitary maintains a striking state of hyperplasia of the thyroid gland. Such a gland might superficially appear to be markedly hyperactive but, in truth, may not be responsible for any hormonal output.

HYPOTHYROIDISM

Hypothyroidism is caused by a deficiency of thyroid hormone. It presents in a wide range of clinical syndromes, depending upon the severity of the hormonal lack and on the age at which the deficiency first appears. *When the hormone lack is present from birth and is severe, it results in cretinism. When the deficiency appears later or is less severe, the hypothyroidism may cause little or no clinical manifestations or, instead, may induce the syndrome known as myxedema.*

CRETINISM

In cretinism, varying levels of physical and mental retardation, or even death, occur, depending on the severity of the hormone lack. When promptly recognized, if irreparable damage has not occurred in utero, it is reversible and can be corrected and controlled by thyroid hormone replacement therapy. The most grave and probably irreversible cause of cretinism is *thyroid aplasia*. However, any disorder which impairs thyroid function may produce this syndrome. A congenital, possibly hereditary, deficiency of one of the many thyroid enzymes necessary for hormonogenesis is an additional, but fortunately rare, cause of cretinism. Such congenital disorders are known generically as *dyshormonogenetic goiters*. Inadequate sources of iodine in the diet of a pregnant woman can induce iodine deficiency in the fetus and result in cretinism. The widespread iodinization of salt and other foods has happily reduced the incidence of this source of cretinism.

The clinical manifestations of cretinism may be difficult to recognize at birth but soon become apparent. The infant fails to thrive and shows progressive retardation in all aspects of physical and mental development. Osseous development is slowed, and so the head appears unusually large. The nose is short and has increased breadth. The eyes are wideset. The tongue is often so enlarged that it protrudes between the lips. Characteristically, the neck is short and thick; the abdomen protruberant; the skin thickened, roughened and dry; and the hair sparse. Mental retardation becomes evident as soon as it can be evaluated. As would be anticipated, the serum PBI and T_4 levels are depressed.

MYXEDEMA

Myxedema is the consequence of thyroid hormone lack in later childhood or adult life. *The causes of myxedema are as varied as the diseases which destroy thyroid structure and function.* Thyroiditis, particularly Hashimoto's chronic thyroiditis, is the most common basis for myxedema. Iodine deficiency or the ingestion of goitrogenic drugs may also induce myxedema. Additional potential causes of myxedema are thyroid atrophy in the aged, extensive amyloid deposits, widespread replacement of thyroid structure by nonfunctioning primary cancers and, of course, ablation of the thyroid either by surgery or irradiation. It is important to recognize that myxedema may not be primary in the thyroid, since severe hypopituitarism may lead to secondary hypothyroidism. In this circumstance, the levels of TSH are abnormally low, while in primary thyroid hypofunction, the opposite applies.

Many patients with mild hypothyroidism go unrecognized because their complaints

—lethargy, easy fatigability, sensitivity to cold and general malaise—are too vague. More overt manifestations include a generally bloated appearance, especially with puffiness of the face; thickened, dry skin; sparse, coarse hair; muscle weakness; slow mentation and hoarseness. The term myxedema alludes to a generalized increase, throughout the body, of interstitial edema which is rich in proteins and mucopolysaccharides. Such edema is most evident in the skin and accounts for some of the physical characteristics just mentioned. The heart is often dilated and flabby and histologically discloses an increased deposition of mucopolysaccharides in the interstitium. Frequently, these patients have cardiac insufficiency and signs of left ventricular failure. Mucoid vacuolation of cardiac, as well as skeletal, muscle occurs in well defined cases. The bone marrow may be hypoplastic and have a proteinous interstitial precipitate similar to that found in other tissues. *Patients with myxedema become hypercholesterolemic and so are prone to the development of accelerated atherosclerosis.* Changes also appear in the anterior pituitary (p. 1363). It should be emphasized that none of the extrathyroidal alterations is pronounced and would easily be missed unless specifically sought.

CONGENITAL ANOMALIES

A variety of anomalies have been briefly cited in the consideration of the normal development of the thyroid gland (p. 1320). Only two are of sufficient frequency and clinical significance to merit further detail.

Thyroglossal Duct or Cyst. A persistent sinus tract may remain as a vestigial remnant of the tubular development of the thyroid gland. Parts of this tube may be obliterated, leaving small segments to form cysts. These occur at any age and may not become evident until adult life. Mucinous, clear secretion may collect within these cysts to form either spherical masses or fusiform swellings, rarely over 2 to 3 cm. in diameter. These are present in the midline of the neck anterior to the trachea. Segments of the duct and cysts that occur high in the neck are lined by stratified squamous epithelium, which is essentially identical with that covering the posterior portion of the tongue in the region of the foramen cecum. Those anomalies that occur in the lower neck more proximal to the thyroid gland are lined by epithelium resembling the thyroidal acinar epithelium. Characteristically, subjacent to the lining epithelium there is an intense lymphocytic infiltrate. It is of interest that this sub-epithelial lymphoid infiltrate is also found in branchial cleft cysts, anomalies that have origin in closely related developmental processes. Superimposed infection may convert these lesions into abscess cavities.

The main significance of these lesions is that (1) they create masses in the neck requiring differentiation from more serious neoplasms; (2) they may communicate with the skin to produce persistent draining sinuses; (3) sometimes the persistent duct drains into the base of the tongue; and (4) these anomalous structures are extremely rare sources for the development of malignancy.

Hypoplasia or Aplasia. Rarely, the thyroid may fail to develop, resulting in total aplasia or in a less severe failure, hypoplasia. These aberrations may be caused by iodine deficiency in the mother. Alternatively, the thyroid may be normal at birth and fail to grow properly and mature, owing to a deficiency of iodine during childhood. In all these circumstances, severe functional insufficiency results in marked retardation of mental and somatic growth described as *cretinism.*

REGRESSIVE CHANGES

Atrophy. Concomitant with the other retrogressive changes that occur in advanced age, the thyroid gland may atrophy. In younger persons, atrophy of the gland may occasionally be the result of panhypopituitarism. In this situation, the loss of the thyrotropic hormone, at first compensated for by hyperplasia of the gland, eventually results in atrophy of the thyroid. By an alternative mechanism, increased pituitary activity will first produce hyperplasia, but if continued for a long time may eventuate in exhaustion atrophy. A shrunken, fibrotic thyroid may also be found as the end-stage of inflammatory involvement of the thyroid. Retrospectively, therefore, it is often impossible to determine the cause of the fibrosis and loss of parenchyma, and the morphologic entity is simply designated as atrophy.

The gland appears as a shrunken, pale gray, firm structure. The contraction is frequently *asymmetrical, producing apparent nodularity*, sometimes confused on clinical examination with a thyroid neoplasm. Usually the encapsulation remains intact and the gland separates readily from surrounding structures. In some postinflammatory fibroses, there may be adherence to surrounding structures. On section, the usual rubbery, red-brown, meaty appearance is replaced by firm, pale gray, homogeneous, apparent connective tissue (Fig. 29–23).

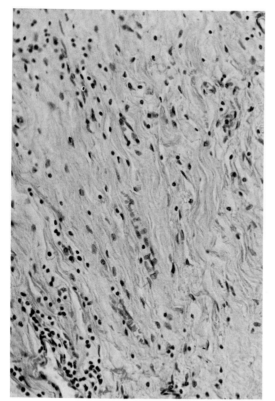

Figure 29–23. Thyroid atrophy. A microscopic field from the center of an atrophying thyroid; no preserved parenchyma is visible.

In the well developed lesion, there is almost total replacement of the parenchymal elements. In less advanced cases, the trapped follicles are distorted and compressed, and are eventually transformed, in some areas, into fused masses of cells having no central follicular space. The epithelial cells undergo marked changes in size and shape. Large pink epithelial cells with abundant granular cytoplasm may appear, so-called *Hürthle cells*. These are usually found in large nests or clusters within the areas of atrophy and fibrosis, and are believed to represent degenerative forms of thyroid epithelium.

It is rare for atrophy in aged individuals to produce clinical thyroid insufficiency. However, in those cases occurring in younger persons, as in association with pituitary insufficiency, the thyroid atrophy may progress to the point of functional insufficiency. Thus, *thyroid myxedema may constitute one element of the clinical syndrome of panhypopituitarism.*

Amyloidosis. In generalized systemic amyloidosis, deposition of amyloid may occur in the thyroid. When these changes are sufficiently severe, there may be an increase in the size and consistency of the gland. This deposi-

tion starts in the stromal connective tissue, chiefly about vessels. In extensive involvement, there may be sufficient pressure upon follicular elements to produce atrophy and some distortion of the gland substance. Usually the deposit is rather minimal in amount, the architecture is not significantly distorted and there is no evidence of functional insufficiency.

Pigmentation. In cases of generalized hemochromatosis, the thyroid gland shares in the deposits of hemosiderin and ferritin together with all the other glands of the body. The more abundant pigment, hemosiderin, is found within the cytoplasm of the thyroid epithelium, as well as within the fibroblasts in the interstitial stroma. Usually the change is of academic interest only, since it produces no impairment of thyroid function.

THYROIDITIS

The term thyroiditis embraces a number of well defined entities, some of which are caused by microbiologic or physical agents, others, which are of presumed immune origin and still others of unknown etiology. These disorders can be classified as in Table 29–1.

TABLE 29–1. THYROIDITIS

I. Due to known agents
    A. Infectious (acute and chronic) due to microbiologic agents
    B. Noninfectious, due to trauma or radiation
II. Due to unknown etiologic agents
    A. Subacute, de Quervain's, granulomatous thyroiditis
    B. Invasive fibrous thyroiditis or Riedel's struma
III. Due to immune reactions (?)
    A. Struma lymphomatosa or Hashimoto's thyroiditis
    B. Lymphocytic thyroiditis

Modified from Strahan, R. W., et al.: Thyroiditis. A classification and review. Laryngoscope, *81*:1388, 1971.

In addition to these better defined entities, there are a variety of nonspecific fibrotic and inflammatory changes sometimes encountered in the thyroid which, for lack of a better designation, are referred to as *nonspecific chronic thyroiditis.* In general, these nonspecific lesions are poorly developed and are not associated with clinical disease.

INFECTIOUS THYROIDITIS (ACUTE OR CHRONIC)

Inflammations of the thyroid gland caused by microbiologic agents are uncommon. The most frequent invaders are group A streptococci, *S. aureus* and pneumococci which reach the thyroid either through the blood stream or by direct extension from neighboring infections. Thyroiditis may develop in the course of measles or chickenpox, and rare cases have resulted from cat-scratch disease. Chronic thyroiditis may appear in the course of disseminated tuberculosis or sarcoidosis.

The anatomic changes vary with the specific causative agent and range from acute neutrophilic interstitial infiltrations, mononuclear interstitial infiltrations, focal suppuration and abscess formation to the characteristic granulomata of tuberculosis and sarcoidosis. As a consequence of the inflammatory changes, the gland becomes somewhat enlarged and tender and produces pain on swallowing. In the usual case, with subsidence of the inflammatory process, the histologic appearance reverts to normal. If focal areas of the gland have been destroyed, scarring may result. Only rarely is thyroid function affected.

THYROIDITIS SECONDARY TO TRAUMA OR RADIATION

Traumatic injuries to the thyroid are not only infrequent, but they rarely cause more than focal hemorrhage which may lead to scars. *Radiation thyroiditis* may, however, be more extensive and clinically significant. The thyroid is relatively resistant to radiation but, of course, has a threshold of susceptibility to beta and gamma rays. Pharmacologic doses of radioiodine, used in place of surgery to reduce thyroid function, can induce injury and, indeed, wipe out thyroid function. It should be emphasized that there is no evidence that radiation injury follows the usual diagnostic dosages of radioiodine. With radiation damage, the thyroid at first shows acute edema, interstitial neutrophilic infiltration and acute injury to follicular epithelial cells, including striking variation in nuclear size and shape readily confused with neoplastic anaplasia. During the phase of acute radiation injury, vascular damage and thromboses may appear within the thyroidal vessels. Months after such therapy, when high dosages have been applied, the glands become shrunken, atrophic and fibrotic. Such follicles as persist are small and distorted, and more often only nests of cells remain trapped within the fibrous scar. The thyroidal vessels are thickened and hyalinized (Friedberg et al., 1952).

Radiation thyroidectomy is only employed in those in middle to later life because of the fear of subsequent neoplasia. As will be discussed later, there is clear evidence that when external radiation was given to the thyroid region of children, as was the practice in former years (p. 1340), it later produced a well defined increase in the incidence of papillary carcinoma in the thyroid gland.

SUBACUTE (de QUERVAIN'S, GRANULOMATOUS) THYROIDITIS

Subacute granulomatous thyroiditis sometimes appears acutely as a painful swelling of the thyroid and, at other times, begins more insidiously with waxing and waning of the discomfort, justifying the designation subacute thyroiditis. It was first described by de Quervain, in 1936, as a febrile disease causing weight loss, lassitude and other systemic reactions. Because of these manifestations, it has long been suspected of being infectious in origin. Numerous investigations have failed to uncover a specific etiologic agent, but there is an increasing tendency to ascribe it to a viral origin. Often the acute thyroid involvement appears to follow an upper respiratory, possibly viral infection (Bergen, 1958). A recent epidemic of mumps was associated with the appearance of a number of these cases, and it was possible in a few to isolate the mumps virus from the thyroid gland. However, the possibility that these cases represented a viremia with coincidental concomitant thyroiditis could not be excluded. More often, the disease occurs sporadically and, in these cases, it is rare to identify a virus. In about half the cases, autoantibodies are present against the constituents of colloid, although antibodies against thyroid cell components are absent. The antibody titers are low and promptly disappear as the disease remits, and it is more reasonable to relate these immunologic changes to a secondary response to thyroid damage than to attribute causal significance to them. Females are affected more often than males in a ratio of about 5 to 1.

The anatomic changes consist of slight to moderate, often asymmetrical enlargement of the thyroid. The capsule may be somewhat bound down by fibrous adhesions to surrounding structures consonant with the inflammatory nature of this condition. Depending upon the duration of the disease, the cut section may bulge above the level of the capsule, if acute edema is present, or may be more firm and nonbulging when there is increased fibrosis.

The diagnostic features are found on histologic examination. Early in the acute stage of the disease, there is a nonspecific acute to subacute inflammatory infiltration surrounding thyroid acini that are obviously damaged. The epithelium lining these acini may be necrotic and desquamated into the central lumen or may have proliferated with the formation of masses of cells that encroach upon the contained colloid. In some areas, the acinar outline may be totally destroyed, leaving only remnants of colloid surrounded by a fairly intense inflammatory reaction. However, the involvement is usually patchy and does not engulf large areas of thyroid substance. **Prominent in this inflammatory infiltrate are large multinucleate giant cells of foreign body type that often contain phagocytized fragments of colloid.** In some instances, the reaction assumes a tubercle-like pattern. The granulomatous lesions probably represent a response to follicle injury and release of colloid into the stroma.

INVASIVE FIBROUS THYROIDITIS (RIEDEL'S STRUMA)

In years past, Riedel's struma was thought to be the fibrotic end-stage of struma lymphomatosa (Hashimoto's disease). In contrast to Hashimoto's disease, fibrous thyroiditis shows no sex preponderance, occurs in a younger age group and has quite different morphologic changes.

The entire thyroid may be normal in size or slightly enlarged, but is usually markedly contracted. **It is stony, hard, pale gray and asymmetrical, having apparent nodularity on clinical palpation.** The capsule is involved in the inflammatory process, producing dense adherence to surrounding structures such as the carotid sheath, trachea and neck muscles—hence, the designation invasive. On section, the tissue is hard and woody.

From the histologic standpoint, there is no specific diagnostic feature of this disorder. In advanced cases, the parenchyma is markedly atrophic and is replaced by masses of dense collagenous fibrous tissue. Scattered throughout this scarring, there is a delicate to moderate lymphocytic infiltration, usually not organized into true lymphoid follicles, such as are seen in Hashimoto's struma. This fibrosis may be so marked as to virtually obliterate the underlying thyroid parenchyma (Fig. 29–24). Such epithelial elements or acini that do remain show varying stages of pressure atrophy and atypicality of cells. Often the trapped epithelial cells resemble those described as Hürthle cells (p. 1326).

The characteristic clinical manifestations of this disease include irregular contraction of the thyroid gland, pressure symptoms, cough and dyspnea. In some patients, the binding of the trachea to the gland evokes the sensation of suffocating. Difficulty in swallowing is another common clinical feature. Thyroid function

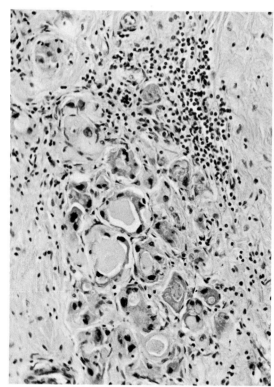

Figure 29–24. A high power view of a Riedel's struma illustrating the extensive fibrosis, scant lymphocytic infiltration and a few residual distorted thyroid follicles.

may be depressed, but it is disproportionately preserved relative to the apparent severity of the fibrosis. Because of the hard asymmetrical distortion and adherence to surrounding structures, the principal differential diagnosis is that of malignant disease. Biopsy or surgical exploration may be required to establish the diagnosis.

HASHIMOTO'S DISEASE (STRUMA LYMPHOMATOSA)

Hashimoto's disease is the most common form of thyroiditis and accounts for about 3 per cent of all thyroid surgical procedures (Statland et al., 1951). It is characterized by:

1. Female preponderance in a ratio somewhere between 30–50 to 1.
2. Peak occurrence at or near the menopause.
3. Symmetrical rubbery enlargement of the thyroid gland.
4. Massive infiltration of the thyroid by lymphoid cells admixed with plasma cells.
5. Transformation of residual thyroid epithelial cells to large, acidophilic Hürthle cells.

6. An abundance of immunologic changes compatible with, but not diagnostic of, an autoimmune disorder.

The incidence of this disorder, as judged by the experience of large clinics, has undergone a remarkable increase in the past three decades (McConahey et al., 1962). Very likely, the increased incidence is spurious and reflects only wider recognition of this entity and better case finding.

Pathogenesis. The evidence supporting an immunologic basis for Hashimoto's disease was discussed in some detail on p. 228. It was pointed out that a variety of humoral and cell-mediated responses to specific thyroid antigens have been identified. In these patients, circulating antibodies have been identified to thyroglobulin, a microsomal fraction and a poorly characterized antigen contained within the follicular colloid. Despite all these circulating antibodies, it is highly likely that cell-mediated reactions are more important and, indeed, in the experimental animal, *thyroiditis cannot be induced in a recipient by transfer of antibodies but only by transfer of sensitized lymphocytes.*

Granting this immunologic evidence, what triggers such a response largely in women in the fourth and fifth decades of life? It was once postulated that thyroglobulin was a sequestered antigen and that some trivial inflammation or injury exposed it to the immune system. It is now clear that minute amounts of thyroglobulin are normally detectable in the circulation and that it is not a sequestered antigen. Some disorder of the basement membrane of the follicles has been vaguely postulated and has been identified in electron micrographs (McConahey, 1972). However, there is a larger body of evidence that the disease is an autoimmune reaction based on some genetic predisposition. Thyroid antibodies can be identified in a significant proportion of apparently normal siblings of patients (Hall, 1960). Identical

spectra of antibodies have been reported in monozygotic twins having this disorder. Hashimoto's thyroiditis frequently coexists with other so-called autoimmune disorders, such as systemic lupus erythematosus, Sjögren's syndrome, rheumatoid arthritis and pernicious anemia (Becker et al., 1963, 1964) (Moore and Neilson, 1963). Thus there is evidence that, on some genetic basis, these patients are predisposed to autoimmune reactions (De-Groot, 1970).

The mere demonstration of circulating and sensitized lymphocytes does not prove an immunologic origin for Hashimoto's disease. Table 29-2 presents an overview of the many disorders in which thyroid antibodies can be found. Could the antibodies merely be secondary to some primary cause of thyroid injury which releases either larger amounts of thyroid antigens or in some way alters them, rendering them antigenic to the host? Uncertainty persists but, on balance, the weight of evidence is in favor of an autoimmune causation.

The relationship of Hashimoto's thyroiditis to Graves' disease (primary hyperthyroidism) is another area of interest and mystery. It is evident from Table 29-2 that antithyroid antibodies occur in both disorders. Patients with Hashimoto's thyroiditis or Graves' disease frequently have close relatives with one or both of these disorders. In some instances, individuals with Graves' disease have, over the course of years and decades, developed the morphologic changes of Hashimoto's disease (McConahey, 1972). Occasional patients with Hashimoto's thyroiditis who are euthyroid have ocular changes typical of those seen in Graves' disease (Wyse et al., 1968). Although most patients with Hashimoto's thyroiditis are hypothyroid, on occasion, they have manifestations indistinguishable from those of Graves' disease. All of this evidence suggests, then, that the two disorders are closely related and, con-

TABLE 29-2. DISORDERS WITH THYROID ANTIBODIES

Disorders	(%) Tests Positive*		
	Precipitin	Tanned Red Cell	Complement Fixing
Hashimoto's disease and chronic thyroiditis	59	80	87
Myxedema	18	72	62
Hyperthyroidism	3	50	64
Nontoxic goiter	1.5	29	9
Subacute thyroiditis	55	50	
Thyroid cancer	9	28	16
No thyroid disease	0	3.3	7.1

*Data derived from Rosenberg, I. N.: Thyroiditis and thyroid antibodies. In Astwood, E. B. (ed.): Clinical Endocrinology. New York, Grune & Stratton, Inc., 1960, p. 185.

ceivably, longstanding Graves' disease may convert into Hashimoto's thyroiditis.

Morphology. **Symmetrical,** firm, rubbery enlargement is the classic appearance of this gland. Increases in size up to three or four times normal may occur. The capsule is intact so that there is no significant adherence. On section, the tissue is firm and pale yellow or gray. Sometimes the enlargement is somewhat asymmetrical.

The dominant histologic pattern is infiltration of the parenchymal substance by large amounts of lymphoid tissue interspersed with plasma cells. In milder cases, there is an overall delicate interstitial fibrosis with a diffuse interstitial infiltration of lymphocytes aggregated in focal areas into lymphoid nests. At a more advanced stage, the aggregates are organized into **lymphoid follicles** surrounded by lymphoid pulp. The replacement may be so extensive as to virtually wipe out the normal thyroid architecture. Histologic sections of such cases may be confused with a lymph node (Fig. 29–25). Commonly, however, small nests of thyroid acini persist, some composed of atrophic cells, but more commonly the cells are large, granular and pink and more or less resemble Hürthle cells. The diffuse increase in the amount of the interacinar connective tissue parallels the severity of the process and is more prominent in advanced cases. The plasma cells, intermingled with the lymphocytes, are interesting in relation to the immune theory of causation of this entity.

Clinical Course. Patients with Hashimoto's thyroiditis come to clinical attention either because of pressure symptoms incident to the glandular enlargement or because of manifestations of hypothyroidism. Common complaints referable to glandular enlargement include fullness in the throat, dysphagia, hoarseness and dysphonia. Although some patients are euthyroid, most have depressed thyroid function. The hypothyroid symptoms and signs are the same as those presented in the discussion of myxedema (p. 1324). Supportive laboratory findings include the demonstration of antithyroid antibodies, decreased serum levels of thyroid hormone and a subnormal uptake of radioactive iodine.

Rare patients with this disorder develop a superimposed cancer. Indeed, in a review of 605 cases, 18 were found to have thyroid cancer and 12 a form of lymphoma—an incidence of 5 per cent of malignancy (Woolner et al., 1959). Many of these thyroidal carcinomas were of microscopic size, and it is reasonable to assume that the incidence of clinically significant cancer in Hashimoto's disease is more nearly 1 to 2 per cent. In its classic expression, Hashimoto's disease occurs as a symmetrical or almost symmetrical enlargement in menopausal females without significant irregular nodularity that would be anticipated in those cases having an underlying cancer.

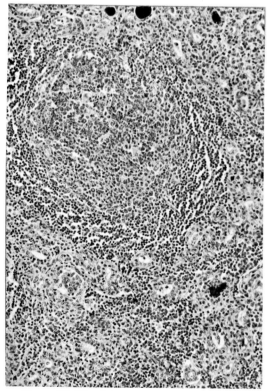

Figure 29–25. *A low power view of a Hashimoto struma illustrating numerous lymphoid follicles and obliteration of the underlying thyroid architecture.*

LYMPHOCYTIC THYROIDITIS

This entity is a first cousin to Hashimoto's thyroiditis but differs insofar as it is encountered in a much younger age group (average 30 years of age) and there are no Hürthle cells in the thyroid gland (Gribetz et al., 1954). There are additional distinctive features which differentiate lymphocytic thyroiditis from Hashimoto's disease. The thyroid enlargement usually develops quite rapidly. While these patients have circulating antibodies, they are usually present in lower quantities than in those with struma lymphomatosa. Despite all of these somewhat distinctive aspects, there is a suspicion that lymphocytic thyroiditis is an early stage of Hashimoto's disease. An alternative theory proposes an abnormal or ineffective thyroid secretory product, resulting in loss of feedback inhibition of the pituitary and consequent increased production of TSH.

Anatomically, the gland is usually diffusely and symmetrically, slightly or moderately enlarged. It may, however, be of normal weight. The lymphocytic infiltration is less extensive than in Hashimoto's disease, and there is less destruction of the thyroid follicles. The epithelial cells are usually unaltered, sometimes slightly hyperplastic, but are not transformed into Hürthle cells.

Most patients are euthyroid adolescents. The PBI is often elevated, which has been attributed to premature release of some abnormal iodinated secretory product from the follicles.

GOITER ARISING IN FUNCTIONAL DERANGEMENTS

The maintenance of the normal functional and anatomic state of the thyroid depends on a host of factors including: adequate dietary supply of iodine, normal levels of TSH, the level of the metabolic demands of the peripheral tissues and normal levels of thyroid-binding globulin (TBG). Excess or deficiencies in the supply of iodides to the gland, stress acting through the hypothalamic-pituitary axis and alterations in the level of TBG all modify thyroid function and structure. For example, estrogens induce increased synthesis of TBG. Thus, more thyroid hormone is bound and less is available to suppress the pituitary, and the resultant increased levels of TSH alter the thyroid structure. So it is that goitrous enlargement of the pituitary may arise through a variety of pathways.

COLLOID (SIMPLE) GOITER

This type of thyroid enlargement is a benign, self-limited condition encountered in females during puberty and pregnancy. It was at one time attributed to work hypertrophy or a deficiency of iodide relative to the increased metabolic demands of puberty and pregnancy. Currently, the view is favored that the colloid storage and goitrous enlargement are the consequence of increased estrogens and elevated levels of TBG (Freedberg et al., 1957). Such a proposition, however, does not explain why the enlarged gland is characterized chiefly by storage of colloid rather than by proliferation of epithelial cells, which would be reasonably anticipated with increased levels of TSH.

The thyroid is modestly, symmetrically enlarged and rarely weighs more than 100 gm. It has an increased firmness and appears to be brittle,

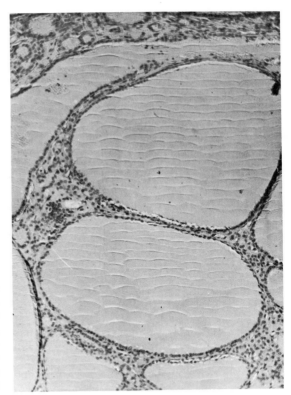

Figure 29–26. *Colloid goiter. The follicles are distended with colloid and the epithelial lining is flattened.*

gelatinous and pale gray-brown on cut section. The enlargement of the follicles can sometimes be identified on gross inspection. The capusle is usually intact and uninvolved.

The histologic pattern depends, to some extent, on the stage at which the gland is examined. In the classic case, large colloid-filled acini lined by flattened epithelial cells are the dominant pattern (Fig. 29–26). Sometimes there are residual foci of small acini lined by cuboidal to columnar cells as residues of the preexisting hyperplasia. There is a scant amount of interacinar connective tissue devoid of significant lymphoid infiltrate. The vascularization is usually diminished, probably because of the increased pressure produced by the distended acini.

The thyroidal enlargement barely merits the designation of a goiter. Rarely, it produces a fullness in the neck which infrequently evokes pressure symptoms. The disorder is usually self-limited and rarely requires treatment. On occasion, it has been evoked by the administration of estrogens.

NODULAR OR MULTIPLE COLLOID ADENOMATOUS GOITER

Nodular enlargement of the thyroid gland is the end result of hyperplasia, asymmetrical focal involution, hemorrhages and scarring of the glandular parenchyma. It is the most common form of goitrous enlargement and produces the most massive increases in size. Women are affected more often than men in a ratio of about 6 to 1.

Pathogenesis. Any cause for goitrous enlargement may eventuate in a nodular goiter as a consequence of uneven focal hyperplasia, involution and scarring. The two most common sequences involve iodine deficiency and ingestion of goitrogens. Certain regions of the world were once characterized as goiter belts because the water supplies and diet in these locales contained little or no iodine. The classic goiter belts were the mountains of central Europe, South America and Asia, and the Great Lakes regions of the United States and Canada. In these areas, the deficiency of dietary iodine prevented the synthesis of adequate amounts of thyroid hormone, resulting in derepression or activation of the adenohypophyseal axis. The widespread addition of iodine to salt and foods in recent years has alleviated this problem in these areas of the world (Weaver et al., 1966). The second pathway involves the ingestion of goitrogenic substances that block thyroid hormone production. Such compounds have been identified in turnip, cabbage, rutabaga, kale and rapeseed. The goitrogen has an action similar to thiouracil and thus blocks the output of thyroid hormone.

Much less frequently, nodular enlargement of the thyroid is encountered in familial disorders characterized by a genetic lack of an enzyme involved in thyroid hormone biosynthesis. These familial goiters are discussed more completely in the following section.

Whatever the underlying mechanism, impaired output of thyroid hormone results in elevated levels of TSH and stimulation of the thyroid which undergoes hyperplasia and becomes enlarged. In time, this diffuse hyperplastic reaction is complicated by focal colloid involution, hemorrhage and scarring, resulting in the multinodularity of these glands.

Morphology. This is the largest form of goiter encountered. Masses of over 1000 gm. have been described. These goiters may enlarge downward behind the sternum and clavicles to produce so-called **intrathoracic** or **plunging goiters**. As the name implies, these goiters are completely **asymmetrical and show multiple nodular masses** on palpation (Fig. 29–27). Usually, the capsule is intact and the gland is not adherent although, in certain areas, adhesion to surrounding structures may be produced by subcapsular hemorrhage. On section, a variegated surface is presented. Areas of

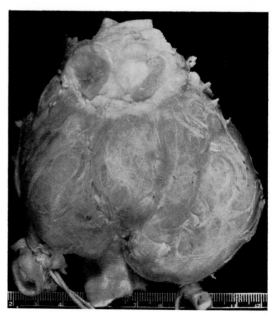

Figure 29–27. *Multiple colloid adenomatous goiter removed with the trachea attached. The asymmetry and enlargement of the gland are apparent.*

meaty, red-brown parenchyma representing probable foci of hyperplasia alternate with other areas of gelatinous granular tissue representing colloid involution. Large cystic softenings may develop and fibrous scarring, hemorrhages and calcification are common.

The histologic pattern conforms to the gross descriptions already given. Perhaps the most important diagnostic feature of this gland is the variable pattern encountered. Nodules of hyperplasia alternate with nodules composed of colloid-filled, dilated follicles. Some are cystically dilated. Interspersed are large hyaline fibrous scars and areas of recent and old hemorrhage (Fig. 29–28). In these scarred areas, hemosiderin, cholesterol clefts and calcifications are common. An important observation is the absence of definite encapsulation of the nodules. They may be surrounded by condensed fibrous tissue derived from the stroma but, with multiple sections, it is apparent that this does not represent a total capsule but simply compression of preexisting trabeculae.

Clinical Course. Nodular goiters most often arise at puberty and during pregnancy when thyroid hormones are in greatest demand. They slowly increase in size over the span of years, and some become large, disfiguring masses which produce severe pressure symptoms (Hermanson et al., 1952). Downward growth behind the sternum into the thoracic inlet often compresses the major neck vessels, trachea and esophagus. In general, the increase in size of these glands is sufficient to

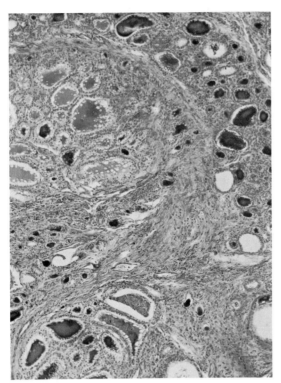

Figure 29–28. Multiple colloid adenomatous goiter illustrating the scarring and variation in size of the follicles.

keep the patients euthyroid with normal levels of serum PBI. Occasionally, a focus within the gland hyperfunctions, producing a *toxic nodular goiter*.

The major complications of nodular goiter are: (1) sudden painful gland enlargement occasioned by an intrathyroid hemorrhage, (2) secondary hyperthyroidism related to a hyperfunctioning focus and (3) the emergence of a carcinoma. The frequency of superimposed carcinoma is a contentious issue. Reported frequencies range from 1 to 11 per cent but, in my experience, a reasonable average would be near the lower limit (Meachim and Stainsby, 1966) (Zacharewicz, 1968).

FAMILIAL GOITER

A variety of inborn errors have been identified, in which there is a congenital lack of a specific enzyme involved in the biosynthesis of thyroid hormone. Some of these disorders are clearly hereditary. Frequently, such infants are the product of consanguineous marriages, and the thyroid lack is so severe it produces cretinism. In other patients, the evidence for a familial trait is less clear. Most familial goiters become evident in the newborn, but the en-

zyme defect might be less severe and only become apparent when thyroid hormone biosynthesis is stressed. Thus, familial goiters tend to become evident during puberty or pregnancy, when there is a lack of iodine in the diet, or when goitrogens complicate the problem.

A number of specific syndromes have been identified (Stanbury, 1963). The following disorders have apparently autosomal recessive modes of transmission:

1. A defect in iodide trapping in which the gland is unable to accumulate adequate amounts of iodine.

2. An inability to convert iodide to organically bound iodine, presumably reflecting a deficiency of peroxidase.

3. An inability to couple MIT and DIT involved in the synthesis of T_3 and T_4. Here again, peroxidases may be lacking.

4. An inability to recapture iodide from iodinated protein byproducts formed in the course of hormone synthesis because of a lack of iodotyrosine dehalogenase.

Other syndromes have been identified with unknown modes of genetic transmission. In Pendred's syndrome, there is an inability to convert iodide to iodine associated with eighth nerve deafness. In yet another syndrome, there appears to be a carrier-protein defect, leading to the formation of an abnormal albumin-bound iodoprotein that is functionally ineffective in the peripheral tissues.

Whatever the specific congenital defect, goitrous enlargement ensues. If the patient survives long enough, a multinodular goiter appears. When this form of goitrous enlargement is discovered in an infant or child, the possibility of a familial trait must be suspected. There have been a number of reports of the development of carcinoma in such cases (Batsakis et al., 1963) (Moore, 1962). However, familial nodular goiters may present considerable epithelial pleomorphism and apparent anaplasia, and so the possibility of overdiagnosis must be guarded against. Indeed, it has been noted in one report that metastases and recurrence are infrequent in these forms of cancer, casting doubt on the diagnosis (Moore, 1962).

IATROGENIC GOITER

The administration of iodide, cyanates, thioureas, as well as other drugs, may induce goiter. Iodide-induced hyperthyroidism is now a well defined entity (Editorial, 1972b). In such patients, the gland exhibits changes to be described as diffuse primary hyperplasia. In other instances, a nodular goiter has developed after long, protracted iodide therapy used as an expectorant in the treatment of asthma or chronic bronchitis. Here it is proposed that the individual develops a goiter because of a particular susceptibility of thyroid peroxidase to iodide inhibition. Goiters may develop in fetuses or appear later in infants when the mother had taken iodide or thioureas during pregnancy. All of these entities are rare but are worthy of note since they represent medically induced disease.

GRAVES' DISEASE (PRIMARY HYPERTHYROIDISM, DIFFUSE PRIMARY THYROID HYPERPLASIA)

Graves' disease is the most common and important cause of hyperthyroidism. In this condition, the hyperthyroidism is associated with striking eye changes, particularly protrusion of the eyeballs, and hence the designation *exophthalmic goiter*. You recall that hyperthyroidism may be produced by nodular goiters or functioning tumors, benign or malignant, but only Graves' disease is regularly associated with exophthalmos. It is apparent, then, that hyperthyroidism is not synonymous with Graves' disease. However, Graves' disease does not invariably cause exophthalmos and, indeed, exophthalmos may be seen in other thyroid disorders associated with hyperthyroidism and even in euthyroid patients (Editorial, 1972a).

Incidence. Primary hyperthyroidism affects females four times as commonly as males. It most often arises in the second to fourth decades of life. A familial predisposition has been identified which may be related to its immunologic causation, as will be discussed below (Werner, 1967).

Etiology and Pathogenesis. Despite an intensive search, the precise origins of this thyroid disorder are still uncertain. Causative mechanisms have been proposed and have gained widespread acceptance, only then to be challenged by new observations. Moreover, the relationship of the exophthalmos to the hyperthyroidism remains an additional area of grayness. Only a brief review of this subject can be presented here.

For many years, it was assumed that the cause of the diffuse thyroid hyperplasia and hyperactivity lay in pituitary hyperfunction and increased levels of TSH. Failure to identify elevations of such thyrotropic hormone in the blood was attributed to insensitive assay techniques. As methods of detecting TSH improved, this theory of causation was more or less discarded (perhaps too soon, as we shall see). More recently, attention has turned to an abnormal thyroid stimulator known as long-acting thyroid stimulator (LATS) (McKenzie, 1972). LATS has been identified as a gamma-G immunoglobulin that directly influences thyroid gland function by stimulation of adenyl cyclase and enhanced production of cyclic AMP. This immunoglobulin has also been imputed to stimulate mitotic division of epithelial cells in the thyroid, possibly by inhibiting or neutralizing control factors such as chalone's (Garry and Hall, 1970). LATS has been identified in 70 to 80 per cent of patients with hyperthyroidism (Chopra et al., 1970).

While enthusiasm for the LATS theory was high only a few years ago, recent observations chip away at its foundations. To begin with, why can it not be identified in at least 20 per cent of patients with Graves' disease despite concentration techniques? Could this reflect only the insensitivity of the bioassay? A more serious attack has been the recent recognition that it is possible to suppress thyroid function in these patients by administration of thyroid hormone (Clark et al., 1970) (Silverstein and Burke, 1970). Such suppression once again suggests a primary pituitary hyperfunction. Since LATS is not involved in the pituitary-thyroid axis, thyroid hormone administration should not affect its pathogenetic role. A third problem with the LATS theory is understanding what initiates the appearance of such an immunoglobulin. Here, genetically determined predisposition to autoimmune disease is invoked. As was cited earlier, Hashimoto's thyroiditis and Graves' disease are closely related, and the former is presently suspected of being an autoimmune disorder. The familial distribution of both Graves' disease and Hashimoto's thyroiditis would be consonant with some genetic defect in immune tolerance. In an attempt to reconcile all these troublesome questions, McKenzie (1972) raises the possibility that LATS alone is not the cause of Graves' disease. Conceivably, it may act in concert with other "permissive" factors in the form of other immunoglobulins.

To confuse the issue even further, recent reports once again raise the specter of TSH and primary pituitary hyperfunction in these patients (Emerson and Utiger, 1972). However, it is by no means clear that TSH is involved in the causation of the preponderance of cases. At the present time, the issue of causation remains in flux, and we must await more data on this intriguing problem.

The ophthalmopathy seen regularly but not invariably in Graves' disease is another area of uncertainty. The eye manifestations include stare, lid retraction, lid lag, delayed blinking and watering but, most importantly, protrusion of the eyeball. There is a good deal of evidence that such ophthalmopathy is not related to LATS, and a suspicion that it is due to pituitary factors (an exophthalmos-producing substance or TSH) (Dobyns and Steelman, 1953) (Editorial, 1972a). Also suggested is another immunoglobulin distinct from LATS that may be related to the ophthalmopathy (Singh and McKenzie, 1971). We cannot delve further into these eye changes, but it must be emphasized that they may attain "malignant" proportions and, indeed, produce blindness.

Morphology. In most cases of diffuse hyperplasia, the gland is usually symmetrical and uniformly but not markedly enlarged. It is **uncommon** to observe **more than threefold** increases in weight up to 80 to 90 gm. The capsule is intact and not adherent. On cut section, the parenchyma has a soft, yielding, red-brown, meaty appearance closely resembling the cross section of normal muscle. Iodine administration preoperatively causes the accumulation of colloid and alters this gross appearance.

The dominant histologic feature is that of excessive cellularity of the parenchyma. This is imparted by two alterations: an increase in the height of the lining epithelial cells to form tall columnar cells, and an increase in the number of the cells, causing them to pile up in papillary buds and encroach upon the acinar spaces (Fig. 29–29 and 29–30). For the most part, these papillae represent **simple, nonbranching** projections, which usually are slightly elevated above the level of the surrounding epithelium. Occasionally, the papillae are sufficiently large to mushroom out and virtually fill the acini. The cells may show slight variation in size and shape, but no striking atypicality is present. Colloid is markedly diminished in amount and, when present, has a thin, pale pink, watery appearance. The interacinar stroma demonstrates a striking increase in the amount of lymphoid tissue and, in some areas, large lymphoid follicles are produced. The accumulation of lymphoid tissue in

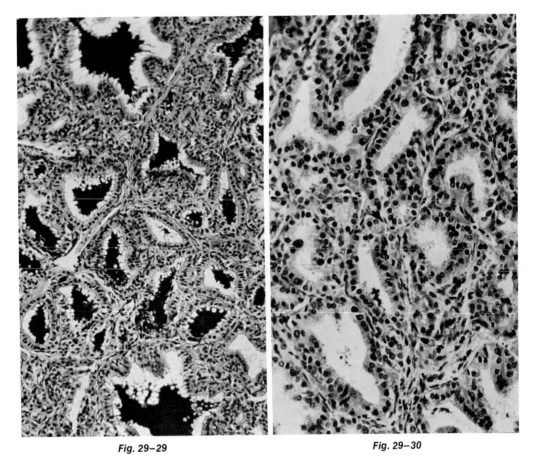

Fig. 29–29   *Fig. 29–30*

Figure 29–29. *A microscopic view of diffuse thyroid hyperplasia. The cellularity of the follicles and resorption of the colloid are evident. High columnar epithelium and small projections into the follicular spaces are visible.*

Figure 29–30. *A high power view of diffuse thyroid hyperplasia illustrating total absence of colloid, increase in height of epithelium and buckling of the lining of the acini into the follicular spaces.*

the thyroid is only one aspect of the generalized lymphoid hypertrophy found throughout the body. There is inevitably a markedly increased vascularization in these glands. This classic histologic pattern may be significantly altered by preoperative medication. Iodine promotes colloid storage, devascularization and involution of the gland, while thiouracil tends to produce marked hyperplasia. Thus, it is impossible to evaluate correctly, from histologic examination, the amount of functional activity of pretreated surgical specimens.

The cause of the exophthalmos, in morphologic terms, includes inflammation and edema of the connective tissue, fat and muscles within the orbit, accompanied by an increase in the mucopolysaccharides of the connective tissue ground substance.

Clinical Course. The clinical features of primary hyperthyroidism stem from three sources: (1) the effects of the excess thyroid hormone, already presented on p. 1323, (2) the thyroid enlargement and (3) the ophthalmopathy present in about 50 to 60 per cent of patients. Goitrous enlargement in Graves' disease tends to be slight. Rarely is it disfiguring and, indeed, it may be so slight as to be imperceptible on clinical palpation. In some patients with more pronounced enlargements, pressure symptoms and some discomfort on swallowing appear. The markedly increased vascularization produces a thyroid bruit which is almost pathognomonic of hyperthyroidism (Kendall-Taylor, 1972). The ocular changes have already been briefly cited. The exophthalmos is one of the most troublesome features of this disease. Protrusion of the eyeballs may occur to the point where the protective action of the eyelids becomes inadequate. The eyes are thus exposed to trauma and infection which can lead to serious ocular damage and loss of vision. Small wonder, then, that extreme examples are called *malignant exophthalmos*. Control of the hyperthyroidism by surgery or radioiodine does not relieve or halt the ocular abnormalities and, in many patients, surgical, orbital decompression is necessary.

As would be expected, the basal metabolic rate, serum PBI and T_4 levels and the radioiodine uptake are all elevated in this disease. When uncontrolled, the hyperthyroid patient may suffer a thyroid storm and die. On the happier side, there is general agreement that diffuse hyperplasia of the thyroid invokes little or no increased risk of the development of cancer.

TUMORS

Relative to their morbidity and mortality, tumors of the thyroid gland have commanded a disproportionate amount of attention. Tumors present as nodules or masses and all nodules are suspected of being cancers. It is important to remember that a palpable nodule in the thyroid in an otherwise euthyroid patient may represent:

1. Hemorrhage into the gland.
2. Lobulation of a normal thyroid.
3. Lobulation of chronic thyroiditis.
4. An intrathyroidal cyst.
5. An adenoma.
6. A carcinoma.
7. Other more rare entities.

In the general population of the United States, thyroid nodules are estimated to be present in as many as 4 to 5 per cent of the population. The overwhelming majority of these nodules represent adenomas or some other form of benign disease.

Thyroid cancers are rare. They account for only 0.4 per cent of all cancer deaths. Furthermore, the most common form of thyroid cancer is the papillary carcinoma, an indolent form of neoplasia which rarely kills. Nonetheless, a mass or nodule in the thyroid evokes alarm, and so thyroid cancers continue to command a great deal of attention. There are only 13 deaths from thyroid cancer per million population per year. If one assumes a 30-year survival for every patient with thyroid cancer, it is evident that its prevalence is on the order of 390 individuals per million population, a far cry from the 5 per 100 incidence (5 per cent) for thyroid nodules in the general population.

Despite all the epidemiologic data, a nodule may, indeed, represent a cancer for the individual patient. The clinical appraisal of nodules is, therefore, a prime diagnostic problem. Regrettably, there are no infallible techniques to differentiate benign from malignant nodules short of histologic examination. The size, shape and consistency are of limited differential value.

One of the most widely used procedures to appraise the nature of a thyroid nodule is the administration of a test dose of radioiodine (RaI) to elicit the level of radioactivity of the nodule based on its iodine uptake. The differential value of the RaI uptake depends on the premise that the greater the RaI uptake, the more well differentiated and functional the nodule, and the better the differentiation, the greater the likelihood of its being benign (McKenney et al., 1972). In usual clinical parlance, the amount of RaI uptake is crudely quantified by the terms hot, warm and cold. Hot nodules have a high RaI uptake and, therefore, are likely to be benign. An additional technique of some value employs suppression of pituitary function by administered thyroid hormone to determine whether the uptake of RaI in a hot or warm nodule will be reduced, indicating dependency on pituitary function. Such dependency is taken to imply that the nodule represents a nodular goiter or a benign tumor. But as every clinician knows, there are no completely reliable diagnostic criteria of thyroid cancer.

An analysis of the validity of clinical diagnosis was reported by a clinic known to be a referral center for thyroid disease (Hurxthal and Heineman, 1958). On pathologic study, 15 cases of cancer were found and confirmed microscopically in 226 thyroid glands containing solitary nodules (Hurxthal and Heineman, 1958). Nine of these cancers were unsuspected clinically. In only six patients was the diagnosis of cancer suspected prior to surgery. Conversely, in 15 other patients thought to have cancer, none was found. The evaluation of a nodule in the thyroid continues to be a problem of great concern to patient and clinician alike.

BENIGN

The most common benign tumor of the thyroid is an adenoma. Adenomas and nodules of multinodular goiter are frequently confused. The latter are not true neoplasms. The criteria which characterize an adenoma are: (1) complete fibrous encapsulation, (2) a clear distinction between the architecture inside and outside the capsule, (3) a uniform histologic architecture within the capsule and (4) compression of the surrounding thyroid substance. For obscure reasons, thyroid adenomas occur far more frequently in females (in a ratio of 7 to 1). Eighty per cent are encountered in patients between the ages of 20 and 60 (Psarras et al., 1972).

Adenomas are divided into two types, follicular and papillary. Sometimes a third wastebasket category is added—atypical adenoma—for those which cannot be fitted into either of the two well defined patterns. The papillary forms will be discussed later. They span a range from well differentiated, orderly, apparently innocent lesions to overt papillary carcinomas. However, even the benign-appearing forms sometimes surprise by recurring or spreading to regional nodes. For these lesions, it is most difficult to predict biologic behavior from their morphology. All papillary lesions will, therefore, be considered together under papillary carcinoma. In the follicular group are placed all adenomas that produce glandular patterns or acini. It therefore includes the former categories of *embryonal, fetal,*

simple and colloid adenomas. This designation also includes both the so-called *microfollicular* and the *macrofollicular* adenomas, based upon size of the acini. Justification for this simplification exists in the fact that, within a solitary adenoma, there is almost invariably a wide variation in the size of acini so that no one dominant pattern can be truly defined.

Follicular Adenoma. This designation includes benign tumors of the thyroid gland that produce simple glandular or acinar patterns. They occur in any age group, more commonly in young adults, in any portion of the thyroid gland.

These adenomas tend to be solitary, discrete, spherical masses, usually less than 3 to 4 cm. in diameter (Fig. 29–31). On occasion, larger lesions up to 10 cm. are encountered (Fig. 29–32). Because of their centrifugal growth within an enclosing capsule, they are more firm than the surrounding thyroid substance. On cut section, they vary from soft gray tissue that bulges above the level of the capsule to a red-brown, somewhat gelatinous tissue. On occasion, small central foci of fibrous scarring or calcification are evident grossly.

Common to all is the production of gland acini. However, there is considerable variation in the size and number of the acini, as well as in the abundance of the interacinar stroma. On the one extreme, tumors may be found which are composed of solid cords of small cuboidal cells separated by a scant fibrous stroma. Acinar production is quite rudimentary and is composed of rare small glands which usually fail to contain colloid. Such tumors were formerly classified as **embryonal adenomas** (Fig. 29–33). At the other extreme are found those tumors that produce large, cystically dilated glands containing abundant colloid and separated by a scant interacinar stroma, formerly categorized as **colloid adenomas** (Fig. 29–34). Between these two extremes, all variations may be found, commonly within a single nodule.

There is, in addition, considerable range in the amount of interacinar stroma present and, in certain follicular adenomas, abundant hyaline collagenous fibrous tissue widely separates small but well formed acini. Formerly such tumors have been called **fetal adenomas** (Fig. 29–35). All adenomas have well developed fibrous capsules (Fig. 29–36).

One additional histologic variation merits mention. Very rarely, adenomas are composed of cells larger and more granular than the usual thyroid epithelium, distributed in poorly defined glands, nests and sheets throughout a fibrous stroma. These so-called Hürthle cells vary quite considerably in size and shape and have abundant, granular, pink cytoplasm with round to oval nuclei. **Hürthle cell adenomas** composed of such cells

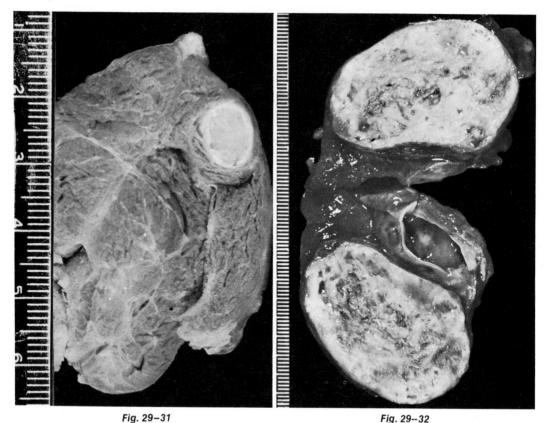

Fig. 29–31   Fig. 29–32

Figures 29–31 and 29–32. Adenomas of the thyroid. View of cross section of the nodules against the background of the darker normal thyroid tissue.

may be difficult to differentiate from a malignancy because of the striking variation in the size and shape of these distinctive cell forms (Fig. 29–37).

About 10 per cent of adenomas show invasive, potentially cancerous, features. Along with capsular invasion, there may be penetration of lymphatic and blood vessel channels about the tumor. Such aggressiveness is most often seen in the embryonal pattern but may be encountered in any of the other patterns mentioned except that they are extremely rare in colloid adenomas. When such invasion is found, the lesion may be designated as an **angioinvasive adenoma** or an **encapsulated follicular carcinoma.**

Follicular adenomas are of clinical significance because: (1) they have the potential of hyperfunction, (2) they comprise nodules which must be differentiated from cancer and (3) they may become malignant or were so from the outset. It is generally held that about 10 per cent of follicular adenomas disclose features of cancer. Whether this represents conversion of a benign adenoma or apparent en-

capsulation of a de novo cancer is unknown and probably academic. Confirming such a frequency in a survey of 692 solitary nodules, 81 proved to harbor cancer (11.7 per cent) (Psarras et al., 1972). This study further revealed that, in persons below the age of 20 and over 60, the nodules were cancerous 2 to 3 times more often than benign, particularly when they occurred in males. The incidence of carcinoma in cold nodules was 12.8 per cent, and in warm nodules, 6.6 per cent. No malignancy was found in a hot nodule or in hyperfunctioning nodules. Even when capsular or vascular invasion is found, these lesions are of low aggressiveness and the local recurrence rate at five years is on the order of 10 per cent.

Teratoma. These are extremely rare, solitary nodules, usually present in the midline, that arise out of vestigial remnants of embryonal tissue. They reproduce the same forms of varied tissues found in teratomas elsewhere and have the same malignant potential.

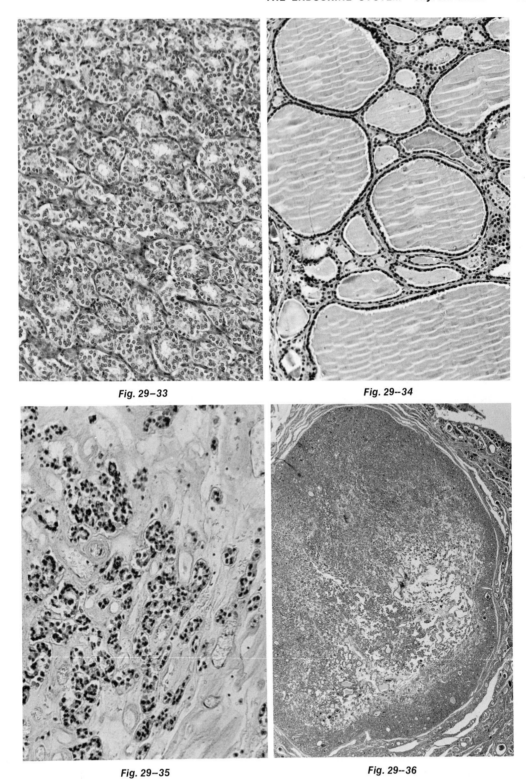

Fig. 29–33

Fig. 29–34

Fig. 29–35

Fig. 29–36

Figures 29–33 to 29–35. *Three types of follicular adenoma illustrating variability in acinar size, colloid content and amount of interstitial connective tissue. Figure 29–35 represents the type formerly referred to as a fetal adenoma.*

Figure 29–36. *A low power view of a follicular adenoma of the thyroid illustrating the discrete encapsulation and demarcation from the surrounding thyroid substance.*

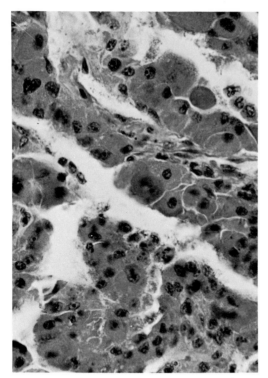

Figure 29–37. *A high power detail of the cells that comprise a Hürthle cell adenoma. Considerable variability in size and shape of cells is evident. The abundant cytoplasm demonstrates a fine granularity.*

MALIGNANT

The rarity of thyroid cancer and its general indolence and low mortality have already been presented (p. 1336).

Little is known about the genesis of these lesions except for two important associations. Ionizing radiation, particularly to the head and neck region, is strongly suspected of predisposing to the later development of thyroid cancer. This relationship is borne out by the increased attack rate of thyroid cancer in patients who have received significant amounts of radiation to the head and neck region during infancy or childhood (Duffy and Fitzgerald, 1950). Thyroid cancer has also been identified in an earlier than anticipated age range in the survivors of the atomic bombs at Hiroshima and Nagasaki (Socolow et al., 1963).

The second pathogenetic mechanism may constitute prolonged TSH stimulation. Williams (1962) proposes that hyperplastic thyroid cells long exposed to TSH may become transformed into autonomous tumor cells having the capacity to produce either benign or malignant neoplasms. While this concept is highly speculative, it does have the support of several observations. It has been possible in rats, by the prolonged administration of thiouracil com-pounds that block thyroid hormone output and induce elevated levels of TSH, to produce progressive hyperplasia and eventually neoplasia of the thyroid epithelium (Purves and Adams, 1960). Moreover, in humans it is often said that thyroid cancers rarely arise in normal glands, and so it is reasonable to assume that antecedent hyperplastic changes may provide the soil on which a neoplasm develops.

Woolner (1971) recently reported an analysis of 1181 thyroid carcinomas seen at the Mayo Clinic during the years 1926–60. His classification of these neoplasms is presented in Table 29–3.

Papillary Carcinoma. Under this designation are included the benign-appearing forms formerly termed papillary adenoma as well as anaplastic lesions. By long custom, these neoplasms are called papillary, but it should be emphasized that almost invariably they contain a follicular component. In some instances, the papillary pattern predominates, while others are predominantly follicular. Irrespective of the relative proportions of these two patterns, all tumors having well defined papillary excrescences are categorized as papillary carcinoma, because all have similar biologic behavior.

Papillary carcinoma is by far the most common category of thyroid cancer as Table 29–3 indicates. In children and young adults less than 40 years of age, these neoplasms account for at least 80 per cent of thyroid cancers. Females are affected more often than males in a ratio of 2.4 to 1. The tumors vary greatly in size, in the dominance of the papillary component and in the extent of involvement of regional lymph nodes. Although for most cancers, these factors would be expected to influence the prognosis, in this pattern of thyroid carcinoma *only the size and local extent of the primary lesion have prognostic significance.* Even metastases within cervical lymph nodes do not seem to influence the curability, because such nodes are readily excised and do not nec-

TABLE 29–3. CLASSIFICATION OF THYROID CARCINOMA

Types of Thyroid Carcinoma	No.	Per Cent
Well differentiated		
Papillary	736	62.3
Follicular	208	17.6
Undifferentiated		
Medullary (solid) with amyloid	77	6.5
Anaplastic	160	13.6
TOTAL	1181	100.0

From Woolner, L. B.: Thyroid carcinoma: pathologic classification with data on prognosis. Seminars Nucl. Med., *1*:481–502, 1971. By permission of Grune & Stratton, Inc.

essarily imply widespread dissemination. For this reason, it has been recommended that papillary carcinoma be subdivided into occult, intrathyroid and extrathyroid (implying direct spread beyond the capsule).

Papillary tumors range from microscopic foci found incidentally in thyroid glands or cervical lymph nodes removed for other reasons to nodules up to 10 cm. in diameter. The microscopic foci are obviously occult and are frequently multicentric. Despite such small size, spread to cervical lymph nodes may be most impressive. Indeed, the well differentiated predominantly follicular metastases gave rise, at one time, to the concept of lateral ectopic or aberrant thyroid glands since the primary was entirely occult. The less well differentiated lesions were interpreted as carcinoma arising in lateral aberrant thyroid tissue. Although aberrant or ectopic thyroids do exist on a developmental basis, in most instances, when found within lymph nodes, an occult primary cancer will be found in the definitive thyroid gland (although it must be admitted

that many investigators still disagree) (Maddox et al., 1971) (Roth, 1965) (Butler et al., 1967).

Larger intrathyroid and extrathyroid invasive papillary lesions may, on cross section, appear solid or cystic and many have an apparent encapsulation. The cut surface may be furry due to the myriads of tiny papillae. Frequently, satellite nodules are found about such discrete tumor masses but usually involvement is confined to one lobe.

The pathognomonic histologic feature of these lesions is a complicated, branching, tree-like pattern most sharply outlined by the papilliform axial fibrovascular stroma (Figs. 29–38 and 29–39). In the benign-appearing so-called adenomas, this framework is covered by a single layer of well oriented regular cuboidal epithelium. Some papillae are cut in cross section to produce apparent isolated islands; elsewhere follicles may be formed, sometimes filled with colloid. All degrees of atypicality and disorientation of cells, piling up of epithelium, invasion of the stalk and capsule and formation of sheets and masses of cells may be encountered in the more obviously malignant lesions

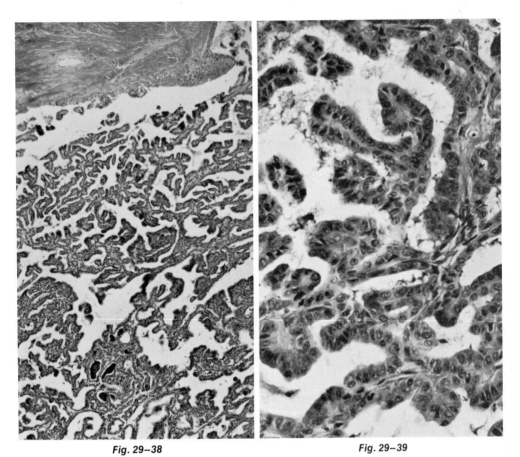

Fig. 29–38   Fig. 29–39

Figure 29–38. A low power view of a papillary cystadenoma of the thyroid illustrating the complex branching pattern of the tumor growth.

Figure 29–39. A high power detail of one microscopic field illustrating the regular alignment of the covering epithelium producing a unicellular layer.

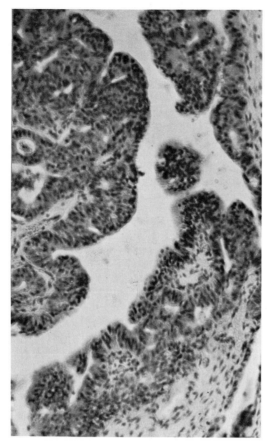

Figure 29–40. *A microscopic field of a papillary cystadenomatous cancer illustrating the irregularity of the epithelium with extension into the connective tissue of the underlying stalk. Comparison of this figure with Figures 29–38 and 29–39 illustrates some of the differences between the benign and malignant-appearing forms of papillary growth.*

(Fig. 29–40). Moreover, a wide range of histologic changes is often found from one microscopic field to another within the same lesion, underscoring the difficulty and impracticality of trying to differentiate so-called adenomas from carcinomas.

In almost all papillary lesions, there is some admixture of follicular architecture. Indeed, they may be dominantly follicular but, as long as one can define papillae having a well defined central fibrovascular stalk covered by epithelium, they should be considered as papillary tumors and will have the clinical behavior and prognosis of such lesions. Foci of calcification or fibrosis are occasionally encountered.

As is evident, papillary lesions span a wide range of cytologic differentiation and size. When they are not occult, they appear as palpable thyroid nodules that are extremely indolent and do not enlarge over the course of months or even years. Rarely, the follicular component may be responsible for hyperfunction and produce hot or warm nodules on isotopic scan. Growth of these tumors can often be suppressed by feeding of desiccated thyroid because of their dependence on TSH. They spread via the lymphatics to the regional nodes in the neck and, overall, such nodal metastasis is found in about 40 per cent, approaching 90 per cent in childhood papillary carcinoma (Hayles et al., 1963). Wider dissemination via the bloodstream is uncommon and is principally encountered in lesions with extrathyroidal extension.

Overall, papillary carcinoma is readily curable by relatively conservative excision of the involved thyroid lobe and suspiciously enlarged lymph nodes. Dessicated thyroid is given following surgery for its suppressive effect. Not infrequently, cervical node metastases spring up months or even years after the thyroidectomy but, once again, excision of the node(s) provides satisfactory control or even cure. With such a regimen, many large surveys have shown that *occult and intrathyroidal lesions have no effect on the normal longevity.* With extrathyroidal extension, the curve of survival is one-third lower than that of normal controls of comparable age and sex (Woolner et al., 1961). Even those with obvious metastases in the lungs may survive for decades and, indeed, die of other causes.

Follicular Carcinoma. This second pattern of well differentiated thyroid carcinoma is characterized by the presence of at least some well developed follicles in some part of the tumor and by the absence of well differentiated papillary structures. They resemble papillary tumors insofar as they are slow-growing and are frequently curable, but they differ in their tendency to spread via the blood stream to distant sites rather than to regional nodes. Thus, follicular carcinomas have a biologic behavior different from that of papillary carcinomas, even those with a large component of follicular architecture.

Anatomically, these tumors take one of two forms: (1) a small nodule apparently encapsulated closely resembling a follicular adenoma and (2) an obvious cancerous mass perhaps occupying an entire lobe. The encapsulated adenomatous lesion has been described earlier as an angioinvasive adenoma which might equally well be called an angioinvasive encapsulated carcinoma. Even these localized lesions have a propensity for invading blood vessels but, for unknown reasons, nodal metastasis is uncommon.

The more common pattern is that of an obvious gross involvement of the thyroid. This type causes irregular enlargement of the gland. The tumorous gray-white tissue overgrows the thyroid, replaces large parts of it and extends through the capsule to become adherent to or invade the trachea, muscles, skin and great vessels of the neck. In this infiltrative progression, the recurrent laryngeal nerves are often trapped. On cut section, the usual red-brown, meaty thyroid substance is involved by gray-white, firm neoplasm (Fig. 29—41). The histologic pattern of adenocarcinoma is readily apparent with characteristic anaplasia of cells, extension beyond the capsule into surrounding structures and invasion of blood vessels (Fig. 29—42). True thyroid follicle formation is present in some very well differentiated tumors, and follicles containing colloid may be faithfully reproduced to the point that differentiation from a normal thyroid is difficult (Fig. 29—43). These extremely well differentiated, colloid-producing adenocarcinomas have in former years been referred to as benign metastasizing struma. On the other hand, the less well differentiated ones grow in sheets of cells, produce only abortive glands and often have little colloid formation.

The prognosis and survival for patients with these neoplasms are largely dependent on the extent of vascular invasion in and about the primary lesion. In general, about half of the follicular carcinomas, irrespective of their size and apparent encapsulation, will show little or only equivocal vascular invasion, and the survival in this group, following adequate excision of the primary tumor, is comparable to a control population. Occasional patients without evidence of significant vascular invasion die, but usually after two or more decades of life. In contrast, when there is well defined vascular invasion, the 10- and 20-year survival rates are on the order of 34 per cent and 16 per cent. Distant metastasis to the lungs and bone and other viscera leads eventually to death, with a mean duration of life after surgery of 6 years.

In general, these masses comprise cold or, at most, warm nodules, as judged by RaI uptake, and they are not suppressable by thyroid treatment. If the lesion takes up RaI, it is sometimes employed in therapeutic doses in an attempt to deliver sufficient irradiation to the cancer, both to its primary site as well as to its metastases.

Medullary Carcinoma with Amyloid Stroma. Although these neoplasms are relatively uncommon in the spectrum of thyroid cancers (7 per cent), they are of great interest because of their association with so many systemic syndromes and their elaboration of a large number of secretory products. For brevity, these associations will be listed:

1. Many medullary tumors are associated with pheochromocytomas, and sometimes both the thyroid and adrenal neoplasms are bilateral.

2. Rare cases are associated with Marfan's syndrome.

3. The association of medullary thyroid carcinoma with pheochromocytomas and parathyroid adenomas comprises the familial multiple endocrine adenomatosis syndrome.

4. Neurofibromatosis and neurofibromas have occurred with medullary thyroid carcinoma.

5. Ganglioneuromas are an additional association.

6. Occasional tumors have elaborated calcitonin.

7. A carcinoid-like syndrome has been identified, accompanied by increased levels of circulating catecholamines.

8. Prostaglandin-induced diarrhea has been encountered with these neoplasms.

9. Occasional patients develop a Cushing-like syndrome, related apparently to the elaboration of increased amounts of ACTH.

It is currently believed that these medullary cancers arise in the parafollicular C cells of the thyroid. Thus, these neoplasms fail to take up RaI and have no dependence on the pituitary.

The designation medullary is something of a misnomer, because these lesions are classically s ony hard due to the large deposits of amyloid within the stroma of the neoplasm. They tend to be sharply circumscribed but unencapsulated. Occasional tumors are small and undetectable clinically, although some are massive lesions and are sometimes bilateral. Histologically, they present nests of cells which sometimes are small and epithelial-appearing, resembling a carcinoid, and at other times are elongated, spindled and resemble a sarcoma. The nests are separated by broad bands of fibrous stroma, in which is found abundant masses of amyloid. In some instances, the amyloid is scant and readily missed unless special stains, such as Congo red or PAS, are employed.

These neoplasms present clinically as masses which are generally readily palpable and are sometimes bilateral. They may arise in the first two decades of life and, under these circumstances, are frequently bilateral and associated with pheochromocytomas, suggesting a familial syndrome. The undifferentiated histologic appearance of these neoplasms belies their generally nonaggressive behavior. In the absence of nodal metastases at the time of surgery, the five-year survival rate is comparable to that of normal controls. With positive cervical nodes, the 10-year survival rate is 42 per cent.

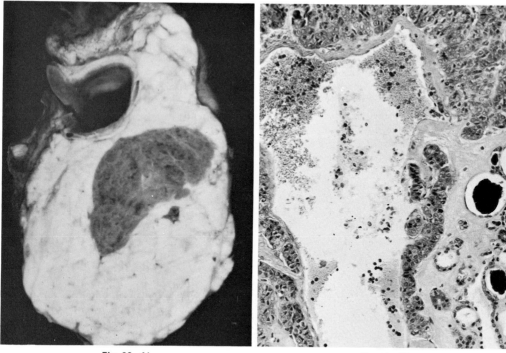

Fig. 29–41

Fig. 29–42

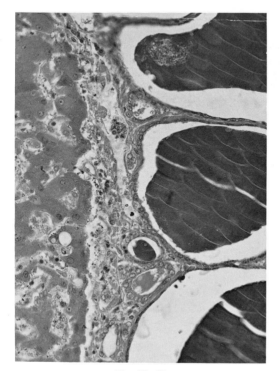

Fig. 29–43

Figure 29–41. *Cross section of gray-white tumor tissue of a thyroid cancer illustrating complete destruction of the gland on one side and persistence of an embedded lobe on the opposite side. The relationship to the trachea is apparent.*

Figure 29–42. *A high power detail of a cancer of the thyroid illustrating extension of the neoplasm through the wall of a vessel. Several small nests of cells are seen lying within the lumen.*

Figure 29–43. *A high power detail of a follicular cancer of the thyroid which has metastasized to the liver. The normal liver cells (on left) can be seen in approximation to extremely well differentiated thyroid tissue demonstrating abundant colloid and deceptively benign-appearing follicular epithelium.*

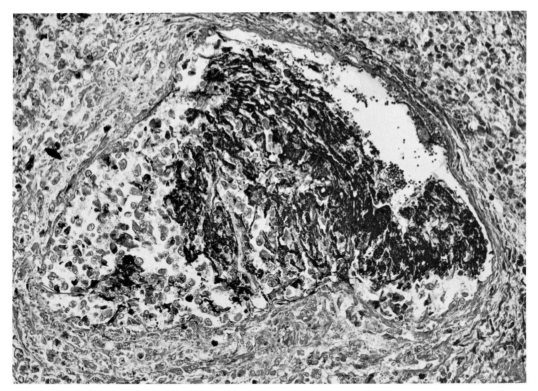

Figure 29–44. *A highly undifferentiated anaplastic cancer of the thyroid showing vascular invasion and thrombosis of the involved vessel.*

Anaplastic Carcinoma. This is a highly malignant form of thyroid cancer growing in a totally undifferentiated pattern. These tumors usually occur in the seventh and eighth decades of life and are among the most malignant tumors in man.

By the time these patients are seen clinically, these tumors have usually extended far beyond the confines of the thyroid gland to produce large, bulky masses obviously invasive of surrounding structures. Growth of the tumor may be apparent within the weeks of observation.

The histologic pattern is that of totally undifferentiated growth, varying from one type that is composed of small, round cells fairly uniform in size and shape and sometimes confused with undifferentiated sarcoma, to other types that present large, anaplastic giant cells with marked variations in cell size and shape and prominent, bizarre, multinucleated giant forms, sometimes called **giant cell carcinomas.** Invasion beyond the capsule, blood vessel involvement and foci of infarct necrosis

caused by rapid growth of the tumor all indicate the truly malignant nature of this lesion (Fig. 29–44).

These neoplasms are among the most lethal in oncology. Irrespective of the mode of treatment, virtually all patients die within one year of diagnosis.

MISCELLANEOUS TUMORS

Squamous cell carcinomas rarely arise within the thyroid gland, usually from metaplastic glandular epithelium. They tend to behave as do squamous cell carcinomas elsewhere.

Sarcomas. A wide variety of sarcomas, including lymphomas, have been described as having arisen in the thyroid. These may originate in the fibrous stroma, blood vessels or lymphoid tissue found in the normal and abnormal thyroid gland. As mentioned earlier, chronic thyroiditis, particularly Hashimoto's disease, is a favored soil for the origin of the lymphomas.

PARATHYROID GLANDS

NORMAL

The parathyroid glands are derived from the branchial pouches—the upper glands from the endoderm of the fourth pouch, and the lower pair from the third pouch. The numerous dorsal and ventral wings of the branchial pouches provide the mechanism for the formation of accessory glands that may be variously located in man from the cricoid cartilage down into the mediastinum.

Normally there are four parathyroids, but more than this number are found in 25 per cent of individuals. Rarely, six are present, equally rarely, fewer than four, and sometimes only two. There is, therefore, hazard in unnecessarily removing even a single gland in a patient who might have only one gland left. In the adult, the parathyroid is a yellow-brown, ovoid, encapsulated nodule weighing approximately 30 mg. It measures between 4 to 6 mm. in length, 2 to 4 mm. in width, and 0.5 to 2 mm. in thickness. It is composed principally of so-called chief cells. However, in adults, with the usual H & E stain, two additional forms are identified; the clear (wasserhelle) cell and the pink granular oxyphil. According to current evidence, the chief cell is the progenitor of the other two forms. It has a diameter of about 7 microns with a centrally placed nucleus that leaves only a thin rim of granular, faintly eosinophilic cytoplasm. Progressive vacuolation gives rise to transitional forms blending into the water-clear cell (wasserhelle). While in the light microscope, the cell membranes in these cells appear quite regular, the electron microscope reveals considerable complexity and tortuosity producing interdigitating cytoplasmic processes. The water-clear cell is larger (10 to 15 microns in diameter) with a similar nucleus but a totally cleared cytoplasm. Oxyphil cells progressively increase in number with age. They are 8 to 15 microns in diameter and have a distinctive acidophilic granularity in their cytoplasm. These granules apparently represent mitochondria (Roth et al., 1962). Elegant electron microscopic details are available in the report of Trier (1958).

In early infancy and in the child, the parathyroids are composed almost entirely of solid sheets of chief cells. With increased age, fat appears in the fibrous stroma to separate the functional cells into strands, cords and nests. This fat accumulates throughout the first three or four decades and, in the middle years, the gland is half fat, half parenchymal cells. In advanced age, the fat again diminishes in amount and oxyphils appear in increased numbers.

Despite many biochemical and electron microscopic studies, it has been difficult to determine which type of cell produces the parathyroid hormone (PTH), and it is probable that all forms have this capability. The cytoplasm of the water-clear cell contains relatively few organelles and abundant cytoplasmic glycogen as well as lipid. Such glycogen storage is usually interpreted as an indication of inactivity. A variety of enzymes has been described in these cells, but not in as rich an abundance as in the oxyphil cell. More active forms of chief cells are richer in mitochondria and enzymes and have less glycogen. Oxyphils contain large numbers of mitochondria. They are also rich in oxidative respiratory enzymes, suggesting a high metabolic level of activity (Balogh and Cohen, 1961). Certainly all types of cells have been associated with hyperparathyroidism and, in the words of Straus and Paloyan (1969): "It becomes evident that the parathyroid parenchymal cell has the ability to switch directly to any of the other two cell forms."

Parathyroid Function and Calcium Regulation. PTH is the principal, but not the only, regulator of serum calcium levels. Calcitonin and vitamin D are also involved in an intricate ballet. Here we shall only briefly review this immensely complex and rapidly evolving subject. PTH is a single-chain polypeptide (molecular weight 8500) which is not stored in parathyroid cells but is synthesized and secreted continuously. Elegant radioimmunoassays are now available for precise quantitation of the circulating levels of this hormone (Berson et al., 1963). PTH elevates serum calcium levels by:

1. Releasing calcium from its major storage depot (the skeletal system), causing, in effect, resorption of bone.

2. Increasing absorption of dietary calcium in the gut.

3. Increasing reabsorption of filtered calcium in the renal tubules.

The serum levels of calcium are reciprocally related to the serum phosphorus levels, and an elevation of one cation lowers the other, maintaining a relatively constant product (serum levels of calcium × serum levels of phosphorus). In the normal state, the serum calcium levels comprise a negative feedback mechanism operating on the parathyroid glands. A decrease in serum calcium stimulates increased secretion of PTH and, conversely, an increase in serum calcium decreases or abolishes secretion of PTH. As will become clear, this oversimplification does not consider the contributions of vitamin D and calcitonin nor the role of magnesium. Hypomagnesemia also stimulates PTH secretion (Sherwood et al., 1970).

It is customary to speak of the action of PTH on the gut, kidney tubules and bone. However, there are many recent observations which raise the question of whether the role of PTH is mediated by metabolites of vitamin D or whether it acts directly and in concert with these metabolites. Significantly, vitamin D is essential for the hypercalcemic effect of PTH (DeLuca, 1971) (Wasserman and Taylor, 1972). Whether directly or indirectly, PTH has an early effect on osteocytes, leading to release of calcium from mature bone crystals into the blood. It has a slower effect on bone turnover and remodeling. This slower action may be mediated by vitamin D. The effect of PTH on the kidneys and on the mucosal cells of the gut is intricately interwoven with vitamin D. It is a known fact that PTH stimulates adenyl cyclase and increased formation of cyclic AMP in the mucosal cells of the gut and the renal tubules. The cyclic AMP turns on the transcription of mRNA involved in the synthesis of increased amounts of calcium-transport protein. Thus, more calcium can be transported across the mucosa of the gut (in other words, can be absorbed) and similarly more calcium can be reabsorbed in the renal tubules (Chase, 1969).

Dietary vitamin D is converted, in the liver, to an active metabolite 25-hyroxycholecalciferol (25-HCC). Recent studies indicate that, in the kidney, 25-HCC is further converted to either a more active metabolite 1,25-dihydroxycholecalciferol (1,25-DHCC) or to a less active 21,25-DHCC. The former metabolite favors the calcification of bone and thus the maintenance of its structure, while the less active 21,25-DHCC favors calcium mobilization, bone resorption and bone disease. PTH acts on the kidney to suppress the formation of 1,25-DHCC and to divert vitamin D metabolism to the formation of 21,25-DHCC, leading to calcium mobilization and bone disease (Editorial, 1972). Thus, the long-term effect of increased levels of PTH on bone may involve the regulation of vitamin D metabolism. Another metabolite of vitamin D enhances calcium transport across the gut. This role of vitamin D is probably mediated or augmented by PTH because, as was pointed out, under the influence of this hormone, calcium-transport protein is synthesized within mucosal cells. It is evident that at the present time it is difficult to segregate the direct and indirect actions of both PTH and vitamin D on bone, the kidney and the gut.

Calcitonin has a well known hypocalcemic effect. This hormone is formed principally in the thyroid gland in parafollicular C cells but is also produced in other mammalian tissues, including the thymus and the adrenals. Calcitonin is a small peptide for which sensitive radioimmunoassays are available. The secretion of calcitonin is directly proportional to serum calcium levels, and calcitonin can be identified in the blood when the serum calcium level exceeds 9 mg. per 100 ml. Apparently, calcitonin acts by inhibiting bone resorption and calcium release. How it exerts this effect is still unclear, but it does not involve the adenyl cyclase system, nor does it require RNA or protein synthesis (Catt, 1970).

New observations on this subject will, unquestionably, evoke a new conception of calcium regulation as research in this area continues. It must suffice for now that the ultimate effects of increased levels of PTH are (1) an increase in the serum calcium level and (2) increased urinary calcium excretion, leading to calcium wastage and, possibly, nephrocalcinosis, urolithiasis and bone disease, as well as other ancillary changes. Conversely, hypoparathyroidism (decreased levels of PTH) induces hypocalcemia, which may lead to the clinical syndrome known as tetany.

PATHOLOGY

Although there are nonfunctioning lesions of the parathyroid glands (tumors, cysts), they are of trivial importance, and so parathyroid pathology is best considered in terms of altered function. *Hypoparathyroidism* is largely a functional metabolic disorder accompanied by a variety of nonspecific anatomic changes save for those related to the parathyroid glands.

Hyperparathyroidism may occur as a primary disease when increased amounts of PTH are produced by hyperplastic or neoplastic parathyroid glands or when nonendocrine tumors secrete PTH or a biologically similar product. In contrast, secondary hyperparathyroidism results whenever there is some cause for chronic hypocalcemia, e.g., chronic renal failure, malabsorption syndromes or dietary rickets. Here it is presumed that the parathyroid hyperfunction represents a compensatory reaction. Increasingly, the question has been raised as to whether some cases of primary hyperplasia and primary adenoma formation are not, in fact, a response to some poorly defined stimulus and, therefore, also a form of secondary hyperparathyroidism. Conceivably, some as yet undiscovered stimulus to parathyroid hyperfunction eventually leads to a proliferative response in the form of hyperplasia. Since the stimulus to such hyperplasia remains unknown, the changes are designated primary hyperplasia. Could continued proliferation within these glands in time give rise to an adenoma and possibly even a carcinoma? Some of these speculative interrelationships are well expressed in Figure 29–45. The occasional cases of hyperparathyroidism exhibiting glandular hyperplasia, as well as one or more adenomas, tend to support such a hypothesis. Similarly, there are reports of patients with apparent secondary hyperparathyroidism who, during the course of their chronic disease, have developed an autonomous functioning adenoma (Davies et al., 1956). Transformation of secondary hyperparathy-roidism to autonomous hyperfunction is now designated *tertiary hyperparathyroidism.*

The segregation of secondary from primary hyperparathyroidism and the separation of morphologic lesions causing primary hyperparathyroidism into hyperplastic and neoplastic categories may be somewhat arbitrary compartmentalizations of a single disorder—namely, parathyroid hyperfunction. Recognizing these uncertainties, we shall consider in the following discussion first hypoparathyroidism and then hyperparathyroidism, utilizing the terminology of primary and secondary forms for lack of better.

HYPOPARATHYROIDISM

The usual cause of hypoparathyroidism is accidental removal of the parathyroid glands in the course of thyroidectomy. The reported frequency of such mishaps ranges from nil to 25 per cent (Hoffenberg, 1972). It should be noted that parathyroid function may also be impaired by the treatment of thyroid disease with therapeutic doses of radioiodine. Idiopathic hypoparathyroidism (noniatrogenic) is much less common. Why parathyroids are sometimes absent or so severely atrophic that they cannot be found remains a mystery. Some instances can be attributed to aplasia or hypoplasia, but in others, as with certain cases of hypothyroidism and hypoadrenalism, the question of autoimmune disease arises. Idiopathic hypoparathyroidism is sometimes associated with Addison's disease, pernicious anemia and chronic thyroiditis, all suspected of being autoimmune disorders (Spinner et al., 1968). Organ-specific antibodies to parathyroid tissue have been reported in approximately 40 per cent of these patients; to gastric tissue, in 20 per cent; and to adrenal tissue, in 10 per cent (Blizzard et al., 1966).

As mentioned previously, hypoparathyroidism is largely a metabolic and clinical disorder with very scant morphologic changes. The most characteristic metabolic derangements are hypocalcemia and hyperphosphatemia. Beyond these biochemical abnormalities, there is a wide range of clinical manifestations and, in some milder cases, the changes may be exceedingly subtle and virtually undecipherable without the help of biochemical determinations. On the other extreme are those patients with frank tetany and its concomitant violent convulsions and laryngospasm which may cause fatal anoxia. More often, the hypocalcemia induces neuromuscular manifestations, including paresthesias, cramps, twitches and carpopedal spasm. The neuromuscular irrita-

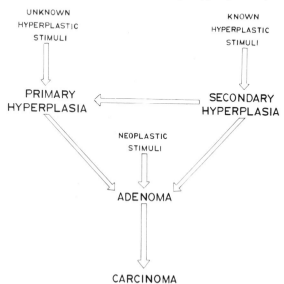

Figure 29–45. *Relationships between the hyperplastic and neoplastic parathyroid conditions. (From Straus, F. H., and Paloyan, E.: The pathology of hyperparathyroidism. Surg. Clin. N. Amer., 49:27, 1969.)*

bility can frequently be evoked by tapping the facial nerve which induces contraction of the eye, mouth or nose muscles (Chvostek's sign). A variety of nervous system abnormalities may be manifested, ranging from psychologic disturbances, and even complete dementia, to epilepsy with tonic spasms and convulsive seizures. The major anatomic features include, in addition to the loss of parathyroid glands, brittle nails, dry scaly skin with a tendency to rashes and, of considerable importance, cataract formation.

The syndrome of *pseudohypoparathyroidism*, originally described by Albright and his colleagues (1942), should be mentioned here. It, too, is characterized by hypocalcemia and hyperphosphatemia, but significantly these biochemical derangements fail to respond to exogenously administered PTH (Lee et al., 1968). Currently, it is believed to be a familial disorder caused by an end organ inability to respond to PTH which, indeed, is secreted in excessive amounts. It is postulated that there is a defect in the membrane-receptor adenyl cyclase system in responsive tissues, such as the kidneys and bone, rendering the role of parathormone ineffective in raising serum calcium levels. Classically, these patients have a variety of somatic defects including shortness of stature, obesity with a rounded face, brachydactyly, mental retardation and subcutaneous foci of calcification or ossification.

PRIMARY HYPERPARATHYROIDISM

In an analysis of 343 cases of this condition, Cope (1966) reported the following distribution of parathyroid lesions:

	Per Cent
Single adenoma	76
Double adenoma	4
Carcinoma	4
Hyperplasia (clear cell)	4
Hyperplasia (chief cell)	12

Not included in this series are the occasional cases of mixed hyperplasia-adenoma or the cases of hyperparathyroidism caused by *nonendocrine* tumors. The variety of cancers of nonendocrine organs which have given rise to hyperparathyroidism, indistinguishable from that caused by disease primary in the parathyroid glands, grows with each passing year (Omenn et al., 1969). Leading the list are undifferentiated carcinoma of the lung and renal cell carcinoma. Recently, a retroperitoneal sarcoma and a hepatic metastasis from a carcinoma of the breast have been implicated (Me-

lick, 1972) In some instances, the secretory product of these tumors, although having PTH-like activity, is not structurally identical with the normal hormone.

Adenomas. These benign tumors are generally extremely small and difficult to locate even at surgical exploration. They may occur in either sex at any age, with a peak incidence in the middle decades of life. As the above listing indicates, they usually occur singly, although occasionally two and even three adenomas are found dispersed among the four glands. In rare cases, they represent only one facet of the multiple endocrine adenomatosis syndrome.

For obscure reasons, most parathyroid adenomas arise in the lower glands. Occasionally, they are found in aberrant parathyroid tissue even within the mediastinum. The usual adenoma is a yellow-brown, soft, somewhat lobular mass ranging in weight between 150 mg. and 5 gm. Extreme weights of over 100 gm. have been reported. The soft, yellowish nodule is usually readily distinguishable from the firm, gelatinous, red-brown substance of the thyroid.

Adenomas are no longer rigidly subclassified on the basis of their cell types. Some are composed of relatively pure cell types, but others display mixed cell populations. The mos common variant is composed principally of chief cells, but many transitional wasserhelle and oxyphil types are often present. The chief cells are frequently slightly larger than normal, with variations in cell and nuclear size. Sometimes hyperchromatic pleomorphic nuclei are present in these benign lesions, wi h occasional binucleate forms—features that are of some importance since they help to distinguish primary adenomas from hyperplasia. In the latter, the cell types are much more uniform. The second most common pattern of adenoma is composed largely of water-clear cells; however, here again chief cells and oxyphils may be found (Fig. 29–46). A functioning adenoma composed largely of oxyphil cells is extremely rare. Whatever the cell type, they are disposed in solid sheets or masses, but occasionally the tumor is separated into apparent nodules by traversing bands of fibrous tissue. At other times, a well vascularized stroma produces cords of cells, and occasionally gland-like patterns are seen. **All adenomas display marked variation in cell composition, with many transitional forms** (Fig. 29–47). The electron microscopy of these adenomas has not revealed great differences between these neoplastic cells and their normal counterparts. Of some interest has been the disclosure that the cells of a large adenoma, presumably undergoing rapid growth, contain a concentric laminated pattern of smooth-faced cisternae,

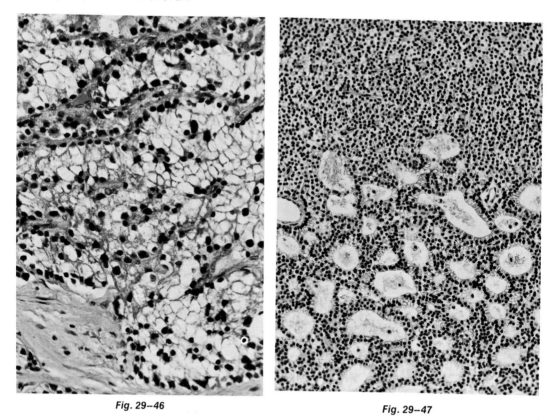

Fig. 29–46   Fig. 29–47

Figure 29–46. *Parathyroid adenoma, chiefly of wasserhelle cell type. Note the slight variability in cell and nuclear size.*

Figure 29–47. *Parathyroid adenoma containing chief cells, oxyphils and a few water-clear cells growing in sheets and glandular patterns.*

termed annulate lamellae, in the region of the Golgi complex (Elliott and Arhelger, 1966). This structure has been identified in many experimental tumors, and there is the suggestion that it is involved in protein synthesis or some other synthetic activity and perhaps accounts for the growth potential of these cells.

No correlation has been noted between the cell type predominating in the adenoma and the level of resultant hyperfunction.

Carcinoma. Carcinoma of the parathyroid glands is a rare cause of primary hyperfunction. While all agree that there are undoubted cases of nonfunctioning carcinomas of the parathyroid glands, the close anatomic similarity between such lesions and carcinomas arising in the thyroid has led to the commonly accepted criterion that the diagnosis of a carcinoma arising in the parathyroid requires the demonstration of hyperfunction (Barnes and Cope, 1961). There is great difficulty in distinguishing between the pleomorphism of adenomas and the mild anaplasia of some carcinomas. As a consequence, it has also been proposed that, for a diagnosis of malignancy,

one of the three following features must be present: (1) metastases, either to regional nodes or to distant organs, (2) capsular invasion or (3) local recurrence following resection.

Most of the carcinomas described have been relatively small and, in fact, some have been less than 1 gm. in weight. They are often irregular in shape and show lobulation and pseudopod formation and sometimes adherence to surrounding structures. They are usually considerably more firm than adenomas. Most commonly, they consist of cords or bands of cells creating a trabecular arrangement. Some have gland patterns, while in others the tumor may be composed of large sheets or masses of cells. **Hyperchromatism, pleomorphism and variation in nuclear size are all present but are not necessarily more marked than that found in some adenomas.** When these lesions metastasize, they usually affect the regional nodes alone. Rarely, they spread to distant organs such as the lungs as well as below the diaphragm.

Survival for many years is not at all uncommon, and death results more often from

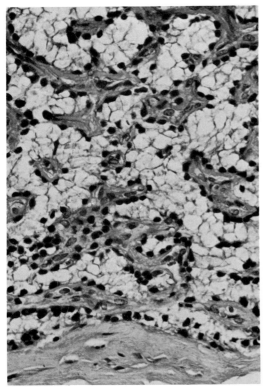

Figure 29–48. *A detail of marked primary parathyroid hyperplasia showing the characteristic wasserhelle cell.*

the complications of hyperparathyroidism than from the malignant nature of the lesion.

Primary Hyperplasia. It has long been known that hyperplasia of all parathyroid glands occurs as a secondary response in any condition associated with chronic hypocalcemia. Only within the past two decades has it become apparent that diffuse hyperplasia may occur as an apparent primary disease. As mentioned earlier (p. 1348), however, it is suspected that some subtle provocation underlies even such so-called primary hyperplasias. For example, it has recently been observed that small decreases in the glomerular filtration rate induce distinct increases in PTH levels long before the serum calcium or phosphate levels are affected (Reiss and Canterbury, 1971).

Whatever its origin, primary hyperplasia causes general enlargement of all of the parathyroid glands. It should be noted that the increase in size may be disproportionate among the four glands, and occasionally one or two glands appear relatively little affected while the others are markedly enlarged. In some patients, the total weight of all glands has been as little as 2 gm, although upper ranges of over 100 gm. have been recorded.

Histologically, two distinctive patterns are encountered: chief cell hyperplasia or, less commonly, clear cell (wasserhelle) hyperplasia. In neither pattern are the glands totally composed of only one cell type. In the chief cell pattern, water-clear cells are often admixed, bu oxyphilic cells are infrequent. The clear cell type likewise displays transitional cell populations, intermediate between water-clear cells and chief cells. Oxyphilic cells are again present but are scanty in number (Straus and Paloyan, 1969). Histologically, the glandular enlargements are made up of sheets of cells sometimes with a tendency toward alveolar and acinar configurations. In contrast to adenomas, the cells are usually qui e uniform in size and cytologic detail (Fig. 29–48).

SECONDARY HYPERPARATHYROIDISM

As previously indicated, hypocalcemia stimulates PTH secretion (Sherwood et al., 1968). Chronic hypocalcemia, whatever its origins, leads in time to secondary hyperparathyroidism. The most important cause is chronic renal insufficiency. However, secondary hyperparathyroidism is also encountered in the malabsorption syndromes and in such calcium wasting disorders as rickets, disseminated metastatic carcinoma and multiple myeloma. The sequence of events in renal insufficiency has been well studied in the experimental animal. By producing progressive renal ischemia, it can be shown that the first critical change is a decrease in the glomerular filtration rate causing an elevation of serum phosphate and a depression of serum calcium levels. Immediately, PTH secretion is increased (Slatopolsky et al., 1968). As the renal disease advances, the complexity of the problem increases. Advanced chronic renal failure induces not only a hyperphosphatemia but also a vitamin D-resistant state, which is likely to be the driving force for increased PTH secretion (Stanbury and Lumb, 1962). Highly sensitive radioimmunoassays reveal elevated levels of PTH in all of these secondary syndromes.

The anatomic changes in the parathyroid glands consist principally of hyperplasia of the chief cells (Fig. 29–49). This usually affects all glands bu , not infrequently, one, two or even three may be spared. The basis for such asymmetrical involvement is obscure. Islands of oxyphils are often present, and the fat is usually largely replaced by hyperplastic cells (Fig. 29–50). But in general more fat remains than in cases of primary hyperplasia.

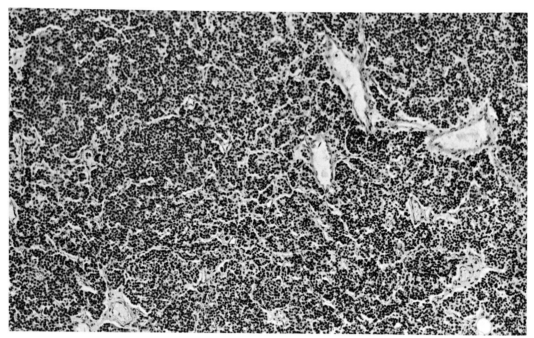

Fig. 29–49

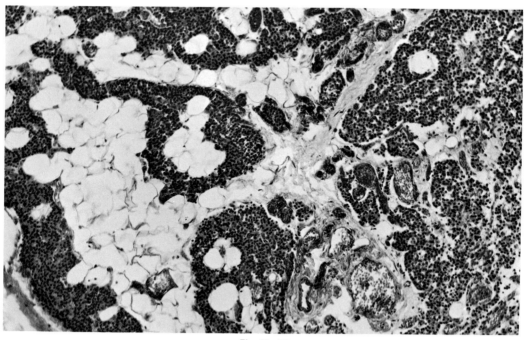

Fig. 29–50

Figure 29–49. Diffuse secondary hyperplasia of the parathyroid illustrating complete replacement and atrophy of the normally contained fat.

Figure 29–50. Normal parathyroid for comparison with Figure 29–49 to illustrate the usual content of fat and abundant connective tissue stroma.

SYSTEMIC EFFECTS OF PARATHYROID HYPERFUNCTION

While primary and secondary hyperparathyroidism present somewhat similar clinical manifestations, they are quite distinctive biochemically. Primary hyperparathyroidism almost always is characterized by hypercalcemia, hypercalciuria and hypophosphatemia. By contrast, in secondary hyperparathyroidism, as for example, with chronic renal disease, the serum calcium levels may be normal or even low, and the phosphate levels are high or normal. It should be noted in passing that primary hyperparathyroidism is not the most common cause of hypercalcemia; it is superseded by excessive bone destruction such as occurs in disseminated cancer. Less frequent causes for increased serum levels of calcium include immobilization, hyperthyroidism, milk-alkali syndrome, vitamin D excess, sarcoidosis as well as other rare conditions (Gordan and Goldman, 1970).

The clinical manifestations of parathyroid hyperfunction, whether primary or secondary, follow, but it should be noted that usually they are more marked in the primary syndromes than in the secondary.

Clinical Manifestations Related to Hyperparathyroidism. In acute hyperparathyroidism, the patient may manifest anorexia, nausea and vomiting, confusion and even coma. With chronic hyperfunction, a variety of mental aberrations appear, including fatigue, listlessness, headache, depression and even psychoses. Muscle weakness, joint pains and arthritis are common. The high serum calcium levels have their effect on cardiac function and produce bradycardia, arrhythmias as well as other ECG abnormalities. Soft tissue lesions may appear in the form of metastatic calcifications found principally in the blood vessels, lungs, stomach and kidneys (p. 52).

Renal Involvement. Prolonged hypercalciuria may result in deposits of calcium in and about the renal tubules (*nephrocalcinosis*). In the course of time, the calciuria may give rise to renal calculi. While hyperfunction of the parathyroid glands should always be suspected when kidney stones are found, overall, this pathway accounts for less than 5 per cent.

Skeletal Involvement. With longstanding hyperparathyroidism, there is progressive calcium wastage and demineralization of bone until eventual structural changes appear. The pattern and magnitude of the skeletal alterations correlate directly with the severity and duration of the hyperparathyroidism and, therefore, are much more pronounced in the primary syndromes than in the secondary.

In the past, it has been customary to refer to the bony alterations in hyperparathyroidism as *osteitis fibrosa cystica (von Recklinghausen's disease)* but, in fact, osteitis fibrosa cystica is the end-stage of advanced parathyroid bone disease. At first, the chronic calcium wastage usually leads only to demineralization of bone which is nonspecific and conforms more or less to the condition known as *osteomalacia*. Continued demineralization results in the development of osteitis fibrosa cystica. In this disease, there is resorption of marrow bone spicules and their replacement by a delicate fibrous tissue containing small or large cystic spaces. Eventually the entire marrow cavity becomes filled with such fibrous replacement, and rarefaction of the cortical bone ensues. Hemorrhages, spontaneous or secondary to microfractures in the weakened bone, create areas of organizing blood clot within the fibrous tissue. The hyperactive osteoclasts and osteoblasts in the areas of organizing hemorrhage produce small, sometimes multiple, reactive giant cell granulomas commonly referred to as brown tumors. Osteitis fibrosa cystica is described in greater detail on p. 1444. The brief description given here is intended to emphasize the point that such advanced changes are only seen in some cases and represent the extreme of skeletal damage. The skeletal changes in hyperparathyroidism are then varied and, until well advanced, nonspecific. Control of the parathyroid hyperfunction, as for example, excision of an adenoma, is usually followed by a striking and amazingly rapid reversion of the bone to normal. If cystic lesions have already developed, however, they may persist for long periods of time.

While advanced skeletal changes are occasionally seen in cases of longstanding chronic renal disease, in most instances of secondary hyperparathyroidism, it is uncommon to find more than minimal skeletal changes. In the past, it has been customary to refer to these secondary skeletal alterations as *renal osteodystrophy* (p. 1444). There is objection to this term since it implies a specific form of bone disease in secondary hyperparathyroidism related to chronic renal disease. As previously mentioned, the skeletal changes in hyperparathyroidism, whatever the cause, reflect only progressive demineralization of bone.

Miscellaneous Changes. Peptic ulcers, usually duodenal, are found in 10 to 15 per cent of patients with hyperparathyroidism. In many of these instances, the patient suffers from multiple endocrine adenomatosis and has a concomitant pancreatic lesion, possibly the Zollinger-Ellison syndrome. There is, however, evidence that even in the absence of pancreatic lesions, hypercalcemia alone may stimulate hypersecretion of gastric acid (Black, 1971). Chronic pancreatitis is also more common in patients with parathyroid hyperfunction, again perhaps related to the effects of the hypercalcemia on pancreatic secretion (p. 1063).

In concluding this consideration of the clinical effects of hyperparathyroidism, it is important to emphasize that it is a disease of enormous variability both in severity and in mode of clinical expression. The patient may

be virtually asymptomatic and only have biochemical alterations or he may have the classic manifestations cited. Occasionally, the hyperparathyroidism is only one facet of a more complex adenomatosis syndrome. While hypercalcemia is classic, the calcium levels may, indeed, be within the normal range, and so the diagnosis of hyperparathyroidism is easily missed unless the wide-ranging ramifications of this disorder are recalled (Keating, 1970).

PITUITARY

NORMAL	adamantinoma)	**Anterior Pituitary Clinical**
PATHOLOGY	Miscellaneous	**Syndromes**
Congenital Anomalies	Malignant	Hyperpituitarism
Lesions Producing Pituitary	Primary	Acromegaly
Insufficiency	Secondary	Gigantism
Inflammations	**Pituitary Changes Incident to**	Hypopituitarism
Infiltrations	**Adrenal, Thyroid and Gonad**	Hypophyseal cachexia or
Vascular lesions	**Dysfunction**	Simmonds' disease
(Sheehan's syndrome)	Adrenocortical hyperfunction	Hypophyseal dwarfism—
Tumors	Adrenocortical hypofunction	Lorain-Levi type
Benign	Thyroid hyperfunction	Froehlich's syndrome
Adenomas	Thyroid hypofunction	(adiposogenital
Craniopharyngioma	Hypergonadism	dystrophy)
(Rathke's pouch tumor,	Hypogonadism	

NORMAL

The pituitary gland weighs between 0.6 and 0.8 gm. in the adult. The glandular portion of the human hypophysis develops from an ectodermal evagination of the oropharynx called Rathke's pouch. The cephalad extension of this pouch brings it into contact with the primitive diencephalon in the early human embryo. This focus of contact with the central nervous system is destined to differentiate into the posterior lobe or neurohypophysis. In animals, but less clearly defined in man, the portion of Rathke's pouch in direct contact with the neurohypophysis forms the pars intermedia of the adenohypophysis. The portion of Rathke's pouch not in contact with the diencephalon enlarges to create the pars anterior.

In man, there is no well developed pars intermedia, and the cells are scattered throughout the anterior lobe, but the region of the pars intermedia is often marked by small microcysts. The cephalad portion of Rathke's pouch is separated from its connection with the oropharynx by an ingrowth of mesenchyme, but often remnants of the lower portion of the pouch remain embedded in the craniopharyngeal canal to constitute the human

pharyngeal pituitary. The neurohypophysis retains its connections with the base of the brain, comprising the pituitary stalk. This neural connection is crucial in the hypothalamic regulation of anterior lobe function.

The histology of the anterior pituitary continues to be an area of confusion engendered by a multiplicity of staining and fixation techniques, variably used terms to denote cell types and the extrapolation of data from animals to man. It is beyond our scope to delve deeply into all of these confusions which have, indeed, led to heated controversy in the literature. Instead, we shall present the classic view as set forth by Russfield (1968) and then cite one of the more important areas of controversy. In the classic view, the anterior pituitary is made up of three cell types: acidophils, basophils and chromophobes. Under optimal conditions, the three cell types can be visualized with H & E staining and more clearly differentiated by Mallory's trichrome technique. Acidophils (eosinophils) comprise about 40 per cent of the anterior lobe. These are polygonal cells with central small nuclei and cytoplasmic granules of growth hormone (GH), which are rose-pink with H & E and impart the acidophilia. Special stains and electron microscopy distinguish two types of acidophils. One is fully granulated and the other contains few but coarse granules (Doniach, 1972).

Basophils having the same shape as acidophils comprise about 10 per cent of the anterior lobe. At least two types can be differentiated on the basis of the distribution and size of the basophilic granules in the cytoplasm. One class is well granulated and the other sparsely granulated. It is widely accepted that basophils secrete thyroid-stimulating hormone (TSH), gonadotropins (FSH and LH) and adrenocorticotropic hormone (ACTH). All these hormones have a high carbohydrate content and, indeed, basophils yield a positive reaction with the PAS stain.

In classic teaching, chromophobes comprise about 50 per cent of the total anterior lobe. In general, they are smaller than the chromophils (acidophils and basophils). While these cells have traditionally been considered to be nonsecretory, in many, electron microscopy reveals widely scattered granules of stored hormone within their cytoplasm (Paiz and Hennigar, 1970).

Thus, we come to one of the more vexing issues involving the anterior pituitary, namely, do *nonsecretory* chromophobes truly exist? The designation chromophobe originates from the days when only H & E stains and light microscopy were available. More sophisticated techniques, as pointed out, disclose secretory granules in many of these cells; immunofluorescent stains reveal small amounts of hormones identical to those in chromophils, and so-called chromophobe adenomas have been found in patients having manifestations of increased GH, TSH or ACTH, implying functional activity of the adenoma (Hamilton et al., 1970) (Dingman and Lim, 1962). So, at the present time some experts hold that chromophobes are not a specific cell type, but only an inactive or secretorily exhausted and degranulated chromophil (McCormick and Halmi, 1971). Whatever their origin and interpretation, a large number of cells in the anterior pituitary contain few granules and appear to be chromophobes. It must be remembered that in man there is no well developed pars intermedia, and these cells are scattered throughout the anterior lobe. They cannot be identified by usual staining techniques and, conceivably, these intermedia cells may appear to be chromophobes, adding to the confusion.

The histology of the neurohypophysis is much simpler, since the posterior lobe is composed of slender neural type pituicytes, dispersed among which are nerve fibers and numerous small anastomosing vascular channels.

Most of the peptide and glycoprotein hormones secreted by the anterior pituitary gland are tropic hormones (i.e., ACTH, TSH, FSH and LH) which stimulate the secretory function of target endocrine organs (i.e., adrenals, thyroid and gonads). Growth hormone and prolactin have direct metabolic effects on tissues. The existence of an additional independent melanophore-stimulating hormone (MSH) has not been unequivocally established in man, although it has been isolated in pigs. An amino acid sequence in human ACTH has been identified which is identical with MSH of porcine origin, providing a possible basis for the melanophore-stimulating activity of ACTH and raising the issue of whether a separate MSH hormone exists in man.

Of posterior pituitary origin are vasopressin (antidiuretic hormone, ADH), which conserves body water by reducing renal excretion of water, and oxytocin, which affects lactation and uterine muscle contraction.

Reference has already been made to the difficulty in assigning specific secretory function to the various cell types in the anterior pituitary. According to presently available evidence, the well granulated acidophils with granules of intermediate size secrete growth hormone. The origin of prolactin appears to be the sparsely, but coarsely, granulated acidophils. Basophils having an abundance of fine granules secrete TSH, and those with sparse, coarser granules secrete gonadotropins. Probably basophils also elaborate ACTH, but there is evidence that chromophobes, perhaps more accurately, sparsely granulated basophils, are also capable of ACTH production (McShan and Hartley, 1965) (Phifer et al., 1970). As mentioned, they may be degranulated because they have exhausted their stores of ACTH. But lest the origin of the pituitary hormones appears to be a settled issue, it should be pointed out that immunofluorescent techniques indicate that occasional basophils appear to contain growth hormone. Moreover, a scattering of chromophobes react in the same fashion (Beck et al., 1966). It is evident, then, that it is still not possible to assign precisely the origin of the various tropic hormones to specific cell types.

Regulation of anterior pituitary function involves three mechanisms: (1) information transfer from the hypothalamus by local products with specific effects upon pituitary hormone release, (2) feedback inhibition by the secretions of the target endocrine organs and (3) local feedback loops of the pituitary hormones themselves. *The hypothalamus stimulates the release of ACTH, TSH, GH, LH and FSH by the production of releasing factors specific for each tropic hormone.* The secretion and release of prolactin and MSH are controlled by inhibitory hypothalamic factors. All hypothalamic regulators are delivered to the anterior pituitary through the so-called adenohypophyseal portal system of vascular sinusoids (Catt, 1970). These vascular channels provide a pathway by which regulators elaborated in the hypothalamus are quickly carried to the anterior pituitary and there diffused widely through an anastomosing vascular network to reach all secretory cells.

It is important to recall that the pituitary gland, like many other organs of the body, has a large factor of functioning reserve. It is estimated that over half of the pituitary can be destroyed without evoking symptoms of insufficiency. Thus, any destructive lesion must be fairly extensive before it will produce detectable symptoms.

PATHOLOGY

In the clinical consideration of pathology of the pituitary, it should be remembered that *symptoms may be produced by primary lesions of this gland in two ways, mechanically and hormonally.* Expanding lesions will produce effects by virtue of their increasing size. These effects may be localized, generalized or both. Thus, in large pituitary tumors, local destructive changes appear within the sella turcica. In more advanced lesions, local pressure on neighboring structures, e.g., the floor of the third ventricle, the hypothalamus or optic chiasm, may produce symptoms. Pressure on the optic chiasm classically evokes a bitemporal hemianopsia. In addition to these local effects, large pituitary tumors act as space-occupying lesions and produce a generalized increase in intracranial pressure. Pituitary tumors may therefore simulate any brain tumor and be responsible for headaches, nausea and vomiting, reflections of elevated spinal fluid pressure.

Inasmuch as the pituitary is the source of numerous hormones, lesions which increase or decrease the production of such hormones will inevitably produce effects upon the dependent endocrine glands. Hyperfunctioning tumors of the pituitary will stimulate the thyroid, adrenals and gonads to excessive activity and, conversely, destruction of the pituitary with the loss of those tropic hormones will be reflected by regressive changes within these glands. Moreover, the target organs of these secondary glands may also become involved. For example, pituitary-induced atrophy of the female gonads leads to regressive changes in the target organs of the gonads, i.e., the uterus and vagina. While both symptom-producing aspects of pituitary diseases are important, the main presenting clinical features of these disorders usually relate to the functional derangements produced by the imbalance of hormones. In an analysis of a series of cases of pituitary tumors, 40 per cent presented with local symptoms, 57 per cent with endocrine and 3 per cent were found by chance (Nabarro, 1972).

The consideration of the following entities is limited to the anatomic aspects of these lesions. The manner in which these disorders alter the fundamental endocrinology of the body is discussed under the clinicopathologic correlation in the concluding sections.

CONGENITAL ANOMALIES

Rests of pituitary cells are rather frequently sequestered high in the pharynx at the site of origin of the pharyngeal contribution to the anterior lobe. The only congenital anomaly of significance involving the pituitary results from the persistence of remnants of Rathke's pouch. These remnants of squamous epithelium, found in about 25 per cent of normal individuals, may give rise to tumors, considered later. While agenesis and hypoplasia have been described, these anomalies are largely limited to fetal "monsters" and are not encountered in clinical medicine.

LESIONS PRODUCING PITUITARY INSUFFICIENCY

Pituitary function may be impaired by a variety of pathologic processes including inflammations, infiltrations, vascular insufficiency and tumors, metastatic or primary. A primary pituitary tumor composed of secretorily inactive cells may progressively destroy the residual pituitary and so induce hypofunction. A hyperfunctioning primary tumor may also lead to pituitary hypofunction. To explain, the adenoma elaborating GH may, as it enlarges, destroy the residual normal gland and then itself undergo ischemic necrosis as the pressure within the sella turcica compresses its blood supply. Alternatively, strategically located minute nodules may impinge on the pituitary stalk and block the adenohypophyseal axis. Pituitary function, of course, may be intentionally reduced by hypophysectomy or radiation, as is sometimes done in patients with breast cancer. Whatever the pathway, no symptoms of pituitary insufficiency become apparent until 70 per cent or more of the anterior lobe is destroyed (Nabarro, 1972).

INFLAMMATIONS

As with all organs, inflammation of the pituitary may be acute or chronic. Acute bacterial infections of the pituitary are rare and arise either from bacteremic seeding or the direct spread of an infection from the leptomeninges, dural sinuses or bone.

The most common chronic inflammatory involvements of the pituitary are seen in systemic sarcoidosis, miliary tuberculosis and congenital syphilis. Indeed, for reasons which are unclear, some patients with generalized sarcoidosis have fairly severe involvement of the posterior lobe or pituitary stalk with resultant diabetes insipidus. Occasionally, granulomatous lesions indistinguishable from Boeck's sarcoidosis are seen in the pituitary in the absence of other manifestations or sarcoidosis elsewhere (Fig. 29–51). Whether this represents a peculiar variant of sarcoidosis or, instead, another granulomatous disorder affecting only the pituitary is unclear. An autoimmune reaction has been proposed and, indeed, similar granulomas may be found in the adrenal glands, suggesting the concurrence of an autoimmune reaction in both endocrine organs. Exceedingly rarely, toxoplasmosis and actinomycosis, as well as other fungal infections, affect the pituitary.

INFILTRATIONS

Amyloid deposits may appear in the pituitary gland in the course of systemic amyloidosis. Usually the deposition is confined to the walls of the vascular channels and the immediate perivascular regions, and only rarely does functional insufficiency appear. In Hand-Schüller-Christian disease, the bony encasement of the pituitary may be significantly involved, encroaching upon and producing some atrophy of the pituitary gland. Generally, the infiltrating lipophages remain confined to the bone, but rarely they may erode the cortex to directly permeate the pituitary, particularly the posterior lobe. In mucopolysaccharidoses (Hunter and Hurler syndromes), the cells of the anterior pituitary may accumulate mucopolysaccharides and become pale, swollen and vacuolated. Pituitary hypofunction is, however, not a common feature of these syndromes.

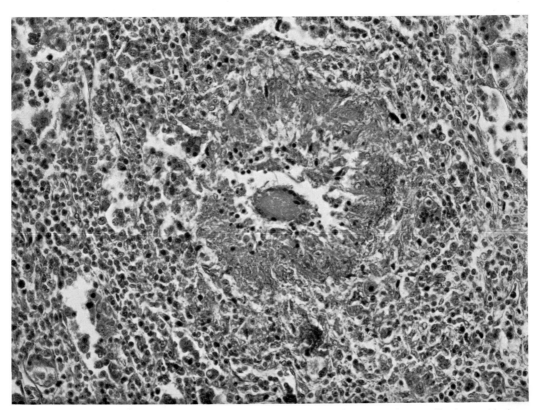

Figure 29–51. *A granuloma in the anterior lobe of the pituitary in a case of generalized sarcoidosis.*

VASCULAR LESIONS

Microscopic foci of necrosis are fairly common in the pituitary gland. Their precise pathogenesis is not clear, but it is likely that they represent minute vascular lesions. More extensive infarction of the pituitary gland may result from generalized atherosclerosis (affecting either the internal carotid artery or its hypophyseal branches) or from thrombosis of the cavernous sinus. Embolic occlusion of the vascular supply of the pituitary is an additional potential mechanism of infarction.

Far more common is massive ischemic necrosis of the anterior lobe secondary to shock. It was estimated in the past that pituitary necrosis of sufficient severity to produce clinical symptoms occurred in half of all women having severe postpartum hemorrhage (Purnell et al., 1964). However, with better control of this obstetric complication, this mechanism of pituitary necrosis occurs far less frequently. The association of postpartum hemorrhage and pituitary damage was accorded the designation *Sheehan's postpartum necrosis.* However, similar pituitary changes have been described in nonpregnant females as well as in males, and so a better term is *Sheehan's syndrome.* The pituitary damage is believed to result from vascular insufficiency or thromboses incident to a sudden drop in the blood pressure, whatever the cause. Thus,

Sheehan's syndrome may follow septic shock, burn shock or massive hemorrhage from any cause. McKay et al. (1953) have postulated that disseminated intravascular coagulation is the mediator of the pituitary necrosis in these situations. However, such pituitary damage is more apt to occur with postpartum hemorrhage than in the other settings described. Other factors connected with pregnancy apparently predispose the pituitary to ischemic injury. It is well documented that the pituitary markedly enlarges during pregnancy, and increases in weight of up to 100 per cent have been recorded. This enlargement is most likely related to hyperplasia of the sparsely granulated basophils, which elaborate prolactin. The large pituitary may compress its own blood supply and thus predispose to infarction with further compromise of the systemic circulation. Thus, disseminated intravascular coagulation is more likely to infarct the enlarged, compressed pituitary of pregnancy.

The gross and histologic changes are fairly standard, irrespective of the initiating event.

In the more extensive early involvement of Sheehan's syndrome, the pituitary may appear either soft, pale and ischemic or hemorrhagic. At a later stage, the ischemic area is resorbed and replaced by fibrous tissue, leading to progressive shrinkage and tough, gray scarring of the anterior lobe. The posterior lobe is rarely affected. In some

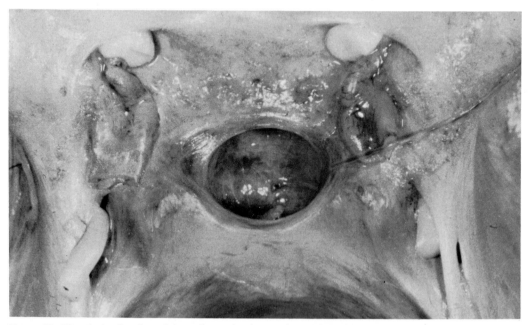

Figure 29–52. *An in situ view of the sella turcica in a patient dying of far advanced pituitary insufficiency following pituitary necrosis. The residual gland substance remains in situ and can be seen as a minute nubbin of tissue protruding from the midline of the posterior wall of the sella (below). No other pituitary substance could be demonstrated at autopsy.*

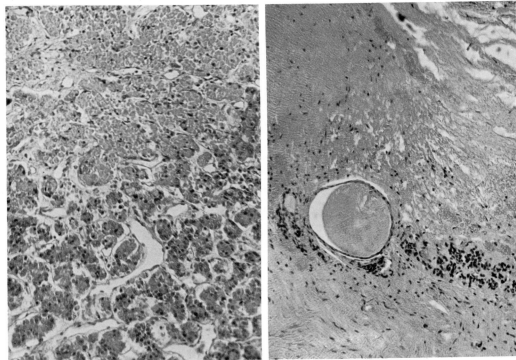

Fig. 29–53

Fig. 29–54

Figure 29–53. *A recent infarct of the pituitary evident as pale-staining shadowy outlines of cells which contrast with the normal nucleated cells immediately below.*

Figure 29–54. *Microscopic view of the anterior lobe of the pituitary illustrated in Figure 29–52. Complete fibrous atrophy of the anterior lobe is evident above the pars intermedia, indicated in the photograph by the cystic space. The posterior lobe is below and appears normal.*

cases first seen years after the acute episode, the gland is reduced to a fibrous nubbin weighing less than 0.1 gm. attached to the wall of the sella turcica (Fig. 29–52). In one postmortem analysis of these cases with manifestations of longstanding pituitary insufficiency, the anterior lobe had been reduced to less than 2 per cent of its normal size in over 60 per cent of the patients (Sheehan, 1968).

The histologic pattern is that of either ischemic or hemorrhagic infarction. It may involve small foci of the gland or the entire substance (Fig. 29–53). If sufficient pituitary remains to maintain life, fibrosis of the infarct will occur (Fig. 29–54). Cells along the margin of the scar may become trapped and destroyed.

While large vascular infarcts in general are uncommon, they are nevertheless one of the most frequent causes of postpartum fatalities. Symptoms of such pituitary failure may not appear for weeks, months or years after the initial damage has occurred, possibly because of the slow but relentless progress of the scarring. In these late-developing cases, it is likely that with this progressive fibrosis additional marginal cells are destroyed until the

threshold of pituitary sufficiency is eventually passed. Unlike Sheehan's necrosis, which tends to be quite extensive, the small focus of infarction frequently found at autopsy comprises only an incidental finding.

TUMORS

Along with Sheehan's syndrome, tumors are the most important pathologic lesions encountered in the pituitary. For obscure reasons, cancers are exceedingly uncommon in this gland and adenomas are of dominant importance.

BENIGN

Adenomas. These benign neoplasms may give rise to either hyperpituitarism or hypopituitarism. Adenomas comprised of acidophils cause gigantism and acromegaly, considered in some detail on p. 1364. Basophil adenomas may cause Cushing's syndrome (p. 1305). Not infrequently, the patient with one of these forms of hyperpituitarism slowly, over the course of years, begins to manifest hypopituitarism. At autopsy of such a case, a necrotic or fibrotic mass may be discovered. As described earlier, presumably the growth of the tumor compressed its own blood supply and caused infarction of the autonomously functioning neoplasm.

Some pituitary adenomas do not evoke an initial phase of hyperfunction but, instead, progressively deplete the normal anterior pituitary function. Classically, such neoplasms have been referred to as chromophobe adenomas and, indeed, some are composed of cells which appear by light microscopy to be devoid of granules. However, as was mentioned earlier (p. 1355), many of these apparent chromophobe adenomas have been shown by electron microscopy to be composed of sparsely granulated cells (Schelin, 1962) (Paiz and Hennigar, 1970). Contrariwise, so-called chromophobe adenomas hve been shown to produce hyperpituitary syndromes (Hamilton et al., 1970) (Dingman and Lim, 1962) (Cassidy, 1960). Indeed, a recent report emphasizing the potential secretory activity of apparent chromophobes denies the finding of a single nonfunctional chromophobe tumor in a series of 145 pituitary adenomas (McCormick and Halmi, 1971). Notwithstanding, the recent literature continues to contain references to chromophobe adenomas (Doniach, 1972). We can leave this vexatious issue with the understanding that the terms chromophobe and chromophobe adenoma are still in use and apply to cells which are either sparsely granulated or completely degranulated. Thus, some chromophobe adenomas are associated with hyperpituitary states, and some are nonfunctional and cause only progressive pressure atrophy of the residual normal pituitary and a hypopituitary syndrome.

Because of the variable use of terms designating cell types, it is impossible to express meaningful data on the relative frequency of adenomas composed of each of the three major cell types in the anterior pituitary. If we include sparsely granulated and degranulated cells, so-called chromophobe adenomas account for more than half of all pituitary adenomas (Kernohan and Sayre, 1956). Next most common is the acidophil adenoma, while basophil adenomas are in general rare. It should be emphasized that 10 to 20 per cent of pituitary adenomas are made up of mixed-cell populations. Altogether, adenomas comprise at least 60 per cent of hypophyseal tumors (Kraus, 1945).

These benign tumors grow slowly and may well begin in a focus of hyperplasia. Indeed, in a postmortem study of 1000 so-called normal pituitary glands, Costello (1936) found foci of basophilic hyperplasia or small adenomas in 12.5 per cent. No information is available as to how long they may be present before they cause enlargement of the sella turcica and produce local pressure changes.

All adenomas appear the same, and are small, spherical, soft, red-brown lesions that are usually well encapsulated and contained within an expanded sella turcica (Fig. 29–55). These lesions may be microscopic in size or may reach a maximal diameter of over 10 cm. In their growth, they may compress and destroy the remaining pituitary substance. Considerable local pressure effects may be produced, with bulging of the diaphragma sellae and erosion of the sella turcica. Progressive centrifugal growth may cause rupture of the capsule and the diaphragma sellae and extension of the tumor outside the sella, with apparent invasion of the cavernous sinuses, nasal sinuses and base of the brain. Occasionally the spread beyond the sella turcica may produce the appearance of malignancy. Pressure atrophy of the optic chiasm or of the optic nerves, producing changes in the visual fields, may be the first clue to the existence of such a lesion (Fig. 29–56). In rare instances, these aggressive but benign lesions may erode into the nasopharynx. Occasionally, chromophobe adenomas are found below the sella turcica, where they presumably arise from sequestered nests of cells along the course of the growth of Rathke's pouch.

The cytologic detail of the usual pituitary cell is produced with considerable faithfulness. The cells are regular and have little variability in size or shape, and mitoses are rare. Although occasionally the growth pattern is papillary or sinusoidal, usually they appear as solid sheets or masses of cells (Fig. 29–57). The identification of the cell type in routine tissue stains may be difficult. Cytologic identification is made more difficult by the common tendency for these tumors to have large areas of infarction necrosis as the result of the progressive development of pressure within the tumor and consequent impairment of blood supply. Special stains cited by Doniach (1972) and electron microscopy may be necessary to identify the cell type of the adenoma. With these studies, it is possible to identify and classify cells on the basis of the tinctorial characteristics and size of the granules. Histologic differentiation of a true adenoma from a focus of hyperplasia or nodular hyperplasia may be difficult at times, but is of no material significance since all these forms of cell proliferation have identical clinical importance.

Craniopharyngioma (Rathke's Pouch Tumor, Adamantinoma).

This is the second most common hypophyseal tumor and occurs

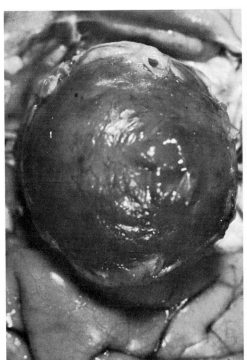

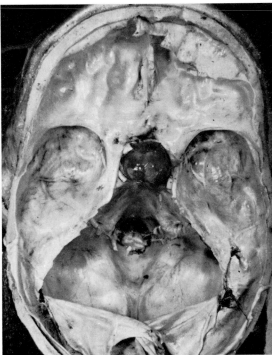

Fig. 29–55   **Fig. 29–56**

Figure 29–55. *A close-up detail of a pituitary adenoma still attached to the brain. Compressed vessels and nerves are apparent above the periphery.*

Figure 29–56. *An in situ view of a pituitary adenoma which has bulged through the diaphragma sellae. Its relationship to the entering internal carotid artery and optic tracts is evident.*

about one-fourth as commonly as the pituitary adenomas. These tumors are derived from vestigial remnants of the craniopharyngeal anlage. Alternatively, it is suggested that they may arise from metaplastic development of the cells of the anterior pituitary. They are most common in children and young adults and are usually completely benign, but occasionally give rise to malignancy.

They may arise in any position along the craniopharyngeal canal and, therefore, some lie within the sella turcica while others lie external to it. They are commonly well encapsulated and grow as either solid or, more commonly, cystic tumors. Occasionally they attain considerable size, up to 8 to 10 cm. in diameter. The cysts may be multiloculated and contain dark brown, oily fluid, in which can be found granular brown debris frequently laden with glittering cholesterol crystals. Over three-fourths of these tumors contain sufficient calcification to be visualized radiographically. As expansile lesions, they often grow enough to compress the pituitary. They may destroy the optic chiasm or nerves and, not infrequently, they bulge into the floor of the third ventricle and base of the brain.

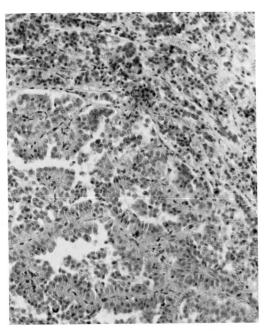

Figure 29–57. *A pituitary adenoma illustrating a tendency to papillary growth and poor demarcation from the surrounding pituitary substance. The tumor cells are uniform in size and compress the adjacent normal gland, above.*

The histologic pattern is variable and presents a wide spectrum of cell types, recalling the cells of the enamel organ of the tooth (Fig. 29—58). These tumors are thus also known as **adamantinomas** or **ameloblastomas.** The solid tumors are made up of stratified squamous epithelium which lacks keratohyaline granules, and columnar epithelium (Love and Marshall, 1950). Nests or cords of stratified squamous or columnar epithelium are embedded in a loose fibrous stroma. These nests of cells may have a peripheral layer of columnar cells which encloses a loose fibrous stroma in the center of which are the squamous cell elements (Fig. 29—59). In the cystic forms, the lining stratified squamous or columnar epithelium may be quite flat and regular, but multiloculated cysts often have papillary projections of epithelium extending into the cystic lumen (Fig. 29—60). Calcification and metaplastic bone formation occur in the necrotic centers of the solid tumors, as well as in the cystic variety, and are of considerable radiologic diagnostic importance. Anaplastic changes in the squamous epithelial cells or the columnar adamantinomatous cells have been described, strangely enough, more commonly in young

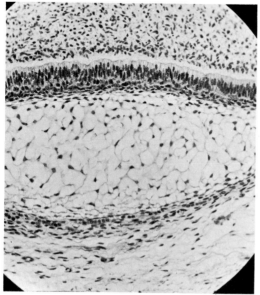

Fig. 29—58

Figure 29–58. *The embryonic tooth bud to illustrate the similarity of cytology to the cells of the adamantinoma.*

Figure 29–59. *Craniopharyngioma (adamantinoma). A nest of cells illustrating the central squamous elements embedded in a loose cellular structure.*

Figure 29–60. *Craniopharyngioma (adamantinoma) growing in a cystic pattern.*

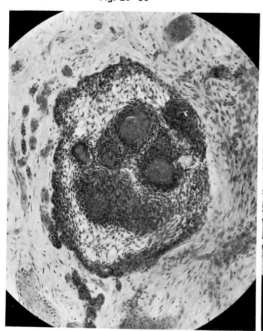

Fig. 29–59

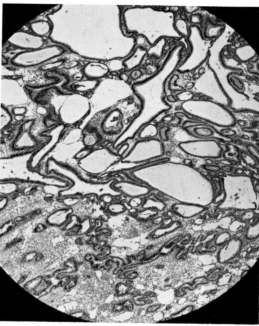

Fig. 29–60

individuals. However, this is infrequent and, as in the adenomas, extension into the surrounding structures does not necessarily imply metastatic potential. Although frank malignancy may occur, it is rare.

Miscellaneous. Other benign tumors have been described within the pituitary. These are all quite rare and include fibromas, hemangiomas and teratomas. Cholesteatomas, essentially identical with dermoid cysts, arise from inclusions of epidermal epithelium. All are rare occurrences in this location.

MALIGNANT

Primary. As has been mentioned, cancers may arise in the anterior lobe, occasionally in preexisting benign adenomas or craniopharyngiomas. They are very rare, however.

A point of importance is that the distinction between an adenoma and a carcinoma of the pituitary may be very difficult. Adenomas have been described as having a tendency to rupture through their capsule and to extend by expansile growth into the adjacent central nervous system tissue and sphenoid sinuses. Thus, these benign lesions produce apparent invasion. This simply represents centrifugal growth and is not true malignant invasiveness. It is said of pituitary lesions that the only true criterion of malignancy is evidence of independent metastatic growth. In the malignant forms which show anaplasia, identification of cell types is extremely difficult, if not impossible.

Secondary. Metastases to the pituitary are quite rare and are seen most often with carcinoma of the breast, lung and thyroid, in the order mentioned.

PITUITARY CHANGES INCIDENT TO ADRENAL, THYROID AND GONADAL DYSFUNCTION

Because the hormones of the adrenals, thyroid and gonads exert feedback inhibition on the corresponding secretory function of the anterior pituitary, alterations in the level of any of these hormones elaborated by target endocrine organs have secondary effects on the anterior lobe. These pituitary changes can largely be deduced from an understanding of the known feedback pathways.

Adrenocortical Hyperfunction. This is the most striking example of the effect of endocrinopathy in a target organ upon the pituitary. Earlier, it was pointed out that Cushing's syndrome is associated with a focus of hyperplasia of basophils or a well defined adenoma in approximately 20 per cent of cases. As was pointed out, most of these tumors are basophil adenomas, but occasionally a so-called chromophobe adenoma is encountered. Moreover, Crooke's hyaline degeneration of basophils is seen in most instances of Cushing's syndrome, whatever its cause (p. 1305). It would be reasonable to expect, then, that the hyalin reflects suppression or derangement of basophil function, and there are hints that the stored ACTH is of altered molecular weight (Currie et al., 1963). Similar basophilic degeneration may be seen in the adrenogenital syndrome and as a result of protracted therapeutic administration of corticosteroids.

Adrenocortical Hypofunction. This is usually accompanied by a marked increase in sparsely granulated basophils. Here the cytology correlates with decreased feedback inhibition of the basophils and increased levels of ACTH secretion. Such changes are seen in Addison's disease. The increased melanin pigmentation of the skin and mucosa in adrenal hypofunction is probably related to the melanocyte-stimulating activity of ACTH augmented possibly by the elaboration of MSH.

Thyroid Hyperfunction. This is not associated with striking changes in the pituitary. Some shrinkage of basophils may be found or, conversely, in rare instances, an increase in the number of basophils may be seen; but these changes do not significantly alter pituitary structure.

Thyroid Hypofunction. This results in a reduction in the number and granularity of the acidophils, as well as in a striking increase in the number of both chromophobes and sparsely granulated basophils. The proliferation of basophils can reasonably be attributed to the increased elaboration of TSH. The reduction in the number of acidophils may be related to the fact that, with a deficiency of thyroid hormone, there is general slowing of metabolism and growth, including the synthesis of growth hormone by the acidophils (Purves and Griesbach, 1946). Why the chromophobes should increase in number and, in fact, be largely responsible for the increase in pituitary size in hypothyroidism is poorly understood; but these cells may represent sparsely granulated basophils.

Hypergonadism. The hypophyseal changes accompanying such forms of gonadal hyperactivity as granulosa cell or Leydig cell tumors are not very striking nor well delineated. In the experimental animal (rats and some strains of mice), prolonged administration of estrogens results first in degranulation of basophils and hyperplasia of sparsely granulated acidophils, presumably the source of prolactin. In time, prolactin-secreting tumors arise in the pituitary. To date, there is no good evidence that prolonged administration of estrogens to patients induces pituitary tumors.

Hypogonadism. This may be associated with striking alterations in the anterior lobe. For the changes associated with the menopause, as well as those encountered during puberty, the menstrual cycle and pregnancy, reference should be made to the excellent review by Russfield (1968). With surgical castration or gonadal agenesis, there is an increase in the number of sparsely granulated basophils. Infrequently, with gonadal agenesis, hyperplasia of the acidophils or an adenoma composed of acidophils or chromophobes has been encountered. Similarly, in Klinefelter's syndrome, the sparsely granulated eosinophils are increased in both number and size. It will be remembered that patients with this syndrome often have elevated urinary gonadotropins, as well as gynecomastia (p. 1293). Conceivably, the latter phenomenon may be related to increased prolactin production. The Laurence-Moon-Biedl syndrome is characterized by hypogonadism. In these patients, there may be a marked increase in the well granulated basophils.

ANTERIOR PITUITARY CLINICAL SYNDROMES

Lesions of the pituitary may be asymptomatic and may be only found incidentally at autopsy. They may make themselves known by local effects (as described earlier), or they may become apparent because of hyper- or hypofunction of the gland.

Hyperpituitarism. The term hyperpituitarism should, in reality, apply to any syndrome resulting from hypersecretion of any one of the tropic hormones. As used clinically, it is generally restricted to those syndromes associated with excessive production of growth hormone by an acidophil adenoma. When the adenoma arises before the epiphyses have closed, i.e., in the child, it produces *gigantism*. In the adult, it induces *acromegaly*.

Acromegaly. This term refers to enlargement of the acral parts (the extremities)—the most distinctive feature of this syndrome. The increased levels of growth hormone in the adult stimulate growth of connective tissue, cartilage and bone (subperiosteal, appositional neo-osteogenesis). Growth of these tissues results in increase in the size of

the skull, prominent cheek bones, protruding jaw and frontal bossing. The fingers and hands become broad and spade-like (Fig. 29–61). The feet also increase in size, particularly in width. Increased growth of subcutaneous tissue of the face produces coarsening of the features, compounded by the hyperplasia and hypertrophy occurring in the cartilages of the nose and ears. The jaw protrudes due to growth of the mandible and the maxilla. Generally, there is no increase in height because, by definition, acromegaly arises in the adult after the endochondral bone formation is completed with fusion of the epiphyses. Almost always in the course of time, osteoporosis (p. 1442) and muscle weakness become evident, and these changes, along with distortion of the articular plate due to bony overgrowth, predispose to osteoarthritis (p. 1470).

Growth hormone has a diabetogenic effect, and approximately 10 per cent of acromegalics have overt clinical diabetes and another 15 per cent, chemical diabetes. Some acromegalics have manifestations suggestive of hyperthyroidism. Laboratory tests usually fail to disclose elevated levels of PBI or RaI uptake, and such manifestations as sweating and excessive sensitivity to heat are attributed to the direct stimulatory effect of growth hormone on metabolism. About a third of males with acromegaly develop impotence, and nearly all women manifest either amenorrhea

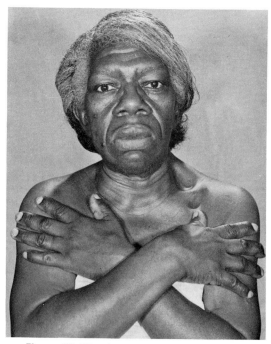

Figure 29–61. *Acromegaly in a 60-year-old woman.*

or menstrual irregularities. Presumably, the expansile growth of the acidophil adenoma destroys or causes atrophy of the marginal native cells of the anterior lobe, so inducing an insufficiency of gonadotropin. In such patients, decreased levels of circulating ACTH may be uncovered, but only rarely is there overt adrenal hypofunction.

Gigantism. Although identical with acromegaly in its pathophysiology, gigantism is manifested by a different clinical appearance. The growth hormone in the growing child leads to excessive, but proportionate, increase in size. Indeed, many of the circus giants who are over 8 feet tall probably represent instances of gigantism. Because both epiphyseal and appositional bone growth occur concomitantly, these patients do not develop the distortions of the acral parts so characteristic of acromegaly. They do, however, suffer from osteoporosis and muscle weakness as much as their acromegalic "first cousins."

Many of the anatomic changes of acromegaly and gigantism are identical. A pituitary adenoma is almost always found, composed of acidophils in approximately 90 per cent of cases. Electron microscopy confirms that the cells in these adenomas are quite usual in appearance and contain cytoplasmic granules ranging from 100 to 500 millimicrons, similar to those in normal cells (Cardell and Knighton, 1966) (Schelin, 1962). In 10 per cent of cases, the tumor is a so-called chromophobe adenoma presumably made up of sparsely granulated acidophils. Rarely, no neoplasm is found, only a microscopic focus of acidophil hyperplasia or an adenoma of microscopic size. There is no linear correlation between size of the neoplasm and the severity of clinical manifestations.

Both pituitary giants and acromegalics have striking splanchnomegaly with enlargement of the liver, spleen, kidneys and other internal organs. In particular, the heart is enlarged and is usually found to have an increase in the size of the myocardial fibers, accompanied by a marked interstitial fibrosis. These patients also suffer from coronary atherosclerosis, perhaps related to a tendency toward hypertension. The interesting issue arises of whether the cardiac hypertrophy is due only to growth hormone or may be related to the somatomegaly and splanchnomegaly. Enlargement of the skeletal system is proportional in the syndrome of gigantism, while in acromegaly the skeletal changes are confined to enlargement of the skull and facial bones and widening of the small bones of the hands and feet. Thyroid enlargement due to multinodular goiter formation and, occasionally, adrenal cortical hyperplasia also occur. In some of these patients, there is

evidence that the pituitary tumors have elaborated not only growth hormone but also ACTH (Mautalen and Mellinger, 1965).

Although the clinical manifestations of acromegaly and gigantism may be obvious in some patients, in others the signs are subtle and develop so insidiously as to be easily missed. The diagnosis may then rest on the demonstration by radioimmunoassay of increased levels of growth hormone in the plasma.

In most patients, both gigantism and acromegaly develop insidiously and often are not noted by the patient or the family until present for years or even decades. The slow progressive changes in appearance and structure appear subtly. Many of these patients ultimately die of cardiac failure. In other instances, however, obvious progression ceases and the disease is said to have "burned itself out." In this circumstance, it may well be that the adenoma has undergone partial or even subtotal ischemic necrosis, reducing the levels of circulating growth hormone. However, cases have been observed in which the somatic alterations plateaued despite the continued presence of excessive levels of growth hormone in the plasma.

Hypopituitarism. This syndrome may be produced by any destructive lesion of the pituitary gland. *The three most common causes are Sheehan's pituitary necrosis, the chromophobe adenoma and the craniopharyngioma.* These three lesions together account for most of the cases of panhypopituitarism. Rarely, other lesions may destroy the pituitary sufficiently to produce inadequacy of function. Among these less common causes are cysts, extrasellar neoplasms, inflammations of the pituitary with particular emphasis upon tuberculosis, sarcoidosis and metastatic malignancy. In some recorded cases, only fibrosis of the pituitary is found, leaving no clue as to the original cause of the pituitary destruction. This subject has been well reviewed by Sheehan and Summers (1949).

The systemic changes which result depend again upon whether the patient is an adult or a child. In the adult, the entity is termed hypophyseal or Simmonds' cachexia or, more properly, panhypopituitarism, since cachexia is not a common clinical feature of these cases. In the child, dwarfism of the Lorain-Levi type or Froehlich's syndrome may result. In any of these syndromes, considerable support for the diagnosis can be obtained from the laboratory. Since the entire pituitary gland is destroyed in these regressive lesions, all the tropic hormones are affected. Thus, the urinary FSH levels are reduced. The first manifestations to appear stem from the insufficiency of gonadotropins, followed by those relating to the growth hormone and TSH. ACTH is usually the last to be affected.

Hypophyseal Cachexia or Simmonds' Disease. This disorder, occurring at any age, is more frequent in adults and has a 2 to 1 preponderance in females. It is quite remarkable that most patients survive many years with an average duration of disease of 30 to 40 years (Escamilla and Lisser, 1942). The systemic manifestations obviously reflect a pluriglandular deficiency. Although there may well be an insufficiency of growth hormone, this is not clinically apparent in most adults. Practically, the clinical syndrome can be best considered as representing that of insufficiency of the gonads, thyroid and adrenals secondary to the loss of their tropic hormones. The precise clinical pattern may reflect atrophy of all three or any combination of these secondary endocrine glands. Perhaps most common is the combination of apparent hypothyroidism and hypoadrenalism. Myxedema resulting from pituitary insufficiency is always to be ruled out in any case of apparent primary thyroid insufficiency (p. 1324).

The addisonian pattern of pituitary origin differs from that of primary adrenal dysfunction in that patients with panhypopituitarism do not have the abnormal pigmentations of the skin and mucous membranes seen in primary adrenal insufficiency. With pituitary destruction, there is loss of the melanocyte-stimulating effect. Moreover, the pituitary gland does not control the formation of aldosterone, and therefore the patient with Simmonds' disease often has no abnormality of salt and water metabolism. In hypopituitarism, weight loss and cachexia may be present, but are commonly absent. The viscera may show brown atrophy with loss of substance. The only constant feature is atrophy of the endocrine glands, particularly the adrenals, thyroid and

gonads, as well as regressive alterations in their target organs. This atrophy of the secondary endocrine glands may become so extreme as to make their identification at autopsy impossible.

Hypophyseal Dwarfism—Lorain-Levi Type. This disorder represents pituitary insufficiency affecting the child in the formative stages and gives rise to a symmetrical dwarf. In these cases, the most common destructive lesion of the pituitary is a craniopharyngioma. However, ischemic necrosis, simple cysts and inflammatory changes have been described as rare causes.

Froehlich's Syndrome (Adiposogenital Dystrophy). This condition is characterized by marked obesity of the eunuchoid type and hypodevelopment of the gonads and genitals. Other findings are lack of secondary sex characteristics, sexual dysfunction and thin, soft skin. The condition usually occurs at an early age and has an equal distribution between the sexes, although the diagnosis in a young female is difficult and perhaps made less often. This entity, which is still not completely understood, has probably been diagnosed too commonly in the past, since it is now recognized that many such cases represent constitutional obesity. Fröhlich's syndrome is a form of panhypopituitarism, reflected chiefly as a deficiency of gonadotropic hormone. Thus, in many cases lesions outside the pituitary are primary, involving the hypothalamic region, infundibulum and floor of the third ventricle, all probably having an influence on the connections between the hypothalamus and the pituitary. These hypothalamic-neurologic lesions may also explain the strange obesity present in these children. For simplicity, the condition is best considered at present as a form of hypopituitarism.

In addition to the functional changes produced in these cases of panhypopituitarism due to destructive tumors, it is to be recalled that local destructive effects and changes secondary to generalized increases of intracranial pressure may also be prominent features.

THYMUS

NORMAL

As is now well known, the thymus is a central lymphoid organ which plays a pivotal role in cell-mediated immunity (p. 203). It is derived from the third and sometimes the fourth branchial pouches. At birth, it weighs approximately 15 to 20 gm. and enlarges to reach a weight of about 30 gm. at puberty. Thereafter, it progressively atrophies, becoming in the adult virtually a fibrofatty pad weighing about 10 to 15 gm. and containing small islands of recognizable thymic tissue.

The thymus is bilobed and enclosed within a loose connective tissue capsule. Each lobe is divided into lobules by fibrous septa. At the periphery of each lobule is the cortex, which encloses the central medulla. The cortex is composed almost entirely of closely packed small lymphocytes belonging to the T-cell system. Scattered among these lymphocytes are larger, paler reticular cells capable of active phagocytosis.

The medulla, in contrast, is largely composed of reticular cells, between which are scattered small lymphocytes. Because the reticular cells have an abundant cytoplasm and pale vesicular nuclei, they are sometimes referred to as epithelial or reticuloepithelial cells. In addition, the medulla contains scattered nests of layered keratinizing epithelial cells—the Hassall's corpuscles.

Passing mention might be made now of the existence of myoid cells in the thymus of the human fetus. This detail will be of further interest in the consideration of the relationship of the thymus to myasthenia gravis. These myoid cells apparently degenerate and disappear during fetal development but provide a possible source for muscle antigens within the thymus (Van de Velde and Friedman, 1970). It should be particularly noted that in the normal thymus there are no lymphoid follicles, and their appearance is interpreted as thymic hyperactivity.

PATHOLOGY

Despite our growing knowledge of the relationship of the thymus to the immune system (discussed in Chapter 7), the thymus remains shrouded in mystery. Rarely does a month go by without the appearance in the medical literature of a new syndrome relating thymic disease to some immunologic, hematologic, endocrinologic, infectious or neoplastic disorder. Sitting in the midst of all this tumult, the thymus displays only a very limited range of morphologic changes which can be categorized as developmental anomalies, hyperplasia and neoplasia.

Developmental Anomalies. Anomalous development of the thymus is responsible for a variety of congenital immunologic deficiency states. These have been considered in detail on p. 215. It is enough here to note that, in diGeorge's syndrome, the thymus may be totally absent (agenesis), or may be hypoplastic with an absence or marked reduction in the number of small lymphocytes, as in thymic alymphoplasia (Good's syndrome) and Swiss-type agammaglobulinemia. Other immunologic deficiency syndromes have been identified as being associated with hypoplasia of the thymus.

Hyperplasia. Thymic hyperplasia causes enlargement of the gland, but it is exceedingly difficult to evaluate this enlargement by weight alone. In the adult, on the average, a weight in excess of 35 gm. may well represent hyperplasia, but many individuals may have persistent and large thymic glands showing completely normal histologic structure, unassociated with any other systemic disorder. Accordingly, *the most reliable criterion of hyperplasia is the appearance of lymphoid follicles within the thymus.* Thymic follicular hyperplasia has been seen in association with myasthenia gravis, Addison's disease, thyrotoxicosis, acromegaly, gonadal hypofunction and, occasionally, in apparently normal thymic glands (Alpert et al., 1971). It is also encountered in many immunologic disorders, particularly those of presumed autoimmune origin, such as lupus erythematosus and dermatomyositis. Indeed, thymic follicular hyperplasia is a relatively constant finding in NZB mice having a variety of autoimmune manifestations closely resembling those seen in systemic lupus erythematosus and autoimmune hemolytic anemia in man. Burnet and Holmes (1964) interpret these follicles in the NZB mice as abnormal "forbidden" clones of lymphoid cells resistant to the normal control processes within the thymus and responsible for the autoimmune manifestations.

In past years, sudden death in infants and children was, in some inexplicable manner, thought to be related to abnormal persistence or hyperplasia of the thymus. Thus arose the diagnosis *status thymicolymphaticus*. Frequently, it was said to be accompanied by hypoplasia of the vascular system. This mythical condition was held in such terror that it was standard practice to obtain chest x-rays in infants about to undergo surgery to measure the size of the thymus. Lamentably, many of these infants with presumed thymic enlargement were administered therapeutic preoperative radiation to shrink the thymus. In the course of time, it became apparent that individuals so treated suffered a significantly increased incidence of thyroid cancer because of coincidental exposure of the thyroid gland to radiant energy (p. 1340). These cancers did not appear until the second or third decade of life. The diagnosis of status thymicolymphaticus has now gone into limbo and, with it, the unfortunate practice of exposing infants and children to needless and damaging radiation for the control of a nonexistent disease.

Tumors of the Thymus. All tumors of the thymus are generically designated as thymomas. While they are rare in clinical practice, they have assumed great interest because, in so many cases, there are neuromuscular, immunologic, endocrinologic and hematologic disorders associated with these neoplasms. In particular, their well known relationship to *myasthenia gravis* makes these tumors a multifaceted enigma.

Thymomas span a gamut of patterns and have been thus the subject of numerous classifications. The simplest essentially divides them into the principal cell types found in the thymus:

    A. Small cell (lymphocytic) thymoma.
    B. Epithelial thymoma.
       1. Spindle cell variant.
    C. Mixed lymphoepithelial thymoma.

Many other terms have been used for specific patterns, but they represent variations of one of these better defined categories just listed. One of these special patterns requires clarification. The term *granulomatous thymoma*, sometimes also called lymphomatous thymoma, has been applied to thymic masses having a histologic architecture identical with that of Hodgkin's disease (usually the nodular sclerosing pattern) (Fig. 29–62). In some of these patients, generalized Hodgkin's disease has later appeared (Katz and Lattes, 1969). Currently, the granulomatous thymoma is con-

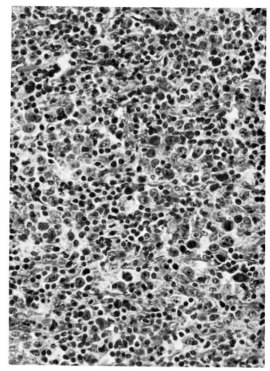

Figure 29–62. *Hodgkin's disease involving the thymus, formerly called "granulomatous thymoma."*

sidered to be an instance of Hodgkin's disease arising within the thymus rather than a valid thymoma. Because many of these granulomatous lesions are of the nodular sclerosing variety, the prognosis for these patients is usually quite favorable (p. 766). An additional variant has been described by Lattes (1962) that is designated as a seminoma or seminomatous thymoma. But the origin of these tumors is uncertain. Since many of these have associated choriocarcinomatous areas and others have teratoid characteristics, it is better to consider this group as teratomas arising in the thymus, having the same significance as teratomas elsewhere. Justification for this concept is the rare case of benign cystic teratoma (dermoid cyst) found in the thymus.

The three principal patterns of thymoma generally appear as sharply circumscribed, apparently encapsulated, firm, gray-white masses varying from several centimeters in diameter to massive lesions up to 15 to 20 cm. in diameter. Some of the more aggressive lesions (approximately one-third) penetrate the capsule to invade adjacent structures. While these aggressive tumors are considered malignant, extrathoracic spread is very uncommon.

Histologically, the **"small cell"** thymoma consists of apparent lymphocytes dispersed in no distinct pattern. These cells may totally obliterate the underlying architecture, but occasionally leave small thymic corpuscles. Plump epithelial cells are usually scattered throughout this sea of lymphocytes. **Hassall's corpuscles are infrequent to rare.** This pattern comprises about 15 per cent of thymomas (Fig. 29–63).

The **epithelial thymomas** are composed of large epithelial cells laid down in small islands and clusters throughout a lymphoid background. The epithelial cells have an abundant pale, acidophilic cytoplasm with vesicular nucleus and appear much larger and paler than the surrounding lymphocytes with their scant cytoplasm. Cystic areas of softening are common. **Hassall's corpuscles are more frequent than in the small cell type, but less frequent than in the spindle cell lesions to be described.**

The **spindle cell variant** of the epithelial thymoma is one in which the cells assume elongated forms resembling fibroblasts. These may form broad bundles of cells or interlacing whorls that **often form mature Hassall's corpuscles.** Many times, these tumors are very vascular and produce strands of cells separated by vascular cords. At other times, they appear lymphangiomatous. The epithelial and spindle cell variants together represent about 20 per cent of thymomas.

The **lymphoepithelial thymoma** is probably

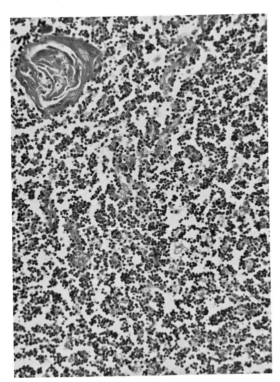

Figure 29–63. "Small-cell" thymoma composed of mature lymphocytes. A Hassall corpuscle is evident in the upper left.

the most common pattern accounting for about half of all thymomas. The neoplasm is composed, as might be expected, of a mixture of well differentiated lymphocytes and scattered cords or clusters of epithelial cells. Which cell population predominates varies from one tumor to another. Hassall's corpuscles are usually rare and often poorly formed.

About one-third of thymomas produce no symptoms and are discovered on routine chest films (Lattes, 1962). About another third cause symptoms related to the expansile mass in the thoracic inlet. In such patients, cough, dyspnea, difficulty in swallowing or signs of compression of the superior vena cava call attention to the lesion (Takita and Mongaya, 1970). In the remaining third, other systemic disorders call the thymus to attention. It is virtually impossible to cite all of the associated systemic disorders, but prominent among them are myasthenia gravis, anemia, pancytopenia, thrombocytopenia, Cushing's syndrome, hypogammaglobulinemia and several forms of so-called autoimmune disease (Lindstrom et al., 1968) (Hirst and Robertson, 1967) (Larsson, 1963) (Rubin et al., 1964) (Schmid et al., 1965) (Dawson, 1972). The underlying mechanisms for these associations are still largely enigmatic but, in some instances, as in the case of anemia, the thymus may elaborate an immune response against erythropoietin (Jepson and Lowenstein, 1966). Often, removal of the thymic tumor has been followed in time (perhaps years) by remission of the associated condition.

The biologic behavior of thymomas is quite variable and difficult to predict from the morphologic examination of the tumor. The most reliable criterion of a favorable prognosis is lack of invasion of the capsule of the lesion and, therefore, confinement of the neoplasm to the thymus (Legg and Brady, 1965). Wilkins et al. (1966) have reported a 100 per cent ten-year survival of patients with encapsulated tumors having no associated systemic disorder such as myasthenia gravis. With capsular invasion, the mean survival time is 2.8 years (Kilman and Klassen, 1971).

The Thymus in Myasthenia Gravis. Myasthenia gravis is a systemic muscular disorder characterized by profound muscle weakness. It is discussed in detail on p. 1426. Here our interest is in the somewhat mysterious association of thymic lesions with myasthenia gravis. The thymus is abnormal in approximately 75 per cent of these cases, representing a thymoma in about one-third and follicular hyperplasia in the remainder, although the precise frequencies vary widely as reported in the literature. Often, follicular hyperplasia is seen in the residual thymic tissue about the margins of a thymoma.

Theories abound as to the pathogenesis of the muscular disorder and the meaning of the thymic lesions associated with it. Numerous observations suggest that myasthenia gravis is fundamentally an immunologic disease. Antibodies can be identified in these patients, which react with antigenic determinants in skeletal muscle and in the thymus (Strauss, 1968). The antibody tends to localize along the I bands of the skeletal muscle, suggesting that the antigens may be either troponin or tropomyosin (Strauss and Kemp, 1967) (van der Geld et al., 1964).

Many attempts have been made to explain the reactivity of antibodies to both thymus and muscle cells. Recall that myoid cells are said normally to be present in the developing fetus. Similar cells are sometimes found in the thymus and thymomas in patients with myasthenia gravis. Conceivably, breakdown of these myoid cells might trigger an immune response, which would then react not only against the myoid cells in the abnormal thymus but also against skeletal muscle (Van de Velde and Friedman, 1970). Alternatively, the appearance of follicular hyperplasia in the thymus

gland of so many patients with the muscle disease might imply the emergence of abnormal clones of lymphocytes reactive against "self" (Alpert et al., 1971). In the experimental animal, it has been possible to produce an apparent myasthenic neuromuscular block by immunization of guinea pigs against thymic or muscular tissue in combination with Freund adjuvant (Goldstein and Whittingham, 1966).

However, it should be emphasized that the mere existence of autoantibodies does not prove that they are of pathogenetic significance. A significant proportion of patients having a thymoma but not myasthenia gravis also have antibodies against thymus and muscle (Strauss, 1968). Children born of myasthenic mothers frequently exhibit transient neonatal myasthenia not associated with demonstrable circulating antibodies, suggesting that other mechanisms were operative in the induction of the transient muscle weakness (van der Geld and Strauss, 1966). Moreover, it must be remembered that only about 33 per cent of patients with myasthenia gravis have demonstrable antimuscle antibodies. Thus it is evident that, although the thymus is frequently abnormal in these patients, the meaning of such changes is unclear as are the nature and cause of myasthenia gravis.

PINEAL GLAND

NORMAL

The pineal gland is a minute structure situated above the posterior extremity of the third ventricle. It is less than 1 cm. in longest diameter, with a weight of approximately 0.1 to 0.2 gm. Histologically, it is composed of a loose connective tissue stroma enclosing nests of large epithelial-appearing cells.

The function of the pineal has come under close scrutiny in recent years and has been well reviewed by Relkin (1966). It elaborates a hormone or hormones that have a variety of effects in animals and man. One is melatonin, derived from serotonin, that antagonizes the melanocyte-stimulating hormone (MSH). The pineal also secretes a substance that inhibits some aspects of gonadal function. It is suspected that this is an additional action of melatonin. Pineal hyperfunction is associated with delayed puberty and hypofunction with precocious puberty. Thus,

certain pineal tumors may be manifested by alterations in sexual maturation and by derangements in sexual behavior. Presumably, the source of these hormones is the epithelial cell of the pineal. In addition, there are scattered neuroglial components within this gland, mainly of the astrocytic type, potential sources of gliomatous tumors.

Calcification of the pineal occurs with age, but recent studies indicate that, despite such calcification, there is no diminution in the secretory activity of the gland. In fact, several analyses indicate that hormonal activity increases during adult life (De Martino et al., 1964).

PATHOLOGY

The only lesions of importance in this gland are tumors. They may be of three types:

1. Pinealomas composed of nests of the large epithelial cells found in the adult pineal. These epithelial clusters are enclosed in a fibrous stroma containing an infiltrate of lymphocytes. The histologic appearance has a remarkable similarity to the seminoma of the testis (p. 1184) and so these pineal neoplasms are sometimes called germinomas (Dayan et al., 1966).

2. Neuroglial tumors producing essentially gliomatous lesions resembling gliomas found in the central nervous system.

3. Teratomas. Because of the midline position of the pineal, residuals of totipotential cells may remain in this site, producing teratomas analogous to those found elsewhere in the body.

REFERENCES

Adrenal Gland

Bill, A. H.: The implications of immune reactions to neuroblastoma. Surgery, 66:45, 1969.

Bongiovanni, A. M., et al.: Disorders of adrenal steroid biogenesis. Recent Progr. Hormone Res., 23:375, 1967.

Bransome, E. D., Jr.: Adrenal cortex. Ann. Rev. Physiol., 30:171, 1968.

Braunstein, H., and Yamaguchi, B. T.: The human adrenal in rapid death and chronic illness. Amer. J. Path., 44:113, 1964.

Brown, J. J., et al.: Hypertension with aldosterone excess. Brit. Med. J., 2:391, 1972.

Catt, A. J.: Adrenal cortex. Lancet, 1:1275, 1970.

Conn, J. W.: Primary aldosteronism. A new clinical syndrome. J. Lab. Clin. Med., 45:6, 1955.

Conn, J. W., et al.: Clinical characteristics of primary aldosteronism from an analysis of 145 cases. Amer. J. Surg., 107:159, 1964.

Crane, W. A., et al.: The role of the adrenal cortex in the aetiology of various diseases. Scot. Med. J., 5:437, 1960.

Cushing, H.: The basophil adenomas of the pituitary body and their clinical manifestations (pituitary basophilism). Bull. Johns Hopkins Hosp., 50:137, 1932.

Decicco, F. A., et al.: Fine structure of Crooke's hyaline change in the human pituitary gland. Arch. Path., 94:65, 1972.

Editorial: Cushing's syndrome in childhood. Lancet, 2:267, 1972.

Eisenstein, A. B.: Addison's disease: etiology and relationship to other endocrine disorders. Med. Clin. N. Amer., 52:327, 1968.

Fränkel, F.: Pheochromocytoma. Virchow Arch. Path. Anat., 103:244, 1886.

Freeark, R. J., and Waldstein, S. S.: Present status of the diagnosis and treatment of Cushing's syndrome. Surg. Clin. N. Amer., 49:179, 1969.

Gabrilove, J. L., et al.: Feminizing adrenocortical tumors in the male: review of 52 cases including a case report. Medicine, 44:37, 1965.

Hartog, M.: Hypoadrenalism. Brit. Med. J., 1:679, 1972.

Hashida, Y., et al.: Ultrastructure of the adrenal cortex in Cushing's disease in children. Hum. Path., 1:595, 1970.

Heinbecker, P., et al.: Functioning and nonfunctioning adrenal cortical tumors. Surg. Gynec. Obstet., 105:21, 1957.

Hutter, A. M., and Kayhoe, D. E.: Adrenal cortical carcinoma. Amer. J. Med., 41:572, 1966.

Jailer, J. W., et al.: Adrenal virilism: diagnostic considerations and treatment. J.A.M.A., 150:575, 1952.

Liddle, G. W., and Shute, A. M.: The evolution of Cushing's syndrome as a clinical entity. Advances Intern. Med., 15:155, 1969.

Liddle, G. W., et al.: Clinical and laboratory studies of ectopic humoral syndromes. Recent Progr. Hormone Res., 25:283, 1969.

Liddle, G. W., et al.: The ectopic ACTH syndrome. Cancer Res., 25:1057, 1965.

Lindgren, S.: Congenital primary adrenal hypoplasia. Acta Path. Microbiol. Scand., 70:541, 1967.

Lipsett, M. B., et al.: Clinical and pathophysiologic aspects of adrenal cortical carcinoma. Amer. J. Med., 35:374, 1963.

Long, J. A., and Jones, A. L.: Observations on the fine structure of the adrenal cortex of man. Lab. Invest., 17:355, 1967.

Loraine, J. A.: The Clinical Application of Hormone Assay. Edinburgh, E. and S. Livingston, Ltd., 1958, p. 244.

Macfarlane, D. A.: Cancer of the adrenal cortex. Ann. Roy. Coll. Surg. Eng., 23:155, 1958.

Moore, F. D., and Ball, M. R.: The Metabolic Response to Surgery. Springfield, Ill., Charles C Thomas, 1955.

Ney, R. L., et al.: Evaluation of pituitary-adrenal function in man. The investigation of hypothalamic-pituitary-adrenal function. In James, V. H. G., and Landon, J. (eds.): Memoirs of the Society for Endocrinology, No. 17. New York, Cambridge University Press, 1967, p. 285.

Omae, T., et al.: Hyperaldosteronism due to adrenocortical adenoma and adenomatous hyperplasia. Endocr. Jap., 17:57, 1971.

Raker, J. W.: Surgery of the adrenal glands. Advances Surg., 5:129, 1971.

Rapaport, E., et al.: Mortality in surgically treated adrenocortical tumors: review of cases reported for 20 year period (1930–1949, inclusive). Postgrad. Med., 11:325, 1952.

Report of the Subcommittee on Childhood Solid Tumor Task Force, National Cancer Institute: Comparison of survival curves 1956 vs. 1962 in children with Wilms' tumor and neuroblastoma. Pediatrics, 45:800, 1970.

Robertson, P. W.: Hyperaldosteronism from adrenal carcinoma. Brit. Med. J., 1:220, 1972.

Russell, R. P., et al.: Adrenal cortical adenomas and hypertension. A clinical pathologic analysis of 690 cases with matched controls and a review of the literature. Medicine, 51:211, 1972.

Selye, H.: The alarm reaction and the diseases of adaptation. Ann. Intern. Med., 29:403, 1948.

Selye, H.: The general adaptation syndrome and diseases of adaptation. J. Clin. Endocr., 6:117, 1946.

Sprague, R. G., et al.: Cushing's syndrome, a progressive and often fatal disease: a review of 100 cases seen between July 1945 and July 1954. Arch. Intern. Med., 98:388, 1956.

Symington, T.: The human adrenal cortex in disease. In Modern Trends in Pathology. London, Butterworth and Co., 1959, p. 248.

Symington, T.: Morphology and secretory cytology of the human adrenal cortex. Brit. Med. Bull., 18:117, 1962.

Symington, T., and Goodall, A. L.: Studies in phaeochromocytoma. I. Pathological aspects. Glasgow Med. J., 34:75, 1953.

Wald, M. K.: Bartter's syndrome in early infancy, physiologic light and electron microscope observations. Pediatrics, Suppl. 2, 47:254, 1971.

Willis, R. A.: The Pathology of the Tumours of Children. London, Oliver and Boyd, 1962, p. 7.

Wuepper, K. D., et al.: Immunologic aspects of adrenocortical insufficiency. Amer. J. Med., 46:206, 1969.

Thyroid Gland

Batsakis, J. G., et al.: Sporadic goitre syndrome. A clinicopathologic analysis. Amer. J. Clin. Path., 39:241, 1963.

Becker, K. L., et al.: Clinical observations on rheumatoid arthritis associated with Hashimoto's thyroiditis. Mayo Clinic Proc., 38:153, 1963.

Becker, K. L., et al.: Morphologic evidence of thyroiditis in myasthenia gravis. J.A.M.A., 187:994, 1964.

Bergen, S. S.: Acute non-suppurative thyroiditis. Arch. Intern. Med., 102:747, 1958.

Butler, J. J. H., et al.: Significance of thyroid tissue in lymph nodes associated with carcinoma of the head, neck or lungs. Cancer, 20:103, 1967.

Chopra, I. J., et al.: Specific and nonspecific responses in the bioassay of long acting thyroid stimulator (LATS). J. Clin. Endocr., 31:382, 1970.

Clark, F., et al.: The response in toxic diffuse goitre to a short course of antithyroid therapy. Clin. Sci., 39:2P, 1970.

Davies, A. G.: Thyroid physiology. Brit. Med. J., 2:206, 1972.

DeGroot, L. J.: Current concepts in management of thyroid disease. Med. Clin. N. Amer., 54:117, 1970.

Dobyns, B. M., and Steelman, S. L.: The thyroid stimulating hormone of the anterior pituitary as distinct from the exophthalmos producing substance. Endocrinology, 52:705, 1953.

Duffy, B. J., Jr., and Fitzgerald, P. J.: Thyroid cancer in childhood and adolescence: a report on twenty-eight cases. Cancer, 3:1018, 1950.

Editorial: Endocrine exophthalmos. Brit. Med. J., *3*:68, 1972*a*.

Editorial: Iodide-induced thyrotoxicosis. Lancet, *2*:1073, 1972*b*.

Emerson, C. H., and Utiger, R. D.: Hyperthyroidism and excessive thyrotrophin secretion. New Eng. J. Med., *287*:328, 1972.

Englund, N. E.: Human thyroid C cells: occurrence and amine formation studied by perfusion of surgically removed goitrous glands. J. Clin. Endocr. Metab., *35*:90, 1972.

Freedberg, I. M., et al.: Thyroid in pregnancy. New Eng. J. Med., *256*:505, 1957.

Friedberg, A. S., et al.: The pathologic effects of I-131 on the normal thyroid gland of man. J. Clin. Endocr., *42*:1315, 1952.

Garry, R., and Hall, R.: Stimulation of mitoses in rat thyroid by long acting thyroid stimulator. Lancet, *1*:693, 1970.

Gribetz, D., et al.: Goitre due to lymphocytic thyroiditis. New Eng. J. Med., *250*:555, 1954.

Hall, R.: Evidence for genetic predisposition to formation of thyroid autoantibodies. Lancet, *2*:187, 1960.

Hall, R.: Hyperthyroidism: pathogenesis and diagnosis. Brit. Med. J., *1*:743, 1970.

Hayles, A. B., et al.: Carcinoma of the thyroid in children. Amer. J. Surg., *106*:735, 1963.

Herman, L.: An electron microscopic study of the salamander thyroid during hormonal stimulation. J. Biophys. Biochem. Cytol., *7*:143, 1960.

Hermanson, L., et al.: The treatment of nodular goiter. J. Clin. Endocr., *12*:112, 1952.

Hurxthal, L. M., and Heineman, A. C.: Nodular goiter and thyroid cancer. New Eng. J. Med., *258*:457, 1958.

Kendall-Taylor, P.: Hyperthyroidism. Brit. Med. J., *2*:337, 1972.

Levey, G. S., and Epstein, S. E.: Myocardial adenyl cyclase activation by thyroid hormones and evidence for two adenyl cyclase systems. J. Clin. Invest., *48*:1663, 1969.

Maddox, W. A., et al.: Carcinoma of the thyroid. Review of 15 years experience. Amer. Surg., *37*:653, 1971.

McConahey, W. M.: Hashimoto's thyroiditis. Med. Clin. N. Amer., *56*:885, 1972.

McConahey, W. M., et al.: On the increasing occurrence of Hashimoto's thyroiditis. J. Clin. Endocr. Metab., *22*:542, 1962.

McKenney, J. F., et al.: The variable nature of the thyroid nodule. Surg. Clin. N. Amer., *52*:383, 1972.

McKenzie, J. M.: Does LATS cause hyperthyroidism in Graves' disease (a review biased toward the affirmative)? Metabolism, *21*:883, 1972.

Meachim, G., and Stainsby, G. D.: The incidence of malignancy in localized thyroid swellings treated surgically. Brit. J. Surg., *53*:788, 1966.

Moore, G. H.: The thyroid in sporadic goitrous cretinism. Arch. Path., *74*:35, 1962.

Moore, J. M., and Neilson, J. McE.: Antibodies to gastric mucosa and thyroid in diabetes mellitus. Lancet, *2*:645, 1963.

Psarras, A., et al.: The single thyroid nodule. Brit. J. Surg., *59*:545, 1972.

Purves, H. D., and Adams, D. D.: Thyroid stimulating hormone. Brit. Med. Bull., *16*:128, 1960.

Randall, L. O.: Reaction of thiol compounds with peroxidase and hydrogen peroxide. J. Biol. Chem., *164*:521, 1946.

Rapoport, B., and DeGroot, L. J.: Current concepts of thyroid physiology. Seminars Nucl. Med., *1*:265, 1971.

Rosenberg, I. N.: Thyroiditis and thyroid antibodies. In Astwood, E. B. (ed.): Clinical Endocrinology. New York, Grune & Stratton, Inc., 1960, p. 185.

Roth, L. M.: Inclusions of non-neoplastic thyroid tissue within cervical lymph nodes. Cancer, *18*:105, 1965.

Schell-Frederick, E., and Dumont, J. E.: In Litwack, G. (ed.): Biochemical Actions of Hormones. Vol. I. New York, Academic Press, 1970, p. 416.

Seljelid, R.: Endocytosis of thyroglobulin and the release of thyroid hormone. Scand. J. Clin. Lab. Invest., Suppl., *22*:106, 1968.

Silverstein, G. E., and Burke, G.: Thyroid suppressibility and long acting thyroid stimulator in thyrotoxicosis. Arch. Intern. Med., *126*:615, 1970.

Singh, S. P., and McKenzie, J. M.: 35-S-sulfate uptake by mouse harderian gland: effect of serum from patients with Graves' disease. Metabolism, *20*:422, 1971.

Socolow, E. L., et al.: Thyroid cancer in man after exposure to ionizing radiation. A summary of the findings in Hiroshima and Nagasaki. New Eng. J. Med., *268*:406, 1963.

Stanbury, J. B.: The metabolic errors in certain types of familial goiter. Recent Progr. Hormone Res., *19*:547, 1963.

Statland, H., et al.: Struma lymphomatosa (Hashimoto's struma): a review of 51 cases with discussion of endocrinologic aspects. Arch. Intern. Med., *88*:659, 1951.

Stein, O., and Gross, J.: Metabolism of 125-I in the thyroid gland studied with electron microscopic radioautography. Endocrinology, *75*:787, 1964.

Sterling, K.: The significance of circulating triiodothyronine. Recent Progr. Hormone Res., *26*:249, 1970.

Strahan, R. W., et al.: Thyroiditis. A classification and review. Laryngoscope, *81*:1388, 1971.

Weaver, D. K., et al.: Surgical thyroid disease. Arch. Surg., *92*:796, 1966.

Werner, S. C.: Two panel discussions on hyperthyroidism. II. Etiology and treatment of hyperthyroidism in the adult. J. Clin. Endocr. Metab., *27*:1763, 1967.

Williams, R. H.: Textbook of Endocrinology. Philadelphia, W. B. Saunders Co., 1962, p. 197.

Woolner, L. B.: Thyroid carcinoma: pathologic classification with data on prognosis. Seminars Nucl. Med., *1*:4, 1971.

Woolner, L. B., et al.: Struma lymphomatosa (Hashimoto's thyroiditis) and related thyroidal disorders. J. Clin. Endocr., *19*:53, 1959.

Woolner, L. B., et al.: Classification and prognosis of thyroid carcinoma. A study of 885 cases observed in a 30 year period. Amer. J. Surg., *102*:354, 1961.

Wyse, E. P., et al.: Ophthalmopathy without hyperthyroidism in patients with histologic Hashimoto's thyroiditis. J. Clin. Endocr. Metab., *28*:1623, 1968.

Zacharewicz, F. A.: Management of single and multinodular goiter. Med. Clin. N. Amer., *52*:409, 1968.

Parathyroid Glands

Albright, F., et al.: Pseudo-hypoparathyroidism: an example of "Seabright-Bantam Syndrome." Endocrinology, *30*:922, 1942.

Balogh, K., Jr., and Cohen, R. B.: Oxidative enzymes in the epithelial cells of normal and pathological human parathyroid glands: a histochemical study. Lab. Invest., *10*:354, 1961.

Barnes, B. A., and Cope, O.: Carcinoma of the parathyroid glands. Report of 10 cases with endocrine function. J.A.M.A., *178*:556, 1961.

Berson, S. A., et al.: Immunoassay of bovine and human parathyroid hormone. Proc. Nat. Acad. Sci. U.S.A., *49*:613, 1963.

Black, B. M.: Primary hyperparathyroidism and peptic ulcer. Surg. Clin. N. Amer., *51*:955, 1971.

Blizzard, R. M., et al.: The incidence of parathyroid and other antibodies in the sera of patients with idiopathic hypoparathyroidism. Clin. Exp. Immunol., *1*:119, 1966.

Catt, K. J.: Hormonal control of calcium homeostasis. Lancet, *2*:255, 1970.

Chase, L.: Mechanism of action of parathyroid hormone. In Auerbach, G. D. (moderator): Polypeptide Hormones and Calcium Metabolism (conference). Ann. Intern. Med., *70*:1243, 1969.

Cope, O.: The study of hyperparathyroidism at the Massachusetts General Hospital. New Eng. J. Med., *274*:1174, 1966.

Davies, D. R., et al.: Hyperparathyroidsim and steatorrhoea. Brit. Med. J., *2*:1133, 1956.

DeLuca, H. F.: Vitamin D. A new look at an old vitamin. Nutr. Rev., *29*:179, 1971.

Editorial: Parathyroid hormone and vitamin D. Lancet, *1*:1000, 1972.

Elliott, R. L., and Arhelger, R. B.: Fine structure of parathyroid adenomas. Arch. Path., *81*:200, 1966.

Gordan, G. S., and Goldman, L.: Hyperparathyroidism. Mod. Treatm., *7*:649, 1970.

Hoffenberg, R.: Disorders of the parathyroid gland. Practitioner, *208*:360, 1972.

Keating, R.: The clinical problem of primary hyperparathyroidism. Med. Clin. N. Amer., *54*:511, 1970.

Lee, J. B., et al.: Familial pseudohypoparathyroidism. Role of parathyroid hormone and thyrocalcitonin. New Eng. J. Med., *279*:1179, 1968.

Melick, R. A.: Parathyroid hormone production and malignancy. Brit. Med. J., *1*:204, 1972.

Omenn, G. S., et al.: Hyperparathyroidism associated with malignant tumors of nonparathyroid origin. Cancer, *24*:1004, 1969.

Reiss, E., and Canterbury, J. M.: Genesis of hyperparathyroidism. Amer. J. Med., *50*:679, 1971.

Roth, S. I., et al.: The eosinophilic cells of the parathyroid (oxyphil cells), salivary (onocytes), and thyroid (Hürthle cells) glands. Lab. Invest., *11*:933, 1962.

Sherwood, L. M., et al.: Parathyroid hormone secretion in vitro: regulation by calcium and magnesium ions. Nature, 225:1056, 1970.

Sherwood, L. M., et al.: Regulation of parathyroid hormone secretion: proportional control by calcium, lack of effect of phosphate. Endocrinology, 83:1043, 1968.

Slatopolsky, E., et al.: Control of phosphate excretion in uremic man. J. Clin. Invest , 47:1865, 1968.

Spinner, M. W., et al.: Clinical and genetic heterogeneity in idiopathic Addison's disease and hypoparathyroidism. J. Clin. Endocr. Metab., 28:795, 1968.

Stanbury, S. W., and Lumb, G. A.: Metabolic studies of renal osteodystrophy. I. Calcium, phosphorus and nitrogen metabolism in rickets, osteomalacia and hyperparathyroidism, complicating chronic uremia and in the osteomalacia of the adult Fanconi syndrome. Medicine, 41:1, 1962.

Straus, F. H., II., and Paloyan, E.: The pathology of hyperparathyroidism. Surg. Clin. N. Amer., 49:27, 1969.

Trier, J.: The fine structure of the parathyroid gland. J. Biophys. Biochem. Cytol., 4:13, 1958.

Wasserman, R. H., and Taylor, A. N.: Metabolic roles of fat soluble vitamins D, E and K. Ann. Rev. Biochem., 41:179, 1972.

Pituitary Gland

Beck, J. S., et al.: Characterisation of an antiserum to human growth hormone and the localization of the hormone in the normal adult adenohypophysis. J. Path. Bact., 91:531, 1966.

Cardell, R. R., Jr., and Knighton, R. S.: The cytology of a human pituitary tumor: an electron microscopic study. Trans. Amer. Micr. Soc., 85:58, 1966.

Cassidy, C. E.: Cushing's disease caused by pituitary chromophobe adenomas in two patients. Metabolism, 9:1139, 1960.

Catt, K. J.: Pituitary function. Lancet, 1:827, 1970.

Costello, R. T.: Subclinical adenoma of the pituitary gland. Amer. J. Path., 12:205, 1936.

Currie, A. R., et al.: Low molecular weight corticotrophin in human pituitary glands in various systemic and endocrine diseases. Acta Endocr., 43:255, 1963.

Dingman, J. F., and Lim, N. Y.: Cushing's syndrome due to an ACTH secreting chromophobe adenoma. New Eng. J. Med., 267:696, 1962.

Doniach, I.: Cytology of pituitary adenomas. J. Roy. Coll. Phys. London, 6:299, 1972.

Escamilla, R. F., and Lisser, H.: Simmonds' disease. J. Clin. Endocr., 2:65, 1942.

Hamilton, C. R., Jr., et al.: Hyperthyroidism due to thyrotropin-producing pituitary chromophobe adenoma. New Eng. J. Med., 283:1077, 1970.

Kernohan, J. W., and Sayre, G. P.: Tumors of the pituitary gland and infundibulum. Fascicle Armed Forces Institute of Pathology, Washington, D.C., 1956, p. 13.

Kraus, J. E.: Neoplastic diseases of human hypophysis. Arch. Path., 39:343, 1945.

Love, J. G., and Marshall, T. M.: Craniopharyngiomas. Surg. Gynec. Obstet., 90:591, 1950.

Mautalen, C. A., and Mellinger, R. C.: Nonsuppressible adrenocortical function in a patient with untreated acromegaly. J. Clin. Endocr., 25:1423, 1965.

McCormick, W. F., and Halmi, N. S.: Absence of chromophobe adenomas from a large series of pituitary tumors. Arch. Path., 92:231, 1971.

McKay, D. G., et al.: The pathologic anatomy of eclampsia, bilateral cortical necrosis, pituitary necrosis, and other fatal complications of pregnancy and its possible relationship to the generalized Shwartzman phenomenon. Amer. J. Obstet. Gynec., 66:507, 1953.

McShan, W. H., and Hartley, M. W.: Production, storage and release of anterior pituitary hormones. Rev. Physiol. Biochem. Exp. Pharmacol., 56:264, 1965.

Nabarro, J. D. N.: Pituitary tumors and hypopituitarism. Brit. Med. J., 1:492, 1972.

Paiz, C., and Hennigar, G. R.: Electron microscopy and histochemical correlation of human pituitary cells. Amer. J. Path., 59:1139, 1970.

Phifer, R. F., et al.: Specific demonstration of the human hypophyseal cells which produce adrenocorticotropic hormone. J. Clin. Endocr., 31:347, 1970.

Purnell, D. C., et al.: Postpartum pituitary insufficiency (Sheehan's syndrome). Review of 18 cases. Mayo Clinic Proc., 39:321, 1964.

Purves, H. D., and Griesbach, W. E.: Studies on experimental goitre. VII: Thyroid carcinoma in rats treated with thiourea. Brit. J. Exp. Path., 27:294, 1946.

Russfield, A. B.: Adenohypophysis. In Bloodworth, J. M. B., Jr. (ed.): Endocrine Pathology. Baltimore, Williams and Wilkins Co., 1968, p. 75.

Schelin, U.: Chromophobe and acidophil adenomas of the human pituitary: a light and electron microscopic study. Acta Path. Microbiol. Scand., Suppl., 158:1, 1962.

Sheehan, H. L.: Neurohypophysis and hypothalamus. In Bloodworth, J. M. B., Jr. (ed.): Endocrine Pathology. Baltimore, Williams and Wilkins Co., 1968, p. 37.

Sheehan, H. L., and Summers, V. K.: The syndrome of hypopituitarism. Quart. J. Med., 18:319, 1949.

Thymus

Alpert, L. I., et al.: A histologic reappraisal of the thymus in myasthenia gravis. Arch. Path., 91:55, 1971.

Burnet, F. M., and Holmes, M. C.: Thymic changes in the mouse strain NZB in relation to the autoimmune state. J. Path. Bact., 88:229, 1964.

Dawson, M. A.: Thymoma associated with pancytopenia and Hashimoto's thyroiditis. Amer. J. Med., 52:406, 1972.

Goldstein, G., and Whittingham, S.: Experimental autoimmune thymitis. An animal model of human myasthenia gravis. Lancet, 2:315, 1966.

Hirst, E., and Robertson, T. I.: The syndrome of thymoma and erythroblastopenic anemia. A review of 56 cases including 3 case reports. Medicine, 46:225, 1967.

Jepson, J. H., and Lowenstein, L.: Inhibition of erythropoiesis by a factor present in the plasma of patients with erythroblastopenia. Blood, 27:425, 1966.

Katz, A., and Lattes, R.: Granulomatous thymoma or Hodgkin's disease of thymus? A clinical and histologic study and a reevaluation. Cancer, 23:1, 1969.

Kilman, J. W., and Klassen, K. P.: Thymoma. Amer. J. Surg., 121:170, 1971.

Larsson, O.: Thymoma and systemic lupus erythematosus in the same patient. Lancet, 2:665, 1963.

Lattes, R.: Thymomas and other tumors of the thymus: analysis of 107 cases. Cancer, 15:1224, 1962.

Legg, M. A., and Brady, W. J.: Pathology and clinical behavior of thymomas. A survey of 51 cases. Cancer, 18:1131, 1965.

Lindstrom, F. D., et al.: Thymoma associated with multiple myeloma. Arch. Intern. Med., 122:526, 1968.

Rubin, M., et al.: Clinical disorders associated with thymic tumors. Arch. Intern. Med., 114:389, 1964.

Schmid, J. R., et al.: Thymoma associated with pure red-cell agenesis: review of literature and report of 4 cases. Cancer, 18:216, 1965.

Strauss, A. J. L.: Myasthenia gravis, autoimmunity and the thymus. Advances Intern. Med., 14:241, 1968.

Strauss, A. J. L., and Kemp, P. G., Jr.: Serum autoantibodies in myasthenia gravis and thymoma: selective affinity for I-bands of striated muscle as a guide to identification of antigen(s). J. Immun., 99:945, 1967.

Takita, H., and Mongaya, R. B.: Thymoma, clinico-pathological observation. New York J. Med., 70:2667, 1970.

Van de Velde, R. L., and Friedman, N. B.: Thymic myoid cells and myasthenia gravis. Amer. J. Path., 59:347, 1970.

van der Geld, H. W. R., and Strauss, A. J. L.: Myasthenia gravis. Immunological relationship between striated muscle and thymus. Lancet, 1:57, 1966.

van der Geld, H. W. R., et al.: Reactivity of myasthenia gravis serum gamma-globulin with skeletal muscle and thymus demonstrated by immunofluorescence. Proc. Soc. Exp. Biol. Med., 115:782, 1964.

Wilkins, E. W., Jr., et al.: Cases of thymoma at the Massachusetts General Hospital. J. Thorac. Cardiovasc. Surg., 52:322, 1966.

Pineal Gland

Dayan, A. D., et al.: Atypical teratomas of the pineal and hypothalamus. J. Path. Bact., 92:1, 1966.

De Martino, C., et al.: Electron microscopic study of impuberal and adult rats, pineal body. Experientia, 20:556, 1964.

Relkin, R.: The pineal gland. New Eng. J. Med., 274:944, 1966.

30

THE SKIN

HERBERT MESCON, M.D.,* AND INTA A. GROTS, M.D.†

NORMAL

The skin is the largest single organ of the body. Its chief functions are concerned with sensation, protection, temperature regulation and control of water output. It is closely associated with the underlying structures, from which and through which it receives its nutrition, and because of its location it is in intimate relation with the external environment. There-

fore, its status is readily affected by general or local diseases of the body (e.g., excoriations seen in systemic Hodgkin's disease) as well as by purely external factors (excessive soap, ultraviolet light or poison ivy resin). More often, it is a combination of systemic and local factors which produces visible skin lesions. A typical example of this would be the drier, thinner, less rapidly growing, atrophic skin of the elderly patient that is more susceptible to the irritative, degreasing action of such agents as soaps, detergents and turpentine. The layers of the skin are, to some extent, continuous with the mucous membranes of the digestive, respiratory and genitourinary tracts. Diseases affecting the skin may also involve the urethra,

---

*Professor of Dermatology, Boston University School of Medicine.

†Assistant Professor of Dermatology, Boston University School of Medicine.

the vagina, the oral and nasal mucosa and the anorectal region. This combined mucosal and skin involvement can be seen in allergic states, such as drug eruptions with or without bullae.

ANATOMIC PHYSIOLOGY

SKIN LAYERS

The skin is composed of three closely related layers (Montagna, 1962). The outermost is called the *epidermis;* the middle layer, the *dermis* or *corium;* and the deepest layer, the *hypoderm* or *subcutaneous tissue.*

Epidermis. This is composed of layers of epithelium. The innermost zone is the *malpighian or prickle layer* and is several cells thick. The lowermost layer of malpighian cells is known as the *basal layer,* and is composed of tall, palisaded, columnar-like cells. The epithelium protrudes downward in finger-like projections, the *rete ridges,* into the upper portion of the dermis. As the prickle cells progress toward the surface, they become granular *(granular layer),* their nuclei become pyknotic and then disappear.

The outermost portion of the epidermis is called the *stratum corneum* or horny layer. Here keratinization, which by electron microscopy has been shown to start in the basal layer, is now complete. The cells have been transformed into scales without nuclei or granules, and cell boundaries are not ordinarily seen with the light microscope on routine sections. Usually this scaling is invisible grossly, but in disease processes, when it is increased or the keratin is abnormal, the scales may become visible. The stratum corneum is porous and loose, is closest to the external environment and tends to lose water. This continuous process of epithelial proliferation to replace the layers lost, and change from basal layer to corneum is known as *keratinization.* In the process of keratinization, hydrophilic lipids are produced which tend to help keep the horny layer from becoming overly dry. Sweat and sebum also tend to prevent dryness. In callus formation and scaling, it is this corneal layer which is thickened or abnormally formed. In some diseases in which scales are prominent, such as psoriasis, the epithelial turnover rate is much more rapid than normal, the scales retain their nuclei and no granular layer is present in the epidermis. This is known as *parakeratosis.* The stratified squamous epithelium of most of the normal mucosa of the lips, oral cavity and vagina has no granular layer and normally has an outer nucleated parakeratotic layer. In certain diseases, irregular keratinization occurs, often in a single cell or group of cells in the malpighian layer. This abnormal keratinization is known as *dyskeratosis.*

The epithelium, especially the basal layer, is continuous with the epithelium of the dermal appendages (hair, sebaceous and sweat glands), which extend into the dermis and hypoderm. There is considerable evidence which indicates that these basal cells and their appendageal extensions are pluripotential, i.e., they can form the surface type of epidermis or one or more appendages. In the healing of skin after a split thickness graft has been removed, or after surgical planing to remove acne scars, the epidermis and appendages will regrow as long as some of the deep portions of the appendages are still present. The basal layer may thus form keratin, sebaceous glands or hair follicles and, conversely, the sweat glands or ducts, sebaceous glands or hair follicle may give rise to surface epithelium (Eisen et al., 1955). Where all the epithelial structures have been destroyed, as by a severe burn, extensive x-radiation damage or full thickness grafts, reepithelialization will take place, usually without regrowth of appendages, by the epithelium which has grown over from the adjacent margins.

Melanocytes, dendritic cells which produce melanin containing organelles (melanosomes), are normally present between the basal cells. The melanosomes migrate into the dendritic processes of the melanocyte between the prickle cells and somehow are transferred from melanocyte to prickle cell.

Dermis. This is composed of a connective tissue stroma containing the blood vessels, nerves, various nerve end organs, lymphatics, arrectores pilorum muscles, and dermal appendages. The upward extensions of the dermis between the epithelial finger-like rete ridges are known as the *dermal papillae.* The connective tissue itself is composed chiefly of collagenous and elastic fibers which play a considerable role in the elasticity of the skin. It is the *elastic fibers* which rupture in pregnancy, Cushing's syndrome and even occasionally in the normal pubertal period to produce striae. The connective tissue fibers degenerate in skin exposed to sunlight for years (solar elastosis).

The direction of the collagen bundles determines which way the skin will "pull" when an incision is made. It must be kept in mind that this direction or line *(Langer's lines)* varies in different parts of the body and in different age groups so that no one pattern is applicable in all cases. Wherever possible, when taking a skin biopsy or excising a skin tumor, the long axis of an ellipitcal incision should parallel the direction of the collagen bundles, or there will be a greater tendency for the wound to pull apart.

Subcutaneous Tissues. These serve as a receptacle for the storage of fat and as the support for the vessels and nerves passing from the tissue below to the corium above. Some of the hair follicles and sweat glands extend into this layer. In the penis, the scrotum, the eyelids and the auricle of the ear, there is no fat. In other areas, fat tends to accentuate the natural body contours. This fat may undergo inflammatory processes. Diseases of the small arterioles or venules in the hypoderm may, by extension, involve the dermis.

APPENDAGES AND SPECIAL STRUCTURES

Hairs. Hairs are specialized keratinous structures produced by the hair bulb. The number of hairs varies in different parts of the body. In examining a slide, we must know what is normal for that area of the skin, as well as the age and sex of the patient.

Hairs grow at different rates (scalp, 0.3 mm. per day) and thicknesses in various parts of the body. Any single hair follicle goes through a cycle with the following stages: (1) growth (anagen); (2) a transitional phase with cessation of active proliferation (catagen); and (3) rest and elimination of the old hair (telogen); then a new cycle starts. In the stage of growth, the hair follicles are located deeper in the dermis than they are in the periods of rest and elimination. In humans, adjacent hair follicles may be in different stages at any given time. Individual hair follicles are more susceptible to disease and damage during the anagen stage of the hair cycle. An example of this is the increased susceptibility of hair follicles to x-radiation or invasion by certain fungi during the stage of active growth. If a growing hair is mechanically plucked, the cycle of growth starts again after a variable period of rest ranging up to four months (Montagna and Ellis, 1958).

In a disease process, if the entire hair follicle and hair-producing bulb are destroyed, there will probably be no regrowth. This may occur in an extensive, deep, local infection with necrosis and deep scarring, or in extensive scleroderma, lupus erythematosus or radiation burns. However, if the destruction of the hair bulb is partial, as with a temporary epilating dose of x-radiation, or in small furuncles or abscesses, hair regrowth is likely. Following certain severe illnesses, i.e., typhoid fever, pneumonia, diphtheria and possibly severe psychogenic trauma, there may be temporary or rarely permanent hair loss, depending upon how severe the insult is to the hair bulb. It must be remembered that there is usually a lag period of two to three weeks before growing hair damaged by disease or radiation will fall out. Again, just as in plucking, there is usually a lag period of several months before hair regrows, if it will.

The hair bulb, in the active stage of growth, is one of the most mitotically active regions of the body. It is thus easy to understand why hormonal, nutritional and "toxic" factors may influence the growth rate to a considerable extent. The best available evidence suggests that, while the cyclic activity of the hair follicles may be modified by hormones, the factors bringing about the changes in the hair cycle are essentially inherent in the follicle itself. All hormones with androgenic activity, regardless of their point of origin, whether from testicles, adrenal cortex or ovaries, have a stimulating effect on the germinative epithelium. However, male baldness after the pubertal period is a well known and frequent occurrence. This does not occur in eunuchs.

Nails. Nails are a modified type of keratin. Growth occurs predominantly from the epithelium beneath the proximal portion of the *nail fold* from a region about 3 mm. proximal to the visible portion of the nail. This is called the *nail matrix.* The nail itself *(nail plate)* is produced at the rate of about 1 mm. a week and, if removed, it takes about three months to be completely replaced. An inflammatory process at the growing portion of the nail may interfere with nail growth temporarily or permanently, depending on the degree of the damage. In temporary damage, such as a local infection extending to involve the growing portion, lasting a week and then healing, it may take an additional few weeks for the damaged nail plate to grow from beneath the nail fold and be visible, manifesting itself as a groove or some other defect. The groove will move distally about 1 mm. a week and, therefore, be visible for about three months. If there is a pigmented lesion beneath the nail fold and the pigment is incorporated into the keratin forming the nail plate, there may then be a pigmented streak along the entire length of the nail. If it were decided to perform a biopsy on the lesion, the place to excise or take the biopsy specimen would be beneath the proximal nail fold and not the distal portion of the nail plate even though that is also pigmented.

Beneath the visible portion of the hard nail plate is the nail bed. This is composed of stratified squamous epithelium, like the rest of the skin. Its keratin layer lies just beneath the nail plate, which glides over it as the nail grows. When we remove a nail by surgical avulsion, we do not remove the underlying keratin of the nail bed. In fungal infections of the nail, the keratin of the nail bed is often also involved. This explains the high rate of recurrence of fungal infections of the nail (onychomycosis) after surgical avulsion of the nail plate, unless the keratin of the nail bed is also removed by energetic curettage. This does not interfere with nail growth if the growing portion of the nail beneath the proximal nail fold is not curetted. The nails, like the hair, are one of the most actively growing portions of the body. Their growth may be easily interfered with by nutritional deficiencies, endocrine or other systemic disease. Striations of the nails which move distally have been seen several weeks following an attack of acute myocardial infarction. In most cases of nail abnormalities, a definite etiologic factor cannot be ascertained.

The nails, like the hairs, are derived from and are part of the epithelium of the skin. In general or local disease of the skin, abnormal nail growth may also be present. In psoriasis, nail changes, clinically not too specific, may rarely precede and often accompany psoriasis of other portions of the skin. In severe exfoliative dermatitis, the nails may be pitted, thickened or even shed just as the remainder of the surface epithelium exfoliates.

Eccrine Sweat Glands. These secrete a watery, salty, clear fluid. They are most profuse on the palms and soles but are also present over most of the remainder of the skin surface and serve chiefly as a means of regulating body temperature by the evaporation of this fluid. The concentrations of urea, ammonia and lactic acid are much greater in sweat than in blood. This high concentration of urea explains the uremic frost (crystals of urea) occurring in a uremic patient whose skin has not recently been washed. Sweat also contains large amounts of chlorides, and in profuse sweating, a large amount of chlorides may be lost. This is partly overcome by the process known as acclimatization, whereby persons in hot environments who sweat profusely tend to have diminution in the sweat chloride concentration, thereby conserving chlorides. In fibrocystic disease of the pancreas, there is increased chloride in the sweat.

These glands are supplied by sympathetic cholinergic nerve fibers so that acetylcholine stimulates them, and the atropine group of drugs inhibit them. A warm environment causes eccrine sweating over most of the body surface except the palms and soles, where sweating is due chiefly to psychic stimulation (mental tension or stress). Sympathectomy stops sweating in sympathectomized areas. Because the eccrine sweat glands are located deep in the dermis and occasionally even in the subcutaneous fat, they are among the most resistant of the dermal appendages to x-radiation. Only deep ulceration destroys them, and because they can produce sweat ducts and surface epithelium, their role in surface wound healing becomes a major one.

Apocrine Sweat Glands. These glands are found chiefly in the axillae, around the nipples and in the periumbilical and anogenital regions, and secrete a milky, opaque, fatty fluid in relatively small amounts. Ordinarily they do not start functioning until puberty and involute at menopause. They are usually stimulated by emotional stress or sexual excitement and are probably under adrenergic control. Contrary to common belief, the fatty secretion itself has little or no odor. However, following bacterial decomposition of the secretion by the bacteria normally found on the skin in those areas, the typical malodor is noticeable.

Sebaceous Glands. These glands are present in the skin over the entire body except the palms and soles and secrete an oily material, sebum. They are most numerous on the face and scalp. Usually they empty into the pilosebaceous follicle. The exact mechanism for stimulation of secretion of these glands is not well understood. They tend to increase in size under androgenic stimulation. Occasionally, they may be seen as yellow-orange pinpoint dots on the buccal or lip mucosa and have no pathologic significance when seen in these regions.

SKIN COLOR

Skin color is due to a combination of several factors (Rothman, 1954). The most important are the following: physical properties of the skin (Tyndall effect); the amount, distribution and oxygenation of the blood; and the amount and distribution of the pigments of the skin, chiefly carotene and melanin.

Physical Properties (Tyndall Effect). Skin is, like many other tissues, a suspension of proteins in water. This suspension tends to *transmit the red* portion of the visible light spectrum, but to *reflect chiefly the blue* wave lengths. Thus, a blood vessel located in the mid-dermis, although it contains red blood, tends to reflect light that is thrown upon it and to appear as a blue vessel. On the other hand, if a light is placed inside the mouth and the cheeks are observed, the *transmitted* color is red. A blood vessel or other structure *very close* to the skin surface might appear its natural red color because there is insufficient overlying skin to have an appreciable Tyndall effect. This is readily seen in tiny, dilated, *superficial* blood vessels (telangiectasia) occurring on the nose of a middle-aged person. A varicose vein deeply *beneath* the skin looks blue. Hemorrhage into the skin, therefore, will vary in color from bright red to purple-blue depending on its depth and, later, its conversion to hemosiderin.

Blood Supply. The amount of blood in the superficial capillaries determines whether the skin looks pale or erythematous. The total blood supply to the skin, usually controlled by deeper arterioles, determines whether it feels warm or cool. If the blood is oxygenated, it will appear redder than if most of the hemoglobin is in the reduced form. An area of stasis or insufficient oxygenation will tend to look blue. Thus, one can have a pale warm extremity, or a cold red extremity or any combination of the two, depending on the patency and blood flow through superficial or deep blood vessels.

Skin Pigments. *Carotene*, related to vitamin A adds a yellow component to normal skin color. It is lipid-soluble and is stored in lipid rich areas of subcutaneous fat as well as in the lipids of keratin. It is present in greater amounts in females and male castrates than in normal males, especially in the breast, abdomen and buttocks. Its presence in keratin tends to account for the yellow tinge of areas of thickened keratin, e.g., palms and soles.

Melanin is an additional pigment whose chemistry and physiology are not completely understood. Melanin formation occurs in the melanocytes, in ultramicroscopic organelles called melanosomes. The enzymically inactive end-stage is the melanin granule. Melanocytes are located chiefly in the basal layer, the retina and the meninges. Tyrosine, the precursor, is converted to dopa dihydroxyphenylalanine, to dopa quinone and, through a series of intermediary steps, to tan (reduced) melanin and black (oxidized) melanin.

The conversion from tyrosine to dopa is facilitated by the enzyme tyrosinase. This enzyme is a copper-protein compound normally present in the skin in an inactivated form. It becomes activated by sunlight or ultraviolet light. It is present in an inactivated form in pigmented nevi, and in an active form in malignant melanoma. This difference has been used with limited success to differentiate between histologically doubtful cases. Tyrosinase is inhibited by sulfhydryl (-SH) groups normally present in the skin. The explanation of increased pigmentation in some inflammatory skin conditions may be that -SH groups are diminished in inflammation and allow tyrosinase to become activated. In heavy metal poisoning, such as arsenic intoxication, the increased skin pigmentation is thought to be due to the local inhibition of -SH groups by the arsenic. This may also account for increased melanin seen in patients with hemochromatosis in which iron is deposited in the skin.

Dopa oxidase converts dopa to melanin. Placing a fresh section of an amelanotic malignant melanoma in a solution of dopa or tyrosine will usually result in pigment formation. This test has sometimes been used to identify amelanotic melanomas when they are anaplastic, do not contain melanin and thus are difficult to identify.

The hormonal control of melanin formation has been discussed on page 1300.

PATHOLOGY

It must be remembered that because the skin can be directly observed, many of the clinical objective findings actually represent the gross pathology of the various dermatologic diseases. Therefore, in the following section, the clinical description usually includes the macroscopic pathology. The clinical picture (gross pathology) as it presents itself to the physician is often a combination of the underlying skin disease modified by four superimposed or complicating factors.

SUPERIMPOSED FACTORS

These are the following: (1) secondary bacterial or fungal infection; (2) miliaria or heat rash; (3) psychogenic factors; and (4) treatment (superimposed allergic sensitivity or irritancy).

Infection. The oozing, serous, crusted or hemorrhagic material that may be present on the surface of an acute dermatitis is largely protein similar to that of blood. This, as well as loose moist keratin, is an excellent culture medium at body surface temperature for many bacteria and fungi. They may easily grow to the point of becoming a major problem in themselves and certainly will complicate the clinical and histologic picture. Coagulase-positive staphylococci may be cultured from the skin of about 40 per cent of normal persons. This increases to over 90 per cent when cultures are taken from patients with various dermatitides. Beta hemolytic streptococci are found on less than 10 per cent of normal skins. This percentage increases to about 40 per cent when dermatitis is present. There have been estimates that the dermatophytic fungi can be cultured from the skin of up to 50 per cent of apparently normal persons without clinical fungus disease. Thus, a positive culture of a bacterium or fungus in itself does not necessarily mean that the organism is the causative agent or in any way contributes to the disease process. The clinician must decide the role of the organisms in the individual case and adjust his therapy accordingly.

Miliaria. As will be pointed out in more detail, in many skin diseases, the application of materials to the skin (even salt water for 12 hours) causes disturbance of the flow or delivery of sweat to the surface. If the body temperature is then elevated either locally or systemically, causing increased production of sweat by the glands, rupture of the sweat duct may occur and result in a secondary heat rash. If the underlying disease process affects the palms, soles or axillae, psychogenic factors will induce sweating which may complicate eruptions in these regions.

Psychogenic Factors. Pruritus (itching) is one of the most common symptoms in dermatologic disease. There is considerable evidence to show that the individual interpretation of the symptom of itching may be influenced considerably by psychogenic factors. The threshold for experimentally produced itching is lower when the patient is emotionally upset than when he is relaxed. In the same patient, the threshold is lower at the end of the day than it is in the morning. This lowered threshold to itching results in greater scratching and, therefore, greater mechanical trauma and excoriations with possible superimposed infection resulting in alteration of the histologic and clinical picture.

Treatment. Many of the materials used in treatment of dermatologic disorders or in routine skin hygiene may, in themselves, irritate an already damaged skin or actually cause local or generalized superimposed allergic eruptions. This may result in more itching and scratching, more trauma, more oozing, more opportunity for superimposed infection, more psychogenic stress and often demands far more extensive and elaborate therapy with the additional possibility of further irritation and sensitivity.

Thus, we see the potential vicious cycle that the four complicating factors may initiate, thereby considerably altering the presenting clinical and histopathologic picture. In order, therefore, to correctly interpret a lesion both clinically and histopathologically, it may be important to know the treatment that has been given, and make this, as well as other pertinent clinical information, available to the pathologist, so that he and the clinician may best evaluate the histopathologic findings. It is also important to select for a biopsy specimen the portion of the lesion that is the most active and, at the same time, has the minimum of the superimposed factors just mentioned, in order to make a more accurate diagnosis of the underlying skin disease. It may often be necessary to bring some of these superimposed complicating factors under control before taking a biopsy specimen.

It must be emphasized that, in most skin diseases, scarring usually does not occur. The depth of the process and its extent, particularly with respect to destruction of tissue, will determine whether any residual scarring will be evident. Most inflammatory skin diseases are relatively superficial. In contrast, in an extensive full-thickness burn in which the skin appendages are completely destroyed, complete repair does not occur and scarring usually results (p. 93).

Because of space limitations, all dermatopathologic entities cannot be covered. In view of the preponderance of certain clinical entities, these will be discussed in more detail, and other less common entities will be mentioned more briefly under etiologic or morphologic groups. Without apology, the rarer disorders are omitted, since they must be relegated more reasonably to specialized texts (Lever, 1967) (Pillsbury et al., 1956).

DEFINITION OF TERMS

Before describing the gross and microscopic pathology of skin, it is important that we define some of our descriptive terms.

MACROSCOPIC PATHOLOGIC TERMS

Macule: circumscribed spot, nonpalpable, not raised above the level of the skin. Example: freckle.

Papule: circumscribed, solid lesion, elevated above the level of the skin, palpable, up to 5 mm. in largest diameter. Example: acne "pimple."

Nodule: circumscribed, solid, elevated lesion of the skin over 5 mm. in diameter. Example: pigmented nevus.

Vesicle: circumscribed, elevated lesion of the skin, containing fluid, up to 5 mm. in diameter. Example: herpes simplex.

Bulla: circumscribed, elevated lesion of the skin containing fluid, over 5 mm. in diameter. Example: large lesion of contact dermatitis due to poison ivy.

Pustule: circumscribed, elevated lesion of the skin, up to 5 mm. in diameter, containing pus. Example: acne pustule.

Wheal: circumscribed, red-white transient elevation of the skin, approximately 0.5 to 10 cm. in diameter, formed by local edema. Example: the common "hives."

Squamous or Scaly: having dried, thin, epithelial, horny lamellae, usually resulting from imperfect cornification. Example: scales of psoriasis.

Lichenification: thickening and exaggeration of normal skin markings and furrows, usually due to persistent scratching. Example: localized neurodermatitis.

Fissure: a crack in the skin, usually extending into the upper corium. Example: crack over knuckles in chronic contact dermatitis of hands.

Excoriation: a self-produced traumatized area, usually "dug out" or linear. Example: scratch mark following a mosquito bite.

Telangiectasis: localized dilatation of individual superficial blood vessels. Example: spider nevus.

MICROSCOPIC PATHOLOGIC TERMS

Hyperkeratosis: thickening of the stratum corneum (horny layer). Example: callus.

Parakeratosis: retention of the nuclei in the stratum corneum (horny layer). Normally seen in true mucous membrane of mouth and vagina. Example: scale of psoriasis.

Acanthosis: thickening of the prickle cell layer. Example: thickening in a wart.

Dyskeratosis: faulty development of the epidermis, resulting in abnormal keratinization often within individual cells of the prickle layer. Example: actinic keratosis.

Acantholysis: loss of cohesion between cells of the epidermis, usually leading to vesicles and bullae. Example: pemphigus.

Pyknosis: darkening and shrinking of nuclei. Example: mycosis fungoides.

Karyorrhexis: fragmentation of nuclei. Example: mycosis fungoides.

Papillomatosis: upward proliferation of the dermal papillae and corresponding intervening downward projection of the rete ridges. Example: exfoliative dermatitis.

FREQUENTLY OCCURRING SKIN DISEASES

ACNE VULGARIS

This disease, which involves a certain type of pilosebaceous unit, the "sebaceous follicle," characterized by *large* sebaceous glands and ducts and small hairs, is one of the most common skin diseases. It affects, at some time of life, to some degree, a majority of the population. It usually occurs during adolescence, involving the face and, less frequently, the upper chest and back.

Although there may be many unknown factors that play a role in acne, the central theme of this disease revolves around sebum, the complex lipid liberated by the breakdown of the sebaceous cells. It differs greatly from other body fats in its high percentage of free fatty acids. The injection of whole sebum into the skin duplicates the pathologic findings of the natural disease of acne. On fractionation of sebum, the free fatty acids, especially the short-chain acids, produce the greatest degree of inflammation. Acne can be viewed basically as a "perifolliculitis" following the rupture of the follicular contents into the dermis. In general, the greater the amount of sebum, the more severe the disease process. However, this is not an absolute rule, for many people with high sebum output do not have acne. Acne is not seen in the absence of large sebaceous glands. Sebum is the fuel, but a "susceptibility" factor must be present. A similar situation exists, for instance, in the case of duodenal ulcers. Hydrochloric acid is a necessary fuel, but ulcers do not occur in everyone with high hydrochloric acid output.

The sebaceous glands are not under nervous control, but are governed by hormones. Because of the necessity for having sebum as the "fuel," the hormonal status of patients assumes an important role. The sebaceous glands of the prepubertal child are tiny masses of undifferentiated lipid-free epithelial cells. Acne does not occur under these circumstances. At the time of puberty, marked glandular hyperplasia with lipid differentiation represents one of the signs in the constellation of androgenic effects. In addition to androgens, which are the prime regulatory substances, large amounts of cortisol also will induce glandular hyperplasia in susceptible subjects, thus explaining the tendency of patients on prolonged high-dose corticosteroid therapy to develop acne. Estrogens do not have any direct effect on the sebaceous glands; only when large unphysiologic amounts, which induce systemic effects, are administered is there any decrease in gland size. Although most authors feel that a high fat diet and psychogenic stress aggravate acne, the roles of diet, skin cleanliness, vitamin A and emotions have probably been overemphasized in the past and are difficult to evaluate.

Grossly, acne is a disease with blackheads (open comedones), whiteheads (closed comedones), papules, pustules, varying sized nodules and scars. The histopathology reflects this pleomorphism. The exact mechanism of the resultant microscopic picture is not definitely settled. In acne, as in any inflammatory process involving the sebaceous glands, the glands may secondarily atrophy or be completely destroyed, they may dedifferentiate toward stratified squamous epithelium even to the point of pseudo-epitheliomatous hyperplasia, or may undergo keratinization and result in keratin cysts or deep keratin crypts. Some of these changes are reversible. Recent work attributes the inflammation to two processes: perforation of the wall of the "sebaceous follicle" with the development of a surrounding perifolliculitis, or rupture of a comedone with perifolliculitis. When the follicular wall is perforated, it causes an inflammatory infiltrate, which varies from polymorphonuclear neutrophilic leukocytes to lymphocytes. It may eventually engulf and destroy the entire follicle, or the epithelium may proliferate and surround the inflammatory zone, suggesting an intrafollicular lesion.

The comedo, which is the only microscopically characteristic lesion of acne, is a dilated follicle with a thin wall and tiny sebaceous glands, filled with an impaction composed of laminated keratin and sebum. Rupture of this lesion leads to inflammatory changes, which usually are of the foreign body type. As healing proceeds, more mononuclear cells and fibroblasts appear, and the process is similar to that described for follicular perforation. The amount of scar tissue is variable.

The bacterial flora of acne are widely disputed. With careful techniques, employing the usual media, most of the lesions appear sterile, and therefore staphylococci are not the major element in the disease. However, *Corynebacterium acnes*, an anaerobic organism that is difficult to culture routinely, can easily be isolated on suitable media and has been seen in tissue sections.

As already stated, with the exception of comedones, most of the changes in acne are nonspecific and represent a perifolliculitis so that the diagnosis is based more on the clinical picture than on the isolated histologic finding of perifolliculitis.

MILIARIA

This disease of the eccrine sweat apparatus is commonly known as heat rash but is seen much more frequently than anticipated from its name, as it may occur in any season of the year. It is thought to be *due to keratinous plugging of the superficial portions of the sweat ducts* (O'Brien, 1950). This can be produced experimentally by the local application for 12 hours of salt, sweat, urine, soaps, salt water, medications or other agents. Even plain tap water applied constantly by a wet patch test for 12 hours results in this plugging. This is only a microscopic plugging without inflammatory reaction and, at first, no abnormality is visible to the naked eye. If the sweat glands are then stimulated in the involved area, the sweat cannot get to the surface, *the sweat duct ruptures and a heat rash develops.* It is commonly seen the day following a sunburn. The ultraviolet light rays act as the irritant to cause plugging of the duct.

The first evidence is a very superficial vesicle in the horny layer filled with clear fluid. Sometimes, with serial sections, the sweat duct can be seen entering the vesicle. At this stage, the disease is called **miliaria crystallina.** The vesicle can be easily brushed off, because the duct rupture is so superficial and the vesicle is contained within the stratum corneum. If the stimulus to plugging of the sweat duct persists, deeper plugging and a deeper vesicle result, usually in the mid or lower epidermis or upper dermis, followed by an inflammatory reaction composed chiefly of lymphocytes and dilatation of the blood vessels causing a small red papule. This stage is called **miliaria rubra.** Because miliaria crystallina is such a superficial and transient disease, biopsies are rarely taken. The diagnosis is usually made clinically. However, if one sees histologically the superficial vesicle with the sweat duct entering it, the slide is diagnostic. Likewise, in miliaria rubra, if one is able to see the ruptured sweat duct entering a zone of edema and inflammation, the diagnosis can be suggested by the pathologist. Even if other skin diseases are present, the pathologist can sometimes visualize the histologic changes described and can suggest miliaria as a complication of the other disease.

The ideal treatment of miliaria is to remove the cause of the plugging of the sweat duct or reduce the stimulus to excessive perspiration. If a warm climate is the cause of excessive perspiration, this is not easy to control and explains the widespread incidence of this disease. In the South Pacific and other tropical areas during World War II, and in the Vietnamese war, miliaria was a very common skin disease *(tropical anhidrosis).* Occasionally, it would interfere with the excretion of sweat to such a degree that body temperature could not be satisfactorily controlled, and the efficiency of the patient was interfered with considerably. Many of the diaper rashes are, in part, a miliaria, the urine acting as the irritant.

This same process accounts for many of the "bed rashes" seen in hospitalized patients. They are washed with soap, which is usually inadequately removed in the small basin of water used to cleanse the patient. These patients are often in overheated wards and frequently lie in one position for long periods of time. This is particularly true of the paralyzed patient in an overheated respirator for extended periods of time. Many of the cases of so-called adhesive tape dermatitis are not true allergic reactions to adhesive tape, but are miliaria developing under the tape which acts as an irritant in an area that is experiencing marked stimulus to sweat due to environmental warmth. It has been shown that if the stimulus is removed, superficial plugging of the sweat duct will resolve in about 12 hours. Inflammatory processes of the skin will often, in themselves, result in plugging of the sweat ducts and may, therefore, superimpose miliaria on the underlying skin disease if the patient is stimulated to sweat excessively. In addition, production of sweat by the eccrine gland itself is interfered with in the involved areas in psoriasis, and this may also occur in other diseases.

SEBORRHEIC DERMATITIS

Seborrheic dermatitis is usually an erythematous, papulosquamous eruption of unknown etiology. The most common and mildest form of the disease is known as "dandruff." The technical name for this mild phase is *seborrhea*. It probably occurs in varying degrees of severity in at least half the adult population. Frequently, the scales and associated oily material may appear matted and yellow. This condition is common in infants and is known as "cradle cap."

The erythematous, raised, scaling lesions may coalesce and form plaques. Often they are pruritic, and secondary excoriations and superimposed local infection may be seen. The lesions usually occur on the scalp, eyebrows, forehead, behind the ears, on the skin of the external ears, face, presternum, axillary and inguinal regions. Rarely, the disease may become generalized and even go on to an exfoliative dermatitis; at other times, it may involute spontaneously. The exact relationship of the sebaceous glands to this disease process is not well understood.

The histologic picture is that of a nonspecific chronic dermatitis (p. 1384) and is not diagnostic. Consistent with the clinical scaling, there is usually hyperkeratosis and parakeratosis. The prickle layer shows moderate acanthosis with some elongation of the rete ridges and slight to moderate, poorly defined edema. The dermal papillae and upper dermis usually contain a mild, scattered, chiefly lymphocytic infiltrate with a few polymorphonuclear neutrophilic leukocytes, as well as some edema. The lower dermis and dermal appendages, including the sebaceous glands, are not remarkable.

Occasionally all variations, both clinically and histologically, may be seen between seborrheic dermatitis and psoriasis.

PSORIASIS

This disease is an erythematous eruption, often in papules or plaques, usually having a white silvery scale. It usually occurs in adults, but children may also be affected. The scalp,

the extensor surfaces of the elbows and knees and the lower portion of the back are the most common sites of involvement, but any part or all of the skin may be involved.

The exact etiology is unknown. Various metabolic and dietary factors have been incriminated in the past, but their exact role is still to be defined. The role of psychogenic factors in this disease may be an important one. Patients with psoriasis have a much greater incidence of a rheumatoid type of arthritis than the general population for unknown reasons. The severity of the disease varies considerably with and without treatment.

The **pathognomonic** histologic picture requires the following features: (1) parakeratosis, (2) acanthosis with thinning of the suprapapillary epidermis, (3) elongation of the rete ridges and dermal papillae, (4) occasional epidermal microabscesses containing polymorphonuclear neutrophilic leukocytes, (5) edema and some clubbing (widening of the upper portion) of the dermal papillae and (6) dilated straight capillaries in the dermal papillae (Figs. 30–1 and 30–2).

This last feature associated with a thin suprapapillary epidermis accounts for the fine bleeding points seen when the scales are scraped. Rarely are all these histologic features seen in one section. When some but not all are present, the lesion may not be diagnostic, and the pathologist may report *psoriasiform dermatitis*. The latter nondiagnostic pattern may be seen in psoriasis but also in other diseases having a nonspecific histologic picture, such as neurodermatitis, exfoliative dermatitis, seborrheic dermatitis, chronic contact dermatitis and others. Occasionally, the disease may become so diffuse as to result in an exfoliative dermatitis. When this occurs in a case of psoriasis, the exfoliative dermatitis will usually retain many of its histologic psoriasiform features and be microscopically suggestive of its origin from psoriasis.

CONTACT DERMATITIS

Contact dermatitis is an inflammatory reaction of the skin caused by contact with something in the external environment. It frequently results in what is called *eczema or eczematous dermatitis*. These latter terms refer to any eruption characterized by oozing, redness, thickening and occasionally fissuring and crusting, and usually passing through an acute to a more chronic phase clinically. The term has been used as a "wastebasket" to include a multiplicity of skin eruptions, some of which

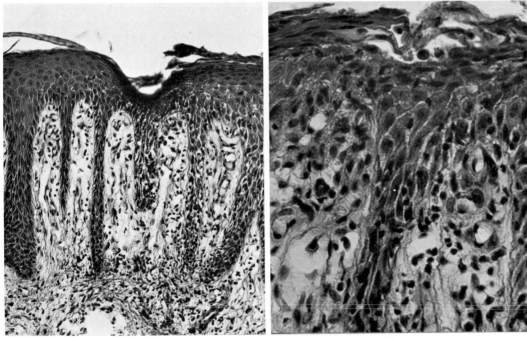

Fig. 30–1   Fig. 30–2

Figure 30–1. *Psoriasis, low power, showing parakeratosis, edematous dermal papillae, thin suprapapillary zone, elongation of rete ridges and mild dermal inflammatory infiltrate.*

Figure 30–2. *Psoriasis, high power. Note parakeratosis, beginning microabscess high in epidermis, and thin suprapapillary zone.*

can now be classified on an etiologic basis. As we come to know more about many of these "eczemas," we should use the term less frequently and employ the more specific etiologic terminology.

Eczema and eczematous dermatitis as well as one of their major prototypes, contact dermatitis, are characterized by a nonspecific, acute, subacute or chronic inflammatory skin reaction histologically. With respect to the nonspecificity of the histologic pattern of reaction, it is important to note that many common diseases, some of which have fairly specific clinical pictures, are nonetheless characterized by equally nonspecific changes. These include atopic dermatitis, localized neurodermatitis, seborrheic dermatitis, exfoliative dermatitis, pityriasis rosea, some drug eruptions and others. To illustrate a histologic nonspecific dermatitis, contact dermatitis has been selected as a prototype and will be discussed in some detail.

Those contactants that cause this disease may be divided into two groups: those that act as primary irritants and those that act as true allergic sensitizers. With more and more chemicals used in our everyday life, both at home and at work, as medications and as constituents of many of our commonly used products, the incidence of contact dermatitis has increased tremendously and is likely to continue to do so. Contact dermatitis is one of the most common causes of industrial skin disease and skin disability. It is noteworthy that about two-thirds of all industrial compensation cases throughout the country are due to dermatologic diseases and that most of these are contact dermatitis. Both groups of contact dermatitis can give rise to acute, subacute or chronic clinical or histologic pictures.

Primary Irritancy. This can be caused by numerous materials, including compounds such as strong alkalis and acids. Many times, minute amounts of these may not be harmful, but higher concentrations or prolonged exposure will result in irritancy in a large segment of the population. Nitric acid and 50 per cent phenol are good examples of such irritants. Occasionally, some of these compounds act indirectly. An example of this is the degreasing action of cutting oils commonly used in industry, or prolonged exposure to soaps or detergents of some housewives. These substances remove the lipids and other hydrophilic material which may be present in the skin or on its surface and cause considerable dryness. If these compounds are stronger or if their use is prolonged, clinical lesions may develop.

One may see all variations from dryness and scaling to oozing, erythema, vesicles, crusting, thickening of the skin and fissuring. When the etiologic agent is removed, the skin will usually tend to repair completely. If there has been sufficient inflammation, some hyperpigmentation or depigmentation may persist for variable periods of time.

Histologically, the picture is not diagnostic and is that of a nonspecific dermatitis, either acute, subacute or chronic.

In **acute dermatitis**, the epidermis contains vesicles and bullae with variable inter- and intracellular epidermal edema. Usually, the vesicle contents will include lymphocytes with some eosinophils and neutrophils. If the edema is of sufficient degree, the basal layer is disrupted and may not be identifiable. There is a moderate upper dermal lymphocytic and, occasionally, neutrophilic infiltrate and edema. Except in severe cases, the lower and mid-dermis are not involved. When the vesicles rupture, crusts composed of precipitated fibrin, necrotic debris, epithelial cells and polymorphonuclear leukocytes can be seen on the surface.

In **subacute dermatitis** the vesicles are smaller and ordinarily not visible to the naked eye, but can be seen with the microscope under low power. There is usually less edema than is found in the acute dermatitis; moderate acanthosis and parakeratosis are usually present. An inflammatory infiltrate, composed chiefly of lymphocytes with some neutrophils and eosinophils, is present in the upper and to a lesser extent the mid-dermis, and often is predominantly perivascular in distribution. The lower dermis is not remarkable (Fig. 30–3).

In **chronic dermatitis**, no vesicles are present. There is moderate to marked acanthosis and variable hyperkeratosis with scattered parakeratosis. The rete ridges are somewhat elongated; the basal layer is usually intact. The edema may not be noticeable or is very minimal. A slight to moderate lymphocytic infiltrate is usually present in the upper and, to a lesser extend, the mid-dermis. Neutrophils are not seen. The lower dermis is not remarkable (Fig. 30–4).

Allergic Contact Dermatitis. Allergic contact dermatitis (dermatitis venenata) is the skin reaction due to true sensitivity to a compound *with which the skin has come in contact.* A common example is dermatitis due to the oleoresin of the poison ivy plant in sensitive persons. Local sensitivity to penicillin ointment or other medications gives a similar picture. The percentage of the population that will develop dermatitis on a sensitivity basis is usually much smaller than those that will develop primary irritancy from a high concentration of an irritant. Previous exposure to the compound or a similar chemically related com-

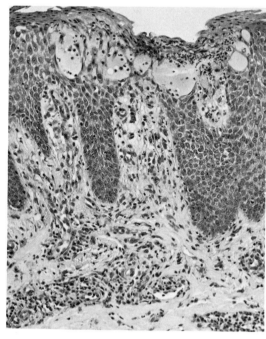

Fig. 30–3

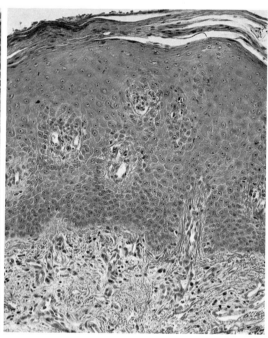

Fig. 30–4

Figure 30–3. Nonspecific subacute dermatitis showing small epidermal vesicles, parakeratosis, acanthosis and inflammatory infiltrate of dermis and epidermis. Note perivascular distribution in dermis.

Figure 30–4. Nonspecific chronic dermatitis. Note hyper- and parakeratosis, acanthosis and mild upper dermal lymphocytic infiltrate.

pound is necessary. This is usually followed by an incubation period of 10 to 14 days after the exposure during which time sensitization develops. Sensitization may occur after a single exposure or may not occur until repeated exposures. After the lag period, any further exposure may be an eliciting one and cause the eruption to occur, usually within hours to a few days after contact with the etiologic agent.

Erythema is usually the first clinical sign, followed by itching, vesiculation or formation of bullae. The vesicles often rupture and form crusts which may become secondarily infected. If the exposure to the allergen is prolonged, thickening of the skin usually occurs and fissures may develop. When the pruritus is severe enough, one may see scratch marks. If the sensitizing agent has not been removed from the skin and is rubbed by scratching into uninvolved areas, new lesions will occur. The inflammatory exudate or blister fluid itself does not contain the sensitizer in amounts sufficient to cause new lesions; if the sensitizer is removed, the eruption will clear completely, usually within a matter of a few weeks. Histologically, the picture is not diagnostic, but rather that of a nonspecific acute, subacute or chronic dermatitis (p. 1384).

Thus, we see that because of the frequent use of irritants and sensitizers in everyday life, contact dermatitides are common. The potential effect of these contactants on diseased skin may superimpose a nonspecific acute, subacute or chronic dermatitis on an underlying skin disease. Indeed, there is some evidence to show that diseased skin is more sensitive to irritants and allows for greater penetration of allergens and hence for more potential systemic as well as local reactions.

SYSTEMIC SENSITIVITY ERUPTIONS (URTICARIA, DRUG ERUPTION AND ERYTHEMA MULTIFORME)

Skin sensitivity to systemically administered allergens may manifest itself in many different ways. Any one drug or sensitizer may cause one of several types of eruptions in the same or different patients at the same or different times. Frequently, no definite allergen can be identified by history. A basophil degranulation or other serologic test may be helpful. The clinical and histologic picture of these eruptions is similar to those that occur when a definite etiology is known. In this section, our discussion will be limited to (1) *urticaria*, (2) *the erythematous papular and papulosquamous sensitivity eruptions so often seen in drug sensitivity* and (3) *erythema multiforme*. It must be

understood that these variants may occur singly or together in individual cases.

Urticaria. The exact incidence of this disease is not known because the majority of the cases of urticaria are extremely mild and never come to the attention of the physician. Usually only the more severely ill patients are seen by the dermatologist or are hospitalized.

Urticaria or "hives" manifests itself by transient erythematous wheals accompanied by pruritus. It may last only for hours or, at other times, persist for days. The lesions may disappear in one focus while reappearing in another. Often they can be extremely firm and well demarcated. In such cases, it is hard to believe that the lesion may not have been there a few hours earlier or that it may be gone a few hours later. In rare cases, the edema may be so marked as to be classified under the term **angioneurotic edema.** Occasionally, it may extend to the glottis and interfere with breathing. This is, however, an extremely uncommon complication. Histologically, moderate to marked dermal edema may be seen. When present in the absence of any other appreciable pathologic change, it is diagnostic. Sometimes in the process of fixation, the overall shrinkage of tissues masks the abnormal tissue spaces produced by the edema so that one is surprised to find no appreciable abnormal picture histologically, even though the biopsy was taken from a clinically typical site. A few lymphocytes, chiefly perivascular in location, may be present in the corium.

Usually the patient will respond to epinephrine, ephedrine, antihistamines or the cortisone group of steroids. The disease is self-limited if the etiologic agent is removed. In most cases of urticaria, particularly when they are persistent, the etiologic agent may never be ascertained. In some cases, however, of acute and particularly chronic recurrent urticaria, psychogenic factors are felt by many to play an etiologic or precipitating role.

Erythematous Papular and Papulosquamous Drug Eruptions. One of the most common types of *drug sensitivity reactions of the skin* is an erythematous papular or papulosquamous nonspecific eruption. This may be localized or generalized. When it is localized and tends to recur in the same site each time the drug is administered systemically, the clinical picture is known as a "fixed drug eruption." Phenolphthalein is a typical offender causing this type of eruption. Most drugs causing a generalized sensitivity eruption do not produce a clinically typical picture, and it is only a combination of the clinical picture with the history, occasionally aided by a biopsy, which will establish the diagnosis. One must constantly keep in mind that most drugs cause several different types of reactions. While it is true that they may cause predominantly an urticarial reaction in some cases, in others, a papulosquamous eruption or even an exfoliative dermatitis may be present. Sensitivity reaction to penicillin is an excellent example of this.

The lesions of the papulosquamous sensitivity eruptions usually start as bright red macules and papules with variable scaling. They may continue to become more widespread, even for several days or weeks after the drug has been stopped. If **new lesions continue to appear** for more than two or three weeks or **the old lesions last longer** than two months after a particular drug has been stopped, the diagnosis of that drug as the etiologic agent should be questioned. Usually the eruption lasts from a few days to two to three weeks but, in very rare cases, it may last up to two months. As the eruption starts to subside, the borders of the individual lesions may be somewhat less discrete and not so bright a shade of red. They usually become darker red to red-purple to salmon-brown and then disappear. In the process of regression, moderate scaling usually occurs. Occasionally, if there has been enough dilatation of the superficial capillaries, some petechiae may be seen, particularly in the dependent areas or over pressure points.

Histologically, the picture is not a diagnostic one, but rather that of a nonspecific subacute to chronic dermatitis previously described (p. 1384) (Fig. 30–5). There is usually some hyper- and variable parakeratosis, acanthosis and papillomatosis. Edema is not marked. A perivascular infiltrate is often seen in the mid-and upper corium, composed chiefly of lymphocytes but occasionally containing eosinophils. The presence of eosinophils suggests an allergic type of reaction.

Erythema Multiforme.

This is the last-mentioned variant of an allergic systemic sensitivity reaction. This reaction may manifest itself as a mild disorder with only focal lesions or, at other times, may be quite severe with widespread generalized involvement. In some cases of erythema multiforme, the disease is self-limited and an etiologic agent is not discernible. In other cases, a definite food or drug may be incriminated or there may be an *underlying infectious* or *malignant disease.*

As the name implies, erythema multiforme causes multiform lesions that may manifest themselves as papules, macules, urticarial lesions, vesicles or bullae. Sometimes there is central clearing and peripheral extension so that an "iris" type of lesion results. The lesions may extend peripherally

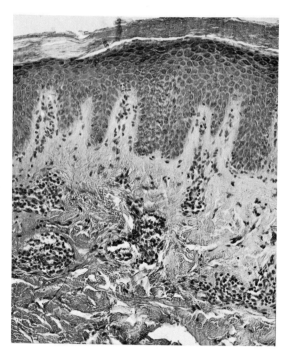

Figure 30–5. *Drug eruption—nonspecific chronic dermatitis. Note hyperkeratosis, acanthosis, elongated rete ridges and perivascular lymphocytic infiltrate.*

and become large and annular. Their margins may be quite distinct, raised, circumscribed or arciform, in which case they have been called **erythema marginatum.** Some investigators feel this latter type is seen only in rheumatic fever. Our experience does not agree with this. Small or large vesicles or bullae may be formed, in which case the disease is called **bullous erythema multiforme.**

Histologically, the picture is not a diagnostic one but rather that of a nonspecific dermatitis, usually subacute or chronic in type. Occasionally, vesicles or bullae may be seen which call for the diagnosis of acute dermatitis. There is perivascular, usually lymphocytic, occasionally eosinophilic, cellular infiltrate in the upper and mid-dermis, which is commonly more marked in degree than in most other nonspecific dermatitides, but not sufficiently so to be diagnostic. The epidermis shows the usual changes of nonspecific dermatitis (p. 1384), that is, hyperkeratosis, acanthosis, variable papillomatosis and edema. When vesicles or bullae are seen, they are usually subepidermal in location, but occasionally appear in the lower or mid-epidermis. The vesicles contain eosinophils, precipitated fibrin and some lymphocytes and polymorphonuclear leukocytes. The floor of the vesicles usually reveals a moderately dense inflammatory infiltrate composed chiefly of lymphocytes, eosinophils and some neutrophils (Fig. 30–6). When the vesicle ruptures, a crust is formed which may contain many polymorphonuclear

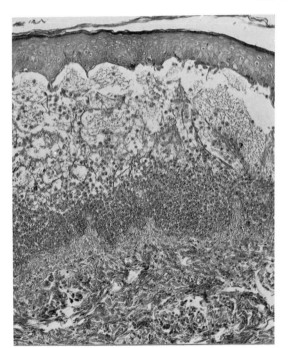

Figure 30–6. *Bullous erythema multiforme. Note that bulla is subepidermal and filled with fibrin, eosinophils and neutrophils. Dermal floor of bulla shows dense infiltrate.*

leukocytes. If the lesion becomes more chronic, some pigmentation may be seen in the upper dermis.

When bullous lesions of erythema multiforme are accompanied by constitutional symptoms, with high fever, prostration and involvement of the conjunctiva or mucous membranes, the syndrome has been referred to as *Stevens-Johnson disease*. The lesions sometimes form crusts and may extend to mucous membranes of the oral or anogenital region. There is some evidence that the gastrointestinal or urethral mucosa may be similarly involved as part of the generalized eruption. Often, in the same patient, the eruption may be predominantly urticarial at one phase and multiform at a later stage. The disease lasts a variable length of time and usually disappears within a few weeks after the systemic allergen is removed.

ATOPIC DERMATITIS AND NEURODERMATITIS

Atopic dermatitis and neurodermatitis are generalized or localized, lichenified, pruritic eruptions of allergic, congenital or psychogenic etiology. Many authors use the term atopic dermatitis as synonymous with widespread neurodermatitis. Almost all agree that localized neurodermatitis has a psychogenic etiology. It is beyond the scope of this book to delve deeply into the extensive arguments that have revolved about the concept of atopy (hay fever, asthma and atopic dermatitis) and the role of congenital factors in the predisposition or causation of this entity. There are disputes as to whether these diseases are attributable to allergic or psychogenic factors or a combination of the two.

The lesions of **atopic dermatitis** usually occur on the flexor surfaces of the elbows and knees, but may occur elsewhere on the skin surface or even be generalized and become an exfoliative dermatitis. Pruritus is usually the chief symptom. The skin appears reddened, thickened and lichenified. As this type of thickened skin does not bend easily, fissures occur over the joints and neck region where folding would normally take place. Usually there is considerable evidence of scratching as indicated by linear scratch marks and excoriations. The patient will frequently be seen rubbing or scratching the areas while a history is being taken. In **localized neurodermatitis,** similar lichenification, excoriations and erythema are seen in a localized area. Common sites for this are the anogenital region, the back of the neck, the dorsal surfaces of the feet and the dorsa of the hands. One or more patches may be seen in a given individual.

Histologically, the picture is that of a nonspecific dermatitis (p. 1384) and, therefore, is not diagnostic. There is hyperkeratosis, acanthosis, variable papillomatosis and moderate to marked edema of the upper corium with a variable inflammatory infiltration, chiefly lymphocytic in type, in the upper dermis. The presence of moderate edema of the upper corium in a chronic dermatitis is somewhat suggestive of neurodermatitis. The mid- and lower dermis are usually not remarkable.

The marked lichenification, accentuation and thickening of the normal skin lines is similar to that which can be produced experimentally with a scratching machine in some patients. There is further experimental work to show that removing several layers of epidermis by stripping them with cellophane tape or adhesive tape will result in thickening of the epidermis and an inflammatory process in the upper dermis within a 24 to 48 hour period. This evidence would tend to support the hypothesis that scratching itself may be a major factor in producing the lesion. Prescribing sedatives so that the patient will not scratch so much or applying a protective dressing to a given area will usually result in marked improvement of any local area. The role of psychogenic stress in itching is important in the genesis of this disorder. In the anogenital region, the localized neurodermatitis is called *pruritus ani* and *pruritus vulvae*. Certainly other factors, such as fungal infection, contact dermatitis, pinworms and local or systemic malignancy, must be excluded as possible causes of local pruritus.

Because the process is relatively superficial, it is easy to understand why complete recovery without scarring occurs during remission even though the disease may be extremely acute, severe and even incapacitating during its exacerbation.

Persons with atopic dermatitis or any extensive dermatitis who usually have not been exposed to herpes simplex virus previously and who come in contact with the virus may develop a generalized herpes simplex infection of the skin called *"eczema herpeticum"* (p. 1391). Similarly, those patients with active and extensive skin eruptions who have never been vaccinated, or not recently vaccinated, may develop a generalized vaccinia called *"eczema vaccinatum"* if they have had contact with the vaccinia virus. Therefore, patients with active atopic dermatitis or extensive skin eruptions should not be vaccinated and should avoid contact with persons recently vaccinated who still have a crust at the vaccination site.

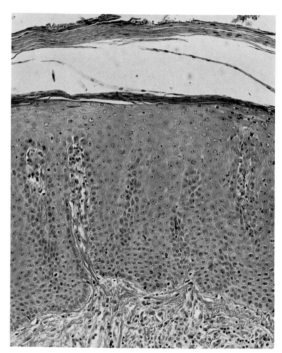

Figure 30–7. *Exfoliative dermatitis—nonspecific chronic dermatitis. Note loose hyper- and parakeratotic scale, which separated in preparing section, acanthosis and elongated dermal papillae and rete ridges.*

EXFOLIATIVE DERMATITIS

This condition is a generalized redness of the skin accompanied by scaling. The etiologic factors are numerous, varied and sometimes unknown. Occasionally, drug eruptions, psoriasis, lichen planus, seborrheic dermatitis, contact dermatitis or other skin diseases may flare and result in a generalized exfoliative dermatitis. Rarely, this disease may be present at birth. Occasionally, it is associated with systemic malignancy, particularly the malignant lymphoma group. There have been some estimates that as many as 25 per cent of all cases of exfoliative dermatitis are associated with the malignant lymphomas. Our experience indicates a much lower incidence.

The course of the disease will vary considerably, depending upon whether or not the etiologic factor is removed or ameliorated. If the basis of the disease is a malignant lymphoma or carcinoma, the skin disease may persist to death. In most cases, however, when malignancy is not associated, and the offending agent is removed or the disease process runs its natural course, improvement may occur. Improvement in many cases is produced or induced by cortisone and related steroid therapy. In the past, elderly patients

who developed this disease were often kept in bed and would develop secondary complications, such as pneumonia, which accounted for many of the deaths in exfoliative dermatitis. During the course of the generalized disease process these people usually cannot perspire and, therefore, are unable to satisfactorily adjust to overheating.

The histologic picture is usually nonspecific (p. 1384) (Fig. 30–7). If, however, the exfoliative dermatitis is secondary to psoriasis, one may often see many of the features of psoriasis persist. When it is secondary to lymphoma, there is a good likelihood of establishing the diagnosis of the lymphoma by the skin biopsy. Usually the lesions reveal a nonspecific subacute to chronic dermatitis. There is hyper- and parakeratosis with variable inter- and intracellular edema. Acanthosis with some papillomatosis is present. Edema and an inflammatory infiltrate are often present in the upper corium. In more chronic cases, the infiltrate and edema are usually less marked.

FUNGAL DISEASES OF THE SKIN

In general, fungal diseases of the skin can be divided into three categories: (1) superficial, those that are chiefly localized to the outer portions of the skin; (2) intermediate, those that may invade both superficial skin and deeper tissues; and (3) deep, those that are predominantly systemic or invade the deeper structures.

Superficial Fungal Diseases. These are caused chiefly by the dermatophytes, resulting in ringworm, athlete's foot (tinea pedis) and "jock" itch (tinea cruris), and *Malassezia furfur*, causing tinea versicolor. In those caused by the dermatophytes, hypersensitivity may play a role, but the allergic phenomena are confined almost entirely to the skin. In general, the superficial fungi cause scaling, erythema and, occasionally, vesicles and fissures. In the nails, they produce thickening and discoloration. The infected hairs may break off close to the scalp. On the smooth glabrous skin of the trunk, there may be one or more circular lesions with central clearing resembling a ring. Rarely, the lesions may become secondarily infected with bacteria.

In this group, the clinical designation will vary depending upon the area of the body involved. When the body is involved, it is known as tinea corporis; when the groin is involved, tinea cruris; the nails, onychomycosis; the scalp, tinea capitis, and so on.

In the dermatophyte group, skin tests with antigen derived from the causative organism or a nonspecific antigen prepared from one of the dermatophytes of the Trichophyton group may be negative or become positive when there is an appreciable inflammatory reaction at the infected site. If the sensitivity reaction is markedly positive, a nonspecific "id" eruption may occur at sites distant from the focus of fungal infection. These secondary "id" sites are usually characterized by tiny vesicles, scaling and minimal erythema and present a nonspecific histologic picture. Fungal cultures of the "id" lesions will be negative, whereas cultures of the acutely inflamed primary focus are usually positive. As the sensitivity to the organism diminishes, the "id" reaction will likewise subside.

Tinea versicolor is a scaling eruption on the trunk, characterized by patches of hypo- and hyperpigmentation with no inflammatory reaction.

In general, the organisms of the superficial mycoses live only in the cornified zone of the epidermis, including the hair and nails. They do not invade the growing portion of the epidermis, nail matrix or hair bulb (Kligman, 1955). Most of them grow best in the presence of moisture. It is, therefore, understandable that the areas of the groin, between the toes, in the armpits and similar sites are commonly involved. It is also understandable that flares occur when there is a recurrence of an environment suitable for good growth. In ringworm of the scalp, hair shafts are invaded down to the zone of keratin formation just above the hair bulb. The diseased hair shafts break off easily above this zone, leaving some of the infected keratin in the follicle. This explains why plucking these diseased hairs is not efficacious in altering the course of this disease. The same process occurs in ringworm of the nails. Since avulsion of a diseased nail plate does not remove all the infected keratin, the new nail growing back is usually reinfected.

Although most cases respond to systemic griseofulvin, the chief reason for culturing the lesions caused by fungal organisms is for prognostic purposes. A good example of this is ringworm of the scalp. If it is caused by the dermatophyte *Microsporum lanosum*, which is commonly the cause of dog and cat ringworm, the majority of human cases will have an inflammatory immune reaction called a *kerion* and will be spontaneously cured in four months. In infections of the scalp due to *Microsporum audouini*, the dermatophyte causing most ringworm of the scalp in children, cure occurs in about 40 per cent of cases in four to six months. In ringworm of the scalp caused by *Trichophyton schoenleini*, which is commonly found in Europe and is fortunately rare in this country, scalp lesions persist for years, and permanent scarring and hair loss are common.

Histologically, a definite diagnosis of superficial fungus infection can usually be made by seeing fungal elements in the sections. However, with the exception of tinea versicolor (see following section), an identification of the specific dermatophyte cannot be made from tissue sections. The corneal layer of the epidermis usually contains spores or mycelial fragments. The remainder of the epidermis and dermis may not be remarkable except for a slight to moderate nonspecific inflammatory reaction. In the stage of acute vesiculation and erythema, edema of the epidermis and upper dermis will be noted, and a greater number of cells, usually lymphocytes with an occasional polymorphonuclear leukocyte, may be seen. Occasionally, a **kerion**, or dense marked inflammatory reaction, occurs, characterized by aggregates of polymorphonuclear leukocytes and occasional giant cells in the dermis. There is an associated folliculitis and perifolliculitis with true abscess formation. During the stage of healing of the kerion, foreign body giant cells can be seen in variable numbers. If fungal elements can be identified in this reaction, a definite histologic diagnosis of kerion can be suggested.

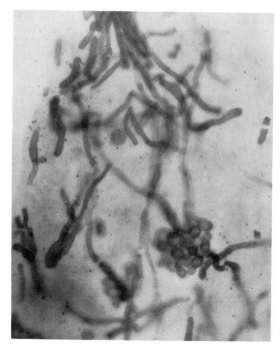

Figure 30--8. *Tinea versicolor. Periodic acid—Schiff stain of skin scrapings. Note clumps of spores and mycelial fragments. Epithelium remains unstained.*

The kerion is not a bacterial superinfection but a local tissue reaction heralding the appearance of immunity to the causative fungus. When this occurs, the prognosis is most favorable.

Of the common superficial fungal diseases, only *tinea versicolor* has diagnostic characteristics which may be seen in superficial scrapings of infected skin (Fig. 30–8). These are clumps of spores, some of which may show minute buds, and numerous mycelial fragments. The other superficial mycotic diseases can only be recognized as fungal diseases and not definitely identified as to the genus or species from smears of scrapings alone.

Intermediate Mycoses. *Moniliasis* is a fungal disease caused by *Candida albicans* which may occur *both as a superficial skin infection and as a systemic disease*. On the skin, it is most commonly found in intertriginous (moist) areas and in the paronychial (edge of nail) regions in persons having their hands exposed to water a good deal. The organism can usually be cultured from or seen on smears of pus from the paronychial region. Moniliasis has been discussed in Chapter 10.

Deep Mycoses. The systemic mycotic diseases, blastomycosis, cryptococcosis, coccidioidomycosis, actinomycosis, mucormycosis and histoplasmosis, have been previously presented (p. 442). Our discussion of the deep

mycoses here will be limited to sporotrichosis and mycetoma, because these principally manifest as dermatologic diseases.

Sporotrichosis is due to the fungus, *Sporotrichum schenckii*. For the most part, this disease affects the skin and subcutaneous tissue and is relatively benign; however, visceral, skeletal and disseminated involvement has been reported.

Usually there is a sporotrichotic "chancre" characterized by an ulcer at the site of inoculation, frequently on the hand. This may be accompanied by multiple subcutaneous nodules appearing proximally along the lymphatics draining the "chancre." This clinical pattern of an ulcer with nodules in a chain-like fashion is sufficient evidence to make a presumptive clinical diagnosis of sporotrichosis. Cultures on Sabouraud's and enriched medium are the most consistently reliable methods of establishing the diagnosis. Periodic acid-Schiff stain on paraffin tissue sections only occasionally establishes the diagnosis. The fungi appear in tissues as small, 3 to 5 micron, variable, fusiform organisms with some budding forms. Routine hematoxylin and eosin stains on paraffin tissue sections will only rarely reveal the organisms in human infections of the skin, because the organisms are missed or confused with nuclear debris. This is one of the deep fungal infections in which routine tissue sections do not usually enable definitive diagnosis.

Histologically, there usually is a dense granulomatous infiltration of the upper and mid-dermis, often with ulceration of the overlying epithelium. At times, pseudoepitheliomatous hyperplasia and deep dermal or subcutaneous abscess formation may be seen. The infiltrate is composed primarily of polymorphonuclear leukocytes with giant cells around the periphery. Occasionally, caseous necrosis may be seen in the sporotrichotic nodule without abscess formation.

Mycetoma is a deep chronic infection with multiple draining sinuses and tumors, usually of the hands and feet, caused by a variety of fungi. At least 26 different etiologic species have been isolated from various cases. *Allescheria boydii*, one of the Ascomycetes, is the most commonly isolated organism in this country. Madurella and Nocardia species may occasionally be found. The disease occurs chiefly in tropical environments in people who usually walk barefoot on the soil.

Usually cutaneous papules and nodules develop, followed by ulceration and often hypertrophic granulation tissue. Occasionally, the underlying bone may be destroyed. Direct smears of the pus of ulcerated lesions may reveal the presence of "grains." These are large granules which, when examined under the microscope in potassium hydroxide preparations, may reveal large clumps of segmented, branched hyphae or, in the case of Nocardia, tangled masses of delicate filaments.

Histologically, in mycetoma one usually sees marked acanthosis with foci of ulceration and numerous abscesses containing polymorphonuclear leukocytes, macrophages, giant cells and fungi in the dermis. Toward the periphery, chronic inflammatory cells are seen, such as lymphocytes, plasma cells and some eosinophils. The appearance of the specific fungus will depend upon the class of organism responsible for the individual case. Usually only a diagnosis of deep fungus infection can be made. The etiologic diagnosis of mycetoma requires correlation of clinical, histopathologic and cultural observations. One of the mycetoma, chromoblastomycosis, can be diagnosed histologically in routine sections by the presence of single or groups of brown rounded or crescent-shaped, thick-walled bodies about 10 microns in diameter. They may be free in the tissues or in giant cells.

HERPES SIMPLEX

Herpes simplex, commonly called "fever blister" or "cold sore," is an acute erythematous and vesicular eruption with grouped lesions on any part of the body, but the lips and genital regions are affected most commonly. Primary infections often occur within the first five years of life, and usually are inapparent or subclinical, nonetheless resulting in specific antibodies of lifelong duration. In less than 1 per cent of persons does the primary infection produce recognizable clinical disease. In this group, acute herpetic gingivostomatitis is the most common clinical syndrome, but central nervous system, liver and other organ involvement may occur, especially in the infant. In a patient with preexisting dermatitis, an extensive vesicular eruption may develop. This is known as eczema herpeticum (p. 1388).

Whether through reinoculation or reactivation of herpes simplex virus already present in the body, recurrent attacks of vesicles may occur throughout life in some persons.

The lesions are characterized by groups of variously sized vesicles, each a few millimeters in diameter, on an erythematous base. The vesicles tend to rupture within days and a crust is formed. Occasionally, secondary infection may be superimposed. Since the histopathologic findings of herpes simplex, herpes zoster and varicella are similar, with multinucleated epithelial giant cells, only a diagnosis of this group of viruses can be made in skin lesions, and no differentiation within the group is possible on a histologic basis. The characteristic features are localized primarily in the epidermis.

The epithelial cells are markedly enlarged and swollen, often becoming separated from each other. At times the cell walls rupture. Some of these cells lose their nuclear detail. The pathognomonic cell is a multinucleated epithelial giant cell usually seen along the base of the vesicle. This alone, in a vesiculobullous disease, is sufficient to make a diagnosis of the simplex-zoster-varicella group. Occasionally one sees intranuclear inclusion bodies which are generally eosinophilic. The dermis beneath the vesicle usually shows a moderately dense polymorphonuclear leukocytic infiltrate with some lymphocytes and monocytes toward the periphery.

It is because of the presence of the multinucleated giant cells that a Tzanck test is of value in this group of diseases. In this test, a relatively clear vesicle must be used. The surface of the vesicle is cut off, the fluid gently blotted with gauze, and the base of the vesicle gently scraped. The material obtained is placed on a slide and stained with Wright's or Giemsa's stain (Blank and Rake, 1955). The presence of multinucleated giant epithelial cells is pathognomonic. It must be remembered that, for both the smear technique and the histologic diagnosis of biopsies, a recent vesicular lesion will reveal the most significant histologic features. Once the vesicle has become cloudy and secondary necrosis and superimposed infection have occurred, the diagnosis is not made as readily (Fig. 30–9).

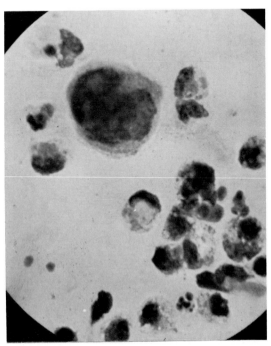

Figure 30–9. Herpes simplex. Tzanck smear of vesicle base stained with Giemsa stain. Note large epithelial multinucleated giant cell.

HERPES ZOSTER

Herpes zoster, commonly known as shingles, is an acute inflammatory disease whose skin manifestations are patches of erythema containing vesicles, usually arranged along the cutaneous distribution of one or more nerves. The disease may occur in any age group and is due to the varicella virus which affects the skin and the peripheral nerves supplying the area. Occasionally, one may see an adult with herpes zoster and a child in the same family developing chickenpox, and vice versa. In children, pain rarely occurs. In adults, particularly the elderly patient, pain may often precede any visible skin lesions by 1 or 2 days.

Erythema and tenderness usually develop first. This is followed by the appearance of vesicles in groups. The lesions tend to coalesce, and the fluid within the vesicles often becomes turbid. Occasionally some hemorrhage occurs into the vesicle. After about a week, the lesions tend to crust, and finally healing occurs. Variable scarring may result, and pain, particularly in the elderly, may persist for weeks or months. Some of the viscera supplied by the same nerve segment may be involved in the process and reveal superficial ulceration. This may account for some of the bizarre symptomatology seen in the disease. Residual scar formation becomes particularly important when the region involved includes the cornea. Partial or permanent disturbance of vision may occur and, for this reason, an ophthalmologic consultation is usually advisable if the region of the eye is involved. Along with the segmental distribution of the vesicles, a rare, isolated, discrete vesicle may occur anywhere on the body without implying an unfavorable prognosis. **Generalized herpes zoster, although rare, is usually associated with systemic malignancy,** often of the lymphoma group. The histologic changes of herpes zoster are similar to those already described for herpes simplex.

The diagnosis of the multinucleated epidermal giant cell group of virus diseases having vesicles (simplex-zoster-varicella) can be made from the section or from a smear of the base of an early vesicle. Differentiation within the group can only be made by means of clinical, cultural and serologic studies.

IMPETIGO

Impetigo is an acute superficial bacterial infection of the skin caused by beta hemolytic streptococci or coagulase-positive staphylococci and characterized by vesicles which later are transformed to crusts. It usually occurs in children. The lesions appear to be autoinoculable and, to some extent, contagious. The exact roles of trauma and malnutrition in this disease have not been thoroughly evaluated.

Usually the lesions start as thin-walled vesicles covering a total area of 2 to 3 cm. in diameter or less. The vesicles rupture, usually within a day or two, and are followed by crusts. The face, particularly the area around the mouth, is a site of predilection, but the ears, neck and hands are also frequently involved. Histologically, the typical picture is a diagnostic one. There is a moderate-sized subcorneal vesicle filled with polymorphonuclear leukocytes with minimal to moderate edema and some inflammatory infiltration of the underlying epidermis and, to a lesser extent, of the upper corium (Fig. 30–10). The mid- and lower dermis are not remarkable. When a biopsy is obtained from an early vesicular lesion, the foregoing picture may be seen. However, once ulceration has taken place, the histologic picture is no longer diagnostic and consists only of a crust composed of fibrin and neutrophils on the surface of the malpighian layer. Scarring practically never occurs because the lesion is so superficially located.

The disease usually responds well to frequent washing and local or systemic antibiotics. Before antibiotics, the disease in infants could become widespread in rare cases and endanger life. When beta hemolytic streptococci are involved, glomerulonephritis may be a complication.

STASIS DERMATITIS OR VARICOSE ECZEMA

Stasis dermatitis refers to chronic inflammatory changes in the skin predisposed to by vascular stasis and edema. When the underlying cause of the stasis is varicosities, the skin changes may be referred to as *varicose eczema*.

The disease usually occurs on the lower extremities when the veins are incompetent. Varicosities, edema, hyperpigmentation, ulceration and fibrosis may be present. The amount of edema will vary with the length of time the extremity has been dependent and the degree of stasis. Some local cyanosis can usually be seen. As the stasis persists, tissue changes characterized by dilatation of superficial blood vessels with some diapedesis of red blood cells and deposition of hemosiderin take place. This will result clinically in varying changes in skin color from red to dark brown. Actual rupture of blood vessels may accentuate this discoloration. With more chronic stasis and hemorrhage, particu-

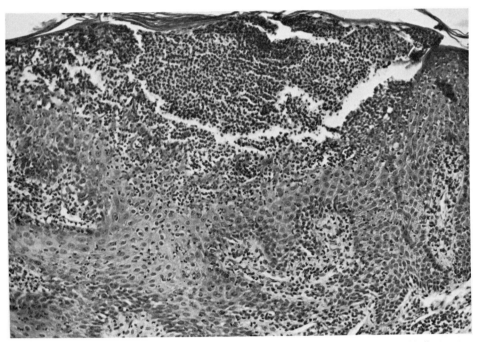

Figure 30–10. *Impetigo. Note superficial subcorneal vesicle filled with neutrophils and inflammatory reaction in the underlying epithelium.*

larly if secondary inflammation is superimposed, some fibrosis of the dermis will result. If these areas of stasis are traumatized or excoriated, they tend to take much longer to heal than skin elsewhere on the body, probably because of their reduced oxygen tension and poor nutrition.

Histologically, the picture is not diagnostic. There is usually a subacute or chronic dermatitis with considerable amounts of hemosiderin present in the dermis. When this is seen, the diagnosis of stasis dermatitis can be suggested by the pathologist. Older lesions may have an increase in fibrous tissue in the dermis. Occasionally, frank occlusion of arterioles or venules is seen. The vessels, both venous and arterial, sometimes show intimal proliferation. In areas of ulceration, the epidermis is destroyed, and the inflammatory infiltrate, composed chiefly of polymorphonuclear neutrophilic leukocytes, as well as some lymphocytes and plasma cells, is intensified. In areas where there is a considerable amount of inflammation of a chronic degree, there may also be some increase in melanin pigmentation in the region of the basal layer and the upper dermis. The skin appendages have usually been destroyed.

Because stasis, even in minimal amounts, may be present in persons of middle age and thereafter, it is generally advisable, if possible, to take skin biopsies from above the thighs to avoid delayed healing in dependent lower ex-

tremities. In many patients with varicosities and stasis, there may also be focal arteriolar changes with obliteration of the arteriolar lumen. This superimposes the factor of local ischemia in a larger area of stasis. For these reasons, areas of stasis dermatitis are particularly vulnerable to trivial injuries and infections. The healing of such lesions is markedly impaired, often leading to persistent ulcerations that are difficult to cure. Therapy must be directed at improving the underlying stasis by elevation of extremities, elastic bandages or stockings, or surgical correction of the incompetent vascular pattern. Treatment directed only locally at the skin site of eczema or ulceration is relatively ineffectual.

WART, CORN, CALLUS, CUTANEOUS HORN

Verruca vulgaris, the common wart, *verruca plantaris*, the wart on the plantar surface or sole, *verruca plana juvenilis*, the juvenile wart, and *condyloma acuminatum*, the venereal wart, are probably variations of the same process caused by a similar etiologic agent modified by the local environmental conditions. These warts are due to a virus and have intranuclear and cytoplasmic inclusion bodies. The exact mechanism of spread and immunology of the causal agent(s) are not understood. In general, these benign lesions tend to occur at sites of trauma and occasionally can be seen along a scratch mark.

Verruca Vulgaris. These lesions are elevated, well circumscribed, papillomatous growths with a keratotic surface. This common epithelial tumor has been attributed to everything from the "touch of the devil" to "touching toads."

They are usually 1 to 2 mm. to 1.0 cm. in largest diameter and raised to about 3 or 4 mm. They are commonly found on the hands.

Histologically, the picture is often a diagnostic one. There is marked hyperkeratosis, parakeratosis and acanthosis with a thickened granular zone. The rete ridges are elongated, and the lateral ones tend to bend toward the center at the base of the lesion. The basal layer of the epidermis is intact. The outstanding diagnostic feature of the epithelium in these lesions is the presence of vacuolated cells in the region of the granular layer. In about 25 per cent of all warts, intranuclear inclusion bodies have been identified in the upper prickle layer or the zone of vacuolization. A variable amount of inflammatory infiltrate may be present in the underlying upper or mid-dermis. The lower dermis is not remarkable (Figs. 30–11, 30–12 and 30–13).

Because they are so superficial, the lesions can be easily removed by surgery or electrosurgery. However, in the region of the nail fold, removal by almost all methods results in frequent recurrence. Many of these warts will disappear of their own accord in a matter of months to years. This must be taken into account in evaluating any therapeutic agent.

Plantar Wart. The plantar wart is similar to the common wart but, because of its location on the sole, it is subject to pressure and therefore as it grows, it is pushed inward into the dermis. Less of it protrudes above the surface of the skin. Because these growths occur chiefly at sites of pressure, there is usually a considerable amount of callus on the surface. Because of their depth and location at sites of pressure, they tend to be painful. Therefore, simple removal of some of the callus affords considerable temporary relief because it allows the lesion to become more superficial. Because these lesions extend deeply, and because of their location, excision may result in tender scar formation. It is estimated in some localities that 25 per cent of all teenagers have plantar warts.

Histologically, they are similar to verruca vulgaris except that there may be more marked hyperkeratosis.

Juvenile Warts. These lesions, also called verrucae planae, are smoother and flatter than ordinary warts and are usually multiple. They occur chiefly on the hands and face of children. *They are similar to verruca vulgaris except that they generally do not have as much overlying keratin or acanthosis, and their rete ridges do not extend as deeply into the dermis.*

Condyloma Acuminatum. Sometimes called "venereal warts," these lesions occur chiefly in the warm, moist, anogenital region. Many of them occur without any sexual contact. However, if the sexual partners of patients with condyloma acuminatum are examined, a high percentage of them will show genital warts.

These growths are usually larger in size than the common wart, varying from a few millimeters to 8 cm. They have a raised rough surface, tending to resemble a cauliflower. Histologically, they are similar to verruca vulgaris except that there is little hyperkeratosis on the surface but rather marked parakeratosis and extreme acanthosis. Vacuolization of the cells of the upper prickle layer is present. In the dermis, there is a slight to moderate lymphocytic infiltrate. When vacuolization of the upper prickle layer, marked acanthosis and parakeratosis are present, a definite diagnosis of condyloma acuminatum can be made.

Clinically, of course, these lesions must be differentiated from condyloma latum, the fungating granulomatous lesion of secondary syphilis that usually contains many spirochetes and is highly contagious. It is, therefore, important to obtain a blood test for syphilis in any questionable case, and a biopsy may be necessary. Treatment with penicillin will produce a dramatic response in condyloma latum but will not affect condyloma acuminatum.

Corns. Warts must be differentiated from corns, calluses and cutaneous horns. The familiar *corns* on the feet are circumscribed horny thickenings, cone-like in shape, with their apex pointing inward and their base on the surface. They occur at the sites of localized friction or pressure and usually disappear spontaneously when the etiologic agent (pressure) is removed. Because they extend inward at sites of pressure, considerable pain may result. Histologically, corns are composed of compressed cornified masses. The remainder of the epidermis may be somewhat atrophic. The basal layer is intact, and a mild lymphocytic infiltrate can be seen in the underlying corium. The diagnosis can be suspected from the microscopic section.

Callus. A callus is an acquired, superficial, circumscribed, yellow-white, flattened,

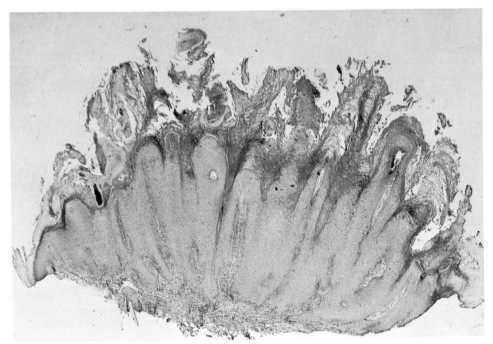

Fig. 30–11

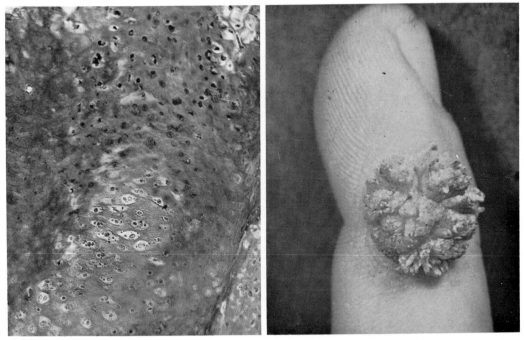

Fig. 30–12   Fig. 30–13

Figure 30–11. *Verruca vulgaris, low power. Note hyperkeratosis, prominent granular layer, marked acanthosis and elongated rete ridges with lateral ones tending to bend toward center.*

Figure 30–12. *Verruca vulgaris, high power. Note marked vacuolization in region of granular layer and suggestion of dark intranuclear inclusion bodies.*

Figure 30–13. *Verruca vulgaris, finger. Note verrucous, papillomatous surface.*

thickened patch of hyperkeratotic material similar to a corn except that there is no central core, and the lesion is more diffusely thickened. These patches are apt to occur over regions of pressure and friction on the hands and feet and are usually not painful.

Histologically, there is increased thickening of the epidermis, particularly of the stratum corneum and the granular layer. The rete ridges may be somewhat atrophic. The dermis is not remarkable. The diagnosis can be suspected histologically.

Cutaneous Horns. These may be confused with warts. Horns are cornified excrescences, varying greatly in size and shape from a few millimeters to several centimeters in length. They are easily palpable as firm, horny projections and may arise from benign lesions such as filiform or fibroepithelial polyps, seborrheic keratoses or verruca vulgaris. However, in some cases they may arise on actinic keratosis or even squamous cell epithelioma. It is for this reason that every time a diagnosis of cutaneous horn is made, the lesion should be excised or a biopsy specimen taken to determine whether it is on a benign or malignant base. The horn does not arise on otherwise normal skin.

Histologically, the horn itself is composed of tremendously thickened stratum corneum with some

scattered areas of parakeratosis. The picture beneath the horn proper will depend on the underlying pathologic process upon which the horn is growing. Often, in preparing sections, the markedly thickened keratinous zone may not cut well, or may be cut obliquely and not be revealed on the slide to its true extent. When it is cut correctly and is present on the slide, the picture is a diagnostic one.

SEBORRHEIC KERATOSIS (BASAL CELL PAPILLOMA)

These are benign superficial epithelial tumors that occur predominantly in middle-aged and elderly patients, usually on the trunk, face and arms. The number may vary from a few to several hundred in an individual patient (Figs. 30–14 and 30–15).

The lesions are raised above the level of the skin, appearing to be "pasted" onto the skin surface, and are sharply circumscribed, varying from light yellow to tan to brown to black. The depth of color varies with the amount of melanin pigment the tumor contains. Usually the lesions are several millimeters in diameter but may extend to several centimeters. When several are present in one patient, all the gradations of size and shades of color just described may be seen.

Histologically, the picture is diagnostic. Under low power or even on examining the slide with a

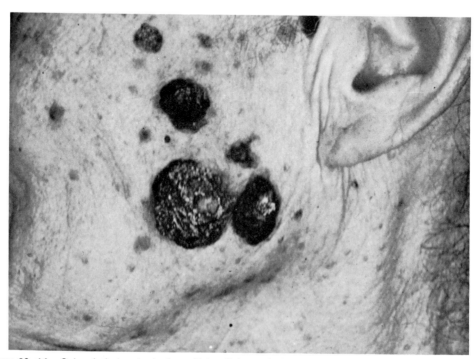

Figure 30–14. Seborrheic keratosis, face. Note all the variations from small, lightly pigmented to larger, dark brown to black lesions.

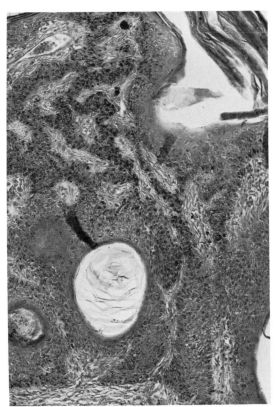

Figure 30–15. *Seborrheic keratosis. Note hyper-keratosis in right upper corner and keratin-filled crypt deep in epidermis. The entire lesion is raised above the level of the adjacent epidermis, a small portion of which is seen in lower right.*

magnifying glass, **the entire process appears to extend above the level of the adjacent epidermis and not into the dermis.** There is marked hyperkeratosis and acanthosis, with melanin pigment present in varying amounts. The keratin extends in projections downward to form crypts in the remainder of the epidermis which, on section, may appear as keratin-filled cysts in the epidermis. The acanthosis is predominantly of the basophilic basal cell type which accounts for one of its alternative names, **basal cell papilloma.** The basal layer is intact, and the dermis is not remarkable. If the lesion has been traumatized or treated, a nonspecific inflammatory infiltrate may occur. If all these features are present, a definite diagnosis can be made.

The superficial location accounts for the clinical finding that much of the tumor can be removed easily with little or no bleeding by scraping with the fingernail, a scalpel or a curette. The patients will often state that they have picked the lesion and it temporarily seemed to disappear. This tumor is not prema-

lignant and does not metastasize. If a patient has many lesions, it would obviously not be feasible or justifiable to remove them all. Certainly a suspicious one that may be confused with a malignant lesion should be excised and sent for examination or, if it is large, a punch biopsy can be taken. Further treatment will depend on the report of the biopsy specimen. Ordinarily, no treatment is needed except for cosmetic reasons.

SENILE (SOLAR) KERATOSIS AND LEUKOPLAKIA

These two diseases are essentially similar, the former occurring on skin, the latter on mucous membrane. They are considered *premalignant squamous cell lesions.*

Senile (Solar) Keratosis. Senile (solar) keratoses are usually located on the sun-exposed portions of the body, such as the face, ears and backs of the hands. These lesions, along with basal and squamous cell carcinomas, are much more common in persons exposed to ultraviolet rays of the sun. The incidence in the southern parts of the United States is much greater than in the northern portions. Farmers and sailors, exposed to the sun for long periods of their lives, and persons in older age groups are much more prone to develop these tumors. They are also more likely to occur in areas of radiodermatitis, sometimes as long as 15 years after the radiation has been given. Many dermatologists and oncologists do not consider roentgen irradiation the treatment of choice in basal cell epitheliomas or squamous cell carcinomas in patients below the age of 50 or 55, when their normal life expectancy is ordinarily beyond 15 to 20 years, because they may later develop senile keratoses and carcinomas secondary to the x-radiation in these areas. However, with newer schedules of fractionated radiation therapy, these secondary complications are much rarer.

In the past, when inorganic arsenical therapy was commonly used in the treatment of many diseases, it was not infrequent to see *arsenical keratoses* develop 10 to 15 years after treatment with arsenic. These arsenical keratoses are multiple and usually occur on the palms and soles, an area where senile (solar) keratosis ordinarily does not occur. Histologically, arsenical keratoses are identical with senile keratosis and their clinical behavior is the same.

Solar keratoses usually occur as scaly or crusted, well circumscribed lesions, often less than 1

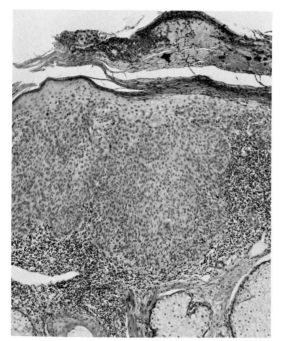

Figure 30–16. Senile keratosis. Note crust and hyperkeratosis on surface and acanthosis. Dyskeratosis not easily identified at this magnification. Moderate upper dermal lymphocytic infiltrate.

cm. in diameter, on an erythematous base. They are often confused with seborrheic keratosis and, not infrequently, both these lesions occur on the same individual. Unlike the benign seborrheic keratosis described previously, the lesions of solar keratosis usually result in some bleeding if the crust is traumatically removed.

Histologically, solar keratosis shows marked hyperkeratosis and acanthosis. Unlike seborrheic keratosis, **the acanthotic epidermis of solar keratosis extends into the corium, showing moderate papillomatosis. There is usually an increase in mitotic activity and some dyskeratosis,** i.e., abnormal keratin formation. Frequently, individual cells in the epidermis will be seen undergoing keratinization in the midst of the prickle layer where keratin ordinarily is not seen. This dyskeratosis and mitotic activity are suggestive of an early intraepidermal malignancy, and it is for this reason that **these lesions are considered by some to represent squamous cell carcinoma, grade one-half.** The basal cell layer is, however, intact, and there is usually a moderately dense lymphocytic infiltrate in the upper dermis. The upper dermal connective tissue may stain faintly basophilic and demonstrate thick, wavy fibers which stain positively with elastic tissue stains (solar elastosis). When these features are present, the slide is a diagnostic one (Fig. 30–16).

Most pathologists do not consider the lesion itself malignant, but feel that some may become true squamous cell carcinomas. Therefore, the preponderance of opinion favors their removal. When a patient has many of them and removal of all of them is impractical, the lesions should be carefully observed. Any change, i.e., bleeding or growth, dictates the need for excision of the affected lesion. As we have discussed earlier in the chapter, a cutaneous horn may develop on a solar keratosis.

Leukoplakia. This lesion, the mucous membrane counterpart of solar keratosis, is an epithelial thickening usually caused by chronic irritation. On the mucous membrane of the lips, tongue and buccal region, it is felt that irritation from hot smoke, pipes, decayed teeth or malfitting dentures may be etiologic. In the mouth, the condition has been called "smokers' patches." Since the patches usually occur in the regions exposed to chronic irritation, these areas of involvement are determined by the way the patient holds his pipe or cigarette. In the past, when the atrophic glossitis of syphilis was more frequently seen, leukoplakia was often present in those patients. Whether the syphilis was causal or purely concidental has been the subject of some dispute. Leukoplakia usually appears as slightly thickened, white patches, rarely crusted, on the lips, tongue, buccal and vaginal mucosa (Fig. 30–17). In the latter area, it is often secondary to senile atrophy of the vulva (p. 1208).

Histologically, leukoplakia takes one of two forms. In one, there is prominent hyperkeratosis with little acanthosis and atypicality of cells. The other pattern is essentially similar to solar kera-

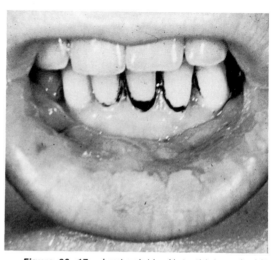

Figure 30–17. Leukoplakia. Note thickened white patches on lower lip.

tosis with the exception that hyperkeratosis is usually less prominent and there is marked to moderate parakeratosis. This is not surprising when we realize that leukoplakia develops in mucous membranes where parakeratotic epithelium is normally present. In addition to parakeratosis, acanthosis and atypicality of the cells of the malpighian layer may be present along with individual cell keratinization and a moderately dense inflammatory infiltrate in the upper portion of the corium extending into the overlying basal layer.

It has been estimated that from 20 to 30 per cent of the cases of untreated leukoplakia go on to squamous cell carcinoma, particularly those cases with atypical cell changes. If the cause is a traumatic one, and is removed, the lesions sometimes disappear spontaneously. If the cause cannot be removed, or if the lesions do not disappear, surgical removal can easily be accomplished because of the superficial nature of the pathologic process. Recurrences are not infrequent, particularly if the cause is not eliminated.

PIGMENTED LESIONS

The following pigmented lesions have been selected for discussion either because they are commonly seen, are malignant or are confused with common or malignant lesions: *the freckle, the lentigo, the mongolian spot, the blue nevus, the pigmented nevus and the malignant melanoma.* These are entities in which there are localized collections of melanin pigmentation or melanin-producing cells in varying locations and concentrations in the skin. There is frequently doubt as to just where the lines of demarcation between some of these conditions should be placed, both clinically and histologically.

Freckles. These are circumscribed, macular collections of pigment. They vary from tan to dark brown in color, and usually range from pinpoint to several millimeters in diameter. They are commonly located on the exposed portions of the body, particularly the hands and face. Upon exposure to the sun, the freckle usually darkens and it tends to fade during the winter months. The lesions are benign. Microscopically, there is increased pigmentation in the region of the basal layer. There is no other abnormality of the epidermis or dermis.

Lentigines. Pigmented macules similar to freckles and not always distinguishable from them are called lentigines. Lentigines tend to occur anywhere on the body, but in older people are more pronounced on the dorsum of the hands and the face. They are benign.

Histologically, the lentigo reveals some elongation, clubbing and melanin hyperpigmentation of the rete ridges with increase of the numbers of melanocytes in the basal layer of these rete ridges. The dermis and remainder of the epidermis are not remarkable.

Mongolian Spots. These circumscribed pigmentations are congenital, nonelevated, nonindurated, dark blue to gray areas, usually on the sacral region, 2 to 10 cm. in diameter, present at birth, and commonly in darker-skinned races. They often disappear spontaneously by the fourth year of life.

Histologically, one can be strongly suspicious of the diagnosis. The skin is not remarkable except for the presence of spindle-shaped and stellate cells in the mid-dermis, containing melanin pigment. The cells are dopa positive. The overlying epidermis and the remainder of the dermis are not remarkable. The blue-gray color of the lesion is due to the depth of the brown melanin pigment seen through the overlying skin.

Blue Nevus. The blue nevus is a well circumscribed nodule, usually several millimeters in diameter, blue to black in color. It is movable over the subdermal structures but not within the dermis of which it appears to be an integral part (Fig. 30–18).

Histologically, the picture is diagnostic. The epidermis and upper dermis are not particularly remarkable. The mid- and lower dermis contain large numbers of stellate and fusiform cells laden with melanin pigment, similar to those seen in the mongolian spot but much more numerous. These cells are also dopa positive. Often the pigment is present in such large amounts that nuclei are not visible. Mitotic figures are not seen. There may also be some melanophores present, that is, macrophages containing melanin. They do not have the stellate appearance but are plumper and shorter than the melanocyte. They are dopa negative. The margins of the blue nevus histologically are not sharply defined, and there is no capsule around them.

The blue-black color is due to the deep location of pigment seen through the overlying skin. Only rarely do the blue nevi undergo malignant degeneration, but they are generally removed in order to be certain that they are not malignant melanomas.

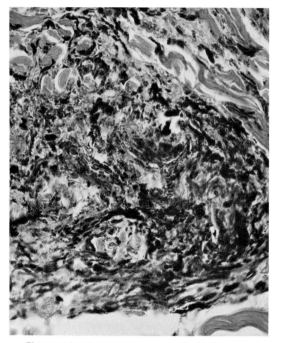

Figure 30–18. *Blue nevus in deep dermis. Note dense aggregates of pigment granules preventing visualization of nuclei.*

Pigmented Cellular Nevi. These are the common pigmented moles present in varying numbers on almost everybody. They are composed of melanocytes, the pigment-producing cells (Figs. 30–19 and 30–20).

The moles vary in size from a few millimeters to several centimeters. They may be nonpalpable to nodular to polypoid. The surface may be smooth or verrucous, depending upon the amount of keratin present. They may contain few to many hairs of varying length, in which case they are sometimes called **hairy pigmented nevi.** Their color varies from flesh color to tan to brown to black, depending upon the amount and location of melanin pigment in the tumor. The closer the pigment to the surface, the darker brown the color.

Histologically, these lesions are diagnostic, and are composed of nevus cells. There has been much discussion in regard to subclassifying the pigmented nevus into the **junctional nevus,** the **intradermal nevus** and the **compound nevus,** based on the location of the nevus cells within the dermis. When these cells are high up in the dermis, **at the dermal-epidermal junction, or in the epidermis,** usually in clumps with some clear spaces between

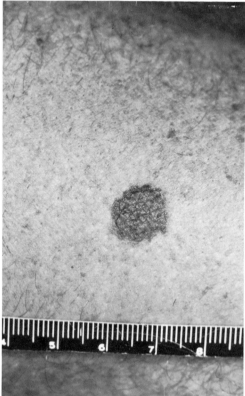

Fig. 30–19

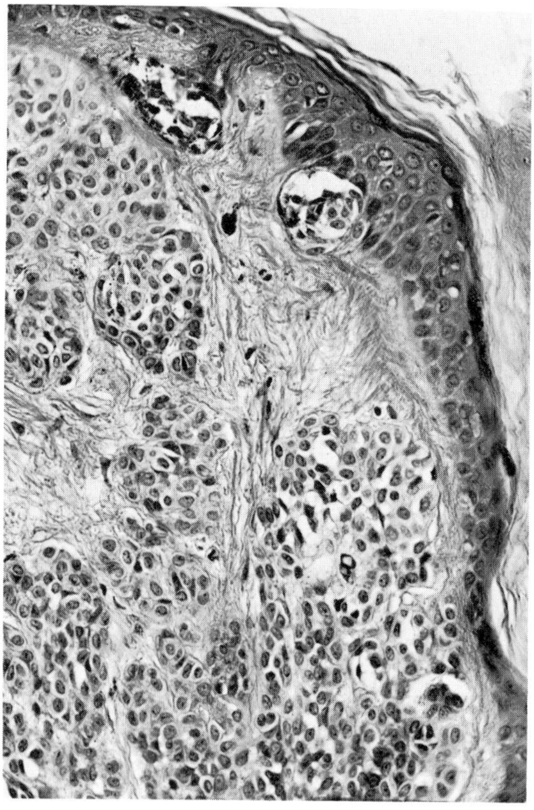

Fig. 30–20

Figure 30–19. *Pigmented cellular nevus (pigmented mole).*
Figure 30–20. *Pigmented cellular nevus, intradermal, with some junctional features at base of epidermis in upper portion of picture.*

and around the individual cells, the lesion is called a **junctional nevus.** Usually, the junctional nevi are smaller and flatter than the other pigmented nevi, but this does not always hold. In the prepubertal age group, almost all pigmented nevi, whether flat or raised, regardless of location, are of junctional type. Since in the adult most nevi are not junctional, it must be assumed that these prepubertal lesions undergo changes. In addition, pigmented nevi on the distal portion of the extremities and on the genital region in all age groups are frequently junctional. This does not connote malignancy. When the nevus cells are located in the dermis and are **not in apposition to the dermal-epidermal junction,** the lesion is known as an **intradermal nevus.** When there is a combination of junctional nevus and intradermal nevus in one lesion, this is called the **dermal-epidermal** or **compound nevus.** There is some question as to the value of making these subdivisions, because all gradations between junctional and intradermal nevi or combinations of them can be seen, often in one lesion. It is interesting to note that if serial sections are made of nevi, nearly all intradermal nevi show some areas of junctional activity. The chief reason why these classifications have persisted is that many authors feel that the junctional nevus is the precursor of the malignant melanoma. We do not believe there is adequate evidence for substantiation of this opinion.

The actual nevus cells vary considerably in appearance. When they contain melanin pigment, identification is easy. The typical cell contains a large, oval, vesicular nucleus and usually a homogeneous, light-staining cytoplasm. They are usually seen in groups dispersed through the dermis in the varying locations cited. Occasionally, several of the cell nuclei appear to gather together and pool their cytoplasm to form a multinucleated nevus giant cell. The nevus cells may occasionally resemble epithelioid cells, or fibroblasts, or cells of the sheath of Schwann. It is, therefore, understandable that there continues to be considerable difference of opinion as to the origin of these cells, i.e., whether epithelial, neural or even mesodermal. Most evidence points toward origin from the ectoderm of the neural crest.

The nevus cells tend to extend deeper into the dermis around the pilosebaceous apparatus, but this is no indication of malignancy. Mitotic figures are very rarely seen in pigmented nevi. If more than one or two mitotic figures are present on a given section of a nevus, the suspicion of a malignant melanoma must be entertained. Usually there is little or no inflammatory reaction in a pigmented nevus, but occasionally a folliculitis or acne lesion may occur in one of the dermal appendages in a nevus and cause an inflammatory reaction and apparent clinical enlargement of a benign lesion. Although a definite capsule is not seen around the pigmented nevus, histologically the clusters of nevus cells are localized to a limited area and end abruptly, so that the margins of the tumor can usually be easily ascertained.

A rare nevus may demonstrate a depigmented zone surrounding the pigmented mass. This is called the halo nevus. Usually this halo heralds spontaneous depigmentation and disappearance of the entire nevus. Histologically, in addition to the nevus cells, there is a dense lymphocytic infiltrate. Rarely, this nonspecific halo has been seen around neurofibromas, malignant melanomas, skin lesions of sarcoidosis, lichen planus and psoriasis.

Malignant Melanoma. This is the malignant lesion of the melanin-producing cell. In the past, some pathologists felt it arose from connective tissue elements and hence it was called *melanosarcoma.* At the present time, the preponderance of opinion is that the tumor is ectodermal in origin and should therefore be called a *melanocarcinoma or malignant melanoma.* Although melanoma technically could mean any tumor containing melanin, most authorities use the term melanoma to mean malignant melanoma.

These tumors are among the most unpredictable in oncology (Allen and Spitz, 1953), because some of them are highly malignant, with the poorest prognosis, whereas others with a similar histologic picture may act in a relatively benign fashion. A particular tumor, formerly believed to represent malignant melanoma in the prepubertal age group on preponderantly histologic grounds but characterized by benign clinical behavior, has received much attention over the past decade or so. This tumor, the *juvenile melanoma,* is now generally felt to represent a histologically recognizable variant of an active compound nevus, hence a benign lesion. Occasionally, however, the histologic findings may be indistinguishable from those seen in malignant melanoma. There is some evidence to show that, in the elderly, malignant melanomas may behave in a more benign fashion also. We have seen lesions that did not grow for many years, and which were removed for cosmetic purposes and revealed a histologic diagnosis of malignant melanoma. There is thus a great deal of discrepancy between the clinical behavior and histologic picture in these tumors. The variations in the behavior of this tumor in the prepubertal age group, the adult and the elderly suggest the role of endocrine factors, possibly the melanocyte-stimulating hormone. Up to the present time, endocrine therapy has not proved efficacious in combating this malignancy.

There is also much controversy about the relationship of pigmented nevi to malignant melanoma (Shaffer, 1956). Do nevi undergo transformation to melanomas, or do melanomas arise de novo from melanocytes? The preponderance of opinion at the present time is that malignant melanomas arise from nevi. This view is partly based on the fact that melanomas usually show considerable junctional activity, particularly when they arise in young people or when the lesion is of short duration. Some of these lesions remain superficial (at the junctional zone) and are relatively less aggressive than the generality of melanomas. The superficial ones are those that extend very little into the epidermis and tend to remain high in the dermis, not extending appreciably below the level of the rete ridges. However, in those malignant melanomas with invasion of the epidermis, there is usually anaplasia and increased mitosis of the tumor cells. In many cases of malignant melanoma, a history of inadequate removal of a pigmented lesion, either by inadequate surgery or inadequate electrosurgery, can be obtained. In the majority of these cases, pathologic examination of the original lesion was not obtained and the question of whether it was a malignant lesion or a benign nevus that became malignant after treatment cannot be definitely ascertained. Certainly all authorities agree that inadequate removal of a pigmented lesion is undesirable even if the lesion is felt to be benign. Although the majority of dermatopathologists question the origin of malignant melanoma from histologically benign nevi, this genesis is supported by most oncologists. It must be kept in mind that malignant melanoma may also arise from other regions of the body where the melanocyte ordinarily occurs. Thus, these tumors have been reported in the retina and the meninges. Malignant melanomas are less common in blacks, but do occur.

The malignant melanoma is usually an enlarging black-brown nodule with some surrounding erythema due to the inflammatory reaction that it generally provokes. Occasionally ulceration may be present. Small satellite lesions, 1 or 2 cm. away from the primary lesion, may be seen. However, it has been pointed out that the lesion may infrequently be deceptively bland-appearing and may not have appreciably changed in size or appearance for years. Most tend to metastasize at an early stage to adjacent skin, to regional lymph nodes and occasionally hematogenously. When lesions enlarge under observation, the clinical diagnosis or index of suspicion is high. However, in a small percentage of cases, the lesions may not contain pigment (amelanotic melanoma) and may be flesh-colored, red or purple due to vascular elements, so that macroscopic diagnosis is difficult if at all possible (Figs. 30–21 and 30–22).

Histologically, the diagnosis of malignant mel-

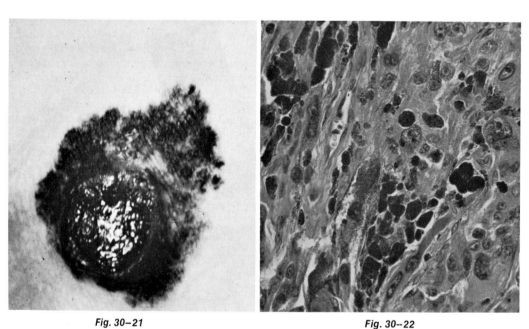

Fig. 30–21   Fig. 30–22

Figure 30–21. *Malignant melanoma. Note marked hyperpigmentation, ulceration and small satellites at upper right portion.*

Figure 30–22. *Malignant melanoma. High power. Note melanin-containing cells and marked anaplasia. Tumor giant cell present at right edge above center.*

anoma can usually be made without too much difficulty. However, in an occasional case when all the criteria are not present, several pathologists may interpret the section differently in regard to its benign or malignant character. Typically, the malignant melanoma usually extends from the region of the dermal-epidermal junction into the dermis for varying distances. There are usually moderate numbers of mitotic figures, anaplasia and an inflammatory infiltrate. Multinucleated bizarre tumor giant cells may be seen. If there are many mitotic figures, anaplasia and melanin pigment, the diagnosis is not too difficult. Occasionally, the tumor cells may be nonpigmented and very anaplastic so that they are hard to distinguish from any other rapidly growing anaplastic malignancy. Stains for activated tyrosinase or dihydroxyphenylalanine (dopa) oxidase will usually be positive in melanomas. The stains are usually satisfactory only on unfixed, relatively fresh tissue. The special stains are of greatest value in the nonpigmented lesions when the melanoma is not suspected clinically. Lymphatic or blood vessel invasion histologically materially worsens the prognosis. Most malignant melanomas occurring in the prepubertal age group tend to have greater numbers of the giant cells and less anaplasia, but cannot be differentiated histologically with certainty from other melanomas by most pathologists.

Until the microscopic sections are examined, a diagnosis cannot be made with certainty. It is for this reason that suspicious lesions, pigmented or not, should be examined preferably by excisional biopsy. Any treatment that is aimed at destroying a growing lesion without examining it histologically may result in not identifying it as a malignant melanoma, possibly in inadequate treatment and in a preventable death. On the other hand, we have seen excellent clinicians suspect malignant melanoma in hyperpigmented verruca vulgaris, seborrheic keratosis, ulcerated hemangioma, and so on. The ultimate diagnosis rests with the pathologist, and his opinion must be obtained before treating a lesion too lightly as well as to prevent needless radical dissection in a lesion which clinically only superficially resembles a malignant melanoma.

WEN, PILONIDAL SINUS

Wen (Sebaceous Cyst, Epidermal Inclusion Cyst). These are epithelium-lined, small (1 to 4 cm.) cysts that usually appear as discrete, doughy, movable, subcutaneous masses. Sometimes a plugged follicle orifice can be seen. Why this plugging occurs is not known. The cyst is usually filled with a cheesy, yellow, fatty substance, some of which may have undergone calcification. The sebaceous cysts and epidermal inclusion cysts are probably variants of the same process. There is considerable experimental evidence to indicate that plugging the sebaceous duct results in change of the sebaceous cells to the squamous type of epithelium with keratin formation inside the cyst instead of sebum. If this is true, the sebaceous cyst may be considered as an earlier form of the epidermal inclusion cyst. If necrosis and abscess formation occur, the cyst may drain spontaneously or can be drained surgically. In the healing process following inflammation, there are varying degrees of fibrosis and scar formation. If there is enough local tissue destruction, the cyst will not recur. If the cyst is partially removed by surgery, recurrence is not infrequent. Malignant degeneration of these cysts has been reported but is extremely rare.

These lesions are usually slow-growing, raised, flesh-colored and attached to, and usually within, the dermis, most frequently occurring on the scalp, face or back. Histologically, the overlying epidermis may be somewhat thin but is otherwise not remarkable. Occasionally the keratin and fat-filled plugged duct may be seen under the microscope. More often, the duct is not visible, and the cyst is seen to be filled with amorphous eosinophilic material, sometimes showing calcification which, under routine hematoxylin and eosin, stains blue. Often concentric lamellae of keratin will fill the entire cyst. In less than 5 per cent of the cases, sebaceous glandular tissue may be identified in the wall of the cyst. When this is present, the outer portion of the cyst wall will contain a layer of basal cells and some fat-laden cells will comprise the remainder of the wall toward the lumen. Usually when sebaceous structures are not identified, typical keratinizing epithelium with the usual transition from basal cell layer through prickle cells to stratum corneum can be seen, the basal layer being outermost (Figs. 30–23, 30–24 and 30–25). These cysts may rupture or become infected and undergo necrosis and abscess formation. Under these circumstances, foreign body giant cells and foreign body granulomas may be present. Sometimes the giant cells contain only fatty debris, but occasionally they contain keratin scales. The surrounding inflammatory reaction is usually composed of polymorphonuclear leukocytes and some lymphocytes.

Pilonidal Sinus (Cyst). A particular form of so-called epidermal inclusion cyst merits special mention, i.e., the *pilonidal cyst*. These lesions consist of subcutaneous inclusions of epithelium in the natal crease between the buttocks in the sacrococcygeal region. They are more common in males and most often cause

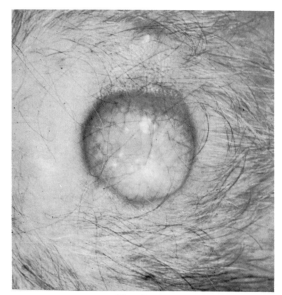

Fig. 30–23

Figure 30–23. *Wen on scalp.*
Figure 30–24. *Wen (keratinous, epidermal inclusion cyst), low power. Note layers of keratin within cyst.*
Figure 30–25. *Wen, high power of wall of cyst. Keratin toward lumen at left of picture. Note epithelial wall similar to epithelium of skin surface but somewhat flattened.*

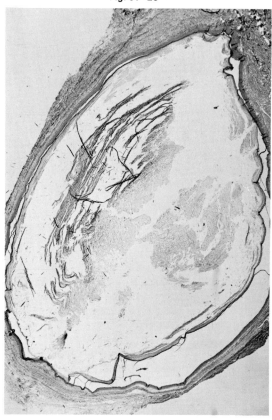

Fig. 30–24

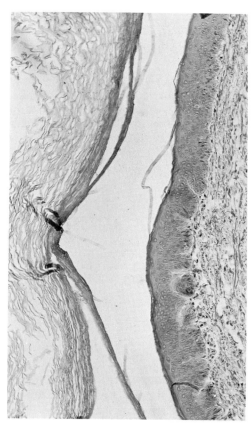

Fig. 30–25

symptoms in the second and third decades of life. The genesis of these buried nests is not well understood. They are attributed to (1) an invagination of the surface epithelium, (2) the ingrowth of hair shafts secondary to inflammation and subsequent inflammatory downgrowths of the surface epithelium, and (3) a vestigial remnant of the primitive medullary canal. Whatever their origin, they have importance because trauma predisposes to bacterial infection, usually to the coliform bacilli and staphylococci.

Anatomically, these lesions may consist sometimes of sinus tracts, **pilonidal sinus,** communicating with the surface through minute (probe diameter) pores; at other times, well developed epidermis-lined cysts, **pilonidal cyst,** that may or may not communicate with the surface; or at still other times, branching, devious, subcutaneous tracts which have poorly developed linings. Common to all these variants are acute and chronic suppurative infections as well as buried hair shafts within these defects. Frank abscesses may develop and often totally destroy all recognizable epithelium. The infection may extend down to the prevertebral fascia and extend laterally through serpiginous tracts into the subcutaneous fat of the buttocks. The histology of these lesions at the time of discovery consists essentially of nonspecific acute and chronic suppuration, only distinctive by the identification of buried stratified squamous epithelium or hair shafts, when these are present. Foreign body giant cells, fatty macrophages and cholesterol debris are frequently prominent.

These defects remain quiescent until the bacterial infection calls attention to their presence by the development of pain, swelling, tenderness and sometimes suppurative drainage. These lesions are readily cured by adequate surgical excision and are more uncomfortable than serious.

BASAL CELL (CARCINOMA) EPITHELIOMA

These are epithelial tumors derived from basal cells or from structures themselves derived from basal cells. The precise limits of what tumors should be included in this group are not well defined and will be elaborated in the discussion to follow. Although they are classically referred to as basal cell carcinomas, there is some question as to whether these are truly malignant tumors. If one adheres to the interpretation of carcinomas or sarcomas as lesions that metastasize, basal cell tumors should probably not be considered as carcinoma, because they rarely, if ever, metastasize

but rather grow by direct extension. For this reason, we have designated them as epitheliomas, realizing that this view is not shared by all oncologists. Basal cell epitheliomas are much more common in the southern portion of the United States and in those persons exposed to considerable sunlight and wind, such as farmers, sailors and year-round sun bathers. People who have been exposed to large doses of x-radiation may develop basal cell epitheliomas as well as squamous cell carcinomas in the irradiated areas and areas of radiodermatitis. In general, basal cell tumors occur predominantly on the face and scalp, and rarely on the palms, soles or mucous membranes. This distribution has led to the belief that they arise in hair follicles and do not occur, therefore, on nonhair-bearing surfaces.

The tumors are usually millimeters to centimeters in diameter, and have a raised pearly border with a central depression. Often there is central ulceration as well as crusting. Telangiectases (dilated blood vessels) are not infrequently seen at the edge of the tumor. Usually these tumors grow by direct extension and local invasion but rarely, if ever, metastasize to distant organs like other carcinomas. Their local aggressiveness is often unappreciated. Mohs (1948), who made large reconstructions from serial sections of recurrent basal cell epitheliomas, showed that, in recurrences, the tumor tended to grow downward often as a single microscopic cord by direct continuity alongside nerves, fascial planes and lymph and blood vessel channels. These single microscopic projections might extend several centimeters deep and would account for the recurrences, even though wide local excision with apparently adequate borders had been performed. The microscopic cord might well be missed in routine sections taken perpendicular to the skin surface. Fortunately the majority of the basal cell epitheliomas grow in a compact mass, and local **adequate** excision or **adequate** destruction by electrocoagulation or x-radiation will result in more than 98 per cent five-year cures.

In the past, before most people were conscious of the benefits of the early treatment of skin tumors, it was not uncommon to see large ulcerating basal cell epitheliomas, "rodent ulcers," which had destroyed a large portion of the patient's face. If death did result, it was usually from direct extension into and destruction of a local vital vessel or structure. Nowadays most of these lesions are seen and treated when they are less than 1 cm. in size.

Microscopically, the picture is diagnostic. The characteristic cell of basal cell epithelioma contains a large blue-staining nucleus with minimal cytoplasm, giving the tumor a basophilic appearance.

The tumor cells at the periphery of any nest or lobule of tumor tissue are arranged with their long axis perpendicular to the edge of that lobule. This lining up of cells gives a "picket fence" appearance to the periphery. Mitotic figures are only occasionally seen in basal cell tumors. Some authors state that basal cell epitheliomas do not contain intercellular bridges. Usually this is so, but these may rarely be seen, probably depending on the degree of differentiation of the tumor. Occasionally, one may see pigment in the tumor which confuses the picture clinically, making one suspicious of a melanoma or nevus, but the presence of it does not alter the prognosis. Rarely, there may be a considerable dermal fibrous tissue response to the tumor so that a fibrosing basal cell epithelioma results. Here the connective tissue proliferation, usually of mature collagenous tissue stroma, is so dense that the basal cells of the tumor are compressed into cords and strands embedded in the stroma. Occasionally, cystic degeneration or even calcification of the tumor cell aggregates may occur (Figs. 30–26, 30–27, 30–28 and 30–29).

We have previously discussed the pluripotentiality of the basal cells (Montagna, 1962) and their capacity to differentiate toward stratified squamous epithelium, hair, sweat glands or ducts or sebaceous structures. It is therefore not surprising to find many histologic patterns in basal cell epitheliomas, varying from sheets of typical basal cells, to those composed chiefly of appendageal cells or any combination of two or three appendages. There is a growing tendency to split these tumors into various clinical and pathologic entities, depending upon which appendage or portion of an appendage predominates. Thus, there are cystic basal cell epitheliomas when many cysts are present, adenoid basal cell epitheliomas when abortive glandular structures are present, trichoepitheliomas when abortive hair structures are present, and calcifying epitheliomas (of Malherbe) when calcification and transformation of the basophilic cells into paler shadow cells are seen. The tumors are called keratinizing basal cell epitheliomas when considerable differentiation toward keratinous cysts is present. This similarity to epithelial "pearls" of squamous cell carcinoma has caused some pathologists to classify them as combined basal-squamous carcinomas.

Tumors have been described specifically for the intraepidermal portion of the eccrine sweat duct (poroma) and others for the clear type of cells and myoepithelial cells of the sweat gland (clear cell myoepithelioma). In general, the specialized differentiation toward one of the skin appendages is associated with a more benign behavior. This, in itself, might justify some of the minute classification of these different forms of tumors. It must be remembered, however, that all variations and combinations between the sheets of typical basal cells and the well differentiated structures can be seen. Most pathologists do not include these well differentiated, relatively benign tumors in the category of basal cell epithelioma, and they are not included in the statistics for cure rates mentioned previously. Often, the well differentiated tumors may be multiple and nevoid, and excision or destruction of all of them is not feasible. In those cases, a biopsy is taken to be certain of the diagnosis and the patient is watched periodically to see if any change occurs.

Two examples among the many other histologically typical, well differentiated, relatively benign epithelial tumors are the following: (1) the syringoma, composed of numerous tiny pinhead-sized nodules on the face, histologically showing small dermal cysts lined by two layers of epithelial cells; and (2) the cylindroma, characterized by multiple nodules on the scalp and face, histologically showing compact dermal islands of two cell types: small, dark-staining ones at the periphery and large, light-staining ones in the center, all embedded in a densely eosinophilic PAS-positive matrix. Again, it must be emphasized that the more well differentiated the tumor is histologically, the more benign it is clinically.

A relatively benign variant of basal cell epithelioma, which has multiple foci of origin and is very superficial, is known as *multicentric superficial basal cell epithelioma*. Usually the patient shows several patches of erythema and scaling varying from one to several centimeters. These may persist for many years (20 to 40), gradually enlarging very slowly at the periphery, and may be clinically misdiagnosed as psoriasis. Only rarely do these superficial tumors start to grow deeper. Usually this is preceded by ulceration and nodularity. Because of their relatively benign nature, considerable discussion arises about their treatment, particularly if they are widespread and of many years' duration when first recognized. The skin of these patients seems to have a predisposition to form these superficial tumors. Often, the surgeon apparently excises a wide border of uninvolved tissues, only to have the pathologist report a single superficial focus at one of the excisional margins. It is because of this that many clinicians advise conservative therapy in this type of tumor and additional biopsies and surgery only when ulceration or nodularity occurs.

SQUAMOUS CELL (PRICKLE CELL, EPIDERMOID) CARCINOMA

In contrast to the basal cell epithelioma, squamous cell carcinoma is unequivocally a malignant epithelial tumor similar to that

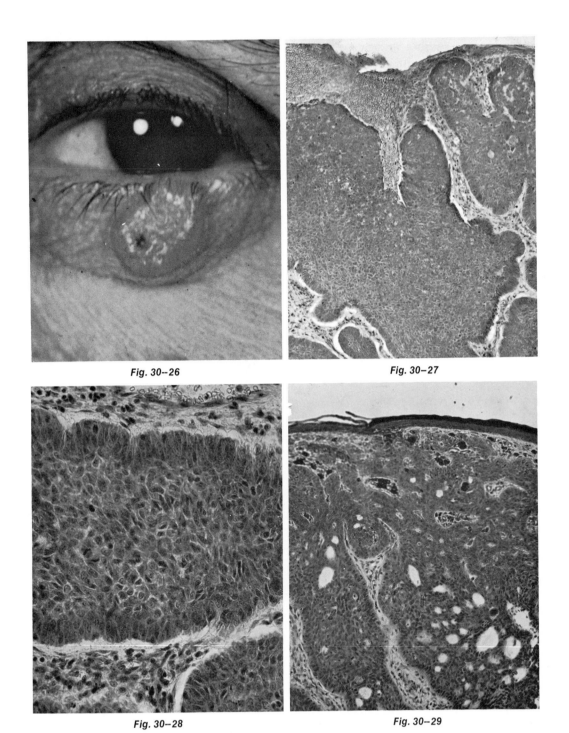

Fig. 30–26

Fig. 30–27

Fig. 30–28

Fig. 30–29

Figure 30–26.   Basal cell epithelioma, lower lid. Note raised pearly border.
Figure 30–27.   Basal cell epithelioma. Note ulceration and sheets of basal cell tumor with columnar arrangement (palisading) of cell at periphery of lobule.
Figure 30–28.   Basal cell epithelioma. High power to show the peripheral palisading seen in Figure 30–27.
Figure 30–29.   Basal cell epithelioma. Note dark melanin pigment granules and abortive adenoid structure of lobules of tumor.

which occurs in many other organs wherever one finds stratified squamous epithelium. It may arise from normal epithelium but is probably predisposed to by senile keratosis, leukoplakia, arsenical keratosis, burn scars or foci of chronic radiodermatitis. Basal cell epitheliomas and squamous cell carcinomas of the skin grouped together are more common than all other malignancies of the body. In Texas, where there is considerable exposure to sunlight, it is estimated that as many as 33 per cent of all cancers are skin cancers. Lower estimates are reported elsewhere. As a rule, men are more often affected than women in a ratio of 2 to 1. Cancer of the skin is rare among blacks. Basal cell epitheliomas are probably more common than squamous cell carcinomas, but the figures vary depending on whether the series are reported by dermatologists or surgeons. The squamous cell carcinomas of the skin tend to occur more commonly in patients above the age of 40.

Usually, the lesions are ulcerated and crusted but they may be raised or verrucous, ranging from millimeters to centimeters in diameter. Histologically, the picture is diagnostic. One finds the surface epithelium acanthotic and irregularly proliferating downward into the dermis. There are variable hyperkeratosis and parakeratosis. The basal layer is usually not intact, and a relatively marked, predominantly lymphocytic inflammatory reaction is seen. The epithelial tumor cells themselves show varying degrees of differentiation. They may vary from anaplastic epithelium with many mitotic figures to relatively well differentiated squamous epithelium, containing numerous epithelial pearl formations and, occasionally, individual cell keratinization (Fig. 30–30). Usually the more mitotic figures and the greater the anaplasia present, the greater the incidence of metastases.

The tumors may be graded from I to IV, according to the proportion of differentiated to atypical cells. Usually many keratinous pearls are present in Grade I. In Grade IV almost all cells are anaplastic and atypical. This classification has definite limitations and varies to some extent with the pathologist. Metastases are rare in squamous carcinoma Grade I but are more common in the higher grades. Exceptions to such behavior based on grades do occur. The regional lymph nodes are generally the first site of metastatic invasion. Later seeding of other organs may result in death. When anaplasia is very marked, the precise diagnosis may be extremely difficult, but there is no doubt about malignancy.

One may see all grades between the premalignant leukoplakia and solar keratosis — with their minimal dyskeratosis, increase in

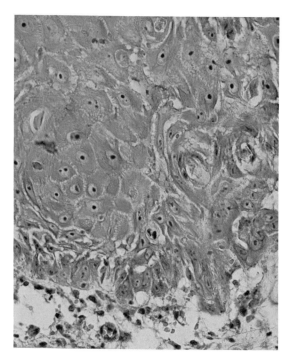

Figure 30–30. *Well differentiated squamous cell carcinoma. Area deep in the dermis. There is slight anaplasia.*

individual cell keratinization, anaplasia and mitotic activity with an intact basal layer — and the malignant, typical, unequivocal squamous cell carcinoma. When the basal layer is still intact but mitotic activity, anaplasia and dyskeratosis are of greater degree than seen in solar keratosis or leukoplakia, and the normal polarity of cells is upset, a diagnosis of *intraepidermal squamous cell carcinoma*, sometimes called *Bowen's disease*, is often made. This may be associated with predisposition to cancer in other internal organs of the patient. When a similar pathologic process occurs on the mucous membranes, usually of the glans penis or vulva, it has been called erythroplasia of Queyrat.

In some chronic, usually ulcerative, inflammatory processes, there may be marked *pseudoepitheliomatous hyperplasia*, in which the differentiation from true squamous cell carcinoma is an extremely difficult one, even by the well trained pathologist. This may occur not infrequently in syphilitic ulcerations, granuloma inguinale, blastomycosis of the skin, bromoderma (fungating reactions to bromide ingestion) and, rarely, in chronic staphylococcal infections. Multiple biopsies and therapeutic trial of antibotic therapy are often necessary to make the proper diagnosis.

LESS FREQUENTLY OCCURRING SKIN PROBLEMS

CONGENITAL

As in most other organs of the body, there are many variations of excessive growth or lack of development of the entire organ or portions of it. Various defects of the skin and the skin appendages (the nails, the teeth, the hair, the eyelids, the sebaceous glands, the sweat glands) or of the connective tissue, blood vessels and nerves may occur on a congenital basis. Ichthyosis and two types of angiomas, port-wine stain and strawberry hemangioma, will be discussed.

Ichthyosis. This is a congenital hypertrophy of the horny layer resulting in hyperkeratosis. This usually produces dryness of the skin with variable amounts of profuse scaling, more noticeable during the cold months. When the scaling is marked, it resembles the scales of fish (ichthyo-), and it is from this that it derives its name. The diagnostic histologic feature of this disease is hyperkeratosis with atrophy or even complete absence of the granular layer.

Port-Wine Stain (Nevus Flammeus). This lesion usually appears as one or multiple, localized or extensive, dull red, nonraised, nonpalpable foci. No uniformly successful treatment is available. Cosmetic preparations are on the market which will cover the lesions and completely hide the presence of the birthmark. Histologically, there is dilatation as well as some increase in the number of capillaries in the dermis. No proliferation of endothelial cells is seen except for the single layer lining the capillary walls.

Nevus Vasculosus (Strawberry Hemangioma). This is an elevated nodule, usually soft, bright red, measuring from a few millimeters to several centimeters in diameter. These lesions are commonly noticed at birth or within a few weeks thereafter and may increase in size for a few months. The majority of them involute spontaneously by seven years of age. When they are located on the exposed portions of the body, there is usually considerable controversy as to whether or not these should be treated and by what means. Histologically, they reveal dilatation and marked increase in the number of capillaries of the dermis, usually associated with considerable proliferation of endothelial cells, which may lie in sheets or around the capillary wall. The lesions are benign.

ATROPHIES

Various atrophic and degenerative changes of the skin occur from unknown etiology as well as from hormonal causes. The somewhat similar atrophic changes seen on the vulva and penis of the aged are only localized manifestations of a generalized atrophic and degenerative process. This section will be confined to a discussion of the changes of senile skin.

Senile Skin. This is more pronounced in skin that is exposed to sunlight, such as the neck and face, but also occurs elsewhere and is characterized by wrinkling, furrowing and thinning. Occasionally, the skin may take on a leathery appearance. Histologically, one usually finds atrophy of the rete ridges and of the collagenous fibers. In skin of older persons exposed to sunlight, basophilic degeneration of the connective tissue can be seen. The most characteristic feature is short, twisted, thick, basophilic staining fibers of the upper third of the corium. These changes in connective tissue manifest themselves by loose skin which, when pinched or stretched, does not return so rapidly as normal skin to its usual contour.

HYPERTROPHIES

Various hypertrophies of the different layers or structures of the skin may occur. Some of these are congenital. Others, such as callus, are due to trauma or other external agents. These are not infrequently seen as signs of a patient's occupation, such as those of the tailor due to holding scissors.

Acanthosis Nigricans. This is a rare disease characterized by large areas of hyperpigmentation and papillary hypertrophy, occurring in three distinct types: (1) a benign type, which is a genodermatosis usually present in childhood; (2) a malignant type in adults, which is associated with internal cancer; and (3) pseudoacanthosis nigricans, which occurs in overweight individuals and is usually reversible when the obesity is corrected. The clinical and histologic aspects of the lesions of all three types are similar. The lesions are usually located in the axilla, the neck and the submammary and the groin regions. Histologically, there is marked hyperkeratosis and papillomatosis with increased pigmentation, usually in the basal layer of cells. Very little acanthosis is present. The chief importance of this disease is that it may signify internal malignancy, especially in adults over 40.

METABOLIC DISEASES OF THE SKIN

In general the skin, being one of the largest organs of the body, readily reflects disturbances of metabolism, often with specific lesions.

Xanthomas. These are localized nodular

tumors of the skin which are composed of large numbers of fat-laden foam cells in the dermis. Because of the large amounts of lipids, they appear grossly yellow or orange colored. Formalin-fixed frozen sections of such lesions stained with fat stains such as Sudan IV or Sudan Black B reveal large amounts of sudanophilic material in these cells. These xanthomas may be widespread and occur in varied forms, such as *xanthoma tuberosum* (increased blood cholesterol and phospholipids, normal blood neutral fats), *biliary xanthomas* (associated with biliary obstruction and jaundice, often disappearing as obstruction is removed) or *xanthoma of idiopathic hyperlipemia* and *secondary hyperlipemia* (severe diabetes, nephrosis, glycogen storage diseases). They may be localized to the eyelids (*xanthelasma palpebrarum*), in which case about half the patients have increased blood cholesterol.

Amyloidosis. This subject has been discussed in Chapter 8 (p. 281). Amyloidosis secondary to other diseases, usually of the chronic debilitating type, rarely involves the skin. Changes in the skin in primary amyloidosis may be of three types: (1) Lichen amyloidosis shows a predilection of papules for the lower extremities. The amyloid is deposited in the skin and no systemic involvement is demonstrable. (2) Localized nodular amyloidosis is characterized by amyloid deposits limited to a single area of skin. (3) Primary systematized amyloidosis has systemic involvement as well as nodular or papular lesions of the skin. Lesions of amyloidosis of the skin do not have a clinically diagnostic picture. Usually they are firm, circumscribed, slightly elevated, flesh-colored lesions. Metachromatic purple staining with crystal violet and green birefringence using polarized light on alkaline Congo red stains are the commonly used techniques on tissue sections to help in diagnosis. The masses of amyloid may be deposited anywhere in the dermis in large foci as well as around the eccrine sweat glands and in the walls of blood vessels.

Calcinosis Cutis. Calcium may be deposited in the skin as a metastatic calcinosis, the result of hypercalcemia (p. 52). It may also be present as a dystrophic calcification as a result of a local disturbance following infection, or in scleroderma or dermatomyositis. Sometimes no previous or concurrent disease can be demonstrated. The gross lesions are not diagnostic. Often, there may be ulcerations with discharge of crumbly material, or firm, sometimes stony hard nodules may be present. Histologic sections are diagnostic. The calcium deposited in the corium stains deeply blue with hematoxylin and eosin stain and black with von Kossa's stain. Foreign body granulomas may be present around the calcium deposits.

Myxedema. Generalized myxedema may be present as a manifestation of hypothyroidism (p. 1324). The skin is thickened but usually does not pit on pressure. The dermal appendages (hairs and sebaceous glands) are also involved. The hair is coarse, and nonoily. Owing to diminution of sebaceous secretion, the general body surface, particularly the legs, is also dry. Localized myxedema usually occurs with, or is preceded by, hyperthyroidism and exophthalmos, and frequently is pretibial in location. A mucinous material, predominantly hyaluronic acid, is present in the corium between collagen bundles and stains light blue with hematoxylin and eosin stains. As a rule, it stains positive with PAS and alcian blue stains.

Addison's Disease. In this disease, diffuse hyperpigmentation of the skin and mucous membranes is present. The increased pigmentation probably results from lack of antagonism by adrenal cortical hormones to the production of MSH and/or ACTH by the pituitary gland (p. 1311). The pigmentation is increased in the basal layer of the epidermis, and moderate numbers of melanophores may be present in the upper dermis. The histologic picture is nondiagnostic and resembles that of the normal skin of blacks.

Hemochromatosis. This has previously been discussed in Chapter 8 (p. 277). Clinically, the skin is diffusely pigmented, similar to that seen in Addison's disease. However, in addition to a slight increase in melanin pigmentation in the basal cells, granules of hemosiderin are sometimes found in dermal macrophages and around sweat glands. The presence of hemosiderin can be confirmed by staining with potassium ferrocyanide, which will reveal granules of Prussian blue color. A biopsy should not be taken from an area where stasis dermatitis or hemorrhage may be present because hemosiderin may be found in those lesions too. Therefore, the lower extremity is clearly not the site of choice for a biopsy to confirm the diagnosis of hemochromatosis.

Ochronosis. The skin is darkened in this inborn disease of tyrosine and phenylalanine metabolism. The darkening of the skin, urine and cartilage is due to the presence of homogentisic acid oxidation products. Sections reveal a light brown pigment in large clumps in the dermis, which appears black following methylene blue staining.

Porphyria. Porphyrias are diseases in which there are inborn or acquired defects in pyrrol metabolism. A monopyrrol, porphobilinogen, is increased in *acute intermittent por-*

phyria. This disorder has no cutaneous signs and is characterized by psychosis, abdominal pain and neurologic disorders. The other porphyrias all show photosensitization sometimes with subepidermal bullae formation and secondary atrophy and scarring. The skin histology is not diagnostic. In all other forms, tetrapyrrols are increased, giving rise to increased uro-, copro- or protoporphyrins in urine, feces or red blood cells. Liver disease from various causes or certain drugs may cause or exacerbate the disease.

Erythropoietic porphyria is rare and recessive and is characterized by accumulations of uro- and coproporphyrins in bone marrow, teeth, red blood cells, urine and feces. Its onset is usually early in life. Bullous fluid, bone marrow and urine may reveal pink fluorescence with the Wood's light (4000 Å). *Porphyria cutanea tarda* usually occurs in adult males in their sixth and seventh decades. Hypertrichosis, hypermelanosis and scarring may occur in the affected areas of skin. Twenty-five per cent of the cases are associated with diabetes mellitus. *Mixed porphyria,* a dominant rare disease, combines photosensitivity with abdominal symptomatology and neurologic disorders. The histopathologic neurologic and abdominal changes are not consistent. The skin changes are similar to those of the other porphyrias. Porphobilinogen can be demonstrated in the urine during acute attacks. *Erythropoietic protoporphyria,* a dominant disease manifesting itself early in life, is also characterized by photosensitivity. The diagnosis can be made often by observing pink fluorescence of red blood cells examined under ultraviolet light. The erythrocyte protoporphyrin levels can be 10 to 30 times normal.

INSECTS AND PARASITES

In different parts of the world and at different times of the year, skin eruptions due to insects and other parasites are frequently seen. This section will be limited to a discussion of papular urticaria, insect bites, scabies and pediculosis.

Papular Urticaria. This is an edematous, papular, pruritic, recurrent eruption, occurring more commonly in the summer months in children usually below the age of seven or eight. The lesions may be few or numerous and may be scattered over the body. Sensitivity to fleas, bedbugs or mosquitoes is probably the cause, and intradermal tests for the specific agent can be performed by the use of suitably prepared antigens. The histologic appearance is not specific. There is usually some acanthosis and intercellular as well as intracellular edema of the malpighian layer. The dermis reveals a moderately dense, chiefly perivascular infiltrate composed predominantly of lymphocytes with some eosinophils. It is felt that not only do lesions occur at the site of recent bites, but that a recent bite may cause a flare at the sites of old bites, where the skin has become sensitized.

Insect Bites. These may be caused by a variety of insects other than those just described. They usually manifest themselves at the site of the bite by a firm papule or nodule, sometimes with ulceration, which may last for several weeks. Histologically, there is a relatively dense infiltrate in the dermis and sometimes in the underlying subcutaneous tissue. It is composed chiefly of eosinophils, lymphocytes and monocytes. Occasionally, parts of the insect may actually be seen in the dermis surrounded by a foreign body reaction. Lymphoid hyperplasia in the skin may also be seen in the sections.

Scabies. This is a contagious pruritic dermatosis caused by the itch mite *Acarus scabiei.* The female mite produces burrows (linear, poorly defined streaks, 2 to 6 mm. in length) on the interdigital skin, the palms, the fingers, the wrists, the periareolar region in women and the genital area in men. Excoriations are commonly seen. Histologically, the burrow traverses the keratin layer and the female mite may be seen in the blind end of the burrow. Usually there is edema of the epidermis in the regions affected. The underlying dermis shows a nonspecific, chronic inflammatory infiltrate composed chiefly of lymphocytes.

Pediculosis. This is caused by the head louse, the crab louse and the body louse. The disease is pruritic and the louse, or the eggs of the louse attached to the hair shafts, can usually be seen with the unaided eye. In pediculosis of the scalp, impetigo and enlarged cervical lymph nodes may be frequent complications in children. The pubic louse may be transmitted through sexual contact. Infection with the body louse is ofttimes known as "vagabond's disease," and is usually characterized by areas of hyperpigmentation and scratch marks. Occasionally, a peculiar bluish pigmentation occurs in spots. The pigmentation is thought to be due to small hemorrhages induced by the bite of the insect. The histologic picture is a nonspecific one.

INFLAMMATIONS OF THE SKIN

The skin is involved in a great many systemic inflammatory diseases. Skin lesions are a prominent feature of syphilis, typhoid fever, rickettsial diseases, lupus erythematosus, dermatomyositis, sarcoidosis and others. These have all been considered in earlier chapters. A few other specific clinical entities will be discussed. These will include eczema in infants, pityriasis rosea, lichen planus, hidradenitis suppurativa, discoid lupus erythematosus and rosacea.

Eczema in Infants. This occurs during the first two years of life and may be localized or generalized, although it is more commonly seen on the face as an erythematous, scaling, occasionally oozing and fissured eruption, often with crusts and secondary infection. The exact etiology is unknown. In the past, this has been felt to be a form of atopic dermatitis or food sensitivity. However, there is considerable evidence that the skin eruption may be caused by a combination of several different factors. These infants frequently drool considerably and sleep face-down in this "pool of drool." This, in itself, would be sufficient to cause a localized miliaria (p. 1381). When partially digested food substances are also regurgitated in the drool, there may be secondary contact dermatitis and superimposed sensitivity. These regions are ofttimes overtreated and further irritated by rubbing or scratching. Because of the varied etiologic factors, it is understandable that treatment is relatively difficult. The histologic picture is that of a nonspecific, acute to subacute to chronic dermatitis (as previously described on p. 1384). Superimposed seborrheic dermatitis is often an additional aggravating factor.

Pityriasis Rosea. This is an erythematous, papulosquamous, self-limited disorder, lasting approximately four to seven weeks, which develops abruptly and usually can be recognized clinically at a glance. It most often is a generalized eruption that does not involve the face, palms or soles. The generalized phase is often preceded by a large herald spot, varying from 2 to 5 cm. in diameter. The diagnostic clinical sign is that many of the individual lesions tend to be oval in shape, with the long axis following the direction of the dermatomes (skin cleavage lines). Itching is the most common symptom. Other signs of sytemic involvement are usually minimal. The disease is thought to be viral in origin, but this has not been proved. Patients are not ordinarily isolated, and usually only one person in the family comes down with the disease. The histologic picture is that of a mild to moderate, nonspecific, chronic dermatitis.

Lichen Planus. This is a subacute or chronic dermatitis, which is usually extremely pruritic, tends to be generalized but may be

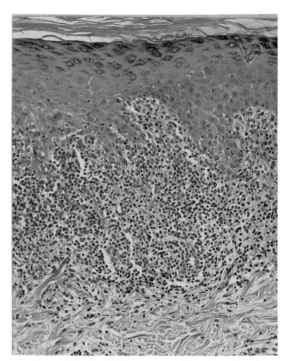

Figure 30–31. *Lichen planus. Note hyperkeratosis, increased granular layer, slight acanthosis, irregularity of rete ridges, poorly visualized basal layer, and a dense sharply delineated lymphocytic infiltrate in the upper corium.*

localized, and is characterized by small, flat-topped, violaceous papules, sometimes with minimal scaling. It is the flat-topped lesions which are diagnostic. The oral mucosa may be involved, usually with a lace-like white pattern, which is not raised or thickened and thus usually easily differentiated from leukoplakia. The cause of this disease is unknown. Sometimes it appears to be caused by sensitivity to drugs. In other cases, the role of psychogenic factors may be a significant one. There is usually hyperkeratosis, increase in thickness of the granular layer, irregular acanthosis with saw-tooth appearance to the rete ridges, destruction of the basal layer, and a dense band-like lymphocytic infiltrate extending from the edematous lower epidermis into the upper dermis, usually sharply demarcated from the midcorium (Fig. 30–31). An occasional melanin-laden macrophage can be seen. When all these features are present, the section is a diagnostic one.

Hidradenitis Suppurativa (Abscesses of the Apocrine Sweat Glands). This is a recurrent persistent disease of the apocrine glands, usually resulting in scarring. Grossly, localized erythematous nodules, varying in number but usually less than 10, tenderness and drainage are present. Most often, it occurs in one axilla but it may occur bilaterally, or be limited to the anogenital region or involve all three locations. Histologically, a mild to moderate inflammatory reaction in or around the apocrine glands is seen, often with abscess formation. Sometimes foreign body giant cells are present.

Chronic Discoid Lupus Erythematosus. Systemic lupus erythematosus (disseminatus) has been discussed in some detail in Chapter 8 (p. 229). In addition to the acute, subacute and chronic systemic forms of lupus erythematosus, there is a type which may clinically be localized to the skin. This is called chronic discoid lupus erythematosus. At present, there is considerable controversy as to whether this is a distinct entity or just an early or more benign form of the systemic disease. The etiology is unknown.

The disease usually affects the face, appearing chiefly on the upper cheeks and over the nose, occasionally occurring on the pinna, the scalp, the vermilion border of the lip and even affecting the buccal mucosa. Rarely, lesions may occur elsewhere on the cutaneous surface. The lesions are usually brightly erythematous; plugging of the follicles may be seen along with adherent scales. With involution of the lesions, atrophy and depigmentation may occur. The disease may be precipitated by exposure to sunlight. The reason for feeling that this disease may be a separate entity from the systemic form is that the majority of these patients have no hematologic or other laboratory evidence of the systemic disease. There is some feeling that those cases with false-positive serologic tests for syphilis may represent cases of the systemic disease. Infrequently the chronic discoid form goes on to unequivocal systemic lupus erythematosus and its severe complications.

The typical histologic picture of chronic discoid lupus erythematosus is hyperkeratosis, keratotic follicular plugging, epidermal atrophy, edema and degeneration of the basal layer, variable edema of the upper corium, some basophilic degeneration of the connective tissue of the upper corium and a perivascular and periappendageal lymphocytic infiltrate. In the advancing edge of a lesion of chronic lupus erythematosus, one may see a more acute process that, histologically, is indistinguishable from the picture seen in the systemic acute or subacute lupus erythematosus (McCreight and Montgomery, 1950). Therefore, only a diagnosis of acute, subacute or chronic lupus erythematosus can be made from the microscopic section. The hematologic work-up and urinalysis, as well as general clinical symptoms, must be taken into account before deciding whether the disease is nonsystemic and limited to the skin, or the systemic type of disease.

Rosacea. This is a chronic disorder, most often of middle age, usually occurring in patients with seborrhea, affecting the central portion of the face and having a superficial resemblance to acne. Usually erythema, papules, pustules and telangiectasia in varying degrees are seen. The etiology is unknown. Histologically, there usually is an inflammatory reaction composed chiefly of lymphocytes with some histiocytes and plasma cells around the hair follicles and sebaceous glands. Occasionally, foci of epithelioid cells and giant cells, indistinguishable from true tubercle formation, can be seen. In these cases, the histologic differentiation from tuberculosis of the skin often cannot be made. Occasionally, intrafollicular abscess formation with pustules and dilatation of capillaries is present. In some cases, hypertrophy of the sebaceous glands and the surrounding connective tissue with inflammation is also present. When this affects the nose and is marked, it is clinically known as *rhinophyma*. In brief, the histologic picture is not diagnostic except in rhinophyma in which it is strongly suggestive.

BULLOUS DISEASES

There are many skin diseases causing vesicles or bullae. Some of the more common ones have been discussed in the previous section and include acute contact dermatitis, impetigo, herpes simplex, herpes zoster, varicella, porphyria and burns. We have discussed the very superficial location of vesicles in miliaria crystallina and impetigo and the relatively deeper subepidermal location in bullous erythema multiforme. In many of the bullous diseases, serial sections of a vesicle or bulla may reveal an intraepidermal vesicle in one section but, if this is followed serially, it may appear to be subepidermal in other sections.

Dermatitis Herpetiformis. This is a chronic, markedly pruritic, noncontagious skin disease having lesions that tend to be grouped, located chiefly on the extensor surfaces of the extremities, the hips and scapular regions, and usually healing with residual pigmentation and some scarring. Vesicles or small bullae may be present only at some stages of the disease. At other times, only papules or pustules may be visualized. The clinical diagnosis can only be suspected unless vesicles are present. The etiology of this disease is unknown but psychogenic factors are felt to play a role. Fortunately, many patients with this disease respond to the administration of sulfapyridine but not to the other sulfonamides. When the disease occurs during pregnancy, it is known as *herpes gestationis*. Frequently, it subsides at the termination of gestation. The histologic picture in this disease is often indistinguishable from that of erythema multiforme. The vesicle or bulla is usually *subepidermal* in location, and numerous eosinophils are usually present both in the vesicle and in the underlying dermis. In the early stages of this disease, before a frank vesicle develops, some investigators have reported suprapapillary microabscesses containing polymorphonuclear neutrophils which they feel are pathognomonic. This is generally but not universally accepted.

Pemphigus. This is a serious bullous disease which usually is generalized, has bullae that break easily and often involves the oral cavity. It had a high fatality rate prior to the use of corticotropin and the cortisone group of steroids. Histologically, the bullae of pemphigus may be diagnostic. They tend to be *intraepidermally* located so that their base is composed of epidermal cells. There is apparently a loss of coherence between the epidermal cells, resulting in acantholysis. This results in clusters of epithelial cells floating in the bulla. The epithelial nuclei become round, swollen and hyperchromatic and tend to have a perinuclear halo. If a Tzanck test is performed similar to that described for herpes simplex (p. 1391), groups of these acantholytic cells can be seen and may be useful for making a rapid, preliminary diagnosis. The dermis beneath the bullae usually contains moderate numbers of eosinophils, which may also be present in the bullae. When the typical picture described is seen, the slide is a diagnostic one.

TUMORS OF THE SKIN

Like other organs of the body, almost any of the structures of the skin can give rise to hypertrophy or to benign or malignant tumors. Therefore, we can observe everything from callosities to squamous cell carcinomas, from fibromas (dermatofibromas) to fibrosarcomas, from neuromas to neurosarcomas, from pigmented nevi to malignant melanomas and from benign lymphocytoses to malignant lymphomas. Some of these have been described in detail and others will be briefly mentioned.

There has been considerable controversy about just when a tumor is a growth of a "congenital rest" or a true neoplastic growth. Certainly all stages of *hamartoma* (overgrowth of a normally occurring structure) of epithelial, ap-

pendageal or mesodermal structures can be seen. Some authors tend to consider as congenital tumors only those occurring at or shortly after birth. Others consider these same types of tumors, even if they occur in adults, as congenital. The explanation offered is that they arose from "congenital rests." Often the word nevus is used to describe these congenital tumors, whether vascular (hemangiomas), pigmented (pigmented nevus) or epithelial (sweat apparatus, hair, sebaceous gland). In general, the word nevus or mole is a loosely used one and, if possible, should be qualified by an adjective, such as hairy, pigmented, vascular, fibrous or the like. Fortunately, these tumors are usually benign and should be treated conservatively. Of course, they can be removed for cosmetic purposes if deemed necessary.

However, the rule must be followed that, in the case of any skin tumor that grows, bleeds or ulcerates, a biopsy should be performed. Whenever feasible, an excisional biopsy should be carried out. Certainly, whether excised completely or not, a biopsy specimen of the tumor should be sent to the pathologist for interpretation and then the tumor promptly treated further, if indicated. Most skin tumors, because they are visible at an early stage, can easily be excised or biopsied. The procedure, either with scalpel or surgical skin punch, is a simple one taking only minutes, and the site need not be sutured if small enough, depending upon its location. There is little or no evidence to show that taking a biopsy of a skin tumor tends to enhance its spread, even if malignant, if the biopsy is followed within a few days by further adequate treatment. We repeat, however, that when feasible, an excisional biopsy is to be advised.

Fibroepithelial Papilloma or Skin Tag. This common lesion is usually 1 to 5 mm. in diameter, flesh-colored to brown, and polypoid in appearance. Microscopically, these structures are usually composed of a loose connective tissue core surrounded by a folded epidermis, which is sometimes acanthotic, sometimes keratotic and occasionally contains melanin. The lesion is benign.

Molluscum Contagiosum. This is a benign, virus-induced, epithelial papular tumor, 3 to 8 mm. in largest diameter, having a diagnostic cytoplasmic inclusion body. The lesion, caused by a virus of the pox group, has an incubation period of three to eight weeks and may occur anywhere on the skin. There may be one or many lesions scattered over the body. The individual papule is smooth-surfaced and hemispheric and has a characteristic central depression or umbilication. Local application

cific inflammatory infiltrate, often containing polymorphonuclear neutrophilic leukocytes. The overlying epidermis is usually flattened

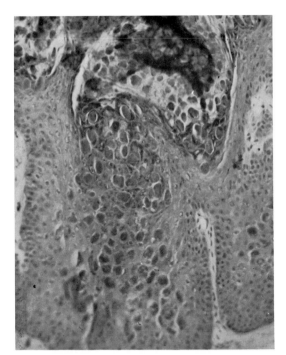

Figure 30–32. Molluscum contagiosum. Note acanthotic epidermis containing large, dark, diagnostic inclusion bodies.

of phenol or nitric acid to the lesion will usually result in its disappearance. Histologically, there is marked acanthosis and downward projection of the epithelium. As the epidermal cells proceed toward the surface, they may be seen to contain a cytoplasmic, usually basophilic, homogeneous inclusion body. The histologic picture is diagnostic (Fig. 30–32).

Granuloma Pyogenicum. This is a solitary, dull red, soft, raised, sometimes pedunculated nodule, which may appear on any part of the body but usually occurs at a site of trauma. Occasionally, it is moist and crusted on the surface and bleeds easily. Usually it varies in size from 5 mm. to 1 or 2 cm. The striking and almost diagnostic clinical feature about the nodule is that it reaches its relatively large size in a very short time, usually a period of about a week. The lesion is a tumor of blood vessels or an overgrowth of granulation tissue and is completely benign but, because of its rapid growth, is often suspected clinically of being a sarcoma or even a malignant melanoma. Excisional biopsy of the lesion usually results in complete cure. The same result will often be obtained even if the tumor is not removed completely (Figs. 30–33 and 30–34).

Histologic examination reveals a relatively circumscribed, pedunculated lesion containing numerous, newly formed capillaries, some endothelial proliferation and usually a nonspe-

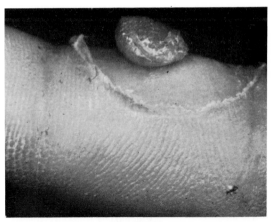

Fig. 30–33

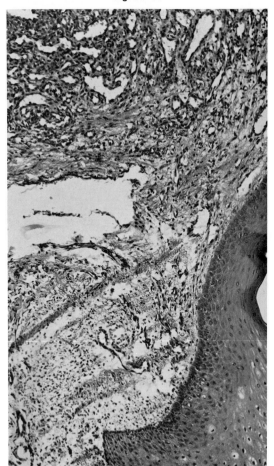

Fig. 30–34

Figure 30–33. Granuloma pyogenicum on finger.
Figure 30–34. Granuloma pyogenicum. Note numerous vascular elements and epithelial collar at base (lower right).

and there may be frank ulceration and crusting. As a rule, the epithelium at the neck of the tumor is thickened to form a collar. The lesion may be diagnosed histologically as a hemangioma or an infected hemangioma and may resemble granulation tissue.

Kaposi's Sarcoma (Multiple Idiopathic Hemorrhagic Sarcoma). This tumor usually presents as several blue-red to brown skin nodules or plaques, sometimes characterized by a verrucous surface. The skin is the most frequent site of involvement but, in about 10 per cent of the cases, visceral lesions are also present. Only rarely are such visceral lesions present without skin nodules. Frequently, one or more lesions occur on the extremities without additional lesions elsewhere. The disease usually lasts for many years and often the patient dies of other causes rather than Kaposi's sarcoma. The preponderant opinion is that the multiple tumors, rather than being true metastases, represent multiple foci, each originating separately. If these were truly metastatic, then once multiple lesions were seen, one would expect rapid progression. This is not the case. Often some of the lesions spontaneously regress and even disappear.

Histologically, there are four components which, when seen in the same section, are diagnostic. They are (1) endothelial proliferation, sometimes as cellular sheets, sometimes as multiple, thin-walled, new vessel formations; (2) hemorrhage, recent or old, manifested by extravascular red blood cells or hemosiderin; (3) fibroblastic proliferation; and (4) an inflammatory reaction usually composed of lymphocytes. In the early stages, the inflammatory granulomatous picture is the more common one. In the later or sarcomatous stage, there is greater fibroblastic proliferation with anaplasia and mitotic activity. The presence of extravasated erythrocytes and hemosiderin differentiates it from fibrosarcoma (Fig. 30–35).

Lymphoma. The many forms of malignant lymphoma have already been discussed in Chapter 18 (p. 752). These may also affect the skin. Often, one of the first recognizable lesions of a systemic lymphoma is a nodule or ulceration of the skin, and the characteristic histologic picture of that particular lymphoma may be obtained on a skin biopsy. On the other hand, some patients with malignant lymphoma may have a nonspecific exfoliative dermatitis, erythema multiforme or other nonspecific erythematous and papulosquamous eruptions. A typical example of this is Hodgkin's disease in which 90 per cent of the generalized skin eruptions occurring as a result of this disease have a nonspecific histologic picture. In 10 per

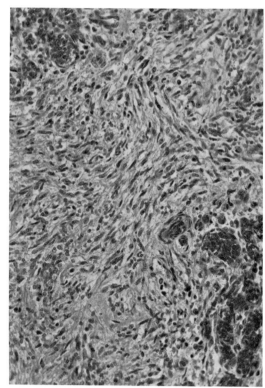

Figure 30–35. *Kaposi's sarcoma. Note multiple blood vessels, hemorrhage (not easily identifiable in black and white photo), fibroblastic proliferation and some inflammation.*

cent, the diagnosis of Hodgkin's disease can be made from the skin biopsy.

One form of lymphoma that characteristically affects the skin first, and later may involve other organs of the body, is known as *mycosis fungoides.* There is some question as to whether or not this is a form of Hodgkin's disease, reticulum cell sarcoma or lymphosarcoma. However, it nearly always has a distinct histologic picture in the skin, and this usually remains true throughout the course of the disease. On the other hand, it may change its characteristics to that of some other form of malignant lymphoma. Clinically, the disease may occur as a diffuse erythema or as well defined elevated plaques or tumors in the skin. It tends to run a course lasting many years (Figs. 30–36 and 30–37).

Histologically, when the following criteria are present, the slide is diagnostic: (1) variable hyper- or parakeratosis; (2) moderate acanthosis with papillomatosis; (3) foci of edema and small microabscesses containing mononuclear cells in the epidermis; (4) moderate edema of the upper dermis; (5) a dense inflammatory infiltrate in the upper and, to some extent, the mid-dermis and extending, to a lesser degree,

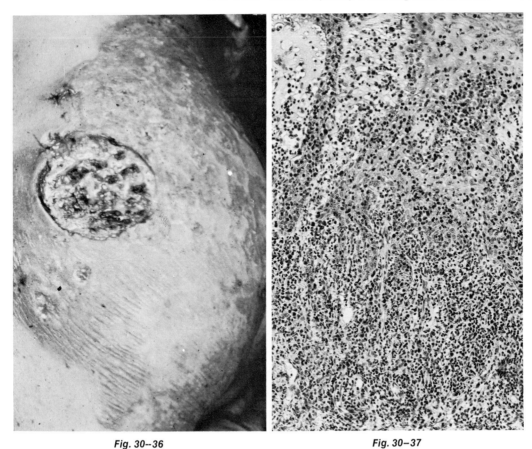

Fig. 30-36   **Fig. 30-37**

Figure 30-36. *Mycosis fungoides. Plaque on hip with ulceration.*
Figure 30-37. *Mycosis fungoides. Note the dense infiltrate and the edema in the dermis extending into the overlying epidermis. Polymorphism and mitoses are not easily seen at this magnification.*

into the overlying epidermis; (6) marked polymorphism of the infiltrate, including giant cells, mitotic figures, some eosinophils, lymphocytes, reticulum cells and some pyknosis and karyorrhexis. Sometimes, before the typical clinical or histologic picture becomes evident, a nonspecific erythematous eruption, plaque-like or generalized, may occur. At this stage, the histologic picture is that of a nonspecific dermatitis. If the lesion eventuates in true mycosis fungoides, the nonspecific picture could be called, with hindsight, the premycotic stage of mycosis fungoides.

Keratoacanthoma. This entity manifests itself as a single or rarely multiple skin nodules, usually with central depressions, 0.5 to 2 cm. in diameter, appearing and reaching maximal size in one to three months. If not treated or only partially removed, it usually regresses completely in a few months. The etiology is unknown. The central crater of the nodule is filled with keratinous material. Histologically, the lesion may be difficult to differentiate from

squamous cell carcinoma, especially if a biopsy specimen is taken from only a portion of the lesion. Keratoacanthoma has probably been included in some series of well differentiated squamous cell carcinomas in the past. When the entire lesion is removed and examined microscopically, it reveals a large, superficial, keratin-filled crater overlying an area of marked acanthosis, papillomatosis and pseudoepitheliomatous hyperplasia. A marked inflammatory reaction, chiefly lymphocytic but containing many neutrophils, is present in the upper dermis and extends into the epidermis so that the basal layer is sometimes not identifiable. Numerous mitotic figures may be seen in the epidermis, but true anaplasia is not present as in squamous cell carcinoma. In many cases, a combination of the history, gross appearance and microscopic findings is necessary to make the diagnosis. Not infrequently, a definitive diagnosis between squamous cell carcinoma and keratoacanthoma cannot be made. In that case, instead of simple local excision, the lesion must be treated as though it were a squamous cell carcinoma.

Urticaria Pigmentosa. This disease has two major clinical variants: a juvenile and an adult type. The juvenile type, characterized by an early onset and a good prognosis, is usually confined to the skin which shows tan to yellow-brown macules and papules occurring as single or multiple lesions. Usually it is asymptomatic, but when a lesion is rubbed, it becomes itchy and forms a wheal. Rarely, purpuric or bullous lesions may occur. It usually appears early in life and diminishes with age, many cases involuting spontaneously by the time of puberty. The adult type usually manifests itself after puberty and may have systemic involvement of varying degree. The skin lesions are essentially similar to those seen in the juvenile type. Occasionally bone, liver, lymph node, thymus and intestinal involvement has been reported. The histologic picture is diagnostic and reveals a tumor composed of large aggregates of tissue mast cells. Giemsa, toluidine blue or periodic acid-Schiff stain may be necessary to identify the mast cell granules. These granules contain histamine, and the release of this substance spontaneously in the adult form may cause urticaria, fainting and dizziness, flushing, dyspnea, headaches, abdominal cramps and diarrhea. Histamine liberators such as polymyxin B or codeine may precipitate these symptoms.

Metastatic Carcinoma. Metastasis of carcinoma to the skin is not common but may occur from any organ. In order of decreasing frequency, the most common sites of primary tumors that metastasize to the skin are the breasts, stomach, uterus, lungs, large intestine and kidneys.

PSYCHOCUTANEOUS DISEASES

The skin may be the site of manifestations of both psychosomatic and psychotic disease. The possible role of psychogenic factors in pruritus, neurodermatitis, atopic dermatitis and urticaria as well as in palmar and plantar hyperhidrosis and superficial vasodilatation in some body areas has already been discussed.

Neurotic Excoriations. These are a result of trauma to the skin due to a "nervous habit." This is similar to the habit of picking the fingers, biting the lip or biting the nails. When the habit is severe, so that the skin is broken in many places and little hemorrhagic crusts are formed, the disease is termed neurotic excoriations. The histologic picture will usually be that of a nonspecific dermatitis with some crusting and ulceration.

Factitial Dermatitis. In this disease, lesions are deliberately produced by the patient and are designed to deceive. In some of these patients, a definite psychosis is present. Material such as acids, alkalis and paraffin has been found injected into the skin. Needles or scissors may be used to traumatize the skin. The picture may be a completely nonspecific one histologically, depending upon the etiologic agent and whether it can be specifically identified on sections.

PIGMENTARY DISEASES

The endocrine control of pigmentation has been discussed in Chapter 29 (p. 1300). A section on color of the skin has been included earlier in this chapter (p. 1377). Two relatively common diseases of increased and decreased pigmentation will be discussed.

Chloasma. The most common type of focal increase of pigmentation, chloasma, usually occurs in adult women around the mouth, the cheeks, the chin and the forehead. It is unaccompanied by any subjective symptoms and is, for the most part, without known significance. It often is more prominent in pregnancy or at specific times of the menstrual cycle. Histologically, there is usually an increase in melanin in the basal layer, which may not be of sufficient magnitude to be recognizable in ordinary hematoxylin and eosin stained sections.

Vitiligo. This is a circumscribed area of depigmentation. The skin is otherwise not remarkable either clinically or histologically. The cause of this disease is not completely understood. Certainly, one may see it after severe inflammation of the skin when the melanin-forming cells have been destroyed. In other cases, there is no history of previous skin disease. Recently, it has been shown that epinephrine locally tends to diminish pigmentation. One of the explanations for the localized foci of depigmentation seen in vitiligo is that there is excessive activity of adrenergic nerve endings, causing local release of epinephrine and, hence, depigmentation. It is interesting to note that, in some patients who have had bilateral vitiligo followed by unilateral sympathectomy or other severe injury, marked diminution of the depigmentation with a return toward normal skin color in the vitiliginous area on the sympathectomized or injured side has been observed.

ALLERGIC DISORDERS OF THE SKIN

These have been discussed earlier in this chapter in the section on sensitivity reactions and contact dermatitis. In addition to those already mentioned, allergic vasculitis and polyarteritis have been discussed in Chapter 7.

Erythema Nodosum. This disease is characterized by symmetrical, erythematous, nodular, painful swellings on the extensor surfaces of the legs or, occasionally, other portions of the body. The etiology cannot always be determined. It may accompany systemic inflammations of varied cause and serious infections such as coccidioidomycosis, sarcoidosis or tuberculosis. In some instances the iodides or bromides as well as other drugs have been incriminated. Histologically, the process is that of a perivascular, relatively dense, inflammatory infiltrate, usually in the mid- and lower corium, often extending into the subcutaneous fat. The infiltrate is composed of polymorphonuclear leukocytes, lymphocytes, histiocytes and, occasionally, eosinophils. The blood vessels may show a true vasculitis with the infiltrate extending directly into the vessel wall. Occasionally necrosis and a granulomatous infiltrate may be present. In older lesions, giant cells and macrophages can be seen. The histologic picture is more often suggestive rather than diagnostic.

REFERENCES

Allen, A. C., and Spitz, S.: Malignant melanoma. A clinicopathological analysis of the criteria for diagnosis and prognosis. Cancer, *6*:1, 1953.

Blank, H., and Rake, G.: Viral and Rickettsial Diseases of the Skin, Eye and Mucous Membranes of Man. Boston, Little, Brown & Co., 1955.

Eisen, A. Z., et al.: Responses of the superficial portion of the human pilosebaceous apparatus to controlled injury. J. Invest. Derm., *25*:145, 1955.

Kligman, A. M.: Survey of the pathogenesis of non-inflammatory tinea capitis. Arch. Dermat. Syph., *18*:231, 245, 1955.

Lever, W. F.: Histopathology of the Skin. 4th ed. Philadelphia, J. B. Lippincott Co., 1967.

McCreight, W. G., and Montgomery, H.: Cutaneous changes in lupus erythematosus. Arch. Dermat. Syph., *61*:1, 1950.

Mohs, F. E.: Chemosurgical treatment of cancer of the skin: a microscopically controlled method of excision. J.A.M.A., *138*:564, 1948.

Montagna, W.: The Structure and Function of Skin. 2nd ed. New York, Academic Press, Inc., 1962.

Montagna, W., and Ellis, R. A.: The Biology of Hair Growth. New York, Academic Press, Inc., 1958.

O'Brien, J. P.: The etiology of poral closure. J. Invest. Derm., *15*:95, 1950.

Pillsbury, D. M., et al.: Dermatology. Philadelphia, W. B. Saunders Co., 1956.

Rothman, S.: Physiology and Biochemistry of the Skin. Chicago, University of Chicago Press, 1954.

Shaffer, B.: Identification of malignant potentialities of melanocytic (pigmented) nevus. J.A.M.A., *161*:1222, 1956.

Strauss, J. S., and Kligman, A. M.: The pathologic dynamics of acne vulgaris. Arch. Derm., *82*:779, 1960.

GENERAL READING

Demis, D. J., et al.: Clinical Dermatology. 4 vols. Hagerstown, Md., Harper & Row, 1972.

Helwig, E. B., and Mostofi, F. K.: The Skin by 30 Authors. Baltimore, Williams and Wilkins Co., 1971.

Jeghers, H., and Mescon, H.: Pigmentation of the skin. In MacBride, C. M. (ed.): Signs and Symptoms: Applied Pathologic Physiology and Clinical Interpretations. 4th ed. Philadelphia, J. B. Lippincott Co., 1964, p. 855.

31

THE MUSCULOSKELETAL SYSTEM

The consideration of the musculoskeletal system will be divided into the following subdivisions: (1) muscles, (2) bones, (3) joints and (4) tendons, fascial and supporting structures.

SKELETAL MUSCLE

NORMAL

The skeletal muscles are derived from mesoderm that becomes set apart early in fetal development into specialized myotomes. In the second month of fetal development, myocytes are formed within these myotomes as elongated hollow tubes with only a scant peripheral cytoplasm and centrally placed ovoid nuclei. By the end of the second month, these hollow tubes become filled with myofilaments embedded within an interfibrillar substance called sarcoplasm. The cross striations characteristic of striated muscle become progressively better defined during the last five months of fetal development. These few comments on the embryogenesis of the myocyte are of significance, because in the various myopathies the regressive changes in muscle cells recapitulate the fetal development of the cells. That is, as the cells degenerate, there is first disappearance of the fibrils and then their sarcoplasm so that ultimately the myocyte reverts to a hollow tube and then the sarcolemmal nuclei disappear. It is these sarcolemmal nuclei that are the vital portion of the cell. As long as these are preserved, regeneration may occur. The myocyte is thus an extremely elongated, truly multinucleated cell.

The muscle cell is a marvelous example of adaptation of structure to function. A wealth of literature is available pertaining to its structural organization (Huxley, 1957, 1963, 1967) (Nelson and Benson, 1963) (Smith, 1966). Remarks here will be limited to those essentials necessary for an understanding of the subsequent discussions. The striated muscle cell has a diameter ranging from 10 to 100 microns and is of considerable length. Indeed, in relatively short muscles, the cell may extend from one tendinous insertion to the other. It is enclosed within a plasma membrane (the sarcolemma) which is separated from an outer basement membrane by a narrow, translucent zone. The myoneural junction constitutes an area of surface specialization. Nerve axon terminals snuggle into indentations of the sarcolemma known as synaptic clefts. The nerve endings are naked, and the narrow space between them and the plasma membrane is filled with an amorphous substance. Small vesicles which contain acetylcholinesterase are found in the muscle cell and in the nerve endings in the region of this junction. This enzyme is important in inactivating the acetylcholine released with each nervous stimulus to the muscle cell.

The nuclei are dispersed along the length of the muscle cell closely approximated to the plasma membrane. The sarcoplasm contains mitochondria, Golgi apparatus, ribosomes, sarcoplasmic reticulum, other tubules and an abundance of myofibrils. The number of contained mitochondria varies with the specific functional activity of the cell. Thus, cardiac muscle cells contain many more mitochondria than the cells of skeletal muscle which have lower oxidative requirements.

Most of the muscle cell mass is made up of a parallel array of myofibrils, which are quite long and may extend the length of the cell. The myofibril, in turn, is composed of an interdigitating array of thick and thin filaments. As is well known, skeletal and cardiac muscle cells are divided into functional contractile units, *sarcomeres*, extending from one Z line to the next. Within the sarcomere, the thick filaments are arranged in register in the central region, creating a broad cross striation known as the A band. Thin filaments, attached at one end to the Z lines, interdigitate at their other ends with the centrally located thick filaments. Where the thin filaments alone lie in register adjacent to the Z lines, light I bands are produced. The thin filaments thus extend through the I band to interdigitate with the central thick filaments.

In the center of the dark A bands where there are no interdigitating thin filaments, there is a slight pallor referred to as the H band, which itself has a central, narrow, darker M band produced by slight thickening of the central regions of the thick filaments as shown in Figure 31–1. Cross bridges which have been noted between the thick and thin filaments are believed to be involved in the transmission of impulses fundamental to the contractile process.

Two systems of tubules are found within the muscle cells. One is essentially a specialization of endoplasmic reticulum known in these cells as *sarcoplasmic reticulum.* The sarcoplasmic tubules run the length of the muscle cell and are interdigitated between (thus surrounding) small clusters of myofilaments. At the junction of the A and I bands in man, the sarcoplasmic reticulum communicates with laterally placed membranous sacs, the terminal cisternae. A second and distinct transverse tubular (T) system traverses the muscle cell, and the lumina

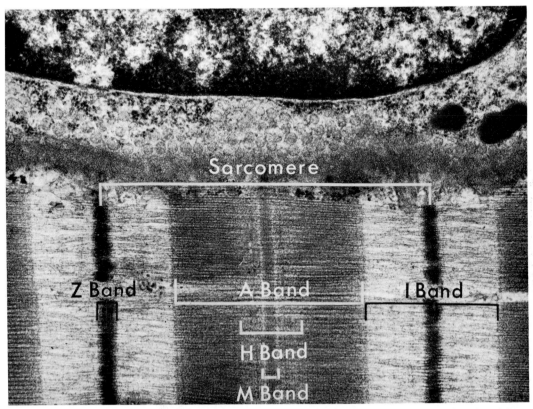

Figure 31–1. *Electron micrograph of parts of two muscle fibers with the nucleus of one (above) and the most superficial myofibrils of the other (below). The principal features of the pattern of cross striations are identified on the figure. × 34,000. (Courtesy of Bloom, W., and Fawcett, D. W.: A Textbook of Histology. 9th ed. Philadelphia, W. B. Saunders Co., 1968, p. 277.)*

appear to be continuous with invaginations of the cell membrane. In effect, the T system is an extension of the interstitial fluid space across the muscle cell. This anatomic detail provides a possible mechanism by which contraction stimuli, initiated at the cell membrane, may spread rapidly across the entire cell, contacting all myofilaments (Nelson and Benson, 1963).

In addition to these structural specializations, the muscle cell often contains lipid droplets, glycogen particles and lipofuscin granules. The lipofuscin is found in increased quantity in the advanced years of life and, as elsewhere, presumably represents a "wear and tear" metabolic residuum (p. 47). In cardiac muscle, the lipofuscin residual bodies are characteristically located at the nuclear poles.

As is well known, the muscle cell is the mover of the body. Its single purpose is contraction which involves the conversion of chemical energy to kinetic energy. ATP is the major source of the chemical energy, and the contractile proteins of the myofilaments, actin and myosin, are the mediators of this transformation of chemical energy. Muscle shortening, according to Huxley (1965), occurs by the sliding of the thin filaments between the thick filaments toward the center of the sarcomere. Since the thin filaments are attached to the Z line at both ends of the sarcomere, a sliding motion toward the central A band causes shortening of the sarcomere, and it is the summation of shortening of all sarcomeres which constitutes contraction of the entire muscle cell.

Muscular contraction is now conceived of as an electrochemical reaction triggered by the release of acetylcholine at the myoneural junction. Involved in such contraction is an energy-consuming interaction between the tadpole-shaped myosin molecule and the reversibly globular-fibrillar actin molecule. The precise sequence of events following acetylcholine release is still a controversial issue and beyond our scope. It is enough to simply indicate that release of acetylcholine results in a flux of sodium and potassium ions along the membrane and through the T system of tubules, transiently depolarizing the membranes. Depolarization is associated with an influx of sodium into the cell, while muscle cell relaxation and repolarization involve an outflow of potassium. The energy consumed in muscular contraction is largely derived from the hydrolysis of ATP by calcium-activated ATPase. Recently, it has been found that in addition to actin and myosin, myofilaments contain two additional proteins, tropomyosin and troponin, which inhibit interaction of actin and myosin and so block contraction. This inhibition is overcome by cal-

cium ions. Further details on the mechanism of excitation-contraction coupling may be found in Sandow (1965).

PATHOLOGY

Disorders of skeletal muscle (myopathies) occur in a variety of systemic diseases as well as in certain primary muscular disorders. In general, these myopathies comprise a relatively small and peripheral area of pathologic practice. To recount all the conditions in which the skeletal muscles may be affected would entail listing a large percentage of all the disorders that have already been presented. For example, in staphylococcic infections, subcutaneous abscesses may secondarily involve adjacent muscle fibers, and hematogenous dissemination of staphylococci may produce multiple foci of suppurative infection within the muscles. Muscular involvement is a prominent feature of scleroderma and dermatomyositis. Muscle cell injury is encountered in typhoid fever. Patients who are long confined to bed or who sustain a fracture with immobilization of an extremity may suffer disuse atrophy of muscles. And so the skeletal muscles are the seat of numerous morphologic changes in a great variety of states.

The present consideration of muscular disease will be largely limited to a description of the basic reactions of muscle to various forms of injury. The number of these morphologic reactions is limited because the same basic reaction may be produced by a variety of etiologies. Thus, atrophy of muscle occurs in immobilization of an extremity, following denervation and in severe malnutrition. To interpret the meaning of one of these reaction patterns, and thus establish a pathogenetic mechanism and a clinical diagnosis of muscular disease, it is necessary to: (1) identify the basic pattern of muscle injury, (2) determine the distribution of muscle involvement and (3) ascertain the coexistence of other organ involvements and possible etiologic mechanisms. A simplified classification of the basic morphologic patterns of muscle injury follows, indicating some of the more common conditions evoking such injury (Table 31–1). Following this overview, some of the more important reaction patterns and a few specific muscle diseases are discussed in greater detail.

MUSCULAR ATROPHY

Atrophic shrinkage, death and disappearance of muscle cells comprise basic reaction patterns to many forms of adverse influence.

TABLE 31-1. CLASSIFICATION OF MYOPATHIES

I. Dysvoluminal Myopathies
  A. Atrophy
    1. Poliomyelitis (or any other form of denervation)
    2. Disuse
    3. Cachexia
    4. Senility
    5. Hyperthyroidism
    6. Panhypopituitarism
  B. Hypoplasia
    1. Amyotonia congenita
  C. Hypertrophy
    1. Myotonia congenita
    2. Hypothyroidism
    3. Hyperpituitarism
    4. Overuse

The major anatomic change in these myopathies involves alteration in size of muscle fibers. The altered volume reflects augmentation or diminution of myofibrils and sarcoplasm.

II. Myopathies Associated with Muscle Cell Necrosis
  A. Primary muscular dystrophies
  B. Specific infections (trichinosis and toxoplasmosis)
  C. Corticosteroid myopathy
  D. Polymyositis and dermatomyositis
  E. Polymyopathy of Meyer-Betz with myoglobinuria

Characteristic of all of these myopathies is necrosis of muscle cells. Usually the whole fiber is not involved, and zones of altered sarcoplasm may be juxtaposed with preserved sarcomeres. In the focus of muscle injury, there is generally a leukocytic infiltrate principally of neutrophils and lymphocytes. Sarcolemmal nuclei may appear shrunken and pyknotic or enlarged and increased in number. In later stages, thin new fibers can be identified as regeneration occurs. If entire fibers are destroyed, foci of fibrosis may result.

III. Myopathies Associated with Distinctive Intracellular Alterations
  A. Familial periodic paralysis
  B. Hyperaldosteronism

In these conditions, the muscle cells contain small hydropic vacuoles, reflecting the accumulation of water.
  C. McArdle's phosphorylase deficiency
  D. Pompe's disease

These two disorders represent glycogen storage diseases in which abnormal accumulations of glycogen appear within lysosomes.
  E. Central core myopathy—The inner part of the fiber contains condensed myofibrils.
  F. Rod-body myopathy—Rod-shaped packets of myosin-like bodies lie beneath the sarcolemma.
  G. Myotonic dystrophy—The main features are peripheral zones of sarcoplasm containing various organelles and isolated myofilaments, some of which form bundles which encircle the longitudinally oriented myofibrils.

IV. Functional Myopathies
  A. Myasthenia gravis
  B. Thyroid myopathies
  C. Tetanus
  D. Addison's disease with contractions

Morphologic examination of muscle may reveal no structural alteration in neurons or muscle fibers in these disorders. Occasionally, intercellular infiltrates of lymphocytes (lymphorrhages) are found, but these are nondistinctive and are often absent.

Atrophy consists essentially of progressive **loss of myofilaments, shrinkage of muscle cells by resorption of sarcoplasm followed later by fibrous replacement of collapsed sarcolemmal sheaths.** The individual myocytes show a progressive diminution in their diameters. The striations are preserved for a long time, but eventually become less distinct. The sarcolemmal or muscle nuclei may appear to increase in number as the fibers lose substance. Eventually, in atrophy, the myocyte shrinks to almost a hollow tube with preservation of only the sarcolemmal nuclei. Up to this stage, there is little increase in the interstitial connective tissue and little evidence of inflammatory reaction. However, the cell may die and be replaced by fibrous tissue and, at this time, a scant lymphocytic interstitial infiltrate appears.

Frequently, in the later stages, golden yellow perinuclear lipochrome pigment becomes apparent within the partially atrophic muscle cells, a change that has already been described as **brown atrophy** (p. 47). The distribution of these atrophic cells is frequently of considerable help in differentiating, for example, disuse, vascular or denervation atrophy from the regressive alterations encountered in the muscular dystrophies. In the pure atrophic process, there is little inflammatory reaction and little evidence of acute necrosis of muscle cells. In general, the atrophic changes tend to affect bundles of cells or whole muscles rather than the random spotty distribution characteristic of the dystrophies to be described.

These alterations, when sufficiently marked, cause shrinkage and flabbiness of the entire muscle mass. Under certain circumstances, as when the atrophy is caused by focal loss of nerve supply, the unaffected adjacent fibers may undergo compensatory hypertrophy and there may be no appreciable loss of muscle mass. The muscle loses its normal redbrown, meaty color and becomes yellow to brown depending upon the amount of deposition of lipochrome pigment. In far advanced cases, the replacement fibrosis imparts a pale gray, fibrous quality to the shrunken muscle.

Causes. The causes of muscular atrophy are legion and vary from the generalized skeletal atrophy encountered in old age to minute foci of atrophy that may affect only a single motor neuromuscular unit when a peripheral nerve fiber is cut. The atrophy of *advanced age* usually produces moderate diminution in the muscle mass without destruction of muscle cells. In this condition, all the muscle fibers tend to be affected equally. *Chronic malnutrition* may produce the same changes. Muscular atrophy which is fairly diffuse throughout the body is also seen in *panhypopituitarism. Ischemia* is an important cause of muscle atrophy and may, in fact, underlie the generalized atrophy of senility. Such ischemia is particularly important in the causation of the atrophy associated with the vascular diseases, such as arteriosclerosis, thromboembolism, Buerger's disease or any other form of vascular narrowing or occlusion.

Muscle cells are entirely dependent upon their motor innervation. On this basis, an important group of muscular atrophies are encountered in *spinal cord or peripheral nerve lesions.* The atrophy that occurs then in poliomyelitis; peripheral neuritis, such as is caused by thiamine chloride deficiency and diabetic neuritis; and in injuries to peripheral nerves follows the pattern of morphologic changes described. The distribution of the atrophy depends upon the pattern of innervation of affected motor nerves. Denervation atrophy may differ slightly from the other forms of atrophy in that, in the plane of section, one may find affected muscle fibers that have lost their innervation adjacent to normal-appearing muscle fibers having an independent nerve supply. The diagnosis of denervation atrophy can frequently be supported by the demonstration of degenerated nerve filaments within the muscle section. This type of apparent denervation atrophy is also encountered in certain specific neuromuscular diseases, i.e., infantile muscular atrophy, amyotonia congenita, progressive muscular atrophy of Aran-Duchenne and amyotrophic lateral sclerosis of Charcot. *Immobilization* of an extremity, either from some central nervous system injury with paralysis of an extremity or by the application of a cast, is followed by atrophy of the muscles.

MUSCULAR DYSTROPHY

The muscular dystrophies comprise a group of genetically determined myopathies characterized by regressive alterations in individual muscle cells that lead to weakness in the affected muscles. The dystrophies have been divided clinically into a variety of types based upon specific patterns of muscle involvement. However, at the level of the anatomic lesion in the individual muscle fiber, the changes are virtually identical in all clinical patterns. A recent classification of the muscular dystrophies is presented in Table 31-2, and a few of these entities are discussed briefly below.

DUCHENNE DYSTROPHY

As is characteristic of all X-linked recessive traits, this disease typically occurs in boys, transmitted through asymptomatic mothers.

TABLE 31-2. CLASSIFICATION OF MUSCULAR DYSTROPHIES

I. Forms Characterized by Proximal Limb Weakness
  A. X-linked recessive diseases
    1. Duchenne dystrophy
    2. Becker dystrophy
  B. Autosomal dominant diseases
    1. Facioscapulohumeral dystrophy
    2. Scapuloperoneal dystrophy
  C. Autosomal recessive diseases
    1. Limb-girdle dystrophies
    2. Congenital muscular dystrophies
II. Forms Characterized by Unusual Distribution of Weakness
  A. Distal muscular dystrophy—? autosomal dominant
  B. Ocular muscular dystrophy—uncertain genetic transmission
III. Forms Characterized by Myotonia
  A. Myotonic muscular dystrophy—autosomal dominant
  B. Chondrodystrophic myotonia
IV. Congenital Myopathies—Uncertain Genetic Transmission, ? Autosomal Recessive, ? Autosomal Dominant
  A. Nemaline myopathy
  B. Central core disease
  C. Centronuclear myopathy
  D. Other forms

From "Muscular dystrophies" by Rowland in Disease-A-Month by Dowling (ed.). Copyright © 1972 by Year Book Medical Publishers. Used by permission.

Occasional cases have been identified in young girls, suggesting an autosomal recessive mode of transmission, but the possibility of spontaneous genetic mutations cannot be ruled out in these instances.

Usually the symptoms of motor weakness do not become apparent until after the first year of life. Thereafter, difficulties become manifest in the form of retarded onset of walking, a waddling gait, inability to run and general lack of motor coordination. All of these problems are due to weakness of the pelvic girdle muscles. Characteristically, the gastrocnemius muscles may appear enlarged, referred to as pseudohypertrophy. Involvement of the arm muscles appears later, but only rarely are the facial and cranial muscles significantly affected.

The disease tends to progress quite rapidly and, by 10 years of age, the motor weakness may be so severe that the patient is confined to a wheelchair. Even sitting becomes difficult and weakness of axial muscles leads to deforming scoliosis. Respiratory movements become progressively weaker as these muscles become affected, predisposing to pulmonary infections. Many of the patients have a lowered intelligence. Electrocardiographic abnormalities indicative of morphologic changes in the cardiac muscle fibers often appear.

Morphologically, in the early stages of the disease, individual fibers are affected and sometimes only several sarcomeres within the cell. The necrotizing lesion may be associated with an infiltrate of neutrophils, lymphocytes and macrophages. In the later stages, when most cases are seen, isolated fiber shrinkage, atrophy and disappearance become evident. Adjacent fibers may be relatively spared or, indeed, hypertrophic, representing a compensatory phenomenon. These hypertrophic cells may disclose proliferation of sarcolemmal nuclei. It is such cellular hypertrophy which gives rise to the so-called pseudohypertrophy of the gastrocnemius muscles. In time, widespread atrophy of muscle cells appears, accompanied by accumulations of fat cells interspersed between the muscle fibers. In these late stages, there may be no well preserved muscle cells, accounting for the generalized atrophy of muscles seen at autopsy. It has been estimated that more than 50 per cent of the cells in a muscle must be involved before clinical evidence of deranged function becomes apparent. Comparable changes may be found in the heart, but they are rarely as advanced as those seen in skeletal muscle (Engel, 1965).

The clinical diagnosis of this condition rests largely on the identification of the distribution of muscle weakness. As would be expected, increased serum levels of GOT, GPT, LDH, CPK, aldolase and myoglobin are present as reflections of leakage of these enzymes from the damaged muscle fibers. Most of the patients die early in life of pulmonary infections related to the progressive involvement of the respiratory muscles.

A "benign" variant of Duchenne dystrophy has been recognized and is referred to as "slow type." The mode of transmission is identical to that of the aggressive form of the disease. In these patients, ability to walk is not lost before middle or even later adult life. Life expectancy is reduced only slightly. These individuals suffer no mental impairment and many have children.

FACIOSCAPULOHUMERAL MUSCULAR DYSTROPHY

In contrast to the Duchenne dystrophy with its invariable pelvic onset, the manifestations of facioscapulohumeral dystrophy begin in the face or shoulder girdle. The pattern of transmission is autosomal dominant, hence both sexes are affected. Symptoms are rarely present before adolescence but, at this age, difficulty in closing the eyes or in whistling becomes manifest. Lifting motions and raising the arms overhead become labored and some-

times impossible. The scapulae appear unusually prominent as the surrounding muscles undergo atrophy. Even though the disorder begins in the upper regions of the body, in time, leg and axial muscle weakness become evident, leading to difficulty both in walking and arising from a sitting position, and in maintenance of an erect stance.

As indicated earlier, the anatomic changes in most muscular dystrophies are quite similar. They vary only in the distribution of muscle involvement. Because facioscapulohumeral muscular dystrophy is, in general, milder than Duchenne dystrophy, the serum enzymes are normal or only slightly increased. The disease usually runs a course of 20 to 40 years and, since it begins in the second or third decade of life, it does not usually significantly shorten the life span.

MICROBIOLOGIC INJURIES TO MUSCLES

Damage to muscle cells may occur from direct invasion by bacteria, viruses, parasites or fungi. In addition, many bacterial toxic products, such as those produced by *Clostridium welchii*, injure muscle cells.

Any of these forms of myopathy, better called myositis, may involve one or many muscles and, in the affected muscles, may present as sharply focalized or diffuse lesions. In the foci of damage, there is usually a fairly prominent inflammatory cell infiltration accompanying the cytologic changes within the muscle cells. Depending upon the underlying cause, injured muscle cells or totally necrotic muscle cells that have undergone fatty changes or coagulative necrosis are found, along with inflammatory white cell infiltration. The leukocytic response comprises neutrophils if the process is acute, or lymphocytes, histiocytes and monocytes if the process is chronic. In later stages, there is more or less fibrous replacement of damaged cells and compensatory hypertrophy of marginal preserved cells. When the muscle is actually invaded by the causative agent (as occurs in abscess formation caused by staphylococci or streptococci, infection by trichinae or the spreading infections of *Clostridium welchii*, toxoplasmosis, cysticercosis or trypanosomiasis), serial studies, special stains and cultural techniques sometimes permit the identification of the underlying etiologic agent at the site of injury.

In the forms of myopathy which are encountered in typhoid fever, influenza, pneumonia and smallpox, the muscle cell injury is usually confined to the sarcoplasmic substance of the muscle cell which may suffer from any of the forms of degeneration or necrosis already mentioned, but in general the sarcolemmal sheath, the interstitial connective tissue and the perimysium are little affected and the inflammatory infiltrate is correspondingly less prominent.

These inflammatory diseases of muscle differ histologically from the muscular dystrophies. In the latter, the inflammatory reaction is more scant, and regenerative activity is minimal, while in the inflammatory conditions, considerable regrowth of injured or partially damaged muscle cells may occur and compensatory hypertrophy of unaffected cells fills in the gap produced by the loss of muscle cells.

In addition to the various diseases already mentioned, inflammatory myositis may be encountered in any of the so-called *connective tissue diseases*, but in these instances the nature of the muscle involvement can be identified only by the characteristic alterations in blood vessels and organs that accompany the muscle changes (Chapter 7). Myositis is one of the most prominent features of *Weil's disease*. An obscure form of primary myositis involving many muscles simultaneously is termed polymyositis. In all forms of myositis, the inflammatory changes are essentially similar and may only be termed myositis. Differentiation of one condition from the other requires a knowledge of associated anatomic changes and the clinical findings.

MYASTHENIA GRAVIS (MG)

Myasthenia gravis is a chronic disease of probable autoimmune origin characterized by abnormal fatigability of skeletal muscles, most likely due to some neuromuscular conduction block. The facial, oculomotor, laryngeal, pharyngeal and respiratory muscles are especially affected. The abnormal muscular fatigability sometimes remains localized to extraocular muscles and remits spontaneously. More frequently, however, it is a progressive disease that sometimes results in death from respiratory failure. Approximately 75 per cent of the cases have some associated thymic abnormality—a thymoma in somewhat less than one-third, and thymic hyperplasia (lymphoid follicle formation) in the remainder. Follicular hyperplasia may also be seen in the residual thymic tissue about the margins of a thymoma (p. 1368) (Castleman and Norris, 1949). The converse also holds; Seybold and his associates (1950) have reported that 75 per cent of patients with thymomas have myasthenia gravis.

Manifestations of MG usually appear in the third and fourth decades of life. Women in this young age group are affected three times more often than men. In most of these young individuals, the thymic lesion takes the form of follicular hyperplasia. When symptoms begin later in life (over the age of 50), there is no sex preponderance, and most of these individuals are likely to have tumors of the thymus (Thomas, 1972). Most of the thymic neoplasms are lymphoepithelial thymomas, but all histologic varieties have been encountered in these patients (Iverson, 1956).

Pathogenesis. The association of thymic lesions with myasthenia gravis and the known importance of the thymus in the immune system have naturally led to the belief that MG is a disease of immunologic origin. While a wealth of immunologic findings have been uncovered, it is by no means clear that these immune reactions impair myoneural conduction. Antibodies reactive against both skeletal muscle and thymic tissue can be demonstrated in the sera of 30 to 75 per cent of patients with MG, the highest frequency being encountered in the most severely affected patients (Strauss, 1968). It is interesting to note that virtually all patients with thymomas have such antibodies. Beutner et al. (1962) believe that there are two types of antibodies. One so-called "S" antibody fixes complement and reacts with an antigen present only in skeletal muscle. The other "Sh" antibody does not fix complement and reacts with an antigen common to skeletal and cardiac muscle. Both antibodies cross react with the thymus. Immunofluorescent studies indicate that, in striated muscle, the antibody binds principally to the I bands (Vetters, 1967). There appears to be considerable specificity to this immunologic response since, with serum dilutions of 1 to 60, no false-positive results were encountered with sera from a host of other disease conditions (Strauss, 1968).

The basis for the cross reactivity of the antibodies in MG between striated muscle and thymic tissue remained mysterious until the rediscovery of the thymic myoid cells. Electron microscopic studies have disclosed cells resembling striated muscle in the thymus glands of many species and in the fetal thymus in man. Goldstein (1966, 1971) proposes that the lymphoid hyperplasia and plasma cell proliferation in the thymus, which he calls "thymitis" are manifestations of some spontaneous loss of tolerance to "self." Abnormal reactivity against the thymic myoid cells might induce antibodies, which would then cross react with striated muscles throughout the body. Thus, the concept has grown that *myasthenia gravis is a form of autoimmune disease.*

It should be noted that the antibodies in MG do not localize at the myoneural junctions.

Indeed, there is no evidence that they participate in the myoneural conduction defect characteristic of this condition. Moreover, some patients with MG fail to have any demonstrable antibodies. It has, therefore, been proposed that the thymus releases a nonimmunologic, humoral substance which, in some way, produces the neuromuscular block. Lymphoid hyperplasia of the thymus gland and impaired neuromuscular transmission can be induced in approximately 50 per cent of animals immunized with saline extracts of heterologous or homologous thymus or striated muscle in Freund's adjuvant. Presumably, when thymitis is present, the gland is more active in elaborating this blocking substance.

The observation that many patients with MG are improved by thymectomy gives support to the view that the thymic lesion, in those with thymic abnormalities, contributes to the muscular dysfunction. The majority of patients with a favorable outcome have simple hyperplasia of the gland and are more likely to be women in whom the onset of symptoms was fairly recent. In many patients, however, even those with a thymoma, removal of the gland and tumor is not beneficial. To date, it has not been possible to predict which patients will be improved and which will not.

The trigger event for the autoimmune reaction is still unestablished. However, there are many hints that some genetic influence predisposes to the development of MG. These individuals appear to have some constitutional predisposition to abnormal immune reactivity. Patients with MG sometimes have thyroid autoantibodies, gastric parietal cell autoantibodies, rheumatoid factor and antinuclear reactivity. Conceivably, the development of a thymic tumor favors the emergence of "forbidden" clones and, indeed, thymic tumors have been identified in patients with SLE, rheumatoid arthritis, scleroderma, Sjögren's syndrome and aplastic anemia (Strauss, 1968). However, as with all autoimmune diseases, the trigger event remains an enigma. In considering all of the foregoing, we must remember that a minority of patients have neither thymic abnormalities nor antibodies, so there are still many unanswered questions relative to the causation of this disease.

Morphology. The thymic changes found in association with myasthenia gravis were described on p. 1369. Seventy-five per cent of patients have thymic hyperplasia accompanied in about one-third of the cases by a thymic tumor. But it should be noted that approximately 25 per cent of patients with MG have normal thymic glands.

In the majority of cases, the muscles appear entirely normal macroscopically. Such atrophy as may be present appears to result from lack of use rather than from any primary cause. Moreover, microscopic examination fails to disclose any defect in the myocytes or supporting stroma. In only a relatively few cases, small focal collections of interstitial lymphocytes (**lymphorrhages**) are found. Usually the muscle cells about these foci appear quite unremarkable. The significance of these lymphoid changes is not clear, but they may possibly be related to the persistence of the thymic gland in cases associated with this abnormality. Lymphocytic infiltrates have also been observed in the liver, thyroid gland, adrenals and other organs.

Clinical Course. The clinical diagnosis usually becomes manifest by the development of abnormal muscular fatigability and weakness, which first becomes evident in the muscles in most active use, i.e., extraocular muscles and those of the face, tongue and upper extremities. The principal danger in this condition is the development of weakness of the respiratory muscles predisposing to inadequate ventilation of the lungs, pulmonary infections and even asphyxia. The disease tends to run a chronic course punctuated by spontaneous remissions, sometimes followed by exacerbations. In a large series of cases followed for up to 35 years, one-third died within six years of the onset of the illness. On the other hand, one-quarter entered a period of complete remission for as long as five years. The prognosis is therefore quite unpredictable. The diagnosis is supported by the demonstration of antibodies against striated muscle and by electromyographic tests confirming impaired neuromuscular transmission. The administration of anticholinesterases and thymectomy sometimes produce gratifying results.

TUMORS AND TUMOR-LIKE DISORDERS OF MUSCLES

Under this heading are included two non-neoplastic disorders that are entirely distinctive, myositis ossificans circumscripta and myositis ossificans progressiva, both having in common replacement of muscle mass by ossifying fibrous tissue, as well as the few, rare, primary neoplasms of muscle.

Traumatic Myositis Ossificans (Circumscripta). In this condition, traumatic injury to muscle, usually accompanied by considerable hemorrhage, is followed by the deposit of fibrous tissue and bone in the site of injury. This type of muscle injury is most apt to occur in young males exposed to heavy strains in the course of their work, athletics or military service. Following the muscle tear or damage, *the hemorrhage is organized by the characteristic formation of granulation tissue and progressive fibrous scarring.* In the course of this process, *cartilage may form and be followed by endochondral ossification. Alternatively, calcification may occur en masse and be followed by ossification.* The origin of the osteoblasts that lay down the bone is uncertain, but they either arise in situ from mesenchymal cells, or are derived from adjacent periosteum which is involved in the muscular injury. Aside from the attendant pain, swelling and tenderness, the major significance of myositis ossificans lies in its possible confusion with a bone tumor. The hard, localized, bony mass, the roentgenographic demonstration of bone density outside the normal bone, and the histologic pattern of proliferating fibroblasts associated with bone formation may all be confused by the unwary with an osteogenic sarcoma or some other type of ossifying bone tumor.

Myositis Ossificans Progressiva. This is an extremely uncommon disease of unknown etiology that tends to affect children or young adults and is characterized by the replacement of muscles, tendons, ligaments, fasciae and aponeuroses by bone. There is some question of its being a congenital, hereditary disorder, since it is accompanied, in a considerable number of cases, by other congenital anomalies, such as absence of digits, congenital hallux valgus, absence of certain teeth and other anomalies. The disorder may affect any of the striated muscles in the body including the heart and diaphragm, but usually it begins in the head and neck region. Its onset is characterized by swelling, redness and tenderness overlying the involved muscle and, as the acute symptoms in the skin subside, the underlying muscle becomes progressively more indurated and finally transformed to bony masses. Histologically, during the acute stages, a diffuse myositis is found that is followed by progressive disappearance of muscle cells and their replacement by collagenous fibrous tissue, which is converted eventually into cartilage and then bone. This sequence of histologic changes begins at one site or in one muscle and, over the course of years, may progressively extend to affect other muscles until eventually death is caused by involvement of the heart or the muscles of respiration.

Desmoid (Musculoaponeurotic Fibromatosis). Desmoid is the name given to a curious fibromatous proliferation that is best considered as a fibrosarcoma Grade 1/2. These lesions do not arise from muscle fibers but rather from the musculoaponeurotic struc-

tures of the body and are, therefore, properly speaking, lesions of the supporting connective tissue of muscle.

They may occur at any age but are most common in the third to fifth decades of life. About 70 per cent occur in women, frequently following pregnancy. The nature of these fibromatoses, which appear histologically benign but are nonetheless locally invasive, is quite mysterious. Two theories are proposed. The first relates the fibrous overgrowth to *trauma*, an association that is borne out by the frequency with which abdominal lesions occur following the violent muscular contractions of parturition. The same relationship to trauma has been established in about one-half of the tumors that occur elsewhere in the body. On the other hand, there is some evidence that desmoids may be caused by *endocrinologic disturbances.* Bio-assays of the tumor tissue have disclosed, in certain cases, a high concentration of estrogenic and pituitary gonadotropic hormones. Moreover, desmoid-like tumors have been produced in guinea pigs by the injection of estrogens. In these experimental animals, the fibromatogenic activity of the estrogens has been blocked by the simultaneous administration of testosterone, progesterone and deoxycorticosterone.

Morphologically, these lesions occur as unicentric, gray-white, firm, unencapsulated, poorly demarcated masses that vary in size from small nodules 1 to 2 cm. in diameter to large masses up to 15 cm. in diameter. Approximately two-thirds of these lesions occur in the musculature or the musculoaponeuroses of the anterior abdominal wall, but virtually every muscle in the body has been affected. The lesions have a rubbery, tough consistency and, on gross inspection, invade between muscles and muscle bundles, separating groups of muscle cells. Histologically, they resemble **a somewhat cellular fibroma,** having an abundance of collagenous fibrous tissue. The individual fibrocytes are usually uniform in size and shape, and only rarely can mitoses or large atypical cells or nuclei be identified. This neoplasia insinuates itself between muscle groups and individual muscle cells and frequently causes destruction and atrophy of trapped myocytes. Often these injured myocytes are transformed to **muscle giant cells.** Histologically, then, the tumor displays the paradoxical qualities of distinct invasiveness but relatively complete cytologic innocence.

Clinically, these tumors appear as slowly developing, firm, subcutaneous masses. Occasionally, pain is associated with their development. It is usually taught that desmoid tumors never metastasize and, therefore, can be successfully cured by adequate surgical excision, but rare cases of local metastasis to regional nodes have been reported. Such biologic behavior clearly indicates that, despite their apparent benign appearance, these tumors are extremely well differentiated, slowly growing, collagenous fibrosarcomas arising in skeletal muscles.

Myoblastoma (Granular Cell Myoblastoma). The myoblastoma is a curious, usually small lesion of uncertain nature and histogenetic origin. It is usually encountered in the skin, mucous membranes or tongue, but may arise in such unusual sites as the breast, larynx, thyroid gland, gallbladder, esophagus, stomach and pituitary gland. In all of these sites, it has an identical gross and microscopic appearance.

These tumors are usually well defined, sharply circumscribed, spherical, gray to yellow-tan nodules that rarely exceed 2 to 3 cm. in diameter. Histologically, the tumors are composed of large, round to polygonal cells that may be arranged in diffuse masses or in cords and narrow columns, separated by a scant connective tissue stroma. The individual **cells have an abundant pink acidophilic cytoplasm** surrounding small, regular, round to ovoid nuclei. The cytoplasm contains numerous coarse and fine granules that make these cells resemble xanthoma cells or lipophages. However, the cytoplasmic material is **not sudanophilic.** The granules are of two sizes. The smaller ones resemble lysosomes, but do not stain with lysosomal markers. The larger ones are more typical of lysosomes and contain, among other enzymes, acid phosphatase (Sobel et al., 1971). In the usual tumor, there are neither mitotic figures nor anaplasia, but rare lesions may show greater cellular and nuclear pleomorphism and have been called malignant granular cell myoblastomas. Such lesions apparently penetrate irregularly into the surrounding normal tissues, but they rarely, if ever, have aggressive infiltrative behavior or metastasize.

The nature and cell of origin of these nodules is still in doubt. The lesion has been variously interpreted as a focal degeneration of cells, a focal storage disease or a tumor of muscle, of histiocytic, fibroblastic or neurogenic origin. Most writers believe that they are tumors but, despite the designation myoblastoma, are not certain that they are of muscle cell origin. Scattered reports suggest that tissue cultures of cells derived from myoblastomas occasionally yield cell forms bearing a striking resemblance to embryonic muscle cells (Bangle, 1952). Alternatively, it has been proposed that they may be derived from fibroblasts or Schwann cells associated with periph-

eral nerves (Sobel et al., 1971). Recently, two reports appeared within the span of a single year, one contending that ultrastructural studies confirmed the Schwann cell origin of the neoplasms (Sobel et al., 1971), and the other contending that there was no evidence that these lesions were neurogenous (Al-Sarraf, 1971).

Whatever their origin, these nodules are usually of little clinical significance and are readily excised and readily cured. Malignant lesions are exceedingly rare and many so reported may not, in reality, represent granular cell myoblastomas. Not infrequently, for obscure reasons, when these tumors occur submucosally or subepithelially, the overlying epithelium undergoes striking hyperplasia (pseudoepitheliomatous), simulating squamous cell carcinoma.

Rhabdomyosarcoma. Rhabdomyosarcomas, although rare, are among the more common malignant tumors of soft parts (muscle, fibrous tissue, fatty tissue). Three distinct histologic and clinical patterns are recognized: (1) adult pleomorphic (10 to 15 per cent), (2) embryonal alveolar (40 to 45 per cent) and (3) embryonal botryoid (40 to 45 per cent).

Adult Pleomorphic Rhabdomyosarcoma. These tumors generally occur in adults between the fourth and seventh decades of life. Only rarely are they encountered in infants and children. Approximately half arise in the lower extremities, but any muscle in the body may be affected, particularly the quadriceps, adductors and biceps.

These tumors vary in size from relatively small to large bulky masses, sometimes over 15 cm. in diameter. Clinically, they are deceptively well circumscribed but, on cross section of the mass, no capsule can be identified. The cut surface varies from pale brown to gray and is often punctuated, in the more rapidly growing lesions, by areas of hemorrhage, cystic softening and pale foci of necrosis.

Microscopically, most are highly undifferentiated, wildly anaplastic tumors. In any single tumor, the cells vary from relatively small, oval to spindled forms with small, darkly chromatic nuclei to huge, irregular masses of cytoplasm containing many large nuclei or one massive multilobed nucleus. Some tumors appear to be made up largely of these tumor giant cells. Vacuoles containing PAS-positive material, presumably glycogen, can sometimes be seen in these giant cells. The entire spectrum of atypical mitotic figures can often be seen in these neoplasms. The tendency for some cells to assume strap-like ribbon or tennis racquet (tadpole) shapes is characteristic of these rhabdomyosarcomas. Longitudinal striations resembling myofilaments can usually be seen within the cytoplasm of the larger cells; but to establish the diagnosis with certainty, it is necessary to delineate cross striations typical of striated muscle (Fig. 31–2).

Just as the tumors span a wide range in cytology, they vary greatly in their growth rate and clinical behavior. Some are slow-growing or even quiescent over a span of years. These lesions are readily excised and cured. Others, however, pursue a fulminating, rapidly progressive course with a dramatic increase in tumor size, invasion into surrounding tissues and ultimate spread to other sites. A common clinical phenomenon is local recurrence after excision, requiring ever more radical surgery and sometimes amputation of the extremity in the hope of thwarting metastatic spread.

Embryonal Alveolar Rhabdomyosarcoma. These occur almost exclusively in children and young adults in the first two decades of life. Common sites for their origin are the upper and lower extremities, although occasionally tumors are encountered in the trunk and, indeed, in any muscle of the body.

These tumors vary widely in size but rarely achieve the massive dimensions of the adult rhabdomyosarcoma. Deceptively localized on clinical examination, they are found on cross section to be

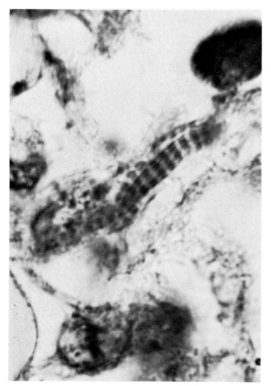

Figure 31–2. *A histologic detail of a well differentiated striated myocyte in a rhabdomyosarcoma.*

circumscribed but unencapsulated. The cut surface is characteristically soft gray and fish-flesh in appearance. Occasionally, areas of cartilaginous consistency and other areas of loose myxoid material can be defined. Microscopically, the tumors are composed of round to oval to occasionally elongated cell forms scarcely resembling adult muscle cells but possibly having some similarity to embryonal forms. The term alveolar refers to the tendency for an abundant fibrous stroma to create numerous interlacing septa which segregate small nests or rosettes of tumor cells. The stroma somewhat reproduces the alveolar pattern of the lung, with the neoplastic cells filling the alveolar spaces. The cells do not align themselves along the fibrous stroma, but rather are loosely attached and sometimes crowded together in a disorderly pattern. Variation in cell and nuclear size is characteristic, but the extremes of anaplasia encountered in the adult forms are rarely seen. Here and there, racquet-shaped cells, strap cells and more differentiated striated elements can be identified. Occasionally, small vacuoles may appear within the cytoplasm, apparently filled with glycogen.

The alveolar rhabdomyosarcoma is an aggressive lesion with a strong tendency toward early metastasis. On the order of 80 to 90 per cent of the patients die of disseminated cancer (blood-borne and lymphatic spread) within a few years of the appearance of the lesion.

Embryonal Botryoid Rhabdomyosarcomas. These lesions are identical to, or close relatives of, the lesions known as sarcoma botryoides encountered in the genitourinary tract (p. 1213). They may, however, arise in other sites, such as the head, neck, orbit, nasopharynx, gallbladder, bile ducts and extremities. They appear to originate in some submucosal location and then spread to involve adjacent muscles. Extragenitourinary lesions are most often encountered in children, but may be found in adults.

The term botryoid (grape-like) refers to the macroscopic appearance of these cancers, which grow as large, polypoid, gelatinous masses having more than a passing resemblance to a cluster of grapes. Thus, they extend into the nasopharynx or gallbladder, for example, as multilobate, pedunculated neoplasms sometimes still covered by intact overlying mucosa. On cross section, they have a soft, jelly-like appearance sometimes marked by focal hemorrhages and areas of cystic softening. Histologically, the predominant cytology is an undifferentiated, small, round cell having a large, hyperchromatic central nucleus and scant cytoplasm. Areas of the neoplasm comprise a loose myxoid stroma having an abundant ground substance in which slender, spindled or stellate cells are scattered. Thus, the botryoid rhabdomyosarcoma is easily confused with a myxosarcoma or a myxoid liposarcoma. With careful searching, racquet shapes and elongated ribbon cells can be found, having an abundant cytoplasm in which cross striations can be discerned.

Patients with botryoid rhabdomyosarcomas have a poor prognosis. Death usually occurs within one to two years of the diagnosis. Only about 10 per cent have a five-year survival. To some extent, the gravity of these lesions arises from their origin in locations not amenable to radical excision, such as the nasopharynx, orbit, genitourinary tract and biliary apparatus. Resection is often followed by recurrence until eventually disseminated blood-borne and lymphatic metastases appear.

BONES

NORMAL
PATHOLOGY
Congenital Disorders
    Osteogenesis imperfecta
        (fragilitas ossium, brittle
        bones)
    Marfan's syndrome
    Dyschondroplasia
    Achondroplasia
    Osteopetrosis (osteosclerosis)
    Gargoylism (Hunter-Hurler
        syndrome)
Infections
    Pyogenic osteomyelitis
    Tuberculosis
    Syphilis
Fractures

Osteoporosis
Osteomalacia
Skeletal Changes in
  Hyperparathyroidism (Osteitis
  Fibrosa Cystica Generalisata,
  von Recklinghausen's Disease
  of Bone)
Osteitis Deformans (Paget's
  Disease)
Hypertrophic (Pulmonary)
  Osteoarthropathy
Fibrous Dysplasia
  (Albright's syndrome)
Tumors
    Osteogenic tumors
      Osteoma
      Osteoid osteoma

      Osteogenic sarcoma
      Fibrosarcoma arising in bone
    Chondromatous tumors
      Exostosis (exostosis
        cartilaginea)
      Enchondroma
      Chondromyxoid fibroma
      Chondrosarcoma
    Giant cell tumors
      Benign chondroblastoma
        of bone
    Angiomatous tumors
      Ewing's sarcoma
    Multiple myeloma (plasma
      cell myeloma)
    Secondary malignancy

NORMAL

Just as the body is dependent on the skeleton for its structural stability and for responding and contributing to changes in blood levels of calcium, so is the skeleton dependent upon the body for its maintenance. Important in this maintenance are: (1) the diet, with an adequate content of minerals and vitamins; (2) normal calcium metabolism, in turn dependent upon the gastrointestinal tract, the kidneys, the parathyroid and thyroid (calcitonin) glands; and (3) a host of biochemical and biosynthetic processes involved in the formation of collagen and cartilage. The complicated interactions involved in normal calcium metabolism were discussed on p. 483 (role of vitamin D) and p. 1346 (role of parathyroids).

The seemingly rigid and unchanging skeletal system is, in reality, a restless tissue, constantly being reworked and remodeled. Unlike predominantly cellular tissues in which renewal takes place largely at the cellular level, renewal of bone occurs at the tissue level. Osteoclastic resorption occurs continuously throughout life and is, in turn, followed by osteoblastic reconstruction and mineralization of the newly created osteoid matrix. Even in the adult, osteoclastic erosion cavities are continually forming and being replaced by new haversian systems. This new bone is as metabolically active as developing bone in the fetus. In contrast, older, well formed bone is quite inactive and contributes little to buffering changes in calcium metabolism. In well formed "old" bone, the turnover of calcium is in the range of 1 to 2 per cent per year.

At the metabolic level, the functioning unit of bone tissue is the osteon. In the words of McLean (1958), this is "...the unit of structure of bone at the microscopic level. This is when fully formed an irregularly cylindrical and branching structure with thick walls and with narrow lumen, the haversian canal. The canal carries one or more capillaries or venules. The cylindrical osteons are usually oriented in the long axis of the bones and their basic structure consists of concentric layers of lamellae, the fibrils of each lamella running spirally to the axis of the canal. The osteon in addition to its canal and its fibrillar structure includes large numbers of lacunae, housing the cells of bone (osteocytes) and interconnected with one another and with the lumen by means of branched canalicules. This circulatory system, poor as it may appear, is the only means for transfer of fluids and dissolved substances between the heart, tissue of bone, and the fluids of the body."

The three characteristic cell types of bone

are the osteoblast, responsible for matrix (osteoid) deposition and for its subsequent mineralization; the osteocyte, confined within its bony lacuna, but communicating with adjacent osteocytes and with vascular channels by means of canaliculi; and the osteoclast, concerned with dissolution of the mineral phase and lysis of bone matrix (Fig. 31–3). The osteocyte appears to be long lived, while the life span of the osteoclast may be limited to not more than a few days. The osteoblast may have a somewhat longer life but does not approach that of the osteocyte. It is evident, then, that in the constant remodeling and reworking of bone, there is a continual renewal of osteoclasts and osteoblasts by mitotic division of progenitors.

Bone formation begins with the secretion of soluble collagen by osteoblasts. In rapidly forming bone, the collagen polymerizes in a random felt-like pattern but, in more slowly forming bone, as occurs with bone remodeling, the collagen fibers are laid down in a highly ordered, regular pattern. Bone matrix is composed almost entirely of collagen fibrils (95 per cent). The remainder of the matrix consists of poorly characterized protein, polysaccharides, glycoproteins and phospholipids. As matrix is elaborated, it appears to undergo some poorly

understood maturation or nucleating configuration. Such mature collagen now embedded within bone matrix appears to bind phosphate. Once this level of maturation has occurred, mineralization proceeds spontaneously in the presence of normal calcium and phosphorus concentrations (Glimcher and Krane, 1968). Mineralization of the bone matrix is still poorly understood. Evidence derived from chemical analysis, x-ray diffraction studies and ion-exchange reactions indicates that the mineral component of bone comprises largely calcium phosphate and calcium hydroxide salts laid down as hydroxyapatite crystals. Small amounts of sodium, potassium and magnesium and trace amounts of zinc are also present in the mineral complexes of bone.

Mineralization of bone requires an adequate blood supply and contact between the mineralizing "front" and extracellular fluid. It is of interest to note that extracellular fluid at the "front" is supersaturated with the minerals found in hydroxyapatite. Hence, once a nucleating configuration has developed in the collagen, continued crystallization of the minerals will occur indefinitely until it is limited by the available space (Glimcher, 1959).

There is evidence that osteoblasts may facilitate mineralization essentially by pumping

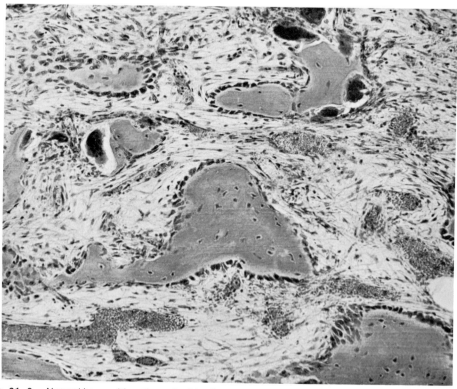

Figure 31–3. *Normal bone with active osteoblastic and osteoclastic activity. There is slight fibrosis of the marrow spaces.*

calcium into the matrix. After a lag period of 6 to 10 days, movement of minerals into new osteoid matrix is initially rapid and may reach 70 per cent full mineralization within a few hours after matrix nucleation. The deposited hydroxyapatite crystals displace the water contained within the matrix. After this initial surge, further mineralization progresses slowly, and the final 30 per cent may take as long as two to three months (Harris and Heaney, 1969). This time sequence is of obvious importance in understanding the progress of healing of fractures.

PATHOLOGY

It is apparent from the foregoing remarks that bone is an exceedingly complex living tissue. It is a composite of protein matrix, hydroxyapatite crystals and living cells, i.e., osteoblasts, osteocytes and osteoclasts and, in addition, contains within its marrow spaces the wide variety of differentiated and primitive cells of the hematopoietic system. It is no surprise, therefore, that the primary diseases of bone are varied and numerous. Any systemic derangement that affects protein synthesis or protein turnover must have its impact on bone. The endocrinopathies are particularly good examples of such. It has already been made clear that the growth and maintenance of bone is intimately dependent upon calcium and phosphorus metabolism with all the numerous factors related to these functions. The development and preservation of bone is further dependent upon the vitality and normal function of the osteoblast and the osteoclast. In addition to all these, the skeletal system is subject to vascular, inflammatory and neoplastic diseases as are the soft tissues of the body. The skeletal tumors may arise from any of the component elements of the bone tissue itself as well as from the RE and myeloid cells contained within the marrow spaces. The bones are also the reluctant hosts to a number of disorders of primary origin elsewhere, such as metastatic tumors.

As if the number of bone diseases were not sufficient, the confusion has been compounded by the zeal that has been displayed in attempting to segregate every involvement of each bone into a distinctive entity and then attaching to these entities an eponymic name. The basic disorder might be the same in all sites, but when aseptic necrosis affects the tibial tubercle, it is called Osgood-Schlatter disease. When this same necrosis affects the navicular bone, it is called Köhler's disease; and when it affects the head of the femur, Legg-Calvé-Perthes disease. In all, ten such eponymic diseases have been created out of a single anatomic derangement. In the face of this complexity, an attempt will be made to select only the more common disorders that represent distinctive morphologic derangements, with omission of many of the eponymic entities. The skeletal system may be affected by virtually every disease "in the book," such as scurvy, leukemia, anemia and brucellosis. The following presentation, therefore, is limited to the principal and primary diseases of bone.

CONGENITAL DISORDERS

Congenital disorders of bone include a variety of relatively innocuous abnormalities that are confined to one or several bones as well as a number of systemic diseases that result in striking skeletal changes and sometimes great morbidity and mortality. Some of the more simple and less serious anomalies consist of failure of development of a bone so that there is congenital absence of a phalanx, rib, clavicle or, more importantly, the femur or other long bone. Occasionally, extra bones are formed, such as supernumerary ribs. Other anomalies take the form of the fusion of two adjacent digits (syndactylism), the duplication of digits resulting in extra fingers or toes (polydactylism) or the development of long spider-like digits (arachnodactylism). The association of this anomaly with Marfan's syndrome will be discussed presently. Other anomalies affect the skull and vertebral column and are frequently of great clinical importance, such as craniorachischisis, failure of closure of the spinal column and skull. This anomaly produces a persistent defect through which the meninges and central nervous system may herniate to produce a meningomyelocele or meningoencephalocele. In addition to these localized developmental defects, there are the following more important systemic disorders.

OSTEOGENESIS IMPERFECTA (FRAGILITAS OSSIUM, BRITTLE BONES)

Osteogenesis imperfecta is an uncommon familial disease characterized by defective synthesis of connective tissue, including, of course, bone matrix (Follis, 1952). The hereditary trait is usually transmitted as an autosomal dominant with variable expressivity. Another distinct form of this disease, with multiple lethal cases in the same family, is thought to be recessively inherited. In this pattern, as many as 25 per cent of the siblings may be affected and the parents are normal (Ibsen, 1967).

The full-blown clinical syndrome is characterized essentially by thin, poorly formed bones, multiple fractures, blue sclerae, deafness, loose-jointedness, scoliosis, a thin skin, a tendency to hernia formation and stunting, with discoloration of the teeth, especially the lower incisors. All of these abnormalities are reflections of a specific defect in collagen synthesis and, therefore, bone matrix formation. Severely affected fetuses with the recessive trait may die at birth; or the infant may survive a short time only to succumb to its multiplicity of fractures. Less severe affliction (the dominant trait) is known as *osteogenesis imperfecta tarda (osteopsathyrosis).* In this less severe form of the disease, the skeletal system is not as weakened, and fractures may not become apparent until the child becomes active in its early years. In those who survive to puberty, fewer fractures appear, perhaps related to better motor coordination and protective instincts.

Morphologically, the skeletal parts are extremely delicate and are often deformed by recent, old and unhealed fractures. Microscopically, the cortical bone is thin to the point of porosity, the cancellous trabeculae are slender, delicate and few in number, and the osteocytes appear to be crowded together by virtue of a lack of intervening matrix. Fractures unite readily, but the bony callus, despite its exuberant nature, is weak, as is the reformed bone. The deafness is the consequence of otosclerosis affecting the middle and inner ear.

Homozygous infants with the recessive trait are most severely affected and, as mentioned, often die within the first years of life. Those who have the autosomal dominant disease have a range of clinical expressions of this condition. Some may have both the skeletal and extraskeletal manifestations, while others may have only mild skeletal changes and, as the only evident involvement, loose-jointedness and blue sclerae.

MARFAN'S SYNDROME

Marfan's syndrome is an interesting hereditary disorder characterized by a basic defect in the formation of elastic fibers. As a consequence, the skeleton, large arteries (principally the aorta and pulmonary artery), suspensory ligaments of the lens and the joint capsules and tendons are affected. This disease is seen in both sexes, and appears to follow the pattern of a *single autosomal dominant although rarely it may occur as a recessive trait.* These people have a slender, elongated habitus with un-

usual height; pectus excavatum; high, arched palate; elongated extremities; loose joints; and spider-like fingers *(arachnodactyly).* The involvement of the ligaments of the lens leads to its displacement and dislocation, sometimes causing blindness. The aortic lesion is the most serious. The deficient formation of elastic fibers is accompanied by the appearance of cystic softening and weakening of the media (cystic medionecrosis). These cysts are usually filled with amorphous ground substance that provides no support for the vasa vasorum that happen to traverse these areas. Rupture of these small vessels leads to dissecting aneurysms, such as occurs in the idiopathic cystic medial necrosis of the aorta (p. 617).

DYSCHONDROPLASIA

Dyschondroplasia refers to *two clinical syndromes* that are characterized by *abnormal cartilaginous growth.* In one, there are abnormal growths of cartilage on the outer surface of the bone producing *multiple cartilaginous exostoses,* while in the other, the deranged cartilaginous growths occur within the bone to produce *multiple cartilaginous enchondroses,* known as *Ollier's disease.*

The pattern characterized by multiple exostoses is a hereditary disease, in which about half the offspring of an affected parent will be involved. The disorder is characterized by many usually symmetrical, bilateral, cartilaginous outgrowths from the metaphysis of bones. Many times, these outgrowths occur more centrally. The long tubular bones are affected most often, particularly the tibia, femur and humerus. The individual lesion consists of a hemispheric or knobby protrusion of quite delicate cancellous bone capped by an outer layer of growing cartilage. It is from this outer layer that endochondral bone is formed progressively to enlarge the lesion (Figs. 31–4 and 31–5). Growth continues throughout childhood, but at the time when the epiphyses close, these lesions cease to enlarge and may even partially regress as the cartilaginous cap is ossified and resorbed. Accompanying these exostoses, there are frequently multiple defects of the skeletal system that generally take the form of shortening or curvature of the long bones. Affected individuals are, therefore, commonly below normal in height. Aside from the deformity and possible discomfort produced by these exostoses, particularly when they occur at sites of weight-bearing or pressure points, the only hazard is the development of a chondrosarcoma in one of the exostoses. Such malignant transformation is rare in those with a solitary exostosis, but represents

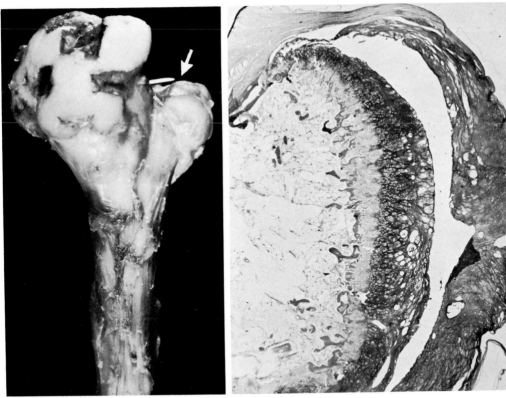

Fig. 31–4   Fig. 31–5

Figure 31–4. Cartilaginous exostosis. The knobby protuberance extends to the right (arrow), *opposite the somewhat deformed irregular femoral head.*

Figure 31–5. Cartilaginous exostosis at low power. The cartilaginous cap has been artefactually lifted off.

a 1 in 10 chance in patients with multiple exostoses.

The other form of dyschondroplasia, known as *Ollier's disease*, is of equally obscure origin, but is nonhereditary. In this condition, *the derangement of cartilaginous growth results in the breaking off, or the incorporation within mature bones, of fragments of epiphyseal plate.* The growth of these cartilaginous fragments gives rise to many enchondroses within the metaphysis. On this basis, a more descriptive designation is *enchondromatosis.* Sometimes these masses of cartilage are more centrally located. Continued growth of these included masses of cartilage may eventually produce expansion of the bone or distortion and disturbance in the growth of the bone. When these skeletal lesions are accompanied by hemangiomas of the skin, the condition is known as *Maffucci's syndrome.*

The long bones are most often affected and, while the disease may be unilateral or affect only a single bone, it is more often bilateral although asymmetrical. In contrast to the distribution of the multiple exostoses described, the hands are most frequently involved (74 per cent in one series of cases). At puberty, the cartilaginous growth usually ceases, and the masses may become totally calcified, producing focal, patchy radiographic densities. The x-ray picture of irregular radiolucent areas representing the enchondroses, flecked with foci of density where ossification has begun, is virtually pathognomonic, particularly when the hands are involved bilaterally. These cartilaginous overgrowths may produce sufficient deformity of bone to seriously impair function and are frequently the cause of pain. As compared with solitary enchondromas (p. 1456), these lesions have a strong tendency to undergo malignant transformation.

ACHONDROPLASIA

Achondroplasia is a hereditary disease having an autosomal dominant mode of transmission characterized by failure of cartilage cell proliferation and premature closure of the growth plates of bones preformed in cartilage. Because the bones of the face, cranium and trunk are produced by membranous bone formation, they are unaffected. Thus eventuates the characteristic "circus" dwarf with head and body too large for shortened arms and legs.

Anatomically, the deranged cartilaginous growth produces thick, knobby epiphyses that calcify early and irregularly. Sometimes exuberant cartilaginous tissue protrudes beyond the contour of the bony cortex. The long bones are abnormally short, but since appositional bone growth is undisturbed, they are relatively thick for their length. Histologically, there is complete disarray of the epiphyseal cartilaginous plates.

Although many of the severely affected fetuses die in utero or soon after birth, other individuals with this same disorder may live to an advanced age in otherwise good health.

OSTEOPETROSIS (OSTEOSCLEROSIS)

Osteopetrosis is also known as *Albers-Schönberg disease* or, more graphically, as *"marble bones" to denote the principal characteristics of overgrowth and sclerosis of bone with resultant marked thickening of the bony cortex and narrowing or even filling of the marrow cavity.* Despite the "too much" bone, the skeleton is abnormally brittle and fractures readily.

This is an uncommon hereditary disorder having two modes of transmission. The autosomal recessive disease is called malignant because, with homozygosity, bony changes appear in utero or in infancy and often result in an early death. In contrast, the pattern having an autosomal dominant mode of transmission is relatively benign (Johnston et al., 1968). While present from birth, the disease is often not recognized until childhood or adult life. Both sexes are affected equally.

The vertebral column, pelvic bones and ribs are most often involved, but any bone in the body may be affected. Membranous bones such as the skull are usually spared. The characteristic morphologic changes consist of extreme density and overgrowth of solid cortical bone. Depending upon the severity and duration of the disease, **the marrow cavity may be narrowed down to a slender central core or, in far advanced cases, the marrow cavity may be obliterated.** However, the bones are not unusually shortened or deformed so that the individuals are of normal stature. Usually the marked overgrowth of bone is manifested by the wideness of the spicules of cancellous bone and the monotonous solidity of the cortical bone. Sometimes within the centers of these solid plates of bone and within the cores of the bone spicules, there is preserved cartilage, suggesting that the normal process of resorp-

tion of cartilage at the time of provisional calcification did not occur. Such marrow space as may be present is frequently extremely fibrotic and virtually no hematopoietic elements are found.

A variety of clinical manifestations are produced by the morphologic changes described. Although the bones are extremely hard and brittle, they have been likened to a stick of peppermint candy that fractures with relatively slight stress. Anemia reflects the replacement of the marrow and is often accompanied by extramedullary hematopoiesis. Visual disturbances and blindness follow the progressive constriction of the foramina of the optic nerve. Deafness reflects the overgrowth of bone within the middle ear and inner ear. Cranial nerve palsies and hydrocephalus are further possible clinical manifestations. The diagnosis of this condition is usually quite obvious from the roentgenograms showing the markedly increased density of the bone, along with the narrowing of the medullary cavity. In the malignant form of the disease, severe encroachment on the marrow spaces may cause death in utero or in infancy, due to profound anemia. The milder, dominant pattern is compatible with a virtually normal life span, although these patients are very vulnerable to even mild trauma and sustain many fractures.

GARGOYLISM (HUNTER-HURLER SYNDROME)

The Hunter and Hurler syndromes are hereditary inborn errors of mucopolysaccharide metabolism. These were discussed previously on p. 304. Here it is only necessary to comment that the abnormal accumulation of mucopolysaccharide-laden storage cells induces skeletal deformities, principally of the skull and facial bones, creating a likeness to the storied gargoyle. Mental retardation, blindness, hepatosplenomegaly and deafness accompany the skeletal deformities.

INFECTIONS

Bacterial infections of bone occur under a variety of circumstances. In any blood-borne systemic disease, such as brucellosis, typhoid fever, the mycoses, tuberculosis and bacterial endocarditis, the bone marrow may be seeded with organisms to produce small foci of infection. Usually these inflammatory lesions are of microscopic size, do not contribute materially to the clinical disease and are of significance only as anatomic findings that aid in establishing the nature of the primary systemic disease. However, in addition to these relatively insignificant lesions, more serious bacterial infections occur in bone. They may affect predominantly the periosteum (*periostitis*), the cortex (*osteitis*) and the marrow (*myelitis*). Both the bone marrow and bone are often affected concomitantly to produce an *osteomyelitis*. The three most serious infections of bone are (1) pyogenic osteomyelitis, (2) tuberculosis and (3) syphilis. However, improved public health control measures and the better therapies of today have made these infections increasingly uncommon clinical problems.

PYOGENIC OSTEOMYELITIS

Osteomyelitis represents a pyogenic infection of the bone and bone marrow. Characteristically, it begins as an acute infection. Many of these infections spontaneously resolve or are aborted by appropriate treatment. Indeed, in the present era of effective antibacterial therapy, most are brought under prompt control. If unrecognized or inadequately treated, however, they may persist to become chronic. One could separate the discussion of acute osteomyelitis from that of chronic osteomyelitis, but since there is no well defined dividing line, it seems better to consider pyogenic osteomyelitis as a single acute or chronic disorder.

Etiology and Pathogenesis. The causative agents reach the bone through one of three pathways: (1) hematogenous seeding, (2) direct extension from a neighboring focus of infection (periapical tooth abscess, soft tissue abscess, suppurative arthritis) or (3) as a consequence of trauma exposing the bone to bacterial contamination (compound fracture, penetrating soft tissue injury). In the majority of the cases, the offending agent is the hemolytic staphylococcus. Less commonly, streptococci, pneumococci, *H. influenzae*, gonococci and coliform bacilli are implicated. Acute hematogenous osteomyelitis occurs principally in children and affects, in order of frequency, the femur, tibia, humerus and radius. In those under two years of age, streptococci are implicated twice as frequently as staphylococci (Green and Shannon, 1936).

Hematogenous osteomyelitis may appear in patients having no clinically detectable primary focus of infection. In only about one-quarter to one-third of the cases can a well defined extraskeletal source of bacterial infection be found. In the remainder, transient bacteremias must have arisen either from unrecognized foci of infection or as fleeting contaminations of the blood demonstrated to occur from such simple origins as chewing, minor trauma to the bowel and virtually insig-

nificant infections about the teeth and upper respiratory tract.

The blood supply to the long bones conditions the localization of hematogenous infections. They frequently begin in the marrow space of the metaphysis, the locus of greatest vascularity, and thus the region most likely to receive blood-borne organisms. The evolution of these infections differs somewhat from those in soft tissues, since the rigidity of the tissue tends to predispose to edematous constriction of blood supply. Once begun, the infection tends to spread widely, cause extensive necrosis and even penetrate the cortex to involve the periosteum and adjacent tissue. Necrosis of fragments of bone (sequestra) produces foreign bodies not easily extruded or digested. In contrast, when infections extend by continuity or arise secondary to some form of trauma, the initial reaction may take the form of a periostitis followed, in time, by osteitis which eventually may trek into the marrow space to evoke a full-blown osteomyelitis.

During the phase of acute osteomyelitis, a characteristic suppurative reaction occurs, which tends to develop considerable exudative pressure and thus extends in both directions within the marrow cavity. The vascular supply is often compromised as the inflammatory pressure builds up. The inflammation **penetrates the endosteum** and enters the haversian and lacunar systems of the bone to reach the subperiosteum. Sometimes it ruptures through this membrane into the surrounding soft tissues. This pattern of penetration of the cortex may occur at one or several points to eventually cause multiple **sinus tracts** through the cortical bone. When spread to the subperiosteum occurs, the infection dissects in this plane to further impair the blood supply in the affected region. The suppurative and ischemic injury may then cause necrosis of a small or large fragment of bone known as a **sequestrum**. This devitalized sequestrum, in the course of time, is sometimes sloughed to form a free foreign body that sometimes dissects through to the skin. In this fashion, or by the direct penetration of the spreading infection, inflammatory **skin sinuses** may develop.

Generally, the epiphyseal cartilaginous plate resists bacterial invasion and, therefore, the osteomyelitis rarely extends into the head of the bone, the epiphysis or the joint cavity. However, when the infection is sufficiently severe, such penetration may occur, or more often spread into the soft tissue and then along the outer or inner surface of the periosteum offering a pathway to the head of the bone and the joint cavity. Such a complicating **suppurative arthritis** may result in extensive destruction of the joint and permanent disability (p. 1465).

Not all instances of acute hematogenous osteomyelitis follow such a spreading destructive pattern as described. In certain instances, the initial infection is localized to a small area, becomes walled off by inflammatory fibrous tissue to create a localized abscess that may undergo spontaneous sterilization or become a chronic nidus of infection (**Brodie's abscess**). In other instances the infection, after having spread through a localized region of the bone, is contained by the natural resistive forces of the host or is controlled by therapy. Although considerable destruction of the cancellous marrow spicules may have taken place, along with some erosion and destruction of cortical bone, no sequestrum is formed and no sinus tracts through the cortical bone are produced. The surrounding soft tissues and periosteum are spared.

In the course of time, all these infections are modified by the reactive reparative responses that come into play even while underlying smoldering infection persists. At this stage, the disease is better called **chronic osteomyelitis.** Osteoblastic activity, particularly from the periosteum, forms new bone subperiosteally (**involucrum**) that encloses and envelops the inflammatory focus. In addition, a considerable amount of new bone is laid down about the focus of infection within the marrow cavity to produce increased density and bony sclerosis at the periphery of the infection. This reaction further localizes the infection. This neo-osteogenesis, if continued for a sufficient period of time, gives rise to a densely sclerotic pattern of osteomyelitis referred to as **Garré's sclerosing osteomyelitis** (Fig. 31–6).

The histologic changes depend entirely upon the stage of the osteomyelitis and its duration. **Basically, two elements can be identified, suppurative and ischemic destructive necrosis and fibrous and bony repair.** In acute osteomyelitis the destructive pattern is most evident. The inflammatory response takes the characteristic pattern of an acute suppurative neutrophilic infiltration accompanied by edema, vascular congestion and small vessel thromboses within the inflammatory focus. In the course of several days, devitalized bone spicules and foci of necrotic cortical bone become evident. The death of such bone is usually recognized by disappearance of the osteocytes and surrounding osteoblasts and osteoclasts as well as by entrance of exudate into the canalicular system. The necrotic bone spicules display fraying and erosion of their margins and granular disintegration of the bone matrix.

With chronicity of the infection, the neutrophilic exudation persists, but is joined by large numbers of lymphocytes, histiocytes and occasional plasma cells. Along with this chronicity, fibroblastic proliferation is evident both as an enclosing membrane and scattered throughout the inflammatory focus. Along with the soft tissue repair, consider-

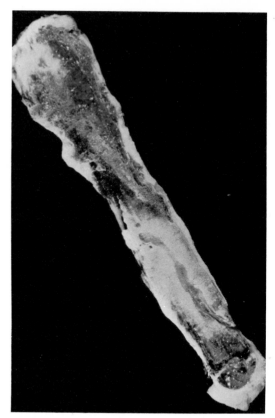

Figure 31–6. *Sclerosing osteomyelitis as evidenced by the dense, sclerotic, pale-appearing area in the shaft.*

able new bone formation is found adjacent to the vital bone. The osteogenesis is manifested by increased numbers of osteoblasts, hypertrophy of these cells and the laying down of new bone lamellae. When sequestration has occurred, such devitalized bone has the histologic characteristics of the necrotic bone spicules already described.

Clinical Course. Hematogenous osteomyelitis usually manifests itself as a sudden, acute, febrile, systemic illness accompanied by symptoms referable to the local lesion. These children have malaise, fever, chills and leukocytosis as well as marked to intense local pain that is frequently described as throbbing in nature. Many times there is redness, swelling and tenderness in the overlying soft tissues. The diagnosis can almost be made from these signs and symptoms, but is confirmed by roentgenologic evidence of bone destruction. It should be cautioned, however, that in the early stages of osteomyelitis, the devitalization and necrosis of bone may not be sufficiently advanced to produce roentgenographic changes. In the majority of instances, blood cultures are positive, particularly during the stage of the development of the bone infection.

In the acute stages, prompt massive antibiotic therapy may successfully abort the infection before much bone necrosis has occurred. If such measures fail, more extensive destruction can be anticipated and it is frequently necessary to resort to surgical drainage and debridement of sequestered fragments. Sometimes the course is complicated by spontaneous fracture of the weakened bone or by the extension of infection into adjacent joints. In addition to the local destruction, osteomyelitis is an important source for the hematogenous dissemination of infection, with the production of pyemic abscesses and focal soft tissue lesions elsewhere in the body, sometimes on the heart valves. The development of osteomyelitis is a feared complication of compound fractures, which seriously delays and prejudices the quality of the eventual repair. Amyloidosis is a potential complication of persistent chronic infections.

TUBERCULOSIS

Clinically, significant tuberculous infections of bone are now rarities. At the present time, the usual osseous infection takes the form of miliary seeding of the marrow cavity in the course of the hematogenous dissemination of this organism. Such miliary tubercles are generally of little consequence to the patient. They are, however, a valuable diagnostic aid in many cases of prolonged fever of unknown origin. Bone marrow biopsy sometimes discloses the nature of the obscure infection by the histologic demonstration of a tubercle. Beyond these relatively innocuous miliary tubercles, spreading serious tuberculous infections of the bone occasionally arise. In general, such infections occur by means of spread, through the circulating blood, of organisms originating in pulmonary tuberculosis but, rarely, they develop by the direct extension of a tuberculous infection from a caseous focus, such as the lymph nodes in the mediastinum, or from those along the aorta in the abdominal cavity. Children are more frequently affected than adults, but not in the great preponderance encountered in the acute pyogenic osteomyelitis described.

Unlike pyogenic osteomyelitis, *tuberculous osteomyelitis tends to arise as an insidious chronic infection that is characteristically much more destructive and resistant to control.* The long bones of the extremities and the spine are the favored sites of localization. Other less favored sites are the skull, hands, feet and ribs. Commonly, the infection extends through large areas of the medullary cavity and causes extensive ulcerative inflammatory necrosis of cortical bone,

with the production of large and multiple sinuses. The necrosis progresses through the periosteum into the soft tissues and frequently produces skin sinuses. Extension through the epiphyseal cartilage into joint spaces and destruction of intervertebral discs make this disease a most disabling one. When it occurs in the spine (*Pott's disease*), compression fractures are prone to develop that result in serious deformities (kyphosis and scoliosis) and often lead to permanent damage as new bone formation fixes the spine in this malalignment. The tuberculous exudation may extend from the vertebral bodies into the paravertebral muscles and, in one characteristic pattern, it extends along the sheath of the psoas muscle to produce a *psoas abscess*. Sometimes these infections present as cold fluctuating abscesses in the inguinal regions and inguinal nodes. The morphologic changes consist of a destructive, caseous, necrotizing osteomyelitis with the characteristic production of large areas of cheesy, granular, necrotic debris that can virtually be recognized as tuberculosis from the macroscopic appearance. Histologically, the characteristic tuberculous destructive and reparative processes are encountered and are, of course, accompanied by the formation of caseous necrosis and tubercles.

The clinical course of tuberculous osteomyelitis tends to be much more insidious and less acute than that of pyogenic osteomyelitis. These infections may first become manifest by the development of local subacute inflammations in soft tissues adjacent to the bone or are sometimes first discovered by slight pain and disability of the affected region. Usually by this time, definite roentgenographic evidence of bone destruction is present. Such an insidious osteolytic inflammatory process is presumptively tuberculous in nature. The control and treatment of these tuberculous infections is much more difficult than that of the pyogenic types and generally consists of the same measures that are applied to pulmonary tuberculosis, i.e., antituberculous drugs and prolonged rest and immobilization.

SYPHILIS

Today, in the United States, syphilitic involvement of bone is indeed an uncommon lesion. It may occur in both congenital and acquired syphilis. In the *congenital form*, the involvement affects principally the junction of the metaphysis and the epiphysis and is designated as *osteochondritis*. When the periosteum, principally of the long bones, is involved alone, it is referred to as *periostitis*. The osteochondritis causes considerable disarray and destruction of the epiphyseal cartilage by the characteristic fibroproliferative inflammatory reaction of syphilis. This invasive granulation tissue may destroy the lateral margins of the epiphyseal plate or invade the epiphyseal plate, sometimes virtually separating the epiphyseal head of the bone from the metaphysis. The inflammatory tissue may extend into the medullary cavity to cause widespread fibrosis.

The characteristic histologic hallmarks of syphilis can be found in this inflammatory response in the form of obliterative endarteritis and striking perivascular mononuclear cell infiltrations, principally of plasma cells. Reactive bone formation occurs from the surrounding vital periosteum. The periostitis produces a similar syphilitic granulation tissue between the cortical bone and the periosteum and is accompanied by the laying down of new bone to produce a characteristic "crew haircut" appearance or sclerosis of the cortex roentgenographically. When this thickening occurs on the tibia, it gives rise to the deformity recognized as *saber shin*.

Acquired syphilis may result in osteochondritis and periostitis, but may also be manifested by the development of a frank syphilitic osteomyelitis, usually by the production of characteristic gummas within the marrow cavity of the bone. In addition to the long bones, the skull and vertebral column are affected in the acquired forms.

FRACTURES

The speed of the healing and the perfection of the repair of a fracture depend upon whether the break has occurred in a previously normal bone or at some site of preexistent disease (*pathologic fracture*). They also depend upon the extent and nature of the fracture. Fractures may be *complete* or *incomplete* (green stick), *closed (simple)* with intact overlying tissue, *comminuted* when the bone has been splintered, and *compound* when the fracture site communicates with the skin surface. Incomplete closed fractures heal most rapidly with virtually complete reconstruction of the preexistent architecture. On the other hand, comminuted and compound fractures heal much more slowly with less satisfactory results. In the former, the devitalized bone splinters constitute impediments to repair, while in the latter, possible infection contributes to bone destruction, impairment of blood supply and stimulates fibrosis which gets in the way of bony healing. On this basis, the morphologic changes that are encountered in the healing of

a fracture depend, to a considerable extent, upon the nature of the fracture and the collateral problems involved. With this understanding, the basic sequence of events in the repair of a simple closed fracture will be presented, since this pattern is followed in the healing of all fractures and is only slowed and more or less impaired by the complications mentioned.

Healing of a fracture represents a continuous process, but it can be divided for convenience into three distinct stages: (1) **organization** of hematoma at the fracture site, leading to a soft tissue so-called **procallus;** (2) conversion of the procallus to fibrocartilaginous callus which more effectively immobilizes the bone fragments; and (3) replacement of the fibrocartilaginous callus by osseous callus which eventually will be remodeled along lines of weight-bearing to complete the repair.

Immediately after a fracture, there is considerable **hemorrhage** into the fracture site from ruptured vessels within the bone as well as from the torn periosteum and surrounding soft tissues. A hematoma is thus formed that fills the fracture cleft and surrounds the area of bone injury. The coagulation of this blood gives rise to a **loose fibrin mesh** that more or less seals off the fracture site and, at the same time, serves as a framework for the ingrowth of fibroblasts and capillary buds. However, the breakdown of this blood acts as a stimulus to a sterile inflammatory reaction. During the first 24 to 48 hours following the injury, the progressive disintegration of red cells provides a continuing inflammatory stimulus that results in significant **edema, vascular congestion and an infiltration of leukocytes, chiefly neutrophils.** After two days have elapsed, the neutrophils are accompanied by large numbers of macrophages that begin the phagocytosis of the tissue and red cell debris. At the same time, fibroblasts from the surrounding connective tissue, the periosteum and the medullary cavity invade the margins of the clot and initiate the reparative process. In this way, fibroblastic repair is begun that forms **a soft tissue callus** in and about the fracture site.

However, the healing of a bone injury differs from the healing of a soft tissue injury from this point on. After the first few days, **newly formed cartilage and bone matrix** are evident in the fibrovascular response. The origin of this osteoid and cartilaginous tissue is somewhat obscure. Some of the osteoblasts and chondroblasts that form it are undoubtedly derived from periosteum and endosteum of the preserved margins of the bone. However, regional fibroblasts may differentiate into osteoblasts and chondroblasts and participate in this activity. By the end of the first week, well developed new bone and cartilage are dispersed through the soft tissue callus (Fig. 31—7). In the course of the suc-

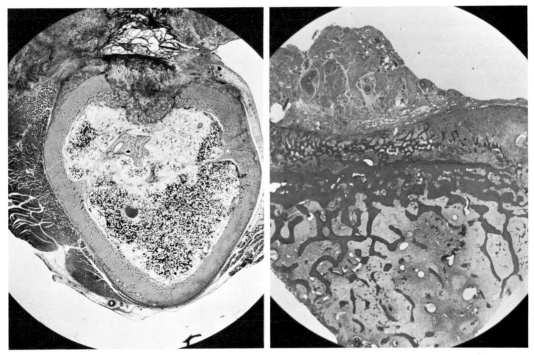

Fig. 31–7

Fig. 31–8

Figure 31–7. *Experimental demonstration of bone repair. The hole drilled in the femur is filled with hemorrhage and granulation tissue. Fibrous tissue fills the adjacent marrow space and bone spicules are found within this soft tissue callus.*

Figure 31–8. *New bone formation (slender spicules) outside the old cortex in the healing of a fracture.*

ceeding days, these bone spicules become sufficiently numerous and aggregated to create a large, fusiform, temporary bony union of the fracture known as the **provisional** or **procallus**. By this time, the inflammatory reaction has largely subsided and the repair is well under way unless bacterial contamination is present.

This provisional callus is considerably wider than the normal diameter of the bone and extends for some distance up over the fractured ends to thus create a spindle-shaped, fairly effective splint (Fig. 31–8). In an uncomplicated fracture, the provisional callus usually attains its maximal size at about the end of the second or third week. Over the subsequent course of time, this provisional callus is increasingly strengthened by the precipitation of bone salts and the widening of the newly formed delicate bone spicules, and is at the same time remodeled by osteoblastic and osteoclastic activity.

The remodeling process is directed by the muscle and weight-bearing stresses imposed upon the bone. If the fracture has been well aligned and the original weight-bearing strains are restored to their original lines, virtually perfect reconstruction of the bone is accomplished. In such reconstruction, the internal callus that fills the marrow space is also resorbed and, at some later date, roentgenograms

may completely fail to demonstrate the site of previous injury.

The influences which dictate architectural reconstruction of bone along lines of weight bearing have always been a mystery. The most appealing postulate suggests the development of electrical fields modifying osteoclastic and osteoblastic activity. It is proposed that both collagen and its associated minerals exhibit piezoelectric properties. Regions under tension act as anodes and compressed regions as cathodes. Electric currents in the millivolt range develop. Bone accumulates about the cathode region, thus spreading the electrical charges over a wider field and, at the same time, lowering the compressive stress per unit of bone. In this fashion, the bone is remodelled along lines of weight-bearing (Bassett, 1968).

Perfect repair may be not only impeded but also blocked by many complications. Malalignment and comminution of the bone are almost inevitably followed by some permanent deformity. Moreover, the devitalized spicules of comminuted bone must be demineralized and the osteoid material resorbed. These processes accentuate the inflammatory reaction, enlarge the provisional callus and favor the formation of an overly large, deforming, permanent callus. Permanent obliteration of the marrow cavity may eventuate. Inadequate immobilization of the bone permits the continuance of twisting, shearing and bending stresses. Under these circumstances, the laying down of an osteoid and chondromatous matrix is slow and, in fact, in many instances is virtually blocked so that the callus may be composed of only fibrous tissue and cartilage which perpetuate the abnormal mobility. An osseous callus may not form under these circumstances and a dense fibrous tissue remains as the end-stage of the repair process producing a **false joint (pseudoarthrosis).** Interposition of soft tissues tends to give rise to such fibrous, inadequate bony union. However, in any of these complications, if the interposed soft parts can be removed at a later date, or adequate immobilization eventually effected, ultimate adequate repair can be anticipated except perhaps in advanced age groups suffering from arterial insufficiency and venous inadequacies.

Systemic derangements may further unfavorably affect the end results. Inadequate levels of calcium and phosphorus, avitaminoses, systemic infections, generalized atherosclerosis that renders the area ischemic and preexistent osteomalacia or osteoporosis (p. 1443) are some of these unfavorable influences. In general, in children and young adults, in whom most uncomplicated fractures are found, practically perfect reconstruction may be anticipated. In older age groups in whom more of the unfavorable influences are prone to complicate the problem, less favorable union occurs.

OSTEOPOROSIS

Osteoporosis is best and most simply characterized as a *reduction in bone mass.* Because it is an almost inevitable accompaniment of advanced age, some writers would prefer to qualify this definition by adding that the reduction in bone mass should only be termed osteoporosis when it induces symptoms of backache and pain associated with objective evidence of fractures (Lutwak, 1969). It is seen clinically in many conditions and may affect the entire skeleton or only part of it.

Hyperparathyroidism, hyperthyroidism, hyperadrenocorticism and acromegaly are well known causes of generalized osteoporosis. It may also occur in association with primary or secondary cancers of the skeletal system. Osteoporosis may be seen in generalized malnutrition, vitamin C deficiency and prolonged bed rest (immobilization). However, the majority of patients are of advanced age and do not have demonstrable underlying causes. In these patients, the condition is termed *senile osteoporosis.* For obscure reasons, women are much more commonly affected, in a ratio of 4 to 1, giving rise to the designation *postmenopausal os-*

teoporosis. Both the senile and/or postmenopausal forms of this disorder are, in the last analysis, idiopathic.

Localized osteoporosis of a specific portion of the skeleton may appear in relation to osteomyelitis, joint disease, such as rheumatoid arthritis, and immobilization of a part of the body.

Pathogenesis. Since time immemorial, the argument has waxed as to whether the reduction in bone mass is due to a primary deficiency of calcium, having secondary effects on bone matrix, or the converse. For years, postmenopausal osteoporosis has been attributed to reduced levels of anabolic steroids and inadequate production of osteoid matrix. In clinically significant osteoporosis, there is a loss of approximately 30 per cent of the mineral content of the skeleton. For such a loss to occur within 10 to 15 years of the menopause, it would require massive losses of bone substance and consequent mobilization of calcium. However, such losses cannot be documented by metabolic balance studies of calcium. Moreover, if loss of ovarian steroids were responsible for postmenopausal osteoporosis, why should the disease not be linearly related to advancing age and what is its explanation in men?

Before proceeding further, we should dismiss the concept of a dietary calcium deficiency. Although still supported by some investigators, most studies fail to document sufficient reduction in calcium intake to adequately explain the reduction in skeletal mass (Garn et al., 1967) (Skosey, 1970). Granted, a deficient diet may be operative in a few patients, but it does not explain the widespread prevalence of osteoporosis in older individuals. Moreover, osteoporotic bone, although reduced in mass, has the same mineral composition as normal bone and shows no evidence of inadequate mineralization.

It may well be that *osteoporosis is not a single disorder but rather a group of disorders of diverse causation all leading to reduction in bone mass.* Cases arising on the basis of hyperadrenocorticism may be the consequence of increased osteoclastic activity and bone resorption. Other cases may be due to malnutrition (proteins, vitamins, minerals). A host of explanations have been offered for the osteoporosis in postmenopausal women and senile men, without commanding evidence for any postulation. Some of the theories invoke increased resorption relative to the skeletal mass, arguing that "normal" levels of calcium turnover are, in reality, increased in the patient with a smaller skeleton. Increased end-organ sensitivity to parathormone and decreased secretion of parathormone have also been suggested (Harris and Heaney, 1969). In conclusion, we must admit that the understanding of the pathogenesis of osteoporosis still leaves much to be desired.

Morphology. With rare exception, osteoporosis is a systemic disorder that affects the entire skeleton. Osteoporosis may occur only in immobilized parts of the skeleton as in fractures or paralyses. In the systemic form, it tends to be most marked in the spine and pelvis and, for obscure reasons, the skull is relatively spared. The bone changes are characterized by thinning of the cortical bone, resorption of cancellous bone spicules, enlargement of the medullary cavity and an overall loss of bone. Compression fractures of the vertebrae are prone to occur together with a generalized predisposition to fracture of all bones. Microscopically, the bone that remains is essentially normal and well mineralized, but new bone formation is usually not evident and the bone cortex is thinned and the trabeculae narrow and delicate.

Clinical Course. Osteoporosis may exist as a clinically undetectable condition. Only when the bone loss has reached the 30 per cent level can it be visualized radiographically. Back pain and predisposition to fractures, particularly of the femoral neck in the aged, are the common overt manifestations. *Serum calcium, phosphorus and alkaline phosphatase levels are characteristically normal*, in contradistinction to osteomalacia (see next section). When a specific cause can be identified, such as immobilization of an extremity or hyperadrenocorticism, the bone loss is reversible. There is no satisfactory treatment for the common forms of senile and postmenopausal osteoporosis, however. The administration of anabolic steroids and a high calcium diet is sometimes but not always helpful.

OSTEOMALACIA

Literally, osteomalacia means "softness of bone." *In essence, it comprises the adult counterpart of childhood rickets and is characterized by inadequate mineralization of bone matrix, resulting in an increase in the relative amount of osteoid tissue and a decrease in the appositional growth rate* (Arnstein et al., 1967) (Winn, 1951). The excess of osteoid is a consequence of the failure of mineralization to keep pace with new synthesis of bone matrix. Hence, the bone displays an increase of osteoid seams, and an abnormally large fraction of the total bone surface is covered by nonmineralized osteoid. Thus, osteomalacia differs from osteoporosis insofar as the former is characterized by a relative deficiency

of mineral and an excess of osteoid, while in the latter, the proportional composition of the bone is essentially normal.

The concept that osteomalacia is merely the result of a dietary deficiency of vitamin D in the adult is simplistic. Dent (1970) cites a constellation of possible mechanisms, all leading to inadequate mineralization of bone. These can be conveniently divided into three large categories. The first represents cases caused by a deficient intake of vitamin D, seen today most commonly in patients with one of the malabsorption syndromes. The second category comprises those cases associated with hypophosphatemia with normal vitamin D intake, principally familial hypophosphatemia (vitamin D-resistant rickets), the Fanconi syndrome and renal tubular acidosis. The third category comprises those instances associated with defective nucleation of preformed matrix without abnormalities of calcium, phosphorus or vitamin D, such as hypophosphatasia and fluoride and strontium intoxication. All three categories produce skeletal changes which cannot be distinguished either grossly or histologically from one another.

Pathogenesis. Whatever the basic defect, osteomalacia is characterized by prolongation of the time interval between osteoid synthesis and mineralization. Instead of the normal delay of 6 to 10 days, the time lag for mineralization in osteomalacia may be as long as two to three months. Moreover, some areas completely fail to mineralize, leaving residuals of osteoid.

Morphology. Osteomalacia is characterized by the inadequate mineralization of newly formed osteoid matrix. With inadequate mineralization, there is some slowing or impairment of the continued formation of matrix so that ultimately the bones are softer and more fragile than normal, as in osteoporosis. Fractures are common as in osteoporosis but, in addition, bending and stress deformities develop because the bones are of decreased brittleness as well as being weaker. Microscopically, there is an excess of osteoid matrix so that, on casual inspection, there appears to be too much bone. However, the inadequate mineralization makes of this matrix a poor substitute for normally ossified bony tissue.

Clinical Course. *The characteristic biochemical alterations of osteomalacia are a normal or, more classically, a low serum calcium, a low serum phosphorus and a high serum alkaline phosphatase* reflecting the normal or even excessive activity of osteoblasts. These blood values help to differentiate osteomalacia from osteoporosis, which is also characterized by increased radiolucency of the skeleton. The urinary calcium is generally low or may even be absent in those instances related to decreased absorption of vitamin D and calcium. In those cases of osteomalacia caused by renal tubular lesions, there is obviously an increased excretion of this mineral. Secondary hyperparathyroidism may be encountered because, in so many of the mechanisms cited, the final common pathway is a decrease in the circulating calcium. Where osteomalacia is due to a dietary deficiency of vitamin D, it promptly responds to diet supplementation. The other forms may or may not respond to pharmacologic doses of this vitamin, coupled with a high calcium intake.

Incomplete fractures are prone to occur in these soft osteoid bones. One special entity has been segregated from the large group of osteomalacias to be designated as *Milkman's syndrome*. The eponym Milkman does not refer to an occupational hazard, but rather to the original writer on this syndrome of bilateral, frequently symmetrical, incomplete fractures that tend to occur in the scapulae.

SKELETAL CHANGES IN HYPERPARATHYROIDISM (OSTEITIS FIBROSA CYSTICA GENERALISATA, VON RECKLINGHAUSEN'S DISEASE OF BONE)

Prolonged or severe hyperparathyroidism, whether primary or secondary, causes progressive resorption and destruction of bone. *While it has always been classically taught that these changes produce a specific anatomic pattern known as osteitis fibrosa cystica, it is now appreciated that many earlier alterations affect the bone that do not fit into this anatomic pattern.* Osteitis fibrosa cystica is the late lesion that only develops in the advanced stages of hyperparathyroidism. The earlier manifestations consist first of demineralization of bone that produces changes very similar to those of osteomalacia-osteoporosis. In time, these may progress to von Recklinghausen's disease of bone.

Pathogenesis. The pathologic physiology of both primary and secondary hyperparathyroidism has already been considered in Chapter 29. For brief review, in the primary disease, an excess of parathormone is produced usually by hyperplasia or neoplasia of the parathyroid gland. The excess parathormone induces an increased mobilization of phosphorus and calcium and progressive demineralization of the skeleton. When this has continued for a period of time, the more classic manifestations of osteitis fibrosa cystica become apparent in the form of increased osteoblastic and osteoclastic activity, leading to generalized resorption and rarefaction of the bone.

The most common cause of secondary hyperparathyroidism is chronic renal insufficiency (Pollak et al., 1959). Much less frequently, such calcium-wasting disorders as rickets, osteomalacia and disseminated cancer of the bone also lead to secondary hyperplasia of the parathyroid glands. In chronic renal disease, the classic mechanism postulated is phosphate retention, abnormal depression of serum calcium and subsequent stimulation of the parathyroids. The chronic metabolic acidosis of the renal failure may contribute to the mobilization of calcium from the bone. The skeletal changes in the cases of secondary hyperparathyroidism are similar to those of primary hyperparathyroidism but are rarely as severe, and the full-blown lesions of osteitis fibrosa cystica are rarely encountered. Collectively, these bony changes in secondary hyperparathyroidism, when caused by renal dysfunction, have been designated as *renal osteodystrophy* or sometimes *renal rickets* because, in the young, not only is the mineralized bone affected but endochondral bone formation is also impaired, producing skeletal changes that, to some extent, resemble rickets.

Morphology. The basic anatomic changes comprise osteoclastic resorption of bone, progressive thinning of the cancellous and cortical bone structure, and fibrosis of the marrow and newly formed spaces. In this way, thinning or even replacement of the cortex with fibrous tissue ensues. Microscopic and gross cysts are formed by this fibroblastic reaction. Focal areas of bony rarefaction may occur at the site of formation of "brown tumors." This misnomer is particularly inappropriate since the lesions are neither brown nor tumors. They represent foci of bony rarefaction which fill with blood and then undergo organization with the accumulation of macrophages and osteoclastic giant cells. The presence of the multinucleate osteoclasts within a fibrous stroma creates more than a passing similarity to true giant cell tumors. However, the lesions in osteitis fibrosa cystica are better referred to as **reparative giant cell granulomas** having none of the neoplastic and malignant potential of the giant cell tumors described on p. 1458.

The extensive destruction and new bone formation in osteitis fibrosa cystica may cause gross bony deformities in the form of irregular abnormal cystic enlargements, fusiform dilatations of the shaft and, with the considerable resorption and softening of the bone, bending and fractures of the more severely affected regions. With such fractures, there is commonly massive bleeding into the cysts and into the soft connective tissue. The brown tumors mentioned are characteristically deeply pigmented by large amounts of old and recent blood pigment.

Histologically, depending upon the severity of the individual case, there is **extensive thinning of the cancellous spicules and replacement of the marrow spaces by fibrous tissue.** In the areas of cyst formation, the bony cortex may be thinned out to the point of complete disappearance. The fibrous tissue that fills the marrow spaces is of a peculiar type, having widely scattered fibroblasts separated by a loose, delicate ground substance. Microcysts are evident within this fibrous tissue (Fig. 31–9). In other areas, the cystic spaces produce the macroscopically visible cysts described. **The overall pattern is one of excessive osteoblastic and osteoclastic activity accompanied by a fibroproliferative response.** For emphasis, it deserves reiteration that such full-blown involvement is only seen late and in severe cases. The earlier alterations are indistinguishable from osteoporosis-osteomalacia.

Clinical Course. The clinical manifestations of von Recklinghausen's disease of bone are almost invariably overshadowed by the accompanying primary hyperparathyroidism or underlying renal failure with secondary hyperparathyroidism. When the bony lesions, how-

ever, become well marked, there is a predisposition to fractures, to skeletal deformities under the stress of weight-bearing and to joint pains and dysfunctions as the lines of normal weight-bearing are disturbed by the skeletal deformity. The diagnosis can usually be made from the biochemical alterations (high serum and urinary calcium, low serum phosphorus and elevated alkaline phosphatase in the primary form, high serum phosphorus and low calcium in the secondary form). The diagnosis is further supported by the rather striking roentgenograms that disclose the irregular bony destruction, cystic formations and overall radiolucency of the skeletal system. Von Recklinghausen's disease of bone due to primary hyperparathyroidism rapidly heals upon surgical removal of the hyperplastic parathyroids or functioning tumor. However, in chronic nephritis, the osseous changes are usually manifested only when severe renal failure is already present and dominates the clinical problem and prognosis of the case.

OSTEITIS DEFORMANS (PAGET'S DISEASE)

Osteitis deformans is an acquired disorder of unknown etiology characterized by hyperactive destruction and formation of bone, with the emphasis upon the *replacement of normal bone by expanded, soft, poorly mineralized, osteoid tissue.* The bony disease occurs in two patterns, monostotic or localized, and polyostotic or generalized. The tibia is the most common site of the monostotic form; the pelvis and sacrum are the first involvements in the polyostotic form. However, even in the generalized pattern, the entire skeletal system is rarely involved and, therefore, it is probable that the etiology of this condition is not that of a systemic metabolic derangement.

Incidence. The disease rarely occurs under the age of 40 and is much more common in males in the ratio of about 2 to 1. Rarely, the disease appears in younger individuals, probably as a familial trait.

Morphology. While it is an uncommon condition, it is encountered in about one in 1000 admissions to a general hospital (Rosenkrantz et al., 1952). The bones affected in decreasing order of frequency are the pelvis, skull, femur, spine, tibia, humerus, scapula and, only occasionally, other bones including the mandible. The bone alterations consist essentially of **resorption and softening of bone, followed by replacement with a poorly mineralized osteoid matrix, accompanied by considerable fibrosis.** The newly created soft tissue and

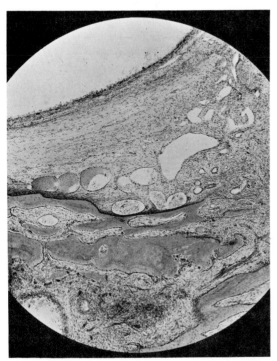

Figure 31–9. Osteitis fibrosa cystica (von Recklinghausen's disease of bone). A histologic detail of the cancellous bone. The wall of a gross cyst appears above and several microcysts are present in the delicate fibrous tissue.

defective bone more than compensate in bulk for the resorptive processes and, as a consequence, **bony enlargement results.** They are, however, soft and are characteristically deformed by the stress of weight-bearing.

Compression of the vertebral bodies gives rise to kyphosis, scoliosis and lordosis, the tibias and femurs bend and the femoral necks may yield under the pressure. While the bones are increased in size, they are **unusually light, soft and porous and almost have the consistency of dry bread.** The outer cortical tables are usually thinned or totally replaced. Paget's disease of the skull is particularly striking by virtue of the irregular thickening of the skull (Fig. 31–10). But the bone can be sliced by a knife and the calvarium, when filled with water, leaks like the proverbial sieve. Similar enlargement, softening and porosity characterize all the bony involvements where they occur. However, during the late, so-called burned-out, stage of Paget's disease, the enlarged bones become well mineralized, thoroughly ossified and densely sclerotic. As was mentioned, this process does not necessarily affect the entire skeleton. Sometimes it is monostotic and, even within a single bone, may involve a sharply localized region well demarcated from the adjacent uninvolved bone.

Histologically, the bone of Paget's disease is characterized by excessive deposition of poorly mineralized new bone in areas of previous osteoclastic resorption. In this irregular, haphazard bone destruction and new bone formation the original haversian lamellar pattern of the bone is destroyed and is replaced by random foci of new bone formation. It is usually possible to identify narrow lines of cement substance between the original bone and the foci of new bone and, with the irregularity of the deposition of bone matrix, **the cement lines create a pathognomonic tile-like or "mosaic" pattern** (Fig. 31–11). **This pathognomonic feature of Paget's is evident in both the cortical and cancellous regions and may completely replace the preexisting structure,** accounting for the porosity and loss of structural strength described. Subperiosteal new bone formation is also of this inadequate, poorly mineralized type and, therefore, merely adds to the overall size of the bone without contributing to its structural integrity. Osteoblasts and osteoclasts are abundant. The former are usually found in apposition to new bone formation, and the latter in lacunar resorptive spaces suggesting marked functional activity. The marrow spaces between the cancellous spicules are filled with a loose fibroblastic connective tissue.

Clinical Course. When multiple bones are involved, Paget's disease usually produces characteristic deformities that are fairly readily identified by simple clinical inspection. Enlargement of the skull, accompanied by bowing of the tibias and femurs, is virtually diagnostic. When concomitant deformity of the trunk occurs due to vertebral column involvement, grotesque, dwarf-like distortions result. Pain is often an early distressing symptom. Radiologically, the affected bones are enlarged, the skull is thickened and weight-bearing bones are bent, but all are characterized by *increased radiolucency.* In the later stages, the deposition of densely sclerotic bone may cause a patchy irregular pattern on the roentgenogram that, in far advanced, burned-out cases, eventuates in

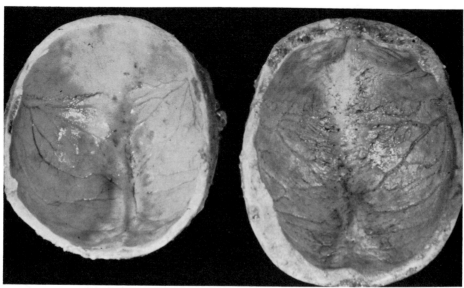

Figure 31–10. *Paget's disease of the skull. The irregular thickening of the right calvarium is well brought out by comparison with the normal control on the left.*

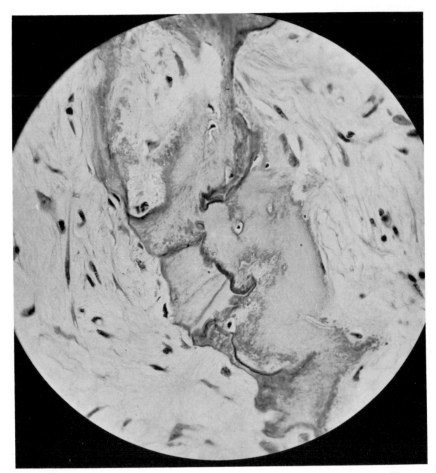

Figure 31–11. *Paget's disease of bone. A histologic detail of a single bone spicule to illustrate the "mosaic" pattern produced by the irregular bone formation.*

an overall increased bone density. As might be anticipated from the marked osteoblastic activity, the serum alkaline phosphatase is characteristically high, often higher than is encountered in any other bony disorder.

In addition to producing bony deformity and predisposing to fracture, Paget's disease of the bone is a prime site for the development of osteogenic sarcomas. This complication is reported to occur in 7.5 to 25 per cent of cases (Freydinger et al., 1963). However, most observers fail to find such high frequencies and cite an average of 1 to 2 per cent of cases (Porretta et al., 1957). The most frequent locations of these sarcomas are, in descending order, the femur, humerus, pelvis, skull, tibia and scapula. When an osteogenic sarcoma arises in advanced age, it is more than likely that it represents a complication of underlying Paget's disease. There is often a markedly increased blood flow in the involved bone, with increased warmth of the overlying skin. These vascular neoformations may act as arteriovenous fistulas, leading to cardiac hypertrophy and sometimes congestive failure (Reifenstein and Albright, 1944).

HYPERTROPHIC (PULMONARY) OSTEOARTHROPATHY

Hypertrophic osteoarthropathy is sometimes erroneously equated with clubbing of the fingers. It has, however, three separate components: *clubbing of the fingers, periosteal proliferation of the distal ends of the long bones, and arthritis manifested by swelling and tenderness of joints.* While these changes are most often associated with pulmonary disease, it has become clear that a host of other clinical disorders may induce this group of lesions.

The changes involved in *clubbing of the fingers* are edema, fibrous overgrowth at the tips of the fingers and an increased vascularization in the nail bed, with rounding or "watch glass" deformity of the nail. The normal inclination of the nail toward the axis of the bone may be altered. The tips of the digits become enlarged and often are dusky or cyanotic. Occasionally, there is some periosteal reaction of the terminal phalanges known as tufting.

These changes in the fingers are found in the following disease states: (1) *Intrathoracic disease*, most importantly bronchogenic carcinoma. It is variously reported that 1 to 10 per cent of patients with these cancers have associated clubbing of the fingers, and there have been instances in which the clubbing has preceded the appearance of the carcinoma by as much as two years. Lung sepsis of whatever type, i.e., lung abscess or bronchiectasis, is also sometimes responsible for clubbing. Arteriovenous aneurysms are rare causes. Surprisingly, pulmonary tuberculosis rarely if ever leads to these changes. (2) *Cardiovascular diseases*, particularly those associated with cyanosis, such as congenital heart disease with a right to left shunt and subacute bacterial endocarditis. (3) *Hepatic disorders*, particularly biliary cirrhosis and liver abscesses. (4) A wide variety of *ulceroinflammatory gastrointestinal diseases* (ulcerative colitis, regional enteritis, the malabsorption syndromes). (5) Certain neoplasias, such as chronic myeloid leukemia, carcinoma of the thymus and mesothelioma of the pleura. About half the patients with mesotheliomas have well defined clubbing of the fingers.

Periosteal bone changes affect the distal radius, ulna, tibia, fibula, metacarpals and proximal phalanges. Periosteal reactions are extremely rare in the terminal phalanges. The amount of bone formation varies from barely radiographically visible tufting to the formation of a complete enclosing layer about the metacarpals and first and second phalanges. While any of the disorders leading to clubbing may produce periosteal proliferation, the dominant cause is bronchogenic carcinoma.

The *pathogenesis* of these skeletal changes, in the wide variety of clinical circumstances in which they are found, has long excited attention. Numerous theories have been proposed involving elaboration of a circulating toxin, peripheral anoxia of the bone, elaboration of some endocrine secretion, autonomic nervous system imbalance, and the production of large amounts of a substance similar to vasodepressor material. All these theories invoke increased blood flow to the skeletal system as the direct mechanism for the bony and nail bed changes described. Of these theories, two are currently favored. Elevated levels of estrogens have been identified in patients with hypertrophic osteoarthropathy (Ginsburg and Brown,

1961). These elevated hormone levels have been found in patients with bronchogenic carcinoma and, surprisingly, removal of the lung tumor leads to a prompt fall in these hormones. It must be assumed that in some way these tumors were responsible, either directly or indirectly, for the steroid secretion. The second theory under intensive scrutiny involves the autonomic nervous system, principally the vagus nerves (Berman, 1963). It has been demonstrated that unilateral or bilateral vagotomy induces reversal of the hypertrophic osteoarthropathy. However, it is difficult to conceive of the pathways followed and how the vagus becomes involved in such random diseases as the malabsorption syndromes and ulcerative colitis.

When the underlying disease is subject to control, the clubbing of the fingers and the periosteal reactions disappear (Skorneck and Ginsburg, 1958) (Hammarsten and O'Leary, 1957).

FIBROUS DYSPLASIA

Fibrous dysplasia of bone is a poorly understood, poorly defined disorder which may affect one bone (monostotic) or multiple bones (polyostotic). Polyostotic fibrous dysplasia is often part of a curious syndrome in which: (1) the bone lesions have a tendency to be unilateral in distribution; (2) scattered areas of melanotic pigmentation of the skin (cafe au lait spots) appear, usually on the same side as the bone lesions; and (3) a variety of endocrinopathies may be present, usually inducing precocious puberty in young females. The concurrence of these widely disparate features is recognized as *Albright's syndrome* (Albright et al., 1937). Polyostotic bone lesions may, however, occur in the absence of skin pigmentation and endocrine disturbances.

In both the monostotic and polyostotic patterns, the bone lesions comprise essentially localized areas of replacement of bony architecture by extensive proliferation of fibrous tissue. Poorly formed and randomly arranged cancellous trabeculae of bone course through this tissue. In some instances, there is little bone formation, and the lesion consists of solid masses of fibrous tissue. Thus the monostotic variant is easily confused with, or may be identical to, nonosteogenic fibroma of bone or ossifying fibroma of bone. Other investigators believe, however, that the solitary lesion is a forme fruste of the polyostotic variant and that, in time, the patient will develop multiple lesions. Certainly, the solitary lesion is much more common than polyostotic fibrous dysplasia with or without the other features of Albright's syndrome.

The etiology of fibrous dysplasia is completely unknown. The multisystem involvement of Albright's syndrome suggests some basic genetic defect arising at an early stage of embryogenesis, but such a defect has never been identified. Endocrine imbalance, deranged bone maturation and abnormal activity of a focus of mesenchymal connective tissue have all been postulated without substantiation (Benedict, 1962) (Lichtenstein and Jaffe, 1947). Whatever its genesis, the anatomic changes suggest a derangement in the normal remodeling of bone with the replacement of resorbed bone by fibrous tissue and poorly formed woven bone. As a consequence, there is progressive increase in size of the fibrous lesion. Since most of the bony remodeling occurs in the intramedullary cancellous bone, these lesions are usually centrally located and are covered by a thin layer of preserved cortex.

Morphology. In most series, the monostotic variant is far more common than the polyostotic. Any bone in the skeleton may be affected, but the most common sites identified by Schlumberger (1946) were the ribs, femur, tibia, maxilla and calvarium, in descending order of frequency. Occasionally, lesions in the skull, face and ribs cause bony deformity. The focal lesion consists of a fibroblastic stroma that has been described by some as delicate with an abundant ground substance, and described by others as fairly tightly compacted with whorling of the fibroblasts. Many believe that the whorling represents a secondary alteration consequent to previous trauma or hemorrhage. **Within this fibrous background, there are laid down trabeculae and masses of a poorly formed membranous bone having no internal lamellar structure.** The osteoid matrix is poorly delimited and, at its margins, matrix projects out into the fibrous stroma in irregular, frayed, tongue-like processes. Much stress is laid upon this poorly formed, membranous, woven bone pattern, as distinctive from the osteogenesis found in osteofibromas and ossifying fibromas (Fig. 31–12). Islands of cartilage, foci of xanthoma cells, hemosiderin pigmentation and occasional giant cells are also present, usually in the lesion that has been previously traumatized or has suffered a hemorrhage. Although these overgrowths remain localized within the shaft of bone and are enclosed within at least a thin shell of cortical bone, they are not encapsulated. Rarely, they erode through to the periosteum.

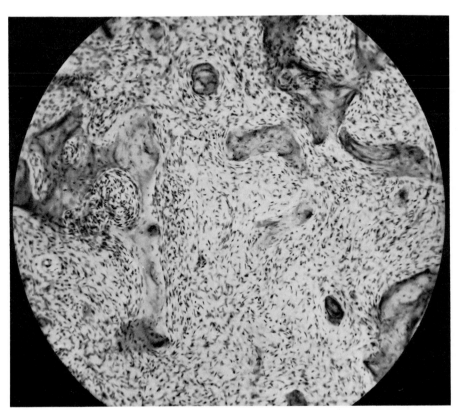

Figure 31–12. Fibrous dysplasia of bone, illustrating the characteristic overgrowth of fibrous tissue within cancellous bone.

Fibrous dysplasia pursues an unpredictable course. The lesions are believed to begin early in childhood, and many appear to become stationary as though arrested in their development. Others progress rapidly to cause bony destruction and disfigurement. When the facial bones are involved, there may be severe distortions of the orbit, nose and jaw. Surgical excision is usually curative, although incomplete removal may be followed by recurrence (Van Horn et al., 1963).

In less than 1 per cent of cases, the lesions of fibrous dysplasia undergo sarcomatous change (Schwartz and Alpert, 1964). In some of these instances, the lesions had been submitted to prior radiation therapy, but malignant transformation has been noted in the absence of such intervention (Huvos et al., 1972).

TUMORS

Although tumors of bones are infrequently encountered in clinical practice, they are nonetheless of great clinical significance because of the possibility that any such lesion may be malignant and because certain of these malignancies are among the most lethal, widely metastasizing cancers of man. The large array of these tumors, their diverse origins from the multiple cell types found in bones, coupled with the tendency of these tumors to produce overlapping anatomic patterns, all make osseous neoplasms a complicated, but highly challenging, area of morphologic diagnosis. Because of these complexities, it has often been said that no anatomic diagnosis of a bone neoplasm should ever be made without full knowledge and consideration of the clinical and roentgenographic features of the lesion. The necessity for such collateral data is perhaps greater with these neoplasms of bone than for any other form of neoplasm in the body.

The wide variety of tumors of bones has led to considerable difficulty in establishing a simple workable classification. Virtually every major writer in the field proposes his own, and has cogent reasons for so doing. Little purpose will be served in further confusing the numerous existing classifications by attempting a new one. Accordingly, the classic approach proposed by Ewing (1939) for the Registry of Bone Sarcoma of the American College of Surgeons will be followed in the present discussion. This classification, as is indicated in the outline to this chapter, essentially divides tumors of bones on the basis of their presumed tissue or cell of origin.

OSTEOGENIC TUMORS

The term osteogenic, when used in relation to tumors, is accorded two different meanings. According to one interpretation, it applies to all tumors *arising* in bone. Such tumors may or may not produce bone, as for example, the fibrosarcoma that arises within bone but produces no osteoid or osseous tissue. In the other intrepretation, osteogenic is used to imply a tumor that *produces* bone, whether it arises in the skeleton or in extraosseous sites. The rare sarcoma arising in metaplastic connective tissue that produces osteoid matrix might be an example of this latter usage. In recognition of this confusion, some writers prefer to use the term osteosarcoma for tumors that produce bone, and reserve the term osteogenic sarcoma for tumors arising out of bone. However, such terminology has not been widely accepted and, in our present consideration, the term osteogenic will be employed to designate tumors that produce bone, whether they arise as they usually do in the skeletal system or from extraskeletal metaplastic soft tissue.

Osteoma. Benign tumors composed of more or less densely sclerotic bone found either within or jutting out from the bone are osteomas (Fig. 31–13). These are uncommon

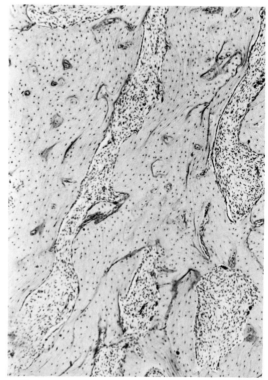

Figure 31–13. Osteoma. Histologic detail to demonstrate broad, well formed, mature bony spicules.

tumors that occur most often in the skull and often project into the orbit or paranasal sinuses. In these locations inside the skull, they are sometimes termed *hyperostosis frontalis interna*. The bone structure that comprises the lesion is usually well developed. In such lesions, there is no evidence of unusual osteoblastic or osteoclastic activity. Other osteomas may be composed of fibrous tissue with only spicules of osseous tissue. Presumably, as these mature, the bony spicules become more densely sclerotic. Such lesions have been followed by x-ray for years with little if any enlargement and, on this basis, their true neoplastic nature is challenged. Possibly some of these lesions are initiated by injury to the periosteum of bone or are formed by the organization of a previous inflammation or hematoma. In strict usage, such reactive bone formations should not be termed osteomas.

Osteoid Osteoma. Osteoid osteoma is a somewhat controversial lesion of bone that is generally interpreted as a small benign tumor composed essentially of fibrous tissue in which are found variable amounts of osteoid or calcified, poorly formed spicules of bone. These lesions were for a long time thought to represent reparative scarring in a focus of previous inflammation or injury. However, it is now believed that they represent a new growth (Jaffe and Lichtenstein, 1940). Tumors are found most often in older children and adolescents and are extremely rare in patients over 30. Males are affected about twice as often as females. Any bone in the body may be involved but, to date, no lesions have been described in the skull and only rarely are the ribs affected. Favorite sites are the femur and tibia, but lesions have been described in the upper extremity and vertebral column.

The characteristic osteoid osteoma is a small, red-brown, fairly discrete firm area rarely over 1 cm. in diameter. It usually arises at the junction of new and old cortex where it causes erosion and resorption of the native bone structure. Immediately surrounding it, there is a zone of delicate porous bone and, about this, a zone of dense reactive sclerotic bone. Frequently, the sclerosis of bone produces sufficient overgrowth to cause external deformity of the bony outline. The tumor itself is composed of highly vascularized fibrous tissue containing osteoid matrix and sometimes poorly calcified spicules of bone. However, these spicules are poorly organized, often producing an irregular, lace-like pattern (Fig. 31–14). Mitoses, cytologic abnormality, hemorrhage and necrosis are conspicuously absent.

The osteoid osteoma is distinctive clinically in several respects. Despite its small size, it is extremely painful, and there may well be localized tenderness over the affected part.

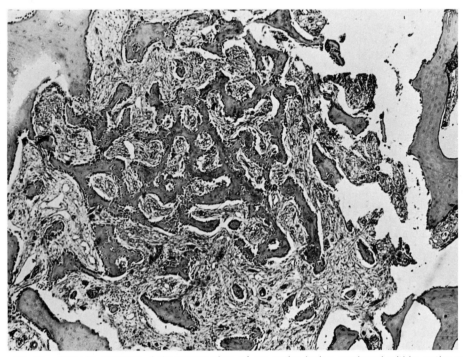

Figure 31–14. Osteoid osteoma. Low power view of an entire lesion enclosed within native wide bone spicules. The lesion is composed of fibrous tissue and numerous anastomosing spicules of osteoid.

The x-ray pattern is quite distinctive and reveals the tumor itself as an osteolytic "nidus" enclosed within densely sclerotic reactive bone. These features in the patient of appropriate age are virtually diagnostic. Relief of pain is prompt following removal of the tumor, and malignant transformation or recurrence is virtually unknown (Patch et al., 1954).

Osteogenic Sarcoma. Osteogenic sarcoma, as the term is used here, refers to a highly malignant tumor characterized by a sarcomatous fibroblastic stroma in which osteoblastic activity has induced the formation of tumor osteoid and bone. Excluded by this definition are the purely fibroblastic and chondromatous sarcomas that arise in bone but do not produce either matrix or bone structure. However, it must be admitted that such a division is unquestionably arbitrary, and many fibrosarcomas arising in bone produce minute amounts of osteoid tissue that make classification difficult. Moreover, it is by no means clear that these fibroblastic and chondromatous tumors arising in bone have any significantly different behavior than the tumors that produce bone.

Although the osteogenic sarcomas have been subdivided by specialists into subvarieties that indicate the amount of vascularization (telangiectatic) or the apparent primary locus of origin (endosteal, medullary), such subdivision is beyond the scope of our present consideration and is not, in fact, widely used. However, these sarcomas tend to grow in one of two patterns that merit mention. About half the tumors form a great deal of osseous neoplastic tissue that further causes considerable reactive bone formation to produce dense eburnated growths designated as *sclerosing osteogenic sarcomas.* The remainder are composed essentially of sarcomatous connective tissue stroma, with only minimal amounts of osteoid matrix and bone designated as *osteolytic osteogenic sarcomas.* It is apparent that these two patterns produce quite different roentgenograms.

Incidence. Next to multiple myeloma, osteogenic sarcoma is the most common malignancy of bone and is certainly the leading form of cancer of the bone in the young. In the very large series reported by McKenna et al. (1966), the peak incidence occurred at about 20 years of age and only rarely were these lesions encountered over the age of 40. Almost invariably, the osteogenic sarcomas that arose in the later decades of life were associated with Paget's disease. In this large series of approximately 300 cases, there were 20 instances in which these cancers were attributed to large doses of irradiation received by these patients for the prior treatment of benign or malignant tumors, and two instances of these lesions in radium dial painters who had apparently absorbed sufficient radioactive material from moistening their brushes with their lips to induce carcinogenesis. In general, males are affected slightly more often than females.

Morphology. These highly malignant cancers almost always occur singly, usually in the long tubular bones, but the skull, mandible, ribs, maxilla, vertebral column, clavicles and small bones of the feet as well as all the other bones of the body have been involved — albeit excessively rarely. In descending order of frequency, the femur, tibia, humerus, ilium, mandible and ribs are favored sites. Approximately 70 per cent of these neoplasms arise in the femur or tibia. For obscure reasons, these tumors tend to occur in the lower end of the femur and upper end of the tibia, i.e., about the knee, while in the upper extremity they tend to affect the upper end of the humerus and lower ends of the radius and ulna, i.e., the "outer" ends of these bones (Coventry and Dahlin, 1957).

In the **sclerosing variety,** when the bone is split longitudinally, a large mass of dense, gray-white, apparent bone is found virtually filling the marrow cavity in the metaphyseal region. The tumor usually extends along a broad front toward the epiphysis and may end abruptly at the epiphyseal cartilage. However, it sometimes penetrates the epiphyseal cartilage to invade the entire head of the bone, but once again the articular cartilage appears to represent a barrier to further spread. The tumor also extends generally in a more conical form toward the diaphysis. Penetration of the cortex is almost invariable, often lifting up the periosteum. The periosteal elevation, in most cases, produces a characteristic acute angle with the underlying cortical bone, referred to as Codman's triangle, an anatomic feature that can be visualized in the roentgenogram and is considered of some diagnostic significance (Fig. 31–15). The tumor may extend through the periosteum into the surrounding tissues. At the same time, this tumor tissue may extend around the head of the bone into the joint capsule and eventually invade the joint space itself. The central regions of the tumor tend to be the most densely sclerotic, and there is considerable increased density to the enveloped cortical bone. At the periphery, the tumor is usually more soft, granular, gray to red and friable.

The **osteolytic variant** tends to be more bulky, presumably because it is more rapidly growing. Medullary involvement is present, similar to that described in the sclerosing tumors, but the tumor in this form tends to be of a more fleshy consistency with areas of hemorrhage, necrosis and cystic softening. More extensive destruction of cortical bone is found, along with greater involvement of the adjacent soft tissues (Fig. 31–16). Small foci of cal-

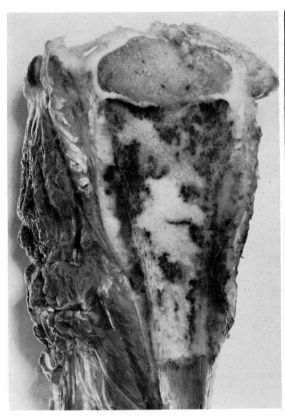 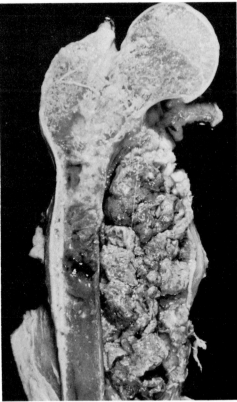

Fig. 31–15   Fig. 31–16

Figure 31–15. Osteogenic sarcoma, sclerosing type, of upper end of tibia. The hard white tumor fills the marrow cavity but has not penetrated the epiphyseal plate. It has infiltrated through the cortex and lifted the periosteum on both lateral aspects.

Figure 31–16. Osteogenic sarcoma, osteolytic type. The tumor has penetrated the cortex to produce a large, soft, necrotic, soft tissue mass.

cification are sometimes encountered in these tumors but, in general, the lesion appears macroscopically as a soft tissue neoplasm.

Histologically, these tumors have **an abundant osteoblastic and connective tissue stroma that is usually frankly sarcomatous and is the component upon which the diagnosis of malignancy is based.** All ranges of anaplasia are encountered, from those which are fairly well differentiated and resemble fibrosarcomatous growths to the other extreme of marked pleomorphism with abundant tumor giant cells and numerous atypical mitotic figures. One should find, dispersed throughout this tumor, trabeculae of tumor osteoid and bone. This osteoid tissue is usually formed directly from osteoblasts within the tumor but, at other times, is transformed from islands of poorly formed masses of cartilage. These features are present in both the sclerosing and osteolytic varieties, but obviously in the former there is greater emphasis upon bone formation along with reactive new bone growth in the enveloped cancellous spicules and cortical bone. In the osteolytic variety, the emphasis is upon resorp-

tion and destruction of preexisting bony architecture (Figs. 31–17, 31–18, 31–19 and 31–20).

Clinical Course. As with most tumors of bone, the presenting clinical complaints are those of pain, tenderness and swelling of the affected parts. Occasionally, however, these tumors remain entirely silent and are called to clinical attention by the sudden fracture of the involved bone. Rapid growth is characteristic of many and may actually cause progressive expansion and enlargement of the limb as the neoplasm enlarges. Usually, these tumors follow a very rapid clinical course and may be observed to increase in bulk under observation. The serum alkaline phosphatase may be elevated, but is usually of no diagnostic significance. Roentgenograms are pathognomonic in a great many instances. The most characteristic feature of the x-ray film is produced by the penetration of the cortical bone with elevation of the periosteum and extension into the soft tissue. This subperiosteal and soft tissue tumor

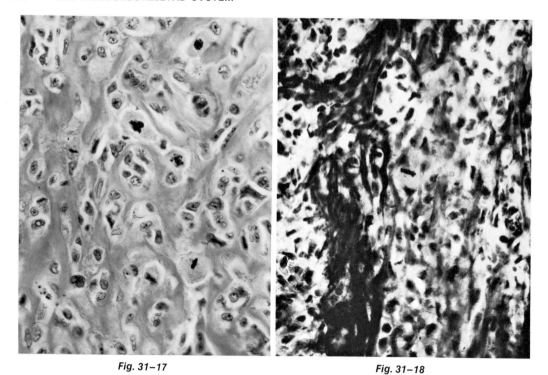

Fig. 31–17 *Fig. 31–18*

Figure 31–17. *The sclerosing pattern with abundant osteoid matrix within the cellular tumor.*
Figure 31–18. *A cellular tumor with irregular black strands of osseomucin.*

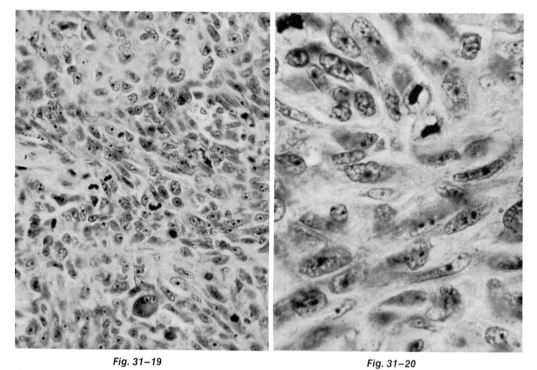

Fig. 31–19 *Fig. 31–20*

Figure 31–19. *The osteolytic pattern with scant osteoid formation. A trapped osteoclast is present in the lower field.*
Figure 31–20. *High power detail of the characteristic spindle cells that make up the bulk of osteogenic sarcomas. Note the mitotic figure.*

with its bony osteoid content produces perpendicular calcified striae that are referred to as ray markings (Fig. 31–21). The radiodensity or radiolucency of the tumor varies according to the extent of bone formation as described previously. While these roentgenographic findings are present in the classic well advanced case, it should be emphasized that the early lesion may, indeed, be difficult to recognize by x-ray examination.

It should be reemphasized that while osteogenic sarcomas usually arise in preexisting normal bone, about 15 per cent arise in previously diseased bone and, exceedingly rarely, these tumors arise in extraosseous soft tissues. The bone diseases associated with osteogenic sarcoma, in order of importance, are Paget's disease (approximately 6 per cent of all osteogenic sarcomas), previously irradiated bone (approximately 4 per cent of all osteogenic sarcomas), hereditary multiple exostosis, polyostotic fibrous dysplasia, and solitary and multiple enchondromas. The origin of osteogenic sarcoma in myositis ossificans is controversial and, while numerous reports of this can be found in the literature, most are currently believed to have arisen in the bone adjacent to the myositis.

The prognosis in these cases is extremely

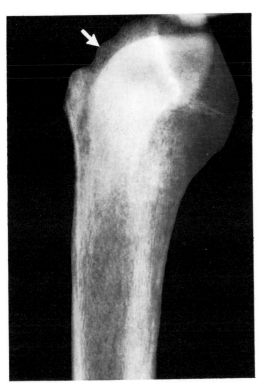

Figure 31–21. Osteogenic sarcoma of the humerus. Note the bone formation visible external to the cortex (arrow).

depressing. Five-year survival rates ranging from 5 to 22 per cent have been reported but, in the experience of most, the lower figure generally prevails (Weinfeld and Dudley, 1962) (Lichtenstein, 1972). The outlook for the patient appears to be quite directly related to the size of the tumor at excision and, in the large report by McKenna et al. (1966), no cures were ever achieved when the neoplasm was greater than 15 cm. in greatest diameter. Death is almost invariably caused by widespread metastasis, principally to the lungs, liver, other bones or virtually any other organ and tissue in the body.

FIBROSARCOMA ARISING IN BONE.

Brief mention should be made of this soft tissue tumor that some prefer to call a variant of osteogenic sarcoma because it arises in bone. Most prefer to designate it as a fibrosarcoma, merely having origin in bone. Histologically, these fibrosarcomas resemble their soft tissue counterparts and presumably take origin from the periosteum, endosteum or fibrous stroma of the medullary cavities. They are much less common than their bone-producing relatives, tend to arise in a slightly older group and have a slightly better prognosis with a five-year survival in the range of 30 per cent.

CHONDROMATOUS TUMORS

Exostosis (Exostosis Cartilaginea). Exostoses are benign new growths that protrude from the outer contour of bones and are characteristically capped by growing cartilage. It will be remembered that such exostoses were described in a hereditary disorder (hereditary multiple cartilaginous exostoses), and thus it is apparent that these lesions may occur singly as apparent isolated defects or multiply as a congenital disorder. Because of the association with this apparently hereditary disorder and because of the extremely indolent course, many prefer to consider the exostosis as an aberration of development rather than a true neoplasm. Those who consider them neoplastic designate these lesions as osteochondromas. Whether these lesions are neoplasms or not, they are tumors in the clinical sense and, therefore, require differentiation from other true neoplasms.

In the multifocal hereditary disorder, the lesions occur in young infants or children and usually cease to enlarge at the time of puberty (p. 1434). The isolated lesions also can occur in young infants, but are occasionally encountered in postadolescence and in adults. At least

80 per cent of the cases are discovered before the age of 21. The isolated lesion is found most often on the lower metaphysis of the femur and the upper metaphysis of the tibia. These may also stop growing and become totally ossified and so, in these late stages, they have been designated as *osteomas*. However, their peripheral location and the orientation of the cartilage over the outer growing surface suggest, rather, that the bony component is derived from endochondral bone formation and not from neoplastic formation of bone. The major clinical significance of these lesions is their potential for malignant transformation with the formation of a chondrosarcoma or osteogenic sarcoma. This hazard appears to be greater with the multiple hereditary disorder than with the solitary lesions.

Enchondroma. Enchondroma is here used to designate a benign tumor occurring within the interior of a bone composed of mature hyaline cartilage. In this sense, the tumor is best designated as an *enchondroma*. Cartilaginous tumors that occur on the surface of bones and jut out from the bony contour almost invariably fall into the pattern of the exostosis cartilaginea and are, therefore, not included within the present category. Solitary chondromas occur in individuals up to the age of 50 but rarely below the age of 10.

As mentioned earlier (p. 1434), enchondromas may occur in multiple sites, often in childhood in a condition that is apparently of familial origin and is designated as *enchondromatosis* or Ollier's disease. When these skeletal lesions are accompanied by hemangiomas of the skin, they have been designated as *Maffucci's syndrome*. The enchondromas of these systemic patterns tend to be somewhat more cellular and somewhat more atypical than the isolated lesions and have a higher incidence of malignant transformation.

Most solitary lesions occur in the small bones of the hands and feet. However, tumors have also been found in the long tubular bones and rarely in the flat bones of the skull and pelvis. These lesions consist of firm, slightly lobulated, rounded, glassy, gray-blue, translucent tissue embedded within the spongiosa of the bone. They abut on and erode the overlying cortical bone. In the small bones of the hand, these lesions may progressively encroach upon the cortex and cause expansion and deformity of the bone. Usually, reactive bone formation, however, maintains a thin outer bony shell. External deformity rarely occurs in the long tubular bones of the extremities.

These gross characteristics are rarely evident in surgical specimens since the standard form of treatment is curettage of the lesion, and all that is received are small granules or rice-like fragments of cartilaginous material, sometimes embedded in spicules of bone where the tumor abuts on the surrounding normal tissue.

Histologically, the tumor is composed of **small masses or islands of hyaline cartilage, separated by a scant, sometimes richly vascularized fibrous stroma.** The cartilage cells are irregularly dispersed through the matrix and are contained within clearly defined lacunar spaces. Not infrequently, one to three nuclei may be found within a single lacuna. Toward the margins of the islands where they abut on the fibrous tissue, the cells become flattened and gradually assume the appearance of spindled fibroblasts so that there is no well defined transition between the cartilage cells and connective soft tissue cells. **Foci of calcification and even ossification are sometimes encountered in the cartilage, but the bone formation is not enclosed within a fibrous stroma,** differentiating such osteoid deposition from that found in osteogenic sarcomas. The innocence of these tumors is established by the regularity of the cartilage cells and by the mature differentiation of the hyaline matrix. Although the tumor is a benign lesion, it erodes adjacent bony structures and may thus appear invasive.

This erosive characteristic may cause pain and swelling, but often the tumors are totally unsuspected until discovered incidentally by roentgenogram or until attention is called to them by a pathologic fracture. Lesions in the small bones of the hands and feet are almost always innocuous and rarely become malignant. Those in the long bones of the extremities have a greater but still only slight tendency to undergo malignant transformation. Cartilaginous tumors in the pelvic bones are often malignant, but it is not certain whether these arise as benign chondromas or were chondrosarcomas from the outset.

Chondromyxoid Fibroma. This is a comparatively newly recognized uncommon lesion principally of young adults that is of importance because it is often misinterpreted as malignant. These tumors tend to occur about the knee joint in the lower metaphysis of the femur, the upper metaphysis of the tibia and the lower end of the fibula. The small bones of the foot may also be affected. As can be seen, this distribution is virtually confined to the lower extremity. Rarely these have been described in the ribs and pelvis. The tumor arises eccentrically within the marrow cavity, and progressively erodes the overlying cortex causing a focus of radiolucency and sometimes total erosion of the cortical bone. They seldom cause obvious clinical deformity and are usually brought to the patient's attention by pain. The neoplasm is firm, gray-white, somewhat rubbery and rarely has a sufficient myxoid element to cause sliminess.

On microscopic examination, it is composed essentially of a loose myxomatous tissue containing characteristic spindled fibroblasts, stellate myxoma cells and, in areas of increased maturity, large amounts of collagenous hyaline fibrous tissue. Some areas may differentiate into cartilage. Usually there is no bone or osteoid formation. The most ominous feature of the tumor is scattered or sometimes aggregated multinucleate giant cells, some of which appear similar to osteoclasts. Other giant cells may have fewer nuclei with considerable hyperchromatism and variation in nuclear size and shape. These cells have the appearance of malignancy and are responsible for the overdiagnosing of these tumors as chondrosarcomas or myxosarcomas. Experience, to date, indicates that these are entirely benign and do not recur after thorough curettement (Jaffe and Lichtenstein, 1948).

Chondrosarcoma. Chondrosarcomas represent only 7.6 per cent of all malignant bone tumors, but it is to be noted that in the reported cures of primary malignant tumors of bone, about half are chondrosarcomas. These neoplasms, therefore, are amenable to surgical removal and cure. They tend to occur in an older age group and are preponderant in males in the ratio of 3 to 1. In many instances,

a history is obtained of a mass present for years, supporting the belief that these lesions arise frequently in preexisting benign tumors.

Because of their origin in benign cartilaginous tumors, they may appear as intramedullary enchondromatous lesions or as lesions arising on the periphery of bone presumably from an exostosis cartilaginea. Many arise from one of the widely scattered, benign, cartilaginous lesions of the congenital Ollier's disease. These sarcomas are frequently large bulky tumors and, as pointed out by O'Neal and Ackerman (1952), when they are large and peripheral and greater than 8 cm. in diameter, they are particularly likely to be malignant. In the same way, large lesions of the pelvis, ribs, sternum and long tubular bones are particularly suspect of malignancy. Erosion of bone, destruction of cortex and extension along broad fronts into the surrounding soft tissues are evident in many (Fig. 31–22).

Histologically, it is sometimes difficult to differentiate chondrosarcomas in which there is some ossification from osteogenic sarcomas that have a considerable component of cartilaginous matrix. In general, the chondrosarcoma presents as an atypical, more cellular enchondroma with islands of mature hyaline cartilaginous matrix interspersed with other areas where the cartilage is poorly developed and contains atypical anaplastic cells. The line of demarcation between cartilage and surrounding soft tissue is very poorly developed in these malig-

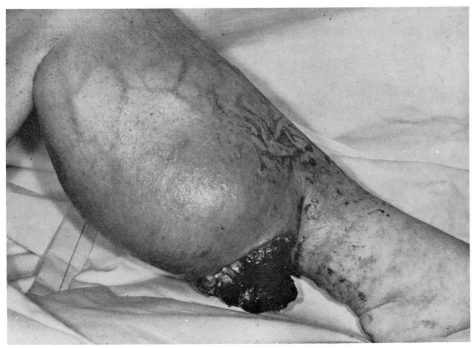

Figure 31–22. Chondrosarcoma of the tibia. The tumor is recurrent after a previous local resection. The bulky lesion has fungated through the skin.

nancies, and the surrounding stroma may, in fact, be atypical and sarcomatous. Such bone as is present appears to be laid down within cartilage in the pattern of endochondral bone formation, differentiating it from the osteoblastic production of the osteogenic sarcoma.

The treatment of these cases poses one of the most difficult problems in surgery. It has been observed that chondrosarcomas, if left alone, may continue to enlarge slowly and remain only locally invasive for years. However, once surgical removal has been attempted and is not complete, local recurrence, more rapid growth rate and greater predisposition to metastasis follow. In the course of time, hematogenous dissemination to distant organs occurs, although usually after a long interval. In adequately excised cases, an excellent prognosis may be expected and, in general, more cures are attained with chondrosarcomas than with any other type of primary bone malignancy.

GIANT CELL TUMORS

Giant cell tumors are also known in the British literature as osteoclastomas, based on the belief that the multinucleate giant cells, which comprise the histologic hallmark of these neoplasms, are osteoclasts. However, because the precise histogenesis of these giant cells is still unclear, the preferred designation is giant cell tumor.

These neoplasms have been the center of a longstanding controversy, both with regard to their differentiation from other lesions bearing giant cells and with regard to their biologic behavior. There are several other lesions replete with similar-appearing giant cells that are not true neoplasms. These include the so-called brown tumors seen in skeletal disease associated with hyperparathyroidism, giant cell granulomas of the gingiva and jaw bones (epuli) and giant cell tumors of synovial or tendon sheath origin. All of these lesions are better known as *reparative giant cell granulomas* and are not true neoplasms despite their histologic resemblance to giant cell tumors of bone. One additional giant cell lesion is the benign chondroblastoma of bone. These neoplasms are best considered as variants of giant cell tumors which have a different clinical course and biologic significance from giant cell tumors.

The other controversy involves the validity of histologic grading of these tumors in an effort to prognosticate their clinical behavior. Many of these tumors are clearly benign histologically and are successfully cured by local resection. Others are unmistakably malignant histologically and behave accordingly. However, many neoplasms having an innocent morphologic appearance display cancerous aggressive behavior and, conversely, some ugly-appearing tumors pursue a benign course. There is then considerable divergence between the morphology and biologic behavior of these tumors, and even those which appear to lack all evidence of anaplasia must be viewed guardedly. Hence, many writers have dropped the term benign as applied to these neoplasms and, instead, divide them into typical and malignant. Even the typical lesions, on recurrence, develop ever more anaplasia and cancerous behavior.

These neoplasms are uncommon and generally occur in the third and fourth decades of life; however, they have been reported in adolescents and in patients of advanced age. Some series have reported a marked female predominance (McGrath, 1972).

The great preponderance (80 to 90 per cent) of giant cell tumors arise near the ends of long bones. The most frequent sites are the lower end of the femur, the upper end of the tibia, the upper end of the femur and the humerus. Over half occur around the knee (Goldenberg et al., 1970) (Dahlin et al., 1970). Sporadic neoplasms have been reported in the skull, pelvis, small bones of the hands and feet and even the patella.

The tumors are almost invariably localized within the end of the long bone and rarely affect the diaphysis. Characteristically, these lesions begin within the center of the shaft of the bone and progressively expand to cause a large club-like deformity of the bone (Fig. 31—23). Since these neoplasms occur in individuals whose epiphyses have already closed, they expand directly up to the articular cartilage, but usually do not erode through it. Despite this great expansion of the external contours of the bone, reactive new bone formation usually maintains a thin enclosing outer shell. The tumor tissue itself is firm, friable and gray-pink to yellow-brown in color. Almost invariably, there are foci of hemorrhage, necrosis and cystic softening. Fine spicules of gritty calcification are often scattered throughout the soft tissue.

Histologically, the tumor is composed of a cellular spindle cell stroma containing numerous, irregularly scattered, large giant cells that resemble osteoclasts or foreign body type giant cells (Figs. 31—24 and 31—25). However, there is some question whether these cells do not, in reality, represent syncytial aggregates of the stromal cells. Areas of hemorrhage, hemosiderin deposition, fibrous scarring, infarct necrosis, inflammatory infiltration and occasional nests of xanthoma cells are sometimes identified in the classic pattern of the giant cell tumor. Bone formation and cartilage are absent or rela-

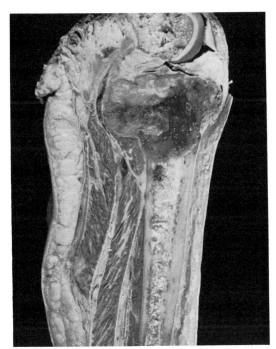

Figure 31–23. *Benign giant cell tumor of upper end of tibia. The tumor has produced an ovoid hemorrhagic mass replacing the entire end of the bone.*

tively inconspicuous, since, as will be shown, these features are presumably pathognomonic of the type now designated as benign chondroblastoma of bone. **The spindle cell stroma of the giant cell tumors requires the most meticulous attention, for it is upon the regularity or anaplasia in these cells that the clinical behavior of the tumor hinges.**

All degrees of cellular atypicality and undifferentiation are encountered, ranging from the well differentiated typical tumors having virtually mature fibroblastic spindle cells with few, if any, mitoses and no tumor giant cells, to the other extreme of cellular pleomorphism, hyperchromasia, abundant mitotic figures and frank sarcomatous changes. Based upon these differences, giant cell tumors have been arbitrarily divided into Grades 1 to 3 (Murphy and Ackerman, 1956) (Jaffe et al., 1940). The Grade 1 neoplasm has the well differentiated stroma and presumably should follow a benign clinical course. The Grade 3 neoplasm with the sarcomatous stroma is the most aggressive and malignant neoplasm (Fig. 31—26). Reference has already been made to the fact that the biologic behavior of the tumor may not necessarily conform to its grade and, therefore, there is a growing tendency to discard the grading system.

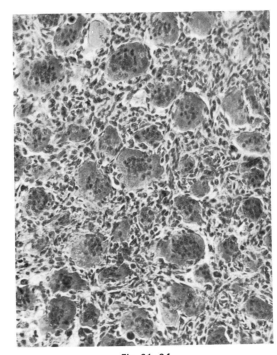

Fig. 31–24

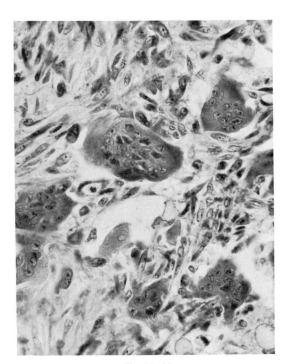

Fig. 31–25

Figure 31–24. *Benign giant cell tumor, illustrating the abundance of multinucleate giant cells.*
Figure 31–25. *A high power detail of the giant cells and well differentiated stroma in the benign form of giant cell tumor. Note the vacuolated lipophages, several in the right lower corner.*

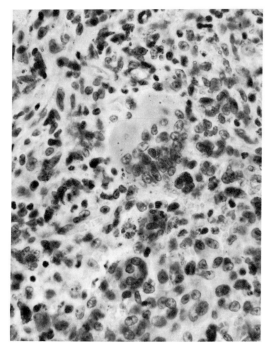

Figure 31–26. Malignant giant cell tumor, illustrating the anaplasia within the spindle cells that comprise the bulk of the neoplasm.

Clinically, these patients present the nonspecific complaints of local pain, tenderness, functional disability and, occasionally, pathologic fractures. However, in a great many instances, the tumors grow insidiously to bulky size and produce externally palpable masses before discovery. Roentgenograms are frequently pathognomonic and show large, roughly spherical, cystic areas of bone rarefaction traversed by irregular strands of calcification. Frequently, multiple cysts create the appearance of a cluster of soap bubbles. A thinned-out but usually preserved cortex surrounds the lesions and, in general, the articular cartilage is preserved and the joint space uninvolved.

In a large series of proved giant cell tumors, approximately one-half are likely to have a favorable outcome irrespective of the treatment, about one-third are likely to be aggressive and recur after simple excision or curettement—a considerable proportion of these may eventually come to amputation—while the remaining 15 per cent will be frankly aggressive, malignant, metastasizing tumors.

On the basis of the data given, it is evident that about half of all giant cell tumors are biologically malignant, ample justification for treating these lesions with due respect. And it will be remembered that one-third of the cases can be cured by adequate removal but are subject to recurrence when incompletely excised. Inadequate removal of these tumors carries the grave risk that, with each recurrence, there is an increased tendency to malignant transformation.

Benign Chondroblastoma of Bone. This neoplasm histologically closely resembles giant cell tumors just described. It differs in several important respects. To begin with, these tumors almost invariably occur in children *under* the age of 20 when the epiphyses probably have not closed. In contrast, giant cell tumors are rare in those under 20 years of age. Their distribution and macroscopic characteristics tend to follow those of giant cell tumors. Histologically, however, these neoplasms often contain *foci of calcification, trabeculae of osteoid tissue and well developed bone as well as more or less well defined areas of deposition of cartilaginous matrix which are not usually present in giant cell tumors.* Additionally, giant cells may be present in these lesions, but usually not in great numbers. In certain instances, they may be almost totally absent. These tumors have been called, in the past, *chondromatous or epiphyseal giant cell tumors or ossifying giant cell tumors.* However, because of the age distribution, the histologic differences, and principally, because *these tumors are virtually always benign, localized lesions that do not recur and do not invade,* there appears to be ample justification for considering them as an entity distinct from the group of giant cell tumors described previously (Lichtenstein and Kaplan, 1949).

ANGIOMATOUS TUMORS

Benign angiomas, both cavernous and plexiform in type, may occur in bone and exactly resemble their counterparts in soft tissue. In the same way, the malignant hemangioendotheliosarcoma does not differ from similar tumors in soft tissues. The only tumor in this group that requires further description is the so-called diffuse endothelioma of Ewing.

Ewing's Sarcoma. Ewing's sarcoma is sometimes referred to as a diffuse endothelioma. Despite this designation and the inclusion of this neoplasm in the angioma category, there is much controversy as to its precise histogenesis (McCormack et al., 1952) (Foote and Anderson, 1941). There is, in fact, no clear validation of the endothelial nature of these tumors. It has alternatively been suggested that the basic cell type represents a fairly undifferentiated mesenchymal tissue cell perhaps closely related to the fibroblasts. A recent ultrastructural study supports this view (Friedman and Gold, 1968). It has even been argued that these tumors are not primary in bone, but represent metastatic neuroblastomas possibly of adrenal medullary origin, or that they fall into the category of lymphomas arising in bone, particularly the reticulum cell sarcoma. The consensus does not support the view that these tumors are metastatic or lymphomatous.

Ewing's sarcoma occurs principally between the ages of 10 and 25 years, an age incidence that corresponds to that of osteogenic sarcoma. However, the lesion is quite rare and is, therefore, much less frequent than the osteogenic sarcomas. There is a well defined male preponderance.

Morphology. Usually these tumors arise in unicentric foci within a single bone but, in occasional cases, multiple lesions within bones are found, and it is not certain whether these represent metastases or multicentric foci of origin. The long tubular bones of the body are the site of origin in about half the cases and the innominate bones in one-fifth as the two major loci of origin. The remaining tumors arise in the pubis, ischium, ribs, skull, clavicle, sternum and in virtually any other skeletal part (Falk and Alpert, 1965). While it has been classically taught that most tumors arise in the diaphysis, recent reviews make clear that metaphyseal origins are more common. Characteristically, by the time the specimen is obtained, the tumor involves large areas of the bone or even the entire medullary cavity. It appears as a soft, gray, often cystic lesion that has eroded and frequently expanded the cortex. Hemorrhages and necroses are common within the tumor tissue. The cortex may be perforated with subsequent widespread subperiosteal expansion and even penetration into the soft tissues. While characteristically it is taught that reactive new bone formation creates a **concentric onion-skin layering** about the tumor, this pattern is not found in more than half the cases. It should be emphasized that these neoplasms are rapidly growing and therefore frequently cause bulky, fleshy masses that are readily palpable in the soft tissues.

Histologically, the tumors are extremely undifferentiated and consist of sheets of small, round, oval or spindle-shaped cells in which principally the nuclei are prominent and the cytoplasm poorly visualized. The nuclei tend to be quite uniform in size and shape and mitotic figures are numerous, but tumor giant cells and pleomorphism are conspicuously absent. This histologic pattern may be modified by large areas of ischemic infarct necrosis (the rapidly growing tumor tends to outgrow its blood supply) so that, in many tumors, the preserved viable cells are found in cords or masses about blood vessels with necrosis of the more remote areas (Fig. 31–27 and 31–28). It is this totally undifferentiated growth that has provided the difficulty in determining the cell type of origin. It should further be

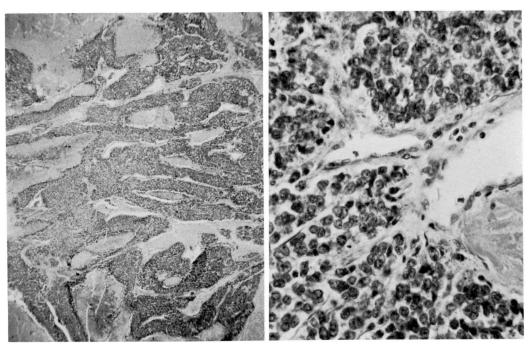

Fig. 31–27   Fig. 31–28

Figure 31–27. *Ewing's sarcoma at low power. The broad bands of cells abut on blood vessels and are created by pale ischemic necrosis of the intervening areas.*

Figure 31–28. *Ewing's sarcoma at high power detail, illustrating the characteristic cytology.*

emphasized that because such cells are completely undifferentiated, the diagnosis of Ewing's sarcoma should not be made without consideration of the possibility that the lesion may represent a metastasis from an undifferentiated carcinoma, undifferentiated sarcoma or neuroblastoma.

Clinical Course. Because of the rapid growth and erosive nature of this tumor, pain is the dominant presenting clinical feature. However, palpable tumor mass, fever, perhaps related to the extensive necrosis of tumor, and tenderness are also frequent findings. The roentgenographic findings are not nearly so characteristic as they are sometimes believed to be. In general, the tumor produces irregular rarefaction and destruction of bone to create a mottled appearaance in the area affected. Lifting of the periosteum may be evident. Subperiosteal new bone formation is rare. All too frequently, by the time the primary tumor is discovered, additional foci are present in other bones and widespread metastatic dissemination is already evident in the lungs, liver, lymph nodes, brain and other viscera. The treatment, which consists of amputation or radical excision when the tumor appears to be localized to the primary site, or irradiation, does not achieve great success. In collected series, less than 15 per cent of patients are alive at five years. These patients usually die of disseminated metastatic cancer within one to two years of the diagnosis. This extremely poor outlook is the highly significant reason for differentiating this lesion from the reticulum cell sarcoma, which permits a 50 per cent survival with appropriate therapy.

MUTLIPLE MYELOMA (PLASMA CELL MYELOMA)

Multiple myeloma is a malignant tumor of plasma cells characterized by (1) multicentric involvement of many sites in the skeletal system; (2) the elaboration of excessive amounts of immunoglobulins; (3) Bence Jones proteinuria; and (4) sometimes extraosseous spread of the plasma cells into various organs or the blood. In an earlier discussion (p. 248), it was pointed out that plasma cell dyscrasias take one of many forms including solitary or multiple osseous lesions (multiple myeloma), soft tissue plasmacytomas and plasma cell leukemias. All are associated with the synthesis of immunoglobulins or fractions thereof (Little and Loeb, 1969).

Multiple myeloma is a disease of the sixth to eighth decades of life. Rare cases occur earlier. Males are affected more often than females in a ratio of 3 to 2. Because this entity has been discussed at some length on page 248, it will be only briefly reviewed here.

Although it has generally been considered a neoplasm of unknown etiology, there has been much speculation that plasma cell neoplasms may be induced by longstanding inflammation or irritation (Clinical Staff Conference, 1963). It is proposed that persistent inflammation may induce a plasma cell inflammatory reaction with active antibody formation. Under this type of continued stimulation, the inflammatory plasma cell might suffer loss of growth controls and assume neoplastic potential. In support of this view, inflammatory *plasma cell granulomas* have been described in the lung, for example, that are considered to be one step removed from overt neoplasia. This concept is still speculative and unsubstantiated.

Morphology. Multiple myeloma characteristically arises in many foci at the same time in various bones of the body (Lichtenstein and Jaffe, 1947). In descending order of frequency, the vertebral column (66 per cent), ribs (44 per cent), skull (41 per cent), pelvis (28 per cent), femur (24 per cent) and clavicle (10 per cent) are affected, and sporadically other sites as well. **Characteristically, these tumors produce soft, red, gelatinous areas of osteolysis within the marrow cavities of the affected bones** (Fig. 31–29). As these foci expand, they may coalesce, erode the cortical bone and sometimes produce through and through defects.

Histologically, the majority of these tumors are composed of fairly well differentiated, readily identified plasma cells (Fig. 31–30). However, as neoplastic cells, they vary in size and shape and are not infrequently binucleate or giant in size. In occasional cases, the cells are more immature and less clearly identifiable as plasma cells. Mitotic activity is readily identified in the more anaplastic variants. In the past, reference has been made to nonplasma cell myelomas, but in all probability these represent the more undifferentiated patterns of plasmacytoma. Necrosis and new bone formation are exceedingly rare, and monotony of plasma cells is characteristic of these lesions.

Clinical Course. The clinical course of these cases is quite characteristic. Most patients present with pain, referred to the osseous lesions. Because the ribs, skull and spine are most frequently involved, the pain is most often referred to the head, chest and back. Weight loss, weakness and a bleeding diathesis are additional major clinical manifestations. Pathologic fractures may develop in bones that are weight-bearing, such as the vertebral bodies and the long bones. As has previously been indicated, the kidney is frequently involved in plasma cell neoplasia in the form of myeloma nephrosis (86 per cent of patients).

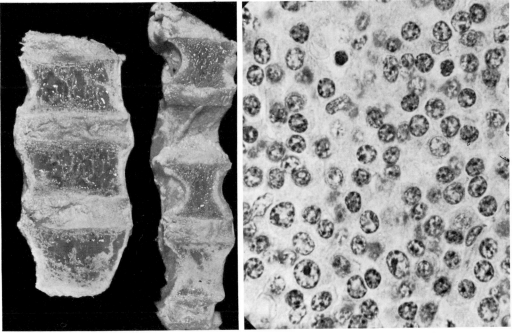

Fig. 31–29   Fig. 31–30

Figure 31–29. Vertebrae from a patient with multiple myeloma. The lesions are diffusely scattered as slightly depressed areas of bone destruction filled with a soft gelatinous tumor.

Figure 31–30. High power detail of fairly regular plasma cells in multiple myeloma.

As a consequence, patients sometimes come to attention in the investigation of renal disease. Proteinuria is present in virtually all patients.

One of the most intriguing and clinically important aspects of plasma cell myelomas is their elaboration of a whole range of immunoglobulins. These are indistinguishable both biochemically and electrophoretically from normal immunoglobulins and may belong to any one of the five major classes. As cited earlier (p. 249), the homogeneity of the elaborated immunoglobulins produces a single, narrow electrophoretic spike referred to as myeloma proteins, M-proteins or paraproteins. In addition, these neoplasms may produce light chain subunits of the immunoglobulins referred to as Bence Jones proteins. These are excreted in the urine, providing one of the important diagnostic tests for this condition. For further details on the synthetic products of these plasma cell tumors and their diagnostic significance, reference should be made to the earlier discussion.

In addition to these immunochemical alterations, the radiographic focal punched-out lesions are virtually pathognomonic (Fig. 31–31). When necessary, the diagnosis can be established more conclusively by aspiration or surgical biopsy of a lesion. To be remembered is the association of amyloidosis with these plasma cell lesions. Some investigators maintain that all primary amyloidosis is due to underlying plasma cell hyperplasia or neoplasia, but most workers in this field do not hold such an extreme position (Osserman, 1959).

Death may be occasioned by intercurrent infection, progressive anemia or the development of renal failure as a reflection of the myeloma nephrosis. The survival time from

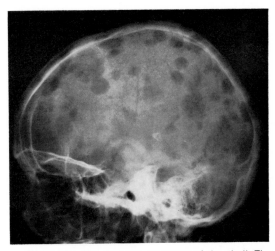

Figure 31–31. Multiple myeloma of the skull. The classic focal osteolytic lesions are readily evident.

diagnosis to death averages six to 12 months. Some success has recently attended the use of chemotherapeutic agents such as urethane and Leukeran, but it is not yet clear that these significantly prolong life.

SECONDARY MALIGNANCY

Metastases to bone from extraosseous primaries are far more common than primary bone tumors. Almost invariably, these secondary growths occur multiply throughout any of the bones of the body and usually they are readily differentiated from the unicentric primary neoplasms of bone. However, considerable difficulty in differential diagnosis may be encountered with multiple myeloma. While most of these secondary tumors produce rarefaction and osteolysis, occasional metastatic tumors provoke considerable reactive bone formation. The most characteristic of these osteoblastic metastases arise in carcinoma of the prostate and, less frequently, the breast. It is impossible to list the primary soft tissue tumors that affect the bone, since it may be said that, in any individual case, any malignancy from any tissue in the body may metastasize to bone, with the possible exception of the primary gliomas of the central nervous system.

The most common sites of metastatic involvement in order of frequency are the vertebral column, ribs, sternum, pelvis, skull, femur, humerus and, only occasionally, the other bones.

JOINTS AND RELATED STRUCTURES

NORMAL	Rheumatoid arthritis variants	**Conditions**
PATHOLOGY	Juvenile rheumatoid arthritis	Synoviosarcoma
Arthritis	Felty's syndrome	Baker's cyst
Suppurative arthritis	Marie-Strumpell disease	Ganglion
Tuberculous arthritis	(ankylosing spondylitis)	**Miscellaneous Lesions**
Arthritis associated with	Osteoarthritis (degenerative	Bursitis
rheumatic fever	joint disease)	Tenosynovitis
Arthritis associated with gout	Villonodular synovitis	Nodular fasciitis
Rheumatoid arthritis (RA)	**Tumors and Tumor-like**	Chordoma

NORMAL

The joints are ideally constructed to serve their function as the hinges of the skeletal system. Each consists principally of two molded, contoured ends of bone shaped to permit motion of one bone upon the other. The bones are connected through a sleeve of dense, collagenous connective tissue, the joint capsule. This capsule is further supported and buttressed by ligaments and tendons. The exposed ends of the bone within the joint space are covered by a thin layer of hyaline articular cartilage that provides a smooth gliding surface. Ease of motion is further provided by a thin, glistening lining epithelium (*the synovial membrane*) and by its secretion, a viscid, clear, white to yellow synovial fluid.

The synovial membrane is derived from mesenchyme. In areas subjected to direct weight-bearing, the membrane consists of a single layer of flattened, virtually inapparent pavement cells resembling, to a considerable extent, the mesothelial lining of the body cavities. In areas subjected to less stress, these cells are cuboidal and more readily visualized and often contain small cytoplasmic vacuoles as indicators of their secretory function. The synovial epithelium is not only secretory, but also serves the important function of transferring fluids and electrolytes into and out of the joint space as well as somewhat larger molecules or particles which may accumulate here as the result of injury or infection.

In this fashion, permanently lubricated hinges are provided. But it is not unanticipated that such structures, in constant use, often subject to excessive strains and stresses, should be the site of frequent injury and degenerative wear and tear.

PATHOLOGY

Diseases of joints are commonplace in clinical medicine. Various surveys indicate that about one in 20 or 30 individuals in the United States suffers from some form of disability of the joints. Young to middle-aged individuals are often afflicted, and the cost of the loss of productive work exceeds hundreds of millions of dollars annually. Despite this staggering significance, we know painfully little about the precise nature of many of these conditions. Our knowledge is particularly deficient in the most important disorders of the joints, namely, the various types of arthritis. Primary attention is devoted in this section to these forms of disabling arthritis as well as to the uncommon but clinically significant tumors that arise in the joints and their investing tissues.

ARTHRITIS

Arthritis is a nonspecific term that refers to any inflammatory involvement of a joint. A number of classifications exist based upon the acuteness or chronicity of the involvement, the etiology of the inflammation, the specific joints involved, as well as upon other considerations. The division employed here is based upon distinctive anatomic features.

SUPPURATIVE ARTHRITIS

Suppurative arthritis refers merely to a suppurative inflammation within a joint space. This type of inflammatory involvement is almost invariably due to direct bacterial invasion. However, very infrequently, physical trauma, bleeding into a joint or a metabolic disorder, such as gout, may evoke a leukocytic infiltrate that resembles, but is not, a valid suppurative arthritis. Bacteria usually seed the joint space in the hematogenous dissemination of an infection localized in some other organ of the body. Much less frequently, bacteria may invade the joint either by the direct spread of a neighboring infection or through a perforating injury. The most common forms of suppurative arthritis are due to the gonococcus, staphylococcus, streptococcus and pneumococcus. These forms of bacterial infection may occur at any age, but are most common in the second, third and fourth decades of life. This age distribution is partially dictated by the fact that bacterial pneumonias, bacterial endocarditis and gonorrheal infections are most prevalent in this age range and are the most common antecedents to suppurative arthritis. For many years, oral sepsis and infected tonsils and sinuses were considered as important causes of suppurative arthritis. However, repeated studies have deemphasized the significance of these focal infections and, in all events, these oral infections are rare antecedents of suppurative infections in the joints.

Any joint may be involved, but those most frequently affected are the large joints, such as the knee, hip, ankle, elbow, wrist and shoulder. For obscure reasons, the sternoclavicular joint is an additional favored site. In most instances, the infection is limited to **a monoarticular involvement.** The anatomic changes consist of a **nonspecific, acute suppurative infection virtually identical with similar infections in other regions of the body.** In early and less severe involvements, the synovial membranes are congested, thickened and edematous, and the joint space contains a thin, cloudy fluid laden with neutrophils (Keefer et al., 1934). Occasionally, bacteria can be identified in the smear of this fluid and often necrotic microorganisms are visible within the cytoplasm of the leukocytes. As the process advances, the inflammatory alterations in the synovial membrane become progressively more severe, and the fluid is transformed to a thick, characteristic pus. **Depending upon the virulence of the causative agent and the chronicity of the infection, the inflammatory synovitis may ulcerate and involve the underlying articular cartilage.** It is, therefore, possible for suppurative arthritis to eventuate in extensive destruction of the joint surfaces and in fibrous bridging scars that seriously hamper the joint function. Calcifications may further limit the mobility, but only infrequently produce permanent ankylosis. In an earlier stage of the disease, the infection may be controlled by appropriate therapy, permitting resolution of the inflammatory changes and restitution of normal structures.

The resultant clinical manifestations are those of any local infection, i.e., redness, swelling, tenderness and pain. Frequently, a systemic constitutional reaction is also present. Because of the destructive tendencies of chronic, persistent, suppurative infections within joint spaces, these conditions require prompt recognition and effective therapy for the preservation of normal joint function. However, overall, suppurative arthritis is an uncommon cause of permanent joint damage.

TUBERCULOUS ARTHRITIS

Tuberculous arthritis is encountered principally in children and is almost invariably a complication of pulmonary tuberculosis. Obviously, however, the initial focus of tuberculous infection may reside in some other site, such as the lymph nodes, kidneys or genital tract. It is usually monoarticular in type. The commonest site of localization is the spine (*Pott's disease or tuberculous spondylitis*). The second most favored site is the hip joint but, in addition, the knee, elbow, wrist, ankle and sacroiliac joints may also be involved.

As in suppurative arthritis, the tuberculous infection follows the pattern of similar infections elsewhere in the body. The initial involvement consists principally of edema, congestion and thickening of the synovial membranes. As the infection advances, the lining membrane becomes studded with small foci of inflammatory granulation tissue harboring solitary and confluent tubercles. Since these infections tend to take a chronic course, the inflammatory tissue creates a thick, felt-like covering over the articular surfaces known as a *pannus.* The caseous necrotizing inflammation may extend from the pannus into the underlying articular surface and thus cause considerable ulceration and destruction as well as erosion into the head of the bone. Sometimes the tuberculous infection erodes into the bone from the margin of the articular cartilage and, thus undermining it, causes it to fragment and slough. Conversely, tuberculous osteomyelitis may trek into the joint space to cause arthritis. *Tuberculous arthritis tends to be a much more destructive process than suppurative arthritis* and frequently eventuates in extensive fibrous bridging and obliteration of the joint space. Late calcification of the inflammatory tissue may lead to ankylosis of the joint. In other instances, the tuberculous infection may erode through the joint capsule to create draining skin sinuses.

The clinical manifestations of these infections are usually slight at first and only become evident when extensive destruction has already occurred. Localized tenderness, swelling, pain on motion, limitation of motion and sometimes surrounding soft tissue inflammation are the principal features of these infections. Tuberculous arthritis cannot be differentiated from the suppurative form by clinical methods. The precise diagnosis requires the identification of the characteristic morphologic tissue reaction or, more positively, the acid-fast bacilli. When a suppurative arthritis fails to yield a common pyogen by means of usual bacterial cultural methods, tuberculosis should be suspected! As a generalization, tuberculous arthritis is usually followed by at least some permanent loss of joint function and often by complete immobilization of the structure.

ARTHRITIS ASSOCIATED WITH RHEUMATIC FEVER

It will be remembered that acute rheumatic fever is classically associated with a *migratory polyarthritis.* Although such joint involvement is a principal clinical manifestation of this disease, the arthritic involvement usually spontaneously or with appropriate therapy subsides to leave no permanent residual. It is the heart that bears the brunt of the destructive effects of this systemic inflammation. For further details on the nature of the joint involvement, reference should be made to Chapter 16.

ARTHRITIS ASSOCIATED WITH GOUT

Acute and chronic involvement of the joints is a characteristic of gout. The articular involvement is the principal and important component of this systemic disorder of uric acid metabolism. In the long chronicity of this disease, deposits of urates in and about the joints may lead to extensive destruction of the articular surfaces and sometimes to permanent loss of joint function. As a systemic metabolic disorder, gouty arthritis has already been described on page 293.

RHEUMATOID ARTHRITIS (RA)

Rheumatoid arthritis is a chronic systemic inflammatory disease of unknown etiology. Although it affects the heart, blood vessels, lungs, eyes, skin, muscles, peripheral nerves and possibly other organs, it primarily causes slowly progressive, disabling arthritis of the small peripheral joints. Typically, the joint involvement is bilaterally symmetrical.

RA is a connective tissue disease closely related to SLE, polyarteritis nodosa, scleroderma, rheumatic fever and dermatomyositis/polymyositis. Both the clinical and anatomic features of RA bear many similarities to, and have many overlaps with, these other connective tissue disorders and, indeed, a synovitis may occur in any of these related disorders which can mimic the joint manifestations of rheumatoid arthritis. Before a diagnosis of RA can be made, it is necessary to rule out closely related conditions (cited below), some of which, indeed, may be variants of RA.

Arthritis associated with agammaglobulinemia

Juvenile rheumatoid arthritis
Felty's syndrome
Ankylosing spondylitis
Psoriatic arthritis
Arthritis associated with ulcerative colitis or regional enteritis
Arthritis encountered in Sjögren's syndrome

In these disorders, the joint involvement is morphologically indistinguishable from RA, but their clinical course or clinical features merit their separation from the parent disease. For example, juvenile rheumatoid arthritis has a much better overall prognosis than RA in adults. Felty's syndrome, on the other hand, like RA is characterized by deforming arthritis, but in this syndrome, it is associated with splenomegaly and leukopenia. The basis for these variations is unknown. Chronic synovitis and arthritis occur, then, in a wide variety of clinical settings and in a range of clinical severities. This diversity has given rise to such qualifying terms as possible, probable, overlapping and borderline rheumatoid arthritis. Recognition of classic RA offers no difficulty, but less well defined joint disease must be considered in the context of the many variants of rheumatoid arthritis and the many connective tissue disorders which can mimic it (Duthie and Alexander, 1968) (Bland; 1968).

Incidence. In 1967, a survey in the United States disclosed an incidence of 0.96 per cent for adults with definite or classic rheumatoid arthritis, rising to 3.2 per cent on inclusion of probable rheumatoid arthritis (Engel and Burch, 1967). The prevalence of this condition rises progressively with increasing age through the seventh decade, affecting women two to three times more often than men. The usual age of onset is in the fourth or fifth decade. While a number of studies have proposed a genetic predisposition to this disease, the evidence so far remains unconvincing (O'Brien, 1967).

Etiology and Pathogenesis. The cause of RA is unknown. Two somewhat related theories of causation dominate present-day thinking: (1) RA is an infectious disease caused by some microbiologic agent or (2) it is a hypersensitivity disease, perhaps autoimmune in origin. Relative to an infectious condition, streptococci, diphtheroids, mycoplasma and viruses have all, at one time or another, been held to be the cause of the chronic synovitis. Experimental mycoplasma infections in cattle, sheep, goats and domestic fowl provide remarkably good models of the disease in man (Thomas, 1973). Recently, arthritis was induced in a strain of mice by suspensions of rheumatoid synovial tissue. Significantly, the disease was passed congenitally to many of the offspring. This finding was interpreted by the authors to mean the existence of a transmissible agent (Warren et al., 1969). On balance, the documentation of an infectious causation is fragmentary and unconvincing (Barnett et al., 1966).

A significant body of data points to an immunologic basis for RA. As mentioned, this disease is closely related to other connective tissue disorders, for example, SLE, of presumed autoimmune origin. The lesions in RA may be proliferative (synovitis, serositis, uveitis), necrotizing (nodules) or vascular (vasculitis in blood vessels of any size)—all highly reminiscent of the changes in known immunologic reactions.

The synovitis is characterized by the accumulation of lymphocytes and plasma cells within the inflammatory synovial membrane. Hypergammaglobulinemia is an almost constant finding in these patients. Finally, and most significantly, *an antibody against IgG, known as the rheumatoid factor (RF), can be demonstrated in the serum of 85 to 90 per cent of these cases.* Rheumatoid factor is an IgM with a sedimentation constant of 19 Svedberg units. In vivo, it circulates as a complex with autologous IgG (7S) to form a soluble 22S macromolecule. RF will cross react with immune globulins of other species. The serum titer of this factor appears to be related to the severity of the disease, and thus it is most elevated in those with severe or widespread involvements. RF can be detected by several specific tests—the latex fixation test, the bentonite flocculation test and the sensitized sheep red cell agglutination test.

What is the origin of rheumatoid factor and what is its significance? It is presumed that it is elaborated by immunocompetent cells in the synovial inflammatory infiltrate and can, in fact, be demonstrated in these cells by immunofluorescent techniques (Rawson et al., 1965) (Tursi et al., 1970). What triggers its appearance is unknown. Some exogenous antigen, such as a microbiologic agent, might possibly possess antigenic similarities to IgG and evoke IgM antibodies recognized as RF (Hamerman, 1968). The involved joints also reveal depressed levels of complement, suggesting the formation of immune complexes with the binding of complement in these areas.

Granting the presence of humoral antibodies, do they evoke the chronic synovitis? Electron microscopy has revealed that the synovial lining cells are of two types, a phagocytic (type A) cell and a cell presumably synthesizing protein-polysaccharides (type B) (Grimley, 1967). A third (type C) cell has also been said to be present in some biopsies, having both synthetic and phagocytic capabilities. It has been proposed that *the phagocytic cells engulf particulate immune complexes and, on their death, release lysosomal acid hydrolases, which evoke the inflammatory synovitis* (Weissmann, 1966) (Ziff, 1973). Immune complexes can, indeed, be visualized within phagocytic synovial cells, as well as in neutrophils within the joint fluid.

Despite all of the evidence of humoral antibodies, the suspicion persists that it is cell-mediated immunity which causes the damage. RF can be identified in low titer in asymptomatic relatives of affected patients. It is also present in a number of other disorders, including SLE, hepatitis, leprosy, syphilis, subacute bacterial endocarditis and chronic tuberculosis, and in these settings, it may well be unassociated with joint disease. You recall that in other immunologic disorders, such as Hashimoto's thyroiditis, it is also believed that, despite the presence of circulating humoral antibodies, cell-mediated immunity actually causes the tissue damage. In rheumatoid arthritis, there is evidence of cell-mediated responses in the involved joints, as for example, detectable titers of macrophage-inhibitory factor (MIF) in the joint fluid. Thus, the ultimate causation of this disorder, the precise role of RF and the trigger events evoking the immune response remain unknown.

Morphology. Joint disease is the cardinal manifestation of RA. The small joints of the hand and feet are usually involved first. In severe progressive disease, the large joints (knees, hips, shoulders and elbows) and, indeed, any joint including the temporomandibular and sternoclavicular may eventually be affected. The joint involvement tends to be symmetrical as mentioned earlier. **The characteristic change is a diffuse proliferative synovitis.** The synovial lining cells become hypertrophied and reduplicated, and the underlying connective tissues undergo reactive hyperplasia. In this manner, the synovial lining is replaced by a highly vascularized, sometimes polypoid mass of inflammatory tissue infiltrated with lymphocytes and plasma cells known as the **pannus.** The mononuclear infiltration may form lymphocytic nodules and is particularly prominent about the newly formed vessels. Foci of necrosis and deposits of fibrinoid may appear within this pannus. In time, the pannus and the inflammatory reaction erode the underlying articular cartilage and eventually invade the bone, causing rarefaction and foci of cystic softening in the juxta-articular bone. At the same time, joint motion causes erosion of the exuberant pannus, leading to bleeding, fibrin clot and the formation of granulation tissue bridges across the joint space. Eventually the total synovial space is obliterated. The eroded, devascularized cartilage may undergo calcification and fragment to produce foreign bodies adding to the inflammatory process. In time, fibrosis and calcification may supervene to yield permanent ankylosis.

As pointed out earlier, immunofluorescent techniques will disclose immune complexes and complement within the reactive cells in the pannus. It should also be pointed out that, before complete destruction of the joint occurs, changes in the joint fluid appear. The fluid aspirated from an involved joint is usually nonviscous and cloudy, and the mucin clot forms poorly in dilute acetic acid. The white cell count in this fluid (predominantly neutrophils) is usually moderately elevated, and many cells contain inclusions, some of which can be shown to be aggregates of rheumatoid factor. It is of interest to note that the white cells within the fluid are neutrophils while those in the pannus are mononuclears.

Chronic inflammatory changes including acute vasculitis (to be described later) and infiltrations of lymphocytes and plasma cells may appear in the periarticular connective tissues and joint capsule.

Subcutaneous rheumatoid nodules appear in about 25 per cent of these patients. They are virtually identical to those encountered in some patients with rheumatic fever and are characterized by a focus of central necrosis surrounded by proliferating connective tissue cells which are usually radially oriented and thus create a well defined palisade (Fig. 31–32). Sometimes the central focus of necrosis contains deposits of fibrinoid. About the palisade, large numbers of lymphocytes and occasional plasma cells accumulate.

Any of the **large or small arteries** of the body may develop an acute necrotizing vasculitis charac-

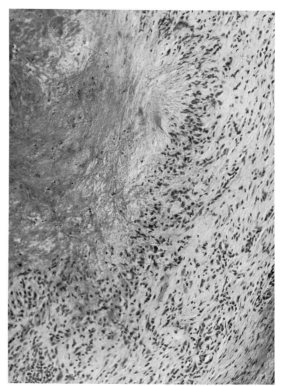

Figure 31–32. *A subcutaneous rheumatoid nodule with an area of necrosis* (upper left) *surrounded by a palisade of fibroblasts and white cells.*

teristic of that seen in other immunologic states such as serum sickness (p. 220). Thrombosis of such involved vessels has been responsible for myocardial infarction, cerebrovascular occlusions, mesenteric infarction and vascular insufficiency in the hands and fingers (Raynaud's phenomenon).

In the **heart,** the pericardium, myocardium and endocardium may be involved (p. 694). The pericarditis is nonspecific and resembles that seen in rheumatic fever, but occasionally typical rheumatoid nodules are present. Myocarditis is seen most frequently in the juvenile form of rheumatoid arthritis and consists of focal necroses and perivascular collections of plasma cells and lymphocytes. Valvular lesions may develop but are indistinguishable from those of rheumatic fever. In addition, endocardial and valvular rheumatoid nodules have been reported (Roberts et al., 1968). Coronary arteritis may lead to myocardial infarction.

In the **lungs,** a variety of changes have been described. Nonspecific fibrinous pleuritis sometimes accompanied by rheumatoid nodules may be found. Nodules may also occur in the lung parenchyma, but more often there is a diffuse chronic interstitial pneumonitis leading to diffuse fibrosis (Martel et al., 1968).

The **eye** may disclose uveitis, keratoconjunctivitis as well as a variety of other manifestations similar to those encountered in Sjögren's syndrome.

Other anatomic changes are also present in the full-blown advanced case, including neuropathy (probably related to vascular disease), inflammatory changes in the skeletal muscles, diffuse lymphadenopathy, splenomegaly and sometimes minimal hepatomegaly. All of these random involvements are minimal and nonspecific, and usually contribute little to the clinical problem.

Clinical Course. As is evident from the widespread distribution of the lesions, RA is a systemic disease of grave nature. Patients generally complain of fatigue, malaise and low-grade fever even before the onset of actual joint pain or swelling. Eventually, however, the nature of this prodrome becomes evident by the appearance of joint stiffness, most pronounced in the morning immediately on waking. Occasionally, the onset is acute with high fever and prostration.

Affected joints are usually enlarged, tender and painful on motion and may be red and warm. With chronicity, these acute manifestations are replaced by progressive induration about the joint and increasing stiffness, until eventually ankylosis causes permanent loss of function. Classically, the enlarged joints have a fusiform tapered appearance with atrophy of the surrounding muscles. In the hands, claw-like deformities sometimes appear, with characteristic flexion contractures or ulnar de-

viation of the immobolized fingers. The overlying skin is often shiny, red and atrophic. It must again be emphasized that such classic joint changes represent the full-blown syndrome and often, at an earlier stage or in other instances, the joint involvement is far more subtle.

As has already been made clear, patients with this disease may develop clinical manifestations of pericarditis, pleuritis, cardiac, pulmonary and vascular involvement as well as the more specific findings relating to the joints.

The diagnosis may be readily evident from physical examination or radiography of the involved joints. But, in addition, there is, characteristically, an elevated erythrocyte sedimentation rate, hypergammaglobulinemia, rheumatoid factor in the serum of most patients and, quite typically, a significant anemia. The source of the anemia is still unclear and has been attributed to oozing of blood into joint membranes or to impaired secretion of erythropoietin. Aspiration of the joint fluid with the demonstration of white cells and poor mucin clot formation is an important part of the diagnostic work-up. The major features which differentiate this form of arthritis from the common osteoarthritis are detailed in Table 31–3.

It is impossible to express a prognosis for this unpredictable disorder. Obviously, those patients with extraskeletal involvements represent a more grave expression of this disease. In general, following appropriate treatment, about 25 per cent of patients are able to return to their former occupation, some never to have further progression of their disease. About 50 per cent have repeated remissions and exacerbations, with varying levels of disability and joint discomfort. The remaining 25 per cent are less fortunate and have fewer remissions and eventually go on to severe debilitation and disability. *Overall, about 15 to 25 per cent of patients with RA will eventually develop systemic amyloidosis.*

RHEUMATOID ARTHRITIS VARIANTS

Juvenile rheumatoid arthritis was formerly called Still's disease. Although it often has an explosive onset with high fever, profound constitutional symptoms and marked joint involvement (more often the larger joints), the prognosis for this form of arthritis is better than that for classic RA. About 50 per cent of patients achieve complete remission, and less than one-sixth progress to severe disability.

Another variant is *Felty's syndrome,* comprising the constellation of rheumatoid arthritis, splenomegaly and leukopenia.

TABLE 31–3. MAJOR DIFFERENCES BETWEEN RHEUMATOID ARTHRITIS AND OSTEOARTHRITIS

	Rheumatoid Arthritis	Osteoarthritis
Age at onset	3rd and 4th decades	5th and 6th decades
Weight	Normal or underweight	Usually overweight
Constitutional manifestations	Present	Absent
Joints involved	Any joint	Mainly knees, spine and peripheral phalanges
Appearance of joint	Soft tissue swelling	Bony swelling
Special deformities	Fusiform finger joint, ulnar deviation	Heberden's nodes
Subcutaneous nodules	Present in 20 per cent	Never present
X-ray	Osteoporosis, erosions	Osteosclerosis, bony spurs
Joint fluid	Increased cells, poor mucin	Few cells, normal mucin
Rheumatoid factor	Present in 85 to 90 per cent	Usually absent
Blood count	Anemia, leukocytosis	Normal
Course	Generally progressive	Stationary or very slowly progressive
Termination	Ankylosis and deformity	No ankylosis
Complicating amyloidosis	15 to 25 per cent	Usually absent

Modified from Cohen, A. S., and Cathcart, E. S.: Arthritis and connective tissue disorders. In Keefer, C. S., and Wilkins, R. W. (eds.): Medicine, Essentials of Clinical Practice. Boston, Little, Brown and Co., 1970. p. 675. © 1970 Little, Brown and Company.

Marie-Strumpell disease or ankylosing spondylitis is chronic arthritis of the spine involving primarily the sacroiliac joints. Since more than 25 per cent of these patients ultimately manifest peripheral joint disease, it appears to be a variant of rheumatoid arthritis affecting primarily the vertebral column. As the name indicates, eventual ankylosis of the spine may cause considerable disability and discomfort, but the overall prognosis is generally good and, in at least half of these patients, peripheral joint disease never develops, nor does the total disability characteristic of classic rheumatoid arthritis.

OSTEOARTHRITIS (DEGENERATIVE JOINT DISEASE)

Osteoarthritis is a noninflammatory disease of joints characterized by deterioration and erosion of articular cartilage and by the formation of new bone at the articular margins sometimes producing so-called spurs. *Osteoarthritis is a disease of articular cartilage, in contrast to rheumatoid arthritis which primarily attacks the synovial membranes.* It is the most common of all forms of arthritis, and it is estimated that it afflicts about 40 million Americans. However, only a small fraction of this number are significantly incapacitated. It is almost as inevitable a concomitant of aging as graying of the hair.

Some experts would restrict the definition of osteoarthritis to degenerative disease affecting movable joints. They would segregate the anatomically similar changes in the vertebral column as a disease primarily of the intervertebral discs, leading to narrowing of the discs. This is followed by abrasion and injury to the anterior margins of the vertebral bodies with secondary spur formation. However, in common clinical practice, these wear-and-tear vertebral changes are generally referred to as osteoarthritis of the spine.

Pathogenesis. Aging is the single most important factor in the development of osteoarthritis. Virtually all persons over the age of 50 have at least traces of this condition. However, it should be pointed out that some aged individuals have little evidence of it, whereas other, relatively young, persons may develop widely disseminated incapacitating arthritis.

The precise nature of the aging influences are uncertain. It has been attributed merely to cumulative stress and mechanical trauma. Indeed, osteoarthritis tends to affect weight-bearing joints and those in constant use (such as fingers) most severely. Recently, attention has turned to some effect of aging on the maintenance of the matrix of articular cartilage. Loss of matrix polysaccharides and particularly loss of chondroitin sulfate have been identified in osteoarthritic cartilage. Conceivably, aging stresses may cause chondrocytes to liberate lysosomal proteases which result in local matrix dissolution. In support of this general proposition, there has been found, about the periphery of areas of matrix degradation, evidence of increased uptake of sulfate, increased synthesis of matrix and increased mitotic activity of chondrocytes, suggesting a compensatory response to matrix loss (Bollet, 1969) (Bollet and Nance, 1966).

Other influences contribute to the pathogenesis of this disease although they are poorly understood. Osteoarthritis tends to appear earlier and to be more severe in patients with diabetes, ochronosis and acromegaly. There are some indications of a familial tendency, but no well defined genetic factors have been identified. It must be admitted that, although a variety of observations have been gathered, the understanding of the fundamental nature of this degenerative joint disease has yielded grudgingly to study.

Morphology. Osteoarthritis may occur as a monoarticular or polyarticular involvement. **The large joints of the body and the spine are principally affected.** The principal anatomic alterations are **degeneration of the cartilage rather than inflammation of the synovia.** The first changes are fissuring and irregularity of the articular cartilaginous surfaces, followed by fibrillation of the cartilage, microfractures and separation of small fragments (Parker et al., 1934). Attendant on these cartilaginous changes is some inflammatory edema and thickening of the synovia, but no significant increased vascularization or leukocytic infiltration that is at all comparable to that described in rheumatoid arthritis. **No true pannus develops.**

With the destruction of the articular cartilage, the underlying bone is exposed. The subarticular bone becomes thickened because of either compression or new bone formation. The marrow spaces in this region are often filled with fibrous tissue and small islands of cartilage that are either driven in by traumatic injury or are formed from the endosteum or connective tissue in the marrow spaces. At the same time, small islands of cartilage, which later become ossified, project above the surface of the articular cartilage, usually about its margins, to produce the characteristic **bony spurs of osteoarthritis.** These spurs are responsible for the "lipping" found in the vertebral body when the spine is affected. When large spurs project from opposing bones, they may come into contact with each other to cause pain and limitation of motion. Rarely, these spurs may fuse to form a solid, calcified bridge, thus destroying all joint motion. As an additional complication of this degenerative process, fragments of cartilage or calcific spurs may break off to form free intra-articular foreign bodies known as **joint mice.** The capsule and ligaments of the joint often undergo calcification to further limit mobility.

Clinical Course. Osteoarthritis is an insidious disease that is usually first noticed as a slight stiffness or decreased mobility in the affected joints. Often a history of repeated microtraumas can be elicited. In this connection, it is generally believed that faulty posture, obesity and occupational stress all predispose to the development of the condition. As the patient ages, the pain, stiffness and limited mo-

tion become more marked. There are no constitutional signs of an inflammatory disease, and the joints rarely have local evidence of inflammation. Crepitus on motion of the joint can sometimes be identified when joint mice are present. There is no satisfactory treatment for this condition, nor any method known for its arrest. Usually, the disorder is slowly progressive over the remaining years of life.

One special form of osteoarthritis should be mentioned, namely, the formation of so-called *Heberden's nodes* about the bases of the terminal phalanges of the fingers. These nodes consist of irregular, firm projections about the joint produced by the calcific spurs formed at the margins of the articular cartilage.

Before concluding this discussion of osteoarthritis, it may be helpful to refer to Table 31–3 on p. 1470 indicating the major differences between rheumatoid arthritis and degenerative joint disease.

VILLONODULAR SYNOVITIS

Villonodular synovitis is, strictly speaking, not a form of arthritis, but merely an inflammation of the synovial membrane of joints or tendon sheaths of unknown cause. It is usually encountered in young adult males and is principally localized to the knee joints. Anatomically, there is nodular thickening of the synovia with the production sometimes of long, slender, filamentous or frond-like processes that project into the joint space. These villi are readily visible macroscopically and often, when the process is advanced, create an appearance that resembles multiple polyposis in the gut. Because the condition is associated with considerable hemorrhage into the synovia, there is an intense deposition of blood pigment within the villi, imparting a yellow to deep brown coloration.

Histologically, the inflammation consists principally of proliferation of subsynovial connective tissue and intense mononuclear leukocytic infiltration, accompanied by extensive deposition of granular hemosiderin pigment within the villous processes (Fig. 31–33). Foci of lipophages in the fibroblastic stroma, hemosiderin pigment and numerous multinucleate foreign body type or osteoclastic giant cells may occur in some instances, producing what is called by some a giant cell tumor. However, these lesions are unquestionably inflammatory reparative granulomas, perhaps a response to old blood and chronic irritation, and do not therefore merit the designation neoplasm. This giant cell pattern is, in fact, much more common in relation to tendon sheaths

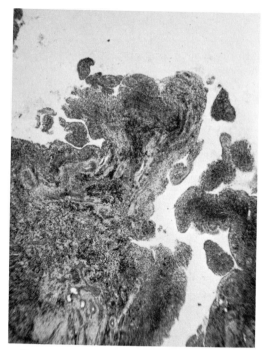

Figure 31–33. *Villonodular synovitis, illustrating the filamentous strands of inflammatory synovia.*

than joint cavities. These so-called *giant cell tumors of tendon sheaths* are so common in the hands and fingers that they are glibly termed "fingeromas." Here they present as yellow, discrete, firm nodules laden with the lipophages described and having the other histologic characteristics already mentioned. Usually there is very little leukocytic element so that the inflammatory origin of these lesions is certainly masked. However, they are never malignant, rarely exceed 1 to 2 cm. in diameter and, in many instances, are removed at a time when they have undergone almost total fibrous replacement, suggesting a natural life history terminating in total fibrosis.

The etiology, then, of both the diffuse synovitis and the localized giant cell granuloma of tendon sheath origin probably rests in some obscure cause for chronic inflammation, such as repeated episodes of hemorrhage. Such an origin would explain the abundant lipid and blood pigment and the essentially reparative characteristic of these lesions. But before concluding, mention should be made of an alternative belief that the giant cell tumor of joint or synovial origin is, indeed, a neoplasm derived from endothelial cells. According to this concept, these giant cell lesions are "first cousins" to the sclerosing hemangioma of capillary origin.

TUMORS AND TUMOR-LIKE CONDITIONS

While a variety of benign and malignant neoplasms have been described in the joints, the only tumor of sufficient frequency to merit citation is the synoviosarcoma.

SYNOVIOSARCOMA

The synoviosarcoma arises in the synovial membrane. This neoplasm is invariably malignant but, notwithstanding, for many years the inappropriate designation of synovioma has been given to it. It usually occurs as a unicentric lesion in middle to later life. Both sexes are affected equally. These neoplasms arise not only in joints but also in tendon sheaths and bursae, all of which contain similar mesenchymally derived synovial cells (Fig. 31–34).

The lesions vary from solitary, well defined, apparently discrete masses several centimeters in diameter up to large, bulky, obviously invasive tumors, 15 or more cm. in diameter. The lower extremity is the site of origin in three-fourths of the cases (Ariel and Pack, 1963). On cross section, the larger lesions often have areas of hemorrhage, cystic necrosis and softening, and they are frequently complicated by spotty calcifications. Histologically, the tumor is quite pleomorphic. The various cell patterns tend to recapitulate the differentiation of cuboidal synovial cells from the more primitive spindle-shaped fibroblasts. The tumor may, therefore, be composed of elongated fusiform cells growing in sheets or cords closely resembling plump fibroblasts. Usually, however, cleft-like spaces are formed that are lined by cuboidal epithelium, suggesting the differentiation of cells into those lining the joint spaces. These gland spaces may contain serous or mucinous secretion similar to the fluid found within the joint spaces. In the better differentiated synoviosarcomas, these spaces form well defined, characteristic glands that create a considerable resemblance to an epithelial glandular carcinoma. Usually, however, a gradual transition can be identified where these cuboidal gland cells merge with the more undifferentiated spindle cells about the gland spaces.

An additional variable histologic pattern is the formation of small papillary projections extending into slit-like or cystic spaces within the tumor (Figs. 31–35 and 31–36). These papillary projections recapitulate the villous projections found in villonodular synovitis. The individual tumor cells display all the characteristics of the anaplasia of malignancy with variation in nuclear size and shape, hyperchromasia and mitotic activity.

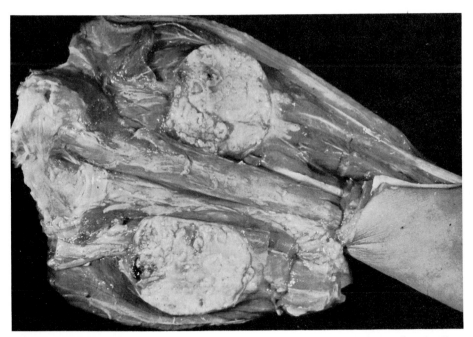

Figure 31–34. *Synoviosarcoma—deceptively discrete mass arising in the tendon sheaths.*

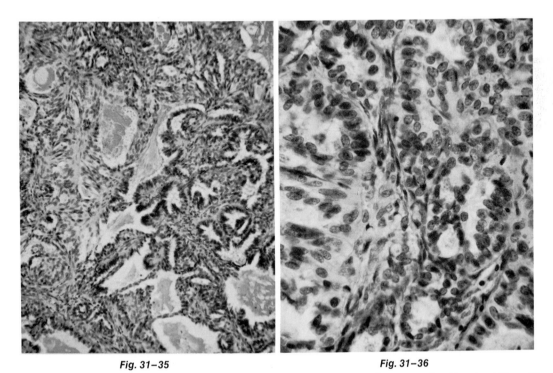

Fig. 31–35   Fig. 31–36

Figure 31–35. *Low power detail of a synoviosarcoma, illustrating cleft-like spaces lined by gland-like epithelium and the formation of papillary projections.*
Figure 31–36. *High power detail of the variable cytologic picture of a synoviosarcoma.*

These tumors are locally invasive, erode into joint spaces and destroy joint function as well as permeate blood vessels and spread to the lungs and other organs. They destroy the adjacent bone by direct penetration. Spread to regional nodes is characteristic and dictates the need for regional node dissection whenever amputation is performed. Even the early well differentiated lesions that appear histologically innocent carry a grave prognosis, and five-year survivals are infrequent (approximately 10 to 25 per cent) (Haagensen and Stout, 1944).

BAKER'S CYST

A Baker's cyst is a non-neoplastic herniation of the synovial membrane of the knee joint into the popliteal space. It usually presents as a round to ovoid subcutaneous mass that may be soft and fluctuant, but more often is firm owing to the tension of the contained fluid. Commonly, these lesions achieve a diameter of 10 to 15 cm. and, by progressive expansion of size, they may dissect beneath the skin into the region of the calf muscles or between the heads of the gastrocnemius muscle. The cyst itself consists of a fibrous wall averaging 2 to 5 mm. in thickness, filled with a limpid or mucoid fluid resembling the joint fluid. The wall may have uneven trabecular thickenings and partial loculation as a point on the cystic circumference weakens and yields to the pressure of the contained fluid. Often it is difficult to identify the communication with the knee joint. Histologically, the wall is composed of dense, collagenous, laminated, fibrous tissue, often mildly infiltrated with lymphocytes. Usually there is no apparent organized synovial lining to the cyst but, in areas, somewhat more cuboidal cells may be identified as representatives of the synovia. This condition is readily cured by surgical excision.

GANGLION

A ganglion is a small cystic swelling that projects from a joint capsule or a tendon sheath. These are found most often on the wrist and are less frequently encountered on the foot or knee. They usually do not exceed 1.5 to 2 cm. in diameter and consist principally of a collagenous, fibrous cyst filled with mucoid fluid. Only infrequently can a synovial cell lining be identified. Usually it is quite difficult if not impossible to identify a communication between the ganglion and the adjacent tendon sheath or joint space.

The genesis of these lesions is obscure. It is postulated that most arise as herniations through a defect in the wall of the joint capsule or tendon sheath. As such, communications should be present in all instances. However, the difficulty in demonstrating such connections raises the possibility that these may arise in displaced rests of synovial tissue or by the transformation of primitive connective tissue into synovial cells that then secrete mucin to create the cystic space. Supporting this local metaplastic concept is the occasional finding of a loose, myxomatous tissue within the ganglion that sometimes assumes an epithelial appearance suggesting differentiation toward the cuboidal cells of the synovia.

MISCELLANEOUS LESIONS

BURSITIS

Bursitis is an inflammation of a bursa. While we may so define the lesion, there is considerable dispute as to the exact nature of the bursa. Standard textbooks of anatomy describe numerous cystic spaces between joints and supporting ligaments and tendon sheaths that are presumed to act as gliding surfaces facilitating the mobility of these supporting ligaments over the adjacent bony prominences. Despite these well ordered descriptions, there is some doubt that bursae are present in the normal individual. According to this view, they arise as pathologic alterations in connective tissue in response to the constant mobility of the connective tissue at sites of pressure. A bursa then may be a pathologic lesion from the outset but, unless further complicated by superimposed inflammation, does not cause symptoms. It is to these further complications that our present interest is directed.

Bursitis tends to be more common in males than in females, perhaps because of greater physical activity. These lesions are most often encountered in the subdeltoid bursa of the shoulder, the olecranon bursa of the elbow, the prepatellar bursa and the radio-humeral bursa of the lateral radial head.

The cause of bursitis is unknown. Trauma is believed to play an important role but whether this acts as an initiating influence or a precipitating factor is still unclear. Bacterial invasion may be responsible for occasional flare-ups but, in the majority of instances, the aspirated fluid is sterile. Most often, no precise initiating influence can be identified except possibly a history of excessive exercise.

In the early acute stages of the inflammatory condition, the bursa is distended with a watery or

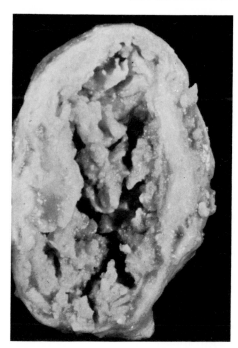

Figure 31–37. Chronic bursitis on cross section to show the markedly thickened wall and shaggy, trabeculated interior.

mucoid fluid. As the chronic stage is reached, the stage at which the lesion is usually excised, the bursal space is filled with a granular, brown, inspissated changed blood heavily admixed with gritty calcific precipitations. The wall is thick, tough and fibrous and is often pigmented by the contained hemorrhage and hardened by calcification. The inner surface is usually shaggy and trabeculated, and often thick, fibrous bridging cords traverse the inner space (Fig. 31–37).

Histologically, the walls are composed of dense, fibrous tissue focally infiltrated by lymphocytes, plasma cells and macrophages. The lining of the bursa is usually composed of granulation tissue or precipitated fibrin. Characteristically, there is marked focal vascularization of the wall of the cyst that often produces small hemangiomatoid collections of capillary channels. Basophilic calcium deposits may be found trapped within the fibrinous lining material and within the wall.

These conditions are more painful than serious and presently are treated by supportive measures, the local instillation of cortisone or similar steroids and, in the calcific stages, by surgical excision.

TENOSYNOVITIS

Tenosynovitis denotes an inflammation of the tendon sheaths and contained tendons. This condition is most often encountered in persons who place great stress upon certain tendons in the course of their occupation. Thus, tenosynovitis is most often encountered in the upper extremities of laborers and artisans, and in the wrists and hands of stenographers. On the basis of this clinical distribution, trauma is believed to play an important role. However, occasionally tenosynovitis may be caused by direct bacterial seeding.

Several anatomic forms of this inflammation are produced by these various causations. *Traumatic synovitis* consists of the accumulation of synovial fluid and fibrin within a tendon sheath. The fibrin may cause a grating sound on motion and may also, in time, become organized to produce fibrous adhesions. Direct bacterial invasion gives rise to a *suppurative tenosynovitis.* The most common offending organisms are the pyogens. Such pyogenic infection may also be initiated by penetrating injuries, as when a surgeon accidentally punctures a tendon sheath in the course of placing sutures. *Tuberculous tenosynovitis* is a very uncommon pattern that usually represents a hematogenous focus of seeding but may occur by direct inoculation of infective material through the skin. These tuberculous infections are characterized by the development of small granulomas on the synovial lining that often protrude and are sloughed off into the fluid of the tendon sheath to produce the characteristic *"rice bodies."* These conditions are extremely painful on motion and cause some disability because of this pain. Adequate rest and other supportive measures usually promote healing. However, sometimes residual fibrous adhesions limit, to some extent, the movement of the tendon. In time, these adhesions usually stretch sufficiently to restore function.

NODULAR FASCIITIS

This is an uncommon but very distinctive tumorous nodule that occurs in any part of the body, principally in the subcutaneous fat and fascia, but may also arise in the deep fascia and contiguous muscle. The major importance of this lesion can be deduced from another of its designations, *"subcutaneous pseudosarcomatous fasciitis."* This lesion is actually a curious, localized overgrowth of fibroblasts that appear to infiltrate. It is therefore apt to be mistaken for a sarcoma. In the words of Price et al. (1961), "the unwary, however, seeing a moderately or highly cellular nodule composed of plump or spindle-shaped connective tissue cells, with nuclei that are often hyperchromatic or in mitosis, lacking a capsule, and sometimes seeming to infiltrate adjacent fat or muscle and to surround nerves and blood vessels is apt to confuse the lesion with a sarcoma." These subcutaneous nodules rarely exceed 3 to 4 cm. in diameter, are obviously infiltrative and often bound to the fascial planes and have a firm, gray to pink, hard cut surface.

Histologically, the distinctive features include a nodular proliferation of plump to spindled fibroblasts without definite encapsulation. Of considerable importance in the differential diagnosis are the features of an inflammatory response in the form of well developed, newly formed blood vessels and an accompanying infiltrate of lymphocytes and other mononuclear cells. Multinucleate giant cells are also present in about half the lesions. Some are obviously foreign body type; others having fewer nuclei are more suggestive of malignant tumor giant cells. The additional presence of mitoses further heightens the similarity to a low-grade fibrosarcoma. One of the useful distinctive features is the tendency for the older, more central regions of the lesion to become collagenized while the more actively growing periphery remains cellular. These lesions have all been successfully treated by local excision, and no recurrences have been reported. It might well be that they would spontaneously collagenize if left alone.

CHORDOMA

These rare neoplasms are presumed to arise from notochordal remnants or rests. Approximately 90 per cent occur in the basisphenoidal or sacrococcygeal areas, but they may also arise from any point along the vertebral column. They usually grow as soft, gray, gelatinous masses that are locally active and slowly invasive. Only infrequently do they metastasize. The range of histologic patterns of these neoplasms encompasses the various stages of embryonic development of the notochord, i.e., spindle cell tumors resembling fibrosarcomas to more classic patterns consisting of large, plump, epithelium-like cells arranged in clusters or sheets. Intra- and extracellular mucus is present to some extent in all forms, but is particularly dominant in the epithelium-like pattern. The intracellular vacuoles often compress the cytoplasm into narrow strands producing distinctive spider web or grapefruit-like trabeculations between the vacuoles (the physaliphorous cell). The extracellular mucus may be so abundant as to create lakes of secretion in which the neoplastic cells float.

REFERENCES

Albright, F., et al.: Syndrome characterized by osteitis fibrosa disseminata, areas of pigmentation and endocrine dysfunction with precocious puberty in females. New Eng. J. Med., 216:725, 1937.

Al-Sarraf, M.: Malignant granular cell tumor. Arch. Path., 91:550, 1971.

Ariel, I. M., and Pack, G. T.: Synovial sarcoma. Review of 25 cases. New Eng. J. Med., 268:1272, 1963.

Arnstein, A. R., et al.: Recent progress in osteomalacia and rickets. Ann. Intern. Med., 67:1296, 1967.

Bangle, R.: A morphological and histochemical study of the granular-cell myoblastoma. Cancer, 5:950, 1952.

Barnett, E. V., et al.: Search for infectious agents in rheumatoid arthritis. Arthritis Rheum., 9:720, 1966.

Bassett, C.A.L.: Biologic significance of piezoelectricity. Calcif. Tissue Res., 1:252, 1968.

Benedict, P. H.: Endocrine features in Albright's syndrome (fibrous dysplasia of bone). Metabolism, 11:30, 1962.

Berman, B.: Pulmonary hypertrophic osteoarthropathy. Arch. Intern. Med., 112:947, 1963.

Beutner, E. H., et al.: Studies on autoantibodies in myasthenia gravis. J.A.M.A., 182:46, 1962.

Bland, J. H.: Rheumatoid arthritis. Med. Clin. N. Amer., 52:477, 1968.

Bollet, A. J.: An essay on the biology of osteoarthritis. Arthritis Rheum., 12:152, 1969.

Bollet, A. J., and Nance, J. L.: Biochemical findings in normal and osteoarthritic articular cartilage. II. Chondroitin sulfate concentration and chain length, water and ash content. J. Clin. Invest., 45:1170, 1966.

Castleman, B., and Norris, E. H.: The pathology of the thymus in myasthenia gravis. Medicine, 25:27, 1949.

Clinical Staff Conference (NIH): Neoplastic plasma cells. Ann. Intern. Med., 58:1073, 1963.

Coventry, M. B., and Dahlin, D. C.: Osteogenic sarcoma: a critical analysis of 430 cases. J. Bone Joint Surg., 39A:741, 1957.

Dahlin, D. C., et al.: Giant cell tumor. A study of 195 cases. Cancer, 25:1061, 1970.

Dent, C. E.: Rickets (and osteomalacia), nutritional and metabolic (1919–1969). Proc. Roy. Soc. Med., 63:401, 1970.

Duthie, J.J.R., and Alexander, W.R.M. (eds.): Rheumatic Diseases. Baltimore, Williams and Wilkins Co., 1968.

Engel, A., and Burch, T.: Chronic arthritis in the United States. Health Examination Survey, Arthritis Rheum., 10:61, 1967.

Engel, W. K.: Muscle biopsy. Clin. Orthop., 39:80, 1965.

Ewing, J.: A review of the classification of bone tumors. Surg. Gynec. Obstet., 68:971, 1939.

Falk, L., and Alpert, M.: The chemical and roentgen aspects of Ewing's sarcoma. Amer. J. Med. Sci., 250:492, 1965.

Follis, R. H., Jr.: Osteogenesis imperfecta congenita: a connective tissue diathesis. J. Pediat., 41:713, 1952.

Foote, F. W., Jr., and Anderson, R. H.: Histogenesis of Ewing's tumor. Amer. J. Path., 17:497, 1941.

Freydinger, S. E., et al.: Sarcoma complicating Paget's disease of bone. Arch. Path., 75:496, 1963.

Friedman, B., and Gold, H.: Ultrastructure of Ewing's sarcoma of bone. Cancer, 2:307, 1968.

Garn, S. M., et al.: Bone loss as a general phenomenon in man. Fed. Proc., 26:1729, 1967.

Ginsburg, J., and Brown, J. B.: Increased estrogen excretion and hypertrophic pulmonary osteoarthropathy. Lancet, 2:1274, 1961.

Glimcher, M. J.: Molecular biology of mineralized tissues with particular reference to bone. Rev. Mod. Phys., 31:359, 1959.

Glimcher, M. J., and Krane, S. M.: Organization and structure of bone and mechanism of calcification. In Ramachandran, G. N., and Gould, B. S. (eds.): Treatise on Collagen. Vol. 2, part B. London, Academic Press, 1968, p. 68.

Goldenberg, R. R., et al.: Giant cell tumor of bone. An analysis of 218 cases. J. Bone Joint Surg., 52A:619, 1970.

Goldstein, G.: Hypophysis, thymitis and myasthenia gravis. Lancet, 2:1164, 1966.

Goldstein, G.: Myasthenia gravis and the thymus. Ann. Rev. Med., 22:119, 1971.

Green, W. T., and Shannon, J. G.: Osteomyelitis of infants. A disease different from osteomyelitis of older children. Arch. Surg., 32:462, 1936.

Grimley, T. M.: Rheumatoid arthritis. Ultrastructure of the synovium. Editorial. Ann. Intern. Med., 66:623, 1967.

Haagensen, C. D., and Stout, A. P.: Synovial sarcoma. Ann. Surg., 120:826, 1944.

Hamerman, D.: Views on the pathogenesis of rheumatoid arthritis. Med. Clin. N. Amer., 5:593, 1968.

Hammarsten, J. F., and O'Leary, J.: The features and significance of hypertrophic osteoarthopathy. Arch. Intern. Med., 99:431, 1957.

Harris, W. H., and Heaney, R. P.: Skeletal renewal and metabolic bone disease. New Eng. J. Med., 280:193, 253, 303, 1969.

Huvos, A. G., et al.: Bone sarcomas arising in fibrous dysplasia. J. Bone Joint Surg., 54:1047, 1972.

Huxley, H. E.: The double array of filaments in cross-striated muscle. J. Biophys. Biochem. Cytol., 3:631, 1957.

Huxley, H. E.: Electron microscope studies on the structure of natural and synthetic protein filaments from striated muscle. J. Molec. Biol., 7:281, 1963.

Huxley, H. E.: Recent x-ray diffraction and electron microscope studies of striated muscle. In The Contractile Process, Proceedings of a Symposium of the New York Heart Association. Boston, Little, Brown and Co., 1967, p. 71.

Huxley, H. E.: Structural evidence concerning the mechanism of contraction in striated muscle. In Paul, W. M., Daniel, E. E., Kay, C. M., and Monckton G. (eds.): Muscle. Oxford, Pergammon Press, Ltd., 1965, p. 3.

Ibsen, K. H.: Distinct varieties of osteogenesis imperfecta. Clin. Orthop., 50:279, 1967.

Iverson, L.: Thymoma: a review and reclassification. Amer. J. Path., 32:695, 1956.

Jaffe, H. L., and Lichtenstein, L.: Chondromyxoid fibroma of bone: a distinctive benign tumor likely to be mistaken especially for chondrosarcoma. Arch. Path., 45:541, 1948.

Jaffe, H. L., and Lichtenstein, L.: Osteoid osteoma: further experience with this benign tumor of bone. J. Bone Joint Surg., 22:645, 1940.

Jaffe, H. L., et al.: Giant cell tumor of bone: its pathologic appearance, grading, supposed variants and treatment. Arch. Path., 30:993, 1940.

Johnston, C. C., Jr., et al.: Osteopetrosis: a clinical, genetic, metabolic and morphological study of the dominantly inherited benign form. Medicine, 47:149, 1968.

Keefer, C. S., et al.: Histologic changes in the knee joint in various infections. Arch. Path., 18:199, 1934.

Lichtenstein, L.: Bone Tumors. 4th Ed. St. Louis, C. V. Mosby Co., 1972, p. 235.

Lichtenstein, L., and Jaffe, H. L.: Multiple myeloma: a survey based on 35 cases, 18 of which came to autopsy. Arch. Path., 44:207, 1947.

Lichtenstein, L., and Kaplan, L.: Benign chondroblastoma of bone, unusual localization in femoral capital epiphysis. Cancer, 2:793, 1949.

Little, J. R., and Loeb, V., Jr.: Immunoglobulin abnormalities and current status of treatment of multiple myeloma. J.A.M.A., 208:1688, 1969.

Lutwak, L.: Symposium on osteoporosis, nutritional aspects of osteoporosis. J. Amer. Geriat. Soc., 17:115, 1969.

Martel, W., et al.: Pulmonary and pleural lesions in rheumatoid disease. Radiology, 90:641, 1968.

McCormack, L. J., et al.: Ewing's sarcoma. Cancer, 5:85, 1952.

McGrath, P. J.: Giant cell tumor of bone. An analysis of 52 cases. J. Bone Joint Surg. (Brit.), 54:216, 1972.

McKenna, R. J., et al.: Sarcomata of the osteogenic series (osteosarcoma, fibrosarcoma, chondrosarcoma, parosteal osteogenic sarcoma and sarcoma arising in normal bones). An analysis of 552 cases. J. Bone Joint Surg., 48:1, 1966.

McLean, F. C.: The ultrastructure and function of bone. Science, 127:451, 1958.

Murphy, W. R., and Ackerman, L. D.: Benign and malignant giant cell tumors of bone: clinical-pathological evaluation of 31 cases. Cancer, 9:317, 1956.

Nelson, D. A., and Benson, E. S.: On the structural continuities of the transverse tubular system of rabbit and human myocardial cells. J. Cell. Biol., 16:297, 1963.

O'Brien, W. M.: The genetics of rheumatoid arthritis. Clin. Exp. Immun., Suppl., 2:785, 1967.

O'Neal, L. W., and Ackerman, L. V.: Chondrosarcoma of bone. Cancer, 5:551, 1952.

Osserman, E. F.: Plasma cell myeloma. Clinical aspects. New Eng. J. Med., 261:952, 1006, 1959.

Parker, F., et al.: Histologic changes in the knee joint with advancing age. Arch. Path., 17:516, 1934.

Patch, D. W., et al.: Osteoid osteoma. Cleveland Clin. Quart., 21:123, 1954.

Pollak, V. E., et al.: Chronic renal disease with secondary hyperparathyroidism. Arch. Intern. Med., 103:200, 1959.

Porretta, C. A., et al.: Sarcoma in Paget's disease of bone. J. Bone Joint Surg., 39A:1314, 1957.

Price, E. B., Jr., et al.: Nodular fasciitis: a clinicopathologic analysis of 65 cases. Amer. J. Clin. Path., 35:122, 1961.

Rawson, A. J., et al.: Studies on the pathogenesis of rheumatoid joint inflammations. II. Intracytoplasmic particulate complexes in rheumatoid synovial fluid. Ann. Intern. Med., 62:281, 1965.

Reifenstein, E. C., Jr., and Albright, F.: Paget's disease: its pathologic physiology and the importance of this in the complications arising from fracture and immobilization. New Eng. J. Med., 231:343, 1944.

Roberts, W. C., et al.: Cardiac valvular lesions in rheumatoid arthritis. Arch. Intern. Med., 122:141, 1968.

Rosenkrantz, J. A., et al.: Paget's disease (osteitis deformans). Arch. Intern. Med., 90:610, 1952.

Rowland, L. P.: Muscular dystrophies. D. M., November 1, 1972.

Sandow, A.: Excitation-contraction coupling in skeletal muscles. Pharmacol. Rev., 17:265, 1965.

Schlumberger, H. G.: Fibrous dysplasia of single bones (monostotic fibrous dysplasia). Milit. Surg., 99:504, 1946.

Schwartz, B. T., and Alpert, M.: The malignant transformation of fibrous dysplasia. Amer. J. Med. Sci., 247:350, 1964.

Seybold, W. D., et al.: Tumors of the thymus. J. Thorac. Surg., 20:195, 1950.

Skorneck, A. B., and Ginsburg, L. B.: Pulmonary hypertrophic osteoarthropathy (periostitis). Its absence in pulmonary tuberculosis. New Eng. J. Med., 258:1079, 1958.

Skosey, J. L.: Some basic aspects of bone metabolism in relation to osteoporosis. Med. Clin. N. Amer., 54:141, 1970.

Smith, D. S.: Organization and function of the sarcoplasmic reticulum and T-system of muscle cells. Progr. Biophys., 16:109, 1966.

Sobel, H. J., et al.: Granular cell myoblastoma Amer. J. Path., 65:59, 1971.

Strauss, A. J. L.: Myasthenia gravis, autoimmunity and the thymus. Advances Intern. Med., 14:241, 1968.

Thomas, L.: Experimental mycoplasmic infections as models of rheumatoid arthritis. Fed. Proc., 32:143, 1973.

Thomas, T. V.: Thymus and myasthenia gravis. Ann. Thor. Surg., 13:499, 1972.

Tursi, A., et al.: An immunofluorescence mixed staining technique for the detection of IgG-rheumatoid factor and IgG-beta-1C complexes in tissues. Clin. Exp. Immun., 6:767, 1970.

Van Horn, P. E., Jr., et al.: Fibrous dysplasia: a clinical-pathologic study of orthopedic surgical cases. Proc. Staff Meet. Mayo Clin., 38:175, 1963.

Vetters, J. M.: Muscle antibodies in myasthenia gravis. Immunology, 13:275, 1967.

Warren, S. L., et al.: An active agent from human rheumatoid arthritis which is transmissible in mice: preliminary report. Arch. Intern. Med., 124:629, 1969.

Weinfeld, M. S., and Dudley, R. H., Jr.: Osteogenic sarcoma. A follow-up study of 94 cases observed at the Massachusetts General Hospital from 1920 to 1960. J. Bone Joint Surg., 44A:269, 1962.

Weissmann, G.: Lysosomes and joint disease. Arthritis Rheum., 9:834, 1966.

Winn, E.: Osteoporosis, osteomalacia, and osteitis fibrosa cystica with special reference to the parathyroid and calcium metabolism. Amer. Pract. Dig. Treatm., 2:921, 1951.

Ziff, M.: Pathophysiology of rheumatoid arthritis. Fed. Proc., 32:131, 1973.

32

THE NERVOUS SYSTEM

JOSEPH M. FOLEY, M.D.*

---

*Professor of Neurology, Case Western Reserve University School of Medicine.

NORMAL CELLS AND THEIR BASIC REACTIONS

All the organs and systems of the body have their own special pathology. The pathology of the nervous system is especially complex for many reasons, the most compelling of which is the anatomic variability of the nervous structures. The brain and spinal cord do not have the relative homogeneity of the liver or the kidneys or the spleen. The student who undertakes the study of a neurologic disorder is confronted not only with the problem of the tissue reaction but also with the problem of location of the tissue reaction in the organ which is his object of study. A tumor of lung, for example, can produce a limited number of symptoms whatever its location in lung. But a tumor of the central nervous system can produce any one or several of an almost indefinite number of symptoms and signs ranging from loss of smell at one end to loss of sphincter control at the other. The study of nervous disease, therefore, requires a knowledge of neuroanatomy. A textbook of pathology cannot attempt to review anatomy in all its detail, and so the student is urged to preface his approach to neuropathology with a review of neuroanatomy, and to revert constantly to his anatomic text while he pursues the study of the disease processes which affect the nervous system.

The histology of nervous tissue also presents a special problem, for although tissue reactions in the nervous system can be analogized with those elsewhere, there are fundamental differences in structure and function that must be understood if the analogies are to be useful (Greenfield, 1958).

THE NEURON

The nerve cell consists of a cell body, a number of smaller processes called dendrites and a larger process called an axis cylinder or axon. There is an enormous variation in size and shape within the range of normal. The most dramatic example of such a difference is in the length of the axis cylinder. Certain large cells in the cerebral cortex, the giant Betz cells in area 4 of the frontal lobe, send axons to the lumbosacral spinal cord, and anterior horn cells of the lumbosacral cord send axons to the feet. At the other extreme, some neurons may have axis cylinders not much longer than the diameter of their cell bodies.

The classic representation of the cell body is a polyhedral structure with a well defined nucleus enclosing a large nucleolus. With chromatic stains such as hematoxylin and eosin, or the basic aniline dyes such as cresyl violet, thionine or toluidine blue, the cytoplasm is represented as containing chunks of material referred to variously as Nissl substance, Nissl bodies, tigroid substance, tigroid bodies or chromidial substance. This material is the endoplasmic reticulum of the nerve cell. When impregnated with reduced silver, the cytoplasm is seen to contain a set of streaming argentophilic fibers which are called neurofibrils, and no Nissl substance is seen. Neurofibrils are found only in nerve cells. They consist of neurofilaments and microtubules. In addition, the nerve cell contains a Golgi apparatus and the mitochondria, lysosomes and inclusions common to other cells.

This traditional diagram of the large cell with well defined Nissl substance in an abundant cytoplasm is a satisfactory representation of only a few of the nerve cells in the central nervous system. The exceptions are too numerous to itemize, but in general there is an enormous variation in size and shape of cell bodies. Some cell bodies are not much larger than astrocyte nuclei and may have no discernible Nissl substance at ordinary magnification with the light microscope. Other nerve cell bodies, such as those in the mesencephalic nucleus of the fifth nerve, are round, and the cytoplasm contains no discrete Nissl bodies but rather a powdery chromatin substance. Some cells, such as those in the locus ceruleus or the substantia nigra, contain black-brown pigment in the cytoplasm. These normal variations in the appearance of the cell body must be kept in mind constantly. When there is doubt about whether a given cell or group of cells is abnormal, it should be compared with the same area and the same stain in a normal brain.

The reactive capacity of the nerve cell in the presence of disease is a limited one. The reaction of the cell body itself generally is seen best in stains such as the Nissl method or hematoxylin and eosin. Injury and repair of the axis cylinder requires study by a silver method, such as the Bodian protargol technique.

In this section we shall be concerned with those morphologic changes which occur in the cell body. The terminology of these various changes in nerve cells (and in glia as well) may seem extremely confusing, but it creates an impression of greater complexity than exists in fact. The student must be warned against regarding the changes described as being radically different from the reactions of cells in other systems and organs.

Axonal Reaction. This is the name applied to that sequence of events which appears in the cell body when its axon is cut or damaged. The axon and covering myelin distal to the lesion ultimately degenerate and, if in the peripheral nervous system, regenerate. In the cell body a change is visible within 24 to 48 hours. It swells slightly and in the perinuclear area the Nissl substance begins to break up. As time goes on, the swelling increases, the cell body loses any angularity it had, the Nissl substance undergoes a progressive peripheral disintegration and the nucleus is displaced to the periphery of the cell (Fig. 32–1, 32–2 and 32–3). This process reaches its maximum at 12 days, and by this time the cytoplasm of the cell has a groundglass appearance except at the very periphery where a few Nissl granules still remain. When the damaged axon is capable of regeneration, as in the peripheral nervous system, there is reconstitution of the cell body to its normal appearance. However, in the central nervous system, especially if the point of section is close to the cell body, there may be no reconstitution of the cell and, in some instances, it may degenerate and disappear completely. The details of axonal reaction differ in various cells of the nervous system, but the general features apply to all.

Whereas the axonal reaction, a retrograde cell change, is an indirect effect, there are many processes which injure the cell body directly. These may be very acute, as in necrosis of infarction, or very chronic, as in a degenerative process like amyotrophic lateral sclerosis, or anywhere between these extremes.

Acute Types of Nerve Cell Change. When the process is acute, the first manifestation is loss of function without any morphologic change as seen by light microscopy. At this stage, the nerve cell is in a state of crisis. Recovery of function may occur with or without any structural change, or the cell may die. The resolution of the crisis in one or the other direction depends upon the intensity and duration of the offending agent. If death occurs in a matter of minutes (as in asphyxiation) or a few hours (as in circulatory collapse), no morphologic changes will be present, even though the cells may have been damaged beyond any possibility of recovery. *The first change visible by light microscopy requires a minimum of 6 to 12 hours of survival.* The cell becomes swollen and any angularity is rounded off. There is dissolution of Nissl substance, and the nucleus swells and is displaced toward the periphery. Such a change is often indistinguishable from an axonal reaction, and probably such a cell is still viable. The next stage is one of hyperchromatism in which the cytoplasm of the cell stains more darkly with the basic dyes, and in which there is some loss of clarity of nuclear structure. The proximal portions of the processes of such a cell may stand out distinctly even without cell stains. Such an appearance probably means a dead cell. The next stage is one of vacuolation and irregular disintegration of the cytoplasmic and nuclear membrane. This is clearly a dead cell, ready for dissolution and phagocytosis.

Another important kind of acute cell change is referred to as "ischemic" because it is seen classically in ischemic disease. This cell is shrunken, its angularity is intensified and the processes stand out prominently and tortuously with cell stains. The nucleus is shriveled, pyknotic and densely basophilic, the nucleolus is no longer distinguishable, and the cytoplasm takes a homogeneous deep basophilia with the Nissl stain or a homogeneous bright eosinophilia with hematoxylin and eosin. This, too, is a dead cell.

Chronic Types of Cell Change. Chronic affection of the cell body is difficult to assess in many cases. Generally, however, the picture is one of cellular atrophy, with reduction in cell size, hyperchromatism of both the cytoplasm and nucleus, and irregularity of the cytoplasmic and nuclear envelopes. By electron microscopy, characteristic and sometimes specific alterations occur in the organelles in all disease states.

In such acute and chronic affections of the nerve cell, there are parallel changes of varying degrees in the glia and the blood vessels. Although there is always an early stage in which such glial and vascular response may be absent, it is a worthwhile rule that *any change in a nerve cell should be viewed with suspicion unless there is evidence of some glial and vascular response.*

Miscellaneous Cell Changes. Some changes in nerve cell bodies do not fit into the categories as given. Occasionally on the edge of a vascular or traumatic lesion, one may see mineralized nerve cells. These are dead cells which for some reason have not undergone phagocytosis and have adsorbed calcium and iron onto their surfaces, becoming in a sense the fossil remains of an old lesion. In the gangliosidoses, there is an abnormal accumulation of lipoid material in the cell cytoplasm. In Alzheimer's disease, appropriate staining with silver techniques demonstrates a tangled, conglutinated arrangement of the neurofibrillar apparatus. In rabies and other viral diseases, inclusion bodies are found within the cytoplasm.

Lipofuscin, or lipochrome, is a lipoidal substance which accumulates within the cytoplasm of many nerve cells. It is more striking as

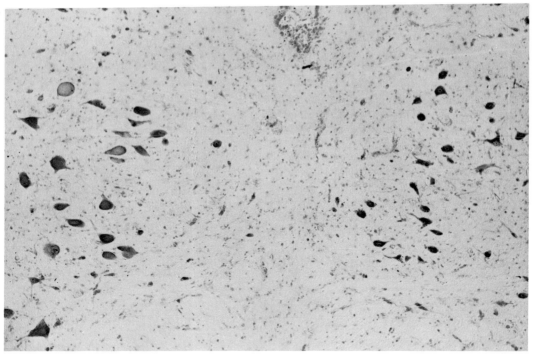

Fig. 32-1

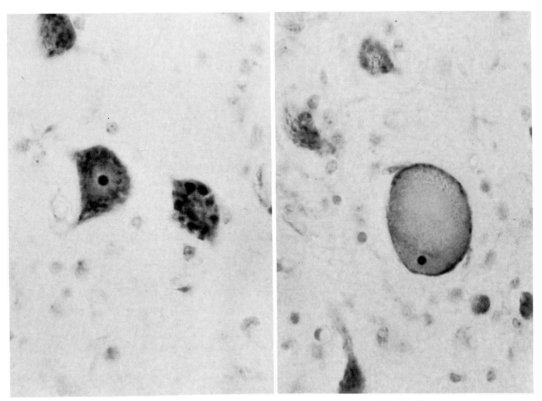

Fig. 32-2

Fig. 32-3

Figure 32-1. *The large motor cells of each hypoglossal nucleus can be seen beneath the floor of the fourth ventricle. Because the twelfth nerve on the left had been cut, there is axonal reaction in the cells of the left side.*

Figure 32-2. *Normal cells from the right hypoglossal nucleus. Cresyl violet stain.*

Figure 32-3. *Axonal reaction in a cell of the left hypoglossal nucleus. Cresyl violet stain.*

age advances. Its chemical nature and its significance are poorly understood, but it is clear that even large quantities may be present in nerve cells without any loss of function. It can be seen by almost any staining method. In the usual cell stains, it presents a granular green or yellow or golden brown accumulation in the cytoplasm.

GLIA

The brain has specialized interstitial cells called glia which subserve certain functions in a supportive, reparative and metabolic capacity. The participation of glia in injury and repair does not exclude the participation of those other elements which operate in the rest of the body. Polymorphonuclear leukocytes, lymphocytes, plasma cells, macrophages and blood vessels have the same role in disease of the nervous system that they have elsewhere. Fibroblasts take no part in the repair of small damage, the network of astrocytes preventing their access to the nervous system. When the astrocytes are destroyed, fibroblasts from the blood vessels or meninges enter the scar.

In reaction to injury, the glia are the special elements of the nervous system. There are three kinds of glial cells. Astroglia (astrocytes) and oligodendroglia (oligodendrocytes) are of ectodermal origin, while microglia are of mesodermal origin.

Astroglia. Astroglia are recognizable in cell stains as rounded or oval nuclei, containing no nucleolus, only a sparse chromatin network, and sometimes a distinct chromatin body called a centrosome. The nucleus is slightly smaller than the nuclei of the larger nerve cells. The processes of astrocytes are visible in chromatic stains, especially in pathologic states, but they are better studied in preparations stained with the gold chloride method of Cajal. On the basis of their processes, astrocytes are either protoplasmic or fibrous. The protoplasmic astrocyte is present only in gray matter; it has relatively short and stubby processes which present a "mossy" appearance and have multiple branchings. The fibrous astrocyte is present in both white and gray matter, although more obvious in white matter, has longer and more sinuous processes and fewer branchings than the protoplasmic astrocyte. In both types of astrocyte, the processes terminate by foot-like extensions upon blood vessels, providing thus an astrovascular supporting framework. The vascular membrane on which the processes terminate is an inward extension of pia about the penetrating blood vessels and so the resultant complex is referred to as the *pia-glial membrane*. It is probably distinct from the true adventitia of the vessel, and the potential space between adventitia and pia-glial membrane is the *Virchow-Robin space*, actually a continuation of the subarachnoid space. The Virchow-Robin space is the site of many perivascular inflammatory reactions.

The reactive capacity of the astrocyte in disease is a function of the duration, the intensity and the quality of the offending agent. Although the astrocyte is less vulnerable to hypoxia than the neuron, it is by no means immune. Sufficient hypoxia may destroy neuron and astrocyte alike; a lesser change will damage only the neurons. Although the astrocyte is never unaffected by nearby disease, it can be remarkably indolent in the presence of secondary degeneration, as when a tract is degenerating after section. The older authors believed that protoplasmic astrocytes underwent transformation to fibrous astrocytes before processes could be produced to form a scar. There is no good proof for this. It is likely that the two cells react to different stimuli—the protoplasmic to toxic and metabolic derangements, the fibrous to those forces which produce discontinuity of tissue or loss of parenchyma.

The terminology of reaction in astrocytes is, if possible, more confusing than that in neurons. Most of this confusion is terminologic, for the facts are relatively simple. When either kind of astrocyte receives a lethal blow from any cause, the cell body swells, the processes fragment and the cell disintegrates and undergoes phagocytosis. When the fibrous astrocyte is capable of effective response, it produces fibers (Fig. 32–4). The cell body swells, the processes elongate, the cell divides amitotically and glial fibers, still attached to their cell bodies, are laid down. This process can be studied very satisfactorily in ordinary cell stains, but the fibers themselves are selectively visualized in such methods as Mallory's phosphotungstic acid hematoxylin. The cell body of the reactive astrocyte may be massive in size with a huge area of distended cytoplasm, on one side of which lies a compressed nucleus. When the lesion is extensive or when it is accompanied by liquefaction, the astrocytes are inadequate for the task, and in this case the fibroblasts enter to aid in the process of restoring supportive integrity. Often, as at the edge of an abscess, the two elements can be found working together, collagen fibers and astrocyte fibers intermingling.

The protoplasmic astrocyte responds by enlargement and division, most obvious in the nucleus. Its fibers are very difficult to stain with the usual methods satisfactory for the fibrous astrocyte.

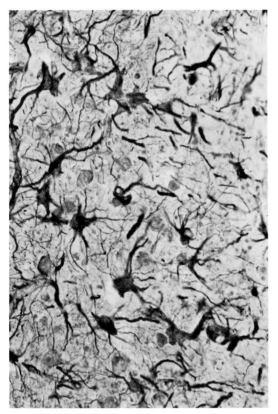

Figure 32–4. *Astrocytes in the wall of a puncture wound in brain. (Cajal gold sublimate stain.)*

Oligodendroglia. Oligodendroglia, like astroglia, arise from neuroectoderm. They are seen in chromatic stains as rounded nuclei containing rather dense clumps of chromatin, and this feature together with their smaller size distinguishes them from astroglia. With silver methods, their cytoplasm is seen as a small crescentic area about the nucleus. Their processes are short and few. They have no vascular attachments. They are found in two locations. First, they are present as satellites about nerve cells, where it is presumed they serve a function relating to fluid and respiratory exchange or to excitability of the cell. They seem to increase in number about a damaged nerve cell, a phenomenon called *satellitosis.* Interfascicular oligodendroglia are found in long streaming rows in white matter, where the myelin sheath can be regarded as a specialized part of the cytoplasm of the cell. There is some evidence that these interfascicular oligodendroglia represent the central equivalent of the Schwann cell.

Oligodendroglia swell with great facility in response to almost any kind of toxic or metabolic change, and such swelling has been regarded as the most sensitive indicator of disease of the nervous system. But this very high sensitivity to almost any stimulus is what makes swelling of oligodendroglia an almost valueless sign in pathologic study. A curious appearance of the nerve cell may result when the satellite oligodendroglia swell. Since the cytoplasm does not stain with cell stains, and yet indents the semifluid neuron, it appears as if rounded bites had been taken out of the nerve cell. This is erroneously referred to as *"neuronophagia."*

Microglia. Microglia, unlike astroglia and oligodendroglia, are derived from mesoderm (Koenigsmark and Sidman, 1963). In chromatic stains, they are seen as small, elongated or crescentic nuclei, about the same size as the nucleus of a capillary endothelial cell, with which they are sometimes confused. There is relatively dense chromatin in the microglia nucleus, less dense than in the oligodendroglia, more so than in the astrocyte. By silver stains, they are seen as small elongated or narrow bodies with many short spiny processes which branch frequently and at right angles.

The microglia are to be regarded as histiocytes, and therefore as part of the reticuloendothelial system. Their principal function appears to be that of phagocytosis, and when the removal of debris is to be undertaken, they become rounded, retract their processes, increase their cytoplasm and behave in the same way as histiocytic macrophages anywhere in the body. These resting cells, the microglia, are not the only source for macrophages. When the task is large enough, they are aided by other macrophages which stream into the area from blood vessels. They are frequently the dominant cell in the reaction. Macrophages, once mobilized, may remain in the area for a long time. It is not unusual to find them in an area of cystic infarction or old trauma several years after the episode.

In more chronic and indolent processes and especially in paretic neurosyphilis, the microglia increase in number, become elongated and have deposits of iron in their cytoplasm. In this form they are known as "rod cells."

Ependymal cells are neuroglia which line the ventricles and the central canal of the spinal cord.

The metabolic functions of the glial cells have been studied extensively. Although uncertainty and controversy continue in these studies, it is reasonably clear that the neuroglia act in part as an extracellular compartment for the nerve cells, for the true extracellular space of the nervous system is much less than for other organs. Yet the brain does have some interstitial space, and passage of material into glia and neurons is from this space, not directly from the plasma.

Synapses. Not subject to adequate study by light microscopy, the synaptic connections of nerve cells and their processes have been clarified greatly by the electron microscope. Clinically important changes, of both function and structure, take place at these sites and represent a new chapter in the understanding of neurologic disease.

The foregoing account of the neurons and the glia is concerned with their appearance in chromatic stains and obviously omits many of the important elements of nervous tissue. Especially neglected is the complex of intertwining and interconnected fibers collectively called the neuropil. Studies of ultrastructure in recent years have demonstrated that there is a complexity of connections even greater than that proposed by the most imaginative anatomists of past generations.

PATHOLOGY

The present chapter illustrates the general principles of interaction between disease and the nervous system. Large gaps, obvious even to the beginner, are due to the restrictions of space; others, to our lack of knowledge about some disease states. Some very rare diseases may seem to get undue attention, but they are included because they may contribute to the understanding of other disease states.

The diseased nervous system does not lend itself as easily as other systems to capsule descriptions of disease. This chapter should be used in conjunction with a clinical text or, better still, in conjunction with repeated and detailed clinical observations of patients with neurologic disorders.

INCREASED INTRACRANIAL PRESSURE

The rigid case of the skull and the dura protects the brain from injury, but sometimes in disease it becomes a liability. Increased intracranial pressure results whenever the volume of the intracranial contents increases beyond the slight leeway allowed for expansion. The causes of such increase in pressure are many and varied. Epidural and subdural hematomas, leptomeningitis with obstruction of outflow of fluid from the ventricles, bleed-

ing or infarct in brain substance, tumors or abscesses of the brain or its coverings, dural sinus thrombosis, and diffuse cerebral edema, such as occurs in lead encephalopathy, are only a few of the conditions which lead to increased intracranial pressure. An understanding of the effects of increased intracranial pressure is therefore necessary to an understanding of a large area of neuropathology.

Papilledema is a noninflammatory swelling of the optic disc. Since the optic nerves are actually prolongations of the brain rather than true nerves, they are surrounded by columns of cerebrospinal fluid. When intracranial pressure is increased, this pressure is transmitted to this part of the cerebrospinal fluid reservoir as well as elsewhere. Stasis occurs in the region of the lamina cribrosa, and the vessels are compressed, producing swelling of the disc. When the pressure is so great or so sudden that there is interference with venous return from the eye, small hemorrhages appear in the retina adjacent to the disc. If the swelling of the nerve head is great enough or is present long enough, the nerve undergoes atrophy and the patient becomes blind.

Papilledema may be the only clinical manifestation of increased intracranial pressure. Headache is an effect not of the pressure per se but of distortion of the pain-sensitive dura and blood vessels. When increased intracranial pressure is relatively symmetrical, distortion does not take place. Vomiting usually signifies increased pressure in the posterior fossa.

Herniation of the brain consists of displacement from one dural compartment to another. The dura lines the inside of the skull and the spinal canal, but has two important extensions. The falx cerebri descends from the vault of the skull into the interhemispheric fissure, descending toward the corpus callosum. The tentorium extends inward from the back of the skull to separate the posterior fossa from the middle fossa. The incisura of the tentorium is the space which allows for easy passage of the brain stem. When things grow tight from increased pressure in one dural compartment, the result is displacement of part of the brain into another compartment. Such displacement means that the local adaptive mechanisms are no longer adequate for the degree of pressure attained.

When something has to yield in the posterior fossa because of pressure increase, one or both tonsils of the cerebellum herniate into the foramen magnum. If this happens suddenly, the medullary centers of respiration and circulation fail as a result of medullary compression, and death is almost instantaneous. Sometimes it happens gradually enough for the medulla to adjust, but even then the adjustment is so delicately balanced that catastrophe can occur at any time.

In asymmetrical pressure increases affecting the cerebral hemispheres, one cingulate gyrus may herniate under the falx cerebri across the midline (Fig. 32–5). The clinical correlation of such subfalcial herniation is not well worked out. Some patients become obtunded. In others, secondary effects referable to the mesial surface of the hemispheres occur as a result of displacement and distortion of the anterior cerebral arteries.

The most complex of the herniations, and the most common, is the displacement of the mesial portion of the temporal lobe through the incisura of the tentorium (Finney and Walker, 1962) (Fig. 32–5). This may be either unilateral or bilateral. Since the oculomotor nerve passes close to the herniating mass of temporal lobe, it is easily compressed, and there is then a transient period of ipsilateral pupillary constriction followed by persistent dilatation. Compression of the midbrain and upper pons by the mass of displaced tissue results in decerebration with loss of consciousness, and these effects are po-tentiated by hemorrhages and infarcts which appear in the midbrain and upper two-thirds of the pons (Fig. 32–5). They are probably due to the shearing force exerted on the perforating branches of the basilar artery when the brain stem is displaced downward while the extraparenchymal arterial trunks remain fixed. Compressions of the aqueduct of Sylvius may increase the pressure in the hemispheres by denying the normal channel of egress of the cerebrospinal fluid. The crowded state of affairs at the incisural opening results in compression of the contralateral cerebral peduncle against the free edge of the tentorium with resulting necrosis and hemiplegia ipsilateral to the side of the displaced temporal lobe. Vulnerable also in this critical state are the posterior cerebral arteries, one or the other of which may be compressed with resultant infarction of the medial surface of the occipital lobe and resultant hemianopsia.

Upward herniation at the incisura occurs when a pressure increase in the posterior fossa displaces the dorsal part of the cerebellum. This tends to obstruct the aqueduct and produce a still greater increase of supratentorial pressure.

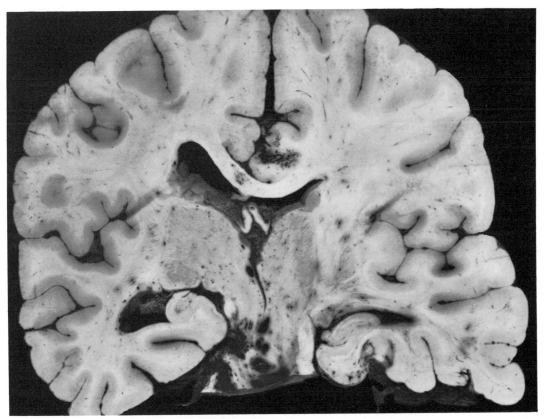

Figure 32–5. *A subdural hematoma (removed on this specimen) had compressed the brain from the right so that the right cingulate gyrus herniated under the falx cerebri and the right temporal lobe through the incisura of the tentorium. Both these herniations have become "strangulated," with hemorrhagic infarction. In the midbrain and pons can be seen a severe grade of the secondary hemorrhages which follow tentorial herniation.*

MALFORMATIONS

Malformations result from an error in the complex development of the nervous system. The etiology of such malformations has excited interest in recent years and, although knowledge is regrettably incomplete, it is known that a variety of influences operating in the early stages of fetal development may result in errors of development (Potter, 1961) (Ford, 1960). Among the known causes are radiation, anoxia, drugs and viral illnesses, especially rubella, in the early months of pregnancy.

A knowledge of embryology is necessary for a detailed understanding of the malformations, but in general the fully developed nervous system is the result of a complex series of fusions and cleavages of the primitive neural structures (Yakovlev and Wadsworth, 1946). The number of possible malformations is very great, and malformations of the nervous system are frequently associated with abnormalities in other parts of the body.

Errors of Fusion. The most extreme degree of failure of closure of the neural tube is *craniorachischisis totalis.* Here the convexity of the skull is absent and the spine is represented only by its bodies with no posterior covering. The nervous system lying in its undeveloped container is equally undeveloped, consisting of blood vessels, glia and scattered unorganized nests of nerve cells and processes. Such a defect is not compatible with extrauterine existence.

At the other end of the scale of incomplete fusion is the failure of closure of the sacral bones, producing *asymptomatic spina bifida occulta.* This is an extremely common defect, usually turned up by roentgenographic examination of the lumbosacral region for some other purpose. Between these two extremes of failure of fusion lie many gradations of defects. The skull may be open and the brain alone poorly developed. This is *cranioschisis.* When the brain is very poorly developed, the term *anencephaly* is applied. When the spinal canal is open, the result is called *rachischisis.*

Some congenital malformations present difficult and interesting problems in care and management. These are the localized outpouchings of brain or spinal cord or its coverings. *Encephalocele* is an outpouching of brain and its coverings through an occipital midline defect. Rarely it may occur in the frontal region. The bony opening is usually very small in comparison with the amount of brain in the sac, and the contents of the sac may become necrotic through interference with its vascular supply. In such cases it is difficult to identify any normal brain within the sac.

Outpouching at the spinal level is much more frequent. It is most common in the thoracolumbar region. Such failure of spinal fusion may be accompanied by a protruding sac of meninges alone, a *meningocele*, or of meninges and spinal cord and roots, a *meningomyelocele* (Fig. 32–6). The latter is so arranged that the roots no longer go to their proper destination, and the infant is usually paralyzed in both the motor and sensory spheres below the level of deformity. There is no neural control of urination and defecation. The protruding sac

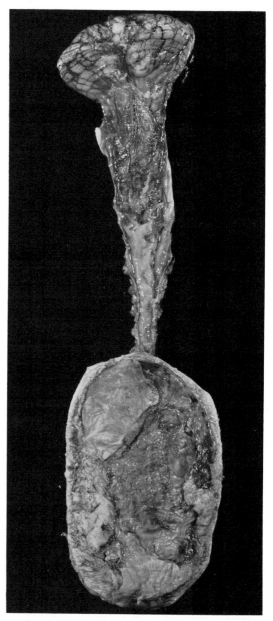

Figure 32–6. *The cord has been removed with the attached mass which contains the meningeal sac, a tangle of nerves and roots, over which lies the skin.*

containing cerebrospinal fluid is likely to be perilously thin, and infection with fatal meningitis is a constant hazard.

Diplomyelia is the result when there has been a failure of fusion of spinal cord of such degree that each half of the spinal cord develops separately over many segments. *Diastematomyelia* is a less extreme degree of such failure, in which each half has only one dorsal and one ventral horn, with an intervening cystic cavity to represent the central canal, and sometimes an intervening bony septum.

Rarely a defect occurs in the vertebral bodies with varying degrees of anterior protrusion of the spinal contents, so-called *spina bifida ventralis.*

The *Arnold-Chiari malformation* actually is a group of different combinations. The generic term is applied to certain deformities of the cerebellum, medulla and cervical cord, usually in association with meningomyelocele. The full deformity is a herniation of the posterior cerebellum, the medulla and the fourth ventricle through the foramen magnum, with an added sharp curvature of the neuraxis at the cervicomedullary junction (Fig. 32–7). There are many variations and many degrees of intensity. Hydrocephalus is frequent, as are platybasia (a flattening of the base of the skull) and basilar invagination (a protrusion of the cervical spinal structures above the foramen magnum). Although the grosser deformity is evident at birth, lesser degrees of change may not become symptomatic until later, even into adult life.

Congenital stenosis of the aqueduct is often present in conjunction with the Arnold-Chiari malformation, but it may occur separately as well. The aqueduct in some cases may be simply smaller than normal with multiple forked outpouchings. Such congenital smallness may be familial. In other cases, when a glial membrane is formed across the cavity of the aqueduct, it is less clearly a malformation, and may be the end result of some antenatal inflammatory process. In either case, the result is an obstructive hydrocephalus, its severity depending upon the degree of obstruction.

Errors of cleavage result in monstrous abnormalities, especially in the brain. The most obvious of these is *cyclopia*, one eye in the middle of a deformed forehead. This arises because of the failure of cleavage of the optic cup. Cyclopia is only part of what is usually a most extensive and multiple anomaly of the central nervous system. It is a component of arrhinencephaly.

Arrhinencephaly is a malformation of the forebrain. The olfactory bulb and tracts are absent in the mildest form of the disorder. In the

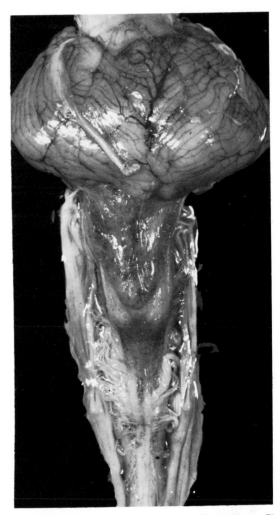

Figure 32–7. *Arnold-Chiari malformation. The cerebellar tonsils are displaced into the cervical canal. The cervical cord seems to be reduplicated, but is actually covered by a downward extension of medulla. This results from preservation of the cervical flexure of the embryo.*

fully developed instance of arrhinencephaly, there is no interhemispheric fissure, only one large ventricular cavity and no commissures. This is the maximal disorder of failure of cleavage.

Complete *agenesis of the corpus callosum* is a component of arrhinencephaly and so is only part of a multiple malformation. It is not uncommon to find a defect of the corpus callosum in the course of a routine autopsy without other anomaly. When such cases are examined carefully, it is seen that there are parts of corpus callosum on either side. The defect is in their failure to meet up in the center. Thus, this is not really an agenesis; it is rather a failure of commissuration.

Errors of Migration. The malformations

discussed up to this point have been errors in fusion or cleavage of the developing brain. Other kinds of malformation result from faulty migration of the neuroblasts from the primitive neural tube. Islands of gray matter may be found within the white matter of the cerebral hemispheres or spinal cord (heterotopias), or well differentiated portions of anatomic structure may be found in anomalous positions (ectopias). An example of the latter is the appearance of a recognizable piece of cerebellum within the cerebral hemispheres.

Three characteristic appearances of the cerebral cortex are also related to faulty migration of neuroblasts. *Status verrucosus* is a wart-like appearance of the cortex produced by a disorderly arrangement of the neuroblasts so that fissuration and sulcation are irregular and unpredictable. The warty appearance is due to excrescences of improperly differentiated clusters of glia and nerve cells. *Pachygyria* is the appearance of large gyri in the cortex due to inadequate differentiation of sulci. This relative absence of sulci gives the brain a smooth appearance, so-called *lissencephaly*. When such a brain is cut, the cortex is seen to be thickened, and the cortical layers obscured. Thus, in pachygyria the neuroblasts get to the cortex but their arrangement is defective after arrival. The same thing is true of *microgyria* in which the secondary fissures are lacking but the individual gyri are excessively sulcated, so that the cortex may look like a pile of earthworms. The lamination of the cortex in microgyria is also disordered and defective.

Status verrucosus, pachygyria and microgyria are often associated with other anomalies. They always result in severe neurologic deficit, and children with such diffuse derangements are always mentally defective.

HYDROCEPHALUS

By hydrocephalus is meant an increased amount of cerebrospinal fluid in the ventriculosubarachnoid pathways of the brain (Russell, 1949).

Pathogenesis. The cerebrospinal fluid is formed, at least originally, by the choroid plexuses of the ventricular system, and is resorbed in large part by the arachnoidal villi which project into the dural venous sinuses. There probably also is some transfer of fluid and electrolytes between blood and cerebrospinal fluid at other levels of the ventriculosubarachnoid system. There is a slow flow from lateral ventricles through the foramina of Monro to the third ventricle, from the third ventricle through the aqueduct of Sylvius to the fourth ventricle, from the fourth ventricle through the centrally placed foramen of Magendie and the laterally placed foramina of Luschka to the subarachnoid space of the brain stem, and thence downward about the spinal cord and upward over the convexity of brain.

The cause of the common hydrocephalus of the antenatal and neonatal period is still controversial. In a large number of cases, the defect would seem to be in the overproduction or under-resorption of cerebrospinal fluid. Stenosis of the aqueduct is not infrequent. Atresia or stenosis of the foramina of Magendie and Luschka is very rare. In those malformations which deform and displace the brain stem structures, such as the Arnold-Chiari malformation, fluid released from the fourth ventricle through the foramina may be prevented from coursing up in the subarachnoid space to the arachnoidal villi.

The Dandy-Walker-Taggart syndrome consists of hydrocephalus in association with a posterior fossa cyst, enlargement of the fourth ventricle and hypoplasia of the cerebellar vermis. It is frequently associated with other developmental abnormalities.

Congenital anomalies are not the only causes of obstructive hydrocephalus in infancy. Infections are of less importance in this era of antibiotics, but even now infectious processes such as the pyogenic meningitides, tuberculous meningitis, and toxoplasmic meningoencephalitis can produce an inflammatory stenosis of the aqueduct, or obliteration of the subarachnoid pathways about the base of the brain. Tumors and abscesses may occur to block the pathway in the infant as well as in the adult.

Tumors and other compressing lesions as well as infections may obstruct the flow of fluid in the child and adult, producing ventricular distention with increased intracranial pressure. Some of the congenital malformations, such as the Arnold-Chiari malformation, may not declare themselves until childhood or adult life. Some people, with chronic hydrocephalus for many years, may compensate for their defect by attaining a kind of hydrodynamic equilibrium despite a degree of anatomic disorder, only to decompensate under the conditions of a generalized infection or metabolic disorder.

When **obstructive hydrocephalus** occurs in the fetus or in the infant before the sutures close, the increased intracranial pressure produces expansion of the brain and its coverings, prying the sutures farther apart, and the entire head increases progressively in size. In extreme cases, the head attains a horribly fantastic size, the peaked small face lying pathetically below, while the scalp veins stand out prominently and the tight skin over the scalp looks ready to burst.

The pressure of the obstructed fluid from within produces a compression of the convexity of the cerebral cortex until only a paper-thin ribbon of cerebral mantle surmounts the distended bag of fluid into which the ventricular system has been transformed (Fig. 32—8). The walls of the ventricles appear corrugated and the septum pellucidum is perforated in many places so that it remains only as a tattered lacework of connective tissue.

Despite such severe degrees of compression of the cerebral cortex, the nerve cells may show a remarkable capacity for survival, and hydrocephalus is not always associated with mental retardation. The fibers of the subcortical white matter are stretched and compressed by obstructed fluid within the ventricles. The fibers from cortex to face and arm, it will be remembered, have a more direct and less vulnerable approach to the internal capsule than do the leg fibers. These latter take their origin from the medial surface of the hemisphere and have to course over and around the dilated ventricle before reaching the internal capsule. Thus, in obstructive hydrocephalus, spastic diplegia of the lower limbs may be present with little or no involvement of the arms and face.

After the sutures have closed and the skull can no longer yield to the pressure of increasing hydrocephalus, the changes in brain tissue are much more destructive.

In the kinds of hydrocephalus already referred to, we have used the term obstructive. **Obstructive hydrocephalus is internal hydrocephalus;** i.e., the internal portion of the fluid pathway is the one that develops the fluid excess. **External hydrocephalus** has only a theoretical existence, implying an excess of fluid in the subarachnoid space without any change in the ventricular system. It is customary to distinguish in internal hydrocephalus between the communicating and the noncommunicating types. In **communicating hydrocephalus,** there is free access of fluid between the ventricles and the lumbar subarachnoid space. Thus, the obstruction must be in the subarachnoid space about the base of the brain so that fluid is permitted to go to the spinal subarachnoid space, but not up and around the cranial subarachnoid space. Communicating hydrocephalus is also present when there is either excessive production or defective absorption. In **noncommunicating hydrocephalus,** access to the spinal subarachnoid space as well as to the cranial subarachnoid space is denied by obstruction at the level of the ventricle's aqueduct, fourth ventricle or the foramina of Luschka and Magendie. For practical purposes, this is determined by injecting a marker into the lateral ventricle and then noting its presence or absence in the fluid withdrawn at lumbar puncture. It will be clear from what has been said that this test has its limitations, depending on the degree of obstruction and the degree of hydrodynamic equilibrium at the time of the test.

Hydrocephalus ex vacuo is a compensatory replacement of volume by fluid. Thus, when a brain is very atrophic from disease, the ventricles become dilated, the subarachnoid spaces become enlarged and the perivascular tissue spaces increase in size. When loss of tissue is localized, as in an old infarct, there is a localized enlargement of the nearby portion of the ventricular and subarachnoid spaces. By this replacement with fluid, the volume of the intracranial contents is preserved, and in focal lesions no shift of midline structures can occur to stretch and distort the rest of the brain.

Clinical Course. The most common form of hydrocephalus compatible with life is that which is associated with meningocele or meningomyelocele. Sometimes these patients die in the first few days or weeks of life, especially if there is obstruction of the aqueduct, for complete aqueductal occlusion does not permit survival. Often, however, they live for years, and may grow into adult life. The head increases in size in the early weeks and months but eventually a hydrodynamic equilibrium is attained. The patient is recognized immediately, even when there are minor degrees of cranial enlargement, by the rounded forehead, the low-slung ears and the triangular face. Subsequent events depend largely on the stability of the hydrodynamic equilibrium. An infection or a metabolic upset may produce acute hydrocephalic attacks, sometimes mistaken for true convulsions. These in fact are episodes of disordered awareness with decerebration. Patients may die in such attacks of increased in-

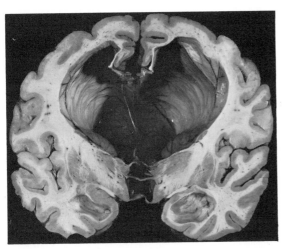

Figure 32—8. Hydrocephalus of moderate degree. This was associated with an Arnold-Chiari malformation. The basal ganglia have been displaced downward and lateralward, and the overlying corpus callosum has been thinned.

tracranial pressure or, if the attacks are prolonged, there may be papilledema going on to optic atrophy. On the other hand, many patients with compensated hydrocephalus may live a full life span. Although some are mentally deficient because of the early brain damage, others are of normal or superior intelligence.

Neurosurgical procedures have been devised for the management of hydrocephalus, the best of them being the ventriculojugular shunts. Their effectiveness depends upon early recognition and the absence of associated prohibitive malformations.

A curious and relatively rare variety of hydrocephalus occurring in middle-aged people is called "normal pressure hydrocephalus" or "low pressure hydrocephalus." There is progressive enlargement of the ventricles as if they were obstructed, but there are no primary changes in the substance of brain. The severe dementia and gait disorder of this condition respond dramatically to the diversion of fluid, as in a ventriculojugular shunt.

INFECTIONS

Almost any pathogenic organism may attack the nervous system or its coverings. Viruses, yeasts, fungi, rickettsiae, bacteria, protozoa and helminths all have their place in the pathology of the nervous system, depending on the part of the world one works in. The majority of infecting agents are amenable to treatment. In almost all instances, the nervous system becomes infected only after infection has started elsewhere, and the best time to treat an infection, if possible, is before it gets to the nervous system. For these reasons, the study of neurologic infections must be correlated with the study of infections in general. The importance of the cerebrospinal fluid examination is considerable in all aspects of neuropathology, but it is of such paramount importance in infections that the student should review all he has learned about it in other courses.

The host element in generalized infections is imperfectly understood. The majority of patients who have a pneumonia, even with septicemia, will not develop a leptomeningitis. Yet a few patients do, and there is no explanation for it. Some patients may come to autopsy with tuberculosis in every organ, but not in the brain or meninges; other patients may have only minimal pulmonary tuberculosis and a fatal tuberculous meningitis. Such examples can be multiplied many times for all classes of infectious agents.

PYOGENIC INFECTIONS

The routes by which suppuration spreads to the nervous system are many and varied. Organisms may be implanted directly, by a dirty crowbar or even by the badly cleaned scalpel. Passage along veins from an infection of the face may set up a dural sinus thrombophlebitis. The arteries to the brain may carry infected emboli from the lungs to produce brain abscesses or from the heart to produce embolic encephalitis. A bacteremia may deposit organisms in the brain or its coverings. The routes of infection must always be ascertained, and in dealing with any infection anywhere, the good physician always considers in advance the prospects of spread to the nervous system, for such spread may mean disaster. If the fuse is kept from burning, the powder keg will not explode.

Leptomeningitis. Almost any pyogenic organism can invade the leptomeninges, but the most common are the pneumococcus, meningococcus and *H. influenzae*. In these cases, the leptomeninges are usually involved in the course of a septicemia. The ventriculo-subarachnoid spaces then act as a pathway for the dissemination of the organisms, and the characteristic inflammatory response is set up, with the cerebrospinal fluid reflecting vividly the account of the battle between the organism and the tissue (Swartz and Dodge, 1965*a*; 1965*b*).

If an autopsy is done at an early stage, the brain and spinal cord are found to be swollen and congested. The subarachnoid space contains exudate which varies in location. In *H. influenzae* meningitis, for example, it is usually basal, but in pneumonococcal meningitis it is more often over the convexity near the longitudinal sinus. From the areas of greatest accumulation of exudate, tracks of suppuration can be followed about the blood vessels (Fig. 32–9). But even in those areas where there is no gross exudate, the leptomeninges are found to be opaque and congested. When the process is fulminant and especially if it is prolonged, there will be inflammation on the ependymal surface, even to the extent of frank suppuration. If the pressure changes are great enough, there may be tentorial or foraminal herniation.

Microscopically, the cellular reaction in the acute stage is polymorphonuclear with varying amounts of fibrin. In the more severely affected areas, the entire subarachnoid space is replaced by the cellular products of inflammation; in less severely affected areas, only the tissue about the leptomeningeal blood vessels contains cells. In a fulminating process, the pial barrier is unable to

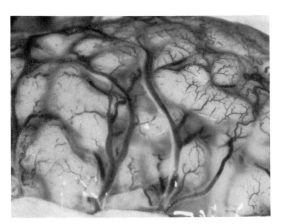

Figure 32–9. Pneumococcal meningitis. There is congestion of the leptomeningeal vessels with suppuration about the veins.

withstand the assault and the process then will extend into the outer layer of brain or cord. In almost all pyogenic leptomeningitides, there is perivascular accumulation of cells in the outer layer of brain or cord.

One of the not uncommon complications of the early stage is thrombophlebitis. When it occurs over the cerebral cortex, the clinical course is punctuated by a convulsion or a series of convulsions. In occlusion of larger veins, a good-sized venous infarct may result, with destruction of the cortex and hemorrhages in subjacent white matter. Arterial resistance to the sepsis is much greater than venous, and so arteritis is not a complication unless the process is very prolonged.

The patient with purulent leptomeningitis has signs of generalized infection, since there is usually a bacteremia. In addition, there are symptoms and signs of meningeal irritation: headache, photophobia, pain on eye movement, stiff neck, stiff back and positive Kernig's sign. Agitation or stupor may be followed by deep coma and death in the inadequately treated case.

The cerebrospinal fluid is under increased pressure. The white cells number thousands of polymorphonuclear leukocytes. The protein is elevated. The sugar is reduced. Bacteria can be seen on smear or cultured easily on appropriate media, sometimes hours before the polymorphonuclear cells appear. Some less common meningitides, such as anthrax, may produce a very hemorrhagic inflammation, and large numbers of red cells may appear in the fluid.

Before the introduction of modern methods of treatment, death was the outcome in the overwhelming majority of cases. Recovery in many cases occurred only after a great deal of destruction of meningeal framework with fibroblastic proliferation succeeding the acute stage so that adhesions appeared between meninges and brain. This resulted in cranial nerve palsies, but the most tragic effect resulted from the production of a basal adhesive arachnoiditis at the base, sealing off the foramina of Magendie and Luschka, or obliterating the subarachnoid space about the brain stem. The result was hydrocephalus, and a lingering death was the usual outcome. Fortunately, such a complication is exceedingly rare with present methods of management and, when it does occur, yields to suitable shunting of the ventricular fluid.

Pachymeningitis. Suppuration of any significance within the cranial *epi*dural space, i.e., between the skull and dura, is rare, as is suppuration in the spinal *sub*dural space. In contrast, spinal epidural and cranial subdural suppuration are relatively frequent.

Suppuration in the cranial subdural space is referred to as *subdural empyema* or, less properly, *subdural abscess* (Kubik and Adams, 1943). Its origin is almost invariably an infection in one of the paranasal sinuses. The subdural space offers no limitation to the spread of infection, and the result is an expanding bag of pus compressing and distorting the cerebral hemisphere, producing headache, convulsions, hemiparesis and eventually death through herniation. In addition, the proximity of the dural sinuses makes them very vulnerable to infection and thrombosis with all the catastrophe this can bring. When the brain is examined, a thick, shaggy, fibrinous exudate remains on the inner surface of the dura and outer surface of the arachnoid after the pus is evacuated. The organisms recovered are usually staphylococcus or pneumococcus. A reflected inflammation is present in the subarachnoid space, accounting for the cellular reaction without organisms found on lumbar puncture. This cellular reaction is usually a mixture of polymorphonuclear cells and lymphocytes and, in contrast to pyogenic leptomeningitis, the sugar is normal.

Infection of the spinal *epidural* space arises as a direct extension from a nearby locus of osteomyelitis in the vertebra and, more rarely, in the absence of bony involvement, from some distant focus (Heusner, 1948). Hemmed in by the epidural fat, the process tends to be granulomatous even though the organism is pyogenic. The seeming indolence of the infection in speed of spread is no indication of the severity of its effect, for it produces cord compression with resulting paraplegia and all that it entails unless surgery is done early. At lumbar puncture, a dynamic subarachnoid spinal block is demonstrable and, as in other infections near the leptomeninges, a sterile inflammatory response is found.

Brain Abscess. Abscesses in the substance of the brain may arise from direct implantation by trauma or surgery, by extension from nearby foci of infection and especially from mastoiditis, or by hematogenous spread, especially from a primary source in lung. Although septic endocarditis may produce miliary multiple abscesses, it does not produce a large purulent collection. Cyanosing congenital heart disease is associated with a high incidence of cerebral abscesses, especially in the parieto-occipital region. This happens only in those patients in whom there is a defect of the sort which removes the bacteria-screening function of the pulmonary vascular system.

Abscess from mastoiditis is usually preceded by an epidural extension from the infecting site, with extension then into either the ipsilateral cerebellar hemisphere or the temporal lobe.

The stage of invasion of an abscess in the brain is like that anywhere. There may be a "cellulitis" of brain substance, which produces severe symptoms and signs and then settles down, leaving a nidus of organisms and necrotic tissue. Adhesions of the

meninges then usually seal off the point of entry from the rest of the subarachnoid space. Gradually, as elsewhere, the abscess expands, destroying and compressing tissues as it grows (Fig. 32–10). A chronic inflammation surrounds it, but an intense polymorphonuclear response continues. Fibrosis and gliosis struggle to contain the advancing edge of suppuration but only rarely do they succeed, and destruction of brain continues. The intensity of the inflammatory reaction is reflected in the cerebrospinal fluid by an increased white cell count and an increase in total protein. No organisms will be present in the fluid unless the mass has ruptured into the ventricle or the subarachnoid space.

Very rarely, an abscess of brain heals spontaneously. Most often, however, unless it is drained, it kills the patient by herniation.

The patient with a brain abscess presents most often with general complaints relating to increased intracranial pressure and focal complaints referable to the area of brain involved. The manifestations of increased pressure occur early in the course of an expanding cerebellar abscess, because of the deformity and compression of the fourth ventricle or aqueduct, but they may be late in abscesses of the frontal or temporal regions. Abscesses are so

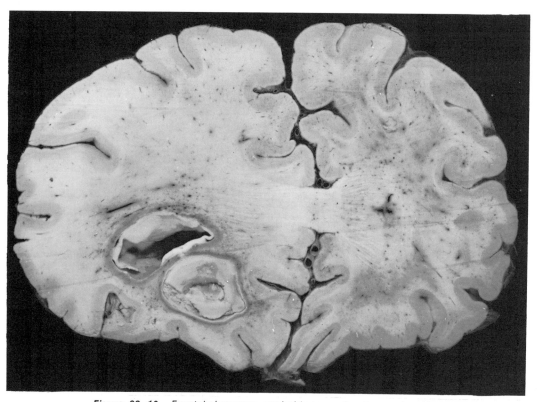

Figure 32–10. Frontal abscesses, probably secondary to pansinusitis.

destructive in their growth that, depending on their location, a clinical deficit is always demonstrable. Hemiparesis, hemianopsia or fits in cerebral abscesses, and cerebellar incoordination in cerebellar abscesses, are among the more dramatic and obvious signs. The cerebrospinal fluid is always under increased pressure, the protein is almost always elevated and rising and the white cells are in excess with a normal sugar. In the diagnosis of abscess of the brain, a source can usually be found, either in the mastoid or other paranasal sinuses, lungs, heart or in a communication through the skull. But a small abscess may be quiescent for many weeks or months, and the activity of the source may have ceased by the time the patient presents with his symptoms of brain involvement.

Abscesses of the substance of spinal cord are exceedingly rare.

TUBERCULOUS INFECTIONS

In terms of its neuropathology, the tubercle bacillus can produce meningitis, spinal epidural granuloma, tuberculoma of brain substance or any combination of these.

Tuberculous Meningitis. Meningitis due to the tubercle bacillus, as might be expected, is of less abrupt onset and of more chronic course than is pyogenic meningitis. The untreated patient may survive, but only very rarely, and usually death comes in less than six weeks.

Grossly, the greatest involvement is at the base of the brain and about the spinal cord, where a shaggy, necrotic, fibrofibrinous yellow exudate compresses the underlying brain and cord and catches the spinal and cranial nerves in a sticky embrace (Fig. 32–11). Frank large areas of caseation may be seen, and about blood vessels there may be tiny discrete tubercles. The histologic reaction is similar to that of tuberculosis elsewhere, with localized caseation and surrounding epithelioid cells and lymphocyst (p. 83). The familiar giant cells are usually sparse. But even in areas where there is no characteristic necrosis, an intense lymphocytic and monocytic response is present.

As with other types of chronic meningeal infection, arteritis is common, sometimes leading to the sudden appearance of infarcts of brain in the course of the illness.

Tuberculous Spinal Epidural Granuloma. Usually associated with tuberculosis of the vertebrae, tuberculous granulomas of the spinal epidural space occur mostly in the thoracic area. They may grow to a considerable size and produce cord compression unless treated surgically.

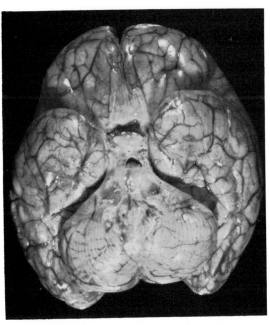

Figure 32–11. *Tuberculous meningitis.*

Tuberculomas of Brain and Cord. In unusual instances, a solitary tuberculoma may appear in the brain or cord. They behave like expanding lesions, simulating brain tumors, since they are for a time at least not associated with tuberculous meningitis. They consist of a large central core of caseation necrosis surrounded by a typical tuberculous histopathologic reaction and a well developed fibrous capsule. Sometimes many large tuberculomas appear in the same brain (Fig. 32–12). It is not rare for the solitary tuberculoma to stop its advance and to calcify, turning up at autopsy many years later as an incidental finding.

FUNGUS INFECTIONS

Many fungi have the capacity for invasion of the brain or leptomeninges. When they become established, they are exceedingly difficult to treat, especially when they occur on the background of severe systemic disease.

The cerebrospinal fluid contains a predominantly lymphocytic cellular response, with variably elevated protein and variably lowered sugar. The organisms may be seen by microscopic examination, and usually they can be cultured in appropriate media.

Coccidioidomycosis is endemic in the southwestern United States. Most often a relatively benign pulmonary process, it infrequently becomes widespread, producing diffuse visceral granulomas. In some of these widespread cases, the nervous system becomes involved.

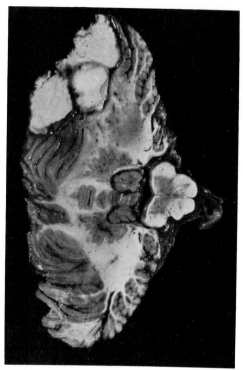

Figure 32–12. Tuberculomas in cerebellum. In addition there were other tuberculomas in the cerebral hemispheres.

The gross appearance is that of a chronic basilar meningitis with or without abscesses in brain substance. The microscopic picture is like that of tuberculosis but is easily differentiated when the organisms are recognized (p. 446).

Histoplasmosis behaves in much the same general way as coccidioidomycosis, but nervous system involvement is far less frequent (p. 447).

Mucormycosis produces leptomeningitis and sometimes focal cerebral abscesses in severe and debilitated diabetics. Usually the patient is in acidosis and there is gross infection of the nasal turbinates and paranasal sinuses.

European blastomycosis is known more commonly as *cryptococcosis* or *torulosis* (Cox and Tolhurst, 1946). It is caused by a blastomyces known as *Cryptococcus hominis* or *Torula histolytica*. Primarily it is a pulmonary infection, but the nervous system is the principal and most important extrapulmonary site of infection (p. 444).

The gross appearance of the brain and cord is variable. There usually is a fibrinopurulent, shaggy exudate on the leptomeninges, more at the base of the brain than over the convexity, looking very much like tuberculous meningitis. In some fatal cases, however, this may be seen only as congestion and opacity.

Microscopically, the process involves both the subarachnoid space and the subjacent superficial layers of the brain and cord. The cellular response is largely lymphocytic and mononuclear with some giant cells, and organisms are easily found. Invasion of blood vessels by the granulomatous exudate may produce a phlebitis or arteritis. A curious feature of cryptococcal meningoencephalitis is the formation of cysts, occasionally large enough to be seen grossly, but almost always present microscopically. These occur especially in the superficial layers of the cortex in the depths of sulci. They contain organisms, and there is little or no reaction about these areas of liquefaction, suggesting that they may be a postmortem change.

The clinical picture is very much like that of tuberculous meningitis, and indeed the coexistence of pulmonary tuberculosis and cryptococcus meningitis is not unusual. An old clinical axiom states that tuberculous meningitis which lasts longer than six weeks is torulosis. The spinal fluid findings are similar to those in tuberculous meningitis except for the identification of the organisms specific for each disease. Ordinarily the cryptococcus can be cultured very easily from the spinal fluid. Many of the reported cases have arisen in patients with preexisting lymphoma or Hodgkin's disease.

NEUROSYPHILIS

The *Treponema pallidum* is an organism of most furtive and insidious habits (p. 378) (Merritt et al., 1946). It is capable of doing mischief almost anywhere, but when it affects the nervous system the results are tragic, since it can deprive a patient of perception, of ambulation and of reason itself. Not all syphilitic patients develop the tertiary stage of neurosyphilis, since the disease may burn itself out spontaneously before it ever gets a foothold in the nervous system or therapy may cure the infection in the primary or secondary stage. All patients who do develop neurosyphilis must pass through a stage of asymptomatic syphilitic meningitis. This stage is recognizable on examination of the cerebrospinal fluid by an increase of white cells with or without a protein increase but with a positive serologic reaction in the fluid.

The implications of this knowledge for therapy are obvious. Syphilis is a treatable disease, but treatment in the sense of a cure is effective only in inverse proportion to the amount of vascular and parenchymal damage that has been allowed to take place. Every case of clinical neurosyphilis represents a mistake on someone's part. If, following a primary infection, a patient does not develop meningeal syphilis within two to three years, he will never develop neurosyphilis from that primary infection. On the other hand, the presence of asymptomatic meningitis does not necessarily mean that the patient will develop clinical neurosyphilis, since the disease may still burn out spontaneously.

Meningeal and Meningovascular Neurosyphilis. Leptomeningeal syphilis is most obvious as a discoloration and thickening of the leptomeninges at the base of the brain, particularly about the optic chiasm and brain stem. There is infiltration with the cell types characteristic of syphilis in other organs: lymphocytes, plasma cells and histiocytes. A more extensive and more intense reaction occurs in acute syphilitic meningitis, with some polymorphonuclear leukocytes and fibrin, and clinically the process may behave like a low-grade pyogenic meningitis, with headache, fever, stiff neck and cranial nerve palsies.

In the more chronic varieties, even without the interposition of an acute exudative attack, fibrosis succeeds to the point of catching up cranial nerves and producing an obstructive hydrocephalus.

In almost all cases of syphilitic meningitis,

there is vascular involvement as well. This is most often due to syphilitic endarteritis, but frequently gummatous lesions of the arterial wall are present. The effect of such blood vessel changes upon the brain and spinal cord depends upon their extent and severity and the coexistence of atherosclerotic disease. Infarcts may occur anywhere, even in the spinal cord.

Paretic Neurosyphilis. General paresis of the insane used to be one of the most common causes of admission to mental hospitals. Like the other symptomatic manifestations of neurosyphilis, it represents a tertiary form of the disease.

Grossly, the brain is atrophic. The meninges are thickened. Ependymal granulations, present in almost all cases of neurosyphilis, are very well developed. They are tiny excrescences upon the ependymal surface, best seen in reflected light. In the advanced cases the sulci are widened, the gyri are narrow, the cortical ribbon is thin and the ventricles are enlarged. Microscopically, the principal lesions are in the cerebral cortex. Widespread loss of nerve cells presents the disordered architecture called the "windswept" cortex. Nerve cells already dead and gone are represented by the tombstones of glial re-

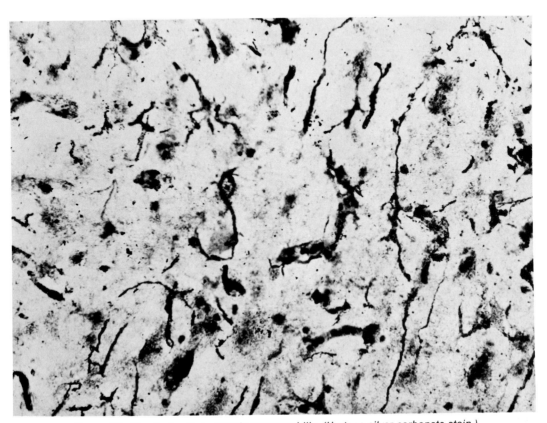

Figure 32–13. Rod cells in paretic neurosyphilis. (Hortega silver carbonate stain.)

placement. The nerve cells which remain are undergoing all degrees of degenerative change. About the blood vessels in the untreated case are the characteristic accumulations of lymphocytes and plasma cells. The microglia are prominent as rod cells, elongated, enlarged, and containing accumulations of iron (Fig. 32–13).

Paretic neurosyphilis, then, is an extension of the destructive effects of the disease to the parenchyma of the brain. This effect is due to the presence of the spirochetes, and with appropriate staining methods it is possible to find them in large numbers throughout the brain. Once this process has begun, it is never spontaneously reversible. Either the patient is treated, or the organisms continue their gruesome work until the patient dies. Since the inflammatory reaction persists, the cerebrospinal fluid always reflects the continuing presence of the disease in the untreated patient.

The early symptoms and signs of paretic neurosyphilis are the subtle changes of an organic intellectual deficit, or dementia. A slight loss of memory, a change in mood and an inappropriateness of language and behavior may be the only hints at the beginning of the illness. Later these symptoms are multiplied and increased to the most extraordinary varieties of dementing psychoses, leaving the patient fit only for the protected life of a hospital for mental disease. Tremors and myoclonic jerkings, especially of the hands and lips, make their appearance along the way.

Tabes Dorsalis. Like general paresis, tabes dorsalis declares itself many years after the primary syphilitic infection. It is also referred to as locomotor ataxia because of the prominence of ambulation difficulties.

The pathogenesis of tabes dorsalis is still very controversial. Some say that it is the consequence of a localized leptomeningeal inflammation of the dorsal roots and the root entry zone. Others blame changes in the dorsal root ganglia. Still others assert that it must represent a toximetabolic disorder of the involved structures. It is remarkable that Treponema organisms are very difficult to demonstrate in the nervous system in this disease.

Tabes dorsalis can be associated with general paresis, or the cord damage can be compounded and confused by an associated meningovascular syphilis.

On gross examination of the cord, the most impressive findings are a smallness of the posterior roots of the lumbar region and a degeneration of the columns of Goll in the posterior part of the cord. It will be remembered that the ascending posterior columns are formed by entering fibers at each segment, which lie laterally as they enter, displacing the fibers of more caudal origin to the medial part of the cord. Thus, in the lumbar region the entire posterior column has the shrunken gray, translucent appearance of atrophy, while in the cervical portion this is restricted to the medial parts of the column.

Microscopically, there is fibrosis about the posterior roots and they are variably atrophic. The leptomeninges over the posterior columns show a fibrous reaction more severe than elsewhere. There is fiber loss and gliosis in the areas of degeneration of the posterior columns (Fig. 32–14). When optic atrophy is present, there is fiber loss, gliosis and interstitial fibrosis of the optic nerve.

Most universal of the symptoms are the lightning pains—sudden jabs of pain in the legs, each one lasting only a fraction of a second, but producing a sustained agony by their confluence in time. Painful paresthesias of the legs or trunk, and infrequently the arms and face, may add to the patient's troubles. Far less common are the so-called visceral crises, bouts of severe cramping abdominal pain and vomiting. Ambulation is affected early, the patient complaining of unsteadiness in walking and especially in the dark or with his eyes closed. Urinary retention is common, and with it the complication of urinary tract infections. The Argyll Robertson pupil, the almost specific pupillary disorder of neurosyphilis, is almost always present in tabes dorsalis. About 10 per cent of all tabetics develop optic atrophy which may progress to total blindness. Deformities of the joints (Charcot joints), painless ulcers of the feet and other trophic disorders appear later in the disease.

On examination of the patient, there is widespread loss of pain sensation, and this is undoubtedly responsible for the Charcot joints and the trophic ulcers. Bands of analgesia and anesthesia in segmental distribution may be present on the trunk or thorax. The position sense defect is responsible for the ataxia of gait and explains why there is so much trouble in the dark and with the eyes closed. Vibration

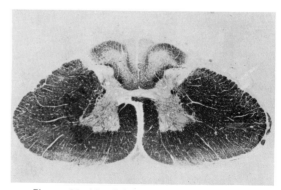

Figure 32–14. *Tabes dorsalis, cervical spinal cord.*

sense is absent. The deep reflexes at the knee and ankle are absent.

In its symptoms and signs, tabes dorsalis is a "sensory disease," accurately reflecting the pathologic involvement of the sensory pathways.

VIRUS DISEASES

The central nervous system can be involved by a multitude of different viruses (Rhodes and van Rooyen, 1968) (Hoeprich, 1972). A systemic infection, which may or may not be symptomatic, precedes the development of neurologic symptoms or signs, and many patients have only the systemic infection without invasion of the nervous system.

A virus may produce disease only in the leptomeninges as in lymphocytic choriomeningitis, largely in the brain as in encephalitis lethargica or largely in the spinal cord as in acute anterior poliomyelitis. In any viral encephalitis or myelitis, there is some reaction of the leptomeninges so that, in the early stages at least, there are inflammatory cells in the cerebrospinal fluid.

There is a degree of histologic uniformity in these lesions of the brain and spinal cord which are due to viruses. Generally the predilection is for gray matter, specifically the nerve cell, which undergoes a change ranging from a reversible dysfunction to destructive necrosis. The neutrophilic response is usually minimal, *the important histologic reaction to destruction being composed of histiocytes and microglia. There is round cell accumulation in the perivascular spaces.*

There are also significant exceptions to these general rules, and differences in histologic character and localization of the process within this group of diseases. Some viruses are capable of eliciting a neutrophilic response in the acute stage, and some can produce white matter lesions. Still other "transmissible agents," probably viruses, can produce unique lesions after prolonged incubation time or chronic progression.

Encephalitis. It is not possible in a volume of this sort to give space to all the viruses which may involve the brain and produce encephalitis. A comment about terminology may mitigate some of the confusion. Encephalitis is a term which should be reserved for those pathologic states of the brain in which inflammation, and especially infection, is predominant. Encephalopathy is a nonspecific term for any more or less diffuse process involving the brain. Thus, a viral encephalitis is an infectious and inflammatory encephalopathy. The same distinctions apply to the terms myelitis and myelopathy and to the combined words encephalomyelitis and encephalomyelopathy.

Encephalitis Lethargica. Encephalitis lethargica is a disease which spread across the world from the Far East in successive epidemics from 1915 to 1926. Some epidemics were associated closely in time with influenza epidemics. Von Economo made an epic study of the Vienna epidemic of 1917, and the disease is often called by his name. The first outbreak in the United States was in 1918. Although an organism was never recovered despite repeated efforts, the pattern of infection was that which one would expect from a communicable disease, and the histologic reaction was similar to that seen in other encephalitides of known virus etiology.

This disease was one of the most destructive scourges of modern civilization. It is frightening to consider the possibility that somewhere in the Orient may be an endemic focus, ready to break out again.

Grossly, the brains showed little change except for swelling. In exceptional cases, there were tiny areas of grossly visible necrosis in gray matter, and small petechial hemorrhages were reported in some cases.

Microscopically, the reaction was a combination of parenchymatous and mesodermal change (Fig. 32–15). Perivascular cuffing in the early stages varied in intensity from place to place, sometimes

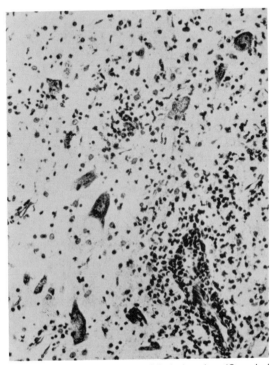

Figure 32–15. *Encephalitis lethargica. (Cresyl violet stain.)*

only a single layer of cells and sometimes a thick collar several layers thick. Nor was the intensity of the perivascular reaction always correlated in degree with the damage to nerve cells. The perivascular reaction in this early stage was usually lymphocytic and histiocytic, and only rarely was a neutrophil to be seen. Nerve cells in the affected areas showed a multitude of degenerating forms, with an intense microglial and, in areas of greater destruction, astroglial reaction to the cell destruction. In the later stages, the tissue showed only little residue of the vascular and perivascular inflammatory reaction, but the areas of affected gray matter were composed of the glial response to the disintegration of the nerve cells.

The illness varied greatly in intensity but was characterized generally by an acute stage with nonspecific prodromata and high fever followed by signs of meningeal irritation, stupor or agitation, or coma, cranial nerve palsies, rigidities, tremors and paralyses. It left many patients with severe consequences: parkinsonian states, spasticities, dystonias, oculogyric crises and dementias. A curious feature of the disease in this regard is that these unfortunate consequences occurred in some cases almost immediately upon the patient's regaining consciousness, while in other cases they were delayed in their onset up to 10 or 12 years after the acute disease was over. The mortality rate was very high, and only a relatively small percentage of patients recovered without having some neurologic deficit.

The long delay in production of certain chronic sequelae has led some investigators to postulate that there is continuing chronic infection by the virus. Others have suggested that the long delay is due to transneuronal degeneration. But neither of these explanations is proved or, at present, provable.

Arthropod-Borne Encephalitides. Outbreaks of encephalitis are most commonly due to arthropod-borne viruses (arboviruses). The infecting agents are different in different parts of the world. The important ones in the Western Hemisphere are eastern equine, western equine, Venezuelan equine, St. Louis and California. In other parts of the world are Japanese B (Siberia, China, Japan, Southeast Asia, India), tick-borne (U.S.S.R. and eastern Europe) and Murray Valley (Australia and New Guinea). All have vertebrate hosts and, except for the tick-borne, all have mosquito vectors. These viruses have many common properties, to the extent that some investigators wish to group them separately as encephaloviruses.

Eastern (Equine) Encephalitis. Eastern equine encephalitis was first described in 1933 as a disease of horses. It was first reported to affect human beings in 1938, when an epidemic among children in Massachusetts followed an epidemic in horses. The disease has always carried a high mortality for those patients who develop clinically obvious encephalitis. It is estimated on the basis of serologic studies that there are 18 people with few or no symptoms for every case of overt disease. Mortality is about 80 per cent. Some patients recover without neurologic defect, but others who survive, especially young children, are left with ghastly residuals.

The lesions are similar in location to those seen in encephalitis lethargica and Japanese B encephalitis, but there is generally more extensive destruction of cerebral cortex. In both eastern and western equine encephalitis, large numbers of polymorphonuclear leukocytes appear in brain and cerebrospinal fluid in the acute stage of the disease. The sugar in the fluid is not decreased even when the cell count is exclusively polymorphonuclear.

Western (Equine) Encephalitis. This disease was first identified as a separate encephalitis in horses with the isolation of the virus in a 1931 epidemic in California. In the late 1930's and early 1940's, it was recognized as a disease in man. A particularly vicious epidemic occurred in 1941 in Canada and the north central United States and involved thousands of people. The mortality rate from western equine encephalitis is not so high as with eastern equine encephalitis, but still it ranges between 8 and 19 per cent.

The pathologic changes are variably severe in the usual sites of predilection for encephalitis, and in addition there is frequent involvement of the upper spinal cord.

Venezuelan (Equine) Encephalitis. Most cases have been endemic or epidemic in northern South America and in Central America, but there have been some cases in the southern United States. Milder than eastern or western, relatively few cases are fatal.

St. Louis Encephalitis. St. Louis encephalitis was first recognized in the midwestern United States where the major epidemic occurred in 1933 in the St. Louis area. The virus was isolated, and the disease was recognized as being distinct from encephalitis lethargica.

The disease may involve any age group. It is usually not severe in infants and children. However, in some outbreaks, very young children were left with substantial neurologic deficits, usually mental retardation and convulsive disorders. Generally, however, complete recovery is the rule in those patients who do not succumb to the acute illness. The fatality rate has varied from 2 to 20 per cent in different epidemics.

The pathologic picture is similar to that

seen in other encephalitides. However, the meningeal reaction is quite prominent, and there is more involvement of the cerebral cortex and spinal cord than in some of the other varieties of encephalitis.

California Encephalitis. This virus is an important cause of a usually mild meningoencephalitis. Cases have been recognized in California, Florida, Indiana, Iowa, Minnesota, North Carolina, Ohio and Wisconsin, but viruses of the California strain have been recovered from rodents, mosquitoes and ticks over a much wider area.

Japanese B Encephalitis. Japanese B encephalitis first appeared in Japan in 1924, affected thousands of people and killed many of them. Tending to occur in summer, it is a continuing public health hazard. It has affected, among others, large numbers of American military personnel stationed in the Far East.

The clinical picture of the acute stage of this disease is similar to that of other kinds of encephalitis. Although signs of general nervous system involvement are present at the beginning of the disease, the patient who recovers makes a complete recovery, and the unhappy consequences of encephalitis lethargica are not seen after Japanese B encephalitis. The disease is fatal in about 8 per cent of cases. In the cases that have come to autopsy there has been severe destruction of gray matter, especially in the basal nuclei, the floor of the fourth ventricle, the cerebellum and the cerebral cortex, with an inflammatory reaction appropriate to the destruction. Concomitant diffuse involvement of the spinal cord is a feature of many cases.

Tick-Borne Encephalitis. These infections may present either as meningoencephalitic forms not unlike other arbovirus encephalitides or as a paralytic form of polioencephalomyelitis. The meningoencephalic form is biphasic, the first phase being a nonspecific febrile syndrome, and the second, a more specifically meningeal and cerebral infection. The polioencephalomyelitic form produces bulbar and upper extremity paralyses, and some epidemics have had 20 to 30 per cent fatalities.

In these viral encephalitides just described, the brain is the principal site of significant infection. There are many other viral diseases in which encephalitis is exceptional or in which it is so mild that its presence escapes clinical detection. Sometimes an organism of the Coxsackie or ECHO group will produce a febrile illness with all the symptoms and signs of encephalitis, but more often any involvement of the nervous system is so mild and transient that the physician is not consulted.

Herpes Simplex Encephalitis. Herpes simplex encephalitis may take many forms, ranging from a relatively mild meningeal inflammation to fulminant, severe, necrotizing encephalitis. The disease may occur in any age group, but is most often seen in children and young adults. The lesions are frequently destructive, with a high tendency to involve the temporal lobes where the focal lesions and severe pressure effects can lead the unwary to a diagnosis of tumor or abscess. Many cases are fatal. Some patients survive with severe dementia, and in particular with a severe memory loss, but some other patients make a complete recovery after a prolonged convalescence.

Antiviral chemotherapy may turn out to be of value, and the struggle to establish a diagnosis may be worthwhile. This may be done by brain biopsy or, less traumatically, by specific immunofluorescence of inflammatory cells in the cerebrospinal fluid.

The lesions are very necrotizing and there are type A inclusions in oligodendroglia and in some nerve cells.

Myelitis. Poliomyelitis. In recent years, immunization has caused a splendid reduction in the number of cases of crippling acute anterior poliomyelitis. There is reason to hope that this disease will never again be a serious threat, but it is still worthy of study because there remain in the population large numbers of patients who have suffered the crippling effects of the disease. Furthermore, the process of infection was well studied clinically and experimentally and can serve as a guide for understanding other viral processes which involve the nervous system.

It is not known where the poliovirus exists in nature outside of man. Outbreaks of the disease occurred principally in summer, although sporadic cases appeared at other times. Although a synonym is "infantile paralysis," in the last several outbreaks older children and adults were more often affected, and some of the most catastrophic paralyses occurred in adults.

Grossly, the brain and cord are congested and edematous, and small hemorrhages may be seen. This is a nonspecific change, seen with some regularity in patients who die with respiratory failure. Cavitation in the anterior horns is a rare finding. In the more chronic state, there will be appropriate atrophy of anterior roots, peripheral nerves and muscle.

Microscopically, in the acute stage a few lymphocytes are found in the leptomeninges, and round cells form cuffs about the blood vessels, both in the meninges and the substance of the brain and cord.

The most important feature is the change in the nerve cell. Experimentally, when the virus gains access to the nerve cell, it produces an alteration in the cytoplasm, with swelling and chromatolysis and nuclear displacement. Presumably, some cells are affected to the degree that their function is lost, but their capacity for recovery remains. About such cells there may be no significant cellular reaction. The next step is cell destruction, and all degrees of swollen and shrunken nerve cells can be seen, their nuclear and cytoplasmic envelopes broken down. Near these cells in some early cases there are many neutrophils, but in other cases only a microglial or histiocytic replacement is present. These diseased and disintegrating cells are eventually replaced by an astroglial scar.

The major site of such destructive and inflammatory changes is the anterior horn of the spinal cord. The motor nuclei of the cranial nerves are involved, but only rarely are there large numbers of destroyed nerve cells as in the cord. Occasionally, in very fulminant cases, there is some overflow of lesions into the posterior horns and even into the white matter of the cord, and in such cases it is not unusual to find some cell loss and inflammatory nodules in the pons, the midbrain and the diencephalon.

In the initial period of viremia, there are nonspecific symptoms of upper respiratory or gastrointestinal involvement and fever. At this point and for days to weeks after, poliovirus may be recovered from the stools. Within a few days after the onset of the generalized symptoms, central nervous system involvement is marked by the development of headache, stiff neck and stiff back. The disease may resolve at this stage or earlier, leaving the patient normal, or signs of central nervous system destruction may appear. These signs are those of a lower motor neuron type of paralysis. Chronic permanent residual paralysis is common in the spinal segments but rare in the cranial nerve (bulbar) distribution. Although the virus of poliomyelitis may affect the nuclei of the diencephalon and even the cerebral cortex, a truly encephalitic picture is very rare. When death occurs, it is usually due to involvement of the nervous mechanisms which control respiration. This may happen as a consequence of involvement of the respiratory center in the medulla or may be due to involvement of the anterior horn cells whence arise the phrenic and intercostal nerves. The only permanent neurologic residue of poliomyelitis is a lower motor neuron paralysis. Rarely, severe myocarditis complicates or terminates the clinical course.

Sometimes Coxsackie viruses (A7, A9, B2–5) cause diagnostic confusion because they may mimic poliomyelitis. The paralysis, however, although it may be severe, is usually transitory.

Rabies. Rabies is one of the most ancient of the virus diseases. It is widespread in nature, and many animals, both domestic and wild, may be affected. In civilized parts of the world, the most frequent animal host is the dog, and the dog is the main vector for man in the United States. It has been well proved that many species of bats can transmit rabies, not only by bite but by respiratory transmission as well.

Rabies is justifiably one of the most feared of all diseases despite its infrequency. It has been uniformly fatal, although the recent recovery of a highly probable case in Ohio gives encouragement that other patients may be saved. The onset is nonspecific, with moderate fever, generalized malaise and varying degrees of headache. The incubation period in man is extremely variable, but usually is about one to three months.

On gross examination, the picture is one of intense edema and vascular congestion. There is extensive and widespread neuronal degeneration, and the severity of this form of encephalitis is attested to by the extension of the inflammatory process out into the white matter. The severity and extent of the inflammatory reaction is greatest in the basal nuclei, the midbrain and the floor of the fourth ventricle, particularly in the medulla. There is likely to be an especially severe inflammatory reaction in those roots and those parts of the brain and spinal cord segmentally related to the site of the wound of entrance of the organism.

Negri bodies are the most characteristic histologic feature. They are found in all neurons but are best seen in the cytoplasm of the large ones. They are eosinophilic and multiple, and are usually rounded, oval or bullet-shaped. They are found most characteristically in Ammon's horn of the temporal lobe but they may be almost anywhere.

In addition to the changes within the brain and cord, there may be involvement also of the dorsal root ganglia and the sympathetic ganglia.

The wound responsible for the entry of the virus is almost always evident. The virus makes its way along nerve pathways from the wound to the central nervous system, and the incubation period varies depending on the distance of the wound from the brain or spinal cord. Paresthesias in the neighborhood of the wound in conjunction with the general symptoms are diagnostic of the disease in its early stage. The patients present a picture of the most extraordinary central nervous system sensitivity. The slightest touch is painful, and the slightest movement sets up a myriad of motor responses which go on to full-blown convulsions. There are periods of alternating mania and stupor. There are signs of meningeal irritation and, as the disease progresses, flaccid paralysis occurs. Eventually the patient succumbs after a period of stupor and coma.

Lymphocytic Choriomeningitis. Lymphocytic choriomeningitis is the best known of those virus diseases of the nervous system which affect the leptomeninges almost exclusively. The virus was identified in 1934. It gets to man from a reservoir in wild mice.

Pathologically, the picture is one of an intense lymphocytic reaction in the leptomeninges and the choroid plexus. The intensity of this reaction is reflected in the cerebrospinal fluid which may show 2000 to 3000 lymphocytes. Such an intensity of lymphocytic cellular reaction in cerebrospinal fluid is almost diagnostic of this disease.

The onset is grippe-like and in many instances, as demonstrated by isolation and neutralization studies, the disease may stop at this point. However, in a certain number of patients, meningeal symptoms and signs then appear and remain severe for seven to ten days. Only rarely is it fatal. Parotitis and orchitis may occur, causing confusion with mumps.

Herpes Zoster. Herpes zoster infection in its most common clinical form is a vesicular, often painful skin eruption in the distribution of one or more spinal or cranial sensory nerve roots (p. 1392). Occasionally, motor paralysis accompanies the sensory change. The skin lesions always are associated with lesions of the corresponding dorsal root ganglion or gasserian ganglion, with varying degrees of spread both distally and proximally in nervous structures. The varicella-zoster virus is recoverable from the lesions either of skin or of nervous tissue.

Grossly, the affected dorsal root ganglion and the nearby root are congested, edematous and often hemorrhagic. Even when there is no corresponding skin lesion, the adjacent ipsilateral ganglia may participate in the pathologic process.

In the acute state, there is inflammatory change of variable degree in the dorsal root ganglion, and there may be complete necrosis of this structure. Polymorphonuclear leukocytes are found about blood vessels, and ganglion cells in varying stages of disintegration are surrounded by small round cells. An inflammatory reaction of lesser degree involves the adjacent spinal ganglia even when there is no skin lesion corresponding to these segments. There is always some inflammatory change in the corresponding spinal nerves.

The process also may extend centrally to affect the anterior and posterior roots, the leptomeninges and the corresponding segments of gray matter of the cord. Finally there may be extension throughout the nervous system to produce an encephalomyelitis.

Sometimes herpes zoster occurs in conjunction with other conditions. It may occur with infections like malaria or pyogenic leptomeningitis, with malignancies, with irradiating or chemotherapeutic treatment of malignancies, or with corticosteroid therapy or immunosuppression.

Slow Viruses. Among the major advances in the understanding of diseases of the nervous system in recent years is the recognition of several diseases caused by transmissible agents with incubation periods measurable in years rather than days or weeks.

Subacute sclerosing panencephalitis (SSPE; Inclusion body encephalitis; Dawson's encephalitis) afflicts children or young adults. Beginning with changes in mental function, sometimes of a subtle sort, the patient becomes delirious and ultimately demented, with myoclonus, convulsions and decerebration and decortication. Some patients die within a few months, while others may go on for years, sometimes with remissions. The cerebrospinal fluid, not usually heavily cellular, contains large amounts of gamma globulin (IgG). The lesions in the brain are always in gray matter but in some cases there is extensive white matter involvement as well. Sclerosis of white matter is seen more often in cases of long duration. There are the usual histologic changes of chronic encephalitis, the distinguishing feature being the presence of intranuclear and intracytoplasmic inclusion bodies in the cortical neurons, seen best in the earlier stages of the process. A measles-like virus has been isolated from the brains of these patients. Unusually high antibody titers to measles are present in both blood and cerebrospinal fluid. The present presumption is that the patient who has had classic measles years before has retained the virus in his tissues or has become peculiarly sensitized to future contact with the virus (Zeman, 1968).

Kuru is a disease of the Fore tribe of eastern New Guinea. It was the cause of death in 50 per cent of the women of the tribe and of some children. Beginning with cerebellar ataxia, the patients went on to develop widespread involvement of forebrain and ultimately died of intercurrent malnutrition and infection within a three to six month period. The brains show extensive neuronal destruction and astrocytic proliferation. A transmissible agent has been recovered from the brains and passed through several generations of chimpanzees which, after a one to two year incubation period, have developed a disease clinically and pathologically similar to Kuru. Since cannibalism has been stopped among the Fore, the disease is dying out. It is likely that the patients were infected by eating diseased brain.

Creutzfeldt-Jakob disease occurs in middleaged people, is not heredofamilial and produces a dementia associated with myoclonus, leading to death over a 6 to 12 month period. The lesions consist of spongiform areas of degeneration in gray matter, especially cerebral cortex, with intense and often disorderly astrocytic reaction. The lesions resemble those seen in some animal diseases, particularly scrapie and mink encephalopathy. In recent years, the disease has been transmitted to chimpanzees by the injection of brain suspensions from affected patients. The incubation period in the chimpanzee is 15 to 24 months.

Progressive Multifocal Leukoencephalopathy. Patients suffering from non-nervous malignant neoplasia may develop a subacute encephalopathy which is generally progressive to death over a period of a few months. There are early alterations of awareness and signs of gross disruption of hemispheric white matter. The brain contains focal areas of demyelination, sometimes confluent. Axis cylinders persist in the less severe lesions. There are enlarged and deformed glial nuclei, probably of both astrocytes and oligodendroglia, which contain type A inclusions. Virus forms have been identified in these lesions, belonging to the papova group. It is probable that the virus, not normally pathogenic for man, is allowed to flourish because of the reduced immune response of the patient with malignant disease.

PROTOZOAL DISEASE

Primary Amebic Meningoencephalitis. A cerebral amebiasis of relatively mild form is sometimes produced by the intestinal parasite *Entamoeba histolytica.* Since 1965, cases have been appearing of a new kind of amebiasis of the central nervous system, designated as primary amebic meningoencephalitis. It is seen in children or young adults who give a history of swimming, within the preceding week, in brackish water during hot weather. The patients develop severe headache with disturbances of smell and taste, and go on to the symptoms and signs of purulent leptomeningitis. Amebas can be seen in the spinal fluid. All patients die in 3 to 5 days. There is no known treatment. The pathologic changes are

of a purulent hemorrhagic leptomeningitis, with hemorrhagic necrosis of the cerebral cortex, especially in the basifrontal and basitemporal regions. The causative organism is always the free-living *Naegleria gruberi* (Duma, 1969).

Toxoplasmosis. *Toxoplasma gondii* is a protozoon which produces an encephalitis in the newborn, characterized by increasing hydrocephalus, convulsions and chorioretinitis (Frenkel and Friedlander, 1951). There are rare cases on record of acute encephalitis in older children due to this organism. The encephalitis of the newborn is acquired prenatally as a consequence of a transient infection, almost always unrecognized, in the mother (p. 455).

The organisms create a very destructive granulomatous inflammation of the leptomeninges, the ependyma, the brain substance and the eye. The organisms are seen as pseudocysts in the granulomas (Fig. 32–16). Obstruction of the flow of cerebrospinal fluid produces hydrocephalus (Fig. 32–17). The lesions tend to calcify early, accounting for the characteristic opacities seen on roentgenograms of the skull.

The outcome is fatal within weeks to months in almost all cases. In those patients who do survive there are profound mental deficiency, convulsive disorder and other evidences of severe destruction of brain tissue.

African Trypanosomiasis. *T. gambiense* and *T. rhodesiense* are parasites of tropical Africa, responsible for large numbers of cases of the vicious African sleeping sickness. The tsetse fly (Glossina) is the vector. When the fly bites a human, an inflammatory response

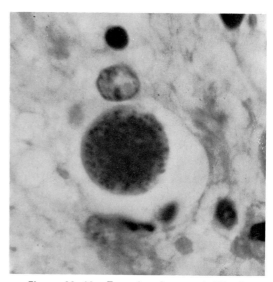

Figure 32–16. *Toxoplasmic encephalitis. A pseudocyst is filled with the organisms.*

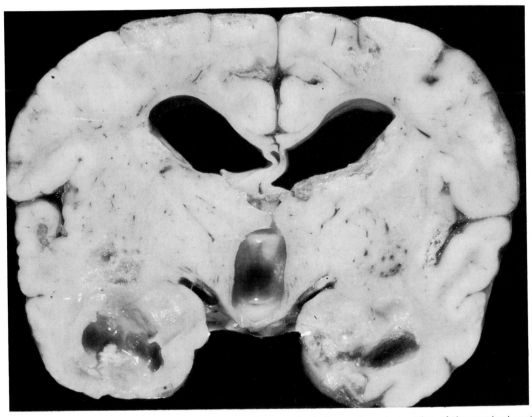

Figure 32–17. *Toxoplasmic encephalitis. There is extensive inflammatory destruction of the cerebral cortex and the periventricular structures.*

occurs locally, followed by local and generalized lymphadenopathy. Disorders of consciousness, involuntary movements, widespread pain, paralysis, gait disorders and reflex changes reflect the involvement of the nervous system. Not all cases are fatal, but death usually comes in several weeks. At autopsy the meninges are thickened by fibrosis, there are destroyed nerve cells at all levels, and the vessels are surrounded by an exudate consisting in large part of plasma cells. The trypanosomes are difficult to visualize in routine autopsy material.

VASCULAR DISEASE

The most common cause of lesions in the brain is disease of the cerebral blood vessels. As elsewhere in the body, hypertension and arteriosclerosis are the principal underlying causes. The form and distribution of a cerebral vascular lesion in any instance is dependent upon a multitude of anatomic and physiologic variables in the cerebral vascular tree itself, in the rest of the circulation, and in the other organ systems of the body.

BLOOD SUPPLY AND VENOUS DRAINAGE OF THE BRAIN

The arterial blood supply of the brain is provided by the two internal carotid arteries and the vertebral arteries.

The internal carotid artery is formed on each side by the bifurcation of the common carotid artery at the upper level of the thyroid cartilage. It ascends to take a curved course through the petrous bone and then traverses the cavernous sinus, finally penetrating the dura on the medial side of the anterior clinoid process. The ophthalmic artery arises from the cavernous portion. Shortly after emerging from the cavernous sinus, the internal carotid artery divides into the posterior communicating, middle cerebral and anterior cerebral arteries. The anterior communicating connects the two anterior cerebrals to form the anterior portion of the circle of Willis.

The vertebral artery, after its origin from the subclavian, runs upward and backward to enter the foramen in the transverse process of the sixth cervical vertebra, and passes upward in the transverse processes of the upper six vertebrae. After leaving the foramen of the atlas, it makes an S-shaped curve rather like that of the internal carotid, and then penetrates the dura at the caudal end of the medulla. Just beyond this point, each vertebral gives off a caudally and medially directed branch, which fuse to form the anterior spinal artery. At the junction of medulla and pons, the vertebral arteries fuse to form the basilar, which continues rostrally to divide at the tentorial opening into the posterior cerebral arteries, which in turn receive the posterior communicating arteries to complete the circle of Willis.

Anomalies of this classic distribution are very common. For example, one vertebral artery may be only a thin thread of a vessel while the other is as large as the basilar artery itself. Sometimes the posterior cerebral artery receives its major supply from the internal carotid artery through an anomalously large posterior communicating artery. Almost any combination of anomalous vascular arrangement may occur. Under normal conditions, such anomalies do not interfere with the effective vascularization of the brain, but when disease of the vessels occurs, the anomaly may result in an atypical and confusing sequence of clinical and pathologic events.

Under normal conditions, blood from one carotid artery or even from one vertebral artery remains on its own side of the brain. However, if one internal carotid artery is occluded in the neck, presuming the rest of the system to be normal, an adequate perfusion of the territory of the occluded vessel is accomplished by a shunting of blood from the opposite internal carotid and the basilar. Such a shunt is the physical consequence of the pressure gradient between the distal portions of the patent and occluded vessels. In addition to this reserve given by the circle of Willis, other anastomotic vessels of smaller order provide an additional margin of safety. These are the anastomotic channels in the leptomeninges of base and convexity between the anterior, middle and posterior cerebral arteries, and between the branches of the vertebral-basilar system in the posterior fossa.

All the major arteries at the base of the brain have a similar plan of branching. From each vessel there arise perforating branches, which provide blood to the midline structures. Short circumferential arteries supply structures out from the midline and long circumferential arteries extend out to the more distant parts of cerebrum and cerebellum.

The finer angio-architecture of the brain is like that elsewhere, a network of arteries, arterioles, capillaries, venules and veins, with generous anastomoses. This is in contrast to some of the older views, which held that the arteries of the brain were end arteries. The density of the capillary bed varies from place to place, and is presumed to be directly proportional to the metabolic activity of the area. As a general rule, although not without its exceptions, capillary density corresponds to density of synaptic connections.

The venous drainage of the brain corresponds roughly to the arterial supply. Large veins course through the leptomeninges and drain into the venous sinuses of the dura mater, all of which then drain into the internal jugular veins. The midline cerebral structures are drained by a system of internal cerebral veins which fuse to form the great vein of Galen, which then proceeds directly into the sinus rectus. There are no valves in the venous system which drains the brain.

Microscopically, the blood vessels of the brain are not much different from those elsewhere in the body. The relation to the glial framework has already been noted. In the arteries there is a well developed internal elastic lamina, but an external elastic lamina is absent. The smaller arteries and arterioles have no distinct elastica at all, and they are difficult and sometimes impossible to distinguish from veins of corresponding size.

PHYSIOLOGY OF THE CEREBRAL CIRCULATION

Certain physiologic data are essential for an understanding of the pathology of cerebral vascular disease (Fields, 1961). The most important consideration is the enormous oxygen requirement of the brain. It has been pointed out that the brain represents only 2 per cent of the body weight, yet in the resting state receives one-sixth of the cardiac output, and is responsible for 20 per cent of the body's oxygen consumption. The responsibility for this disproportionately high requirement of the brain oxygen belongs principally to the nerve cell, by which is meant not only the nucleus and cytoplasm seen under ordinary magnification with traditional staining, but also the axonal and dendritic surfaces and connections. Deprivation of oxygen results first in a loss of function followed by destruction. The survival time of a nerve cell depends upon the duration and intensity of hypoxia under different circumstances, but experimentally it would appear that the nerve cell can resist total deprivation of oxygen for no longer than a few minutes.

The cerebral circulation does not follow

passively the changes in systemic blood pressure. Cerebral blood flow is maintained, even when the blood pressure drops drastically, by alteration of cerebrovascular resistance, a result obtained through the intervention of several metabolic and reflex homeostatic mechanisms. It would appear that cerebral blood flow is more dependent upon cardiac output than upon systemic blood pressure per se.

The brain can resist loss of function or structure if a noxious circulatory change occurs sufficiently gradually. Acutely reduced levels of oxyhemoglobin, whatever the cause, can produce more change in nervous tissue than the same levels attained gradually. In the same way acute ischemia, as in vascular occlusion, is more likely to produce symptoms and signs than when the occlusion develops more slowly. Such mechanisms of adaptation and compensation, although poorly understood, are important in the degree of neuropathologic change consequent upon a disease process.

Not included to any appreciable degree among the protective mechanisms is autonomic nervous control of vascular constriction and dilatation. Whereas spasm of cerebral vessels can occur in response to certain nonphysiologic stimuli, such as direct percussion of a vessel, stimulation of the sympathetic ganglia produces in the intracerebral circulation only one-eighth the degree of vasoconstriction which is attainable in the extracranial circulation. Further, autonomic stimulation produces only an insignificant vasodilating effect. Low oxygen tension or high carbon dioxide tension can produce powerful vasodilatation, and high oxygen or low carbon dioxide tension can produce a moderate vasoconstriction.

ANOXIC ENCEPHALOPATHY

The mechanisms which are operative to protect the brain against hypoxia become ineffective in the more extreme degrees of change and in the presence of preexisting disease of the cerebral blood vessels. In the normal person, the systolic blood pressure may go acutely as low as 70 mm. Hg without necessarily producing symptoms and signs of brain dysfunction. In a person with severe atherosclerosis of the cerebral vessels, or in a person with well established hypertension, a lesser degree of fall in systolic pressure may produce anoxic change.

Pathogenesis. Any process which reduces the effective *oxygenated* perfusion of the brain can result in anoxic (or hypoxic) encephalopathy (Plum and Posner, 1972). Systemic hypotension, reduced cardiac output, respiratory failure due to muscular or pulmonary causes, and depletion of oxyhemoglobin due to anemia or intoxication are the most common causes. Anoxic encephalopathy is rightly the most feared effect of any medical or surgical disease or procedure.

The changes in the brain in hypoxia depend on the duration and intensity of the hypoxia and upon the duration of survival. In cases with only a few minutes or a few hours' survival, no change is seen regardless of the severity of the insult. When the insult has been very slight, the nerve cells may recover function and no anatomic change may occur. The first demonstrable anatomic change, seen after a survival of 12 to 24 hours, is in the nerve cells. Most vulnerable are the large cells in Sommer's sector of the hippocampus, followed by the Purkinje cells of the cerebellum. The primary motor areas and receptive areas are relatively spared in contrast to the severe involvement of the association areas. If the areas of destruction are extensive, the brain may be swollen, and a muddy discoloration of the affected parts can be seen with some loss of the usual demarcation between gray and white matter.

Microscopically, the cells show ischemic cell change, although some may be swollen rather than shrunken. In the cortex, the process is widespread but not complete; clusters of damaged cells lie near unaffected cells, even in the same cortical lamina. In very severe cases there may be lengthy areas of confluence of the damaged cells, and in such areas the staining capacity of the tissue is reduced or lost. As time goes on, the anatomic changes correspond to what one would expect from the early lesions. The nerve cells drop out, to be replaced by glia. Frank necrosis followed by glial scarring occurs in the areas of greater destruction so that a "laminar necrosis" interrupts the normal continuity of the cerebral cortex. The degree of cortical atrophy in the long-term case is proportional to the amount of nerve cell destruction.

In some instances there is patchy destruction of the immediately subcortical white matter. In others there is symmetrical necrosis of the globus pallidus.

Clinical Course. The effect of cerebral hypoxia upon the patient depends upon its intensity and duration and upon the maintenance of an effective systemic circulation. When the deprivation of oxygen has been slight, there may be an early euphoria, followed by listlessness, drowsiness, apathy and defective judgment. This sequence of events is seen, for example, in people exposed to the low oxygen tension of high altitudes. When the deficit is severe and especially when it is sudden, unconsciousness and convulsions may occur. The patients develop the clinical appearance of decortication, with the head retracted, the arms and hands flexed and the legs held in rigid extension. When the brain swelling produces herniation, the picture of decerebration may appear. Patients who recover are often left with a considerable deficit. They are often demented, have bilateral spasticity, and some of them have a liability to recurrent convulsions. Visual agnosia is a not uncommon end result.

INFARCTION OF THE BRAIN

Infarction of the brain *(encephalomalacia)* is the consequence of the deprivation of blood supply to a localized area. When there is deprivation of blood to the totality of brain, as in cardiac arrest, the result is either death or the more diffuse change already discussed as anoxic encephalopathy.

Etiology and Pathogenesis. Although infarcts are the most common lesions of brain substance, much remains to be learned about their pathogenesis. Certain propositions are worth presenting at the outset, since they are helpful in approaching some of the areas of controversy and uncertainty.

1. Sudden complete occlusion of a vessel, as by an embolus, usually results in infarction of the tissue in the distribution of supply of the occluded vessel.

2. Gradual occlusion of a vessel, as in the concentric obliteration of a vascular lumen by an atheroma, does not necessarily produce infarction.

3. Infarction may occur under certain circumstances in the territory of a vessel which is stenosed but not completely occluded.

4. When the structural integrity of an area of the brain is threatened by ischemia resulting from vascular occlusion or stenosis, the fixed collaterals must be utilized for adequate blood flow through the threatened area. If these collaterals are adequate and if blood flow can be restored in time, infarction does not occur. If they are inadequate for any reason, the result is infarction.

The collaterals of which we speak are fixed channels; the time interval in which they must respond occupies seconds or minutes, not hours or days. Whenever the integrity of a given area of brain is threatened by ischemia, there is an interval of crisis, called by Denny-Brown (1945) the *cerebral hemodynamic crisis.* A crisis by definition cannot continue indefinitely, and the resolution of a cerebral hemodynamic crisis is favorable if the collaterals succeed, and unfavorable if they fail.

The principal causes for the ultimate development of infarcts in brain are emboli to cerebral vessels, arteriosclerotic vascular disease and the inflammatory arteritides.

Emboli to cerebral vessels come chiefly from the heart, either from atrial thrombi in fibrillation, from ventricular mural thrombi in myocardial infarction or from the valvular accumulations of bacterial or nonbacterial endocarditis. Some emboli may come from thrombi in the great vessels of the aortic arch and its branches, and sometimes a detached particle of atheroma may be the emblous. Fat emboli may come from broken bones and air emboli whenever air enters the general circulation. Even amniotic fluid emboli have been described in the brain.

Infarctions in the inflammatory arteritides arise when thrombi form in the lumen of inflamed vessels. Infectious arteritis leading to infarcts occurs in the longstanding meningitides, such as tuberculosis and influenza. In addition, angiitis and thrombotic vascular occlusion may occur with other processes, such as Boeck's sarcoid, hyperergic angiitis, polyarteritis nodosa, lupus erythematosus and other disorders. Giant cell arteritis (temporal arteritis), although most often encountered in the scalp vessels, may involve the arteries of the brain as well.

Atherosclerosis produces infarction in the brain by vascular changes similar to those in the coronary circulation which produce myocardial infarction. Thrombi may form on an atheromatous plaque, or intravascular clotting may occur in an area of stenosis in which the stream is slowed or where eddying occurs. These mechanical obstructions in vessels are obvious causes of infarction in atherosclerosis, but there are some cases of infarction in which no thrombus may be found, or in which the demonstrated thrombus is not adequate to explain the distribution or duration of the infarction. There are also cases in which fresh infarction has occurred in the territory of a vessel which appears to have been totally occluded for weeks or months or even years. In such cases, more dynamic concepts must be invoked to explain why the infarct occurred when it did.

The territory of an artery which is occluded or severely stenosed depends for its structural integrity upon the functional capacity of the collaterals, which depends in turn largely upon their relative patency and the state of the general circulation. These hemodynamic concepts have already been explained in detail in the consideration of the genesis of infarcts of all tissues (p. 343) and in the development of myocardial infarcts. To summarize, four factors govern the development of an infarct:

1. The general status of the cardiovascular system.
2. The anatomic pattern of the vascular supply.
3. The collateral circulation.
4. The vulnerability of the tissue to ischemia.

Review of these factors makes clear the genesis of a fresh infarct in an area supplied by a markedly narrowed vessel—precipitated, for example, by a drop in systemic blood pressure. Neither are paradoxic infarcts unknown to the brain, as, for example, when collaterals from the right internal carotid artery maintain a marginal area ordinarily supplied by the left internal carotid. Occlusion then of the right internal carotid leads to infarction in the distribution of the left.

Grossly, an infarct may be either ischemic or hemorrhagic. The original mechanism is the same for each—deprivation of blood to a given area. The infarct which becomes hemorrhagic at a later stage was originally ischemic, but blood flow was once again restored to vessels which had been rendered abnormally permeable by ischemia, so that diapedesis of blood surrounded the blood vessels in the infarct (Fig. 32–18). A hemorrhagic infarct therefore can occur in embolism, if the embolus moves distally from its original point of stenosis or occlusion when the collaterals restore flow into the ischemic area.

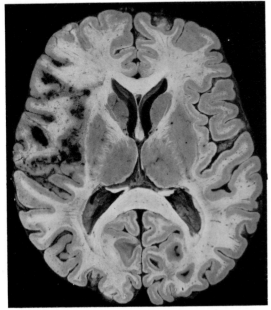

Figure 32–18. *Hemorrhagic infarct in part of the supply of the middle cerebral artery.*

The gross pathology of infarction of the brain is not demonstrable with any certainty before about five to six hours of survival. The earliest change is a slight discoloration of the affected area, so that the gray matter takes on a muddy color (Fig. 32–19) and the white matter loses its normal fine-grained appearance. There is fuzziness of the usual clear border between gray and white matter. Within 48 to 72 hours, necrosis is well established and there is mushy disintegration of the ischemic area (Fig. 32–20), with a stage of pronounced swelling which produces herniation in lesions of sufficient size. Eventually, if the lesion is of sufficient size, there is liquefaction and cyst formation, the cyst being traversed by trabeculations of blood vessels and surrounded by a firm glial barrier. The leptomeninges, if in contact with the infarct, become thickened and opaque, and often form the outer wall of a cyst (Fig. 32–21). In hemorrhagic infarction, the sequence of events in the gross is the same except that there is blood in the beginning, and the orange-brown discoloration of hemosiderin in macrophages is prominent beyond the early stages.

The first histologic change, seen after about 6 to 12 hours of survival, is a diffuse reduction of the staining power of the tissue. In chromatic stains, **the first discrete change is in the nerve cell body which becomes swollen, with disarrangement and disintegration of chromatin substance of nucleus and cytoplasm.** In addition, but probably following the initial swelling of the cell, there are large numbers of cells showing **classic ischemic cell change: shrunken, tortuous cell bodies with pyknotic nuclei and, in combined stains, bright eosinophilic cytoplasm.** Myelin sheath or axis cylinder stains at this stage show interruption and disintegration of these structures.

At about 48 hours, the blood vessels stand out prominently and some polymorphonuclear leukocytes begin to pass through the vessel wall and extend out into the tissue. Infrequently this response is so intense as to simulate a septic infarct, but usually it is replaced at 72 to 96 hours by the prominent appearance of histiocytes about blood vessels. From this stage on, the histiocytes are the dominant cell of reaction, attaining their maximum at about two weeks. After this they diminish gradually, but even years later histiocytes are still found in the interstices of old infarcts. In ischemic infarcts they are fat-filled; early in hemorrhagic infarcts they may contain red cells, but in the end they are filled with hemosiderin.

The oligodendroglia are next in vulnerability to the neuronal elements, and in the usual infarct they disappear almost completely. The astrocytes also are destroyed in severe lesions, but they are more resistant than the oligodendroglia. The astrocytes at the edge of the lesion show prominent activation at five to seven days and, becoming

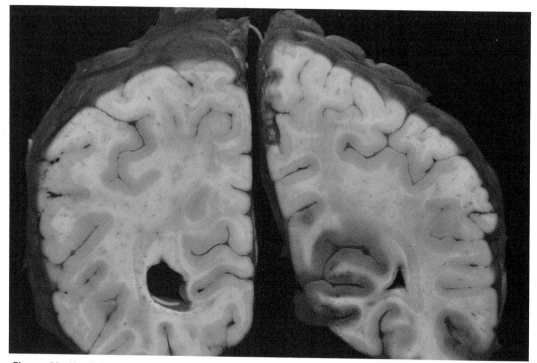

Figure 32–19. *Infarction (on the right) in partial distribution of the posterior cerebral artery. There is slight swelling; the cortex is discolored.*

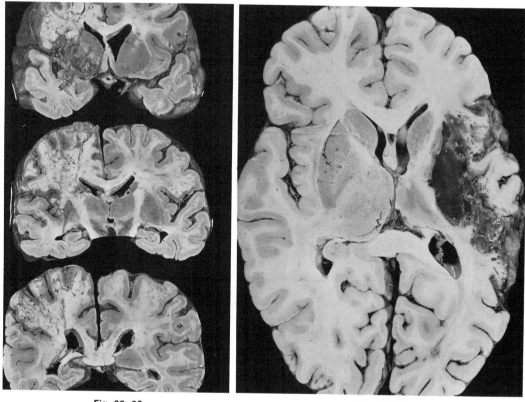

Fig. 32–20

Fig. 32–21

Figure 32–20. *Extensive infarction (on the left) in the distribution of the middle cerebral artery. The usual landmarks are obscured as the infarcted tissue reaches the state of disintegration.*

Figure 32–21. *Old cystic infarction with scar formation.*

hypertrophied, they proliferate, send out fibers and form the ultimate astroglial scar.

There are dozens of variations on this classic theme of response to infarction, depending upon the intensity and the distribution of the ischemic process. These variations can be understood if the order of descending vulnerabilities of the elements is kept in mind: nerve cell, axis cylinder and myelin sheath, oligodendroglia, astrocytes and blood vessels.

Very common in hypertensive patients, but occurring also in some diabetics and some very elderly people, are small lesions of a few millimeters or less, which are called lacunar infarcts. They are the consequence of occlusions in very small arteries. A frequent clinical association is the syndrome of pseudobulbar palsy.

Clinical Course—the Arterial Syndromes.
The symptoms and signs of infarction of the brain depend upon the size of the lesion and the structures involved. Generally it is possible to designate the specific artery on the basis of the clinical picture. A few general observations are of some assistance in understanding the variations.

Loss of consciousness in infarction is generally correlated with the amount of brain involved. For example, hemiplegia, hemianesthesia and hemianopsia may result from a lesion in the total distribution of the middle cerebral artery, a very large area, and loss of consciousness always occurs. But these same manifestations may occur without loss of consciousness in a lesion of the anterior choroidal artery, since the area involved is so small.

Convulsions at the onset of an infarct are uncommon. They are more frequent in embolism. In some cases, as in internal carotid artery lesions, they represent a diffuse cerebral ischemia of sudden onset. Convulsions as a late consequence of infarcts are relatively common, and they can usually be correlated with old scars in cerebral cortex.

The Internal Carotid Artery. The supply of this vessel is the combination of the supply of the anterior and middle cerebral arteries as well as the ophthalmic artery. In chronic occlusion of the vessel, intermittent episodic losses of function with recovery in one or other parts of its total supply occur repeatedly. There may be transient faciobrachial or crural hemiplegia, transient episodes of monocular blindness or other manifestations. On one final occasion, recovery may fail to occur and an infarct in a localized part of the distribution of the vessel is found. Acute occlusion, as in embolism, produces unconsciousness and complete loss of function of the opposite side of the body, and is almost always fatal. Herniation of the swol-

len hemisphere under the falx or through the tentorium adds more damage and complicates the clinical findings.

The Anterior Cerebral Artery. This vessel supplies the anterior part of the anterior limb of the internal capsule by a small branch (Heubner's artery) which penetrates the anterior perforated space. It supplies a large part of the orbital surface and the tip of the frontal lobe, the entire mesial surface of the hemisphere back to the parieto-occipital junction, a thin rim of contiguous parasagittal convexity, the ipsilateral part of the corpus callosum and the anterior portion of the caudate nucleus.

A complete infarct produces unconsciousness at the onset, mental symptoms, a hemiplegia involving mostly the leg and a cortical sensory deficit in the leg. Incomplete lesions may produce any one or any combination of these effects.

The Middle Cerebral Artery. The area of supply of this artery is enormous. The cortical branches extend up from the sylvian region to supply the entire convexity except for the small areas at the frontal and occipital poles and the parasagittal rim of the anterior cerebral distribution. In addition, the cortex of the lateral orbital frontal surface and the tip of the temporal lobe fall within the territory of this vessel. Penetrating branches supply the internal capsule, the caudate, the lenticular nucleus and the anterior thalamus.

Infarction in the total distribution of this vessel produces a functional deficit similar to that seen in total internal carotid lesions. The patient is unconscious, there is a dense loss of all motor, sensory and visual function contralateral to the lesion, and the massive swelling with herniations produces an additional complexity to the clinical picture. If the patient lives and regains consciousness, the neurologic deficit is severe, complex and permanent. If the lesion is in the dominant hemisphere, aphasia, apraxia or agnosia is added. The clinical manifestations of parietal lobe dysfunction appear in some form, regardless of the side of the lesion.

Incomplete degrees of infarction in the distribution of the middle cerebral artery are more common, and a complete documentation is not possible without a prolonged discussion of the anatomy and physiology of the cerebral hemispheres. But it should be remembered that infarction in the territory of this artery is the most common cause of hemiplegia, and that the vessel has been called "the artery of aphasia."

The Posterior Cerebral Artery. By recurrent and penetrating branches from near the point of its formation from the basilar artery, the posterior cerebral artery supplies the midbrain and the superior cerebellar peduncle, the posterior part of the thalamus, including the lateral geniculate body, and the most posterior part of the internal capsule. Coursing around the cerebral peduncle on its way to the occipital lobe, it gives off branches to the base and all but the most anterior part of the medial surface of the temporal lobe. The posterior part of the corpus callosum (splenium) receives branches, and finally there is a large distribution to the medial surface of the occipital lobe.

Infarction in the total distribution is very infrequent. In portions of this territory, infarctions produce some characteristic and interesting symptoms. Involvement of the thalamus and lateral geniculate body gives contralateral hemianopsia and hemianesthesia. A lesion in or about the subthalamic nucleus gives contralateral hemiballismus. Damage to the medial surface of the occipital lobe produces quadrantanopsia or hemianopsia. Oculomotor palsy with contralateral tremor (Benedikt's syndrome) is due to involvement of the red nucleus and third nerve fibers. Oculomotor palsy with contralateral hemiplegia (Weber's syndrome) is due to involvement of third nerve fibers and the basis pedunculi.

The Vertebral-Basilar System. The arteries of the vertebral-basilar system supply the structures of the posterior fossa (medulla, pons, midbrain, cerebellum) before the basilar bifurcates into the posterior cerebral arteries. Clinically, chronic occlusion or stenosis of the vertebral-basilar system produces intermittent manifestations similar to those of the internal carotid lesions, but with cranial nerve, cerebellar and bilateral corticospinal tract manifestations.

Complete infarction in the vertebralbasilar distribution is incompatible with life, and in fact almost never occurs, there being effective collaterals in the form of anastomoses between the posterior inferior cerebellar artery (a branch of vertebral) and the anterior inferior and superior cerebellar arteries (branches of basilar). Incomplete infarction may occur as a consequence of occlusion of individual branches from the main trunk or as a localized effect distal to the point of occlusion. Thus an infarct in the distribution of the left posterior cerebral artery may be due to an occlusion in the left vertebral artery, or an occlusion in the caudal part of the basilar artery may produce only irregular patchy infarction in either pons, midbrain, thalamus, or basal-medial temporal or occipital cortex.

The Posterior Inferior Cerebellar Artery Syn- **drome.** Lesions of this artery produce an infarction of the dorsolateral medulla which is characterized by dysarthria, dysphagia, ipsilateral Horner's syndrome, ipsilateral cerebellar signs, ipsilateral loss of pain and temperature on the face and contralateral loss of pain and temperature on the body. The syndrome of the *anterior inferior cerebellar artery* is the same except that instead of dysarthria and dysphagia there is ipsilateral seventh nerve weakness. In the syndrome of the *superior cerebellar artery*, the motor manifestations are in the extraocular muscles, and there is contralateral loss of pain and temperature on the face and body. The raison d'être of these syndromes can be understood by simple recourse to an anatomy text.

HEMORRHAGE IN THE BRAIN

Hemorrhage into brain substance is caused by hypertensive cerebral vascular disease, by trauma, by rupture of aneurysms, by angiomas, by blood dyscrasias and by bleeding into tumors. Atherosclerosis without hypertension is not a cause. Hypertension is the most common cause, being 10 to 20 times more frequent than all the other causes in routine autopsies in a large general hospital.

Hypertensive hemorrhage into the brain is the most common cause of death in the group of cerebral vascular diseases. Whereas infarcts are more common, they do not cause death unless they are massive, while recovery after hypertensive hemorrhage, although possible, is very infrequent.

The mechanism of this common lesion is not understood, although certain facts are generally agreed upon. It occurs in patients who have had significant systolic-diastolic elevation for at least several years. The vessel which is the source of the bleeding is in the brain substance, not in the leptomeninges. The occurrence of the hemorrhage is usually related to at least mild exertion; it almost never happens during sleep. The idea that miliary aneurysms of the small arteries were produced by hypertension and then ruptured is no longer accepted. Some have theorized that vascular spasm in a group of vessels leads to infarct necrosis which, in turn, leads to rupture of the damaged blood vessels. The fact is that there is no good explanation of the pathogenesis. What is known is that a blood vessel may burst within the brain substance in a hypertensive patient.

It is important to distinguish between a true hemorrhage and a hemorrhagic infarct. A hemorrhagic infarct corresponds to the supply of a given artery; **a hemorrhage may overlap arterial sup-plies.** In a hemorrhagic infarct, the architecture of the tissue remains, with diapedesis of red blood cells into the tissue surrounding the blood vessels; in a hemorrhage, the architecture is destroyed to be replaced by blood. Under some circumstances, an infarct may be so hemorrhagic that one has some trouble distinguishing it from a true hemorrhage.

Hypertensive hemorrhage has certain areas of predilection. About 80 per cent are in the cerebral hemispheres, 10 per cent in the pons or midbrain, and 10 per cent in the cerebellum. Of the hemorrhages in the hemisphere, the largest number occur in the lateral ganglionic region, i.e., the putamen and claustrum. Next in frequency are those in the thalamus, and finally a small number occur in the white matter of the hemispheres. Although there is no doubt that a hemorrhage into white matter can be the result of hypertension, such a location always demands a search for another etiology, especially angioma, trauma or blood dyscrasia.

Most hemorrhages are of very large size. Infrequently one sees a relatively small slit-like lesion in the lateral ganglionic region or a small rounded lesion in the thalamus (Fig. 32—22) or cerebellum, but for the most part hypertensive hemorrhage is a massive lesion, occupying 50 to 80 per cent of the entire hemisphere (Fig. 32—23). The tissue in the path is wiped out by the bleeding, and about the edge the remaining tissue is compressed, distorted and discolored. Ring hemorrhages of small and large size are common, and infarction, either arterial or venous, is not unusual in those parts of the hemisphere which have not been destroyed by the hemorrhage itself. Edema is massive, the ventricles are displaced, the ipsilateral one compressed. Herniations are the rule: tentorial and subfalcial in cerebral hemorrhage, foraminal in brain stem and cerebellar hemorrhage. Rupture into the ventricle occurs in almost all large ones, and into the subarachnoid space in many. From this gross appearance, it can be appreciated that hypertensive hemorrhage is the most destructive and most final nontraumatic lesion which can affect the brain.

Histologically, the sequence of events is what one might expect. The surrounding tissue is ringed with multiple smaller perivascular hemorrhages. In the early stages there is intense congestion of the blood vessels with exudation of polymorphonuclear neutrophils from their wall. At about 3 to 4 days, the histiocytes become activated, phagocytizing red cells, and eventually, in large numbers, becoming filled with hemosiderin, persisting in diminishing numbers for years. The astrocytes become very active at about the seventh or eighth day and form a dense scar in which fibroblasts also play a significant part.

Hypertensive cerebral vascular disease is essentially a disorder of smaller arteries and arterioles. Therefore, in hypertensive hemorrhage the

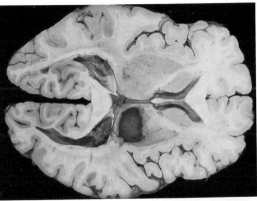

Fig. 32-22

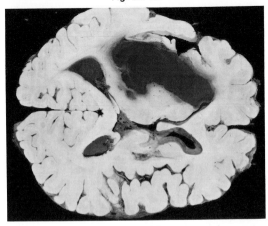

Fig. 32-23

Figure 32-22. Hypertensive hemorrhage, thalamus.

Figure 32-23. Hypertensive hemorrhage, massive, probably beginning in lateral ganglionic region but becoming widespread and rupturing into lateral ventricle.

characteristic changes are seen: thickening of the walls of these vessels, increase in cellularity of some, hyalinization, sometimes with necrosis, of others. Although in many cases of hypertension there is concomitant severe atherosclerosis, this is not a necessary association. In many cases of hypertensive hemorrhage, there is no atherosclerosis of the vessels of the circle of Willis or of the smaller vessels.

Clinical Course. The typical clinical history of hypertensive hemorrhage is of sudden onset with collapse, but there are some cases in which the onset is less apoplectic, beginning with headache and small focal signs before the final collapse. In supratentorial cerebral hemorrhage, there is usually a massive flaccid hemiplegia at the outset, and eventually decerebration and cranial nerve signs appear as a consequence of tentorial herniation. In cerebellar hemorrhage, intractable vomiting is

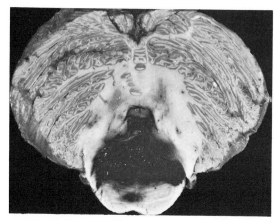

Fig. 32–24

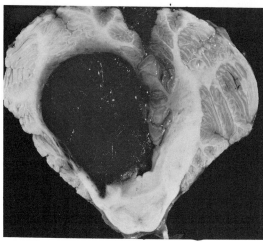

Fig. 32–25

Figure 32–24. Hypertensive hemorrhage, pons.
Figure 32–25. Hypertensive hemorrhage, cerebellum, with rupture into fourth ventricle and distortion and displacement of brain stem.

common. In pontine hemorrhage, there are pupillary and extraocular muscle disturbances. In cerebellar and pontine hemorrhage, with rupture into the fourth ventricle and foraminal herniation (Figs. 32–24 and 32–25), death may occur within a few hours, whereas in cerebral hemorrhage the patient usually survives for several days. In all cases there is blood in the cerebrospinal fluid.

Hemorrhages which occur into the brain substance from blood dyscrasias, such as leukemia, thrombocytopenia and other states, may be as massive as hypertensive hemorrhage but usually are less extensive, less destructive, and curiously likely to be in occipital white matter.

HYPERTENSIVE ENCEPHALOPATHY

Hypertensive encephalopathy occurs in hypertensive vascular disease as an acute clinical condition in which there is a severe and usually abrupt elevation of systolic and diastolic blood pressure, headache, clouding of consciousness and convulsions, leading to stupor or coma. There are usually retinal changes with papilledema, exudates and hemorrhages, and a degree of renal failure is also present. The patient may die or may recover.

The pathogenesis is related to acute, severe increases in intravascular pressure. Longstanding hypertension is not necessary for its development, since it can occur in eclampsia and other acute hypertensive episodes, and can be produced experimentally in animals. In addition, lowering of the blood pressure can produce the most extraordinary relief of the signs and symptoms.

Since this is essentially an acute disturbance in the hemodynamics of smaller arteries and arterioles, it is not surprising that there is no consistent clinicopathologic correlation. A few findings are relatively constant at autopsy. The brain is very swollen, even to the production of herniation. Microscopically, there are the changes of hypertensive disease in patients with longstanding hypertension, and in some of these patients there may be fibrinoid necrosis of some vessel walls. Microinfarcts and petechial hemorrhages appear in some cases. There may be perivascular deposits of high-protein fluid, or fibrin, or round cells in longer-lasting cases. But it is important to remember that this is a functional disorder which may kill the patient before any of these morphologic changes appear.

ANEURYSMS OF THE VESSELS OF THE BRAIN

Aneurysms of the vessels of the brain are of three sorts: mycotic, arteriosclerotic fusiform, and congenital saccular (Walton, 1956).

Mycotic aneurysms are the result of infected emboli, which produce a septic degeneration of the elastic and muscular coats of the vessel wall with resultant rupture and subarachnoid hemorrhage. They are far less common than when subacute bacterial endocarditis was a frequent clinical and pathologic occurrence, but still are seen in patients whose artificial valves have become foci of infection from which septic emboli arise.

Arteriosclerotic fusiform aneurysms are the result of a combination of severe hypertension and severe atherosclerosis of the vessels of the circle of Willis. In longstanding hypertension, even without associated atherosclerosis, the vessels of the circle become tortuous and sometimes dilated. This is best seen in the vertebral-basilar system and is seen almost as well in the carotid-middle cerebral tree. When atherosclerosis is associated with this change, elongated fusiform dilatations of the vessels may occur, with irregular points of constriction and ectasia. The extreme degree of this change is seen in the vertebral-basilar system, where the vertebrals may fuse far laterally in the cerebellopontine angle, giving rise to a tortuous, dilated, fusiform basilar artery which runs diagonally across the base of the pons, grooving the pontine base (Fig. 32–26). The firm aneurysmal dilatations in this system may compress cranial nerves, and in the carotid system, the optic nerves or chiasm may be compressed. Rupture of such aneurysms with resulting subarachnoid hemorrhage or carotid-cavernous communication is an infrequent complication.

Congenital saccular aneurysms are far more common than either of the conditions just mentioned, and are the most common cause of uncomplicated subarachnoid hemorrhage. They appear as saccular dilatations on the vessels of the circle of Willis, most often at bifurcations. They vary greatly in size; some are so small they can be seen well only with a hand lens, while others are 2 to 3 cm. in diameter. Although they can occur anywhere in the circle, they are most frequent in the anterior portion, 70 per cent being on the internal carotid, middle cerebral and anterior cerebral arteries. They may be multiple.

Their pathogenesis is still a matter of some controversy.

The rupture of a saccular aneurysm has little to do with its size. Indeed, the most catastrophic hemorrhages may come from very small aneurysms. Rupture may occur at any age, rarely in infancy and childhood, most commonly in young and middle-aged adults, and with a greater than usually realized frequency in old age. Hypertension seems to predispose to the fact and the severity of rupture. It usually but not always follows some exertion and, regrettably, sexual intercourse seems to be a common precipitant. The whole subarachnoid space is flooded with blood, which accumulates especially about the site of the aneurysm, and lumbar puncture always yields bloody fluid. Rupture may occur not only into the subarachnoid space, but into the brain substance as well (Fig. 32–27). In the very common aneurysms of the anterior cerebral and anterior communicating arteries, the hemorrhage may burst right through the brain and into the ventricle. Sometimes a rupture may break the arachnoid and produce a sizable subdural hematoma.

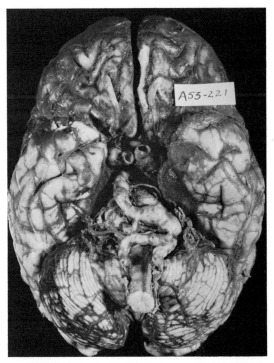

Figure 32–26. *Arteriosclerotic fusiform aneurysm of the vertebral-basilar sytem. The dilated, deformed vessel is displaced into the cerebellopontine angle on one side.*

In addition to rupture, aneurysms may increase in size by successive bleeding into the vessel wall, simulating a tumor of the base of the brain. Sometimes a clot forms within the sac, either before or after rupture, producing infarction in the supply of the vessel.

The classic picture of ruptured saccular aneurysm is the sudden onset of a very severe occipital headache which then becomes generalized. Nausea, vomiting and prostration supervene rapidly in severe hemorrhage. The third nerve, lying as it does so close to some of the commonly affected vessels, especially the carotid, the posterior communicating and the posterior cerebral, is frequently paralyzed. If recovery occurs, the patient may be prone to a second or third rupture, his chances for recovery diminishing with each one.

VASCULAR MALFORMATIONS

A not uncommon finding in routine autopsies is a *telangiectasis*, a cluster of thin-walled vessels, no more than 1 or 2 mm. in size (Cushing and Bailey, 1928). These are often mistaken in the gross for small petechial hemorrhages. In the brain they tend to occur in white matter and probably have no clinical sig-

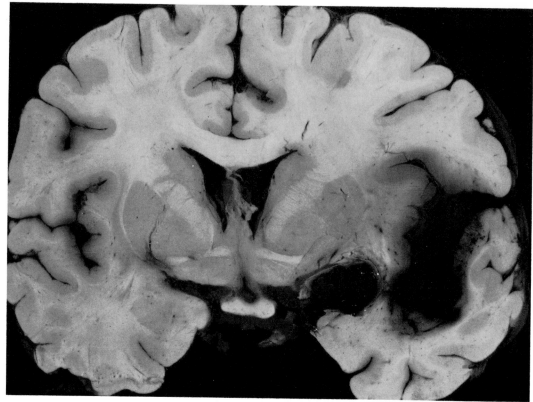

Figure 32–27. *Meningocerebral hemorrhage subsequent to rupture of an aneurysm on the middle cerebral artery.*

nificance. In the brain stem, they may occupy one-half of the pontine base and tegmentum, normal brain tissue lying between the vessels. Rarely, by bleeding in the brain stem, telangiectases may produce clinical effects.

Angiomas. Although these lesions are termed angiomas, they are not true neoplasms. They are malformations of the vascular system, and many are probably hamartomatous. They are traditionally divided into venous and arteriovenous types. They may involve the leptomeninges or the brain substance or both. The majority are in the distribution of the middle cerebral artery, but they may occur anywhere, including the posterior fossa. They are supplied by large arterial channels and drained by large veins. The so-called venous angiomas consist entirely of thin-walled vessels, but in the arteriovenous type there are many channels with a muscular coat, some of them communicating directly with larger veins without going through a capillary net.

In the leptomeninges, they vary in size from a small varicose cluster to a huge deforming mass covering an entire hemisphere. Calcification occurs to a radiologically demonstrable degree in the underlying cortex. Such leptomeningeal angiomas are sometimes associated with cutaneous angiomas in the distribution of the fifth cranial or the cervical spinal nerves. This association is called Sturge-Weber disease, has occurred in families and is frequently associated with mental retardation.

In the brain substance, the common angioma is wedge shaped, its apex at the ventricle and its base upon the convexity, nervous tissue lying between the abnormal vascular channels. Thrombosis or hemorrhage in the malformation may result in destruction of the nervous tissue within or nearby the lesion.

The clinical picture is one of convulsive disorder and recurrent subarachnoid hemorrhage, with or without signs of focal brain damage. The convulsions may be present for years before subarachnoid hemorrhage occurs, or recurrent subarachnoid hemorrhage may appear before the convulsions.

TUMORS OF THE BRAIN

There are two quite different categories of "tumors of the brain"—those intracranial tumors which are inside and those outside brain substance (Russell and Rubinstein,

1963) (Rubinstein, 1972). Inside the brain substance are found the gliomas and the tumors of blood vessels. Outside the brain substance are found the meningiomas, the acoustic neurinomas and the tumors of the pituitary region. Metastatic tumors may be either inside or outside or both.

Of all intracranial tumors in routine autopsies in a general hospital, metastatic tumors represent at least one-third. This figure is lower in neurosurgical centers and in hospitals with a population in the younger age groups. Of the group of primary brain tumors, those within the brain are more frequent in all series than those outside the brain, the comparative figures being about 5 or 6 to 1. Almost all of the group of primary tumors within the brain substance are gliomas.

The effects of an intracranial tumor are local and generalized. The *local effects* are those due to the irritative, depressive or destructive effect of the tumor itself upon that part of the brain in or near which it lies. Thus, jacksonian seizures beginning in the contralateral foot occur with parasagittal posterior frontal meningiomas, contralateral homonymous hemianopsia with temporal and occipital gliomas, staggering with tumors of the cerebellar midline, or simply unilateral anosmia with a meningioma of the olfactory groove. Any symptom or sign of localized stimulation or depression of the brain substance may occur.

The *generalized effects* are due to increased intracranial pressure, cerebral edema and distortion of structure. The effects of increased intracranial pressure have already been considered in a separate section. It should be noted that increased intracranial pressure may occur from the added volume of the tumorous mass, from obstruction of the ventricular system and from the cerebral edema which occurs with tumors.

This cerebral edema is a diffuse swelling of a large area adjacent to the tumor mass. As might be expected, it is generally maximal in large, rapidly growing tumors of brain substance. This general rule has its frequent exceptions and even a relatively small metastasis within the brain substance may produce edema throughout an entire cerebral hemisphere. The edema of cerebral tumors is of the vasogenic rather than the cytotoxic types (Klatzo, 1967). It is a lesion largely of white matter and includes gray matter only for the variable amount of myelinated material within the cortical ribbon and gray nuclear masses. The extracellular space of the fiber bundles becomes distended with fluid and solutes, which escape through the abnormally permeable vessel walls.

METASTATIC TUMORS

The most common primary sites of intracranial metastatic tumors are bronchus and breast, and between them these two sources contribute 40 to 50 per cent of such tumors. Almost all carcinomas or sarcomas elsewhere in the body have the capacity for metastasis to the brain or its coverings. Particularly aggressive in this regard, in addition to the two carcinomas mentioned, are melanocarcinoma, embryonal carcinoma, chorioepithelioma and renal cell carcinoma. Carcinomas of the prostate and of the cervix uteri only infrequently go to brain substance, although they may involve the overlying dura or skull.

The clinical picture is a varied one, depending on the variations in the pathology. Only infrequently are metastases single, and it is not exceptional to find dozens or scores of metastatic nodules in the same brain.

Some metastases are localized to the leptomeninges, where they produce a clinical picture of chronic meningitis with headache, signs of meningeal irritation, cranial nerve palsies and cells in the cerebrospinal fluid. The cells proliferating within the subarachnoid space result in a lowering of the sugar content of the fluid, again in this regard resembling a bacterial or fungal meningitis.

The gross appearance of tumor metastases is usually characteristic. The small ones are almost perfectly spherical, their centers at the junction of gray and white matter, the edges seemingly well demarcated from the normal brain about them. Frequently necrosis and hemorrhage appear at the center. As the tumors enlarge, they are restrained in their external growth by the pia, or by the ependyma, but their extension into the brain is relentless and uniform, terminating only with the death of the patient. Infrequently a single metastatic tumor grows irregularly through the brain substance, becoming necrotic or hemorrhagic or both, and simulating a malignant glioma.

Microscopically, the structure of the primary tumor is reproduced. The precise demarcation of the gross lesion is found to be fraudulent, for tiny malignant fingers are found stretching out into the surrounding brain, which may look normal, compressed or edematous. When necrosis or hemorrhage occurs, the cells immediately next to the blood vessels survive.

It is not unusual for patients to present with their neurologic symptoms, the primary tumor being discovered only on investigation or at autopsy. The rarely occurring single metastasis can be removed if it is in a suitable area of brain. Corticosteroids, while in no sense curative, have been very valuable in relieving symptoms and signs and increasing life span.

GLIOMAS

The gliomas are those tumors within the brain substance which arise from glial cells. In this group are the astrocytoma, oligodendroglioma, ependymoma and medulloblastoma. The rare primary reticulum cell sarcoma of the brain might be thought of as a microglioma.

The numerical frequency of these tumors depends on the clinic which reports them, and no helpful purpose can be served by adding further figures to the literature. The group of astrocytomas is by far the most common. Medulloblastoma is one of the most frequent gliomas of childhood. Oligodendroglioma and ependymoma can be expected to turn up every now and then, but primary reticulum cell sarcoma of brain is a rarity.

In a structure like the brain, the malignancy of a tumor must be thought of in two senses: the aggressiveness of its cellular constituents and the strategic importance of its location. An astrocytoma of the tip of the right frontal lobe may be as benign in its cytology as an astrocytoma of the hypothalamus. The tip of the right frontal lobe can be amputated; the hypothalamus cannot.

The terminology of the tumors which compose the glioma group is as pleomorphic as some of the tumors themselves. Bailey and Cushing (1926), in the early work on gliomas, utilized a diagrammatic histogenetic basis for identification, and brought some order out of the chaos. Many authors have insisted on retaining an elaborate complex of terms which single out a freakish feature of a given tumor to endow it with a separate name and an identity of its own, distinct from all others.

Newer techniques of ultrastructural and histochemical analysis may in the next several years give the data which will provide a rational basis for a generally acceptable classification. In the meantime, the beginning student is less likely to suffer pain or error from oversimplification than from overcomplexity (Kernohan and Sayre, 1952).

Astrocytoma. This glioma arises from the astrocyte. There are four grades of malignancy, depending on cellular appearance and prognosis, the usual custom being followed so that Grade I is the least and Grade IV the most malignant. Whatever their degrees of malignancy, all are invasive, some subtly, some obviously.

Although the more benign forms are found somewhat more often in children and young adults, and the more malignant forms occur more often in middle life and old age, there is no absolute difference in terms of age.

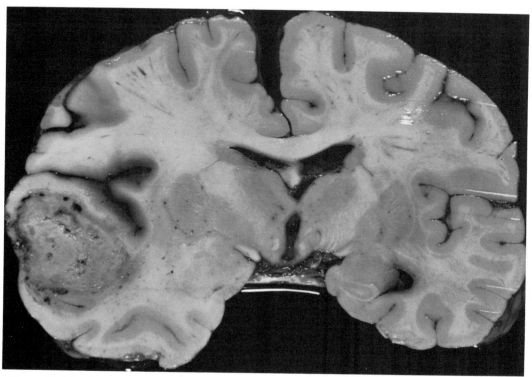

Figure 32–28. Astrocytoma, Grade I. The tumor is in the temporal lobe. The hemisphere is enlarged. The ventricular system is displaced away from the lesion and the ipsilateral ventricle is compressed. The cingulate gyrus has herniated under the falx cerebri.

The gross appearance of an astrocytoma depends largely upon its degree of malignancy. Some of the very slowly growing, well differentiated tumors may be hard to recognize in the gross, producing only a fullness and ivory whiteness of the part affected without distorting architecture to any serious degree. They vary considerably in size. Some are only a few centimeters in size (Fig. 32–28). Others may occupy the whole of a lobe, or a hemisphere, or even spread to the opposite side. They may be particularly difficult to recognize when they are restricted to the white matter. Since the tumor is firmer than the surrounding brain, the palpating finger may tell more than the eye. Generally hemorrhage and necrosis and intense edema occur in and about the more rapidly growing astrocytomas, producing a multicolored, ragged, viciously invasive appearance (Fig. 32–29). Especially in the cerebellar astrocytomas of childhood, cystic change may occur in some of the more slowly growing tumors (Fig. 32–30). A small nubbin of viable tumor (the "mural nodule") may sit projecting itself into the relatively large cyst cavity. The fluid in such cysts reaccumulates rapidly after simple evacuation, and the tumor itself must be excised to give any result resembling a cure. None of the astrocytomas are encapsulated.

Astrocytoma, Grade I, is called fibrillary astrocytoma or protoplasmic astrocytoma in the older classification. It will be remembered that protoplasmic astrocytes occur only in gray matter. The microscopic appearance is that of an excess of astrocytic cell bodies and fibers, the individual cells looking normal or almost normal (Fig. 32–31). The nuclei may be a little larger than normal, or more densely chromatinized than normal, and the processes may be thicker and more abundant than normal. Pleomorphism is minimal; there are no mitoses and no tumor giant cells. The blood vessels may be more numerous, but they lack the proliferative appearance seen in the more malignant grades of tumor. With these characteristics, it is understandable that the pathologist may be unable with limited material, as in a biopsy, to distinguish such benign astrocytomas from astrocytic proliferation in the repair of some pathologic process.

Astrocytoma, Grade II, is the astroblastoma of the older literature. It differs from Grade I only in a quantitative way. The cells are more abundant, and there is a small but definite difference in size and shape of nuclei. Mitoses are completely absent or very rare. The nuclei stain more densely, and the processes are thicker. Some of the blood vessels have a suggestion of active proliferation, and the walls are thickened as a consequence. Necrosis and hemorrhage do not occur.

Astrocytoma, Grades III and IV, are the tumors called **glioblastoma multiforme** in the older and no so old literature. The older term does not die easily, and perhaps it should not. It is a mellifluous designation which makes the lesion sound as impressive and important as it really is. Even the most enthusiastic proponents of the newer numerical terminology find themselves using the venerable Latin name. These grades of malignant astrocytoma are the most common of all gliomas, accounting for from 40 to 60 per cent in various published series. They are by far more common in the cerebral hemispheres than elsewhere in the brain. They may attain the most incredible size, and may even appear multifocal in the gross, although microscopic isthmuses of communication are demonstrable when sought with care.

Astrocytoma, Grade III, still contains some cellular elements clearly recognizable as astrocytes, but there is now considerable variation in size and shape and a denser chromatism to the nuclei than in the lower grades. The cell processes are shorter and thicker and more disorganized. Mitoses are present but must be sought, and tumor giant cells are prominent. The walls of the blood vessels look active, with proliferating adventitial and endothelial cells, but the blood supply falls behind the rapid growth of the tumor, and areas of necrosis and small hemorrhage are many and confluent.

Astrocytoma, Grade IV, is one of the most unrestrained of all tumors. Only an infrequent cell is recognizable as an astrocyte. There are all sizes and shapes of nuclei, but all are hyperchromatic, and a field can hardly be found in which mitoses and giant cells are absent (Fig. 32–32). Newly formed blood vessels, with very cellular walls and many mitoses in the walls, stand out everywhere. Necrosis and small hemorrhages are even more prominent than in Grade III tumors.

In all tumors of the astrocyte series, astrocytic fibers can be demonstrated with appropriate stains. The gold sublimate method (Cajal) is favored by some, but phosphotungstic acid

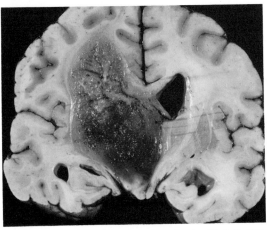

Figure 32–29. Astrocytoma. Grade IV (glioblastoma multiforme).

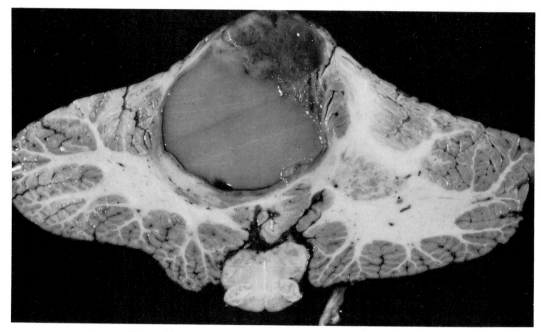

Figure 32–30. *Astrocytoma, cystic, in the cerebellum.*

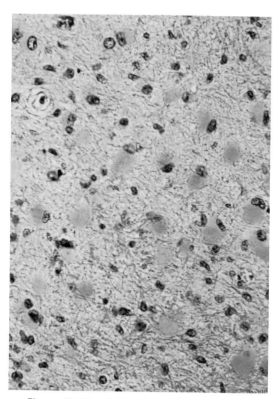

Figure 32–31. *Astrocytoma. Grade I. The cells look like reactive astrocytes. (Hematoxylin and eosin stain.)*

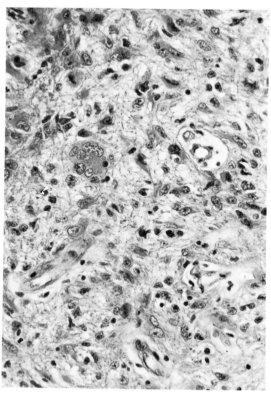

Figure 32–32. *Astrocytoma. Grade IV (glioblastoma multiforme). (Phloxine-methylene blue stain.)*

hematoxylin (Mallory) is the one most commonly used. With the Mallory method, the fibers are seen as a delicate, blue, interlacing network. They are found with great ease in the lesser degrees of malignancy, but in the greater degrees of malignancy it may be necessary to search through many fields to find the telltale fibers.

As should be clear from the microscopic description of the various grades of astrocytoma, **a tumor is graded by its most malignant part.** One may find Grade I or Grade II patterns in a tumor which is ultimately classed as more malignant in other sections. A biopsy of the tumor at one point in its development may show only a minor grade of malignancy, and several years later only Grade III or Grade IV elements may be found at operation or autopsy.

The prognosis for life in all the astrocytomas is poor. Although there are exceptional situations, the usual survival after operation for the more benign astrocytomas is measured in terms of a few years, and for the more malignant ones, in terms of a few months. Efforts at radical excision are palliative rather than curative. The effectiveness of radiation therapy is variable and unpredictable in any given case. As in metastatic tumors and other gliomas, the corticosteroids allow some symptomatic relief and increased duration of life.

Ependymoma.   The ependymoma is derived from the ependymal cell and as might be expected, therefore, occurs along the ventricular pathways. When the tumor is not in obvious contact with the ventricular surface, the presumption is that it has taken its origin from the not infrequently seen nests of displaced ependyma. Of the cerebral ependymomas, 70 per cent are in the fourth ventricle. Their usual proximity to the ventricle makes them particularly liable to produce obstructive symptoms and signs. They occur most frequently in children and young adults, and in most series represent the second most common glioma.

Grossly, ependymoma can be suspected when an infiltrating tumor is found in proximity to the ventricular pathway. But even in those ependymomas that are not in such a situation, the tumor has a gray and fleshy appearance quite different from that of the astrocytoma. Some ependymomas may protrude themselves into the lateral ventricle and reach an enormous size. Others, as in the fourth ventricle, may produce severe symptoms even when they are relatively small. Cystic degeneration is more common than in the astrocytoma, but necrosis and hemorrhage are very rare.

Microscopically, there are three varieties of ependymoma: epithelial, papillary and cellular.

The epithelial ependymoma is composed of ependymal cells arranged about canals. It is densely cellular with little or no stroma. The papillary ependymoma is composed of a branching stroma which is lined by ependymal epithelium. The myxopapillary ependymoma of the lower spinal canal is not seen in brain. The cellular ependymoma is composed of tumorous ependymal cells without either of the patterns described.

All three types of ependymoma can be graded into four categories of malignancy similar to those for astrocytoma. It is quite possible that some instances of glioblastoma multiforme began as ependymomas. The microscopic diagnosis of ependymoma is not always simple for the pathologist. The hallmarks are the arrangement into rosettes and the cytoplasmic basal bodies of ciliary shafts called blepharoplasts. These hallmarks are not easily found in all ependymomas.

The outcome of ependymoma is not much happier than in astrocytoma. The proximity of these tumors to the ventricle makes surgical extirpation technically difficult. The survival postoperatively depends largely on the grade of malignancy, and corresponds generally to the survival for comparable grades of astrocytoma.

Oligodendroglioma.   The oligodendroglioma arises from the oligodendroglia. Five to 10 per cent of gliomas are in this category. Although the tumor may occur in any age group, it is rare in the very young and in the elderly. Its most frequent site is the white matter of the centrum semiovale, but it may involve the cortex secondarily and may even penetrate into the subarachnoid space over the surface of the cerebrum.

Grossly, the tumor is gray, fleshy and soft. There is great variation in size. About one out of five is cystic and small hemorrhagic foci are common. Microscopically, the characteristic appearance makes it one of the easiest tumors to diagnose. It is densely cellular with little or no stroma. The nuclei are small and regular, like the nuclei of normal oligodendroglia in size and shape. The cell membrane takes the stain but the cytoplasm does not stain, so that each nucleus seems to sit in the middle of its own little compartment.

Efforts to grade the malignancy of the oligodendrogliomas have not been successful. There is, however, a variant, a more malignant form called an oligodendroblastoma. It is similar in gross appearance to the oligodendroglioma, but microscopically there is a moderate pleomorphism with less orderly arrangement, frequent mitoses and proliferative change in the blood vessels.

Of especial interest in both oligodendroglioma and oligodendroblastoma is the appearance of calcification. Although calcification may appear in other gliomas, only rarely is it sufficiently marked to permit x-ray visualization. In the oligodendroglial tumors, about 40 to 50 per cent contain enough calcification to permit this finding to be an important preoperative or premortem diagnostic aid.

Prognostically, patients with oligodendroglial tumors do better than those with other gliomas. Some patients have had their tumors for many years before surgery and it is not unusual to see patients survive for many years following operation. Yet, in other instances, the tumors move more swiftly and more violently, and no correlation of histology and clinical course seems to work.

Medulloblastoma. The cell of origin of the medulloblastoma is one of the interesting controversies of modern pathology. One of the more attractive ideas about the origin of the medulloblastoma is that it arises from the cells of the external granular layer of the cerebellar folia. This layer is present in the infant in well developed form for the first several months of life and is thought by some to contribute in a kind of bipotential way to the neuronal and glial population of the deeper layers of the infant's developing cerebellum.

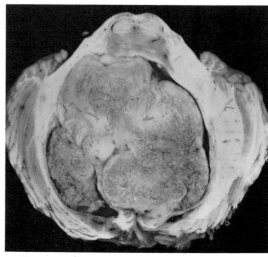

Figure 32–33. Medulloblastoma of the cerebellum, extending into the fourth ventricle, distorting and compressing the brain stem and obstructing the ventricular pathway.

However they may originate, these growths are always in the cerebellum. About two-thirds of medulloblastomas occur in children, and these are principally in the midline; another one-third in the 15 to 35 age group, and they are principally in the lateral lobes of the cerebellum.

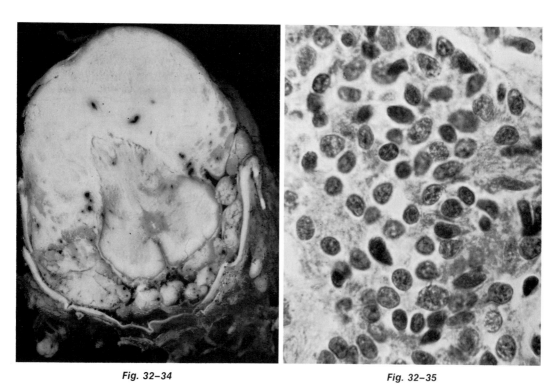

Fig. 32–34

Fig. 32–35

Figure 32–34. Medulloblastoma seedings surrounding the spinal cord.
Figure 32–35. Medulloblastoma. (Hematoxylin and eosin stain.)

Grossly, the midline medulloblastoma expands into the fourth ventricle, and its major clinical manifestations are related to the obstruction of the ventricular system (Fig. 32–33). It is a fleshy gray mass, always connected to the cerebellum as it hangs down into the ventricle, and the entire ventricular pathway above it is dilated. It does not become necrotic or hemorrhagic, but more than any other glioma, it has a habit of seeding through the subarachnoid space, giving a kind of frosted appearance to the brain and cord and enveloping even the roots of the cauda equina (Fig. 32–34).

Microscopically, this tumor is very densely cellular with practically no stroma and few blood vessels (Fig. 32–35). There is great variation in cell appearance from one tumor to another. Classically, the cells are small, the nuclei oval or elongated and the cytoplasm tapering at one end so that they are often called "carrot-shaped." Characteristically, also, they may group about a blood vessel to form incomplete rosettes. Mitoses are usually abundant.

The laterally placed tumors are usually on the dorsal aspect of the cerebellar hemisphere. They are smooth or slightly nodular and are distinct from adjacent cerebellar folia. They have the same unhappy seeding and spreading habits as the midline tumors.

The medulloblastoma has some treacherous clinical habits. For a period of some weeks, the only symptoms in the child may be morning vomiting, until eventually staggering and headache appear. By the time the child gets to the physician, there is usually severe papilledema from increased intracranial pressure.

Although they are radiosensitive in the beginning, these tumors carry a grim prognosis and total recovery is very rare, although radiation and surgery may delay the last act of the tragedy for several years.

Other Parenchymatous Tumors. All gliomas are not of pure cell type; there are *tumors of mixed cell types* which are difficult to classify. *Polar spongioblastoma* is a rare tumor of early life, which is found around the third or fourth ventricle; its behavior is as malignant as its histology is primitive. The *ganglioglioma-ganglioneuroma* tumors of young people are probably related to the neuroblastomas. The *reticulum cell sarcoma-microglioma* group poses difficult problems of cytogenesis and pathogenesis; they may be simple or multifocal in brain; they may be only in brain or they may be associated with histiocytic (reticulum cell) lymphomas elsewhere in the body.

BLOOD VESSEL TUMORS

There are many malformations of blood vessels which are sometimes included in the literature under tumors (Cushing and Bailey, 1928). The only true tumor of blood vessels in the brain is the hemangioendothelioblastoma, sometimes called hemangioblastoma or angioblastoma.

These are generally tumors of early middle life and, although they may occur in the cerebral hemispheres, they are more frequent in the cerebellum. Among brain tumors they are rare, representing probably no more than 1 per cent.

Grossly, they are cystic lesions, often red and hemorrhagic, and in the cerebellum they are always in a lateral lobe. A small mural nodule is generally present in the cyst. Microscopically, they consist of small vascular channels lined by endothelium. There is very little interstitial tissue, but most characteristic of the tumor are foamy cells, probably histiocytes, the cytoplasm of which is positive for fat stains.

These tumors may have some interesting associations. Von Hippel described a small hemangioendothelioblastoma of the eye, and Lindau later pointed out the association of this with the cerebellar tumor. The combination is eponymically known as Lindau-von Hippel disease. In addition there may be similar tumors of the spinal cord along with cystic disease of the pancreas and kidneys. About 20 per cent are heredofamilial. When treated by total extirpation, the cerebellar tumor permits a good prognosis.

MENINGIOMA

Meningiomas constitute about 15 per cent of all brain tumors, are far more common in adults than in children and are about twice as common in women as in men. The type cell of the meningioma is the arachnoidal fibroblast. Normally arachnoidal tissue is invaginated into dura in the arachnoidal villi of the venous sinuses. In addition, displaced arachnoidal cells can sometimes be found in the dura. Presumably it is from such invaginations and displacements that the tumors arise. Their enormous importance lies not so much in their comparative frequency as in the fact that most of them are amenable to surgical removal. They are outside the brain substance and they are slow growing. The heart of the neurologic surgeon, so often in despair with other tumors, leaps up when he finds a meningioma.

Intracranial meningiomas have certain favored locations: Kernohan and Sayre, in a study of 794 cases, found over 50 per cent in a few specific sites: 184 in the parasagittal regions, 73 on the sphenoid ridge, 26 in the basifrontal or olfactory groove area, 61 near the sella turcica and 55 in the cerebellopontine angle. Intraventricular meningiomas do occur; they arise at the areas of arachnoidal contributions to the tela choroidea and the choroid plexuses. Each one of these groups has its own characteristic clinical picture.

Grossly, although meningiomas vary considerably in appearance, they have certain similarities. They are grayish white and nodular, always attached to dura, and compress but are rarely invasive (Fig. 32–36). They are usually encapsulated. As they expand, they displace and compress brain substance. Some are very small, and are found only incidentally at autopsy, especially in elderly people. Others may grow to enormous size, occupying one-sixth of the volume of the cranial cavity. Some are rounded, uniformly displacing and compressing the brain as they grow, and others are flattened on the surface (meningioma en plaque). Calcification is common and often is great enough to be visualized by roentgenogram of the skull. Another feature of diagnostic value in those near bone is the tendency to excite an osteoblastic reaction, also easily seen by x-ray. Infrequently malignant transformation results in invasion rather than compression of adjacent brain substance. These tumors may be locally aggressive and invade the overlying bone, but this growth is not necessarily an indication of malignancy in the generally understood meaning of the term.

Probably the simplest classification of the meningiomas is into three types: meningotheliomatous, psammomatous and fibroblastic. It is likely that the cell type is the same in all three, and indeed there are overlapping and intermediate forms. The variation in appearance is related to mechanical and temporal factors of growth rather than to different cells of origin.

The meningotheliomatous meningioma consists of clusters of cells with varying amounts of stroma. The cells are almost identical with those in the outer layer of arachnoid. They are large, with moderately chromatic oval or round nuclei and finely granular cytoplasm. On ordinary cell stains, the cytoplasmic membrane is indistinct. The stroma is collagenous or hyalinized, and contains large numbers of blood vessels.

The psammomatous meningioma has the same type of cell and the same general features and variability of stroma (Fig. 32–37). The cells are arranged in whorls, and in the center of the whorls there appears at first a tiny dot of hyalinization, which enlarges concentrically in lamellar fashion,

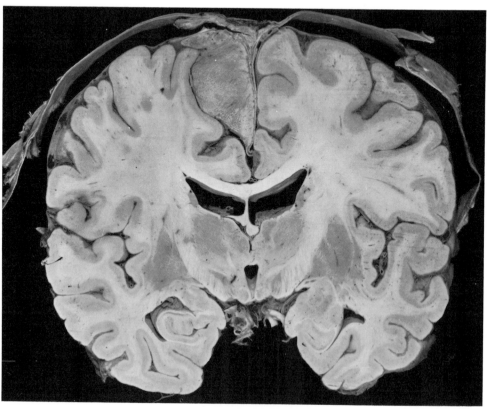

Figure 32–36. *Parasagittal meningioma.*

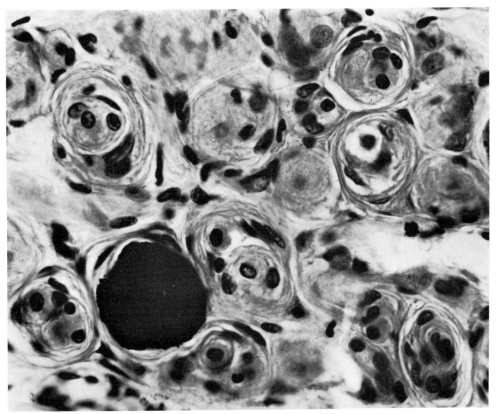

Figure 32–37. Meningioma, psammomatous. (Hematoxylin and eosin stain.)

later becoming calcified. These balls of hyalinization and calcification are referred to as psammoma bodies. They probably take their origin in a degenerating cell or group of cells in the center of a whorl.

The fibroblastic meningioma looks much like a fibroblastic tumor anywhere else in the body, except that diligent search will usually reveal meningotheliomatous elements. This variety of meningioma is less common than the other two and is thought by some to arise from a different cell of origin.

Malignant change in a meningioma is indicated by anaplasia, mitoses and tumor giant cells. Invasion of bone is not of itself indicative of malignancy, the truly malignant lesion producing osteoclastic rather than osteoblastic change. Rarely, a malignant meningioma metastasizes outside the cranial cavity.

ACOUSTIC NEUROMA

The most important of the neuromas of the cranial cavity are those which take origin from the root of the eighth nerve. A rare neuroma may involve the fifth or seventh nerves or even ninth or eleventh, but neuromas of the eighth nerve are said to constitute as high as 8 to 9 per cent of all brain tumors in some series, especially in neurosurgical centers where biopsy material is included. They do not occur in children.

Their location in the angle formed by the pons, medulla and cerebellum accounts for the commonly used synonym of **cerebellopontine angle tumors** (Fig. 32–38). They probably take origin from the vestibular rather than the auditory portion of the eighth nerve. They are encapsulated and, like meningiomas, they distort and compress rather than invade the brain. As they grow, they compress the fifth and seventh nerves which also lie in the cerebellopontine angle. Ultimately the pons and medulla become compressed and distorted to the extent of obstruction of the flow of cerebrospinal fluid, both in the fourth ventricle and in the subarachnoid space about the brain stem, with resulting obstructive hydrocephalus. In addition to this effect of inward growth upon the brain, the outward growth produces a dilatation and erosion of the internal auditory meatus. This change in the temporal bone is seen even with very small and early tumors. The tumors probably originate at the point of penetration of the nerve into the meatus, which is also the point at which the glial framework is replaced by Schwann cells and fibroblasts.

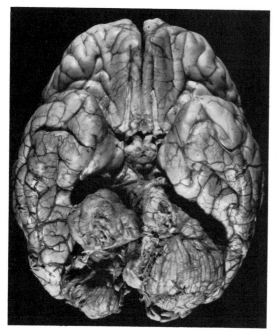

Figure 32–38. *Acoustic neuroma.*

On the external surface, the tumor is irregular in outline by virtue of firm nodules and small thin-walled cysts. On cut section, these cysts may occupy a large area of the tumor mass, but more often they are small and few. Both the solid and the cystic parts of the tumor may have patches of orange-yellow discoloration.

Microscopically, the tumor consists of slender elongated cells with little chromatin in the nuclei. These cells and fibers are arranged into groups in roughly parallel fashion, each group going in a different direction so that they interlace. So-called palisading of nuclei, in which they lie side by side in rows separated by fibers or hyalin, is very diagnostic but not very frequent. Interrupting this arrangement are variably frequent clusters of loose reticular tissue. Within foci of degeneration there are frequent hemosiderin-filled macrophages.

Although there is still no unanimity of opinion about it, the cell type probably is the perineurial fibroblast or the Schwann cell (Harkin and Reed, 1969).

The tumor is slow growing. The patient develops tinnitus first because of eighth nerve involvement. Later a degree of deafness appears and the labyrinth is found to be unresponsive to stimulation. The fifth nerve is compressed before the seventh, loss of the very sensitive corneal reflex being the first evidence. Facial weakness, or less often facial spasm, is the result of seventh nerve involvement. But usually the patient presents because of increased intracranial pressure or because of signs relating to distortion and compression of the brain stem. By the time the patient comes to surgery, the tumor is often large and the problem of removal is difficult so that this benign tumor outside the brain carries a rather high mortality even with the best surgical efforts.

TUMORS OF THE SPINAL CORD

The most useful pathologic and clinical classification of spinal cord tumors is by location in reference to the dura, that is, extradural and intradural, and in the intradural group in reference to the cord, that is, intramedullary or extramedullary. In contrast to the situation in brain, the majority of tumors which affect the spinal cord are attached to the meninges or to the roots of the spinal nerves.

Kernohan and Sayre (1952) found the following distribution in 979 primary neoplasms within the spinal canal:

	Cases	%
Neurofibromas	293	29.9
Meningiomas	254	25.9
Intramedullary gliomas	220	22.5
Sarcomas	110	11.2
Extramedullary hemangiomas	57	5.8
Chordomas	35	3.6
Dermoids	10	1.0

Of this group, 18 per cent were in the cervical region, 48.5 per cent thoracic, 25.5 per cent lumbar, 6 per cent sacral and 1 per cent at multiple levels. These figures do not include metastatic tumors, which are almost nonexistent in the spinal cord itself but quite common in the epidural space because of involvement of contiguous vertebrae.

INTRAMEDULLARY TUMORS

Since the spinal cord contains the same histologic elements as the brain, it is to be expected that the same kinds of tumors would occur, and indeed they do, but with important dissimilarities of frequency. Spinal oligodendroglioma is extremely rare. Whereas in the brain astrocytoma is far more frequent than ependymoma, the reverse is true in the cord, where ependymomas are over twice as common. The largest number of ependymomas occur caudally, in the conus medullaris and the filum terminale, and they are usually of the papillary type with extensive myxoid degeneration of the stroma.

The astrocytomas of the spinal cord are frequently slow growing, and it is not unusual to find this tumor when symptoms have been present as long as four or five years.

EXTRAMEDULLARY TUMORS

The most common tumor in this group is the neurofibroma. It arises most often from the posterior root and can be quite elongated within the subarachnoid space, or can emerge through the intervertebral foramen to attain a dumbbell shape. Histologically, the spinal neurofibroma is similar to that elsewhere, except perhaps that palisading of the nuclei is a more constant and conspicuous feature.

Meningiomas also fall into this category. They usually occupy only a short cephalocaudal extent but may grow slowly to great size at a given level. Histologically, they are usually of the psammomatous type.

It should be emphasized that these two tumors are the most common of all those which affect the spinal cord. They are benign and operable and, if removed in time, they may not produce any permanent damage.

EXTRADURAL TUMORS

The most common extradural tumor is metastatic. From a focus of metastatic deposit in a vertebra, and sometimes independently of such a focus, the metastasis expands within the narrow extradural space, compressing the cord as it grows. Pelvic carcinomas, especially those of the prostate, seem to have a high affinity for the spinal extradural space, but primary sources in breast, lung and the gastrointestinal tract as well as others are not uncommon.

Those tumors which lie within the substance of the spinal cord can invade, destroy and replace the nuclear masses and the fiber pathways. The common pathologic feature of all tumors within the spinal canal is cord compression. There is little room for expansion in the canal, and as a tumor grows, whether inside or outside the cord, eventually there occurs a critical level of pressure at which the blood vessels can no longer perfuse the cord substance adequately. This results in ischemic change, first in the gray matter and then in the white matter, so that in the extreme but unfortunately not rare case, there may be complete necrosis of the cross section of the cord with irreversible loss of function below the level of the compression.

The symptoms and signs of spinal cord tumors depend in large part upon the level of involvement. The manifestations are multitudinous. Root pain is likely to occur when there is compression and distortion of the root. In extradural lesions, especially, there may be tenderness and limitation of movement. Tumors of the caudal end of the cord are attended by bladder and bowel symptoms. Intramedullary tumors in the cervical region may simulate syringomyelia with dissociated loss of pain and temperature, amyotrophy and reflex loss.

The cerebrospinal fluid protein is usually elevated, even in the absence of a complete dynamic block. When a complete dynamic block has taken place, the fluid below the level of the block is loculated and, on removal from the lumbar theca, is yellow, clots spontaneously and has a very high protein content, often as much as 1000 or 2000 mg. The presence of a block means that the circulatory supply of the cord is in peril, and decompression is then an emergency.

From the pathology, it can be seen that the treatment of spinal tumors is effective more often than that of brain tumors. The prognosis for the benign extramedullary lesions is excellent as long as compression has not done severe damage to the cord itself. Prognosis for relief from symptoms and prevention of paraplegia is generally good even in some epidural metastatic lesions. Some of the gliomas of the cord respond to radiation therapy up to a point, but generally the prognosis is poor.

TRAUMA OF THE BRAIN

Trauma to the head is important in proportion to the effect it has on the brain (Denny-Brown, 1945). Certain physical effects of blows on the head are essential to an understanding of the pathogenesis of the different kinds of damage produced. The brain, having a weight different from that of the skull, is not displaced at the same time as the skull when a blow lands on the head. Some blows to the head fracture the skull; others may damage the brain without skull fracture. A skull fracture may occur without any effect on the brain. When a blow produces a rotary effect, there is a shearing action upon blood vessels, not only in the coverings of the brain but at points of different consistency of tissue in the brain substance.

Concussion. A concussion may be defined as the loss of consciousness and loss of reflex activity which result when a sudden blow is applied to the head. It has been shown that a degree of acceleration or deceleration is necessary to produce concussion, and the resulting diffuse and transient neuronal paralysis results from the inequality of movement by the brain and skull, in the course of which the brain is thrust suddenly and violently against its bony covering. If acceleration or deceleration is prevented by holding the head immobile, a blunt heavy blow, even when it does not fracture the skull, can produce damage to the brain and cranial nerves without loss of consciousness.

It is generally agreed there are no morphologic changes in concussion. The few minor changes mentioned by some investigators are difficult to evaluate. Recovery is the rule, although there may be troublesome symptoms for weeks to months after.

Contusion. A contusion is a traumatic lesion in which the architecture of the tissue has been preserved, but into which there has occurred perivascular bleeding. If the head is struck forcibly by a small object, there is momentary depression of the skull with or without fracture, and a contusion may appear in the superficial part of the brain under the site of the blow. If the injury is by a larger object, then the brain is displaced at a rate unequal to that of the skull. The skull moves first so that the brain pushes against the site of the blow, its opposite pole pulling away from the skull. At this point of pulling away, the leptomeninges, and especially the pia with its blood vessels, may be torn, with resultant wedge-shaped infarction in the underlying cortex and hemorrhage in the subpial layer (Fig. 32–39). Common sites of such *contrecoup* lesions are in the tips of the frontal and temporal lobes in falls on the back of the head, and in the tips of the occipital lobes in falls on the front of the head.

Laceration. A laceration is defined as a traumatic lesion in which there is interruption of the continuity of tissue (Fig. 32–40). In severe *contrecoup* lesions, the effect may be laceration of brain substance rather than contusion. In some shearing lesions of the brain, the continuity of tissue can be interrupted at the junction of gray and white matter to produce

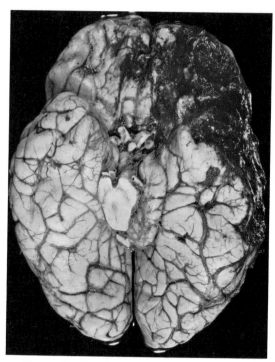

Figure 32–40. *Severe laceration of brain with herniation of temporal lobe.*

intracerebral hemorrhage. Laceration is frequent with crushing injuries to the skull. Penetrating lesions of brain substance, of course, produce laceration by definition. When laceration occurs, there is inevitable flooding of the subarachnoid space by blood. It is noteworthy that some penetrating injuries, by not displacing the skull and brain, may not produce unconsciousness.

Whether the injury is a contusion or laceration, some brain damage occurs and must be repaired. In the course of a contusion, a certain amount of necrosis occurs. The expected sequence of histologic events takes place, with scar formation by astrocytes and fibroblasts, and large numbers of hemosiderin-filled macrophages in and about the area. As the scar retracts, there remains a depressed area of orange-yellow discoloration at the summit of a gyrus or group of gyri, referred to as a "plaque jaune."

A more severe contusion or a laceration, especially if there has been a tear in the leptomeninges, forms a meningocerebral cicatrix, a tight union of scarred brain with overlying thickened dura. Such scars distort the nearby cortex, and are exceedingly epileptogenic. "Plaques jaunes" and meningocerebral cicatrices are the usual pathologic findings in cases of post-traumatic epilepsy.

Epidural Hematoma. Fracture of the

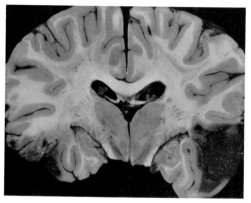

Figure 32–39. *Contusion and laceration.*

skull in a location to damage the middle meningeal artery results in bleeding into the epidural space. The blood cannot disseminate easily and freely throughout the whole area, and continues to accumulate in a relatively localized manner, producing a tense compression of the dura which in turn compresses the brain (Fig. 32–41). Clinically there may be no effects immediately after the trauma, but when the hematoma builds up to a critical level in several hours, events move rapidly. The patient becomes progressively more stuporous and progressively more hemiparetic, convulsions appear, and unless the mass of blood is evacuated, herniation through the tentorium occurs and the patient dies.

Subdural Hematoma. An *acute subdural hematoma* is the consequence of laceration of the brain with a tear in the arachnoid so placed that blood and cerebrospinal fluid go into the subdural space. If there is more cerebrospinal fluid than blood, the accumulation is callled a subdural hygroma. An acute subdural hematoma is an added element in a very severe head

injury. By its size and position it increases the complexity of the injury, compressing and distorting an already damaged and edematous brain. Acute subdural hematomas may occur infrequently in ruptured saccular aneurysm or even in hemorrhage of the brain if there has been tearing of the arachnoid over the hemorrhagic source.

A *chronic subdural hematoma* has a different pathogenesis. Generally associated with closed head injuries, it arises as the consequence of tearing of the bridging veins, especially those leading into the sagittal sinus. This results in a slow leakage of blood into the subdural space, with gradual increase in size of the clot. Blood in the subdural space, having no easy access by blood vessels, remains there and gradually a fibroblastic and vascular membrane grows in from the edges of the dura between the hematoma and the arachnoid so that the mass becomes encapsulated (Fig. 32–42). By osmosis, the hematoma then picks up fluid and increases in size still more. The result is a tight large mass in the subdural space which com-

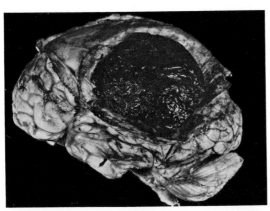

Fig. 32–41

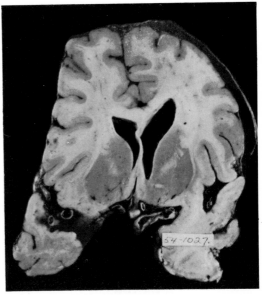

Fig. 32–43

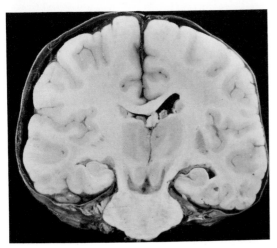

Fig. 32–42

Figure 32–41. Epidural hematoma, result of laceration of the middle meningeal artery by fracture of skull.

Figure 32–42. Subdural hematoma. The thin inner membrane can be seen between the clot and the leptomeninges.

Figure 32–43. Compression of brain by a subdural hematoma. The dura and clot have been removed from the specimen.

presses the brain and eventually produces herniation, decerebration and death (Fig. 32–43). Some few chronic subdural hematomas become resorbed and only the thickened dura, with a hemosiderin-discolored membrane attached, is found incidentally at autopsy. When the brain has been compressed for any period of time by a chronic subdural hematoma, it does not regain its full original volume and a small hemisphere with a dilated ipsilateral ventricle may be found after the clot has been resorbed or evacuated.

The symptoms and signs of a chronic subdural hematoma do not develop for weeks or months following a head injury. The patient complains of headache, and there is a gradually progressing stupor and hemiparesis but no sign of destruction of brain substance. Eventually a dilating pupil, fixed to light, heralds the onset of tentorial herniation. Although it is true that some patients recover spontaneously without herniation, there is only one treatment: the clot must be evacuated. If treatment is undertaken in time, the results are among the most dramatic and most gratifying in all medicine.

Infection as a Complication of Head Injury. Penetrating head injuries are obvious sources for the introduction of sepsis to the brain and its coverings. Subdural or epidural empyema, leptomeningitis and brain abscess are all too familiar complications, especially when the acute craniocerebral injury has not been properly managed.

A more subtle septic complication is that which results from the imperfect closure of a fracture through a paranasal sinus. This may manifest itself by repeated bouts of leptomeningitis, and the clue is given when the patient has transient episodes of cerebrospinal fluid rhinorrhea.

TRAUMA OF THE SPINAL CORD

Injury to the spinal cord is usually the result of injury to the covering spinal column. Sometimes the cord can be "concussed" as by a fall, leading to a transient reversible paralysis for which there is no certain morphologic change.

A crushing or penetrating wound of the spinal column and spinal cord can produce a laceration of the cord with complete interruption of continuity. Hemorrhage into cord substance may occur (hematomyelia), tearing up the gray matter over several segments.

The most common cause of spinal cord injury, however, is compression by dislocation or fracture-dislocation of the vertebrae. Some-

times the dislocation is abrupt and transient, in the course of which the cord is percussed with resulting contusion. A severe dislocation, especially with introduction of bone fragments, may even lacerate and transect the cord (Fig. 32–44).

Compression by the dislocated vertebra, if maintained over any period of time, may produce infarct necrosis over several segments by compression of the blood vessels. Because of the peculiarities of blood supply of the cord, the infarction may be at a distance from the point of compression.

Bleeding into the epidural space may produce an acute compression analogous to the effect of cranial epidural hemorrhage.

The symptoms and signs of cord compression are of vital importance. The patient develops paresthesias and weakness distally at first, with extension upward. A sensory level may or may not be present. Other evidences of long tract involvement, as manifested by corticospinal and posterior column signs, make their appearance. The proof of compression is made by the demonstration of a dynamic spinal fluid block on lumbar puncture. Such a

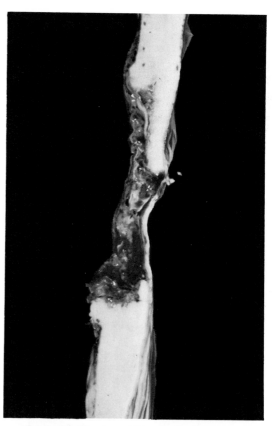

Figure 32–44. *Laceration and almost complete transection of spinal cord by trauma.*

block can be shown by the absence of a rise of pressure in the lumbar manometer when the jugular veins are compressed in the neck. The site of block can be demonstrated by myelography with a radiopaque dye. From a practical point of view, when there is serious concern that a spinal subarachnoid block is present, the clinican goes directly to myelography.

DISORDERS OF PERIPHERAL NERVES

Peripheral nerve is limited in the number of ways in which it can react to injury by any agent, and yet the pathogenetic and morphologic problems of peripheral neuropathy are among the most difficult in all pathology. Part of the reason for this lies in the long time and great expense necessary to undertake a complete postmortem study of any given case, requiring as it does sections of brain and spinal cord, roots, ganglia, large numbers of peripheral nerves and muscles and sensory endings in skin. Biopsies, properly studied, can give some limited useful information but, of necessity, must be restricted to small sensory nerves.

Some of our knowledge of reactions in nerve has come from studies in animals, but many kinds of neuropathy which affect man are associated with disease states which are not reproducible in animals.

The function of a nerve is to conduct impulses. A peripheral nerve will still conduct after being compressed to one-quarter its diameter or stretched to twice its length if the compression or stretch is made gradually.

Wallerian, or secondary degeneration is the process by which the distal stump of a sectioned peripheral nerve undergoes dissolution and resorption. The events which affect the cell body have been described as axonal reaction (p. 1480). When the nerve is sectioned, there is degeneration of the axis cylinder and covering myelin proximally over the distance of a few nodal segments, and distally the entire nerve trunk and its terminal arborizations undergo simultaneous degenerative change. The axis cylinder swells and becomes deformed and fragmented before it disappears. The myelin sheath begins to degenerate shortly after the beginning of the process in the axis cylinder and breaks up into the globules which are ingested by macrophages which appear after several days. As the myelin degenerates, a complex series of biochemical changes takes place, leaving behind neutral fat within the macrophages, which then are resorbed over several weeks.

Pari passu with degeneration, regeneration is already taking place. At the cut edge, endoneurial fibroblasts proliferate to form a framework for the regenerating nervous elements. If the fibroblasts cannot bridge the gap, they are likely to form an "amputation neuroma," a bundle of fibroblasts which can prevent further efforts at regeneration. But if the gap is bridged successfully, Schwann cells proliferate to form the hollow tube into which the axis cylinders advance from the proximal end of the stump. Reconstitution of the nerve, with its axis cylinders, myelin sheaths and terminal arborizations takes three to six months, depending upon the distance involved and upon the metabolic and nutritional state of the patient.

A less well studied mode of reaction in peripheral nerve is the so-called segmental degeneration of Gombault. This occurs in certain of the metabolic, toxic and nutritional neuropathies. There is dissolution of myelin over segments of the nerve, with preservation of the structural integrity but probably temporary functional loss of the axis cylinder. As the myelin breaks up, it is ingested by macrophages and, if the local and general circumstances are right, remyelination takes place.

Neuropathies may be divided into mononeuropathies and polyneuropathies. A group of mononeuropathies in the same patient is referred to by the hybrid name of mononeuropathy multiplex.

Mononeuropathy. Sharp objects will lacerate and blunt objects will contuse a nerve. External compression may damage exposed nerves. The patient who has attempted suicide with barbiturates may emerge from the narcosis with a lesion of the common peroneal nerve. An alcoholic in an acute bout may fall asleep on a park bench, his arm over the back, to awaken with a radial nerve palsy. Internal compression has a damaging effect in many different ways. The median nerve may be caught in the carpal tunnel in rheumatoid arthritis, in pregnancy, in myxedema or in certain occupational stresses. Tumors, tophi, other masses and bony displacements of any sort may produce internal compression. Hemorrhage into a nerve may occur in blood dyscrasias, and infarction of a nerve in diabetes and collagen disease. The third cranial nerve and the femoral nerve are especially likely to be infarcted in diabetics, but almost any mononeuropathy may occur. Leprosy on a worldwide basis is one of the commonest causes of multiple mononeuropathies. In the later stages of leprosy, there is an interstitial or subepineurial leprous granuloma which produces an indolent chronic reaction in the nerve. The ulnar nerve is especially vulnerable. In another form of leprous neuritis, the small cutaneous nerves are involved, and the resulting sensory disorder is responsible for the fiercely destructive trophic lesions of leprosy. For a large group of mononeuropathies, there is no easy explanation. A facial nerve paralysis is common in sarcoidosis even in the absence of uveoparotid fever. Bell's palsy is a paralysis of the seventh cranial nerve of unknown cause. Less frequently, other cranial nerves for no obvious reason will suffer temporary or permanent functional loss. Lead may produce a localized motor neuropathy, notably in radial nerve.

Herpes zoster ("shingles") is properly a primary lesion not of peripheral nerve but of the dorsal root ganglion. It produces a vesicular eruption in the distribution of a cranial or spinal sensory root. The lesions ultimately become scarred and, especially in older people, there may be intense and long-lasting pain. Inflammatory changes, frequently destructive, occur in the dorsal root ganglia, in the spinal cord and, to a varying degree, in the corresponding peripheral nerves. Sometimes the anterior horn cells become involved, with resulting muscular paralysis and atrophy.

Likewise so-called "brachial neuritis" may be more a lesion of root. Usually unilateral and very painful, there is sensory, motor or sensorimotor involvement in one or more roots which form the brachial plexus. The lesion is demyelinative and its mechanism uncertain. In the old days, it frequently followed injections of tetanus antitoxin, but at present it is seen following banal infections or with no apparent precipitant. Some families have a predisposition to this lesion.

Polyneuropathy. Idiopathic polyneuritis (acute infective polyneuritis, postinfectious polyneuritis, Guillain-Barré syndrome) may be the equivalent in the peripheral nervous system of postinfectious encephalomyelitis (Asbury et al., 1969). Frequently an enteric or respiratory infection precedes it by a few days to a few weeks. A condition which very greatly resembles it has been produced in animals by inoculating peripheral nerve myelin with Freund adjuvant. This disease is an especially paralytic disorder of acute or subacute evolution, which produces only mild sensory symptoms. The paralysis in limbs is more proximal than distal, one or both of the facial nerves are involved, and the nerves to the muscles of respiration are very vulnerable. Death may result from respiratory failure. The protein in the cerebrospinal fluid is often very elevated.

There is a well developed cellular inflammatory reaction in all parts of the peripheral nervous system, even in the very early stages of the disease. The neuropathy involves extensive segmental demyelination with many focal areas of perivascular lymphocytes. If the lesions are destructive to the axis cylinder, Wallerian degeneration will occur. It is a cell-mediated immunologic disorder in which peripheral myelin is attacked by specifically sensitized lymphocytes.

The polyneuropathy of malnutrition is common in those parts of the world where near-starvation is a way of life. It was common in prisoners of war in Asian prison camps in World War II. In medical practice in so-called civilized countries, it is most often seen in chronic alcoholism, but there are some cases in patients who are depressed or who have conditions predisposing to vomiting or absorption problems. Onset may be sudden or gradual. Manifestations are most often sensory, often asymptomatic but sometimes very painful. Paralyses, especially distal in the legs, occur in some cases. The pathologic changes are distal, in the form of Gombault's segmental demyelination. In the cases of rapid onset, there may be severe destructive changes and subsequent Wallerian degeneration.

Polyneuropathy is common in some metabolic disorders. One of the commonest is due to diabetes mellitus. Whereas the mononeuropathy of diabetes may be looked upon as a vascular complication of the disease, the bilateral symmetrical polyneuropathy must be regarded as part of or another intrinsic manifestation of the disease, even though the mechanism of its production is not understood. Uremic polyneuropathy has become much more common as more patients with renal failure are kept alive. It is bilaterally symmetrical, distal and frequently severe. It is principally a demyelinative reaction in nerve, and is reversible with renal transplantation, less frequently with hemodialysis.

Acute intermittent porphyria produces a very severe acute polyneuropathy, largely motor and mostly proximal. The respiratory muscles become paralyzed in some cases. Frequently there is coexisting encephalopathy. The lesions may be present in the anterior roots as well as the nerves, and paralysis may be profound and prolonged.

Certain disease states associated with dysproteinemia, including primary amyloidosis. Waldenström's macroglobulinemia, sarcoidosis, immune diseases and multiple myeloma produce a chronic, severe, usually relentlessly progressive bilateral symmetrical polyneuropathy. It involves both motor and sensory nerves, begins distally and extends proximally. The mechanism is unknown.

Carcinoma, especially of the lung, in some obscure way, and without tumorous involvement of the nerves themselves, may produce a sensory or a sensorimotor neuropathy, characterized by degeneration of the distal fibers of the nerves (Brain and Norris, 1965).

Toxic Disorders. A multitude of intoxicants, organic and inorganic, of agricultural, industrial or pharmaceutical origin, can produce polyneuropathy. It is by no means a homogeneous group, either clinically or pathologically, but generally toxic polyneuropathy is sensorimotor, distal, nonfatal except in its complications, and usually reversible. The usual pathologic change is a distal segmental degeneration. Lead neuropathy is likely to be predominantly motor and frequently localized. Arsenic is present in pesticides, and accidental ingestion still occurs. It has a long history of use in a criminal attempt to settle marital maladjustments. Triorthocresyl phosphate (TOCP), as a vehicle for medication, as with Jamaican ginger, or as a contaminant in food containers, as in a Morocco epidemic, has affected thousands of patients with a severe and generally recoverable polyneuropathy but with an associated, usually irreversible, myelopathy.

Heredofamilial Disorders. In this category of polyneuropathies are relatively rare but probably distinct entities. In most patients, the disease does not become evident until adolescence or adult life. Peroneal muscular atrophy *(Charcot-Marie-Tooth disease)* is a progressive, predominantly motor lesion which begins in the peroneal muscles but goes on to involve the other leg and lower thigh muscles as well as the forearm and hand muscles. It is of varying severity and irregular progression. The muscular atrophy is secondary to degeneration in the peripheral nerves.

Hypertrophic interstitial polyneuritis (Dejerine-Sottas disease) evolves much as does peroneal muscular atrophy. The primary change is a bulbous proliferation of the neural fibroblasts, resulting in gross thickening of the nerve, and destructive compression of the nerve fibers.

Hereditary sensory radicular polyneuropathy was described by Denny-Brown (1951*b*) who emphasized degenerative changes in the dorsal root ganglia. The patients suffered from trophic ulcers, lightning pains and deafness.

Heredopathia atactica polyneuritiformis (Refsum's disease) combines polyneuritis with ichthyosis, degenerative retinopathy, deafness and anosmia. The polyneuritis is of the hypertrophic interstitial variety. The ataxia is due to a combination of the polyneuritis and varying degrees of central nervous fiber degeneration. There is a persistent elevation of protein in cerebrospinal fluid. Patients with this disease have been found to have phytanic acid (3,7,11,15-tetramethylhexadecanoic acid) in the cholesterol esters and other lipoid fractions of their tissues.

Secondary Degeneration in Peripheral Neuropathy. In addition to the primary changes in the nerve itself in lesions of the peripheral nervous system, there are other morphologic phenomena which are secondary. The integrity of the myelin sheath depends upon the integrity of the axis cylinder and, whenever the axis cylinder undergoes degeneration, the myelin sheath will disintegrate. The reverse is not true—an axis cylinder can retain its structural integrity after it has lost its myelin sheath. The factors which permit or prevent axonal function after demyelination are not yet fully understood, but of probable importance are the length of the demyelinated segment, the suddenness of onset, and the intensity of the associated inflammatory reaction. In some of the peripheral neuropathies, a segmental demyelination without axis cylinder loss is the only change.

When the afferent nerve fiber degenerates in neuropathy, there are changes in the cells of dorsal root ganglia and autonomic ganglia. In addition there is degeneration of fibers in the dorsal funiculi of the spinal cord, since some of these fibers are continuous with nerve without the interposition of a synapse. Distally the specialized sensory endings of skin and muscle also undergo degeneration.

Degeneration of the efferent fiber produces the changes in anterior horn cells described as axonal reaction (p. 1480), unitary loss of muscle fibers and loss of somatic and visceral effector end-organs.

DEMYELINATIVE DISEASES

Demyelination, in the loose sense of myelin loss, is a property common to many pathologic processes of the central nervous system, but the use of the term should be restricted to loss of myelin without proportionate loss of axis cylinders. A demyelinative disease is one which has as its most important attribute a tendency to produce such an effect. There are only three important diseases which closely correspond to this strict definition: postinfectious encephalomyelitis, multiple sclerosis and progressive multifocal leukoencephalopathy. Frequently, other processes are listed as demyelinative because of their localization in white matter. Prominent in this group are the so-called leukoencephalopathies, which are usually progressive and destructive, and acute or subacute necrotizing lesions of white matter of brain or cord.

Postinfectious Encephalomyelitis. Within a few to many days after the onset of certain exanthems, such as measles, German measles, chickenpox or smallpox, or after inoculation for prevention of smallpox or rabies, a diffuse disorder of the nervous system may appear which produces severe manifestations of cerebrospinal disease, even to the extent of producing coma, decortication, decerebration or paraplegia for a period of days to weeks. It is sometimes fatal, but is most often followed by complete or almost complete recovery of function (Miller et al., 1956).

The pathogenesis of this disorder would seem to be related to an autoimmune ("isoallergic") reaction against nervous tissue, and much experimental work in this direction has been done in the past 20 years. Injection of brain tissue and adjuvants, such as mineral oil and dead tubercle bacilli, can set up a reaction in the central nervous system of experimental animals, which has a marked resemblance to postinfectious encephalomyelitis. There is less evidence for the theory that postinfectious encephalomyelitis is the result of invasion of the central nervous system by the modified original virus.

The gross pathology is largely one of hyperemia of the brain and cord. Microscopically, the lesions are characteristically in the white matter, and consist of perivascular, largely perivenous accumulations of cells. In the early stages a few polymorphonuclear leukocytes may be seen, but mostly the cells are lymphocytes and plasma cells, with histiocytes appearing at a later stage when myelin disintegration requires their activation. Myelin sheath and axis cylinder stains show a loss of myelin without corresponding loss of axis cylinders. Indeed there may be no effect upon the axis cylinders at all.

The profound neurologic symptoms and signs of postinfectious encephalomyelitis are due to the widespread loss of function in the axis cylinders during the period of acute inflammation. Recovery is due to the restoration of function in the denuded axis cylinders.

Multiple Sclerosis. Also called *disseminated sclerosis,* this is a remitting and relapsing disease of the nervous system, principally affecting white matter (McAlpine et al., 1972). It is one of the most frequent nonvascular causes of neurologic disability. It affects men and women about equally, and generally begins in early adult life, although cases are known of onset in children and in the sixth and seventh decades.

The pathogenesis of multiple sclerosis remains a mystery. It is not significantly heredofamilial, but there is some suggestion that patients with some serotypes may be especially susceptible. No biochemical difference of a causative sort has been found in the brain, or specifically in the myelin, of the patient with multiple sclerosis. Toxic, nutritional and metabolic factors have been sought without success. The facts in regard to pathogenesis are more suggestive of an infectious or immune origin. The polar and equatorial regions have not been studied well but, apart from these extremes, the disease is much more common in the higher latitudes and much less common in the lower latitudes in both the northern and southern hemispheres. There are exceptions, as in Japan, where at any latitude the disease is uncommon. Preadolescents who move from a low-risk to a high-risk area are as likely to get the disease as if they had been born in the high-risk area. This suggests than an infectious agent acquired in early life is the determining factor, and the best such candidate is a virus. Either a virus becomes latent and is activated intermittently to produce recurrent attacks, or the virus provides an immunity which acts to protect against multiple sclerosis later in life. The measles virus and other myxoviruses are currently the object of much research attention as this hypothesis is being explored (Weiner et al., 1973).

The lesions of multiple sclerosis vary in size from 0.1 to several centimeters in size. They have a particular predilection for the optic nerves, the periventricular areas of the anterior and posterior parts of the lateral ventricles, the brain stem, the cerebellar peduncles and the dorsal half of the spinal cord (Fig. 32–45), but they may occur anywhere in white matter. When there are lesions in gray matter, they are usually the result of an extension from a white matter lesion. This is especially true in the subcortical lesions of the cerebral hemispheres. The lesions may have a very sharp differentiation from surrounding normal brain or may merge indistinctly into normal brain. The older lesions are white and rather translucent and the tissue retracted, the fresh lesions are pink and congested, and there are all gradations between. Cavitation is very infrequent.

Microscopically, the acute lesions are often in relation to congested veins, and there is likely to be a cuff of lymphocytes and plasma cells about the veins. Characteristically, the myelin breaks up within the lesion, but the axis cylinders are preserved. The degenerating myelin calls forth histiocytic macrophages which become for a time the domi-

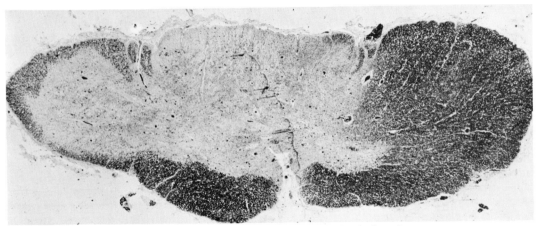

Figure 32–45. Multiple sclerosis, cervical spinal cord.

nant cell in the lesion. Eventually gliosis appears, still sparing the axis cylinders at least in part. Some lesions, however, are more destructive, and in them a certain number of axis cylinders disappear as well. When this occurs over any considerable area, ascending and descending degenerations appear.

The natural clinical history of multiple sclerosis is very variable, and so, of course, are the pathologic findings. Some patients may have only a few brief episodes of slight dysfunction of the nervous system, with rapid recovery. Other patients may progress rapidly, with a course measured in weeks or months, to death, and there are all variations in between. Common manifestations in the early stages are paresthesias, diplopia, central scotomata, mild sensory or motor disorder of a limb or cerebellar incoordination. Remission of symptoms is one of the hallmarks of the disease but, as more and more nervous tissue is involved by subsequent attacks, there is less left for effective remission. The end stage is too often characterized by dementia due to cerebral white matter lesions, blindness due to bilateral retrobulbar neuritis, ataxia due to cerebellar disease, and incontinence and paraplegia in flexion due to spinal cord disease. Fortunately not all patients reach this tragic degree of utter helplessness.

Devic's disease (neuromyelitis optica) is regarded by some as a manifestation of multiple sclerosis, and by others as a distinct clinical and pathologic entity. There are very destructive, usually cystic lesions, of spinal cord and one or both optic nerves, occurring simultaneously or within a few weeks of one another.

Subacute Sclerosing Panencephalitis (Dawson's Encephalitis, van Bogaert's Encephalitis, Subacute Inclusion Encephalitis).

This relatively rare disease was discussed earlier on p. 1501 as a slow virus infection by the measles agent. It is brought up again in the present section because it has a demyelinative component which is reminiscent of certain aspects of multiple sclerosis. By analogy, multiple sclerosis, which is the classic prototype of a demyelinative disease, may ultimately also be of viral origin.

The brain is involved in a heavy panencephalitic process, with inflammatory infiltrates about vessels, scattered demyelination and inclusion bodies in the nuclei of neurons and glial cells. Measles antibodies are increased in the serum and cerebrospinal fluid of all cases, and structures resembling paramyxovirus nucleocapsids have been found in the intranuclear inclusions. A virus which almost certainly is a modified measles virus has been recovered by serial subculture and cocultivation with other cell types.

Progressive Multifocal Leukoencephalopathy.

This is a unique demyelinating lesion of the brain which occurs in patients with extraneural malignant disease, especially lymphoma and Hodgkin's disease, and in other disorders of immunologic competence such as sarcoid, tuberculosis and immunosuppressive drug therapy. The patients develop gross signs of hemisphere white matter disease, such as hemiplegia or hemianopsia, and go on inevitably to die with persisting and progressing neurologic symptoms and signs in weeks to months.

The lesions are demyelinating, multifocal and usually confluent. Within the lesions, oligodendroglia have disappeared with the myelin, and there are multinucleated or mitosing astrocytes. Outside the lesions, the oligodendroglial nuclei show inclusion bodies which, on electron microscopy, have the characteristics of papovaviruses, in particular, the SV 40-polyoma subgroup. These viruses and an additional one, the JC virus, have been identified by culture of the lesions in several cases.

The mechanism of the demyelination seems clear. The virus attacks the nucleus of the oligodendroglial cell, which then disappears, along with the segment of myelin which it supports.

Leukoencephalopathies. There is a group of relatively rare diseases which occur in infancy or childhood, in which the principal lesion or lesions are in the white matter of the brain and especially of the cerebral hemispheres. Generically, this group is referred to as the leukoencephalopathies. The term leukodystrophy is applied to some of them, especially those which occur early in life and which are thought of as representing a congenital defect in the formation or maintenance of myelin.

Metachromatic leukodystrophy (sulfatide lipidosis) is a progressive disorder, generally beginning in the 5 to 10 age group and producing death in three to five years from onset. Both central and peripheral nervous systems are involved, so that the patient becomes mute, blind, deaf and quadriplegic. Although the disease is most dramatic and destructive in its neurologic effects, it is a generalized process, and there are lesions in kidney, testis and gallbladder. Sulfatide, which is metachromatic, is normally present in myelin. It accumulates to excess not only in myelin, but also in glia and neurons, because there is a deficiency of arylsulfatase-A, without which the degradation to cerebroside cannot occur. Diagnosis can be made with biochemical methods, in particular by demonstrating the reduction of aryl-sulfatase-A in the urine, or by appropriate histochemical study of biopsied sural nerve, intestinal mucosa or brain.

Globoid cell leukodystrophy (Krabbe's disease) has its origin in late infancy. The infants become disinterested, and development ceases. Myoclonus, decerebration, decortication and episodic opisthotonus are the signs of the severe destructive process. Phagocytic cells of a multiloculated and globoid appearance are present in large numbers in white matter of the brain and spinal cord and, to a lesser degree, in peripheral nerves. The enzyme defect is thought to be galactosyl ceramide-beta-galactosyl-hydrolase (beta-galactosidase), with a resultant abnormal accumulation of galactocerebroside.

Pelizaeus-Merzbacher disease is a familial disorder of early life, which runs a protracted course into adolescence. The lesions in white matter are separate and scattered, and the axis cylinder is likely to be spared. It is likely that degeneration occurs after the myelin has been completely and normally formed.

TOXIC, NUTRITIONAL AND METABOLIC DISORDERS

The overlap between intoxications, metabolic derangements and nutritional disorders is such that proper categorization with respect to the nervous system is not always possible in a given instance. Intoxications and nutritional disorders produce an ultimate metabolic disorder at a cellular level. Some intoxications produce their effect through lack of a given essential nutritional substance.

Running through this group of disorders, either as a determining or a complicating event, is cerebral hypoxia, the effects of which have been considered in the section on vascular disease of the brain. Some of the most common of the intoxicants of the central nervous system, such as the sedative drugs, produce only a biochemical lesion in the brain, producing no specific pathologic appearance. The common change in the central nervous system in the fatal case is that due to the secondary hypoxic effect of such drugs. In the same way, nutritional and metabolic disorders may be complicated by hypoxia on the basis of a failing respiration or circulation.

INTOXICATIONS

Carbon Monoxide. Carbon monoxide poisoning is seen most frequently as the result of accidental or deliberate exposure to illuminating gas or the exhaust fumes of an automobile. It has become a distressingly common method of attempting suicide. The effect of monoxide is the consequence of the displacement of effective oxygen transport by carboxyhemoglobin. The important pathologic effects are those of anoxic encephalopathy (p. 1505). A curious feature in some cases (but by no means in all) is the development of symmetrical necrosis of the globus pallidus. Some investigators have regarded this as specific for carbon monoxide intoxication, but there are many cases in which it does not occur, and it may be found in cases of hypoxia of other cause.

Ethyl Alcohol. No medical student needs to be told that ethyl alcohol can produce intoxication. Yet it is problematic whether this drug can produce any specific morphologic change in brain or spinal cord (Victor and Adams, 1953). When morphologic changes occur in alcoholic brains, they are rather the result of a complicating hypoxia, a complicating liver disease or a nutritional deficiency.

Polioencephalitis haemorrhagica superior is the name given by Wernicke to an encephalopathy characterized clinically by mental confusion, nystagmus, extraocular palsies, prostration and death. It has been shown to be a consequence of thiamine deficiency and, in the early stages, its manifestations are reversed completely by the administration of thiamine (p. 497). It occurs most often in chronic alcoholics, but is seen also in pernicious vomiting of pregnancy, carcinoma of the stomach and other states accompanied by severe malnutrition (Victor et al., 1971).

The lesions in the nervous system are most constant and most impressive in the mammillary bodies, but important lesions may also be present in the structures in the walls of the third ventricle (Fig. 32—46), about the aqueduct of Sylvius, and in the floor of the fourth ventricle. The nuclei of the extraocular muscles, the vestibular nuclei and the dorsal motor nuclei of the vagi are commonly involved. Grossly, the lesions are those of congestion with a brownish gray discoloration. Frank hemorrhages, prominently described in the older literature, are not so frequent in our own material. Microscopically, there is a vacuolated appearance of the affected structures. Severe loss of nerve cells is infrequent. The most impressive and probably the most important change is in the smaller blood vessels, which are only slightly increased in number but stand out prominently by virtue of the increased cellularity of their walls. This cellular increase affects the endothelium most strikingly, the lumen of the vessels being narrowed by the protrusion of the swollen and proliferating endothelial cells. Glial and his-tiocytic response is in proportion to the amount of destruction the disease produces in the affected nuclear masses.

Korsakoff's dementia is the result of thalamic lesions developing as a part of Wernicke's encephalopathy. The determining lesions for the memory defect are probably in the medial dorsal nuclei. The mentally crippling effect of severe memory loss with confabulatory reaction is frequently irreversible.

Alcoholic cerebellar degeneration is probably also a nutritional disorder (Victor et al., 1959). The patient develops a severe ataxia of gait, which is found to be a combination of truncal ataxia with cerebellar tremor of the legs, and only mild, if any, tremor in the arm. Pathologically, there is gross atrophy of the anterodorsal midline of the cerebellum, with severe loss of Purkinje cells and granule cells.

Methyl Alcohol. Methyl alcohol intoxication is usually the result of ingestion of denatured alcohol by poverty-stricken or otherwise desperate alcoholics. It produces blindness and delirium. The change responsible for the delirium is not known. There may be some hypertrophy and proliferation of the endothelium of small vessels, but nerve cells of the brain itself are not visibly affected, and the mental change is quite reversible. The lesions responsible for the blindness are in the ganglion cells of the retina, and there is resulting atrophy of the optic nerves (p. 519).

Lead. Peripheral neuropathy due to lead intoxication may appear at any age, but is rare in infancy. On the other hand, encephalopathy due to lead is almost exclusively a disease of infants and very young children (p. 524). It generally occurs as an episode, usually a fatal one, in a patient with lead absorption. It is often precipitated by an infection, with resulting acidosis and acute mobilization of the lead stored in bones. The usual history given by the patient's family is that the child has been nibbling the paint from window sills or from a crib. Then over a period of hours, he complains of headache, becomes lethargic, develops severe seizures and becomes decerebrate or decorticate.

If the patient dies in the first few days, the brain is pale and swollen. The swelling frequently is great enough to produce herniations. Microscopically, there is almost always a degree of anoxic change. In addition, there may be tiny petechiae and microinfarcts. About some blood vessels, there is high protein fluid, presumably the result of an altered permeability. There is proliferation of the cellular elements, especially the endothelium, in the vessels of smaller size. In some patients who

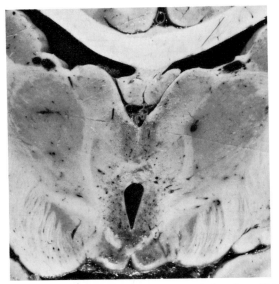

Figure 32–46. *Wernicke's encephalopathy. The wall of the third ventricle is discolored and there are many small hemorrhages.*

survive for a few days, there may be a polymorphonuclear and lymphocytic response about the blood vessels in the brain or subarachnoid space, a finding which correlates with the frequent appearance of cells in the cerebrospinal fluid.

Although the disease still carries a high mortality, many patients now survive without mental or neurologic defect if the process is diagnosed early enough to permit the use of agents which chelate the lead and reduce cerebral edema.

Arsenic. The neuropathology of arsenic poisoning is complex because of the complicating metabolic effects of the generalized disorder it produces. For example, there are severe gastrointestinal, hepatic and renal lesions (p. 525). Formerly, treatment of syphilis with arsenicals or the management of many illnesses with arsenic solutions was a common cause. At present, the few cases seen arise either from homicidal intent or the accidental ingestion of arsenic in insecticides.

As in lead encephalopathy, the onset of encephalopathy due to arsenic is likely to be acute. The changes in the brain are largely hemorrhagic, with multiple petechial hemorrhages scattered throughout white matter. These would appear to be the consequence of a necrotizing effect of the intoxicant upon the walls of smaller blood vessels. Survival after the hemorrhagic encephalopathy of arsenic is rare and, as in lead encephalopathy, there is usually a severe neurologic deficit.

Other Heavy Metals. The neuropathology of manganese poisoning has never been well studied even though it is a not uncommon industrial hazard. Mercury, thallium, selenium and other compounds, in both organic and inorganic forms, are capable of producing clinical and pathologic effects on the nervous system, but again the knowledge of pathogenesis and morphology is incomplete and confused by the effects of the intoxicants in other tissues and organs.

NUTRITIONAL DISORDERS

In many nutritional diseases, the nervous system is affected by a biochemical disorder which does not produce morphologic changes. In others, it is affected indirectly through the intervention of primary damage to another tissue or organ. Thus, hypocalcemic tetany from vitamin D depletion is a reversible state which has no morphology of its own. Subdural hematoma may occur with less than usual trauma in the scorbutic as a local manifestation of a diffuse change in the connective tissue of blood vessels. It goes without saying that there may be some neurologic diseases of etiology unknown at present, which will prove to be due to a nutritional defect.

The most important nutritional diseases which produce morphologic change in the nervous system are those due to deficiencies of B vitamins. The polyneuropathy of vitamin B deficiency (p. 1530) and the encephalopathy of thiamine deficiency are considered elsewhere (p. 498).

Pellagra. In clinical practice, pellagra is a disease difficult to define, and probably represents a complex deficiency of more than one factor, although depletion of niacin seems to be the determining factor (p. 500). The neurologic manifestations are those of a dementing or confusional psychosis. The changes in the nervous system are in the nerve cell body, which undergoes a cloudy swelling that is presumably reversible. Degeneration in the posterior columns of the spinal cord is probably secondary to lesions in peripheral nerves and dorsal roots and ganglia.

Subacute Combined Degeneration. The manner in which *pernicious anemia* exerts its effect on the spinal cord is still not completely understood. Surely it is not the anemia itself, since other anemias of equivalent magnitude, even macrocytic anemias, do not have any effect, and improvement of the anemia by folic acid will not prevent the cord disease. It is clearly related to the deficiency of vitamin B_{12}, since the symptoms and signs of the early stages of cord disease can be cured by the administration of vitamin B_{12} (p. 715).

The essential spinal cord change involves the posterior columns. Grossly, the change in the well developed case is found to be an atrophy of the posterior columns, which appear small and grayish white. A similar change usually affects the lateral columns as well, by the time the posterior column disease is well advanced and, in very severe cases, the rest of the white matter of the cord may show some small degree of change.

Microscopically, the principal change seen in early cases consists of a series of focal areas of vacuolated demyelination in the posterior columns of the lower cervical and upper thoracic regions (Fig. 32–47). When these foci of change are more severe or of longer duration, a variable degree of axis cylinder destruction takes place. The focal lesions have a rough but not absolute symmetry, and extend caudally and rostrally so that ultimately the entire area of the dorsal column is involved. In the meantime, the lesions have begun in the lateral columns, and may even extend into the other long tracts. The gray matter is spared. The histologic re-

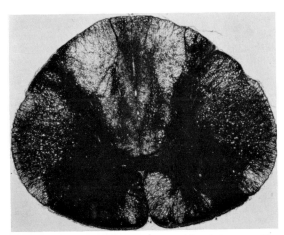

Figure 32–47. Subacute combined degeneration due to pernicious anemia. (Loyez stain for myelin sheaths.)

action is the expected one for foci of demyelination or necrosis, the exception being the reluctance of the astrocytes to react to any significant degree until treatment has been instituted.

The question of whether there is a true peripheral neuropathy due to pernicious anemia is still unsettled. The neuropathic picture seen in the disease may be the manifestation of an associated deficiency, but many patients with true subacute combined degeneration show no evidence of neuropathy.

Clinically, the patient with subacute combined degeneration develops paresthesias in the hands and feet and, on examination at this stage, may be found to have only loss of vibration sense and absent knee and ankle jerks. In more severe cases, a sensory ataxia develops, which is related to proprioceptive loss. Then there appear varying degrees of spasticity with extensor plantar responses but still with absent knee and ankle jerks. This spasticity indicates that the corticospinal tracts have been involved. The combination of corticospinal and dorsal column disease finally results in the deforming end result, a paraplegia in flexion with severe flexor spasms. Fortunately, the prognosis is good if the disease is treated in time.

In the rare case, foci similar to those described in the cord make their appearance in the white matter of the cerebral hemispheres, with resulting confusion and dementia.

METABOLIC DISORDERS

Disorders of metabolism may affect the nervous system profoundly without producing any primary structural change. The convulsions of insulin reaction and the coma of diabetic acidosis are alike capable of recovery without lesions. In a sense, every metabolic disorder has an effect on nervous tissue, although it is not necessarily a direct effect or an effect with specific morphologic features. Therefore, the selection of certain metabolic disorders for inclusion in a section of this sort is arbitrary and incomplete. The conditions included here have been chosen either because of their frequency, their obvious morphology or an increasing understanding of their mechanisms.

Hypoglycemia. The nervous system is totally dependent upon glucose for its energy metabolism. When the many protective reflex and hormonal mechanisms are insufficient to maintain effective blood levels of glucose, symptoms and signs of hypoglycemia appear. Sweating, pallor and tachycardia appear when the threat is a gradual one—these are responses to released epinephrine. When blood sugar drops abruptly, convulsions occur. The usual clinical causes are treatment with hypoglycemic drugs, pancreatic adenoma and functional hyperinsulinism. After the onset of hypoglycemia, the outcome is recovery, death or survival with irreversible nerve cell damage. The gross and histologic effects are much like those of anoxic encephalopathy.

Hepatic Encephalopathy. Patients with severe liver disease are subject in the course of their disease to a neurologic disorder characterized by reduction of awareness, mental agitation and a characteristic disorder of movement, terminating in deep coma (p. 991) (Adams and Foley, 1953) (Victor et al., 1965). It may run a rapid course over a few days to death, may produce recurrent episodes or may produce a chronic state lasting for months or years. Such changes may occur in patients with portacaval shunts who do not have liver disease, and the appearance of the disorder is correlated in most cases but probably not directly related to an increase in the level of blood ammonia (p. 993).

The changes in the brain in fatal cases are largely in the protoplasmic astrocytes, which undergo hypertrophy and hyperplasia. Enlarged, deformed and proliferating protoplasmic astrocytes are found everywhere in gray matter, but especially in the lenticular nucleus, thalamus, red nucleus, substantia nigra and deeper layers of the cerebral cortex. In uncomplicated cases, there are no morphologic changes in the nerve cells themselves, although they must be suffering a biochemical lesion as judged by the clinical effects.

Such changes in the protoplasmic astrocytes are by no means specific for hepatic encephalopathy. To a lesser degree, they appear in uremia, hypoxia and some of the intoxications.

Amino Acid Disorders. There are many amino acid disorders which have an effect on nervous tissue. Only two are mentioned here, because of their relative frequency and remediability. *Phenylketonuria* is a heredofamilial defect in the metabolism of phenylalanine. Diagnosis can be made early by the quantitative demonstration of excess phenylalanine and tyrosine in the serum, and phenylketones in the urine. There is reason to believe that a diet low in phenylalanine will prevent the mental retardation which is a part of the syndrome. In some instances, there is no gross or histologic change despite the presence of a mental defect; but in other cases, extensive demyelination and white matter destruction have been noted in brain and cord. Treatment has been so effective that some patients have grown with normal intelligence but, still hyperphenylalaninemic, have produced offspring with mental retardation and malformations.

Maple syrup urine disease is the quaint name given to a disorder which makes its appearance in the third to fifth postnatal day, with vomiting, muscular hypertonicity and the presence of ketoacids in the urine. The patients fail progressively and die rapidly, with fits and paralyses. Myelin never gets properly formed, and there is spongy degeneration of the white matter of the cerebral hemispheres. Treatment is directed to a diet low in the branched-chain amino acids.

Lipid Storage Diseases. Tay-Sachs disease, formerly referred to as amaurotic family idiocy, is the best known and the most common of a group of disorders which have in common a disorder of lipid metabolism resulting in the accumulation of abnormal lipopigment within the cell bodies of neurons. Zeman and Dyken (1969) recognized two broad categories, the gangliosidoses and the neuronal ceroid-lipofuscinoses. Gangliosidoses occur when there is a lack of certain genetically controlled lysosomal enzymes. G_{m2}-gangliosidosis, which group includes Tay-Sachs disease, is related to deficiencies of B-d-N-acetyl-galactosaminidase; G_{m1}-gangliosidosis results from a β-galactosidase deficiency. The biochemical defect in the ceroid-lipofuscinoses is not yet clear.

If the child dies in an early stage of Tay-Sachs disease, the brain is likely to be more full than usual, a manifestation of the enlargement of individual nerve cell bodies by the accumulation of the ganglioside. More often at autopsy, the gross appearance is one of widespread atrophy, as the affected nerve cells undergo progressive degeneration and disappear. Histologically, every remaining nerve cell body in the brain, cord, dorsal root ganglia and autonomic ganglia is found distended with a foamy vacuolated material which fills the cytoplasm, enlarging the cell to many times its normal size and flattening and displacing the nucleus to one corner of the cell. The abnormal cytoplasmic inclusions stain positively with periodic acid-Schiff reagent and with almost any fat stain. Degenerating forms are intermingled with cells showing the full-blown change, and in most areas there is extensive nerve cell loss with glial replacement. The electron microscope reveals the inclusions to be curled-up double membrane structures.

The clinical picture is one of progressive dementia, blindness, epileptic myoclonus and decortication, and death comes eventually through inanition or infection. In the infantile form, the one properly called Tay-Sachs disease, there is a "cherry red spot" about the macula, the result of degeneration of retinal ganglion cells.

Other varieties of lipid storage diseases may occur in older children, and some even in adult life. They are, like Tay-Sachs disease, heredofamilial, and they produce widespread neurologic dysfunction and neuronal destruction.

Other "Storage" Diseases. *Hand-Schuller-Christian complex* does not involve nerve cells. Its neuropathologic importance is related to the granulomatous lesions of the skull, which can involve cranial nerves and the basal structures so that diabetes insipidus, deafness, exophthalmos and other changes may be present (p. 305).

Gaucher's disease is also a diffuse systemic disease with some incidental findings in the nervous system in the form of infrequent lipoid inclusions in nerve cells (p. 299).

Gargoylism is the name given to another genetically determined, diffuse systemic storage disease (p. 304). Although it is very rare in its fully developed form, there are many "formes frustes," lesser degrees of severity, which are compatible with long life and minimal disability. The inclusions in the nerve cells in gargoylism are never so total as in Tay-Sachs disease. A cluster of affected cells may lie beside a group of normal cells. The material within the nerve cell is thought to be a combination of a ganglioside and a cerebroside, whereas in the viscera it is largely mucopolysaccharide. The neurologic manifestations of gargoylism are nonspecific; mental retardation and convulsive disorder are most prominent.

Whipple's Disease. In some patients

with Whipple's disease, even in the absence of an obvious defect in intestinal absorption, there may appear a progressive neurologic disorder characterized by dementia and paralyses of cerebral origin. In such cases, and even in some neurologically asymptomatic cases, there have been found in cerebral white matter PAS-positive substances identical with those found in the intestines (p. 947) (Smith et al., 1965).

DEGENERATIVE DISEASES

Traditionally the term "degenerative" has been applied to those nervous diseases which have in common a slow but progressive evolution, an unknown pathogenesis, and unresponsiveness to any known treatment. For almost all the diseases generally listed under this rubric, some new facts have emerged as the result of research in recent years. The decision to list some diseases as degenerative rather than metabolic is an arbitrary one.

Wilson's Disease. Wilson's disease is used to open this account of the degenerative diseases because, except for some few clues, it would be no better understood and no more responsive to treatment than any of the other conditions to be discussed. The aura of hopelessness which has lain about these disorders for many years is being dissipated by the discovery of new facts.

The inheritance of hepatolenticular degeneration requires consanguinity of parents, since the trait is an autosomal recessive and the gene is an uncommon one. The predominant features are a characteristic corneal discoloration (the Kayser-Fleischer ring), liver disease and brain disease. The liver disease always precedes the brain disease, and may kill the patient before the brain disease has a chance to develop (p. 1037). The brain disease usually begins in early adolescence, but its onset may be delayed until adult life.

Although the pathogenesis is by no means clarified, studies in recent years have contributed a large (but somewhat controversial) body of knowledge about this disease which only a short time ago was as imperfectly understood as the other degenerative diseases. The important data might be summarized as follows:

1. There is a defect in gastrointestinal absorption, which allows copper to be taken up in excessive amounts.

2. Copper is massively increased in the tissues, clinical signs probably not appearing in liver or brain or cornea until the intracellular copper has exceeded a critical level.

3. Ceruloplasmin, the essential copper-containing protein of plasma is decreased, although albumin-bound copper is increased.

4. There is a renal tubular reabsorption defect which results in excessive urinary excretion of amino acids, peptides, proteins, glucose, uric acid and phosphates.

5. Substances which mobilize copper from tissues and increase excretion (such as penicillamine) can cause remarkable improvement in the neurologic symptoms and signs.

Clinically and pathologically, two types of hepatolenticular degeneration should be distinguished. In both there is liver disease and in both Kayser-Fleischer rings are present. In the so-called *Westphal-Strümpell* variety ("pseudosclerosis"), there is usually a later onset of less disabling neurologic manifestations, with little or no dementia, and a predominant tremor. In the so-called *Wilson* type, there is onset, at adolescence, of a rapidly progressing dystonia with dementia and little or no tremor.

The neuropathologic changes are not restricted to the lenticular nucleus, but are widespread throughout the brain, justifying the term "hepatocerebral degeneration" used by some authors. In the dystonic variety of early onset and rapid evolution (Wilson), there are always gross changes. The most dramatic finding is cavitation in the lenticular nucleus, the tips of the frontal lobes and rarely in the dentate nucleus of the cerebellum. When cavitation is not present, there is a brownish discoloration with some atrophy of the nuclear masses at the base. In the Westphal-Strümpell variety of late onset and less rapid deterioration, the brain may be grossly normal, or there may be a mild atrophy and discoloration of the basal nuclei.

In both forms, the histologic changes are widespread, but are maximal in the lenticular nucleus, especially in the putamen. The thalamus, red nucleus and dentate nucleus of the cerebellum are prominently affected. The important histologic change is in the protoplasmic astrocytes. They are increased in size and in number, and many are multinucleated. In regions where these multinucleated forms are prominent, there is evidence of degeneration of nerve cells, many of them already disappeared. The cavitation appears to be related to the confluence of areas of intense degeneration of astrocytes and nerve cells.

Alzheimer's Disease. There are, in the central nervous system of the aged person, many changes which represent the accumulated involution of the years. Arteriosclerotic cerebral vascular disease, although more common in the aged, cannot be regarded as due to aging itself, and the tendency to blame all clinical and pathologic events of the senium upon the blood vessels is to be deplored. The major cause of organic mental change in the elderly is Alzheimer's disease (Wolstenholme and O'Connor, 1970).

The dura in Alzheimer's disease becomes adherent and thin, and the leptomeninges thickened and opaque. The reticular framework of blood vessels becomes more prominent. There is fibrosis and calcification of the arachnoidal villi. The dorsal root ganglia lose some of their cells and the dorsal columns some of their myelinated fibers, especially those from the lower segments. The brain is atrophic, especially in its frontal regions, frequently in the parietal regions and, to a lesser degree, in the temporal and occipital regions. Because of this atrophy of the cerebral cortex, the white matter may be smaller and firmer than usual, and the ventricles are dilated by a hydrocephalus ex vacuo. The atrophy does not spare the basal nuclei, but it is less striking here than in the cortex.

Microscopically, the atrophic portion of the cerebral cortex is found to have lost many nerve cells, and an excess of astroglia and microglia appears in these areas of cell loss. But more specific for Alzheimer's disease are two pathologic findings: the senile plaque and neurofibrillar degeneration (Margolis, 1959).

The senile plaque can be seen in the usual chromatic stains, but it is best studied with the periodic acid-Schiff method or with silver impregnation. There is a smudged core of amorphous material with a circular or ray-like ring about it, consisting variously of fibrous and cellular elements (Fig. 32–48). Probably the most complete and satisfactory representation is given by the PAS method. Plaques occur only in gray matter, and vary greatly in number from case to case. They are especially abundant in the hippocampus. They may occur in any cortical layer, and vary in size from 20 to 150 microns in diameter. Their pathogenesis is not understood, but their occurrence only in gray matter and only in areas of nerve cell degeneration suggest that the core is formed by a degenerate nerve cell or its fiber or its satellite oligodendroglia, the peripheral part of the plaque being a tissue reaction to the degenerate material of the center.

Neurofibrillar degeneration is an alteration of the neurofibrillar apparatus of the nerve cell in such a way that the fibrils become thickened and tortuous, forming a tangled skein within the cell (Fig. 32–48) (Terry, 1963). Although this change may obscure the nucleus, it does not necessarily destroy it. The small pyramidal cells of the outer laminae are most likely to be affected by this degeneration.

Although in general the number of cells showing neurofibrillar degeneration is directly proportional to the number of senile plaques, there is no absolute correlation, and one kind of change may

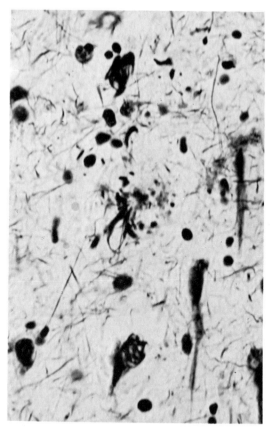

Figure 32–48. Alzheimer's disease. A senile plaque is in the center, and two cells showing neurofibrillar degeneration lie nearby. (v. Braunmühl's stain.)

be present to the almost complete exclusion of the other. Although such degenerative changes are present to a degree in all patients with senile dementia, and indeed in almost all aged people, there is no necessary quantitative correlation between the degree of the dementia and the degree of pathologic change.

The parenchymal lesions of the senium, with cortical atrophy, nerve cell loss, neurofibrillar degeneration and senile plaques, may appear earlier in life without any of the other manifestations of advanced age. The clinician calls this condition presenile psychosis or presenile dementia, and the pathologist calls it presenile atrophy. There is some tendency to familial occurrence. It usually begins in the fifth or sixth decade, but may begin even earlier with general impairment of higher intellectual functions or sometimes with localized symptoms of aphasia, agnosia or apraxia. Convulsive disorder may be prominent. Progression is steady to the end result of total dementia. It is essentially a disease of the cerebral cortex, and the transcortical functions are the ones which are lost.

Pick's Disease. Lobar atrophy or sclerosis, although far less frequent, is considered in clinical neurology as a companion disease of Alzheimer's presenile atrophy because of its occurrence in the presenium and because of the frequently indistinguishable clinical symptoms and course. It affects women more than men, has an occasional familial occurrence and generally begins in middle or late middle life, with symptoms and signs of local cerebral cortical disease which then become submerged in a "sea of mindlessness."

There is severe atrophy of the cortex of the frontal or temporal lobes or both, with frequent asymmetry. In the frontal lobes, the precentral cortex is spared, and in the temporal lobe the hippocampus and the transverse gyrus of Heschl (the primary auditory receptive area) are spared. In the atrophic gyri, there is nerve cell loss and a corresponding degree of glial activation and replacement. The remaining nerve cells may show curious argentophilic cytoplasmic bodies, but these are unlike the neurofibrillar degeneration of Alzheimer's disease. Senile plaques are not part of the process.

Huntington's Chorea (Huntington's Disease). This strongly heredofamilial disease is characterized by the onset, in adult life, of a dementia and choreoathetosis, progressively advancing to a degree of mental and physical incapacity (Denny-Brown, 1962). Nothing is known of its pathogenesis. There are no visceral lesions as in hepatolenticular degeneration. Treatment is symptomatic only.

The changes in the brain are widespread in the cerebral cortex and in the basal ganglia, with predominant affection of the head of the caudate, which may be atrophied to only a thin ribbon, losing its normal convex protrusion into the ventricle (Fig. 32–49). The cerebellum, pons and medulla are not involved. The cerebral cortex, especially the frontal cortex, is always affected, some authors reporting maximal change in the deeper layers, others in the middle layers. Histologically, there is derange-

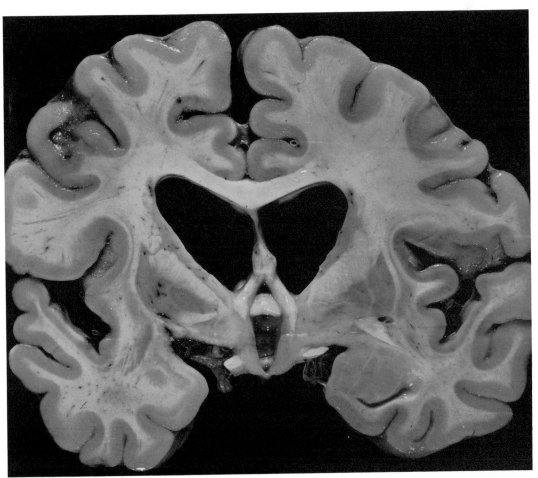

Figure 32–49. Huntington's chorea. There is diffuse atrophy, but the caudate nuclei are most affected.

ment of the cellular architecture of the involved structures by loss of nerve cells and replacement gliosis. Those cells which remain are in varying stages of chronic cell change. There is no significant reaction by blood vessels or histiocytes.

Parkinson's Disease (Paralysis Agitans).
Parkinson's disease is a unique neurologic entity, probably of still unknown cause. Its most important manifestations are a characteristic tremor, a cogwheel rigidity, a slowness of movement and disorganization of movement referred to as bradykinesia or akinesia and, in some cases, an inability to remain still, referred to as akathisia. It generally develops in late middle life or in old age, but there are many exceptions to this. Onset below the age of 40 is exceptional, and below the age of 30, is rare. It is progressive but varyingly so over the years. Not fatal in itself, it produces an immobility with attendant problems of malnutrition, infection and thromboembolism.

There are other disorders which have parkinsonian features but which are distinguishable from paralysis agitans. In this group are Wilson's disease, the postencephalitic state of encephalitis lethargica, carbon monoxide poisoning, anoxic encephalopathy, pseudobulbar palsy and manganese poisoning. Certain drugs, particularly reserpine and the phenothiazines, produce a disorder in some patients which is quite indistinguishable from classic paralysis agitans.

The mechanism of symptom production in paralysis agitans is poorly understood despite large advances over the last 15 years. A system of dopaminergic neurons is present in putamen, caudate, globus pallidus and substantia nigra. Well proved in animals, and highly probable in man, is a nigrostriatal dopamine pathway. Reserpine depletes the brain of its dopamine; phenothiazine drugs probably block the dopamine receptors in the striatum. In paralysis agitans, the dopamine content of the putamen, caudate, globus pallidus and substantia nigra is reduced. Levodopa, which is transformed to dopamine within the cell, produces improvement in the symptoms and signs of the disease. This dopaminergic neuron hypothesis, although incomplete, explains the disease from a pharmacologic point of view. The mechanism by which dopamine is depleted and the cells destroyed, as prominently in the substantia nigra, remains unknown.

The pathology of paralysis agitans is as mysterious as its clinical features, and is a great deal more controversial. There is reduction or loss of pigment in substantia nigra. Some investigators point to a smallness of the lenticular nucleus, especially of the pallidal part, and an atrophy of the ansa lenticularis. Histologically, there is controversy about the location of the important lesions. Although all investigators agree that there are histologic changes, the great difference of opinion concerns the relative significance of the lesions in the globus pallidus and substantia nigra. There is no doubt that there are lesions in the substantia nigra in the form of nerve cell loss and degeneration. There are, in many of the nigral cells, rounded intracytoplasmic inclusions which are called Lewey bodies. The lesion in the globus pallidus, and there is probably some lesser degree of such change in the putamen and caudate as well, is a loss of nerve cells with degenerative changes in those cells which remain.

Cerebellar and Cerebellar Pathway Degeneration. There is a group of diseases in which the most prominent clinical disturbance is in cerebellar function. Some are sporadic and some are heredofamilial; for most of them, there is no clue to their biochemical pathogenesis. A useful way of categorizing them is in terms of those which involve the afferent pathways to the cerebellum, those which involve the cerebellum itself and, in particular, the cerebellar cortex, and those which involve the pathways efferent from cerebellum.

The *spinocerebellar degenerations* are predominantly spinal diseases, with atrophy of the spinocerebellar pathways, the dorsal and lateral funiculi. The most frequently discussed disease in this group is Friedreich's ataxia, even though it is by no means the most common. At present, there is controversy about the purity of the spinocerebellar syndromes. Some investigators insist that Friedreich's disease at least is unique; others claim that there are a multitude of variations within the Friedreich cases and even speak of a "spectrum" which would unite such seemingly diverse diseases as Charcot-Marie-Tooth disease, hereditary spastic paraplegia and the spinocerebellar degenerations. At present, there seems insufficient reason to unify these processes under one category; further research into pathogenesis and more extensive genetic studies will be necessary before this difficult group can be clarified.

Friedreich's Ataxia. This is a heredofamilial disease of the nervous system which begins at or near adolescence and runs a progressive course to severe neurologic disability within a few years of onset. Nothing is known of its pathogenesis.

Pathologically, the impressive gross change is a smallness of the spinal cord which is due to an atrophy of the posterior columns, the corticospinal tracts and the dorsal spinocerebellar tracts (Fig. 32–50). In addition,

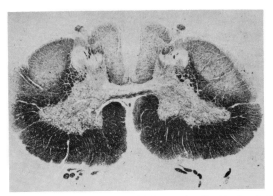

Figure 32–50. Friedreich's ataxia. Cervical spinal cord. (Loyez stain.)

there is smallness of the posterior roots. These changes are most pronounced in the more caudal portion of the cord, becoming less obvious rostrally. The medulla, pons and cerebellum are usually normal. An important and sometimes fatal association is an interstitial myocarditis.

The child with Friedreich's ataxia begins to have disabling symptoms and signs at adolescence or in the preadolescent period. A foot deformity, pes cavus, is present in all patients and there is some degree of kyphoscoliosis. There is a cerebellar type of ataxia compounded by a sensory ataxia on the basis of the posterior column deficit. Within a few months to years, the disability increases to the point of a bed and wheel chair existence.

Ataxia-telangiectasia is a complex disorder, involving much more than cerebellar function, but is of interest because of the immunologic disorder which underlies it and the implications this might have in understanding some of the other disorders of cerebellum. A very rare disorder, the Bassen-Kornzweig syndrome, also produces a clinical neurologic state which has resemblances to Friedreich's ataxia. These patients have a celiac syndrome, pigmentary retinal degeneration, acanthocytosis and an a-betalipoproteinemia.

Carcinomatous Cerebellar Degeneration. This disorder is a not infrequent clinical process which produces cell loss throughout the cerebellar cortex as a nonmetastatic effect of carcinoma, most often of lung or ovary (Brain and Norris, 1965). In some cases, there is also involvement of dorsal funiculi, lateral funiculi and spinocerebellar tracts of spinal cord, so that the result is a combined cerebellar and spinocerebellar degeneration.

Alcoholic cerebellar degeneration is another example of a primary disorder of cerebellar cortex.

Olivopontocerebellar degeneration is an example of a combined cerebellar cortical and efferent pathway disorder. It occurs sporadically in middle life and is always fatal, producing a combined cerebellar and basal ganglionic clinical picture. Some patients have orthostatic hypotension and others autonomic disturbances. Probably this is the so-called Shy-Drager syndrome.

It must be reemphasized that the conditions listed above are only a few examples of the multitudinous syndromes which are included in the disorders of cerebellum and cerebellar pathways.

Motor Neuron Disease. *Progressive spinal muscular atrophy, amyotrophic lateral sclerosis and progressive bulbar palsy constitute a triad of disease states in which there is a difference in distribution of the lesions but in which the basic pathologic process is a degeneration of corticospinal or corticobulbar pathways and of motor nerve cells of the spinal cord and brain stem. The disease is most common in early middle life, affects males and females about equally and has no significant association. The pathogenesis is unknown.*

Pathologically, the changes are in muscle, which undergoes the atrophy of denervation, in the motor roots of the spinal and cranial nerves, which are thin and gray, and in the corticospinal tracts. Microscopically, the important changes are in the large cells of the cranial motor nuclei and anterior horns of the spinal cord and in the corticospinal tracts. In progressive muscular atrophy and amyotrophic lateral sclerosis, the greatest degree of change is in the spinal cord and, in progressive bulbar palsy, the most severe lesions are in the motor nuclei of the bulb. There is no hard and fast differentiation, and by the time the disease has progressed to fatality, there are lesions in both spinal and pontomedullary areas. The degeneration of the corticospinal tracts is never complete, and is best seen on myelin sheath or fat stains, since a number of histiocytic macrophages are always present to ingest the products of myelin degeneration. Even in progressive bulbar palsy it is difficult to identify degeneration in the corticospinal tracts above the medullary pyramids. There is a moderately intense glial response to the tract degeneration. In affected nuclear areas there is a reduction in the number of the large motor cells, with corresponding glial replacement. The remaining cells are small and shrunken, or some have a great excess of lipofuscin, or some others have intracytoplasmic vacuoles. There is nothing specific about the manner of the cellular disintegration. In addition to these expected sites of involvement, there may be loss of giant Betz cells in the motor cortex.

Clinically, progressive muscular atrophy and amyotrophic lateral sclerosis are no more sharply distinguished than they are pathologically, the categorization depending on whether at a given time there are symptoms and signs of corticospinal involvement. If there are, the condition is called amyotrophic lateral sclerosis; if not, it is called progressive muscular atrophy. There is progressive weakness and atrophy of muscle without sensory disorder. Fascicular contractions of the muscles at rest are characteristic. The disease may begin anywhere and even asymmetrically but usually involves the distal muscles first. The course of the illness to death from inanition or bulbar muscle involvement is measured in terms of a few years. In bulbar palsy, the prominent manifestations from the beginning are in the bulbar muscles so that chewing, swallowing, talking and breathing are compromised from the start. This bulbar onset is generally associated with a similar process in the distribution of the higher cervical segments. The prognosis is much worse than in progressive muscular atrophy and amyotrophic lateral sclerosis.

Syringomyelia. A chronic disease of variable and intermittent progression, syringomyelia is of unknown cause. Its pathogenesis is unknown, and it has been considered at one time or another a congenital malformation, an inflammatory reaction, a tumor or a primary degeneration of astroglia. It has no familial association and is about equally frequent in males and females.

The cyst of syringomyelia has its greatest size most often in the cervical region. At autopsy, the cord is tense and full over several segments if there is fluid in the cyst, or collapsed if the fluid has been extruded. The overlying leptomeninges may be thickened and opaque. On cross section, the cord contains a cyst with yellow fluid about which there is scar tissue (Fig. 32–51). The cyst in extreme examples may occupy almost the entire cross section of the cord, compressing the few remaining structures out to the periphery. In early cases, the only cyst is a small one in a ventral or dorsal horn or immediately dorsal to the central canal. Ascending and descending degenerations depend upon the cross section extent of the cyst and the gliosis. Although the cervical cord is the usual site of the process, it may be lumbar or there may be separate cavities in cervical and lumbar regions. Extension to or separate involvement of the medulla is called syringobulbia, a slit-like cavity running obliquely across the lateral part of the medullary tegmentum.

Microscopically, the cyst has no necessary connection with the central canal and has no ependymal surface. The important pathologic change is a gliosis which precedes cyst formation. The gliosis is relatively acellular and there is no significant inflammatory change or vascular reaction in the wall of the cyst. In some few cases, a glioma or hemangioblastoma is found in the wall of the cyst (Poser, 1956).

Tuberous Sclerosis (Epiloia, Bourneville's Disease). Tuberous sclerosis is even more difficult to categorize than is syringomyelia. It is characterized clinically by a combination of mental retardation, fits and sebaceous adenomas of the skin. Its pathogenesis is unknown, but it is frequently associated with visceral lesions, rhabdomyoma of the heart, or kidney or pancreatic cysts. It is often heredofamilial. It begins in infancy or childhood and may progress intermittently or only up to a given point of disability. The fully developed case is relatively rare, but there probably are many "formes frustes."

In the fully developed form, there are on the cortical surface nodules of firm whitish tissue of

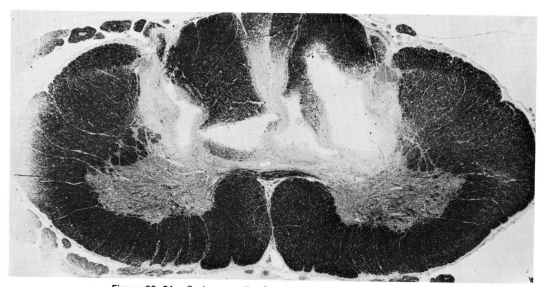

Figure 32–51. Syringomyelia. Cervical spinal cord. (Loyez stain.)

pinhead to thumbnail size or even larger. Overgrowth and protrusion of subependymal glia produce an appearance of "candle dripping" on the surface of the ventricles. Microscopically, the nodules in the cortex are characterized by loss or distortion of the usual cytoarchitecture, with an excess of glia and many deformed, often enlarged nerve cells. These nerve cells have no definable chromatin and their processes are poorly developed. Frequently, they are multinucleated. Calcification within the nodules is often sufficiently intense to permit x-ray visualization.

EPILOGUE

It is evident at the conclusion of this brief overview of the diseases of the nervous system that, in number and complexity, they rival the myriad complexities of the nervous system itself. It can be hoped that the capsule descriptions of the less common disorders, if nothing else, provide a glossary of terms and an appreciation of the range of problems which daily confront the neurologist and neuropathologist.

REFERENCES

Adams, R. D., and Foley, J. M.: The neurological disorder associated with liver disease. Assn. Res. Nerv. & Ment. Dis. Proc., 32:198, 1953.

Asbury, A. K., et al.: The inflammatory lesion in idiopathic polyneuritis. Medicine, 48:173–215, 1969.

Bailey, P., and Cushing, H. W.: Classification of the Tumors of the Glioma Group on a Histogenetic Basis with a Correlated Study of Prognosis. Philadelphia, J. B. Lippincott Co., 1926.

Brain, W. R., and Norris, F. H. (eds.): The Remote Effects of Cancer on the Nervous System. New York, Grune & Stratton, Inc., 1965.

Cox, L. B., and Tolhurst, J.: Human Torulosis. Melbourne and London, Melbourne University Press, 1946.

Cushing, H. W., and Bailey, P.: Tumors Arising from the Blood Vessels of the Brain. Angiomatous Malformations and Hemangioblastomas. Springfield, Ill., Charles C Thomas, 1928.

Denny-Brown, D.: Cerebral concussion. Physiol. Rev., 25:296, 1945.

Denny-Brown, D.: The Basal Ganglia and Their Relation to Disorders of Movement. London, Oxford University Press, 1962.

Denny-Brown, D.: Treatment of recurrent cerebrovascular symptoms and question of "vasospasm." Med. Clin. N. Amer., 35:1457, 1951a.

Denny-Brown, D.: Hereditary sensory radicular neuropathy. J. Neurol. Neurosurg. Psychiat., 14:237, 1951b.

Dodge, P. R., and Swartz, M. N.: Bacterial meningitis. II. Special neurologic problems, postmeningitic complications and clinicopathological correlations. New Eng. J. Med., 272:954–960, 1965.

Duma, R. J., et al.: Primary amoebic meningoencephalitis. New Eng. J. Med., 281:1315–1323, 1969.

Fields, W. S. (ed.): Pathogenesis and Treatment of Cerebrovascular Disease, Springfield, Ill., Charles C Thomas, 1961.

Finney, L. A., and Walker, A. E.: Transtentorial Herniation. Springfield, Ill., Charles C Thomas, 1962.

Ford, F. R.: Diseases of the Nervous System in Infancy, Childhood, and Adolescence. 4th ed. Springfield, Ill., Charles C Thomas, 1960.

Frenkel, J. K., and Friedlander, S.: Toxoplasmosis: Pathology of Neonatal Disease, Pathogenesis, Diagnosis and Treatment. Washington, D.C., Public Health Service Publication No. 141, 1951.

Greenfield, J. G.: Greenfield's Neuropathology. 2nd ed. Blackwood, W., et al. (eds.). Baltimore, Williams & Wilkins, 1963.

Harkin, J. C., and Reed, R. J.: Tumors of the Peripheral Nervous System. Fasc. 3. 2nd Series. Atlas of Tumor Pathology. Washington, D. C., Armed Forces Institute of Pathology, 1969.

Heusner, A. P.: Nontuberculous spinal epidural infections. New Eng. J. Med., 239:845, 1948.

Hoeprich, P. D. (ed.): Infectious Diseases. Hagerstown, Md., Harper & Row, 1972.

Kernohan, J. W., and Sayre, G. P.: Tumors of the Central Nervous System. Section X, Fasc. 35, Atlas of Tumor Pathology. Washington, D.C., Armed Forces Institute of Pathology, 1952.

Klatzo, I.: Neuropathological aspects of brain edema. J. Neuropath. Exp. Neurol., 26:1, 1967.

Koenigsmark, B. W., and Sidman, R. L.: Origin of brain macrophages in the mouse. J. Neuropath. Exper. Neurol., 22:643, 1963.

Kubik, C. S., and Adams, R. D.: Subdural empyema. Brain, 66:18, 1943.

Margolis, G.: Senile cerebral disease. A critical survey of traditional concepts based upon observations with newer techniques. Lab. Invest., 8:335, 1959.

McAlpine, D., et al.: Multiple Sclerosis: A Reappraisal. Baltimore, The Williams & Wilkins Co., 1972.

Merritt, H. H., et al.: Neurosyphilis. New York, Oxford University Press, 1946.

Miller, H. G., et al.: Parainfectious encephalomyelitis and related syndromes: a critical review of the neurological complications of certain specific fevers. Quart. J. Med., 25:427, 1956.

Plum, F., and Posner, J. B.: Diagnosis of Stupor and Coma. Philadelphia, F. A. Davis Co., 1972, pp. 166–176.

Poser, C. M.: The Relationship Between Syringomyelia and Neoplasm, Springfield, Ill., Charles C Thomas, 1956.

Potter, E. L.: Pathology of the Fetus and Infant. 2nd ed. Chicago, Year Book Publishers, 1961.

Rhodes, A. J., and van Rooyen, C. E.: Textbook of Virology. Baltimore, The Williams & Wilkins Co., 1968.

Rubinstein, L. J.: Tumors of the Central Nervous System. Fasc. 6. 2nd Series. Atlas of Tumor Pathology. Washington, D.C., Armed Forces Institute of Pathology, 1972.

Russell, D. S.: Observations on the Pathology of Hydrocephalus. London, His Majesty's Stationery Office, Series G. B., Medical Research Council, Special Report Series No. 265, 1949.

Russell, D. S., and Rubinstein, L. J.: Pathology of Tumors of the Nervous System. 2nd ed. Baltimore, The Williams & Wilkins Co., 1963.

Smith, W. T., et al.: Cerebral complications of Whipple's disease. Brain, 88:137, 1965.

Swartz, M. N., and Dodge, P. R.: Bacterial meningitis. I. General clinical features, special problems and unusual meningeal reactions mimicking bacterial meningitis. New Eng. J. Med., 272:842–848, 1965.

Terry, R. D.: The fine structure of neurofibrillary tangles in Alzheimer's disease. J. Neuropath. Exp. Neurol., 22:629, 1963.

Victor, M., and Adams, R. D.: The effect of alcohol on the nervous system. Ass. Res. Nerv. Ment. Dis. Proc., 32:526, 1953.

Victor, M., et al.: The acquired (non-wilsonian) type of chronic hepatocerebral degeneration. Medicine, 44:345, 1965.

Victor, M., et al.: A restricted form of cerebellar cortical degeneration occurring in alcoholic patients. Arch. Neurol., 1:579, 1959.

Victor, M., et al.: The Wernicke-Korsakoff Syndrome. Philadelphia, F. A. Davis Co., 1971.

Walton, J. N.: Subarachnoid Hemorrhage. London, E. and S. Livingstone, 1956.

Weiner, L. P., et al.: Viral infections and demyelinating diseases. New Eng. J. Med., 288:1103–1110, 1973.

Wolstenholme, G. E. W., and O'Connor, M.: Alzheimer's Disease and Related Conditions. London, J. and A. Churchill, 1970.

Yakovlev, P. I., and Wadsworth, R. C.: Schizencephalies: a study of the congenital clefts in the cerebral mantle. J. Neuropath. Exp. Neurol., 5:116, 1946.

Zeman, W., and Dyken, P.: Neuronal ceroid-lipofuscinosis (Batten's disease). Relationships to amaurotic family idiocy? Pediatrics, 44:570–583, 1969.

Zeman, W., et al.: Measles virus and subacute sclerosing panencephalitis. Neurology, Suppl., 18:part 2, January. 1968.

INDEX